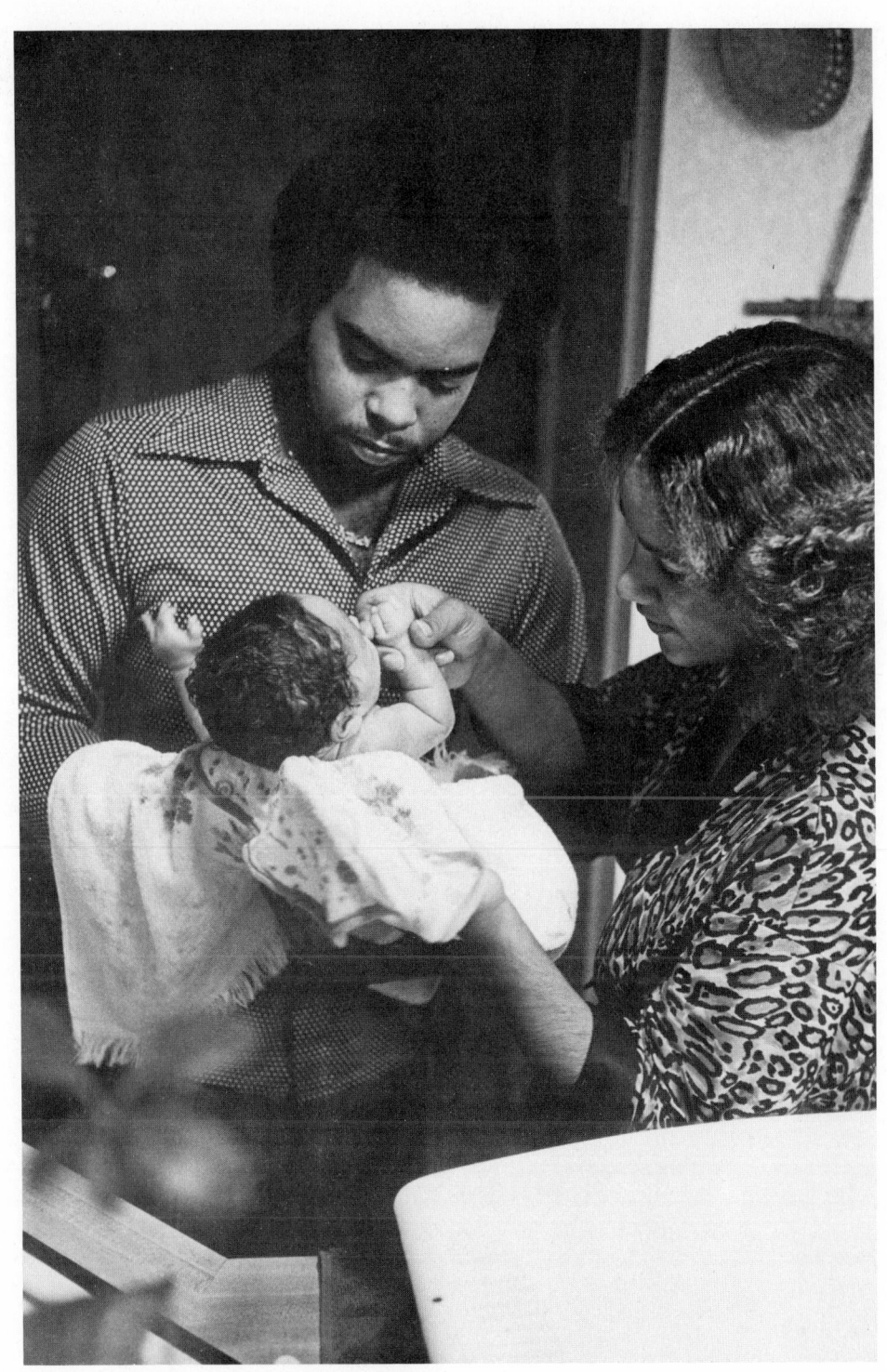

MATERNAL-NEWBORN NURSING
A Family-Centered Approach

SECOND EDITION

MATERNAL-NEWBORN NURSING

A Family-Centered Approach

FORMERLY OBSTETRIC NURSING

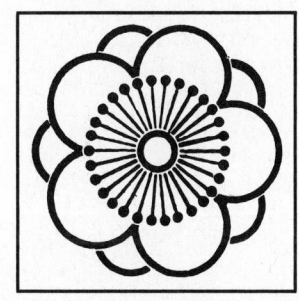

SECOND EDITION

Sally B. Olds, R.N., M.S.
Marcia L. London, R.N., M.S.N., N.N.P.
Patricia A. Ladewig, R.N., M.S.N., N.P.

ADDISON-WESLEY PUBLISHING COMPANY

Nursing Division • Menlo Park, California
Reading, Massachusetts • London • Amsterdam
Don Mills, Ontario • Sydney

Sponsoring Editor: Deborah Gale
Production Editor: Betty Duncan-Todd
Copy Editor: Adrienne Mayor
Production Team: Polly Koch (Proofreader), Janet Bollow (Page layout), Elliot Simon (Pagechecker), and Elinor Lindheimer (Indexer)
Book Design: Julie Kranhold
Cover Design: Michael A. Rogondino
Artist: Jack Tandy
Photographers: William Thompson, George B. Fry III, and Suzanne Arms

Formerly **Obstetric Nursing**

Library of Congress Cataloging in Publication Data
Olds, Sally B., 1940–
    Maternal–newborn nursing.

    Bibliography: p.
    Includes index.
    1. Obstetrical nursing.   I. London, Marcia L.   II. Ladewig,
Patricia A.   III. Obstetric nursing.   IV. Title.
[DNLM: 1. Obstetrical nursing. WY 157 0124]
RG951.038   1984   610.73′678   83–14461
ISBN–0–201–12797–0

BCDEFGHIJ–MU–8987654

The authors and publishers have exerted every effort to ensure that drug selection, dosage, and composition of formulas set forth in this text are in accord with current formulations, recommendations, and practice at the time of publication. However, in view of ongoing research, changes in government regulations, the reformulation of nutritional products, and the constant flow of information relating to drug therapy and drug reactions, the reader is urged to check product information or composition on the package insert for each drug for any change in indications of dosage and for added warnings and precautions. This is particularly important where the recommended agent is a new and/or infrequently employed drug.

Addison-Wesley Publishing Company

Nursing Division
2725 Sand Hill Road
Menlo Park, California 94025

To our families, who were patient, supportive, and always there.
Joe, Scott, and Allison Olds
David, Craig, and Matthew London
Tim, Ryan, and Erik Ladewig

PREFACE

The first edition of this book, *Obstetric Nursing,* reflected our commitment to a family-centered approach to maternity nursing, and the nursing community responded in an overwhelmingly positive manner. We received numerous letters from nurse educators, practicing nurses, and students expressing the belief that ours was an up-to-date, sensitive, and readable *nursing* text. However, they found it difficult to reconcile a title reflecting a medical model in a book that so strongly emphasized the nursing model and a family-centered approach. In response to these concerns and in line with our own feelings that a new title would better reflect the nursing emphasis of the book, the title of the text has been changed to *Maternal–Newborn Nursing: A Family-Centered Approach.*

We have also changed our terminology to reflect our belief that the woman is an active participant in her own health care. We have used the word "client" when discussing women with essentially normal pregnancies, but to maintain a bridge with more traditional approaches we have retained the term "patient" in high-risk situations.

In the second edition, we continue our efforts to promote the use of the nursing process as the framework for client care. To achieve this, our detailed assessment guides have been expanded and updated to reflect current practice. In addition, the nursing care plans have been revised and expanded.

New Features

Several new features have been added to this edition to meet the specific needs of both nurses and students of nursing. These include:

- **Drug guides** compiled from a variety of sources provide pertinent and in-depth information on the physiologic actions of and nursing implications of drugs commonly administered to the maternity client or the newborn.
- **Color plates** contain photographs of some common and some not so common clinical situations found in the maternity setting.
- A section identifying possible **nursing diagnoses** that might be appropriate has been added to each of the nursing care plans.
- A section entitled **Client/Family Educational Focus** has also been added to each nursing care plan. This section highlights major areas of teaching on which the nurse might focus.
- A list of **national resource groups** at the end of certain chapters provides information about support groups that aid childbearing families who require information or assistance.

New Content

To remain current with the state of the art, all the chapters have been revised and updated. However, the following additions deserve special mention.

- Coverage of adolescent pregnancy and cultural considerations has been expanded. In keeping with our belief that both developmental and cultural factors influence the entire childbearing cycle, this content has been integrated throughout rather than covered in isolated chapters.
- Additional content on physiologic and pathophysiologic processes has been added, with an entire new chapter devoted to the specialized area of newborn physiology (Chapter 21).
- Chapter 1, "Current Perspectives of Maternal–Newborn Nursing," retains its historical content but has

been refocused to consider pertinent perinatal issues of today such as technology, the expanded role of nurses, and legal and ethical considerations.

- New Chapter 2, "Tools for Maternal–Newborn Nursing Practice," describes tools that are useful to professional nurses in providing effective care, such as the nursing process (including nursing diagnosis), nursing research, and descriptive and inferential statistics.

Applications

The logical sequencing of content and the inclusion of nursing skills where appropriate makes this text invaluable for students in all types of programs. Faculty members can select those chapters that are most useful in the course they offer. For example, those programs incorporating genetics in the maternity nursing course will find Chapter 7, "Genetic Counseling," an accurate resource. For students in programs that cover this content elsewhere, this chapter serves as a reference for specific situations that may arise in the clinical area. By the same token, some programs cover the high-risk infant in detail and will appreciate the comprehensiveness and currentness of Chapters 24 and 25 ("The High-Risk Newborn: Needs and Care" and "Complications of the Neonate"). For those who do not include this content, it remains available for reference, and all the information they might need on the normal newborn is available in Chapters 22 and 23. Chapter 13, "Diagnostic Assessment of Fetal Status," covers new, exciting trends in diagnostic testing and will be useful for all.

The step-by-step description of common maternal and neonatal procedures remains a useful tool for both students and practitioners, as do the physical assessment guides. The chapters devoted to families, crisis intervention, parenting, and attachment expand the psychosocial nursing base and enable nurses to consider the childbearing family more holistically.

Pedagogical Aids

Many of the learning tools of the first edition have been retained in the second in an updated form. The learning objectives at the beginning of each chapter, the glossary, appendices, references, and additional readings all serve to guide learning. Procedures, drug guides, and nursing care plans will be helpful for quick reference.

Numerous new photographs and line drawings, new or updated tables, and color plates do more than make the text visually appealing. They enhance the reader's understanding of complex processes, conceptual relationships, and clinical skills.

Complete Teaching–Learning Package

Nursing faculty will find several tools available for their use. The *Instructor's Manual* has been completely revised and expanded. In addition, a packet of 79 transparencies is available. The *Transparency Resource Kit* contains transparencies of material not available in the text as well as transparencies of important text figures. *Maternal–Newborn Nursing Care: A Workbook* may also be used to supplement the main text.

We were pleased and awed by the fine reception given the first edition of this text. It inspired our commitment to maintain the same high quality in the second edition that was apparent in the first. We believe that in this revised and expanded text we have succeeded.

Acknowledgments

It would be impossible to undertake a book of this magnitude without the help and support of many people. We wish first to thank the many members of the nursing community who wrote to tell us what they found most useful in the text and to share their suggestions for changes or additions. These letters gave us invaluable information and ideas, and most importantly, a place to start.

A special acknowledgment goes to the following people. They contributed significant content to the first edition, and the foundation they helped establish is still evident in the second edition: Elizabeth M. Bear, Laurel Freed, Sandra L. Gardner, Pauline Goolkasian, Loretta C. Cermely Ivory, Janet Kennedy, Eleanor Latterell, Mary Ann McClees, Caryl E. Mobley, Carol Freeman Rosenkranz, and Marcia Vavich.

We wish to thank the many nursing educators and practicing clinicians who reviewed content or contributed to this edition. We believe that having reviewers and contributors from all over the United States and Canada helped us avoid regionalization in focus or approach.

We wish to extend a special word of appreciation to Thomas Purdon, M.D., F.A.C.O.G., Colorado Springs, Colorado, for reviewing the chapters on diagnostic assessment, and antepartal/intrapartal complications. Other reviewers who contributed their criticisms, praise, and suggestions are as follows: Nora Biegler, St. Joseph Mercy School of Nursing, Sioux City, Iowa; Mary Lou Cheatham, Ball State University, Muncie, Indiana; Bruce D. Clayton, University of Nebraska Medical Center, Omaha, Nebraska; Pramilla Dahya, Portland Community College, Portland, Oregon; Mary Jo Eoff, Indiana University, Indianapolis, Indiana; Eileen Fishbein, University of Maryland, Baltimore, Maryland; Juanita Flint, Brookhaven College, Farmers Branch, Texas; Sue Hall, Rogue Community College, Grant's Pass, Oregon; Peggy W. Harris, Southeastern Louisiana University, Baton Rouge, Louisiana; Kimberly Hubbell, University of Washington, Seattle, Washington; Renee Korbach, San Jacinto College North, Houston, Texas; Nancy K. Lowe, Northern Illinois University, DeKalb, Illinois; Crystal Mahoney, Ball State University, Muncie, Indiana; Susan Marchessault, Northeastern University,

Boston, Massachusetts; Judy McAulay, Okanagan College, Kelowna, British Columbia; Phyllis L. Neff, University of Maryland, Baltimore, Maryland; Thomas F. Purdon, M.D., OB/GYN, Private Practice, Colorado Springs, Colorado; Marilyn J. Robertson, Seattle University, Seattle, Washington; Constance L. Slaughter, University of Portland, Portland, Oregon; Karen Stevens, Catholic University, Washington, D.C.; Frann B. Teplick, Albert Einstein Medical Center, Philadelphia, Pennsylvania; Louise Timmer, California State University, Sacramento, California; Betsy Todd, Cabrini Hospice, New York, New York; Barbara West, Broward Community College, Fort Lauderdale, Florida; Sally Wicklund, *Nurses Drug Alert,* New York, New York; and Sheila Zerr, Faculty of Health Sciences, University of Ottawa, Ottawa, Ontario.

Suzanne Arms' and William Thompson's special photographic skills are evident in the clarity and sensitivity of many of the photos used throughout the text. In addition, we wish to thank Paul Winchester, M.D., Director, Intensive Care Nursery, Memorial Hospital, Colorado Springs, Colorado, for providing some of the photographs used in the chapters on the high-risk newborn. We are indebted, too, to the many individuals and families who, by consenting to be photographed, shared themselves and their experiences.

We value the efforts of Cynthia L. McMahon, who developed the nursing diagnoses found in the care plans. We also appreciate the patience and skill of Beverly Watson in typing this manuscript.

We have developed a special fondness and tremendous respect for the many people with whom we have worked in the Nursing Division of Addison-Wesley Publishing Company. They are a creative, supportive, and enthusiastic group committed to producing high-quality nursing textbooks. While it is not possible to name everyone who has worked to make this book successful, we would like to acknowledge the following individuals:

• Deborah Gale served as our developmental editor on the first edition and our sponsoring editor on this edition. She is very gifted and creative, and we would be

lost without her wonderful sense of humor, large measure of tact, and special feeling for this book.

• Betty Duncan-Todd was our production editor for this edition. She is tremendously organized and amazingly calm and got us through on schedule. More than that, she is a very likeable person, and we appreciate her efforts.

• Pat Franklin Waldo was Special Projects Manager when we started this edition but also served as our sponsoring editor for a time on the first edition. She has a warmth and a joy in living that can hardly be matched, and she shared this with us, to our delight.

• Wayne Oler, executive vice-president, is a caring man who is always willing to lend encouragement or support. We look forward to and enjoy our visits with him.

• Nick Keefe, General Manager of the Nursing Division, is a special friend. He is enthusiastic, creative, and willing to try new things. He inspires us.

• Adrienne Mayor served as copy editor for this edition. Her sharp eye and flair for precision were invaluable.

A word of appreciation goes to our artist, Jack Tandy. The illustrations he did for both editions were wonderful, but more than that, working with him is a creative experience.

Finally, special thanks to our families. They gave us support and encouragement when we needed it; physical assistance in typing, sorting, and arranging when necessary; and the knowledge that they believed in us and were proud of what we were attempting. Without their giving, unique love, we might not have persevered.

Sally B. Olds
Marcia L. London
Patricia A. Ladewig

AUTHORS

Sally B. Olds, R.N., M.S.
Coordinator, Maternal–Child Nursing
Beth-El School of Nursing
Colorado Springs, Colorado

Marcia L. London, R.N., M.S.N., N.N.P.
Neonatal Nurse Practitioner
Intensive Care Nursery
Memorial Hospital
Colorado Springs, Colorado

Patricia A. Ladewig, R.N., M.S.N., N.P.
Assistant Professor
Loretto Heights College
Denver, Colorado
and
Doctoral Candidate
University of Denver
Denver, Colorado

Joan Edelstein, R.N., P.N.P., M.S.N., M.P.H.
Doctoral Candidate
Assistant Professor, Family Health
San Jose State University
San Jose, California
Contributed to Chapters 14, 15, 16, and 29

Ann Havenhill, R.N., M.N.
Associate Professor, Division of Nursing
Graceland College
Independence, Missouri
Contributed to Chapter 15

Louise Westberg Hedstrom, R.N., C.N.M., M.S.N.
Assistant Professor, Department of Nursing
North Park College
Chicago, Illinois
Contributed to Chapter 12

Linda Andrist Hereford, R.N., M.S.N., N.P.
Assistant Professor
Massachusetts General Institute of Health Professions
Boston, Massachusetts
Contributed to Chapters 11, 16, and 27

E. JoAnne Jones, R.N., M.Ed., M.S.N.
Doctoral Candidate
Associate Professor
School of Nursing
Norfolk State University
Norfolk, Virginia
Contributed Chapter 17

Joy M. Khader, R.N., M.S.N.
Assistant Professor, Department of Nursing
Westminster College
Salt Lake City, Utah
Contributed to Chapters 24 and 25

CONTRIBUTORS

Virginia Gramzow Kinnick, R.N., C.N.M., M.S.N.
Assistant Professor, School of Nursing
University of Northern Colorado
Greeley, Colorado
Contributed Chapter 11

Nancy Ellen Krauss, R.N., M.S.
Assistant Professor
School of Nursing
University of Maryland
Baltimore, Maryland
Contributed to Chapters 3, 10, 16, and 27

Joan Kub, R.N., M.S.
Instructor, School of Nursing
University of Maryland
Baltimore, Maryland
Contributed to Chapters 3, 10, 16, and 27

Mary Ann Leppink, R.N., M.S.
Instructor,
Department of Nursing
Westminster College
Salt Lake City, Utah
Contributed to Chapters 24 and 25

Anne L. Matthews, R.N., M.S.
Doctoral Student, School of Nursing
University of Colorado Health Sciences Center
Denver, Colorado
Contributed Chapter 7

Nancy McCluggage, R.N., C.N.M., M.A.
Program Instructor, Maternal-Newborn (Nurse Mid-Wifery) Program
Yale University School of Nursing
New Haven, Connecticut
Contributed Chapter 13 and contributed to Chapter 15

Cynthia A. McMahon, R.N., M.S.N.
Instructor of Nursing
Beth-El School of Nursing
Colorado Springs, Colorado
Contributed to Chapter 2

Anne Garrard McMath, R.N., M.S.N., P.N.P.
Maternal-Child Nursing Instructor
Loretto Heights College
Denver, Colorado
Contributed to Chapters 23 and 27

Donna Rae Meirath Moriarty, R.N., M.S.N.
Assistant Professor, Parent-Child Nursing
School of Nursing
Creighton University
Omaha, Nebraska
Contributed to Chapter 19

Karen Rooks Nauer, R.N., B.S.
Maternal–Child Educator
Memorial Hospital
Colorado Springs, Colorado
Contributed to Chapter 23

Sally J. Phillips, R.N., M.S.N.
Doctoral Candidate
Assistant Professor, School of Nursing
University of Colorado Health Sciences Center
Denver, Colorado
Contributed to Chapter 20

Lovena L. Porter, R.N., M.S.
OB/GYN Nurse Clinician
Colorado Springs Medical Center
Colorado Springs, Colorado
Contributed to Chapters 6 and 10 and contributed Chapter 9

Joanne F. Ruth, R.N., M.S.
Maternal-Child Nursing Instructor
Beth-El School of Nursing
Colorado Springs, Colorado
Contributed to Chapter 23

M. Carole Schoffstall, R.N., M.S.
Department of Nursing
Beth-El School of Nursing
Colorado Springs, Colorado
Contributed to Chapter 30

Constance Lawrenz Slaughter, R.N., B.S.N.
Assistant Professor, Maternal-Child Nursing
University of Portland
Portland, Oregon
and
Staff Nurse
Bess Kaiser Hospital
Portland, Oregon
Contributed to Chapters 3, 18, and 21

Mari Lou Steffen, R.N., Ed.D.
Chairperson, Nursing Department
Westminster College
Salt Lake City, Utah
Contributed Chapter 8 and contributed to Chapter 26

Elvira Szigeti, R.N., M.N.
Doctoral Student
Associate Professor
Loretto Heights College
Denver, Colorado
Contributed to Chapter 28

Janel N. Timmins, R.N., M.A.
Maternal-Child Nursing Instructor
Beth-El School of Nursing
Colorado Springs, Colorado
Contributed to Chapter 20

Bette Blome Winyall, R.N., M.S.N.
Assistant Professor
School of Nursing
University of Maryland
Baltimore, Maryland
Contributed Chapters 4 and 5

FIRST EDITION CONTRIBUTORS

Martha Cox Baily, R.N.

Elizabeth M. Bear, C.N.M., M.S.

Irene Bobak, R.N., C.N.P., M.N., M.S.N.

Sallye P. Brown, R.N., M.N.

Penelope Childress, R.N.

Pamela Crispin, R.N.

Marilynn Doenges, R.N., M.A.

Nancy Donaldson, R.N., M.S.N.

Mildred R. (Holly) Emrick, R.N., M.S.N.

Jack Ford, M.D., F.A.C.O.G.

Laurel Freed, R.N., P.N.P., M.N.

Sandra L. Gardner, R.N., P.N.P., M.S.

Pauline Goolkasian, R.N., M.S.N.

Ann Kelley Havenhill, R.N., M.N.

Loretta C. Cermely Ivory, R.N., C.N.M., M.S.

L. Jean Johns, R.N., M.S.

E. JoAnne Jones, R.N., M.Ed., M.S.N.

Emma K. Kamm, R.N.

Janet Kennedy, R.N., D.N.Sc.

Jean Theirl King, R.D., B.S.

Virginia Gramzow Kinnick, R.N. C.N.M., M.S.N.

Eleanor Latterell, R.D., M.S.

Eileen Leaphart, R.N.C., M.N.

Anne Lamphier Matthews, R.N., M.S.

Mary Ann McClees, R.N., M.S.

Nancy McCluggage, R.N., C.N.M., M.A.

Caryl E. Mobley, R.N., M.S.N.

Irene L. Nielsen, R.N., C.N.M., M.S.

Lovena L. Porter, R.N., M.S.

Carol Freeman Rosenkranz, R.N., M.N.

Joanne F. Ruth, R.N., M.S.

Paula Shearer, R.N., M.S.N.

Mari Lou Steffen, R.N., Ed.D.

Marie Swigert, R.N., M.S.N.

Marcia Vavich, R.N., M.A.

Janet Veatch, R.N., M.N.

Betty Blome Winyall, R.N., M.S.N.

ACKNOWLEDGMENTS

For photographs used as unit and chapter openers and for the color plates, the publisher and authors would like to acknowledge the following photographers.

Unit Openers

I	William Thompson	IV	Suzanne Arms ©
II	George B. Fry III	V	George B. Fry III
III	Suzanne Arms ©	VI	Rosyln Banish ©

Chapter Openers

1	George B. Fry III	16	Suzanne Arms ©
2	William Thompson	17	George B. Fry III
3	George B. Fry III	18	William Thompson
4	George B. Fry III	19	William Thompson
5	William Thompson	20	Suzanne Arms ©
6	William Thompson	21	Suzanne Arms ©
7	George B. Fry III	22	George B. Fry III
8	George B. Fry III	23	George B. Fry III
9	William Thompson	24	George B. Fry III
10	William Thompson	25	George B. Fry III
11	William Thompson	26	William Thompson
12	William Thompson	27	William Thompson
13	George B. Fry III	28	George B. Fry III
14	Suzanne Arms ©	29	George B. Fry III
15	William Thompson	30	George B. Fry III

Color Plates

I	Suzanne Arms ©
II–XII	William Thompson

Addison-Wesley, Nursing Division, and the authors would also like to thank the nurses and staff of W3A and the Labor and Delivery room of Stanford University Hospital and Sequoia Hospital for their cooperation.

CONTENTS IN BRIEF

UNIT I □ INTRODUCTION TO FAMILY-CENTERED MATERNITY NURSING   1

1 Current Perspectives of Maternal–Newborn Nursing   2

2 Tools for Maternal–Newborn Nursing Practice   18

3 Dynamics of Family Life   30

UNIT II □ HUMAN REPRODUCTION AND DEVELOPMENT   55

4 Human Reproductive System   56

5 Sexual Development and Sexuality   87

6 Family Planning   109

7 Genetic Counseling   133

8 Conception and Fetal Development   156

UNIT III □ PREGNANCY   189

9 Physical and Psychologic Changes of Pregnancy   190

10 Antepartal Nursing Assessment   209

11 The Expectant Family: Needs and Care   244

12 Complications of Pregnancy   309

13 Diagnostic Assessment of Fetal Status   365

UNIT IV □ LABOR AND DELIVERY   393

14 Processes and Stages of Labor and Delivery   394

15 Intrapartal Nursing Assessment   423

16 The Family in Childbirth: Needs and Care   465

17 Obstetric Analgesia and Anesthesia   509

18 Complications of Labor and Delivery   534

19 Elective Obstetric Procedures   584

20 Birthing Options   612

UNIT V □ THE NEONATE   633

21 Physiologic Responses of the Newborn to Birth   634

22 Nursing Assessment of the Newborn   659

23 The Normal Newborn: Needs and Care   708

24 The High-Risk Newborn: Needs and Care   732

25 Complications of the Neonate   784

26 Congenital Anomalies   847

UNIT VI □ THE PUERPERIUM   899

27 The Postpartal Family: Assessment,
    Needs, and Care   900

28 Attachment   951

29 Complications of the Puerperium   972

30 Families in Crisis and the Role of
    the Nurse   991

APPENDICES   1021

A   PREGNANT PATIENT'S BILL OF RIGHTS 1021

B   UNITED NATIONS DECLARATION OF
    THE RIGHTS OF THE CHILD   1022

C   EVALUATION OF FETAL WEIGHT AND
    MATURITY BY ULTRASONIC
    MEASUREMENT   1024

D   CLINICAL ESTIMATION OF
    GESTATIONAL AGE   1025

E   NATIONAL CENTER FOR HEALTH
    STATISTICS: PHYSICAL GROWTH
    PERCENTILES   1027

F   CONVERSIONS AND EQUIVALENTS   1031

GLOSSARY   1032

INDEX   1055

CONTENTS IN DETAIL

UNIT I ■ INTRODUCTION TO FAMILY-CENTERED MATERNITY NURSING   1

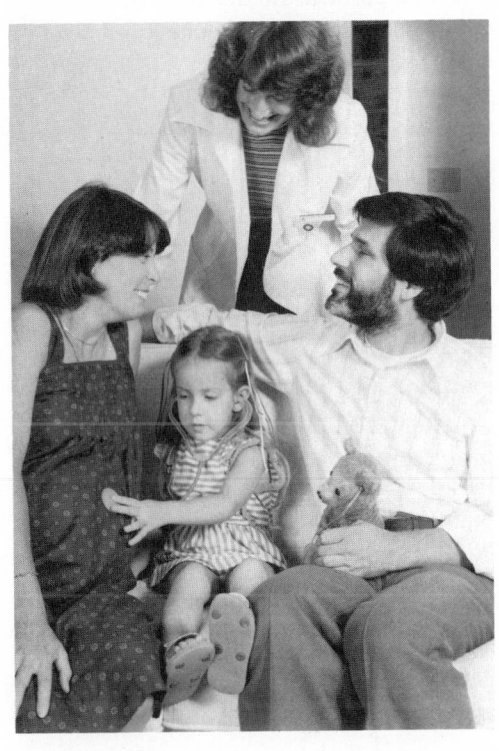

European Developments   3

Developments in the United States   4

Development of Nurse-Midwifery   5
Nurse-midwifery in Europe □ Nurse-midwifery in the United States

OVERVIEW OF CONTEMPORARY MATERNITY CARE   8

State of the Art   8
Ultrasonography □ Amniocentesis □ Electronic fetal monitoring □ Fetal surgery □ In vitro fertilization □ Scientific advances or medical excesses

Ethical Issues   10
Abortion □ Passive euthanasia □ Amniocentesis for sex determination □ Intrauterine fetal surgery □ In vitro fertilization and surrogate childbearing □ Implications for nurses

The Changing Health Care Environment   12
Development of family-centered care □ Birth alternatives □ Implications for nurses

CHAPTER 1
CURRENT PERSPECTIVES OF MATERNAL–NEWBORN NURSING   2

HISTORICAL OVERVIEW OF OBSTETRICS AND MATERNITY NURSING CARE   3

Early Recorded Developments   3

THE EXPANDING ROLE OF NURSES IN MATERNITY CARE   14

Roles and Settings for Nurses   14

Legal Aspects of Maternal–Newborn Nursing   14

Nurses and Physicians   15

SUMMARY   16

CHAPTER 2

TOOLS FOR MATERNAL–NEWBORN NURSING PRACTICE   18

KNOWLEDGE BASE   19

NURSING PROCESS   19

Assessment   19

Nursing Diagnoses and Planning   19

Nursing Interventions   20

Evaluation   20

COMMUNICATION   20

STATISTICS   20

Descriptive Statistics   21
Birth rate □ Age of mother □ Weight at
birth □ Infant mortality □ Maternal mortality

Implications for Nursing   23

NURSING RESEARCH   26

Application of Research   26
Example 1 □ Example 2

APPLICATIONS OF TOOLS FOR NURSING
PRACTICE   27

SUMMARY   28

CHAPTER 3

DYNAMICS OF FAMILY LIFE   30

THE CONTEMPORARY FAMILY   31

Structural Configurations   32
Other Emerging Family Structures   32

FAMILY PROCESSES   35

Functions   35

Roles   35

THEORETICAL APPROACHES TO
UNDERSTANDING THE FAMILY   36

Developmental Approach   36
Developmental stages and tasks □ Psychosocial
development of family members

Other Approaches to the Family   41

FACTORS AFFECTING FAMILY STRUCTURES
AND PROCESSES   41

Socioeconomic Factors and Life-Style   41

Societal Trends   42
Changing status of women □ Value of children

Ethnic and Cultural Influences   43
Mexican American family □ American Indian
family □ Black American family □ Oriental
families

Environmental Factors   46

NURSING IMPLICATIONS   46

The Family as Client   47

Family Assessment   47

Nursing Diagnosis and Planning   49

Intervention   49

Evaluation   50

Application of the Nursing Process:
A Case Example   50

SUMMARY   52

UNIT II ▪ HUMAN REPRODUCTION AND DEVELOPMENT

55

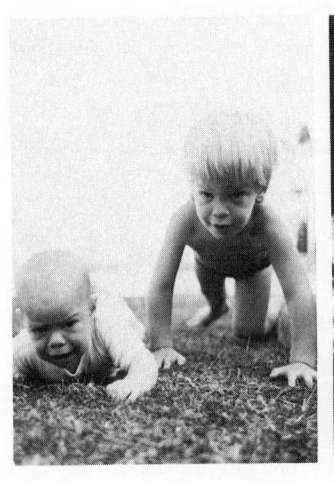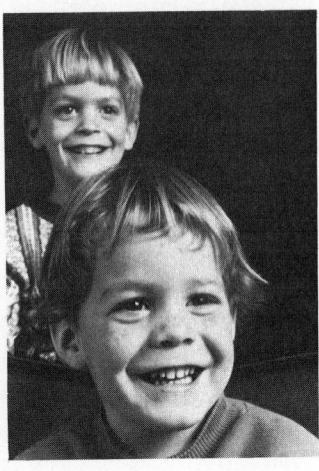

CHAPTER 4

HUMAN REPRODUCTIVE SYSTEM   56

**EMBRYOLOGIC DEVELOPMENT OF THE
REPRODUCTIVE SYSTEM   57**

  Ovaries and Testes   57

  Other Internal Genitals   57

  External Genitals   57

MALE REPRODUCTIVE SYSTEM   59

  External Genitals   59
  Penis □ Scrotum

  Internal Genitals   61
  Testes □ Epididymides □ Vas deferens
  □ Ejaculatory ducts □ Urethra

  Accessory Glands   63
  Seminal vesicles □ Prostate gland
  □ Bulbourethral and urethral glands

  Semen   64

  Breasts   64

FEMALE REPRODUCTIVE SYSTEM   65

  Bony Pelvis   65
  Bony structure □ Pelvic floor □ Pelvic
  division □ Types of pelves

  External Genitals   71
  Mons pubis □ Labia majora □ Labia minora
  □ Clitoris □ Urethral meatus and paraurethral
  glands □ Vaginal vestibule □ Perineal body

  Internal Genitals   73
  Vagina □ Uterus □ Uterine ligaments □
  Fallopian (uterine) tubes □ Ovaries

  Breasts   84

SUMMARY   86

CHAPTER 5

SEXUAL DEVELOPMENT
AND SEXUALITY   87

COMPONENTS OF HUMAN SEXUALITY   88

DEVELOPMENT OF SEXUALITY   89

  Infancy to Late Childhood   89

  Adolescence   89

  Adulthood   90

PUBERTY   91

  Major Physical Changes   91

  Physiology of Onset   92

  Effects of Male Hormones   93

  Effects of Ovarian Hormones   93
  Estrogen □ Progesterone □ Role of
  prostaglandins

MENSTRUAL CYCLE   94

  Female Reproductive Cycle   96

  Ovarian Follicular Changes   96

  Ovulation   98

  **Endometrial and Cervical Mucosal
  Changes   98**

  Premenstrual Tension Syndrome   99

  Dysmenorrhea   100

  Menstrual Cycle Variations   100

CLIMACTERIC   101

  Psychologic Aspects of Menopause   101

  Physical Aspects of Menopause   101

  Sexual Activity in the Climacteric   102

  Interventions   102

COITUS (SEXUAL INTERCOURSE)   102

Psychosocial Aspects   102

Physiology of Sexual Response   103

Neurologic Control of Sexual
Response   104

IMPLICATIONS FOR NURSES   105

Children's Sexuality Counseling   105

Sexual History Assessments   106

SUMMARY   106

CHAPTER 6

FAMILY PLANNING   109

INFERTILITY   110

Essential Components of Fertility   110

Preliminary Investigation   111

Tests for Infertility   115
Ovulatory function □ Cervical mucosal
tests □ Sperm adequacy tests □ Tubal
patency tests

Methods of Infertility Management   118
Pharmacologic methods □ Artificial insemination □ In vitro fertilization □ Adoption

The Nurse's Role   119

CONTRACEPTION   120

Fertility Awareness Methods   120

Mechanical Contraceptives   122

Oral Contraceptives   125

Injectable Contraceptives   127

Spermicides   127

Operative Sterilization   127

Induced Abortion   128
Factors influencing the decision to seek
abortion □ Counseling □ Methods
□ Nursing management

SUMMARY   131

CHAPTER 7

GENETIC COUNSELING   133

CHROMOSOMES AND CHROMOSOMAL
ABERRATIONS   135

Autosome Abnormalities   136
Abnormalities of chromosome number
□ Abnormalities of chromosome structure

Sex Chromosome Abnormalities   140

PATTERNS OF INHERITANCE   142

Autosomal Dominant Inheritance   142

Autosomal Recessive Inheritance   143

X-Linked Recessive Inheritance   144

X-Linked Dominant Inheritance   145

Polygenic Inheritance   145

Nongenetic Conditions   145

PRENATAL DIAGNOSIS   146

POSTNATAL DIAGNOSIS   148

GENETIC COUNSELING: THE NURSE'S ROLE   150

What Can Families Expect?   150

Appropriate Referrals   151

Alternatives to Increased Risks   151

Prerequisites of Counseling   152

Principles in Counseling   152
Accurate diagnosis □ Nondirective counsel-
ing □ Confidentiality □ Truthfulness □ Timing
□ Team approach □ Follow-up counseling

SUMMARY   154

CHAPTER 8

CONCEPTION
AND FETAL DEVELOPMENT   156

OVERVIEW OF GENETIC PROCESSES   157

Chromosomes and Genes   157

Cellular Division   157
Mitosis □ Meiosis

Maturation of Gametes   160
Ovum □ Sperm

Sex Determination   160

FERTILIZATION   160

CELLULAR MULTIPLICATION   162

IMPLANTATION   162

CELLULAR DIFFERENTIATION   163

INTRAUTERINE ORGAN SYSTEMS   165

  Placenta   165
  Development □ Circulation □
  Functions □ Transport mechanisms

  Fetal Circulation   171

  Fetal Heart   171

**EMBRYO AND FETAL DEVELOPMENT AND
ORGAN FORMATION**   171

Preembryonic Stage   173

Embryonic Stage   173
Third week □ Fourth week □ Fifth
week □ Sixth week □ Seventh week □ Eighth
week

Fetal Stage   179
9–12 weeks □ 13–16 weeks □ 17–20
weeks □ 21–24 weeks □ 25–28 weeks □ 29–
32 weeks □ 33–36 weeks □ 37–40 weeks

**Factors Influencing Embryonic and Fetal
Development   183**

TWINS   185

SUMMARY   185

UNIT III ■ PREGNANCY   189

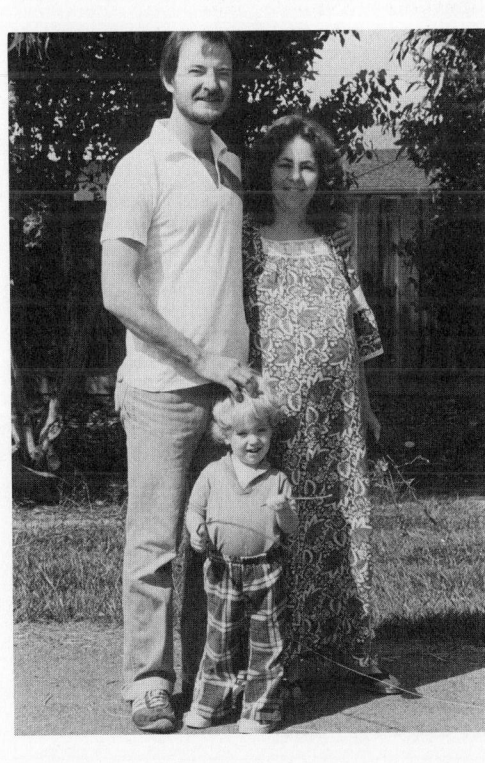

CHAPTER 9

PHYSICAL AND PSYCHOLOGIC CHANGES OF PREGNANCY   190

SUBJECTIVE (PRESUMPTIVE) CHANGES   191

OBJECTIVE (PROBABLE) CHANGES   192

PREGNANCY TESTS   194

  Immunoassay   194

  Radioreceptor Assay (RRA)   194

  Bioassay   194

  Over-the-Counter Pregnancy Tests   195

DIAGNOSTIC (POSITIVE) CHANGES   195

**ANATOMY AND PHYSIOLOGY OF
PREGNANCY**   195

  Reproductive System   195
  Uterus □ Cervix □ Ovaries □ Vagina
  □ Breasts

Respiratory System   197

Cardiovascular System   198

Gastrointestinal System   198

Urinary Tract   199

Skin   199

Skeletal System   199

Metabolism   200
Weight gain □ Water metabolism □ Nutrient
metabolism □ Mineral and vitamin metabolism

Endocrine System   201
Thyroid □ Parathyroid □ Pituitary □
Adrenals □ Pancreas □ Placental hormones
□ Prostaglandins in pregnancy

EMOTIONAL AND PSYCHOLOGIC CHANGES
OF PREGNANCY   203

Ambivalence   203

Acceptance   203

Introversion   204

Emotional Lability   204

Body Image   204

CULTURAL VALUES AND REPRODUCTIVE
BEHAVIOR   204

Health Beliefs   205

Health Practices   206

SUMMARY   207

CHAPTER 10

ANTEPARTAL NURSING ASSESSMENT   209

CLIENT HISTORY   210

Definition of Terms   210

Client Profile   211

Obtaining Data   211

Prenatal High-Risk Screening   213

INITIAL PHYSICAL ASSESSMENT   213

DETERMINATION OF DELIVERY DATE   236

Nägele's Rule   236

Uterine Size   236
Physical examination □ Fundal height
□ Quickening □ Fetal heartbeat

Ultrasound   237

INITIAL PSYCHOLOGIC ASSESSMENT   238

SUBSEQUENT PHYSICAL ASSESSMENT   238

SUBSEQUENT PSYCHOLOGIC ASSESSMENT   240

ROLE OF THE NURSE   243

SUMMARY   243

CHAPTER 11

THE EXPECTANT FAMILY:
NEEDS AND CARE   244

PREGNANCY AND THE EXPECTANT FAMILY   246

Pregnancy as Crisis   246

Pregnancy as a Developmental Stage   247

THE EXPECTANT FAMILY'S RESPONSES TO
PREGNANCY   247

The Mother   247

The Father   249
First trimester □ Second trimester □ Third
trimester □ Couvade

Siblings   250

Grandparents   251

COMMON DISCOMFORTS OF PREGNANCY   252

First Trimester   252
Nausea and vomiting □ Nasal stuffiness and
epistaxis □ Ptyalism □ Urinary frequency and
urgency □ Breast tenderness □ Increased
vaginal discharge

Second and Third Trimesters   256
Heartburn (pyrosis) □ Ankle edema
□ Varicose veins □ Hemorrhoids
□ Constipation □ Backache □ Leg
Cramps □ Faintness □ Shortness of breath

Nursing Responsibilities   259

COMMON CONCERNS DURING PREGNANCY   260

Breast Care   260

Clothing   260

Bathing   261

Employment   261

Travel   261

Activity and Rest   261

Exercises   262
Abdominal musculature □ Perineal
musculature □ Tailor sitting

Sexual Activity   263

Dental Care   265

Immunizations   265

Teratogenic Substances   265

Medications   266

Smoking   268

Alcohol   268

NUTRITION   269

Maternal Weight Gain   269

Nutritional Requirements   270
Calories □ Protein □ Fat □ Carbohydrates
□ Minerals □ Vitamins

Vegetarianism   279

Factors Influencing Nutrition   281
Lactose intolerance □ Pica □ Food
myths □ Cultural, ethnic, and religious
influences □ Psychosocial factors

Nursing Responsibilities   285

ANTEPARTAL NURSING MANAGEMENT   285

**Assessment: Establishing the
Data Base   285**

Interventions   286
Support of family unit □ Cultural
considerations in pregnancy □ Anticipatory
guidance for the pueperium □ Teaching
communication skills

**Classes for Family Members During
Pregnancy   291**
Prenatal education □ Prepared sibling
programs □ Classes for grandparents

**SELECTED METHODS OF CHILDBIRTH
PREPARATION   293**

Read Method   293

Psychoprophylactic (Lamaze) Method   294

Bradley Method   295

Hypnosis   295

**PREPARING THE ADOLESCENT FOR
CHILDBIRTH AND CHILDREARING   296**

Physical Changes of Adolescence   296

Psychosocial Effects of Adolescence   296

The Pregnant Teenager   297
Physiologic risks of the pregnant
teenager □ Psychologic risk of
pregnancy □ Sociologic risk

The Adolescent Father   301

**Parents' Reaction to Adolescent
Pregnancy   301**

**Nursing Management of the Pregnant
Adolescent   302**
Assessment: Establishing the data
base □ Nursing responsibilities

Prenatal Education for the Adolescent   305

SUMMARY   305

CHAPTER 12

COMPLICATIONS OF PREGNANCY   309

PREGESTATIONAL MEDICAL DISORDERS   310

Cardiac Disease   310
Classification □ Clinical manifestations □
Fetal–neonatal implications □ Interventions

Diabetes Mellitus   313
Classification of diabetes mellitus □ Influence of
pregnancy on diabetes □ Influence of diabetes
mellitus on pregnancy outcome □
Maternal implications □ Fetal–neonatal
implications □ Tests for diabetes
mellitus □ Interventions □ Labor □
Postpartum

Thyroid Dysfunction   321
Hyperthyroidism (thyrotoxicosis)
□ Hypothyroidism

**Other Medical Conditions and
Pregnancy   326**
Anemia

**MEDICAL DISORDERS ASSOCIATED
WITH PREGNANCY   328**

Hyperemesis Gravidarum   328
Interventions

Bleeding Disorders   328
General principles of nursing intervention
□ Spontaneous abortion □ Ectopic
pregnancy □ Hydatidiform mole □ Placenta
previa □ Abruptio placentae

Incompetent Cervix   335

HYPERTENSIVE DISORDERS IN PREGNANCY 336

**Pregnancy-Induced Hypertension
(Preeclampsia and Eclampsia) 336**
Incidence ☐ Etiology ☐ Normal physiology and
pathophysiology of PIH ☐ Clinical manifestations ☐ Fetal–neonatal implications ☐ Interventions—mild preeclampsia ☐ Interventions—severe eclampsia ☐ Interventions—
eclampsia ☐ Labor and delivery ☐
Postpartum

Chronic Hypertensive Disease 347

RH SENSITIZATION   347

Fetal–Neonatal Implications 347

Nursing Management 347
Maternal and paternal screening ☐ Prenatal
assessment and interventions ☐ Prenatal
interventions ☐ Postpartal interventions

SURGICAL PROCEDURES DURING
PREGNANCY   351

Appendicitis 351

Cholecystitis and Cholelithiasis 351

Carcinoma of the Breast 352

Carcinoma of the Cervix 352

ACCIDENTS AND TRAUMA   352

INFECTIONS   353

Urinary Tract Infections 353
Lower urinary tract infection ☐ Upper urinary
tract infection

Sexually Transmitted Diseases 354
Syphilis ☐ Gonorrhea ☐ Chlamydial
infections ☐ Condylomata accuminata

Vaginal Infections 355
Monilial (yeast) infection ☐ Trichomonas
infection ☐ Other vaginal infections ☐
Listerial infection

TORCH 357
Toxoplasmosis ☐ Rubella ☐ Cytomegalovirus ☐ Herpesvirus type 2

DRUG USE AND ABUSE   360

Drug Addiction 360

Alcoholism 362
Maternal implications ☐ Fetal–neonatal
implications

SUMMARY   362

CHAPTER 13
DIAGNOSTIC ASSESSMENT
OF FETAL STATUS   365

ULTRASOUND   366

Procedure 367

Clinical Application 368
Early pregnancy detection ☐ Measurement of
biparietal diameter of fetal head ☐ Measurement of crown-to-rump length ☐ Measurement
of femur length ☐ Abdominal measurements
☐ Head-to-abdomen ratios ☐ Detection of
fetal abnormalities ☐ Fetal growth determination ☐ Fetal breathing movements ☐
Localization of placenta ☐ Placental grading
☐ Risks of ultrasound

MATERNAL ASSESSMENT OF FETAL
ACTIVITY   372

NONSTRESS TESTING   373

Interpretation of NST 373

Procedure 374

Prognostic Value 374

CONTRACTION STRESS TEST   374

Indications and Contraindications 375

Procedure 376
CST with intravenous oxytocin ☐ Breast
self-stimulation test

Clinical Application 376

ESTRIOL DETERMINATIONS   379

Estriol Metabolism 379

Patterns of Excretion 379

Urinary Estriol Determinations 380
Procedure ☐ Serial determinations

**Urinary versus Plasma (Serum) Estriol
Determinations 381**

HUMAN PLACENTAL LACTOGEN   381

AMNIOTIC FLUID ANALYSIS   381

Amniocentesis 381
Procedure ☐ Nursing interventions

Clinical Application 382
Evaluation of Rh-sensitized pregnancies
☐ Optical density

Evaluation of Fetal Maturity   384
L/S ratio □ Lung profile □ Shake test (foam
stability test) □ Creatinine level □ Cytologic
examination of fetal cells

Identification of Meconium Staining   387

Antenatal Genetic Screening   387

AMNIOSCOPY   387

X-RAY EXAMINATION   387

FETOSCOPY   388

**IMPLICATIONS OF PRENATAL TESTING
FOR DELIVERY**   388

SUMMARY   388

UNIT IV ▪ LABOR AND DELIVERY   393

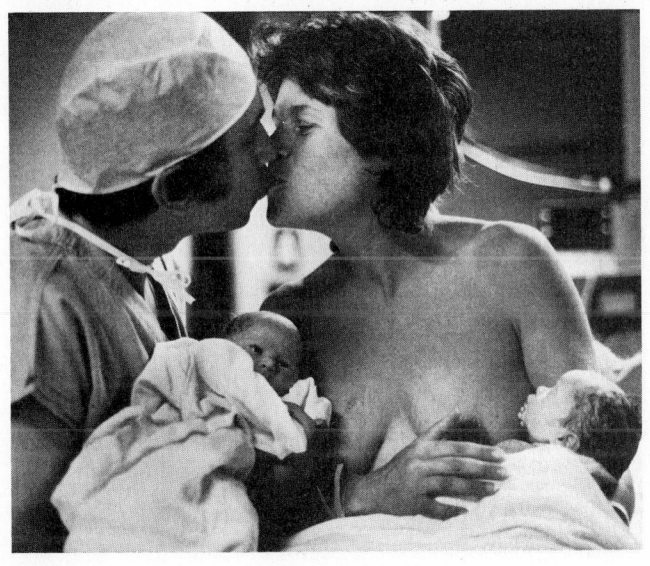

CHAPTER 14

PROCESSES AND STAGES OF
LABOR AND DELIVERY   394

CRITICAL FACTORS IN LABOR   395

The Passage   396
Types of pelves

The Passenger   397
Fetal head □ Fetal attitude □ Fetal lie □ Fetal
presentation □ Fetal position

The Powers   404
Uterine response

The Psyche   405
Coping mechanisms □ Support systems □
Preparation for childbirth

PHYSIOLOGY OF LABOR   406

Possible Causes of Labor Onset   406
Oxytocin stimulation theory □ Progesterone
withdrawal theory □ Estrogen stimulation
theory □ Fetal cortisol theory □ Fetal membrane phospholipid–arachidonic acid–prostaglandin theory □ Distention theory

Biochemical Interaction   407

Myometrial Activity   407

Intraabdominal Pressure   408

**Musculature Changes in the
Pelvic Floor   408**

MATERNAL SYSTEMIC RESPONSE TO LABOR   408

Cardiovascular System   408

Blood Pressure   408

Fluid and Electrolyte Balance   408

Gastrointestinal System   408

Respiratory System   408

Hemopoietic System   408

Renal System   408

Response to Pain 410
Theories of pain ☐ Pain during labor ☐ Factors affecting response to pain

FETAL RESPONSE TO LABOR   413

Biomechanical Changes 414

Cardiac Changes 414

Hemodynamic Changes 414

Positional Changes 414

PREMONITORY SIGNS OF LABOR   415

Lightening 415

Braxton Hicks Contractions 415

Cervical Changes 415

Bloody Show 415

Rupture of Membranes 415

Sudden Burst of Energy 416

Other Signs 416

Differences Between True and False Labor 416

STAGES OF LABOR AND DELIVERY   416

First Stage 417
Latent phase ☐ Active phase

Second Stage 418
Spontaneous delivery (vertex presentation)

Third Stage 419
Placental separation ☐ Placental delivery

Fourth Stage 420

SUMMARY   421

CHAPTER 15

INTRAPARTAL NURSING ASSESSMENT 423

MATERNAL ASSESSMENT   424

History 424

Intrapartal High-Risk Screening 425

Intrapartal Physical Assessment 425

Assessment of Pelvic Adequacy 426
Pelvic inlet ☐ Pelvic cavity (midpelvis) ☐ Pelvic outlet

Intrapartal Psychologic Assessment 433

Methods of Evaluating Labor Progress 433
Contraction assessment ☐ Cervical assessment ☐ Evaluation of labor progress

FETAL ASSESSMENT   441

Determination of Fetal Position and Presentation 441
Inspection ☐ Palpation ☐ Vaginal examination and ultrasound

Evaluation of Fetal Status During Labor 443
Auscultation of FHTs ☐ Electronic monitoring ☐ Telemetry

Fetal Heart Rate Patterns 450
Baseline rate ☐ Baseline changes ☐ Tachycardia ☐ Bradycardia ☐ Baseline variability ☐ Periodic changes ☐ Accelerations ☐ Decelerations ☐ Reassuring and nonreassuring FHR patterns

Value of Electronic Fetal Monitoring 458

Psychologic Reactions to Electronic Monitoring 459

Nursing Care and Responsibilities 460
Interpretation of FHR tracings

Additional Assessment Techniques 461
Monitoring of fetal acid–base status ☐ Fetal blood sampling procedure

SUMMARY   463

CHAPTER 16

THE FAMILY IN CHILDBIRTH: NEEDS AND CARE   465

NURSING MANAGEMENT OF ADMISSION   466
NURSING MANAGEMENT OF LABOR   469

Cultural Considerations 469
Modesty ☐ Pain expression ☐ Role of the father

The Adolescent During Labor and Delivery 471

Management of Pain Relief 482
Assessment ☐ Intervention

Nursing Care Plan 487

MANAGEMENT OF SPONTANEOUS DELIVERY 487

Birthing Room 487

Delivery Room 488

Nursing Interventions 488
Preparing the woman and the coach for delivery ☐ Assisting the physician/nurse-midwife

Physician/Nurse-Midwife
Interventions   490

IMMEDIATE CARE OF THE NEWBORN   492

Apgar Scoring System   492

Care of Umbilical Cord   495

Physical Assessment of Newborn by
Delivery Room Nurse   495

Newborn Identification Procedures   497

MANAGEMENT OF THE THIRD AND FOURTH
STAGES OF LABOR   497

Third Stage   497

Use of oxytocics ☐ Controlling postpartal
hemorrhage

Fourth Stage   500

FACILITATION OF ATTACHMENT   502

DELIVERY IN LESS-THAN-IDEAL
CIRCUMSTANCES   503

Precipitous Delivery   503

Delivery of infant in vertex presentation
☐ Delivery of infant in breech presentation

Out-of-Hospital Births   505

Nursing management of the expectant
mother ☐ Nursing management of the
newborn ☐ Facilitation of parent–infant
bonding

SUMMARY   507

CHAPTER 17
OBSTETRIC ANALGESIA AND
ANESTHESIA   509

METHODS OF PAIN RELIEF   510

Systemic Drugs   510

Administration of analgesic agents ☐ Narcotic
administration ☐ Narcotic
Agonists ☐ Ataractics ☐ Sedatives

Regional Analgesia and Anesthesia   513

Regional anesthetic agents ☐ Adverse maternal
reactions ☐ Interventions

Paracervical Block   516

Technique ☐ Nursing implications

Peridural Block—Epidural and
Caudal   517

Technique for lumbar epidural
block ☐ Technique for continuous lumbar
epidural block ☐ Technique for caudal block

Subarachnoid Block (Spinal, Low Spinal,
Saddle Block)   525

Technique ☐ Nursing implications

Pudendal Block   527

Technique

Local Anesthesia   528

Technique

GENERAL ANESTHESIA   528

Inhalation Anesthetics   529

Nitrous oxide ☐ Methoxyflurane
(Penthrane) ☐ Halothane (Fluothane)

Intravenous Anesthetics   529

Thiopental sodium (Pentothal) ☐ Ketamine
(Ketalar, Ketaject)

Balanced Anesthesia   530

Complications of General Anesthesia   530

Fetal depression ☐ Uterine
relaxation ☐ Vomiting and aspiration

Medical Interventions for Acute Respiratory
Obstruction   531

SUMMARY   531

CHAPTER 18
COMPLICATIONS OF LABOR AND
DELIVERY   534

COMPLICATIONS INVOLVING THE PSYCHE   535

Interventions   536

COMPLICATIONS INVOLVING THE POWERS   536

General Principles of Nursing
Intervention   536

Dysfunctional Labor Patterns   537

Hypertonic labor patterns ☐ Hypotonic labor
patterns ☐ Prolonged labor ☐ Precipitous labor

Friedman's Classification of Dysfunctional
Labor   544

Dystocia Due to Uterine Rings   545

Physiologic retraction rings ☐ Pathologic
retraction rings

Premature Rupture of Membranes   546

Preterm Labor   547

Ruptured Uterus   550

COMPLICATIONS INVOLVING THE PASSENGER   551

Fetal Problems   551

Malpositions □ Malpresentations

Developmental Abnormalities   556

Macrosomia □ Hydrocephaly □ Other fetal malformations

Multiple Pregnancies   557

Identification of multiple gestations □ Three or more fetuses

Fetal Distress   560

Intrauterine Fetal Death (IUFD)   560

Placental Problems   561

Abruptio placentae □ Placenta previa □ Complications associated with bleeding □ Other placental problems

Problems Associated with the Umbilical Cord   574

Prolapsed umbilical cord □ Umbilical cord abnormalities

Problems Associated with Amniotic Fluid   576

Amniotic fluid embolism □ Hydramnios □ Oligohydramnios

COMPLICATIONS INVOLVING THE PASSAGE   577

Contractures of the Inlet   577

Contractures of the Midpelvis   578

Contractures of the Outlet   578

Implications of Pelvic Contractures   578

COMPLICATIONS OF THIRD AND FOURTH STAGES   578

Postpartal Hemorrhage   578

Uterine atony □ Retained placenta □ Retained placental fragments □ Placental accreta □ Lacerations

Inversion of Uterus   579

Genital Tract Trauma   580

Hematoma □ Perineal lacerations

COMPLICATED CHILDBIRTH: EFFECTS ON THE FAMILY   580

Nursing Management   580

SUMMARY   581

CHAPTER 19

ELECTIVE OBSTETRIC PROCEDURES   584

VERSION   585

External Cephalic Version   585

Internal or Podalic Version   585

Nursing Interventions   586

AMNIOTOMY   586
INDUCTION OF LABOR   587

Contraindications   587

Labor Readiness   588

Fetal maturity □ Cervical readiness

Methods   588

Amniotomy □ Oxytocin infusion □ Nursing interventions

Prostaglandin Administration   595

EPISIOTOMY   595

Nursing Interventions   596

FORCEPS DELIVERY   596

Types of Forceps   597

Indications   597

Complications   597

Prerequisites for Forceps Application   598

Trial or Failed Forceps Delivery   598

Nursing interventions

VACUUM EXTRACTION   598

Nursing Interventions   599

CESAREAN BIRTH   599

Indications for Cesarean Delivery   600

Maternal Mortality and Morbidity   605

Types of Cesarean Deliveries   605

Uterine Incisions   605

Low-segment transverse incision □ Classic cesarean incision □ Low classic incision

Elective Repeat Cesarean   606

Nursing Interventions for Family Having Cesarean Birth   606

Preparation for cesarean birth □ Preparation for repeat cesarean birth □ Preparation for emergency cesarean delivery □ Delivery

Analgesia and Anesthesia   609

Immediate Postpartal Recovery Period   609

SUMMARY   609

CHAPTER 20
BIRTHING OPTIONS 612

BIRTHING OPTIONS 613
Siblings at Birth 613
Alternative Positions 614
The Leboyer Method 617

Birth Centers 618
Case study
Early Discharge 628
Home Births 628
Assessment □ Antepartal interventions □ Labor
and delivery at home □ Indications for
hospitalization
SUMMARY 631

UNIT V ■ THE NEONATE 633

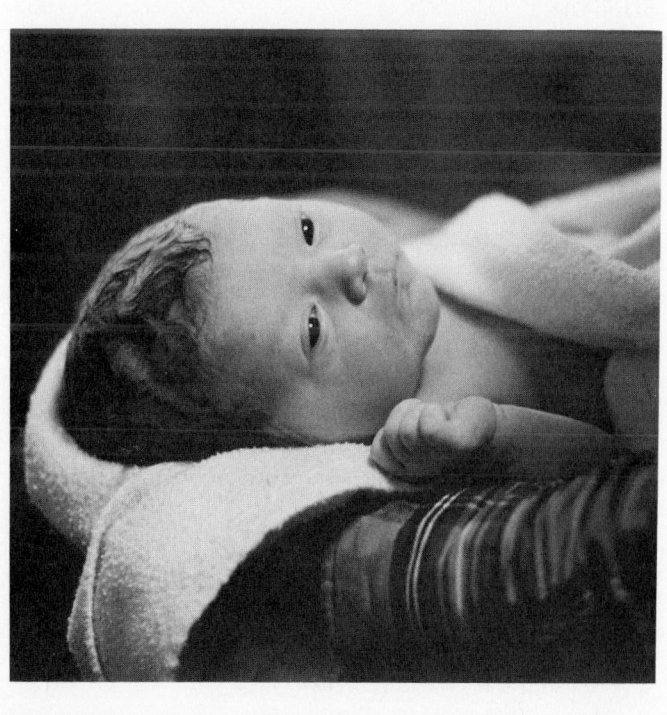

CHAPTER 21
PHYSIOLOGIC RESPONSES OF THE NEWBORN TO BIRTH 634

RESPIRATORY ADAPTATIONS 635
Initiation of Breathing 636
Chemical stimuli □ Thermal stimuli □ Sensory
and physical stimuli □ Mechanical events
Neonatal Pulmonary Physiology 637
Characteristics of Neontal Respiration 639

CARDIOVASCULAR ADAPTATIONS 639
Embryology 639
Fetal–Neonatal Transition Circulation 640
Characteristics 641
Heart rate □ Blood pressure □ Heart murmurs
□ Cardiac output
Oxygen Transport 642

HEMATOPOIETIC SYSTEM 643
Neonatal Hematology 644

TEMPERATURE REGULATION   645

   Heat Loss 646

   Heat Production (Thermogenesis) 647
   Response to heat

HEPATIC ADAPTATION   648

   Iron Storage and Red Blood Cell
   Production 648

   Carbohydrate Metabolism 648

   Physiologic Jaundice—Icterus
   Neonatorum 648
   Breast-feeding jaundice

   Coagulation 650

GASTROINTESTINAL ADAPTATION   650

   Functional Development 651

   Digestion of Carbohydrates 651

   Digestion of Proteins 651

   Digestion of Fats 651

GENITOURINARY ADAPTATION   652

   Kidney Development and Function 652

   Genital Development 653

IMMUNOLOGIC ADAPTATIONS   653
NEUROLOGIC AND SENSORY/PERCEPTUAL
FUNCTIONING   654

   Motor Activity 654

   Sensory Capacities of the Newborn 655
   Auditory capacity □ Olfactory capacity
   □ Taste □ Tactile capacity □ Sucking

   States of the Newborn 655
   Sleep states □ Alert states

   Neurologic Adaptations 657

SUMMARY   657

CHAPTER 22

NURSING ASSESSMENT OF THE
NEWBORN   659

ESTIMATION OF GESTATIONAL AGE   660

   Assessment of Physical
   Characteristics 661

   Assessment of Neurologic Status 669

PHYSICAL EXAMINATION   674

   General Appearance 674

   Posture 675

   Weight and Measurements 675

   Temperature 676

   Skin 677

   Head 678
   General Appearance

   Face 678
   Eyes □ Nose □ Mouth □ Ears

   Neck 681

   Chest 682

   Cry 682

   Respiration 682

   Heart 682

   Abdomen 683

   Genitals 684
   Male infants □ Female infants

   Anus 684

   Extremities 684
   Arms and hands □ Legs and feet

   Back 685

   Neurologic Status 685

NEONATAL PHYSICAL ASSESSMENT   687

NEONATAL BEHAVIORAL ASSESSMENT   687

SUMMARY   706

CHAPTER 23

THE NORMAL NEWBORN: NEEDS
AND CARE   708

NURSING OBSERVATIONS AND CARE:
THE FIRST 24 HOURS   709

   Nursing Management of the Newborn at
   Admission 709

   Periods of Reactivity 711

   Subsequent Nursing Management 712

DAILY NEONATAL OBSERVATIONS
AND CARE   714

   Handling and Positioning 714

   Nasal and Oral Suctioning 714

   Wrapping the Newborn 716

   Safety Considerations 716

NEWBORN FEEDING　716

Initial Feeding in the Hospital　716

Nutritional Needs of the Newborn　717

Breast or Bottle?　717
Decision making □ Breast milk: nutritional aspects □ Formula: nutritional aspects

Establishing a Feeding Pattern　718

Nutritional Assessment of the Infant　719
Nutritional assessment tool

Supplemental Foods　721

Weaning　721

CIRCUMCISION　722

SLEEP AND ACTIVITY　723

Sleep–Wake States　724
Crying

ENHANCING INTERACTION BETWEEN PARENTS AND INFANT　725

Early Experiences and Needs at Home　725

THE NEWBORN SCREENING PROGRAM　725

PARENT EDUCATION　725

Positioning and Handling　726

Oral and Nasal Suctioning　726

Stools and Voids　726

Bathing　727
Sponge bath □ Tub baths

Nail Care　728

Dressing the Newborn　728

Temperature Assessment　728

Safety　729

Discharge Planning　730

SUMMARY　731

CHAPTER 24

THE HIGH-RISK NEWBORN: NEEDS AND CARE　732

IDENTIFICATION OF HIGH-RISK INFANTS　733

NURSING MANAGEMENT OF HIGH-RISK INFANTS　735

PRETERM (PREMATURE) INFANTS　737

Preterm Infant's Physiologic Adaptations　737

Respiratory Physiology and Considerations　737

Cardiovascular Physiology and Considerations　739
Thermoregulation

Nutrition and Fluid Requirements　740
Digestive physiology and enzymatic activity □ Formulas for preterm neonates □ Methods of feeding □ Nutritional requirements □ Schedule of feedings

Renal Physiology　746
Fluid requirements □ Nursing management

Hepatic Physiology and Considerations　748

Immunologic Physiology and Considerations　748

Hematologic Physiology and Considerations　748

Reactivity Periods and Behavioral States　749

Central Nervous System Physiology and Considerations　749
Apnea and other complications

Long-Term Needs and Outcome　758

POSTTERM NEONATE　758

LARGE-FOR-GESTATIONAL-AGE INFANT　760

SMALL-FOR-GESTATIONAL-AGE INFANT　761

Etiology　761

Patterns of Intrauterine Growth Retardation　762
Complications

Long-Term Outcome and Needs　762

INFANT OF DIABETIC MOTHER　763

INFANTS OF MOTHERS WITH CARDIAC OR HYPERTENSIVE CARDIOVASCULAR DISEASE　768

Infant of Mother with Cardiac Disease　768

Infant of Mother with Hypertensive Cardiovascular Disease　769

ALCOHOL- OR DRUG-ADDICTED NEONATES　769

Alcohol Dependency　770
Long-term outcomes

Drug Dependency　770
Long-term outcomes

PARENTING THE HIGH-RISK NEONATE   772

   Attachment   772

   Adjustment   772

   Nursing Interventions   774
Intensive care □ Touching and caretaking
□ Nurse–parent interactions □ The role of the
family

   Predischarge Care   779

SUMMARY   780

CHAPTER 25

COMPLICATIONS OF THE NEONATE   784

ASPHYXIA   786

   Pathophysiology   786

   Resuscitation   786
Identification of infants in need of
resuscitation □ Nurse's role □ Equipment and
medications □ Initial resuscitative management
□ Drug therapy

RESPIRATORY DISTRESS   792

   Idiopathic Respiratory Distress Syndrome
   (Hyaline Membrane Disease)   792
Pathophysiology □ Clinical
manifestations □ Interventions

   Transient Tachypnea of the Newborn (Type
   II Respiratory Distress Syndrome)   797

   Meconium Aspiration Syndrome   798
Clinical manifestations □ Management at
delivery □ Management in the nursery

   Complications of Respiratory Therapy   815
Retrolental fibroplasia □ Bronchopulmonary
dysplasia □ Interstitial pulmonary
emphysema □ Pneumothorax □ Other
pulmonary complications □ Cardiac
complications

COLD STRESS   817

   Interventions   817

HYPOGLYCEMIA   818

   Treatment   818

HYPOCALCEMIA   821

   Diagnosis and Treatment   821

NEONATAL JAUNDICE   822

   Mechanism of Bilirubin Conjugation   822

   Pathologic Jaundice   823
Hyperbilirubinemia □ Kernicterus

   Nursing Management   824

HEMOLYTIC DISEASE OF THE NEWBORN   824

   Rh Incompatibility   824
Laboratory data

   ABO Incompatibility   826
Laboratory data

   Prognosis   826

   Neonatal Assessment   827

   Treatment of the Neonate and Nursing
   Responsibilities   827
Exchange transfusion □ Phototherapy □ Drug
therapy

   Support of the Family   830

NEONATAL ANEMIA   830

   Clinical Manifestations and Diagnosis   835

   Management   835
Nursing interventions

POLYCYTHEMIA   835

   Therapy   836

HEMORRHAGIC DISEASE   836

INTRAVENTRICULAR HEMORRHAGE   836

   Interventions   836

**DISSEMINATED INTRAVASCULAR
COAGULATION**   837

NECROTIZING ENTEROCOLITIS   837

   Clinical Manifestations and Diagnosis   837

   Complications   838

   Interventions   838

INFECTIONS   841

   Sepsis Neonatorum   841
Clinical manifestations and diagnosis □ Nursing
management

   Group B Streptococcus   842

   Syphilis   843

   Gonorrhea   844

Herpesvirus Type 2   844

Monilial Infection (Thrush)   844

SUMMARY   845

CHAPTER 26

CONGENITAL ANOMALIES   847

INFANT WITH A DEFECT:
CRISIS FOR THE FAMILY   848

INFANT WITH FEEDING PROBLEMS   850

Pierre Robin Syndrome   850
Physiology and pathophysiology □ Clinical
manifestations □ Differential
diagnosis □ Interventions □ Prognosis

Cleft Lip and Palate   851
Physiology and pathophysiology □ Clinical
manifestations □ Interventions

Choanal Atresia   852

INFANT WITH INBORN ERRORS OF
METABOLISM   857

Phenylketonuria   857

Maple Syrup Urine Disease   858

Homocystinuria   858

Galactosemia   859

Other Metabolic Disorders   859

Congenital Hypothyroidism   859

INFANT WITH GASTROINTESTINAL DEFECT   859

Esophageal Atresia and Tracheoesophageal
Fistula   85
Physiology and pathophysiology □ Clinical
manifestations □ Interventions □ Complications
of surgery □ Prognosis

Diaphragmatic Hernia   861
Physiology and pathophysiology □ Clinical
manifestations □ Interventions □ Nursing
management □ Prognosis

Omphalocele (Exomphalos)   867
Physiology and pathophysiology □
Clinical manifestations □ Interventions
□ Prognosis

Aganglionic Megacolon   868
Physiology and pathophysiology □ Clinical
manifestations □ Differential diagnosis □
Interventions □ Nursing management □
Prognosis

Imperforate Anus   871
Physiology and pathophysiology □ Clinical
manifestations □ Interventions □ Nursing
management □ Complications □ Prognosis

Intestinal Obstruction   872
Physiology and pathophysiology □ Clinical
manifestations □ Differential
diagnosis □ Interventions □ Nursing
management

INFANT WITH GENITOURINARY DEFECT   874

Exstrophy of the Bladder   874

INFANT WITH DISTURBANCE OF
LOCOMOTION   875

Talipes Equinovarus (Clubfoot)   875
Physiology and pathophysiology □ Clinical
manifestations □ Interventions □ Prognosis

Dysplasia of the Hip   876
Physiology and pathophysiology □ Clinical
manifestations □ Differential
diagnosis □ Interventions □ Prognosis

Spina Bifida: Failure of Closure of the
Neural Axis   878
Physiology and pathophysiology □ Clinical
manifestations □ Interventions

CONGENITAL HEART DEFECTS   881

Overview of Congenital Heart Defects   881

Acyanotic Lesions   881
Patent ductus arteriosus □ Atrial septal
defects □ Ventricular septal defects □
Endocardial cushion defects □ Coarctation
of the aorta

Cyanotic Lesions   889
Tetralogy of Fallot □ Pulmonary
stenosis □ Transposition of the great
vessels □ Anomalous venous return of the
pulmonary veins □ Hypoplastic left heart
syndrome

Congestive Heart Failure   893
Physiology and pathophysiology □ Clinical
manifestations □ Interventions

DEVELOPMENTAL CONSEQUENCES OF
CONGENITAL ANOMALIES   894

SUMMARY   895

UNIT VI ■ THE PUERPERIUM   899

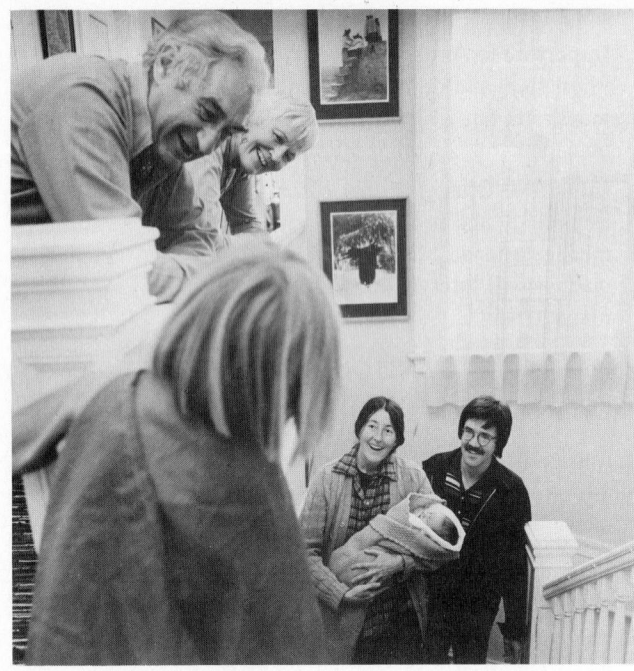

CHAPTER 27

THE POSTPARTAL FAMILY: ASSESSMENT, NEEDS, AND CARE   900

PUERPERAL PHYSICAL ADAPTATIONS AND PSYCHOLOGIC ADAPTATIONS   901

Reproductive Organs   901
Involution of uterus □ Lochia □ Cervical changes □ Vaginal changes □ Perineal changes □ Recurrence of ovulation and menstruation

Abdomen   905

Lactation   905

Gastrointestinal System   905

Urinary Tract   905

Vital Signs   906

Blood Values   906

Weight Loss   906

Postpartal Chill   906

Postpartal Diaphoresis   907

Afterpains   907

Puerperal Psychologic Adaptations   907

POSTPARTAL NURSING ASSESSMENT   907

Risk Factors   907

Physical Assessment   907
Breasts □ Abdomen and fundus □ Lochia □ Perineum □ Lower extremities □ Vital signs □ Nutritional status □ Elimination □ Rest and sleep status

Psychologic Assessment   913

Cultural Influences   914

POSTPARTAL NURSING CARE   914

Promotion of Comfort and Relief of Pain   915

Promotion of Rest and Graded Activity   916
Postpartal exercises □ Resumption of activities

Promotion of Maternal Psychologic Well-Being   916

Promotion of Successful Infant Feeding   921
Cultural considerations in infant feeding □ Lactation □ Suppression of lactation in the non-nursing mother □ Bottle-feeding □ Breast-feeding □ Medications and breast-feeding □ Potential problems in breast-feeding □ Breast-feeding and the working mother

Promotion of Effective Parent Education   938
Assessment and nursing diagnosis □ Planning □ Implementation □ Evaluation

Promotion of Family Wellness   939
Rooming-in □ Reactions of siblings □ Sexual relations between parents □ Family planning □ Discharge instructions

POSTPARTAL NURSING CARE AFTER CESAREAN BIRTH   941

Facilitation of Parent–Infant Interaction after Cesarean Birth   942

THE ADOLESCENT ON THE POSTPARTAL UNIT   942

THE FOURTH TRIMESTER   943

Nursing Management   944
Two- and six-week examinations □ Follow-up care

SUMMARY   949

CHAPTER 28
ATTACHMENT   951

NATURE OF ATTACHMENT   952

WHAT THE MOTHER BRINGS TO THE FIRST INTERACTION   952

Life History   952

Personality   953

Sexual-Reproductive Experience   953

Present Pregnancy   954

WHAT THE NEWBORN BRINGS TO THE FIRST INTERACTION   954

Appearance   954

Behaviors   954

THE SETTING   955

Physical Environment   955

Human Environment   955

Condition of the Interactors   955

MOTHER-INFANT INTERACTIONS   956

Introductory Bonding   956

Acquaintance Phase   958

Phase of Mutual Regulation   959

Reciprocity   960

Attachment Behaviors in the Adolescent Mother   962

FATHER-INFANT INTERACTIONS   962

SIBLINGS AND OTHERS   964

ASSESSMENT AND INTERVENTIONS IN MOTHER-INFANT RELATIONSHIPS   964

Assessment of Early Attachment   965

Guidelines for Intervention   965

Assessment of Bonding   966

COMPLICATIONS OF MATERNAL-INFANT ATTACHMENT   969

SUMMARY   970

CHAPTER 29
COMPLICATIONS OF THE PUERPERIUM   972

PUERPERAL HEMORRHAGE AND HEMATOMAS   973

Postpartal Hemorrhage   973
Subinvolution

Hematomas   974

Discharge Planning   974

PUERPERAL INFECTIONS   974

Causative Factors   975

Pathophysiology   975
Localized infections ☐ Endometritis ☐ Salpingitis and oophoritis ☐ Pelvic cellulitis (parametritis) and peritonitis

Interventions and Nursing Care   977

Discharge Planning   977

THROMBOEMBOLIC DISEASE   977

Superficial Leg Vein Disease   981

Deep Leg Vein Disease   982
Treatment of deep vein thrombosis

Pulmonary Embolism   982

PUERPERAL CYSTITIS AND PYELONEPHRITIS   983

Overdistention   983

Cystitis   987

Pyelonephritis   987

Interventions and Nursing Care   987

DISORDERS OF THE BREAST AND COMPLICATIONS OF LACTATION   987

Mastitis   987

Breast Abscess   988

Persistent Abnormal Lactation   988

Postdelivery Anterior Pituitary Necrosis   989

PUERPERAL PSYCHIATRIC DISORDERS   989

SUMMARY   990

CHAPTER 30

FAMILIES IN CRISIS AND THE
ROLE OF THE NURSE　991

FAMILIES AND CRISIS　992

CRISIS INTERVENTION　994

Assessment　995

Planning Therapeutic Intervention　996

Intervention　996

Evaluation　997

THE ROLE OF THE MATERNITY NURSE
DURING CRISIS　997

FAMILIES AT RISK　998

LOSS AND GRIEF　999

CRISIS INTERVENTION DURING
POSTPARTAL PERIOD　1002

Loss of Newborn　1002
Nursing intervention

Preterm Birth　1006
Nursing intervention

Defective Newborn　1010

CRISIS INTERVENTION DURING
POSTPARTAL FOLLOW-UP CARE　1010

Attachment Problems　1011
Nursing interventions □ Promoting attachment
when the newborn is hospitalized

Unwanted Pregnancy and
Relinquishment　1014
Nursing intervention

Child Abuse　1014
Nursing intervention

The Adolescent Parent　1016
Nursing intervention

Single-Parent Families　1018
Nursing intervention

SUMMARY　1018

APPENDICES　1021

A　PREGNANT PATIENT'S BILL OF RIGHTS　1021

B　UNITED NATIONS DECLARATION OF
THE RIGHTS OF THE CHILD　1022

C　EVALUATION OF FETAL WEIGHT
AND MATURITY BY ULTRASONIC
MEASUREMENT　1024

D　CLINICAL ESTIMATION OF
GESTATIONAL AGE　1025

E　NATIONAL CENTER FOR HEALTH
STATISTICS: PHYSICAL GROWTH
PERCENTILES　1027

F　CONVERSIONS AND EQUIVALENTS　1031
GLOSSARY　1032

INDEX　1055

NURSING CARE PLANS

Diabetes Mellitus in Prenatal, Intrapartal, and Postpartal Periods   322

Preeclampsia-Eclampsia (PIH)   337

Labor and Delivery   472

Immediate Care of the Newborn   498

Regional Anesthesia   521

Fetal Distress   538

Hemorrhage   569

Induction of Labor   591

Cesarean Birth   601

AGA and LGA Preterm Infants   750

SGA infants   764

Respiratory Distress Syndrome   801

Jaundice   831

Necrotizing Enterocolitis   839

Cleft Lip and Palate   853

Tracheoesophageal Fistula   862

Meningocele/Meningomyelocele   882

Postpartal Period   917

Puerperal Infection   978

Thrombophlebitis and Pulmonary Embolism   984

Stillbirth   1004

PROCEDURES

10-1   Auscultation of Chest   231

10-2   Breast Self-Examination   232

10-3   Cardiac Examination   233

10-4   Assisting with Pelvic Examination   235

12-1   Intrauterine Transfusion   350

13-1   Amniocentesis   383

15-1   Intrapartal Vaginal Examination   436

16-1   Delee Suction   500

18-1   Double Setup Examination   565

24-1   Gavage Feeding   743

25-1   Tracheal Intubation   791

25-2   Umbilical Catheterization   811

25-3   Endotracheal Suctioning   812

25-4   Dextrostix   819

25-5   Exchange Transfusion   825

27-1   Methods of Bottle Sterilization   928

ASSESSMENT GUIDES

Initial Prenatal Assessment Guide   216

Initial Psychologic Assessment Guide   238

Subsequent Physical Assessment Guide   239

Subsequent Psychologic Assessment Guide   241

Intrapartal Physical Assessment Guide: First Stage of Labor   428

Intrapartal Psychologic Assessment Guide   435

Postpartal Home Visit Assessment Guide   624

Neonatal Physical Assessment Guide   688

Postpartal Physical Assessment Guide: 2 Weeks and 6 Weeks after Delivery   945

Psychologic Assessment Guide   948

DRUG GUIDES

Magnesium Sulfate ($MgSO_4$)   345

Meperidine Hydrochloride (Demerol)   512

Betamethasone (Celestone Solupan)   547

Ritodrine (Yutopar)   549

Oxytocin (Pitocin)   590

Erythromycin (Ilotycin)—Ophthalmic Ointment   711

Vitamin K_1 Phytonadione (AquaMEPHYTON)   711

Sodium Bicarbonate   793

Naloxone Hydrochloride (Narcan)   793

Methylergonovine Maleate (Methergine)   903

Bromocriptine (Parlodel)   926

MATERNAL-NEWBORN NURSING

A Family-Centered Approach

SECOND EDITION

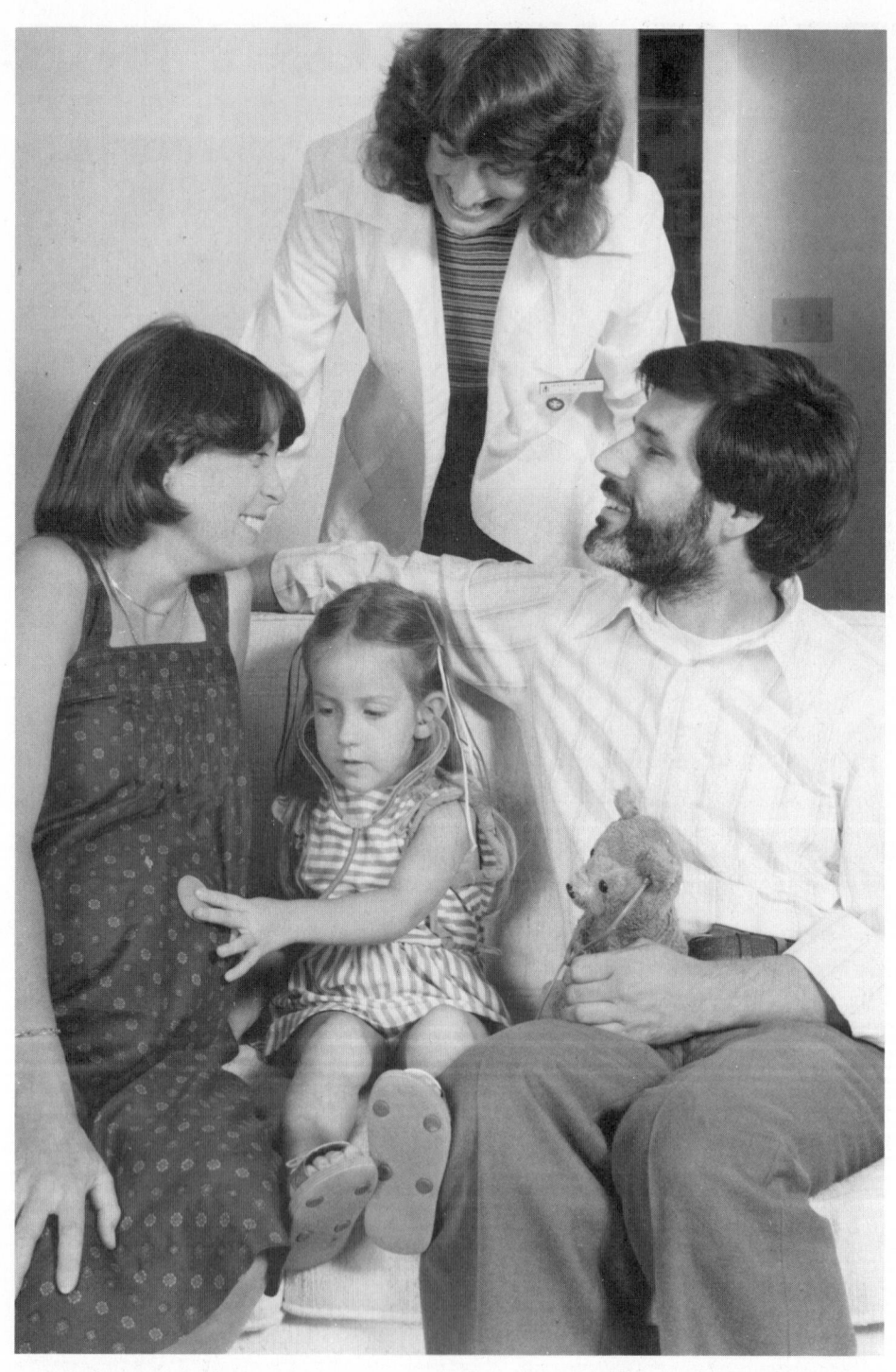

■ 1 ■

INTRODUCTION TO FAMILY-CENTERED MATERNITY NURSING

Chapter 1 ■ Current Perspectives of Maternal–Newborn Nursing

Chapter 2 ■ Tools for Maternal–Newborn Nursing Practice

Chapter 3 ■ Dynamics of Family Life

■ 1 ■

CURRENT PERSPECTIVES OF MATERNAL–NEWBORN NURSING

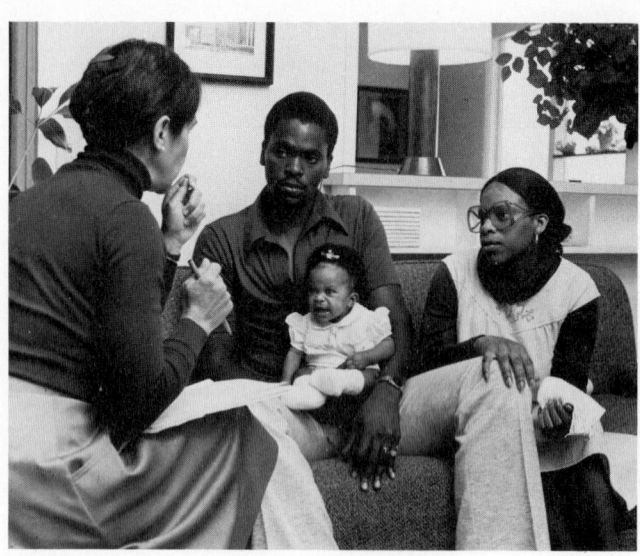

■ CHAPTER CONTENTS

HISTORICAL OVERVIEW OF OBSTETRICS AND MATERNITY NURSING CARE

    Early Recorded Developments

    European Developments

    Developments in the United States

    Development of Nurse-Midwifery

OVERVIEW OF CONTEMPORARY MATERNITY CARE

    State of the Art

    Ethical Issues

    The Changing Health Care Environment

THE EXPANDING ROLE OF NURSES IN MATERNITY CARE

    Roles and Settings for Nurses

    Legal Aspects of Maternal–Newborn Nursing

    Nurses and Physicians

■ OBJECTIVES

- Identify pertinent historical developments in obstetrics.

- Describe the role of the nurse-midwife in providing maternity care.

- Briefly discuss selected "state of the art" advances in the care of the childbearing family.

- Compare the opposing arguments advanced for specific ethical issues affecting maternity care.

- Describe significant changes that have occurred in the health care environment.

- Identify current maternity nursing roles.

At the moment a child is born, the quality of his or her future depends on many factors, not the least of which are the physical and psychologic health of the parents. The maternity nurse contributes to the quality of the child's life by providing expert care to both parents and child throughout the entire time that the family is expanding.

The quality of care provided to the childbearing family is a product of the professional's skill and knowledge. This skill and knowledge evolved over thousands of years. This chapter will consider the past, the present, and the future of obstetrics, maternity nursing, and related fields.

HISTORICAL OVERVIEW OF OBSTETRICS AND MATERNITY NURSING CARE

Early Recorded Developments

The earliest known records are found in the Egyptian papyruses. The Ebers papyrus (circa 1550 BC), a comprehensive papyrus scroll dealing primarily with obstetrics and gynecology, documents practices relating to abortion, augmentation of labor, menstruation, diseases peculiar to women, and methods of treatment.

Egyptian religious beliefs prohibited the practice of dissecting the dead body. Even though knowledge of anatomy was therefore scant, the Egyptians' ability to see causal relationships is illustrated by their tests to determine pregnancy and fetal sex. The woman's urine was used to water wheat and barleycorns. If the plants grew rapidly, pregnancy was confirmed; if the barley grew faster than the wheat, the unborn child was a female. Modern day replication of this practice, based on knowledge of pituitary and ovarian hormonal influences on plant growth and germination, has produced results with very high accuracy.

Operative obstetrics had its beginnings in these ancient times. In ancient India Hindu religious edicts forbade the mutilation of a dead body. However, it was thought that an unborn child possessed no spirit until some time after birth, so the baby could be extracted by crude forceps or by severing various limbs until the entire infant was re-

moved. Although women from royal families or with malpresentations were attended by a physician, most deliveries were handled by midwives. Birthing stools were common.

Little is written about obstetrics in Greek history. Athenian law required pregnant women to be attended by midwives—Greek women who had borne children and were past the childbearing age. Midwives and physicians performed abdominal palpations and vaginal examinations, noted cervical changes during pregnancy, and used vaginal speculums, irrigations, and dilators. Pessaries were commonly used for uterine support and other gynecologic problems but could not be used to induce an abortion, which was absolutely forbidden under the Hippocratic oath.

In ancient Rome, a Greek physician named Soranus specialized in gynecology and obstetrics. He became known as the father of obstetrics, and is best known for the use of podalic version.

With the decline of Rome, interest in the medical sciences also waned. During the ensuing Dark Ages, most aspects of progress were paralyzed until the fifteenth century, when the transition from the medieval to the modern world began in Europe.

European Developments

The invention of movable type by Gutenberg in 1450 heralded the end of the oral tradition, which had limited knowledge as well as misinterpreted it. Renaissance art became the forerunner of the new scientific age. Artists such as Leonardo da Vinci (1452–1519) and Michelangelo Buonarroti (1475–1564) did human dissections and accurately illustrated every aspect of the human body.

The anatomic studies of the human body of Andreas Vesalius (1514–1564) radically changed medical science and thus influenced the development of obstetrics. Ambroise Paré (1517–1590), a French physician, wrote two books on obstetrics and in one described the technique of podalic version, which had been lost from the time of Soranus. It replaced the crude and usually fatal practice of cesarean delivery. Paré used cervical dilatation to induce labor in women who were bleeding, described fetal move-

3

ment on abdominal palpation, and proposed the use of a nipple shield. His contribution to the science of obstetrics was perhaps the turning point that shifted the responsibility of the management of pregnancy and birth from midwives to trained physicians.

The sixteenth and seventeenth centuries produced several men whose influence on obstetrics is still felt. Peter Chamberlen (1560–1631) is credited with the invention of the obstetric forceps, which was modified for practical use in the eighteenth century by Leuret and Smellie. William Harvey (1578–1657), the discoverer of the circulatory system, developed the scientific field of embryology and set the pattern for the evolution of the midwifery schools in England. He is thus often referred to as the father of British midwifery.

Francois Mauriceau (1637–1709) was the first to observe that puerperal fever was epidemic. He described a mechanism for breech extraction, refuted the idea that the pubic bones separated during labor, advocated suturing tears of the perineum, instituted the routine use of a bed for delivery rather than a birth stool, and tried to dispel the ancient idea that a fetus had some control over birth. (It was believed that the fetus would attempt to be born at 7 months' gestation; if unsuccessful, it would attempt again at 8 months' gestation but would be weakened by the first efforts. The general belief was that a fetus born at 7 months was stronger and would be healthier than a fetus delivered at 8 months. Some lay people still believe this myth.)

A Dutch physician, Hendrik van Deventer (1651–1724) was the first to accurately describe the pelvis. He identified several different types of pelves and the axis of the birth canal and noted deformities that could delay or impede delivery of the infant. His writings on midwifery were widely accepted. He is known as the father of modern midwifery.

During the 1700s, two British physicians, William Smellie (1697–1763) and William Hunter (1718–1783), had significant influence on obstetric practice. Smellie observed and recorded the mechanisms of labor, used manikins for teaching, measured the diagonal conjugate, invented the curved and locked forceps, and advocated a conservative third stage of labor. Hunter discovered the separate nature of maternal and fetal circulations and established the first lying-in ward in London.

Sir Fielding Ould introduced the episiotomy in the middle of the eighteenth century, despite the lack of anesthetics. It was used sparingly and only when indicated.

Of major importance to obstetrics was the discovery of anesthesia in the nineteenth century. The use of anesthesia was extremely controversial. Scientists viewed it as an end to pain; moralists declared it the work of the devil and a violation of scripture. The arguments continued for several years and finally ceased when Queen Victoria delivered Prince Leopold after receiving chloroform.

Many techniques, procedures, and clinical findings used in modern practice bear the names of Europeans who devoted their practice to obstetrics and gynecology: John Braxton Hicks (Braxton Hicks contractions, p. 415), Friedrich Wilhelm Scanzoni (Scanzoni maneuver or operation, p. 551), Alfred Hegar (Hegar's sign, p. 192), Franz Nägele (Nägele's rule, p. 236), and Karl Credé (Credé method).

Credé and his contemporary, Ignaz Philipp Semmelweis (1818–1865), used their clinical observations, the newly established germ theory, and independent research to produce two simple techniques with overwhelming significance: eye prophylaxis and hand-washing.

A paper published by Credé in 1884, called "The Prophylactic Treatment of Ophthalmia Neonatorum," described in detail the administration of a 2% silver nitrate solution to a newborn infant's eyes. Only the advent of antibiotic ointments and the use of 1% silver nitrate solution have altered the basic procedure, which has prevented blindness due to gonorrhea in countless numbers of newborns.

The story of Semmelweis is famous. During the 1840s, while serving as a physician at Vienna General Hospital, he noted the low mortality in the ward run by midwives and the high number of deaths in the ward managed by obstetricians. Then a colleague died of septicemia after receiving a cut from an infected scalpel used to examine a woman who had died from puerperal fever. This incident confirmed for Semmelweis his belief that puerperal sepsis was passed from one woman to another by the contaminated hands of physicians and medical students coming from the cadaver laboratory. Semmelweis immediately instituted a policy of hand-scrubbing in a chloride of lime solution before examining any woman in labor or performing a delivery or postpartum examination. The results were conclusive: the incidence of sepsis dropped from almost 12% to 3.8% in a year and to 1.2% the following year. Later, in a controlled study at another hospital, Semmelweis further reduced deaths to 0.39% (Graham, 1951).

Semmelweis continued to replicate his studies, moving from one institution to another, trying to gain acceptance for his discovery. Despite his dramatic findings, Semmelweis could not convince his colleagues to wash their hands. He continued to be ridiculed and ignored by the majority of physicians throughout Europe.

Developments in the United States

During the early colonization period, maternity care was based on the different traditions and practices of the European settlers. Midwives or neighbors helped with deliveries, breast-feeding was assumed, and home care was the only option.

William Shippen, a pupil of Smellie and Hunter, established a school for midwifery in Philadelphia in 1762, designed to be attended by both men and women. However, few, if any, women entered the school, and "man-midwifery" had its start in the United States. Shippen's school eventually became part of the University of Pennsylvania, and the curriculum became known as "obstetrics" rather than midwifery.

Samuel Bard, educated abroad and trained in midwifery, helped establish King's Medical College (known today as Columbia University) and wrote the first American obstetrics textbook. Valentine Seaman established the first school of nursing in New York in 1798 to train women in midwifery and the care of children. A Philadelphia physician, Joseph Warrington, also began a school of midwifery but soon extended it to all kinds of care of patients with medical and surgical conditions.

During the nineteenth century, obstetrics and midwifery were greatly influenced by William Dewees. He brought into practice the lithotomy position for delivery, insisted on relieving pain during labor, and advocated judicious use of forceps. Many consider him the person who made obstetrics a science in the United States and refer to him as the father of American obstetrics.

The American Medical Association, founded in 1847, established a section on obstetrics, women's diseases, and children in 1873.

As in Europe, the need for hand-washing prior to obstetric procedures was viewed with skepticism and doubt by physicians in the United States. A paper written in 1843 by a young Harvard physician, Oliver Wendell Holmes, titled "On the Contagiousness of Puerperal Fever," was not well received by the medical world. However, eventually the importance of asepsis was recognized, and hand-washing and other aseptic measures became standard procedures.

By the end of its first hundred years, the United States was well on the way to having an organized system of medical and nursing care that would part from the European tradition and become institutionally oriented.

Prior to 1900 few infants were delivered in hospitals. Only the very poor or unwed women went to a hospital for confinement. After a hospital delivery, newborns remained with their mothers; hammocklike cribs were placed at the foot of the bed where, with some help from a nurse, the mother could tend her infant. However, wards became noisy and crowded, and many women were too ill to care for their infants. To remedy this situation, the Boston Lying-in Hospital established a night nursery in 1898 to prevent infants from disturbing the patients and personnel on the ward. This proved satisfactory. Indeed, many of the physicians and nurses were of the opinion that newborns should remain in a nursery at all times to maintain the quiet and tidiness of the ward.

Early in the twentieth century, a real need for newborn nurseries appeared. Outbreaks of diarrhea, scarlet fever, diphtheria, and other communicable diseases caused a large number of infant and maternal deaths. Physicians stressed the need for separate care as a control method for preventing the spread of infection, and nurseries became essential.

By midcentury, hospital deliveries had steadily increased, with a concomitant decrease in mortality. The newborn nursery—and thus the separation of mother and child—became a firmly entrenched practice, heralding an era of rigid schedules, formula feedings, and strict asepsis. Minimal thought was given to the psychologic effects of this practice on the childbearing family (see the section on Development of Family-Centered Care, p. 12).

More than 50 years ago, the federal government became involved in improving the quality of maternity care. The Sheppard-Towner Act of 1921 was the first federal legislation to provide funds for state programs in maternal and child health; this act was in force until 1929. In 1935 came the Social Security Act, which provides federal grants for health and welfare programs, with extensive services in the maternal–child health area.

In 1964, as a result of an amendment to Title V of the Social Security Act, the Maternity and Infant (M&I) Care Projects were begun by the Public Health Service of the Department of Health, Education, and Welfare in 56 areas where maternal and infant mortality rates were significantly higher than the national average. The states recently assumed management of these projects, although they are still federally funded.

The purpose of these projects is to provide good maternity care to high-risk women thereby reducing maternal and infant mortality and preventing or decreasing prematurity, birth traumas, and mental retardation. Services include medical care, dental care, social services, infant care, nutrition services, client education, family planning services, nursing care, and special services to pregnant adolescents. The efficacy of the program has been demonstrated by reduced rates of prematurity and maternal and infant mortality (Wallace, 1975). The most significant contributions of the M&I Care Projects for the professional have been the emphasis on early prenatal care, a humanizing approach to public clinics, and utilization of the health team as a functional unit.

The WIC program, a supplemental food program for Women, Infants, and Children, was established in 1975 to provide supplemental food and nutrition counseling to low-income families during important periods of growth and development. WIC is handled by local agencies and has been significant in promoting the nutritional well-being of women and small children.

Development of Nurse-Midwifery

Throughout history, most societies have used some form of birth attendant or midwife. Midwifery is an honored profession, evolving distinct characteristics as it has developed throughout the ages. Even today, 80% of the world's population is attended in childbirth by a midwife.

Midwifery and nursing are distinct disciplines; in fact, the training, regulation, and practice of the professional midwife were instituted before organized professional nursing came into existence in 1871. However, they are complementary disciplines, and this has led to the development of another health professional—the nurse-midwife.

The history of the establishment of nurse-midwifery as an accepted and respected profession is briefly reviewed here. It is interesting to note how the professional development of midwifery and nurse-midwifery have differed in Europe and the United States.

NURSE-MIDWIFERY IN EUROPE

The Scandinavian countries led Europe in providing a sound basis for the development of the professional midwife. As early as 1673, in Denmark midwives were given examinations to determine their competency. Finland and Sweden also emphasized training and competency of midwives beginning in the eighteenth century.

By the early 1800s schools of nursing were being established throughout Europe. In 1860 Florence Nightingale founded St. Thomas School of Nursing in London. She advocated the training of a "better class" of women as nurses and midwives to provide services to women, and she even wrote a book on the subject, *Introductory Notes on Lying-in Institutions Together with a Proposal for Organizing an Institution for Training Midwives and Midwifery Nurses.* She probably influenced the founding of the Ladies' Obstetrical College (1864), which was attended by women who were daughters of professional men and who wished to become midwives.

Nightingale attempted to establish a school of nurse-midwifery in 1867, but unfortunately an epidemic of puerperal sepsis forced the closing of the program. Her emphasis on training had its effect, however, and in 1872 the Obstetrical Society of London began issuing certificates to qualified midwives. In 1881, Rosalind Paget, one of "Miss Nightingale's Young Ladies," founded the Midwives Institute (now the Royal College of Midwives) to register midwives and promoted a bill to ensure proper education and control. In 1902 the English Midwives Act was passed, and state registration became mandatory. The act also brought into existence the Central Midwives Board, a statutory body controlling the training and practice of midwives in England. The original act of 1902 has been revised several times, most recently in 1951. It requires the training period for midwives to be one year for trained nurses and two years for those untrained. The act clearly states that it gives "statutory recognition to the position of the midwife as a professional practitioner in her own right" (Central Midwives Board, 1962).

Throughout the Continent, the option still exists to become either a midwife or a nurse-midwife; each is considered a professional. The settings for practice vary extensively from nation to nation, with births being conducted in family dwellings, maternity homes, and hospitals.

NURSE-MIDWIFERY IN THE UNITED STATES

□ *HISTORICAL STATUS OF MIDWIFERY* Early records indicate that the midwife was an important person in settlements and towns throughout the colonies. However, in strongly Puritan communities she was frequently suspected of witchcraft. The most infamous midwife of the time was Anne Hutchinson. She came to Boston from England in 1634 and soon established her skill as a midwife, but she was suspect because of her so-called heretical religious views. When she delivered an anencephalic child, the community had its confirmation that she was a witch. Hutchinson was banished from Massachusetts by the General Court and was excommunicated as well.

Midwifery was unattractive in America as a result of economic problems related to educating midwives and of strong religious pressures and superstitions affecting the practice of midwifery. There were no effective licensing regulations or training programs (recall that Shippen established a school for midwifery in 1762 that attracted only men). The different ethnic groups had their own traditions and myths about childbirth. It also became the fashion for middle-class women to seek the care of a physician or male attendant. All these factors made trained midwifery a less than highly esteemed profession in the United States.

Although great numbers of midwives were practicing in the United States, no professional advances occurred in over 200 years. In 1905 there were over 3000 midwives delivering approximately 40% of all the children born in New York City. Only a small percentage of these midwives had any formal training, and even fewer had medical support. This prompted an investigation of midwifery in New York City in 1906 by the Public Health Commission of the Association of Neighborhood Workers in conjunction with the New York City Health Department. The report described midwives as ignorant, untrained, incompetent, and dirty women. The published results were devastating to midwifery throughout the United States. States passed laws prohibiting or restricting the practice of midwifery and placed the control of midwives under physicians within the state health departments.

By state law (1907) the New York City Board of Health became responsible for the regulation and practice of midwifery, and in 1911 a school for midwives was opened at Bellevue Hospital. The city's Sanitary Code of 1914 required that all midwives applying for a permit to practice must graduate from a school approved by the Board of Health. Thus in New York City the number of practicing midwives decreased from 3000 in 1905 to approximately 850 licensed midwives in 1932. The Bellevue School was forced to close in 1936, and three decades later no more licensed midwives were practicing in New York City.

□ *GROWTH OF NURSE-MIDWIFERY* Despite the prevailing attitudes toward midwifery, public health and obstetric nurses recognized their responsibility to provide services and care to pregnant women, newly delivered mothers, and their infants. One such nurse was Mary Breckinridge. After World War I, she went to Europe where she was introduced to French midwives and saw how effectively they provided care in villages, small farm communities, and areas destroyed by the war. She found that although competent midwives in France were not nurses and competent nurses in the United States were not midwives, the English had combined the two successfully. Breckinridge realized that nurse-midwifery was the answer to inadequate maternity and child care in the rural areas of the United States.

She received training as a nurse-midwife in 1923 in England and returned to the United States to practice in rural Kentucky. In 1925 she established the first nurse-midwifery program in this country, the Kentucky Committee for Mothers and Babies. The name was changed to the Frontier Nursing Service in 1928, and a 28-bed hospital was constructed in Hyden, Kentucky, that year.

The excellent work and accomplishments of the nurse-midwives of the Frontier Nursing Service were soon recognized. Infant and maternal mortality dropped significantly, and the families received quality health care.

The Frontier Graduate School of Midwifery was founded in 1939. In 1970 a certificate program to prepare family nurses was developed in coordination with the nurse-midwifery curriculum to produce a broadly prepared primary care nurse for rural areas. The school changed its name to the Frontier School of Midwifery and Family Nursing. Since its inception the school has trained approximately 500 nurse-midwives.

While Breckinridge was proving the value of nurse-midwives in a rural setting, women's groups, nurses, and physicians joined forces in New York City in an attempt to reduce the high number of maternal and infant deaths. In 1918 the Maternity Center Association was founded. The goal of this organization was and still is to work "to assure that every baby born will be wanted and welcomed, and will have the high quality of care needed before, during and after birth" (Maternity Center Association, 1975). Dr. Ralph W. Lobenstein was the first chairman of the Medical Advisory Board for the Maternity Center Association, and his name was given to a midwifery clinic and to the first nurse-midwifery school established in the United States. The Lobenstein School began in 1931 under the auspices of the Association for the Promotion and Standardization of Midwifery and merged (along with the clinic) with the Maternity Center Association in 1934. The intent of this educational program was "to teach midwifery to qualified public health nurses so they might supervise the untrained midwives now practicing throughout the country and, also, under the direction of obstetricians, bring skilled care to the mothers in isolated rural areas" (Maternity Center Association, 1975). In the early years, the Maternity Center Association program graduated approximately a dozen nurse-midwives a year. The Maternity Center Association

is currently allied with the State University of New York at Downstate Medical Center.

Other nurse-midwifery programs have since been established. Currently there are 27 nurse-midwifery programs in the United States approved by the American College of Nurse-Midwives. Some are certificate programs, which provide additional training for RNs; the others are master's degree programs. As of August, 1982, there were 2598 certified nurse-midwives in the United States.*

The official professional organization is the American College of Nurse-Midwives. Established in 1969, it evolved from the desire of nurse-midwives for an organization that would meet the needs of the practitioner, that would assure quality of care, and that would maintain standards for safe, effective care that meet the individual needs of childbearing families. This professional body determines the functions, standards, and qualifications for the practice of nurse-midwifery. It is also the official agency for approving educational programs and certifying graduates of these programs. The National Certification Examination, first administered in 1971, assures that an individual is capable of safe, effective practice as a nurse-midwife. The initials CNM indicate that one is a certified nurse-midwife.

The basic beliefs and commitments of nurse-midwives are well reflected in the philosophy of the American College of Nurse-Midwives:

> Every childbearing family has a right to a safe, satisfying experience with respect for human dignity and worth; for variety in cultural forms; and for the parents' right to self-determination.
>
> Comprehensive maternity care, including educational and emotional support as well as management of physical care throughout the childbearing years, is a major means for intercession into, and improvement and maintenance of, the health of the nation's families. Comprehensive maternity care is most effectively and efficiently delivered by interdependent health disciplines.
>
> Nurse-midwifery is an interdependent health discipline focusing on the family and exhibiting responsibility for insuring that its practitioners are provided with excellence in preparation and that those practitioners demonstrate professional behavior in keeping with these stated beliefs.†

Nurse-midwifery made a major advance in 1981, when Congress authorized medicaid payments for the services of nurse-midwives.

---

*Information provided by the American College of Nurse-Midwifery, Washington, D.C. in March 1983.

†American College of Nurse-Midwives. 1972. *Statement of philosophy*. Washington, D.C.: The College.

OVERVIEW OF CONTEMPORARY MATERNITY CARE

State of the Art

In the past few years, tremendous technologic strides have been made in maternity and newborn health care. The medical and nursing knowledge base is increasing, and as a result more services are available to health care consumers.

With these technologic advances have come several clinical and research specialties that focus on various aspects of childbearing, fetal development, and newborn care. *Perinatology* is a hybrid of obstetrics and pediatrics. Perinatal specialists are concerned with the diagnosis and treatment of high-risk obstetric or fetal conditions to prevent or reduce negative outcomes of childbearing and child development. The pregnant woman, fetus, and newborn are the perinatal specialist's clients.

Neonatology is usually considered a pediatric subspecialty, since it deals with children, albeit newborn children. The neonatal specialist is concerned with the management of high-risk conditions in the newborn.

Nurse and physician clinical and research specialists in obstetrics, pediatrics, perinatology, neonatology, and other related fields are continually striving to develop diagnostic and treatment tools that will enhance the longevity and quality of both mother and child's lives. Some of these developments are discussed in the following sections.

ULTRASONOGRAPHY

Prior to the advent of ultrasound, radiography was a primary tool for assessing the fetus in utero, although the inherent risks to the fetus meant it was seldom used unless absolutely necessary. Ultrasonography represents an apparently safe means of fetal assessment that can be used in a variety of ways, including the diagnosis of uterine pregnancy, ectopic pregnancy, or multiple pregnancy; estimation of gestational age, fetal growth, and fetal weight; recognition of certain congenital anomalies; localization of the placenta; and confirmation of hydatidiform mole. In addition, the knowledge ultrasound provides about fetal and placental location has facilitated the development of other specialized procedures such as amniocentesis, intrauterine transfusions, and even intrauterine surgery.

Research to date has failed to demonstrate any side effects, although the long-term side effects of ultrasound may not yet be known. However, the rapidly growing popularity of ultrasound as a valuable diagnostic tool and the ready availability of both formal ultrasound and portable real-time scanners have led to its widespread use for prenatal clients in most of the United States. (See Chapter 13 for further discussion.)

AMNIOCENTESIS

Amniocentesis is a diagnostic tool with tremendous existing and potential value. With the availability of ultrasonography to localize the placenta and fetus, amniocentesis has become a relatively safe and simple procedure that can provide information about the genetic makeup of the fetus, its health status, and its maturity. (See Chapters 7 and 13 for further discussion.)

ELECTRONIC FETAL MONITORING

Electronic fetal monitoring, a procedure originally designed to assess the status of the fetus during labor, has gained widespread acceptance in the past two decades. Initially electronic fetal monitoring was used primarily for women considered to be high risk, but increasingly it is used to monitor low-risk labors. Most obstetric units have electronic fetal monitoring equipment available. It is also used in conjunction with fetal scalp blood sampling to accurately assess evidence of hypoxia.

The availability of electronic fetal monitoring has led to the development of techniques such as the nonstress test (NST) and contraction stress test (CST) to serially monitor the status of the fetus and to attempt to determine its ability to withstand the stress of labor. (See Chapter 13.)

FETAL SURGERY

Fetal surgery, one of the most exciting obstetric ventures of the 1980s, is a logical step in the progression of technology. Ultrasonography led to the early diagnosis of certain serious congenital anomalies, and efforts to correct these problems followed predictably. Currently, in utero surgical activities focus on certain conditions such as hydrocephalus and hydronephrosis. Using ultrasound for guidance, the physician attempts to place shunts to drain excess fluid—in the first case, cerebrospinal fluid and in the second, urine—to prevent the progression of tissue damage the excessive fluid could produce in the fetus.

Experimental in utero surgery is also developing in other areas. For example, congenital diaphragmatic hernia has traditionally been repaired in the neonatal period. However, because herniation of the viscera occurs in utero, pulmonary hypoplasia is often a problem. As a result, 50%–80% of affected newborns die because of pulmonary insufficiency. It has been demonstrated on fetal lambs that surgery in utero during the third trimester to correct the defect permits the lung to grow and develop enough to support life (Harrison et al., 1981). It seems only a matter of time before such surgery is attempted on a human fetus. In addition, in 1981, physicians in San Francisco made an incision in a pregnant human uterus, partially removed the fetus, performed surgery to remove a urinary tract blockage, and then replaced the fetus in the uterus. The pregnancy continued to term but the infant died shortly after birth because of pulmonary complications (Henig, 1982). It seems logical to assume that this is only the beginning of such surgical efforts.

IN VITRO FERTILIZATION

Technology stirred the imagination and sparked countless debates in 1978 with the report of the birth of Louise Brown, the world's first "test-tube" baby. The in vitro procedure was developed to deal with the problem of infertility resulting from blockage of the fallopian tubes in women with functioning ovaries. A mature ovum is collected from the woman and fertilized in vitro by sperm from her partner. The embryo is then transferred to the woman's uterus and allowed to implant. In the United States, Norfolk, Virginia, was the site of the first clinic licensed to perform in vitro fertilization, although several others are now so authorized.

SCIENTIFIC ADVANCES OR MEDICAL EXCESSES?

The "good" that these technologic advances have done is undeniable. Because of these advances, a healthy baby was delivered in a San Francisco hospital from a brain-dead mother whose body was kept functioning for over two months until the fetus was viable. More lives, maternal and neonatal, are being saved daily; more families are being helped to live better lives. Yet concern is growing that the reliance on technology in obstetrics is excessive and that in some cases the risks of certain procedures outweigh the advantages of their use. For example, amniocentesis is fatal to fetuses in 1.5% of cases (Science News, 1979a). Elective induction of labor may lead to maternal and fetal morbidity. Other medical procedures are also being scrutinized for their potential negative effects.

The controversy about electronic fetal monitoring is representative of the larger issue of excessive technologic involvement in obstetrics. In the United States, nearly 65% of all labors are monitored by electronic equipment (Science News, 1979b). Some health care professionals advocate monitoring all labors (Butler and Parer, 1976). In this way, cases can be identified that were prenatally categorized as low risk but that are adversely affected by labor.

Yet there are situations in which external or internal electronic monitoring adversely affects the laboring woman or her fetus. Although data about maternal and fetal complications due to invasive fetal monitoring are conflicting, maternal infection, uterine perforation, and other soft tissue trauma have been reported. The newborn may suffer scalp abscesses from clipping of the electrode on soft tissue (Gee and Ledger, 1976).

The increasing incidence of cesarean births has been attributed to the routine use of fetal monitoring. When fetal distress is indicated by abnormal fetal heart rate patterns, the infant is frequently delivered by cesarean birth.

However, the National Institutes of Health warns that "abnormal fetal heart rate patterns do not always mean that a fetus is in distress" (Science News, 1979b). Thus, the decision to perform a cesarean delivery may in fact be based on misleading data from the electronic monitoring equipment. The woman is then subjected to a surgical procedure that is not really needed, and the couple is deprived of the emotional satisfaction of a more natural delivery.

Fetal monitoring equipment may interfere with the childbirth experience. The couple prepared for the childbirth may find the equipment and the staff's concern with the technical aspects of labor and delivery limiting and a symbol of their lack of control in this matter. In addition, the couple may suffer from unwarranted anxiety about the well-being of the fetus because of the complexity and noise of the machinery.

One nursing research study found parents responding positively to fetal monitoring (McDonough, Sheriff, and Zimmel, 1981). It is important to point out that the actions of the nursing staff may have influenced this outcome. The nurses at the hospital studied provided clear explanations about how the monitor worked, coaching fathers were taught how to "read" the monitor tracing to identify the onset of a contraction before the woman felt them, and the laboring client was the nurse's primary object of attention, not the monitor.

Does intrapartal fetal monitoring or similar procedures in cases of low-risk labor and delivery constitute excessive medical practice? There are those who argue that every pregnancy and delivery carries with it potential medical problems, and therefore maternity clients must be managed intensively to prevent complications and to ensure the well-being of both woman and child. To that end, the use of any tool in the medical repertoire is justified. Others support the notion that pregnancy and childbirth are natural, normal processes and should not be managed in the same rigorous way as pathophysiologic abnormalities. Medical intervention is perceived as an unnecessary and costly interference in low-risk cases.

Opinion is growing that more stringent screening of clients receiving certain services should be done. Because of the high cost of certain procedures, insurance companies are becoming involved in this issue, as are consumers who are questioning the necessity and compulsory nature of particular medical procedures. Many expectant couples are responding to the increase in technologic interventions by seeking alternatives to the health care system's traditional management of childbirth.

□ *IMPLICATIONS FOR NURSING* Consumers and health care professionals are increasingly supportive of the idea that medical and nursing actions should be dependent on the maternity client's level of risk. Nursing has recognized the need for rigorous evaluation of all clients, and all nurses are being encouraged to develop their assessment skills. In this textbook, entire chapters are devoted to assessment during the maternity cycle, and in-depth physical and psychologic assessment guides and high-risk screening tools are provided.

The increasing technology of the health care system has had an additional effect on the educational and occupational aspects and opportunities available to nurses. Many nurses are participating in related research; others are administering highly specialized services that require stringent training. This trend will probably continue, since the need for highly skilled staff is growing.

Those nurses who choose to provide general health maintenance services to maternity clients must be aware of the current "state of the art" if they are to provide the best possible care for expectant families. To that end, information about available and developing technology and related nursing actions is provided in this textbook.

The increasing sophistication of high-risk obstetric and neonatal technology raises several questions regarding the direction of nursing, however, and today's student—tomorrow's nurse—may be called upon to answer these questions. For example, will the trend toward specialization result in further fragmentation of client care? If the nurse becomes a technician, who will provide continuity of care to the expectant mother and her family? Does the concept of specialization run counter to the nursing philosophy of caring for the whole client? Indeed, these are difficult questions, but they should be kept in mind by nursing educators as they further refine the theories and philosophy of the profession.

Research by nurses will help clarify the relationship of technology, the health care professional, and the client/family. Studies of the attitudes of nurses and physicians about diagnostic and treatment tools, how they are administered, and how the results are translated into action should be undertaken. (See Chapter 2.)

Ethical Issues

While ethical dilemmas confront us in all areas of nursing, those involving pregnancy, childbearing itself, and/or the resulting infant seem especially difficult to resolve. These conflicts range from abortion to passive euthanasia to intrauterine surgery.

ABORTION

In 1973 the U.S. Supreme Court rendered its decision in the case of *Roe* v. *Wade*. It stated that during the first trimester the decision to terminate a pregnancy rested with the attending physician (in consultation with the client) without state regulation.

The Court decision further fueled a debate that had raged for years and continues with increasing hostility more than a decade later. Opponents of abortion, the "pro-life" group, support one moral principle—the right of the unborn fetus to life. Their efforts, begun at the grass-

roots level, have been vigorous and effective, and have resulted in the blocking of public funding for abortion (Arras and Hunt, 1983).

Proponents of abortion, the "pro-choice" group, support the moral principle that a woman has the ultimate right to control her own body and reproductive activity. Some advocates of abortion have also advanced the argument that the fetus is not yet a human being. Others suggest that while the fetus may be genetically human, it has not yet achieved personhood and is, therefore, not a member of the moral community (Arras and Hunt, 1983).

PASSIVE EUTHANASIA

Other moral problems besides abortion are receiving increasing attention. Passive euthanasia occurs when someone is allowed to die because of inaction or lack of treatment. Maternity nurses are confronted with this issue most frequently when the decision is made to allow a severely handicapped newborn to die by withholding necessary medical treatment, surgery, or even food. A famous example, the "Johns Hopkins Case," involved the decision made at the request of the parents to withhold corrective surgery from a child born with Down syndrome and an intestinal obstruction, and sparked countless debates about the rights of the parents, the rights of infants, and the quality of life for severely impaired children.

Ethical arguments on passive euthanasia take three main positions (Beauchamp and Walters, 1978):

1. All life should be saved if possible because everyone has an overriding right to life and no one person should be permitted to make life-or-death decisions for another.

2. The quality of an individual's life, should he or she survive, should be weighed against the suffering he or she would probably endure. This is referred to as the patient-oriented standard, and advocates the use of an impartial proxy to make an anticipatory evaluation for the affected individual (in this case, the infant).

3. Decisions regarding treatment or withholding treatment for infants or those deemed incompetent (such as the comatose) should consider and possibly be determined by familial and broader social concerns. This approach encourages the determination of the benefits/harm ratio of allowing a severely handicapped individual to die.

For those supporting the first position, treatment is always indicated. Those supporting the second and third positions must deal with related issues such as the severity of the defect, the fact that decisions must often be made hastily or without complete medical and social information, and the possibility that withholding treatment could be considered illegal and subject to prosecution as child abuse (Robertson, 1981).

Legally some flexibility exists about the use of maximum treatment in all cases. "The presumption in favor of life and treatment can be overridden when a neutral appraisal shows that further life is not in the child's interests" (Robertson, 1981, p. 8). Perhaps the issue will be best managed by identifying guidelines specifying those cases when treatment would always be indicated, those in which treatment could always be withheld, and those less clearcut cases in which the specific circumstances should be reviewed.

AMNIOCENTESIS FOR SEX DETERMINATION

The new technology has raised other controversial questions. For instance, with amniocentesis it is generally possible to determine the sex of the fetus. Is it morally permissible to perform amniocentesis solely for the purpose of sex determination followed by abortion if the fetus is not of the desired sex even though no sex-related adverse conditions exist? Proponents of amniocentesis for sex determination suggest that it is illogical to legally support a woman's right to decide her own reproductive activity and then withhold information she needs to make the decision about continuing a pregnancy (Fletcher, 1980). Opponents suggest that such an approach makes poor use of limited existing facilities for genetic information and has overtones of genetic engineering. In addition, if one assumes that the majority of women would elect to continue the pregnancy if the fetus is male, it places women in the unusual position of having guaranteed to them ". . . the right of self-determination for the purpose of discriminating against their own kind by either doing away with the fetuses of their own sex or by choosing male children as their firstborns" (Lenzer, 1980, p. 18).

Prenatal clinics vary in their approach to the issue but usually include some counseling about the risks of amniocentesis to woman and fetus, and the psychologic and physical implications of abortion for the woman. Other factors considered include the couple's cultural and religious preferences, the emotional implications should a child of an unwanted sex be born, and whether the couple will terminate the pregnancy anyway if sex selection is not permitted. Currently the Genetics Research Group of the Hastings Center (1979) supports the view that the use of amniocentesis solely for determining fetal sex should be discouraged but not legally restricted.

INTRAUTERINE FETAL SURGERY

Intrauterine fetal surgery also has many ethical ramifications. Does the possibility of surgery change the moral status of the fetus? Does the fetus have the absolute right to treatment? Is the fetus a patient? What are the rights of the fetus versus the rights of the pregnant woman? Can a woman be required to undergo surgery to ensure a better quality of life for her fetus? What if a woman knowingly continues a pregnancy involving a damaged fetus without taking advantage of available treatment?

Recognizing the numerous ethical issues associated with their pioneering surgery, the team at the University of Colorado Health Sciences Center, who performed the first intrauterine brain shunt procedure, consulted with the Human Subjects Committee and also appointed two advocates for fetuses that are potential candidates for intrauterine surgery—one, a theologian, and the other, a neonatologist. Others suggest that those engaging in fetal surgery enlist the aid of a compassionate ethicist and an overseeing body of uninvolved professional colleagues (Ruddick and Wilcox, 1982).

Those involved are very aware of the need to consider the interests of both the woman and her fetus, but it seems likely that countless additional questions will be raised as techniques advance and new procedures are developed.

IN VITRO FERTILIZATION AND SURROGATE CHILDBEARING

In vitro fertilization and surrogate childbearing may be viewed as the major moral dilemmas of the decade. In vitro fertilization offers hope for women with tubal obstruction. The woman's egg is surgically removed, fertilized with her partner's sperm, and then, at the appropriate time, returned to the woman's uterus and allowed to implant. Surrogate childbearing occurs when a woman agrees to become pregnant for a childless couple and then release the infant to the couple. In both cases fertilization is by artificial insemination, usually with the sperm from the man who desires the child. The need for candidate selection, the religious objections to such artificial conception, the question of who will assume financial and moral responsibility for a defective child born following both these approaches, and the spectre of genetic engineering must all be considered and weighed in light of existing information.

IMPLICATIONS FOR NURSES

Today nurses often find themselves confronted by a variety of ethical and moral issues involving conflicting opinions of rights, needs, and responsibilities. In their role as client advocates nurses may find their views in conflict with the physician caring for a client or with the choices the client has made.

Nurses must learn to anticipate ethical dilemmas and to develop some basic beliefs about the issues. This can be done by reading literature on bioethical issues and by attending courses and workshops on ethical topics pertinent to one's area of practice. It also requires the development of skills in logical thinking and critical analysis.

Nurses must thoughtfully assess their convictions and identify any clinical situations in which they feel they could not function. For example, a nurse who is totally opposed to abortion should not accept a position requiring her to assist in the procedure. By the same token, it is important to differentiate personal biases from ethical beliefs in order to avoid imposing personal standards on others without sufficient justification.

The Changing Health Care Environment

Over the past two decades, attitudes of those utilizing health care services have changed radically. The feminist and self-help movements provided the impetus for women and men outside and inside the health care system to appraise its practices. No longer do people believe that "the doctor always knows best." Clients are asking for complete information about medical practices—what, why, and how much. Entrants into the health care system are looking at traditional medical methodology and philosophy with new eyes. They are finding that the costly services offered by the system are not always meeting their needs. Women are also realizing that sexism in the health care system does affect the way they are treated by health care professionals and possibly affects the quality of care received.

Obstetrics may be one of the most highly criticized specialties because of the traditional methods of management of pregnancy and labor and delivery. In the past, labor and delivery was treated as a medical problem, controlled by the obstetrician and the hospital staff. Many types of analgesic agents were given during labor, and general anesthesia was administered for delivery. Some of these agents were harmful to the fetus. During labor and delivery, the father sat in the waiting room. After the delivery the father saw his child through the window of the nursery. Frequently, the mother was separated from her infant for hours after the delivery, and maternal–infant contact was dependent on hospital routine and schedule. Postpartal stays for mother and child were usually about 10 days, and infant care classes were unknown.

Increasingly, it is being acknowledged that pregnancy is not a disease but a normal process. Women are realizing that the successful outcome of pregnancy usually has more to do with their role and activities than those of the obstetrician. Typically, the maternity client enters the health care system not because of ill health but because she and the expectant father want to optimize their chances of having a healthy child. Couples are seeking assistance from physicians and nurses—not control. Fathers often desire to be participants, not passive bystanders. Each couple wants their childbearing experience to be special and meaningful.

The outcry from health care consumers and health care professionals regarding the management of pregnancy and childbirth has resulted in the development of the concept of family-centered care and the modification of hospital policies and practices.

DEVELOPMENT OF FAMILY-CENTERED CARE

As already discussed, hospitalization for labor and delivery became a common practice in North America. The childbirth experience was dictated by strict hospital rules. Parents were separated during labor and delivery, and mothers and infants were separated at birth to prevent and control infections. Infants were placed in newborn nurseries where routine care was characterized by strict aseptic procedures, rigid feeding schedules, and formula feedings.

In the early 1940s, parents began to question the necessity of the rigid rules and routines of the hospital. Social scientists and health care professionals began analyzing the effects of these practices on family relationships and on individual members. Studies revealed that the quality of the early mother–child relationship was a critical factor in child development. Psychologists and psychiatrists stated that it was important to a new mother's emotional security that she handle her infant and meet his or her physical and psychologic needs. Breast-feeding, which was thought to provide psychologic satisfaction for both mother and infant, had decreased with the separation of mother and infant in the hospital, and it was believed that the rigid feeding schedules in newborn nurseries contributed to many of the feeding problems that later developed.

Increasingly, psychologic and social problems were being attributed to the rigid practices advocated by hospitals. It became evident to some individuals that more personalized and family-oriented maternity care was essential, and they began advocating changes in the kind of care given during the childbearing experience. These advocates included Grantly Dick-Read (1953), who in the 1940s introduced the concept of childbirth preparation and participation of the father in labor and delivery; Arnold Gesell, who supported the practice of rooming-in in which newborns remain with their mothers after birth; and John Bowlby, (1953) who described the tragic effects of maternal deprivation on children.

The movement toward family-centered care during the childbearing experience was furthered in the late 1950s by the Family-Centered Maternity Care Program established at St. Mary's Hospital in Evansville, Indiana. This program was based on the notion that a hospital could provide professional services to mothers, fathers, and infants in a homelike environment that would enhance the integrity of the family unit.

The success of St. Mary's Hospital's maternity program has been followed by a movement in other hospitals to extend the family-oriented approach to other areas besides the maternity unit. For example, many hospitals encourage parents or other family members to participate in the care of sick children in pediatric units.

Nurses and other health professionals are well aware that a client's needs generally go beyond the purely physical and that these other needs must be met for the client to achieve optimum health. Others who are affected by that individual's life, such as family members, also have needs that must be satisfied. The physical and emotional status of the expectant woman is strongly influenced by that of her partner, and the physical and emotional development of the child is strongly influenced by those who are rearing him or her. These interrelationships make family-centered care a necessity.

BIRTH ALTERNATIVES

Alternatives to conventional institutional childbirth are being offered to low-risk clients by some hospitals. Labor and delivery rooms are being remodeled to convey a homelike atmosphere. Some hospitals are establishing outpatient birth centers.

The goal of birth rooms within hospitals is to promote a meaningful experience for the family. The father and persons important to the expectant mother are permitted to participate in the birth. Medical intervention is minimal. In some in-hospital birth rooms, siblings are permitted to be present during the labor and delivery.

Those birth facilities that are being established outside the hospital are usually associated with a nearby hospital and are often managed jointly by physicians and nurse-midwives (Lubec and Ernst, 1978; Norwood, 1978). Occasionally the birth center is established and managed by nurse-midwives solely, and support services include physician consultation. Nurse-midwives are the staff in attendance during labor and delivery. If a complication arises during labor or delivery, clients are transferred quickly to a health care facility that is equipped to handle the situation. These birth centers attempt to offer high-quality care to low-risk clients at low cost. Medical interventions such as episiotomies and anesthetics are not standard procedures. Fathers are permitted to assist during the delivery. The family and health care staff work together.

Despite the changes in maternity services, some expectant families feel that the health care system has not responded suitably or quickly enough to their demands. They object to the increase in technologic interventions and regard certain conventional medical practices more a matter of physician convenience than client safety. These families may choose to deliver their children at home and may engage a midwife or nurse-midwife to attend the birth. It is infrequent that a physician will perform an elected home delivery, since many regard home birth as a potentially dangerous practice.

The data concerning the safety of home births are conflicting. One study has found that the risk of fetal mortality is two to five times greater for babies born out of the hospital than those born in a hospital (*J. Obstet. Gynecol. Neonatal Nurs.*, 1978). Other evidence suggests that home birth is a safe alternative for medically screened healthy women (Mehl et al., 1977).

A primary focus of this textbook is nursing care during in-hospital births, simply because the majority of births occur in hospitals. However, alternative modes of childbirth are considered in Chapter 20.

IMPLICATIONS FOR NURSES

The traditional phrase "patient–health care professional relationship" has implied a specific pattern of interaction. The patient placed faith and trust in the professional's expertise, and the professional assumed the role of primary decision maker for the patient in matters of health and sickness (Reeder, 1978). The patient usually took the passive, dependent role in this relationship.

The phrase "consumer–health care provider relationship" denotes a different perspective. A consumer purchases services or goods from the providers of these services or goods and expects quantity and quality for his or her money. Faith and trust are not the bases of the relationship between consumer and the providers of health care. Satisfaction with services rendered determines the continuation of this relationship.

The phrase "client–health care professional relationship" carries yet another connotation. The term "client" implies an active role, not passive. The client seeks assistance from individuals who have special skills and knowledge that the client does not. Information and suggestions for a plan of action regarding the client's particular problem are offered to the client by the health care professional. It is understood that the client can choose not to accept the professional's advice and that the health care professional cannot proceed with the plan of action without the client's consent. In this relationship, the client assumes responsibility for his or her decisions.

The nursing profession has been at the forefront in its recognition that people who are able to should take an active role in their health care, and the term "client" best fits this concept. Nurses involved in a maternity client–health care professional relationship must understand that it is their professional expertise and skill that is being sought; they should not make decisions for their clients.

An important role of nurses is that of client advocacy. According to Kohnke (1982), the nurse advocate informs the client and then supports the decision made by the client. The maternity nurse advocate informs clients by clearly delineating all the options available as well as the risks of each one, by explaining simply but completely the nursing actions, and by answering all questions with facts and not personal opinions. The maternity nurse advocate then supports the client's decision by adhering to it and ensuring that others do the same.

The advocacy role of the nurse can enhance the consumer–health care provider relationship by providing individuals with complete information about the services desired so that the consumer's expectations are realistic. The client–health care professional relationship can also be enhanced by helping individuals understand that their participation in their health care is desired and indeed necessary.

The nursing profession is meeting consumer and client demands in obstetrics in other important ways. Nurses are usually the instructors of prenatal and postpartal education classes. Many nurse practitioners and nurse-midwives are providing the kind of alternatives to conventional institutional obstetric management that many families are seeking. Nurses are frequently the primary caregivers in clinics and birth centers that emphasize family-centered health. Maternity clients and their families are finding that nursing's orientation toward education, self-care, and health maintenance meshes with their desire for participation in and decision making about the childbirth experience.

The expanded role of nurses in obstetrics is discussed further in the next section, but it is important to note that the obstetric consumer's demand for alternatives has aided the nursing profession in its striving for autonomy and recognition for its unique role in the health care system. The demand for choices by clients and their families has provided nurses with more choices of specialization, work setting, and degree of involvement in client care.

THE EXPANDING ROLE OF NURSES IN MATERNITY CARE

Professional options are growing for nurses. This section considers the various roles and settings for nurses in obstetrics and also explores some of the issues that have developed from the expansion of nursing practice.

Roles and Settings for Nurses

Nursing is unique in its adaptability and flexibility in providing maternity care in various settings. Maternity nurses are found in the obstetric department of acute care facilities, in physicians' offices, in public health department clinics, in college health services, in family planning clinics, in school nursing programs dealing with sex education or adolescent pregnancies, in volunteer community health services, in abortion clinics, and in any other setting where a client has a need for maternity care. The depth of nursing involvement in various settings is determined by the qualifications and role/function of the nurse employed. Many different titles have evolved to describe the professional requirements of the nurse in various maternity care roles.

• *Professional nurses* are graduates of an accredited basic program in nursing who have successfully completed the nursing examination (NCLEX) and are currently licensed as a registered nurse. Professional nurses utilize the nursing process and employ their clinical skills in a variety of settings to provide basic nursing care. Today's nurse assumes a collaborative role in dealing with the physician and other members of the health care team, and is competent, assertive, and willing to take risks in the role of client advocate.

• *Nurse practitioners* are professional nurses who have received specialized education in either a master's degree program or a continuing education program. They function in a newer, expanded role, most often as providers of ambulatory care services. They focus on physical and psychosocial assessment, including health history, physical examination, and certain diagnostic tests and proce-

dures. "Based on clinical impressions, the nurse practitioner will initiate treatments within his or her defined scope of competence, seek physician recommendations, and assume responsibility for the clinical management of patients in the stable phase of their illness, while recognizing those deviations that require consultation or referral" (Keen, 1979).

• *Clinical nurse specialists* are master's degree prepared professional nurses, with additional specialized knowledge and competence in a specific clinical area. They assume a leadership role within their specialty and work to improve client care both directly and indirectly.

• *Certified nurse-midwives* (CNM) are educated in the two disciplines of nursing and midwifery and possess evidence of certification according to the requirements of the American College of Nurse-Midwives. Nurse-midwifery practice is the independent management of care of essentially normal newborns and women, antepartally, intrapartally, postpartally, and/or gynecologically, occurring within a health care system that provides for medical consultation, collaborative management, or referral and is in accord with the *Functions, Standards, Qualifications* for nurse-midwifery practice as defined by the American College of Nurse-Midwives (1979).

The nurse-midwife practices within the framework of a medically directed health service. The CNM functions as a member of the obstetric team in medical centers, institutions, universities, and community health projects with active programs of nurse-midwifery.

Legal Aspects of Maternal–Newborn Nursing

Nurses are legally bound to perform their duties according to the scope of nursing function, specified standards of care, and their recognized level of skill and training. The scope of nursing function is basically spelled out in each state's Nurse Practice Act. Although these acts vary somewhat from state to state, they are usually broadly written, especially in describing acts the nurse may do, and more specifically written in identifying functions and actions beyond the scope of nursing. The trend is toward increased flexibility in describing functions in the acts, especially in light of the varied backgrounds, educational levels, and competence of today's nurses. Many current Nurse Practice Acts also address the issues of qualifications and scope of practice for nurses in expanded roles, especially nurse practitioners, certified nurse-midwives, and nurse anesthetists.

Nurses in expanded roles, by reason of their training and experience, often find it necessary to make decisions formerly seen as being in the realm of medicine. These nurses generally work under "protocols" or accepted guidelines for practice, which may be viewed as equivalent to "standing orders." The nurse makes judgments about client care using the protocols as guidelines. "If the professional nurse has been educated to make this type of judgment (even though the education came from the institution's staff development department, rather than from formal academic institutions), the nurse is legally capable of making such *medical* decisions" (Bille, 1980). This also protects nurses working in highly technical areas such as neonatal or adult intensive care units.

Specified or accepted standards of care form the second basis by which all nurses are legally held accountable. Standards of care may be specified by the employing agency in its Policies and Procedures Manual, by the standards of the Joint Commission on Accreditation of Hospitals (JCAH), and by accepted community practices and policies. Negligence may exist if it can be established that the nurse ". . . is doing something or failing to do something contrary to what a reasonable, prudent nurse would do under all the facts and circumstances, in accordance with prevailing professional standards in the community or in similar communities under like circumstances" (Southwick, 1978).

As the role of nurses expands, so do their legal accountabilities. Nurses who are careless, who perform their professional duties below the acceptable standards of care, or who behave unprofessionally place their clients at risk. If a client suffers loss or damage because of faulty nursing action, the nurse and employing institution may be held liable in a civil suit action.

Informed consent is another legal concept that has great significance for nurses. Basically, the policy protects a client's right to autonomy and self-determination by specifying that nothing may be done to a client without her understanding and freely given consent. While this concept is usually adhered to for major procedures such as surgery or regional anesthesia, in actuality it pertains to *any* nursing, medical, or surgical intervention. To touch a client without consent (except in an emergency) constitutes battery. Frequently in the past, labor and delivery was viewed as an emergency situation in which informed consent may be waived. Currently this view is not acceptable in a normal, uncomplicated labor when the woman has time to give consent (Trandel-Korenchuk, 1982). Informed consent requires that the woman understand the usual procedures, their rationale, and any associated risks. She should also understand any possible birthing alternatives, so that she is truly an active participant in decision making about her care.

While the physician is bound by the doctrine of informed consent with regard to any diagnostic or treatment activities performed, the nurse is responsible for client education about any nursing care provided. Prior to each nursing intervention the woman should be informed of what to expect to ensure her cooperation and obtain her consent. When client teaching is done, the nurse should document it and the learning outcomes in the woman's medical record. The importance of clear, concise, and complete nurs-

ing records cannot be overemphasized. These records are evidence that a nurse obtained consent, performed prescribed treatments, reported important observations about the client to the appropriate staff, and adhered to acceptable standards of care.

In summary, the nurse's role in the health care system is growing. Underlying the concept of professional autonomy is the concept of responsible, thoughtful action. Clearly, nurses must render care of the highest quality to every patient. However, they must do so with their legal limitations in mind.

Nurses and Physicians

The nurse-midwife and nurse practitioner are becoming major providers of health services during the prenatal, intrapartal, and postpartal periods. Family planning and general health clinics are being established and run by nurse practitioners. These nurses are assuming the responsibilities of genetic counseling, family planning guidance, and health maintenance. Clients are referred to physicians as necessary.

Nurse-midwives are often the primary caregivers in birth centers. Frequently, the facility is run independently of physician control, although physicians are consulted when necessary. The nurse-midwives provide education to clients and serve as the delivery attendants. In addition, nurse-midwives are called upon to attend the family during home births in some states.

Many physicians are supporting the increasing autonomy of nursing professionals. Joint practices in which physicians and nurse practitioners or nurse-midwives are equal partners have been established. Physicians serve as consultants and provide support services to clinics and birth centers. These physicians are showing their endorsement of the expanded role of nurses by their participation in and encouragement of this development.

Other physicians support the theory behind expansion of nursing roles but find the practice less palatable. In theory, the physician will have more time to care for seriously ill patients if other health care professionals assume the responsibility of caring for individuals who are not seriously ill or who are essentially healthy and want to maintain that state (Tomich, 1978). The low-risk maternity client fits this last category, and nurse practitioners and nurse-midwives are adequately trained to care for this person.

The reaction of many physicians to actual independent nursing practice is less than supportive. Physician organizations have blocked clinics run by nurse practitioners (Beason, 1978; *RN*, 1979). Birth centers have also been under attack. Physicians in New York petitioned the state government unsuccessfully to deny a license to a birth center in Manhattan (Norwood, 1978). Regulations were proposed in New Jersey that would have hampered home birth by nurse-midwives and that would have made physician presence necessary during certain procedures performed by nurse-midwives in birth centers (*New York Times*, April 1978). Some nurse-midwives have been denied hospital privileges (*Nursing Careers*, 1982).

The reason usually cited for the negative reaction of many physicians is the threat that these alternatives pose to client safety. Certainly this is a legitimate concern, and quality control is a necessity in all health care facilities. However, other reasons for this negative response by physicians have been proposed. As Tomich (1978) points out, "The emergence of new roles in nursing may be considered as a set of challenges to the primacy of the physi-

cian." Consumers are also challenging the status of the medical profession and are making choices between conventional physician management and nursing services. Some physicians may feel threatened economically, which may provide further motivation for their nonsupportive attitude.

It is only natural that those desiring change will be opposed by those fearful of it. In obstetrics, the role of nurses is expanding and some physicians are opposing this change. Even so, physicians and nurses are becoming colleagues in the health care system, and nurses are continuing their development as autonomous professionals.

SUMMARY

Integration of historical data about obstetrics and maternity care allows the professional nurse to understand the evolution of modern-day nursing care. The foundation for modern family-centered maternity care was laid in ancient times, and the difficulties experienced by midwives and nurses through the ages have influenced the current practice of nurse-midwifery and maternal–newborn nursing.

The advances in medical technology have led to exciting developments in the field of obstetrics but have created new, more complex ethical and moral dilemmas. Consumers are becoming more vocal about their needs and ability to make their own choices, which has brought about major changes in the health care delivery system. Today's professional nurse, in the forefront of this movement in the role as advocate, is a competent, assertive, and actively functioning member of the health care team.

References

American College of Nurse-Midwives. 1972. *Statement of philosophy*. Washington, D.C.: The College.

American College of Nurse-Midwives. 1979. *What is a nurse-midwife?* Washington, D.C.: The College.

Arras, J., and Hunt, R. 1983. *Ethical issues in modern medicine*. 2nd ed. Palo Alto, Calif.: Mayfield Publishing Company.

Beason, C. Oct. 1978. Nurse practitioners: the flak from doctors is getting heavier. *RN*. 41:27.

Beauchamp, T. L., and Walters, L. 1978. *Contemporary issues in bioethics*. Belmont, Calif.: Wadsworth Publishing Company, Inc.

Bille, D. A. Fall 1980. Legal considerations in nursing service. *Nurs. Admin. Q*. 5:73–82.

Bowlby, J. 1953. *Child care and the growth of love*. Baltimore: Penguin Books.

Butler, J. M., and Parer, J. T. Sept./Oct. 1976. Is intensive intrapartum monitoring necessary? *J. Obstet. Gynecol. Neonatal Nurs*. 5(supp.):45.

Central Midwives Board. 1962. *Midwives Act, 1951: handbook*. London: Wm. Clowes & Sons, Ltd.

Dick-Read, G. 1953. *Childbirth without fear*. Rev. ed. New York: Harper & Row Publishers, Inc.

Fletcher, J. C. Feb. 1980. Ethics and amniocentesis for fetal sex identification. *Hastings Center Report*. 10:15.

Gee, C. L., and Ledger, W. J. Sept./Oct. 1976. Maternal and fetal morbidity associated with intrapartum monitoring. *J. Obstet. Gynecol. Neonatal Nurs*. 5(supp.):65.

Genetics Research Group of the Hastings Center. 1979. Guidelines for the ethical, social and legal issues in prenatal diagnosis. *N. Engl. J. Med*. 300:168.

Graham, H. 1951. *Eternal Eve*. New York: Doubleday and Co., Inc.

Harrison, M. R.; Golbus, M. S.; and Filly, R. A. Aug. 1981. Management of the fetus with a correctable congenital defect. *J.A.M.A*. 246:774.

Henig, R. M. 1982. Saving babies before birth. *New York Times Magazine*, Feb. 28, 1982.

J. Obstet. Gynecol. Neonatal Nurs. May/June 1978. Editorial. 7:5.

Keen, M. A. June 1979. The nurse practitioner in ambulatory gynecologic services. *Clin. Obstet. Gynecol*. 22:445.

Kohnke, M. F. 1982. *Advocacy: risk and reality*. St. Louis: The C. V. Mosby Co.

Lenzer, G. Feb. 1980. Gender ethics. *Hastings Center Report*. 10:18.

Lubec, R. W., and Ernst, E. K. N. 1978. The childbearing center: an alternative to conventional care. *Nurs. Outlook*. 26:754.

Maternity Center Association. 1975. *Log 1915–1975*. New York: The Association.

McDonough, M.; Sheriff, D.; and Zimmel, P. Jan./Feb. 1981. Parents' responses to fetal monitoring. *MCN* 6:32.

Mehl, L. E., et al. 1977. Outcome of elective home births: a series of 1,146 cases. *J. Reproduc. Med.* 19:281.

New York Times. April 6, 1978 (II:24); April 20, 1978 (XI:6).

Norwood, C. May 1978. Birth centers: a humanizing way to have a baby. *Ms.* p. 89.

Nursing Careers. March/April 1982. Nurse-midwives fight. 3:8.

Reeder, S. J. 1978. The social context of nursing. In *The nursing profession: views through the mist,* ed. N. L. Chaska. New York: McGraw-Hill Book Co.

RN. Feb. 1979. Nursing news. 42:14.

Robertson, J. A. Oct. 1981. Dilemma in Danville. *Hastings Center Report.* 11:5.

Ruddick, W., and Wilcox, W. Oct. 1982. Operating on the fetus. *Hastings Center Report.* 12:10.

Science News. 1979a. A safer alternative to amniocentesis. 115:230.

Science News. 1979b. NIH on electronic fetal monitoring. 115:183.

Southwick, A. F. 1978. *The law of hospital and health care administration.* Ann Arbor, Mich.: Health Administration Press.

Tomich, J. H. 1978. The expanded role of the nurse: current status and future prospects. In *The nursing profession: views through the mist,* ed. N. L. Chaska. New York: McGraw-Hill Book Co.

Trandel-Korenchuk, D. M. Nov./Dec. 1982. Informed consent. *J. Obstet. Gynecol. Neonatal Nurs.* 11:379.

Wallace, H., ed. 1975. *Health care of mothers and children in national health services.* Philadelphia: Ballinger Publishing Co.

Additional Readings

Evans, M. I., and Dixler, A. O. June 1981. Human in vitro fertilization. *J.A.M.A.* 245:2324.

Fagerhaugh, S.; Strauss, A.; Suczek, B., et al. Nov. 1980. The impact of technology on patients, providers, and care patterns. *Nurs. Outlook.* 28:666.

Fletcher, J. C. Aug. 1981. The fetus as patient: ethical issues. *J.A.M.A.* 246:772.

Guillemin, J. June 1981. Babies by cesarean: who chooses, who controls. *Hastings Center Report.* 11:15.

Kalisch, J. J. Nov./Dec. 1980. From medical care helper to health care provider: perspectives on the development of maternal child nursing. *MCN* 5:377.

Levine, M. E. 1980. The ethics of computer technology in health care. *Nurs. Forum.* 19:193.

Marsh, F. H., and Self, D. J. June 1980. In vitro fertilization: moving from theory to therapy. *Hastings Center Report.* 10:5.

Mauksch, I. G. June 1981. Nurse–physician collaboration: a changing relationship. *J. Nurs. Admin.* 11:35.

Ross, M. G. Nov./Dec. 1981. Health impact of a nurse midwife program. *Nurs. Res.* 30:353.

Schlotfeldt, R. M. May 1981. Nursing in the future. *Nurs. Outlook.* 29:295.

Silverman, W. A. Dec. 1981. Mismatched attitudes about neonatal death. *Hastings Center Report.* 11:12.

Simmons, R. S. and Rosenthal, J. June 1981. The women's movement and the nurse practitioner's sense of role. *Nurs. Outlook.* 29:371.

■ 2 ■

TOOLS FOR MATERNAL–NEWBORN NURSING PRACTICE

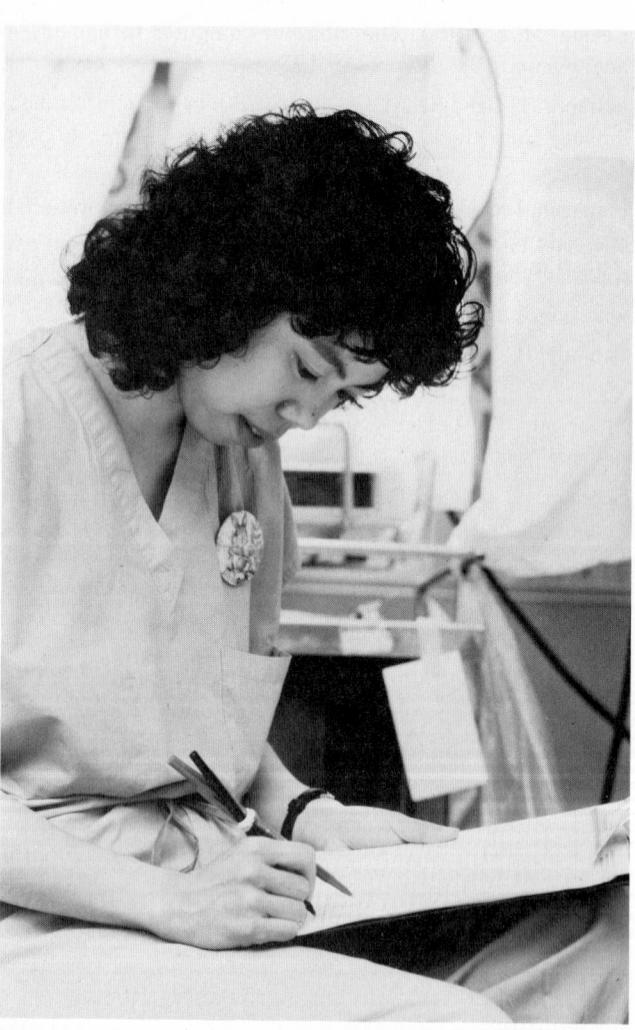

■ CHAPTER CONTENTS

KNOWLEDGE BASE

NURSING PROCESS
    Assessment
    Nursing Diagnoses and Planning
    Nursing Interventions
    Evaluation

COMMUNICATION

STATISTICS
    Descriptive Statistics
    Implications for Nursing

NURSING RESEARCH
    Application of Research

APPLICATION OF TOOLS FOR NURSING PRACTICE

- Discuss selected tools and the implications of each for maternity nursing practice.
- Describe the application of the nursing process in the maternity setting.
- Compare descriptive and inferential statistics.

- Discuss the possible use of statistical data in formulating further research questions.
- Discuss the application of nursing research in the maternity clinical setting.

Professional maternity nurses incorporate a variety of "tools" in everyday practice that enable them to deliver high-quality nursing care. The first of these tools, an adequate knowledge base that incorporates information from a variety of disciplines, is absolutely necessary to the practice of professional nursing. With a firmly established knowledge base the nurse is able to utilize the nursing process in planning and providing care to clients in a variety of settings. Knowledge about the client and care provided must be shared with all members of the health care team if it is to be truly effective. The *problem-oriented medical record* method is a pertinent yet succinct communication approach.

Bodies of statistics are often overlooked or underestimated as useful tools available to nurses. Descriptive statistics provide key factual data designed to answer a specific question. Inferential statistics explore possible causes and ramifications of the information obtained. Nursing research is essential to provide a scientific basis for nursing practice and to ensure the recognition of nursing as a respected profession. Whether this research is theoretical or conducted in a clinical setting, it must be relevant to the practice of nursing.

This chapter is not designed to give a complete explanation of nursing tools but to highlight them and explore ways in which the maternity nurse may use them in providing high-quality care.

KNOWLEDGE BASE

Current knowledge and theories form the basis for nursing activities. They are subject to change if proven wrong or modified by new discoveries. Change also occurs if statistics reveal alterations in the relationships between variables. New technology is discovered and implemented at a rapid rate in our society—change is inevitable. Nurses find it a challenge to keep their understanding current with this explosion of new knowledge; therefore specialization has become prevalent.

NURSING PROCESS

The nursing process, built on a comprehensive knowledge base, represents a logical approach to problem identification and resolution, and serves as the framework for nursing. Whether it consists of four or five steps (some authors separate the making of a diagnosis from the planning phase), the nursing process is an analog of the problem-solving process used by nurses since Florence Nightingale.

Assessment

The nurse gathers both subjective and objective data about the health status of the client. Subjective information is obtained from the client and family members and includes their perceptions of the health impairment or problem and its management. Objective data are more measurable and include physical assessment findings, laboratory test results, and observations noted by other health team members.

Nursing Diagnoses and Planning

The second step in the process is the assimilation and clustering of assessment data into relevant categories from which *nursing diagnoses* are derived. Each nursing diagnosis describes a specific health problem, its etiology, and the associated signs and symptoms. The making of a nursing diagnosis is the crucial step in the process, for the resultant plan of care is based on what the nurse perceives to be the problem. In contrast to the medical diagnosis, which generally remains the same throughout the client's health problem, the nursing diagnosis will reflect the changing *response* of the client as her condition improves or worsens, and as she and her family adjust to those changes.

Once established, the nursing diagnoses serve to direct the nursing plan of care. Expected outcomes (goals) and priorities of care are identified. Nursing interventions necessary to achieve the specified goals are also identified. Nursing interventions are directed at altering or eliminating the cause (or etiology) of the health problem, and the related signs and symptoms serve as a baseline for evaluation of the effectiveness of care.

Nursing Interventions

In the third step of the nursing process, the nursing actions or treatments identified in the planning step are performed according to assessment data.

Evaluation

The client's progress or lack of progress toward the identified expected outcomes (goals) is evaluated by the client and the nurse. These questions are asked: Have expected outcomes been met? Is reassessment needed? Are new problems present? Are changes in any part of the process necessary? Do new priorities need to be identified? Is revision of the plan of care required?

The following brief example illustrates the application of the nursing process.

> A client with preeclampsia is found to have pedal edema, hypertension, and proteinuria. The nurse makes a diagnosis of "intravascular fluid volume deficit related to loss of protein" and lists the supporting signs and symptoms. Nursing interventions will include measuring intake and output and urine protein, ascertaining daily weights, monitoring blood pressure, observing peripheral edema, and instituting measures to reduce the dependent edema and prevent skin breakdown. The effectiveness of these actions will be evaluated by the achievement (or nonachievement) of outcomes related to normal fluid balance.

COMMUNICATION

The problem-oriented medical record (POMR) system allows for the systematic documentation and retrieval of information about the client's care and progress. Although originally intended for use with medical diagnoses, POMR can be adapted for documentation of nursing care using nursing diagnoses. POMR is a system of charting observations and interventions using the SOAP format. The acronym SOAP stands for the four components of each charting entry: Subjective data, Objective data, Analysis (sometimes called Assessment), and Plan. The subjective and objective data come from the nursing assessment (the first step in the nursing process) and are recorded under the appropriate problem number (each nursing diagnosis is listed numerically on a problem sheet kept on the chart). The analysis entry represents the nurse's conclusions

about the client's progress, based on the data collected (for example: Do the intake and output along with the daily weight change indicate fluid retention? Has the blood pressure remained elevated despite antihypertensive medications?). Finally, the plan of care is continued or changed in accordance with the data analysis.

The importance of the POMR system for nursing is that the SOAP format, when used correctly, provides readily accessible data and ongoing evaluation of the effects of nursing care. The response to treatment can be evaluated regularly and as frequently as the client's condition dictates, and the plan for nursing care can be altered.

STATISTICS

Evaluation of the health care system relies on *statistics*, the collection and analysis of pertinent numerical data. Health-related statistics provide an objective basis for projecting client needs, planning for utilization of resources, and analyzing new data for evaluation of effectiveness of treatment.

There are two major types of statistics—descriptive and inferential. Descriptive statistics describe or summarize a set of data: they report the facts—what *is*—in a concise and easily retrievable way (an example is the birth rate in the United States). How the data are compiled and presented is determined by the question being asked. Although no conclusion may be drawn about *why* some phenomenon has occurred from these "vital" statistics, certain trends can be identified, high-risk "target groups" delineated, and research questions generated that will provoke further investigation using more sophisticated statistical testing.

Inferential statistics allow the investigator to draw conclusions or inferences about what is happening between two or more variables in a population and to establish or refute causal relationships between them. For example, descriptive statistics show that the infant mortality rate in the United States has declined over the past decade. Exactly *why* that trend has occurred cannot be answered by simply looking at these data, however. More data and inferential statistics, using smaller samples of the population of pregnant women, are needed to determine whether this finding is due to earlier prenatal care, improved maternal nutrition, use of electronic fetal monitoring during labor, and/or any number of factors potentially associated with maternal–fetal survival.

Descriptive statistics are the starting point that allows the formulation of research questions. Inferential statistics answer specific questions and generate theories to explain relationships between variables. Theory applied in nursing practice can help make changes in the specific variables that may be causing or contributing to certain health problems. The following section deals primarily with descrip-

Table 2-1   Live Births, Birth Rates, and Fertility Rates, by Race of Child, United States, 1960–1980*

	Number	Birth rate[†]				Fertility rate[†]			
				All other				All other	
Year	All races	All races	White	Total	Black	All races	White	Total	Black
Registered births									
1980[‡]	3,612,258	15.9	14.9	22.5	22.1	68.4	64.7	88.6	88.1
1979[‡]	3,494,398	15.6	14.5	22.2	22.0	67.2	63.4	88.5	88.3
1978[‡]	3,333,279	15.0	14.0	21.6	21.3	65.5	61.7	87.0	86.7
1977[‡]	3,326,632	15.1	14.1	21.6	21.4	66.8	63.2	87.7	88.1
1976[‡]	3,167,788	14.6	13.6	20.8	20.5	65.0	61.5	85.8	85.8
1975[‡]	3,144,198	14.6	13.6	21.0	20.7	66.0	62.5	87.7	87.9
1974[‡]	3,159,958	14.8	13.9	21.2	20.8	67.8	64.2	89.8	89.7
1973[‡]	3,136,965	14.8	13.8	21.7	21.4	68.8	64.9	93.4	93.6
1972[‡]	3,258,411	15.6	14.5	22.8	22.5	73.1	68.9	99.5	99.9
1971[§]	3,555,970	17.2	16.1	24.6	24.4	81.6	77.3	109.1	109.7
1970[§]	3,731,386	18.4	17.4	25.1	25.3	87.9	84.1	113.0	115.4

*Modified from National Center for Health Statistics: Advance report of final natality statistics, 1980. *Monthly vital statistics report,* Vol. 31, No. 8, Supp. DHHS Pub. No (PHS) 83-1120. Public Health Service, Hyattsville, Md. November 1982.
[†]Birth rates per 1000 population in specified group. Fertility rates per 1000 women aged 15–44 years in specified group. Population enumerated as of April 1 for census years and estimated as of July 1 for all other years. Beginning 1970 excludes births to nonresidents of the United States.
[‡]Based on 100% of births in selected states and on a 50% sample of births in all other states.
[§]Based on a 50% sample of births.

tive statistics, although inferential considerations are addressed through the use of possible research questions that may assist in identifying relevant variables.

Descriptive Statistics

BIRTH RATE

Birth rate refers to the number of live births per 1000 population. A related statistic, the *fertility rate,* is the number of births per 1000 women aged 15–44 years in a given population.

Table 2-1 compares live births, birth rates, and fertility rates by race for 1960–1980. After a peak of the birth rate for all races of 25.0 in 1955, there has been a decline until the rate remained constant in 1975 and 1976—14.6 live births per 1000 population. This is the lowest recorded birth rate in the history of the United States. Since 1975–1976 there has been a small yearly increase in the birth rate.

Comparison of live birth rate between white and black populations in the United States reveals a decrease until 1976, when it was 13.6 for white women and 20.5 for black women. Since then there has been an increase. In

Table 2-2   Canada: Live Births, Birth Rates, and General Fertility*

Year	Live births[†]	Birth rate[‡]	General fertility[§]
1980	370,709	15.5	57.9
1979	366,064	15.5	58.2

*Modified from *Vital statistics.* Vol. I. Births and deaths. 1980. Canada Health Division Vital Statistics and Disease Registry. Cat. 84-204. Minister of Supply and Services. May 1982. Table 1, p. 2.
[†]Live births = per 1000 population
[‡]Live birth rate = per 1000 population
[§]General fertility rate = birth rate per 1000 women 15–49 years

1980 the live birth rate was 14.9 for white women and 22.1 for black women.

Live births, birth rate, and general fertility for Canada are presented in Table 2-2. The birth rate remains similar to the United States; however, the fertility rate is lower.

□ *INFERENTIAL CONSIDERATIONS* The "postwar baby boom," which followed World War II and resulted in a marked increase in the birth rate, has been in evidence for several years. The impact of this larger number of babies had implications for the number of maternity care facilities needed in the middle to late 1940s; for public school systems as the children entered and progressed through school; and again for maternity care as the postwar babies reached childbearing age.

Additional inferences about birth rates may be identified by posing some of the following research questions:

- Is there an association with changing societal values?
- Is the difference in birth rate between various age groups reflective of education? Or does it represent availability of contraceptive information?

AGE OF MOTHER

In looking at 1980 total birth rates for all races in the United States, the highest birth rate (115.1) for the first child was in women 20–24 years of age, followed by a birth rate of 112.9 for women 25–29 years of age. Teenagers in the 15–19 age group had a total birth rate of 53.0 for first births (Table 2–3).

Of all the age groups, the smallest increase, less than 1%, occurred in teenage girls 15–17 years of age. The birth rate of 1.1 for all races in the 10–14 age range is low;

however, its existence is of concern to health care providers and educators.

Women in the 30–34 age range had a birth rate of 61.9 in 1980. As in recent years, the largest increase in births is observed in this age range. The increase was 2.7% higher in 1980 than 1979. In comparing 1975 and 1980, there was a 60% increase. In recent years, a trend of increase in first-order births for women in their 30s is obvious. The rate for second-order births also showed large increases in the woman 30–44 years of age.

□ *INFERENTIAL CONSIDERATIONS* The identification of variables that affect the birth rate of different age groups and races may be addressed by posing the following research questions.

- Is there an association with changing societal values? With changing roles of women? With changing national economic conditions and financial status?
- Is there a correlation between years of education? Availability of contraceptive information for different age groups and races?

Table 2–3   Birth Rates by Age of Mother, Live-Birth Order, and Race of Child, United States, 1980*

| | | | **Age of mother** | | | | | | | | |
| | | | **15–19 years** | | | | | | | | |
Live-birth order and race of child	15–44 years[†]	10–14 years	Total	15–17 years	18–19 years	20–24 years	25–29 years	30–34 years	35–39 years	40–44 years	45–49 years
All races											
Total	68.4	1.1	53.0	32.5	82.1	115.1	112.9	61.9	19.8	3.9	0.2
First child	29.5	1.1	41.4	28.5	59.7	57.3	38.2	12.8	2.6	0.3	0.0
Second child	21.8	0.0	9.8	3.6	18.6	39.8	41.9	20.7	4.2	0.5	0.0
White											
Total	64.7	0.6	44.7	25.2	72.1	109.5	112.4	60.4	18.5	3.4	0.2
First child	28.4	0.6	36.0	22.7	54.8	57.2	39.6	12.8	2.5	0.3	0.0
Second child	21.0	0.0	7.6	2.3	15.1	37.8	42.6	20.7	4.0	0.4	0.0
All other											
Total	88.6	3.9	94.6	68.3	133.2	145.0	115.5	70.8	27.9	6.5	0.4
First child	35.6	3.7	68.3	57.1	84.9	57.5	30.0	12.6	3.2	0.5	0.0
Second child	26.2	0.1	20.8	9.9	36.8	50.3	37.8	20.8	5.6	0.7	0.0
Black											
Total	88.1	4.3	100.0	73.6	138.8	146.3	109.1	62.9	24.5	5.8	0.3
First child	35.2	4.2	71.8	61.3	87.3	55.9	24.3	9.1	2.4	0.3	0.0
Second child	25.7	0.1	22.3	10.9	39.0	51.2	35.6	16.8	4.2	0.5	0.0

*Based on 100% of births in selected states and on a 50% sample of births in all states. Rates are live births per 1000 women in specified age and racial groups. Live-birth order refers to number of children born alive to mother. Modified from National Center for Health Statistics: Advance report of final natality statistics. 1980. *Monthly vital statistics report.* Vol. 31, No. 8, Supp. DHHS Pub. No. (PHS) 83–1120. Public Health Service, Hyattsville, Md. November 1982.

[†]Rates computed by relating total births, regardless of age of mother, to women aged 15–44 years.

WEIGHT AT BIRTH

In 1980, the median birth weight of infants was 3360 g (7 lb, 7 oz). The newborn posing the most concern to health professionals is the low-birth-weight (less than 2500 g) infant. In the United States in 1980, low-birth-weight infants comprised 6.8% of all births. This rate is a slight decrease from the 1976 rate of 6.9%. However, as in previous years, a substantial racial difference persists, with 5.7% for white births, 12.5% for black births, and 11.5% for all other races. Teenagers and women between 40–49 years of age are most likely to bear low-birth-weight infants. In 1980 the rate of low-birth-weight infants to teenagers under 15 years of age was 2.5 times the number born to women aged 25–29 and 30–34 years (Table 2–4).

Canadian statistics for 1980, presented in Table 2–5, reveal that the highest percentage of low-birth-weight infants occurs in women in the under 20 and 40–44 age range.

□ *INFERENTIAL CONSIDERATIONS* The review of the descriptive statistical data reveals discrepancies between differing age ranges and between races. To gain further data the following research questions may be addressed:

• Are there factors that affect different age and racial groups? Nutritional status before and during pregnancy? Educational level? Length of time between pregnancies? Availability of prenatal care? Desire and ability to seek prenatal care? Physical health of the mother? Presence of environmental factors such as high pollution levels, or high altitude?

INFANT MORTALITY

The *infant death rate* is the number of deaths of infants under 1 year of age per 1000 live births in a given population. *Neonatal mortality* is the number of deaths of infants less than 28 days of age per 1000 live births. *Perinatal mortality* encompasses both neonatal deaths and fetal deaths per 1000 live births. (Fetal death is death in utero at 20 weeks or more gestation.) For statistical purposes the period from 28 days to 11 months of age is designated the *postneonatal period*. Table 2–6 delineates infant mortality by age. Although the United States ranked the fifteenth highest among nations in infant deaths in 1980, with few exceptions there had been a steady decline in neonatal and postneonatal deaths within the United States since 1940.

Infant mortality for 1979 and 1980 in Canada is presented in Table 2–7. Comparison of Canadian and U.S. infant mortality reveals a lower rate for Canada.

Among the principal causes of infant death are causes originating in the perinatal period; congenital anomalies; sudden infant death syndrome; respiratory distress syndrome; and disorders relating to preterm and low-birth-weight infants.

□ *INFERENTIAL CONSIDERATIONS* Currently, some researchers predict the infant mortality may rise due to worsening economic situations. Newland (1982), in her study on infant mortality and the health of societies, points out that the infant mortality "reflects not simply per capita stocks of food, clean water, medical care, and so forth, but the actual availability of such amenities to all segments of a population."

Additional factors may be identified by considering the following research questions:

• Does infant mortality correlate with a specific maternal age?

• Is it associated with the time in pregnancy that the woman seeks prenatal care? Number of prenatal visits?

• Is there a difference between racial groups? If so, is it associated with educational level? Availability of prenatal care?

MATERNAL MORTALITY

Maternal mortality rate is the number of deaths from any cause during the pregnancy cycle (including the 42-day postpartal period) per 100,000 live births.

The maternal death rate in the United States has decreased steadily in the last 25 years (Table 2–8). The 1980 estimated maternal mortality of 6.9 is almost two-thirds less than the 1970 rate of 21.5. In 1980, 250 women died of causes listed as complications of pregnancy, childbirth, and puerperium. In Canada, the maternal death rate for 1980 was 8.0.

□ *INFERENTIAL CONSIDERATIONS* Factors influencing the decrease in maternal mortality include development of obstetrics and gynecology as a recognized medical specialty; the increased use of hospitals and specialized health care personnel for antepartal, intrapartal, and postpartal care of the maternity client; the establishment of high-risk centers for mother and infant care; the prevention and control of infection with antibiotics and improved techniques; the availability of blood and blood products for transfusions; lowered rates of anesthesia-related deaths; and the application of research for the prevention of maternal deaths (Danforth, 1982).

Additional data may be identified by asking:

• Is there a correlation with age? Availability of health care? Economic status?

Implications for Nursing

The successful implementation of the nursing process depends on the appropriate application of statistics. Nurses can make use of statistics in a number of ways. For example, statistical data may be used to:

• Determine populations at risk

• Assess the relationship between specific factors

• Help establish a data base for different client populations

Table 2–4 Number and Percent Low Birth Weight, by Age of Mother and Race of Child, United States, 1980*

Age of mother and race of child	Percent low birth weight	Total	Birth weight†				
			Under 500	500–999	1000–1499	1500–1999	2000–2499
All races							
All ages	6.8	3,612,258	3,591	15,903	21,936	47,680	157,182
Under 15 years	14.6	10,169	32	162	150	326	812
15–19 years	9.4	552,161	663	3,516	4,955	10,285	32,401
20–24 years	6.9	1,226,200	1,223	5,263	7,325	16,100	54,689
25–29 years	5.8	1,108,291	980	4,212	5,569	12,219	41,282
30–34 years	5.9	550,354	515	2,075	2,879	6,252	20,580
35–39 years	7.0	140,793	153	571	854	2,068	6,166
40–44 years	8.3	23,090	24	100	187	403	1,192
45–49 years	9.2	1,200	1	4	17	27	60
White							
All ages	5.7	2,898,732	2,120	9,755	14,079	31,788	107,074
Under 15 years	11.2	4,171	10	46	50	117	241
15–19 years	7.7	388,058	329	1,897	2,830	5,901	18,869
20–24 years	5.7	982,526	694	3,142	4,607	10,633	36,924
25–29 years	5.0	933,159	643	2,837	3,881	8,843	30,572
30–34 years	5.1	459,151	334	1,394	2,018	4,566	15,142
35–39 years	6.2	113,124	95	371	566	1,413	4,486
40–44 years	7.4	17,652	14	65	117	295	806
45–49 years	7.7	891	1	3	10	20	34
All other							
All ages	11.5	713,526	1,471	6,148	7,857	15,892	50,108
Under 15 years	17.1	5,998	22	116	100	209	571
15–19 years	13.5	164,103	334	1,619	2,125	4,384	13,532
20–24 years	11.8	243,674	529	2,121	2,718	5,467	17,765
25–29 years	10.0	175,132	337	1,375	1,688	3,376	10,710
30–34 years	9.7	91,203	181	681	861	1,686	5,438
35–39 years	10.5	27,669	58	200	288	655	1,680
40–44 years	11.3	5,438	10	35	70	108	386
45–49 years	13.4	309	—	1	7	7	26
Black							
All ages	12.5	589,616	1,381	5,748	7,208	14,463	44,662
Under 15 years	17.2	5,793	22	115	96	203	558
15–19 years	14.0	150,353	323	1,568	2,038	4,182	12,828
20–24 years	12.6	209,596	508	2,010	2,547	5,085	16,245
25–29 years	11.2	135,680	311	1,248	1,534	2,977	9,112
30–34 years	11.1	64,369	156	603	687	1,390	4,307
35–39 years	11.7	19,631	53	173	242	537	1,287
40–44 years	12.2	3,990	8	31	61	83	302
45–49 years	15.8	204	—	—	3	6	23

*Based on 100% of births in selected states and on a 50% sample of births in all other states. Modified from National Center for Health Statistics: Advance report of final natality statistics, 1980. *Monthly vital statistics report.* Vol. 31, No. 8, Supp. DHHS Pub. No. (PHS) 83-1120. Public Health Service, Hyattsville, Md. November 1982.

†Equivalents of the gram weight in terms of pounds and ounces are as follows:
  Under 500 g = 1 lb, 1 oz or less
  500–999 g = 1 lb, 2 oz–2 lb, 3 oz
  1000–1499 g = 2 lb, 4 oz–3 lb, 4 oz
  1500–1999 g = 3 lb, 5 oz–4 lb, 6 oz
  2000–2499 g = 4 lb, 7 oz–5 lb, 8 oz

Table 2-5   Canada: Live Births by Birth Weight, Sex, and Age of Mother (Excluding Newfoundland), 1980*

Age of mother		% 2500 g or less†
Under 20	Males	7.2
	Females	7.9
20-24	Males	5.9
	Females	7.0
25-29	Males	4.9
	Females	6.1
30-34	Males	5.1
	Females	5.9
35-39	Males	6.1
	Females	7.4
40-44	Males	7.7
	Females	8.4

*Modified from *Vital statistics.* Vol. I. Births and deaths. 1980. Canada Health Division Vital Statistics and Disease Registry. Cat. 84-204. Minister of Supply and Services. May 1982. Table 1, p. 2.
†Based on stated birth weights

Table 2-6   Infant Mortality Rates by Age: United States, 1950, 1960, 1965, and 1970-80*

Year	Under 1 year	Under 28 days	28 days-11 months
1980 (est.)	12.5	8.4	4.1
1979 (est.)	13.0	8.7	4.2
1978	13.8	9.5	4.3
1977	14.1	9.9	4.2
1976	15.2	10.9	4.3
1975	16.1	11.6	4.5
1974	16.7	12.3	4.4
1973	17.7	13.0	4.8
1972†	18.5	13.6	4.8
1971	19.1	14.2	4.9
1970	20.0	15.1	4.9
1965	24.7	17.7	7.0
1960	26.0	18.7	7.3
1950	29.2	20.5	8.7

*For 1979 and 1980, based on a 10% sample of deaths; for all other years, based on final data. Rates per 1000 live births. From National Center for Health Statistics. Advance report of final natality statistics. 1981. *Monthly vital statistics report.* Vol. 29. No. 13. Public Health Service, Hyattsville, Md. Sept. 17, 1981.
†Based on a 50% sample of deaths.

Table 2-7   Canada: Infant Mortality (Total Infant Death Rate per 1000 Live Births)*

Year	Under 1 year (infant)	Under 28 days (neonatal)	28 days-11 months (postneonatal)
1980	10.4	6.7	3.8
1979	10.9	7.2	3.7

*Modified from *Vital statistics.* Vol. I. Births and deaths. 1980. Canada Health Division Vital Statistics and Disease Registry. Cat. 84-204. Minister of Supply and Services. May 1982. Table 1, p. 2.

Table 2-8   U.S. Maternal Mortality Rate per 100,000 Live Births*

Year	Rate	Year	Rate
1980 (est.)	6.9	1969	22.5
1979 (est.)	7.8	1968	24.5
1978	9.6	1967	28.0
1977	11.2	1966	29.1
1976	12.3	1965	31.6
1975	12.8	1964	33.3
1974	14.6	1963	35.8
1973	15.2	1962	35.2
1972	18.8	1961	36.9
1971	18.8	1960	37.1
1970	21.5	1950	83.3

*From National Center for Health Statistics: Advance report of final natality statistics. 1981. *Monthly vital statistics report.* Vol. 29. No. 13 Public Health Service, Hyattsville, Md. Sept. 17, 1981.

- Determine the levels of care needed by particular client populations
- Evaluate the success of specific nursing interventions
- Determine priorities in case loads
- Estimate staffing and equipment needs of hospital units and clinics

Descriptive statistics may also be used to help decide whether a problem actually exists. For example, a nurse working in a large maternity center that has 60,000 births per year (500 births per month) notes that 20 babies with diaphragmatic hernia have been born in the last year. She wonders whether this number is reflective of the projected incidence and whether the rate is higher than normal.

A method of obtaining an answer has been illustrated by Layde and Rubin (1982). The rate of the defect would be determined by dividing the number of cases by the number of births.

$$\frac{20 \text{ (number of cases)}}{60,000 \text{ (number of births)}} = 0.0003 \text{ (rate)}$$

By calculating the hospital's rate, the nurse can demonstrate that although the number of cases has seemed excessive, it is within the "normal" rate or incidence, which is 1:3000 live births (rate 0.0003).

If the rate had been higher than normal, then additional questions would need to be asked. Is there a correlation with a particular maternal age? Diet? Illness during pregnancy? Place of residence? Treatment during pregnancy? Exposure to toxic materials?

Statistical information is available through many sources, including professional literature; state and city health departments; vital statistics sections of private, county, state, and federal agencies; special programs or agencies (family planning agencies); demographic profiles of specific geographic areas. Nurses who make use of this information will find themselves well prepared to protect the health needs of maternity clients and their families.

NURSING RESEARCH

Research is a vital step toward establishing a science of nursing. It is also a means to improve client care and to establish nursing as a true profession, with its own unique knowledge base. Many nursing leaders have voiced the same sentiments as Fawcett (1980): "If nursing practice is to be more than action based on rituals and myths; if it is to be professional practice, then research must be its prime directive, for only research can generate, refine, and expand the scientific knowledge needed to move nursing toward a truly professional status." For this to occur, the research that is done must be translated into clinical practice—it must be made useful to nurses taking care of clients.

This gap between research and practice is being narrowed by activities that involve publication of research findings in popular nursing journals; establishment of departments of nursing research in hospitals; and collaborative research activities between nurse researchers and clinical practitioners. Specific efforts, such as the CURN (Conduct and Utilization of Research in Nursing) Project in Michigan (from which a series of volumes have been published, each of which organizes the research related to a specific nursing care problem and discusses the practice changes indicated by the results) have been especially helpful in correlating research and practice (Horsley, Crane, and Bingle, 1978). In addition, numerous journal articles giving "how-to" information for translating research into practice have been published within the last few years (Jaecox and Prescott, 1978; Fawcett, 1980; Loomis and Krone, 1980; Moore, 1980; King, Barnard, and Hoehn, 1981; Davis, 1981; Hunt, 1981; and Lewandowski, 1981).

Success in this effort ultimately depends on the willingness and ability of practitioners to transfer research-generated knowledge into practical nursing interventions. How is this done? By taking completed research studies of relevance to the specific health problem or need, and trying out methods that worked for the investigator. Of course, this is a gross oversimplification, but the process of applying research findings to improve client care should be made a relatively simple exercise in problem solving; otherwise, the gap between research and action will remain wide.

Application of Research

The best way to begin the application of research to daily practice is to read research studies relevant to the practice setting. The following two brief examples specific to maternal–child nursing help illustrate how the findings of a research study might be applied to improve client care. Nursing diagnoses will be used to help clarify that concept.

EXAMPLE 1

As the benefits, in terms of nutritional and immunologic advantages, of human breast milk over cow's milk or soy-based formulas are recognized, mothers are increasingly being encouraged to breast-feed their infants. Nurses have the opportunity to play a major role in increasing the success of breast-feeding through client education. One of the first complications a nursing mother may experience is sore nipples. Atkinson (1979) investigated the effectiveness of a prenatal nipple-conditioning regimen to determine whether nipple soreness can be prevented.

The nipple-conditioning regimen consisted of nipple rolling twice a day for 2 minutes each time; providing gentle friction against the nipple with a terrycloth towel for 15 seconds once a day; and nipple airing for 2 hours a day, allowing outer clothing to rub against the nipple. This program was started 6 weeks before the expected date of delivery; each woman in the study served as her own control, conditioning one nipple but not the other. Seventeen primigravida women successfully completed the study. Although the sample was very small, significant results were obtained. Results showed that the prenatal nipple-conditioning program significantly reduced the amount of total nipple pain experienced during the first few days of breastfeeding, and the amount of extreme pain experienced on the conditioned nipple was significantly reduced compared with the control nipple. In addition, it was found that fair-skinned women reported more nipple soreness on unconditioned nipples, and olive-complected women reported significantly less nipple soreness on unconditioned nipples.

To demonstrate the use of this research in the clinical setting, a nursing diagnosis of "knowledge deficit related to techniques of nipple conditioning" would be made by the nurse in the prenatal setting in which a nipple-conditioning regimen could be initiated 6 to 8 weeks before the expected date of birth. If the nipple-conditioning regimen is successful, then problems with breast-feeding (related to nipple soreness) can be decreased and infant feeding and the mother's feelings of success can be enhanced. In this way, the possible need for a nursing diagnosis such as "impairment of skin integrity related to cracked nipples" has now been negated.

EXAMPLE 2

Prenatal education is not a new idea; classes are commonly offered by hospitals with obstetric units. But what difference does prenatal education make? Is it worth the time and effort to offer such information on a formal basis? How do women who attend such classes differ from women who don't?

Timm (1979) found that women who attended a prenatal class program required significantly less medication during labor than women exposed to other structured programs during pregnancy. The classes provided general information on fetal development, pregnancy, prenatal nutrition, labor and delivery, analgesics and anesthetics in labor and delivery, and the postpartal period. A second variable, infant birth weight, was not demonstrated to be affected by attendance at the prenatal education series. Timm's findings were consistent regardless of age, race, and parity and suggest the value of prenatal education in reducing levels of medication required by women during labor.

The results of this study support what is already known about the interrelationship between the phenomena of "knowledge deficit," "fear," and "alteration in comfort" in clients. In this instance, prenatal teaching made a difference in the amount of pain medication needed by women during labor. It may be postulated that the women's anxiety about the unknown experience of childbirth was alleviated through learning what to expect. They were thus less fearful and more relaxed, thereby decreasing the need for analgesics.

Because analgesic agents have the capacity to cross the placental blood barrier, there are implications for the fetus as well. The fetal "potential for ineffective breathing patterns" diagnosis exists due to the depression of the fetal central nervous system (CNS) by certain medications used for maternal pain relief. Timm also found studies that showed the most powerful and persistent depressive effect to be on the sucking rate of the infant, which remained depressed throughout the first 4 days of postnatal life.

If this CNS depression occurred, there would be a potential nursing diagnosis of "alteration in nutrition: less than body requirements of the newborn related to inadequate intake of nutrients." In addition, the newborn might not be able to take in adequate fluids, resulting in "fluid volume deficit." The consequences of medicating the woman (and subsequently, her infant) during labor are not insignificant. If prenatal education can reduce the need for maternal analgesia, thereby reducing the risk to woman and infant, why not initiate such a program in the obstetric setting?

These examples are meant to illustrate how a practitioner may begin to think about using nursing research to improve maternal care. There is, of course, much time and work between an idea and its implementation. Change must be regarded in terms of the costs and benefits before old ways are discarded for new.

APPLICATION OF TOOLS FOR NURSING PRACTICE

Each of the tools—knowledge, nursing process, nursing diagnosis, statistics, nursing research—can exist separately, but in practice they overlap with and yet build upon each other. For example, the maternity nurse uses a knowledge base to utilize the nursing process, yet as one proceeds through the nursing process and evaluates the client response, one's knowledge base is affected.

Each of these tools for practice may be implemented in a variety of ways, as the obstetric nurse provides care for the childbearing family. An example of just one possible situation is presented in the following case study.

Two labor and delivery nurses express concerns to each other about the seemingly high numbers of adolescents who have been delivering in their unit.

At the next staff meeting, they voice their concerns and raise questions about whether the number of teenage mothers seen in their unit is higher than normal. After discussion, the nurses decide that they need to formulate a plan to gather more information. Each nurse volunteers to pursue a particular aspect of a plan of action.

Their plan includes contacting the local public health department for local and national statistics on this age group; looking at the availability of health care for adolescents in their community; investigating the particular health problems of the pregnant teenager and risks to their infants; checking the availability of prenatal education groups for adolescents; finding out whether their community has school health programs and what the program content is; looking at national statistics regarding when adolescents seek prenatal care; talking with community nurse-midwives, physicians, and prenatal clinic personnel to see if the national statistics apply to their community; collecting information about current legislative issues affecting adolescent health care; seeking further information about the needs of adolescents during pregnancy and delivery by doing a library search; and looking for continuing education programs dealing with the pregnant adolescent client.

At subsequent staff meetings each nurse shares information and other areas are investigated as the need is identified. How they evaluate the data and apply them will depend on the requirements of their maternity unit and the unique needs of their community.

Possible outcomes may include developing a research study; working as a volunteer in local adolescent clinics; developing and teaching prenatal classes for adolescents; volunteering to teach in community school health programs; organizing a continuing education program on the adolescent mother for community hospitals; and forming a network within their professional nursing organizations to stay informed about legislative issues pertaining to adolescents.

As the case study demonstrates, the application of tools for nursing practice helps define a problem, guides the collection of data, and provides a framework for intervention.

SUMMARY

Various tools for maternity practice are available that assist nurses to identify and define a problem, guide collection of data, facilitate the implementation of care, and finally, enhance the evaluative process. All these tools work together, complementing and supplementing each other as the professional nurse works with the childbearing family to provide maternity care of the highest quality possible.

References

Atkinson, L. D. 1979. Prenatal nipple conditioning for breastfeeding. *Nurs. Res.* 28:267.

Danforth, D. N., ed. 1982. *Obstetrics and gynecology.* 4th ed. Philadelphia: Harper & Row.

Davis, M. Z. 1981. Promoting nursing research in the clinical setting. *J. Nurs. Adm.* 11:22.

Fawcett, J. 1980. A declaration of nursing independence: the relation of theory and research to nursing practice. *J. Nurs. Adm.* 10:36.

Horsley, J. A.; Crane, J.; and Bingle, J. D. 1978. Research utilization as an organizational approach. *J. Nurs. Adm.* 8:4.

Hunt, J. 1981. Indicators for nursing practice: the use of research findings. *J. Advanced Nurs.* 6:189.

Jaecox, A. and Prescott, P. 1978. Determining a study's relevance for clinical practice. *Am. J. Nurs.* 78:1882.

King, M. J.; Barnard, K. E.; and Hoehn, R. 1981. Disseminating the results of nursing research. *Nurs. Outlook.* 29:164.

Layde, P. M., and Rubin, G. L. Dec. 1982. Counting diseases and deaths—meaningfully. *Contemp. OB Gyn.* 20:87.

Lewandowski, L. A., 1981. Research. It doesn't pertain to me—or does it? *Focus.* 8:27.

Loomis, M. E., and Krone, K. P. 1980. Collaborative research development. *J. Nurs. Adm.* 10:32.

Moore, F. 1980. Research in a clinical setting: promises and potential. *Supervis. Nurse.* 11:36.

Newland, K. 1982. *Infant mortality and the health of societies.* Worldwatch Institute: Washington, D.C.

Timm, M. M. 1979. Prenatal education evaluation. *Nurs. Res.* 28:338.

Additional Readings

Alexander, M. F. June 1982. Integrating theory and practice in nursing. Part 1. *Nurs. Times.* 78:65.

————. June 1982. Integrating theory and practice in nursing. Part 2. *Nurs. Times.* 78:69.

Barnard, K. 1982. Measurement: descriptive statistics. *MCN* 7:235.

Chase, B. A. July/Aug. 1982. Nursing service standards as context for self-assessment. *J. Contin. Educ. Nurs.* 13:26.

Cox, C. L. Oct. 1982. An interaction model of client health behavior: theoretical prescription for nursing. *ANS* 5:41.

Dickinson, S. June 1982. The nursing process and the professional status of nursing. *Nurs. Times.* 8:61.

Dickson, G. L. et al. Oct. 1982. Nursing theory and practice: a self care approach. *ANS* 5:29.

Fawcett, J. June 1982. Utilization of nursing research findings. *Image.* 14:57.

Fuller, E. O. June 1982. Selecting a clinical nursing problem for research. *Image.* 14:60.

Ellis, R. 1982. Conceptual issues in nursing. *Nurs. Outlook.* 30:406.

Jackson, N. E. 1982. Choosing and using a statistical consultant. *Nurs. Res.* 31:248.

Munhall, P. L. 1982. Nursing philosophy and nursing research: in apposition or opposition? *Nurs. Res.* 31:176.

Tamarisk, N. K. Aug. 1982. The computer as a clinical tool. *Nurs. Manage.* 13:46.

■ 3 ■

DYNAMICS OF FAMILY LIFE

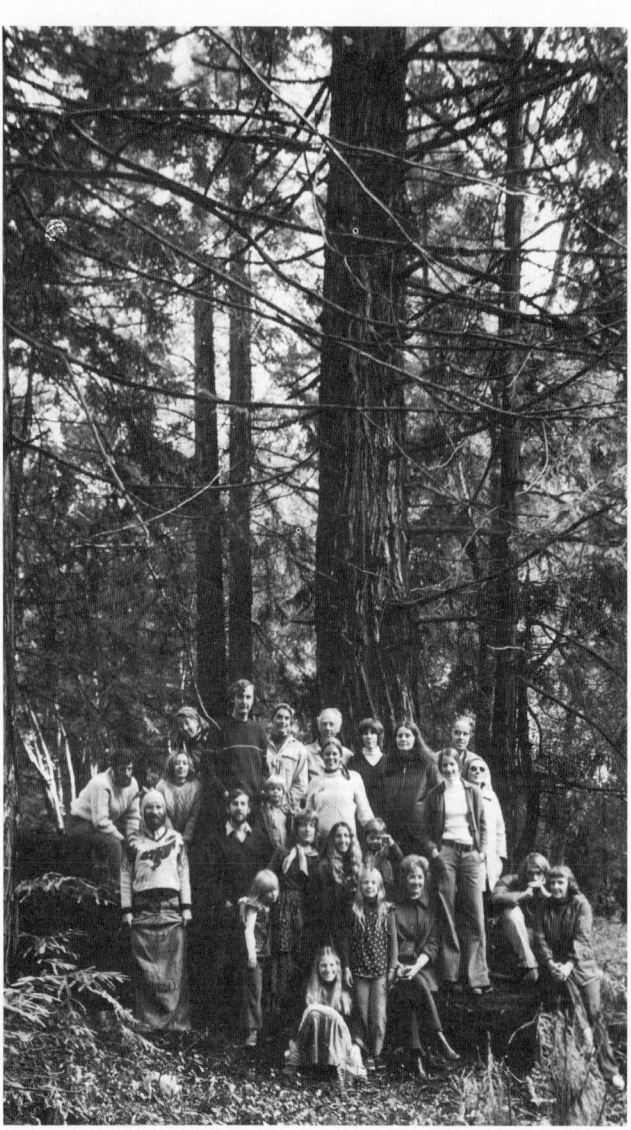

■ CHAPTER CONTENTS

THE CONTEMPORARY FAMILY
   Structural Configurations
   Other Emerging Family Structures

FAMILY PROCESSES
   Functions
   Roles

THEORETICAL APPROACHES TO UNDERSTANDING THE FAMILY
   Developmental Approach
   Other Approaches to the Family

FACTORS AFFECTING FAMILY STRUCTURES AND PROCESSES
   Socioeconomic Factors and Life-Style
   Societal Trends
   Ethnic and Cultural Influences
   Environmental Factors

NURSING IMPLICATIONS
   The Family as Client
   Family Assessment
   Nursing Diagnosis and Planning
   Intervention
   Evaluation
   Application of the Nursing Process: A Case Example

■ OBJECTIVES

- Discuss the application of family theory as it relates to the interaction and communication between the nurse and various family members.

- Explain the best measures that a nurse can use in determining the degree of family wellness.

- Identify the main features of a family.

- Contrast the family's developmental stages with the psychosocial stages of family members.

Family health, long the domain of public health professionals, is becoming a primary concern of all health care professionals. This emphasis on family-centered health care is a result of many factors. As people become better educated, they desire not only increased knowledge about themselves, but also more information about the purpose and consequences of health care services for themselves and their families. Changing value systems and the high cost of health care have generated considerable consumer demand for alternative services and personnel. Growing awareness of the interdependence of stress and illness as well as physical fitness and health has contributed to the increasing interest in individual and family self-care.

Family-centered care is also widely endorsed by health care professionals, who recognize the family as the primary source of physical and emotional support for its members as well as the primary influence on its children's development. Research on childbearing families has shown that family involvement during pregnancy and birth can enhance the delivery experience, attachment between parents and infants, and parenting skills.

Many hospitals have responded to these forces and have modified the hospital environment and procedures. For example, many hospitals provide alternative birth rooms besides the traditional labor and delivery rooms for those couples who wish to be in a homelike setting. Nurse-midwives are on the staff of many hospitals, providing an alternative to the physician-managed birth. Rooming-in programs as well as early discharge for mothers are common in many hospitals.

Recognition by health care professionals and consumers that effective health care of individuals requires the involvement of their support network has necessitated an expanded role for the nurse. Including the family in health teaching, explanations of medical and surgical interventions, and coordination of health care activities has become the responsibility of the nurse. In addition, the family can provide important information about the client that affects the nurse's plan of care. The ability to work with family members requires knowledge about family dynamics. This chapter examines the family unit, the role and function of each member, and the importance of the family in effective maternity nursing.

THE CONTEMPORARY FAMILY

What (or who) is the "typical" family? In the 1950s and the early 1960s that phrase evoked an image of a happily married couple with their two or three children. As portrayed in many television shows, this family was white and middle class. The man was the breadwinner, working to support the family. The woman was a housewife, taking care of the children and home. The children were well behaved and well adjusted. The teenagers danced and drank soda pop at parties. Divorce was infrequent because it was socially unacceptable. An aura of stability, contentment, and complacency surrounded this family.

The political and social upheaval of the late 1960s and 1970s drastically altered the image of the typical family, however. The civil rights demonstrations, the antiwar protests, and the women's liberation movement revealed that many people were not content but extremely dissatisfied and angry. Long-held values, traditions, and assumptions about social, racial, political, and gender matters became subjects for debate. Self-examination and personal development became important and accepted activities.

During this period of redefinition and change, our assumptions and beliefs about the family and the roles and tasks of its members also were held up for examination. Individual members' frustration with stereotyped gender roles or behavioral and social expectations resulted in family stress and conflict. Many families emerged intact, although changed, from this crisis. Other families suffered irreparable damage, resulting in divorce of the parents and/or estrangement of the children.

People have learned some valuable lessons from this chaotic time. Clearly, a great difference exists between the typical family as created from statistical information (or wishful thinking) and real families. Real families are dynamic and unique. Many families do indeed consist of two adults and two or three children. However, the couple may not necessarily be married or white or middle class. The woman may be the breadwinner, and the man may be a "house-husband." It is not unlikely that one or both adults have been or will be divorced. The children may be siblings by marriage (that is, stepsiblings), not by blood ties. Television and other media expose children to a broad range of

31

world events, technology, and life-styles that far exceeds that experienced by their counterparts 15 years ago. This has resulted in an accelerated childhood in some cases. If the children are teenagers, they probably have been exposed to and may have used one or more so-called recreational drugs.

Contemporary family life is not simple and easy. There is little room for complacency. What is typical about the typical family is that its members are faced with the difficult but usually gratifying task of coexisting with one another and their environment. To provide effective and holistic health care, nurses must understand that such coexistence is critical to an individual's well-being, and this requires knowledge about the variety of families that exist.

Two or more individuals who are emotionally involved and live in geographical proximity comprise a *family* (Friedman, 1981). This broad definition recognizes the existence of a variety of traditional and nontraditional contemporary family forms. *Familism* is "the interdependence of, and attachment to, family members" (Friedman, 1981).

Structural Configurations

Many trends and changes in attitudes have contributed to the increase in the kinds of family configurations. Longevity has increased. The average age of persons marrying has increased, with most marriages now occurring between persons in their early 20s.

Fewer children are being born in North America, particularly in the middle- and upper-class families. Concerns about population control and the economic costs of providing children with educational and social opportunities have made large families less feasible. The feminist movement has encouraged women to extend their interests and energies beyond the home and to consider other roles besides those of wife and mother. In fact, many couples delay childbearing or decide not to have children so that both partners can pursue their career goals without the burden of children. With the high number of divorces and remarriages (or other cohabitational arrangements), single parent and blended families are common.

According to Hymovich (1980) and Friedman (1981) most families belong to one of the following types of family configurations:

Single adult. According to Friedman's definition, the unmarried adult living alone is not considered to be a family configuration because the proximity, interaction, and support that are part of family life may not be present. The person living alone must perform functions typically ascribed to the family, however, such as finding suitable housing and income and organizing relationships with the extended family and community.

A variation of the single adult family configuration is the unmarried parent family, usually consisting of a mother

and child. For these parents, marriage either is not desired or is impossible. With society's increasingly liberal attitudes toward sexuality, the option of keeping a child rather than giving it up for adoption is being chosen by a greater number of unmarried women. In addition, an increasing number of single adults are adopting children. This family configuration is the same as that of the single-parent family, discussed later, with the important exception that the latter involves a disrupted family, in which one of the parents is no longer living in the immediate geographical area.

Nuclear dyad. Frequently referred to as the *beginning family,* the nuclear dyad consists of a husband and wife living in a single family residence (Figure 3–1). One or both partners have a career, and either there are no children or, in the case of an older couple, there are no children at home.

Single-parent families. One-parent family types are becoming far more prevalent as the rate of divorces and separations continues to rise. One adult is left alone (by separation, divorce, or death) to raise minor children in a separate household with no other adults. If no other source of family income exists or if the adult prefers, he or she may seek a career, adding even more responsibilities to family life. Many single parents eventually remarry, creating a need for additional role changes for both the former and newly formed family units.

Nuclear family. The most common configuration in our society is the nuclear family. It includes husband, wife, and all minor children living together in a single household. A dual career may or may not be a component of this family. In this chapter the nuclear family is generally the unit referred to, although many of the concepts discussed can be applied to other family types.

Three-generation family. In the three-generation structure, one or more dependent grandparents live in a single household with either a single-parent family or a nuclear family. The parents have authority over the household and care for the grandparents.

Kin network (or extended family). The extended family type includes two or more nuclear or unmarried households or any of the previously described configurations living in proximity, exchanging goods, and looking to each other for interaction and support. Although the adults have authority within their single household, the elder adults are consulted for advice, support, and authority in intrafamily affairs.

Other Emerging Family Structures

Family structures that break from the more traditional ones have emerged in recent years. Some authorities theorize that they are the outgrowth of disorganization within the traditional family units. The causes of this disorganization seem to be increased mobility, movement to cities, increased economic independence of women, and de-

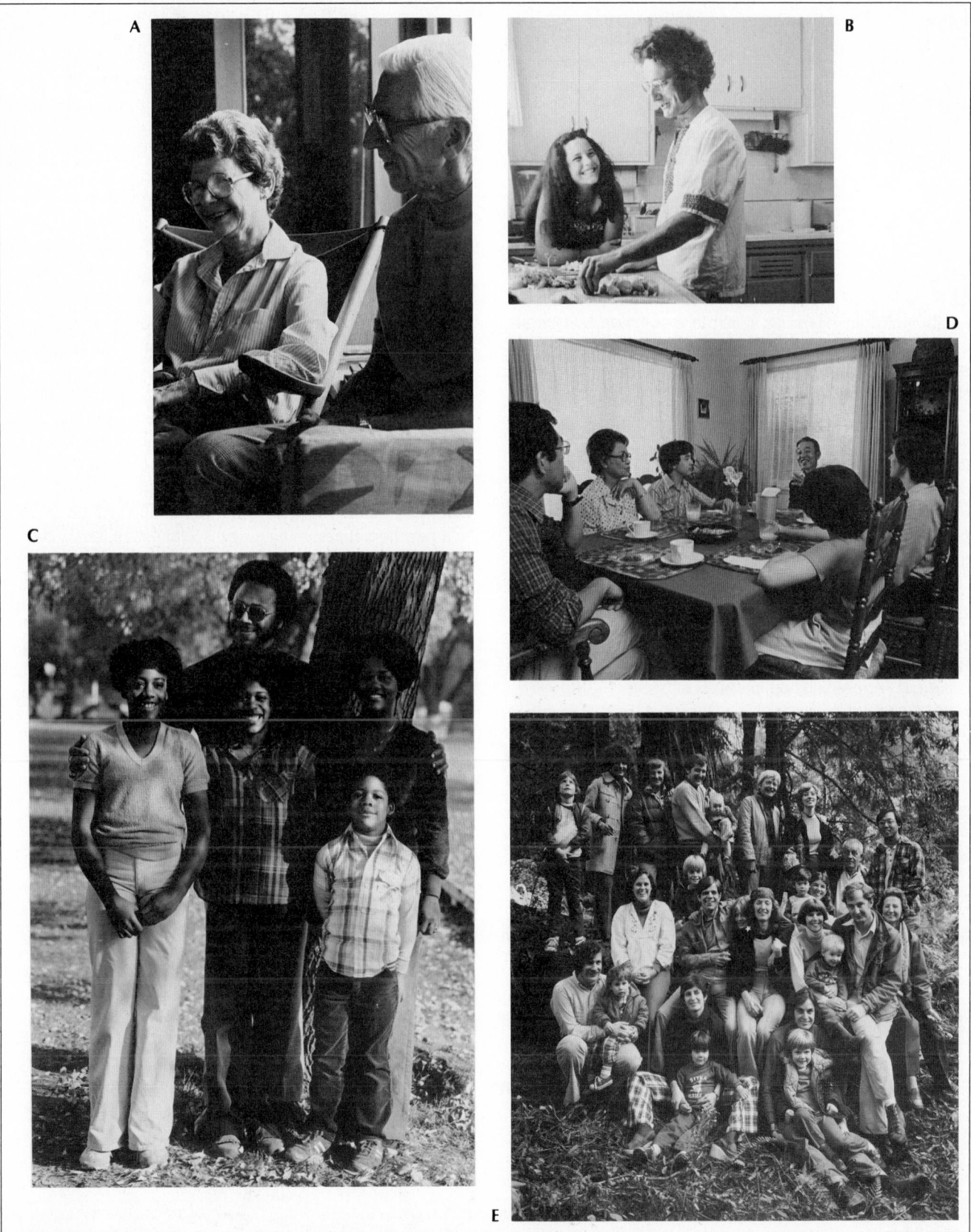

FIGURE 3–1 A, Nuclear dyad. **B,** Single-parent family. **C,** Nuclear family. **D,** Three-generation family. **E,** Kin network.

creased control of the kin network and the traditional family style (Mowrer, 1927). The resulting emerging family structures include the communal family, the common-law family, and the homosexual family (Hymovich and Barnard, 1973):

The communal family. Communal families vary in organization and philosophy. One type of communal family is made up of more than one married couple, with or without children, sharing a common household with its facilities and resources and participating in common experiences and childrearing responsibilities. Each family retains its legal identity within the larger community. This style is best typified by the kibbutzim in Israel. In another type, adults and their offspring, living in a common household, merge in a "group marriage" arrangement (Figure 3–1). All adults are considered parents to all children and share childrearing responsibilities.

Common-law family. The common-law marriage, in which a man and a woman live together sharing companionship and responsibilities without the legal commitment of marriage, is not a recent form of family structure. However, the number of couples choosing this arrangement is increasing. Children may be conceived by the couple or informally adopted.

Homosexual family. This type of family, in which two adults of the same sex choose to live together in a sexual relationship and share responsibilities, has received a great deal of publicity within recent years. Children from a previous marriage may live with the couple, or children may not be present.

The concept of family is changing. Many conceptual and structural differences are found among groups calling themselves families. A family has a discernible structure with many facets. Figure 3–2 is a conceptual diagram of a family and its field of influence. The center, or nucleus, is the small group that makes up the *nuclear family,* with one or more adults and possibly one or more children. The arrows between family members denote interaction—emotional and intellectual communication. This interaction is necessary for the maintenance of the family unit.

On the outside of the wheel are the concrete and abstract forces that exert power and influence over the family. Culture has the greatest impact, as it prescribes expected behaviors, including family traditions, childrearing practices, and methods of handling illness. Social changes that bring about changes within the family include moving to a new home, assuming a new social status, birth, death, and marriage. Interaction with the environment takes

FIGURE 3–2 Conceptual framework of a family unit. Arrows indicate interactional patterns and the influence of the family on its environment and the influences of the environment on the family.

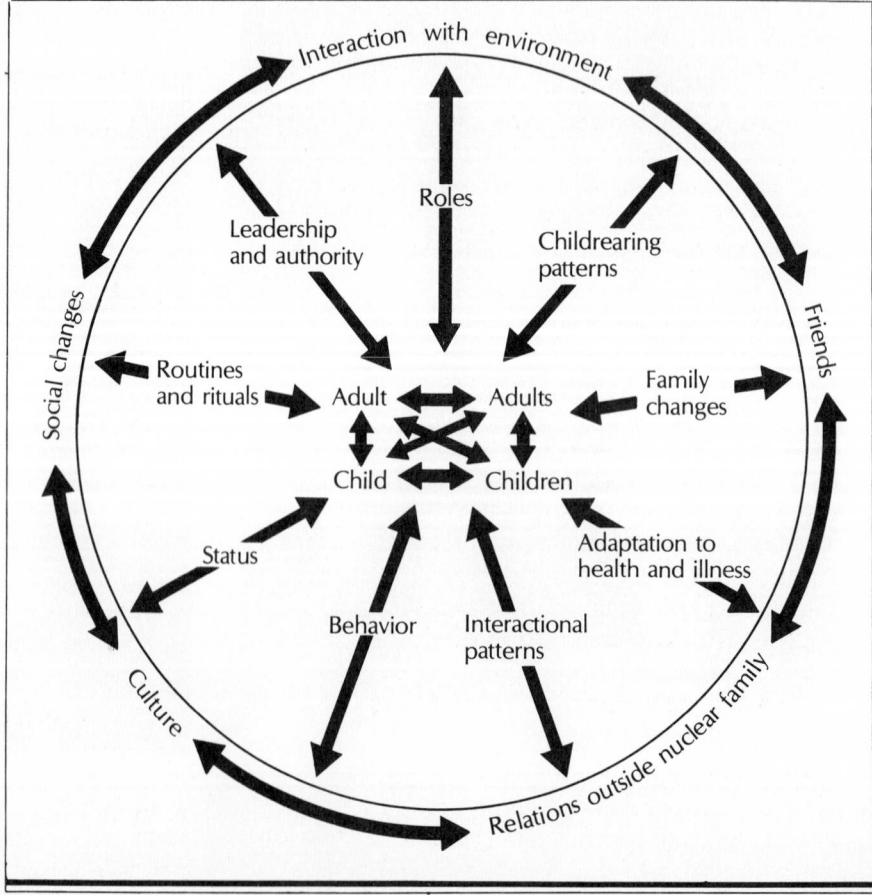

place as people change their surroundings to meet their needs. Friends and relatives outside the nuclear family also have direct and indirect influences on it. In many cases they are the ones who impart cultural and social standards to the family.

Between the nucleus and the outside of the wheel are spokes representing facets of the family that are influenced by culture, social change, environmental interaction, and friends and relatives. Roles, status, and behavior are specific to each family member, and a member's change in any one area can effect a like change in another member.

No matter what type of structure a family has, its primary objective generally is to support the emotional and physical health of its members through stability, comfort, reassurance, encouragement, and empathy and to provide warm and intimate relationships.

FAMILY PROCESSES

Functions

Because the family occupies a position between the individual and society, its purpose is twofold—to meet the needs of the individual and to meet the needs of the society. The specific primary functions of the family include the following (Friedman, 1981):

1. *Care and rearing of children.* Although childrearing functions have become less important in some families as a result of population control and individual desire not to have children, procreation remains a vital family function. Many young couples bear children and rear them in the traditions and with the values of their parent cultures.

2. *Socialization and social placement, including transmission of cultural values and/or rituals from one generation to another.* Primary socialization, which is frequently shared with outside institutions (such as school), is directed toward making family members productive members of society as well as conferring social status. As children are told about and participate in cultural activities, traditions are passed from generation to generation. Children learn much of their behavior, including the values of right and wrong, by imitating parents or significant others. The desired outcome is "an adult whose personality characteristics are compatible with the demands and expectations of the society of which he is a member" (Kenkel, 1977).

3. *Provision for physiologic needs.* The family meets members' basic physical needs by providing sufficient food, shelter, clothing, comfort, and health care. The family has the additional responsibilities of allocating its eco-nomic resources appropriately and promoting the safety of its members.

4. *Affective function (personality maintenance).* The family provides for the psychologic needs of the family members according to the requirements of the individual or the unit.

5. *Family coping.* The family is continually confronted with internal and external demands and expectations that it is supposed to fulfill. To ensure family survival, stability, and growth, the family must use effective problem-solving mechanisms to cope with environmental requirements.

Roles

A *role* is a cluster of interpersonal behaviors, attitudes, and activities that are associated with an individual in a certain situation or position. The behaviors tend to be learned through interactions with parents and siblings. *Attitudes* are expectations of the society in which the child is raised; they affect and can be modified by the individual's behaviors. Role activities are governed by expectations and behavior patterns of friends, relatives, and others outside the individual (Burgess, 1971). Role behaviors, attitudes, and activities are learned to a large extent through the process of socialization.

Each family must define its role in the community and the roles of its individual members within the family unit. These roles are learned through interaction and imitation.

Each member has a number of positions: the woman may be wife, mother, wage earner, housekeeper, and cook, with additional positions in the community; the man's roles may include husband, father, wage earner, gardener, and mechanic; each offspring is a child and perhaps a sister or brother, with responsibilities for some household or family tasks. These roles, determined partially by culture and partially by the family and the individual, prescribe what persons do, to whom they are obligated, and upon whom they have a rightful claim (Robischon and Scott, 1969). For each role in the family, there is a complementary role: husband–wife, parent–child, sister–brother. Each individual must learn about the role of his or her complement to understand and perform his or her own role properly. Adult relationships are determined by the roles the partners assume. Each child has to work out his or her own identity within the network of family relationships.

Children learn the roles of their parents while learning their own roles and form their self-concepts on the basis of how well they execute their own roles. The roles that children assume affect their psychosocial development into adulthood.

Earlier research on birth order tended to focus on the characteristics of children in different positions in the family, but it does not appear that any position is especially preferable. The primary value of examining the influence of birth order and the roles of children in the family is to enhance one's sensitivity to the subtle patterning of relationships within the family.

Roles are not static; they change from time to time as circumstances and events precipitate a change. Within the family a person may shift roles many times; for example, a woman becomes a wife with marriage and adds the role of mother when she has her first child.

Once the roles of family members are developed, family processes usually continue in a predictable pattern. If there are interruptions in the expected personal roles, family processes will also be interrupted. In most cases, one person will assume the other's role. For example, when the wage earner is disabled for a period, the spouse may need to find a job to replace the lost income and the children may have to add more household duties and responsibilities to their roles.

THEORETICAL APPROACHES TO UNDERSTANDING THE FAMILY

Developmental Approach

The study of family development involves tracing the family life cycle from its inception with the newly married couple, through its developmental stages, to the family's termination by the death of one or both spouses or by divorce if no children are involved. The developmental pattern is not rigid. For example, some families may decide not to have children, thus skipping those stages that involve childbearing and childrearing; in other families, adoption of older children may result in omission of particular steps in the developmental process.

The following is a summary of the principles governing family development (Duvall, 1971):

1. Development is orderly, sequential, and predictable. Life in the traditional family usually follows a regular pattern from marriage, to bearing children, to raising children, to having them establish their own homes, to eventual death. Crises may alter this pattern, but in most instances family development continues.

2. Developmental stage time periods vary within certain stages according to the individual family's needs. Family members determine the duration of developmental stages. Generally a family moves through the early stages in a few years, with each successive stage becoming longer.

3. Socially prescribed expectations order the major events of development. Although marriage is certainly not a biologic prerequisite for bearing and rearing children, it is expected in society that a couple will have a courtship period followed by a period of adjustment to marriage before bringing children into the world.

4. Family development proceeds in a specific direction from a known beginning to an expected end, with the anticipated endpoint of each developmental stage serving as family goals. Attainment of short-term and long-term family goals brings a sense of fulfillment and success to members.

5. When certain developmental tasks are successfully accomplished, further tasks evolve. For example, following the birth of a child, the couple prepares for the task of rearing the child.

6. Only the family can complete the developmental tasks it faces. The family relies on social interaction and internal resources and knowledge to direct the achievement of its goals.

DEVELOPMENTAL STAGES AND TASKS

Duvall (1977) has identified eight family tasks as being essential for the survival of the family unit, for continuity of family development, and for growth of the individual and his or her family. The specific manner in which the following goals are met is determined by each family according to the developmental stage at which it finds itself:

- *Physical maintenance.* Providing shelter, food, clothing, and health care and meeting other fundamental physiologic needs of the family.

- *Allocation of resources.* Ascertaining which family needs will be met and achieved financially and distributing material goods, space, authority, and affection.

- *Division of labor.* Determining who will procure needed income, manage the household, and care for the children.

- *Socialization of family members.* Guiding the internalization of acceptable, increasingly mature patterns of behavior and physical functioning.

- *Reproduction, recruitment, and release of family members.* Bearing of children, adoption of children, adding new members by marriage, and establishing policies for the inclusion and release of other family members or friends into the family circle.

- *Maintenance of order.* Devising and using effective means of communication and patterns of interaction and affection, expressing sexuality and aggression acceptably, determining and clearly defining right and wrong, and attaining a certain degree of conformity within the group.

- *Placement of members into the larger society.* Determining in which social institutions family members wish to participate (church, school activities, political and social groups), protecting the family from undesirable outside influences, and establishing policies for including in-laws, relatives, guests, and friends.

- *Maintenance of motivation and morale.* Satisfying needs of family members, providing rewards as positive feedback, giving encouragement when needed, dealing with crises, and inculcating a sense of family loyalty.

Duvall (1977) has also identified stages in the family life cycle in which these eight tasks are accomplished by a variety of methods. The two major phases in the family life cycle are the *expanding family,* from the beginning of the marriage until the children leave home, and the *contracting family,* from the launching of the children to the death of one or both spouses. These two major stages are further divided into the following eight stages, which are based on plurality patterns, the age of the eldest child, school placement of the eldest child, and the function and status of the family before children are born and after they leave home:

1. Married couples/beginning families (without children)
2. Childbearing families (eldest child 30 months)
3. Families with preschool children (eldest child 2½–6 years)
4. Families with schoolchildren (eldest child 6–13 years)
5. Families with teenagers (eldest child 13–20 years)
6. Families launching young adults (first child gone from home to the last child leaving home)
7. Middle-aged parent families ("empty nest" to retirement)
8. Aging family members (retirement to the death of both spouses)

The first two stages, married couples/beginning families and childbearing families, are discussed in the next sections.

□ *MARRIED COUPLES/BEGINNING FAMILIES* The first stage of Duvall's developmental family life cycle is the married couple/beginning expectant family stage, which starts when the couple enters marriage and ends with the birth or adoption of the first child. Prior to marriage each couple has started to work on the tasks involved in the first stage; however, the intimate relationship of marriage accentuates the importance of these tasks and their evolution. The transition from single to married life involves a variety of changes including new roles to learn, new situations to deal with, and new relationships with people. Success in this period depends on completion of developmental tasks as a single person and in large measure on past family experience.

The primary family tasks of the married couple/beginning family are establishing a mutually satisfying marriage relationship, forming a new household, and deciding whether or not to become parents. For the remarried, an additional critical task is acceptance of the termination of

the previous marriage in order to establish a healthy conjugal relationship with a new mate.

Open, honest communication on both intellectual and emotional levels provides a basis for mutually satisfying marriage. When conflict results, the couple must find appropriate methods to deal with the situations before they interfere with the marriage relationship. Successful conflict resolution and decision making are more likely if both partners are able to be empathetic, to display reciprocal respect, to acknowledge individual differences, and to be mutually supportive.

A couple may experience difficulty in sexual adjustment because of inaccurate or incomplete information resulting in unrealistic expectations of each other. The degree of sexual experience, particularly the amount of factual knowledge the partners bring to the marriage, affects their adaptation to the relationship. Marriage partners who recognize each other's varying needs and expectations are able to cooperate to achieve a mutually fulfilling sexual relationship.

The formation of a new household occurs in conjunction with the couple's combining resources, altering roles, and assuming new family functions. These circumstances may be stressful unless the partners are willing to make mutually agreeable decisions about the home and the social responsibilities they will accept. With the selection of a home, the critical issues for the couple become financial planning, including budgeting, and the division of household and other duties.

Socially, the couple must establish patterns of communications with friends and others in the community. They may find that they have more in common with groups or other couples than with single people. Demands of work or other concerns may arise. Whatever the pressures, each couple needs to agree on ways to cope.

The couple's families of origin continue to be important, but relationships with them change. No longer is each partner a member of one family; each now has relationships with three families—the family of origin of each partner and the couple's own developing family. The young couple may maintain close ties with their original families, choose to keep distant from their families for fear of interference, or establish a satisfying degree of involvement with both families.

Heterosexual couples face the decision about bearing children. Family planning and the use of contraceptives have received widespread acceptance in our society. Many couples are choosing not to have children; many more are limiting the size of their families because of economic concerns or the desires of the woman to pursue a career or other interests. A small proportion of couples are unable to conceive a child despite their desire to have one and may seek medical help for a solution to their reproduction problem.

Another task involves working out a philosophy of life

as a couple. Optimally, each individual enters marriage with a philosophy of life, which must be correlated with that of the partner. They may disagree on particular issues, but they must be able to live with or accept these differences with compromises. The philosophy they develop will identify them and reflect their attitudes and priorities. In addition, it will provide a framework for later decision making.

The early stage of the married couple phase is a precarious period; the marriage is vulnerable to many stresses that could destroy it. The tasks just described may not be completed within the first few years of marriage or indeed may never be completed. However, the greater the success in meeting the demands of these tasks, the more likely the marriage is to be mutually satisfying to both partners.

In the latter part of the first stage in the family life cycle, a couple's expectations of having their own child may be fulfilled. This marks the *beginning family phase.* Although this phase may cover the shortest time span in the cycle, this period is filled with many intense and diverse feelings. When the couple is told that conception has occurred, they may either accept or reject the pregnancy. Some pregnancies are unplanned, although either partner may subconsciously desire it. Others are planned and may even have been anticipated for months or years before conception actually takes place.

After their initial reactions to the fact that the wife is pregnant, the couple must accomplish certain tasks that are an offshoot of those from the earlier part of the married couple phase. For example, arrangements must be made for the physical care of the baby. These arrangements may mean drastic changes for the family if they have to move into larger quarters or to a place where children are accepted.

In the beginning family period, the couple must make adjustments in patterns of earning and spending. Generally, the man is in the early phase of his career, when his salary may be low. The woman's salary, which may be a necessary part of the family income, may come to an end during the pregnancy. Many women who have worked during the early part of their marriage stop work during pregnancy or when the baby is born—a time when there is greater monetary outlay for shelter, food, clothing, and other supplies for the baby. Even if the mother chooses to return to work after the baby is born, child care is a costly item in the budget. Health care during the pregnancy and birth also requires large amounts of money, especially with rising medical costs.

Work loads and designation of authority in the household also change out of necessity during pregnancy. The husband may assume more of the heavy household chores, as it is difficult for his pregnant wife to bend and move about. At the same time, pregnant women do not find that their physical state prohibits them from pursuing many of the activities they enjoy, such as working, entertaining, or even participating in sports.

Sexual activities are another aspect of marital interaction that must be altered to accommodate both physical and emotional changes of pregnancy. The pregnancy may have positive, negative, or no effects on the couple's sexual relationship. Husbands are as likely to feel changes in their sexual responses as their wives are. Because of changes in breast and abdominal size, the couple will need to reorient their normal sexual activities.

As soon as the couple knows they are expecting a child, a new focus of interaction becomes evident, enlarging their need for and use of communication. The couple is about to enter Erikson's developmental stage of generativity versus stagnation (p. 41), and with this stage come the motivations that help them work together to prepare for their child. Most couples feel a sense of fulfillment as they feel pride in their ability to conceive a child, as the wife starts to show signs of pregnancy, and as they make plans for the child's arrival. Husband and wife undergo changes in self-concepts in terms of masculinity, femininity, and parenthood. All of these tasks are accomplished with greater ease if the husband and wife develop communication patterns that help them cope with new responsibilities.

Communication with relatives also takes on a new perspective. Close relatives may have a prominent role in helping the young couple with their baby after birth; they can give physical and emotional support to the wife as she undertakes the new tasks of child care. On the other hand, family members can interfere with the couple's adjustment to pregnancy and childbirth with the telling of "old wives' tales" and possibly frightening myths. Reorienting relatives to the kind of relationship that is most desirable for new parents and their child is a major task of the beginning expectant family.

Reorientation must also occur in relationships with friends and in community activities. Recreational and social activities can continue to be a major part of the couple's life and may be curtailed only to the extent that the pregnancy decreases the woman's ability to participate. The mother-to-be may be more sensitive to her husband's activities because his mobility is not affected. She may believe that he is seeking outside interests as she becomes more introspective about the birth of the child. The man may feel left out of many of his wife's activities as she has frequent visits to the physician and attends groups to discuss the care and rearing of children. If they plan joint activities that help them remain with each other while continuing to respect each other's needs for autonomy, the couple can make a comfortable transition to the complementary relationship that will be needed in future years.

The expectant couple needs to acquire a great deal of knowledge about pregnancy, labor and delivery, and child care. Their background knowledge may be based more on hearsay than on fact. They may have had little or no experience with infants and small children. Pregnancy is a period when an expectant couple is open to and anxious for knowledge. The more highly educated the couple, the more likely that they desire in-depth knowledge about this event.

The final task of the expectant couple—maintenance of morale—can be accomplished if each partner meets the other's needs for acceptance, support, and affection. They must deal with questions of whether they are prepared to bring a child into their lives, of how the baby will fit into their pattern of living, and of how they will alter their lifestyle for their child. As mentioned earlier, both partners feel emotions that are new to them and seek understanding from their partners. The more one partner is able to meet the other's emotional needs, the more love each will be able to give to their child.

□ *CHILDBEARING FAMILY* The arrival of the first child marks a time of both great joy and crisis for the young family. Again, the family faces a period of reorganization. During the childbearing family stage (from the birth of the first child until that child is 30 months old), the baby and family become stabilized in their schedules and relationships with each other. The parents feel great joy about the birth of their first child and share their joy with their family and friends; the new mother feels a sense of accomplishment and is ready to relax and let others care for her and her baby for a few days. At the same time, the young couple has a feeling of great responsibility for their child's growth and development.

The first task of the childbearing family is to arrange the home to meet the needs of the infant. The reality of the baby in the home setting necessitates tailoring the already-prepared accommodations to most easily meet the needs of the infant and parents. The primary responsibility of the parents is to provide a safe, comfortable environment for the child. A primary need of the newborn infant is a quiet, clean place to sleep. As children grow and become more mobile their immediate environment enlarges, even though they are still unable to protect themselves from many of its dangers. Eventually curiosity leads them to explore, and their parents have to "childproof" the home, setting limits within which the child can function safely.

Costs of raising a child are drastically increasing, creating additional problems for a couple already dealing with the increased costs of daily living. Even in the United States, where prosperity is relatively common, many families are below poverty level and children are raised with a minimum of economic expenditure.

The crisis of the first child's birth requires a reworking of responsibility and accountability patterns. A baby requires round-the-clock care, much of which is assumed by the mother, particularly if she is breast-feeding the child. The husband must assume more of the household tasks, such as shopping and running errands outside the home, during the mother's confinement with child care. Both partners share in seeking solutions to problems arising during the day. The child also has accountability to parents as he or she grows older. The approval or disapproval of parents teaches him or her what parents consider good and bad, and he or she recognizes good acts as pleasing ones. While young children are in Erikson's stage of autonomy versus shame and doubt (see p. 40), they develop a sense of accountability to themselves as they learn to control bodily functions.

Reestablishing a satisfying sexual relationship with one's partner is another task of the childbearing family stage. Sexual activity usually decreases or ceases during the postnatal period. The new mother becomes absorbed in her child, and her close physical relationship with the baby may decrease her sexual needs. Her husband may feel rejected as the new mother focuses on the baby's needs instead of those of her husband. A great deal of mutual patience and understanding is necessary as the couple strives to reunite to meet each other's needs.

Two stresses occur in the childbearing family period that can hinder or further the development of effective communication. The first stress comes from the type of communication that a newborn must use to express his or her needs—crying. Until the new parents can interpret what the various types of cries mean and until they learn to anticipate their infant's needs, the crying can be extremely disconcerting. When the parents believe they have met the needs of their child and the crying continues for no apparent reason, their frustration increases. However, as the parents attempt to meet the baby's needs lovingly, the baby's trust in them increases, and other methods of communication emerge, such as smiling, cooing, and eventually talking. The other strain on effective communication is decreased sharing between the parents. Their tasks may be more separately defined as the husband works outside the home while his wife remains busy caring for their new baby and the house. They participate in different activities and have less time to be alone together. Instead of the one relationship of husband–wife, three relationships have developed to include the infant in the family circle. However, even though the parents may have distinct tasks, they can share more as they watch their baby grow.

Dealing with relationships with relatives is also a facet of the development of the family with a very young child. The new parents will receive a great deal of advice on how to care for the child. If they are mature and have successfully completed their previous developmental tasks, they are able to sift through this information and use what is most meaningful to them. The greater the difference between the two parental families, the greater the likelihood of conflicting advice, because each set of grandparents will want the child to be raised according to the traditions of their family. And, of course, the parental families can also supply a great deal of support and comfort to the new parents who are endeavoring to establish their own traditions.

The young family must participate in community activities to establish relationships outside the home. They are more involved in their home life than they were prior to their baby's birth and must find suitable babysitting arrangements if they desire to go out together. Their interests may change as they seek out congenial couples with young children who can share similar experiences.

A further task of the childbearing family is to decide whether or when to have more children and to take appropriate measures. Having children in quick succession may prove to be a tremendous strain for both parents although some couples may choose to have their children close together to allow the mother to resume her career as soon as possible. If the first child is defective or dies shortly after birth, the decision about whether or when to have another child becomes paramount.

Maintenance of motivation and morale of the childbearing family may become difficult. The repetitious tasks of everyday child care may overshadow the basic satisfactions of parenthood. Values placed on material objects may need to be changed, becoming dependent on what is good for the young child. The parents need to continue their independence as a couple while recognizing the child's dependence on them. The developmental needs of the child and those of the parents may be in conflict, so priorities must be set. The young family may need to accept assistance from relatives and friends at a time when they are still striving to be a separate unit.

The early childbearing and childrearing years have a significant influence on the ultimate strength of the family unit. Many crises occur that can either divide or unite the family. A division or conflict may not be evident while the children are still dependent but may manifest itself after the children have left home and there is little else to hold the parents together. Yet these same stresses can unite the family more solidly if they are faced as mutual problems and if individual needs and priorities are taken into account in family interrelationships.

PSYCHOSOCIAL DEVELOPMENT OF FAMILY MEMBERS

The stages of the family life cycle are listed in Table 3–1 with the probable corresponding developmental stages of the individual members. Clearly development of the individual and the family are interdependent phenomena and one influences the well-being of the other. Erikson (1963) described the psychosocial development of an individual as occurring in eight stages. Successful resolution of each of these stages results in the emergence of a predominant positive quality, whereas unsuccessful handling of each stage produces negative qualities. These stages are as follows:

- *Basic trust versus basic mistrust (early infancy: birth to 1 year).* If infants' needs are met consistently and if there is constancy in their surroundings and their caretakers, they will develop a sense of certainty and predictability about their external and internal environments.

- *Autonomy versus shame and doubt (late infancy: 1–3 years).* As a result of muscular maturation, the child develops a sense of control over bodily functions and environment. The child begins to realize that he or she is a person apart from the parents. Overcontrol by others can result in a loss of self-esteem.

Table 3–1 Stages of Individual and Family Development

Erik Erikson's stages	Evelyn Duvall's stages
1. Adult: intimacy vs. isolation	Married couple/beginning family
2. Adult: generativity vs. stagnation Child: trust vs. mistrust autonomy vs. shame and doubt	Childbearing family phase
3. Adult: generativity vs. stagnation Child: initiative vs. guilt	Families with preschool children stage
4. Adult: generativity vs. stagnation Child: industry vs. inferiority	Families with schoolchildren stage
5. Adult: generativity vs. stagnation Child: identity vs. role confusion	Families with teenagers stage
6. Adult: generativity vs. stagnation Child: intimacy vs. isolation	Families launching young adults stage
7. Adult: generativity vs. stagnation Child: generativity vs. stagnation	Middle-aged parent families stage
8. Adult: integrity vs. despair Child: generativity vs. stagnation	Aging families stage

- *Initiative versus guilt (early childhood: 4–5 years).* During this stage, the quality of purpose emerges. The child undertakes or plans to achieve activities that seem desirable. Depending on external influences or parental sanctions, the child may feel guilt about the goals or acts he or she contemplates.

- *Industry versus inferiority (middle childhood: 6–11 years).* The child develops skills and learns to use tools to a productive end. Feelings of inadequacy may arise in children about their abilities or about what they produce.

- *Identity versus role confusion (puberty and adolescence: 12–20 years).* The major developmental task at this stage is to integrate how one sees oneself with how one is perceived by others. Adolescents' attempts to determine their place in the world may lead to overidentification with groups, ideologies, or individuals.

- *Intimacy versus isolation (early adulthood: 20–30 years).* The young adult manifests a readiness to commit himself or herself to others and to situations. The individual who is afraid of ego loss avoids such experiences, leading to separation and isolation.

- *Generativity versus stagnation (early and middle adulthood: 30–64 years).* Primary motivations during this period of life are productivity and creativity. For many persons, this involves reproduction and readying the next generation for its life.

- *Ego integrity versus despair (late adulthood: 65 years and older).* One accepts how one has lived one's life, how one will continue to live it, and the fact that it will end in this stage.

Just as Erikson's stages serve as guidelines for evaluating the development of the individual, those for the family serve as guidelines for analyzing the nuclear family. During each stage, certain key needs of the family must be met. The differences among these needs are a result of the varying developmental stages of the individuals within the family. As Duvall (1977) points out, the success of the family and the developmental stages of the individuals within it depends on close, nurturing interrelationships among all members of the family.

The developmental approach is useful to nurses dealing with expectant and childbearing families. Nurses can better identify the goals of the maternity client and her family, anticipate family crises, and meet client and family needs after determining the developmental stage of the family and its members.

Other Approaches to the Family

Although the focus of this chapter is on the developmental approach to understanding families, brief recognition should be given to alternative methods of studying families. Chief among these is the systems approach. Use of the systems theory to study individuals and groups such as families, health care professionals, and communities is increasing. The focus is on the interaction among interdependent parts of the identified system. Sedgwick (1981) has identified characteristics of the family as a system and described the mutual interaction and interdependence of the family members as they function within the family and with other systems.

Three other methods in common use are the structural-functional approach, the interactional approach, and the institutional-historical approach. References describing these theories are included at the end of the chapter.

FACTORS AFFECTING FAMILY STRUCTURES AND PROCESSES

The family, regardless of its structure, does not function in isolation. The well-being of a family can be promoted or hindered by the acts or policies of other persons or institutions. Inherent characteristics such as race or a less common family configuration may have implications for the family in terms of social status, income level, and community acceptance.

Religion often has a strong influence on the values, beliefs, and moral concepts of the family. Many religions also dictate behavioral codes, rituals, and traditions of family life.

The implications of these and other factors differ for each family. In addition, members within each family can be affected to varying degrees. For the purposes of this chapter, socioeconomic, cultural, and environmental factors are explored in more depth.

Socioeconomic Factors and Life-Style

Although the class system among whites and blacks is similar, there are some basic differences in orientations, values, and beliefs. In general, values in the middle class focus on self-direction, whereas those in the working class emphasize conformity.

The following analysis of the class system focuses on general characteristics; note that within these broad categories there are many persons whose life-styles or beliefs do not necessarily correspond to those typically ascribed to their socioeconomic level.

In the white upper class, family groupings are usually made up of extended patriarchal families. Men carry high prestige, and sons are highly desired to carry on the family name. Women have lower prestige and usually no career, but they are highly refined and maintain an influential life-style through household management and entertaining.

The white upper middle class is populated with professionals who are achievement- and college-oriented. Families think in long-term goals. Because of the high degree of mobility in this group, the nuclear family predominates. However, there is strong extended family support despite the distance separating the nuclear family from the family of origin. The wife may work, but the husband is still considered head of the household. Children are raised to value self-discipline, to take responsibility, and to show initiative; aggression is permitted only as needed for self-defense.

White-collar, skilled, and semiskilled workers make up the white middle class. Most middle-class adults achieve a high school education but desire more for their children. They live in nuclear families, but mobility is less than in the upper middle class, and close relatives frequently live in the same community. Women often work to supplement their husband's income, but few have actual careers. The husband continues to be the head of the household, but the wife keeps the budget and maintains finances.

The white lower class is also divided into two segments. The upper lower class comprises semiskilled and skilled laborers, many of whom are foreign born and some of whom have high school educations. This group is characterized by nuclear families with strong kinship ties, and women fulfill the traditional tasks of homemaking and child care. Success for the upper lower class is thought of in terms of material goods and possessions; job security is of greater priority than upward mobility—an attitude that leads to job stagnation and dissatisfaction. Children are expected to work and supplement the family income after high school; a college education is considered of little value.

Impoverishment, poor housing with inadequate health and safety facilities, poor education, and unskilled, sometimes seasonal jobs mark the lives of the poverty-level white family. Life takes on an aura of hopelessness and despair, leading to distrust of the social system. Families are larger, with more children being born out of wedlock than in the other classes. There is no motivation to marry, and fatherless children are readily accepted into the mother's family. Although the number of one-parent families in this class is large, a high proportion of two-parent families is still prevalent. Extended families supply emotional support but are unable to give economic aid.

As is true for most groups, variations in the black American family exist and are influenced by economics and education. Among black people, the upper class consists of professionals, many of whom become wealthy with the help of the wife's income. Many blacks enter this class from the middle and lower classes through fame in athletics, entertainment, or other highly paid endeavors. Black upper-class families live in nuclear households and have close relations with their extended families, but these relationships are not as close as in the white upper class.

Middle-class black American families are characterized by a sense of teamwork, with both husband and wife as wage earners. The family size may be smaller for economic purposes (Spradley and McCurdy, 1980). They work in the same occupations as the white middle class and are widely involved in community affairs.

The working-class black family requires cooperation of all its members. This family tends to be larger, and education may be limited to high school. Although the extended family is valued and often live near, work schedules may be so demanding that there may be little time for social and family affairs.

The lower-income black family may have a fatalistic approach to life. Mutual help by all family members is necessary. Family living arrangements may vary for expedience. For example, a younger child may be sent to a childless relative to be reared. Frequent moves, unemployment, and distrust may characterize these families. Fathers may be only marginally involved in the family in some instances, since lack of trust also deters the development of a positive female–male relationship (Martin and Martin, 1978). The black lower class is similar to the white lower class except that it is highly matriarchal.

Societal Trends

CHANGING STATUS OF WOMEN

The traditional role for a woman in our society gave her dominance in the home. This role had value for the family but did not have prestige. The lack of prestige made it a safe role for women, one in which their husbands would not intervene. Thus the home became the stronghold for women. However, division of labor within the home changed greatly as women found that they were able to fulfill other roles without being subjected to culturally defined boundaries.

Similarly, the husband has traditionally been considered the head of the household, and the status and lifestyle of those within the home have depended to a large extent on him. But now more women are becoming part of the work force to supplement family income, to satisfy chosen career goals, or to work voluntarily in charitable organizations. As women move out into the working world and find fulfillment, they are gaining more status for themselves within their family and the community, in addition to supplementing the income so that their family can enjoy a higher standard of living. Their increase in status has confirmed the importance of women in the household and is increasing their privileges and responsibilities, especially for women in the middle and upper classes.

VALUE OF CHILDREN

The value of children varies greatly, depending on the meaning each society attaches to children. In addition, the reaction of individual family members to a child is personalized and subjective. Historically, the motivations for having children have been religious, political, and cultural. Some individuals want children for their own gratification—to have someone to guide and control, to reap economic gains, to improve one's status, to ensure one is cared for in old age, to satisfy cultural requirements, or to provide a means of personal immortality (Berelson, 1976).

In industrial societies the degree to which children are wanted seems to depend somewhat on the state of the economy. For example, during the economic recession of the 1970s, the birth rate in the United States dropped and continued to decline until zero population growth was reached in 1976. This trend can be contrasted to the post-World War II "baby boom," which occurred in a thriving economy.

Many historical changes have influenced the importance of children in society. In agrarian societies, children are valued for the economic gain they bring to their family and society. Industrialization and urbanization in North America have reduced the economic necessity of having children. As a result, children have become less "valuable" and more valued.

Among the events that have stimulated many persons to reevaluate their childbearing function are (a) lower death rates, which threaten to drastically accelerate population growth; (b) the "sexual revolution," which has resulted in the separation of sexuality from reproduction and has liberalized sex roles; and (c) the women's liberation movement, which promoted the realization that childbearing and childrearing are not necessarily the only roles for women.

The decision for many couples today is not *when* to have a child but *whether* to have a child. They are thoughtful about the consequences of childbearing—the effects that the presence of children will have on their relationship or career goals and the cost of children in terms of money and time—and about their ability to raise a well-adjusted, well-provided-for child.

Ethnic and Cultural Influences

Culture has been viewed as "a blue-print for man's way of living, behaving, and feeling" (Friedman, 1981, p. 271). Culture and family must be viewed simultaneously for, regardless of the family type, it remains the basic unit of society and influences human development over the life span.

Extended and three-generation families are preferred in many cultures. The older adults in these families often have significant roles in health and child care, household maintenance, and decision making. Multiple caretakers are available to help with childrearing and discipline.

Socialization is an early family function. Socialization includes all the learning experiences of early life. For the health professional, the acquisition of beliefs and ideas about health and illness, maintenance, prevention, and cure are of particular significance. Home remedies and folk care practices for prevention of illness, maintenance of health, and curative purposes remain primary sources for most families, regardless of ethnic and cultural backgrounds. It is only after these remedies are ineffective that alternatives are sought.

Communication patterns are influenced by a family's culture. To be effective, the nurse must be aware of these cultural patterns, such as appropriate situations for communication, tempo of conversation, taboo topics, display of emotion, use of eye contact, and physical proximity (Brownlee, 1978).

Religious beliefs and practices are part of cultural and familial heritage and influence health care behaviors. For example, the Jewish religion emphasizes wellness and health and permits dietary restrictions and proscribed activities on the Sabbath to be altered if one's health requires such changes.

Family roles, size, structure, and values change over time. Moving to an alien environment can speed changes by forcing the family to stretch its coping resources and cultural beliefs. For example, the Vietnamese family who left a tropical climate to settle in Colorado must adjust to extreme environmental differences. This move may have necessitated an occupational change for the parents and a decrease in economic and social status. Children may assume a role of greater importance as they act as translators for their parents who may not have mastered the new language as quickly as the child attending school. As the child becomes acculturated, the parents may be faced with dissension when they try to maintain the valued ways of their ancestors. Implications for the physical and mental well-being of family members are clearly evident under such conditions.

The American Indian has a similar situation. Moving between the greater environment and the tribal culture poses problems. The American Indians' values of cooperation and group support are immediately at odds with the greater society's emphasis upon independence and competitiveness.

Such factors affect the family regardless of cultural practices. Therefore, emphasis must be placed upon an in-depth assessment of the individual to help the professional avoid the problems of stereotyping and generalization.

North America contains a rich variety of ethnic and cultural groups, with certain areas containing greater numbers of certain groups. This text focuses on Mexican American, Native American (American Indian), black, and Oriental cultures in the United States (Table 3–2).

The Hispanic (Spanish-speaking) population is the most rapidly growing minority in the United States, and 60.6% of Spanish people in the United States are of Mexican background.

Black Americans comprise 11.7% of the population in

Table 3-2   Population in the United States by Race by Percent Distribution*

Group	1980	1970
White	83.2%	87.5%
Black	11.7	11.1
American Indian, Eskimo, Aleut	0.6	0.4
Asian and Pacific Islanders	1.5	0.8
Other (includes Cambodian, Laotian, and Thai)	3.0	0.3

*Adapted from resident population by race and Spanish origin, in *Population Characteristics, Series P-20.* June 1981. Washington, D.C.: Bureau of Census, U.S. Government Printing Office.

the United States. Even though acculturation has been great, the beliefs and attitudes of this group have been influenced over the centuries by slavery, racism, and a rich cultural heritage.

The American Indian makes up 0.6% of the population. Over 200 different tribes exist, each with its own language and culture. Therefore, where possible, specific tribal affiliations are noted, although some attitudes and values are common across tribes.

The term *Oriental* is used for a number of cultural groups. Although differences exist among the various Oriental cultures, the influence of the Chinese upon neighboring lands over hundreds of years has produced similar behaviors and beliefs within several groups. Whenever possible the specific Oriental group will be noted. In recent years, immigration by some groups (Koreans, Laotians, Vietnamese, and Cambodians) has added to the Oriental population. Other cultural and ethnic groups are also important to recognize, but space does not allow discussion of all of them. However, it is the responsibility of the nurse professional to develop cultural awareness and to seek information about other cultures whenever this knowledge is necessary to provide high-quality care.

MEXICAN AMERICAN FAMILY

The Mexican American family is a strong social unit characterized by familism. Family needs supersede individual needs, and a sense of obligation pervades in the family. This provides a sense of belonging as well as support and resources to all members. The Mexican American is people- and present-oriented rather than goal- and future-oriented. Responding to conflicts and dilemmas of others may take precedence over other responsibilities such as appointments or a particular task.

Religion affects the orientation to the present, since it is believed that God (rather than self) controls all events. The beliefs and rituals of the Roman Catholic church play a major role in family life (Henderson and Primeaux, 1981).

The traditional Mexican American family is large. Parents cherish and indulge their young children. Children learn that family is the most important unit in life, and respect and obedience to elders are expected (Branch and Paxton, 1976). The kinship network extends to grandparents, cousins, and in-laws, and includes the "compadre" system. Jackson (Branch and Paxton, 1976) defines compadre as co-parent or one who will assume the parenting role if necessary. The compadre may be formally announced, for example through the ritual of baptism, or agreed on informally.

Family roles are clearly defined. The man heads the household and is the authority figure and decision-maker. The ideal machismo requires that the Mexican American man appear strong, reliable, aggressive, and intelligent, especially outside of the family. It may also allow for extramarital sexual relationships by the male (Friedman, 1981; Henderson and Primeaux, 1981). The father is expected to provide for his family and is proud to do so.

The woman has specific caretaking roles. She is to be loving and self-sacrificing to her husband and children. Her husband's decisions are to be accepted. The Mexican American woman may have limited knowledge about her body and human sexuality. Modesty is valued, and sexual behavior may be circumscribed by prohibitions and inhibitions. It has been noted that the Mexican American woman may be ambivalent about her role (Friedman, 1981). Since family structure is a dynamic entity, one might anticipate changes as the feminist movement continues and acculturation occurs, especially in the single-parent urban family.

Family elders are accorded respect and have authority over younger members. Grandparents provide wisdom, support, and warmth. The advice of elderly women may be sought for illnesses prior to seeking other forms of health care. Older children frequently help care for younger siblings. Children, especially girls, may also be expected to help with household chores. Boys may help by providing additional income. Communication follows the line of authority. Older adults and males are approached with respect, and their authority is unquestioned. Children communicate more readily with their mothers since fathers are more distant and demanding (Friedman, 1981).

The Mexican American family faces discrimination and biases. Poverty, lack of English fluency, and minimal education can compound problems for these families.

AMERICAN INDIAN FAMILY

"To be really poor in the Indian world is to be without relatives" (Backup, 1979, p. 82). Traditionally, for most American Indian tribes the extended family is of utmost importance. Tribal members may also be considered family (Henderson and Primeaux, 1981). Children and grandparents are the most important groups in the family. Tradition teaches that they are safe within the universe and are watched by the Great Spirit (Backup, 1979).

Children are considered assets to the family. The elderly, who are respected and loved, share their wisdom and knowledge through story telling and direct counsel. Grandparents also assume significant roles in child care and rearing (Henderson and Primeaux, 1981).

The woman's role may vary. Many tribes are matrilineal (for example, Hopi and Navajo). Women may have much power and authority. The woman is held in high regard, for she is able to conceive and bear children (Higgins and Wayland, 1981). Generally, the woman is instrumental in maintaining the family, its traditions, and its cohesiveness.

The male role traditionally has been to provide goods and services for the family and the tribe or community. Unemployment, poverty, and reduced need for traditional skills have negatively affected the male role. This has led to decreased self-esteem, conflicts, and inability of the Native American male to provide role models for offspring.

The American Indian respects and values the freedom and independence of the individual. This has impact upon behaviors such as communication, interpersonal relationships, and childrearing (Farris, 1976; Backup, 1979). The American Indian traditionally depends on a communal approach to meeting basic needs such as food, shelter, and survival. Generosity, sharing, and giving are highly valued. Competition, confrontation, and challenging or questioning others are contrary to American Indian beliefs and are considered bad manners.

Harmony extends beyond relationships with people to all aspects of nature and the universe. The American Indian's religious beliefs and practices incorporate the value of self in harmony with the universe.

American Indians who live outside the tribal community may find their attitudes and values to be in conflict with those of the predominant culture. Adaptation may lead to acculturation and a loss of traditional customs. Some may attempt to follow tribal customs despite the cultural conflicts that may arise. Others may seek to maintain their "Indianness" and join forces with other Indians, regardless of tribal heritage.

BLACK AMERICAN FAMILY

The black American family has been described and labeled in several ways. It has been called a matriarchy, a "pathologic disorganized structure," and an adaptive, strong unit that maintains the race. The extended black family is now recognized as the primary family unit, affected by its location and socioeconomic variations.

The extended black family is characterized by three elements. First, the extended family base is multigenerational and interdependent. It may extend over great geographic distances, especially as family members migrate to seek employment opportunities. Second, it includes subextended families, which may appear as single-parent or nuclear families. The subextended family is attached by the dominant leadership base and by a sense of obligation to the extended family. The dominant leader is often an older family member. The position may be shared by husband and wife, or it may be held by an elderly woman who has outlived her husband. Such a position gives the aged members a sense of worth, fulfillment, and family respect, as well as additional responsibility. The third element is the mutual support system, whose function oversees economic and emotional security, group direction and identity, and overall welfare and survival (Martin and Martin, 1978).

The extended black family system functions more successfully in rural areas. It is present in urban areas but is threatened by certain characteristics and demands of urban living. For example, adequate and affordable living space that will accommodate the number of family members who may come to the dominant household in times of need is difficult to find. High rates of unemployment and the necessary government assistance interfere with the goals of the extended family. Childrearing may be more difficult without the support and education provided by members of the extended family, especially older relatives.

In rural areas, neighbors help "watch out" for children. This sense of community is often lost in urban settings. An urban environment encourages characteristics that seem to blend best with society's nuclear family orientation. These include individualism, materialism, and secularism (Martin and Martin, 1978). Occasionally black families in the city send their children to relatives in rural areas to avoid the hazards in the urban ghetto.

Since the single-parent family may actually be a subextended family, one must be careful not to assume a lack of a consistent male figure in the home. Strong support may be provided by an uncle, cousin, brother, or grandparent from the extended family. Informal adoption by members of the extended family is common. Aunts or grandmothers who assume childrearing roles may be called "Mamma," although children are clearly taught who their natural parents are. In the past, black families have been large because children are highly valued. Although out-of-wedlock pregnancy is not encouraged or welcomed, the child born out of wedlock is welcomed, cherished, and reared without prejudice.

Children are expected to show respect to their elders. Survival in, and adaptation to, the white world is taught; special help is necessary to learn to deal with the prejudice of the greater society. Because individual family member's problems become the extended family's problems, obedience is stressed. Religion in the black American community is often a source of help and support. Moral strength and social cohesion are offered through the church and its community.

ORIENTAL FAMILIES

The history of some Oriental groups in the United States spans several generations. The Japanese, for example, span as many as four generations. Each generation has a specific name (Issei, Nisei, Sansei, and Yansei) as well as special characteristics due to acculturation, varying experiences, education, and economic levels.

Many Oriental cultures value the extended family and familism. Worship of ancestors is part of this heritage, although an exception is the Cambodian family, which does not trace lineage through the paternal side (*Cambodia—the land and its people,* 1976). The marital union is a function of Oriental familism too. The wife enters her husband's household to serve her husband, his mother, and his family. Traditionally, the husband remains in or near his family's home to serve his father and family. The contemporary Oriental couple may not reside in the paternal family house, but close ties are maintained with frequent calls and visits. Grandparents and elderly relatives may live in the couple's home.

Family roles and functions are clearly defined. The senior household member serves as advisor and decision-maker. Filial piety and respect are expected. Grandparents function as disciplinarians and guides for their grandchildren's upbringing. Women may be wage earners. However, in the traditional family, women remain subservient to men, despite their career status.

Children are valued, and a male child is preferred as the first born to maintain family lineage. The dutiful child obeys parental laws. Children are expected to achieve success in some aspect of life, for to do so brings honor to the family (Ho, 1976).

Problems may arise for immigrants in an alien society. When the extended family is fragmented or lost, it becomes increasingly difficult to maintain role modeling across generations. Traditional roles and behaviors of family members become vulnerable; family distress may occur as old values and customs are challenged or rebuked in the new home. New ways may also cause shame and guilt for the member who strays from filial piety (Ho, 1976).

The Oriental values harmony in relationships (Chang, in Henderson and Primeaux, 1981). To achieve a state of harmony the individual may communicate in a restrained, reserved manner. Confrontation is avoided, and self-blame may be employed to avoid embarrassing another. Overt expressions of emotions may be inhibited by the traditional value of self-control in emotional situations. Failure to achieve harmony disgraces not only oneself but also the family, and family disgrace is avoided at all costs. The Japanese proverb, "Life is for one generation; a good name is forever," reflects this Oriental ideal. In general, gentleness, modesty, patience, reserve, and social sensitivity are emphasized (Fong, 1973, p. 120).

Environmental Factors

Environmental factors influencing the family are closely interrelated with cultural and socioeconomic factors discussed previously. The environment includes outside forces that may alter the behaviors and activities of the family member and family group. Forces such as relatives, friends, and significant others; home, neighborhood, and community settings; and social, religious, and governmental institutions within the community all have impact.

In childbearing families, environmental factors are most significant in terms of their effects on parents. Parents, based on their experience and background, interpret to their children the meaning of the interaction between environmental forces and the family. If their explanations are positive, they transmit to their children feelings of security, stability, and well-being. However, if the parents feel negative toward or threatened by their surroundings, they impart feelings of danger, hostility, and anger to their children. The nature of the family's interaction with its milieu is likely to have a direct effect on ability to meet members' needs, individually and collectively.

The physical setting in which the family resides has a pronounced effect on family functioning. Poor housing may adversely influence family and member attitudes, behaviors, motivational levels, and self-esteem, which in turn increases stress and the risk of illness and accidents. The physical design of a home may interfere with privacy and result in unfavorable childrearing and housekeeping practices. Chaotic, disorganized homes may produce children with developmental delays or deviancies, which may or may not be permanent. If family functioning continues to be impaired as the child's environment expands to settings outside the home, problems may become evident in the child's ability to communicate, solve problems, and form relationships.

Within the neighborhood and community, healthy families tend to associate freely with community groups and institutions to identify resources and receive services as needed by them. The ability of the healthy family to seek help through contact with others appears related in part to the family's perception of itself as a part of a whole and to their successful dealings with the larger community in meeting physical, psychologic, and social (biopsychosocial) requirements. The less healthy family, on the other hand, accepts assistance passively or relies on others to initiate the helping process.

NURSING IMPLICATIONS

A major goal of family-centered maternity care is to help each member of expectant families achieve optimal health by preventive, maintenance, and restorative measures. Nurses have the additional role of assisting families to accomplish appropriate developmental tasks at each family stage.

The success of the family depends on the achievement of these tasks. At times the family may find that success comes easily; at other times, they must overcome delay or failure. Since failure tends to follow failure just as success follows success, the nurse may need to intervene to break a family's cycle of failures in performing tasks and to guide them toward success.

When a member of the family becomes ill, that individual becomes dependent on others, thereby increasing stress and perhaps temporarily or permanently impeding the ability of the family to perform its tasks, depending on the severity and length of the illness. The nurse can help the other family members devise methods of taking on added responsibilities and of finding outside resources to support family functioning; by doing so the nurse may prevent further complications for the ill individual or the family.

When giving care to a client, the nurse should keep in mind the long-term, intimate relationships among family members. The person receiving care has performed a unique role within the family group that must be acknowledged if the family is to function optimally. Thus, families have the right to examine the kind of care and service a family member is receiving, to complain when the service is unsatisfactory, and to seek other sources of services when they are dissatisfied.

To ensure the provision of holistic, individualized care, the maternity nurse uses the nursing process as the framework for planning and implementing responsible health care.

The Family as Client

Because the individual develops as a member of a family unit, the nurse must acquire understanding of the family to understand the individual. This is especially important in the maternity setting because the nurse is directly responsible for the well-being of two members of the same family—mother and child.

The concept of the family as a client is one of the most important components of family-centered maternity nursing. Ideally the family gives each member love, trust, and response consistently so that he or she may mature into an individual who is able to give these qualities to others.

Friedman (1981) identifies the family unit as being the critical resource for the delivery and success of health care services for the following reasons:

1. In a family unit a dysfunction of one or more family members generally affects each individual as well as the family unit. If the nurse considers only the individual, the nursing assessment is fragmented rather than complete and holistic.

2. Assessing the family facilitates the nurse's understanding of the individual functioning within his or her primary social context. With the expectant and childbearing family, the nurse is able to assist the prospective parents to prepare for the new family member.

3. A strong interrelationship exists between the health status of a family as a unit and that of the individuals who constitute the family. The nurse, by emphasizing health promotion and maintenance in the family, should have a positive effect not only on the individuals in the family but on the family unit. Health education becomes a primary learning modality for families.

4. In considering the family as a whole, potential risk factors can be identified, thereby assisting the nurse's role in illness prevention.

5. When illness occurs, the family is instrumental in seeking medical assistance and in determining members' sick-role behaviors.

In family-centered maternity nursing, the nurse generally focuses on health promotion and maintenance and prevention of illness, primarily within the beginning or childbearing family. The nurse uses a *biopsychosocial* approach, recognizing the influence of the prenatal environment and the quality of parenting on the growth and development of the child. The nurse considers how variables such as cultural beliefs, community resources, and health beliefs affect the family's response to health care.

It is imperative that the nurse do the following:

• Reevaluate one's personal cultural beliefs and values.

• Recognize one's own biases and beliefs about a particular culture (stereotyping).

• Assess the individual/family carefully and openly without judgment.

• Avoid generalizations and assumptions based upon personal ideas and knowledge about a particular culture. There is diversity *within* every culture.

In view of these suggestions, it is a good idea to tactfully validate any inferences made regarding the particular culture or group by speaking with the individual or family. To do otherwise might compromise the nurse's goal of giving excellent care based upon a complete biopsychosocial assessment that has included a cultural component.

Through the assessment process (discussed next), the nurse identifies risk factors that may precipitate illness. Planning with the family determines health goals that may or may not necessitate the involvement of other health team members.

Family Assessment

Assessment of the beginning or childbearing family's status is the first step in determining the family's level of functioning. Data may be gathered in a variety of settings, including the home, clinic, and hospital. When assessing the family of a maternity client, the nurse should be comprehensive but focused on areas of particular relevance to the family. In-depth data collection is necessary in those areas that pose a problem for the family or are of concern to the nurse.

To collect valid, pertinent data, the nurse must establish a positive relationship with the client, a family member, and/or the family group. The use of empathy, positive regard, and active listening enables the nurse to gather complete, yet selective, information about the family.

Basic identifying information should be obtained, including the names, ages, gender, and relationships of all family members. Religious and cultural associations are determined, along with type of family configuration. Similar data about the members of the extended family who are closest to the nuclear family may be important, especially if they reside nearby and form a strong support group for each other. Individual and family developmental history may also be incorporated at this time.

A health history of the entire family is recorded, since family health problems have potential effects on children born or unborn. The nurse gathers information about the extended and nuclear family regarding past acute and chronic illnesses, congenital defects, mental health, and such alterations as obesity or the occurrence of accidents. A family pedigree may be helpful in summarizing this information visually (see Chapter 7 on genetic counseling). With the beginning expectant family or the childbearing family, data about all pregnancies become significant. Past experiences of family members with health care delivery systems or hospitalization are important in ascertaining which approach to the family will be most helpful.

Data about the current health status of each family member must be obtained. With the beginning and childbearing family, the nurse assesses the family's strengths and limitations in promoting and maintaining health by eliciting such information as the family's definitions of health and illness, their nutritional status, attitudes toward medicine use (prescription and nonprescription), recreational and exercise activities, exposure to environmental hazards, and sleep and rest practices. When a client is pregnant, prenatal assessment is essential (Chapter 10). Other important information includes data on each member's allergies, health problems requiring prescription medications, environmentally and genetically related illnesses, the family's knowledge about these disorders, and treatments recommended and implemented.

Assessing the competency of the family to promote and maintain health, care for ill members, and carry out health care instructions is vital in determining the nurse's interaction with the family. Many families use preventive health measures such as obtaining routine medical, dental, hearing, and ophthalmic examinations and immunizations; and participating in other screening programs. If the family does not use such preventive measures, questions should arise about their availability or the family's knowledge about them. The nurse may find it necessary to identify health care facilities that are accessible to the family and how they are utilized.

A valid assessment of the family may require several home visits. Some families may feel that a home visit by a nurse is an invasion of privacy but most become more amenable as rapport is established. When assessing the characteristics of a home, the nurse must make objective observations; personal standards and values should not be allowed to distort evaluation of the living conditions. Living space that provides all family members with privacy and comfortable sleeping arrangements and permits each person to pursue interests and needs is important. If an additional family member is expected, preparation for arrival should be evident. Facilities for ill and convalescent family members should also be evaluated. Adequate heat, light, cooking facilities, water, storage facilities, and hygienic equipment are necessary for maintaining the well-being of all family members. Toys, books, and other recreational and educational equipment should be available for the children. Play areas should be away from safety hazards and should be adequately supervised. Safety hazards such as peeling paint, exposed electrical wiring, rugs that are not held in place, and exposed heating equipment can be of great danger, particularly to small children and the elderly. The distance of the home from health care facilities and the availability of transportation to them should also be investigated.

Appraisal of the home environment gives only some indication of the economic status of the family. Knowledge about the sources and amounts of family income and about the work skills of individual members aids in assessing health behavior and needs. Information about the allocation of income to shelter, clothing, food, savings, insurance, education, recreation, and health care reveals the family's economic priorities and its ability to meet the needs of all family members.

The assessment may also include observations of the population characteristics and resources of the neighborhood and the larger community in which the family resides, taking into account the family's associations and transactions within the community. How parents view their interaction with their neighborhood and community is significant in that their children tend to relate in a similar fashion. Certain health problems can also affect many within a community; for example, diseases can be transmitted by children to other children in schools and from them to the rest of the family. After identifying such situations, a nurse can make recommendations to help families cope with such problems.

Interaction among members is vital to the maintenance of a healthy, well-adjusted family. Observing the various roles members have in the family, the flexibility of the roles, and the sources of authority within the family reveals underlying relationships among members. In couples beginning a family, another important observation concerns each member's response to the incorporation of the new role of mother or father. Assessing communication patterns provides further validation of family relationships.

A simple technique the nurse may use is to pay attention to who says what to whom, how it is said, and what the consequence seems to be (Sedgwick, 1981). The emotional atmosphere of the family unit may be assessed by the nurse by noting degree of comfort in self-disclosure, willingness to disagree, positive statements verbalized, and use of touch. Identification of family coping mechanisms provides the nurse with insight about the family's response to stress. The nurse should identify any stressors (divorce, separation, death, or other significant changes) that are affecting family function. Value conflicts, if evident, are assessed for their impact on the health status of the family. Other important aspects for the nurse to consider are the parents' childrearing practices, rationale for using particular procedures, attitudes toward health and the health care delivery system, intellectual interests, religious practices and beliefs, and sociocultural reference groups. Interaction with members of the extended family and the types and amount of support they give each other should also be explored.

Nursing Diagnosis and Planning

After completing the assessment of the family, the nurse analyzes the data to formulate nursing diagnoses. Goals based on each nursing diagnosis are then established for the family. These are divided into short- and long-range goals and should be a joint enterprise between the family and the nurse. Without this cooperative interaction, the goals may not meet those needs that the family believes are important, may not be realistic for the family, or may not be accepted by the family as its responsibility.

The priority of these goals must then be determined. This is a highly individualized process; input from the family continues to have great importance. A severe illness, an unplanned child, and lack of funds for a needed purchase can all be crucial matters. However, the family may consider obtaining funds to be the most pressing goal, the nurse may believe that accepting the child should receive immediate attention, and the physician may think that the treatment of the illness should be given top priority. Factors that affect setting priorities include the family's perceptions of its needs, the number of problems that require attention, the feasibility of goals set, the readiness of the family to meet the goals, and the amount of preparation or education necessary before the goals can be met (Sobol and Robischon, 1970). Working with the family, the nurse must validate the goals and their importance to gain the family's support in achieving them.

Planning interventions is the next step in the nursing process. The nursing care plan must be based on the goals set in consultation with the family. There are generally many approaches to every problem, and the nurse must identify the one that seems most likely to work in the family's particular framework of attitudes, beliefs, and values. Family participation in the decision about the approach can be valuable, because the family is aware of its ability to deal with the situation. In any event, the nursing plan must be accepted by the family prior to putting it into action.

During the planning stage, decisions must be made about those health care workers, other professionals, and community agencies that will be of greatest value to the family. The services available from these agencies are then explained to the family. The family's needs may be best satisfied through the participation of several agencies, which requires interagency cooperation and coordination of efforts. The nurse may serve as the coordinator of these activities, assuring continuity of services to the family. One long-range goal for the family should be to strengthen its knowledge of community resources to meet its own health needs.

Intervention

In implementing a care plan, the nurse must constantly keep in mind the short- and long-range goals that have been set for the family. Therapeutic interaction continues to be of primary importance. Changes in family needs often produce stress on some or all members. The recommendations and teaching of the nurse or other professionals may cause more stress, as any change always causes some tension and anxiety. Family members may feel guilty about having certain needs and may be concerned about how these needs will be accepted by others. Any serious difficulties have probably already disrupted the family, and its members may have had to take on roles and responsibilities with which they are unfamiliar; this can modify the family's life-style. The nurse must be aware of any situations that arise as the nursing plan is implemented. Further resources may need to be consulted to help in dealing with any problems.

When working with beginning and childbearing families, the nurse assumes many roles, including teacher, counselor, coordinator, researcher, and advocate. In these roles, the nurse is careful to communicate in a manner that is understandable and meaningful to the family. Knowledge of the family's developmental level, internal processes, socioeconomic status, and cultural background helps in determining the most effective method to use. For learning to occur, a collaborative effort is involved. The nurse assists the family to define change strategies and the family decides how to apply the learning primarily through their own resources. In some circumstances, the nurse supports the family's position or initiates plans to foster further development, thus ensuring continued learning on the part of the family.

The nurse acts primarily as a teacher, counselor, and advocate in helping a couple determine their family-planning needs. The nurse offers information in a manner that the family can understand and use, demonstrating understanding and respect for needs and belief systems. Some families may be hesitant to use family planning techniques because of fears or dislike of, or misconceptions about, contraception; because of worries that they cannot afford family planning; or because of beliefs that others are trying to limit the size of their social group.

The nurse's responsibilities to the beginning expectant family include preparing the couple for the woman's physical and emotional condition and needs, and planning for the man's desires for involvement. Teaching expectant couples about pregnancy, labor, and delivery, and counseling them about child care and the parental role are important components of nursing responsibilities.

After the child is born, a primary concern of the nurse is to make sure that the family can meet the needs of the newborn infant. The nurse assumes the roles of teacher and counselor when discussing the needs of the infant and demonstrating infant care to the parents. In addition, the nurse acts as the family advocate by giving emotional support to new parents and by providing guidance on effective use of health care professionals.

The nurse can serve as a resource person to parents with children of various ages who need guidance and who desire knowledge about their children's developmental tasks, appropriate toys for each age group, safety in the household, health care needs, adjustments to school or the mother's return to work, and the child's gradual separation from the family.

Families with an elderly member may require counseling on his or her physical and emotional needs and their responsibilities in meeting these needs. The nurse can help coordinate health care for the older family member and can teach the family how to meet his or her health care needs.

Evaluation

To interpret the success or failure of the nursing care plan, the nurse must take into account the goals set for the family and the effects produced. Again, the family should play an important part in this evaluation, as it has in other steps of the nursing process. Members must be encouraged to respond freely and openly.

If a goal has been fully achieved, the nursing interventions have been successful. If a goal has not been attained, the nurse should explore the reasons for the failure and devise a new plan that might meet with greater success. If a goal has been partially achieved, the nurse and family ascertain whether the plan is realistic and simply needs more time or whether modifications are necessary. The nurse may find that changes in the family necessitate adjustments and adaptations in the nursing care plan at any point during its implementation. Even when all goals appear to have been attained, periodic reevaluation and encouragement are necessary for the family to continue to function at the best level.

Application of the Nursing Process: A Case Example

The following example demonstrates the effective use of the nursing process with a family (Figure 3-3). Mr. Johnston (30 years old) and Mrs. Johnston (27 years old) have been married for 5 years. This couple has two children, Jeffrey, 3 years old, and Jennifer, 7 months old. Both parents are high school graduates. Mrs. Johnston was employed before having children, but now is primarily responsible for the management of the home and children. She plans to return to work when both children are in school. Mr. Johnston is the manager of a local grocery store.

Mrs. Johnston and Jennifer were attending a well-baby examination when Mrs. Johnston mentioned that she was concerned that Jennifer was not yet sitting by herself. She noted that Jeffrey was sitting by 6½ months of age and that several neighbors had been surprised at Jennifer's inability to sit alone. Through further exploration the nurse learned that Jeffrey had been caught several times treating Jennifer roughly and had tried to pick her up by her legs a number of times.

The nurse formulated two tentative nursing diagnoses: (a) anxiety related to Jennifer's perceived developmental lag, and (b) sibling rivalry related to the integration of a new family member. To obtain additional data for further documentation and to determine the priority of concerns, the nurse's plan was to allow Mrs. Johnston to express her anxieties freely. The nurse also decided to ask pertinent questions about Jeffrey's behavior and other family member's reactions to it.

The nurse discovered that this behavior began shortly after Jennifer was born. At first Jeffrey ignored his new baby sister, but he began to pat her after about a week. His parents accompanied his touching her with remarks that he should pat her gently because she was only a baby and could be easily harmed. Jeffrey was usually kept away from Jennifer, but several times he got into her room and was caught hitting her. As he became more aggressive, Mr. Johnston spanked him, and Mrs. Johnston yelled at him. Neither form of punishment alleviated Jeffrey's problem, but rather accentuated it. When his parents found him holding Jennifer up by the legs, they were afraid that her spine had been injured; this fear seemed validated by Jennifer's slow motor development.

After allowing Mrs. Johnston the opportunity to express her concerns, the nurse selected a teaching strategy as a means to reduce Mrs. Johnston's anxiety about Jennifer's perceived developmental lag. The nurse explained to Mrs. Johnston that all babies develop at their own rate, even within the same family. A Denver Developmental Screening Test showed that Jennifer was functioning within the normal limits for her age. These results were explained to Mrs. Johnston, and several books on child devel-

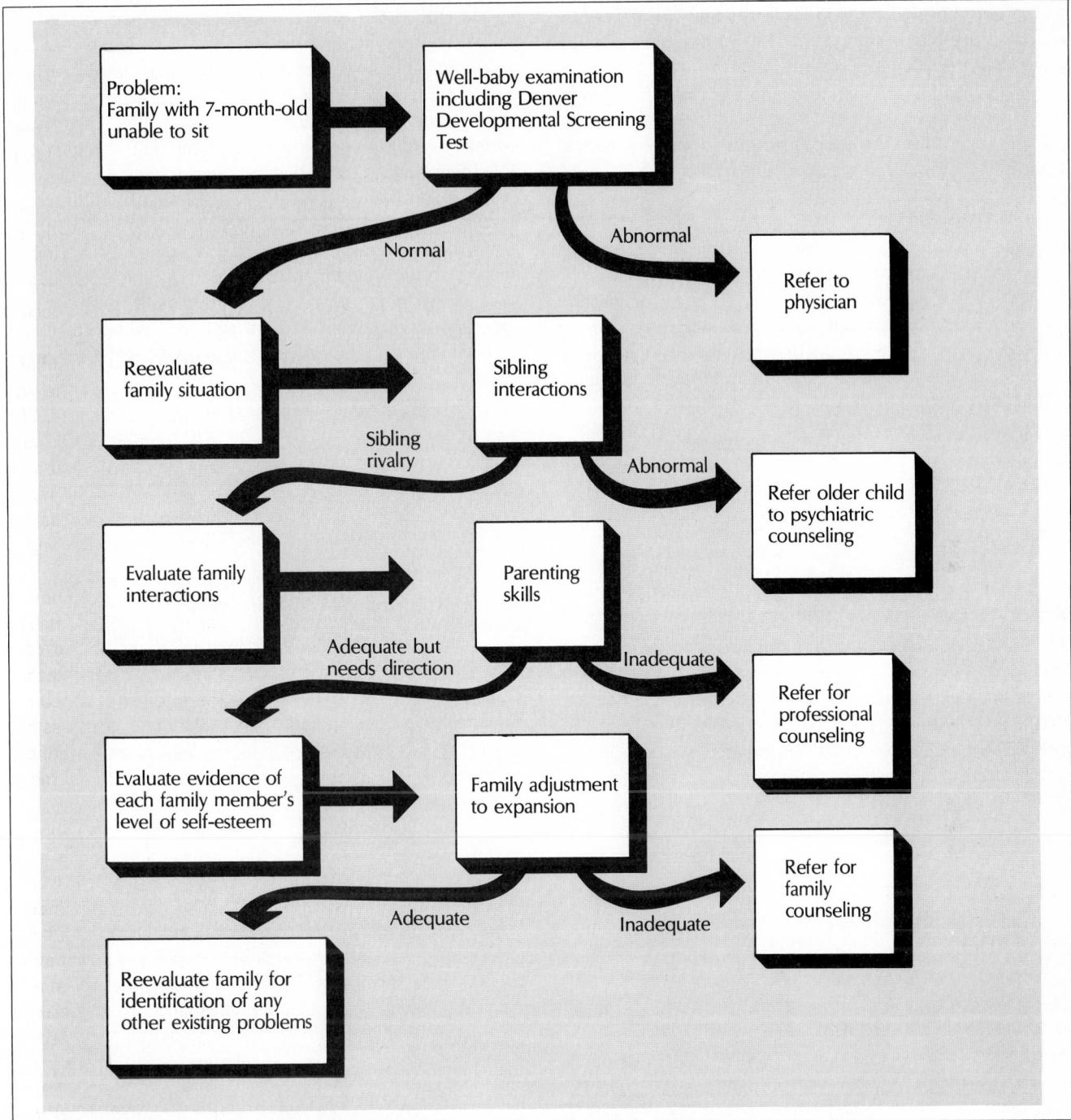

FIGURE 3–3 Flow chart.

opment were suggested to her. Mrs. Johnston was advised that although Jennifer's motor development was coming along fine and the physician had determined that there were no residual effects from Jeffrey's rough treatments, they both might enjoy infant physical stimulation classes that were offered through a local agency.

Mrs. Johnston was still concerned about Jeffrey's possible future physical harm to Jennifer. As teacher and counselor, the nurse explained that behavior like Jeffrey's is a frequent reaction of an older sibling to the birth of a baby and that he probably felt that Jennifer had usurped his place of importance within the family. Mrs. Johnston was asked to bring Jeffrey in, as it was time for his routine examination. His developmental abilities were assessed, along with his sleep and activity patterns, eating, elimination, communication, temperament, and dependence-independence patterns. He was found to have occasional temper tantrums when he was tired and to wet his bed at night. Otherwise, he demonstrated no difficulties in adapting to his surroundings.

The nurse suggested that Jeffrey be included in the care of Jennifer when possible and that the parents set aside a special time period each night, possibly after Jennifer was in bed, devoted entirely to Jeffrey's needs and desires. Mrs. Johnston was advised to set up an area in Jeffrey's room with a hammering board and tools where he could retreat to take out his frustrations in a more acceptable manner.

Several weeks later, during Jennifer's next routine examination, the nurse evaluated the effectiveness of the suggestions. Mrs. Johnston reported that Jeffrey continued to have angry outbursts but that he was sent to his room, where he had learned to work out his feelings. He seemed to enjoy playing with Jennifer now that she was able to appreciate his antics; he had not been caught being overly rough with her in the previous month, although he liked to jostle her while she laughed back at him. Jennifer had shown progress in sitting and remained sitting for indefinite periods and had also started crawling. The nurse's roles of teaching, support, encouragement, and reassurance had worked well through planned, thoughtful intervention, based on the selective assessment of the Johnston family.

SUMMARY

The family is a unit of simple origin but complex makeup. Many of the family's needs for assistance in accomplishing developmental tasks and for health care can be met by the nurse. By means of supportive intervention, the nurse can assume therapeutic roles that maintain or restore health as well as prevent illness within families.

Resource Group

Parents Without Partners. A listing is usually available in any telephone book. The group provides support and social activities for single parents of either sex raising children.

References

Backup, R. W. 1979. Implementing quality health care for the American Indian patient. *Washington State J. Nursing.* Supplement: 20.

Berelson, B. B. 1976. The value of children: a taxonomical essay. In *Raising children in modern America: problems and prospective solutions,* ed. N. B. Talbot. Boston: Little, Brown & Co.

Branch, M. F., and Paxton, P. P. 1976. *Providing safe nursing care for ethnic people of color.* New York: Appleton-Century-Crofts.

Brownlee, A. T. 1978. *Community, culture and care: a cross-cultural guide for health workers.* St. Louis: The C. V. Mosby Co.

Burgess, E. W. 1971. *The family: from traditional to companionship.* New York: Van Nostrand Reinhold Company.

Cambodia—the land and its people. 1976. Lutheran Immigration and Refugee Service. Lutheran Council in the USA.

Duvall, E. M. 1971. *Family development.* Philadelphia: J. B. Lippincott Co.

Duvall, E. M. 1977. *Marriage and family development.* 5th ed. Philadelphia: J. B. Lippincott Co.

Erikson, E. H. 1963. *Childhood and society.* 2nd ed. New York: W. W. Norton & Co., Inc.

Farris, L. S. March/April 1976. Approaches to caring for the American Indian maternity patient. *MCN* 1:80.

Fong, S. L. M. 1973. Assimilation and changing social roles of Chinese-Americans. *J. Social Issues.* 292:115.

Friedman, M. M. 1981. *Family nursing theory and assessment.* New York: Appleton-Century-Crofts.

Henderson, G., and Primeaux, M. 1981. *Transcultural health care.* Menlo Park, Calif.: Addison-Wesley Publishing Co.

Higgins, P. G., and Wayland, J. September 16, 1981. Labour and delivery in North America. *Nursing Times Midwifery Supplement.*

Ho, M. K. March 1976. Social work with Asian Americans. *Social Casework.* 57:195.

Hymovich, D. P. 1980. *Child and family development implications for primary health care.* New York: McGraw-Hill Book Co.

Hymovich, D. P., and Barnard, M. U. 1973. *Family health care.* New York: McGraw-Hill Book Co.

Kenkel, W. F. 1977. *The family in perspective.* 4th ed. New York: Appleton-Century-Crofts.

Martin, E. P., and Martin, J. M. 1978. *The black extended family.* Chicago: University of Chicago Press.

Mowrer, E. R. 1927. *Family disorganization: an introduction to a sociological analysis.* Chicago: University of Chicago Press.

Robischon, P., and Scott, D. July 1969. Role theory and its application in family nursing. *Nurs. Outlook.* 17:52.

Sedgwick, R. 1981. *Family mental health theory and practice.* St. Louis: The C. V. Mosby Co.

Sobol, E. G., and Robischon, P. 1970. *Family nursing: a study guide.* St. Louis: The C. V. Mosby Co.

Spradley, J. P., and McCurdy, D. W. 1980. *Conformity and conflict; readings in cultural anthropology.* 4th ed. Boston: Little, Brown & Co.

Additional Readings

Allan, H. 1981. *Ethnicity and medical care.* Cambridge, Mass.: Harvard University Press.

Anderson, G., and Tighe, B. 1973. Gypsy culture and health care. *Am. J. Nurs.* 73:282.

Davies, M., and Yoshida, M. March 1981. A model for cultural assessment. *Can. Nurse.* 77:22.

DeGracia, R. T. 1979. Cultural influences on Filipinos. *Am. J. Nurs.* 79:1412.

Henderson, G. 1979. *Understanding and counseling ethnic minorities.* Springfield, Ill.: Charles C Thomas, Publisher.

Jacobsen, D. S. Jan./Feb. 1980. Stepfamilies. *Child. Today.* 9:2.

Kitano, H. H. L. 1976. *Japanese Americans, the evolution of a subculture.* 2nd ed. Englewood Cliffs, N.J.: Prentice-Hall, Inc.

Leininger, M. March 1977. Cultural diversities in health and nursing care. *Nurs. Clin. North Am.* 12:1.

Olness, K. 1979. Cultural aspects in working with Lao refugees. *Minn. Med.* 62:871.

Red Horse, J. G., et al. Feb. 1978. Family behavior of urban American Indians. *Social Casework.* 59:67.

Rosenblum, E. H. 1980. Conversation with a Navajo nurse. *Am. J. Nurs.* 80:1459.

Schlegel, A. 1972. *Male dominance and female autonomy: domestic authority in matrilineal societies.* New Haven, Conn.: Human Relations Area Files Press.

Sowell, T. 1981. *Ethnic America—a history.* New York: Basic Books, Inc.

Whall, A. L. Oct. 1980. Congruence between existing theories of family functioning and nursing theories. *ANS* 3:59.

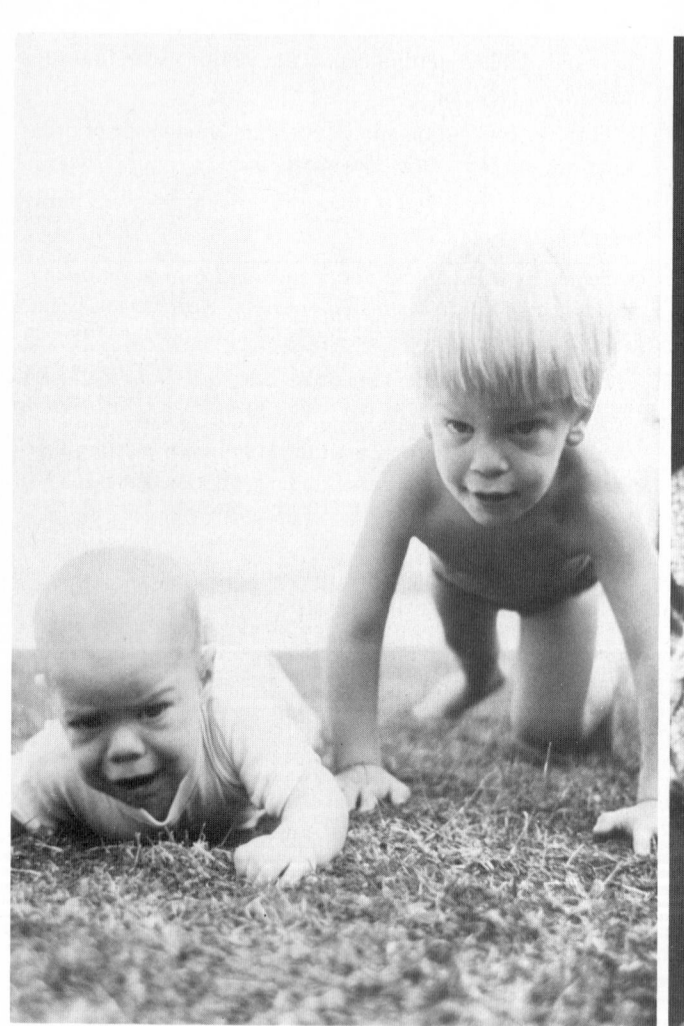
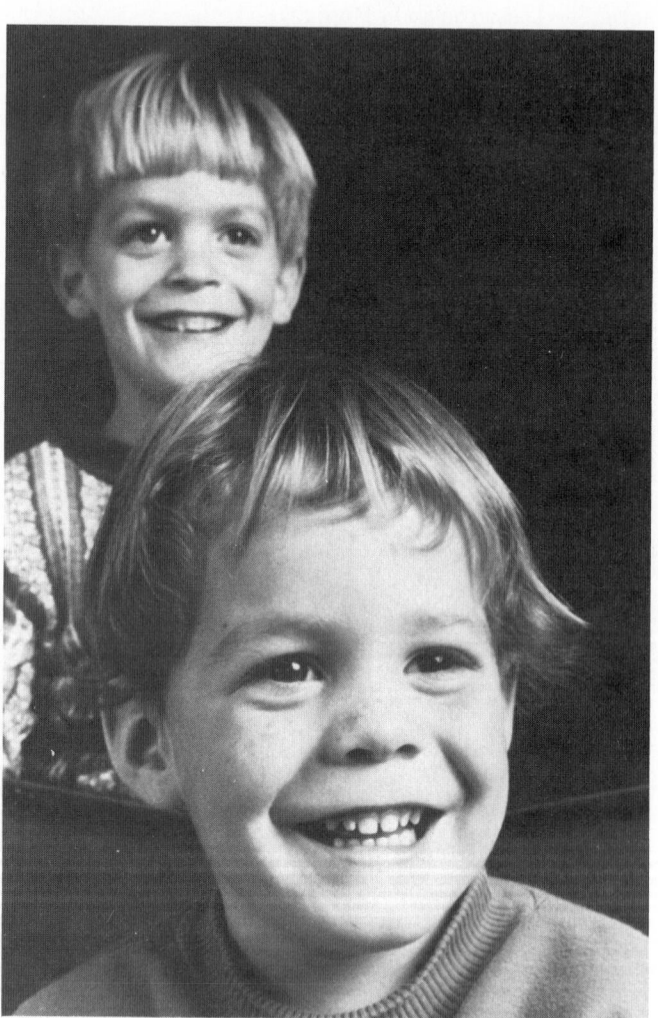

▪ II ▪

HUMAN REPRODUCTION AND DEVELOPMENT

Chapter 4 ▪ Human Reproductive System

Chapter 5 ▪ Sexual Development and Sexuality

Chapter 6 ▪ Family Planning

Chapter 7 ▪ Genetic Counseling

Chapter 8 ▪ Conception and Fetal Development

■ 4 ■

HUMAN REPRODUCTIVE SYSTEM

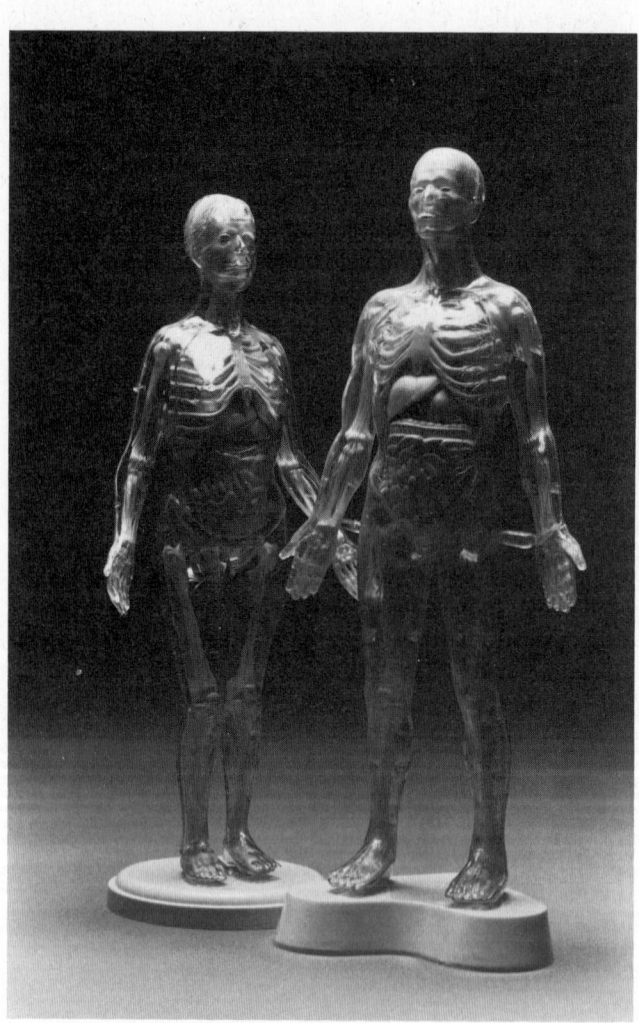

■ CHAPTER CONTENTS

EMBRYOLOGIC DEVELOPMENT OF THE REPRODUCTIVE SYSTEM

    Ovaries and Testes

    Other Internal Genitals

    External Genitals

MALE REPRODUCTIVE SYSTEM

    External Genitals

    Internal Genitals

    Accessory Glands

    Semen

    Breasts

FEMALE REPRODUCTIVE SYSTEM

    Bony Pelvis

    External Genitals

    Internal Genitals

    Breasts

• Relate information about the embryologic development of the human reproductive system to reproductive functions.

• Review the anatomy and physiology of the male and female reproductive systems.

• Correlate anatomic and physiologic information to provide basis for implications of nursing care.

Any logical account of prenatal development must start with a consideration of the phenomena that initiate it. Understanding life before birth requires more than knowledge of the structure of the conjugating sex cells. One needs information about germ cell production and the extraordinary provisions that ensure the union of egg and sperm in a given place and at such a time that each is capable of discharging its function. One also needs an understanding of the changes in the woman's body that provide for the embryo's nutrition during its intrauterine existence and for breast-feeding after birth. But before proceeding to these matters, it is necessary for one to become familiar with the embryologic development and main structural features of the male and female reproductive organs.

EMBRYOLOGIC DEVELOPMENT OF THE REPRODUCTIVE SYSTEM

Knowledge of the embryologic development of the human reproduction system greatly facilitates understanding of the correlations among anatomy, physiology, and function. This section provides a brief overview of the development of the internal and external genitals. Chapter 8 contains a more complete discussion of fetal development.

The male and female reproductive organs are homologous; that is, they are fundamentally similar in structure and function. The genetic sex of the embryo is determined at fertilization (Chapter 8). However, the developing fetus exhibits no sexual differentiation until the eighth week. This early period is known as the *indifferent stage*.

Ovaries and Testes

A *gonad* is an organ that produces sex cells. The female gonad is the ovary, which produces ova; the male counterpart is the testis, which produces sperm. During the fifth week of gestation, a primitive gonad arises from the medial aspect of the urogenital ridge. The gonads develop a medulla and cortex as primary sex cords appear in the underlying mesenchyme. In genetic males, during the seventh and eighth week the medulla develops into a testis, and the cortex regresses. In genetic females, the cortex

develops into an ovary, recognizable about the tenth week, and the medulla regresses. All primordial follicles, which contain the primitive ovarian eggs (oogonia), are formed during prenatal life.

Figure 4–1 illustrates the embryologic development of the gonads and other internal reproductive organs.

Other Internal Genitals

During the indifferent period, two pairs of genital ducts develop: the *mesonephric* and *paramesonephric* ducts. These ducts are complete at the seventh week. The paramesonephric ducts meet in midline to form the Y-shaped uterovaginal primordium. At its dorsal end is the urogenital tubercle or sinus. In genetic males, the fetal testes secrete two hormones: testosterone stimulates the mesonephric ducts to develop into the male genital tract, and the other hormone (müllerian regression factor) suppresses development of the paramesonephric ducts, which would otherwise develop into the female genital tract.

With further differentiation of the mesonephric ducts comes development of the efferent ductules, vas deferens, epididymides, seminal vesicles, and ejaculatory ducts. Both the prostate and the bulbourethral glands develop from endodermal outgrowths of the urethra (see Figure 4–1).

In genetic females, the uterine tubes are formed from the unfused portions of the paramesonephric ducts, and the fused portions give rise to the epithelium and uterine glands. The endometrial stroma and the myometrium develop from the adjacent mesenchyme.

The vagina is derived from more than one embryologic structure. The vaginal epithelium develops from the endoderm of the urogenital sinus, and the musculature, from the uterovaginal primordium.

The urethral and paraurethral glands develop from outgrowths of the urethra into the surrounding mesenchyme. Bartholin's glands arise from similar structures.

External Genitals

In the fourth week a genital tubercle develops ventrally to the cloacal membrane. On each side of the cloacal membrane, labioscrotal swellings and urogenital folds develop. The genital tubercle lengthens and is called a *phallus* in

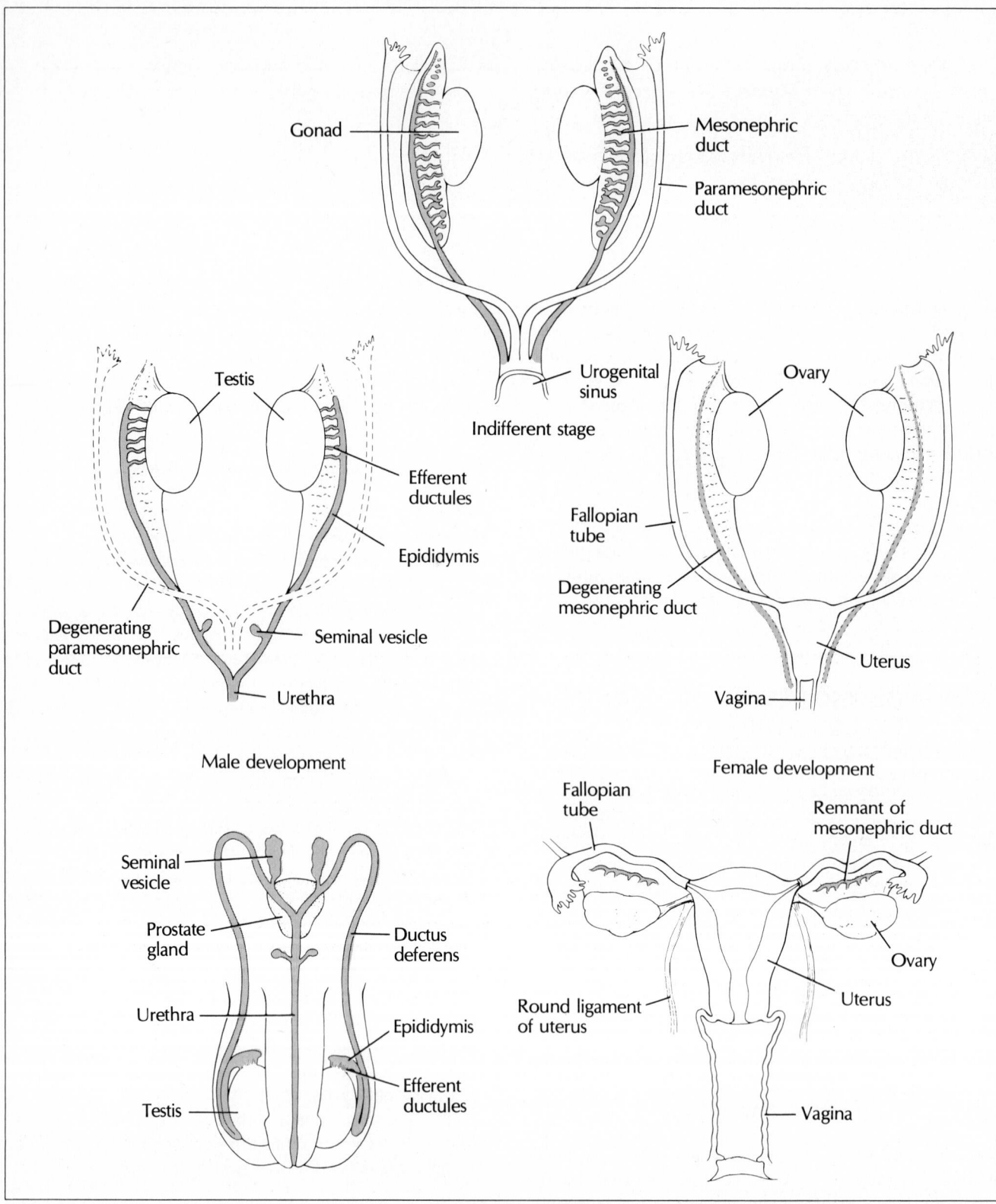

FIGURE 4–1 Embryologic differentiation of male and female internal reproductive organs. (From Spence, A. P., and Mason, E. B. 1983. *Human anatomy and physiology.* 2nd ed. Menlo Park, Calif.: Benjamin/Cummings Publishing Co., p. 728.)

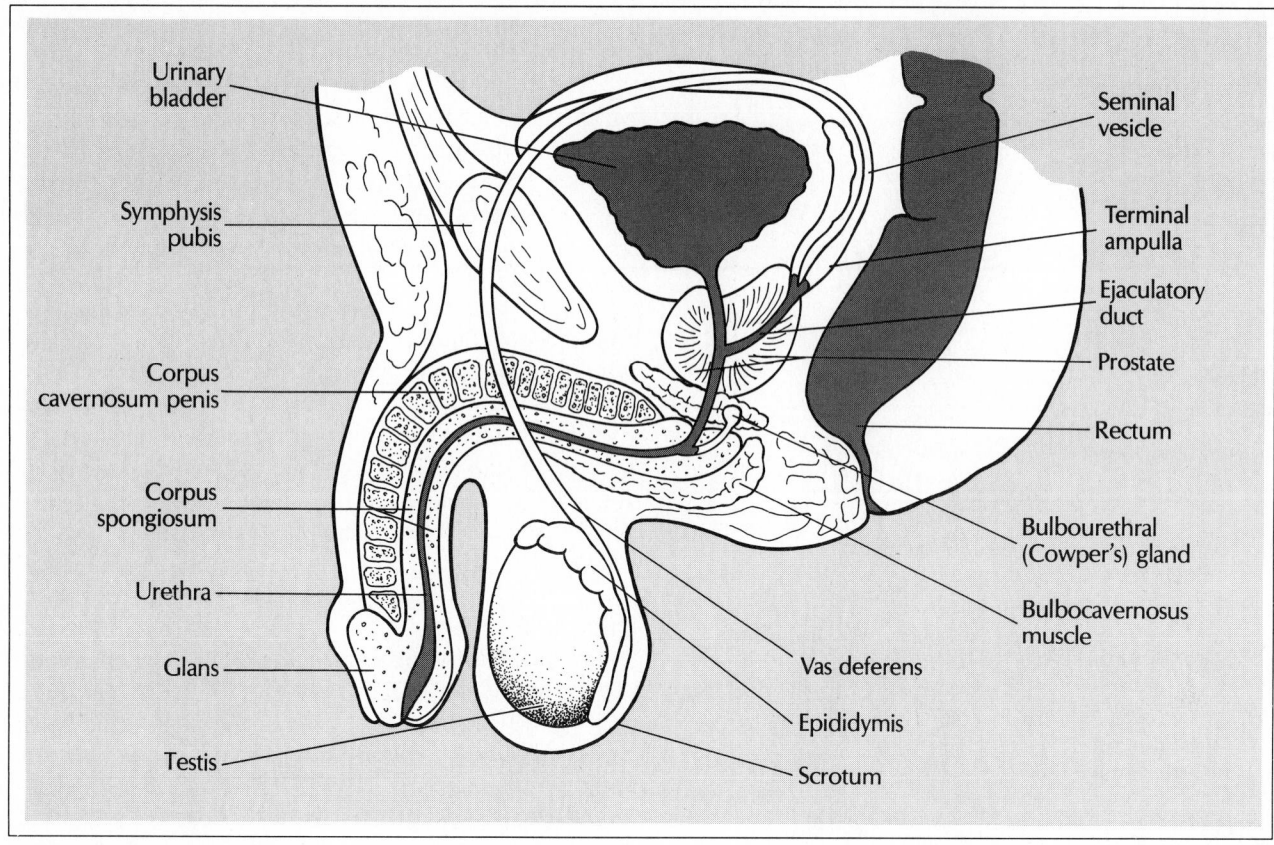

FIGURE 4–2 Male reproductive system.

both males and females. On the ventral side of the phallus, a urethral groove develops. Genetic males and females possess the same external genitals until the end of the ninth week. By the twelfth week, differentiation of the external genitals is complete.

Under the influence of the fetal testes' production of dihydrotestosterone, the indifferent external genitals become masculine. The phallus elongates, forming the penis. The fusion of the urogenital folds on the ventral surface of the penis forms the penile urethra, with the urethral meatus moving forward toward the glans penis.

In the absence of fetal testosterone, feminization of the indifferent external genitals occurs. The phallus becomes the clitoris, and the urogenital folds remain open, forming the labia minora. The labioscrotal folds form the labia majora.

MALE REPRODUCTIVE SYSTEM

Andrology is the study of the male reproductive organs. To date, the male organs have not been studied to the same depth as their female counterparts. New techniques are being applied to research and the clinical study of the role of males in such areas as infertility, contraception, congenital anomalies, and reproduction in general. Particular emphasis has been placed on neurohormonal control and the role of prostaglandins (Hafez, 1980; Caldwell and Behrman, 1981).

The male reproductive system consists of the external and internal genitals (Figure 4–2). Because the breasts seem related to the purely sexual aspects of the reproductive system, they will be considered as accessory organs.

External Genitals

The two external reproductive organs are the penis and the scrotum.

PENIS

The *penis*, or copulatory organ, is an elongated, pendant structure consisting of a body, termed the *shaft*, and the *glans* (Figure 4–3). It is attached to the front and sides of the pubic arch and lies anterior to the scrotum.

The shaft of the penis is made up of three longitudinal columns of erectile tissue: the paired *corpora cavernosa penis* and a third, the *corpus spongiosum penis*. These columns are covered by a dense fibrous connective tissue called the *tunica albuginea* and then enclosed by an elastic

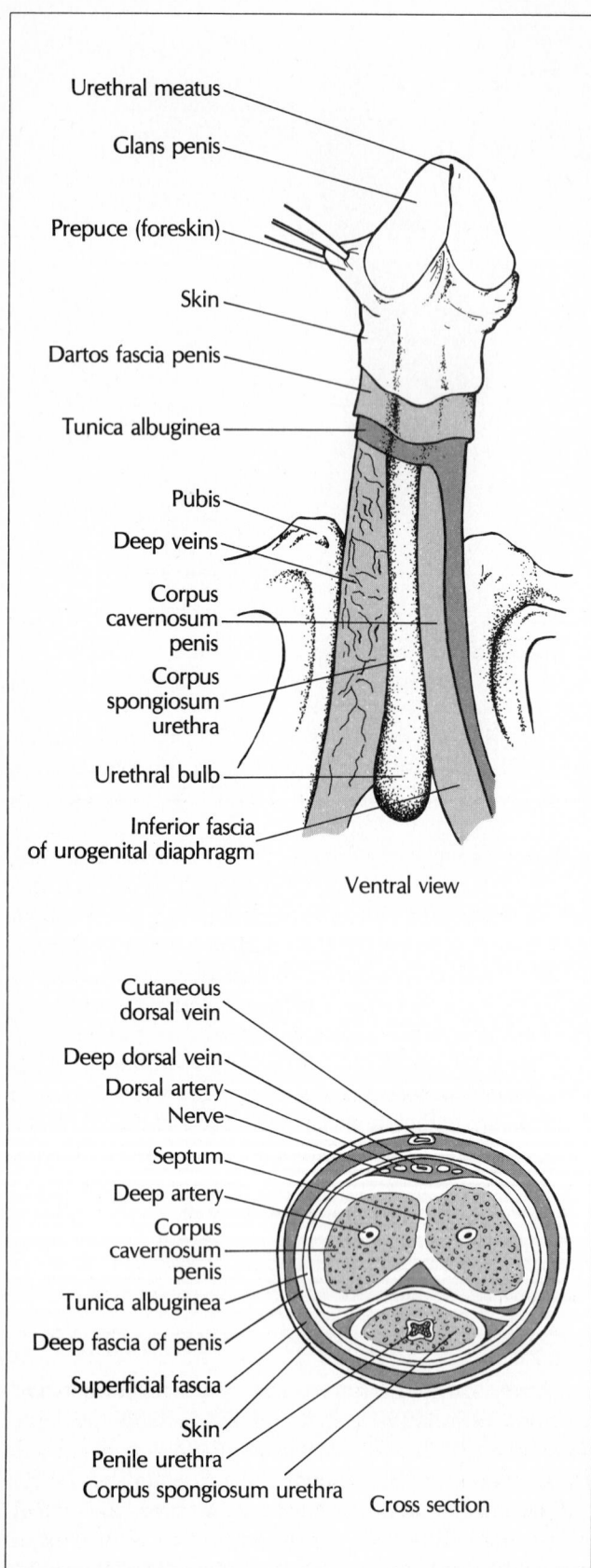

Ventral view

Cross section

FIGURE 4-3 Anatomy of the penis.

areolar tissue, the *fascia penis*. The penis is covered by an outer layer of skin with a very thin epithelium continuous with that covering the pubic region anteriorly, the perineum laterally, and the scrotum posteriorly.

The paired corpora cavernosa penis are side by side on the dorsal surface of the organ. The third column, the corpus spongiosum penis (also known as the corpus cavernosum urethra), lies ventral to the others, contains the urethra, and extends beyond the corpora cavernosa to become the glans at the distal end of the penis. The urethra widens within the glans to form the *fossa navicularis* and terminates in a slitlike orifice, located in the tip of the glans, called the *urethral meatus*. A circular fold of skin arises just behind the glans and covers it. Known as the *prepuce,* or foreskin, it is frequently removed by the surgical procedure of circumcision (Chapter 23). If the corpus spongiosum does not surround the urethra completely, the urethral meatus may occur on the ventral aspect of the penile shaft (hypospadias) or on the dorsal aspect (epispadias).

The suspensory ligament is the main attachment and support for the penis. It extends from the symphysis pubis and merges with the deep fascia of the penis. Additional support is given by the urethra, the muscles around the crura, and the bulb.

The blood supply to the penis is a parallel system of internal and external pudendal arteries and veins. Blood to the cavernous sinuses is provided by two branches of the penile artery.

The penile substance is supplied by the dorsal nerve of the penis from the pudendal nerve. Sympathetic fibers come from the hypogastric and pelvic plexuses, while parasympathetic fibers from the third and fourth sacral nerves form the splanchnic nerves. When the parasympathetic fibers are stimulated, the penis becomes erect because the contraction of the ischiocavernous muscle prevents the return of venous blood from the cavernous sinuses, resulting in engorgement of the blood vessels.

The penis serves both the urinary and reproductive systems. Urine is expelled through the urethral meatus. However, the primary function of the penis is the depositing of sperm in the female vagina during sexual intercourse to provide for fertilization of the ovum.

As the procreative functions of men and women have become minimized, the penis has assumed increasing importance as provider of sexual pleasure. To many men, the penis is a symbol of virility and masculinity, and its loss or altered function results in a lessening of their self-esteem.

SCROTUM

The *scrotum* is a pouchlike structure suspended from the perineal region (Figure 4–4). It hangs anterior to the anus and posterior to the penis and may extend below it. Composed of skin and the *dartos,* which contains fascial connective tissue with smooth muscle fibers, the scrotum shows increased pigmentation and scattered hairs. The sebaceous glands open directly onto the scrotal surface; their secretion has a distinctive odor. Because of the rugae caused by the dartos and the cremasteric muscle, the scrotum appears rough and wrinkled. The degree of wrinkling is greatest in young men and at cold temperatures and is least in older men and at warm temperatures. Contraction of the dartos and cremasteric muscles shortens the scrotum and draws it closer to the body, thus wrinkling its outer surface.

Inside the scrotum are two lateral compartments separated by a medial septum derived from the dartos muscle. In each compartment is a testis with its related structures. Because the left spermatic cord grows longer during embryologic development, the left testis and its scrotal sac hang lower than the right. A ridge (raphe) on the external scrotal surface marks the position of the medial septum. This raphe continues anteriorly on the urethral surface of the penis but disappears in the perineal area.

Scrotal innervation is concentrated and is derived from the genitofemoral, pudendal, posterior femoral cutaneous, and ilioinguinal nerves and the hypogastric plexus.

The function of the scrotum is to protect the testes and the sperm by maintaining a temperature lower than that of the body. Spermatogenesis will not occur if the testes fail to descend, thus remaining at body temperature. By being sensitive to touch, pressure, temperature, and pain, the scrotum serves as a defense against potential harm to the testes. Innervation of the anterior third of the scrotum is supplied mainly from the first lumbar segment of the spinal cord, whereas the posterior two-thirds are supplied mainly from the third sacral segment. Thus spinal anesthetic agents must be injected much higher up to anesthetize the anterior rather than the posterior portion of the scrotum.

Internal Genitals

The male internal reproductive organs include the gonads (testes or testicles), a system of ducts (epididymis, vas deferens, ejaculatory duct, and urethra), and accessory glands (seminal vesicles, prostate gland, bulbourethral glands, and urethral glands).

TESTES

The *testes* are a pair of bilateral, oval, compound glandular organs contained in the scrotum (Figure 4–5). In the sexually mature male, they are the site of spermatozoa production and the secretion of several male sex hormones (androgens). *Testosterone* is the most prevalent and potent; it is considered the primary male sex hormone. The testes are abdominal organs, whereas the penis is a pelvic organ. Each testis is 4–6 cm long, 2–3 cm wide, and 3–4 cm deep and weighs about 10–15 g. It is covered by a serous membrane known as the *tunica vaginalis.* Under this membrane is the *tunica albuginea,* which is a tough, white, fi-

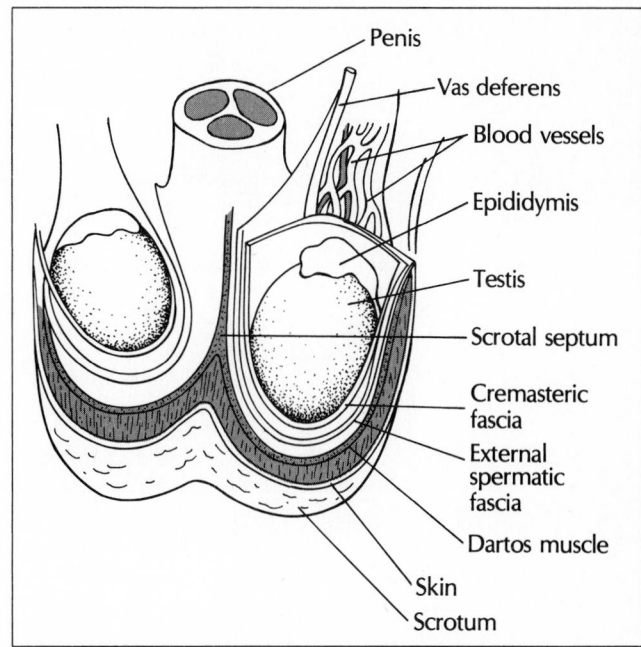

FIGURE 4–4 Anatomy of the scrotum.

brous capsule covering each testis. The tunica albuginea sends projections inward to form septa, thereby dividing the testis into 250 to 400 lobules. Each lobule contains one to three tightly packed, convoluted seminiferous tubules containing sperm cells in all stages of development, arranged in layers. The seminiferous tubules are surrounded by loose connective tissue, which houses abundant blood and lymph vessels and the Leydig's (interstitial) cells, producers of testosterone. The interstitial cells of Leydig make up about 20% of the bulk of the adult testes.

The connective tissue septa extend from the tunica albuginea to the posteriorly positioned mediastinum. In this area a system of collecting ducts begins, with smaller ducts forming larger ducts, which in turn form even larger ducts. The multitudinous seminiferous tubules come together to form the 20 or 30 straight tubules, or tubuli recti, which in turn form an anastomosing network of thin-walled spaces, the *rete testis.* At the upper border of the mediastinum, the rete testis forms 10 to 15 efferent ducts that perforate the tunica albuginea and empty into the duct of the epididymis. Prior to this, the efferent ducts enlarge and become convoluted.

Most of the cells lining the seminiferous tubules undergo a process of maturation called *spermatogenesis.* (See Chapter 8 for further discussion of spermatogenesis.) These cells are located between the basement membrane and the lumen of the tubule, with the most immature cells on the basal membrane. Sperm production varies among and within the tubules, with cells in different areas of the same tubule undergoing different stages of spermatogenesis.

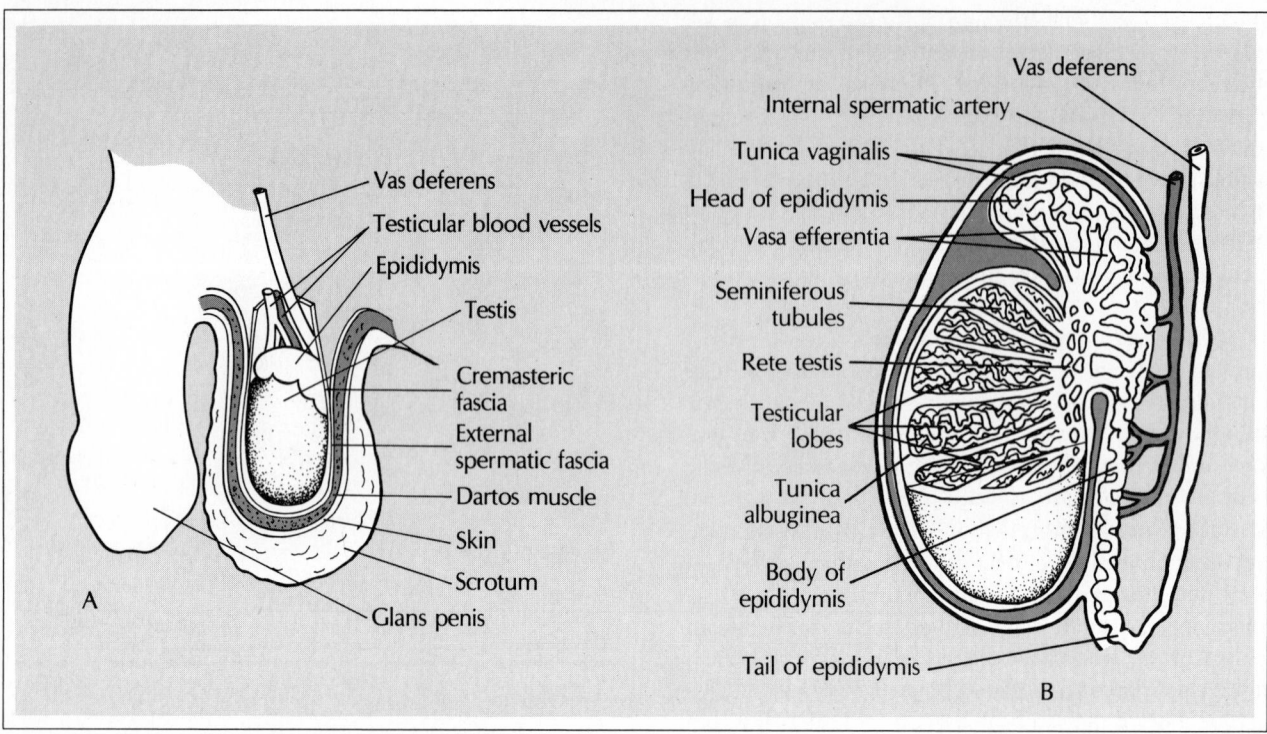

FIGURE 4–5 The testes. **A,** External view. **B,** Sagittal view showing interior anatomy.

After the onset of puberty, spermatogenesis occurs continually to provide the large numbers of sperm necessary for unlimited ejaculations over the mature life span. Estimates of the time required for the complete process range from 2–10 weeks. Spermatogenesis is primarily under the control of the central nervous system. The process is complex. Briefly, afferent impulses are integrated in the hypothalamus, which in turn secretes releasing factors. These stimulate the anterior pituitary to release the gonadotropins, hormonal substances that stimulate the activity of the gonads (see Chapter 5 for further discussion of hormonal activity and the reproductive system). These hormones in turn cause the testes to produce testosterone, which maintains spermatogenesis, increases sperm production by the tubules, and stimulates production of seminal plasma. The mature sperm is discussed on p. 64.

The seminiferous tubules also contain Sertoli's cells, which provide nutrients and protection for the germ cells. Sertoli's cells undergo specific cyclic changes with each generation of spermatozoa, beginning with the spermatogonia and ending as the mature sperm are released into the lumen.

The blood supply of the testes originates at the kidney level. Each testis is supplied by the internal spermatic artery, which branches from the dorsal aorta near the kidney. The spermatic veins lead from the testes, the right entering the vena cava, the left entering the left renal vein.

Both artery and vein pass through the inguinal canal and reach the testis by way of the spermatic cord.

Lymphatic vessels are prolific in the interstitial tissue and drain with those of the epididymis into those in the spermatic cord. They eventually empty into the lumbar nodes near the kidney or into those surrounding the aorta.

The testes are supplied with parasympathetic fibers from the vagus nerve and with sympathetic fibers from the tenth thoracic spinal cord segment via the testicular plexus. Visceral afferent fibers transmit impulses to the central nervous system.

In summary, the testes are the site of spermatogenesis and the production of testosterone. The spermatozoa that are released from the testes must undergo a process of maturation in the duct system before ejaculation.

EPIDIDYMIDES

As the initial part of the excretory duct system of the testis, an *epididymis* lies posterior to each testis (Figure 4–5). Consisting of a head, body, and tail, the epididymis is about 5.6 m long, although it is convoluted into a compact structure about 3.75 cm long. The head sits on top of the superior aspect of the testis, firmly attached to it by the efferent ductules. The body, made up of the tightly coiled portion, descends posteriorly along the testis. The tail narrows slightly, becomes less convoluted with a wider lumen, and turns back on itself to become the vas deferens (discussed in the next section).

The tail of the epididymis provides a reservoir where spermatozoa can survive for a long period of time. The secretory epithelium of the epididymis provides a nutritional fluid for the maturing sperm. When discharged from the seminiferous tubules into the epididymis, the sperm are immotile and incapable of fertilizing an ovum. The spermatozoa remain in the epididymis for 2–10 days, until the process of maturation is complete.

VAS DEFERENS

The *vas deferens*, also known as the *ductus deferens,* is about 40 cm long and connects the epididymal lumen with the prostatic urethra. One vas deferens ascends the posterior border of each testis (Figure 4–5). It joins the spermatic cord, passing through the inguinal canal and entering the abdominal cavity. The vas deferens passes over the bladder, and between the ureter and the posterior surface of the bladder, then bends medially along the seminal vesicle until it meets the vas deferens from the opposite side. Turning downward to the base of the prostate gland, it forms the ejaculatory duct as it joins the duct from the seminal vesicle. Prior to its entrance into the prostate, the vas deferens becomes enlarged and tortuous. This enlargement is called the *terminal ampulla* and serves as the primary storehouse for spermatozoa and tubule secretions.

The vas deferens can be divided into five portions: the sheathless epididymal portion within the tunica vaginalis; the scrotal portion; the inguinal portion; the retroperitoneal or pelvic portion; and the ampulla. The scrotal portion is usually the surgical site of a vasectomy, the male sterilization procedure.

The three layers of smooth muscle that make up the vas deferens are the middle circular and the outer and inner longitudinal layers. The duct is capable of vigorous peristaltic motion. The ductal lumen is lined with epithelium lying on a basement membrane. Thick connective tissue surrounds the muscle layers.

Stored sperm remain relatively immotile, although mature. No doubt this is because of the metabolic production of carbon dioxide by the sperm, creating an acidic environment that inhibits motility. Also, the vas deferens secretions do not provide high-energy nutrients, which can be metabolized into lactic acid (Odell and Moyer, 1971).

Innervation is through the hypogastric plexus of the autonomic nervous system. There are pain receptors in the sheath of the vas deferens in the scrotal portion.

The spermatic cord is made up of the vas deferens and the pampiniform plexus of veins, arteries, lymphatic vessels, and nerves. Held together by connective tissue, this cord extends from the tail of the epididymis to the abdominal inguinal ring and is enclosed by the cremaster muscle and layers of fascia issuing from the abdominal wall.

EJACULATORY DUCTS

The vas deferens and a seminal vesicle duct unite to form the *ejaculatory duct.* Each of the two ejaculatory ducts enters the posterior surface of the prostate gland. After a distance of about 2.5 cm, they terminate in the prostatic urethra. These ducts serve as passageways for semen and for fluid secreted by the seminal vesicles.

URETHRA

The male urethra is a common passageway for urine and semen. The epithelium tissue throughout the urethra is specific to the urethral section.

The urethra begins a little posterior to the midpoint of the inferior aspect of the bladder and courses through the prostate gland, where it is called the *prostatic urethra.* The surrounding connective tissue is highly vascular and contains glands, elastic fibers, and smooth muscles arranged in an inner longitudinal layer and an outer circular layer. These circular fibers form the internal urethral sphincter.

The urethra emerges from the prostate gland to become the *membranous urethra.* As it passes through the urogenital diaphragm, skeletal muscle fibers form the external urethral sphincter.

The *spongy urethra* is contained in the corpus spongiosum penis. In the penile urethra, discussed on p. 60, goblet secretory cells are present, and smooth muscle is replaced by erectile tissue.

Accessory Glands

SEMINAL VESICLES

The *seminal vesicles* are two lobulated glands, each about 7.5 cm long, situated between the bladder and rectum and immediately superior to the base of the prostate. A fold of peritoneum forming the rectovesical pouch separates them from the rectum, and nerves are supplied from the hypogastric plexus. Secretory columnar epithelium lines the diverticula of the seminal vesicles and secretes an alkaline, viscid, clear fluid rich in high-energy fructose, prostaglandins, fibrinogen, and proteins that becomes mixed with the sperm during ejaculation. This fluid assists in providing an environment favorable to optimal sperm motility and metabolism. It is believed that prostaglandins aid fertilization (Guyton, 1981) while fibrinogen increases the viscosity of the semen.

PROSTATE GLAND

The *prostate gland* surrounds the upper part of the urethra and lies inferior to the neck of the urinary bladder and superior to the fascia of the urogenital diaphragm. Made up of several lobes, it measures about 4 cm in diameter and weighs 20–30 g. A dense capsule of muscle fibers encloses this gland, which is made up of both glandular and muscular tissue.

The two ejaculatory ducts are located between the middle and lateral lobes of the prostate gland and join the prostatic urethra.

Prostatic glandular tissue consists of 30 to 50 branched tubular glands with ducts opening into the prostatic urethra. There are mucosal, submucosal, and external (main) glands. The mucosal glands are the smallest and frequently hypertrophy in older men, causing urinary distress because of pressure on the prostatic urethra. The submucosal glands circle the mucosal glands, and the external glands form the major portion of the prostate.

The prostate secretes a thin, milky, slightly acidic fluid (pH 6.5) containing high levels of zinc, calcium, citric acid, and acid phosphatase. The daily secretion averages 4–6 mL. This fluid protects the sperm from the acidic environment of the female vagina and male urethra (Polakoski et al., 1976). The enzyme fibrinolysin, capable of dissolving fibrin, is also present. Unlike the seminal vesicle ejaculate, the prostate fluid does not contain fructose (Eliasson and Lindholmer, 1976).

BULBOURETHRAL AND URETHRAL GLANDS

The *bulbourethral or Cowper's glands* are a pair of small round lobulated structures within the urogenital diaphragm on either side of the membranous urethra. Each gland, about 1 cm in diameter, has a terminal excretory duct, about 2.5 cm long, opening into the base of the corpus spongiosum penis. These glands secrete a clear, viscous, alkaline fluid rich in mucoproteins that becomes part of the seminal plasma. It is thought that this secretion also lubricates the penile urethra during sexual excitement as well as neutralizing the acid in the male urethra and female vagina, thereby enhancing sperm motility.

The *urethral or Littre's glands* are tiny mucous-secreting glands found throughout the membranous lining of the penile urethra. Their secretions add to those of the bulbourethral glands.

In summary, the male accessory glands are specialized structures under endocrine and neural control. Each secretes a unique and essential component of the total seminal plasma in an ordered sequence. The continuing study of the physiology of these ejaculates will lead to an increased understanding of male fertility and infertility and to potential methods of modifying both.

Semen

The male ejaculate *semen* is made up of spermatozoa and seminal plasma, which is composed of the secretions of the accessory sex glands in a specific pattern. Seminal fluid contains the greatest level of prostaglandins in the entire male body (Caldwell and Behrman, 1981). The bulbourethral and urethral glands, prostate, epididymides, and seminal vesicles contribute components to the seminal plasma, which serves to transport viable and motile sperm to the female reproductive tract. Effective transportation of sperm requires adequate nutrients, a pH of 7.2–7.8, a specific concentration of sperm to fluid, and an optimal osmolarity (Polakoski et al., 1976). While prostaglandins are thought by many investigators to be essential to sperm transport, there is no consensus that the seminal level of prostaglandins directly relates to sperm activity (Caldwell and Behrman, 1981).

Sperm may be stored in the male genital system for a period of several hours to 42 days, depending primarily on the frequency of ejaculations. The average volume of ejaculate following continence for several days is 2–5 mL but may vary from 1–10 mL. Repeated ejaculation results in decreased volume.

The chemical composition of semen is complex and still under investigation. Over 60 components have been identified. Semen tends to clot and then liquefies in about 15 minutes. This liquefaction is thought to be due to the presence of fibrinolysin.

Once deposited in the female vagina, sperm travel at about 3 mm/min through the female genital tract. Sperm transport is complex and is discussed further in Chapter 8.

A spermatozoon is made up of a head and a tail that is divided into the middle piece, principal piece, and endpiece (Figure 4–6). The head's main components are the acrosome, nucleus, and nuclear vacuoles. The head carries the haploid number of chromosomes (23), and it is the part that enters the egg at fertilization (Chapter 8). The tail, or flagellum, is uniquely specialized for optimal motility in each of its parts. Figure 4–7 shows a scanning electron micrograph of human spermatozoa.

Breasts

Although the male breast remains dormant throughout the life span (Donovan, 1977), it is a site of sexual arousal and pleasure for the male. Given no particular sexual connotation in American society, male breasts are bared without notice. They can provide exquisite sensation if stimulated during sexual activity. Such stimulation is frequently accompanied by spontaneous erection of the penis.

Occasionally, bilateral or unilateral gynecomastia will occur during adolescence. This hypertrophy of rudimentary mammary tissue occurs in response to increased hormonal levels and may cause embarrassment. If spontaneous remission does not occur, reduction surgery usually achieves excellent cosmetic and psychologic results (Donovan, 1977).

Less than 1% of all breast cancer in the United States occurs in men (Urban, 1977). Inspection of the breasts for dimpling, discharge, inverted nipples, or other unusual changes should be routine, and abnormalities should be investigated immediately.

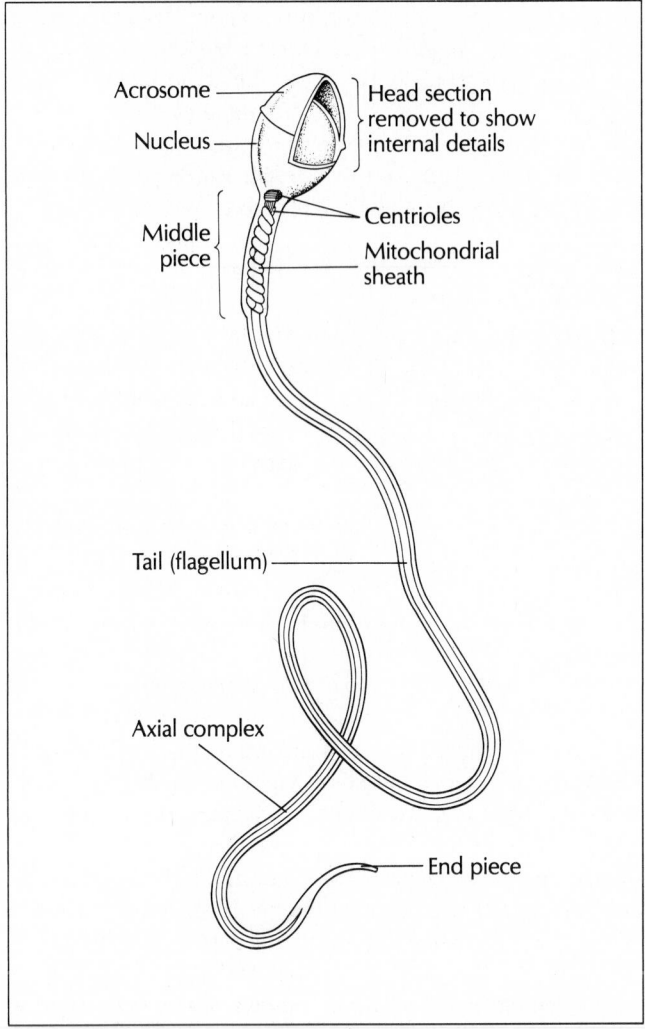

FIGURE 4–6 Schematic representation of mature spermatozoon.

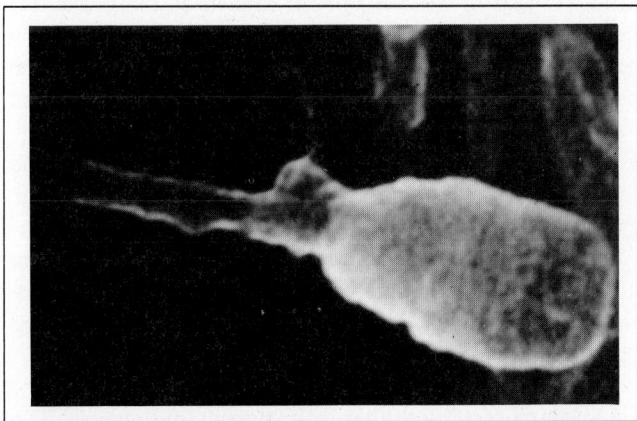

FIGURE 4–7 Scanning electron micrograph of human spermatozoa. (Courtesy Dr. Landrum B. Shettles.)

FEMALE REPRODUCTIVE SYSTEM

The female reproductive system consists of the external and internal genitals and the accessory organs of the breasts, or mammary glands. Also important to the female system is the bony pelvis with its structures, which have important obstetric implications.

Bony Pelvis

In addition to supporting the weight of the upper torso and distributing it to the lower body, the female *bony pelvis* has the unique functions of supporting and protecting the pelvic contents as well as forming the relatively fixed axis of the birth passage. For these reasons, structural aspects of the pelvis important to childbearing must be understood clearly.

BONY STRUCTURE

The pelvis, which resembles a bowl or basin, is made up of four bones: two innominate bones (os coxae), the sacrum, and the coccyx. The innominate or hip bones comprise the anterior and lateral framework, and the sacrum and coccyx provide the posterior section. Lined with fibrocartilage and held tightly together by ligaments, the four bones articulate at the symphysis pubis, the two sacroiliac joints, and the sacrococcygeal joints (Figure 4–8).

The *innominate bones* are made up of three separate bones whose junctions are calcified at puberty: the ilium, the ischium, and the pubis. The fusion of these bones forms an articular circular cavity, the *acetabulum*, which articulates with the head of the femur.

The *ilium*, which makes up a large portion of the acetabulum, is the broad upper part of the innominate bone. Its anterior prominence, palpated as the foremost angle of the innominate bone, is the anterior iliac spine. The iliac crest extends backward and is convex, thickened, and rough.

The *ischium* is the strongest bone and is inferior to the ilium and below the acetabulum. It consists of a body and a ramus. The ramus joins the inferior ramus of the pubis. At its posterior point the ischium terminates in a marked protuberance, the ischial tuberosity, upon which the weight of the body rests when in a seated position. The ischial spines arise from the posterior border of the ischium and jut into the pelvic cavity. Between the ischial spines is the shortest diameter of the pelvic cavity. The ischial spines can be palpated during rectal or vaginal examination, and they can serve as a guide during labor to evaluate the descent of the fetal head into the birth canal.

The *pubis* consists of a superior ramus, body, and inferior ramus and forms the slightly bowed anterior portion of the innominate bone. It contributes to the anteromedial one-fifth of the acetabulum. The ischial and pubic inferior

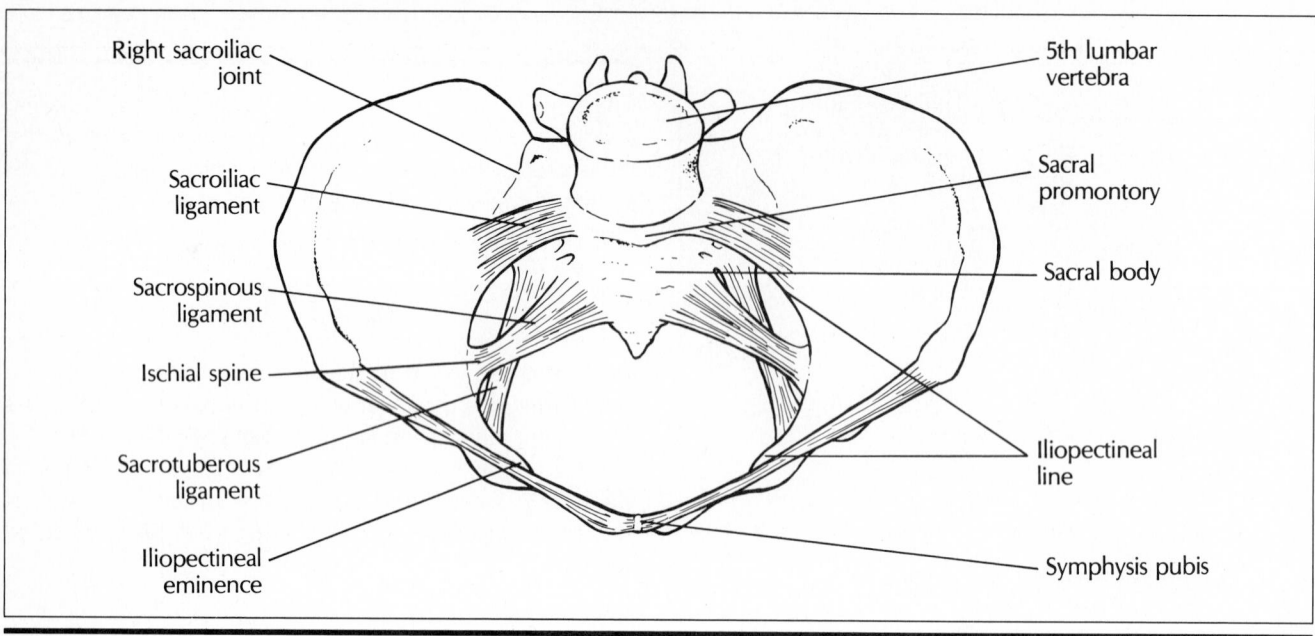

Right sacroiliac joint

Sacroiliac ligament

Sacrospinous ligament

Ischial spine

Sacrotuberous ligament

Iliopectineal eminence

5th lumbar vertebra

Sacral promontory

Sacral body

Iliopectineal line

Symphysis pubis

FIGURE 4–8 Bony pelvis with ligaments.

rami form a large triangular aperture, the *obturator fora-men*, in the lower half of the hip bone. A strong membrane of thin fibrous tissue is attached to its boundary. The pubis extends medially from the acetabulum to the midpoint of the bony pelvis, where it forms the symphysis pubis at its junction with the other pubis. The triangular space below this junction is known as the pubic arch. The baby's head passes under this arch during birth. The symphysis pubis is formed by heavy fibrocartilage and the superior and inferior pubic ligaments, with the latter designated as the *arcuate pubic ligament*. The mobility of the arcuate pubic ligament increases during pregnancy and to a greater extent in mul-tiparas than in primigravidas.

The sacroiliac joints also have a degree of mobility that increases at term as the result of an upward gliding move-ment. The pelvic outlet may be increased by 1.5–2 cm in the dorsal lithotomy position. These relaxations of the joints are induced by the hormones of pregnancy.

The *sacrum*, a wedge-shaped bone formed by the fu-sion of five vertebras, becomes smaller toward the inferior portion. On the anterior upper portion of the body of the first sacral vertebra is a marked projection into the pelvic cavity, known as the *sacral promontory*, that can be palpat-ed vaginally and is another obstetric guide in determining pelvic measurements. The inner surface of the sacrum is concave in both the lateral and vertical aspects.

The *coccyx*, a small triangular bone that is the last on the vertebral column, is formed by the union of four rudi-mentary vertebras. Its course is downward and slightly for-ward from the lower sacral border, and it articulates with the sacrum at the sacrococcygeal joint. Generally, there is

an intervertebral disk between the sacrum and the coccyx. In its absence, the two bones are partially or completely fused together, making them immovable. The coccyx usu-ally moves backward during labor to provide the fetus with more room.

PELVIC FLOOR

A complementary structure of the bony pelvis is its muscu-lar *pelvic floor* which is designed to overcome the force of gravity exerted on the pelvic viscera and, to a lesser ex-tent, on the abdominal viscera. It acts as a buttress to the irregularly shaped pelvic outlet, thereby providing stability and support for surrounding structures and organs.

Deep fascia and the levator ani and coccygeal muscles form the part of the pelvic floor known as the *pelvic dia-phragm*. Superior to it is the pelvic cavity; inferior and posterior to it is the *perineum*. Laterally, the walls of the pelvis are composed of the obturator internus muscles and fascia which form a band called the arcus tendineus. The sacrum is located posteriorly. Lateral and anterior to the sacrum are the many nerves of the sacral plexus, also cov-ered with parietal pelvic fascia.

The sheetlike *levator ani muscle* makes up the major portion of the pelvic diaphragm and consists of four mus-cles: ileococcygeus, pubococcygeus, puborectalis, and pubovaginalis.

Forming a sling for the pelvic structures, the levator ani is interrupted by the urethra, vagina, and rectum. The coccygeal muscle is a thin muscular sheet overlying the sacrospinous ligament and assists the levator ani in giving support to the abdominal and pelvic viscera (Figure 4–8).

Table 4–1 Muscles of the Pelvic Floor

Muscle	Origin	Insertion	Innervation	Action
Levator ani	Pubis, lateral pelvic wall, and ischiadic spine	Blends with organs in pelvic cavity	Inferior rectal, second and third sacral nerves, plus anterior rami of third and fourth sacral nerves	Supports pelvic viscera; helps form pelvic diaphragm
Iliococcygeus	Pelvic surface of ischial spine and pelvic fascia	Central point of perineum, coccygeal raphe, and coccyx		
Puboccocygeus	Pubis and pelvic fascia	Coccyx		
Puborectalis	Pubis	Blends with rectum; meets similar fibers from opposite side		Forms sling for rectum, just posterior to it; raises anus
Pubovaginalis	Pubis	Blends into vagina		Supports vagina
Coccygeus	Ischial spine and sacrospinous ligament	Lateral border of lower sacrum and upper coccyx	Third and fourth sacral nerves	Supports pelvic viscera; helps form pelvic diaphragm; flexes and abducts coccyx

The origins, insertions, innervations, and actions of these muscles are presented in Table 4–1.

Endopelvic fascia covers the pelvic diaphragm. Benson (1976) points out that these component parts function as a whole, yet are able to move over one another. This provides an exceptional capacity for dilatation during parturition and involution in the puerperium (Figure 4–9).

The *urogenital triangle* (diaphragm) is external to the pelvic diaphragm, in the triangular area between the ischial tuberosities and the hollow of the pubic arch. It is made up of superficial and deep perineal membranes extending from the rami of the ischial and pubic bones. Most important in this region are the deep transverse perineal muscles, which are flat bands of muscle arising from the ischiopubic rami and intertwining in the midline to form a seam, or raphe. These muscles are modified to encircle both the urinary meatus and the vaginal orifice, forming the urethral and vaginal sphincters.

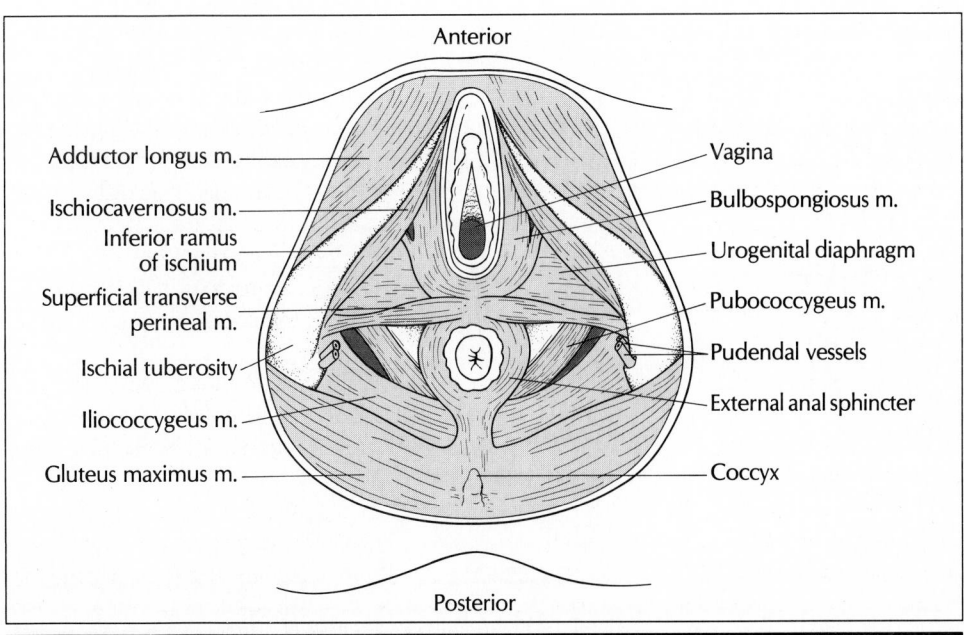

FIGURE 4–9 Muscles of the pelvic floor.

The ischiocavernosus and bulbocavernosus are the muscles of the external genitals and form external coverings for the vestibular bulbs and crus of the clitoris. The fibers of the bulbocavernous muscle do not articulate with each other on either side of the vagina; they are separate.

PELVIC DIVISION

The pelvic cavity is divided into the false pelvis and the true pelvis (Figure 4–10,A).

False pelvis. The false pelvis, also known as the *major* or *greater pelvis*, is the portion above the pelvic brim, or linea terminalis, bounded by the lumbar vertebras posteriorly, the iliac fossae laterally, and the lower abdominal wall anteriorly. Its functions are to support the weight of the enlarged pregnant uterus and to direct the presenting fetal part into the true pelvis below.

True pelvis. The true pelvis, also called the *minor* or *lesser pelvis*, lies below the pelvic brim and is bounded superiorly by the promontory and alae of the sacrum and the upper margins of the pubic bones and inferiorly by the pelvic outlet. The true pelvis represents the bony limits of the birth canal. It measures about 5 cm at its anterior wall at the symphysis pubis and about 10 cm at its posterior wall. When a woman is standing upright, the upper portion of the pelvic cavity or canal is directed downward and backward and its lower portion, downward and forward. This forms an axis or curved canal through which the presenting part of the baby must pass during birth (Figure 4–10,B). The inclination of the pelvis is the angle formed by two planes, a horizontal one through the tip of the coccyx and the superior border of the symphysis pubis and an inclined one through the sacral promontory and the superior border of the symphysis pubis. This pelvic angle of inclination usually measures 50°–60° (Figure 4–11).

The bony circumference of the true pelvis is made up of the sacrum, coccyx, and innominate bones below the linea terminalis. This area is of paramount importance in obstetrics because its size and shape must be adequate for normal fetal passage during labor and at delivery. The relationship of the fetal head to this cavity is of critical importance.

The true pelvis is considered to have three parts: the inlet, the pelvic cavity, and the outlet. The pelvic planes are imaginary flat surfaces drawn across the three parts of the true pelvis at strategic levels (Figure 4–12). Associated with each part are distinct obstetric measurements that aid in the evaluation of the adequacy of the pelvis for childbearing:

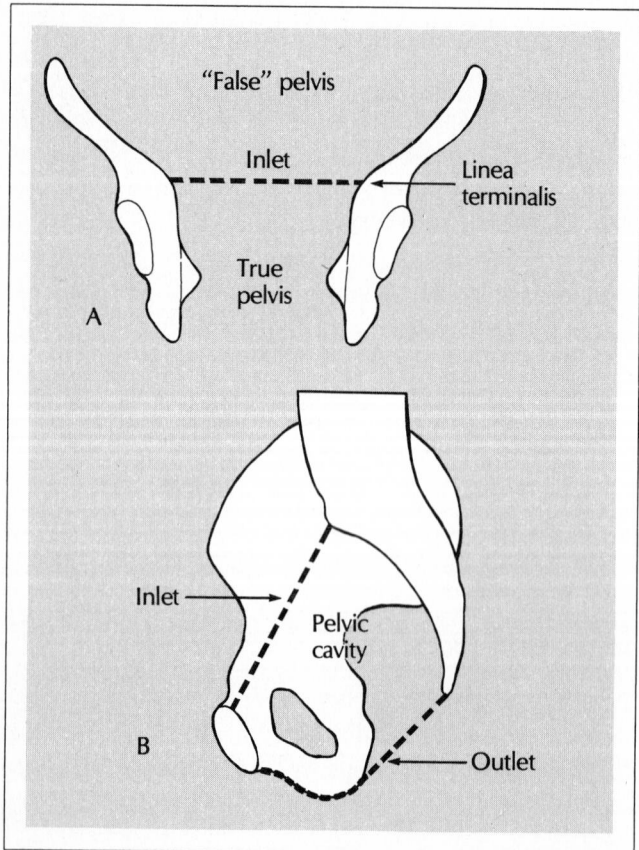

FIGURE 4–10 Female pelvis. **A,** False and true pelves. **B,** Pelvic cavity.

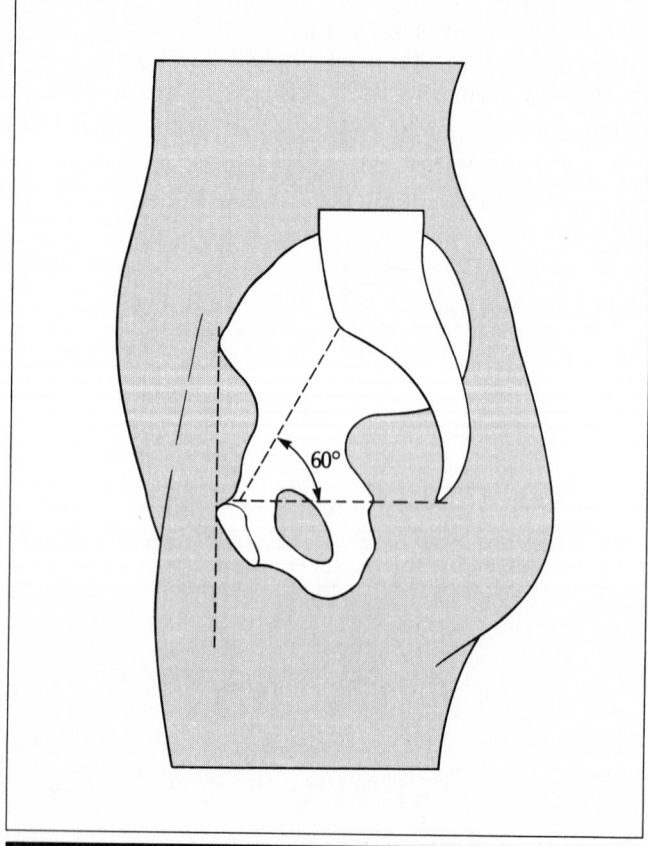

FIGURE 4–11 Pelvic angle of inclination while woman is standing.

A. Pelvic inlet
  1. Anteroposterior diameters
    a. True conjugate
    b. Obstetric conjugate
    c. Diagonal conjugate
  2. Transverse diameter
  3. Right and left oblique diameters
B. Pelvic cavity
  1. Plane of greatest dimensions
  2. Plane of least dimensions
    a. Anteroposterior diameter
    b. Transverse (interspinous) diameter
    c. Posterior sagittal diameter
C. Pelvic outlet
  1. Anteroposterior diameters
    a. Anatomic
    b. Obstetric
  2. Transverse (intertuberous) diameter
  3. Anterior sagittal diameter
  4. Posterior sagittal diameter

The dimensions of the true pelvis and their obstetric implications are described here. Measurement techniques are discussed in Chapter 14. The effects of inadequate or abnormal pelvic diameters on labor and delivery are further considered in Chapter 18.

The *pelvic inlet,* also referred to as the *superior strait,* is the upper border of the true pelvis and is bounded posteriorly by the promontory and alae of the sacrum, laterally by the linea terminalis, and anteriorly by the upper margins of the pubic bones and symphysis pubis. The female pelvic inlet is typically round.

The anteroposterior, transverse, and right and left oblique diameters of the inlet are of obstetric importance (Figure 4–13). The anteroposterior diameter is the distance between the symphysis pubis and the sacrum. It is the shortest of the inlet diameters and therefore the most significant, because its inadequacy is the most common cause of inlet contraction. The true (anatomic) conjugate, or conjugata vera, extends from the middle of the sacral promontory to the middle of the pubic crest (superior surface of the symphysis).

The obstetric conjugate extends from the middle of the sacral promontory to the posterosuperior margin of the symphysis, or about 1 cm below the pubic crest. In reality, it is through this diameter that the fetus must pass, and its size determines whether engagement of the fetal head will occur upon entering the superior strait.

The diagonal conjugate extends from the subpubic angle to the middle of the sacral promontory. The transverse diameter is the largest diameter of the inlet and is measured from one side to the other using the lineae terminales as the points of reference. This diameter assists in determining the shape of the inlet. It and the true conjugate lie at right angles to each other.

The suboccipitobregmatic diameter of the fetal head (see Chapter 14) usually presents parallel to the transverse diameter because it is longer than the anteroposterior diameter. If the transverse or anteroposterior diameter is too short, the baby's head cannot enter the pelvis.

The right oblique diameter extends from the right sacroiliac joint to the left linea terminalis eminence. The right and left oblique diameters have the same measurement.

Occasional mention is made of the posterior sagittal

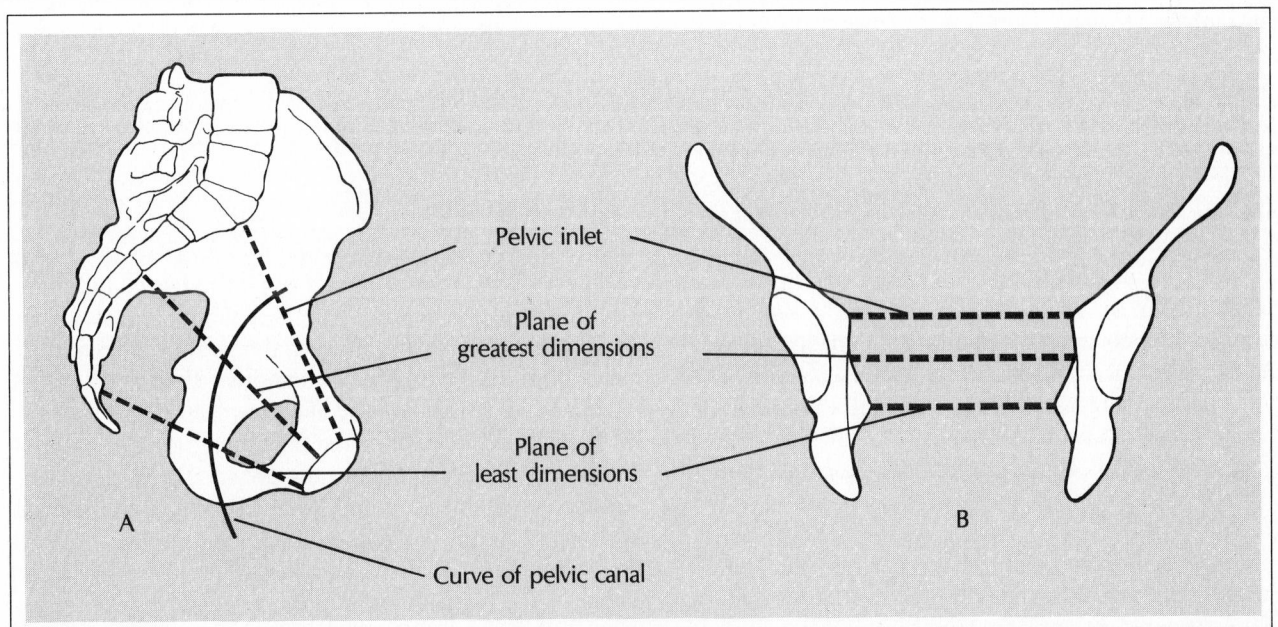

FIGURE 4–12 Pelvic planes. **A,** Sagittal section. **B,** Coronal section.

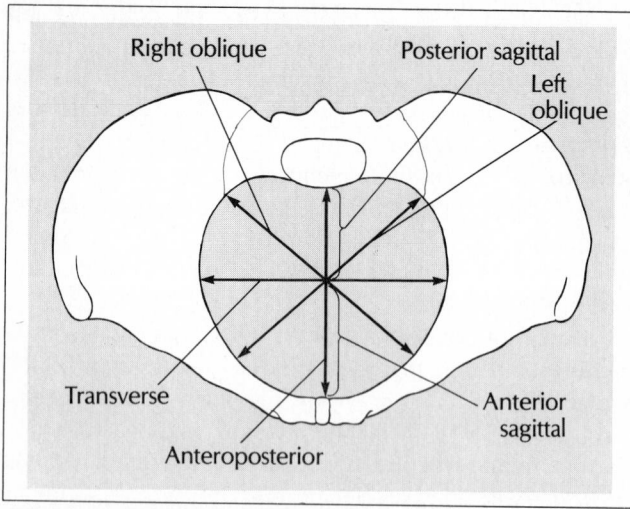

FIGURE 4–13 Diameters of pelvic inlet.

diameter, which extends from the intersection of the anteroposterior and transverse diameters to the middle of the sacral promontory (Figure 4–13).

The *pelvic cavity* (canal) has varying diameters. The largest part of the pelvis is called the *plane of the greatest dimensions* (Figure 4–12). It is bounded by the junction of the second and third sacral vertebras posteriorly, the upper and middle thirds of the obturator foramen laterally, and the midpoint of the posterior surface of the pubis anteriorly. It is a curved canal with a longer posterior than anterior wall. A change in the lumbar curve can increase or decrease the pelvic inclination and can influence the progress of labor, because the fetus has to adjust itself to a curved path as well as to the different diameters of the true pelvis (Figure 4–10,A).

The smallest part of the pelvis is called the *plane of the least dimensions*, or the midpelvic plane (Figure 4–12). Arrest of labor occurs most frequently because of contracture in this plane, so its diameters are of great importance. The plane extends from the lower margin of the symphysis pubis, through the ischial spines, to the junction of the fourth and fifth sacral vertebras. Its anterior and posterior borders are bounded by the lower margin of the symphysis pubis, and fascia covering the obturator foramen, the ischial spines, the sacrospinous ligaments, and the sacrum. The anteroposterior diameter extends from the lower margin of the symphysis pubis to the junction of the fourth and fifth sacral vertebras. The transverse (interspinous) diameter extends between the ischial spines and measures about 10.5 cm; it is the shortest pelvic diameter. The posterior sagittal diameter extends from the bispinous diameter to the junction of the fourth and fifth sacral vertebras (Figure 4–13). At the midpelvic plane, the curve of the pelvic canal begins, and the axis of the birth canal changes. The

fetal head, until it reaches the ischial spines, descends in a straight line. Then it curves forward toward the pelvic outlet (Figure 4–12A).

The *pelvic outlet*, also called the *inferior strait*, is at the lower border of the true pelvis. It can be thought of as being composed of two triangles with a common base but in different planes. The common base as well as the most inferior part is the transverse diameter between the ischial tuberosities. The anterior triangle has as its apex the lower margin of the symphysis pubis, and the posterior triangle, the tip of the sacrum (Figure 4–12).

The anteroposterior diameter extends from the inferior margin of the symphysis to the tip of the coccyx. This is the anatomic diameter. The obstetric anteroposterior diameter extends to the sacrococcygeal joint (see Chapter 15). The anteroposterior diameter increases during delivery as the presenting part pushes the coccyx posteriorly at the mobile sacrococcygeal joint. Decreased mobility, a large fetal head, and/or a forceful delivery can cause the coccyx to snap. As the infant's head emerges, the long diameter of the head (occipital frontal) parallels the long diameter of the outlet (anteroposterior).

The transverse diameter (bi-ischial or intertuberous) extends from the inner surface of one ischial tuberosity to the other. It is the shortest diameter of the pelvic outlet and becomes shorter as the pubic arch narrows. The anterior sagittal diameter extends from the middle of the transverse diameter to the suprapubic angle. The posterior sagittal diameter extends from the middle of the transverse diameter to the sacrococcygeal junction. This is the most significant diameter of the outlet because it is the smallest diameter through which the infant must pass as it descends through the pelvic canal. The pubic arch has great importance, because the baby must pass under it. If it is narrow, the baby's head may be pushed backward toward the coccyx, making the extension of the head difficult. This situation is known as *outlet dystocia*, and forceps (outlet) delivery is required.

TYPES OF PELVES

The Caldwell-Moloy classification of pelves is widely used to differentiate types of bony pelves (Caldwell and Moloy, 1933). Gynecoid, android, anthropoid, and platypelloid are the four basic types. However, variations in the female pelvis from plane to plane are so great that classic types are not usual. An imaginary line drawn through the greatest transverse diameter of the inlet divides it into anterior and posterior segments, and the pelvis type is always determined on the basis of the posterior segment of the inlet. With the posterior segment determining the type, the anterior segment of the inlet names variations. For example, an android pelvis with an anthropoid variation means that the posterior segment of the inlet is android and the anterior segment is anthropoid. These four types of pelvis are de-

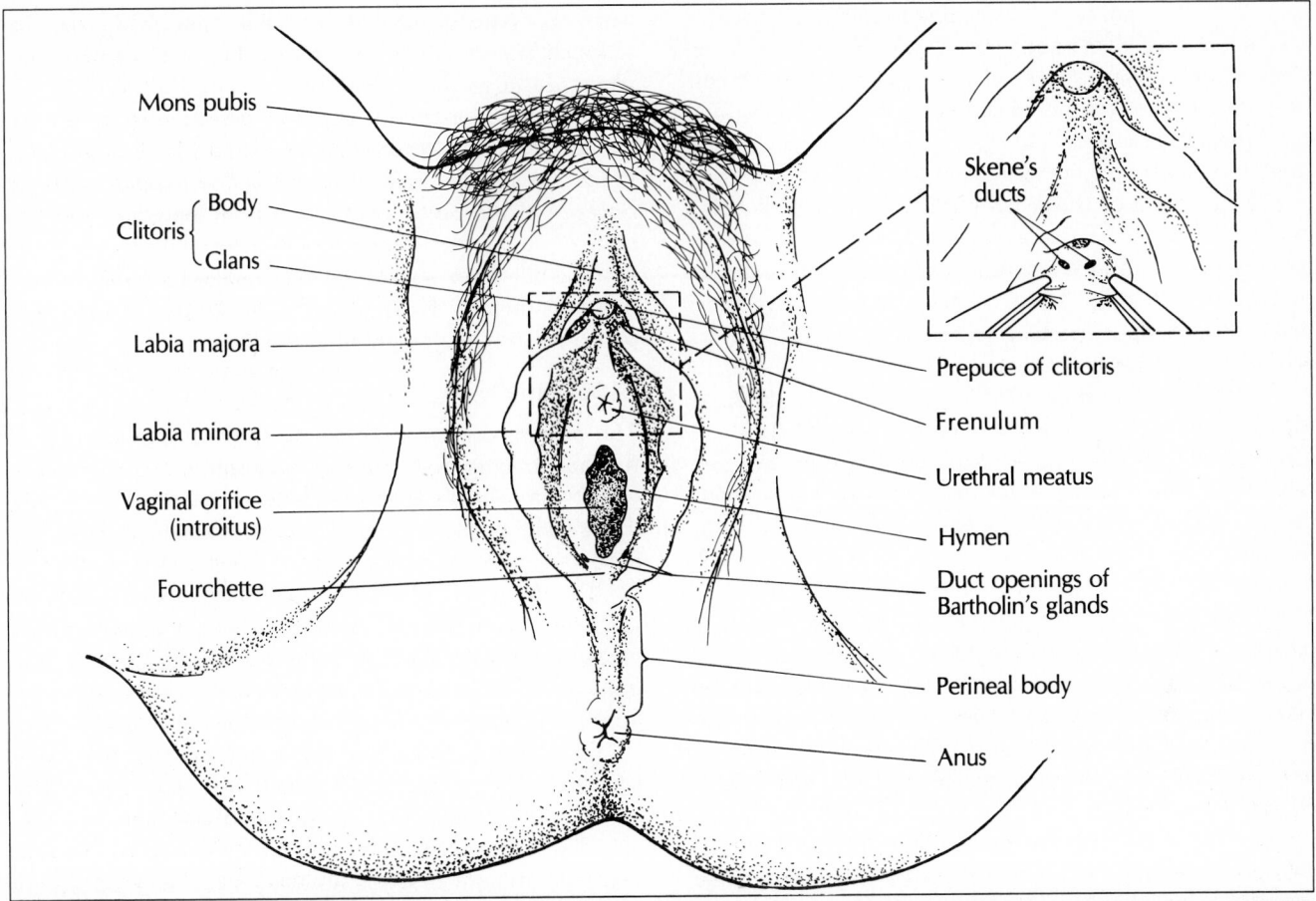

FIGURE 4–14 Female external genitals, longitudinal view.

scribed further in Chapter 14. Each type has certain implications for labor and delivery, which are discussed in Chapter 18.

External Genitals

The female external genitals, referred to as the *vulva* or *pudendum,* include the following structures (Figure 4–14):

1. Mons pubis
2. Labia majora
3. Labia minora
4. Clitoris
5. Urethral meatus and paraurethral (Skene's) glands
6. Vaginal vestibule
   a. Vaginal orifice
   b. Vulvovaginal (Bartholin's) glands
   c. Hymen
   d. Fossa navicularis
7. Perineal body

Although not true parts of the female reproductive system, the urethral meatus and the perineal body will also be considered here because of their proximity and relationship to the vulva. All the external reproductive organs except the glandular structures can be directly inspected.

A composite structure, the vulva is a functional unit. Its organs, targets for estrogenic hormones throughout a woman's life (Beller et al., 1980), are endowed with a generous blood supply and complex innervation. With advancing age and decreased hormonal activity, these organs atrophy and are subject to a variety of lesions.

The size, color, and shape of these structures vary extensively among races and individuals. Racial characteristics, body size, and patterns of pigmentation all influence their appearance (Benson, 1976).

MONS PUBIS

A softly rounded mound of subcutaneous fatty tissue beginning at the lowest portion of the anterior abdominal wall, the *mons pubis* (also known as the *mons veneris*) covers the anterior portion of the symphysis pubis (Figure 4–14). It is covered with hair in a typically female pubic pattern of distribution, with the hairline forming a transverse line across the lower abdomen. Approximately 75% of women display this pattern. The remaining 25% have hair extending toward the umbilicus along the linea alba. The hair is short and varies from sparse and fine in the Oriental woman to heavy, coarse, and curly in the black woman.

The function of the mons pubis is threefold. It helps protect the pelvic bones, especially during coitus. It contributes to the rounded contours of the feminine body. And finally, although it has no actual reproductive function, the mons appears to be sensually important (Masters and Johnson, 1966).

Because of the amount of loose connective tissue in the mons pubis, the incidence of edema is high relative to its occurrence in other parts of the body (Bloom and Van Dongen, 1972). During pregnancy, edema of the mons may accompany severe preeclampsia–eclampsia.

LABIA MAJORA

The *labia majora* are longitudinal raised folds of deeply pigmented skin, one on either side of the vulval cleft (Figure 4–14). As the pair descend, they narrow, enclosing the vulval cleft, and merge posteriorly to form the posterior commissure of the perineal skin. The *vulval cleft* includes the clitoris, urethral meatus, vaginal vestibule, and vaginal orifice.

The labia majora are homologues of the unfused halves of the scrotum. With each pregnancy they become less prominent, so that in multiparous women they may be obliterated as distinct structures. The labia majora are covered by stratified squamous epithelium containing hair follicles and sebaceous glands with underlying adipose and muscle tissue. Immediately under the skin is a sheet of dartos muscle called the *dartos muliebris,* which is responsible for the wrinkled appearance of the labia majora as well as for their sensitivity to heat and cold.

The subcutaneous tissues of the labia majora contain a great deal of loose connective tissue, which, as with the mons pubis, partially explains why edema occurs to a greater extent here than in any other part of the body, except the eyelids (Bloom and Van Dongen, 1972).

Arterial blood is supplied by the internal and external pudendal arteries, with numerous anastomoses. The venous drainage is composed of an extensive plexus in the area, in communication with the veins of the clitoris, labia minora, and perineum. Because of the extensive venous network in the labia majora, varicosities may occur during pregnancy, and obstetric or sexual trauma may cause hematomas of these structures.

The lymphatics of the labia majora are shared with other related structures of the vulva. They are extensive, diffuse, and a key to understanding malignancies of the female reproductive organs.

The labia majora are supplied with an extensive network of nerve endings that make them extremely sensitive to touch, pressure, pain, and temperature. The nerves supplying the area are mainly from the central nervous system: the anterior third is supplied primarily from the first lumbar segment of the spinal cord, and the posterior two-thirds are supplied mainly from the third sacral segment. Because of the central nervous system innervation of this area, certain regional anesthesia blocks will affect it.

The chief function of the labia majora is protection of the components of the vulval cleft. Similar to the mons pubis, they have a potential erotic function.

LABIA MINORA

The *labia minora,* or nymphae, are soft folds of skin within the labia majora that converge both inferiorly and posteriorly (Figure 4–14). The labia minora are homologues of the unfused penile urethra of the male. Maldevelopment or fusion suggests anomalous sexual differentiation.

Toward their upper extremity each labium minus divides into two lamellas. The upper two merge to form the prepuce of the clitoris, and the lower pair fuse to form the frenulum of the clitoris. Inferiorly the labia minora unite to form the *fourchette,* a fold of skin below the vaginal orifice.

Each labium minus has the appearance of shiny mucous membrane, moist and devoid of hair follicles. The labium minus is covered with stratified squamous epithelium, devoid of hair follicles but rich in sebaceous glands. The labia minora tissue is erectile, containing loose connective tissue, blood vessels, numerous large venous spaces, and involuntary muscle tissue. Because the sebaceous glands do not open into hair follicles but directly onto the surface of the skin, sebaceous cysts commonly occur in this area. Vulvovaginitis in this area is very irritating because of the many tactile nerve endings.

The functions of the labia minora are to lubricate and waterproof the vulvar skin, to provide bactericidal secretions, and to heighten sexual arousal and pleasure.

CLITORIS

The *clitoris* is the most erotically sensitive part of the genital tract and is known to many females early in life as the site of masturbation. The term is derived from the Greek word *cleitoris,* meaning "key"; the ancients perceived it as the key to female sexuality. The clitoris is homologous to the male penis and is sometimes called the *penis muliebris,* or penis of woman (Bloom and Van Dongen, 1972). However, it contains no corpus spongiosum or urethral meatus.

The clitoris is at the anterior juncture of the labia minora (Figure 4–14), which form the prepuce anteriorly and the frenulum posteriorly. The clitoris consists of the glans, the corpus or body, and two crura. The glans is partially covered by the prepuce at the distal end, and this area often appears as an opening to an orifice. Attempts to insert a catheter here produce extreme discomfort.

Visible between the folds of the labia minora, the clitoris is about 5–6 mm in length and 6–8 mm in diameter. Its tissue is essentially erectile, because of the large amounts of involuntary smooth muscle surrounding numerous venous channels. The clitoris has exceedingly rich blood and nerve supplies.

Clitoral innervation is through the terminal branch of the pudendal nerve, which lies next to the dorsal artery. Its branches terminate in the glans and prepuce. Heightened clitoral sensation may be dependent on an abundance of Dogiel, Krause, and Ruffini corpuscles (specialized genital receptor nerve endings). The incidence of free nerve endings is thought to be most prevalent in the prepuce of the clitoris (Benson, 1976). Overall, the clitoris is endowed with a nerve supply more plentiful than that of the male penis.

The clitoris exists primarily for female sexual enjoyment. In addition, it produces smegma. Along with other vulval secretions, smegma has a unique odor that may be erotically stimulating to the male.

URETHRAL MEATUS AND PARAURETHRAL GLANDS

The *urethral meatus* is 1–2.5 cm beneath the clitoris in the midline of the vestibule (Figure 4–14). At times the meatus is difficult to see because of the presence of blind dimples, small mucosal folds, or wide variance in location. Its appearance is often puckered and slitlike.

The *paraurethral glands*, or *Skene's ducts*, open into the posterior wall of the female urethra close to its orifice (Figure 4–14). The paraurethral glands are homologous to the male prostate glands. Skene's ducts can become infected with gonococcus.

VAGINAL VESTIBULE

The *vaginal vestibule* is a remnant of the urogenital sinus of the embryo. It is bordered anteriorly by the clitoris and urethra, laterally by the labia minora, and posteriorly by the fourchette (Figure 4–14). The vaginal vestibule is a boat-shaped fossa, visible when the labia majora are separated. Part of its contents, the vaginal introitus, has special significance, because it is the border between the external and internal genitals.

The junction of the vaginal orifice with the vestibule is limited by a thin, elastic membrane called the *hymen*. Its strength, shape, and size vary greatly among individuals and can change within the same individual as a result of age, coitus, and parity. The belief that the intact hymen is a sign of virginity and that it is perforated at first sexual intercourse with resultant bleeding is not valid. The hymen is essentially avascular. Intact hymens are found in heterosexually active and parous women, whereas virgins may possess broken hymens. The hymen may be broken through strenuous physical activity, masturbation, men-

struation, or the use of tampons. Once it is broken, the irregular tags that remain are called *carunculae myrtiformes,* or hymenal caruncles.

External to the hymenal ring at the base of the vestibule are two small papular elevations containing the orifices of the ducts of the *vulvovaginal (Bartholin's) glands.* They lie under the constrictor muscle of the vagina. Generally, the vulvovaginal glands are not palpable upon examination, being placed deep in the perineal structures. Their ducts measure 1.5–2 cm in length and about 0.5 cm in diameter. The mucous secretion is clear and viscid, with an alkaline pH, all of which enhance the viability and motility of the sperm deposited in the vaginal vestibule.

The *fossa navicularis* is a slight depression or pitted area between the fourchette and the hymen.

Innervation of the vestibular area is mainly by the perineal nerve from the sacral plexus. The area is not sensitive to touch generally, although the hymen contains numerous free nerve endings as receptors to pain.

PERINEAL BODY

The *perineal body* is a wedge-shaped mass of fibromuscular tissue, measuring about $4 \times 4 \times 4$ cm, found between the lower part of the vagina and anal canal (Figure 4–14). In obstetrics and gynecology, this area between the anus and the vagina is referred to as the *perineum.*

The muscles that meet at the central tendon of the perineum are the external sphincter ani, both levator ani, the superficial and deep transverse perineal, and the bulbocavernosus. These muscles mingle with elastic fibers and connective tissue in an arrangement that allows a remarkable amount of stretching. The perineum is much larger in the female than in the male and is subject to laceration during childbirth. Without proper repair, such damage may produce weakness of the pelvic floor, or dyspareunia. It is the site of episiotomy during delivery.

Internal Genitals

The female internal reproductive organs are highly specialized in structure and function. The target organs for estrogenic hormones—the vagina, uterus, uterine or fallopian tubes, and ovaries—play a unique part in the reproductive cycle. They are shown in Figure 4–15. Each of these organs can be palpated manually or bimanually and can be observed through instrumentation with a speculum, laparoscope, or culdoscope. Radiography and sonography of these organs have contributed greatly to the study and diagnosis of the reproductive process and related functions. In addition, the recent techniques of transmission electron microscopy and scanning electron microscopy have yielded extremely detailed microphotographs of the cells and tissues of the reproductive organs (Ferenczy and Richart, 1974).

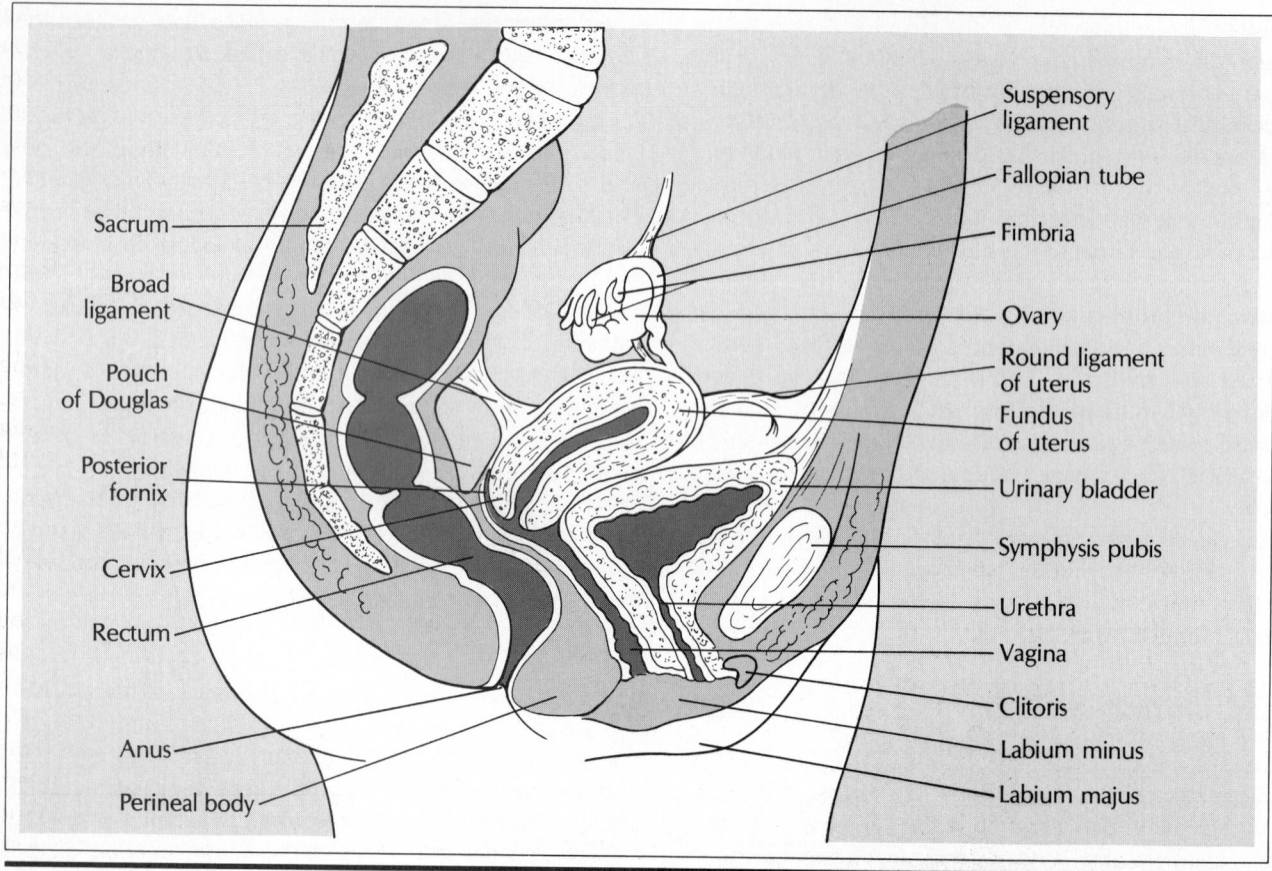

FIGURE 4–15 Female internal reproductive organs.

VAGINA

The *vagina* is a musculomembranous tube that connects the external genitals with the center of the pelvis (Figure 4–15). Its passage superiorly and posteriorly from the vulva to the uterus is in a position nearly parallel to the plane of the pelvic brim. This direction is optimal for coitus. The vagina also forms the lower part of the axis through which the fetal head (or presenting part) must negotiate during its passage at birth.

Because the cervix of the uterus projects into the upper part of the anterior wall of the vagina, the anterior wall is approximately 2.5 cm shorter than the posterior wall. There is great individual variation in vaginal size. Measurements range from 6–8 cm for the anterior wall and from 7–10 cm for the posterior wall. The cervical projection (portio vaginalis cervicis) into the upper part of the vagina (vaginal vault) also creates a recess or hollow around the cervix, which for descriptive purposes is divided into four arches, referred to as the *vaginal fornices.* The anterior vaginal fornix is shallow, the two lateral fornices are deeper, and the posterior fornix is the deepest. These fornices are separated from surrounding organs by a single layer of connective tissue; the walls of the vaginal vault are very

thin. Such structure enhances examination of the pelvic contents in a pelvic examination. Through the anterior fornix, the body of an anteverted uterus as well as the bladder, when distended with urine, can be palpated. Through the posterior fornix, the body of a retroverted uterus, recto-uterine pouch (pouch of Douglas, or cul-de-sac) and any contents, uterosacral ligament, and rectum can be palpated. Through the lateral fornices, the ovaries, appendix, cecum, colon, and ureters can be palpated. Many examiners confuse the round ligament with the uterine tube, which usually cannot be palpated unless it is enlarged.

When a woman lies on her back, the space in the posterior fornix favors the pooling of semen after coitus. This space is called the *receptaculum seminis* and may enhance the chances of impregnation by the collection of large numbers of sperm close to a favorable cervical environment.

The vagina is divided into the lower, middle, and upper (vaginal vault) portions. Each portion is supported by ligaments and muscles attached to the vaginal wall by pelvic fascia. The upper vaginal portion is supported by the levator ani muscles and transverse cervical, pubocervical, and sacrocervical ligaments. The middle vaginal portion is supported by the urogenital diaphragm, and the lower vaginal portion, especially the posterior wall, is supported by the perineal body.

Generally, the anterior and posterior walls of the vagina are in approximation, so that the resting vagina has an **H** shape on transverse section. The embryologic development of the vaginal canal involves canalization and fusion of two separate halves of the paramesonephric ducts. Any interference with these processes can produce congenital malformations, frequently involving the presence of superfluous septa.

Extending into the lumen from the medial surface of the lower two-thirds of the vaginal anterior and posterior walls are prominent longitudinal ridges called *anterior* and *posterior vaginal columns*. Almost at right angles to these columns are the *rugae vaginales*, transverse ridges of the mucous membrane. Although these ridges are numerous at the midline, they almost disappear at the lateral walls. This patterned surface is present after menarche and is often obliterated with multiple pregnancies. These rugae allow for the profound vaginal stretching during the descent of the fetal head and may provide some additional friction or grasping effect for the erect penis during intercourse.

The noncornified, stratified, squamous epithelium lining of the vagina proliferates under the influence of estrogenic hormones and is an even more sensitive index of steroid hormonal effects than the uterine endometrium (Beller et al., 1980). Its structure parallels that of the skin, although there are no sweat glands, sebaceous glands, or hair follicles to weaken it. Immediately under the epithelial layer, the connective tissue is arranged to provide the epithelium with optimal nourishment by approximating a great number of mature basal cells with the underlying blood capillaries. The connective tissue layer has a profuse blood supply, occasional lymphoid nodules, and few somatic nerve endings. The rich blood supply is needed to maintain a high glycogen content in the epithelial cells as well as to nourish the underlying musculofascial layer, through which the vaginal vault gains strong attachments to the cervix. The two-layered smooth muscle component of the musculofascial layer is continuous with the superficial muscle fibers of the uterus. The outer layer is composed of longitudinal muscle fibers, and the inner layer is composed of circular muscle fibers. The outermost vaginal layer is a dense sheet of connective tissue, containing the larger vaginal arteries and venous plexus. A thin band of striated muscle, the sphincter vagina, is found at the lowest extremity of the vagina. However, the levator ani is the principal muscle that closes the vagina.

During a woman's reproductive life, a vaginal pH range of 4–5 is normal, with the lowest pH at midcycle and the highest premenstrually. Transudate of the vaginal epithelium provides a moist environment. The acidic pH is maintained by a symbiotic relationship between the lactic acid-producing Döderlein bacillus (lactobacillus) and the vaginal contents. The bacilli depend on the desquamation of vaginal epithelial cells containing high levels of glycogen. Ovarian hormones regulate not only the glycogen content of these cells but their sloughing and renewal as well. The bacilli break down the glycogen enzymatically to simple sugars and finally to lactic acid. Figure 4–16 illustrates this process. Any interruption of this cycle can destroy the normal self-cleansing action of the vagina. Such interruption may be caused by antibiotic therapy, douching, or use of vaginal sprays or deodorants.

The acidic vaginal environment is normal only in the mature reproductive years and in the first days of life, when maternal hormones are operating in the infant. The relatively neutral pH of 7.5 is normal from infancy until puberty and after menopause.

Each third of the vagina is supplied by a distinct vascular pattern. Its upper third is supplied by the cervicovaginal branches of the uterine arteries; its middle third by the inferior vesical arteries (bladder arteries); its lower third by the internal pudendal and the middle hemorrhoidal arteries (rectal arteries). The venous drainage is accomplished by a closely interwoven, intercommunicating venous network. Because these venous plexuses also anastomose with the vertebral venous plexus, it is possible for a pelvic embolism or carcinoma to bypass the heart and lungs and lodge in the brain, spine, or other remote part of the body (Bloom and Van Dongen, 1972).

Lymphatic drainage of the vagina follows a direct pattern. The upper third drains into the external and internal iliac nodes; the middle third, into the hypogastric nodes; and the lower third, into the inguinal glands. The posterior wall drains into nodes lying in the rectovaginal septum. Any vaginal infection follows these routes.

The vagina is a relatively insensitive organ, with meager somatic innervation to its lower third by the pudendal nerve and virtually no special nerve endings. Therefore sensation during sexual excitement and coitus is minimal and pain during the second stage of labor is less than if somatic innervation were greater. Nervous supply to the vagina is predominantly autonomic. Sensation arises in the vagina and terminates at the S2-3-4 level.

Serving as the copulatory and parturient passage, the vagina is frequently called the *birth canal*. It also enables the discharge of menstrual products from the uterine endometrium to the outside of the body. Finally, the vagina protects against coital trauma and infection from pathogenic organisms.

UTERUS

Throughout the ages, the *uterus*, or womb, has been endowed with a mystical aura. As the core of reproduction and hence continuation of the human race, the uterus and its bearer have received particular attention and treatment. Numerous customs, taboos, mores, and values have

FIGURE 4–16 Scheme of biology of vagina: Reciprocal influence of the vaginal epithelium and Döderlein bacilli on maintenance of acidic vaginal milieu. (From Beller, F. K., et al. 1974. *Gynecology: a textbook for students.* 2nd ed. New York: Springer Verlag New York, Inc., p. 220.)

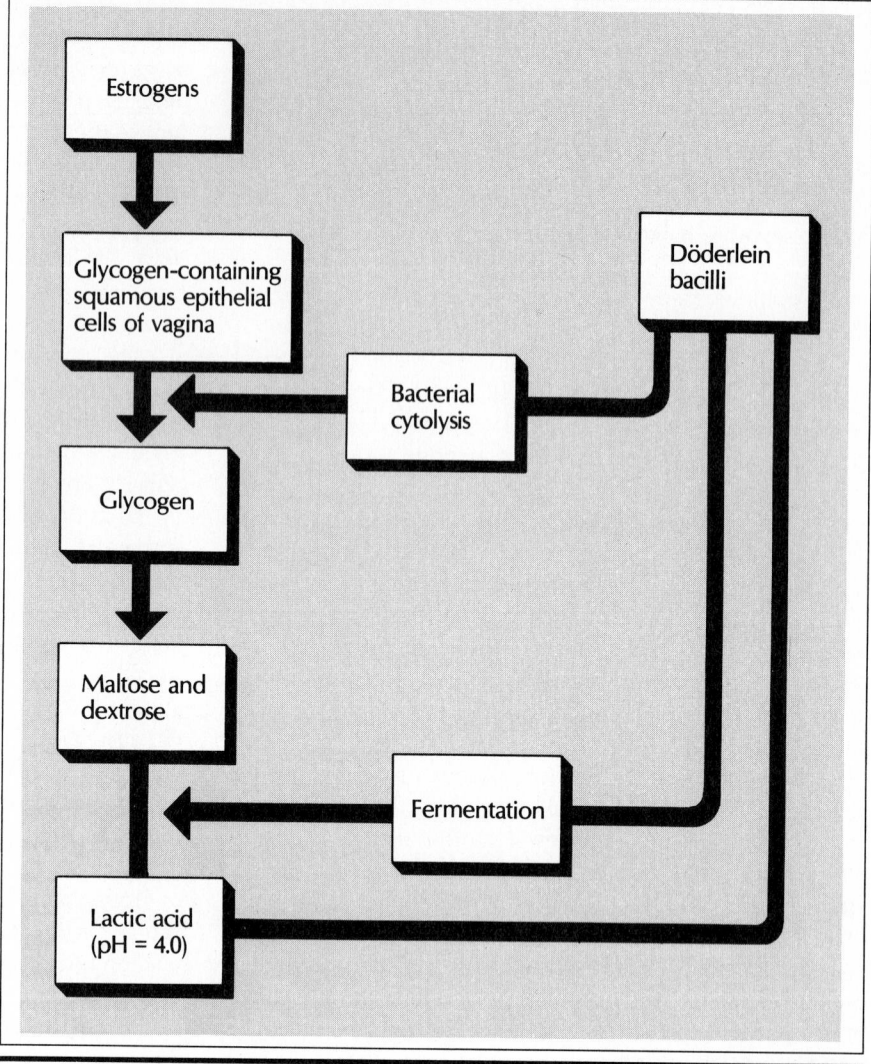

evolved about women and their reproductive function. Although scientific knowledge has replaced much of this folklore, remnants of old ideas and superstitions pervade the thinking of many who seek or provide maternal health care. The nurse must be able to recognize and deal with such attitudes and beliefs so that application of the nursing process is most effective.

The uterus is a hollow, muscular, thick-walled, pear-shaped organ lying central in the pelvic cavity between the base of the bladder and the rectum and above the vagina (Figure 4–17). It is level with or slightly below the brim of the pelvis, with the external os about the level of the ischial spines. Its anterior and posterior surfaces are in opposition, making its cavity potential rather than actual. Although the anterior or vesical (bladder) surface is almost flat, the posterior surface is convex. Because the body of the uterus is flattened, the lateral diameter is greater than the anteroposterior diameter. Loops of the bowel are usu-

ally superior to the uterus. The mature organ weighs about 60 g and is approximately 7.5 cm long, 5 cm wide, and 1–2.5 cm thick. Clinical approximation of size is inaccurate; uterine sounding is needed for a more exact measurement.

As Heinrich von Waldeyer, a Berlin anatomist, pointed out, "The uterus has one typical, but many normal positions" (Bloom and Van Dongen, 1972). Posture, parity, bladder and rectal fullness, and even normal respiratory patterns influence the position of the uterus; only the cervix is anchored laterally. The body of the uterus can move freely in the anteroposterior plane. The axis also varies. Generally, the uterus forms a sharp angle with the vagina. There is a bend in the area of the isthmus; from there the cervix points downward. This is the so-called normal anteversion or angulation of the uterus.

The uterus is kept at its normal level in the pelvis by three sets of supports. The upper supports are the broad and round ligaments. The middle supports are suspensory

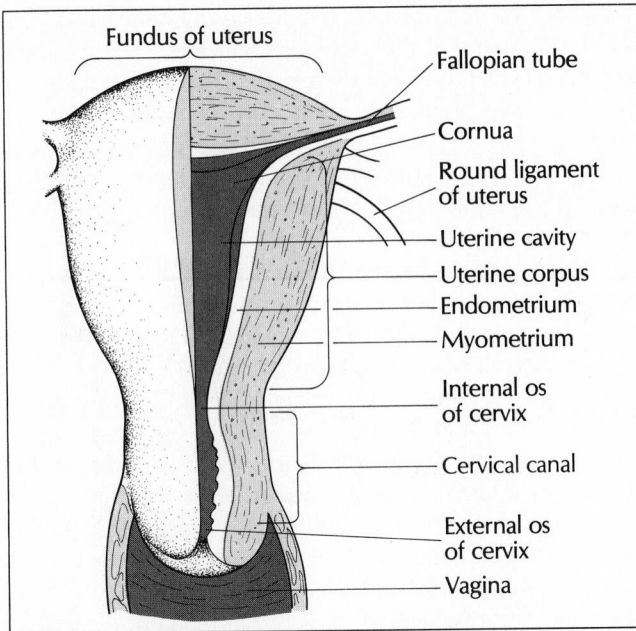

FIGURE 4–17 Anatomy of the uterus. (Modified from Spence, A. P., and Mason, E. B. 1983. *Human anatomy and physiology*. 2nd ed. Menlo Park, Calif.: Benjamin/Cummings Publishing Co., p. 742.)

and consist of the cardinal, pubocervical, and uterosacral ligaments. The lower supports are those structures considered to be the pelvic muscular floor.

Many uterine anomalies are thought to be congenital and can be understood more easily by reviewing the embryologic development of the uterus. Between the sixth and ninth week of embryonic development, the two paramesonephric ducts, which are adjacent to the mesonephric ducts, grow caudally. Their ultimate fusion gives rise to the fallopian tubes, uterine fundus, cervix, and upper vagina. A normal uterus therefore requires two symmetrical, parallel, equal-sized paramesonephric ducts to meet in the midline. Anomalies represent the absence of either one or both of the ducts, degrees of failure to fuse, or canalization defects. Figure 4–18 illustrates the normal uterus as contrasted with the common types of malformations (Jarcho, 1946). The bicornuate and didelphys uterine malformations are found most frequently.

In cases of habitual abortion, a hysterogram should be done to evaluate the normalcy of the uterus. Because both the urinary and reproductive systems develop from the common urogenital fold in the embryo, anomalies in one system are frequently accompanied by anomalies in the other. Problems of infertility and premature labor and delivery are common.

A slight constriction called the *isthmus* divides the uterus into two unequal parts. The upper two-thirds is the triangular body, or *corpus,* composed mainly of myome-

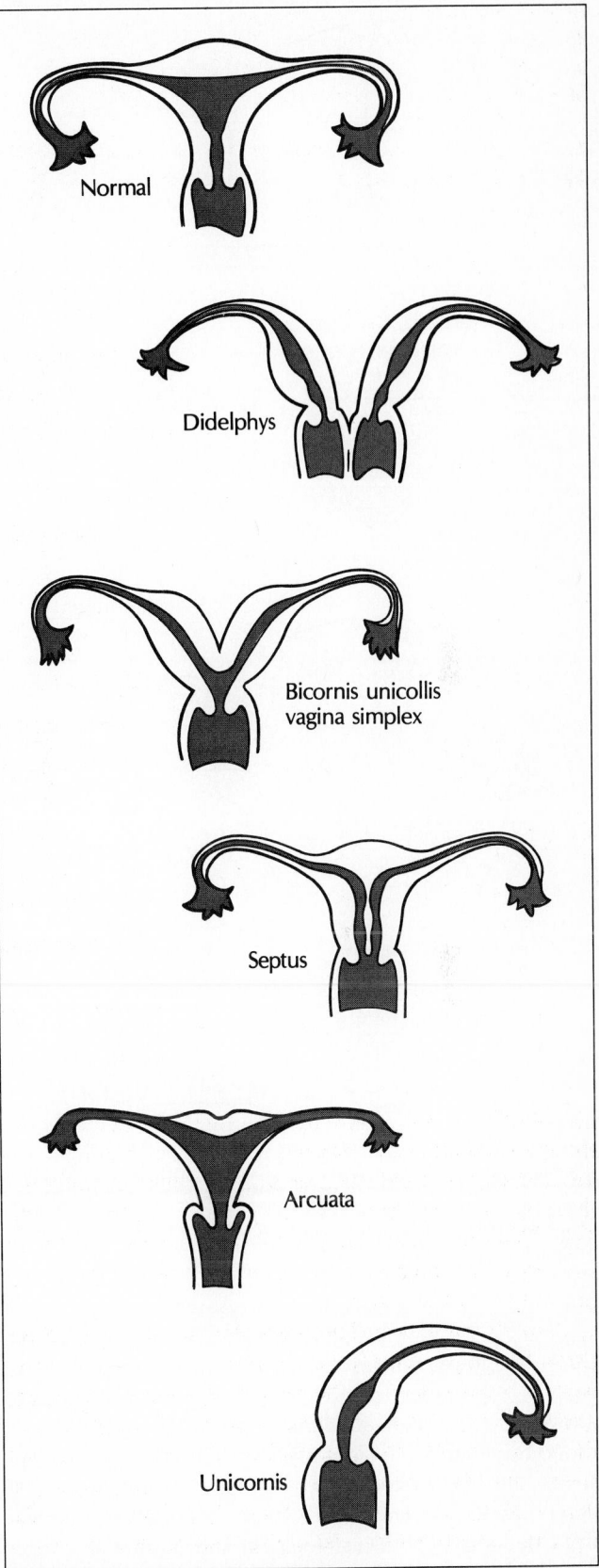

FIGURE 4–18 Congenital malformations of the uterus.

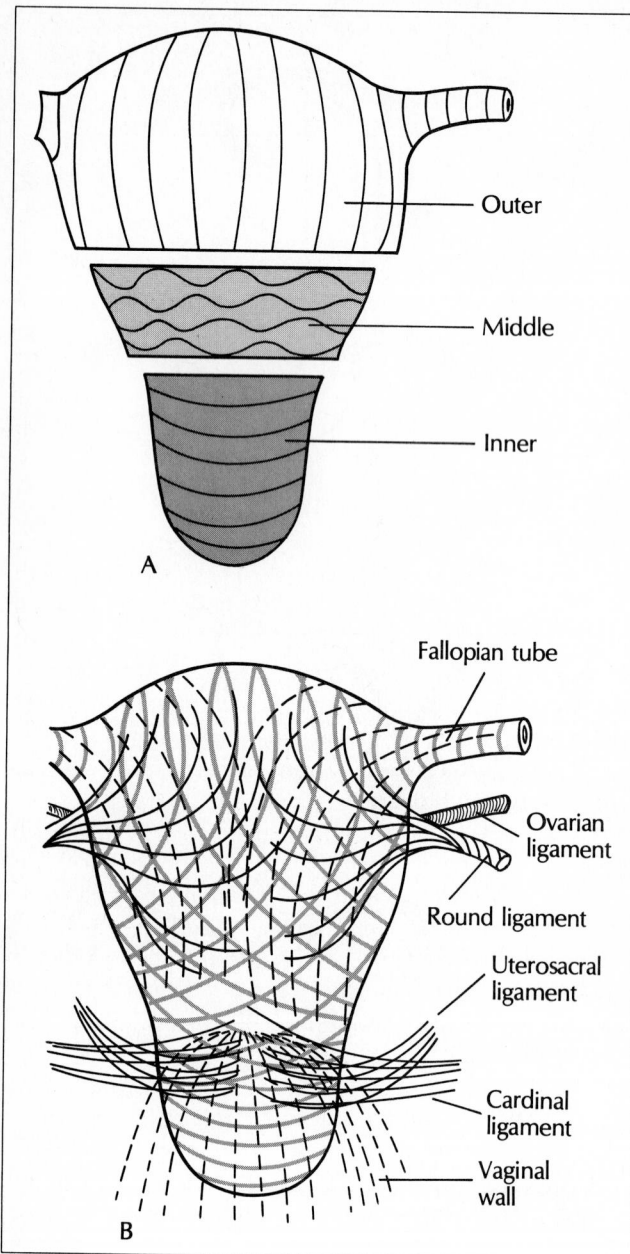

FIGURE 4–19 Uterine muscle layers. **A,** Muscle fiber placement. **B,** Interlacing of uterine muscle layers.

The isthmus is about 6 mm above the internal os, and it is in this area that the uterine endometrium changes into the mucous membrane of the cervix. The isthmus takes on significance in pregnancy, because it becomes the lower uterine segment. With the cervix, it is a passive segment and not part of the contractile uterus. At delivery, this thin lower segment, situated behind the bladder, is the site for lower-segment cesarean deliveries.

The corpus of the uterus is made up of three layers: outermost, or serosal (perimetrium); middle, or muscular (myometrium); and innermost, or mucosal (endometrium). Each layer is distinct in makeup and function.

The *serosal layer* is peritoneum, which passes down from the anterior abdominal wall onto the bladder surface, runs directly onto the anterior surface of the uterus at the level of the internal os, and continues over the fundus and down over the posterior surface of the corpus. As it covers the superior surface of the posterior vaginal fornix, it forms the anterior wall of the rectouterine pouch (pouch of Douglas). The two-layered folds of peritoneum, extending from the lateral uterine margins to the lateral pelvic walls, make up the broad ligament.

The *muscular uterine layer* has, in turn, three indistinct layers. It should be noted that myometrium is continuous with the muscle layer of the fallopian tubes as well as with that of the vagina. This helps these organs to present a unified reaction to various stimuli—ovulation, orgasm, or the deposit of sperm in the vagina. These muscle fibers also extend into the ovarian, round, and cardinal ligaments and minimally into the uterosacral ligaments, which helps explain the vague but disturbing pelvic "aches and pains" reported by many pregnant women.

Figure 4–19 shows the three layers of uterine involuntary muscle. The outer layer, distributed mainly over the fundus, is made up of longitudinal muscles, especially suited for their expulsive function during the birth process. The middle layer is thick and made up of interlacing muscle fibers in figure-eight patterns. These fibers surround large blood vessels, and their contraction produces a hemostatic action. The inner muscle layer is made up of circular fibers, sparse over the fundus but concentrated to form sphincters at the uterine tube attachment sites (tubia ostia) and at the internal os. The internal os sphincter inhibits the expulsion of the uterine contents during pregnancy. An incompetent cervical os can be caused by a torn, weak, or absent sphincter at the internal os. The sphincters at the tubia ostia prevent the regurgitation of menstrual blood into the uterine tubal lumen from the uterus.

Although each layer of muscle has been discussed as having a unique function, it must be remembered that the uterine musculature works as a whole. The uterine contractions of labor are responsible for the dilatation of the cervix and provide the major impetus for the passage of the fetus through the pelvic axis and vaginal canal at birth.

The *mucosal* or *innermost layer* of the uterine corpus is

trium; the lower third is the neck, or *fusiform cervix*. The rounded uppermost portion of the corpus that extends above the points of attachment of the uterine tubes is called the *fundus*. The lateral elongation of the uterus into which the uterine tube opens is called the *cornua*. The cervix, about 2.5 cm in both length and diameter, differs from the corpus both histologically and physiologically. It is canallike, with its exit into the vagina called the *external os* and its entrance into the corpus, the *internal os* (Figure 4–17).

the endometrium, a single layer of columnar epithelium, glands, and stroma. From menarche to menopause, the endometrium undergoes monthly degeneration and renewal in the absence of pregnancy. As it responds to a governing hormonal cycle and prostaglandin influence as well, the endometrium varies in thickness from 0.5–5 mm.

Covering the endometrial surface are simple, tubular-type glands lined with columnar cells, which are continuous with those covering the surface of the endometrium. The glands produce a thin, watery, alkaline secretion that keeps the uterine cavity moist. Not only is this "endometrial milk" capable of assisting the sperm on their journey to the uterine tubes, but it provides nourishment to the blastocyst prior to implantation (Chapter 8).

During the late luteal (secretory) phase of the menstrual cycle (Chapter 5) or in early pregnancy, the endometrium is composed of three layers. Beginning with the luminal surface, the zona compacta is in the region of the mouth of the glands. The zona spongiosa is the next deeper layer. Its glands are dilated and extremely tortuous. The deepest layer, adjoining the myometrium, is the *zona basalis*. The zona compacta and zona spongiosa are frequently combined to be called *zona functionalis*. These two layers are shed at menstruation.

The unique blood supply to these three layers is important. In the myometrium, the radial arteries branch off from the arcuate arteries at right angles. Approaching the endometrial border, the radial arteries branch extensively. Once inside the endometrium, they become the basal arteries, supplying the zona basalis, ultimately becoming the coiled arteries, supplying the zona functionalis. The straighter basal arteries are smaller than the coiled arteries; they are not sensitive to cyclic hormonal control. Hence the zona basalis remains intact and is the site of new endometrial tissue generation. The coiled arteries are extremely sensitive to cyclic hormonal control. Their response is alternate relaxation and constriction during the ischemic or terminal phase of the menstrual cycle.

When pregnancy occurs and the endometrium is not shed, the reticular stromal cells surrounding the endometrial glands become the decidual cells of pregnancy. The stromal cells are highly vascular, channeling a rich blood supply to the endometrial surface.

The *cervix* is a protective portal for the body of the uterus as well as the connection between the vagina and the uterus. The cervix is divided by its line of attachment into the vaginal and supravaginal areas. The *vaginal cervix* includes about one-fourth of the anterior cervix and one-half of the posterior cervix. It projects into the vagina at an angle of 45°–90°. The *supravaginal cervix* is surrounded by the attachments that give the uterus its main support: the uterosacral ligaments posteriorly, the transverse ligaments of the cervix (ligaments of Mackenrodt) laterally, and the pubocervical ligaments anteriorly.

The vaginal cervix appears pink and is covered by pale

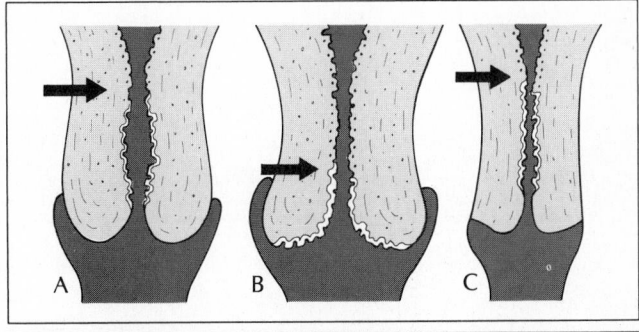

FIGURE 4–20 Changes in squamocolumnar junction (*arrow*) at various stages of life. **A,** Childhood. **B,** Reproductive years. **C,** Old age. (Modified from Beller, F. K., et al. 1974. *Gynecology: a textbook for students.* 2nd ed. New York: Springer Verlag New York, Inc., p. 34.)

squamous stratified epithelium, which is continuous with the vaginal lining. The vaginal cervix ends at the external os. The cervical canal appears rosy red and is lined with tall columnar ciliated epithelium containing many branching mucus-secreting glands. Most cervical cancer begins at this squamocolumnar junction. Its exact location varies with age and parity. Figure 4–20 shows this junction at various stages of a woman's life.

Elasticity is a chief characteristic of the cervix. Its ability to stretch is made possible by the high fibrous and collagenous content of the supportive tissues and by the arrangement of vast numbers of folds and plications in the cervical lining. As in the vagina, anterior and posterior ridges with rugae branch off obliquely in the cervix. Thus the actual area is increased tremendously. About 10% of the cervix is composed of muscle cells.

The cervical mucosa has three functions: (a) to provide lubrication for the vaginal canal, (b) to act as a bacteriostatic agent, and (c) to provide an alkaline environment to shelter deposited sperm from the acidic vagina. At ovulation, cervical mucus is clearer, more viscous, and higher in alkalinity.

Both the body of the uterus and the cervix are changed permanently by pregnancy. The body never returns to its nulliparous size, and the external os changes from a circular opening of about 3 mm to a transverse slit with irregular edges. Figure 4–21 illustrates the changes in size of the uterus and the external os during the life span of a parous woman.

The ovarian artery arise from the abdominal aorta below the renal arteries and can supply the ovary, fallopian tube, and upper third of the uterus. The uterine artery arises from the hypogastric branch of the internal iliac artery and supplies the lower two-thirds of the uterus. There are numerous anastomoses between the ovarian and uterine arteries and their branches. The uterine veins are arranged in a pattern similar to those of the uterine, ovarian, and tubal arteries (Figure 4–22).

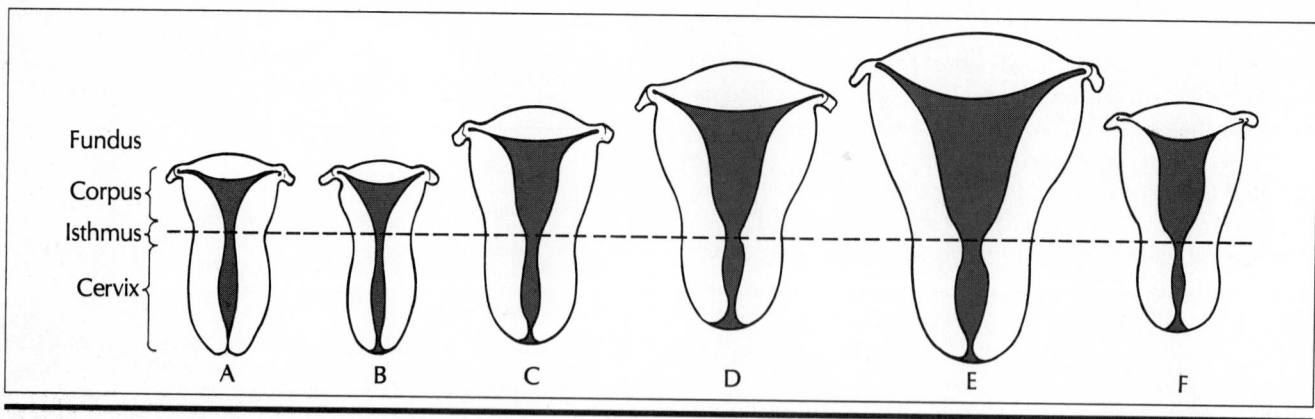

FIGURE 4–21 Changes in size of uterus and external os during a woman's life. **A,** Neonate: corpus ⅓ and cervix ⅔; length varies from 2.5–3.5 cm. **B,** Childhood (preschool): same proportion; has elongated slightly. **C,** Puberty: corpus ½ and cervix ½; length varies from 5–6 cm. **D,** Adulthood (nulliparous): corpus ⅔ and cervix ⅓; length varies from 6–8 cm. Weight varies from 50–70 g. **E,** Adulthood (multiparous): corpus ⅔ and cervix ⅓; length varies from 9–10 cm. Weight about 80 g or more. **F,** Postmenopause: corpus ⅔, cervix ⅓; decrease in size and weight.

Lymphatic drainage from the cervix moves in three areas: (a) external iliac nodes, (b) internal iliac nodes, and (c) sacral nodes. The body of the uterus is drained by a scant system for each of its three layers. One set of collecting vessels follows the broad ligament and ovarian vessels to end in the para-aortic nodes, another follows the round ligaments to terminate in the inguinal lymph glands, and the third set merges with lymphatics of the cervix into the external iliac nodes.

Innervation of the uterus is entirely by the autonomic nervous system and seems to be more regulatory than primary in nature. It is helpful to recall that generally sympathetic fibers stimulate muscle contraction and vasoconstriction; parasympathetic fibers inhibit contractions and stimulate vasodilatation. There is adequate contractility of the uterus without an intact nerve supply, as illustrated by the fact that hemiplegic patients have adequate uterine contractions (Beller et al., 1980).

Uterine parasympathetic fibers arise from the second, third, and fourth sacral nerves to form the pelvic nerves. Sympathetic fibers enter the pelvis through the hypogastric plexus. Although the sympathetic and parasympathetic fibers enter the pelvis separately, they become mixed in the uterovaginal plexus of Frankenhäuser.

Both the sympathetic and parasympathetic nerves contain motor fibers and a few sensory fibers. Pain of uterine contractions is carried to the central nervous system by the eleventh and twelfth thoracic nerve roots. Pain from the cervix and upper vagina passes through the ilioinguinal and pudendal nerves. The motor fibers to the uterus arise from the seventh and eighth thoracic vertebras. Because the sensory and motor levels are separated in this manner,

caudal and spinal anesthesia can be utilized during labor and delivery.

The uterine functions are designed to provide a safe environment for fetal development. The uterine lining is cyclically prepared by steroid hormones for nidation (implantation of the embryo). Once implanted, the developing fetus is protected until it is expelled.

UTERINE LIGAMENTS

The uterine ligaments are shown in Figure 4–23.

Broad ligament. The broad ligament, or *mesosalpinx*, is a double mesenteric layer continuous with the abdominal peritoneum. The peritoneum may be thought of as being draped over the bladder, over and around the uterus and extending uterine tubes, and down the posterior uterine border. Thus this double sheet of peritoneum, extending from the lateral margins of the uterus outward to the pelvic wall, enfolds the fallopian tubes and the round and ovarian ligaments at the upper border of the broad ligament. At its lower border, its fasciomuscular composition becomes more dense to form the cardinal ligaments. Laterally, beyond the uterine tubes, the broad ligament continues as the infundibulopelvic or suspensory ligament.

Between the folds of the broad ligament are large amounts of connective tissue, small amounts of involuntary muscle, blood vessels, lymph channels, and nerves. The broad ligament, with its specialized areas, keeps the uterus and tubes centrally placed and provides stability within the pelvic cavity.

Round ligaments. Each of the round ligaments arises below and anterior to the uterine tube insertion and courses outward between the folds of the broad ligament

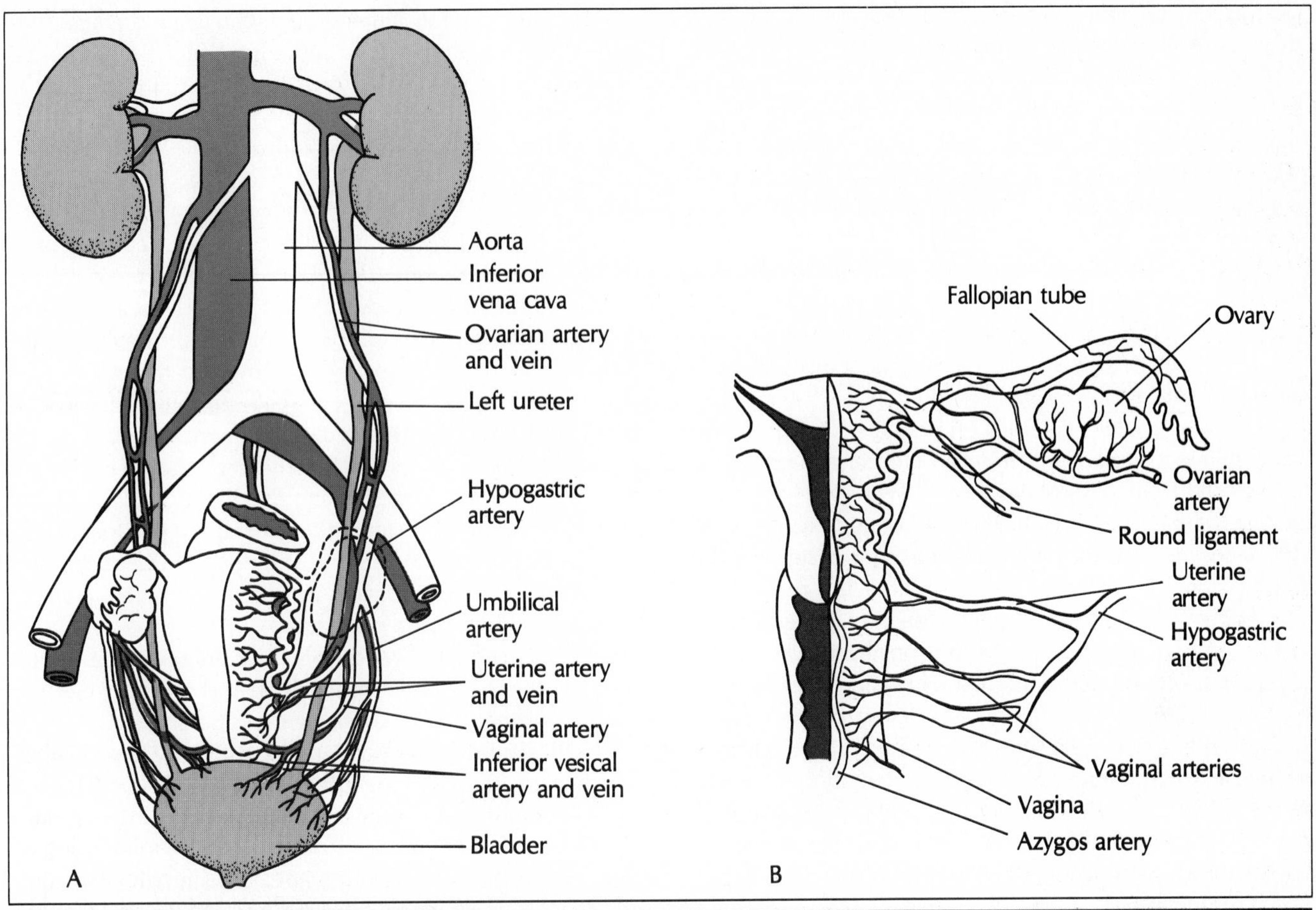

Aorta

Inferior vena cava

Ovarian artery and vein

Left ureter

Hypogastric artery

Umbilical artery

Uterine artery and vein

Vaginal artery

Inferior vesical artery and vein

Bladder

A

Fallopian tube

Ovary

Ovarian artery

Round ligament

Uterine artery

Hypogastric artery

Vaginal arteries

Vagina

Azygos artery

B

FIGURE 4–22 Blood supply to internal reproductive organs. **A,** Pelvic blood supply. **B,** Blood supply to vagina, ovary, uterus, and fallopian tubes.

in a curved and tortuous manner, passing through the inguinal ring and canal, to fan out and fuse with the connective tissue of the labia majora. Made up of involuntary longitudinal muscle, which is continuous with that of the uterus, the round ligament hypertrophies during pregnancy. Although it shows signs of contractility and tonus, it probably does not contribute support to the uterus. However, during labor, the round ligaments steady the uterus, pulling downward and forward so that during the first stage the presenting part is forced into the cervix with encouragement to descend into the birth canal during the second stage (Bloom and Van Dongen, 1972).

Ovarian ligaments. The ovarian ligaments are short, round fibromuscular cords that anchor the lower pole of the ovary to the cornu of the uterus. Structurally, the ovarian and round ligaments are the same and are homologous to the male gubernaculum testis. Although they begin as continuous structures in embryologic life, their continuity is interrupted by the developing uterus.

The contractile ability of the ovarian ligament allows it to influence the position of its ovary to some extent, thus

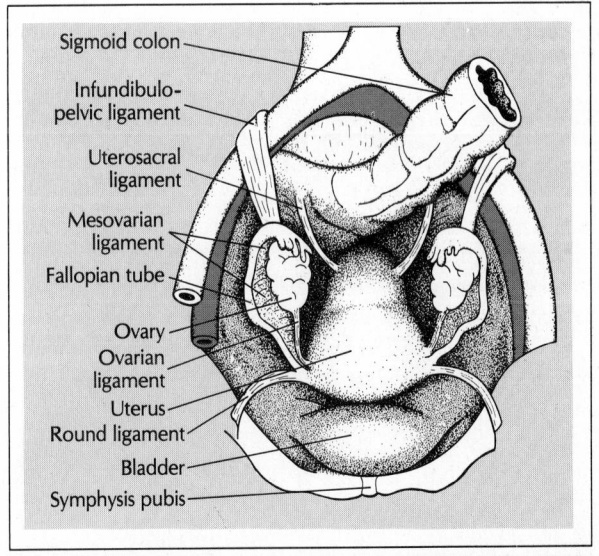

Sigmoid colon

Infundibulo-pelvic ligament

Uterosacral ligament

Mesovarian ligament

Fallopian tube

Ovary

Ovarian ligament

Uterus

Round ligament

Bladder

Symphysis pubis

FIGURE 4–23 Uterine ligaments.

assisting the fimbriae of the uterine tubes in "catching" the ovum each month as it is released.

Cardinal ligaments. The cardinal ligaments, also known as *Mackenrodt's ligaments* or the *transverse cervical ligaments,* originate on the lateral pelvic walls and terminate in attachments to the lateral vaginal fornices and the supravaginal cervix. This thickened base of the broad ligament is continuous with the connective tissue of the pelvic floor and is made up of longitudinal smooth muscle fibers. It is the strongest band of the pelvic floor and the chief uterine support, suspending the uterus from the lateral walls of the true pelvis, and prevents uterine prolapse. It also supports the upper vagina.

Infundibulopelvic ligament. The outer third of the broad ligament, extending from the fimbriated end of the uterine tube to the lateral pelvic wall, forms the infundibulopelvic, or suspensory, ligament. It contains the ovarian vessels and nerves and serves to suspend and support the ovaries.

Uterosacral ligaments. The uterosacral ligaments arise on each side of the pelvis from the posterior wall of the uterus at the level of the internal os, sweep back around the lower third of the rectum, and insert on the lateral borders of the first and second sacral vertebras. These peritoneal folds make up the lateral boundaries of the pouch of Douglas. With the cardinal and pubovesical ligaments, the uterosacral ligaments make up a fibromuscular tissue support system extending from the pelvic wall to the uterus near the internal os.

The uterosacral ligaments contain smooth muscle fibers, connective tissue, blood and lymph vessels, and nerves. Providing support for the uterus and cervix at the level of the ischial spines, they also contain sensory nerve fibers that contribute to dysmenorrhea.

FALLOPIAN (UTERINE) TUBES

Derived embryologically from the paramesonephric ducts, the *fallopian* or *uterine tubes* (also known as the *oviducts*) arise laterally from the cornua of the uterus and progress almost to the side walls of the pelvis, where they turn posteriorly and medially toward the ovaries (Figure 4–24). Each tube is approximately 8–13.5 cm long, lying in the superior border of the broad ligament (mesosalpinx). These tubes are not inert, rigid structures; they are dynamic and restless, constantly seeking the ovum to be released from the ovary. The fallopian tubes link the peritoneal cavity with the external environment by way of the uterus and vagina, an arrangement that increases a woman's biologic vulnerability to disease processes.

A short section of each fallopian tube is intrauterine. Lying within the uterine muscular wall, its opening into the uterus (uterine ostium) is only 1 mm in diameter.

Each tube may be divided into three parts: the isthmus, the ampulla, and the infundibulum (fimbria). The isthmus is straight and narrow, with a thick muscular wall and a lumen 2–3 mm in diameter. It is the site of tubal ligation. Adjacent to the isthmus is the curved distal ampulla, comprising the outer two-thirds of the tube. Fertilization of the

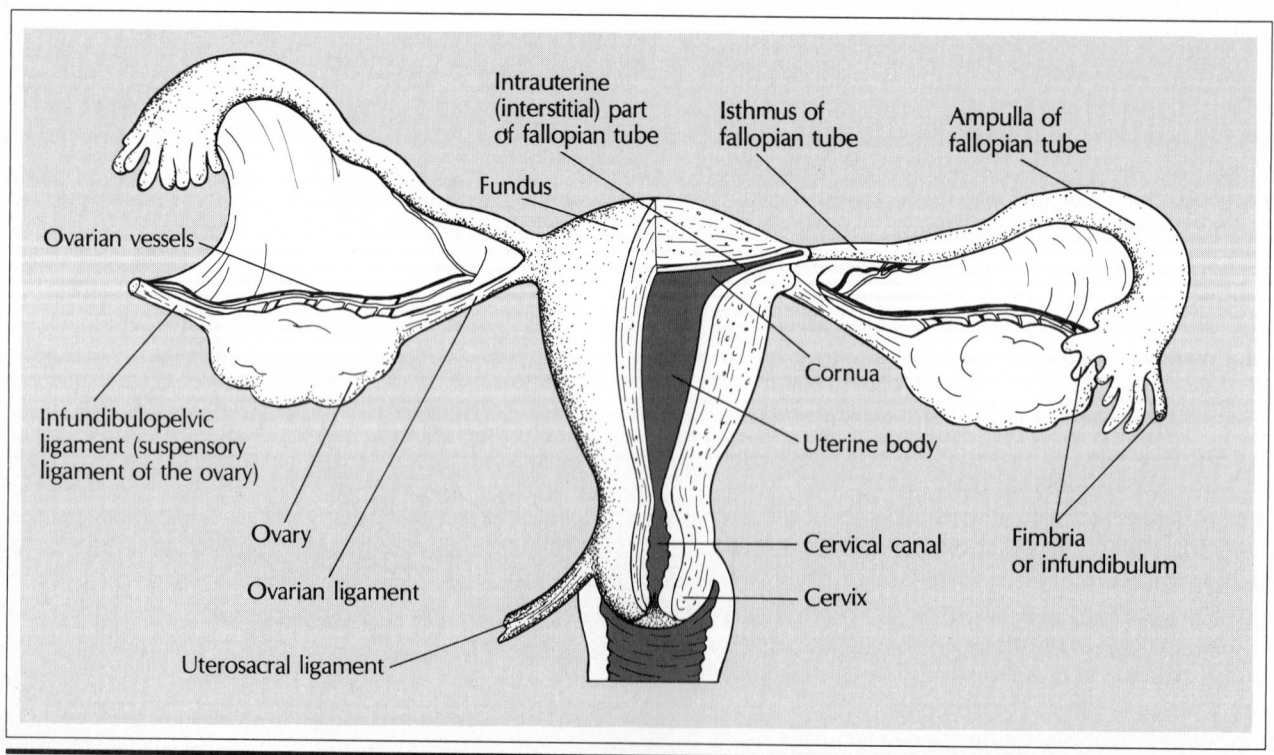

FIGURE 4–24 The fallopian tubes (oviducts or uterine tubes) and ovaries.

ovum by a spermatozoon usually occurs here. The ampulla has the widest lumen, and its muscular wall is thin and distensible. It terminates into the infundibulum, which is a funnel-like enlargement with many moving fingerlike projections (fimbriae) reaching out to the ovary. The longest of these, the fimbria ovarica, is attached to the ovary to increase the chances of intercepting the ovum as it is released.

The wall of the fallopian tube is made up of four layers: peritoneal (serous), subserous (adventitial), muscular, and mucous tissues. The peritoneum of the broad ligament covers the tubes and becomes continuous with the mucous membrane lining the tube in the infundibular area. The subserous layer contains the blood and nerve supply, and the muscular layer is responsible for the peristaltic movement of the tube, created by the outer longitudinal and inner circular smooth involuntary muscle fibers. The mucosal layer, immediately adjacent to the muscular layer, is continuous with the uterine endometrium although less sensitive to hormonal cyclic changes. This layer is arranged in longitudinal folds, or plicae, which are few in number in the isthmus but increase in number and complexity in the ampulla so that they extend beyond the ampulla as the fimbriae. The mucosal layer is composed of ciliated and nonciliated columnar epithelium, with the number of ciliated cells increasing at the fimbria. Nonciliated cells are goblet cells, which secrete a protein-rich, serous fluid that nourishes the ovum. The constantly roving tubal cilia create currents moving toward the uterus. Because the ovum is a large cell, this ciliary action is needed to augment the tubal peristalsis of the muscular layer. It is apparent that any malformation or malfunction of the tubes could result in infertility or even sterility.

In addition to physical problems, psychologic disturbances may influence fertility adversely. Bloom and Van Dongen (1972) report that a tense woman, with resultant autonomic nervous hyperactivity, may have spastic or tense fallopian tubes, causing reduced contractility and patency of the tubes. A well-functioning tubal transport system involves active fimbriae in close proximation to the ovary; peristalsis of the tube created by the muscular layer; ciliated currents beating toward the uterus; and the proximal contraction and distal relaxation of the tube caused by different types of prostaglandins (Marshall and Ross, 1982).

A double blood supply serves each oviduct. Branches of the uterine and ovarian arteries anastomose, creating a rich network in the mesosalpinx. Thus the uterine tubes have an unusual ability to recover from any inflammatory process. Venous drainage occurs through the pampiniform plexus and the ovarian and uterine veins. Lymphatic drainage occurs through the vessels close to the ureter into the lumbar nodes along the aorta.

Both parasympathetic and sympathetic motor and sensory nerves from the pelvic plexus and ovarian plexus supply the uterine tubes. The ampulla is supplied from ovarian

branches, and the isthmus is supplied by the uterine branches. Pain arising from the tubes is referred to the area of the iliac fossae, because both areas are served by the same segmental skin innervation.

The functions of the uterine tubes are to provide transport for the egg from the ovary to the uterus; to act as a site for fertilization; and to serve as a warm, moist, nourishing environment for the egg or zygote (Chapter 8). The time needed for transport through the uterine tubes varies between 3–4 days.

OVARIES

The *ovaries* are two almond-shaped glandular structures lying on the posterior surface of the broad ligament, just below the pelvic brim and near the infundibulum (Figure 4–24). Their size varies among individuals and with the stage of the menstrual cycle. Right and left ovaries vary in size, weighing approximately 6–10 g and measuring 1.5–3 cm in width, 2–5 cm in length, and 1–1.5 cm in thickness. During fetal life, they develop from the germinal epithelium of the urogenital ridge of the posterior abdominal wall and descend into the pelvis much as the testes do (Beller et al., 1980). The ovaries are small in childhood but increase in size after puberty. They also change in appearance: From a dull white, smooth-surfaced organ, the ovaries become a pitted gray because of scarring following ovulation.

The typical position of each ovary is in the upper part of the pelvic cavity at the lateral wall in a fossa created at the external iliac vein and ureteral junction. It is rare that both ovaries are at the same level. The ovary is connected to the uterus by the ovarian ligament, to the back of the broad ligament by the mesovarium, and to the lateral pelvic wall by the infundibulopelvic ligament (Figure 4–24). Blood vessels, nerves, and lymphatics enter the ovary through the hilum.

There is no peritoneal covering for the ovaries. Although this assists the mature ova to erupt, it also enhances the spread of malignant cells from cancer of the ovaries. A single layer of cuboidal epithelial cells, called the *germinal epithelium*, covers the ovaries. Three additional layers comprise the ovaries: the tunica albuginea, the cortex, and the medulla. The *tunica albuginea* is dense and dull white and serves as a protective layer. The *cortex* is the main functional part because it contains graafian follicles, corpora lutea, atretic follicles, and corpora albicantia held together by the ovarian stroma. The *medulla* is completely surrounded by the cortex and contains the nerves and the blood and lymphatic vessels.

The ovary is a crucial component of reproduction. Even a small part of a functioning ovary will ovulate, providing an ovum for fertilization monthly. Every oocyte available for maturation within a woman's reproductive life is present at birth. No oogenesis occurs after fetal development. Close to a million oocytes are locked in the first meiotic division at birth. (See Chapter 8 for a discussion of meiosis and maturation of ova.) Because of follicular atretic processes, about 300,000 oocytes remain in a girl of 7 years, and about 30,000 are present at puberty (Bloom and Van Dongen, 1972). Almost 400 ova are actually extruded over the reproductive years. In spite of prepubescent bursts of pituitary activity that incite large numbers of follicles to attempt to ripen, they do not. The maturation of graafian follicles and the release of a mature ovum are discussed in Chapter 5.

The motor and sensory parasympathetic and sympathetic nerves that accompany the ovarian artery from the abdomen cross over the infundibulopelvic ligament to reach the ovarian hilum. The ovaries are relatively insensitive unless they are squeezed or distended. Ovarian cancer usually originates in the germinal epithelium and is relatively painless (Bloom and Van Dongen, 1972). *Mittelschmerz*, or midcycle pain, is frequently noted and is due to irritation of the peritoneum caused by fluid or blood escaping along with the ovum. Pain can also be caused by follicular cysts.

The unique and vital function of the ovaries is to release a mature ovum monthly for fertilization (Chapter 8). When no more follicles remain in the ovary, resulting in the cessation of ovarian activity (usually in women aged mid-40s to early 50s), menopause occurs. Should this cessation occur in a woman in her 30s, it is called *premature menopause*. If sufficient viable follicles are not present in the 20s, gonadal or ovarian failure has occurred.

Breasts

Embryologically the breasts (mammae), which develop from ectoderm and mesoderm, appear about the sixth week of life along the mammary ridge. Although several mammary buds may appear on each ridge, only one develops. Solid cords evolve in the pectoral breast by the fifth month, and during the last trimester these cords become lumina, which ultimately are the chief ducts of the breast. Rudimentary acini are present at birth; the inverted nipple

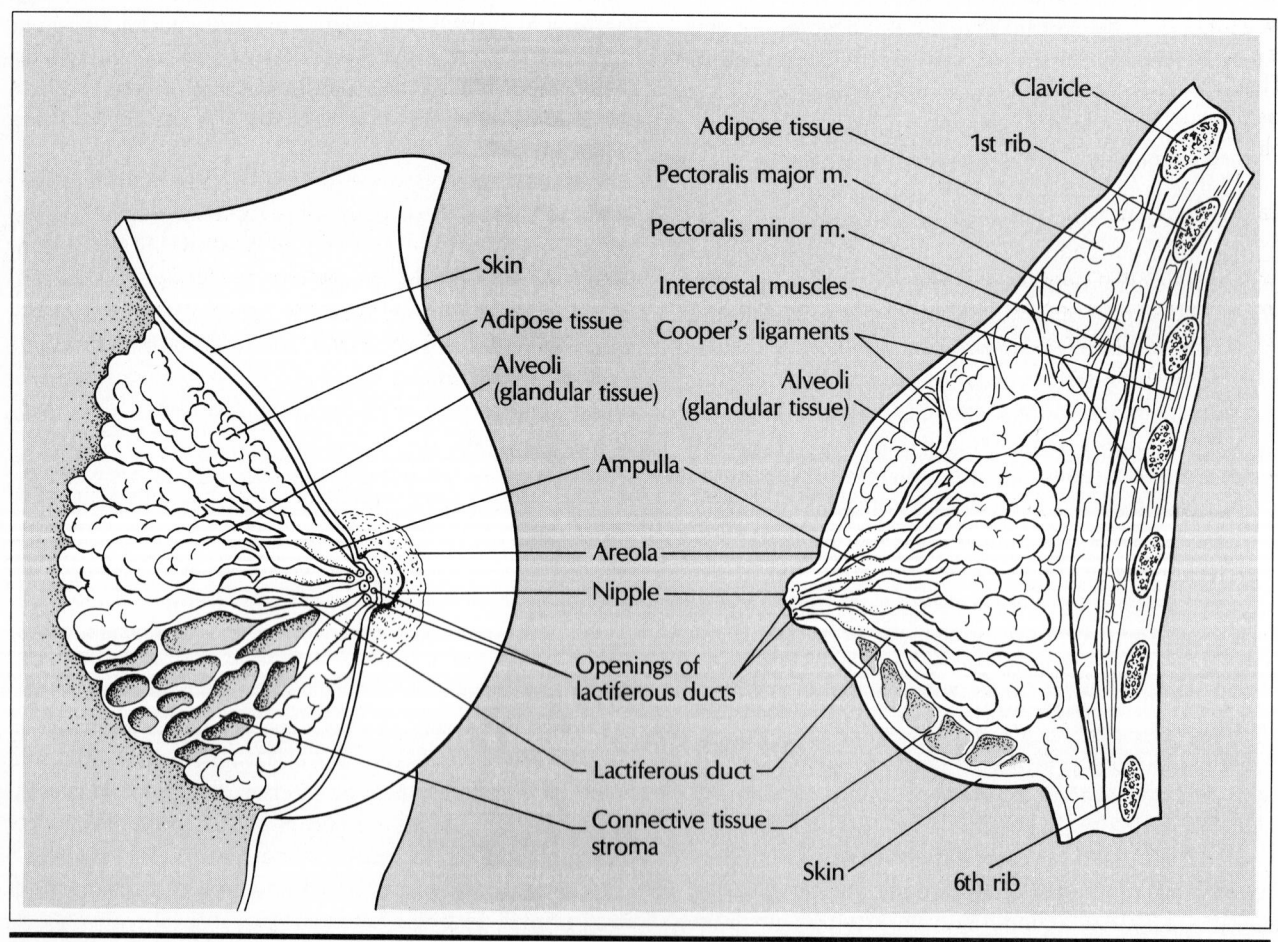

FIGURE 4–25 Anatomy of the breast. **A,** Anterior view of partially dissected left breast. **B,** Sagittal view. (Modified from Spence, A. P., and Mason, E. B. 1983. *Human anatomy and physiology.* 2nd ed. Menlo Park, Calif.: Benjamin/Cummings Publishing Co., p. 747.)

everts, and the areolar tissue is noticeable shortly after birth.

The breasts are considered accessories of the reproductive system and are specialized sebaceous glands known as *racemose* or *compound glands*. They appear in pairs and are symmetrically placed on the sides of the chest between the second and sixth ribs and the sternal edge and midaxillary line. Each breast, conical in shape, is separated from the underlying greater pectoral and anterior serratus muscles by a bed of connective tissue. The weight of each breast is about 200 g (Lawrence, 1980). Generally breast tissue extends into the axilla from the outer margin of normal breast tissue, called the *tail of Spence*. Frequently, the left breast is larger than the right.

In the center of each mature breast is the nipple, a protrusion about 0.5–1.3 cm in diameter. The nipple is composed largely of erectile tissue and becomes more rigid and prominent during the menstrual cycle, sexual excitement, pregnancy, and lactation. The nipple is surrounded by the heavily pigmented areola, 2.5–10 cm in diameter. Both the nipple and areola are roughened by small papillae called *tubercles of Montgomery*. These tubercles are sebaceous glands that secrete a lipoid material during an infant's suckling that helps lubricate and protect the breasts.

The breasts are composed of glandular, fibrous, and adipose tissue. The glandular tissue consists of acini or alveoli (Figure 4–25), which are arranged in a series of 15 to 24 lobes. These lobes are in a radial pattern and are separated from one another by varying amounts of adipose and fibrous tissue. Fibrous tissues called *Cooper's ligaments* extend from the deep fascia overlying the chest wall muscles through the alveolar tissue and eventually fuse with the superficial fascial layer just under the skin. They suspend the breasts.

Each lobe of the breast is made up of several lobules, which in turn are made up of large numbers of alveoli in grapelike clusters around minute ducts. They are lined with a single layer of cuboidal epithelium, which secretes the various components of milk. The ducts from several lobules combine to form the larger lactiferous ducts or sinuses. Each lactiferous duct opens separately on the surface of the nipple and may be seen as a tiny isolated orifice. The smooth muscle of the nipple causes erection of the nipple on contraction.

Cyclic hormonal control of the mature breast is complex. Essentially, estrogenic hormones stimulate the growth and development of the ductal epithelium. Progesterone, in association with estrogen, is responsible for the acinar and lobular development during the luteal phase of menstruation. In addition, adrenal corticosteroids, prolactin, somatotropin (growth hormone), and thyroxine are necessary for estrogen and progesterone to act.

The arterial, venous, and lymphatic systems communicate medially with the internal mammary vessels and laterally with the axillary vessels. Therefore, in cancer of the breast metastasis follows the vascular supply both medially and laterally (Figure 4–26).

The cutaneous nerve supply to the upper breast is from the third and fourth branches of the cervical plexus, whereas the supply to the lower breast is from the thoracic intercostal nerve.

The biologic function of the breasts is to provide nourishment and protective maternal antibodies to infants through the lactation process. Additionally, they are a source of much pleasurable sexual sensation. In Western culture the breasts have become a sexual symbol; their size and sexual qualities receive more attention than their lactogenic functions.

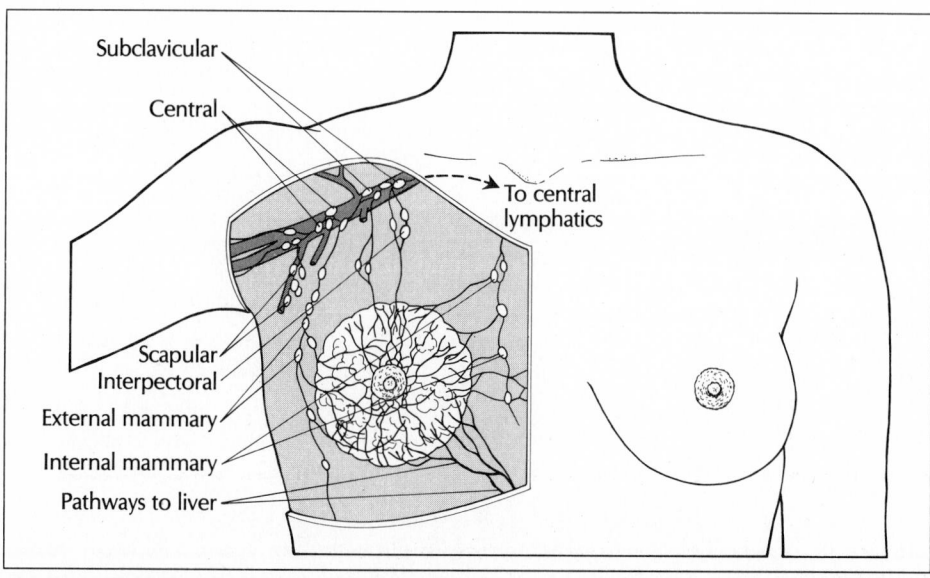

FIGURE 4–26 Lymphatic drainage of the breast.

Subclavicular

Central

To central lymphatics

Scapular
Interpectoral

External mammary

Internal mammary

Pathways to liver

SUMMARY

The miracle of life begins with the fusion of the egg and sperm in the woman's body and continues with the embryologic development of the zygote. This chapter presented a discussion of the differences and similarities between the male and female reproductive organ development, blood supply, lymph supply, innervation, and functioning.

Many changes occur in a woman's body during the process of fetal growth. The foundation of knowledge necessary for understanding these numerous changes has been provided here, through presentation of the embryologic development, anatomy, and physiology of the female and male reproductive systems.

References

Beller, F. K., et al. 1980. *Gynecology: a textbook for students.* 3rd ed. New York: Springer Verlag New York, Inc.

Benson, R. C. 1976. *Current obstetric and gynecologic diagnosis and treatment.* Los Altos, Calif.: Lange Medical Publications.

Bloom, M. L., and Van Dongen, L. 1972. *Clinical gynaecology: integration of structure and function.* London: William Heineman, Ltd.

Caldwell, B. V., and Behrman, H. R. 1981. Prostaglandins in reproductive processes. *Med. Clin. North Am.* 65:927.

Caldwell, W. E., and Moloy, H. C. 1933. Anatomical variations in the female pelvis and their effect on labor with a suggested classification. *Am. J. Obstet. Gynecol.* 26:479.

Donovan, A. J. 1977. The breast: anatomy, physiology, and benign lesions. In *Rhoad's textbook of surgery: principles and practice,* 5th ed., ed. J. D. Hardy. Philadelphia: J. B. Lippincott Co.

Eliasson, R., and Lindholmer, C. 1976. Functions of male accessory glands. In *Human semen and fertility regulation in men,* ed. E. S. E. Hafez. St. Louis: The C. V. Mosby Co.

Ferenczy, A., and Richart, R. M. 1974. *Female reproductive system: dynamics of scan and transmission electron microscopy.* New York: John Wiley & Sons, Inc.

Guyton, A. C. 1981. *Textbook of medical physiology.* 6th ed. Philadelphia: W. B. Saunders Co.

Hafez, E. S. E. 1980. *Human reproduction: conception and contraception.* 2nd ed. Hagerstown, Md.: Harper & Row.

Jarcho, J. 1946. Malformations of the uterus. *Am. J. Surg.* 71:106.

Lawrence, R. A. 1980. *Breastfeeding: a guide for the medical profession.* St. Louis: The C. V. Mosby Co.

Marshall, J. R., and Ross, J. 1982. Other aspects of the endocrine physiology of reproduction. In *Obstetrics and gynecology,* 4th ed., ed. D. N. Danforth. Philadelphia: Harper & Row.

Masters, W. H., and Johnson, V. E. 1966. *Human sexual response.* Boston: Little, Brown & Co.

Odell, W. D., and Moyer, D. L. 1971. *Physiology of reproduction.* St. Louis: The C. V. Mosby Co.

Polakoski, K. L., et al. 1976. Biochemistry of human seminal plasma. In *Human semen and fertility regulation in men,* ed. E. S. E. Hafez. St. Louis: The C. V. Mosby Co.

Urban, J. A. 1977. Malignant lesions of the breast. In *Rhoad's textbook of surgery: principles and practice,* 5th ed., ed. J. D. Hardy. Philadelphia: J. B. Lippincott Co.

Additional Readings

Budd, K. 1977. Variations in response to hysterectomy—basis for individual care to women. In *Nursing of women in the age of liberation,* ed. N. A. Lytle. Dubuque, Iowa: William C. Brown Co.

Embrey, M. P. 1981. Prostaglandins in human reproduction. *Br. Med. J.* 238:1563.

Fogel, C. I., and Woods, N. F. 1981. *Health care of women: a nursing perspective.* St. Louis: The C. V. Mosby Co.

Ganong, W. F. 1981. *Review of medical physiology.* 10th ed. Los Altos, Calif.: Lange Medical Publications.

Gold, J. J., and Josimovich, J. B., eds. 1980. *Gynecologic endocrinology.* 3rd ed. Hagerstown, Md.: Harper & Row.

Greisheimer, E. M., and Wideman, M. P. 1972. *Physiology and anatomy.* 9th ed. Philadelphia: J. B. Lippincott Co.

Hafez, E. S. E., and Ludwig, H. 1982. Scanning electron microscopy of human reproduction. In *Obstetrics and gynecology,* 4th ed., ed. D. N. Danforth. Philadelphia: Harper & Row.

Kolstad, P., and Stafl, A. 1977. *Atlas of culposcopy.* Baltimore: University Park Press.

Macdonald, R. R., ed. 1978. *The scientific basis of obstetrics and gynecology.* 2nd ed. Edinburgh: Churchill Livingstone.

Novak, E. R., et al. 1980. *Novak's textbook of gynecology.* 10th ed. Baltimore: The Williams & Wilkins Co.

Romney, S. L., et al., eds. 1981. *Gynecology and obstetrics: the health care of women.* 2nd ed. New York: McGraw-Hill Book Co.

Tyler, S. L., and Woodall, G. M. 1982. *Female health and gynecology: across the life span.* Bowie, Md.: Robert J. Brady Co.

■ 5 ■

SEXUAL DEVELOPMENT AND SEXUALITY

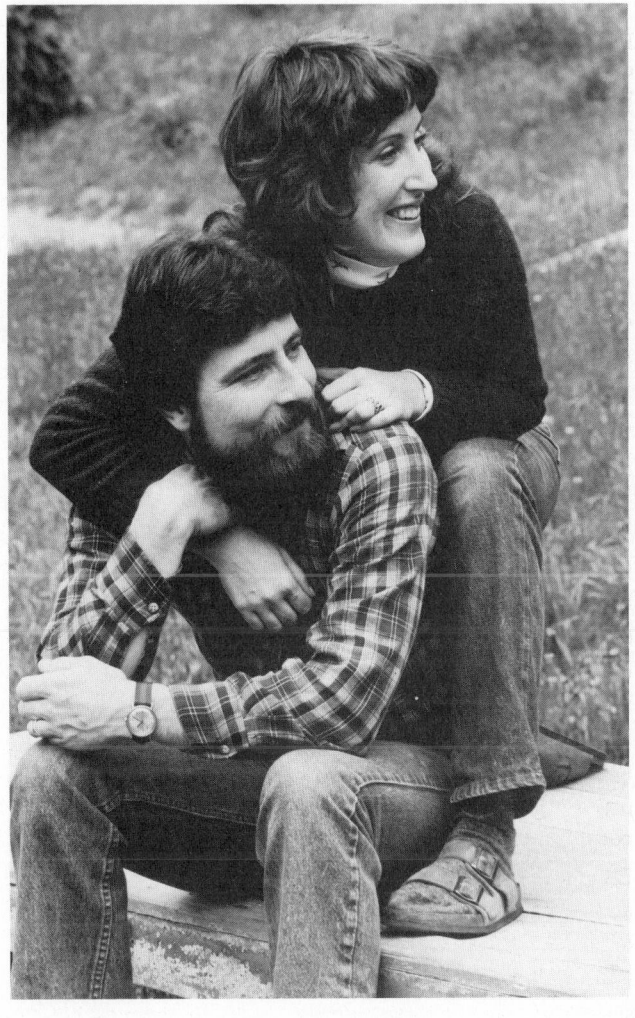

■ CHAPTER CONTENTS

COMPONENTS OF HUMAN SEXUALITY

DEVELOPMENT OF SEXUALITY
  Infancy to Late Childhood
  Adolescence
  Adulthood

PUBERTY
  Major Physical Changes
  Physiology of Onset
  Effects of Male Hormones
  Effects of Ovarian Hormones

MENSTRUAL CYCLE
  Female Reproductive Cycle
  Ovarian Follicular Changes
  Ovulation
  Endometrial and Cervical Mucosal Changes
  Premenstrual Tension Syndrome
  Dysmenorrhea
  Menstrual Cycle Variations

CLIMACTERIC
  Psychologic Aspects of Menopause
  Physical Aspects of Menopause
  Sexual Activity in the Climacteric
  Interventions

COITUS (SEXUAL INTERCOURSE)
  Psychosocial Aspects
  Physiology of Sexual Response
  Neurologic Control of Sexual Response

(Continued)

■ OBJECTIVES

- Describe the components and development of sexuality.

- Discuss puberty and the changes that the adolescent experiences.

- Explain the physical and psychologic aspects of the menstrual cycle.

- Identify the physical and emotional changes of the climacteric.

- Describe the physical and emotional aspects of coitus.

COMPONENTS OF HUMAN SEXUALITY

Sexuality is a dynamic force that is active throughout each person's life. And because its psychosocial and biologic components are intertwined and interdependent, sexuality is a forceful determinant of personality and behavior. Lief (1981) has developed a sexual system that emphasizes the pervasiveness of sexuality in our lives. The components of this sexual system are:

Biologic sex	Chromosomes; hormones; primary and secondary sex characteristics
Sexual identity (or core-gender identity)	Sense of maleness and femaleness
Gender identity	Sense of masculinity and femininity
Gender role behavior	
Sex behavior	Behavior motivated by desire for sexual pleasure, ultimately orgasm (physical sex)
Gender behavior	Behavior with masculine and feminine connotations*

*From Lief, H. I. 1981. Sexual counseling. In *Gynecology and obstetrics: the health care of women,* 2nd ed., ed. S. L. Romney et al. New York: McGraw-Hill Book Co.

Biologic sex is determined at conception (this process is discussed in Chapter 8). A female embryo develops ovaries, and a male embryo develops testes. Generally, infants are born with clearly defined primary sex characteristics. Secondary sex characteristics develop at puberty. When primary sex characteristics are ambiguous at birth, the sex assigned to the child will be the determining factor in his or her ultimate concept of sexual identity.

Sexual identity (core-gender identity) is an individual's inner feeling of maleness or femaleness over a period of time. Lief (1981) suggests that a secure sense of maleness or femaleness is established in a child by age 3 years as a result of consistent parental and social reinforcements. Sex-appropriate clothing (for example, pink-colored clothes for girls and blue for boys) and verbal reinforcers ("That's my big strong boy"; "That's my sweet baby girl") are among the most obvious methods parents use to assign sexual identity. This term is defined differently by other theorists. For example, Hyde (1982) sees sexual identity as a person's concept of herself or himself as a heterosexual, homosexual, or bisexual.

Gender identity refers to the broader, stereotypical ideas of masculinity and femininity that are the sex roles prescribed by society. Traditionally, masculinity has been associated with courage, strength, stoicism, aggression, sexual assertiveness, rational thinking, stability, intelligence, and career achievement. Femininity has been associated with dependence, passivity, motherhood, tenderness, nurturance, and submission. Gender identity is learned over time through reinforcement. Some self-doubts and conflicts about gender identity are normal, especially during adolescence and middle age. Serious deviations in gender identity can lead to sexual behavior such as fetishism, promiscuity, or excessive competitiveness in nonsexual pursuits (Lief, 1981). Homosexuality was once classified as a deviation in gender identity. However, it is currently viewed as a variation. Insecurity in one's gender identity may lead to poor adjustment with the opposite sex. Impotence may occur in the male; lack of arousal and response may occur in the female.

Gender role behavior has two components: physical sex behavior and gender behavior. The act of coitus (sexual intercourse), physiologic responses, and sexual dysfunctions are aspects of physical sex behavior; gender behavior is reflected in the sexual relationships between individuals. These two components of gender role behavior do not stand isolated in life: they merge within the individual.

Many researchers are currently evaluating traditional sexual roles and relationships to determine what is biologically inherent and what is societally imposed. Some are questioning whether these sexual roles stifle rather than encourage an individual's quest for personal development and psychologic well-being. Many social critics promote the discarding of stereotyped roles; others encourage their modification. In our society many of the rigid aspects characteristic of sexual roles have given way to increased flexibility.

DEVELOPMENT OF SEXUALITY

The evolvement of sexuality begins at conception and continues through adulthood. The development of sexuality is modified and influenced by all life experiences—biologic, psychologic, sociocultural, and ethical. During the prenatal period, biologic sex is determined by the complex interaction of neurohormonal, genetic, and physiologic factors (Wolman and Money, 1980). In addition, other senses and systems are developing that enable the infant at birth to react to sexual stimuli. For example, touch, which is fundamental in the development of sexuality, is highly developed by 8 weeks' gestation.

Infancy to Late Childhood

Tactile stimulation is essential for normal growth, development, and maternal–child bonding. Thus an infant responds positively to cuddling, holding, and touching. Adults demonstrate an identical need to be held, to be fondled, and to be physically close to a loved or cherished person. It should be noted that male and female children have traditionally been treated differently in our society with regard to physical affection. Males usually receive less tactile stimulation after infancy than do females, which certainly has implications for the development of gender role behaviors.

Many sexual stereotypes are perpetuated by parents. Children's gender identity is established in part by the manner in which they are treated by parents and others, the toys they are given, the way they are disciplined, and the expectations others have for their behavior, education, and career. In addition, children are influenced by parental attitudes toward elimination, nakedness, and touching. A child senses parental embarrassment or reluctance to answer questions related to sexuality. The expectations that begin early in life influence a child's self-esteem regarding sexual functioning.

Sexual identity is also established by the functioning of the child's body. Male genitals are evident and responsive. Penile erections occur frequently, and masturbation begins early. Boys are taught to be proud of their genitals, which are occasionally given nicknames such as "the family jewels." Subtle innuendoes regarding boys' sexuality may confuse masculinity and sexuality (for example, a macho man is sexy).

Female genitals are less obvious, and the beginning of sexual feelings is more diffuse. Girls, for example, are not accustomed to the daily touching of genitals. Well-meaning mothers may slap girls' hands and tell them "not to touch down there." Menstruation may be considered dirty, so that girls may grow up not understanding their own sexuality and feeling less worthy than boys.

Parents build self-esteem in their children by actively listening to them, taking them seriously, treating them as important loved people, and letting them know they are genuinely needed. Such children will grow up with positive feelings of self-worth and dignity. In response to questions about sexuality, parents must be honest, answer questions when they are asked, and be available to talk and establish rapport with their children. Open lines of communication begin early in the parent–child relationship, not when the child reaches 13 years old.

Adolescence

Adolescence is perhaps the most critical period for the awakening of sexual feelings. The change in one decade of life from prepubertal child to psychosexually mature adult is overwhelming to adolescents and parents alike. For both sexes, the occurrence of puberty heightens sexual feelings and thoughts. Adolescence finds sexually mature young persons trying to cope with new situations and sensations while they are still psychologically immature. Sexual experimentation begins in various ways. Masturbation accompanied by fantasy is prevalent. Homosexual experiences may occur in the form of exploratory erotic play, fondling, or bodily examination; and mutual masturbation for boys is not uncommon. These activities are transient and do not signify a homosexual tendency. Heterosexual contacts progress over 4 or 5 years from initial kissing and fondling to mutual bodily exploration and masturbation to sexual intercourse.

The "problem" of adolescent sexuality is not new, although it has received widespread attention in the last decade. Society is witnessing a change in attitudes toward sexuality. There is an increased visibility of sexuality and sexually active adolescents. It is the exceptional young person who does not have sexual intercourse during the teenage years. On the average, the age of first intercourse is 16 years (Guttmacher, 1981). The problems inherent in adolescent sexuality are pregnancy and sexually transmitted disease. The goal of health care providers, parents, and society must be to assist adolescents in responsible sexual decision making.

Sexually active *young adolescents* (under 15 years old) are often products of a troubled home life, school failure, or severe depression. Sex for this age group is not within normal limits of psychosocial development. Their participation in sexual activity often has underlying motives, whether conscious or subconscious, such as to rebel or to counteract feelings of worthlessness. These youngsters are rarely involved in positive relationships, but use sex as a way to obtain rewards such as love or attention and to punish family or school. Their knowledge of reproduction and contraception is minimal; they represent the highest risk group for problems should they become pregnant. Sexually active young adolescents need expert counseling by professionals who can assist the youngsters in finding out and resolving the conflicts that are the true motives behind their behavior.

The peer group is the paramount authority among adolescents and it gives them the security to experiment with independent decision making. Adolescent rebellion becomes a vehicle to accomplish this as well as other developmental tasks. Limit testing and risk taking are prevalent as these young people work through their rebellion. If peer pressure is strong, sexual experimentation will probably be considered an accepted practice.

Girls may perceive sex as a requisite for dating or solidifying a relationship. Many girls think that to be popular, they must engage in sexual intercourse. In reality, many girls may not want to have intercourse as much as the rewards of intercourse: being caressed, held, and loved. The double standard of virginity and "nice girls don't" is still strong but is schizophrenic in nature.

Boys too are under pressure to have intercourse. Peer pressure is important and encourages sexual experimentation. Boys are expected to know how to perform sexually, creating even more pressure and, perhaps, damage to self-esteem. Boys may see intercourse as a way of achieving adulthood and being a man. Men have "natural drives" that they must "satisfy." These myths can be particularly damaging to young men in their adjustment to sexual identity.

Many incidents of first intercourse are unprotected. Reasons vary from "I didn't expect it," to "I didn't think I'd get pregnant," to "contraceptives weren't available," to "I thought it was the wrong time of the month." Lack of knowledge regarding sexual reproduction is a major factor in teenage pregnancy; the other major factor is adolescents' inability to foresee the consequences of their actions.

Middle adolescents begin to think more abstractly and can begin to see consequences. While they may be ignorant of reproductive anatomy and physiology, their use of contraception is generally more widespread than that of younger adolescents. Frequently, however, the methods they use are among the most ineffective contraceptives. Withdrawal and "Coke" douches may be relied on until the teen either experiences a pregnancy scare or comes to grips with his or her sexual activity and consciously seeks family planning.

Adolescents must confront a number of factors prior to seeking contraception. Admitting to being sexually active is perhaps the most difficult barrier. Overcoming the guilt associated with intercourse; being mature enough to understand the consequences of pregnancy; and dealing with the fear of parental recrimination take a great deal of intellectual work on the part of the adolescent.

Late adolescence is associated with a more mature attitude toward oneself and one's life. This attitude may manifest itself in educational or career pursuits or in the search for a marriage partner and entrance into parenthood. The culmination of this stage is a unified sense of self. The ending of the adolescent period varies greatly and is influenced by the sociocultural and economic status of the family.

Adulthood

Adult sexuality is practiced within and outside of marriage. Gagnon (1977) states that 80%–90% of the adults in the United States marry. Even though it is estimated that one divorce occurs in every third or fourth marriage, divorced persons remarry at a high rate. Sexual expression has the most legitimacy within marriage in our society (Hyde, 1982); hence marital sex is one of the most frequent forms of sexual expression for adults. Hyde reports that coital behavior is more frequent, of longer duration, and more varied now than 40 years ago. It is clear that new lifestyles, changing morality, and effective contraceptive methods have separated sexual expression from its reproductive functions. Indeed, in the young adult period (age 20–35 years) the major developmental tasks may include learning to give and receive pleasure, making decisions about childbearing, and developing a sexual value system while learning tolerance for the values of others (Mims and Swenson, 1980).

Both advantages and disadvantages have resulted from these new sexual freedoms. For many adults, they have been a positive contribution in the development of a meaningful, mutually satisfying, and pleasurable sexual life. For others, unrealistic sexual expectations, sexual exploitation of one partner by another, meaningless sexual encounters, and overemphasis on sexual performance for its own sake have created serious problems. Most authorities agree that the majority of adults experience sexual acts within meaningful, responsible, and committed relationships.

There has been unfounded belief that as men and women grow older they cease to be sexual beings. Perhaps this notion takes seed as young people observe the behavior of their parents and other adults, many of whom think that expression of sexual feelings in front of children is inappropriate. Children begin to believe that their parents and similar-age persons are incapable of experiencing passion and intense sexual urges and desires. Fortunately, most adults do not believe this, and expression of their sexuality adds great joy and dimension to their lives.

Many people view sexual activity among elderly persons as unseemly. Caretakers of the elderly in nursing homes discourage expression of sexuality among residents. The fact that sexual activity can and does continue well after the 60s and 70s—even into the 90s (given an attentive partner and reasonable health) must receive recognition and planning. Positive attitudes toward the sexuality of the elderly as well as privacy for sexual expression should be encouraged.

PUBERTY

The term *puberty* refers to the transitional and developmental period between childhood and the attainment of adult sexual characteristics and functioning. Its onset is never sudden, although it may appear so to parents or to the young person who is not prepared for the bodily and emotional changes of puberty. Generally, boys mature physically about two years later than girls. The average age of onset is 14 years in boys and 12 years in girls, although there is wide individual variation. The onset of puberty ranges in boys from 10–19 years of age, and in girls from 9–17 years of age. Puberty occurs over a period of time ranging from 1½ years to 4 or 5 years and involves profound physical, psychologic, and emotional changes. These changes result from the interaction of the central nervous system (CNS) and the endocrine organs.

Closely associated with puberty is the period of *adolescence*. Adolescence is initiated by puberty and ends with the attainment of young adulthood. Early adolescence begins one to two years before puberty occurs.

Major Physical Changes

In both boys and girls, puberty is preceded by an accelerated growth rate called the *adolescent spurt* (Gold and Josimovich, 1980). Widespread systemic changes occur, as well as maturation of the reproductive organs. One correlation between physical and sexual maturation can be seen: The broadening of the female hips and new distribution of adipose tissue and the broadening of the male shoulders and increasing muscularity of the body are associated with sexual maturation. These patterns occur prior to and during the maturation of the secondary sexual characteristics.

Tanner (1962) described a normal clinical progression of three significant somatic changes that occur during puberty in British children. These somatic changes involve development of the breast, pubic hair, and male external genitals. Zacharias and colleagues (1970) confirmed no significant variations in development of these same somatic changes in other industrialized countries. Although individual maturational patterns vary widely, usually males first note such changes as an increase in the size of the genitals; the appearance of pubic, axillary, and facial hair; the deepening of the voice; and nocturnal seminal emissions without sexual stimulation (mature sperm are usually not contained in the earliest emissions). Females experience a broadening of the hips, then budding of the breasts, the appearance of pubic and axillary hair, and the onset of menstruation. The maturation process spans approximately 4.5 years, as identified by the earliest recognizable somatic changes (breast buds and growth spurt) to full maturity. Average time between breast development and menarche is 2.3 years (Stone, 1981). A wide physiologic variation exists in the chronologic appearance and progression of the somatic puberty changes and there is considerable overlapping of events.

Figure 5–1 shows the signs of puberty in females correlated with age of onset. These variations are a result of different degrees of response of the gonads and adrenal gland to hypothalamic–pituitary stimulation and the target organ's cellular sensitivity to sexual steroids.

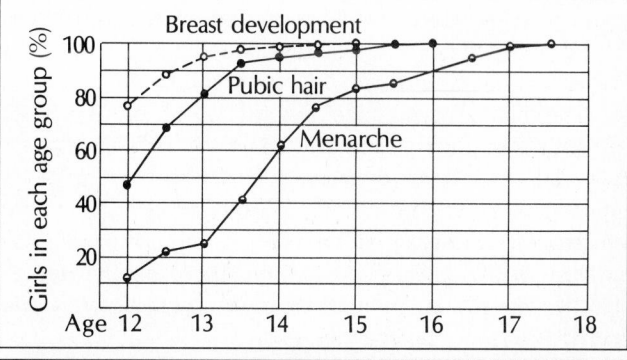

FIGURE 5–1 Signs of puberty in females according to age. (From Beller, F. K., et al. 1974. *Gynecology: a textbook for students.* 2nd ed. New York: Springer Verlag New York, Inc., p. 69.)

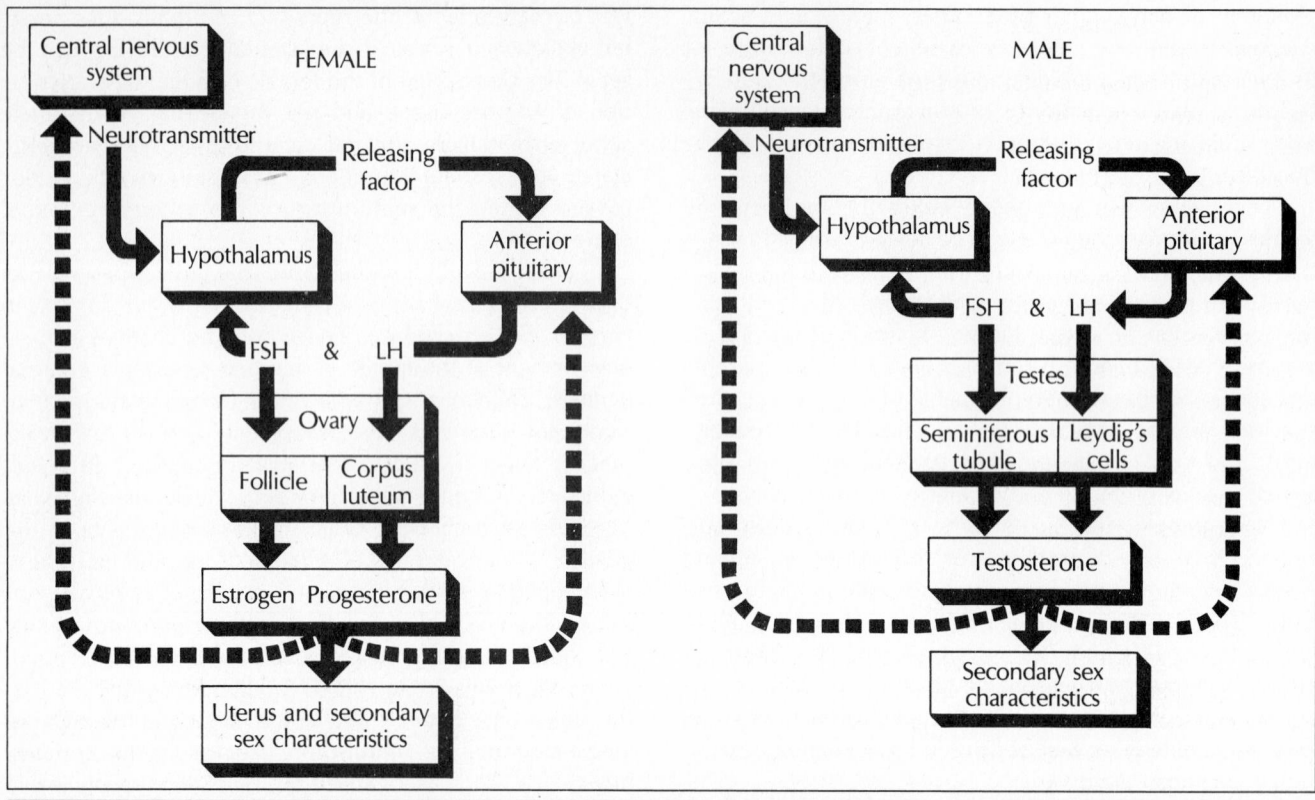

FIGURE 5–2 Positive feedback is illustrated with solid lines and negative feedback is illustrated with a broken line. Through a neurotransmitter, the CNS stimulates the hypothalamus, which in turn produces a gonadotropin-releasing factor that causes the anterior pituitary to produce gonadotropins (FSH or LH). These hormones stimulate specific structures in the gonads to secrete steroid hormones (estrogen, progesterone, or testosterone). The rise in pituitary hormone production increases hypothalamus activity in a positive feedback relationship. Elevated steroid hormone levels stimulate the CNS and pituitary gland to inhibit hormone production in a negative feedback relationship.

Physiology of Onset

Puberty is initiated by the maturation of the hypothalamic–pituitary complex (*gonadostat*) and the input of the CNS. The process, which begins in fetal life, is sequential and complex. For example, the critical rise of adrenal androgens around 8 years of age in both boys and girls is probably one precursor essential to the maturation of the gonadostat (Ducharme et al., 1976). Following prepubertal progressive rises in the levels of *follicle-stimulating hormone* (FSH) and *luteinizing hormone* (LH), and in response to the gonadostat maturation, the hypothalamus is triggered, and pubertal changes begin.

The hypothalamic nuclei synthesize and release *gonadotropin-releasing factor* (GnRF), which is transmitted by a portal system to the anterior pituitary. There it causes the synthesis and secretion of FSH and LH. Prior to puberty,

the gonads do synthesize and secrete small amounts of androgens and estrogens, which are thought to inhibit production of GnRF. This inhibitory activity is decreased at puberty, and a new equilibrium is established in the hypothalamic–pituitary–gonad complex, whereby increased amounts of androgens and estrogens are required to inhibit the production of GnRF. Meanwhile, increased FSH and LH are released (Blum, 1982). Figure 5–2 illustrates this neuroendocrine regulation of gonadal maturation or gonadostat.

Other hormones are involved in the onset of puberty. Their action, although less direct, is essential. Abnormally high or low levels of adrenocorticotropic hormone (ACTH), thyroid hormone, or somatotropic (growth) hormone (STH) can cause disruptions in the occurrence of normal puberty.

Effects of Male Hormones

In addition to being essential for spermatogenesis, *testosterone* is responsible for the development of secondary male characteristics and for certain behavioral patterns. These androgenic effects include structural and functional development of the male genitals and accessory glands, emission and ejaculation of seminal fluid, distribution of bodily hair, and the hypertrophy of the vocal cords. The action of testosterone on the CNS is thought to produce aggressiveness and sexual drive. Testosterone also stimulates the sebaceous glands' production of sebum, which contributes to the development of acne, and it assists in the lessening of subcutaneous fat deposits. The anabolic activity of testosterone increases muscle mass, promotes growth and strength of the long bones, and enhances the rate of erythrocyte production. The resulting male characteristics of greater strength and stature, as well as a higher hematocrit than females, generally develop over a period of 4 or 5 years (Ticky and Malasanos, 1975). The action of testosterone is constant; it is not cyclic, nor is it limited to a certain number of years.

Along with testosterone and the other androgens, FSH maintains the spermatogenic function of the testes. LH is called *interstitial cell-stimulating hormone* (ICSH) in males because it stimulates the interstitial cells of the testes (Leydig's cells) to synthesize testosterone from cholesterol. Testosterone in turn inhibits the secretion of ICSH by the anterior pituitary. Most of the circulating testosterone is converted in the liver to 17-ketosteroids, which are secreted in the urine. About one-third of these ketosteroids are metabolized from testicular testosterone; the rest is adrenal in origin. (Figure 5–2).

In addition to the testes, the prostate and seminal vesicles are major target organs for testosterone.

Effects of Ovarian Hormones

Having experienced menarche, a female undergoes a cyclic pattern of ovulation and menstruation (if pregnancy does not occur) for a period of 30–40 years. This cycle is an orderly process under neurohormonal control: Each month one ovum matures, ruptures, and presents itself for fertilization. The ovary, vagina, uterus, and fallopian tubes are major target organs for female hormones. Each organ undergoes changes indicative of the exact point in time of any menstrual cycle.

Like the testes, the ovaries produce mature gametes and secrete hormones. These activities are controlled by the continuous feedback system shown in Figure 5–2. Ovarian hormones include the estrogens, progesterone, and testosterone. The ovary is sensitive to FSH and LH. The uterus is sensitive to estrogen and progesterone. The relative proportion of these hormones to each other controls the events of both the ovarian and uterine cycles.

ESTROGENS

Estrogens are associated with those characteristics contributing to "femaleness." Although the six natural estrogens are usually not differentiated from each other, the major estrogenic effects are due primarily to three classical estrogens: estrone, β-estradiol, and estriol. β-estradiol is the major estrogen. Estrogens are secreted in large amounts by the ovaries in nonpregnant women; minute amounts are secreted by the adrenal cortex.

Estrogens control the development of the female secondary sex characteristics: breast development, the widening of the hips, and the adipose deposits in the buttocks and mons pubis. Certain characteristics, such as a high-pitched voice, occur because of low androgen levels, although the adrenal cortex supplies sufficient androgens to cause hair growth. The female pattern of hair growth is influenced by estrogens. Estrogens assist in the maturation of the ovarian follicles and cause the endometrial mucosa to proliferate following menstruation. The amount of estrogens is greatest during the proliferative (follicular or estrogenic) phase of the menstrual cycle (p. 97). Estrogen also causes the uterus to increase in size and weight because of increased glycogen, amino acids, electrolytes, and water. Blood supply is augmented as well. Under the influence of estrogens, myometrial contractility increases in both the uterus and the fallopian tubes, and there is increased uterine sensitivity to oxytocin. The vaginal epithelium becomes thicker. More sodium and chloride are retained by the kidneys, causing mild edema and body weight increase. Estrogens inhibit FSH production and stimulate LH production.

Estrogens have effects on many hormones and other carrier proteins. This explains, for example, the increased amount of protein-bound iodine in pregnant women and in women who use oral contraceptives containing estrogen (Little and Billiar, 1981)

Estrogens may increase libidinal feelings in humans. They decrease the excitability of the hypothalamus, which may cause an increase in sexual desire and contribute to so-called feminine behavior.

For many years estrogens have been considered a preventive factor for coronary artery disease in women up to menopause, in the absence of diabetes or hypertension. Both lipoprotein and triglyceride metabolism are altered by estrogens. Although low estrogen levels do decrease serum cholesterol and β-lipoprotein levels and increase phospholipids and α-lipoprotein levels, numerous other factors must be considered in the development of coronary artery disease. Persistently high stress levels coupled with specific types of personality patterns, diet, smoking, obesity, and lack of exercise seem influential in today's rising incidence of coronary artery disease in women. Currently, there is no reliable evidence for administration of estrogen in either males or females to reduce coronary artery disease (Little and Billiar, 1981).

PROGESTERONE

Progesterone is secreted by the corpus luteum and is found in greatest amounts during the secretory (luteal or progestational) phase of the menstrual cycle. It decreases the motility and contractility of the uterus caused by estrogens, thereby preparing the uterus for implantation after fertilization of the ovum. The endometrial mucosa is in a ready state as a result of estrogenic influence. Progesterone causes the uterine endometrium to further increase its supply of glycogen, arterial blood, secretory glands, amino acids, and water. This hormone is often called the *hormone of pregnancy* because its effects on the uterus allow pregnancy to be maintained.

Under the influence of progesterone, the vaginal epithelium proliferates and the cervix secretes thick, viscous mucus. Breast glandular tissue increases in size and complexity. Progesterone also prepares the breasts for lactation.

The temperature rise of about 0.35C (0.5F) that accompanies ovulation and persists throughout the secretory phase of the menstrual cycle is probably due to progesterone. Historically, progesterone has been thought to cause passive behavior and to have a calming effect.

ROLE OF PROSTAGLANDINS

Prolific research is underway to determine the definite and complete role of *prostaglandins* (PGs) in human reproduction (Caldwell and Behrman, 1981; Wilhelmson et al., 1981). Many PGs have been identified and classified according to their molecular structure. They are complex lipid compounds, rapidly synthesized throughout the body from arachidonic acid. They have a very short half-life. Being tissue hormones rather than humoral, only very small amounts circulate (Lackritz, 1981). Their actions are more varied than any other naturally occurring compound in the body (Hall and Behrman, 1981). To date, the majority of the research on PGs has been done with animals. Reports of human research are increasing; however, lack of agreement exists in many of the reported results.

Certain PGs are known to have a major role in the regulation of the reproductive processes. In the female, PGE_2 and $PGF_{2\alpha}$ are the most important. Generally, PGEs relax smooth muscles and are potent vasodilators; PGFs are potent vasoconstrictors and increase the contractility of muscles and arteries. While their primary actions seem antagonistic, their basic regulatory functions in cells are achieved through an intricate pattern of reciprocal events. The discussion here will summarize briefly their role in ovulation and menstruation.

Authorities differ about the precise mechanisms by which PGs control and/or mediate ovulation. PG formation increases during follicular maturation and is essential to ovulation. Extrusion of the ovum, resulting from the increased contractility of the smooth muscle in the theca layer of the mature follicle, is thought to be caused by $PGF_{2\alpha}$. Significant amounts of PGs are found in and around the follicle at the time of ovulation. A possibility exists that PGs may act as intracellular regulators in hormone action (Little and Billiar, 1981). $PGF_{2\alpha}$ receptors have been demonstrated in the human corpus luteum (Hall and Behrman, 1981), and $PGF_{2\alpha}$ is known to cause luteolysis. While the exact mechanism by which the corpus luteum regresses remains obscure, $PGF_{2\alpha}$ is postulated to induce progesterone withdrawal, the nadir of which coincides with the onset of early menses.

Endometrium and menstrual fluid are known to be rich sources of PGs. It is thought that estrogen acts on the uterus primed by progesterone to produce PGs. Vijayakumar and colleagues (1981) suggest that the ratio of PGF to PGE is a critical factor in the endometrial cycle. Both PGE and PGF peak during the proliferative phase, but PGE peaks at a higher level, which increases through vasodilatation the blood supply for the regenerating endometrium. The level of PGE then steadily falls during the secretory phase while the $PGF_{2\alpha}$ level rises. Only during the late secretory phase is the level of $PGF_{2\alpha}$ higher than that of PGE. This event results in an increase in vasoconstriction and contractility of the myometrium which contributes to the ischemia preceding menstruation. High concentration of PGs may also account for the vasoconstriction of the endometrium venous lacunae allowing for platelet aggregation at vascular rupture points, thereby preventing a rapid blood loss during menstruation. The menstrual flow's high concentration of PGs may also facilitate the process of tissue digestion, which allows for an orderly desquamation of the endometrium during menstruation.

MENSTRUAL CYCLE

Menarche—the onset of menstruation—occurs at approximately 12–13 years of age. Early cycles are often anovulatory and irregular in frequency, amount of flow, and duration. Within several months to 2–3 years, a regular cycle becomes established.

Menstrual parameters vary greatly among individuals. Generally, menses occur every 28 days, plus or minus 5–10 days. Approximately 60% of women experience menses every 25–30 days, but 1% menstruate as frequently as every 20 days or less and another 1% have periods 36–40 days apart. Emotional and physical factors such as illness, excessive fatigue, and high levels of stress or anxiety can alter the cycle interval. In addition, certain environmental factors such as temperature and altitude may influence the cycle.

The duration of menses is from 2–8 days, with the blood loss averaging 30–100 mL and the loss of iron averaging 0.5–1 mg daily.

Menstruation may be defined as cyclic uterine bleeding in response to cyclic hormonal changes. The menstrual discharge or flow is composed of blood mixed with fluid, cervical and vaginal secretions, bacteria, mucus, leukocytes, and partially autolyzed cellular debris. The menstrual discharge is dark red and has a distinctive odor. It results from physiologic tissue necrosis caused by ischemia and anoxia of the endometrium. Menstruation occurs when the ovum is not fertilized.

A review of the endometrium and its arterial blood supply will provide further understanding of this process.

Blood flow from the spiral arterioles in the superficial endometrium is reduced, with resultant ischemia and anoxia, which in turn produce necrosis and discharge of the superficial endometrium (menses). Concurrently, the straight arterioles provide the basal endometrium with sufficient blood flow to maintain it and the endometrial glands or seeds that are responsible for the regeneration of the endometrium in the next female reproductive or menstrual cycle (Figure 5–3). Bleeding is controlled by vasospasm of the straight basal arterioles, resulting in coagulative necrosis at the vessel tips.

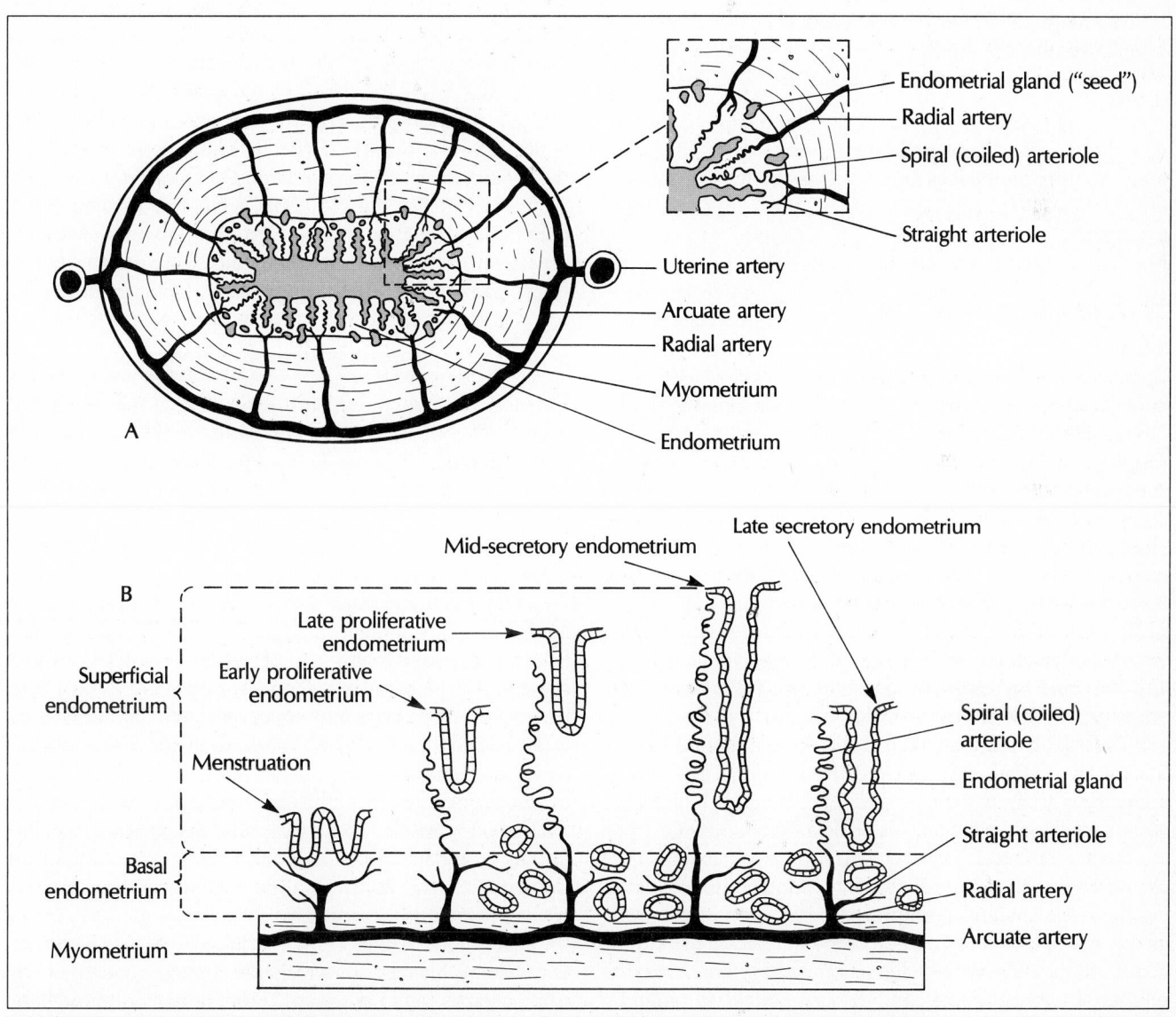

FIGURE 5–3 A, Blood supply to the endometrium (cross-section view of the uterus). **B,** Schematic representation of blood supply during complete menstrual cycle. (Modified from Bloom, M. L., and Van Dongen, L. 1972. *Clinical gynaecology: integration of structure and function.* London: Williams Heinemann Medical Books Ltd., pp. 144–145.)

Female Reproductive Cycle

It has been customary to call the monthly rhythmic changes in sexually mature females "the menstrual cycle." A more accurate term is the *female reproductive cycle* (FRC). The FRC is comprised of the ovarian cycle (ovulation) and the uterine cycle (menstruation), which occur simultaneously (Figure 5–4). In turn, the ovarian and uterine cycles have particular phases.

1. Ovarian cycle
   a. Follicular phase (Days 1–14)
   b. Luteal phase (Days 15–28)
2. Uterine cycle
   a. Menstrual phase (Days1–5)
   b. Proliferative phase (Days 6–14)
   c. Secretory phase (Days 15–16)
   d. Ischemic phase (Days 27 and 28)

The FRC is mediated by complex interactions between neurohormonal systems and their target tissues. This hierarchial neurohormonal system involves the hypothalamus, anterior pituitary, and the ovaries; their functions are reciprocal.

The hypothalamus controls anterior pituitary hormone production by secretion of gonadotropin-releasing hormone (GnRH). This releasing hormone is often called both luteinizing hormone–releasing hormone (LHRH) and follicle stimulating hormone–releasing hormone (FSHRH). Recent studies have shown some basis for the belief that the GnRH molecule combines both LHRH and the FSHRH (Guyton, 1981). Therefore, the term GnRH is used interchangeably with either LHRH and/or FSHRH.

In response to the hypothalamic-releasing hormone GnRH, the anterior pituitary secretes gonadotropic hormones: follicle-stimulating hormone (FSH) and luteinizing hormone (LH). The ovaries contain specialized FSH and LH receptor cells. These receptor cells activate the production of adenylcyclase, causing increased cell growth and hormone secretion through the cyclic adenosine monophosphate (cAMP) mechanism.

The FSH is primarily responsible for the maturation of the follicle. During this process, the maturing follicle secretes increasing amounts of estrogen, which enhance the growth and maturation of the follicle. (Concurrently, the excessive amounts of estrogen also are responsible for the rebuilding/proliferation phase of the endometrium following its desquamation during menses.) In spite of the rich supply of FSH, final maturation of the follicle will not come about without the synergistic action of LH. The anterior pituitary's production of LH increases sixfold to tenfold. About 18 hours after the peak production, ovulation occurs. Additionally, LH is responsible for the "luteinizing" of the theca and granulosa cells of the ruptured follicle (described in the next section). As a result, estrogen production is reduced and progesterone secretion is continued. Thus estrogen levels fall a day before ovulation; tiny

amounts of progesterone are in evidence. Ovulation takes place following the very rapid growth of the follicle, as the sustained high level of estrogen diminishes, and progesterone secretion is begun.

The ruptured follicle undergoes rapid change; luteinization is accomplished and the mass of cells becomes the corpus luteum. The lutein cells secrete large amounts of progesterone with smaller amounts of estrogen. (Concurrently, the excessive amounts of progesterone are responsible for the secretory phase of the uterine cycle.) After 7 or 8 days following ovulation, the corpus luteum begins to involute, losing its secretory function. The production of both progesterone and estrogen is severely diminished. The anterior pituitary responds with increasingly large amounts of FSH; a few days later LH production begins. As a result, new follicles become responsive to another ovarian cycle.

As has been described, hypothalamic releasing hormones, anterior pituitary gonadotropic hormones (FSH and LH), and ovarian estrogen and progesterone comprise the neurohormonal hypothalamic–pituitary–ovarian axis system controlling the FRC. The hormones are secreted in continuously fluctuating amounts throughout the female reproductive cycle in precarious and miraculous interrelationships, which are still incompletely understood.

Ovarian Follicular Changes

FSH induces the growth and maturation of the primordial follicle. Within it, the oocyte grows. Follicular cells increase in number, and a fluid space (antrum) appears and increases in size. Under the dual control of FSH and LH, as previously described, a mature *graafian follicle* appears about the fourteenth day. Figure 5–5 shows a mature graafian follicle in diagrammatic form.

In the mature graafian follicle, the cells surrounding the antral cavity are granulosa cells. The oocyte and follicular fluid are enclosed in the cumulus oophorus. The stromal elements of the ovary are condensed around the follicle in two layers: the *theca interna,* a vascular, hypertrophied layer; and the *theca externa,* an avascular layer of connective tissue. The theca interna cells resemble the luteal cells of the corpus luteum. The zona pellucida (oolemma), a thick elastic capsule, develops around the oocyte. The fully mature graafian follicle is a large structure, measuring about 5–10 mm. With maturity the follicle produces increasing amounts of estrogen.

Just before ovulation the mature oocyte completes its first meiotic division, in which the diploid number of 46 chromosomes found in somatic cells is reduced to the haploid number of 23. As another result of this division, the first polar body and the secondary oocyte are formed (see Chapter 8). This process is usually completed as ovulation is completed. It is not until after sperm penetration of the ovum that the second meiotic division occurs and the second polar body is formed.

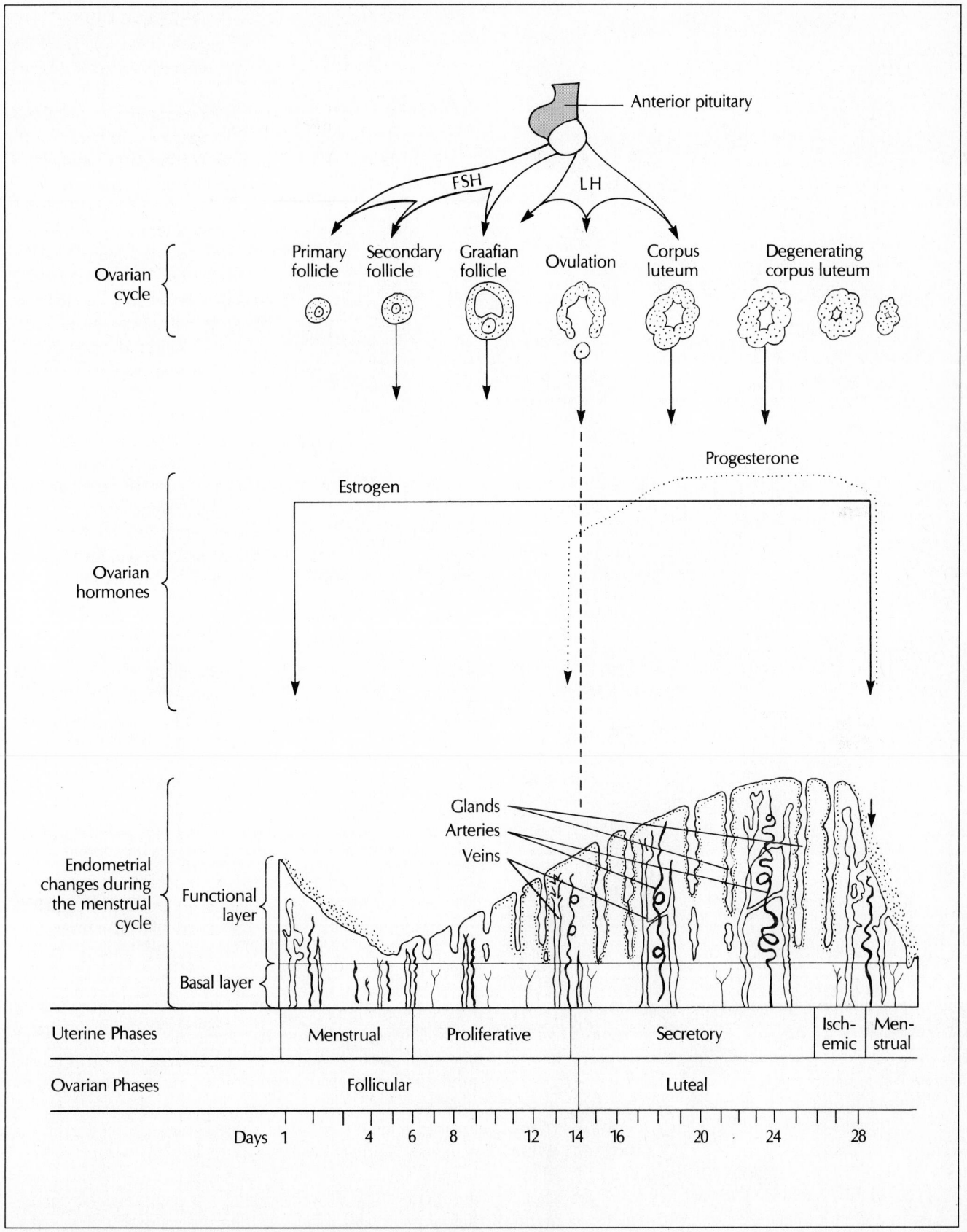

FIGURE 5–4 Female reproductive cycle: Interrelationships of hormones and the four phases of the uterine cycle and the two phases of the ovarian cycle.

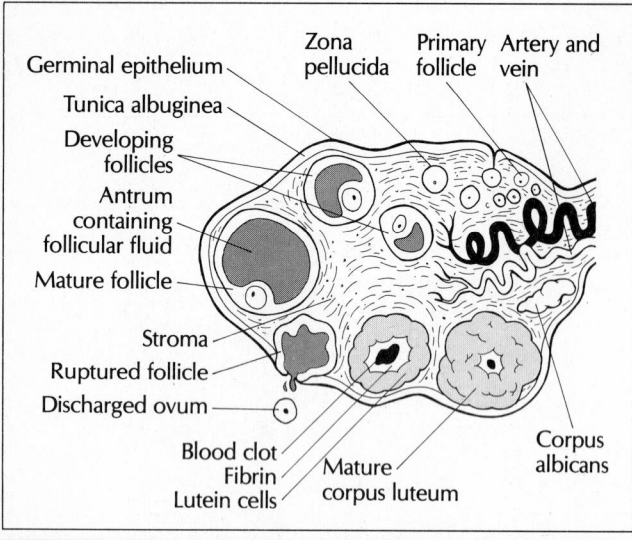

FIGURE 5–5 Various stages of development of the ovarian follicles.

Ovulation

As the graafian follicle matures and enlarges, it comes close to the surface of the ovary. The ovary surface has a blisterlike protrusion 10–15 mm in diameter, and the follicle's walls become thin. Extrusion of the ovum is aided by proteolytic enzyme formation by the theca externa and prostaglandin secretion into the follicular tissues. Thus the secondary oocyte, the polar bodies, and the follicular fluid are extruded. The egg carries with it the cumulus oophorus. Discharged near the fimbriated end of the fallopian tube, the egg is pulled into the tube and begins its journey through it. Occasionally ovulation is accompanied by midcycle pain, known as *mittelschmerz*, which may be caused by a thick ovarian tunica albuginea or by a local peritoneal reaction to the expelling of the follicular contents.

Vaginal secretion may increase during ovulation, and a small amount of blood (midcycle spotting) may be discharged as well. The body temperature increases about 0.3–0.6C (0.5–1.0F) at the time of ovulation or shortly thereafter and remains elevated throughout the secretory phase. There may be an accompanying sharp temperature drop just before the increase. These temperature changes are useful clinically to determine the approximate time of ovulation (see Chapter 6).

Ovum transport is important to fertility. Because the ovum is thought to be fertile for only 6–24 hours, any delay in transport causes difficulty. Generally, the ovum takes several minutes to travel from the ruptured follicle to the fallopian tube opening. The contractions of the fallopian tube smooth muscle and ciliary epithelial action propel the ovum through the tube. The ovum remains in the ampulla where it may be fertilized and cleavage can begin. It

reaches the uterine lumen 72–96 hours after extrusion. By then, denudation of the cumulus oophorus is completed.

Under the effects of increasing amounts of LH, the corpus luteum develops from the ruptured follicle as a result of the luteinization of the granulosa cells. Following the disappearance of the antral cavity, the granulosa cells secrete steroids, primarily progesterone. Within 2 or 3 days the corpus luteum becomes yellowish and spherical and increases in vascularity. If the ovum is fertilized, followed by implantation of the resultant blastocyst in the endometrium, the blastocyst begins to secrete human chorionic gonadotropin (hCG), which is needed to maintain the corpus luteum. If fertilization does not occur, within 8 days after ovulation the corpus luteum begins to degenerate and becomes the corpus albicans, which has a dull white appearance. Approximately 14 days after ovulation (in a 28-day cycle), in the absence of pregnancy, menstruation begins again.

Endometrial and Cervical Mucosal Changes

During menstruation and the sloughing of the functional endometrial layer, some of the remaining tips of the endometrial glands (seeds) begin to regenerate while other areas are being shed. Following menstruation, the endometrium is in a resting state. Its stromal cells are dense and compact, the epithelium is cuboidal, and the endometrial glands are short and straight. Estrogen levels are low. The endometrium is 1–2 mm deep. The cervical mucosa during this part of the cycle is scanty, viscous, and opaque.

In response to increasing amounts of estrogen, the glands hypertrophy, becoming tortuous and longer. The blood vessels become prominent and dilated and the endometrium increases sixfold to eightfold. This gradual process reaches its peak just before ovulation. Under the influences of estrogen, the cervical mucosa becomes thin, clear, and watery, which is more favorable to spermatozoa. The cervical mucosal pH increases from slightly below 7.0 to 7.5 at the time of ovulation. The fernlike pattern of cervical mucus increases during the preovulatory phase, becoming full and complete and most pronounced at the time of ovulation. This fern pattern is a useful aid in assessment of ovulation time.

Following ovulation, the endometrium, under estrogenic influence, undergoes slight cellular growth. Progesterone causes such marked swelling and secretory growth that the epithelium is thrown into folds (Figure 5–6). Increased amounts of tissue glycogen are present, and the glandular epithelial cells begin to fill with cellular debris, become tortuous or like a corkscrew in appearance, and are increasingly dilated. The glands secrete small quantities of endometrial fluid. During the secretory phase, the endometrium is prepared for a fertilized ovum, providing optimal conditions for the protection and nurturance of the

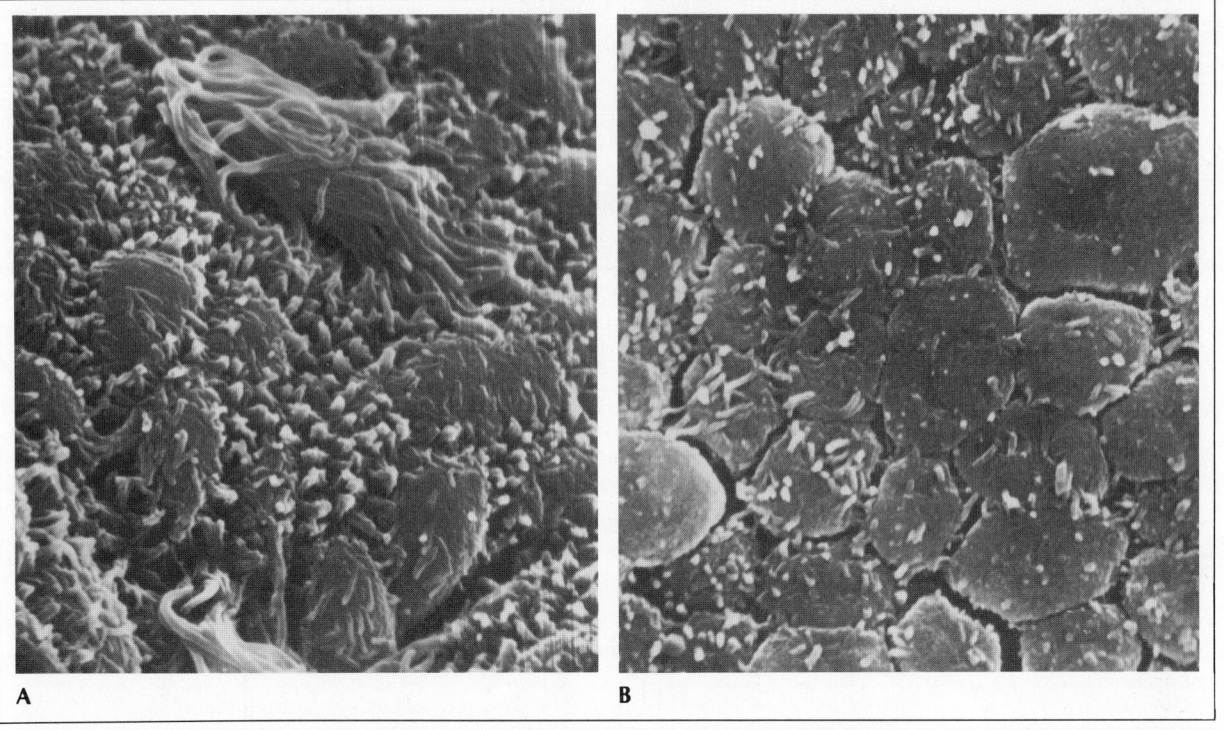

FIGURE 5–6 Scanning electron micrographs of the uterine lining during different phases of the uterine cycle. During the luteal phase **(A),** some of the cells have cilia and some are secreting droplets. The secreting cells are covered with microvilli. In the secretory phase **(B),** microvilli are still present on the surfaces of the secreting cells, but the general surface of the lining has a more lumpy appearance than during the proliferative phase, and the cilia appear shorter and less numerous. The named phases refer to the uterine condition at the time the photographs were taken. (Courtesy Dr. E. S. E. Hafez, Wayne State University, Detroit, Mich.)

developing embryo. The vascularity of the entire uterus increases greatly, providing a succulent bed for implantation. Hypertrophy and hyperplasia of the myometrium occur. The postovulation cervical mucosa pattern is cellular, as progesterone appears. If implantation occurs, the endometrium, under the influence of progesterone, continues to develop and becomes even thicker (Figure 5–7).

If fertilization does not occur, the corpus luteum shows early signs of degeneration, resulting in withdrawal of both estrogen and progesterone. Small areas of necrosis appear under the epithelial lining. As the levels of progesterone fall, extensive vascular changes occur. Small blood vessels rupture and the spiral arteries constrict and retract, causing a deficiency of blood in the functional endometrial layer. The endometrium becomes pale. This ischemic phase is characterized by the extravasation of blood into the stromal cells and is followed by the menstrual flow. The basal layer remains, so that the tips of the glands can regenerate the new functional endometrial layer. These endometrial changes, as well as the ovarian follicular changes in response to hormone levels, are illustrated in Figure 5–4.

Premenstrual Tension Syndrome

Progesterone withdrawal and a decreased progesterone to estrogen ratio with its resultant physiologic and metabolic changes in the late luteal/secretory phase may produce a cluster of symptoms known as *premenstrual tension* (PMT) syndrome. It has been estimated that from 30%–40% of all ovulating women have mild or severe episodes of some or all of the following symptoms: pelvic fullness, abdominal weight gain, bloating, headache, irritability, depression, anxiety, fatigue, exhaustion, food craving, nausea, vomiting, diarrhea, and constipation (Chihal, 1982). These cyclic symptoms are most pronounced 2 or 3 days before the onset of menstruation and subside as the flow begins, with or without treatment. It is less well known that some women experience feelings of heightened creativity, increased powers of concentration, and more productive activity—both mental and physical (Fogel and Woods, 1981).

Although PMT syndrome seems to be based more on empirical reports rather than on controlled physiologic studies, it is real. After diagnosis by clinical evaluation,

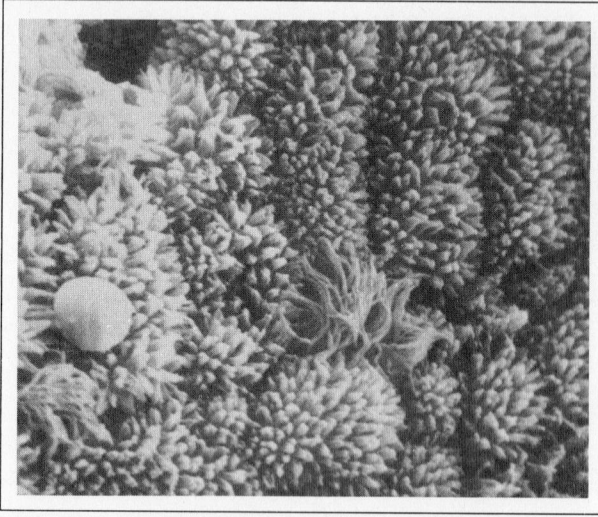

FIGURE 5-7 Scanning electron micrograph of the inner lining of the uterus at the time of implantation of the blastocyst. The blastocyst is an embryo at an early stage of development (see Chapter 8 for further discussion). (Courtesy Dr. E. S. E. Hafez, Wayne State University, Detroit, Mich.)

PMT management may include dietary restriction of salt and sugar with increases of complex carbohydrates, a balance between rest periods and a program of aerobic exercise such as race walking, jogging, and aerobic dancing.

Two widely accepted pharmaceutical treatments are progesterone supplementation by means of vaginal or rectal suppositories and spironolactone (a progesterone agonist) orally. Some researchers support pyridoxine (vitamin B_6) supplementation. An empathetic relationship with a health professional in which a woman may freely discuss her concerns is highly beneficial. It is likely that premenstrual tension is related to other personality and physical traits.

Dysmenorrhea

Dysmenorrhea, or painful menstruation, occurs at or a day before the onset of menstruation and disappears by the end of menses. Halbert (1981) reports 90% of women experience some pain with menses, 50%–60% require analgesia some of the time, and 10% report lost time from work or school due to their incapacitation.

Dysmenorrhea is classified as primary or secondary. Primary or essential dysmenorrhea usually appears 2 or 3 years after menarche, is present for the first 1 or 2 days of menstrual flow, is absent when ovulation does not occur, and occurs without demonstrable organic disease. Its causative factors seem to be intrinsic to the uterus itself. Nulliparous teens and women under 25 years of age experience it most frequently.

Hypercontractility of the uterus (and the gastrointestinal tract as well) may be caused by excessive prostaglandin F_2. Treatment of physiologic primary dysmenorrhea includes hormonal therapy, dilatation of the cervix, and aspirin and codeine (Gold and Josimovich, 1981).

Dysmenorrhea may be psychologic in origin, resulting from an inability or unwillingness to cope with the sexual and reproductive meanings of the menses. Depending on the degree of conflict within the woman, some form of long-term counseling or psychotherapy may be needed to help uncover such feelings.

Secondary dysmenorrhea is associated with pathology of the reproductive tract and usually appears after menstruation has been established. Conditions that most frequently cause secondary dysmenorrhea include endometriosis, residual pelvic inflammatory disease, and anatomic anomalies such as cervical stenosis, imperforate hymen, or uterine displacement (Fogel and Woods, 1981). Because primary and secondary dysmenorrhea may coexist, accurate differential diagnosis is essential for appropriate treatment.

Menstrual Cycle Variations

Amenorrhea, the absence of menses, is classified as primary or secondary. Primary amenorrhea is said to occur if menstruation has not been established by age 18 years. Secondary amenorrhea is said to occur when an established menses (of longer than 3 months) ceases.

Primary amenorrhea necessitates a thorough assessment of the young woman to determine its cause. Identified causes include congenital obstructions, congenital absence of the uterus, testicular feminization, or absence or imbalance of hormones. Successful treatment is limited by causative factors. Many causes are not curable, and infertility will persist (Fogel and Woods, 1981).

Secondary amenorrhea is caused most frequently by pregnancy. Additional causes include lactation, hormonal imbalances, poor nutrition (anorexia nervosa, malnutrition, obesity, fad dieting), ovarian lesions, extreme athletic regimens (long-distance runners), debilitating systemic disease, stress of high intensity and/or of long duration, oral contraceptives, the phenothiazine and chlorpromazine group tranquilizers, and syndromes such as Cushing's and Sheehan's. Treatment is dictated by the causative factors (Fogel and Woods, 1981).

An abnormally short menstrual cycle is termed *hypomenorrhea*; an abnormally long one is called *hypermenorrhea*. Excessive, profuse flow is called *menorrhagia*, and bleeding between periods is known as *metrorrhagia*. Infrequent and too frequent menses are termed *oligomenorrhea* and *polymenorrhea*, respectively. Such irregularities should be investigated to rule out any disease process.

CLIMACTERIC

The *climacteric* is thought to occur in both men and women. It is commonly called the *change of life*. In women, it is associated with *menopause*, or cessation of menstruation, and with distinct hormonal changes leading to the inability to bear children. In men, there are no identifiable physical signs, and the vasomotor and psychologic disturbances reported in men age 45–52 may simply reflect a maturational crisis over the aging process. Therefore, the following discussion of the climacteric will be limited to its occurrence in women.

Psychologic Aspects of Menopause

Menopause is to the climacteric as menarche is to puberty —one indication of a larger, complex process. In addition to the normal physiologic cessation of ovarian function in women at about the age of 50, menopause can appear prematurely or can be surgically induced. Menopause is a turning point in any woman's life because it marks the end of her reproductive function—a meaningful event for a woman whether or not she has borne children.

A woman's approach to the climacteric is influenced by social forces in her culture. It is important to determine if she has internalized Victorian beliefs about reproductive and sexual behaviors. Does she believe that sex should be limited to procreative purposes only? Is she intimidated by stereotypes of "older women" portrayed in the media? Is she bound by the traditional double standard? Is she ashamed or bewildered by an increased libido? These and other questions may help nurses understand a particular woman's response to this stage in her life. Spurred by the feminist movement, research is increasing in the area of adjustment and behaviors during, before, and after menopause. Fogel and Woods (1981) present an excellent summary of numerous studies. Of particular interest is a study by Uphold and Susman (1981). The results stress the importance of the quality of marital relationships as correlated with the reporting of climacteric symptoms. The most frequent and severe symptoms were reported by women whose marital adjustment was low. Symptoms were not related to the "empty nest" stage of childrearing as has often been assumed. Further research needs to consider the presence of and satisfaction with the support systems in women's lives.

Physical Aspects of Menopause

The physical aspects of menopause are difficult to distinguish clearly, because subjective symptoms reported by women are much more extensive than those documented in the literature. However, certain physical findings are significant.

Menopause usually occurs between 45 and 52 years of age. The age of onset may be influenced by nutritional, cultural, or genetic factors. The physiologic mechanisms initiating its onset are not known exactly. The onset of menopause is probably due to the progressive decrease in activity of the corpus luteum.

Generally, ovulation ceases 1 or 2 years prior to menopause. However, individual variation does exist; as much as 6–8 years of transition prior to menopause has been noted. The change is usually gradual, and normal menstrual irregularities do not include menorrhagia or metrorrhagia. Atrophy of the ovaries occurs gradually; FSH levels rise permanently. With the endometrium in a persistent state of proliferation, an increased tendency toward uterine fibroids and endometriosis is noted. The increased incidence of Down's syndrome in infants of mothers over 40 years of age is attributed partly to the lowered quality of the ova released.

Contrary to popular thought, low levels of estrogen are maintained in about 40% of postmenopausal women. Estrone, produced by the adrenal glands, is the chief circulating estrogen.

The uterine endometrium and myometrium atrophy, as do the cervical glands. The uterine cavity becomes stenosed. The fallopian tubes atrophy extensively. The vaginal mucosa becomes smooth and thin and the rugae disappear, leading to loss of elasticity. As a result, painful intercourse, or *dyspareunia*, may occur. Dryness of the mucous membrane can lead to burning and itching. Vaginal pH level increases as the number of Döderlein's bacilli decreases.

Vulval atrophy occurs late, and the pubic hair thins, turns gray or white, and may ultimately disappear. The labia shrivel and lose their heightened pigmentation. Pelvic fascia and muscles atrophy, resulting in decreased pelvic support. The breasts become pendulous and decrease in size and firmness.

In most menopausal women, certain vasomotor disturbances occur that are clearly related to the cessation of menstruation and to hormonal changes. Although the physiologic mechanism has not yet been clearly delineated, 75% of women report symptoms of heat arising on the chest and spreading to the neck and face, sweating (mild to drenching), sleep disturbances, and occasional chills. This cluster of symptoms is often referred to as *hot flashes*. There may be 20–30 of these a day, lasting 3–5 minutes. Dizzy spells, palpitations, and weakness are also reported.

Long-range physical changes may include osteoporosis, a decrease in the bony skeletal mass. The bones become more brittle and thus can more easily be broken. This change is thought to occur in association with lowered estrogen and androgen levels, lack of physical exercise, and a chronic low intake of calcium. The occurrence of diabetes mellitus increases at this age. Loss of protein from the skin and supportive tissues causes wrinkling. Frequently, postmenopausal women gain weight, which may be due to excessive caloric intake rather than to a change in adipose deposits.

Endocrine changes include a decrease in the steroid hormones produced by the ovary, and decreased estrogen levels cause the anterior pituitary to produce more FSH. The underlying causes of such endocrine changes are not clear.

Sexual Activity in the Climacteric

Masters and Johnson (1966) reported that sexual function persists into old age, with many persons in their 60s and 70s sexually active in a manner satisfactory to both partners. It is known that while all aspects of the sexual response are still present, they occur more slowly at a less intense degree and are of shorter duration. Men are able to control ejaculation more easily, enabling longer-lasting penile penetration before climax. Atrophy of the vagina may cause painful intercourse; this may be overcome with the use of lubricating gel or saliva. Women are still multiorgasmic. Men need a longer time to recover before they are able to become erect again and the amount of ejaculate decreases. These changes influence coital activity but in no way necessitate a decrease in its occurrence or enjoyment. In fact, sexual activity may bloom at this time, as the need for contraception disappears and personal growth and awareness increase. Unopposed circulating testosterone may also contribute to rises in the libido. The notion that sexual interest and activity decrease as a natural correlate of the aging process is a myth.

In addition to the erroneous stereotype that older people are asexual, the belief exists that only the young can enjoy sexual and intimate contact. Nothing is further from the truth. When a couple has shared a lifetime of being together, they often experience an exquisite and overwhelming quality to their love and its sexual expression, which includes closeness, touching, knowing, and caring.

Interventions

Until recently, menopausal symptoms were commonly treated with supplementary estrogen. However, estrogen therapy has been challenged in recent years. It has been determined that only vasomotor symptoms and vaginal atrophy are related to low estrogen levels. Also, sustained high-dosage estrogen therapy has been reported to predispose women to malignancy of the reproductive tract. Currently, the prescription of short-term, low-dose estrogenic therapy for extensive troublesome vasomotor disruptions and of intravaginal estrogenic creams for vaginal atrophy are preferred treatment measures.

Counseling menopausal women to assist them in successfully adjusting to this developmental crisis of life is receiving increased attention. Reaction to menopause is determined to a large extent by the kind of life the woman has lived, by the security she has in her feminine identity, and by her feelings of self-worth and self-esteem.

Nurses or other health professionals can help the menopausal client achieve high-level functioning at this time in her life. Of paramount importance is the nurse's ability to understand and provide support for the client's views and feelings. Whether the woman expresses "relief and delight" or "tearfulness and fear," the nurse needs an empathetic approach in counseling, health teaching, or providing physical care. The importance of touch and caring as nursing measures may enhance the self-actualization of both nurse and client.

A woman at menopause looks forward to about 30 more years of life. As she accomplishes the developmental tasks of the climacteric period and adjusts to changes through incorporation of role transitions, she can affirm her worth and go on to an exciting and challenging time of her life. Maturity has many rewards.

COITUS (SEXUAL INTERCOURSE)

Among the numerous terms used to describe the sexual mating of a sexually mature female and male are coitus, coition, sexual intercourse, copulation, making love, and the sex act. *Coitus* may be defined as the insertion of the erect male penis into the female vagina. After repeated thrusting movements of the penis, the man experiences ejaculation of semen (seminal fluid) concurrent with orgasm. Ejaculation is the expulsion of semen from the genital tract to the exterior of the urethral meatus through the rhythmic contraction of the penile muscles. Orgasm is the involuntary climax or apex of the sexual experience, involving a series of muscular contractions, profound physiologic bodily response, and intense sensual pleasure. Orgasm may be achieved by other methods of sexual stimulation besides coitus, such as masturbation and oral stimulation. Orgasm in the absence of ejaculation can occur, usually in aged men.

Although the basic events of coitus are the same for all couples, wide variation exists in sexual positions, technique, duration, intent, meaning, and reactions among individuals.

Psychosocial Aspects

Coitus is a personal act between two consenting adults. Its performance can signify a variety of feelings, beliefs, and attitudes.

The traditional purpose of coitus is procreation. However, with the availability of contraceptive methods and with changing social mores, sexual intercourse is also becoming accepted as a pleasurable and personally gratifying experience in itself. The sexual union of two individuals may reflect their mutual commitment and caring, or it may be a more immediate interaction, for the purpose of personal pleasure or merely temporary companionship. In our society, sexual intercourse ideally is the sharing of two persons' minds and bodies in a uniquely intimate way that represents the larger sharing of their lives together. Such sexual interactions are the result of mutual caring and love.

According to Fromm (1956), love has four essential components: labor, responsibility, respect, and understanding. If one person is willing to evaluate the consequences of one's behavior as it affects the other and choose accordingly; if one does not exploit but enables the other to become; if one tries to understand the other's feelings, hopes, and desires—then one person may be considered to love the other. Sexual interaction is an important way for individuals to express their love, and it is in this context that coitus can be most meaningful to the participants.

Physiology of Sexual Response

Masters and Johnson (1966) have identified and described the physiology of the sexual response in both males and females. Sexual response occurs in four phases: excitement, plateau, orgasm, and resolution. Essentially, the male and female sexual response is the same, involves the total body, and is a continuous process. Individual variation does occur.

All the responses can be classified as either vasocongestive or myotonic. *Vasocongestion* involves the congestion or engorgement of blood vessels and is the most common physiologic response to sexual arousal. *Myotonia*, a secondary physiologic response, is increased muscular tonus, which produces tension.

The sexual responses of female reproductive organs are given in Table 5–1; the male response is given in Table

Table 5–1   Summary of Female Sexual Response

Organ	Excitement (foreplay)	Plateau (entry and coital movements)	Orgasm (climax)	Resolution (relaxation)
Labia minora	Vasocongestion of erectile tissue occurs; color darkens; extension of tissue	Increases		Return to normal size and color
Labia majora	Vasocongestion and swelling occurs; nulliparous: flatten and widen; multiparous: widen by movement from vaginal introitus	Increases		Return to normal size and color
Clitoris	Size of glans increases; engorgement of dorsal vein occurs; shaft elongates	Glans retracts under hood after erection	Rhythmic muscular contractions occur, ranging from intense to mild	Returns to normal; no refractory period; multiple orgasms possible
Vagina	Vaginal lubrication appears; in 10–30 seconds, widens and lengthens 1 cm; walls become purplish; progressive distention occurs; upper portion "tents"; rugae become smooth	Engorgement occurs; outer third of vagina swells; "orgasmic platform" develops; interior lumen decreases to "grasp" penis	Outer third has spasm, then rhythmic contractions; perivaginal muscles contract	Outer third relaxes after clitoris returns to normal; remaining portion returns to normal
Cervix	Moves upward and backward posteriorly	Cervical os opens slightly		Returns to normal position; os closes in 20–30 minutes
Uterus	Moves upward and backward posteriorly	Increases in size	Rhythmic contractions from fundus to cervix occur	Returns to precoital size slowly
Breasts	Areolae increase in size; nipples become erect and size increases; sex flush may appear		Sex flush most pronounced	Slow return to normal; sex flush disappears

Table 5-2   Summary of Male Sexual Response

Organ	Excitement (foreplay)	Plateau (entry and coital movements)	Orgasm (climax)	Resolution (relaxation)
Scrotum	Skin thickens; scrotal sac elevates and flattens against body (spermatic cord contracts)	Remains tense and close to body		
Seminal vesicles			Semen is discharged into urethral bulb	
Urethra	Moistened with mucus	Mucus increases; becomes distended with semen just before orgasm	Semen ejected with force as bulb contracts	Minor contractions persist even after semen is ejected
Prostate			Contracts, expelling fluid into urethral bulb	
Testes	Elevate with scrotum	May increase in size by 50%; remain elevated		
Penis	Engorgement and erection is rapid; size increases; position changes: angle of protrusion created	Coronal ridge size increases; glans becomes purplish	Contracts	Becomes flaccid; refractory period: erection may not be experienced
Bulbourethral glands		Few drops of fluid may be discharged (contain sperm)		
Breasts	Nipple erections; sex flush may appear		Sex flush most pronounced	Slow return to normal; sex flush fades slowly

5-2. Several responses are shared by both women and men. The *sex flush* consists of a maculopapular rash that may begin in the epigastric area and spread quickly to the breasts. Less than half of men experience this, whereas more than half of women do. Heart rate and blood pressure increase in proportion to the degree of sexual excitement. The intercostal and abdominal muscles may tense. This tension, beginning in the excitement phase, intensifies during the plateau phase and may involve the buttocks and anal sphincter. Hyperventilation occurs just before and during orgasm. At orgasm, muscle tension is extreme. The face may be contorted, while muscles of the neck, extremities, abdomen, and buttocks are tightly contracted. There may be uncontrollable moans, murmurings, or outcries. Grasping motions by each partner are not uncommon. There is a feeling of total surrender to bodily responses, and acute pleasure and relief are felt.

The male physical response is relatively constant, resulting in orgasm if erection and sexual stimulation are maintained. Female sexual response varies considerably. Not all women experience orgasm consistently; they are influenced by their subjective psychologic state, their health, their current sexual motivation, and environmental distractions. Therefore, a woman may not experience or-

gasm during a particular act of coitus, or she may experience one or multiple orgasms of varying intensity. Such variation is usual in a woman of "normal" sexual activity, interest, and response. Figure 5-8 illustrates the cycle of sexual response for the male and female.

Neurologic Control of Sexual Response

Cortical influences (limbic system and hypothalamus), peripheral nerves, autonomic pathways, spinal cord pathways, and reflex centers share the control of the sexual response.

In the male during the excitement phase, psychogenic or physical stimuli are transmitted by ascending sensory pathways or descending corticomotor pathways. Stimuli from pressure or tension in the pelvic organs or from touch of the external genitals create impulses carried by the pudendal and pelvic afferent fibers to the sacral cord. There they synapse with the parasympathetic efferent fibers to the pelvis. Reflex erection may result, as these fibers cause dilatation of the penile arteries and some constriction of the penile veins, with resultant vasoconstriction.

Heightened sexual arousal stimulates reflex centers of the spinal cord, which send out sympathetic impulses to the genital organs to initiate ejaculation. When the urethra is full of semen, impulses are transmitted to the sacral regions of the cord. The efferent fibers carry rhythmic impulses from the cord to the skeletal muscles surrounding the erectile tissue, inducing rhythmic contractions. Sexual stimulation can arise from tubal fullness or irritation—the so-called morning erection is caused by fullness of the bladder.

A similar neurologic pattern is found in females. Tactile or psychogenic stimuli may cause sexual arousal. Local sexual sensations are carried to the spinal cord through the pudendal nerve and sacral plexus and are referred to cerebral centers. Reflexes associated with female orgasm seem to be associated with the lumbar and sacral regions of the cord. As in the male, erectile tissue is controlled by parasympathetic nerves.

Neural control of the female orgasm follows the same pathways as in the male.

To summarize, sympathetic innervation of sexual response causes vasoconstriction and orgasm in both sexes and ejaculation in the male. Parasympathetic innervation controls vasodilatation and erection of sex organs.

IMPLICATIONS FOR NURSES

Because sexuality is an intrinsic part of life from birth to death, people have many problems, needs, and questions concerning sex roles, sexual behaviors, family planning, sex education, sexual inhibitions, and other related areas. The nurse is frequently confronted with these concerns by clients and thus may need to assume the role of sexual counselor. For nurses to assume this role, they must be secure about their own sexuality. Although this advice is given to nurses repeatedly, few suggestions are made to assist nurses to feel "comfortable" with their own sexuality. Continuing education for the practicing nurse and incorporation of appropriate courses in undergraduate and graduate nursing education programs may help nurses achieve this sense of self-security. Courses designed to teach nurses about sexual values, attitudes, alternative lifestyles, cultural factors, misconceptions, and myths provide a fuller knowledge of sexual behavior and function in health and illness (Nelson, 1977; Keller, 1982). It is imperative that each client's needs be met with appropriate information without embarrassment or judgment and referral initiated as required.

Children's Sexuality Counseling

The health care profession, parents, and society must make a commitment to educate young people about sexuality. Whether given at home or school, sex education is necessary. Nurses can advise parents how, what, and when to teach their children about sexuality.

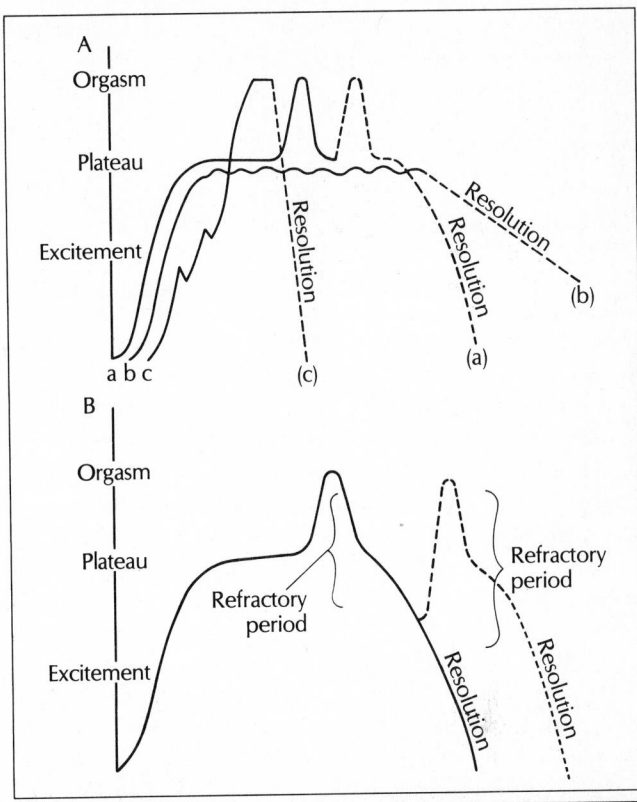

FIGURE 5–8 A, Cycle of female sexual response: a, reaction pattern with single or multiple orgasms; b, reaction pattern without orgasm; c, reaction pattern without distinct plateau. B, Cycle of male sexual response. (From Masters, W. H., and Johnson, V. E. 1966. *Human sexual response.* Boston: Little, Brown & Co. p. 55.)

Although sexual functioning emerges in adolescence, the antecedents are present during infancy and childhood, as discussed earlier in this chapter. The atmosphere in which the child is raised will affect future attitudes and behaviors. Sex education for parents is an integral part of the nurse's teaching and can begin in the nursery. Discussions about erections in male newborns and the presence of smegma in the vaginas of female newborns can precipitate discussions about toddlers touching and exploring their bodies. Although this information will not necessarily be remembered, the seed will be planted to introduce parents to the normalcy of sexual behavior in their children. The nurse may also work with teachers and PTA groups as well as community organizations to develop appropriate sex-education programs and materials.

The adolescent clinic is another area in which sexuality discussion is important. Assessing each adolescent's adjustment to the trying teenage period naturally includes sexuality assessments. The nurse can promote self-esteem, correct misconceptions, and even give the adolescent permission to say "No" to intercourse.

In assessment of an adolescent, the nurse must find out

how each adolescent perceives himself or herself. Five areas should be addressed:

- Self-esteem
- Body image
- Social skills
- Decision making
- Coping skills

Information gathered about these areas of concern will give the nurse an idea about how to counsel the adolescent.

The young adolescent (11–14 years) needs firm, direct support and limit setting in simple, concrete choices. By being a caring adult, and treating the adolescent with respect, the nurse gains the trust of the client. Encouraging these youngsters to say "No" to sexual intercourse is important. Young adolescents, more than any other age group, need counseling and guidance if they are sexually active.

The middle adolescent probably needs more guidance in problem solving. The nurse may act as a sounding board to help the teenager negotiate choices, while also gently confronting the adolescent about consequences and responsibility. Paying attention to peer norms in this age group is important. Some peer support groups might encourage waiting until the adolescent is responsibly mature to have sex. Youngsters should know that the rewards for delaying intercourse include peace of mind, energy to devote to goals, self-protection, and family approval.

Teaching adolescents about anatomy and physiology of reproduction and responsible sexual decision making alleviates the problems associated with adolescent sexuality. Decreasing the incidence of adolescent pregnancy and sexually transmitted diseases will benefit all of society.

Sexual History Assessments

As nurses extend their expertise in the area of sexuality, taking a sexual history will become a standard procedure in the assessment phase of the nursing process. While Mims and Swenson (1980) warn against the gathering of personal information for which there is no use, they urge the nurse to make logical assessments appropriate to each client's developmental level, educational level, and cultural background.

Information related to the sexual history can be easily gathered when obtaining reproductive information about the female client, or genitourinary system information about the male client. Initial questions can be introduced by "giving the client permission" to talk about sexual matters. A "universality statement" (Mims and Swenson, 1980) may put the client at ease: When clients discover that many persons their age or stage have questions or problems in certain areas, they may feel more willing and able to speak of their own feelings.

A more complete history will be obtained if the nurse makes an effort to do the following (Block et al., 1981):

- Provide privacy
- Build trust and confidence
- Assure confidentiality
- Progress from less sensitive areas to more sensitive areas
- Progress from less threatening areas to more threatening areas

Although no consensus exists concerning the level of counseling appropriate for a professional nurse without additional preparation in the area of sex education and counseling, some judgment is necessary for appropriate referrals to be made. Most writers agree that the greater the level of intervention, the greater professional skill is needed (Watts, 1979).

Rather than judging sexual behavior by predetermined standards of so-called normal behavior, the nurse should allow each individual or couple to evaluate their own sexual activities. Each person or couple should determine their own patterns and preferences. If nurses are to satisfactorily meet the needs of their clients, they must acknowledge personal differences in sexual behaviors and provide support or information whenever requested.

SUMMARY

The development of sexuality is a function of societal, biologic, and physical factors. Society dictates many of the norms forming the framework for core-gender identity. Biologic factors are first established at conception and then are influenced by hormonal processes. Physical factors are influenced by hormonal levels and by an intricate feedback mechanism with the body.

The expression of sexuality is a learned process, and research has identified specific physiologic responses to sexual stimulation. Understanding the development and processes of sexuality will enable the nurse to interact with and counsel patients more appropriately as the role of the nurse expands in this area.

Resource Groups

Center for Population Options (2031 Florida Avenue, N.W., Suite 301, Washington, DC 20008). Develops programs and materials designed to encourage teens to be sexually responsible. Works with youth-serving agencies to help develop sexuality education programs.

Institute for Family Research and Education (Syracuse University, 760 Ostrom Avenue, Syracuse, NY 13210). Sponsors National Family Sex Education Week. Supports research and programs in sex and parent education.

Planned Parenthood Federation of America (810 Seventh Avenue, New York, NY 10019). Publishes family planning pamphlets for teens. Community educators available in some localities who visit classrooms and community groups.

References

Block, G. J., et al. 1981. *Health assessment for professional nursing: a developmental approach.* New York: Appleton-Century-Crofts.

Blum, R. W., ed. 1982. *Adolescent health care: clinical issues.* New York: Academic Press.

Caldwell, B. V., and Behrman, H. R. 1981. Prostaglandins in reproductive processes. *Med. Clin. North Am.* 65(4):927.

Chihal, H. J. 1982. Painful periods and preludes. *Emergency Medicine* 14(17):33.

Ducharme, J. R., et al. 1976. Plasma adrenal and gonadal sex steroids in human pubertal development. *J. Clin. Endcrinol. Metab.* 42:468.

Fogel, C. I., and Woods, N. F. 1981. *Health care of women: a nursing perspective.* St. Louis: The C. V. Mosby Co.

Fromm, E. 1956. *The art of loving.* New York: Harper & Row.

Gagnon, J. H. 1977. *Human sexualities.* Glenview, Ill.: Scott, Foresman.

Gold, J. J., and Josimovich, J. B., eds. 1980. *Gynecologic endocrinology.* 3rd ed. Hagerstown, Md.: Harper & Row.

Alan Guttmacher Institute. 1981 *Teen pregnancy: the problem that hasn't gone away.* 360 Park Avenue, New York, NY 10010.

Guyton, A. C. 1981. *Textbook of medical physiology.* 6th ed. Philadelphia: W. B. Saunders Co.

Halbert, D. R. 1981. Dysmenorrhea. In *Gynecology and obstetrics,* vol. 5, ed. J. J. Sciarra et al. Hagerstown, Md.: Harper & Row.

Hall, A. K., and Behrman, H. R. 1981. Prostaglandins: basic chemistry and action. In *Gynecology and obstetrics,* vol. 5, ed. J. J. Sciarra et al. Hagerstown, Md.: Harper & Row.

Hyde, J. S. 1982. *Understanding human sexuality.* 2nd ed. New York: McGraw-Hill Book Co.

Keller, M. C. 1982. Teaching sexuality as a nursing elective. *Nursing and Health Care.* 3(6):311.

Lackritz, R. M. 1981. Prostaglandins in pregnancy. In *Gynecology and obstetrics,* vol. 5, ed. J. J. Sciarra et al. Hagerstown, Md.: Harper & Row.

Lief, H. I. 1981. Sexual counseling. In *Gynecology and obstetrics: the health care of women,* 2nd ed., ed. S. L. Romney et al. New York: McGraw-Hill Book Co.

Little, A. B., and Billiar, R. B. 1981. Endocrinology. In *Gynecology and obstetrics: the health care of women,* 2nd ed., ed. S. L. Romney et al. New York: McGraw-Hill Book Co.

Masters, W. H., and Johnson, V. E. 1966. *Human sexual response.* Boston: Little, Brown & Co.

Mims, F. H., and Swenson, M. 1980. *Sexuality: a nursing perspective.* New York: McGraw-Hill Book Co.

Nelson, S. E. 1977. All about sex education for students. *Am. J. Nurs.* 77(4):611.

Stone, S. C. 1981. Physiology of puberty. In *Gynecology and obstetrics,* vol. 5, ed. J. J. Sciarra et al. Hagerstown, Md.: Harper & Row.

Tanner, J. M. 1962. *Growth of adolescents.* 2nd ed. Oxford, Engl.: Blackwell Scientific Publications, Ltd.

Ticky, A. M., and Malasanos, L. J. Nov./Dec. 1975. The physiological role of hormones in puberty. *Am. J. Mat. Child Nurs.* 1:384.

Uphold, C. R., and Susman, E. J. March/April 1981. Self-reported climacteric symptoms as a function of the relationship between marital adjustment and childrearing stage. *Nurs. Research.* 30(2):84.

Vijayakumar, R., et al. 1981. Myometrial prostaglandins during human menstrual cycle. *Am. J. Obstet. Gynecol.* 141(3):313.

Watts, R. J. 1979. Dimensions of sexual health. *Am. J. Nurs.* 77(9):1568.

Wilhelmson, L., et al. Aug. 1981. Effects of prostaglandins on the isolated uterine artery of the non-pregnant woman. *Prostaglandins.* 22(2):223.

Wolman, B. B., and Money, J., eds. 1980. *Handbook of human sexuality.* Englewood Cliffs, N.J.: Prentice-Hall, Inc.

Zacharias, L., et al. 1970. Sexual maturation in contemporary American girls. *Am. J. Obstet. Gynecol.* 108:833.

Additional Readings

Beach, R. K. April 1982. Adolescent sexual decision making and sexual responsibility: perspectives for professionals in the 1980's. Paper presented at Adolescent Pregnancy: New Directions for the 80's, Rocky Mountain Chapter Society for Adolescent Medicine, Denver, Colorado.

Broude, G. J. 1981. The cultural management of sexuality. In *Handbook of cross-cultural human development,* ed. R. H. Munroe; R. L. Munroe; and B. B. Whiting. New York: Garland Press.

Carter, B., and McGoldrick, M., eds. 1980. *The family life cycle.* New York: Gardner Press.

Delaney, J., et al. *The curse: a cultural history of menstruation.* New York: New American Library.

Eskins, B. A., ed. 1980. *The menopause: comprehensive management.* New York: Massom Publishing.

Kart, C. S., et al. 1978. *Aging and health: biologic and social perspectives.* Menlo Park, Calif.: Addison-Wesley Publishing Co.

Katchadourian, H. Feb. 1980. Adolescent sexuality. *Pediatr. Clin. North Am.* 27:17.

Leach, A. M. 1982. Threat to nurses' sexual identity. In *Comprehensive psychiatric nursing,* 2nd ed., ed. J. Haber et al. New York: McGraw-Hill Book Co.

Lewis, M., and Lewis, H. 1980. *The parents' guide to teenage sex and pregnancy.* New York: St. Martin's Press.

Lion, E. M., ed. 1982. *Human sexuality in nursing process.* New York: John Wiley & Sons.

Marks, A. 1980. Understanding adolescent pregnancy. In *Psychological aspects of pregnancy, birthing and bonding,* ed. B. L. Blum. New York: Human Sciences Press.

Mims, F. H. 1982. Psychosexual issues. In *Comprehensive psychiatric nursing,* 2nd ed., ed. J. Haber et al. New York: McGraw-Hill Book Co.

Page, E. W., et al. 1981. *Human reproduction: essentials of reproduction and perinatal medicine,* 3rd ed. Philadelphia: W. B. Saunders Co.

Tanner, J. M. 1975. Growth and endocrinology of the adolescent. In *Endocrine and genetic disease of childhood and adolescence,* 2nd ed., ed. L. I. Gardner. Philadelphia: W. B. Saunders Co.

Thornburg, H. S. A. 1981. Source of information on sex. *School Health.* 63(4):274.

Urban, D. J., et al. May/June 1982. Nurse specialization in reproductive endocrinology. *J. Obstet. Gynecol. Neonatal Nurs.* 11(3):167.

Whitney, M. P., and Willingham, D. 1978. Adding a sexual assessment to the health interview. *J. Psychiatr. Nurs. Ment. Health Serv.* 16(4):17.

Zabin, L. and Clark, S. Sept./Oct. 1981. Why they delay: a study of teenage family planning clinic patients. *Fam. Plan. Perspec.* 13:205.

■ 6 ■

FAMILY PLANNING

■ CHAPTER CONTENTS

INFERTILITY
- Essential Components of Fertility
- Preliminary Investigation
- Tests for Infertility
- Methods of Infertility Management
- The Nurse's Role

CONTRACEPTION
- Fertility Awareness Methods
- Mechanical Contraceptives
- Oral Contraceptives
- Injectable Contraceptives
- Spermicides
- Operative Sterilization
- Induced Abortion

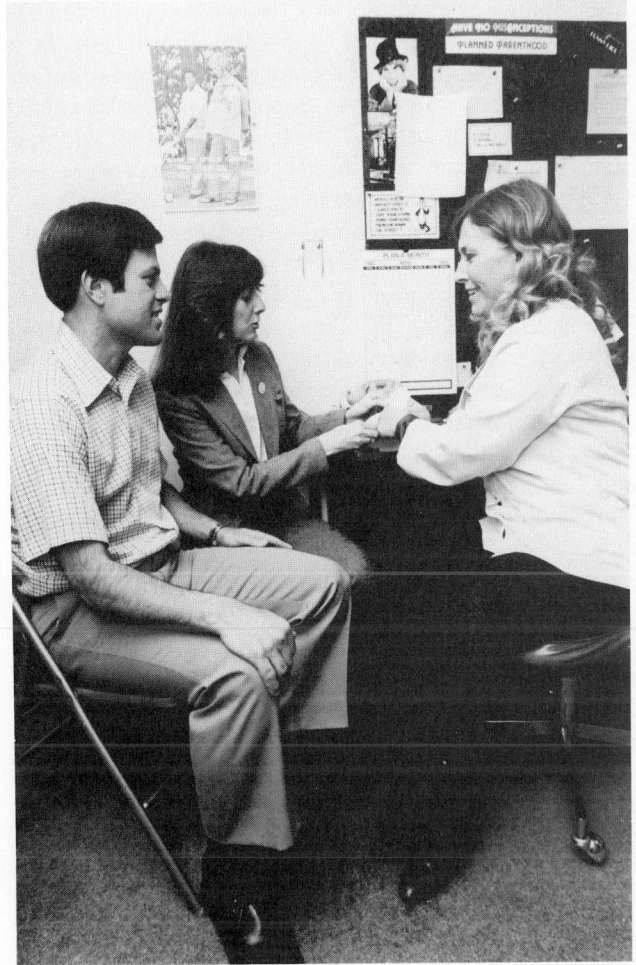

- Identify the three main reasons for couples to seek family planning.
- Discuss infertility and its effect on couples.
- Compare various methods of contraception.
- Describe the various types of abortions.

Control of reproduction has always been one of the foremost concerns of both men and women. Couples have eagerly sought fertility and freedom from risk of conception at various times and under chosen circumstances. The man–woman relationship and the woman's self-concept have been greatly affected by the development of reliable methods for the control of reproductive functions. Motherhood has become a matter of choice, and birth control methods have reinforced the concepts of freedom of choice and the individual's right to self-determination.

The terms "family planning," "birth control," and "contraception" are used interchangeably. Usually, the term *family planning* is the broadest concept and includes voluntary interruption of pregnancy, seeking solutions to infertility, controlling the timing of pregnancies, and assessing the social, psychologic, economic, physical, and theologic concerns of couples making decisions about having children. *Contraception* and *birth control* generally refer to the methods employed to space or avoid pregnancies.

Family planning is the responsibility of the involved couple. The health care professional can assist by providing clear, specific, and accurate information with which the couple may make informed decisions. Before they can reach a decision, the couple must evaluate sociocultural, economic, religious, physical, and psychologic factors in relation to their beliefs and values. After they reach a decision about which contraceptive method to use, the variables that contribute to acceptability of a method must be evaluated. Selection of the method of birth control requires information about cost, effectiveness, procedure for use, previous history of use or friends' use of a given method, personal objections and desires for use, and medical contraindications for a given couple. Health care professionals must be careful not to influence a couple's decision making according to their own preferences, because such persuasion is likely to reduce the effectiveness of the contraceptive method.

The reasons for a couple to engage in family planning are threefold: (a) to identify and correct causes of infertility; (b) to control the number of children in the family; and (c) to predetermine the interval between desired children. Besides contributing to psychologic health by giving increased mastery over an important life event, family planning has physical benefits. It is well documented that the state of a woman's health is often negatively influenced by too frequent or too numerous pregnancies or by the absence of pregnancy. Given these facts, nurses have a responsibility to provide information related to the various methods of family planning in an objective and nonjudgmental manner.

INFERTILITY

Although the phrase "family planning" has come to imply planned limitation of pregnancies, an important aspect of family planning addresses itself to increasing the chances of conception, or to identifying couples for whom conception may be difficult or impossible.

Infertility can be defined as the inability of a couple to produce a living child as a result of failure to conceive or of failure to carry a conceptus to a viable state. Primary infertility indicates those women who have never conceived, whereas secondary infertility identifies the client who has formerly been pregnant but has not conceived during one or more years of unprotected intercourse (Coulam, 1982). *Sterility* is a term applied when there is an absolute factor preventing reproduction. The incidence of infertility appears to be increasing, which may be related to the trend in delaying marriage and postponing childbearing until the couple has passed the age of optimal fertility (24–25 years). Other factors in infertility include increased risk of prolonged anovulation following the use of birth control pills, infections associated with use of intrauterine devices or following abortions, and obstructive diseases of the male and female reproductive systems caused by sexually transmitted diseases.

Essential Components of Fertility

Understanding the elements essential for normal fertility can help the nurse in identifying the many factors that may cause infertility. The following essential components must be present for normal fertility:

Male partner:

1. The testes must produce spermatozoa of normal quality and quantity.
2. The male genital tract must not be obstructed.
3. The male genital tract secretions must be normal.

4. Ejaculated spermatozoa must be deposited in the female genital tract in such a manner that they reach the cervix.

Female partner:

1. The cervical mucus must be favorable for survival of spermatozoa.

2. There must be clear passage between the cervix and the fallopian tubes.

3. Fallopian tubes must be patent and have normal peristaltic movement to allow ascent of spermatozoa and descent of ovum.

4. Ovaries must produce and release normal ova.

5. There must be no obstruction between the ovaries and the fimbriae of the fallopian tubes.

6. The endometrium must be in a normal physiologic state to allow implantation of the blastocyst and to sustain normal growth.

Correlation of these necessary normal findings with possible cause of deviations is found in Table 6–1.

In addition to these specific conditions, general physiologic and psychologic conditions must be such as to support conception.

With intricacies of timing and environment playing such a crucial role, it is an impressive natural phenomenon that approximately 85% of couples in the United States are able to conceive. Of the remaining 15%, for every 100 couples about 40 will show a male deficiency, 10 to 15 a female hormonal defect, 20 to 30 a female tubal disorder, 5 a cervical defect, and 10 to 20 couples have no discernible cause of their infertility (Coulam, 1982). In 35 of the couples multiple etiologies will be identified. Professional intervention can assist approximately 30% of infertile couples to achieve a pregnant state.

Couples present concerns about infertility following their inability to conceive after at least one year of attempting to achieve pregnancy. At the age of 25 years, which is identified as the couple's most fertile time, the average length of time needed to achieve conception is 5.3 months. For every 100 couples, 25 will achieve pregnancy after 1 month of unprotected intercourse, 63 by the end of 6 months, 75 by the end of 9 months, and 80 by the end of 12 months (Shane, Schiff, and Wilson, 1976).

Preliminary Investigation

Evaluation and preliminary investigation should be available for couples seeking help for infertility. Extensive testing is avoided until data confirm that the timing of intercourse and the length of coital exposure have been adequate.

Preliminary evaluation that includes a comprehensive

Table 6–1 Possible Causes of Infertility

Necessary norms	Deviations from normal
Male	
Normal semen analysis	Congenital defect in testicular development, mumps after adolescence, cryptorchidism, varicocele, infections, gonadal exposure to X rays, smoking, alcohol abuse, malnutrition, chronic or acute metabolic disease, medications (for example, morphine and cocaine), constrictive underclothing
Unobstructed genital tract	Infections, tumors, congenital anomalies, vasectomy
Normal genital tract secretions	Infections, autoimmunity to semen, tumors
Ejaculate deposited at the cervix	Premature ejaculation, hypospadias, retrograde ejaculation (for example, if diabetic), neurologic cord lesions
Female	
Favorable cervical mucus	Cervicitis, immunologic response, ``hostile'' mucus, use of coital lubricants
Clear passage between cervix and tubes	Myomas, adhesions, adenomyosis, polyps, endometritis, cervical stenosis, endometriosis, congenital anomalies (for example, septate uterus)
Patent tubes with normal motility	Pelvic inflammatory disease, peritubal adhesions, endometriosis, IUD, salpingitis (for example, tuberculosis), neoplasm, ectopic pregnancy, tubal ligation
Ovulation and release of ova	Primary ovarian failure, polycystic ovarian disease, hypothyroidism, pituitary tumor, lactation, periovarian adhesions, endometriosis, medications (for example, oral contraceptives), premature ovarian failure
No obstruction between ovary and fimbria	Adhesions, endometriosis, pelvic inflammatory disease
Endometrial preparation	Anovulation, luteal phase defect, IUD

history and physical examination for assessment of any obvious causes of infertility is done before a costly, time-consuming, and emotionally trying investigation is initiated. During the first visit for preliminary investigation, the requirements for a basic infertility investigation (the five basic tests) are explained and the foundation for a trusting relationship is established between the health professionals and the infertile couple.

It is never easy to discuss one's sexual activity, especially when potentially irreversible problems with fertility may exist. The mutual desire to have children is the basis of many marriages. A fertility problem is a deeply personal, emotion-laden area in a couple's life. The self-esteem of one or both partners may be threatened if the inability to conceive is perceived as a lack of virility or femininity. The nurse can provide comfort to the client by offering a sympathetic ear, a nonjudgmental atmosphere, and appropriate information and instructions. Since counseling includes discussion of very personal aspects, nurses who are comfortable with their own sexuality are more capable of establishing rapport and eliciting relevant information.

Health care interventions in cases of infertility are illustrated in Figure 6–1. Following the initial interview with the infertile couple, a complete history is taken and a comprehensive physical examination is conducted. The historical data base for the couple should include the following information.

A. Female
   1. Menstrual history
      a. Age of menarche; interval, duration, and quantity of menses
      b. Ovulation
         1. Symptoms, including PMT (premenstrual symptoms such as mood changes, breast tenderness, acne), mittelschmerz (midcycle ovulatory pain), intermenstrual spotting, increased midcycle discharge, and dysmenorrhea
      c. Date of last menstrual period
      d. Current lactation (amenorrhea)
   2. Medical history
      a. Diabetes
      b. Genital tuberculosis
      c. Tailed intrauterine device use may cause increased bacterial growth on endometrial surfaces
      d. Pelvic inflammatory disease
      e. Sexually transmitted disease (gonorrhea, syphilis, herpes)
   3. Surgical history
      a. Appendectomy—appendicitis may cause tubal obstruction or adhesions
      b. Reproductive surgery
      c. Endometriosis

      d. Intra-abdominal surgery that resulted in inflammatory complications
      e. Abortions
   4. Fertility history
      a. Length of time without contraception
      b. Duration of infertility
      c. Fertility testing in the past
      d. Previous pregnancy: number and age at time of conception
      e. Family reproductive history
      f. Contraception use (type, duration, complications, time without contraception)
      g. Previous labor or postpartum circumstances surrounding pregnancy loss
   5. Sexual history
      a. Frequency of intercourse
      b. Sexual techniques
      c. Fertility with the other partners
      d. Number of partners—over a period of time multiple partners can create cervical antibody reactions against different men's semen
   6. Occupation
      a. Exposure to toxic substances (X rays, lead, chemicals, anesthetic gases)
      b. Irradiation may cause ovarian failure
   7. Medications
      a. Oral contraceptives, or other medications affecting fertility
   8. Personal habits
      a. Alcohol consumption
      b. Smoking
      c. Strenuous exercise (long-distance running or professional dancing may cause reversible amenorrhea)
      d. Douching, lubricants, vaginal deodorants
      e. Weight history, especially if amenorrhea has resulted from weight loss
      f. Use of "recreational drugs" (such as marijuana)

B. Male
   1. Age (sperm count decreases with age)
   2. Occupation (some occupations expose the scrotum to excessive heat, which is harmful to spermatogenesis, for example, cross-country truck driving)
   3. Medical history
      a. Mumps after adolescence
      b. Diabetes
      c. Tuberculosis
      d. Venereal disease, epididymitis, orchitis, hypospadias, or other medical conditions
   4. Surgical history
      a. Accidental damage to testes
      b. Previous hernia repairs, cryptorchidism, circumcision, hypospadias, or other conditions requiring surgical intervention

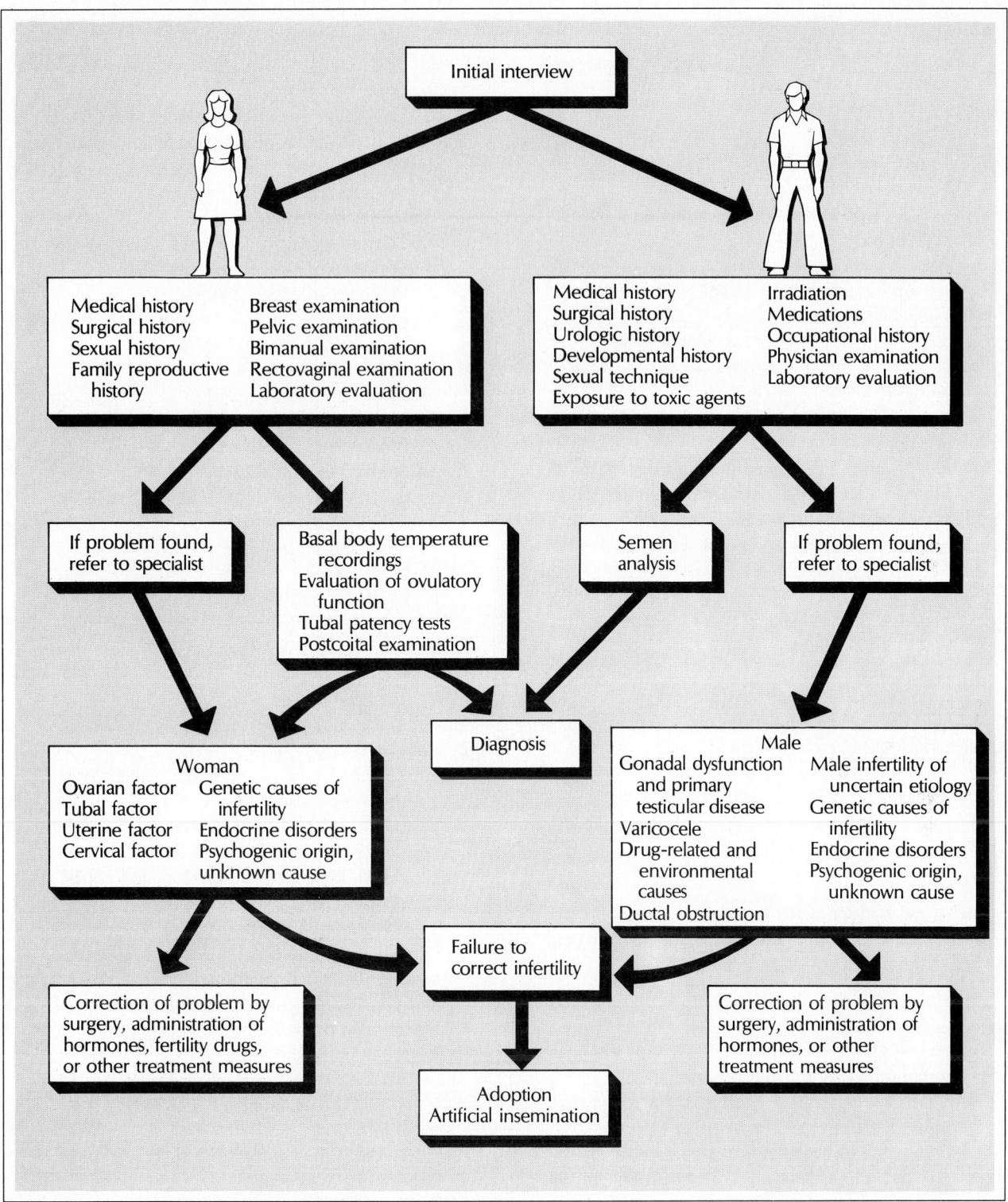

FIGURE 6–1 Flow chart for management of the infertile couple.

5. Developmental history
   a. Endocrine diseases
   b. Age when growth spurt occurred; acne; appearance of facial hair
6. Sexual history
   a. Sexual technique
   b. Frequency of intercourse
   c. Adequacy of erection
   d. Presence of orgasm during coitus and ejaculation with orgasm
   e. Previous fathering of other children with different sexual partner
   f. Family reproductive history
7. Exposure to toxic substances or irradiation
   a. Toxic substance exposure (such as X rays, lead, chemicals)
   b. Irradiation in work place or for genital cancer
8. Medications
   a. Drugs affecting potency (such as narcotics, alcohol, tranquilizers, monoamine oxidase inhibitors, and guanethidine and methyldopa, which interfere with the autonomic nervous system and cause retrograde ejaculation)
   b. Drugs affecting spermatogenesis (including amebicides, antimalarial drugs, nitrofurantoin, and methotrexate)
9. Personal habits
   a. Smoking and alcohol consumption
   b. Type of underwear worn (tight underwear may raise scrotal temperature)
   c. Bathing habits (hot baths and saunas may harm sperm)
   d. Use of recreational drugs (marijuana may depress androgen levels)

Following completion of the couple's histories, a complete physical examination of each partner is performed. At this time the following areas are evaluated:

A. Female
   1. Physical examination
      a. Assessment of height, weight, blood pressure, temperature, and general health status
      b. Endocrine evaluation of thyroid for exophthalmos, lid lag, tremor, or palpable gland
      c. Optic fundi evaluation for presence of increased intracranial pressure especially in oligomenorrheal or amenorrheal women
      d. Reproductive features (including breast and external genital area)
      e. Physical ability to tolerate pregnancy
   2. Pelvic examination
      a. Papanicolaou smear
      b. Culture for gonorrhea
      c. Signs of vaginal infections (see Chapter 10)
      d. Shape of escutcheon (for example, does pubic hair distribution resemble that of a male?)
      e. Size of clitoris (enlargement caused by endocrine disorders)
      f. Evaluation of cervix: old lacerations, tears, erosion, polyps, condition and shape of os, signs of infections, cervical mucus (evaluate for estrogen effect of spinnbarkeit and cervical ferning)
   3. Bimanual examination
      a. Size, shape, position, and mobility of uterus
      b. Presence of congenital anomalies
      c. Presence of endometriosis
      d. Evaluation of adnexa: ovarian size, cysts, fixations, or tumors
   4. Rectovaginal examination
      a. Presence of retroflexed or retroverted uterus
      b. Presence of rectouterine pouch masses
      c. Presence of possible endometriosis
   5. Laboratory examination
      a. Complete blood count
      b. Sedimentation rate
      c. Serology
      d. Urinalysis
      e. Rh factor and blood grouping
      f. If indicated (incomplete list), thyroid function tests, glucose tolerance test, 17-ketosteroid assay, 17-hydrocorticoid assay, urine pregnanediol level
B. Male
   1. Physical examination
      a. General health (assessment of height, weight, blood pressure)
      b. Endocrine evaluation (for example, presence of gynecomastia)
      c. Visual fields evaluation for bitemporal hemianopia
      d. Abnormal hair patterns
   2. Urologic examination (includes presence or absence of phimosis; location of urethral meatus; size and consistency of each testis, vas deferens, and epididymis; presence of varicocele)
   3. Rectal examination
      a. Size and consistency of the prostate, with microscopic evaluation of prostate fluid for signs of infection
      b. Size and consistency of the seminal vesicles
   4. Laboratory examination
      a. Complete blood count
      b. Sedimentation rate
      c. Serology
      d. Urinalysis
      e. Rh factor and blood grouping
      f. Semen analysis
      g. If indicated (incomplete list), testicular biopsy, buccal smear

Tests for Infertility

Five general areas are investigated during a fertility evaluation: ovulatory function, cervical mucosal adequacy/receptivity to sperm, sperm adequacy, tubal patency, and the general condition of the pelvic organs. The tests to investigate these functions are designed to evaluate the anatomy, physiology, and sexual compatibility of the couple.

OVULATORY FUNCTION

One basic test is the *basal body temperature* recording (BBT). At the initial visit, the woman is instructed in the technique of recording basal body temperature, which may be taken with a BBT thermometer. This special thermometer measures temperature between 96F and 100F and is calibrated by tenths of a degree, thereby enabling easier identification of slight temperature changes. The woman may choose the site to obtain the temperature. Possible sites include oral, axillary, rectal, or vaginal, and the same site should be used each time. For best results the thermometer should be kept beside the bed and the woman should take her temperature upon awakening, before any activity. After obtaining her temperature, she shakes the thermometer down to prepare it for use the next day. This step is important, as even the activity of shaking the thermometer immediately before use can cause a small increase in the basal temperature. Other factors that may produce temperature variation are sleeplessness, digestive disturbances, illness, fever, and emotional upset. Daily variations should be recorded on the temperature graph. The temperature graph and the readings are used for detecting ovulation and timing intercourse.

Basal temperature for females in the preovulatory phase is usually below 98F (36.7C). An ovulatory menstrual cycle is characterized by a biphasic basal body temperature pattern. As ovulation approaches, production of estrogen increases and at its peak may cause a drop in the basal temperature. When ovulation occurs, progesterone is produced by the corpus luteum causing a 0.5–1.0F (0.3–0.6C) rise in basal temperature. Figure 6–2 shows a BBT chart. The rise in BBT is associated with increased ovarian progesterone production. It does not predict the day of ovulation but provides supportive evidence of ovulation 2 or 3 days after it has occurred. Actual release of the ovum probably occurs 24–36 hours prior to the first temperature elevation (Coulam, 1982). With the additional documentation of coitus, serial BBT charts can be used to indicate if, and approximately when, the client is ovulating and if intercourse is occurring at the proper time to achieve conception. A proposed schedule for intercourse based on serial BBT charts might be to recommend sexual intercourse every other day in the period of time beginning 3–4 days prior to and continuing for 2–3 days following the expected time of ovulation.

Hormonal assessments of ovulatory function tests are available but used infrequently because they are often too expensive and time-consuming. These tests fall into three categories:

1. *LH assays.* Daily samplings of serum LH at midcycle can detect the LH surge. Estimated ovulation is within less than 24 hours of the LH peak in 75% of cycles and within 48 hours in all cycles (WHO, 1978). The day of the LH surge is believed to be the day of maximum fertility. LH assay tests are still being refined.

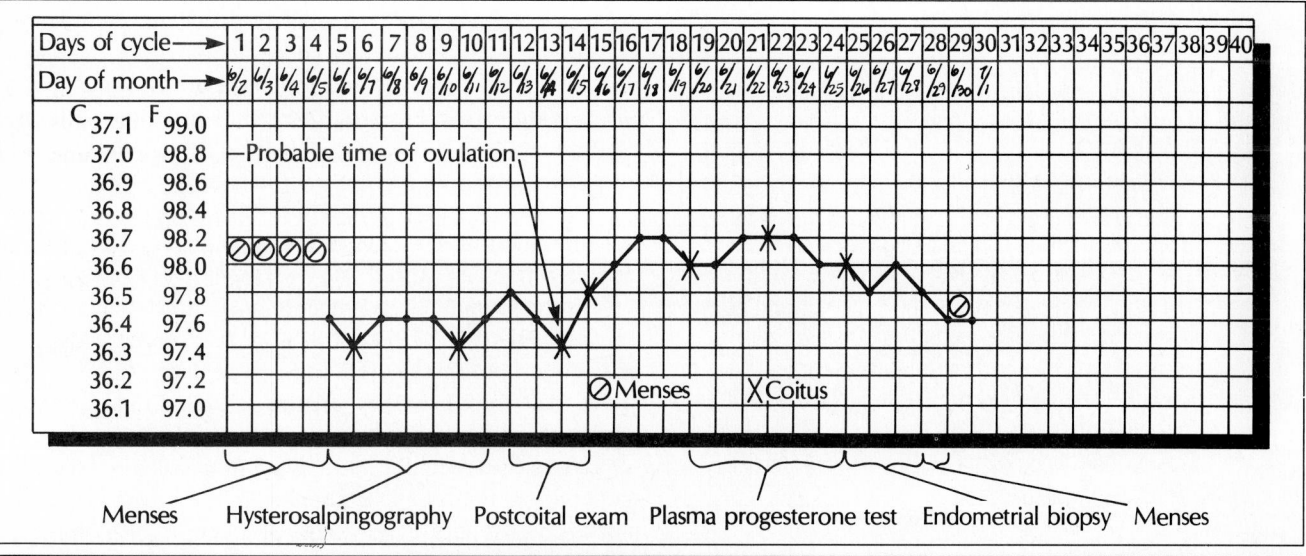

FIGURE 6–2 Basal body temperature chart with different types of testing and the time in the cycle that each would be performed.

2. *Estrogen assay.* Serum estradiol measurement at mid-cycle can estimate time of ovulation. Estrogen peaks approximately one day before the LH surge and 37 hours before ovulation. With urinary estrogen assays, the preovulatory peak is 40–100 ng/24 hours. More direct assays are being perfected.

3. *Progesterone assays.* Progesterone levels furnish the best evidence of ovulation and corpus luteum functioning. Plasma progesterone levels begin to rise with the LH surge and peak about 8 days after the LH surge. Two blood samples, on days 8 and 21, showing an increase of from less than 1 ng/mL to greater than 5 ng/mL indicate ovulation (Ross et al., 1970). Urinary pregnanediol reaches levels of 4–6 mg/24 hours after ovulation; a level of 2 mg/24 hours or greater indicates ovulation.

Hormonal determinations, once perfected, will assist in validation of commonly performed methods of ovulation detection.

Further evaluation of ovulatory function is made by performing a *biopsy of the endometrium*, which provides information regarding the effects of progesterone produced after ovulation by the corpus luteum. A sample of endometrium from the fundal area of the uterus is obtained by use of a special small tubular curet (Novak), which is attached to either electric, water, or syringe suction. The biopsy is usually performed 2–6 days before menstruation as this is the time of the greatest luteal function. The endometrial biopsy is performed in a physician's office. The client should be informed that she may experience cramping similar to menstrual cramps at the time the actual specimen is taken.

CERVICAL MUCOSAL TESTS

The *postcoital examination* (Sims-Huhner's test) is performed 1 or 2 days prior to the expected date of ovulation. The couple is asked to have intercourse 2–4 hours before the examination. The evaluation consists of examining the cervical mucus and the number and motility of sperm present at the endocervix. A small plastic catheter, attached to a 10-mL syringe, is placed in the cervix. Mucus is aspirated from the internal and external os, measured, and examined microscopically for signs of infection, number of active spermatozoa per high-powered field, and number of spermatozoa with poor or no activity.

The cervical mucus, which is produced by the mucous-secreting cells of the endocervix, consists predominantly of water. As ovulation approaches, increased secretion of estrogen by the ovary causes a change in cervical mucus. The amount of mucus increases greatly, and the water content rises significantly. Elasticity, or *spinnbarkeit*, increases and the viscosity decreases. Excellent spinnbarkeit exists when the mucus can be stretched 5 cm or longer (Coulam, 1982). This is accomplished by using two glass slides (Figure 6–3,A) or by grasping some mucus at the external os and stretching it in the vagina toward the introitus.

The *ferning capacity* (Figure 6–3,B) of the cervical mucus also increases as ovulation approaches. Ferning, or crystallization, is caused by increased levels of salt and water interacting with the glycoproteins in the mucus during the ovulatory period and is thus an indirect indication of estrogen production. To test for ferning, mucus is obtained from the cervical os, spread on a glass slide, allowed to air dry, and examined under the microscope.

Research directed at detection of ovulation is focusing on determination of cyclic changes in the various cervical mucus constituents. At present, BBT, biophysical (ferning and spinnbarkeit) and biochemical constituents of cervical mucus, and endometrial biopsy for endometrial morphol-

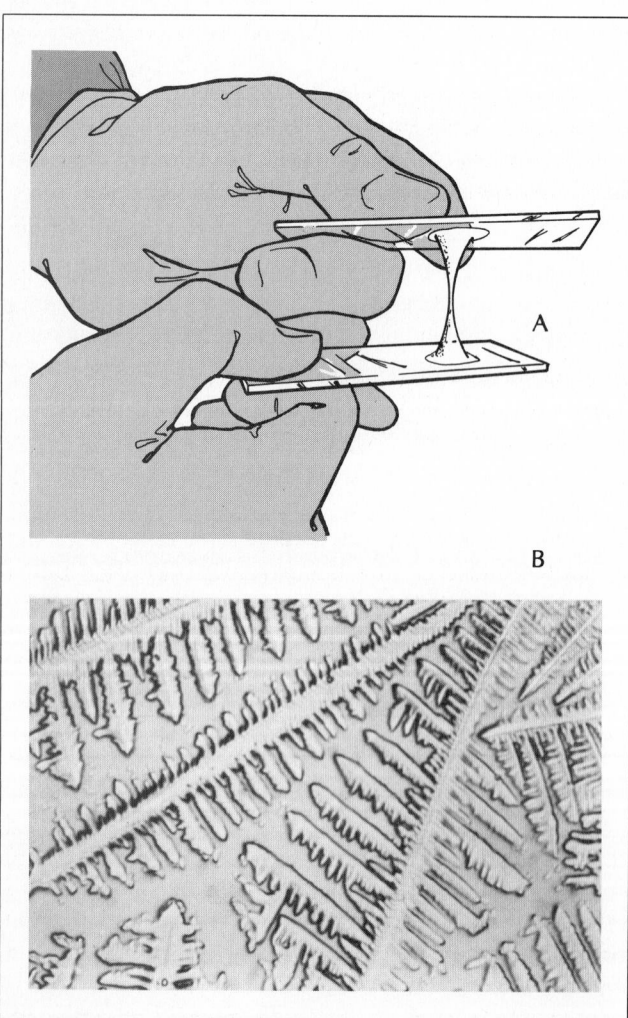

FIGURE 6–3 A, Spinnbarkeit (viscosity). B, Ferning. (Courtesy of Lovena L. Porter.)

ogy studies are the most practical methods of ovulation detection.

Cervical mucus "hostile" to sperm survival can result from several causes, some of which are treatable. For example, estrogen secretion may be inadequate for the development of appropriately elastic mucus. Therapy with supplemental estrogen for approximately 6 days before expected ovulation permits the formation of suitable spinnbarkeit. Cervical infection, another cause of mucosal "inhospitality" to sperm, can be treated, depending on the type of infection. The cervix can also be the site of secretory immunologic reactions in which antisperm antibodies are produced causing agglutination of the semen. A combination plasma–semen–mucous test is under investigation that will help diagnose this problem. Corticosteroid therapy for immunosuppression has been attempted with positive reports.

SPERM ADEQUACY TESTS

Many physicians replace the postcoital examination for sperm analysis with a *semen analysis*, which can be done anytime in the investigation and is the most important initial diagnostic study of the male. Optimum results are obtained when a specimen is collected after 2 days of abstinence. The specimen should be placed in a glass container and brought to the laboratory within an hour, if possible, marked with the time of collection and date of previous ejaculations. It should be maintained at body temperature.

Sperm analysis can provide information about sperm motility and morphology as well as a determination of the absolute number of spermatozoa present. A normal semen analysis may be defined as one that shows at least 50 million sperm per milliliter, semen volume of 2–5 mL, pH level of 7.2–7.8, sperm motility of greater than 60% (within 2 hours of collection) with normal progression, and at least 70% normal sperm forms. The chance to impregnate is remote if the semen analysis reveals less than 10 million sperm per milliliter, less than 50%–60% active sperm, or less than 70% normal sperm forms. Recent studies document the occurrence of autoimmunity to sperm. Spermatozoa has been shown to possess intrinsic antigens that may provoke immunologic infertility. Therapy has been attempted with immunosuppressive agents and insemination techniques (Dondero et al., 1979).

TUBAL PATENCY TESTS

Tubal patency is confirmed with either tubal insufflation with carbon dioxide gas (Rubin's test) or hysterosalpingography. The cervical os is sealed off and carbon dioxide gas is passed through a cannula into the uterine cavity, fallopian tube, and if patent, into the abdominal cavity. Determination of patency is dependent on the gas pressure registered at insufflation. It can be further assessed by auscultation of the abdomen for gas movement, a "jet"

sound, and shoulder pain in the client when she is placed in a sitting position. This pain is referred from the peritoneum, which is irritated by the subdiaphragmatic collection of gas.

Tubal insufflation gives presumptive evidence of tubal patency, but its advantages are otherwise limited. The procedure does not tell whether one or both tubes are patent and gives no information about the contour of the uterine cavity, about uterine anomalies, or about distortion of one or both tubes as a result of pelvic adhesions.

Hysterosalpingography, or *hysterogram*, is an instillation of a radioopaque substance into the uterine cavity. The filling of the uterus and tubes, and spilling into the peritoneal cavity is viewed with roentgenographic techniques. It can reveal tubal patency and any distortions of the endometrial cavity. This procedure has also been known to have a therapeutic effect. Pregnancy is frequently achieved within the first three cycles following the test. This effect may be caused by the flushing of debris, by breaking of adhesions, or by induction of peristalsis by the media.

Both tubal insufflation and hysterosalpingography cause moderate discomfort. Thus the more informative of the two, hysterosalpingography, should be utilized. The hysterosalpingography should be performed in the proliferative phase of the cycle to avoid interrupting an early pregnancy and also to avoid the lush secretory changes in the endometrium that occur after ovulation, which may prevent the passage of the dye, presenting a false picture of cornual obstruction.

Culdoscopy is also used to assess tubular function. The client is given heavy analgesia and is placed in the kneechest position. The posterior cul-de-sac is infiltrated with local anesthetic and entered with a metallic trocar. Culdoscopic examination of pelvic structure is accomplished by direct visual inspection. Indigo carmine or similar dyes can be injected through a cannula inserted into the cervix, and the patency of the fallopian tubes can thereby be evaluated.

Laparoscopy is replacing culdoscopy for the direct viewing of pelvic organs. With this procedure the woman usually is given a general anesthetic. Entry is made through an incision in the area of the umbilicus and occasionally suprapubically. The peritoneal cavity is distended with carbon dioxide gas, and the pelvic organs can be directly visualized. Tubular function can be assessed and evaluation for endometriosis, adhesions, organ fixations, pelvic inflammatory disease, tumors, and cysts is done by instillation of a dye into the uterine cavity from below. Visualization is best when the procedure is performed in the early follicular stage of the cycle. The intraperitoneal gas is usually manually expressed at the end of the procedure (Figure 6–4). Routine preanesthesia instructions should be given. The client is told she may have some discomfort from organ displacement and shoulder and

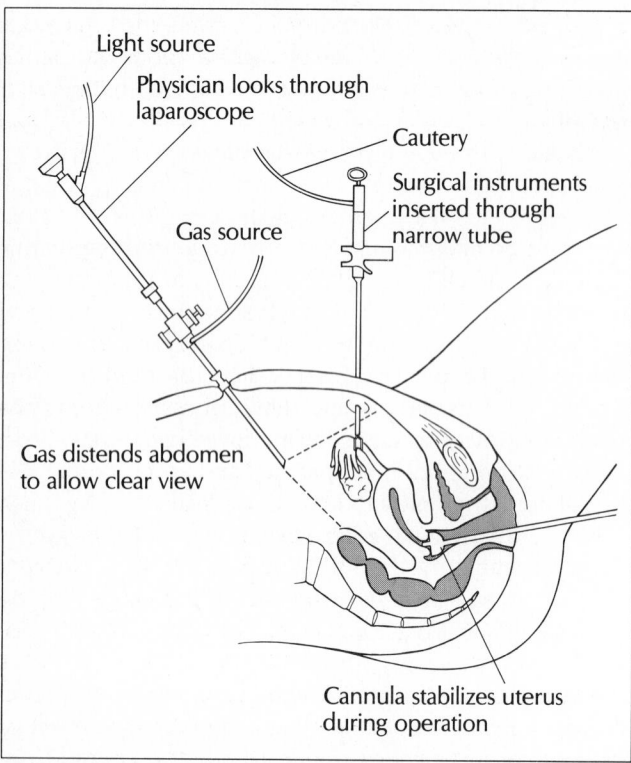

Light source

Physician looks through
laparoscope

Cautery

Surgical instruments
inserted through
narrow tube

Gas source

Gas distends abdomen
to allow clear view

Cannula stabilizes uterus
during operation

FIGURE 6-4 Laparoscopy with laporoscope inserted through an incision at the umbilicus and instruments through a suprapubic incision after the peritoneal cavity is distended with carbon dioxide gas.

chest pain caused by anesthesia and by gas in the abdomen lasting 24–48 hours after the procedure. She should be informed that after resting for about 2 days she can resume normal activities.

Methods of Infertility Management

PHARMACOLOGIC METHODS

If a defect in ovulation has been detected in the fertility testing, the treatment depends on the specific etiology of the problem. In the presence of normal ovaries and an intact pituitary gland *clomiphene citrate* (Clomid) is often used. This medication induces ovulation in 70%–80% of women by actions at both the hypothalamic and ovarian levels. The woman is instructed to take the medication daily beginning day 5 of the menstrual cycle and is informed that if ovulation occurs it will be on the eighteenth to twentieth cycle day. The presence of ovulation and evaluation of response to therapy should be assessed by BBT, plasma progesterone, or cervical mucus and vaginal cytology studies, then clomiphene administration should be discontinued. Pregnant rat studies show dose-dependent in-

crease in malformations when clomiphene is given during organogenesis (Cantor, 1982). The client should be evaluated pelvically to rule out ovarian enlargement or the presence of pregnancy before another cycle is begun. Ovarian enlargement and abdominal discomfort may result from follicular growth and development and multiple corpus luteum formation. Persistence of ovarian cysts is a contraindication for further clomiphene administration. An increase in dose may be necessary to induce ovulation. Augmentation of the midcycle LH surge to cause ovulation may be accomplished by intramuscular administration of a hCG on cycle day 12–14. Supplemental low-dose *estrogen* may be given to insure appropriate quality and quantity of cervical mucus, as clomiphene has been shown to inhibit mucous production.

Human menopausal gonadatropin (hMG), a potent hormone, is capable of causing mild to severe reactions. It is a combination of FSH and LH obtained from postmenopausal women's urine and administered intramuscularly for 9–12 days in the first half of the cycle to stimulate follicular development. To effect ovulation, hCG must also be given. Hyperstimulation syndrome may develop with this form of therapy. Follicle size and number can be monitored by real-time ultrasound, and the hCG can be administered accordingly to match the LH surge. Multiple birth rate is reported to be about 20%, with 15% twins. Medication with hMG is not in common use, and women who elect this form of therapy usually have passed through all other forms of management without conceiving. Strong emotional support is needed because of the expense, the numerous office visits each month, and the stress within the client's relationship.

When hyperprolactinemia accompanies anovulation, the infertility may be treated with *bromocriptine*. This medication acts directly on the prolactin-secreting cells in the anterior pituitary. High prolactin levels may impair the glandular production of FSH and LH and/or block their action on the ovaries. BBT shows a biphasic pattern with the medication. The drug should be discontinued if pregnancy is suspected or at the anticipated time of ovulation.

When endometriosis is determined to be the cause of the infertility, *danazol* (Danocrine) may be given to suppress ovulation and menstruation, and effect atrophy of the ectopic endometrial tissue. It has an antigonadatropin effect and suppresses both FSH and LH. Temporary suppression has been shown to result in healing of the endometriosis. The treatment regime may last for 3–8 months or longer, depending on the severity of the disease. The return of menstrual function and fertility is prompt after discontinuation of danazol, with the first menstrual period occurring within 4–6 weeks. (This same suppression can be achieved with the continuous use of oral contraceptives. However, troublesome side effects are much more frequent and symptomatic relief is less.) The client is instructed to begin the danazol on day 1 of the menstrual cycle and take it daily for 3–8 months.

ARTIFICIAL INSEMINATION

Artificial insemination, with either the husband's semen (AIH) or that of a donor (AID), is the depositing of semen at the cervical os by mechanical means. The conception rates are approximately 30% for AID with 15% for AIH. AIH is used in cases of too small or large semen volume, oliozoospermia or polyzoospermia, low levels of spermatozoal motility, anatomic defects accompanied by inadequate deposition or penetration of semen, or retrograde ejaculation.

AID is considered in cases of total lack of sperm motility or combination of inadequate motility and viability of sperm, recurrent abortions resulting from male cytogenetic abnormality, or male homologous translocation carrier. AID is not appropriate therapy in cases of women with antibodies, since they have antibodies against antigens common to all human sperm cells, not just to their husband's sperm.

Numerous factors need to be evaluated before AID is performed. Has every possible effort been made to diagnose and treat the cause of the male infertility? Do tests indicate normal fertility and sperm/ovum transport in the woman? Is each member psychologically stable? Is this a voluntary decision on the part of the male partner? Are there any religious contraindications?

Artificial insemination is accomplished by collecting semen from the male in a glass container. The semen then is drawn into a syringe and placed into a small plastic cervical cup. The cup is put in place at the cervical os, and the woman remains in the supine position with the hips elevated for about 30 minutes. Since the timing of artificial insemination may be delayed until the BBT has been obtained for several months, the semen may need to be frozen.

IN VITRO FERTILIZATION

Human oocytes have been collected by aspiration at laparotomy or laparoscopy for *in vitro fertilization* and implantation after early cell division when tubal factors have been the cause of infertility. The birth of an infant girl was reported in Great Britain in 1978 and in the United States in 1981 using this technique. However, there is not enough experience in this area to make judgments about the feasibility of this procedure to resolve infertility problems. (See Chapter 1 for discussion of related ethical issues.)

ADOPTION

The adoption of an infant is not as satisfactory an alternative to infertility today as it was in the past. A waiting period of as long as 5–7 years to even begin the adoption process is not uncommon. Many out-of-wedlock infants are being reared by their mothers instead of surrendered for adoption as in the past, and many unwanted pregnancies are being terminated by elective abortion. Some couples seek international adoptions or consider adopting older children, those with handicaps, or children of mixed parentage.

The Nurse's Role

Approximately 4–5 million Americans are unable to conceive or carry a pregnancy to term even after years of medical evaluation and treatment. The couple may incur tremendous emotional and physical stress, as well as financial expense. Years of effort and numerous evaluations and examinations may take place before a conception occurs, if it occurs at all. In a society that values children and considers them to be the natural result of marriage, such couples may face myriad tensions.

The nurse must be constantly aware of the emotional needs and sometimes irrational thoughts and fears of the couple with a fertility problem. Constant attention to temperature charts and instructions about their sex life from a person outside the relationship naturally affects the spontaneity of a couple's interactions. Their relationship will be stressed by these and other intrusive but necessary measures. The tests may heighten feelings of frustration or anger between the partners. In addition, the introduction of other parties to the problem in this intimate area of a relationship may precipitate feelings of guilt and shame. Throughout the evaluations and strains one or both partners may undergo at this time, the nurse has a major responsibility for teaching and offering emotional support.

Correction of infertility may require surgery, administration of hormones, or other treatment measures. The role of the nurse is to provide information and emotional support to the infertile couple throughout the procedures. It is in this emotionally laden atmosphere that infertility evaluation and management must take place.

Infertility may be perceived as a loss by one or both partners, and as in the loss of a loved one who dies, this situation is attended by feelings of grief and mourning. Each couple passes through several stages of feelings, not unlike those identified by Kubler-Ross: surprise, denial, anger, isolation, guilt, grief, and resolution (Menning, 1980). Nonjudgmental acceptance and a professional caring attitude on the nurse's part can go far to dissipate the negative emotions the couple may experience while going through this process. This is also a time when the nurse may assess the quality of the couple's relationship—are they able and willing to verbally communicate and share feelings? Are they mutually supportive? The answers to such questions may help the nurse to identify areas of strength and weakness that will assist in the construction of an appropriate plan of care. At times, individual or group counseling with other infertile couples may facilitate the couple's resolution of feelings brought about by their own difficult situation.

CONTRACEPTION

Gaining control over the number of children they will conceive and spacing their children are two motivating factors in a couple's decision to use a contraceptive measure. In choosing a specific method, consistency of use outweighs the absolute reliability of a given method. Consideration of the risk factors and contraindications for use of a particular contraceptive method is important if the nurse is going to assist the couple in selecting a contraceptive method that has practical application and that is compatible with the couple's health and physical needs.

Women seeking contraception should have a history taken and a screening physical examination with minimal laboratory tests done before choosing a method of contraception. The history should include immediate family incidences of diabetes, bleeding or clotting problems, heart problems or high blood pressure, migraine headaches or seizure disorders, kidney or liver disease, anemia, tuberculosis, stroke, cancer, or mental problems. This information provides a baseline of risk factors that could influence or contraindicate the prescription of oral contraceptives. A past medical and surgical history is completed, as is a detailed menstrual and obstetric history. The data base should also include information on previous use of and experience with contraceptives, history of allergies, and information about smoking habits and use of "recreational drugs."

A precontraception physical examination should include, as a minimum, a breast check, a pelvic examination and a Pap smear, and some type of health screen. Weight, age, and blood pressure can indicate risk factors that may preclude prescribing certain forms of birth control.

Minimal laboratory testing includes a hemoglobin/hematocrit analysis; urinalysis for sugar and protein; Pap smear; endocervical culture for *Neisseria gonorrhoeae;* serologic test for syphilis; pregnancy test, if indicated; and any other test identified during the history or physical as being appropriate.

The couple's decisions about contraception should be made voluntarily, with full knowledge of options, advantages, disadvantages, effectiveness, side effects, and long-range effects; with access to alternatives; without pressure by health professionals; and with the strictest confidentiality. Many outside factors influence a couple's choice, including cultural influences, religious beliefs, personality, cost, effectiveness, misinformation, practicability of method, and self-esteem. Different methods of contraception may be appropriate at different times in the couple's life.

Following is a review of the major contraceptive meth-

ods available, with an examination of their advantages and disadvantages and effectiveness (Table 6–2).

Fertility Awareness Methods

Increasing numbers of couples are becoming interested in methods of contraception that do not use artifical devices or substances. These methods have been called "natural family-planning" methods. Recently, there has been much debate over what is "natural" and therefore what may appropriately be called "natural family-planning." Strict proponents believe that a natural method cannot include any alternate means of birth control (such as condoms or diaphragm) during the fertile period of the cycle. Others wonder whether avoiding intercourse at a time in the menstrual cycle when the women physiologically and psychologically may be most interested in having intercourse is really "natural." Some question the sole reliance on natural methods since contraceptive failures which occur when the ova and sperm involved in the fertilization process are relatively aged may increase the incidence of pregnancy loss and congenital anomalies (Hatcher et al., 1982a). Because of these debates and a belief that all clients or couples have a right to fertility information, many authors are now calling natural family-planning techniques *fertility awareness methods.*

The methods of fertility awareness based on the woman's menstrual cycle are basal body temperature, calendar rhythm, ovulation, and symptothermal. Periodic abstinence from sexual intercourse is a requirement of all four methods, as is the recording of certain events during the menstrual cycle; hence cooperation of the partner is important. Advantages of the natural methods include an increased awareness of one's body and avoidance of artificial substances.

The *basal body temperature method* to detect ovulation requires that the woman take her BBT every morning and record the readings on a temperature graph. The completed graph then provides data to identify the safe and unsafe periods of the menstrual cycle. Intercourse is avoided on the day of temperature rise and for the following 3 days. Not all temperature curves are interpretable, however, so many abstain from intercourse for an extended period of time, between days 12 and 18 in a cycle, to ensure safety.

The *calendar rhythm method* first requires the recording of each menstrual cycle for at least 6 months so that the shortest and longest cycles can be identified. The first day of menstruation is the first day of the cycle. The fertile phase "extends from and includes the 18th day before the end of the shortest likely cycle through the 11th day before the end of the longest likely cycle" (Hatcher et al., 1982b). For example, if a woman's cycle lasts from 24–28 days, the fertile phase would be calculated as day 6 through 17. Once this information is obtained, the woman

Table 6-2 Advantages, Disadvantages, and Effectiveness of Different Forms of Contraception*

	Theoretical effectiveness†	Use effectiveness†	Inexpensive	No major side effects	No medical exam or follow-up	Protects against VD	Disposable	Partner cooperation needed	Increased body awareness	Avoidance of "artificial substances"	Can predispose to major health problems	Can cause major infections	Can cause minor irritations	Can be expelled or dislodged	Can initiate menstrual problems	Can cause discomfort to wearer	Coital related	Must manipulate genitals
Tubal ligation	0	0.04									X							
Vasectomy	0	0.15									X							
Oral contraceptives	0.1	0.3									X		X		X			
IUD	2	5									X	X	X	X	X	X		X
Diaphragm with spermicide	3	15	X							X		X	X				X	X
Condoms	1	5	X	X	X	X	X	X		X			X				X	X
Foams or jellies	5	20	X	X	X	X	X			X			X				X	X
Rhythm (calendar)	14	35-40	X	X	X			X	X	X								
Withdrawal	3	15-23	X	X	X			X	X	X							X	X
Mucous (ovulation method)			X	X	X			X	X	X								X
Cervical cap	3	15	X							X		X	X			X		X
Douche		35-40	X	X	X		X			X			X				X	X

*Adapted from Romney, S. L., et al. 1975. *Gynecology and obstetrics: the health care of women.* New York: McGraw-Hill, Blakiston, p. 552, and modified from Tatum, H. J., and Connell-Tatum, E. P. July 1981. Barrier contraception. *Fertil. Steril.,* p. 5
† Number of pregnancies per 100 woman-years of use.

can identify the fertile and infertile phases of her cycle and, for effective use of the method, she must abstain from intercourse during the fertile phase.

Rhythm is a variation of the calendar rhythm method previously discussed. It is based on identification of the "unsafe period" of a menstrual cycle, which is a period of time immediately before and after ovulation. Theoretically, conception may occur on only 3 days in each cycle, but women who have irregular cycles find it difficult to pinpoint the time of ovulation (see Figure 6-2). The irregularity of menses during the postpartum period and lactation is an obvious limitation of the rhythm method of contraception.

The *ovulation method,* sometimes called the *Billings method,* involves the assessment of cervical mucus changes that occur during the menstrual cycle. The amount and character of cervical mucus change as a result of the influence of estrogen and progesterone. Type E mucus is predominant at the time of ovulation and is the re-

sult of the effect of estrogen on the approximate 100 mucous secretory units present in the cervix. Type G mucus predominates during the luteal phase and is the result of the effects of progesterone.

As ovulation approaches, the amount of cervical mucus increases, and it becomes clearer and more stretchable. This type E mucus consists of "96.7% water, 1% protein, 0.8% NaC1, 1.5% mucin, and a few cells" (Britt, 1977). Type E mucus shows a fern pattern that becomes apparent when the mucus is placed on a glass slide and is allowed to dry (Figure 6-3,*B*).

The stretchability (spinnbarkeit) of the cervical mucus is greatest at the time of ovulation and may vary from 5-20 cm. Spinnbarkeit may be assessed by obtaining mucus from underwear, from the labia, or from the vagina and then stretching the mucus between two glass slides or between two fingers.

Type E mucus allows increased permeability to sperm and enables sperm to pass through the cervix because of the presence of mucin fibers that lie parallel to each other. At ovulation, type E mucus is greatest in amount and stretchability. The woman notices a feeling of wetness around the vagina.

During the luteal phase, the characteristics of the cervical mucus change. It becomes thick and sticky and forms a network in the cervical canal that traps the sperm and makes their passage more difficult. This type G mucus consists of "90.2% water, 3% protein, 0.8% NaCl, 6% mucin, and an abundance of cells" (Britt, 1977).

To use the ovulation method, the woman should abstain from intercourse for the first menstrual cycle. Cervical mucus should be assessed for amount, ferning, and spinnbarkeit on a daily basis as the woman becomes more familiar with varying characteristics. After a pattern has been established, abstinence from intercourse is necessary when type E mucus predominates and for four days following ovulation.

The *symptothermal method* consists of various assessments that are made and recorded by the couple. They use a chart to record information regarding cycle days, coitus, cervical mucous changes, and secondary signs such as increased libido, abdominal bloating, mittelschmerz, and basal body temperature. Through the various assessments, the couple learns to recognize signs that indicate ovulation. This combined approach tends to improve the effectiveness of fertility awareness birth control approaches.

Situational contraceptives also fall under the heading of natural family planning. These methods involve no prior preparation of the couple but involve motivation to abstain from intercourse or to interrupt the sexual act prior to the ejaculation of the sperm into the vagina. *Coitus interruptus,* or withdrawal, is the oldest method of contraception but has limited effectiveness as a birth preventive. This method depends on the male's ability to time his ejaculation. In the male partner experiencing premature ejaculation, timed withdrawal is a problem. Moreover, in the plateau phase of arousal, a few drops of sperm-containing fluid may be discharged.

Douching after intercourse is an ineffective method of contraception. It may actually facilitate conception by pushing the sperm farther up the birth canal. Furthermore, sperm have been identified in the fallopian tubes as soon as 90 seconds after ejaculation.

Mechanical Contraceptives

Mechanical contraceptive methods act either as barriers preventing the transport of sperm to the ovum or by preventing implantation of the ovum/zygote. *Condoms,* although originally developed to protect against sexually transmitted disease, offer a viable means of contraception when used consistently and properly (Figure 6–5). Acceptance has been increasing as a growing number of men are assuming responsibility for regulation of fertility. Condoms are applied to the erect penis, rolled from the tip to the end of the shaft, before vulvar or vaginal contact. A small space must be left at the end of the condom to allow for collection of the ejaculate so that the condom will not break at the time of ejaculation. Vaginal jelly should be used if the condom and/or vagina are dry to prevent irritation and possible condom breakage. Care must be taken in removing the condom after intercourse. For optimum effectiveness, the penis should be withdrawn from the vagina while still erect and the condom rim held to prevent spillage. If after ejaculation the penis becomes flaccid while still in the vagina, the male should hold onto the edge of the condom while withdrawing from the vagina to avoid spilling the semen and to prevent the condom from slipping off. The effectiveness of condoms is largely determined by their use. The condom is small, lightweight, disposable, and inexpensive; has no side effects; requires no medical examination or supervision; offers visual evidence of effectiveness; and protects against venereal diseases. Breakage, displacement, possible perineal or vaginal irritation, and dulled sensation are frequently cited as disadvantages.

The *diaphragm* (Figure 6–6) offers a good level of protection from conception and must be used with spermicidal creams or jellies. The client must be fitted with a diaphragm and instructions given by trained personnel. The diaphragm should be rechecked for correct size after each childbirth and if a client has a weight gain or loss of 20 pounds or more.

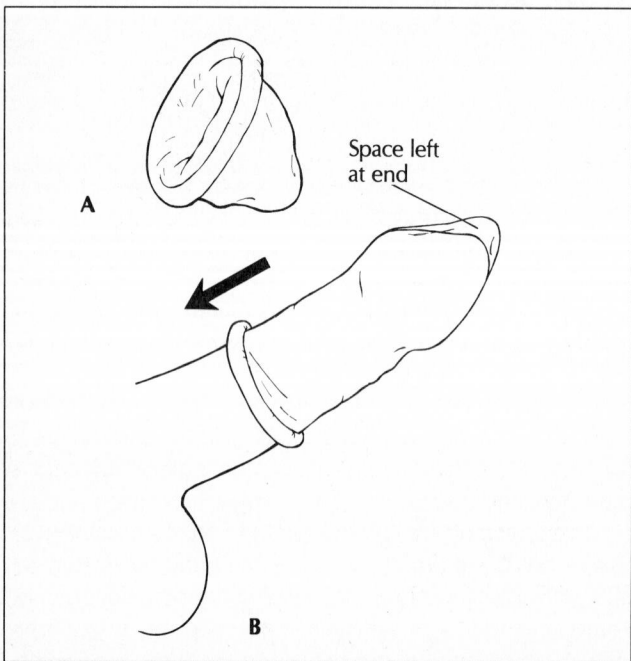

Space left at end

A

B

FIGURE 6–5 A, Condom. **B,** Condom applied to penis. Note space left at end to allow collection of ejaculate.

FIGURE 6–6 A, Diaphragm and jelly. Jelly is applied to the rim and center of the diaphragm. **B,** Insertion of diaphragm. **C,** Rim of diaphragm is pushed up under the symphysis pubis. **D,** Checking placement of diaphragm. Cervix should be felt through the diaphragm.

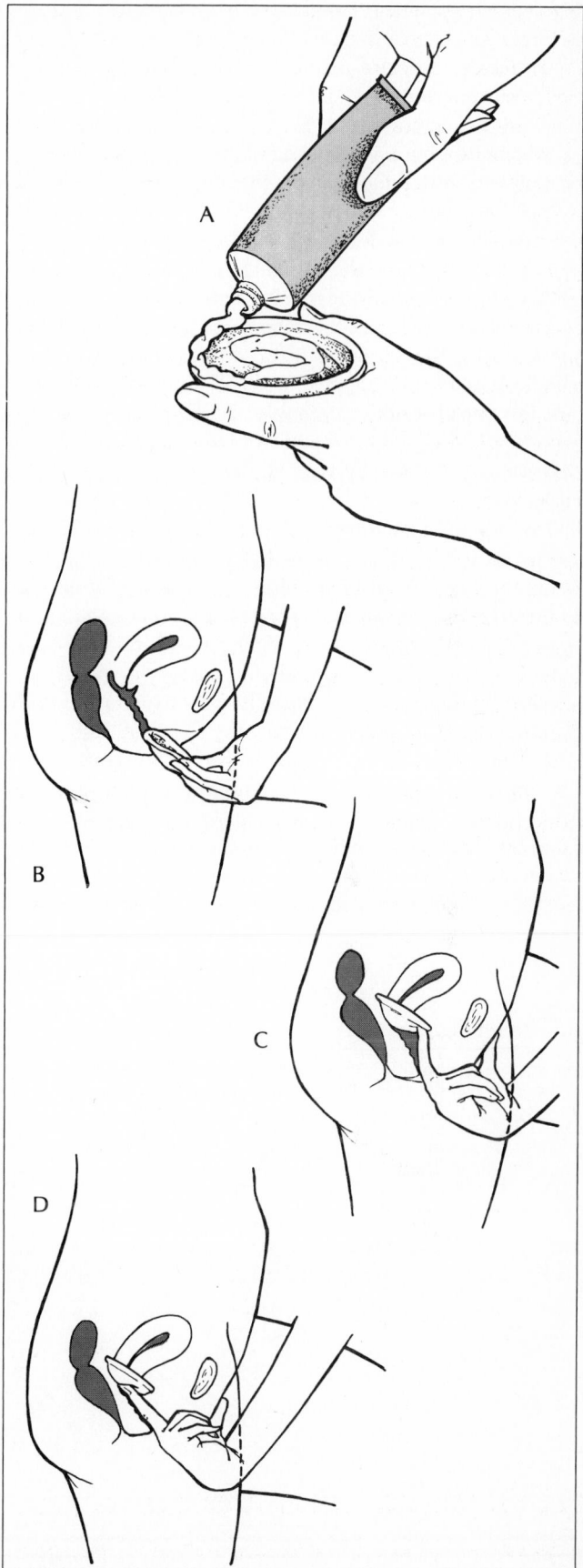

The diaphragm must be inserted prior to intercourse, with approximately 1 teaspoonful (or 1½ inches from the tube) of spermicidal jelly placed around its rim and in the cup. This serves as a chemical barrier to supplement the mechanical barrier of the diaphragm itself. The diaphragm is inserted through the vagina and covers the cervix. The last step in insertion is to push the edge of the diaphragm under the symphysis pubis, which may result in a "popping" sensation. When fitted properly and correctly in place, the diaphragm should not cause discomfort to the wearer or her partner. Correct placement of the diaphragm can be checked by touching the cervix with a fingertip through the cup. The cervix feels like a small rounded structure and has a consistency similar to that of the tip of the nose. The center of the diaphragm should be over the cervix. Women who have chronic urinary tract infections or those who object to manipulation of the genitals for insertion, determination of correct placement, and removal may find this method offensive. If more than 4 hours elapse between insertion of the diaphragm and intercourse, additional spermicidal cream should be used. It is necessary to leave the diaphragm in for 6 hours after coitus. Some couples feel that the use of a diaphragm interferes with the spontaneity of intercourse. It can be suggested that the partner insert the diaphragm as part of the foreplay to overcome this idea. If intercourse is again desired within the next 6 hours, another type of contraception must be used or additional spermicidal jelly placed in the vagina with an applicator, taking care not to disturb the placement of the diaphragm. The diaphragm should be periodically held up to a light and inspected for tears or holes. Diaphragms are an excellent contraceptive means for women who cannot or do not desire to use the pill (hormonal contraceptives), who wish to avoid exposure to the increased risk of pelvic inflammatory disease associated with intrauterine devices, or who wish to be sexually active for several years prior to starting her family (Hatcher et al., 1982b).

The *cervical cap* is a cup-shaped "diaphragm" placed over the cervix that stays in place by suction. The degree of suction is dependent upon the tightness of the fit between the cap and the cervix. The fitting must be meticulous, with best results from custom-made caps. A gynecologist and a dentist have developed a technique using an impressing technique, as is done for denture fitting. Since pregnancies have occurred without cap displacement, spermicidal jelly should be used in the cap. It can remain in place for one or more days. Caps with a one-way valve have been theorized. At present the FDA prohibits their use outside specific test sites, and the only manufacturer is in Great Britain (Tatum and Connell-Tatum, 1981).

Intracervical devices made of either plastic or metal are under current investigation. Expulsion rates are unacceptable, but new models offer promise.

Vaginal sponges constructed of natural collagen fibrous protein with and without a spermicide incorporated in the matrix have been studied since 1976. The preliminary data indicate a need for modifications in design: Complaints concern size, dyspareunia, and vaginal dryness. The contraceptive vaginal sponge currently under consideration is a small (6 cm diameter by 1.5 cm thick) pillow-shaped synthetic sponge with a concave dimple on one side (an indention or cupping area). The sponge is inserted into the vagina prior to intercourse and placed near the cervical os. It is held in place by the vaginal walls, and the concave cup fits snugly over the cervical os, which decreases the chance of the sponge's dislodgement during intercourse. The contraceptive sponge can be placed in the vagina no sooner than 1 week before coitus and must be removed within 6–48 hours after intercourse (Tatum and Connell-Tatum, 1981). The sponge is absorbent enough to be worn during menstruation. (Sponges, which have been used in the past for menstruation, contain no spermicide and are reusable. Some women have attached a string to artist sponges and have used them as menstrual sponges.) Proposed advantages of the sponge are: professional fitting not required as for the diaphragm; may be used for multiple coitus up to 48 hours unlike the single-use condom, one size fits all, and it is both barrier and spermicide (when spermicide is added to the sponge matrix). Based on clinical trials, a spermicide must be incorporated into the

the sponge to ensure an acceptable degree of contraception. This method is now FDA approved.

Intrauterine devices (IUDs) come in many types and shapes, but primarily work by producing a local reaction in the endometrium. It is generally accepted that the IUD produces a local sterile inflammatory reaction. The inflammatory reaction increases the number of uterine leukocytes whose tissue break-down products are toxic to the sperms and the blastocyst. Nidation is inhibited if fertilization occurs (Danforth, 1982).

Possible adverse reactions to the IUD include discomfort to the wearer, increased bleeding during menses, pelvic inflammatory disease, perforation of the uterus, intermenstrual bleeding, dysmenorrhea, expulsion of the device, and ectopic pregnancy. Advantages include convenience, no coital-related activity, and duration of effectiveness.

The IUD is inserted into the uterus with its strip or tail protruding through the cervix into the vagina. Four types are currently in use: the loop, double coil, copper 7, and progesterone-releasing T. The copper 7 and the T-shaped IUD are smaller and have a lower incidence of pain after insertion, and therefore are used more frequently in nulliparous women (Figure 6–7).

The copper 7 continuously releases a small amount of copper and has to be replaced every 3 years. Progesterone-releasing IUDs must be replaced each year. Plastic IUDs may also have to be replaced on a regular basis. When they have been in place more than a year, calcium salts may become deposited on the plastic. This forms a rough surface that irritates the endometrium and can cause ulceration and bleeding. If these symptoms occur, the IUD should be removed and replaced.

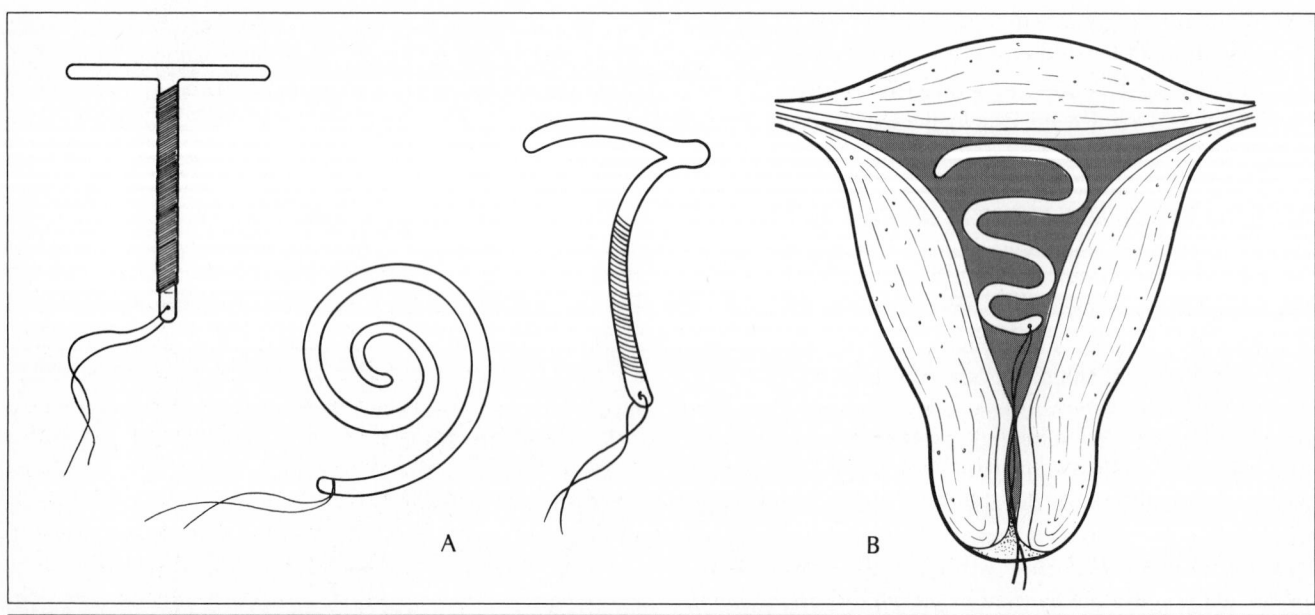

FIGURE 6–7 A, Types of intrauterine devices. *Left,* Progeste-sert; *center,* coil; *right,* copper 7. **B,** Lippes loop in place within the uterus.

The IUD may be inserted at the fourth-to-sixth week postpartum check or during a menstrual period. After insertion, the woman should be instructed to check for the presence of the string once a week for the first month and then after each menses. She is told that she may have some cramping and/or bleeding intermittently for 2–6 weeks and her first few menses may occur in an irregular fashion. Follow-up examination is suggested 4–8 weeks after insertion.

Oral Contraceptives

The use of hormones, specifically the combination of estrogen and progesterone, succeeds as a birth control method by inhibiting the release of an ovum and by maintaining type G mucus, which interferes with the passage of sperm through the cervix.

Numerous oral contraceptives are available, as shown in Table 6–3. The dosage regimen consists of taking one tablet daily beginning on the fifth cycle day (the first day of menstruation is cycle day 1) and continuing for 20–21 days. In most cases, menstrual bleeding will occur 1–4 days after the last tablet.

Some pharmaceutical companies have added seven "blank" tablets so that the woman can continue to take one tablet daily and still maintain the monthly dosage regimen. With the 21-day package, the woman goes off the pill 7 days and restarts taking the pill without waiting until the fifth day of the cycle. The oral contraceptives or birth control pills recommended for general usage are the low-dose (35 mg or less) estrogen preparations. The majority of the more serious side effects from oral contraceptives appear to be estrogen dose-related (Danforth, 1982). The woman should establish a routine in taking the tablets. For example, she may take a tablet daily with breakfast or may prefer to take it with supper. Establishment of a regular routine reduces the chance of forgetting a day and causing intermenstrual bleeding with possible ovulation. If the client should forget a pill, she is instructed to take it as soon as it is discovered, even if it means taking two pills in one day. If she misses two daily pills, she is instructed to take two pills a day to catch up, continue medication on schedule, and use another method of contraception until the next menses.

Although highly effective, oral contraceptives may produce side effects ranging from break-through bleeding to thrombus formation. Regulation of dosages has reduced many of the side effects, but the threat of potential risk is sufficient to deter some women from using oral contraceptives.

Another oral contraceptive is the seldom-used progesterone-only pill, also called the *mini-pill*. It is used primarily with women who have a contraindication to the estrogen component of the combination preparation, such as history of thrombophlebitis, but are strongly motivated toward

---

Side Effects of Oral Contraceptives*

Estrogen component

Altered lipid metabolism
Altered convulsive threshold
Leukorrhea, cervical erosion, or polyposis
Headache
Excessive menstrual flow
Hypertension
Altered carbohydrate metabolism
Altered clotting factors—thrombophlebitis
Chloasma
Breast tenderness or engorgement
Venous or capillary engorgement (spider nevi)
Irritability, nervousness
Edema and cyclic weight gain
Nausea, bloating

Progestin component

Oligomenorrhea
Amenorrhea
Acne
Hirsutism
Breast regression
Anabolic weight gain
Increased appetite
Fatigue
Depression and altered libido
Moniliasis
Loss of hair

*Modified from Kreuther, A. K. K., and Hollingsworth, D. R. 1978. *Adolescent obstetrics and gynecology.* Chicago: Year Book Medical Publishers, Inc., pp. 369, 372.

---

this form of contraception. The major problems with this preparation are amenorrhea or irregular spotting and bleeding patterns. Most women want a monthly period to assure them of nonpregnancy. This same hormone can be given in injectable form every 3 months, but it has the same drawbacks and is not released at this time for this use by the FDA.

Contraindications of the use of oral contraceptives include pregnancy, previous history of thrombophlebitis or thrombolic disease, acute or chronic liver disease of cholestatic type with abnormal function, presence of estrogen-dependent carcinomas, undiagnosed uterine bleeding, heavy smoking, hypertension, diabetes, toxemia, age over 40, lack of regular menstrual cycles for at least 1–2 years in adolescents, and hyperlipoproteinemia. In addition, women with the following conditions who use oral contraceptives should be examined every 3 months: migraine headaches, epilepsy, depression, oligomenorrhea, and amenorrhea. Women who choose this method of contraception should be fully advised of potential side effects. See the above boxed material for side effects of oral contraceptives.

Table 6–3 Relative Potency of Oral Contraceptive Steroids Currently Marketed in the United States

Relative potency of identical doses*		Estrogens (μg)		Gestagens (mg)						
		1.0	1.7–2.0	1	1.09	2	15	30	
						Norethin-drone acetate	Ethyn-odiol diacetate		Potency ratio†
Brand name	Company	Mes-tranol	Ethinyl estradiol	Norethin-drone	Norethy-nodrel			Norges-trel	(E/G × 10⁻³)
Combination									
standard or high dose									
Demulen	Searle		50				1.0		6.7
Enovid-E	Searle	100			2.5				36.7
Enovid-5	Searle	75			5.0				13.8
Norinyl 1/50	Syntex	50		1.0					50.0
Norinyl 1/80	Syntex	80		1.0					80.0
Norinyl 2	Syntex	100		2.0					50.0
Norlestrin 1	Parke-Davis		50			1.0			50.0
Norlestrin 2.5	Parke-Davis		50			2.5			20.0
Ovcon 50	Mead/Johnson		50	1.0					50.0
Ovral	Wyeth		50					0.5	6.7
Ovulen	Searle	100					1.0		6.7
Ortho-Novum 1/50	Ortho	50		1.0					50.0
Ortho-Novum 1/80	Ortho	80		1.0					80.0
Ortho-Novum 2	Ortho	100		2.0					50.0
Ortho Novum 10	Ortho	60		10.0					6.0
Low dose									
Brevicon	Syntex		35	0.5					140.0
Loestrin 1/20	Parke-Davis		20			1.0			20.0
Loestrin 1.5/30	Parke-Davis		30			1.5			20.0
Lo-Ovral	Wyeth		30					0.3	6.7
Modicon	Ortho		35	0.5					140.0
Norinyl 1/35	Syntex		35	1.0					70.0
Ortho Novum 1/35	Ortho		35	1.0					70.0
Ovcon 35	Mead/Johnson		35	0.4					175.0
Gestagen only									
Micronor	Ortho			0.35					
Nor-Q-D	Syntex			0.35					
Ovrette	Wyeth							0.075	

From Danforth, D. N. 1982. *Obstetrics and gynecology.* 4th ed. Philadelphia: Harper & Row, p. 258.

*Estrogens, based on uterine volume analysis by histometric technique in human females (Delforge, J. P., and Ferin J. 1970. *Contraception* 1:57); gestagens, based on a delay in menses test in human females (Greenblatt, R. B. 1967 *Med. Sci.* 18:37).

†A dimensionless number calculated by converting the estrogens to mg and using the relative potency of 2.0 for ethinyl estradiol. This number should be used with caution, since some gestagens are inherently estrogenic (e.g., norethynodrel), while others have antiestrogenic effects (weak: e.g., norethindrone; strong: e.g., norgestrel and norethindrone acetate).

Injectable Contraceptives

Two injectable steroid contraceptives are available and marketed only in Europe at present. Depomedroxyprogesterone acetate (Depo-Provera) is a microcrystalline suspension of progestins, and Norethindrone Enanthate is an oily suspension with a shorter duration than Depo-Provera.

The drugs inhibit secretion of gonadotropins including midcycle LH release. In one study resumption of ovulation and fertility occurred in the majority of women within 1 year of discontinued treatment (WHO, 1977).

Prolonged amenorrhea or increased uterine bleeding or both have occurred during and after steroid contraceptive use (Cheng et al., 1974), and thromboembolism has also been noted (Schwallie, 1974). Return of fertility is delayed until the effects of the injected progestin have elapsed.

Spermicides

A variety of creams, jellies, foams, and suppositories, inserted into the vagina prior to intercourse, destroy sperm or neutralize vaginal secretions and thereby immobilize sperm. Spermicides that effervesce in a moist environment offer more rapid protection and coitus may take place immediately after they are inserted. Suppositories may require up to 30 minutes to dissolve and will *not* offer protection until they do so. The woman should be instructed to insert these spermicide preparations high in the vagina and maintain a supine position. Spermicides are minimally effective when used alone, but in conjunction with a diaphragm or condom, their effectiveness increases. They provide a high degree of protection from exposure to several sexually transmitted diseases, especially gonorrhea (Tatum and Connell-Tatum, 1981).

Operative Sterilization

Before sterilization is performed on either partner, a thorough explanation of the procedure should be given to both. Each should understand that sterilization is not a decision to be taken lightly or entered into when psychologic stresses, such as separation or divorce, exist. Even though male and female procedures are theoretically reversible, the permanency of the procedure should be stressed and understood. All forms of reversible contraception should be explained and discussed in detail to assist the client in making an informed decision.

Male sterilization is achieved by a relatively minor procedure called a *vasectomy*. Under local anesthesia, a 2–3 cm incision is made over the vas deferens on each side of the scrotum. The ducts are isolated; severed; and occluded by ligation of the ends, by coagulation of the lumen, by burial of the cut ends, or by use of clips or polyethylene tubing with a stopcock for potentially reversible procedures (Figure 6–8). Absorbable sutures are used to close

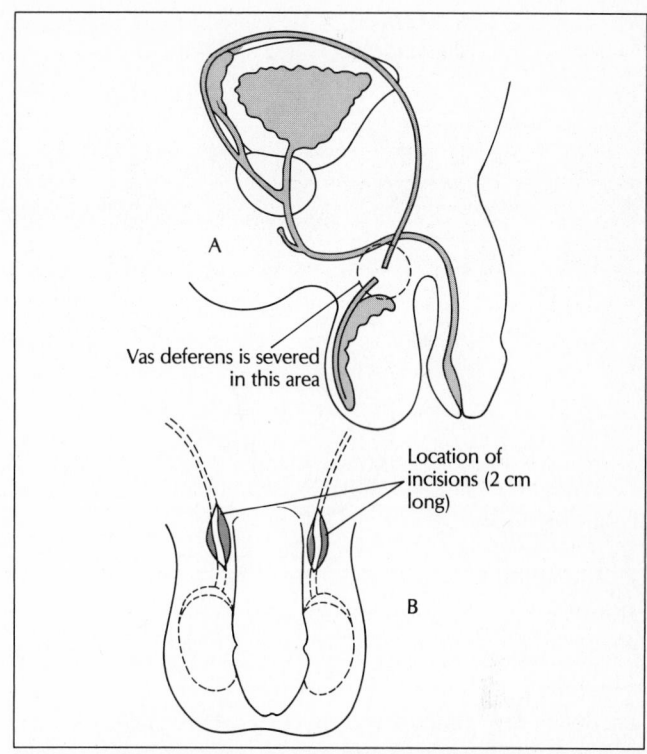

FIGURE 6–8 Vasectomy. **A,** Ligation of the vas deferens. **B,** Location of incisions at either side of the scrotum.

the skin, and the patient is instructed to apply ice when pain or swelling occurs and to use a scrotal support for a week. It takes about 4 to 6 weeks and 6 to 36 ejaculations to clear remaining sperm from the vas deferens. During that period, the couple is advised to use another method of birth control and to bring in two or three sperm samples for a sperm count. The man is rechecked at 6 and 12 months to insure that fertility has not been restored by recanalization. Side effects of a vasectomy include hematoma, sperm granulomas, and spontaneous reanastomosis.

Vasectomies can be reversed with the use of microsurgery techniques, but the fertility reestablishment rate is only approximately 14%–55%. The primary factor appears to be an autoimmune response developed by a man to his own sperm during the period of suppression, as the vasovasostomy reestablishes patency of the vas deferens in 85% of cases (Pabst et al., 1979).

Female sterilization can be accomplished by several abdominal and vaginal procedures. In most cases the fallopian tubes are transected. Figure 6–9 shows *tubal ligation*, which has been the most common method. The postpartal laparotomy is done 1–3 days after delivery, under general anesthesia and usually with a small subumbilical incision. The tubes are isolated and may then be crushed, ligated, or plugged (in the newer reversible procedures). The interval minilaparotomy uses a suprapubic incision with similar techniques for interrupting tubal patency and requires about 2 days of hospitalization. Local anesthesia can be

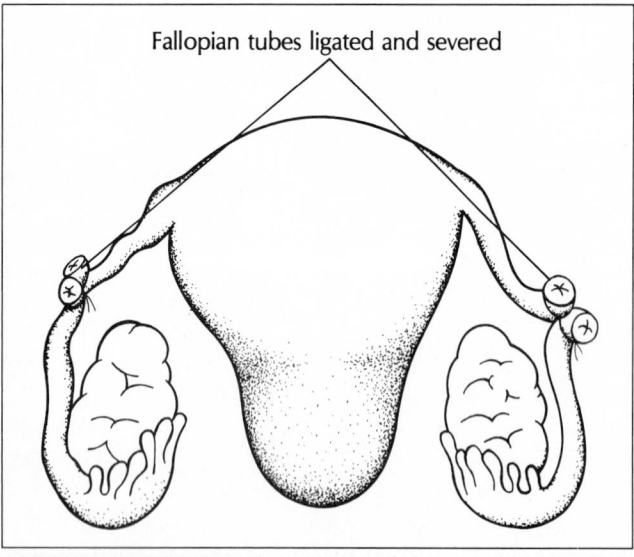

Fallopian tubes ligated and severed

FIGURE 6–9 Pomeroy-method tubal ligation. Both fallopian tubes are ligated and severed, which interrupts continuity of the tube.

used for the minilaparotomy in certain cases. A new method, laparoscopic sterilization, may be done at any time. One or two incisions in the subumbilical area are made. The abdomen is distended with carbon dioxide gas, the laparoscope is introduced through a trocar, and the fallopian tube is visualized. The isthmic portion of the tube is grasped and coagulated and may be transected. The procedure is repeated on the other tube.

Complications of female sterilization procedures include coagulation burns on the bowels, bowel perforation, infection, hemorrhage, and adverse anesthesia effects. Reversal of a tubal ligation depends on many factors, including the portion of the tube excised, the presence or absence of the fimbriae, and the length of the tube remaining. With microsurgical techniques, a pregnancy rate of approximately 70% is possible (Siber and Cohen, 1980).

A reversible form of sterilization is currently being investigated, which incorporates the use of a hysteroscope for direct visualization of the tubal openings into the uterus. The openings are injected with a silicone substance which hardens and occludes the cornual section of the fallopian tube. Hysterosalpingography confirms the success of the procedure and a thread is left in the uterine cavity for future removal.

Induced Abortion

Probably one of the most debated of all contraceptive measures is abortion by voluntary means. For centuries, abortion was illegal according to church and public law. Nevertheless, many women still sought to terminate their pregnancies, and illegal abortions became the single highest cause of maternal death in this country. In 1973, as a result of action by the United States Supreme Court, in-

duced abortion became a legal option. Under this ruling, an induced abortion may be performed legally during the first 3 months of pregnancy. All legal abortions must be performed by a licensed physician. It is left to individual states to determine what restrictions should be placed on abortions after the first trimester.

Although legalized abortion has been in effect for several years, controversy over the moral and legal issues continues (see Chapter 1 for additional discussion). This controversy is as readily apparent in the medical and nursing professions as among other groups. Not all physicians will perform the procedure, and some who have decided to provide the service have not reached the decision on a moral level and therefore offer little, if any, psychosocial support to the woman.

Some nurses, too, find the abortion issue threatening to their basic values. Ambivalence results for nurses who perceive an incompatibility between their professional goal of helping to preserve life and the professional act of assisting clients who choose the option of abortion. Each nurse must decide according to individual moral codes whether to participate in nursing care concerning abortions. In making such a decision, the nurse must consider the necessity of providing psychosocial support to clients who have had an abortion. If the nurse cannot provide empathetic, compassionate support for the woman seeking an abortion, the nurse should see that the client gets appropriate support from another member of the health team.

Many issues surrounding abortion still require clarification. Whether a minor can obtain an abortion without parental consent is under controversy in many states. The rights of the male partner in relation to the decision to terminate pregnancy are also being discussed. Another issue being debated is the "inappropriate" use of abortion as a contraceptive method. Continued education and counseling are needed to resolve these issues. It has been documented that as many as one out of ten normal pregnancies are terminated by therapeutic abortion. In 1980 an estimated 155 million legal abortions occurred compared to about 3.6 million live births in the United States (Tietze, 1982). These figures emphasize the continued need for more adequate contraceptive counseling.

FACTORS INFLUENCING THE DECISION TO SEEK ABORTION

A number of factors influence a woman's decision to seek an abortion, most of them relating to socioeconomics and interpersonal relationships. More specifically, the woman's self-concept and self-esteem and the couple's communication and relationship patterns enter into the decision. Many researchers have demonstrated that a breakdown in these areas can predispose to rejection of the pregnancy.

COUNSELING

Preabortion counseling is important and is most effective when it occurs before the evaluation exam. This often incorporates the use of values-clarification techniques: What stage is she in her life at the present time? What does she want to do? What does a child mean to her now? The initial health assessment includes biologic data, such as medical history; laboratory tests of urine, blood type and cross-match, blood count, and Rh factor (for determination of RhoGAM use); and culture for gonorrhea. The nurse should also obtain psychosocial data about the woman's decision-making process in seeking an abortion and her support systems.

METHODS

Most induced abortions are performed in the hospital on a "same-day discharge" basis, although some states allow abortions on a hospital outpatient basis or as outpatient surgery in a physician's office. The decision about which method should be employed to terminate pregnancy is based primarily on the number of elapsed weeks of gestation. The gestational periods and the method of abortion specified for each period are shown in Table 6–4.

□ *FIRST TRIMESTER* Several methods can be utilized at this time.

Morning-after pill. This method requires the administration of relatively high doses of a synthetic estrogen during the first 3 days after possible conception. The drug causes the endometrial lining to be shed. The patient may experience nausea and vomiting following this procedure.

Vacuum aspiration. Pregnancies of less than 10 weeks' gestation may be terminated by vacuum aspiration (menstrual extraction) using a cannula and suction. Prior to suctioning, the cervix must be dilated. Dilatation to accommodate the cannula may be accomplished by one of two methods: use of a laminaria tent (the dried stem of a seaweed, fashioned in the shape of a cone, which swells and slowly dilates the cervical os, usually overnight) or introduction of increasingly larger sounds. In very early pregnancies, a 4–5 mm cannula can be used, and suction is accomplished with a closed-suction system. Later in pregnancy, a 6–10 mm cannula is necessary, and a small suction pump is used to remove the products of conception.

The woman, who may be premedicated, is placed in a lithotomy position. A vulval and vaginal prep is performed using an antiseptic solution and sterile technique. The client is draped. To facilitate control of the uterus, the cervix is stabilized with a tenaculum. A paracervical block may be administered using 1% Xylocaine or another anesthetic agent. "Supportive anesthesia" may be utilized in place of a blocking agent. In this case, the physician and nurse or another individual should provide emotional and physical support during the procedure. The abortion is usually performed in less than 5 minutes. Following suction, a curet may be introduced into the uterine cavity to assess completeness of the procedure.

During vacuum aspiration the woman may experience cramping or discomfort due to positioning. After the procedure, she should experience little or no discomfort and

only slight vaginal bleeding, which should stop prior to her discharge. She may have a light menstrual-type flow for several days. The length of stay varies from setting to setting but is usually 1–4 hours. On discharge the client is counseled to watch for signs of unusual bleeding or signs of infection, which include high temperature, foul-smelling discharge, or general malaise; and an appointment is set up for a postabortion checkup.

Prostaglandin. Two prostaglandin preparations have been approved and are currently used to terminate pregnancy. Their action is similar to oxytocin in that they cause smooth muscle tissue to contract and the action has a stimulating effect on the contractility of the myometrium. PG is used to terminate pregnancy after 15 weeks' gestation, or for late first-trimester or second-trimester abortion. Side effects are nausea and vomiting and marked constriction of bronchial musculature. Therefore, PG use is contraindicated in women with asthma or other respiratory problems. PG can be instilled vaginally in 20-mg suppository form into the cul-de-sac, or administered intra-abdominally into the amniotic sac. The time required to expel the products of conception varies with the length of gestation. The mean time is approximately 24 hours. Side effects of the vaginal suppository method are gastrointestinal problems and fever; other side effects are similar to intrauterine PG described next.

Intra-amniotic injection involves the injection of 40 mg of $PGF_{2\alpha}$. A small test dose of 1 mL is injected slowly over 5 minutes. If no side effects occur, the remainder of the dose of about 8 mL of 40 mg $PGF_{2\alpha}$ is given slowly. If side effects do occur, recovery takes about 30 minutes because of the short half-life of PG and the minimal test dose.

Clients should be prepared for the possibility of expulsion of a live fetus. Following expulsion of the fetus the placenta may be retained; a curet may be used to extract it. Additional side effects of this procedure include chills, vomiting, diarrhea, cervical lacerations, and tissue reaction at the site of injection.

Dilatation and curettage. This procedure is performed prior to 12 weeks' gestation. If the technique is used after the first trimester, a danger of uterine perforation and hemorrhage exists because of the thinning uterine wall and increased blood supply. Dilatation and curettage involves preparation of the woman similar to that mentioned for vacuum aspiration. A regional or general anesthetic may be used. The cervix is dilated with sounds, and a curet is introduced into the uterus to scrape the products of conception from the uterine wall. Intravenous therapy may be utilized, and an oxytocic medication may be included to assist in the contraction of the uterus after the abortion. Following this procedure, the patient may experience some cramping with minimal vaginal bleeding. She may be discharged in one day with self-care instructions and an appointment to return for a postabortion checkup.

□ *SECOND TRIMESTER* In general, the more advanced the pregnancy, the greater the possibility of physiologic prob-

Table 6-4   Abortion Methods

Gestational age	Abortion method	Possible side effects	Facility required
Week 5 to 7	Menstrual extraction (endometrial aspiration, menstrual regulation, miniabortion)	Allergic reactions, mild cramping, minimal vaginal bleeding, or incomplete removal of tissue	Physician's office or family planning clinic
Week 7 to 12	Vacuum aspiration (suction curettage) or dilatation and curettage (D&C)	Mild cramping and minimal bleeding after vacuum aspiration Uterine or cervical trauma, incomplete evacuation, or infection following D&C	Physician's office, family planning clinic, or hospital
Week 13 to 15	Prostaglandin vaginal suppository	CNS reaction including vomiting, diarrhea, or temperature elevation	Hospital
Week 16 to 24	Prostaglandin intra-amniotic injection	Headache, vomiting, or diarrhea; retained placenta with hemorrhage; cervicovaginal fistula; allergic reaction to drug; bronchial constriction; hypotonic uterus	Hospital
	Urea intra-amniotic injection	Dehydration or alteration in coagulation factors	Hospital
	Saline injection	Hypernatremia resulting from infiltration into tissues Vascular system leakage may result in abdominal pain, severe headache, backache, tachycardia, drowsiness, confusion, seizures Ascending infection from vagina with external rupture of membranes When used with an oxytocin infusion; water intoxication, confusion, drowsiness, headache, cervical tear, uterine rupture	Hospital
	Hysterotomy	Future pregnancies may require repeat cesarean delivery	Hospital
After 24 weeks	Abortion is inadvisable		

lems related to abortion. Thus the methods discussed in this section are considered a greater risk to the woman's health than first-trimester methods are.

Saline induction. Saline abortion procedure is utilized only after 16 weeks' gestation, when the uterus is high enough and the amniotic fluid sufficient for safe amniocentesis. Hospitalization is required. The patient empties her bladder and is given an enema to decrease pressure when the fetus is expelled. The abdomen is shaved and cleansed

and 1% Xylocaine is used to anesthetize the site of amniocentesis. A small amount of amniotic fluid is withdrawn and tested with nitrazine paper to be sure that the amniotic sac has been penetrated. Next, up to 250 mL of amniotic fluid is withdrawn, and a test dose of 10 mL of 20% hypertonic saline is injected. If severe side effects occur, such as tinnitus, tachycardia, dryness of the mouth, severe headache, or flushing, the procedure is terminated and 5% dextrose in water is administered intravenously to prevent cerebral dehydration. If no side effects are experienced, 200–240 mL of 20% hypertonic saline fluid is infused into the amniotic sac. This solution can be infused either in a short time or by the drop method. The needle is withdrawn carefully to avoid a spill of hypertonic solution into the peritoneal cavity. This could cause hypernatremia by drawing fluid from the serum and the extracellular tissues. Following the procedure, the patient may experience cramping and a feeling of fullness. Fetal death usually occurs within an hour of injection.

Some physicians may start an infusion of intravenous oxytocics about 6 hours after injection to speed up labor; others believe that this is unnecessary because labor begins by itself in about 12–24 hours. The client should be throughly informed prior to the procedure. Explanation of the procedure should be repeated two or three times so that any misconceptions can be clarified. Many people are unaware that this method necessitates labor to deliver the fetus. Labor generally lasts about 22 hours, and may cause considerable discomfort to the woman. The woman has the same assessment needs as any laboring patient; that is, vital signs to assess for possible reactions to the saline injection, help with breathing and relaxation techniques, help with voiding, and so on. When delivery is imminent, the woman should not be alone. Delivery usually occurs soon after spontaneous rupture of the membranes. The woman should be informed, in advance, that the body of the fetus is often expelled first and it may take further cervical dilatation to expel the larger after-coming head. The placenta is usually spontaneously aborted 1–2 hours later. Occasionally the placenta is retained, and curettage is necessary to remove it. Postabortion hemorrhage and infection must be watched for carefully during the postpartum period.

Saline induction has many hazards, including hypernatremia, cardiovascular shock, hypertension, peritonitis, acute pulmonary edema, inadvertent intravascular injection of the saline solution, retention of placental fragments, or consumption coagulopathy.

Hysterotomy. The hysterotomy method involves an in-cision into the uterus. This abortion technique is primarily used when other methods are contraindicated or when the woman also wants a tubal ligation for the purpose of sterilization.

NURSING MANAGEMENT

Perhaps the major contributing factor to high-quality nursing care for a woman undergoing abortion is the nurse's objective understanding and acceptance based on an adequate self-assessment. With this foundation a nurse can effectively understand the biologic and psychosocial needs of women undergoing abortion and plan to meet them. The nurse may be able to apply crisis theory to the abortion client, since in times of crisis one experiences a decrease in defenses and this aids in establishment of new, more appropriate, coping mechanisms. Nurses also use psychiatric nursing principles, such as remaining silent and letting the client take the lead at times. One cannot assume that all people want to talk about their problems with strangers.

Important aspects of care surrounding abortion include allowing for verbalization by the patient; support before, during, and after the procedure; monitoring of vital signs, intake, and output; preparing the client for potential pain and discomfort during the procedure; providing for physical comfort and privacy throughout the procedure; and health teaching regarding self-care, the importance of the postabortion checkup, and contraception review. Upon release after the procedure, the woman should be given the telephone number of local helping agencies to whom she could turn for help if needed. If she has been told to anticipate a normal depression, these feelings will not be frightening. The grief period following an abortion lasts from 2–3 months (Hymovich and Barnard, 1973). The postabortion checkup is, perhaps, the most important aspect of counseling in these situations. The client's emotional adjustment can be assessed, and she can be assisted in planning positively for her future. This type of involved, understanding nursing care can help the client achieve an optimum level of health.

SUMMARY

Understanding a couple's desire to plan fertility for appropriate times and under chosen circumstances is important for the health care provider. Nurses can assist a couple in identifying and correcting causes of infertility or help them control the number and interval of children only when they disseminate contraceptive knowledge in an objective, nonjudgmental manner. Risk factors related to the woman's health, influences of culture and religion, psychosocial pressures, personal choices, and economic considerations are determining factors in the selection of a contraceptive method.

Resource Groups

RESOLVE, Inc. A national organization with chapters throughout the United States, offers counseling, referral, and support for the infertile couple.

Planned Parenthood. A national group with offices throughout the United States, offers contraceptive information and counseling services.

References

Britt, S. S. March/April 1977. Fertility awareness: four methods of natural family planning. *J. Obstet. Gynecol. Neonatal Nurs.* 6:9.

Cantor, B. 1982. Induction of ovulation with clomiphene citrate. In *Gynecology and obstetrics*, vol. 5, ed. J. J. Sciarra et al. Hagerstown, Md.: Harper & Row.

Cheng, M. C. E., et al. 1974. Six monthly Depo-Provera injections as a contraceptive agent: its acceptability in Singapore. *Aust. NZ. J. Obstet. Gynecol.* 14:231.

Coulam, C. B. 1982. The diagnosis and management of infertility. In *Gynecology and obstetrics*, vol. 5, ed. J. J. Sciarra et al. Hagerstown, Md.: Harper & Row.

Danforth, D. N., ed. 1982. *Obstetrics and gynecology*, 4th ed. Philadelphia: Harper & Row.

Dondero, F., et al. 1979. Treatment and follow up of patients with infertility due to spermagglutinins. *Fertil. Steril.* 31:48.

Hatcher, R. A., et al. 1982a. Fertility awareness methods. In *Gynecology and obstetrics*, vol. 6, ed. J. J. Sciarra et al. Hagerstown, Md.: Harper & Row.

———. 1982b. *Contraceptive technology 1982-1983.* 11th ed. New York: Irvington Publishers, Inc.

Hymovich, D. P., and Barnard, M.U. 1973. The woman and her family in therapeutic abortion. In *Family health care.* New York: McGraw-Hill Book Co., p. 377.

Menning, B. E. 1980. The emotional needs of the infertile couple. *Fertil. Steril.* 34(4):313.

Pabst, R., et al. 1979. Is the low fertility rate after vasectomy caused by nerve resection during vasectomy? *Fertil. Steril.* 31(3):316.

Ross, G. T., et al. 1970. Pituitary and gonadal hormones in women during spontaneous and induced ovulatory cycles. *Recent Prog. Horm. Res.* 26:1.

Schwallie, P. C. 1974. Experience with Depo-Provera as an injectable contraceptive. *J. Reprod. Med.* 13:113.

Shane, J. M.; Schiff, I.; and Wilson, E. A. 1976. The infertile couple. *Clin. Symp.* 28(5): 2.

Siber, S. J., and Cohen, R. 1980. Microsurgical reversal of female sterilization: role of tubal length. *Fertil. Steril.* 33(6):598.

Tatum, H. J., and Connell-Tatum, E. B. July 1981. Barrier contraception. *Fertil. Steril.* 36(1):1.

Tietze, C. 1982. Induced abortion: epidemiological aspects. In *Gynecology and obstetrics.* vol. 6, ed. J. J. Sciarra et al. Hagerstown, Md.: Harper & Row.

World Health Organization (WHO). May 1977. Expanded programme of research development and research training in human reproduction: task force on long-acting systemic agents for the regulation of fertility. *Contraception.* 15:513.

———. 1978. Special programme of research, development and research training in human reproduction. *Seventh Annual Report*, p. 67.

Additional Readings

Ansari, A. H. 1979. Diagnostic procedures for assessment of tubal patency. *Fertil. Steril.* 31(5):469.

Billings, J. 1972. *Natural family planning, the ovulation method.* Collegeville, Minn.: Liturgical Press.

Blandau, R. J. 1980. In vitro fertilization and embryo transfer. *Fertil. Steril.* 33(1):3.

Boston Women's Health Book Collective. 1976. *Our bodies, ourselves.* New York: Simon & Schuster.

Collingh Bennink, H. J. T. 1979. Intermittent bromocriptine treatment for the induction of ovulation in hyperprolactinemic patients. *Fertil. Steril.* 31(3):267.

Dmowski, W. P. 1979. Endocrine properties and clinical application of danazol. *Fertil. Steril.* 31(3):237.

Gibbs, C. E.; Martin, H. W.; and Gutierrez, M. Jan. 1974. Patterns of reproductive health care among the poor of San Antonio, Texas. *Am. J. Public Health* 64:37.

Hilgers, T. W. 1980. Natural family planning II. Basal body temperature. *Obstet. Gynecol.* 55(3):333.

Huppert, L. C. 1979. Induction of ovulation with clomiphene citrate. *Fertil. Steril.* 31(1):1.

Jones, W. R. 1980. Immunologic infertility—fact or fiction? *Fertil. Steril.* 33(6):577.

McCusker, S. 1977. NFP and the marital relationship: The Catholic University of America Study. *Int. Rev. Natural Fam. Plann.* 1:331.

Robbie, M. O. July/Aug. 1978. Contraceptive counseling for the younger adolescent woman: a suggested solution to the problem. *J. Obstet. Gynecol. Neonatal Nurs.* 7(4):29.

Rutledge, A. L. March 1979. Psychomarital evaluation and treatment of the infertile couple. *Clin. Obstet. Gynecol.* 22:255.

Sabaugh, G. Jan. 1980. Fertility planning of Chicano couples in Los Angeles. *Am. J. Public Health.* 70:56.

Swanson, J. M. 1981. Birth planning in Cuba: a basic human right. *International J. Nurs. Studies.* 18:81.

Strickland, O. L. Jan. 1981. In vitro fertilization: dilemma or opportunity? *ANS* 3(2):41.

Taylor, C. 1978. Cultural aspects of human sexuality. In *Human sexuality for health professionals*, ed. M. U. Barnard; B. J. Clancey: and K. E. Krantz. Philadelphia: W. B. Saunders Co.

Wiehe, V. R. July/Aug. 1976. Psychological reaction to infertility: implications for nursing in resolving feelings of disappointment and inadequacy. *J. Obstet. Gynecol. Neonatal Nurs.* 5:28.

■ 7 ■

GENETIC COUNSELING

■ CHAPTER CONTENTS

CHROMOSOMES AND CHROMOSOMAL ABERRATIONS
- Autosome Abnormalities
- Sex Chromosome Abnormalities

PATTERNS OF INHERITANCE
- Autosomal Dominant Inheritance
- Autosomal Recessive Inheritance
- X-Linked Recessive Inheritance
- X-Linked Dominant Inheritance
- Polygenic Inheritance
- Nongenetic Conditions

PRENATAL DIAGNOSIS

POSTNATAL DIAGNOSIS

GENETIC COUNSELING: THE NURSE'S ROLE
- What Can Families Expect?
- Appropriate Referrals
- Alternatives to Increased Risks
- Prerequisites of Counseling
- Principles in Counseling

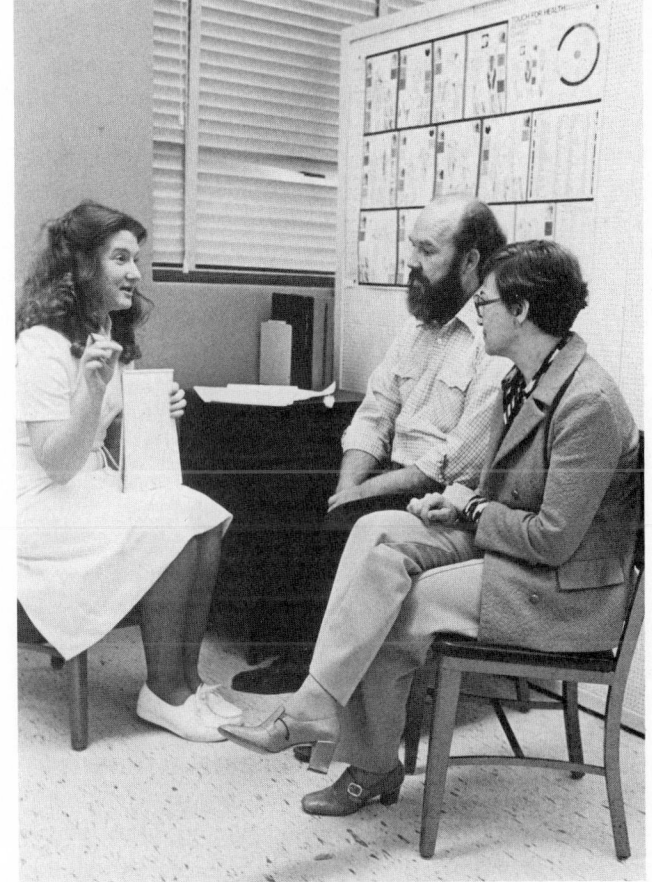

■ OBJECTIVES

- Identify indications for chromosomal analysis.

- Differentiate between Down syndrome caused by trisomy 21 and Down syndrome caused by a translocation.

- Discuss the significance of the Barr body in identifying sex chromosomal abnormalities.

- Identify general characteristics of an autosomal dominant disorder.

- Compare autosomal recessive disorders with X-linked (sex-linked) recessive disorders.

- Compare prenatal and postnatal diagnostic procedures that may be utilized to determine the presence of genetic disease.

- Explain the nurse's responsibility in genetic counseling.

- Discuss the use of a family pedigree as a screening tool in genetic counseling.

The desired and expected outcome of any pregnancy is the birth of a healthy, "perfect" baby. In most cases, when parents gaze at their new son or daughter, they can sigh with relief at the ending of a 9-month period that was filled with hope, concern, and joyful anticipation. Unfortunately, a small but significant number of parents experience grief, fear, and anger at this moment, when they discover that their baby has been born with a defect or a genetic disease. Such an abnormality may be evident at birth or may not appear for some time. The child may have inherited the same genetic disease that one of his parents has, creating more guilt and strife within the family. The child may be mentally retarded and require institutional care.

Regardless of the type or scope of the problem, parents will have many questions: "What did I do?" "What caused it?" "Will it happen again?" The professional nurse must anticipate the parents' questions and concerns and be able to guide, direct, and support the family. To do so, the nurse must have a firm basic knowledge of genetics and genetic counseling. Many congenital malformations and diseases are genetic or have a strong genetic component. Others are not genetic at all. The genetic counselor attempts to categorize the problem and answer the family's questions. Professional nurses can help expedite this process if they already have an understanding of the principles involved and are able to direct the family to the appropriate resources.

Is the magnitude of the problem great enough to warrant the nurse's time and effort? The problem of genetic disease can be likened to an iceberg—only the tip is immediately apparent. With the enormous strides and rapid increase in our understanding of heredity, more disease processes are now considered to be genetic, and their genetic components have been well—or reasonably well—established. Statistics indicate that:

1. Each couple has a 3%–5% risk of having a child with a major congenital abnormality.

2. Approximately 30%–50% of all spontaneous abortions are caused by gross chromosomal defects.

3. Approximately 0.5%–1.05% of all live newborns have a chromosomal abnormality.

4. Approximately one-third of all hospitalized pediatric patients have a genetic disease.

5. Of the 3% of the U.S. population who are mentally retarded, about four-fifths are believed to carry a genetic component.

6. There are over 2000 *known* inherited diseases (U.S. Department of Health, Education, and Welfare, 1976).

None of these statistics or estimations take into account the many diseases or conditions that have either been recently shown to have a genetic component or are strongly suspected to have one. Included among these are heart disease, cancer, and mental illness.

What of the cost of genetic disease? How do the costs of untreated genetic diseases compare with the costs of prevention and therapy? One can look at two well-known genetic problems—Down syndrome and phenylketonuria (PKU). It has been estimated that the lifetime cost of maintaining a severely retarded individual who needs institutionalization is $250,000. The incidence of Down syndrome is approximately 1 per 600 to 800 live births every year. If we take the mean, 1 per 700 live births, there are approximately 5000 children born with Down syndrome each year. Thus, per year, the lifetime committed expenditure for Down syndrome alone is approximately $1.25 billion.

However, with available technology, including prenatal diagnosis, it is possible to prevent the birth of a high proportion of such affected infants. It has been estimated that if fetuses of high-risk (older) pregnant women were screened in utero for Down syndrome, approximately 1000 cases per year might be prevented—a savings of about $250 million in lifetime care. To detect 1000 cases, approximately 96,000 pregnancies would have to be monitored. The cost of such monitoring is estimated to be between $15 million and $25 million, less than a tenth of the cost of lifetime care.

Even the screening of fairly rare diseases such as PKU (1 per 14,000 births) appears to benefit society. The test to screen a newborn for PKU costs about $1.25, or approximately $17,000 to detect each case. If an additional $8000–$16,000 is spent for dietary therapy, the cost of care to prevent severe mental retardation is approximately $33,000 per child. Compare this to the $365,000 it would cost to care for an untreated severely retarded child (50 years in an institution at $20 per day). The costs of detection and prevention are one-tenth that of lifetime care.

It would appear that the detection, treatment, and prevention of genetic disease does indeed save a great deal of money. What cannot be accurately estimated in dollars and cents is the emotional and psychologic savings to the afflicted individual and family when such genetic diseases are prevented or treated.

What is of most importance is that many genetic diseases can be either prevented or successfully treated to prevent irreversible damage. In some cases, to prevent the disease one must prevent the birth of an affected individual. This might be accomplished by a family deciding not to have any children, by using artificial insemination, or by prenatal diagnosis and elective termination of pregnancy. Some genetic diseases such as PKU and galactosemia are treatable with dietary modifications if detected early. Frequently, avoidance of substances that are toxic in certain genetic diseases is appropriate, such as the avoidance of copper in Wilson's disease.

Thus, even though more disease processes are being found to have a genetic basis, more methods of prevention and therapy are also being utilized. Nurses find it imperative to be well informed so they can help families reach their maximum level of wellness and productivity. This chapter examines the principles of genetic counseling and the scientific data on which those principles are based.

CHROMOSOMES AND CHROMOSOMAL ABERRATIONS

As will be discussed in detail in Chapter 8, all hereditary material is carried on tightly coiled strands of DNA known as chromosomes. The chromosomes carry the genes, the smallest unit of inheritance. Although human chromosomes were described as early as the 1870s, it was not until 1956 that the normal human chromosome constitution was identified. All somatic cells contain 46 chromosomes, which is the diploid number, while the sperm and

egg contain 23 chromosomes, or the haploid number. There are 23 pairs of homologous chromosomes (a matched pair of chromosomes, one inherited from each parent). Twenty-two pairs are known as autosomes (non-sex chromosomes), and one pair are the sex chromosomes, X and Y. A normal male, in standard notation, has a 46,XY chromosome constitution; the normal female is 46,XX (Figures 7–1 and 7–2).

The karyotype, or pictorial analysis of chromosomes, is usually performed on peripheral blood lymphocytes. These cells are stimulated to undergo mitosis and are arrested during metaphase. This preparation is stained, and the chromosomes can be seen (Figure 7–3). Although use of peripheral blood is an easy, convenient method for obtaining chromosomes, almost any tissue can be examined to get this information. Skin, bone marrow, and organ tis-

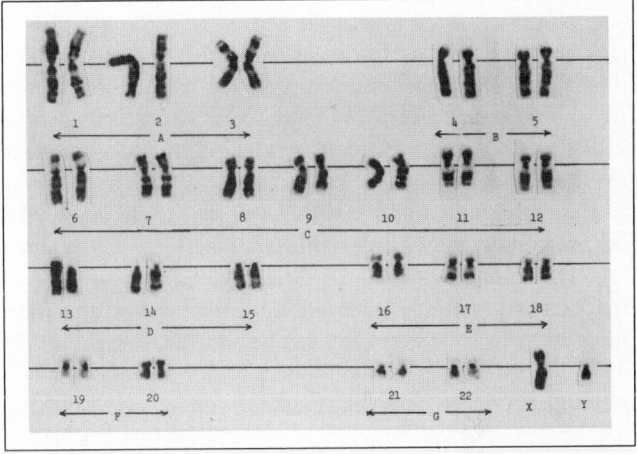

FIGURE 7–1 Normal male karyotype. (Courtesy Dr. Arthur Robinson, National Jewish Hospital and Research Center.)

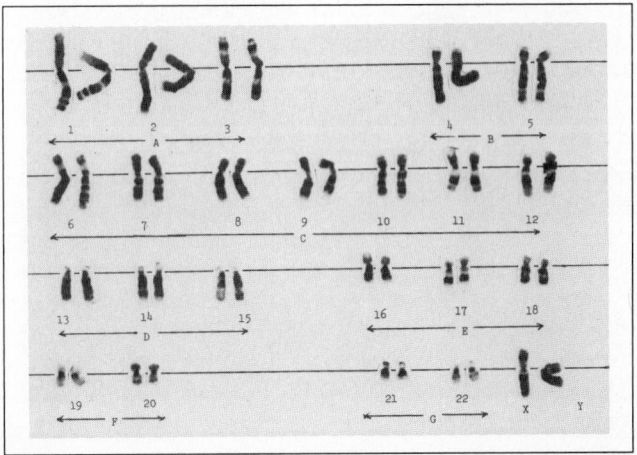

FIGURE 7–2 Normal female karyotype. (Courtesy Dr. Arthur Robinson, National Jewish Hospital and Research Center.)

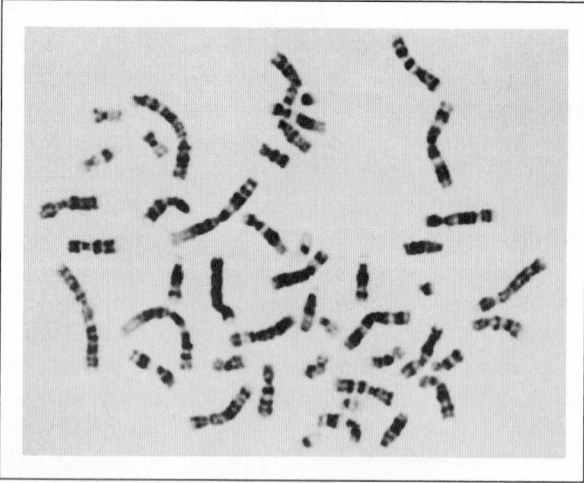

FIGURE 7-3 Chromosomes in metaphase spread. (Courtesy Dr. Arthur Robinson, National Jewish Hospital and Research Center.)

sue can be used. In the case of a stillbirth or perinatal death in which there are multiple congenital abnormalities and there is a question of diagnosis or cause, karyotypes of cells in the thymus can be examined if it has not been fixed in formalin.

Chromosome abnormalities can occur in either the autosomes or the sex chromosomes and can be divided into two categories: abnormalities of number and abnormalities of structure. With the advent of quinacrine mustard staining of chromosomes, begun by Caspersson in 1970, it has been possible to identify not only those cases in which an entire chromosome has been added or deleted

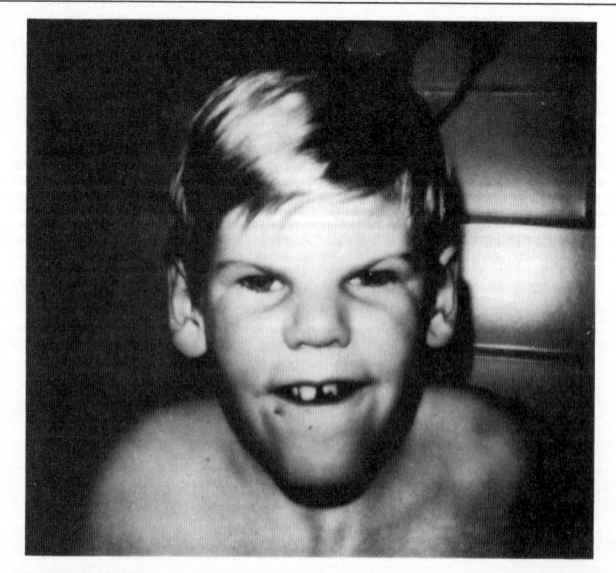

FIGURE 7-4 Ten-year-old boy who has a partial trisomy for the short arm of chromosome number 4; he is mentally retarded and has minor abnormalities.

but also those in which the addition or deletion of chromosomal material has been very small. Many children who received chromosomal analysis prior to this test were said to have normal chromosomes. But when examined with the new banding techniques, many were found to have additions or deletions of chromosomal material.

Even small aberrations in chromosomes can cause abnormalities, especially those associated with slow growth and development or with mental retardation. The child need not have obvious major malformations to be affected (Figure 7-4). In addition, some of these abnormalities can be passed on to other offspring. Thus, in some cases chromosomal analysis is appropriate even if clinical manifestations are mild. Whatever the case, too much or too little genetic material usually produces adverse effects on normal growth and development.

Indications for chromosomal analysis include:

- Chromosome syndrome suspected (or clients with a clinical diagnosis of Down syndrome)
- Mental retardation and congenital malformations
- Abnormal sexual development (primary amenorrhea, lack of secondary sex characteristics)
- Ambiguous genitals
- Multiple miscarriages
- Possible balanced translocation carrier

Autosome Abnormalities

ABNORMALITIES OF CHROMOSOME NUMBER

In 1959 Lejeune described the presence of an extra chromosome 21 in children with *Down syndrome,* also referred to as *mongolism.* The child with Down syndrome has a chromosome constitution of 47,XX(or XY),+21; referred to as *trisomy 21* (Figure 7-5). This is by far the most common trisomy (Turpin and Lejeune, 1969).

Abnormalities of chromosome number are most commonly seen as trisomies, monosomies, and as mosaicism. In all three cases, the abnormality is most often caused by *nondisjunction.* Nondisjunction occurs when paired chromosomes fail to separate during cell division. If nondisjunction occurs before fertilization in either the sperm or egg (meiotic nondisjunction), the resulting zygote will have an abnormal chromosome constitution in all cells (trisomy or monosomy). If nondisjunction occurs after fertilization (mitotic nondisjunction), the zygote will have cells with two or more different chromosome constitutions, evolving into two or more different cell lines (mosaicism).

Trisomies are the product of the union of a normal gamete (egg or sperm) with a gamete that contains an extra chromosome. The individual will have 47 chromosomes and is trisomic for whichever chromosome is extra. Down syndrome is an example of nondisjunction that produces a trisomy, specifically trisomy 21. *Monosomies* occur when a normal gamete unites with a gamete that is missing a chromosome. In this case, the individual will have only 45 chromosomes and is said to be monosomic. Monosomy of an entire chromosome is incompatible with life. The only exception is in the sex chromosomes. A female can survive with only one X chromosome; this condition is known as *Turner syndrome.*

As already noted, Down syndrome is the most common trisomy abnormality seen among children. The presence of the extra chromosome 21 produces distinct clinical features in the child (Figure 7–6). Those clinical features most commonly seen include:

CNS: Mental retardation
        Hypotonia at birth
Head: Flattened occiput
        Depressed nasal bridge
        Mongoloid slant of *eyes*
        Epicanthal folds
        White speckling of the iris
           (Brushfield's spots)
        Protrusion of the tongue
        High arched palate
        Low-set ears
        Broad, short neck
Hands: Short fingers
        Abnormalities of finger and foot dermal
           ridge patterns (dermatoglyphics)
        Transverse palmar crease (simian line)
Other: Congenital heart disease

Congenital heart disease is seen in approximately one-half of those affected. With the advent of antibiotics and improved techniques in heart surgery, children with Down syndrome are now living into adulthood. In fact, it is not uncommon for these individuals to survive into their fifth or sixth decade of life.

Trisomies can occur among other autosomes, the two most common being trisomy 18 and trisomy 13. Children with trisomy 18 have the following characteristics (Figure 7–7):

CNS: Mental retardation
        Severe hypertonia
Head: Prominent occiput
        Low-set ears
        Corneal opacities
        Ptosis (drooping of eyelids)
Hands: Third and fourth fingers overlapped by
           second and fifth fingers
        Abnormal dermatoglyphics
        Syndactyly (webbing of fingers)
Other: Congenital heart defects
        Renal abnormalities
        Single umbilical artery
        Gastrointestinal tract abnormalities

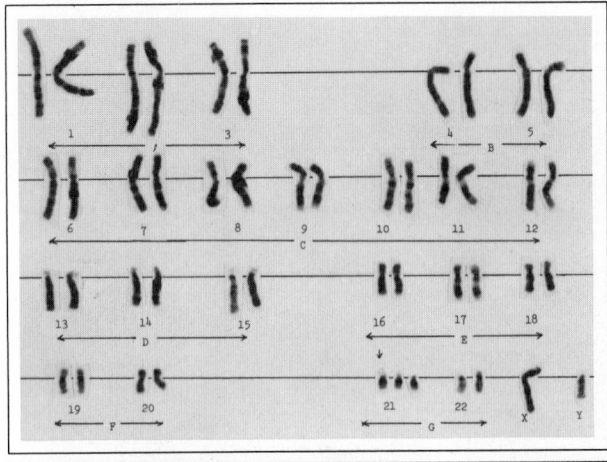

FIGURE 7–5 Karyotype of a male who has trisomy 21, Down syndrome: note extra 21 chromosome. (Courtesy Dr. Arthur Robinson, National Jewish Hospital and Research Center.)

        Rocker-bottom feet
        Cryptorchidism
        Various malformations of other organs

A child born with trisomy 13 usually exhibits the following clinical characteristics (Figure 7-8):

CNS: Mental retardation
        Severe hypertonia
        Seizures
Head: Microcephaly
        Microphthalmia and/or coloboma
        Malformed ears
        Aplasia of external auditory canal
        Micrognathia
        Cleft lip and palate

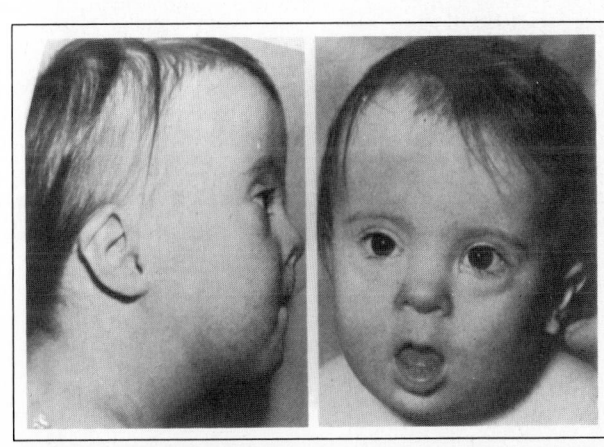

FIGURE 7–6 A child with Down syndrome. (From Smith, D. W. *Recognizable patterns of human malformations.* © 1982 by the W. B. Saunders Company, Philadelphia, Pa.)

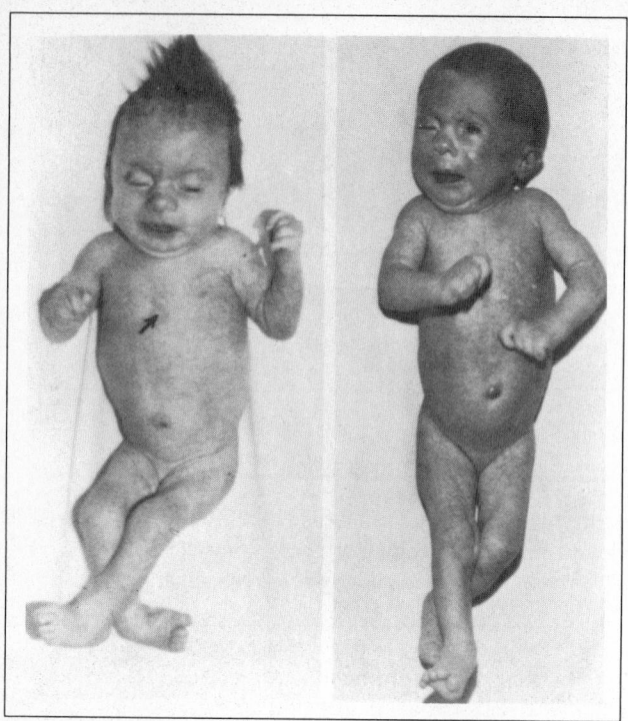

FIGURE 7–7 Infants with trisomy 18. In the child shown on the left an arrow denotes the lower end of the sternum. (From Smith, D. W. *Recognizable patterns of human malformations.* © 1982 by the W. B. Saunders Company, Philadelphia, Pa.)

Hands: Polydactyly (extra digits)
          Abnormal posturing of fingers
          Abnormal dermatoglyphics
Other: Congenital heart defects
          Hemangiomas
          Gastrointestinal tract defects
          Various malformations of other organs

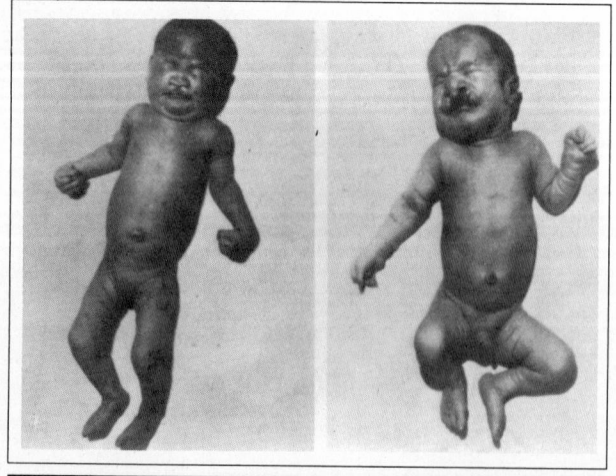

FIGURE 7–8 Infants with trisomy 13. (From Smith, D. W. *Recognizable patterns of human malformations.* © 1982 by the W. B. Saunders Company, Philadelphia, Pa.)

The prognosis for both trisomy 13 and 18 syndromes is extremely poor. Most children (70%) die within the first 3 months of life. A very few children with trisomy 18 have survived into childhood, although this is rare. The major cause of death is usually secondary complications related to cardiac and respiratory abnormalities. The incidence of trisomy 18 is about 1 per 3000 live births. Trisomy 13 occurs less frequently, about 1 per 5000 live births.

Mosaicism, the other common abnormality caused by nondisjunction, occurs after fertilization and results in an individual who has two different cell lines, each with a different chromosomal number. Mosaicism tends to be more common in the sex chromosomes, but when it does occur in the autosomes, it is most common for Down syndrome. Depending on when mitotic nondisjunction occurs after fertilization, different tissues may have different chromosome constitutions. Or the tissue may have a mixture of cells and the ratio of normal to abnormal cells may vary from one tissue to the next. For instance, in Down syndrome, one cell line may contain the normal 46 chromosomes while the other cell line contains 47 chromosomes, that is, an extra number 21. Or within a single tissue, some of the cells may be normal whereas others may contain the extra chromosome 21.

Clinical signs and symptoms may vary if mosaicism is present. In Down syndrome, the clinical signs may be classic, minimal, or nonapparent, depending on the number and location of the abnormal cells. An individual with many classic signs of Down syndrome but who has normal or near normal intelligence should be investigated for the possibility of mosaicism. More than one tissue may have to be examined to make the diagnosis. The peripheral blood may contain 46 chromosomes while the skin fibroblasts contain 47, +21. The frequency of mosaicism among children with Down syndrome is approximately 1%.

ABNORMALITIES OF CHROMOSOME STRUCTURE

Abnormalities of chromosome structure involving only parts of the chromosome generally occur in two forms: translocation and deletions and/or additions. Both types of structural abnormalities can produce distinct clinical signs and symptoms. Over 100 such abnormalities have been described in the literature. Again, Down syndrome is one of the most common syndromes described.

Not all children born with Down syndrome have trisomy 21. Instead, they may be the victims of an abnormal rearrangement of chromosomal material known as a *translocation*. Clinically, the two types of Down syndrome are indistinguishable. What is of major importance to the family is that the two different types have different risks of recurrence. The only way to distinguish the two is to do a chromosome analysis.

The translocation occurs when the carrier parent has 45 chromosomes, usually with one of the number 21 chromosomes fused to one of the number 14 chromosomes

(Figure 7–9). The parent has one normal 14, one normal 21, and one 14/21 chromosome. Since all the chromosomal material is present and functioning normally, the parent is clinically normal. This individual is known as a *balanced translocation carrier*. When this person mates with a person with a structurally normal chromosome constitution, there are several possible outcomes (Figure 7–10). The offspring can receive the carrier parent's normal number 21 and normal number 14 chromosomes in combination with the noncarrier parent's normal chromosomes 21 and 14. In this case the offspring is chromosomally normal. Or the child may receive one of the balanced translocations, thus becoming a carrier like the carrier parent—chromosomally abnormal but clinically normal. If, however, the offspring receives the carrier parent's normal number 21 chromosome and the 14/21 chromosome and the noncarrier parent's normal chromosomes, the offspring receives two functioning number 14 chromosomes and three functioning number 21 chromosomes (Figure 7–11). Although the offspring has at first glance 46 chromosomes, on careful analysis he is discovered to have an extra chromosome 21. Thus he has an *unbalanced translocation* and has Down syndrome.

In Down syndrome, if the mother is a carrier of a 14/21 balanced translocation, there is a 10%–15% risk of having an affected offspring. If the father carries the balanced translocation, there is a 2%–5% risk. Other types of translocations can occur. But regardless of the chromosome involved, any person having a balanced chromosome rearrangement (translocation) has the potential of having a

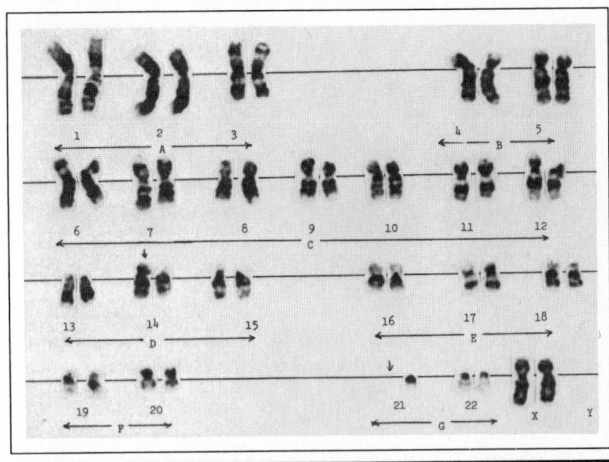

FIGURE 7–9 Karyotype of a female who is a balanced translocation carrier for chromosomes number 14 and 21: note chromosome 21 is translocated to chromosome 14. (Courtesy Dr. Arthur Robinson, National Jewish Hospital and Research Center.)

child with an unbalanced chromosome constitution. This usually means a substantial adverse effect on normal growth and development.

The other type of structural abnormality seen is caused by *additions and/or deletions* of chromosomal material. Any portion of a chromosome may be lost or added, generally leading to some adverse effect. Depending on how much chromosomal material is involved, the clinical effects may be mild or severe. Many types of additions and deletions have been described and new syndromes identified.

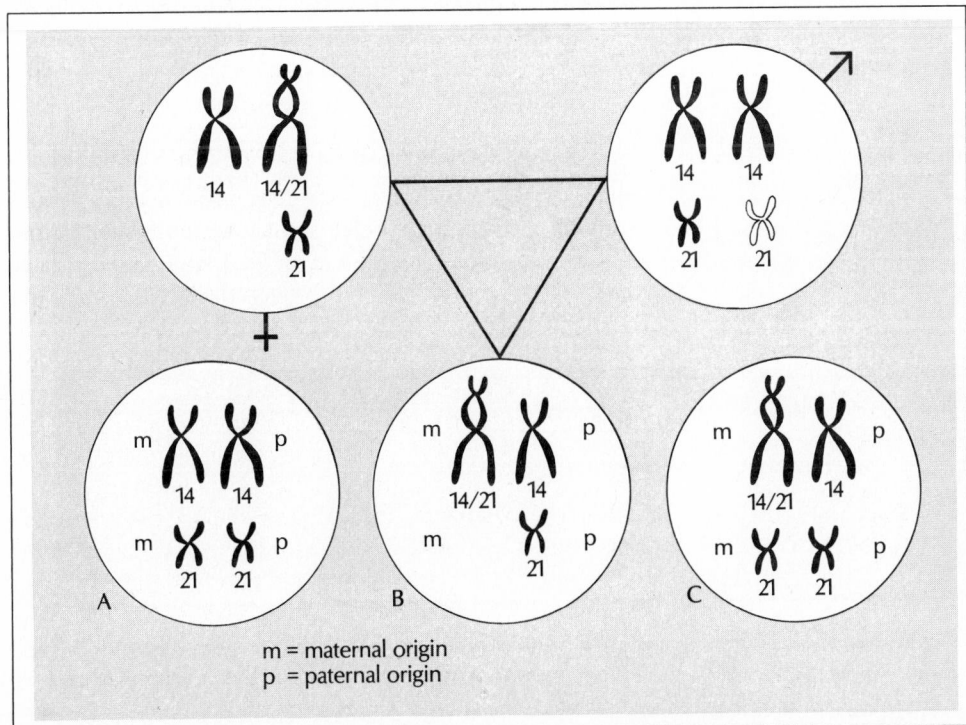

m = maternal origin
p = paternal origin

FIGURE 7–10 Diagram of various types of offspring when mother has a balanced translocation between chromosomes 14 and 21 and father has the normal arrangement of chromosomal material. **A,** Normal offspring. **B,** Balanced translocation carrier. **C,** Unbalanced translocation. Child has Down syndrome.

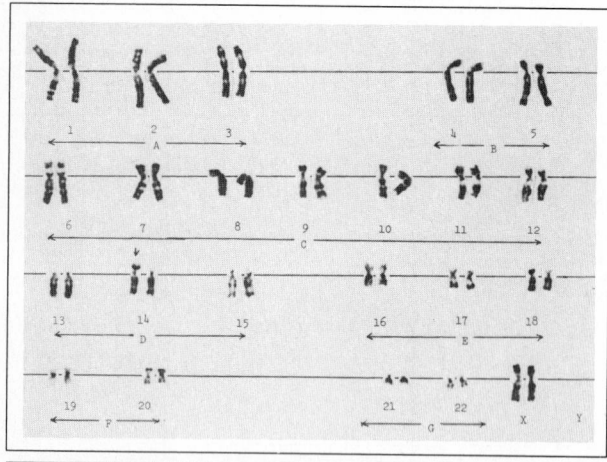

FIGURE 7–11 Karyotype of a female who has Down syndrome as a result of an unbalanced translocation: note extra chromosome 21 attached to chromosome 14. (Courtesy Dr. Arthur Robinson, National Jewish Hospital and Research Center.)

The cri du chat (cat cry) syndrome is associated with the deletion of one of the short arms of chromosome 5. Clinical features are severe mental retardation, a catlike cry in infancy, failure to thrive, microcephaly, hypertelorism, epicanthal folds, low-set ears, and various other organ malformations.

A deletion of the long arm of chromosome 18 usually results in severe psychomotor retardation, microcephaly, stenotic ear canals with conductive hearing loss, and various other organ malformations.

Sex Chromosome Abnormalities

To better understand normal X chromosome function and thus abnormalities of the sex chromosomes, the nurse should have a basic understanding of the *Lyon hypothesis.* This well-established principle states that in females, at an early embryonic stage, one of the two normal X chromosomes becomes inactive, that all descendants of that cell will have the same X chromosome inactivated, and that inactivation is random and independent in each cell (Lyon, 1962). Thus, on an average, 50% of X chromosomes of maternal origin and 50% of X chromosomes of paternal origin become inactivated. The inactive X chromosome forms a dark staining area known as the *Barr body,* or *sex chromatin body* (Figure 7–12).

The Barr body may be observed by examining the cells scraped from the inside of a client's mouth. This procedure, the *buccal smear,* will show the number of inactivated X chromosomes or Barr bodies present. The normal female has one Barr body, since one of her two X chromosomes has been inactivated. The normal male has no Barr bodies, since he has only one X chromosome to begin with. The number of Barr bodies seen on the buccal smear is always one less than the number of X chromosomes present in the client's cells.

This same technique may also be used to examine the Y chromosome. The cells are stained with a fluorescent stain, which under the fluorescent microscope shows the Y chromosome to be a bright body within the nucleus. The number of Y bodies present is equal to the number of Y chromosomes present. Males should have one Y body and females none (Figure 7–13).

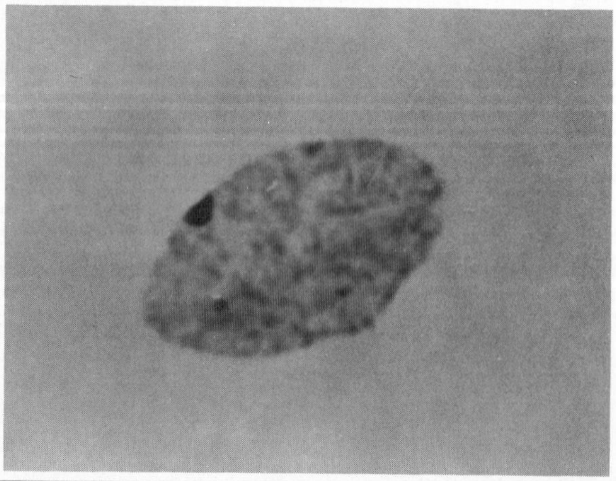

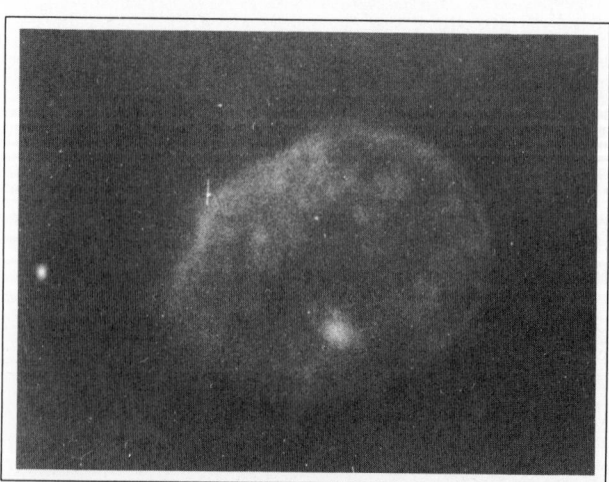

FIGURE 7–12 Nucleus with one Barr body; the patient is sex chromatin positive. (Courtesy Dr. Arthur Robinson, National Jewish Hospital and Research Center.)

FIGURE 7–13 Nucleus with a Y body present. (Courtesy Dr. Arthur Robinson, National Jewish Hospital and Research Center.)

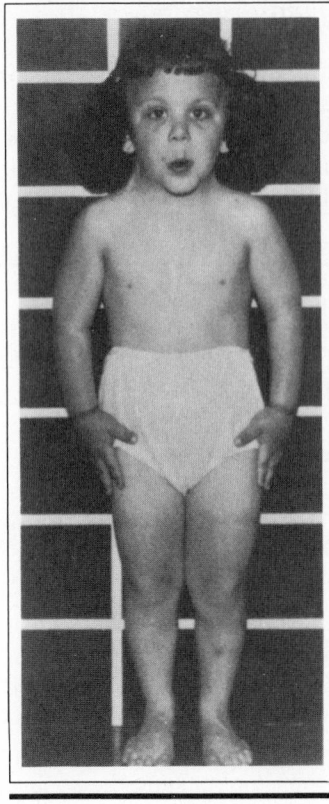

FIGURE 7-14 Girl with Turner syndrome: 45,X karyotype. (From Smith, D. W. *Recognizable patterns of human malformations.* © 1982 by the W. B. Saunders Company, Philadelphia, Pa.)

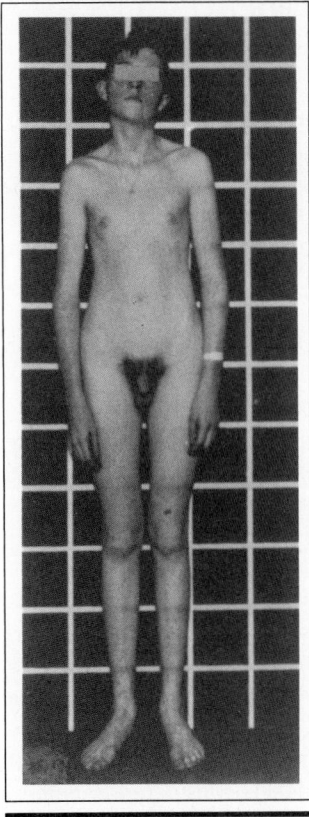

FIGURE 7-15 Boy with Klinefelter syndrome: 47,XXY karyotype. (From Smith, D. W. *Recognizable patterns of human malformations.* © 1982 by the W. B. Saunders Company, Philadelphia, Pa.)

The female with Turner syndrome (Figure 7–14), on chromosomal analysis, is found to have only 45 chromosomes, with one X chromosome missing. No Barr body is present, since she is sex chromatin negative. During the newborn period, clinical signs and symptoms of Turner syndrome are lymphedema of the dorsum of the hands and feet and excessive skin in the neck. Other features seen later in life are short stature, webbed neck, low hairline, cubitus valgus (increased carrying angle of arm), excessive nevi, broad shieldlike chest with widely spaced nipples, and underdeveloped secondary sex characteristics. The female external genitals and uterus are normal, but the ovaries are fibrous streaks. Primary amenorrhea is a striking symptom, and these individuals are usually infertile. There are often renal anomalies, and the most common cardiac malformation is coarctation of the aorta. The patient with Turner syndrome usually is not intellectually impaired, although she may have some perceptual difficulties. Turner syndrome has an incidence of about 1 per 3000 to 7000 live female births.

When a female's cells contain two Barr bodies, this condition is known as *triplo X.* She has a chromosome constitution consisting of 47,XXX. Few physical features are usually associated with this chromosomal abnormality, and recent studies have shown that intellectual impairment is inconsistent; that is, she may or may not be impaired

(Burns, 1976). The incidence of triplo X is approximately 1 per 1000 to 1200 live female births.

Klinefelter syndrome is one of the most common sex chromosome abnormalities among males (Figure 7–15). The male has a chromosome constitution of 47,XXY and is chromatin positive (one Barr body present). Clinical signs associated with Klinefelter syndrome include small, soft testes; eunuchoid body proportions; occasional gynecomastia (breast development); mild mental retardation; and underdeveloped secondary sex characteristics. These males are usually sterile. The incidence is approximately 1 per 1000 live male births. Approximately 1%–2% of institutionalized males have Klinefelter syndrome.

Another sex chromosome abnormality among males is 47,XYY. In the past it was believed that these males were always very tall, aggressive or criminally inclined, and mentally retarded. Recent studies have not borne out this notion (Lubs and Lubs, 1975). However, the occurrence of mental retardation and psychiatric problems may be increased with this syndrome. There are no characteristic clinical findings.

Other sex chromosome abnormalities may occur. Whether there is an increased number of X chromosomes or Y chromosomes or both, the affected individual generally has an increased number of abnormalities and increased severity of mental retardation.

PATTERNS OF INHERITANCE

Not all genetic disorders are caused by abnormalities of the chromosomes. Many inherited diseases are produced by an abnormality in a single gene or pair of genes. In such instances the chromosomes are grossly normal, but the defect is at the gene level and cannot be detected by present laboratory techniques. The pattern of inheritance for a particular disease or defect is determined by two methods: (a) a close examination of the family in which the disease appears and (b) a knowledge of how the disease has been previously inherited as reported in the literature.

There are two major categories of inheritance: mendelian, or *single-gene, inheritance,* and nonmendelian, or *polygenic, inheritance.* Each single-gene trait is determined by a pair of genes working in concert. These genes are responsible for the observable expression of the trait, referred to as the *phenotype.* The total genetic endowment or constitution is referred to as the *genotype.* One of the genes for a trait is inherited from one's mother; the other, from one's father. The gene pairs are located on homologous (paired) chromosomes, and the place that each gene occupies is known as its *locus.* An individual who has two identical genes at a given locus is considered to be *homozygous* for that trait. An individual is considered to be *heterozygous* for a particular trait when he or she has two different *alleles* (alternate forms of the same gene) at a given locus on a pair of homologous chromosomes.

The well-known modes of single-gene inheritance are autosomal dominant, autosomal recessive, and X-linked (sex-linked) recessive. There is also an X-linked dominant mode of inheritance that is less common.

Autosomal Dominant Inheritance

An individual is said to have an autosomal dominantly inherited disorder if the disease trait is heterozygous. That is, the abnormal gene overshadows the normal gene of the pair, and the individual is thus affected. Autosomal dominant disorders have several distinctive characteristics:

1. An affected individual generally has an affected parent. Thus, the family pedigree usually shows multiple generations having the disorder (Figure 7–16).

2. The affected individual has a 50% chance of passing on the abnormal gene to each of his or her offspring, regardless of the genes of the other parent (Figure 7–16).

3. Both males and females are equally affected, and a father can pass the abnormal gene on to his son. This is an important principle when distinguishing autosomal dominant disorders from X-linked disorders.

4. A mutation or a change of a normal gene into a dominant abnormal gene is possible. In this case, this is the first time the disorder is seen in the family; an affected child is born to parents who are unaffected. In such instances, there is not an increased risk for future children of the same parents to be affected. The child, however, now has a 50% chance of passing the abnormal gene on to each of his or her offspring.

5. An unaffected individual in most cases cannot transmit the disorder to his or her children.

6. Dominant disorders may be clinically milder, since many affected individuals are able to reproduce and pass on the abnormal gene to their offspring.

FIGURE 7–16 A, Autosomal dominant inheritance. One parent is affected. Statistically, 50% of offspring will be affected, regardless of sex. **B,** Autosomal dominant pedigree.

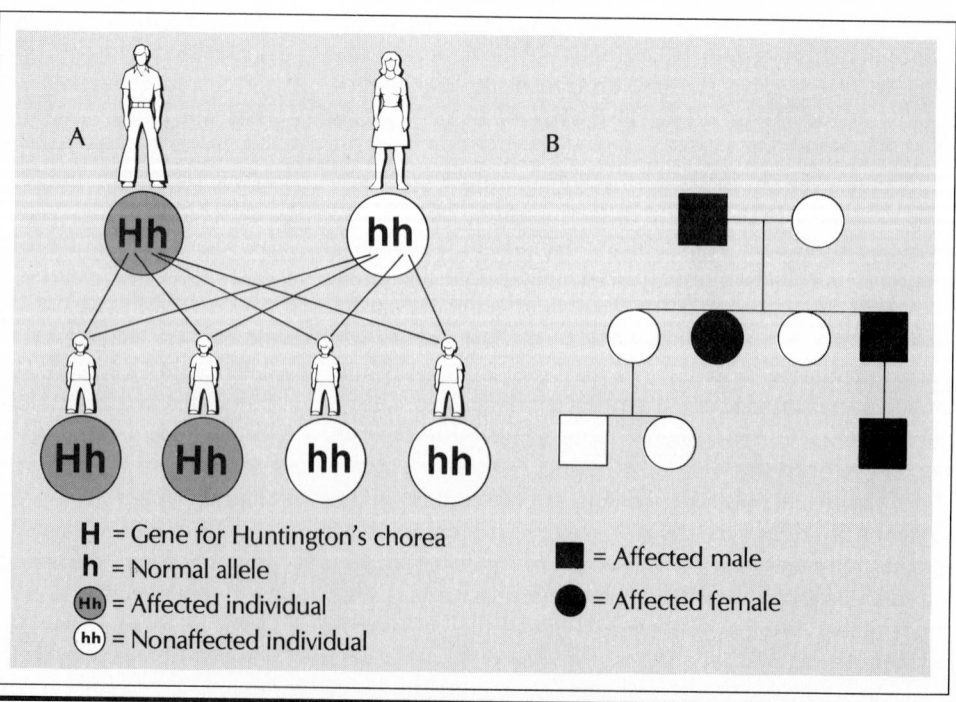

H = Gene for Huntington's chorea
h = Normal allele
Hh = Affected individual
hh = Nonaffected individual

= Affected male
= Affected female

7. Dominantly inherited disorders tend to have a variable pattern in their expression or observable characteristics. They may be more evident or more severe in one individual in the family than in others. This is an important factor when counseling families concerning autosomal dominant disorders. A parent may have a mild form of the disease, whereas his child may have a more severe form. Unfortunately, there is no method for predicting whether a child will be only mildly affected or more severely affected. The physician–geneticist must be thorough in the examination of family members to discern whether any of those individuals are indeed affected. They may express the disease in such a mild form that a cursory examination may miss clinical signs of the disease.

Some common autosomal dominantly inherited disorders are Huntington's chorea, polycystic kidney disease, neurofibromatosis (von Recklinghausen disease), and achondroplastic dwarfism.

Autosomal Recessive Inheritance

An individual has an autosomal recessively inherited disorder if the disease manifests itself only as a homozygous trait. That is, because the normal gene overshadows the abnormal one, the individual must have two abnormal genes to be affected. The notion of a *carrier state* is appropriate here. An individual who is heterozygous for the abnormal gene is clinically normal. It is not until two individuals mate and pass on the same abnormal gene that

affected offspring may appear. Characteristics of autosomal recessive disorders include:

1. An affected individual has clinically normal parents, but they are both carriers of the abnormal gene (Figure 7–17,A).
2. Parents who are both carriers for the same abnormal gene have a 25% chance of both passing the abnormal gene on to any of their offspring (Figure 7–17,A).
3. If the offspring of two carrier parents is clinically normal, there is a 50% chance that he or she is a carrier of the gene (Figure 7–17,A).
4. Both males and females are equally affected.
5. The family pedigree usually shows siblings affected in a horizontal fashion (Figure 7–17,B). Future generations are not affected unless both parents carry the same abnormal gene.
6. There is often an increased incidence of consanguineous matings. Parents who have a common ancestor are more likely to have the same genes in common than two parents who are unrelated.
7. Recessively inherited disorders tend to be more severe in their clinical manifestations. Clinically normal carrier parents pass on the disorder, and the affected offspring will often not reproduce. If an affected individual does reproduce, all the offspring will be carriers for that disorder.
8. For some autosomal recessively inherited disorders, the presence of the abnormal gene in a normal carrier parent can be detected. For instance, Tay-Sachs dis-

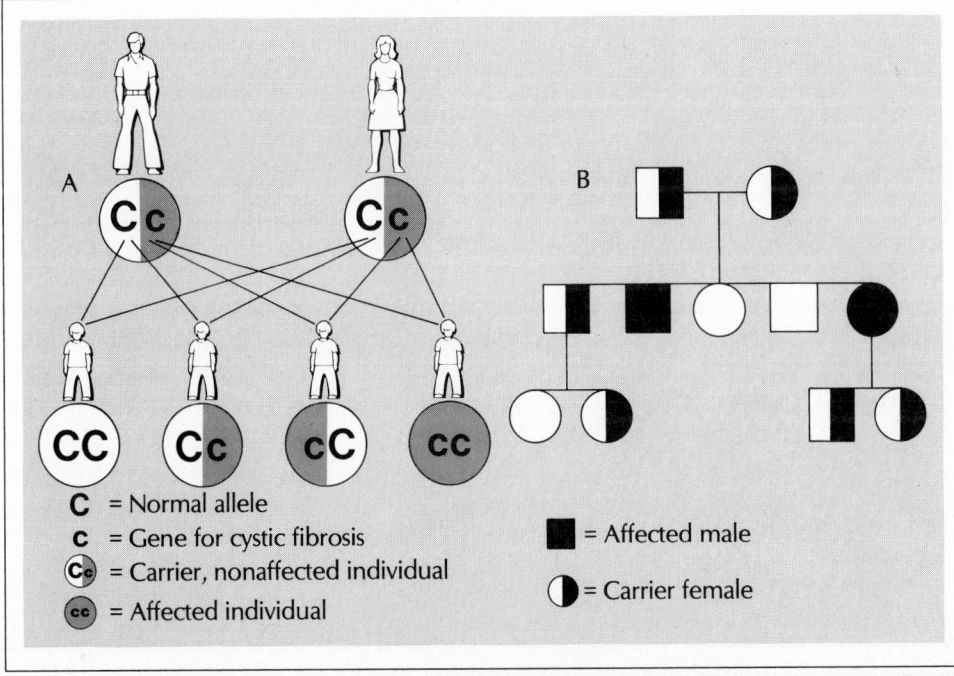

FIGURE 7–17 A, Autosomal recessive inheritance. Both parents are carriers. Statistically, 25% of offspring are affected, regardless of sex. B, Autosomal recessive pedigree.

ease is caused by an inborn error of metabolism—that is, a deficiency of the enzyme hexosaminidase A. An affected individual has little or no enzyme activity present, whereas a carrier parent usually has 50% normal enzyme activity present. Thus, biochemically the carrier is abnormal, and the heterozygous state can be detected, even though it is asymptomatic.

Some common autosomal recessive inherited disorders are cystic fibrosis, PKU, galactosemia, sickle cell anemia, Tay-Sachs disease, and most metabolic disorders.

X-Linked Recessive Inheritance

X-linked or sex-linked disorders are those for which the abnormal gene is carried on the X chromosome. A female may be heterozygous or homozygous for a trait carried on the X chromosome, since she has two X chromosomes. A male, however, has only one X chromosome, and there are some traits for which no comparable genes are located on the Y chromosome. The male in this case is considered to be *hemizygous,* having only one allele instead of a pair for a given trait or disorder. Thus an X-linked disorder is manifested in a male who carries the abnormal gene on his X chromosome. His mother is considered to be a carrier when the normal gene on one X chromosome overshadows the abnormal gene on the other X chromosome.

The major distinguishing feature of X-linked disorders is that there is *no* male-to-male transmission. Males pass only their Y chromosomes to their sons and only their X

chromosomes to their daughters. Thus a son always receives his X chromosome from his mother and his Y chromosome from his father. Daughters receive one of their mother's X chromosomes and their other X chromosome from their father.

Other characteristics seen in X-linked recessive disorders include the following:

1. The family pedigree is viewed in an oblique fashion (Figure 7–18). Affected males are related through the female line.

2. There is a 50% chance that a carrier mother will pass the abnormal gene on to each of her sons, who will thus be affected. There is a 50% chance that a carrier mother will pass the normal gene on to each of her sons, who will thus be unaffected. Finally, there is a 50% chance that a carrier mother will pass the abnormal gene on to each of her daughters; thus the daughters become carriers like their mother (Figure 7–18).

3. Fathers affected with an X-linked disorder cannot pass the disorder on to their sons. Conversely, *all* their daughters become carriers for the disorder.

4. Occasionally a female carrier may show some symptomatology of an X-linked disorder. This situation is probably due to random inactivation of the X chromosome carrying the normal allele (Lyon hypothesis). Thus, a heterozygous female may show some manifestation of an X-linked disorder.

Common X-linked recessive disorders are hemophilia, Duchenne muscular dystrophy, and color blindness.

FIGURE 7–18 A, X-linked recessive inheritance. Mother is carrier. Statistically, 50% of male offspring are affected and 50% of female offspring are carriers. **B,** X-linked pedigree.

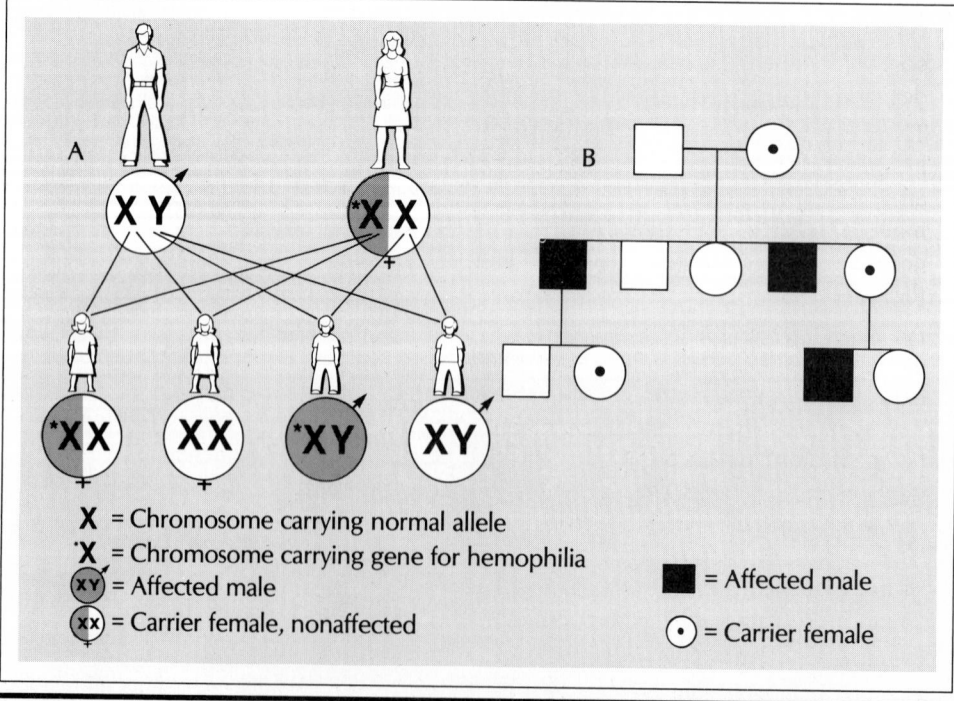

X = Chromosome carrying normal allele
˙X = Chromosome carrying gene for hemophilia
(XY) = Affected male
(XX) = Carrier female, nonaffected

■ = Affected male
⊙ = Carrier female

X-Linked Dominant Inheritance

X-linked dominant disorders are extremely rare, the most common being vitamin D–resistant rickets. When X-linked dominance does occur, the pattern is similar to X-linked recessive inheritance except that heterozygous females are affected. Since the abnormal gene is dominant, it overshadows the normal gene on the female's other X chromosome. Again, the major feature distinguishing this pattern from autosomal dominant inheritance is that there is no male-to-male transmission. An affected father will have affected daughters, but none of his sons will be affected.

Polygenic Inheritance

Many common congenital malformations, such as cleft palate, heart defects, spina bifida, dislocated hips, clubfoot, and pyloric stenosis, are not inherited in specific single-gene patterns but are caused by an interaction of many genes and an environmental influence on those genes. Instead of a single gene or a pair of genes being responsible for the manifestation of a disease or malformation, many genes appear to be coded to produce the defect. It is commonly hypothesized that each individual has a threshold above which such a defect will be manifested (Riccardi, 1977).

Several features are characteristic of polygenic inheritance:

1. The malformations are usually seen along a continuum from mild to severe. For example, spina bifida may range in severity from mild, as spina bifida occulta; to more severe, as a myelomeningocele; to its most severe state, anencephaly. It is believed that the more severe the defect, the more genes are present for that defect.

2. There is often a bias of sex. Clubfoot is more commonly seen in males, whereas cleft palate is more common among females. Thus, when a member of the less commonly affected sex manifests this type of condition, a greater number of genes must be present to manifest the defect.

3. An environmental influence (such as seasonal changes, altitude, irradiation, chemicals in the environment, or exposure to toxic substances) may be present. For example, suppose that it takes a certain number of genes to produce cleft lip and palate. If both parents pass on genes coded for cleft lip and palate and their offspring receives a particular number of genes above the threshold, he or she is affected. If, however, some environmental influence is present, it may take fewer genes to manifest the defect in the offspring.

4. In contrast to single-gene disorders, there is an additive effect in polygenic inheritance. The more first-degree relatives affected with a malformation, the greater the risk for the next pregnancy to also be affected (Table 7–1).

5. Risk figures are empirical. They are determined by the distribution of cases found in the general population as reported in the literature. In general, the risk of recurrence is usually 2%–5% for all first-degree relatives if one family member is affected; the recurrence figure continues to decrease with second-degree relatives and so forth.

Although most congenital malformations are polygenic traits, a careful family history should always be taken, since occasionally cleft lip and palate, certain congenital heart defects, and other malformations can be inherited as autosomal dominant or recessive traits. Other disorders thought to be within the polygenic inheritance group are diabetes, hypertension, some heart diseases, and mental illness.

Nongenetic Conditions

Not all disorders or congenital malformations are inherited or have an inherited component. Malformations present at birth may represent an environmental insult during pregnancy, such as exposure to a drug or an infectious agent (see Chapter 12). Some malformations are considered to be developmental in nature and represent an abnormality of embryonic development that is not explained by known or possible genetic mechanisms or by known teratogens (Riccardi, 1977). Thus, a couple who has a child with pho-

Table 7–1 Risk of Recurrence of Spina Bifida or Anencephaly*

Family history of spina bifida and/or anencephaly	Estimated recurrence risk (%)
One sibling affected	5
Parent and sibling affected	13
Two siblings affected	13
Three siblings affected	21
One sibling and 2nd-degree relative affected	9
One sibling and 3rd-degree relative affected	7
One sibling affected, no other family history	4

*From Smith, C. 1973. Implications of antenatal diagnosis. In *Antenatal diagnosis of genetic disease*, ed. A. Emery. Edinburgh: Churchill Livingstone, p. 137.

comelia (abnormality of the limbs), in the absence of any other problems or family history, may be reassured that the problem is developmental in etiology and the risk for future pregnancies is low. Such reassurance is also appropriate for families concerned about a child's seizures or developmental delays, which can be attributed to an acquired problem. If the child was hypoxic during a difficult labor and delivery or had spinal meningitis, the resulting developmental delays can be attributed to the postnatal insult and not to a genetic mechanism.

PRENATAL DIAGNOSIS

Prenatal diagnosis of genetic disease is one of the most exciting and significant advances in preventive medicine in recent years. The ability to diagnose certain genetic diseases by various diagnostic tools, such as amniocentesis, carries with it enormous implications for the practice of preventive health care. Since parent–child and family-planning counseling have become a major responsibility of professional nurses, it is imperative that nurses have the most current knowledge available concerning prenatal diagnosis.

Several methods are available for prenatal diagnosis, although some are still being used on an experimental basis. The use of *ultrasound*, a sonarlike procedure, involves directing sound waves over the abdomen. In areas of high density, such as bone, the sound waves are deflected and are picked up by the machine and projected on a screen. Information obtainable from the ultrasound includes the presence of a fetal head (from which fetal size and gestation can be approximated), localization of the placenta, the size of the uterus, the presence of twins, and structural abnormalities. As ultrasound technology has improved, the number of structural abnormalities being detected has greatly increased. Craniospinal defects (anencephaly, microcephaly, hydrocephalus), gastrointestinal malformations (omphalocele, gastroschisis), renal malformations (dysplasias or obstruction), and skeletal malformations are only some of the disorders that have been diagnosed in utero by ultrasound (Sabbagha et al., 1981). There has been no evidence of harmful effects to either mother or fetus from exposure to ultrasound.

X-ray examination at approximately 20 weeks of pregnancy can be used to determine gross limb or generalized bone abnormalities. An x-ray film on an oblique axis can be used to rule out such inherited disorders as metatropic

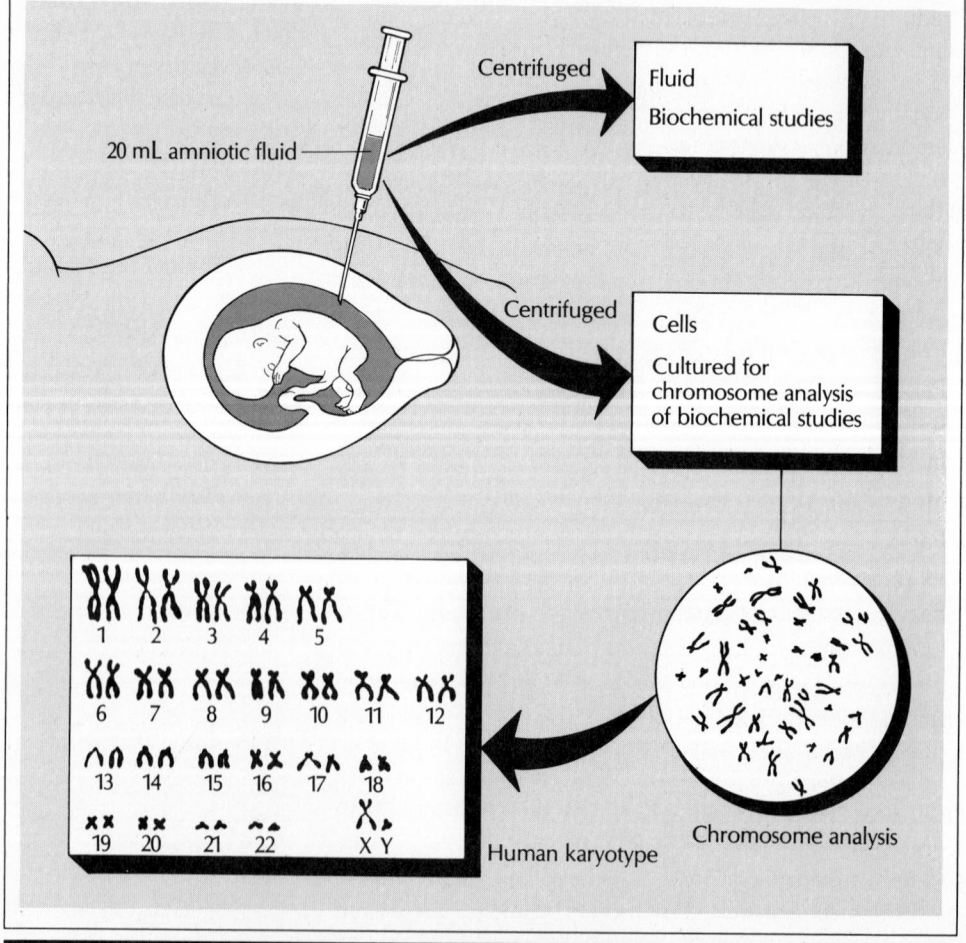

FIGURE 7–19 Genetic amniocentesis for prenatal diagnosis is done at about 14–16 weeks' gestation. (Modified from Richie, D. D., and Carola, R. 1979. *Biology.* Reading, Mass.: Addison-Wesley Publishing Co., p. 302.)

dwarfism and hypophosphatasia. Unfortunately, x radiation may produce unwarranted effects on the fetus. However, if the risk and burden of a genetic disease are higher than the risk of problems due to x-ray exposure, then the use of x-ray examination should be considered.

Amniography (the instillation of dye into the amniotic cavity to outline the fetus) and *amnioscopy* (direct visual presentation of the fetus by a scope) are two methods of prenatal diagnosis that are not yet available for generalized clinical use. These methods are used primarily to observe the fetus for major structural abnormalities or to obtain fetal blood and tissue. Because the risks of these methods have not yet been determined, they remain experimental tools. Researchers continue to look for alternate methods by which to make the diagnosis of some disorders.

The major diagnostic method for prenatal diagnosis is *genetic amniocentesis*. This procedure, available for general clinical use since the early 1970s, differs from amniocentesis done late in pregnancy for Rh incompatibility in that it is performed early in pregnancy to diagnose a variety of genetic disorders. The fourteenth to sixteenth week of pregnancy (based on last menstrual period) appears to be the optimal time for the procedure, based on uterine size, volume of fluid, and the number of viable cells present in the fluid. After ultrasound is performed to localize the placenta and to estimate gestational size, a 22-gauge spinal needle is inserted through the abdomen (the puncture point is anesthetized) into the uterus. Approximately 30 mL of amniotic fluid is removed. This fluid contains sloughed fetal skin and mucous-membrane cells, which can then be grown in culture or tested biochemically (Figure 7-19). The procedure is usually done on an outpatient basis, with no need for restriction of activities after the tap. (See Chapter 13 for an in-depth description of the procedure and specific nursing interventions.)

The indications for genetic amniocentesis include:

- Previous child with a chromosomal abnormality
- Parent carrying a chromosomal abnormality (balanced translocation)
- Increased maternal age (age 37 and over)
- Mother carrying an X-linked disease
- Parents carrying an inborn error of metabolism that can be diagnosed in utero
- Family history of neural tube defects (anencephaly or spina bifida)

Young couples who have had a child with trisomy 21 have approximately a 1%-2% risk of a future child having a chromosome abnormality. Although no statistics of recurrence risks for other chromosome abnormalities have been established, genetic amniocentesis is made available to any couple who has already had a child with a chromosome abnormality. In addition, any couple in which one of the partners is a carrier of a balanced translocation should be considered for prenatal diagnosis. Although the person

with the chromosome rearrangement is clinically normal, he or she has the potential for conceiving a child with an unbalanced chromosome constitution, which usually has substantial adverse effects on normal development. For example, a woman who carries a balanced 14/21 translocation has a risk of approximately 10%-15% that her offspring will be affected with the unbalanced translocation of Down syndrome; if the father is the carrier, there is a 2%-5% risk (Henry and Robinson, 1978).

One of the major indications for genetic amniocentesis is increased maternal age, since any woman age 37 or older is at greater risk for having children with chromosome abnormalities. This maternal age effect is most pronounced for trisomy 21. For women between 35 and 40 years of age, the risk for having children with Down syndrome is 1%-3%; between 40 and 45 years, the risk is 4%-12%; after 45 years, it is 12% or greater.

The occurrence of other autosomal trisomies (trisomy 13 and 18) also shows a correlation with increasing maternal age, although it is not as marked as in trisomy 21. The mechanism underlying the increased occurrence of nondisjunction (resulting in too many or too few chromosomes) is not known, but it is thought to be in some way related to the fact that women are born with their entire complement of eggs. The eggs are arrested in a stage of meiosis until ovulation and are subject to all the environmental factors that a given woman experiences.

In families in which the woman is a known or possible carrier of an X-linked disorder such as hemophilia or Duchenne muscular dystrophy, genetic amniocentesis may be an appropriate option for the family. These disorders are not routinely diagnosable in utero. However, because they usually affect only males, the sex of the fetus can be determined and termination of pregnancy considered when it is found to be male. For a known female carrier, the risk of an affected male fetus is 50%. The decision to abort a possibly normal male fetus must be discussed and made within each family. Similarly, couples in which the father is affected with an X-linked disorder may elect to have only male children so that the gene would not be continued in the family; all females (who would have to be carriers) could be aborted. Since many males with X-linked disorders, especially hemophilia, are surviving to reproduce as greater advances in medical treatment become available, genetic amniocentesis for these reasons may become more common.

Another fairly common indication for genetic amniocentesis occurs when both parents carry a gene for the same autosomal recessive disorder, which is usually one of the biochemical inborn errors of metabolism. Presently, over 70 inherited metabolic disorders have been diagnosed in utero.

Metabolic disorders detectable in utero include (partial list):

Argininosuccinicaciduria	Fabry disease
Cystinosis	Galactosemia

Gaucher disease   Metachromatic leukodystrophy
Homocystinuria   Methylmalonic aciduria
Hunter syndrome   Niemann-Pick disease
Hurler disease   Pompe disease
Krabbe disease   Sanfilippo syndrome
Lesch-Nyhan syndrome   Tay-Sachs disease
Maple syrup urine disease

When both parents are carriers of an autosomal recessive disease, there is a 25% risk for each pregnancy that the fetus will be affected. Diagnosis is made by testing the cultured amniotic fluid cells (either enzyme level, substrate level, or product level) or the fluid itself.

Most recently, genetic amniocentesis has been made available to those couples who have had a child with neural tube defects or who have a family history of these conditions, which include anencephaly, spina bifida, and myelomeningocele. Neural tube defects are usually polygenic traits. In cases in which the family history is otherwise negative, an empiric recurrence risk is approximately 5% for the couple with a previously affected child (Table 7-1). Regardless of the statistical risk for a given family, whether for an isolated neural tube defect or a disorder in which a neural tube defect is a constant feature, the risk of recurrence can be reduced (possibly by as much as 90%) through α-fetoprotein (AFP) determination of the amniotic fluid. Normally α-fetoprotein is a substance found in high levels in a developing fetus and in low levels in maternal serum and in amniotic fluid. In pregnancies in which the fetus has an open neural tube defect, α-fetoprotein leaks into the amniotic fluid and levels are elevated. Elevation of α-fetoprotein may also occur in cases of fetal distress, imminent or actual fetal death, and several other disorders. Thus, genetic amniocentesis allows those families for whom the risk of a neural tube defect is increased the opportunity to choose whether to have a child affected with such a high-burden disorder.

Great strides have been made in the field of prenatal diagnosis in the past few years. The greatest research to date has been in the diagnosis of hemoglobinopathies. Both sickle cell anemia and β-thalassemia have been diagnosed using fetal blood samples obtained by amnioscopy (Alter et al., 1976). Hemophilia A has also been diagnosed in fetal blood by measuring the ratio of factor VIII coagulant to factor VIII-related antigen (Firshein et al., 1979). Creatinine phosphokinase (CPK) activity in fetal blood for the diagnosis of Duchenne muscular dystrophy has been attempted a number of times. Unfortunately, because the analysis of CPK activity remains unreliable, it is not appropriate for the prenatal diagnosis of this disorder (Golbus et al., 1979).

Perhaps one of the most promising break-throughs is the prenatal diagnosis of cystic fibrosis. Walsh and Nadler (1980) have reported quantitative and qualitative differences in 4-methylumbelliferyl quanidinobenzoate (MUGB)-

reactive proteases in normal control and cystic fibrosis amniotic fluid samples. In five pregnancies that resulted in children with cystic fibrosis, amniotic fluids were significantly reduced in MUGB-reactive proteases when compared with over 1000 control fluids. If these findings continue to be confirmed, the prenatal diagnosis of cystic fibrosis may become a reality.

With the advent of diagnostic techniques such as amniocentesis, couples who would not otherwise have additional children because of the risk or burden can decide to conceive. The percentage of therapeutic abortions after amniocentesis is small; most couples find peace of mind throughout the remainder of the pregnancy after prenatal diagnosis.

Prenatal diagnosis offers an alternative to having children affected with certain genetic diseases. For many couples it is not an acceptable option, as the only method of preventing a genetic disease is preventing the birth of an affected child. This decision is an individual one to be made by the family. Most genetic centers do not require or even solicit an agreement or irrevocable decision regarding termination of pregnancy upon detection of an abnormal fetus. Genetic counselors do, however, discuss with the family all available options if an abnormal fetus is discovered or suspected.

Prenatal diagnosis cannot guarantee the birth of a normal child. It can only determine the presence or absence of specific disorders (within the limits of laboratory error). Nonspecific mental retardation, cleft lip and palate, and PKU are a few of the disorders that are not amenable to intrauterine diagnosis. A couple is at the same risk as the general population or at the risk calculated for their individual cases based on their family history for any other disorder. It becomes imperative, then, that preamniocentesis counseling precede any procedure for prenatal diagnosis. Many questions and points must be considered if the family is to reach a satisfactory decision.

In the future, if cure or treatment of diagnosable disorders is possible, prenatal diagnosis may allow for treatment to be initiated during the pregnancy, thus possibly preventing irreversible damage. For other disorders, effective postnatal treatment may make prenatal diagnosis unnecessary. The capability of diagnosis of many diseases in utero is realized every day. In light of the philosophy of preventive health care, this information should be made available to all couples who are expecting a child or who are contemplating pregnancy.

POSTNATAL DIAGNOSIS

Questions concerning genetic disorders, cause, treatment, prognosis, and so on are most often first discussed in the newborn nursery or in the first few months of life. When a child is born with anomalies, has a stormy neonatal period, or does not progress as expected, a genetic evaluation may well be warranted. To assist the primary health care provider in making an accurate diagnosis and directing appropriate care for the child, data from the following sources must be collected and evaluated: complete, detailed histories; thorough physical examination; laboratory analysis; consultation with other specialists; and a review of the literature.

History. As will be discussed in more detail later, a careful and detailed history should be obtained that includes a pedigree; conception, pregnancy and delivery history; and neonatal and developmental history. This may help to determine whether the problem is of prenatal (congenital) or postnatal onset, or whether the trait is familial, and/or may suggest a possible etiology.

Physical examination. The physical examination is paramount in helping to establish the diagnosis. The geneticist must attend to minute details and look for specific patterns of abnormalities. Two major questions should be kept in mind: Is just one organ system involved or are multiple systems involved? Does the abnormality have a prenatal or postnatal onset? If only a single malformation is present, such as cleft palate, or only one organ system is involved (the skin), the geneticist tends to think in terms of polygenic, single-gene disorders, or developmental etiologies. If multiple malformations are present, chromosomal and teratogenic etiologies are often the first causes to consider. Many chromosomal abnormalities and single-gene disorders have a specific pattern of malformations associated with them. Thus, the geneticist must have expertise in syn-

drome recognition to be able to arrive at an accurate diagnosis (Riccardi, 1977).

Another area that can be extremely helpful in delineating the etiology is *dermatoglyphic* analysis. Dermatoglyphics are the patterns of the ridged skin found on the fingers, palms, toes, and soles (Thompson and Thompson, 1980). Although each individual has a unique ridge pattern, specific types of patterns exist that can be systematically classified. Since differentiation of dermal ridges is complete by the end of the fourth month of gestation, many genetic disorders that affect multiple systems also affect the dermatoglyphics. Thus, a child with a chromosomal abnormality often exhibits certain characteristic dermatoglyphics.

Pattern combinations and frequencies considered together are more significant than pattern types alone. In Down syndrome or any other abnormality, any one of the particular specific patterns seen can also be found in normal individuals. It is when these patterns are in *combination* that they are associated with a specific disorder, such as Down syndrome.

The dermal patterns in Down syndrome are some of the more well-known abnormalities found. Children with Down syndrome often have a single flexion crease (simian line) on the palms, an increased number of ulnar loops on the fingertips (often on all ten fingers), and a characteristic pattern on the soles of the feet (the hallucal pattern), known as an arch tibial (Figure 7–20). Children with trisomy 13 are found to have an increase in the number of arch patterns on the fingertips and also single flexion creases of the palms (Thompson and Thompson, 1980). Chromo-

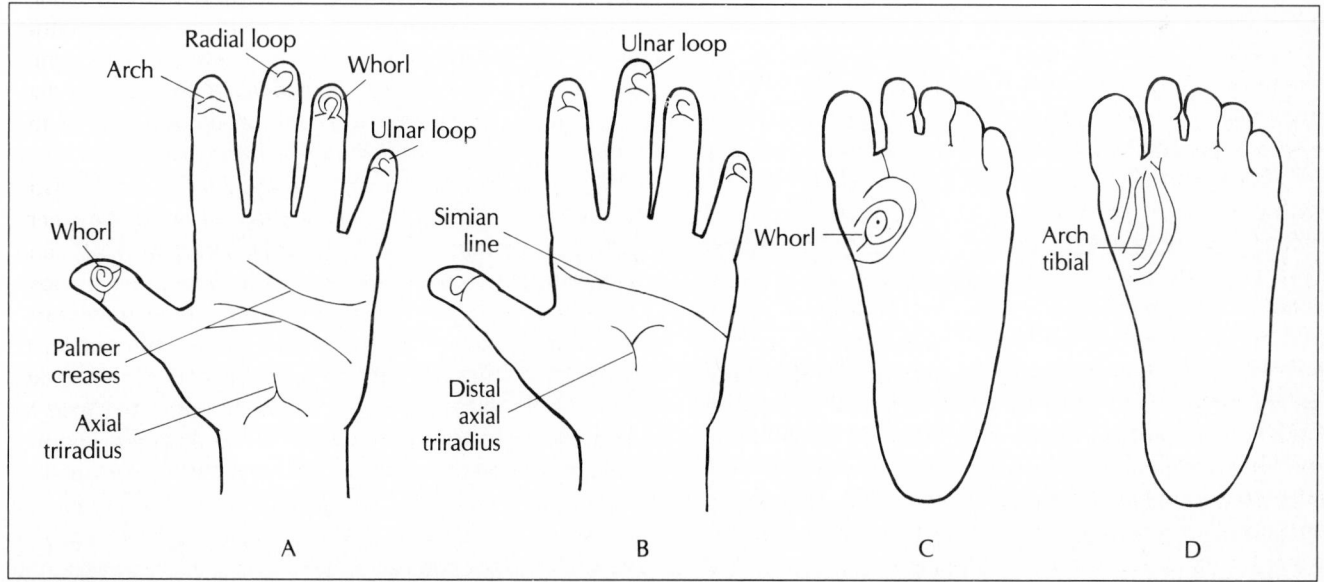

FIGURE 7–20 Dermatoglyphic patterns of the hands and feet in a normal individual (**A** and **C**) and those commonly found in a child with Down syndrome (**B** and **D**). Note the simian line, distally placed axial triradius, increased number of ulnar loops, and the arch tibial pattern on the hallucal area of the foot.

some abnormalities are only one area in which unusual dermatoglyphics have been described and can be associated with other single-gene or polygenic disorders.

Laboratory screening. Beyond the many laboratory analyses that are performed on ill newborns (blood counts, electrolytes, biopsies, x-ray films, and so on), laboratory tests are also directed specifically at establishing a genetic diagnosis. Laboratory screenings include chromosome analysis, enzyme assays, and antibody titers. As already discussed, there are a number of indications for initiating a *chromosome analysis.* It should always be considered in light of multiple malformations.

Enzyme assays for the diagnosis of inherited metabolic diseases usually follow if the result on newborn screening is abnormal or if the child has any combination of the following: nausea and vomiting, enlarged viscera, poor feeding, lethargy, and/or seizures. Metabolic abnormalities should also be considered in any child who does well during the neonatal period with normal developmental milestones, but then deteriorates, particularly in CNS functioning. The major assays done are of amino and organic acids. Other specific enzyme assays are performed only if the clinical picture warrants doing them. Thus, it is important to inform the biochemical geneticist of the child's clinical course so the appropriate tests may be carried out.

As mentioned, some newborns are identified to have a genetic disorder on newborn screening. Since the early 1960s, most states have passed legislation requiring the screening of all newborns for PKU. Many institutions now screen for five other inborn errors of metabolism: galactosemia, hypothyroidism, sickle cell anemia, maple syrup urine disease, and homocystinuria. These five tests use the same dried blood spot used in PKU screening. The major purpose of these screening programs is to identify affected newborns as soon as possible after birth so that medical treatment may be instituted *prior* to irreversible damage. (See Chapter 26 for further discussion of these conditions.)

Another area of laboratory analysis that may be appropriate are *serologic* and *microbiologic studies* to identify infectious teratogens, such as a serum TORCH screen. The TORCH screen tests the child's serum for antibodies against TOxoplasmosis, Rubella, Cytomegalovirus, and Herpesvirus type 2 (see Chapter 12).

With collection of all the data from histories, laboratory analyses, and physical examination, the geneticist may then consult colleagues and the current literature in evaluating all the available information before arriving at a diagnosis and plan of action.

GENETIC COUNSELING: THE NURSE'S ROLE

Genetic counseling is a communication process in which the genetic counselor tries to provide a family with the most complete and accurate information on the occurrence or the risk of recurrence of a genetic disease in that family. The goals inherent in this definition are threefold. First, genetic counseling allows families to make informed decisions about reproduction. Second, it assists families in assessing the available treatments, examining appropriate alternatives to decrease the risk, learning about the usual course and outcome of the genetic disease or abnormality, and dealing with other psychologic and social implications that often accompany such problems. Finally, it is hoped that genetic counseling will help decrease the incidence and impact of genetic disease.

What Can Families Expect?

The process of genetic counseling usually begins after the birth of a child diagnosed as having a congenital abnormality or genetic disease. After the parents have been referred to the genetics clinic, they are sent a form requesting information on the health status of various family members. This type of previsit information form is used in many genetic centers throughout the country. At this time the nurse can be helpful to the family and the genetic counselor by discussing the form with the family or clarifying the information needed to complete it. It may be beneficial for the parents to write or telephone relatives to gather additional data. Perhaps someone in the extended family will recall pertinent events, such as the birth of a related child with spina bifida. In addition, medical records are requested for family members who may be similarly afflicted.

At the initial genetic counseling visit, an extensive family history is taken in the form of a pedigree. The counselor gathers additional information about the affected child, pregnancy, growth and development, and the family's understanding of the problem. Generally, a physical examination is performed on the affected individual. Other family members may also be examined. If any laboratory tests, such as chromosomal analysis, metabolic studies, or viral titers, are indicated, they are performed at this time. The genetic counselor may then give the family some preliminary information based on the data in hand.

When all the data have been carefully examined and analyzed, including any laboratory results, the family returns for a follow-up visit. At this time the parents are given all the information available, including the medical facts, diagnosis, probable course of the disorder, and any available management; the inheritance pattern for this particular family and their risk of recurrence; and the options or alternatives for dealing with the risk of recurrence. The remainder of the counseling session is spent discussing the course of action that seems appropriate to the family in view of their risk and family goals.

The family may return a number of times to allow ample time for airing their questions and concerns. It is most desirable for the nurse working with the family to attend many or all of these counseling sessions. Since the nurse has already established a rapport with the family, the nurse can act as a liaison between the family and the genetic counselor. Hearing directly what the genetic counselor discusses with the family is useful in helping family members formulate their questions.

When the parents have completed the counseling sessions, a letter is sent to them and to their physician stating what was said during the sessions. This written document of the counseling session should be kept for the family to refer to as needed.

Appropriate Referrals

Genetic counseling is an appropriate course of action for any family wondering "Will it happen again?" Referrals to the genetic counseling clinic may be made by anyone interested in helping the family answer this question. Occasionally families contact the clinic independently; most often their physician refers them. Increasingly, however, it is the nurse who makes the referral. Nurses who are aware of families at an increased risk are in an ideal position to make the referral. The nursery nurse frequently has the first contact with the family of a child born with a congenital abnormality. The pediatric nurse, school nurse, or nurse practitioner often is the first to observe problems in growth and development or in perceptual and sensory functioning. The public health nurse has a rapport with the entire family and may be the only health professional with whom families are comfortable in relating their questions and concerns. The family nurse practitioner or family-planning nurse is in an excellent position to reach at-risk families *before* the birth of an abnormal child.

Which families, then, should the nurse refer for genetic counseling? The major categories of indications that aid in determining referrals are:

1. *Congenital abnormalities, including mental retardation.* Any couple who has had a child or a relative with a congenital malformation may be at an increased risk and should be so informed. Also, if mental retardation of unidentified cause has occurred in a family, they may be at an increased risk of recurrence. With the appropriate data, the genetic counselor will try to identify the risk.

   In many cases the genetic counselor will identify the cause of a malformation as a teratogen (see Chapter 12). The family should be aware of teratogenic substances or exposures so they can be avoided with the next pregnancy.

2. *Familial disorders.* Families should be told that certain diseases may have a genetic component and that the risk of their occurrence with a particular family may be higher than that for the general population. Such disorders as diabetes, heart disease, cancer, and mental illness fall into this category.

3. *Known inherited diseases.* Families may know that a disease is inherited but not know the mechanism or the specific risk for them. A couple may be affected or may have a relative or child who is affected with an inherited disease and may wish to know the specific risk for passing the disorder on to other offspring. An important point to remember is that family members who are not at risk for passing on a disorder should be as well informed as those family members who *do* have an increased risk.

4. *Metabolic disorders.* Any families at risk for having a child with a metabolic disorder or biochemical defect should be referred. Because most inborn errors of metabolism are autosomal recessively inherited, a family may not be identified as at risk until the birth of an affected child. The three most common metabolic disorders for which families can be screened are PKU, sickle cell anemia, and Tay-Sachs disease. Infants are screened for PKU at birth, and an affected child can be treated by diet. However, no carrier test is available to identify parents before the birth of a PKU child.

   Carriers of the sickle cell trait can be identified before pregnancy is begun, and the risk of having an affected child can be determined. Prenatal diagnosis of an affected fetus is available on an experimental basis only.

5. *Chromosomal abnormalities.* As discussed previously, any couple who has had a child with a chromosomal abnormality may be at an increased risk of having another child similarly affected. This group would include families in which there is concern for a possible translocation.

6. *Prenatal diagnosis.* Prenatal examination and diagnostic procedures can point out those families at risk, as discussed earlier in this chapter.

Alternatives to Increased Risks

During the genetic counseling session, an important area of discussion concentrates on availability of alternatives for a family with an increased risk. Based on the family history, the inheritance pattern of the disease, and the disease process, none, one, or several alternatives may be appropriate for the family to consider. Among those options that may be considered are adoption, artificial insemination, delayed childbearing, prenatal diagnosis, and early detection and treatment.

If the risk of occurrence is high within the family or if the burden of the disease is high, a couple may choose not to have any of their own children but to *adopt*. In this case, the disease would not be passed on; the couple would not have the agonizing burden of caring for a chronically handicapped child. Their needs as parents would be fulfilled, and a parentless child would have a loving family. Unfortunately healthy and young adoptive children are not as available today as they were in the past.

The family may consider *artificial insemination by donor* (AID), discussed in Chapter 6. This alternative is appropriate in several instances; for example, if the male partner is affected with an autosomal dominant disease, AID would decrease the risk of having an affected child to zero, since the child would not inherit any genes from the affected parent. If the man is affected with an X-linked disorder and does not wish to continue the gene in the family (all his daughters will be carriers), AID would be an alternative to terminating all pregnancies with a female fetus. If the man is a carrier for a balanced translocation and if termination of pregnancy is against family ethics, AID is the most appropriate alternative. AID is also appropriate if both parents are carriers of an autosomal recessive disease. AID lowers the risk to a very low level or to zero if a carrier test is available. Finally, AID may be appropriate if the family is at high risk for a polygenic disorder.

Couples who are young and at risk may decide to *delay* childbearing for a few years. Medical science and medical genetics are continually making break-throughs in early detection and treatment. These couples may find in a few years that prenatal diagnosis will be available or that a disease can be detected and treated early to prevent irreversible damage.

Prerequisites of Counseling

Taking the family history and constructing the pedigree are the fundamental steps that must be taken before initiating any counseling session. The overall goal of eliciting a history is to identify families for which the risk and burden is so high that they may wish to alter their reproduction plans based on this information.

Once a family has been identified as being at risk, the family history serves three additional purposes. First, even if a specific diagnosis cannot be made, the family history may indicate the mode of inheritance. If a family is afflicted with a neuromuscular degenerative disorder and the pedigree displays an autosomal dominant pattern of inheritance, a specific *recurrence* figure can be given to the family even if a specific name cannot be given to the disease.

Second, the history and pedigree allow the genetic counselor to identify other areas that should be of concern to the family. Take the example of a pregnant woman, 45 years of age, who comes for preamniocentesis counseling and learns that she is at risk for having a child with a neural tube defect. This additional information may help to prevent a tragic situation.

Finally, the pedigree and history allow the genetic counselor to identify other family members who might also be at risk for the same disorder. The family being counseled may wish to notify those relatives at risk so that they, too, can be given genetic counseling. When done correctly, the family history and pedigree become one of the most powerful and useful tools that the genetic counselor can use in determining a family risk.

The pedigree is a fairly easy and productive method for screening families. The nurse can obtain the necessary information and draw a screening pedigree in approximately 15 minutes. Information that should be obtained when drawing the family pedigree includes names (maiden names if appropriate) and birth dates of members of the immediate family; names and ages of the remainder of the family (including deceased members), with a description of their health status; causes of death of family members; and any other information the family feels is significant. In discussing the affected individual, the nurse should obtain information on the pregnancy history of the mother (including miscarriages), medications and drugs taken during pregnancy, x-ray exposure, infections or illness during pregnancy, the type of birth control used prior to pregnancy, and the method used to diagnose the pregnancy. A complete delivery history should be taken, including a description of any complications. It is also appropriate for the nurse to ask the family when the problem was evident to them or was diagnosed.

The nurse should inquire about the affected child's growth and development, including developmental milestones, growth in comparison to siblings or other children the same age, symptoms of a problem, school records, and any previous testing.

Finally, information concerning ethnic background, family origin, and/or religion should be elicited. Many genetic disorders are more common among certain ethnic groups or more commonly found in particular geographic areas. For example, the Ashkenazi Jewish population are at higher risk for being carriers of Tay-Sachs disease; the black population has a high incidence of sickle cell anemia; families from the British Isles are at higher risk of having children with neural tube defects; and there is a higher incidence of thalassemias in people of Mediterranean stock.

A screening pedigree generally includes the affected individual, siblings, parents, aunts and uncles, and grandparents (Figure 7–21). If the family does not have all the necessary information at hand, the nurse can urge them to obtain the information in time for their first genetic counseling session, when a more extensive pedigree will be taken.

Principles in Counseling

For genetic counseling to be an effective avenue of health care, geneticists and health professionals must adhere to certain principles to guide them in their clinical practice. Seven major principles govern genetic counseling: accurate diagnosis, nondirective counseling, confidentiality, truthfulness, timing, team approach, and follow-up counseling.

ACCURATE DIAGNOSIS

Before any information can be given to a family, an accurate diagnosis must be established. The ability to provide

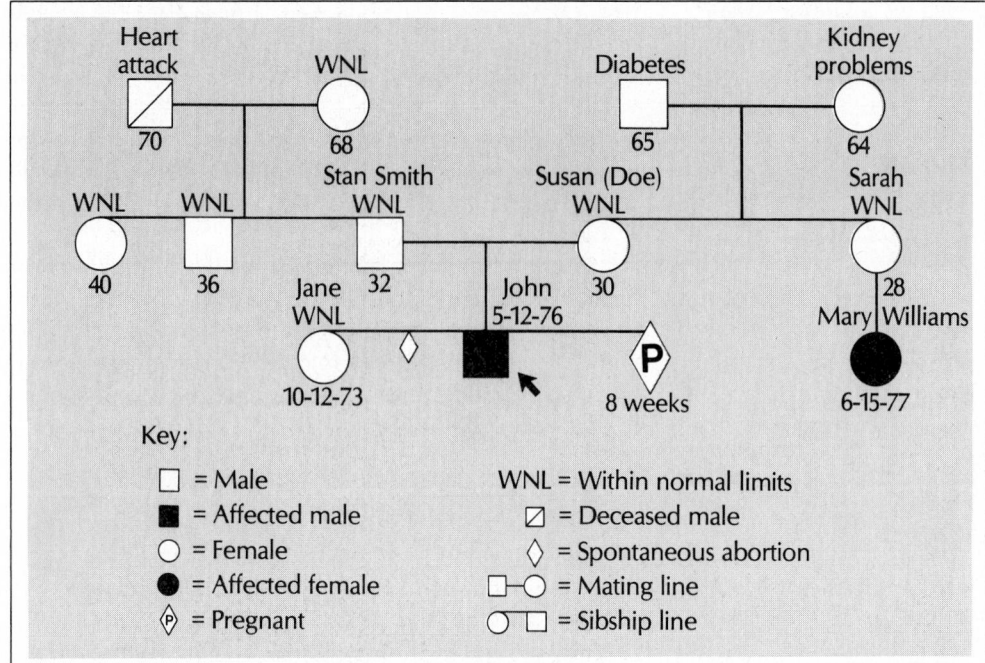

FIGURE 7-21 Screening pedigree. *Arrow* indicates the nearest family member affected with the disorder being investigated. Basic data have been recorded. Numbers refer to the ages of the family members.

information on the risk of recurrence, on the course of the disease process, on appropriate options, and on treatment modalities is based on an accurate diagnosis. Thus, special care and consideration must be given to establishing that diagnosis. When either confirming or establishing a diagnosis, the genetic counselor examines past medical records and the results of laboratory tests, requests photographs, reviews the literature, looks for minute details and subtleties on physical examination, and consults with colleagues. Only after the correct diagnosis has been confirmed or established does the genetic counseling process continue.

Unfortunately, a diagnosis is not always possible. Even more grave, the family may be given an inaccurate diagnosis. If data are insufficient—if there are no medical records or if the syndrome has not been described previously—the genetic counselor may not be able to proceed with specific facts and figures. Instead, the counselor must speak in terms of "if" and must be acutely aware of the dilemma being created for the family. Fortunately, this situation is not common and affects only a small percentage of families.

NONDIRECTIVE COUNSELING

Although it is impossible for the genetic counselor to be completely unbiased and unopinionated, he or she must strive to create a nonthreatening, noncoercive atmosphere in which families can make decisions for themselves. The counselor's role is to provide information and to assist and support families in their decisions, not to make the decision for them. What the counselor can and should provide to each couple is assistance in realizing what their personal priorities are and how their decisions may affect those priorities. Once they have decided on the course of action they wish to pursue, both the genetic counselor and the nurse should assist them as much as possible in accepting that decision and seeing it through.

CONFIDENTIALITY

As with any client–professional relationship, confidentiality and trust are paramount to genetic counseling. Families should be assured that information they provide about their relatives' health status will not be indiscriminately discussed or shared.

However, the issue of confidentiality is not clear cut. For example, what is the genetic counselor's moral obligation if an autosomal dominant disorder is diagnosed in a client and the client refuses to share this information with siblings, who are at 50% risk of being similarly affected? This situation is rare, and it is hoped that the geneticist can persuade the individual to share as much information with relatives as possible.

TRUTHFULNESS

Occasionally truthfulness in counseling becomes an issue. A counselor may be tempted to dilute or hide certain facts from a couple to protect them from undue anxiety or blame and guilt. While one does not have to dwell on all the "gruesome" facts concerning the disease process, the family does have a right to know what to expect. Similarly, the genetic counselor should discuss with the family members the problem of blaming someone in the family for passing on the disease and the ways the family can best deal with this problem.

On occasion, the genetic counselor may know of potentially damaging information, such as laboratory results that clearly dispute paternity. In this case, the counselor must weigh truthfulness against family solidarity and survival. To divulge the truth in this instance may not be appropriate.

TIMING

Timing is an important aspect of the counseling process. When should genetic counseling be initiated? Preferably, counseling should be *prospective*—before the birth of an affected child. Increasing numbers of young couples who are contemplating childbearing are seeking genetic counseling to discover their risk of having children with an abnormality or genetic disease. However, many genetic diseases do not present themselves until after an affected child is born. Genetic counseling in this case is *retrospective*.

In retrospective genetic counseling, time is a crucial factor. One cannot expect a family who has just learned that a child has a birth defect or has Down syndrome to assimilate any information concerning future risks. However, the couple should never be "put off" from counseling for too long a period, only to find that they have borne another affected child. Here the nurse can be instrumental in directing the parents into counseling at the appropriate time. At the birth of an affected child, the nurse can inform the parents that genetic counseling is available before they attempt having another child. Often, asking one or two members of a genetics team to introduce themselves to the family is enough to bring up the subject of genetic counseling. When the parents have begun to recover from the initial shock of bearing a child with an abnormality or when they begin to contemplate having more children, the nurse can persuade the couple to seek counseling.

TEAM APPROACH

Because genetic counseling is a complex and multidimensional process, it cannot be done efficiently or effectively in isolation. The genetics team consists of health professionals and scientists from a variety of backgrounds and exper-

tise. The genetics unit itself usually includes a medical geneticist, a genetic associate, and/or a nurse-geneticist. Often a social worker is directly involved. This group works closely with cytogeneticists, biochemists, and other specialty groups to clarify the situation for families. Many genetics groups also work closely with clergy and family support groups to provide the family with additional resources.

The genetics team continually makes efforts to inform and assist the primary health care provider before, during, and after counseling. Ideally, the primary physician or nurse clinician will feel free to consult the genetics team as a resource group for information, assistance, and support in the care of their clients.

FOLLOW-UP COUNSELING

Perhaps one of the most important and crucial aspects of genetic counseling in which the nurse is involved is follow-up counseling. The nurse who has the appropriate knowledge in genetics is in an ideal position to help families review what has been discussed during the counseling sessions and to answer any additional questions they might have. As the family returns to the daily aspects of living, the nurse's extensive background in family dynamics will enable the nurse to assist the family in making adjustments to living with and caring for a child with a handicap. The nurse can provide helpful information on the day-to-day aspects of caring for the child, answer questions as they arise, support parents in their decisions, and act as a resource for the family to other health and community agencies.

If the couple is considering having more children or if siblings want information concerning their affected brother or sister, the nurse should recommend that the family return for another follow-up visit with the genetic counselor. At this time, appropriate options can again be defined and discussed, and any new information available can be given to the family. Many genetic centers have found the public health nurse to be the ideal health professional to provide such follow-up care.

SUMMARY

Throughout the genetic counseling process, the nurse serves as the vital link between the genetic counseling team and those families at risk. With a full knowledge base and resource information, the nurse can be involved in case finding, referral, and preparation of the family for counseling. Nurses act as a liaison during counseling sessions and as resource persons after counseling sessions have been completed. Thus, it has become imperative that professional nurses have a sound background in the principles of genetics and genetic counseling to provide families

with the benefits of this rewarding aspect of preventive health care.

Resource Groups

March of Dimes Birth Defects Foundation, 1275 Mamaroneck Avenue, White Plains, NY 10605

National Genetics Foundation, 9 West 57th Street, New York, NY 10019

National Self-Help Clearinghouse, 184 5th Avenue, New York, NY 10010

Cystic Fibrosis Foundation, 3379 Peachtree Road, N.E., Atlanta, GA 30326

Down's Syndrome Congress, P.O. Box 1527, Brownwood, TX 76801

National Association of Sickle Cell Disease, Inc., 945 South Western Avenue, Los Angeles, CA 90006

In addition, there are support groups for most disease conditions. Information about them often may be obtained from the family physician. The National Self-Help Clearinghouse will generally be able to refer people to an appropriate support group.

References

Alter, B. P.; Modell, C. D.; Fairweather, D., et al. 1976. Prenatal diagnosis of hemoglobinopathies. *N. Engl. J. Med.* 295:1437.

Burns, G. 1976. *The science of genetics: an introduction to heredity.* 2nd ed. New York: The Macmillan Co.

Firshein, S. I.; Joyer, L. W.; Lazarchick, J., et al. 1979. Prenatal diagnosis of classic hemophilia. *N. Engl. J. Med.* 300:937.

Golbus, M. S.; Stephens, J. D.; Mahoney, M. J., et al. 1979. Failure of fetal creatine phosphokinase as a diagnostic indicator of Duchenne muscular dystrophy. *N. Engl. J. Med.* 300:860.

Henry, G. P., and Robinson, A. 1978. Prenatal genetic diagnosis. *Clin. Obstet. Gynecol.* 21:329.

Lubs, H. A., and Lubs, M. L. 1975. Genetic disorders. In *Medical complications during pregnancy,* ed. G. N. Burrow and T. S. Ferris. Philadelphia: W. B. Saunders Co.

Lyon, M. F. 1962. Sex chromatin and gene action in mammalian X-chromosome. *Am. J. Hum. Genet.* 14:135.

Riccardi, V. M. 1977. *The genetic approach to human disease.* New York: Oxford University Press.

Sabbagha, R.; Tamura, R. K.; Dal Compo, S. 1981. Antenatal ultrasonic diagnosis of genetic defects: present status. *Clin. Obstet. Gynecol.* 24:1103.

Thompson, J. S., and Thompson, M. W. 1980. *Genetics in medicine.* 3rd ed. Philadelphia: W. B. Saunders Co.

Turpin, R., and Lejeune, J. 1969. *Human afflictions and chromosomal aberrations.* (English translation of *Les chromosomes humaines,* 1965.) Elmsford, N.Y.: Pergamon Press, Inc.

U.S. Department of Health, Education, and Welfare. 1976. *What are the facts about genetic disease?* Publication No. (NIH) 76–370. Washington, D.C.: U.S. Government Printing Office.

Walsh, M. M. J., and Nadler, H. L. 1980. Methylumbelliferyl quanidinobenzoate-reactive proteases in human amniotic fluid: promising marker for the intrauterine detection in cystic fibrosis. *Am. J. Obstet. Gynecol.* 137:978.

Additional Readings

Ampola, M. G. 1982. *Metabolic diseases in pediatric practice.* Boston: Little, Brown & Co.

Carter, C. O. 1973. Multifactorial genetic disease. In *Medical Genetics,* ed. V. McKusick and R. Claiborne. New York: H. P. Publishing Co., Inc.

Erbe, R. W. 1976. Current concepts in genetics. *N. Engl. J. Med.* 294:381.

Jacobs, P., et al. 1974. A cytogenetic survey of 11,680 newborn infants. *Ann. Hum. Genet.* 37:359.

Leonard, M., et al. 1974. Early development of children with abnormalities of the sex chromosomes: a prospective study. *Pediatrics.* 54:208.

McKusick, V. A. 1982. *Mendelian inheritance in man.* 6th ed. Baltimore: Johns Hopkins University Press.

Milunsky, A., ed. 1975. *The prevention of genetic disease and mental retardation.* Philadelphia: W. B. Saunders Co.

———. 1979. *Genetic disorders and the fetus.* New York: Plenum Press.

Milunsky, A., and Atkins, L. 1974. Prenatal diagnosis of genetic disorders. *JAMA* 230:232.

Smith, D. W. 1982. *Recognizable patterns of human malformations.* 3rd ed. Philadelphia: W. B. Saunders Co.

Stanbury, J. et al. 1982. *The metabolic basis of inherited disease.* 5th ed. New York: McGraw-Hill Book Co.

Whaley, L. 1974. *Understanding inherited disorders.* St. Louis: The C.V. Mosby Co.

■ 8 ■

CONCEPTION AND FETAL DEVELOPMENT

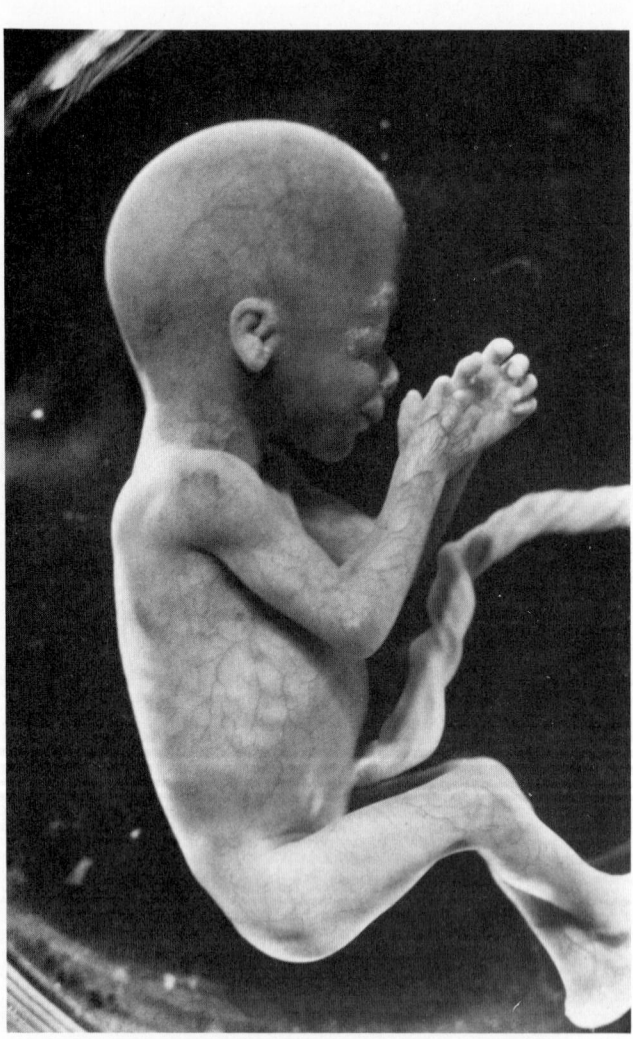

■ CHAPTER CONTENTS

OVERVIEW OF GENETIC PROCESSES
- Chromosomes and Genes
- Cellular Division
- Maturation of Gametes
- Sex Determination

FERTILIZATION

CELLULAR MULTIPLICATION

IMPLANTATION

CELLULAR DIFFERENTIATION

INTRAUTERINE ORGAN SYSTEMS
- Placenta
- Fetal Circulation
- Fetal Heart

EMBRYO AND FETAL DEVELOPMENT AND ORGAN FORMATION
- Preembryonic Stage
- Embryonic Stage
- Fetal Stage
- Factors Influencing Embryonic and Fetal Development

TWINS

■ OBJECTIVES

- Discuss meiotic cellular division and how it differs from mitotic cellular division.

- Describe the structure and functions of the umbilical cord and placenta during intrauterine life.

- Identify the significant changes in growth and development of the fetus in utero at 4, 8, 12, 16, 20, 24, 36, and 40 weeks' gestation.

- Identify the vulnerable periods in which malformations of various organ systems may occur and describe the resulting congenital malformations.

OVERVIEW OF GENETIC PROCESSES

Each person is unique. At the basis of this uniqueness are the physiologic mechanisms of heredity, which are reflected in the structure and function of cells and organ systems as determined by chromosomes and genes and the processes of cellular division.

Chromosomes and Genes

The somatic cells of each individual contain within their nuclei threadlike bodies known as *chromosomes,* which are composed of strands of deoxyribonucleic acid (DNA) and protein. *Genes* are regions in the DNA strands that contain coded information used to determine the unique characteristics of the individual; they are arranged in linear order on the chromosomes.

As the storage place for genetic information, DNA does not leave the cell nucleus. The DNA strand splits apart and forms the basis for a ribonucleic acid (RNA) molecule. The RNA passes out of the nucleus and carries coded information to the cytoplasm of the cell. A single error in the "reading" of the code can cause a change that may have serious effects on the functioning of the organism. For example, the alteration of one amino acid in the hemoglobin molecule produces abnormal hemoglobin, causing a disorder called sickle cell anemia. This type of genetic error is referred to as a *gene mutation.* Gene mutations can be induced by exposing cells to certain chemicals or to certain kinds of radiation.

Each chromosome contains two longitudinal halves called *chromatids,* which are joined together at a point called the *centromere.* Each animal species tends to have a constant number of chromosomes. Human beings have 46 chromosomes divided into 23 pairs: 22 pairs of autosomes and one pair of sex chromosomes. Each member of a pair carries either similar genes referred to as *homologous,* or dissimilar, allelic, genes referred to as *heterozygous* (Figure 8–1,*A*).

The chromosomes are classified according to their length and to the position of their centromere (Figure 8–1,*B*). When the centromere is centrally located, the longitudinal halves are divided into arms of approximately equal length, and the chromosome resembles an X. Such a chromosome is termed *metacentric.* If the centromere is located nearer one end of the chromosome than the other, the arms are of unequal length, and the chromosome resembles a Y. This configuration is termed *submetacentric.* A third type of chromosome (*acrocentric*) has a terminally located centromere at the distal end, where a second constriction occurs, referred to as a *satellite* (Figure 8–1,*B*). Satellites are often found in relation to abnormalities and can be induced by exposure to certain chemicals (Whaley, 1974).

Cellular Division

Although humans are multicellular animals, they begin life as a single cell. This cell reproduces itself, each of the new cells also reproduces, and so the process continues. The new cells must be basically similar to the cells from which they came.

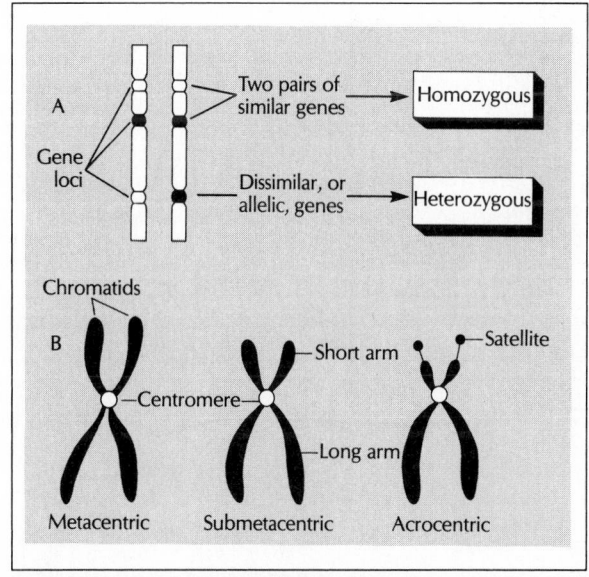

FIGURE 8–1 A, Pair of chromosomes with similar (homozygous) and dissimilar (heterozygous) genes. **B,** Classification of chromosomal joining. (From Whaley, L. F. 1974. *Understanding inherited disorders.* St. Louis: The C. V. Mosby Co., pp. 6, 8.)

Cells are reproduced by two different but related processes. The process of *mitosis* results in the production of additional body cells. Mitosis makes growth and development possible, and in mature individuals it is the process by which cells continue to divide and replace themselves. The other process of cell reproduction, *meiosis,* leads to the development of a new organism.

MITOSIS

Although mitosis is a continuous process, it is generally divided into five stages: interphase, prophase, metaphase,

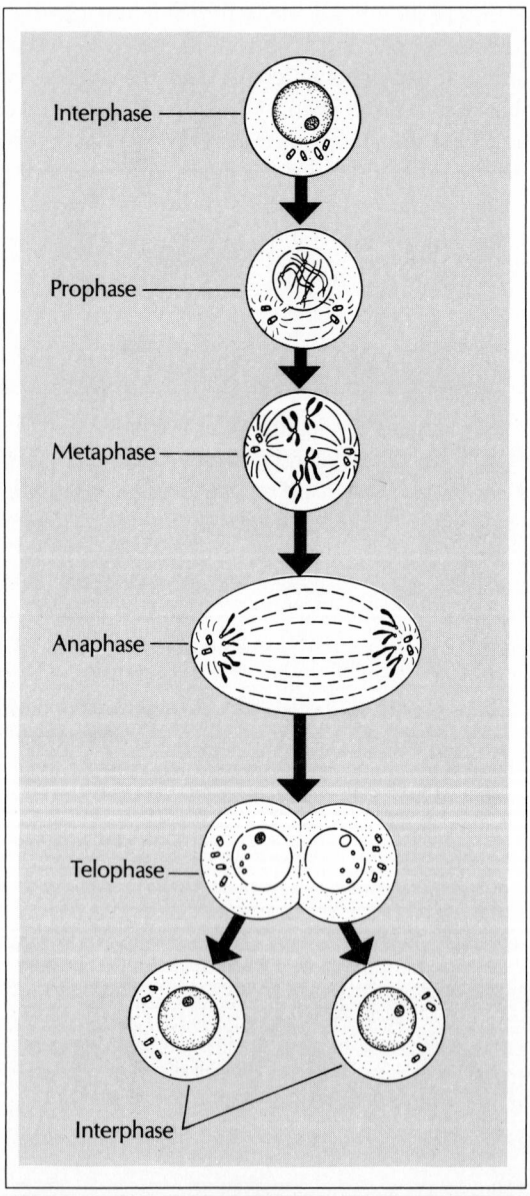

FIGURE 8-2 Somatic cell undergoing mitosis. Only four chromosomes are illustrated. (From Whaley, L. F. 1974. *Understanding inherited disorders.* St. Louis: The C. V. Mosby Co., p. 11.)

anaphase, and telophase (Figure 8-2). During *interphase,* cell division is not taking place, but DNA is replicating itself within the chromosomes so that the genes will be doubled. Mitosis actually begins when the cell enters the *prophase.* The strands of chromatin shorten and thicken, and the chromosomes reproduce themselves by doubling the strands of chromatin. Next comes the appearance of a mitotic apparatus known as a *spindle,* in which fine threads extend from the top and bottom poles of the nucleus. At each pole of the spindle, a body known as the *centriole* is formed, so that the threads of the spindle extend from one centriole to the other. Next the nuclear membrane, which separates the nucleus from the cytoplasm, disappears; the nucleus thus disappears, and the cell enters metaphase. During *metaphase,* the chromosomes line up at the equator (midway between the poles) of the spindle. Metaphase is followed by *anaphase,* in which the two chromatids of each chromosome separate and move to opposite ends of the spindle, where they cluster in masses near the two poles of the cell. *Telophase* is essentially the reverse of prophase. A nuclear membrane forms, separating each newly formed nucleus from the cytoplasm. The spindle disappears, and the centrioles relocate outside of each new nucleus. Within the nucleus the nucleolus again becomes visible, and the chromosomes lengthen and become threadlike. As telophase nears completion, a furrow develops in the cytoplasm at the midline of the cell and divides it into two *daughter cells.* Daughter cells have the same diploid number of chromosomes and the same genetic makeup as the cell from which they came (Winchester, 1966). In other words, after a cell with 46 chromosomes goes through mitosis, the result is two identical cells, each of them having 46 chromosomes.

MEIOSIS

Meiosis occurs during *gametogenesis,* the process by which germ cells, or *gametes,* are produced. The male gamete (sperm) is produced in the seminiferous tubules of the testes by the process of spermatogenesis (Chapter 4 and p. 160). Oogenesis takes place in the graafian follicle of the ovary and results in the production of the female gamete (ovum) (p. 160). To maintain genetic balance, the chromosomes, through meiosis, are reduced by either reduction division or extrusion to form a gamete with 23 chromosomes (22 autosomes and 1 sex chromosome), the haploid number.

Meiosis consists of two successive cell divisions, each of which includes the stages of interphase, prophase, metaphase, anaphase, and telophase (Figure 8-3). The chromosomes are replicated early in meiosis, although exactly when this occurs is not known, and the chromatids of each homologous pair of chromosomes are joined together at the centromere. At this point, an essential difference between mitosis and meiosis becomes apparent. Whereas the replicated chromosomes function independently in mi-

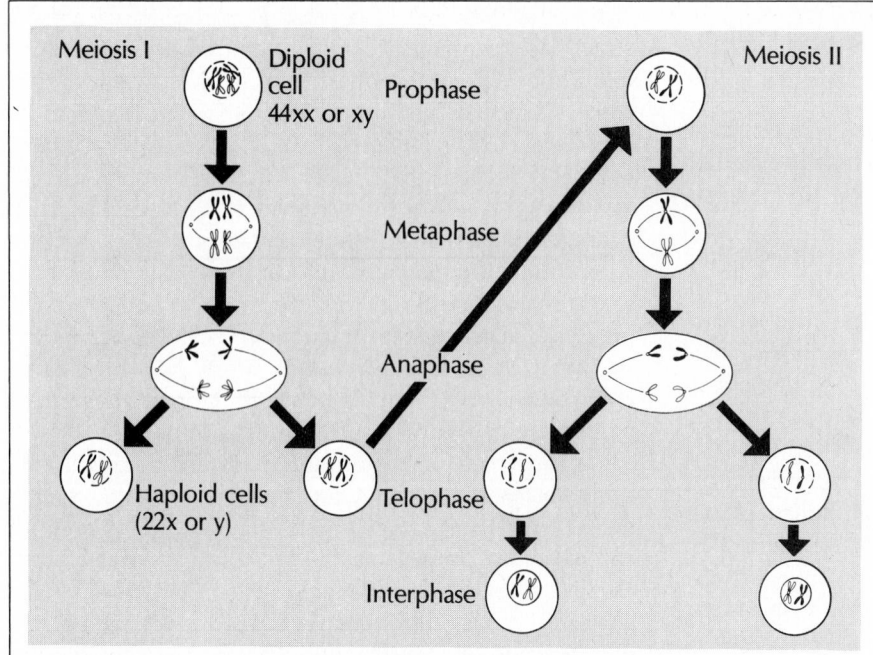

FIGURE 8–3 Meiosis in a germ cell. This illustration indicates the behavior of two pairs of homologous chromosomes. (From Whaley, L. F. 1974. *Understanding inherited disorders.* St. Louis: The C. V. Mosby Co., p. 13.)

tosis, they become closely associated in meiosis. They often become entwined, forming a bundle of four chromatids referred to as a *tetrad*. At this stage an exchange of parts between chromatids, known as *crossing over,* often takes place (Figure 8–4). At each point of contact, there is physical exchange of genetic material between the chromatids. New combinations are provided by the newly formed chromosomes, accounting for the wide variation of traits seen in individuals. The replicated pairs of chromosomes line up at the equator of the spindle, and each member of a pair moves toward an opposite pole of the spindle. (In mitosis, the chromatids of each chromosome move together toward the poles.)

One of the members of each chromosome pair came originally from the father and the other, from the mother. At the end of the first meiotic division, the maternal and paternal chromosomes are randomly distributed between two separate daughter cells. Each of these cells contains half the usual number of chromosomes (haploid number), but these chromosomes are still made up of two chromatids.

At the beginning of the second meiotic division, the chromosomes of each daughter cell line up along the equator of the spindle. The centromeres split, and the chromatids of each chromosome separate and move to opposite poles. The result of the second division is the formation of four cells, each containing the haploid number of chromosomes. In other words, an ovum (or sperm) begins the process of meiosis with 23 chromosomes, and ends as a cell with 23 chromosomes.

Occasionally during the second meiotic division, two of

the chromatids may not move apart rapidly enough when the cell divides. The still-paired chromatids are carried into one of the daughter cells and eventually form an extra chromosome. This condition is referred to as an *autosomal nondisjunction* (chromosomal mutation) and is harmful to the offspring that may result should fertilization occur. The implications of nondisjunction are discussed in Chapter 7.

Another type of chromosomal mutation can occur if chromosomes break during meiosis. If the broken segment is lost, the result is a shorter chromosome; this situation is known as *deletion*. If the broken segment becomes attached to another chromosome, it is called *translocation*, which often results in harmful structural mutations (Whaley, 1974). The effects of translocation are described in Chapter 7.

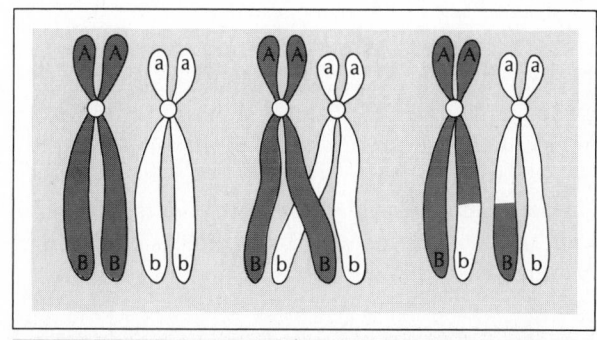

FIGURE 8–4 Phenomenon of crossing over. (From Spence, A. P., and Mason, E. B. 1983. *Human anatomy and physiology.* 2nd ed. Menlo Park, Calif.: Benjamin/Cummings Publishing Co., p. 77.)

Maturation of Gametes

OVUM

As discussed in Chapter 4, the ovaries begin development early in the fetal life of the female, and all the ova that an individual will produce are formed by about the sixth month of fetal life. The germinal epithelium of the outside of the ovary gives rise to oogonial cells, which develop into oocytes. Meiosis takes place within the oocytes, and meiotic division begins in all oocytes before the child is born. Meiosis stops just prior to the first meiotic metaphase in all oocytes and remains retarded until puberty. During puberty, the mature primary oocyte proceeds through the first meiotic division through the process of oogenesis.

The first meiotic division gives rise to two cells of unequal size—a result of unequal division of the cytoplasm. These two cells are a *secondary oocyte* and a minute *polar body*—the end of the spindle and its pole with half of the chromosomes are actually extruded outside the cell membrane of the secondary oocyte. When fertilized by a sperm, the secondary oocyte proceeds rapidly through the second meiotic division. The second meiotic division is similar to the first, except that the chromatids separate *before* migrating to opposite poles. Division is again not equal, producing an ovum with the haploid number of chromosomes and another extrusion of chromosomes into a second polar body. In addition, the first polar body has divided producing two additional polar bodies. As a result of meiosis, four haploid cells have been produced: three small polar bodies, which eventually disintegrate, and one ovum, which will be functional (Figure 8–5).

SPERM

When a boy reaches puberty, at about 14 years of age, the germinal epithelium in the seminiferous tubules of the testes begins the continuous process of spermatogenesis, which will continue until senescence. As the diploid spermatogonium enters the first meiotic division, it is referred to as a *primary spermatocyte*. During the first meiotic division it forms two haploid cells, termed *secondary spermatocytes*, each of which contains 22 autosomes and either an X sex chromosome or a Y sex chromosome. They will divide during the second meiotic division and form four *spermatids* with the haploid number of chromosomes. The spermatids undergo a series of changes during which they lose most of their cytoplasm. The nucleus becomes compacted into the head of the sperm, which is covered by a cap called an *acrosome*, and a long tail is produced from one of the centrioles (Figure 8–5).

Sex Determination

The two chromosomes of the twenty-third pair (either XX or XY) are called *sex chromosomes*. The larger of the sex chromosomes has a centrally located centromere and is designated the *X chromosome*. The smaller sex chromosome has a terminally located centromere and is designated the *Y chromosome*. Females have two X chromosomes, and males have an X and a Y chromosome. Because male cells contain both an X and a Y chromosome, meiosis produces two gametes with an X chromosome and two gametes with a Y chromosome from each primary spermatocyte. The sex chromosomes in oocytes are both X, and thus the mature ovum can have only one type of sex chromosome, an X. For the resulting child to be female, she must get an X chromosome from her mother and an X chromosome from her father. For the resulting child to be a male, he must get an X chromosome from his mother and a Y chromosome from his father.

When genes for two or more traits are situated on the same chromosome, the term *linkage* is used to describe their tendency to travel together during cell division. Y chromosomes contain mainly genes for maleness, but X chromosomes carry several genes other than those for sexual traits. These other traits are termed sex-linked because they are controlled by the genes on the sex chromosome. Hemophilia and color blindness are examples of sex-linked traits.

As discussed in Chapter 7, it is postulated that one X chromosome in every somatic cell of the female becomes genetically inactivated. This inactive X chromosome is pressed to the edge of the nucleus, where it remains as a tightly coiled small mass of material. This small mass of material, called the *sex chromatin* or *Barr body,* is discussed on p. 140.

FERTILIZATION

The mature ovum and a spermatozoon must unite within a brief period of time, as their life span is limited. Ova are thought to be fertilizable for about a 24-hour period after ovulation. Sperm, although they may survive in the female genital tract for up to 72 hours, are believed to be healthy and highly fertile for about 24 hours (Silverstein, 1980).

The process of *fertilization* takes place in the ampulla of the fallopian tube. The high estrogen level at the time of ovulation increases the contractility of the fallopian tube, propelling the ovum through its passageway. This high estrogen level also causes an increase in cervical mucus, which becomes less viscous (less sticky) and more readily penetrated by spermatozoa.

The ovum's cell membrane is surrounded by two layers of tissue. The layer closest to the cell membrane is called the *zona pellucida.* It is a clear, noncellular layer whose function is not known. Surrounding the zona pellucida is a ring of elongated cells, called the *corona radiata* because they radiate from the ovum like the gaseous corona around the sun. These cells are held together by hyaluronic acid.

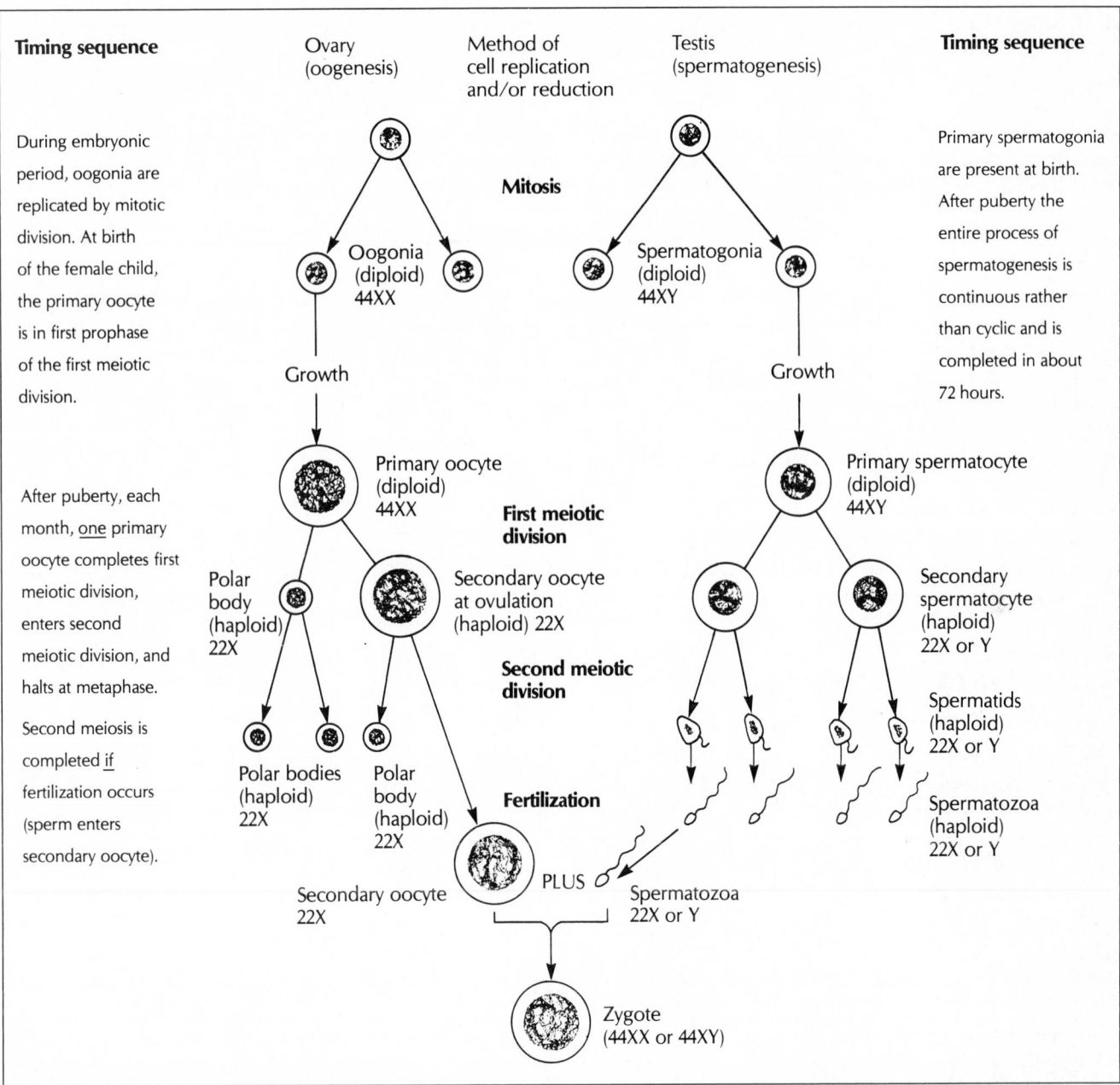

Timing sequence

During embryonic period, oogonia are replicated by mitotic division. At birth of the female child, the primary oocyte is in first prophase of the first meiotic division.

After puberty, each month, <u>one</u> primary oocyte completes first meiotic division, enters second meiotic division, and halts at metaphase.

Second meiosis is completed <u>if</u> fertilization occurs (sperm enters secondary oocyte).

Timing sequence

Primary spermatogonia are present at birth. After puberty the entire process of spermatogenesis is continuous rather than cyclic and is completed in about 72 hours.

FIGURE 8–5 Gametogenesis involves meiosis within the ovary and testis. Note that during meiosis, each oogonium produces a single haploid ovum, whereas each spermatogonium produces four haploid spermatozoa. (Modified from Spence, A. P., and Mason, E. B. 1983. *Human anatomy and physiology.* 2nd ed. Menlo Park, Calif.: Benjamin/Cummings Publishing Co., pp. 739, 748.)

A single ejaculation deposits about 2.0–5.0 mL of semen, containing approximately 200–400 million spermatozoa, in the vagina. The spermatozoa ascend the female tract by means of the flagellar action of their tails and the assistance of uterine contractions (Danforth, 1982). The prostaglandins in the semen may increase uterine smooth muscle contractions, thereby assisting the transport of the sperm (Spence, 1982). The fallopian tube has dual ciliary action in both directions, facilitating movement of the ovum down and propelling the sperm up the tube (Pritchard and MacDonald, 1980). The ovum has no inherent power of movement.

The *capacitation process* of the spermatozoa must precede the acrosomal reaction involved in fertilization of the ovum. During capacitation, the plasma membrane overlying the spermatozoa's acrosomal area loses seminal plasma proteins and its glycoprotein coat. Capacitation occurs in the female reproductive tract and is thought to take about 7 hours (Langman, 1981).

The acrosome covering the head of the spermatozoon is believed to contain the enzyme hyaluronidase. As several million spermatozoa surround the ovum, they deposit their minute amount of hyaluronidase. This activity is called *acrosomal reaction;* it breaks down enough hyaluronic acid in the outer layer of the ovum for one spermatozoon to penetrate it (DeCoursey, 1974). Only the head and neck of the spermatozoon enter the ovum; the tail becomes detached and remains in the ovum's outer membrane (Figure 8–6). Simultaneously with penetration, a cellular change occurs in the ovum that renders it impenetrable to other spermatozoa; thus only one spermatozoon enters a single ovum.

At the moment of penetration the second meiotic division is completed in the nucleus of the ovum, and the second polar body is extruded. Each gamete contains a haploid number of chromosomes (23 chromosomes); at their union, the diploid number is restored, for a total of 46

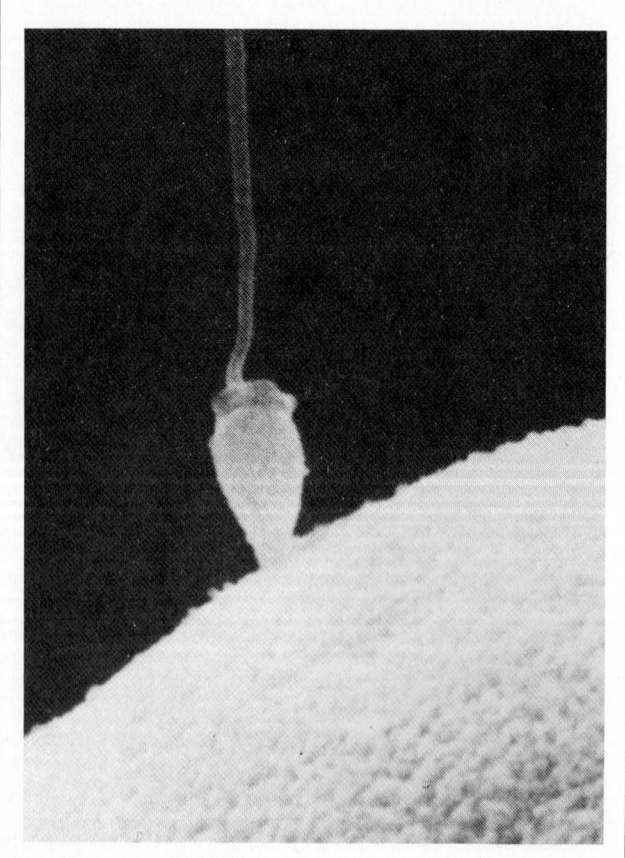

FIGURE 8–6 Electron micrograph of a sperm about to penetrate the surface of an ovum. (From Bloom, W., and Fawcett, D. W. 1975. *A textbook of histology.* 10th ed. Philadelphia: W. B. Saunders Co.)

chromosomes. At this moment the sex of the offspring is also established. As the male and female nuclei approach each other, a mitotic spindle forms between them, their nuclear membranes disappear, and their chromosomes pair up along the equatorial zone of the newly formed spindle apparatus. Thus a new cell is formed from the union of a male and a female gamete. This cell, referred to as the *zygote,* contains a new combination of genetic material, resulting in an individual different from either parent and from anyone else in the world.

Intrauterine human development after fertilization can be divided into three phases: cellular multiplication, cellular differentiation, and development of organ systems. These phases and the process of implantation will be discussed next.

CELLULAR MULTIPLICATION

Cellular multiplication begins as the recently fertilized ovum is transported through the fallopian tube into the cavity of the uterus. This transport takes about three or more days (Pritchard and MacDonald, 1980; Danforth, 1982) and is effected mainly by a very weak fluid current in the fallopian tube resulting from the beating action of the ciliated epithelium that lines the tube.

The zygote enters a period of rapid mitotic divisions called *cleavage,* in which it divides into two cells, four cells, eight cells, and so on. The cells that are produced during this period are called *blastomeres* and are so small that the developing mass is only slightly larger than the original zygote. The blastomeres are held together by the zona pellucida and eventually form a solid ball of cells referred to as the *morula.* After reaching the uterus, the morula floats freely for a few days, undergoing changes that result in the development of a cavity within the mass of cells. The inner, solid mass of cells is called the *blastocyst,* and the outer layer of cells forming the cavity and replacing the zona pellucida is referred to as the *trophoblast.* Eventually the trophoblast develops into one of the embryonic membranes, the chorion. The blastocyst develops into the embryo and the other embryonic membranes.

The journey of the fertilized ovum to its uterine destination is illustrated in Figure 8–7.

IMPLANTATION

While floating free in the uterine cavity, the blastocyst derives its nutrition from the uterine glands, which secrete a mixture of mucopolysaccharides, lipids, and glycogen. After the loss of the zona pellucida, the newly formed trophoblast must attach itself to the surface of the endometrium for further nourishment. The trophoblast most often selects a site for implantation in the upper part of the posterior uterine wall (Figure 8–7) and then burrows between the columnar epithelial cells, penetrating down toward the maternal capillaries. Between day 7 to 9 after fertilization, the blastocyst implants itself in the uterus by sinking down into the uterine lining until it is completely covered. The lining of the uterus thickens below the implanted blastocyst and the cells of the trophoblast grow down into the thickened lining, forming processes called *villi.*

The endometrium, under the influence of progesterone, has undergone changes to prepare for implantation and nutrition of the ovum. Its vascularity and thickness are greatly increased. After implantation, the endometrium is referred to as the *decidua.* The portion of the decidua that overlies the blastocyst is called the *decidua capsularis;* the portion directly beneath the implanted blastocyst is the *decidua basalis;* and the portion that lines the rest of the uterine cavity is the *decidua vera* (parietalis). The maternal portion of the placenta develops from the decidua basalis, which contains large numbers of blood vessels.

CELLULAR DIFFERENTIATION

At the time of implantation, the embryonic membranes begin to form (Figure 8–8). These membranes protect and support the embryo during its growth and development within the uterus.

The first membrane to form is the *chorion,* the outermost embryonic membrane, which encloses the amnion, embryo, and yolk sac. It is a thick membrane that develops

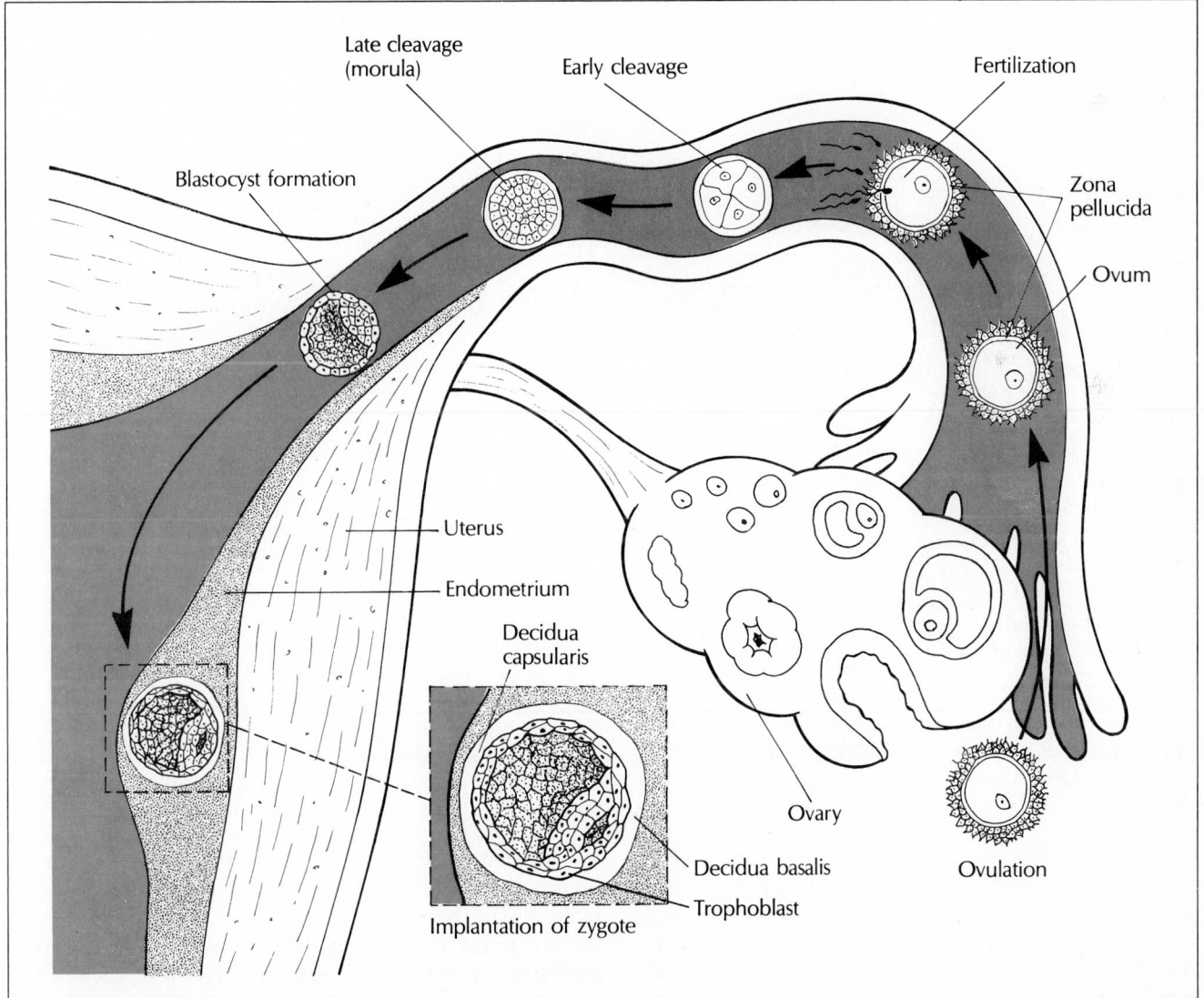

FIGURE 8–7 Fertilization generally occurs in the outer third of the fallopian tube. Illustrated is the cellular development of the ovum as it progresses to implantation in the uterus.

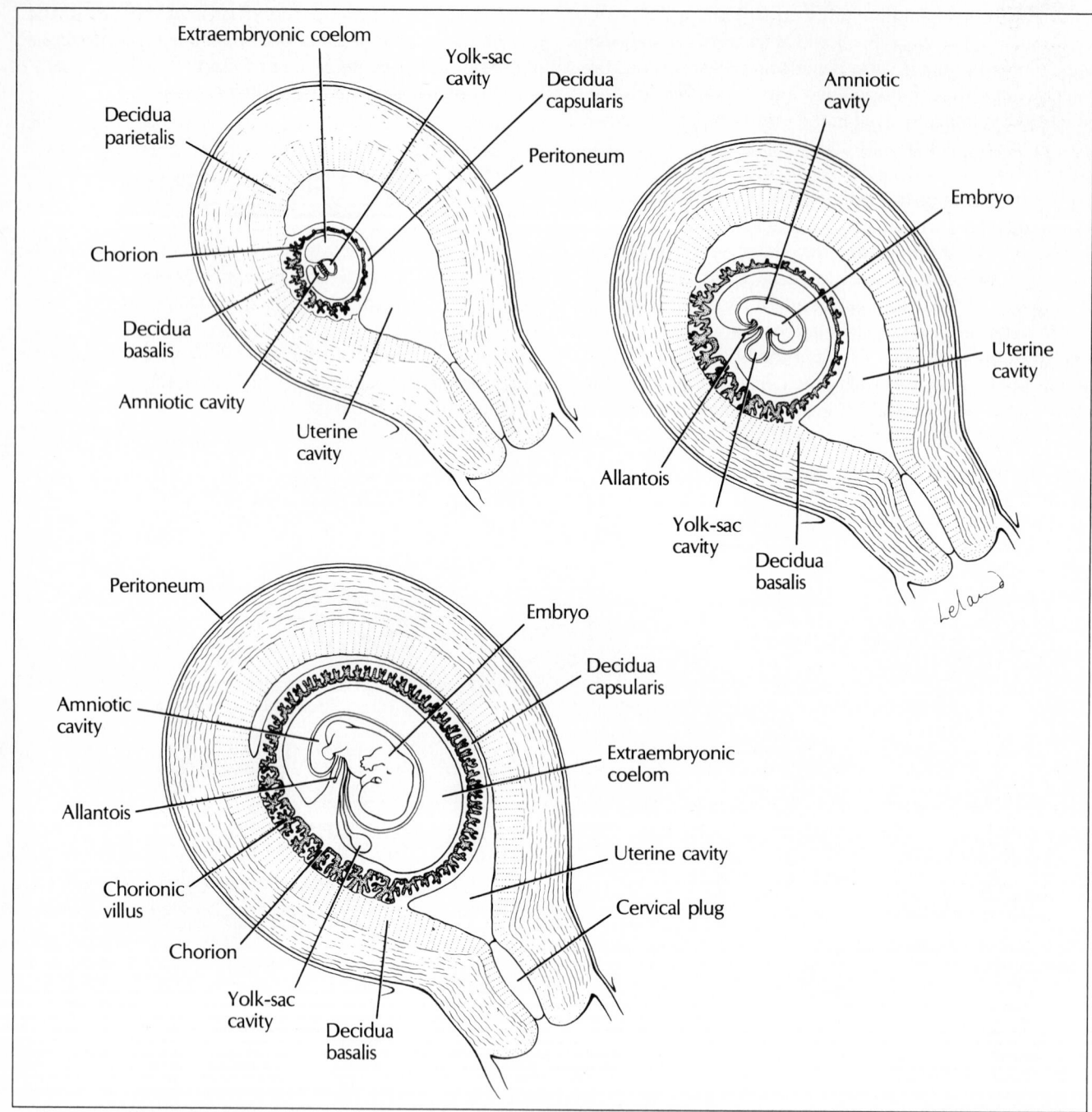

FIGURE 8–8 Early development of the embryonic membranes. (From Spence, A. P., and Mason, E. B. 1983. *Human anatomy and physiology.* 2nd ed. Menlo Park, Calif.: Benjamin/Cummings Publishing Co., p. 767.)

from the trophoblast, with numerous fingerlike projections over its surface called *chorionic villi.* Soon after development, the villi begin to degenerate, with the exception of those immediately beneath the embryo, which continue to grow and branch, fitting into depressions in the uterine wall and forming the embryonic portion of the placenta. By the fourth month of pregnancy, the surface of the chorion is smooth except at the place of attachment to the uterine wall.

The second membrane, the *amnion,* originates from the ectoderm during the early stages of embryonic development. It is a thin protective membrane that contains amniotic fluid. The space between the membrane and the embryo is the *amniotic cavity.* The spaces in the extraembryonic mesoderm fuse, creating a fluid-filled cavity (extraembryonic coelom or chorionic cavity) surrounding the amnion and yolk sac; except where the germ layer (developing embryo) disk attaches to the trophoblast by the connecting stalk (Langman, 1981).

The amnion expands as the embryo grows, until it fills the extraembryonic cavity and comes into contact with the chorion. These two slightly adherent membranes form a fluid-filled sac, and the embryo literally floats within this protective envelope. The amniotic fluid acts as a cushion to protect against mechanical injury, helps control the embryo's temperature, prevents adherence of the amnion, and allows freedom of movement so the embryo can change position.

It is not known how amniotic fluid originates in early pregnancy. Moore (1977) postulated that amniotic fluid was formed by the amniotic membrane. Numerous researchers have suggested that amniotic fluid is a transudate of maternal plasma or a transudate of fetal plasma, since a close relationship exists between fetal size and amount of amniotic fluid up to 20 weeks' gestation. Current evidence indicates that the major pathway for intrauterine water accumulation in pregnancy is across the chorion between the maternal and fetal compartments. Presumably this water transfer from the mother occurs in response to a very small intermittent chemical potential gradient (Seeds, 1980).

The volume of amniotic fluid increases from about 30 mL at 10 weeks' gestation to 350 mL at 20 weeks' gestation (Moore, 1977). After 20 weeks, the volume ranges from 500–1000 mL. The amniotic fluid volume constantly changes as a result of fluid movement in both directions through the placental membrane. Later in pregnancy the fetus contributes to the volume of amniotic fluid by excretion of urine, and it absorbs up to 400 mL/24 hr through its gastrointestinal tract by swallowing amniotic fluid. Amniotic fluid is slightly alkaline and contains albumin, urea, uric acid, creatinine, lecithin, sphingomyelin, bilirubin, fat, fructose, epithelial cells, leukocytes, enzymes, and lanugo hair.

About the eighth or ninth day, the yolk sac forms as a second cavity in the blastocyst. The yolk sac is small and functions only during early embryonic life. In animals other than mammals, the yolk sac is the source of nourishment. In humans, the yolk sac forms primitive red blood cells during the first 6 weeks of development until hematopoiesis begins in the liver of the embryo. As the embryo develops, the yolk sac is incorporated in the umbilical cord, where it can be identified as a degenerate structure.

About the tenth to fourteenth day, simultaneously with the development of the embryonic membranes, the once homogeneous mass of cells begins to differentiate. Three primary germ layers are formed: the ectoderm, mesoderm, and endoderm (Figure 8–9). From these three primary cell layers, all the tissues, organs, and organ systems will differentiate (Table 8–1).

How and why differentiation occurs are not clearly understood, although it is believed to be a gene-directed phenomenon that originates in the DNA of the zygote and that is carried out in the cytoplasm by an elaborate set of chemical reactions caused by the RNA-controlled synthesis of specific enzymes.

INTRAUTERINE ORGAN SYSTEMS

Placenta

The *placenta* is the means of metabolic exchange between embryonic and maternal circulation.

DEVELOPMENT

Whereas the other embryonic membranes are formed during the time of implantation or shortly thereafter, true pla-

Table 8–1 Derivation of Body Structures from Primary Cell Layers

Ectoderm	Mesoderm	Endoderm
Epidermis	Dermis	Respiratory tract epithelium
Sweat glands	Wall of digestive tract	Epithelium (except nasal), including
Sebaceous glands	Kidneys and ureter (suprarenal cortex)	pharynx, tongue, tonsils, thyroid,
Nails	Reproductive organs (gonads, genital	parathyroid, thymus, tympanic cavity
Hair follicles	ducts)	Lining of digestive tract
Lens of eye	Connective tissue (cartilage, bone, joint	Primary tissue of liver and pancreas
Sensory epithelium of internal and	cavities)	Urethra and associated glands
external ear, nasal cavity, sinuses,	Skeleton	Urinary bladder (except trigone)
mouth, anal canal	Muscles (all types)	Vagina (parts)
Central and peripheral nervous systems	Cardiovascular system (heart, arteries,	
Nasal cavity	veins, blood, bone marrow)	
Oral glands and tooth enamel	Pleura	
Pituitary glands	Lymphatic tissue and cells	
Mammary glands	Spleen	

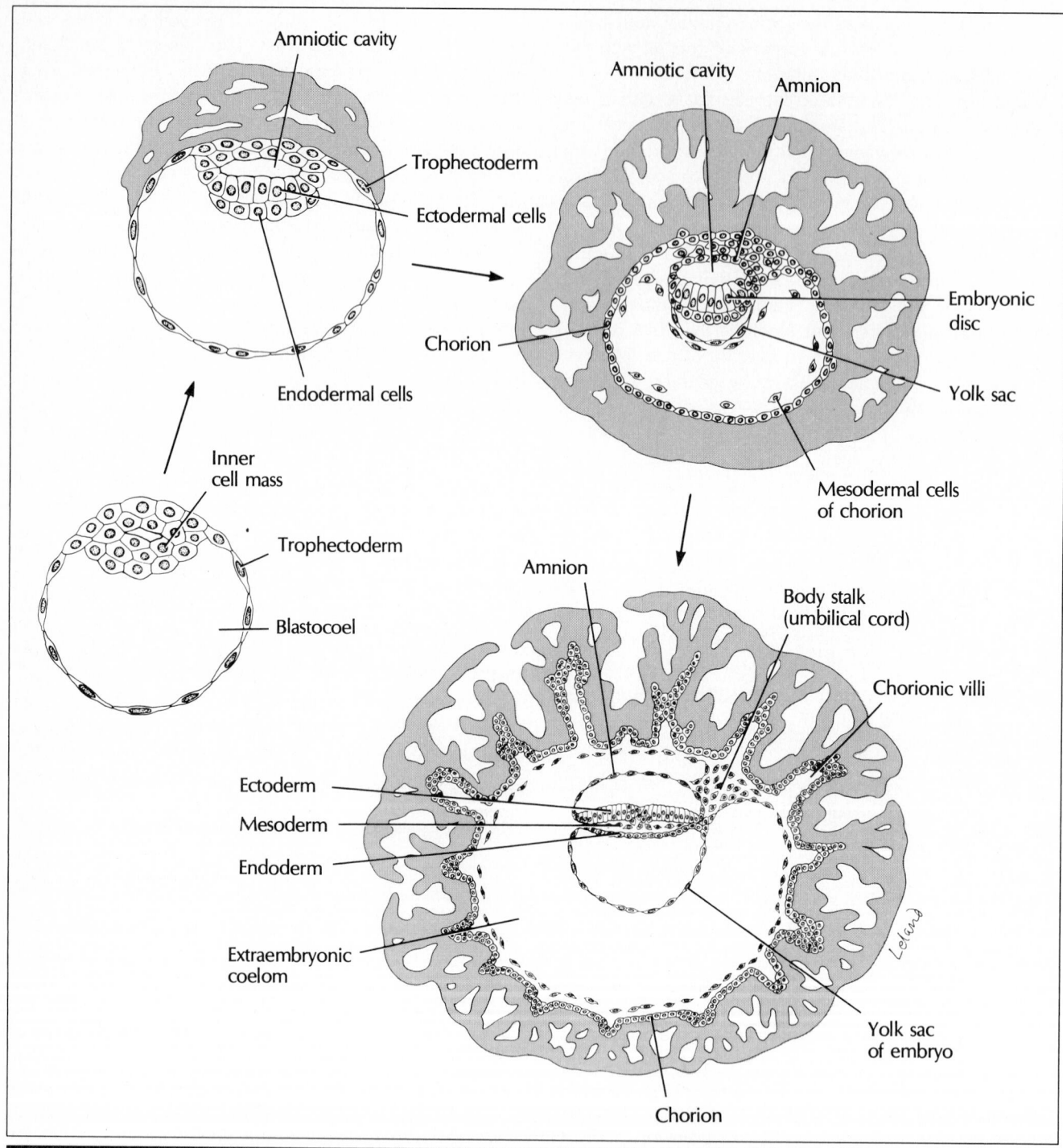

FIGURE 8–9 Formation of primary germ layers. (From Spence, A. P., and Mason, E. B. 1983. *Human anatomy and physiology.* 2nd ed. Menlo Park, Calif.: Benjamin/Cummings Publishing Co., p. 766.)

cental formation does not begin until the third week of development. The placenta forms at the place of attachment of the developing embryo to the uterine wall. The process begins with the chorionic villi.

Both the chorion and the uterus have extensive circulatory systems. The trophoblast cells of the chorionic villi

form spaces in the tissue of the decidua basalis. These spaces fill with maternal blood, and it is into these spaces that the chorionic villi grow. As the chorionic villi proliferate, two distinct trophoblastic layers appear: an outer layer, called the *syncytium* (consisting of syncytiotrophoblasts) and an inner layer, known as the *cytotrophoblast*

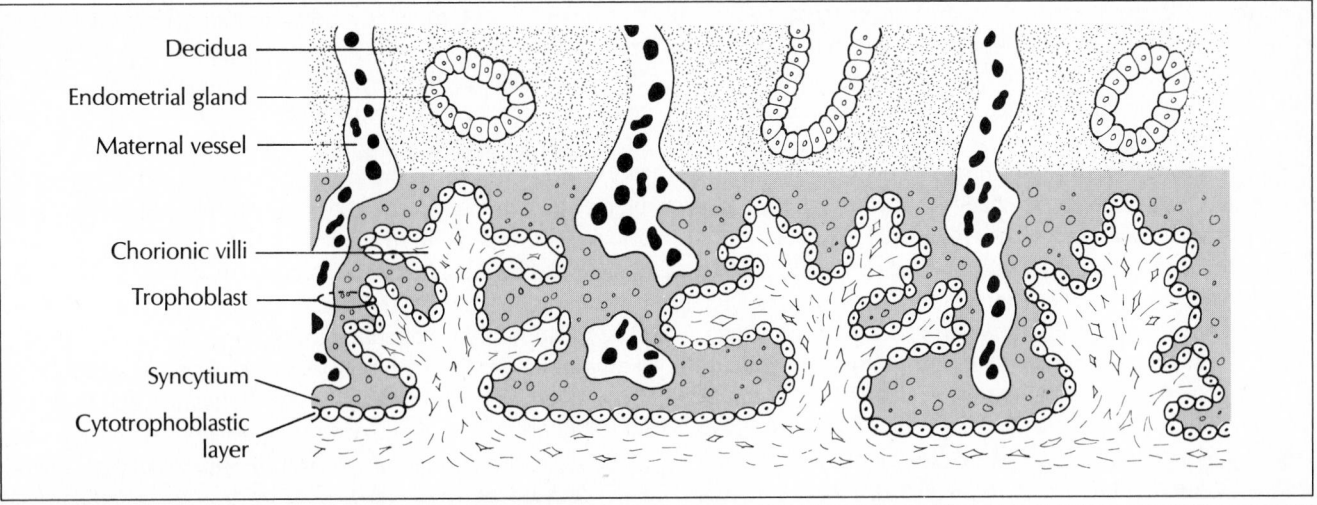

Decidua

Endometrial gland

Maternal vessel

Chorionic villi

Trophoblast

Syncytium

Cytotrophoblastic layer

FIGURE 8–10 Longitudinal section of placental villus. Spaces formed in the maternal decidua are filled with maternal blood; chorionic villi proliferate into these maternal blood-filled spaces and differentiate into a syncytium layer and cytotrophoblast layer.

(Figure 8–10). Both layers are present during the first 5 months of pregnancy, but later the cells of the cytotrophoblast become fewer and eventually disappear, so that during the last half of pregnancy only a single layer of syncytium covers the chorionic villi.

Placental permeability is relatively slight during the early months of development because the villous membranes have not yet been reduced to their minimum thickness. Its permeability increases progressively until about the last month of pregnancy, when it begins to decrease again because of deterioration of the placenta with age. A third, inner layer of connective mesoderm develops in the chorionic villi and grows through the cell columns, forming anchoring villi. These anchoring villi eventually form the septa (partitions) of the placenta. The maturing placenta is divided by the well-developed septa into 15 to 20 segments called *cotyledons*. In each cotyledon the branching villi form highly complex vascular systems through which the exchange of gases and nutrients takes place.

Expansion of the placenta continues until about the twentieth week, at which time it covers one-half of the internal surface of the uterus. After 20 weeks, the placenta grows only in thickness, not in width. At 40 weeks' gestation, the placenta is a discoid organ about 15–20 cm (5.9–7.9 in.) in diameter and 2.5–3.0 cm (1.0–1.2 in.) in thickness and weighs about 400–600 g (14–21 oz).

The placenta is composed of two portions. The maternal portion is made up of the decidua basalis and its circulation. Its surface is red and fleshlike. The fetal portion consists of the chorionic villi and their circulation. The fetal surface is covered by the adherent amnion, which eventually gives it a shiny grayish appearance (see Color Plate III).

As the placenta is developing, the umbilical cord is also being formed. The developing embryo is connected to the yolk sac by an area of tissue known as the *body stalk*. A chain of vessels that communicate with the gut of the developing embryo develops in the body stalk. The chorion and the amnion are also attached at this structure. To obtain more nourishment, the chain of vessels in the body stalk extends into the chorionic villi. The body stalk then fuses with the embryonic portion of the developing placenta to provide circulatory pathways connecting the chorionic villi and the embryo. The body stalk elongates and becomes known as the *umbilical cord*, or *funis*. The vessels in the cord are reduced to one large vein and two smaller arteries. About 1% of umbilical cords have only two vessels, an artery and a vein; this condition is associated with congenital fetal malformations.

A specialized connective tissue known as *Wharton's jelly* surrounds the blood vessels. This tissue, plus the high blood volume pulsating through the vessels, prevents intrauterine compression of the umbilical cord.

At term, the cord averages 2 cm (0.8 in.) in diameter and is about 55 cm (22 in.) in length, extending from the umbilicus of the fetus to the fetal surface of the placenta. The attachment of the umbilical cord in the placenta is eccentric, having either a central or peripheral (battledore) insertion. In rare circumstances the cord inserts away from the placenta so that vessels run along the membranes from the site of cord insertion to the surface of the placenta. This configuration is called a *velamentous placenta*.

CIRCULATION

After implantation of the blastocyst, the cells distinguish themselves into fetal cells and trophoblastic cells. The proliferating trophoblast successfully invades the decidua basalis of the endometrium, first opening uterine capillaries and later the larger uterine vessels. The placental villi are an outgrowth of the blastocystic tissue. As these villi continue to grow and divide, the fetal vessels begin to form. The intervillous spaces in the decidua basalis develop as the endometrial spiral arteries are opened.

By the fourth week, the placenta has begun to function as a means of metabolic exchange between embryo and mother. The completion of the maternal–placental–fetal circulation occurs about 22 days after conception when the embryonic heart begins functioning (Martin and Gingerich, 1976). By the fourteenth week, it is a discrete organ.

Recall that the trophoblastic tissue of the villi is divided into the cytotrophoblast and the syncytium. The syncytium, an outgrowth of the cytotrophoblast and the functional layer of the placenta, is in direct contact with the maternal blood at the intervillous space. It also secretes the placental hormones of pregnancy.

The cotyledons of the maternal surface contain branches of a single placental mainstem villus, allowing for some compartmentalization of the uteroplacental circulation. Each cotyledon is a natural vascular unit containing branching vessels distributed throughout that particular lobule and partially separated from other lobules by the cotyledon's thin septal partitions.

In the fully developed placenta, fetal blood in the villi and maternal blood in the intervillous spaces are separated by three to four thin layers of tissue. The capillaries of the villi are lined with an extremely thin endothelium and are surrounded by a layer of mesenchymal (connective) tissue that is covered by chorionic epithelium consisting of cytotrophoblast and syncytiotrophoblast (see Figure 8–10). As previously discussed, one of the layers of the chorionic epithelium, the cytotrophoblast, thins out and disappears after the fifth month.

Fetal blood flows through the two umbilical arteries to the capillaries of the villi, and back through the umbilical vein into the fetus. During late pregnancy a soft blowing sound (*funic souffle*) can be heard over the location of the umbilical cord of the fetus. The rate of the sound is synchronous with the fetal heartbeat and the flow of fetal blood through the umbilical arteries.

Maternal blood, rich in oxygen and nutrients, flows from the spiral uterine arteries into the intervillous spaces in spurts. These spurts are produced by the maternal blood pressure. The spurt of blood is directed toward the chorionic plate, and as the blood flow loses pressure, it becomes lateral (or spreads out). Fresh blood continually enters and exerts pressure on the contents of the intervillous spaces, pushing blood toward the exits in the basal plate. Blood is then drained through the uterine and other pelvic veins (Figure 8–11). A uterine souffle is also heard during the last months of pregnancy. It is identified as a loud blowing murmur or swishing sound heard just above the symphysis pubis and timed precisely with the mother's pulse. This sound is caused by the augmented blood flow entering the dilated uterine arteries.

Circulation within the intervillous spaces depends on maternal blood pressure producing a gradient between arterial and venous channels. The lumen of the spiral uterine artery is narrow when it pierces the chorionic plate and enters the intervillous space, resulting in an increased blood pressure. The pressure in the arteries forces the blood into the intervillous spaces and bathes the numerous small villi in oxygenated blood. As the pressure decreases the blood flows back from the chorionic plate towards the decidua where it enters the endometrial veins. Naeye (1981) found uteroplacental blood flow to be low and term neonates underweight when maternal blood pressure did not exceed 110/65 mm Hg during pregnancy. Rankin and McLaughlin (1979) postulated that prostaglandins are implicated in the regulation of uterine and placental blood flow because of their vasoconstrictive and vasodilatative effects.

Braxton Hicks contractions (Chapter 9) are believed to facilitate placental circulation by enhancing the movement of blood from the center of the cotyledon through the intervillous space (Reynolds et al., 1968).

FUNCTIONS

Placental exchange functions occur only in those fetal vessels in intimate contact with the covering syncytial membrane. In these villi, the syncytium has brush borders containing many microvilli, which greatly increase the exchange rate between maternal and fetal circulation (Langman, 1981).

The placental functions, many of which begin soon after implantation, include fetal respiration, nutrition, and excretion. To carry out these functions, the placenta is involved in metabolic and transfer activities. In addition, it has endocrine functions and special immunologic properties.

Endocrine functions. The placenta produces hormones that are vital to the survival of the fetus. The syncytium is believed to be the site of hormone production. Four hormones are known to be produced by the placenta: two protein hormones—human chorionic gonadotropin (hCG) human placental lactogen (hPL)—and two steroid hormones, estrogen and progesterone.

Biochemically, hCG is similar to pituitary luteinizing hormone (LH), and its most important function is to prevent the normal involution of the corpus luteum at the end of the menstrual cycle. The hCG causes the corpus luteum to secrete increased quantities of estrogen and progesterone. If the corpus luteum ceases functioning before the eleventh week of pregnancy, spontaneous abortion occurs. After the eleventh week, the placenta produces enough progesterone and estrogen to maintain pregnancy. In the male fetus, hCG also exerts an interstitial cell-stimulating effect on the testes, resulting in the production of testosterone. This small secretion of testosterone during embryonic development is the factor that causes male sex organs to

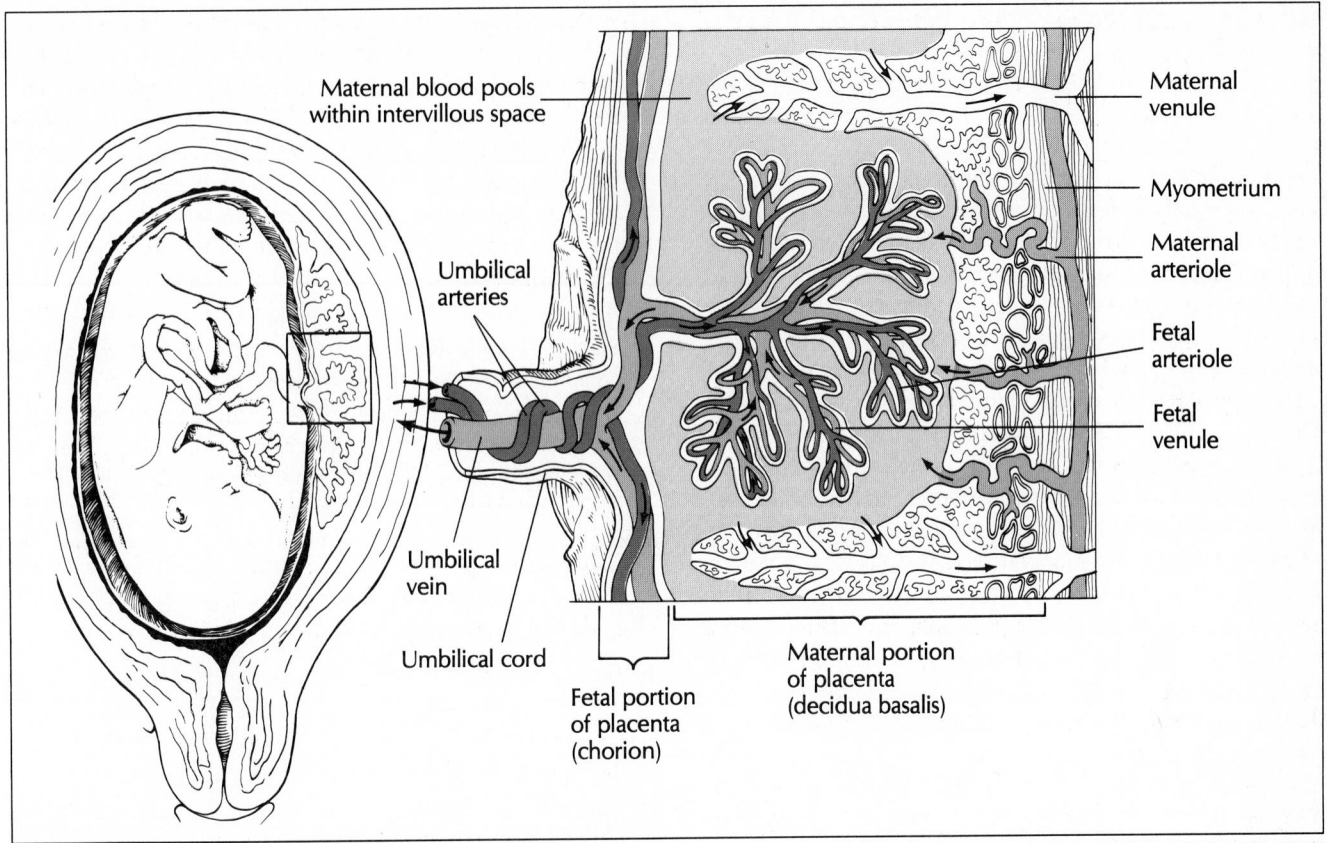

Maternal blood pools within intervillous space

Umbilical arteries

Umbilical vein

Umbilical cord

Fetal portion of placenta (chorion)

Maternal portion of placenta (decidua basalis)

Maternal venule

Myometrium

Maternal arteriole

Fetal arteriole

Fetal venule

FIGURE 8–11 Vascular arrangement of the placenta. *Arrows* indicate the direction of blood flow. Maternal blood flows through the uterine arteries to the intervillous spaces of the placenta and returns through the uterine veins to maternal circulation. Fetal blood flows through the umbilical arteries into the villous capillaries of the placenta and returns through the umbilical vein to the fetal circulation. (From Spence, A. P. and Mason, E. B. 1983. *Human anatomy and physiology.* 2nd ed. Menlo Park, Calif.: Benjamin/Cummings Publishing Co., p. 764.)

grow. The hCG also stimulates fetal steroidogenesis (Serón-Ferré et al., 1978).

The hCG is present in maternal blood serum 8–10 days after fertilization, just as soon as implantation has occurred, and is detectable in the maternal urine a few days after the missed menses. Chorionic gonadotropin reaches its maximum level at 50–70 days' gestation and then begins to decrease as placental hormone production increases.

Progesterone is a hormone essential for pregnancy. It increases the secretions of the fallopian tubes and uterus to provide appropriate nutritive matter for the developing morula and blastocyst. Progesterone causes decidual cells to develop in the uterine endometrium, and it must be present in high levels for implantation to occur. It also decreases the contractility of the uterus, thus preventing uterine contractions from causing spontaneous abortion.

The production of progesterone by the corpus luteum prior to stimulation by hCG reaches a peak about 8 days after ovulation. Implantation occurs at about the same time as this peak. At 10 days after ovulation, progesterone reaches a level between 15 and 30 ng/mL of body plasma and continues to rise slowly in subsequent weeks (Vande

Wiele et al., 1976). After the tenth week of pregnancy the placenta (syncytiotrophoblast) takes over the production of progesterone and secretes it in tremendous quantities, reaching levels late in pregnancy of more than 250 mg per day (Simpson and MacDonald, 1981).

By the seventh week of pregnancy, more than 50% of the estrogens in the maternal circulation are produced by the placenta. Estrogens serve mainly a proliferative function, causing enlargement of the uterus, breasts, and breast glandular tissue. Estrogens also have a significant role in increasing vascularity and vasodilatation, particularly in the villous capillaries near the end of pregnancy. Placental estrogens increase markedly toward the end of pregnancy, to as much as 30 times the daily production in the middle of a normal monthly menstrual cycle. The primary estrogen secreted by the placenta is different from that secreted by the ovaries: the placenta secretes mainly estriol, whereas the ovaries secrete primarily estradiol. The placenta by itself cannot synthesize estriol. Essential precursors are provided by the adrenal glands of the fetus and are transported to the placenta for the final conversion to estriol. Therefore, measurement of the presence of estriol can be a test for both fetal well-being and placental functioning.

The hormone hPL (sometimes referred to as human chorionic somatomammotropin or hCS) is biochemically similar to human pituitary growth hormone. Secretion of this protein hormone can be detected about the fourth week of pregnancy (Batzer, 1980). Placental lactogen stimulates key maternal metabolic adjustments ensuring more protein, glucose, and minerals are available for the fetus.

Immunologic properties. The placenta is a transplant of living tissue within the same species and is therefore considered a *homograft.* Ordinarily, homografts are destroyed by the host within a week or two. The placenta and embryo, however, seem to be exempt from their host's immunologic reactivity. In fact, a totally unrelated embryo will grow after being transferred to a second uterus. One theory used to explain this phenomenon postulates that trophoblastic tissue is immunologically inert. It may contain a cell coating that masks transplantation antigens and that repels sensitized lymphocytes (Beer and Billingham, 1974). Recent data suggest that there is a suppression of cellular immunity during pregnancy effected by the placental hormones, specifically progesterone and hCG (Gusdon and Sain, 1981).

Metabolic activities. The placenta is believed to have a metabolic rate comparable to that of an adult liver or kidney. Glycogen, cholesterol, and fatty acids are continuously synthesized by the placenta for fetal usage and hormone production. The placenta also produces the numerous enzymes necessary for fetoplacental transfer, and it breaks down certain substances such as epinephrine and histamine by enzymatic deamination. In addition, it functions as a storage unit for glycogen and iron.

TRANSPORT MECHANISMS

The placenta is no longer considered to be an inert barrier with pores that prevent the transfer of large molecules and that permit the transfer of small molecules. It is a functional membrane that controls the transfer of a wide range of substances by five major mechanisms:

1. *Simple diffusion.* This type of transport requires no energy output. Molecules move from an area of higher concentration to an area of lower concentration until an equilibrium is established. Substances that transfer across the placental membrane by simple diffusion are water, electrolytes such as sodium and chloride, carbon dioxide, anesthetic gases, and drugs. Recent studies suggest that the rate of oxygen transfer across the placental membrane is greater than that allowed by simple diffusion, indicating that oxygen transfers by facilitated diffusion of some type (Martin and Gingerich, 1976).

2. *Facilitated transport.* This type of transport involves a carrier system to move molecules from an area of greater concentration to an area of lower concentration, thereby speeding up the transfer of certain substances through the placental membrane. Among molecules carried by facilitated placental transport are glucose, galactose, and some oxygen. The glucose level in the fetal blood ordinarily is approximately 20%–30% lower than the glucose level in the maternal blood because glucose is being metabolized rapidly by the fetus (Vorherr, 1982). This, in turn, causes rapid transport of additional glucose from the maternal blood into the fetal blood.

3. *Active transport.* This type of transport requires energy, involves an enzymatic pathway, and can work against a concentration gradient, with molecules moving from an area of lower concentration to an area of higher concentration. Amino acids, calcium, iron, iodine, water-soluble vitamins, and glucose transfer across the placental membrane by active transport. The measured amino acid content of fetal blood is greater than that of maternal blood, and calcium and inorganic phosphate occur in greater concentration in fetal blood than in maternal blood (Aladjem and Lueck, 1982).

4. *Pinocytosis.* In this type of transport, materials are engulfed by amebalike cells forming plasma droplets. This mechanism is important for transferring large molecules, such as albumin and gamma globulins, across the placental membrane.

5. *Bulk flow.* Water and some solutes are transported across the placental membrane by hydrostatic and osmotic pressures. Most fetal water comes from the mother.

Other modes of transfer exist. For example, fetal red blood cells pass into the maternal circulation through breaks in the placental membrane, particularly during labor and delivery. Certain cells, such as maternal leukocytes, and microorganisms, such as viruses and *Treponema pallidum* (which causes syphilis), can also cross the placental membrane, but the exact mechanism is not known. Some bacteria and protozoa infect the placenta by causing lesions, and then entering the fetal blood system.

Parer (1974) and Dilts (1981) have identified several factors that affect transfer rate: (a) molecular size, (b) electrical charge, (c) lipid solubility, (d) placental area, (e) diffusion distance, (f) maternal–fetal–placental blood flow, (g) blood saturation with gases and nutrients, (h) pka of the substance, and (i) maternal–placental–fetal metabolism of the substance. Substances that have a molecular weight of 1000 daltons or more have difficulty crossing the placenta by simple diffusion. Therefore, heparin with a molecular weight above 6000 does not cross the placenta, while warfarin sodium (Coumadin) has a molecular weight in the 300 to 400 range and crosses easily (Dilts, 1981).

Electrically charged molecules pass across the placenta more slowly. An example is the muscle relaxant, succinylcholine. A lipid-soluble substance moves quickly across the placenta into the fetal circulation. Reduction of the placental surface area, as with abruptio placentae, will lessen the area that is functional for exchange. Placental diffusion distance also affects exchange; in conditions such as diabetes and placental infection, edema of the villi increases the diffusion distance, thus increasing the distance the substance has to be transferred.

The placental concentration gradient is altered by the concentration of substances in the maternal and fetal blood, by the placental blood flow from the fetus and the intervillous space blood flow from the mother, by the ratio of blood on each side of the placenta, and by the functioning of the carrier molecules in binding and dissociating. Decreased intervillous space blood flow is seen in labor and with certain maternal disease conditions such as hypertension. Mild hypoxia in the fetus increases the umbilical blood flow, and severe hypoxia results in decreased blood flow.

As the maternal blood picks up fetal waste products and carbon dioxide, it drains back into the maternal circulation through the veins in the basal plate. Fetal blood is hypoxic; it therefore attracts oxygen from the mother's blood. In addition, affinity for oxygen increases as the fetal blood gives up its carbon dioxide, which also decreases its acidity.

Fetal Circulation

Because the fetus must maintain the blood flow to the placenta to obtain oxygen and nutrients and to remove carbon dioxide and other waste products, the circulatory system of the fetus has several unique features.

The lungs of the fetus do not carry out respiratory gas exchange in utero. Therefore, a special circulatory system is required to bypass the blood supply to the lungs. The placenta assumes the function of the lungs by allowing carbon dioxide to be excreted by the fetus and carried off by the maternal blood, and allowing oxygen as well as nourishing products to be acquired by the fetus. The blood from the placenta is carried through the umbilical vein, which penetrates the abdominal wall of the fetus. It divides into two branches, one of which circulates a small amount of blood through the liver and empties into the inferior vena cava through the hepatic vein. The other larger branch, called the *ductus venosus*, empties directly into the vena cava. The blood then enters the right atrium, passes through the *foramen ovale* into the left atrium, and pours into the left ventricle, which pumps it into the aorta. Some blood returning from the head and upper extremities by way of the superior vena cava is emptied into the right atrium and passes through the tricuspid valve into the right ventricle. This blood is pumped into the pulmonary artery, and a small amount passes to the lungs, to provide nourishment only. The larger portion of blood passes through the *ductus arteriosus* into the descending aorta, thus bypassing the lungs. Finally, blood returns to the placenta through the two umbilical arteries, and the process is repeated (Figure 8–12).

The mean P_{O_2} of the maternal blood in the placental sinuses is approximately 50 mm Hg while the mean P_{O_2} in the blood leaving the villi and circulating to the fetus is about 30 mm Hg. At term, the fetus receives oxygen from maternal circulation at the rate of 20–30 mL/min (Langman, 1981). The fetus is able to obtain sufficient oxygen due to special fetal hemoglobin, which carries as much as 20%–30% more oxygen than mature hemoglobin. Also, the hemoglobin concentration in the fetus is about 50% greater than that of the mother. For further discussion see Chapter 21. The fetal circulatory pathway provides the highest available oxygen concentration to the head and neck, brain, and coronary circulation while a lesser degree of oxygenation and blood goes to the abdominal organs, and the lower body (Koffler, 1981).

Fetal Heart

The heart of the fetus, as of the adult, is under the control of its own pacemaker. The sinoatrial (S-A) node sets the rate and is supplied by the vagus nerve. Bridging the atrium and the ventricle is the atrioventricular (A-V) node. It is also supplied by the vagus nerve. Baseline variability of the fetal heartbeat has been shown to be under the influence of this nerve. Atropine will block this effect.

Under the influence of the sympathetic nervous system, norepinephrine is released when the fetus is stressed, causing an increase in the fetal heart rate. To counteract the increase in blood pressure, baroreceptors, which respond to stretch, are present in the vessel walls at the junction of the internal and external carotid arteries. When stimulated these receptors, under the influence of the vagus and glossopharyngeal nerves, cause the fetal heart rate to slow.

Chemoreceptors in the fetal peripheral and central nervous systems respond to decreased oxygen tensions and to increased carbon dioxide tensions, leading to fetal tachycardia and an increase in blood pressure. In studies conducted with the fetal lamb and monkey, it was concluded that the CNS also has control over heart rate. Increased activity of the lamb in a wakeful period was exhibited in an increase in the beat-to-beat variability of the fetal heart baseline. Sleep patterns demonstrated a decrease in the beat-to-beat baseline variability. In cases of severe hypoxia, increased levels of epinephrine and norepinephrine act on the fetal heart to produce a faster and stronger rate.

EMBRYO AND FETAL DEVELOPMENT AND ORGAN FORMATION

Pregnancy is calculated to have an average of 10 lunar months, 40 weeks, or 280 days. This period of 280 days

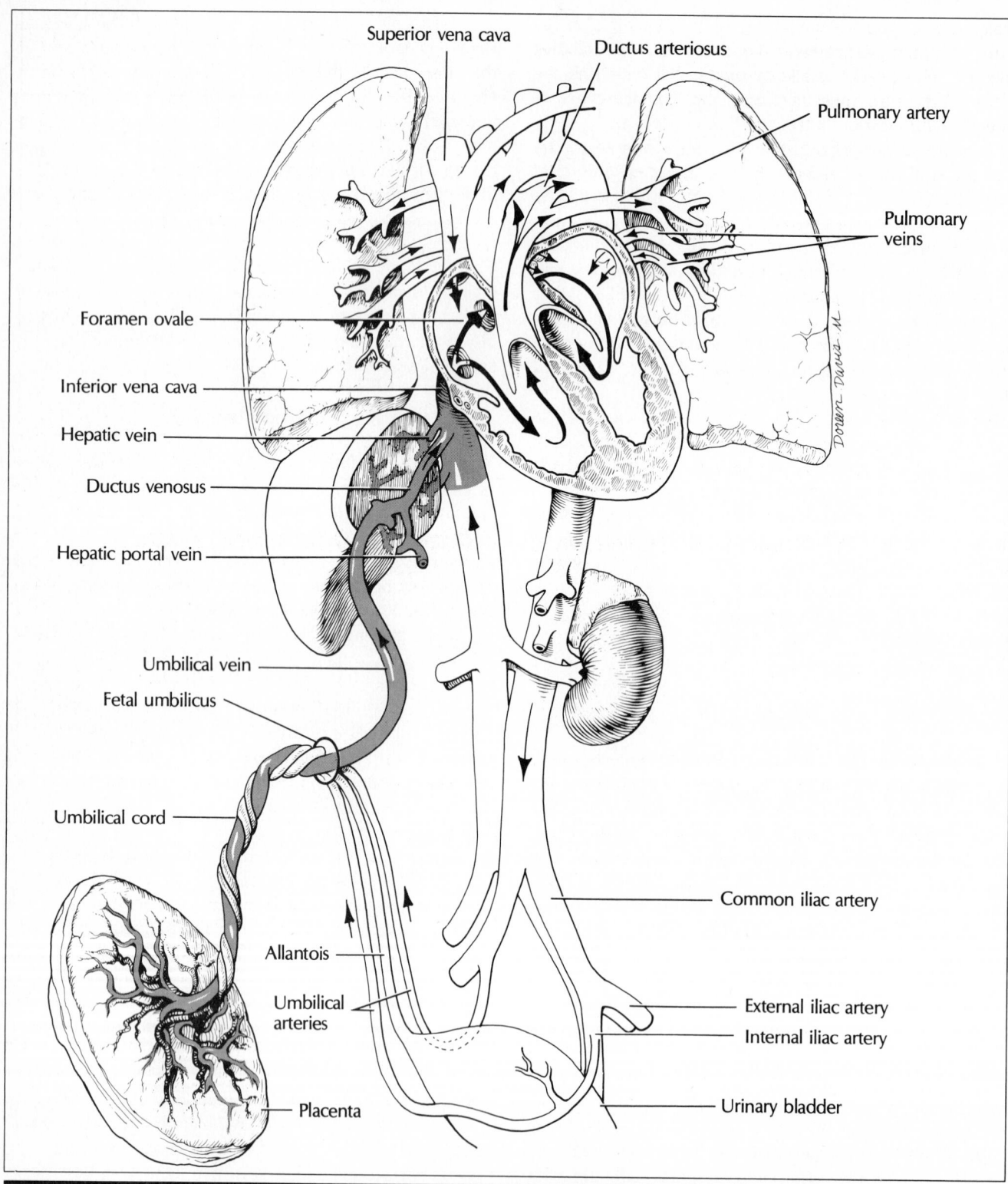

FIGURE 8–12 Fetal circulation. Blood leaves the placenta and enters the fetus through the umbilical vein. After circulating through the fetus, the blood returns to the placenta through the umbilical arteries. The ductus venosus, the foramen ovale, and the ductus arteriosus allow the blood to bypass the fetal liver and lungs. (From Spence, A. P., and Mason, E. B. 1983. *Human anatomy and physiology.* 2nd ed. Menlo Park, Calif.: Benjamin/Cummings Publishing Co., p. 776.)

is calculated from the beginning of the last menstrual period to parturition. Calculating the gestational age of the embryo or fetus, which is about 2 weeks less or 266 days or 38 weeks, is more accurate because it measures from the time of fertilization of the ovum or conception.

The basic events of organ development in the embryo and fetus are outlined in Table 8–2 on pp. 174–179.

Preembryonic Stage

The first 14 days of human development, starting on the day the ovum was fertilized (conception), are referred to as the *preembryonic stage,* or the *stage of the ovum.* This period is characterized by extremely rapid cellular multiplication and differentiation and the establishment of the embryonic membranes and germ layers, as discussed in detail earlier in this chapter.

Embryonic Stage

The stage of the embryo begins the third week after conception or fertilization and continues until approximately the eighth week or until it reaches a crown-to-rump length of 3 cm or 1.2 in. This length is usually attained about 49 days after fertilization. The embryonic stage is a period of differentiation of tissues into essential organs and the development of the main external features.

THIRD WEEK

In the third week the embryonic disk becomes elongated and pear-shaped, with a broad cephalic end and a narrow caudal end (Figure 8–13). The ectoderm has formed a long cylindrical tube for brain and spinal cord development. The gastrointestinal tract, created from the endoderm, appears as another tubelike structure communicating with the yolk sac. The most advanced organ is the heart. At 3 weeks, a single tubular heart forms just outside the body cavity of the embryo and by the end of 28 days it is beating at a regular rhythm and pushing its own primitive blood cells through the main blood vessels.

FOURTH WEEK

The interval between day 21 and day 32 is characterized by *somite* formation. Somites are a series of mesodermal blocks that form on each side of the midline of the embryo. By the twenty-eighth day, between 30 and 40 pairs of somites are present, appearing in a craniocaudal sequence. The vertebras that form the spinal column will develop from these somites. Arm and leg buds are not yet visible, but the tail bud is present. By this time four pairs of pharyngeal arches and five pairs of pharyngeal pouches have developed. The first arch will form the lower jaw (mandibular arch), the second arch will form the hyoid bone, and the third and fourth arches will form cartilage

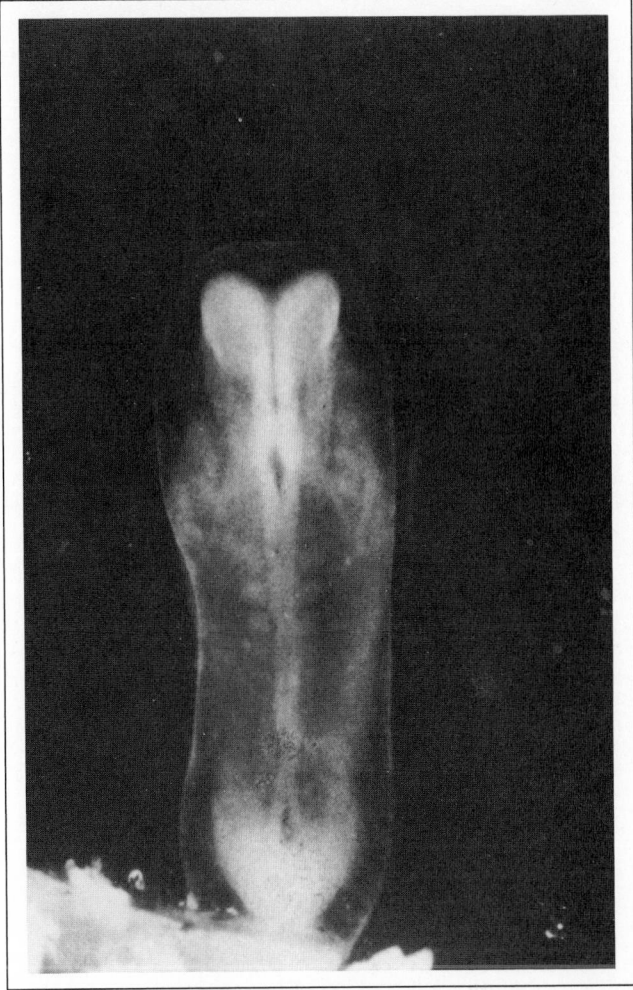

FIGURE 8–13 Third week. (Courtesy Drs. Roberts Pugh and Landrum B. Shettles.)

for the larynx. The first pouch, located just below the first arch, will form the eustachian tube and the cavity of the middle ear. The second pouch takes part in the formation of tonsils, and the third and fourth pouches contribute to the formation of the parathyroid and thymus glands. The fifth pouch is rudimentary and does not persist in the human embryo. The primordia of the eye and ear are also present. By about day 30, the arm and leg buds become prominent and, by day 35, they are well developed, with paddle-shaped hand and foot plates.

FIFTH WEEK

During the fifth week, the optic cups and lens vesicles of the eye form and the nasal pits develop. Partitioning in the heart occurs with the dividing of the atrium. The embryo has a marked C-shaped body, accentuated by the rudimentary tail and the large head folded over a protuberant trunk

(Text continues on p. 178.)

Table 8–2 Classification of Organ System Development

Gesta-tional age*	Length†	Weight	Nervous system	Musculoskeletal system	Cardiovascular system	Gastrointestinal system
Conception 2–3 weeks	2mm C–R		Groove is formed along middle of back as cells thicken; neural tube formed from closure of neural groove		Beginning of blood circulation; heart begins to form during third week	
4 weeks	4 mm C–R	0.4 g	Anterior portion of neural tube closes to form brain; closure of posterior end forms spinal cord	Noticeable limb buds	Tubular heart is beating at 24 days and primitive red blood cells are circulating through fetus and chorionic villi	Mouth: formation of oral cavity; primitive jaws present; esophagotracheal septum begins division of esophagus and trachea Digestive tract: stomach forms; esophagus and intestine become tubular; ducts of pancreas and liver forming
5 weeks	8 mm C–R	Only 0.5% of total body weight is fat (to 20 weeks)	Brain has differentiated and cranial nerves are present	Developing muscles have innervation	Atrial division has occurred	
6 weeks	12 mm C–R			Bone rudiments present; primitive skeletal shape forming; muscle mass begins to develop; ossification of skull and jaws begins	Chambers present in heart; groups of blood cells can be identified	Oral and nasal cavities and upper lip formed
7 weeks	18 mm C–R				Fetal heartbeats can be detected	Mouth: tongue separates; palate folds Digestive tract: stomach attains final form

Table 8–2   Classification of Organ System Development Cont'd   175

Genitourinary system	Respiratory system	Skin	Specific organ systems	Sexual development
Formation of kidneys beginning	Nasal pits forming		Endocrine system: thyroid tissue appears Eyes: optic cup and lens pit have formed; pigment in eyes Ear: auditory pit is now enclosed structure Liver function begins	Determination of sex
	Trachea, bronchi, and lung buds present		Ear: formation of external, middle, and inner ear continues Liver begins to form red blood cells	Embryonic sex glands appear
Separation of bladder and urethra from rectum	Diaphragm separates abdominal and thoracic cavities		Eyes: optic nerve formed; eyelids appear but are fused shut; thickening of lens	Differentiation of sex glands into ovaries and testes begins

Table 8–2 Classification of Organ System Development Cont'd

Gestational age*	Length†	Weight	Nervous system	Musculoskeletal system	Cardiovascular system	Gastrointestinal system
8 weeks	2.5–3 cm C-R	2 g		Digits formed; further differentiation of cells in primitive skeleton; cartilaginous bones show first signs of ossification; development of muscles in trunk, limbs, and head; some movement of fetus is now possible	Development of heart is essentially complete; fetal circulation follows two circuits — four extraembryonic and two intraembryonic	Mouth: completion of lip fusion Digestive tract: rotation in midgut; anal membrane has perforated
10 weeks	5–6 cm C-H	14 g	Neurons appear at caudal end of spinal cord; basic divisions of the brain present	Fingers and toes begin nail growth		Mouth: separation of lips from jaw; fusion of palate folds Digestive tract: developing intestines enclosed in abdomen
12 weeks	8 cm C-R, 11.5 cm C-H	45 g		Clear outlining of miniature bones (12–20 weeks); process of ossification is established throughout fetal body; appearance of involuntary muscles in viscera		Mouth: completion of fusion of palate Digestive tract: appearance of muscles in gut; bile secretion begins; liver is major producer of red blood cells
16 weeks	13.5 cm C-R, 15 cm C-H	200 g		Teeth: beginning formation of hard tissue that will become central incisors. Mother can detect fetal movement		Mouth: differentiation of hard and soft palate Digestive tract: development of gastric and intestinal glands; intestines begin to collect meconium
18 weeks				Teeth: beginning formation of hard tissue (enamel and dentine) that will become lateral incisors	Fetal heart tones audible with fetoscope at 16–20 weeks	
20 weeks	19 cm C-R, 25 cm C-H	435 g (6% of total body weight is fat)	Myelination of spinal cord begins	Teeth: beginning formation of hard tissue that will become canine and first molar Lower limbs are of final relative proportions		Fetus actively sucks and swallows amniotic fluid; peristaltic movements begin

Table 8–2 Classification of Organ System Development Cont'd   177

Genitourinary system	Respiratory system	Skin	Specific organ systems	Sexual development
			Ear: external, middle, and inner ear assuming final structure forms	External genitals appear similar
Bladder sac formed Urine formed			Endocrine system: islets of Langerhans differentiated Eyes: development of lacrimal duct	
	Lungs acquire definitive shape	Skin pink, delicate	Endocrine system: hormonal secretion from thyroid Immunologic system: appearance of lymphoid tissue in fetal thymus gland	
Kidneys assume typical shape and organization		Appearance of scalp hair; lanugo present on body; transparent skin with visible blood vessels	Eye, ear, and nose formed Sweat glands developing	Sex determination possible; descent of testes into inguinal canal at 12–24 weeks
	Final cellular structure of alveoli	Lanugo covers entire body; brown fat begins to form; vernix caseosa begins to form	Immunologic system: detectable levels of fetal antibodies (IgG type normally) Blood formation: iron is stored and bone marrow is increasingly important	

Table 8-2 Classification of Organ System Development Cont'd

Gestational age*	Length†	Weight	Nervous system	Musculoskeletal system	Cardiovascular system	Gastrointestinal system
24 weeks	23 cm C-R, 30 cm C-H	780 g	Structure of brain; looks like mature brain	Teeth: beginning formation of hard tissue that will become second molar		
28 weeks	27 cm C-R, 35 cm C-H	1250 g	Nervous system begins regulation of some body functions			
32 weeks	31 cm C-R, 40 cm C-H	2000 g	More reflexes present			
36 weeks	35 cm C-R, 45 cm C-H	2750 g		Distal femoral ossification centers present		
40 weeks	40 cm C-R, 50 cm C-H	3200+ g (16% of total body weight is fat)				

*Refers to gestational age of fetus/conceptus; postconception age.
†C-R = crown-rump; C-H = crown-heel

(Figure 8-14). The heart, circulatory system, and brain show the most advanced development. The brain has differentiated into five areas, and ten pairs of cranial nerves are recognizable.

SIXTH WEEK

At 6 weeks, the head structures are more highly developed and the trunk is straighter than in earlier stages (Figure 8-15). The upper and lower jaws are recognizable, and the external nares are well formed. The trachea has developed, and its caudal end is bifurcated for beginning lung formation. The upper lip has formed, and the palate is developing. The ear is developing rapidly, as are the other postbranchial body parts. The arms have begun to extend ventrally across the chest, and both arms and legs have digits, although they may still be webbed. There is a slight elbow bend in the arm, and the arm is more advanced in development than the leg. The embryo at this time has a prominent tail, but beginning at this stage, the tail will regress. The heart now has most of its definitive characteristics, and fetal circulation begins to be established. The liver begins to produce blood cells.

SEVENTH WEEK

At the seventh week the head of the embryo is rounded and nearly erect (Figure 8-16). The eyes have shifted from their original lateral position to a forward location, where they are closer together, and the eyelids are beginning to

Table 8–2 Classification of Organ System Development Cont'd   179

Genitourinary system	Respiratory system	Skin	Specific organ systems	Sexual development
	Respiratory movements may occur (24-40 weeks) Nostrils reopen Alveoli appear in lungs and begin production of surfactant; gas exchange possible	Skin reddish and wrinkled, vernix caseosa present	Immunologic system: IgG levels reach maternal levels Eyes structurally complete	
		Adipose tissue accumulates rapidly; nails appear; eyebrows and eyelashes present	Eyes: eyelids open (28-32 weeks)	Testes descend into scrotal sac
		Skin pale; body rounded; lanugo disappearing; hair fuzzy or woolly; few sole creases; sebaceous glands active and helping to produce vernix caseosa (36-40 weeks)	Ear lobes soft with little cartilage	Scrotum small and few rugae present; descent of testes into upper scrotum to stay (36-40 weeks)
	At 38 weeks, L/S ratio approaches 2:1	Skin smooth and pink; vernix present in skinfolds; moderate to profuse silky hair; lanugo hair on shoulders and upper back; nails extend over tips of digits; creases cover sole	Ear lobes stiffened by thick cartilage	Males: rugous scrotum Females: labia majora well developed

form. The palate is nearing completion, and the tongue also develops in the formed mouth. The gastrointestinal and genitourinary tracts undergo significant changes during the seventh week. Prior to this time, the rectal and urogenital passages formed one tube that ended in a blind pouch; they now separate into two tubular structures. At this point, the beginnings of all essential external and internal structures are present.

EIGHTH WEEK

At the eighth week the embryo is approximately 3 cm (1.2 in.) long and clearly resembles a human being (Figure 8–17). Face and features continue their development. External genitals appear but are not discernible, and the rectal passage opens, with the anal membrane now perforated. The circulatory system through the umbilical cord is well established. Long bones are beginning to form, and the large muscles that have developed are capable of contracting. By the end of the embryonic period, all major organ systems and external structures have been started, or have become completely established.

Fetal Stage

By the end of the eighth week the embryo has moved so far along in development that it can no longer be called an embryo and is now called a *fetus*, an offspring. No further primordia will form, every structure is present that will be

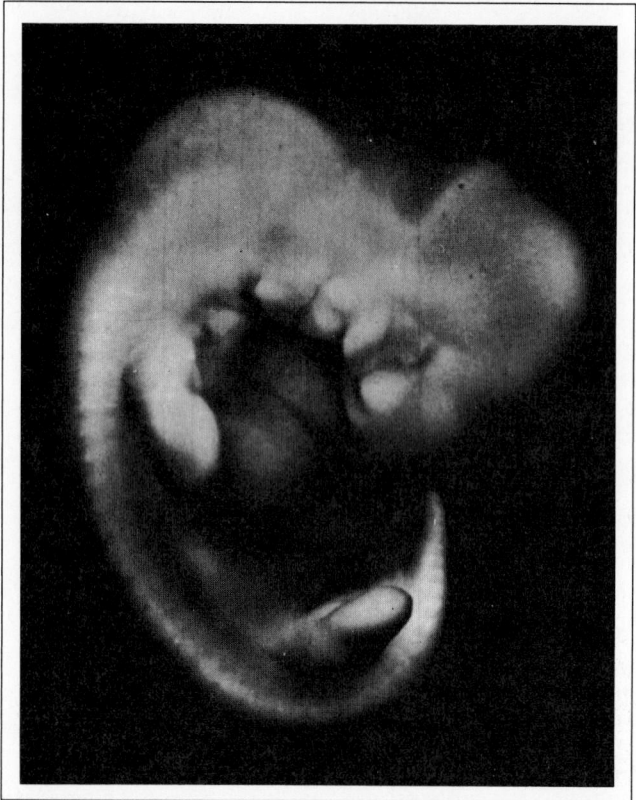

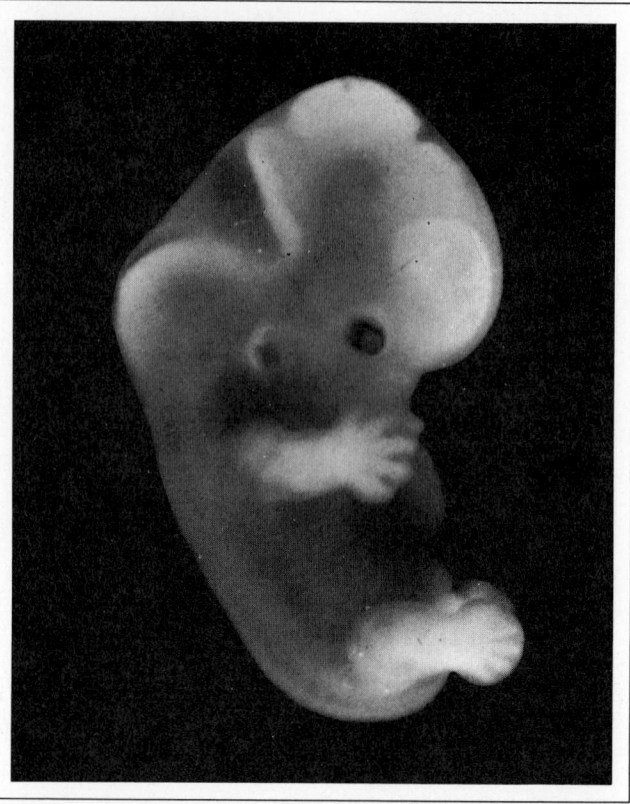

FIGURE 8–14 Fifth week. (Courtesy Drs. Roberts Pugh and Landrum B. Shettles.)

FIGURE 8–15 Sixth week. (Courtesy Drs. Roberts Pugh and Landrum B. Shettles.)

found in the full-term neonate. The rest of the gestational period is devoted to refinement of structures and organization and perfection of function.

9–12 WEEKS

The fetus by 10 weeks reaches a crown-to-rump length of 5 cm (2 in.) and probably weighs about 14 g. The head is large and comprises almost half of the fetus's entire size (Figure 8–18). The neck is distinct from the head and body, and both the head and neck are straighter than in previous stages of development. The face is well formed, with the nose protruding, the chin small and receding, and the ear acquiring a more adult shape. The eyelids close at about the tenth week and will not reopen until about 28 weeks. Some reflex movements of the lips suggestive of the sucking reflex have been observed at 3 months. Tooth buds now appear for all 20 of the child's first teeth (baby teeth). The limbs are long and slender, with well-formed digits. The fetus can curl the fingers toward the palm and make a tiny fist. The legs are still shorter and less developed than the arms. The urogenital tract completes its development, well-differentiated genitals appear, and the kidneys begin to produce urine. Red blood cells are pro-

duced primarily by the liver. Spontaneous movements of the fetus now occur.

13–16 WEEKS

At 13 weeks the fetus weighs 55–60 g and is about 9 cm (3.6 in.) in crown-to-rump length. Downy *lanugo hair* begins to develop, especially on the head. The fetal skin is so transparent that blood vessels are clearly visible beneath it. More muscle tissue and body skeleton have developed, which tend to hold the fetus more erect. Active movements are present—the fetus stretches and exercises its arms and legs. It makes sucking motions, swallows amniotic fluid, and produces meconium in the intestinal tract. Bronchial tubes are branching out in the primitive lungs, and sweat glands are developing. The liver and pancreas now begin production of their appropriate secretions.

17–20 WEEKS

Growth is rapid during the 17–20 week period. The fetus almost doubles its length and at 20 weeks now measures about 20 cm or 8 in. With this great increase in size, fetal weight increases to between 435 and 460 g. Lanugo cov-

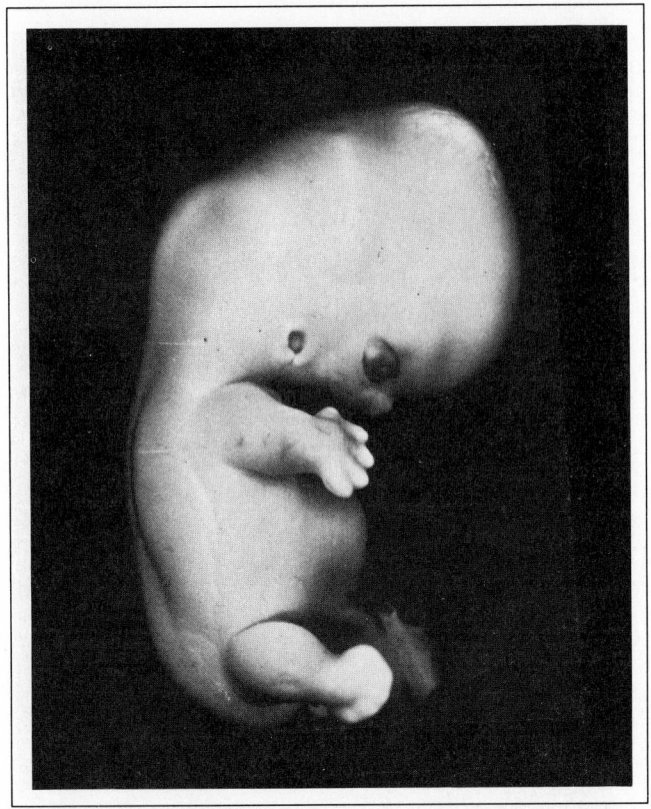

FIGURE 8–16 Seventh week. (Courtesy Drs. Roberts Pugh and Landrum B. Shettles.)

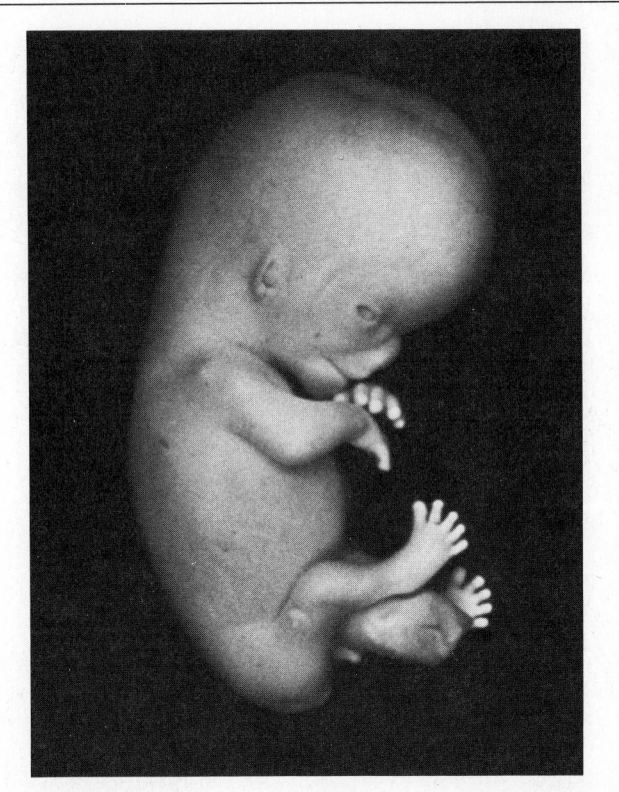

FIGURE 8–17 Eighth week. (Courtesy Drs. Roberts Pugh and Landrum B. Shettles.)

ers the entire body and is especially prominent on the shoulders. Subcutaneous deposits of brown fat have made the skin a little less transparent. Nipples now appear over the mammary glands. The head sports fine, "woolly" hair, and the eyebrows and eyelashes are beginning to form. The fetus has nails on both fingers and toes. Muscles are well developed, and the fetus is active. Fetal movement, known as *quickening*, is felt by the mother. The heartbeat is audible with the use of a stethoscope. Quickening and fetal heartbeat can assist in reaffirming maternal estimated delivery date.

21–24 WEEKS

The fetus at 24 weeks reaches a crown-to-heel length of 28 cm (11.2 in.). It weighs about 780 g (1 lb, 11 oz). The hair on the head is growing long, and eyebrows and eyelashes have formed. The eye is structurally complete and will soon open. The fetus has a reflex hand grip (grasp reflex), and by the end of the sixth month will have a startle reflex. Skin covering the body is reddish and wrinkled, with little subcutaneous fat. Skin on the hands and feet has thickened, with skin ridges on palms and soles forming distinct footprints and fingerprints. The skin over the en-

tire body is covered with a protective cheeselike fatty substance secreted by the sebaceous glands called *vernix caseosa*. The alveoli in the lungs are just beginning to develop.

25–28 WEEKS

At 6 calendar months the fetus has the appearance of a little old man; the skin is still red, wrinkled, and covered with vernix caseosa. During this time the brain is developing rapidly, and the nervous system is complete enough to provide some regulation of body functions. The eyelids open and close under neural control. If the fetus is a male, the testes begin to descend into the scrotal sac. Respiratory and circulatory systems have developed sufficiently. Week 28 has traditionally been considered the earliest period of extrauterine viability. In some current literature, it has been suggested that extrauterine viability begins as early as 24 weeks' gestational age (Ziegel and Cranley, 1979). However, very few infants delivered at this gestational age survive, no matter how expert their care is. At 28 weeks' gestation the lungs are still immature, and the fetus requires intensive specialized care to survive. The fetus at 28 weeks (Figure 8–19) is about 35–38 cm (14–

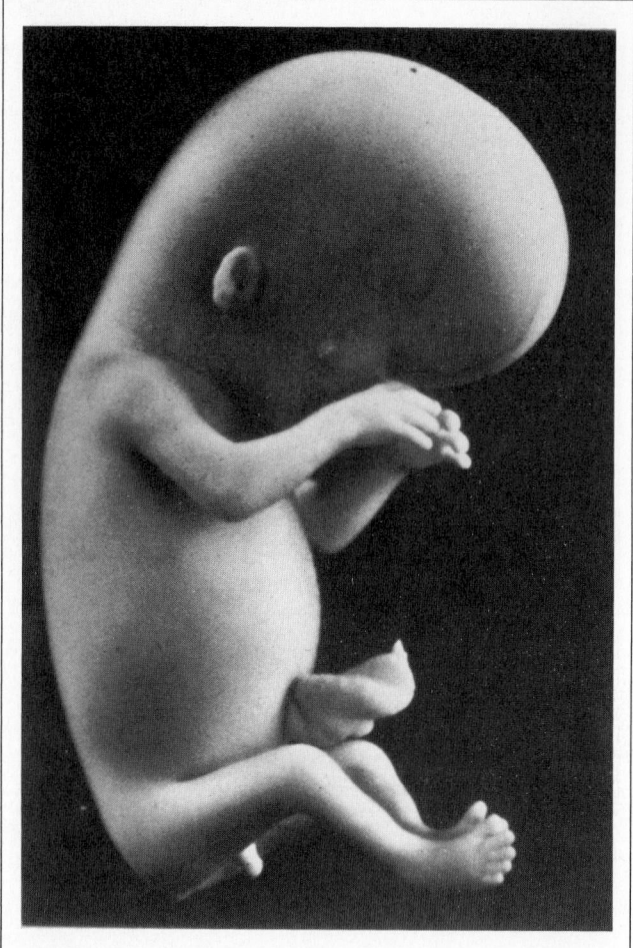

FIGURE 8-18 Ninth week. (Courtesy Drs. Roberts Pugh and Landrum B. Shettles.)

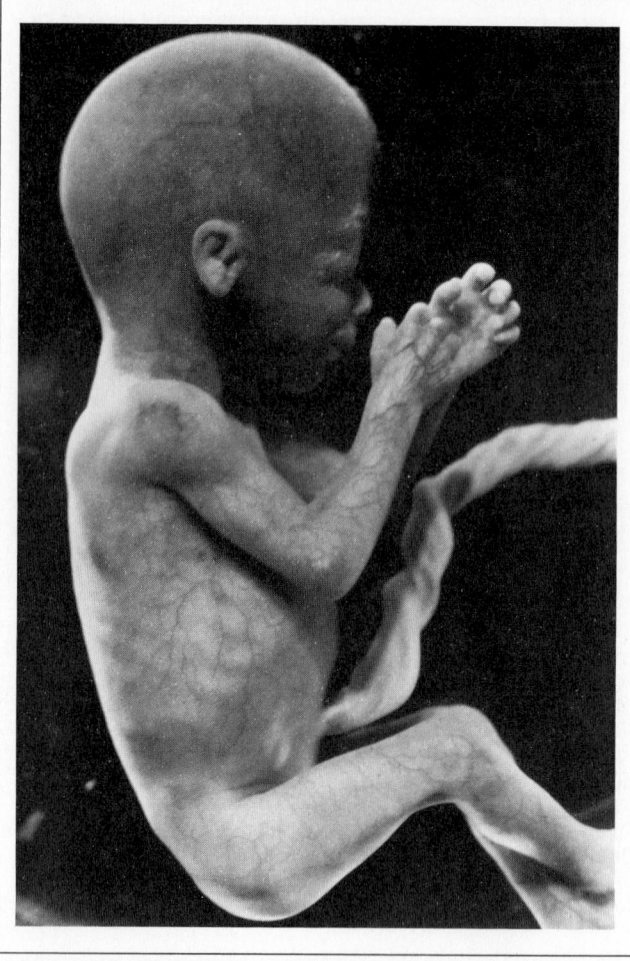

FIGURE 8-19 Twenty-eighth week. (Courtesy Drs. Roberts Pugh and Landrum B. Shettles.)

15 in.) long crown to heel and weighs about 1250 g (2 lbs, 15½ oz).

29-32 WEEKS

The fetus is gaining weight from an increase in body muscle and fat and weighs about 2000 g (4 lb, 6.5 oz) with a length of about 38–43 cm (15–17 in.) by 32 weeks of age. If born during this time, the infant has about a 60% chance of surviving with special care. The CNS has matured enough to direct rhythmic breathing movements and partially control body temperature. However, the lungs are not yet fully mature. Bones are now fully developed but are soft and flexible. The fetus begins storing minerals—iron, calcium, and phosphorus. In males, testicles may be located in the scrotal sac but are often still high in the inguinal canal.

33-36 WEEKS

The body and extremities of the fetus are "filling out" by 33–36 weeks. The fetus is beginning to get plump, with

less wrinkled skin covering the deposits of subcutaneous fat. Lanugo hair is beginning to disappear, and the nails have grown so they reach the edge of the fingertips. By 36 weeks of age the weight is usually 2600–2750 g (3 lb, 12 oz–6 lb, 1 oz) and the length of the fetus is about 42–48 cm (16–19 in.) long from crown to heel. If born at this time, the infant has a good chance of surviving but still requires some special care.

37-40 WEEKS

The fetus is considered full term at 38 weeks. Crown-to-heel length varies from 48–52 cm (19–21 in.) with males usually longer than females. Males also usually weigh more than females. The weight at term is about 3000–3600 g (6 lb, 10 oz–7 lb, 15 oz). The skin is pink and smooth with a polished look. The only lanugo hair remaining is on the upper arms and shoulders. On the head, the hair is no longer woolly but coarse and about an inch long. Vernix caseosa is still present but varies in amount, with heavier deposits remaining in creases and folds of the skin. The

Table 8-3   Developmental Vulnerability Timetable*

Weeks since conception	Common site of action of tetratogen	Potential malformation
3	Central nervous system	Ectopia cordis
		Ectromelia
		Sympodia
	Gastrointestinal tract	Omphalocele
4	Gastrointestinal tract	Omphalocele
		Tracheoesophageal fistula
	Central nervous system	Ectromelia
		Hemivertebra
	Heart, eye	Heart defects
5	Gastrointestinal tract	Tracheoesophageal fistula
	Central nervous system	Hemivertebra
	Eye	Nuclear cataract
		Microphthalmia
	Face	Facial clefts
	Arms and legs	Carpal or pedal ablation
6	Central nervous system	Congenital heart disease
	Heart	Gross septal or aortic abnormalities
	Ear and eye	Microphthalmia
		Lenticular cataract
	Teeth and mouth	Cleft lip, agnathia
	Arms and legs	Carpal or pedal ablation
7	Heart	Congenital heart disease
		Interventricular septal defects
		Pulmonary stenosis
	Arms and legs	Digital ablation
	Palate	Cleft palate, micrognathia
	Eye	Epicanthus
	Central nervous system	Brachycephaly
	External genitalia	Mixed sexual characteristics
8	Heart	Congenital heart disease
		Persistent ostium primum
	Face	Nasal bone ablation
	Central nervous system	Brachycephaly
	Arms and legs	Digital stunting

*Modified from Danforth, D. N. 1982. *Obstetrics and gynecology.* 4th ed. Philadelphia: Harper & Row, p. 265.

body and extremities are plump, with good skin turgor, and the fingernails extend beyond the fingertips. The chest is prominent but still a little smaller than the head, and mammary glands protrude in both sexes. The testes are in the scrotum or are palpable in the inguinal canals. As the fetus enlarges, amniotic fluid diminishes to about 500 mL or less, and the fetal body mass fills the uterine cavity. The fetus assumes what is referred to as its *position of comfort*, or *lie*. Generally, the head is pointed downward, because of the shape of the uterus and also possibly because the head is heavier than the feet. The extremities and often the head are well flexed. After the fifth month, feeding patterns, sleeping patterns, and activity patterns become established, so that at term the fetus has its own body rhythms and individual style of response.

Factors Influencing Embryonic and Fetal Development

Among factors that may affect embryonic development are the quality of the sperm or ovum from which the zygote was formed and the genetic code established at fertilization.

In addition, the adequacy of the intrauterine environment is important for optimal growth. If the environment is unsuitable before cellular differentiation occurs, all the cells of the zygote are affected. The cells may die, resulting in a spontaneous abortion, or growth may be slowed, depending on the severity of the situation. When differentiation is complete and the fetal membranes have formed, an injurious agent has the greatest effect on those cells undergoing the most rapid growth. Thus, the time of injury is critical in the development of anomalies.

Because organs are formed primarily during embryonic development, the growing organism is considered most vulnerable to noxious agents during the first months of pregnancy. Table 8–3 (p. 183) lists potential malformations related to the time of insult. Chapter 12 discusses the

effects of specific teratogenic agents on the developing fetus. Any agent, such as a drug, virus, or radiation, that can cause development of abnormal structures in an embryo is referred to as a *teratogen*.

The adequacy of the maternal environment is also extremely important to embryonic and fetal development. Those substances required for growth of a particular structure must be readily available at its time of development. In general, raw materials for development come from the mother's diet and not from her bodily reserves. Thus temporary deficiencies in the mother's diet, which may cause no manifest symptoms in her, may affect the developing embryo or fetus.

Research studies on animals have found that poor nu-

FIGURE 8–20 A, Formation of identical twins. **B,** Formation of fraternal twins.

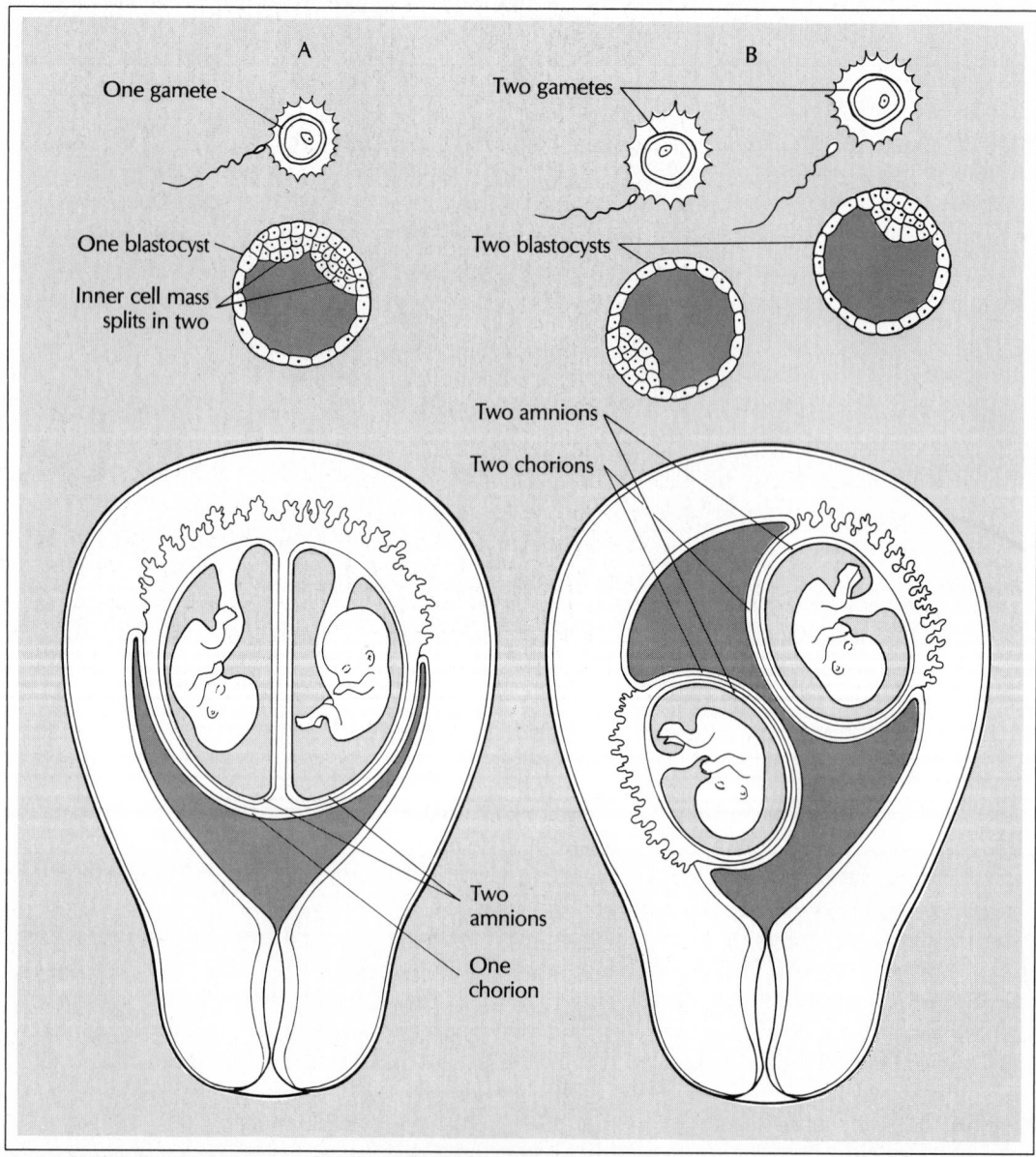

TWINS

trition produces specific developmental anomalies (Moore, 1977). Such research has not been conducted on humans, so generalizations about the effects of diet on human development are of limited validity. Data concerning infants born to mothers with reportedly deficient diets during pregnancy indicate smaller intrauterine growth and more susceptibility to infections, particularly respiratory infections, during the first year of life. It is believed that barely adequate maternal nutritional intake may sustain growth and development during early pregnancy but may not meet the needs of the rapidly growing fetus during late pregnancy.

The period of maximum brain growth begins with the fifth lunar month before birth and continues during the first 6 months after birth. Amino acids, glucose, and fatty acids are considered to be the primary dietary factors in brain growth. A subtle type of damage that affects the associative capacity of the brain, possibly leading to learning disabilities, may be caused by nutritional deficiency at this stage and is the subject of current research.

Maternal nutrition during pregnancy is discussed in Chapter 11.

Twins may be either fraternal or identical. If they are fraternal, they are *dizygotic*, which means they arise from two separate ova fertilized by two separate spermatozoa. They have two placentas, two chorions, and two amnions; however, the placentas sometimes fuse together and look as if they are one. Despite their birth relationship, they are no more similar to each other than they would be to siblings born singly. They may be the same or different sex.

Identical, or *monozygotic*, twins develop from a single fertilized ovum. Consequently, they are of the same sex and have the same genotype. Division of the single fertilized ovum into two units does not occur at the first cleavage division, as was once believed, but only after the embryo consists of thousands of cells. Complete separation of the cellular mass into two parts is necessary for twin formation. Identical twins have a common placenta and a single chorion but always two separate amnions (Figure 8–20).

Twins have been reported to occur more often among black than among white women and more often among white individuals than Orientals. Among all groups, as parity increases so does the chance for multiple births. In the United States, 2% of births are plural.

SUMMARY

From a single fertilized cell, through an orderly series of events, a complex human being develops and begins his or her existence. This process is one of the most dynamic events in nature. The period of embryonic and fetal development is characterized by rapid cellular division, multiplication, and differentiation and by formation of the structures necessary for intrauterine development in the placenta, fetal membranes, and umbilical cord.

It is essential that the nurse comprehend the processes and mechanisms of embryonic, fetal, and placental development to understand the various critical influences that timing of cellular division and environment have on the successful completion of this complex process.

References

Aladjem, S., and Lueck, J. 1982. Placental physiology. In *Gynecology and obstetrics*, vol. 3, ed. J. J. Sciarra et al. Hagerstown, Md.: Harper & Row.

Batzer, F. R. July 1980. Hormonal evaluation of early pregnancy. *Fertil. Steril.* 34(1):1.

Beer, A. E., and Billingham, R. E. April 1974. The embryo as a transplant. *Sci. Am.* 230:36.

Danforth, D. N. 1982. *Obstetrics and gynecology.* 4th ed. Philadelphia: Harper & Row.

DeCoursey, R. M. 1974. *The human organism.* 4th ed. New York: McGraw-Hill Book Co.

Dilts, P. V. June 1981. Placental transfer. *Clin. Obstet. Gynecol.* 24(2):555.

Gusdon, J. P., and Sain, L. E. March 1981. Uterine and peripheral blood concentrations and human chorionic gonadotropin and human placental lactogen. *Am. J. Obstet. Gynecol.* 39(2):705.

Koffler, H. June 1981. Fetal and neonatal physiology. *Clin. Obstet. Gynecol.* 24(2):545.

Langman, J. 1981. *Medical embryology.* 4th ed. Baltimore: Williams & Wilkins.

Martin, C. B., and Gingerich, B. Sept./Oct. 1976. Uteroplacental physiology. *J. Obstet. Gynecol. Neonatal Nurs.* 5 (suppl.):16.

Moore, K. L. 1977. *The developing human: clinically oriented embryology.* 2nd ed. Philadelphia: W. B. Saunders Co.

Naeye, R. L. Dec. 1981. Maternal blood pressure and fetal growth. *Am. J. Obstet. Gynecol.* 141(7):780.

Parer, J. T. 1974. Uteroplacental and fetal physiology. In *A clinical approach to fetal monitoring*. San Leandro, Calif.: Berkeley Bio Engineering, Inc.

Pritchard, J. A., and MacDonald, P. C., 1980. *Williams obstetrics*. 16th ed. New York: Appleton-Century-Crofts.

Rankin, J. H. G., and McLaughlin, M. K. Feb. 1979. The regulation of the placental blood flow. *J. Develop. Physiol.* 1:3.

Reynolds, S. R. M.; Freese, A. E.; Bueniarz, J.; and Caldeyro-Barcia, R. 1968. Multiple simultaneous intervillous space pressures recorded in several regions of the hemochorial placenta in relation to functional anatomy of the fetal cotyledon. *Am. J. Obstet. Gynecol.* 102:1128.

Seeds, A. E. Nov. 1980. Current concepts of amniotic fluid dynamics. *Am. J. Obstet. Gynecol.* 138(5):575.

Serón-Ferré, M.; Lawrence, C. C.; and Joffe, R. B. 1978. Role of hCG in the regulation of the fetal tone of the human fetal adrenal gland. *J. Clin. Endocrinol. Metab.* 46:834.

Silverstein, A. 1980. *Human anatomy and physiology*. New York: John Wiley & Sons.

Simpson, E. R., and MacDonald, P. C. 1981. Endocrine physiology of the placenta. *Ann. Rev. Physiology* 43:163.

Spence, A. P. 1982. *Basic human anatomy*. Menlo Park, Calif.: Benjamin/Cummings Publishing Co.

Vande Wiele, R. L., et al. 1976. Progesterones in pregnancy. In *Diabetes and other endocrine disorders during pregnancy and in the newborn*, ed. M. I. New and R. H. Fiser. New York: Alan R. Liss, Inc.

Vorherr, Helmuth. March 1982. Factors influencing fetal growth. *Am. J. Obstet. Gynecol.* 142(5):577.

Whaley, L. F. 1974. *Understanding inherited disorders*. St. Louis: The C. V. Mosby Co.

Winchester, A. M. 1966. *Heredity: an introduction to genetics*. New York: Barnes & Noble, Inc.

Ziegel, E., and Cranley, Mecca. 1979. *Obstetric nursing*. 7th ed. New York: Macmillan Co.

Additional Readings

Abramovich, D. R. 1981. Interrelation of fetus and amniotic fluid. *Obstet. Gynecol. Ann.* 10:27.

Anderson, D. F., et al. July 1980. Prediction of fetal drug concentration. *Am. J. Obstet. Gynecol.* 137(6):735.

Baker, H., et al. 1981. Role of placenta in maternal–fetal vitamin transfer in humans. *Am. J. Obstet. Gynecol.* 141(7):792.

Battaglia, F. C., and Meschia, G. 1981. Fetal and placental metabolism: their interrelationship and impact upon maternal metabolism. *Proc. Nutr. Soc.* 40(1):99.

Challis, J. R. G., and Patrick, J. E. 1980. The production of prostaglandins and thromboxanes in the feto-placental unit and their effects on the developing fetus. *Seminars in Perinatology.* 4(1):23.

Everett, R. B., and MacDonald, P. C. 1979. Endrocinology of the placenta. *Ann. Rev. Medicine.* 30:473.

Falkner, F. April 1981. Maternal nutrition and fetal growth. *Am. J. Clin. Nutrition.* 34:769.

Martin, C. B. 1981. Behavioral states in the human fetus. *J. Reprod. Med.* 26(8):425.

Nilsson, L., et al. 1975. *A child is born*. New York: Dell Publishing Co., Inc.

Rudolph, A. M., et al. April 1981. Fetal cardiovascular responses to stress. *Seminars in Perinatology.* 5(2):109.

Sadovsky, E. April 1981. Fetal movements and fetal health. *Seminars in Perinatology.* 5(2):131.

Van den Berg, B. J. April 1981. Maternal variables affecting fetal growth. *Am. J. Clin. Nutrition.* 34:722.

Varner, M. W., and Hauser, K. S. April 1981. Current status of human placental lactogen. *Seminars in Perinatology.* 5(2):123.

Young, M. April 1981. Placental factors and fetal nutrition. *Am. J. Clin. Nutrition.* 34:738.

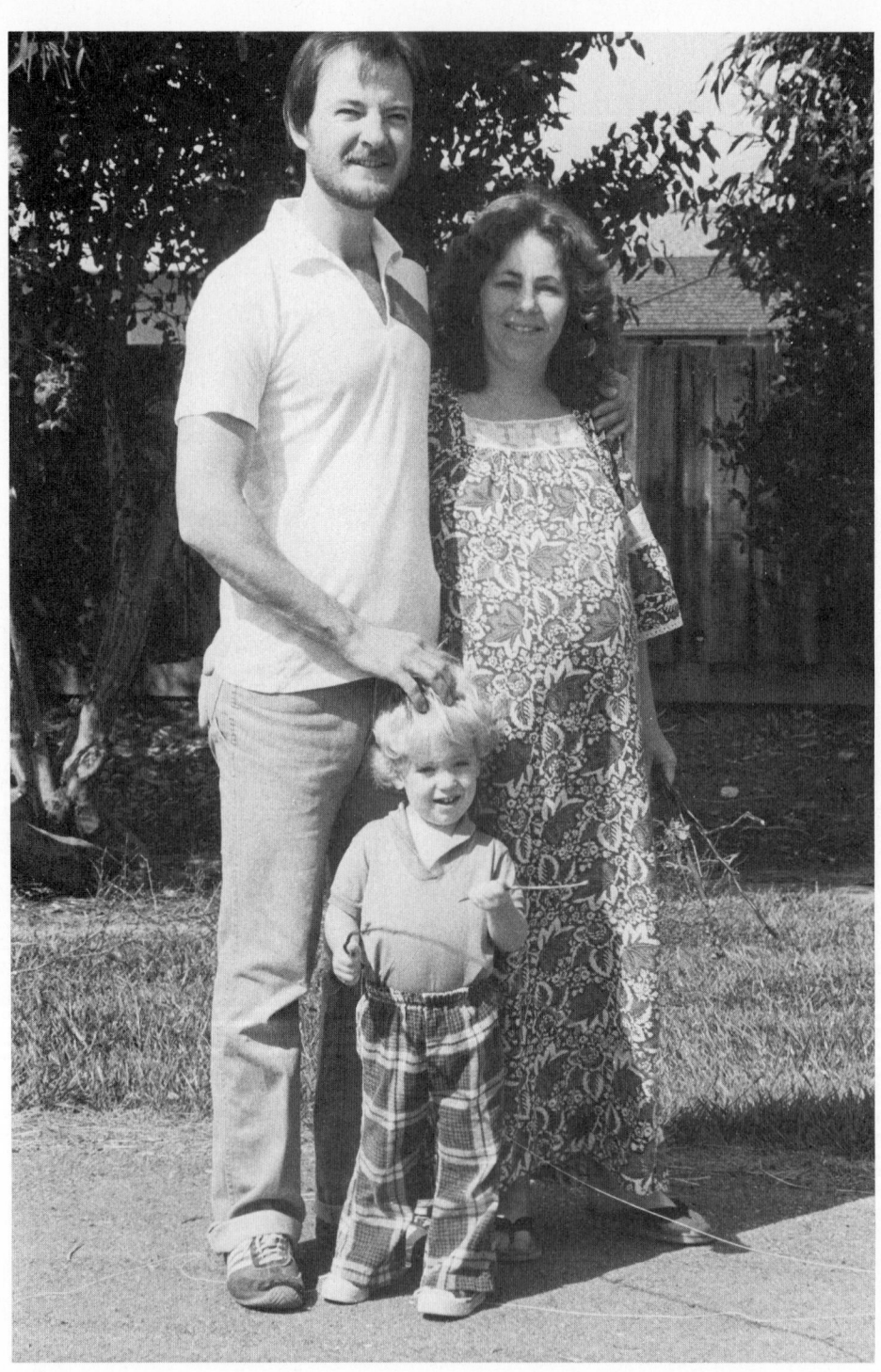

III

PREGNANCY

Chapter 9 ■ Physical and Psychologic
Changes of Pregnancy

Chapter 10 ■ Antepartal Nursing Assessment

Chapter 11 ■ The Expectant Family: Needs and Care

Chapter 12 ■ Complications of Pregnancy

Chapter 13 ■ Diagnostic Assessment of Fetal Status

■ 9 ■

PHYSICAL AND PSYCHOLOGIC CHANGES OF PREGNANCY

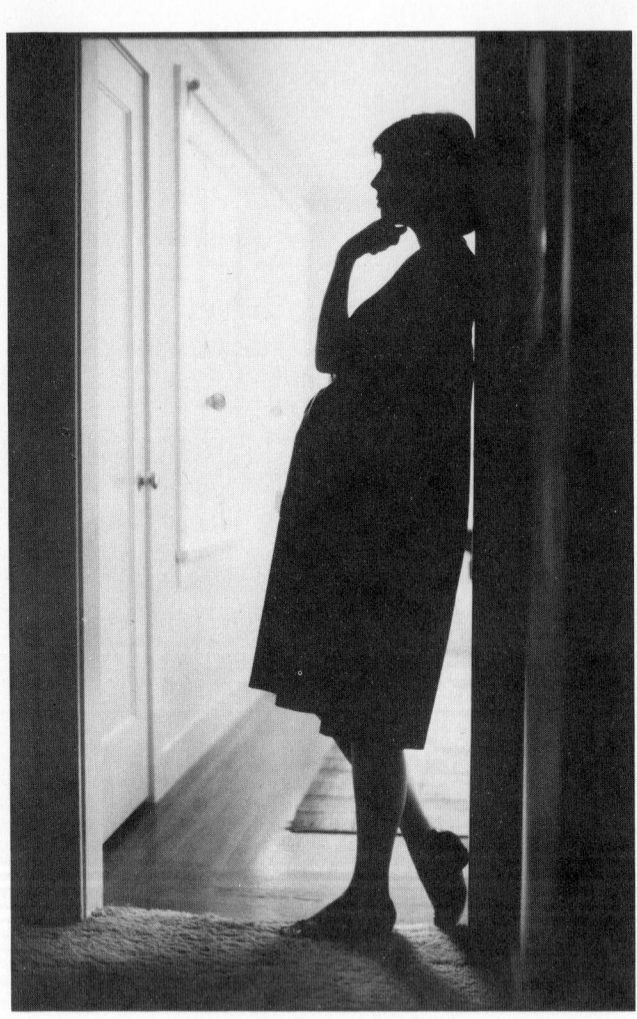

■ CHAPTER CONTENTS

SUBJECTIVE (PRESUMPTIVE) CHANGES

OBJECTIVE (PROBABLE) CHANGES

PREGNANCY TESTS
> Immunoassay
> Radioreceptor Assay
> Bioassay
> Over-the-Counter Pregnancy Tests

DIAGNOSTIC (POSITIVE) CHANGES

ANATOMY AND PHYSIOLOGY OF PREGNANCY
> Reproductive System
> Respiratory System
> Cardiovascular System
> Gastrointestinal System
> Urinary Tract
> Skin
> Skeletal System
> Metabolism
> Endocrine System

EMOTIONAL AND PSYCHOLOGIC CHANGES OF PREGNANCY
> Ambivalence
> Acceptance
> Introversion
> Emotional Lability
> Body Image

CULTURAL VALUES AND REPRODUCTIVE BEHAVIOR
> Health Beliefs
> Health Practices

■ OBJECTIVES

• Compare subjective (presumptive) and objective (probable) changes of pregnancy.

• Describe the various types of pregnancy tests that may be used to determine pregnancy.

• List the diagnostic (positive) changes of pregnancy.

• Relate the physiologic changes that occur in the body systems as a result of pregnancy to the signs and symptoms that develop.

• Discuss the emotional and psychologic changes that commonly occur in a woman during pregnancy.

• Identify cultural factors that may influence a family's response to pregnancy.

The duration of human pregnancy is 9 calendar months, 10 lunar months, 40 weeks, or 280 days. The dating of a pregnancy is estimated from the first day of the last menstrual period (LMP), making the actual gestation period about 266 days, with considerable variation possible. Ovulation occurs approximately two weeks before the menstrual period begins. The last menses provides the most specific time for dating a pregnancy, since the times of ovulation and fertilization are usually unknown. The commonly used method for estimating the length of pregnancy is Nägele's rule. (This and other methods to determine the delivery date are discussed in Chapter 10).

Pregnancy is divided into three trimesters, each a 3-month period. Each trimester has its own predictable developments, both fetally and maternally.

Generally, the diagnosis of pregnancy is not difficult for the clinician. In most cases the woman is fairly certain of the diagnosis when she presents herself for the initial office visit. For a woman with regular menstrual periods, the absence of one or more menses usually confirms the diagnosis. The objective diagnosis is based on the subjective symptoms of the pregnant woman and on certain clinical signs, which can be noted on physical examination and through laboratory procedures. Pregnancy causes both obvious and subtle changes involving the psyche and every organ system of the body.

SUBJECTIVE (PRESUMPTIVE) CHANGES

The subjective changes of pregnancy can be caused by other conditions (Table 9–1) and therefore are inconclusive and not diagnostic of pregnancy. The following can be diagnostic clues when other signs and symptoms of pregnancy are also present.

Amenorrhea is the earliest symptom of pregnancy. In a healthy woman whose menstrual cycles are regular, one missed menstrual period leads to the consideration of

pregnancy. The missing of successive menstrual periods increases the diagnostic value of this symptom.

Table 9–1 Differential Diagnosis of Pregnancy— Subjective Changes

Subjective changes	Possible causes
Amenorrhea	Endocrine factors: early menopause; lactation; thyroid, pituitary, adrenal, ovarian dysfunction Metabolic factors: malnutrition, anemia, climatic changes, diabetes mellitus, degenerative disorders Psychologic factors: emotional shock, fear of pregnancy or venereal disease, intense desire for pregnancy (pseudocyesis) Obliteration of endometrial cavity by infection or curettage Systemic disease (acute or chronic), such as tuberculosis or malignancy
Nausea and vomiting	Gastrointestinal disorders Acute infections such as encephalitis Emotional disorders such as pseudocyesis or anorexia nervosa
Urinary frequency	Urinary tract infection Cystocele Pelvic tumors Urethral diverticula Emotional tension
Breast tenderness	Premenstrual tension Chronic cystic mastitis Pseudocyesis Hyperestrinism
Quickening	Increased peristalsis Flatus (``gas'') Abdominal muscle contractions Shifting of abdominal contents

Nausea and vomiting are experienced by almost half of all pregnant women during the first 3 months of pregnancy and result from elevated hCG levels and changed carbohydrate metabolism. The woman may feel merely a distaste for food or may suffer extreme vomiting. These symptoms frequently occur in the early part of the day and disappear within a few hours and hence are commonly referred to as *morning sickness*. Some women may complain of nausea or vomiting in late afternoon and evening, especially in association with fatigue. This gastrointestinal disturbance usually appears about the end of the first month of pregnancy and disappears spontaneously 6–8 weeks later, although it may be prolonged in some instances.

Excessive fatigue may be noted within a few weeks after the first missed menstrual period and may persist throughout the first trimester.

Urinary frequency is experienced during the first tri-

Table 9–2   Differential Diagnosis of Pregnancy— Objective Changes

Objective changes	Possible causes
Changes in pelvic organs	Increased vascular congestion
Goodell's sign	Estrogen–progestin oral contraceptives
Chadwick's sign	Vulvar, vaginal, cervical hyperemia
Hegar's sign	Excessively soft walls of nonpregnant uterus
Uterine enlargement	Uterine tumors
Braun von Fernwald's sign	Uterine tumors
Piskacek's sign	Uterine tumors
Enlargement of abdomen	Obesity, ascites, pelvic tumors
Braxton Hicks contractions	Hematometra, pedunculated, submucous and soft myomas
Uterine souffle	Large uterine myomas, large ovarian tumors or any condition with greatly increased uterine blood flow
Pigmentation of skin	Estrogen–progestin oral contraceptives
Cholasma	
Linea nigra	Melanocyte hormonal stimulation
Nipples/areola	
Abdominal striae	Obesity, pelvic tumor
Ballottement	Uterine tumors/polyps, ascites
Pregnancy tests	Increased pituitary gonadatropins at menopause, choriocarcinoma, hydatidiform mole
Palpation for fetal outline	Uterine myomas

mester. In the early weeks of pregnancy, the enlarging uterus is still a pelvic organ and exerts pressure on the bladder. The increased vascularization and pelvic congestion which occurs in each pregnancy can also cause frequent micturition. This symptom decreases during the second trimester, when the uterus is an abdominal organ, but reappears during the third trimester when the presenting part descends into the pelvis.

Changes in the breasts are frequently noted in early pregnancy. Some women report significant breast changes prior to missing their first menses. Engorgement of the breasts due to the hormonal-induced growth of the secretory ductal system results in the subjective symptoms of tenderness and tingling, especially of the nipple area. Some women may report increased pigmentation of the areola and nipple and changes in Montgomery's glands.

Quickening, or the mother's perception of fetal movement, occurs about 18–20 weeks after the LMP. Quickening is a fluttering-type sensation in the abdomen that gradually increases in intensity and frequency. As with all the other symptoms of pregnancy, it can be simulated by other conditions.

OBJECTIVE (PROBABLE) CHANGES

The objective changes that occur in pregnancy are more diagnostic than the subjective symptoms. However, their presence does not offer a differential diagnosis of pregnancy (Table 9–2).

Changes in the pelvic organs are the only physical signs detectable within the first three months of pregnancy and are caused by increased vascular congestion. These changes are noted on pelvic examination. There is a softening of the cervix, referred to as *Goodell's sign. Chadwick's sign* is the deep red to purple or bluish coloration of the mucous membranes of the cervix, vagina, and vulva due to increased vasocongestion of the pelvic vessels. Pritchard and MacDonald (1980) consider Chadwick's sign a presumptive sign while Danforth (1982) considers it an objective sign. *Hegar's sign* is a softening of the isthmus of the uterus, the area between the cervix and the body of the uterus, which occurs at 6–8 weeks of pregnancy. This area may become so soft that on a bimanual exam there seems to be nothing between the cervix and the body of the uterus (Figure 9–1). *Ladin's sign* is a soft spot anteriorly in the middle of the uterus near the junction of the body of the uterus and cervix (Figure 9–2,A). *MacDonald's sign* is an ease in flexing of the fundus of the cervix.

The uterus assumes an irregular globular shape during the early months of pregnancy. Irregular softening and enlargement at the site of implantation, known as *Braun von Fernwald's sign,* occurs about the fifth week (Figure 9–2,B). Occasionally an almost tumorlike, asymmetrical enlargement occurs, called *Piskacek's sign* (Figure 9–2,C).

Generalized enlargement and softening of the body of the uterus are present after the eighth week of pregnancy. The fundus of the uterus is palpable just above the symphysis pubis at approximately 10–12 weeks' gestation and at the level of the umbilicus at 20–22 weeks' gestation (Figure 9–3).

Enlargement of the abdomen during the childbearing years is usually regarded as evidence of pregnancy, especially if the enlargement is progressive and is accompanied by a continuing amenorrhea. However, since obesity or a pelvic tumor can also cause such an enlargement, this change cannot be relied on exclusively as a diagnostic sign.

Braxton Hicks contractions are painless contractions of the uterus occurring at irregular intervals throughout pregnancy but felt most commonly after the twenty-eighth week. They are not a positive sign of pregnancy, since they have been noted in pathologic states also, as in cases of hematometra and pedunculated myomas. (See p. 415 for further discussion.)

Uterine souffle may be heard when auscultating the abdomen over the uterus. It is a soft blowing sound at the same rate as the maternal pulse and is due to the increased uterine vascularization and the blood pulsating through the placenta.

Changes in pigmentation of the skin and the *appearance of abdominal striae* are common cutaneous manifestations in pregnancy. The pigmentation of the nipple and areola may darken, especially in the primigravida and the dark-haired individual. The Montgomery tubercles, which are sebaceous glands of the areola, become enlarged. The skin in the midline of the abdomen may develop a pigmented line, known as the *linea nigra* (Color Plate II), which may also include the umbilicus and surrounding area. These pigmentation changes are hormonally induced. As the uterus enlarges, reddish, irregular, wavy, depressed streaks (striae) appear on the abdomen and buttocks as the underlying connective tissue breaks down. These changes occur in about one-half of all pregnant women.

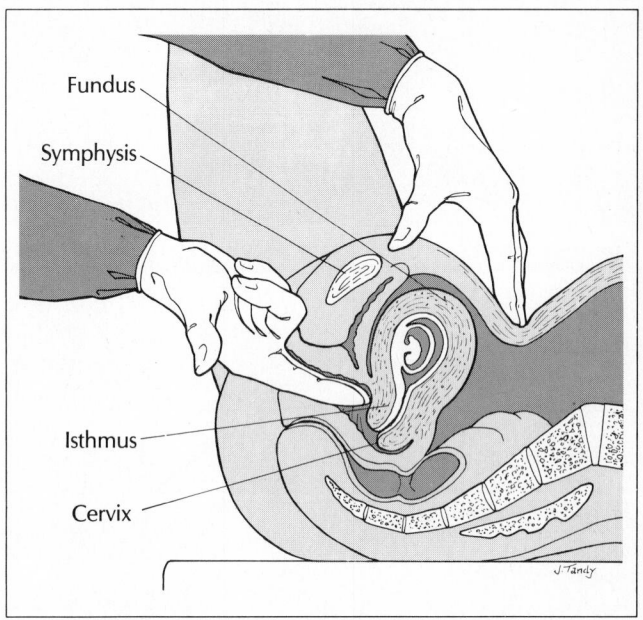

FIGURE 9–1 Hegar's sign.

Facial *chloasma* (also referred to as "mask of pregnancy"), or darkening of the skin over the forehead and around the eyes, occurs in varying degrees in pregnant women after week 16. This condition is aggravated with exposure to the sun. It is hormonally induced and usually fades after pregnancy.

The *fetal outline* may be identified by palpation in many pregnant women after 24 weeks of gestation, becoming easier to distinguish as term approaches. Uterine myomas may be mistakenly diagnosed as the fetal head or small parts. Hence, positive diagnosis of pregnancy cannot be made by palpation alone.

Ballottement is the passive fetal movement elicited by tapping the lower pole of the uterus/cervix with two fin-

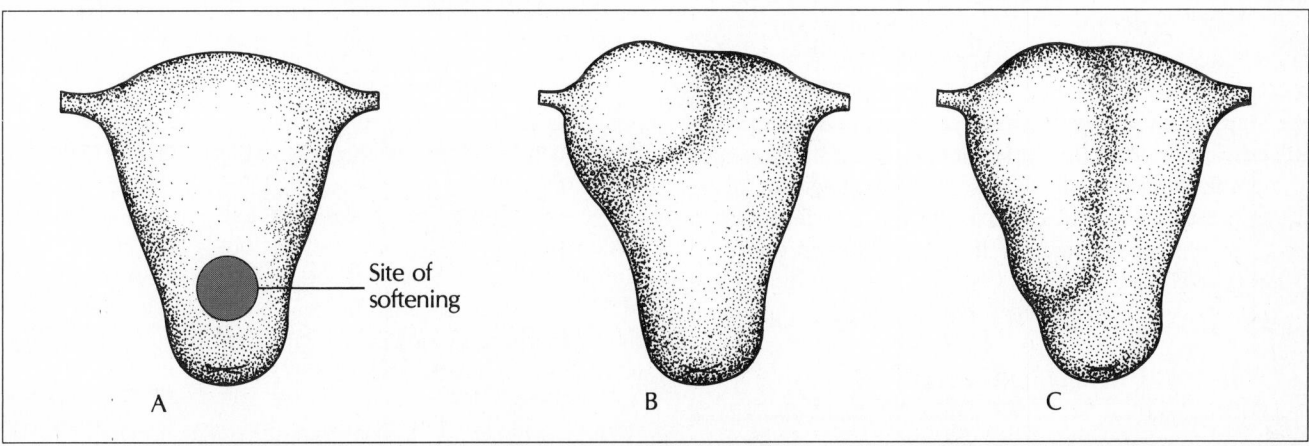

FIGURE 9–2 Early uterine changes in pregnancy. **A,** Ladin's sign. **B,** Braun von Fernwald's sign. **C,** Piskacek's sign.

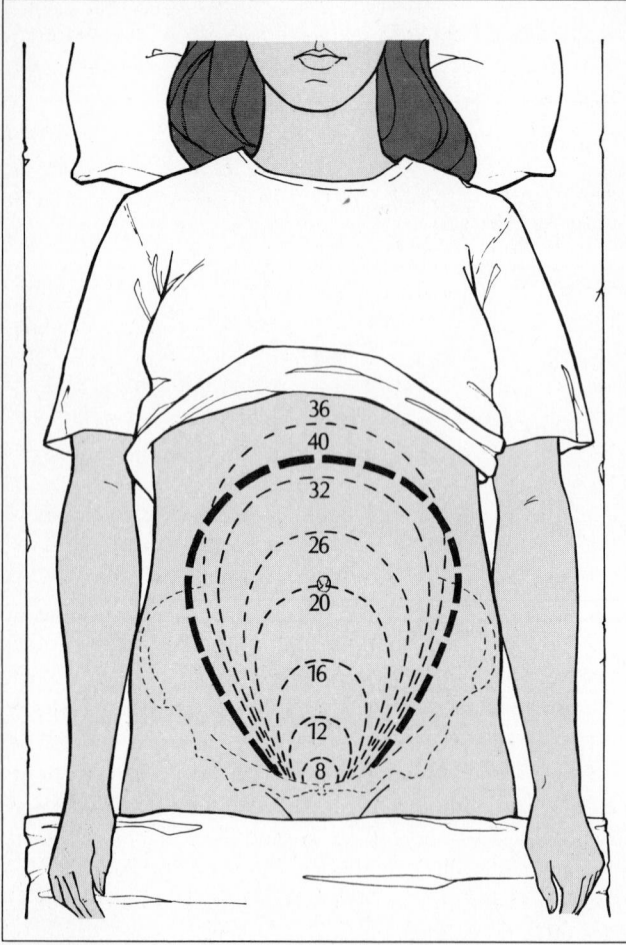

FIGURE 9-3 Approximate height of the fundus at various weeks of pregnancy.

gers inserted in the vagina. This pushes the fetal body up and, as it falls back, a bump or rebound is felt by the examiner.

Pregnancy tests are based on analysis of maternal blood or urine for the detection of human chorionic gonadotropin (hCG), the hormone secreted by the trophoblast. These tests are not considered positive signs of pregnancy because the similarity of hCG and the pituitary-secreted LH occasionally results in cross reactions. In addition, certain conditions other than pregnancy, such as the presence of a hydatidiform mole, cause elevated levels of hCG. While the levels of hCG tend to be much higher with a mole than in pregnancy, in the first 100 days after a missed period confusion may develop because higher levels may also occur initially in a multiple pregnancy.

PREGNANCY TESTS

The endocrine pregnancy tests are divided into three types: immunoassay, radioreceptor assay, and bioassay. Immunoassay and radioreceptor assay are reliable and the

results are quickly available, while the bioassay tests are subject to false results, require meticulous procedures, and take several days to obtain the results. Consequently, bioassays are seldom used and are described here primarily for historical value.

Immunoassay

The immunologic pregnancy tests are chemical urine tests that utilize the antigenic property of hCG. The tests are of three types:

1. *Hemagglutination-inhibition test (pregnosticon R)*. No clumping of cells occurs when the urine of a pregnant woman is added to the hCG-sensitized red blood cells of sheep.

2. *Latex agglutination tests (Gravidex and pregnosticon slide test)*. Latex particle agglutination is inhibited in the presence of urine containing hCG.

These two tests have an accuracy of approximately 95% in the diagnosis of pregnancy and 98% in determining the absence of pregnancy. The tests become positive approximately 10–14 days after the first missed menstrual period. The specimen utilized for the tests is the first early morning midstream urine because it is adequately concentrated for accuracy. The presence of protein substances (such as blood) in the specimen should be avoided because false positive results may occur.

3. *Solid-phase radioimmune assay or RIA (hCG and Preg/ Stat ß-hCG)*. This test, the newest development in the area of immunologic tests, utilizes an antiserum with specificity for the ß subunit of serum hCG in blood plasma. This means no cross reaction occurs with the ß subunit of LH, as with other tests. Thus, greater accuracy is possible. This radioisotope procedure requires about 1 hour to complete and becomes positive a few days after presumed implantation, thereby permitting earlier diagnosis of pregnancy. This test is also used in the diagnosis of ectopic pregnancy or trophoblastic disease.

Radioreceptor Assay (RRA)

Radioreceptor assay (Biocept-G) utilizes radio-iodine labeled hCG. It is a sensitive test and can be quickly performed in 1 hour, but because it fails to distinguish between hCG and LH, cross reactions may occur. This limitation may be overcome by setting the test sensitivity at 200 mIU/mL serum. Because this level is higher than the midcycle peak of LH (175 mIU/mL serum) confusion is avoided (Danforth, 1982).

Bioassay

The *Aschheim-Zondek test*, regarded as 98%–99% accurate, is the oldest and most reliable of the bioassay tests.

The urine of the presumably pregnant woman is injected into an immature female mouse. The mouse is then killed and the ovaries inspected for significant follicular change, which would indicate a pregnancy.

Friedman's test, a modification of the Aschheim-Zondek test, uses a virgin rabbit as the test animal. The test urine is injected into the animal on 2 successive days, with the animal being killed on the third day. The ovaries are inspected for follicular changes. Friedman's test is approximately 97% accurate.

The *male frog test* is a simple, rapid test based on the ability to induce the emission of spermatozoa by the male frog through injection with the urine of a pregnant woman. The test is positive if spermatozoa are detected in the urine of the frog ½–3 hours after the injection.

In the *female frog test*, the animal is injected with the urine of the presumed pregnant woman. The test is positive if the frog extrudes ripe eggs within 18 hours of injection.

The *Kupperman* or *rat hyperemic test* is less reliable than other bioassay tests. A female rat's ovaries are inspected for changes 2 hours after the injection of the woman's urine. The color changes, from pale pink to pink to dark red, are noted. Since the endpoint of color change is not sharp, a 10% rate of false negative results has been reported.

Over-the-Counter Pregnancy Tests

Over-the-counter pregnancy tests are available at the local pharmacy or drugstore for approximately $10. These tests, performed on urine, employ the hemagglutination-inhibition principle. The false positive rate of these tests is ≃5% while the false negative rate is ≃20% (Pritchard and MacDonald, 1980). Opinion varies about the advisability of making these tests available to nonprofessionals. Proponents suggest that the results will encourage women to seek care earlier in the event of pregnancy. Opponents suggest that once a woman has her pregnancy confirmd she may delay seeking care. They also believe that false results may lead to unnecessary anxiety or, more importantly, to a false sense of security or even relief.

DIAGNOSTIC (POSITIVE) CHANGES

The positive signs of pregnancy are completely objective, cannot be confused with pathologic states, and offer conclusive proof of pregnancy, but they are usually not present until after the fourth month of pregnancy.

The *fetal heartbeat* can be detected and counted by approximately week 17 to 20 of pregnancy. With the electronic Doppler device, it is possible to detect the fetal heartbeat as early as week 10 to 12 of pregnancy. The fetal heart rate is between 120 and 160 beats/min and must be counted and compared with the maternal pulse for

differentiation. Auscultation of the abdomen may reveal sounds other than that of the fetal heart. The maternal pulse, emanating from the abdominal aorta, may be unusually loud or a uterine souffle may be heard.

Fetal movements are actively palpable by a trained examiner after about the eighteenth week of pregnancy. They vary from a faint flutter in the early months to more violent movements late in pregnancy.

Radiologic examination is usually not possible until after the fourth month of pregnancy and depends on a variety of factors, such as the thickness of the abdominal wall and the radiologic technique used. Foci of ossification have been demonstrated as early as week 14, but a true fetal skeletal outline is not visible until week 16 of gestation (Pritchard and MacDonald, 1980). X-ray examinations are of special value in determining the death of a fetus or in differentiating a pregnant uterus from an abdominal tumor. This technique is not used to diagnose pregnancy per se, because of the possibility of causing gonadal damage and genetic abnormalities.

Fetal electrocardiographic evidence has been recorded as early as day 84 of pregnancy and offers proof of a living fetus. The failure to detect fetal cardiac electrical activity does not exclude an early pregnancy, nor does it necessarily indicate the death of a fetus.

Ultrasonic echosound is a technique that can be utilized as early as the sixth week of pregnancy for a positive diagnosis. The gestational sac can be observed by 5–6 weeks' gestation (3–4 weeks after conception); fetal parts and fetal heart movement can be seen as early as 10 weeks.

Fetal movement can be detected with the real-time methods at approximately 12 weeks after the LMP (10 weeks after conception). (See Chapter 13 for further discussion.)

ANATOMY AND PHYSIOLOGY OF PREGNANCY

Reproductive System

The changes in the body during pregnancy are most obvious in the organs of the reproductive system.

UTERUS

The changes in the uterus during pregnancy are phenomenal. Before pregnancy, the uterus is a small, semisolid pear-shaped organ measuring approximately 7.5 × 5 × 2.5 cm and weighing about 60 g (2 oz). At the end of pregnancy the dimensions are approximately 28 × 24 × 21 cm, with an organ weight of approximately 1000 g (2.2 lb). This growth represents an estimated 500- to 1000-fold increase in capacity.

The enlargement of the uterus is primarily a result of

hypertrophy of the preexisting myometrial cells (Figure 9–4). Individual cells have been shown to increase 17 to 40 times their prepregnant size as a result of the stimulating influence of estrogen and the distention caused by the growing fetus. The amount of fibrous tissue between the muscle bands increases markedly, which adds to the strength and elasticity of the muscle wall.

The uterine walls are considerably thicker during the first few months of pregnancy than during the nonpregnant state. The initial changes are stimulated by the increased estrogen and progesterone levels and not by mechanical distention by the products of conception. After approximately the third month, intrauterine pressure begins to be exerted by the uterine contents. The myometrial hypertrophy ceases at about the fifth lunar month and the musculature begins to distend, resulting in a thinning of the muscle wall to a thickness of about 5 mm or less at term. The ease of palpating the fetus through the abdominal wall attests to this thinning.

The circulatory requirements of the uterus increase as the uterus enlarges and the fetus and placenta develop. By the end of pregnancy, one-sixth the total maternal blood volume is contained within the vascular system of the uterus.

The irregular, painless Braxton Hicks contractions of the uterus, which occur intermittently throughout the menstrual cycle, continue during pregnancy. They are stimulated by increasing amounts of estrogen and increasing distention of the uterus. These contractions occur despite the inhibiting effect of progesterone. They may be felt through the abdominal wall beginning about the fourth month of pregnancy. During a contraction, the previously relaxed uterus becomes firm or hard and then returns to its previously relaxed state. It is postulated that these contractions stimulate the movement of blood through the intervillous

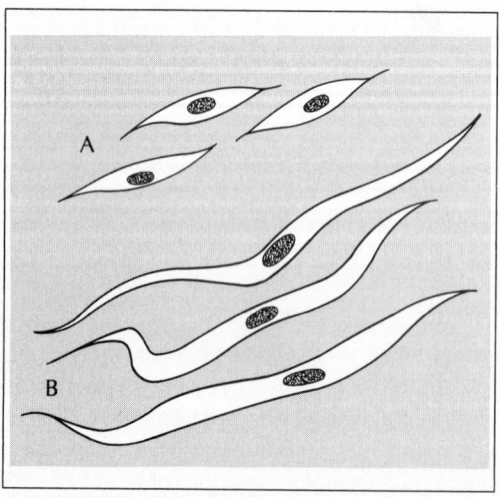

FIGURE 9–4 Hypertrophy of preexisting myometrial cells. **A,** Nonpregnant state. **B,** Pregnant state.

spaces of the placenta (Danforth, 1982). Some mothers report that Braxton Hicks contractions late in pregnancy are more uncomfortable than early labor contractions. Multigravidas tend to report greater incidence of Braxton Hicks contractions than do primigravidas.

CERVIX

The mucosa of the cervix undergoes marked changes during pregnancy. The glandular tissue becomes hyperactive and proliferates in number as well as in secretions. These increases are estrogen-induced. The endocervical glands occupy about half the mass of the cervix at term, as compared to a small fraction in the nonpregnant state. They secrete a thick, tenacious mucus, which accumulates and thickens to form the mucous plug that seals the endocervical canal and prevents the ascent of bacteria or other substances into the uterus. This plug is expelled when cervical dilatation begins. The hyperactive glandular tissue also causes an increase in the normal physiologic mucorrhea, at times resulting in extreme discharge. Increased vascularization causes both softening and the blue-purple discoloration of the cervix (Chadwick's sign). Increased vascularization is a result of hypertrophy and engorgement of the vessels below the growing uterus.

OVARIES

The ovaries cease ovum production during pregnancy. Many follicles temporarily develop but never to the point of maturity, because the appropriate hormonal stimulation is absent. The cells lining these follicles, the thecal cells, become active in hormone production and have been called the *interstitial glands of pregnancy.*

The corpus luteum persists and produces hormones until about week 10 to 12 of pregnancy. It engulfs approximately a third of the ovary at its peak of hypertrophy. By the middle of pregnancy, it has regressed to almost complete obliteration. Progesterone secretion by the corpus luteum increases and decreases in relation to its size, maintaining the endometrial bed until adequate progesterone is produced by the placenta to maintain the pregnancy.

VAGINA

The vaginal epithelium undergoes hypertrophy, increased vascularization, and hyperplasia during pregnancy. As with the cervical changes, these changes are estrogen-induced and result in a thickening of mucosa, a loosening of connective tissue, and an increase in vaginal secretions. The secretions are thick, white, and acidic (pH 3.5–6.0). The acid pH plays a significant role in preventing the invasion of pathogenic microorganisms. However, it also favors the growth of yeast organisms, resulting in moniliasis, a common vaginal infection during pregnancy.

As in the uterus, the smooth muscle cells of the vagina become hypertrophied, with an accompanying lessening of the supportive connective tissue. By the end of pregnancy, the vaginal wall and perineal body have become sufficiently relaxed to permit passage of the infant.

The increased vascularization of the uterus and cervix is also observed in the vagina. Within a short time after conception, the characteristic bluish purple color of Chadwick's sign is also seen in the vaginal mucosa.

BREASTS

Soon after the first menstrual period is missed, estrogen- and progesterone-induced changes are noted in the mammary glands. Increases in breast size and nodularity are the result of glandular hyperplasia and hypertrophy in preparation for lactation. By the end of the second month, superficial veins are prominent, nipples are more erectile, and pigmentation of the areola is obvious. Hypertrophy of Montgomery's follicles is noted within the primary areola. Striae may develop as the pregnancy progresses. Breast changes are often most noticeable in the primigravida.

Colostrum, a yellow secretion, may be expressed or leaked from the breast during the last trimester of pregnancy. This substance has more protein and minerals but less sugar and fat than mature milk. The antibody-rich colostrum persists for about 2–4 days after delivery, gradually undergoing conversion to milk.

Respiratory System

Pulmonary function is modified throughout pregnancy (Table 9–3). Pregnancy induces a small degree of hyperventilation as the tidal volume (amount of air breathed with ordinary respiration) increases steadily throughout pregnancy. There is a 30%–40% rise from nonpregnant values in the volume of air breathed each minute. Between weeks 16 and 40, oxygen consumption increases by approximately 15%–20%. The vital capacity increases throughout pregnancy while lung compliance and pulmonary diffusion remain constant. Measurements of airway resistance show a marked decrease in pregnancy in response to elevated progesterone levels. This permits increases in oxygen consumption, carbon dioxide production, and in the respiratory functional reserve (Aladjem, 1980).

The diaphragm is elevated and the substernal angle is increased as a result of pressure from the enlarging uterus. This change causes the rib cage to flare, with a decrease in the vertical diameter and increases in the anteroposterior and transverse diameters. The circumference of the chest may increase by as much as 6 cm. The increase compensates for the elevated diaphragm, and there is no significant loss of intrathoracic volume. Breathing changes from abdominal to thoracic as pregnancy progresses, and descent of the diaphragm on inspiration becomes less possible.

Nasal "stuffiness" and epistaxis are not uncommon. They occur because of estrogen-induced edema and vascular congestion of the nasal mucosa.

Table 9–3 Measurable Pregnancy Changes*

Parameter	Increase (%)	Decrease (%)	Unchanged
Respiratory system			
Tidal volume	30–40		
Respiratory rate			X
Resistance in tracheo-bronchial tree		36	
Expiratory reserve		40	
Residual volume		40	
Functional residual capacity		25	
Vital capacity			X
Respiratory minute volume	40		
Cardiovascular system			
Heart			
Rate	0–20		
Stroke volume	X		
Cardiac output	20–30		
Blood pressure			X
Peripheral blood flow	600		
Blood volume	48		
Blood constituents			
Leukocytes	70–100		
Fibrinogen	50		
Platelets	33		
Carbon dioxide		25	
Standard bicarbonate		10	
Proteins		15	
Lipids	33		
Phospholipids	30–40		
Cholesterol	100		
Gastrointestinal system			
Cardiac sphincter tone		X	
Acid secretion		X	
Motility		X	
Gallbladder emptying		X	
Urinary tract			
Renal plasma flow	25–50		
Glomerular filtration rate	50		
Ureter tone		X	
Ureteral motility			X
Metabolism			
Nitrogen stores	X		
Sodium stores	X		
Potassium stores	X		
Calcium stores	X		
Oxygen consumption	14		

*From Danforth, D. N., ed. 1982. *Obstetrics and gynecology.* 4th ed. Philadelphia: Harper & Row, p. 339.

Cardiovascular System

As the growing uterus exerts pressure on the diaphragm, the heart becomes displaced upward and to the left and is lengthened in the longitudinal and transverse diameters. Blood volume progressively increases beginning in the first trimester, increasing rapidly in the second trimester and slowing in the third to peak at term at 30%–50% above the pregestational level. This increase is related to a complex series of renal and cardiac factors and also to the elevated levels of estrogen found during pregnancy. Estrogen stimulates the adrenal secretion of aldosterone with resulting salt and water retention. Ultimately this interplay of factors leads to increased total body water and increased blood volume (Aladjem, 1980).

During pregnancy, organ systems receive additional blood flow according to their increased work load. Thus, blood flow to the uterus and kidneys is increased while hepatic and cerebral flow remains unchanged.

Frequently, the pulse rate increases during pregnancy, although the amount varies from almost no increase to an increase approaching 20%, or 10–15 beats/min, at term. The blood pressure remains relatively unaltered, with the lowest levels occurring during the second trimester and the highest levels during the last week of pregnancy.

The femoral venous pressure slowly rises as the uterus exerts increasing pressure on return blood flow. There is an increased tendency toward stagnation of blood in the lower extremities, with a resulting dependent edema and tendency toward varicose vein formation in the legs, vulva, and rectum late in pregnancy. The pregnant woman is more prone to develop postural hypotension because of the increased blood volume in lower extremities.

Pressure of the expanding uterus on the vena cava when the pregnant woman lies supine, the *supine hypotensive syndrome*, may produce marked decrease in the blood pressure with accompanying symptoms of dizziness, pallor, and clamminess. This may be prevented to a certain extent by the development of collateral circulation in the woman's back and abdominal wall.

Because the veins surrounding the spinal cord dura mater also increase in size, the cerebral spinal fluid space decreases. Consequently, a pregnant woman undergoing spinal anesthesia may experience a higher level of anesthesia and a greater drop in blood pressure than a nonpregnant woman (Aladjem, 1980).

The erythrocyte count declines slightly as a result of hemodilution. Although the concentration is lower, the total red blood cell volume actually increases about 33%. The hematocrit decreases by an average of about 7%, but the total amount of hemoglobin increases by an average of 12%–15% above prepregnancy levels. This increase is less than the plasma volume increase, so there is a decrease in hemoglobin concentration, which results in the *physiologic anemia of pregnancy (pseudoanemia)*. Even though the gastrointestinal absorption of iron is moderately increased during pregnancy, it is usually necessary to add supplemental iron to the diet to meet the expanded red blood cell and fetal needs.

Leukocyte production equals or is slightly greater than the increase in blood volume. The average cell count is 10,000–11,000/mm³, with an occasional woman developing a physiologic leukocytosis of 15,000/mm³. During labor these levels may reach 25,000/mm³. Although an estrogen-related cause has been suggested, the reason for this dramatic increase remains unknown.

The fibrin level in the blood is increased by as much as 40% at term, and the plasma fibrinogen has been known to increase by as much as 50%. The increased fibrinogen accounts for the nonpathologic rise of the sedimentation rate. Although the clotting time of the pregnant woman does not differ significantly from that of the nonpregnant woman, blood factors VII, IX, and X are increased so that pregnancy becomes a somewhat hypercoagulable state. When these changes are coupled with venous stasis in late pregnancy, it becomes obvious that the pregnant woman has an increased risk of developing venous thrombosis.

The body's physiologic response to reduce risks associated with pregnancy includes: (a) coagulation/fibrinolysis equilibrium, (b) increased blood volume, (c) increased red blood cells, and (d) increased oxygenation of tissues.

Gastrointestinal System

Many of the discomforts of pregnancy are attributed to the changes in the gastrointestinal system. Nausea and vomiting, so common during early pregnancy, are associated with the hCG secreted by the nidated ovum and with a change in carbohydrate metabolism that occurs in early pregnancy. Peculiarities of taste and smell are also common and can further aggravate gastrointestinal discomfort. Gum tissue may become softened and may bleed when only mildly traumatized. Oral and gastric secretions are altered with hypersalivation, or ptyalism, sometimes becoming excessive; decreased gastric acidity is the most noteworthy change.

In later months of pregnancy, numerous gastrointestinal symptoms are attributable to the pressure of the growing uterus. Anatomically, the intestines are displaced laterally and posteriorly and the stomach superiorly. Heartburn (pyrosis) is caused by the reflux of acidic secretions from the stomach into the lower esophagus as a result of relaxation of the cardiac sphincter. Gastric emptying time and intestinal motility are delayed, leading to frequent complaints of bloating and constipation, which can be aggravated further by smooth muscle relaxation stimulated by the high level of placental progesterone and by increased electrolyte and water reabsorption in the large intestine. Hemorrhoids frequently develop in late pregnancy from the pressure on vessels below the level of the uterus.

Only minor liver changes occur with pregnancy. Because of the effects on the liver of high levels of circulating estrogen and progesterone, symptoms of cholestasis and pruritus gravidarum may occur, but they subside after delivery. Plasma albumin concentrations and serum cholinesterase activity decrease with normal pregnancy as with certain liver diseases. Spider nevi and palmar erythema, also seen with hepatic diseases, may occur transiently during pregnancy.

The emptying time of the gallbladder is prolonged during pregnancy as a result of smooth muscle relaxation from progesterone. Hypercholesterolemia may follow, and it can predispose the woman to gallstone formation.

Urinary Tract

The kidneys, ureters, and bladder undergo striking changes in both structure and function. The growing uterus puts pressure on the bladder and bladder irritation is present until the uterus rises out of the pelvis. Near term, when the presenting part engages in the pelvis, pressure is again exerted on the bladder. This pressure can impair the drainage of blood and lymph from the hyperemic bladder, rendering it more susceptible to infection and trauma. The bladder, normally a convex organ, is rendered concave from the external pressure, and its retention capacity is greatly reduced.

Dilatation of the kidney and ureter may occur, most frequently on the right side, above the pelvic brim, due to the lie of the uterus. This dilatation is accompanied by an elongation and curvature of the ureter. There appears to be no single factor accounting for this anatomic variation but rather a combination of ureteral atonia and hypoperistalsis, possibly caused by the placental progesterone and by pressure from the enlarging fetus. The same type of hydroureter and bladder relaxation can be produced in the nonpregnant female with massive doses of progesterone.

The glomerular filtration rate (GFR) and renal plasma flow (RPF) increase early in pregnancy. The RPF increases rapidly in the first trimester by 25%–50%; little change occurs in the second trimester; and a drop to near normal levels occurs by term. The GFR rises by as much as 50% by the beginning of the second trimester and remains elevated until delivery. The mechanism for these rises remains unclear, but hPL may play a part as it possesses properties similar to the pituitary growth hormone and has been shown experimentally to produce rises. The influence of posture on GFR and RPF is unclear, with different studies producing varying and contradictory results.

An increased renal tubular reabsorption rate compensates for the increased glomerular activity. Glycosuria is not uncommon or necessarily pathogenic during pregnancy but is merely a reflection of the kidneys' inability to reabsorb all of the glucose filtered by the glomeruli. However, pregnancy can be diabetogenic, so the possibility of diabetes mellitus cannot be disregarded.

The increased renal function during pregnancy results in an increased clearance of urea and creatinine and in a lowering of the blood urea and nonprotein nitrogen values. Because of this, measurement of creatinine clearance provides an accurate test of renal functioning during pregnancy.

Skin

Changes in skin pigmentation commonly occur during pregnancy, in various areas of the body, stimulated by elevated levels of melanocyte-stimulating hormone, which may, in turn, result from the increased estrogen and progesterone (Pritchard and MacDonald, 1980). In a fair-complexioned woman the nipple and areolar areas of the breasts darken. The abdominal wall frequently develops linea nigra and striae. Striae may occur as a result of reduced connective tissue strength due to elevated adrenal steroid levels. The cervix, vagina, and vulva become darker. Pigmentation of the cheeks, forehead, and nose may also occur. This facial chloasma is more prominent in dark-haired women and is occasionally disfiguring. Fortunately, it fades, or at least regresses soon after delivery when the hormonal influence of pregnancy has stopped. In addition, the sweat and sebaceous glands are frequently hyperactive during pregnancy.

Vascular spider nevi may develop on the chest, neck, face, arms, and legs. They are small bright-red elevations of the skin radiating from a central body. This condition frequently occurs in conjunction with palmar erythema and is of no clinical significance. Both usually disappear shortly after the termination of pregnancy, when there is a decrease in estrogen levels within the tissues.

Skeletal System

No demonstrable changes in the teeth of the pregnant woman occur. No demineralization takes place. The fairly common occurrence of dental caries during pregnancy has led to the myth, "A tooth for every pregnancy." James's research showed that a dog maintained on a calcium-poor diet during pregnancy has a resultant decalcification of its bone but that its teeth show no change (Worthington et al., 1977). The dental caries that may accompany pregnancy are more often caused by a slight decrease in salivary pH and by inadequate oral hygiene and dental care.

With a well-balanced diet, the pregnant woman's calcium and phosphorus requirements of 1.2 g/day can be met. This is an increase of 0.4 g over the needs of the nonpregnant body.

The sacroiliac, sacrococcygeal, and pubic joints of the pelvis relax in the later part of the pregnancy, presumably as a result of hormonal changes. The result is often a waddling gait. A slight separation of the symphysis pubis can often be demonstrated on radiologic examination.

As the pregnant woman's center of gravity gradually

FIGURE 9-5 Postural changes during pregnancy.

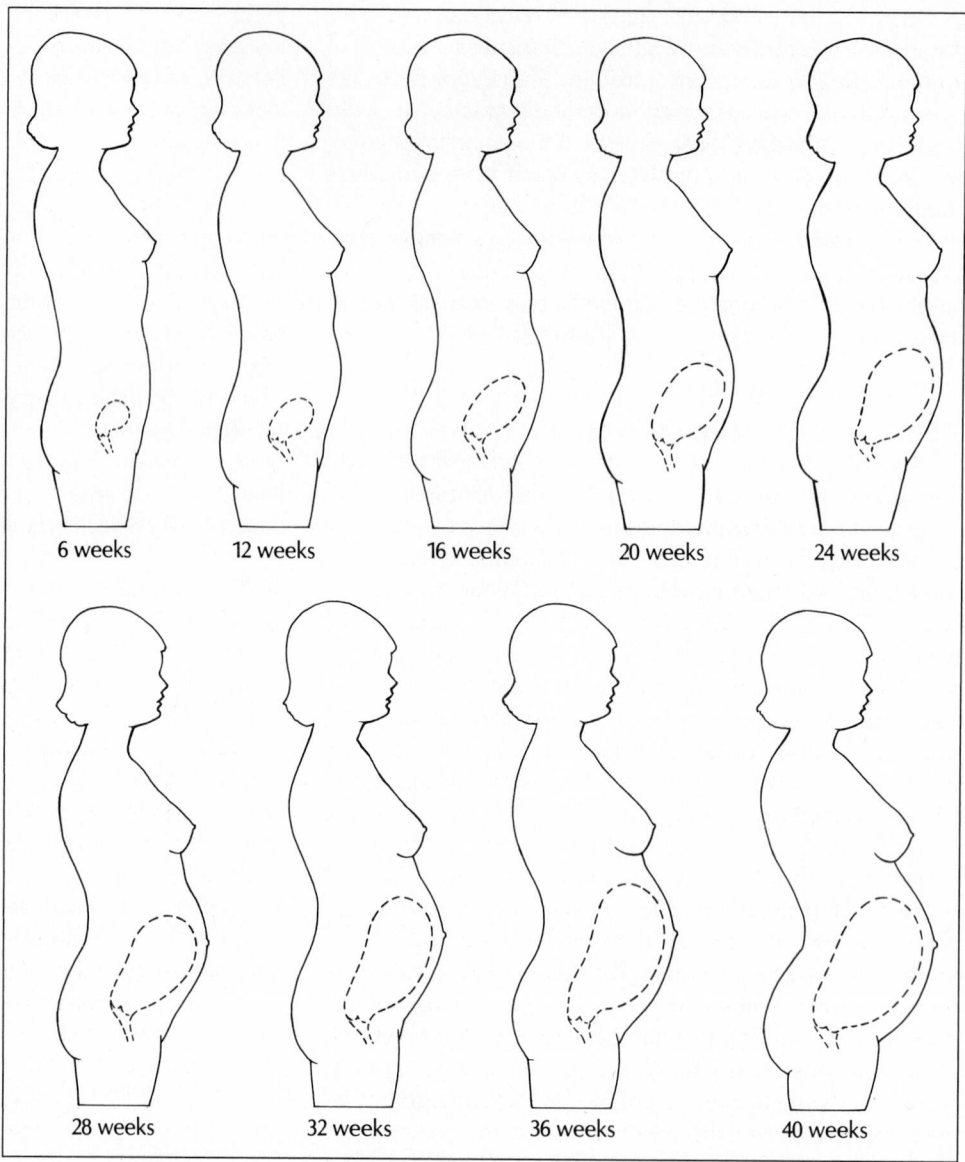

| 6 weeks | 12 weeks | 16 weeks | 20 weeks | 24 weeks |

| 28 weeks | 32 weeks | 36 weeks | 40 weeks |

changes, there is an accentuation of the lumbodorsal spinal curve and a posture change (Figure 9–5). This posture change compensates for the increased weight of the uterus anteriorly and frequently results in low backache. Late in pregnancy, neck, shoulder, and upper extremity aching may occur from shoulder slumping and anterior flexion of the neck accompanying the lumbodorsal lordosis.

Metabolism

Most metabolic functions accelerate during pregnancy to support the additional demands of the growing fetus and its support system. The expectant mother must meet her own tissue replacement needs, those of the conceptus, and those preparatory for labor and lactation.

WEIGHT GAIN

The average weight gain during a normal pregnancy is 25–30 lb or 11.0–13.6 kg. Weight may decrease slightly during the first trimester due to nausea, vomiting, and food intolerances of early pregnancy. But the lost weight is soon regained, and an average increase of 3, 12, and 12 lb occurs in the first, second, and third trimesters, respectively. The total weight gain may be accounted for as follows: fetus, 7½ lb; placenta and membranes, 1½ lb; amniotic fluid, 2 lb; uterus, 2½ lb; breasts, 3 lb; and increased blood volume, 2–4 lb. The remaining 4–9 lb is extravascular fluid and fat reserves.

WATER METABOLISM

Increased water retention is one of the basic chemical alterations of pregnancy. Several interrelated factors cause this phenomenon. The increased level of steroid sex hormones affects sodium and fluid retention. The lowered serum protein also influences the fluid balance, as does the increased intracapillary pressure and permeability. The products of conception—fetus, placenta, and amniotic fluid—account for an average increase of 3.5 L of water. Another increase of 3.5 L is contained within the mother's hypertrophied organs and augmented blood volume and interstitial fluids. The extracellular fluid is distributed primarily below the uterus, the area of elevated venous pressure.

NUTRIENT METABOLISM

The fetus makes its greatest protein and fat demands during the last half of gestation; it doubles in weight in the last 6–8 weeks. The increased nitrogen (*protein*) retention that begins in early pregnancy is initially utilized for hyperplasia and hypertrophy of maternal tissues, such as the uterus and breasts. Nitrogen must be stored during pregnancy to maintain a constant level within the breast milk and to avoid depletion of maternal tissues.

Fats are more completely absorbed during pregnancy, resulting in a marked increase in the serum lipids, lipoproteins and cholesterol, and decreased elimination through the bowel. Fat deposits in the fetus increase from about 2% at midpregnancy to almost 12% at term. The excess nitrogen and lipidemia are considered to be a preparation for lactation.

Carbohydrate needs increase, especially during the last two trimesters. Ketosis can be a problem, especially with the diabetic woman, due to glycosuria, reduced alkaline reserves, and lipidemia. Intermittent glycosuria is not uncommon during pregnancy. When it is not accompanied by a rise in blood sugar levels, glycosuria is a physiologic entity secondary to the increased glomerular filtration rate. Fasting blood sugar levels tend to fall slightly to an average of 80–85 mg/dL, returning to more normal levels by the sixth postpartal month. The oral glucose tolerance test shows no change with pregnancy.

The possibility of *diabetes* must not be overlooked during pregnancy. Plasma levels of insulin are increased during pregnancy, and rapid destruction of insulin takes place within the placenta. Insulin production must be increased by the mother, and any marginal pancreatic function becomes apparent. The diabetic woman often experiences increased exogenous insulin demands during pregnancy.

MINERAL AND VITAMIN METABOLISM

The demand for *iron* during pregnancy is accelerated, and the pregnant woman must guard against anemia. Iron is necessary for the increase in erythrocytes, hemoglobin, and blood volume, as well as for the increased tissue demands of both woman and fetus.

Iron transfer takes place at the placenta in only one direction: toward the fetus. It has been demonstrated that approximately five-sixths of the iron stored in the fetal liver has been assimilated during the last trimester of pregnancy. This stored iron in the fetal liver compensates in the first four months of neonatal life for the normal inadequate amounts of iron available in breast milk and non-iron-fortified formulas.

The progressive absorption and retention of *calcium* during pregnancy has been noted. The maternal plasma concentration of bound calcium decreases as the levels of bindable plasma proteins fall. Approximately 30 g of calcium is retained in maternal bone for fetal deposition late in pregnancy.

Pregnancy produces little change in the metabolism of most other minerals other than retention of amounts needed for fetal growth.

Vitamin metabolism does not change appreciably with pregnancy (see p. 270 for requirements of minerals and vitamins).

Endocrine System

THYROID

Pregnancy influences the thyroid gland's size and activity. Often a palpable change is noted, which represents an increase in vascularity and hyperplasia of glandular tissue. The accompanying rise in the amount of iodine in the blood is in the form of thyroxine, with thyroxine-binding capacity increasing as early as the third week of pregnancy and continuing until term. Increased thyroxine-binding capacity is represented by the change in serum protein-bound iodine (PBI) from a nonpregnant level of 4–8 μg/dL to a pregnant level of 7–12 μg/dL. The presumable cause is the increase in circulating estrogens; the same situation can be simulated by the exogenous administration of estrogens, including oral contraceptives, to the nonpregnant woman.

The basal metabolism rate (BMR) rises to a +25% level in late pregnancy. Blood studies and BMR indicate the existence of hyperthyroidism, but it is not present clinically. Within a few weeks after parturition, all thyroid function is within normal limits. It should be noted that, in the presence of hypothyroidism, spontaneous abortion often occurs.

PARATHYROID

The concentration of the hormone secreted by the parathyroids and the size of the glands increase, paralleling the fetal calcium requirements. Parathyroid hormone concentration reaches its highest level between 15 and 35 weeks of gestation, returning to a normal or even subnormal level before parturition.

PITUITARY

Enlargement of the pituitary gland is greatest during the last month of gestation, but it returns to normal size after delivery. There is no significant change in the posterior lobe of the gland, although the anterior lobe increases in weight with each successive pregnancy. On rare occasions the enlarged anterior lobe causes pressure on the optic chiasm, resulting in restriction of the visual field. Visual impairment subsides spontaneously postpartally as the gland recedes in size.

Pregnancy is made possible by the hypothalamic stimulation of the anterior pituitary hormones: FSH, which stimulates ova growth, and LH, which effects ovulation. Pituitary stimulation prolongs the corpus luteal phase of the ovary, which maintains the secretory endometrium for development of the pregnancy (see Chapter 8). Two additional pituitary hormones, thyrotropin and adrenotropin, alter maternal metabolism to support the pregnancy. Prolactin, also an anterior pituitary secretion, is responsible for initial lactation. (Continued lactation depends on the suckling of the infant.)

The posterior pituitary contains the mechanism for the release of oxytocin and vasopressin, which exert three physiologic effects: oxytocic, vasopressor, and antidiuretic. The main effects of oxytocin are the promotion of uterine contractility and the stimulation of milk ejection from the breasts. Vasopressin causes vasoconstriction, which results in increased blood pressure; it also has an antidiuretic effect and plays an important role in the regulation of water balance. Vasopressin secretion is controlled by changes in plasma osmolarity and blood volume.

ADRENALS

The adrenal cortex hypertrophies during pregnancy in response to the hyperestrogen state. There is an increase in the circulating cortisol levels which regulate carbohydrate and protein metabolism. These substances are concentrated in the placenta but are not synthesized by the placenta. A normal level resumes 1–6 weeks postpartum.

PANCREAS

Because insulin needs are increased in the pregnant woman and the blood glucose drop is diminished when an insulin load is administered, the islets of Langerhans of the pancreas are stressed during pregnancy and a latent deficiency state will become more apparent in a pregnant woman. Placental lactogen (hPL), by its diabetogenic effect, increases maternal insulin requirements during pregnancy.

PLACENTAL HORMONES

□ *HUMAN CHORIONIC GONADOTROPIN* The "pregnancy hormone" hCG was first described by Aschheim and Zondek in 1927. Secreted by the trophoblast in early pregnancy, it stimulates progesterone and estrogen production by the corpus luteum to maintain the pregnancy until the placenta is developed sufficiently to assume that function.

□ *HUMAN PLACENTAL LACTOGEN* Also called human chorionic somatomammotropin, hPL is synthesized in the syncytiotrophoblast. The hPL promotes lipolysis which increases the circulation of free fatty acids for maternal cellular metabolic use and decreases maternal metabolism of glucose and amino acids. Because placental lactogen is a physiologic antagonist of insulin, it is considered the principal maternal diabetogenic factor. Placental lactogen also plays a role in the growth of the breasts and other maternal tissue during pregnancy.

□ *RELAXIN* Relaxin is a hormone detectable in the serum of a pregnant woman by the time of the first missed menstrual period. Although the exact source is unknown, relaxin acts to inhibit uterine activity and aids in the softening of the cervix. It can also diminish the strength of myometrial contractions. Studies on the effects of relaxin on the connective tissue of women have not as yet been done (Szlachter et al., 1982).

□ *ESTROGEN* Estrogen, secreted originally by the corpus luteum, is generated primarily by the placenta as early as the seventh week of pregnancy. It stimulates hypertrophy and hyperplasia of the uterus to provide a suitable environment for the developing fetus. Estriol, the predominant estrogen in pregnancy, may play a role in bringing about the increased uteroplacental blood flow found during pregnancy (Aladjem, 1980). It also promotes the development of the ductal system of the maternal breasts in preparation for lactation.

□ *PROGESTERONE* Progesterone, also a product initially of the corpus luteum and then of the placenta, is the hormone most responsible for the maintenance of the pregnancy. During the second half of the menstrual cycle, progesterone stimulates the endometrium to change from primarily proliferative to secretory in preparation for potential implantation of a fertilized ovum. This environment is ideal for support of the ovum. The continued high levels also prevent the sloughing of the endometrial lining as menses. Because progesterone inhibits spontaneous uterine contractility, it prevents early spontaneous abortion induced by uterine activity. In addition, under the stimulation of progesterone, the cervical mucus becomes hostile to sperm and prevents their penetration.

Progesterone is responsible for the development of the acini and lobules of the breasts in preparation for lactation. Hence, it is apparent that estrogen and progesterone work in concert to promote many of the changes necessary for a successful pregnancy, and for breast-feeding after delivery.

PROSTAGLANDINS IN PREGNANCY

Prostaglandins are lipid substances that can arise from most body tissues but occur in high concentrations in the female reproductive tract and are present in the decidua during pregnancy. The exact functions of PGs during pregnancy are still unknown, but they are believed to play a role in the initiation of labor.

EMOTIONAL AND PSYCHOLOGIC CHANGES OF PREGNANCY

Pregnancy is a condition that causes alterations in the internal body milieu, hormonal balance, and external body image, necessitating a reordering of social relationships and changes in roles of family members. Any one of these situations produces stress. In pregnancy, they are present in concert. The way a particular woman meets the stresses of pregnancy is influenced by her emotional makeup, her sociologic and cultural background, and her acceptance or rejection of the pregnancy.

Ambivalence

Initially, even if the pregnancy is planned, there is an element of surprise that conception has indeed occurred. This feeling is generally coupled with a feeling that the timing is wrong, that pregnancy is desirable "some day" but "not now" (Rubin, 1970). The reasons women cite may vary widely—long-term plans, job commitments, financial stress, the needs of an existing child—but the feeling that one is not ready to have a child at this time remains. This feeling accounts for much of the ambivalence commonly experienced by women during early pregnancy. Ambivalence may also be related to the need to modify personal relationships or career plans, to fear coupled with excitement about assuming a new role, to unresolved emotional conflicts with one's own mother, and to fears about pregnancy, labor, and delivery. Such fears may be even more pronounced in the event of an unplanned or unwanted pregnancy. Ambivalence may be verbalized by the woman or may be expressed as denial or rejection of the pregnancy, as depression, nausea, and vomiting, or in the form of somatic complaints.

During the early months the pregnant woman may seriously consider the possibility of an abortion if the pregnancy is unwanted. In the event of religious conflicts about induced abortion, the woman may experience guilt feelings about her thoughts or may tend to focus on the possibility of spontaneous abortion (miscarriage). Colman and Colman (1971) point out that even when the pregnancy is consciously planned and desired, thoughts of abortion and miscarriage arise. The idea that the baby might be lost has a certain emotional appeal because it represents the possible relief of fears and ambivalence.

Acceptance

During the first trimester, evidence of pregnancy is limited to amenorrhea and to the word of the caregiver that the pregnancy test was positive. In an effort to verify her condition, a woman may become minutely conscious of changes in her body that could validate the pregnancy. She closely watches for thickening of her waist, breast development, and weight increase. Morning sickness, though unpleasant, offers further corroboration. During the first trimester the woman's baby does not seem real to her and she focuses on herself and her pregnancy (Colman and Colman, 1971).

The second trimester is relatively tranquil. Morning sickness generally passes, the threat of spontaneous abortion diminishes, and the woman begins to accept the reality of her pregnancy. It is not unusual for enthusiastic primagravidas to don maternity clothes at the beginning of this trimester even when it is not truly necessary. The clothing serves as a verification of her pregnant state. During this time some women may seek to give substance to their baby by shopping for a crib or baby clothes, while other women may find they are not yet ready for that degree of preparation and involvement.

The highlight of the second trimester is quickening, which generally occurs about the twentieth week—midway through the pregnancy. (With the increased use of the Doppler to verify fetal heart tones during the last portion of the first trimester, the woman's acceptance of her baby's existence may occur earlier than it has in the past.) Actual perception of fetal movement frequently produces dramatic changes in the woman. She now perceives her baby as a real person and generally becomes excited about the pregnancy even if she hasn't been prior to this time.

As quickening and her altered physical appearance confirm her pregnant state, the woman adjusts to the idea of change and begins to prepare for her new role and her new set of relationships—with her partner and family, with the child-to-be and with other children, with friends, and with loved ones. She also takes pleasure in the sensations of pregnancy and attempts to picture her baby in order to know him or her better. Women may avidly delve into folklore regarding the child's sex and may carefully study photos of herself and her partner to gain some clues about her child's appearance. She may ask her friends about childbirth and seek out other women who are pregnant or who have recently given birth. She is eager to learn and to share. She feels well, is excited, and may exhibit the "glow" so often attributed to pregnant women.

The third trimester combines a sense of pride with anxiety about what is to come in order for the child to be born. During this time the special prerogatives of pregnancy may be most marked. As her protruding abdomen proclaims her advanced pregnancy, the woman may find that others become more solicitous, that a chair may be offered in a crowded room, that others may carry her parcels. The woman may actually need this help, she may simply enjoy it as a privilege of pregnancy, or she may reject it if she fears that such gestures indicate she is helpless.

During the final trimester physical discomforts again increase, and adequate rest becomes a necessity. The woman, eager for the pregnancy to end, wonders if her expected date of delivery is accurate. She makes final preparation for the baby and may spend long periods considering names for the child.

Rubin (1970) points out that during this time the woman feels very vulnerable to rejection, loss, or insult. She may worry about a variety of things and hesitate to go out unless accompanied by someone she is certain cares about her. She may withdraw into the security and quiet of her home. Toward the end of this period there is often a burst of energy as the woman prepares the "nest" for her expected infant. Many women report bursts of energy in which they vigorously clean and organize their home.

Introversion

Introversion, or turning in on one's self, is a common occurrence in pregnancy. An active, outgoing woman may become less interested in previous activities and more concerned with increased need for rest and time alone. This concentration of attention permits the woman to plan, adjust, adapt, build, and draw strength in preparation for her child's birth (Rubin, 1975). As she becomes more aware of herself, her partner may feel she is being overly sensitive. He may perceive her introversion and passivity as exclusion of him, and may in turn become unable to interact with her, either verbally or physically, and unable to provide the affection, support, and consideration she requires (Stickler et al., 1978). This change in relationships may result in disequilibrium and stress for the entire family. It is essential that the couple work together to establish new, mutually acceptable patterns of response in order to overcome these blocks to communication.

Emotional Lability

Throughout pregnancy the emotions of the woman are characterized by mood swings, from great joy to deep despair. Frequently the woman will become tearful, with little apparent cause. When asked why she is crying, she may find it difficult or impossible to give a reason. The situation is extremely unsettling for the partner, causing him to feel confused and inadequate. Because the man may feel unable to handle the woman's tears, he often reacts by withdrawing and ignoring the problem. Since the pregnant woman needs increased love and affection, she may perceive his reaction as unloving and nonsupportive. Once the couple understands that this behavior is characteristic of pregnancy, it becomes easier for them to deal with it more effectively—although it will be a source of stress to some extent throughout pregnancy.

Body Image

Body image refers to "the picture of our own body which we form in our mind, that is to say, the way in which the body appears to ourselves" (Schilder, 1950). It involves personal attitudes, feelings, and perceptions and may be influenced by environmental, cultural, temporal, physiologic, psychologic, and interpersonal factors. Thus, it is dynamic and ever-changing.

Pregnancy produces marked changes in a woman's body, resulting in major alterations in body configuration within a relatively short period of time (Fisher, 1972). These alterations result in a change in the pregnant woman's body image. The degree of this change is related to personality factors and attitudes toward pregnancy (Fawcett, 1978).

In the second trimester, the woman becomes aware that her body is widening and requires more body space. By the third trimester she is very aware of her increased size and may feel ambivalent about the changes that have occurred in her figure (Jessner et al., 1970).

Body boundary is another aspect of body image. It is the "perceived zone of separation between self and nonself" (Fawcett, 1978). When the body boundary is definite, the body is seen as firm, strong, and distinct from its environment. Body boundary vulnerability occurs when the body boundary is perceived as delicate, capable of being penetrated, and not readily distinguishable from its environment. Recent studies suggest that the pregnant woman feels both increased body boundary definitions and body boundary vulnerability during pregnancy, which suggests that the woman may perceive her body as vulnerable and yet as a protective container (Fawcett, 1978).

Research has long shown that the man experiences changed body image and sympathetic symptoms during his partner's pregnancy. Fawcett's (1978) findings suggest that "wives and husbands demonstrate statistically similar patterns of change in perceived body space from the eighth month of pregnancy through the twelfth postpartal month." Fawcett suggests that men may be more involved in the course of pregnancies than it appears and that identification plays a role in promoting these changes in body image for the man.

Changes in body image are normal but can be a cause of real concern to the pregnant woman and may even contribute to the crisis aspect of both pregnancy and parenthood (Russell, 1974). Expectation of the physiologic changes, coupled with discussion of alterations in body image for both woman and man, may help decrease the stress associated with this aspect of pregnancy.

Changes in a pregnant woman's sexuality also occur and are discussed in Chapter 11.

CULTURAL VALUES AND REPRODUCTIVE BEHAVIOR

Reactions to pregnancy are often dependent on the social meaning of the event for the individual and group. No culture ignores pregnancy or treats it with total indifference. Pregnancy evokes numerous emotions and reactions, including feelings of shyness, shame, reticence, pride, or joy (Mead and Newton, 1967). See Chapter 3 for further discussion of cultural factors.

Knowledge of specific cultural values fosters understanding of various reactions and emotions about childbearing. The relationship between values, customs, and practices, and reproductive behavior is schematized by Richardson and Guttmacher (1967). Values often underlie customs, practices, and behavior.

$$\boxed{\text{Values}} \rightleftarrows \boxed{\begin{array}{c}\text{Customs and}\\\text{Practices}\end{array}} \rightleftarrows \boxed{\begin{array}{c}\text{Reproductive}\\\text{Behavior}\end{array}}$$

The identification of cultural values is useful in predicting reactions. An understanding of male–female roles, family life-styles, or the meaning of children in a culture may explain reactions of joy or shame. Pregnancy is a joyful event in a culture that highly values children. In some cultures pregnancy may be a shameful event if it occurs outside of marriage.

Health values and beliefs are also important in understanding reactions and behavior. If a culture views pregnancy as a sickness, certain behaviors can be expected, whereas if pregnancy is viewed as a natural occurrence, other behaviors may be expected. Prenatal care may not be a priority for women who view pregnancy as a natural phenomenon.

Generalizations about cultural characteristics or cultural values are difficult since these characteristics may not be exhibited by every individual within a culture. Just as variations are seen between cultures, variations are also seen within cultures. For this reason, a general knowledge of cultural values and practices in addition to an individual assessment usually lead to an accurate understanding of a client's behavior.

Variation within a culture is seen in the black community where three classes—upper, middle, and lower—are recognized (Stokes, 1977). Many factors, which are primarily social and economic, influence the way the black woman regards pregnancy. Pregnancy is usually seen as a state of wellness. Acceptance of the pregnancy may depend upon the marital and social situation and whether the pregnancy is planned (Carrington, 1978).

Pregnancy, viewed as a natural condition, is usually desired as soon as possible in the traditional Mexican American family (Kay, 1978). The importance of family is one factor influencing this behavior. Moreover, the role of the traditional Mexican American woman is one of complete devotion to her husband and children (Murillo, 1978). Children are an important part of the Mexican American family; they assure continuation of the family and cultural values.

Machismo or manliness is another cultural concept that influences the reproductive behavior in this group. The term *macho* represents various definitions, with the most frequent being "virile." Research suggests that male individualism and large family size are evidence of machismo (Tamez, 1981).

Traditional practices may change with time. As in the black family, social and economic factors also influence Mexican American practices. Today middle-class Mexican American couples are not starting their families right away (Ehling, 1981). Gender roles also may be changing. In addition, a reduced fertility pattern is found among Mexican American women who participate in the labor force (Johnson, 1976).

Since there are hundreds of different American Indian tribes, it becomes difficult and hazardous to generalize Indian beliefs and practices. It is noted, however, that most of the Indian population considers pregnancy a normal process (Farris, 1978). Children are desired and admired.

Pregnancy and birth are significant times for the Oriental family. In the traditional Chinese family, the wife's status improves with the birth of a child, especially the birth of a son because a son assures the continuation of a family name. Pregnancy has been referred to among Orientals as "happiness in her body" (Rose, 1978). It is considered a normal and natural process, but is also a time of anticipation and anxiety (Char, 1981).

Health Beliefs

Two major explanations of illness have been proposed by Foster and Anderson (1978). The first is the view that illness is the result of the intervention of an agent that may be a supernatural, a nonhuman, or a human being. Beliefs in witches, evil spirits, or God as primary factors in health are part of this view. The second explanation conforms to an equilibrium model of health. For example, health may be viewed as a balance between hot and cold. When this equilibrium is disturbed, illness results.

Although pregnancy is perceived as a natural occurrence in many cultures, it may also be viewed as a time of increased vulnerability. For individuals within groups who adhere to beliefs in evil spirits, certain protective precautions are often followed. For example, pregnant Vietnamese women are admonished to avoid funerals, places of worship, and streets at noon and five o'clock in the afternoon since spirits are present at these times (Stringfellow, 1978). In the Mexican American culture, the concept of *mal aire* or bad air is sometimes related to evil spirits (Baca, 1969). It is thought that air, especially night air, may enter the body and cause harm. Preventive measures, such as keeping the windows closed or covering the head, are used.

Most of the taboos stemming from the belief in evil spirits exist for fear of injuring the unborn child. They arise from a general belief that the unborn infant is the weakest of all beings and is at the mercy of the mother's prenatal behavior. Taboos also emanate, however, from the fear that a pregnant woman has evil powers (Brown, 1976). For this reason, women are sometimes prohibited from taking part in certain activities. For example, the pregnant Vietnamese woman cannot attend a wedding for fear of bringing bad luck to the newlyweds (Hollingsworth et al., 1980).

The equilibrium explanation of health is often associated with so-called humoral pathology, based on the Greek concepts of the four bodily humors (blood, phlegm, black bile, and yellow bile) with their associated qualities (hot, cold, moist, and dry) (Foster and Anderson, 1978). A correct proportion of all these substances and qualities defines health. Many of these same ideas still are retained in folk beliefs, although with less emphasis on moist and dry and more emphasis on hot and cold. The hot–cold classification is seen in cultures in Latin America, the Near East, Far East, and Asia. The dimensions and meanings of this classification may vary, however, and require further investigation (Messer, 1981).

Mexican Americans often consider illness to be an excess of either hot or cold. To restore health, imbalances are often corrected by the proper use of foods, medications, or herbs. These substances are also classified as hot or cold (Murillo-Rohde, 1979). For example, an illness attributed to an excess of coldness will only be treated with hot foods or medications. The classification of foods is not always consistent but it does conform to a general structure of traditional knowledge (Messer, 1981). Certain foods, spices or herbs, and medications are perceived to cool or heat the body. These perceptions do not necessarily correspond to the actual temperature; some hot dishes may be said to have a cooling quality.

Variations in the classification of pregnancy as a hot or cold condition for the Hispanic population are prevalent. Mexicans often view the body as unusually warm in pregnancy and avoid cold foods (Currier, 1978). These beliefs are upheld throughout the entire pregnancy and will therefore affect behavior throughout this period. An understanding of the hot–cold dichotomy may also explain the fear of *mal aire* since air is a main source of cold.

Variations in the classification of pregnancy also exist in the Asian culture. For example, Malays view pregnancy as a hot state while the Vietnamese consider it a cold state (Manderson, 1981).

Oriental health beliefs also reflect the equilibrium concept. Chinese medicine evolved from an Eastern philosophy that stresses duality. According to these beliefs, "The energy for regulating the universe is composed of two opposing forces, the Yin and the Yang." The Yin "represents the female, negative force; darkness, cold, and emptiness," while Yang is the "male and positive force; producing light, warmth, and fullness." In this philosophy "an imbalance is thought to cause catastrophe and illness" (Campbell and Chang, 1973). The concepts of equilibrium and hot–cold forces are as important in understanding health and illness in Oriental health beliefs as in Mexican American folk beliefs. Proper foods and herbs are also used to maintain and restore a balance.

The concepts of hot and cold are not as important in American Indian or black American beliefs. There are some similarities, however, in all of these groups because of the emphasis upon a balance in nature. Black Americans believe that health is a harmony with nature and a balance between good and evil, while the American Indians have traditionally seen health as harmony with nature (Henderson and Primeaux, 1981).

Health Practices

Health care practices during pregnancy are influenced by numerous factors, such as the prevalence of traditional home remedies and folk beliefs, the importance of indigenous healers, and the influence of professional health care workers. In an urban setting, the age, length of time in the city, marital status, and strength of the family may affect these patterns (Hessler et al., 1975). Socioeconomic status is also important since modern medical services may be more accessible to those who can afford it.

An awareness of alternative health sources is crucial for health professionals since these practices affect health outcomes. Many Mexican American mothers are strongly influenced by familism and will seek and follow the advice of their mothers or older women in the childbearing period (Tamez, 1981).

Indigenous healers are also important to specific cultures. In the Mexican American culture the healer is called a *curandero*. In some American Indian tribes, the medicine man may fulfill the healing role. Herbalists are often found in Oriental cultures and in the black culture faith healers, root doctors, and spiritualists are sometimes consulted.

The importance of assessing health care practices becomes evident in looking at current maternal and infant mortality rates. Although the overall maternal mortality has decreased over the past 50 years, it still remains a problem. A study in Michigan found that hemorrhage, infection, and toxemia were leading causes of maternal death and that the rates of these among nonwhites were more than four times greater than among whites (Schaffner et al., 1977). A large prospective study (1959–1966) showed that the perinatal mortality in the United States for whites was 34 deaths per 1000 total births, for blacks 51 per 1000, for Puerto Ricans 41 per 1000, and for Orientals 23 per 1000. Disorders responsible for these differences included premature rupture of the membranes, placental growth retardation, amniotic fluid infections, and major congenital malformations (Naeye, 1979).

Many of these conditions are preventable with prenatal

care. In providing nursing care to women of different cultural backgrounds, the professional must be aware of cultural values, health beliefs, and specific health practices. Every effort must be made to encourage prenatal care. This may be accomplished by working with healers respected in other cultures. It is hoped that elimination of barriers, including communication difficulties and economic factors, will lead to trust and use of the professional health care system. Certainly, an overall cultural sensitivity would result in greater understanding between health professionals and clients of all cultures.

SUMMARY

Although each pregnancy is unique physiologically and emotionally, certain functional and structural changes are common to all normal pregnancies. Deviations from normal anatomic and physiologic alterations may indicate pathology, and the nurse must be able to detect these abnormalities during prenatal care so that the nurse can institute appropriate interventions. A basic understanding of physical and psychologic changes of pregnancy, along with knowledge of significant cultural influences, forms a foundation from which the nurse can more effectively assess (Chapter 10) and intervene in (Chapters 11 and 12) the health problems of the expectant woman.

References

Aladjem, S. 1980. *Obstetrical practice.* St. Louis: The C. V. Mosby Company.

Baca, J. E. 1969. Some health beliefs of the Spanish speaking. *Am. J. Nurs.* 69:2172.

Brown, M. S. Sept./Oct. 1976. A cross-cultural look at pregnancy, labor, and delivery. *J. Obstet. Gynecol. Neonatal Nurs.* 5:35.

Campbell, T., and Chang, B. April 1973. Health care of the Chinese in America. *Nurs. Outlook.* 21:245.

Carrington, B. 1978. The Afro American. In *Culture childbearing health professionals,* ed. A. L. Clark. Philadelphia: F. A. Davis Company.

Char, E. I. 1981. The Chinese American. In *Culture childbearing,* ed. A. L. Clark. Philadelphia: F. A. Davis Company.

Colman, A., and Colman, L. 1971. *Pregnancy: the psychological experience.* New York: Herder and Herder, Inc.

Currier, R. L. 1978. The hot–cold syndrome and symbolic balance. In *Hispanic culture and health care,* ed. R. A. Martinez. St. Louis: The C. V. Mosby Company.

Danforth, D. N., ed. 1982. *Obstetrics and gynecology.* 4th ed. Philadelphia: Harper & Row.

Ehling, M. B. 1981. The Mexican American (el Chicano). In *Culture childbearing,* ed. A. L. Clark. Philadelphia: F. A. Davis Company.

Farris, L. 1978. The American Indian. In *Culture childbearing health professionals,* ed. A. L. Clark. Philadelphia: F. A. Davis Company.

Fawcett, J. July/Aug. 1978. Body image and the pregnant couple. *Am. J. Mat. Child Nurs.* 3:227.

Fisher, S. 1972. *The female orgasm: psychology, physiology, fantasy.* New York: Basic Books.

Foster, G. M., and Anderson, B. G. 1978. *Medical anthropology.* New York: John Wiley & Sons.

Henderson, G., and Primeaux, M., eds. 1981. The importance of folk medicine. In *Transcultural health care.* Menlo Park, Calif.: Addison Wesley Publishing Co.

Hessler, R. M.; Nolan, M. F.; Ogbru, B.; New, P. K. 1975. Intraethnic diversity: health care of the Chinese Americans. *Hum. Organization.* 34:253.

Hollingsworth, A. O.; Brown, L. P.; Brooten, D. A. November 1980. The refugees and childbearing: what to expect. *RN.* 43:45.

Jessner, L., et al. 1970. The development of parental attitudes during pregnancy. In *Parenthood: its psychology and psychopathology,* ed. E. J. Anthony and T. Benedek. Boston: Little, Brown & Co.

Johnson, C. A. 1976. Mexican American women in the labor force and lowered fertility. *Am. J. Public Health.* 66:1186.

Kay, M. A. 1978. The Mexican American. In *Culture childbearing health professionals,* ed. A. L. Clark. Philadelphia: F. A. Davis Company.

Manderson, L. 1981. Roasting, smoking and dieting in response to birth: Malay confinement in cross-cultural perspective. *Soc. Sci. Med.* 15B:509.

Mead, M., and Newton, N. 1967. Cultural patterning of perinatal behavior. In *Childbearing—its social and psychological aspects,* ed. S. A. Richardson and A. F. Guttmacher. Baltimore: Williams & Wilkins.

Messer, E. 1981. Hot–cold classification: theoretical and practical implications of a Mexican study. *Soc. Sci. Med.* 15B:133.

Murillo, N. 1978. The Mexican American family. In *Hispanic culture and health care,* ed. R. A. Martinez. St. Louis: The C. V. Mosby Company.

Murillo-Rohde, I. 1979. Cultural sensitivity in the care of the Hispanic patient. *Washington State J. Nurs.* (Special Suppl): 25.

Naeye, R. 1979. Causes of fetal and neonatal mortality by race in a selected U.S. population. *Am. J. Public Health.* 69:857.

Pritchard, J. A., and MacDonald, P. C. 1980. *Williams obstetrics.* 16th ed. New York: Appleton-Century-Crofts.

Richardson, S. A., and Guttmacher, A. F., eds. 1967. *Childbearing—its social and psychological aspects.* Baltimore: Williams & Wilkins.

Rose, P. A. 1978. The Chinese American. In *Culture childbearing health professionals,* ed. A. L. Clark. Philadelphia: F. A. Davis Company.

Rubin, R. March 1970. Cognitive style in pregnancy. *Am. J. Nurs.* 70:502.

————. Fall 1975. Maternal tasks in pregnancy. *MCN* 4:143.

Russell, C. S. May 1974. Transition to parenthood: problems and gratifications. *J. Marriage Fam.* 36:294.

Schaffner, W.; Federspiel, C. F.; Fulton, M. L.; Gilbert, D. G.; and Stevenson, L. B. 1977. Maternal mortality in Michigan—an epidemiologic analysis, 1950–1971. *Am. J. Public Health.* 67:821.

Schilder, P. 1950. *The image and appearance of the human body.* New York: International Universities Press.

Stickler, J., et al. May/June 1978. Pregnancy: a shared emotional experience. *Am. J. Mat. Child Nurs.* 3:153.

Stokes, L. G. 1977. Delivering health services in a black community. In *Current practice in family-centered community nursing,* ed. A. M. Reinhardt and M. D. Quinn. St. Louis: The C. V. Mosby Co.

Stringfellow, L. 1978. The Vietnamese. In *Culture childbearing health professionals,* ed. A. L. Clark. Philadelphia: F. A. Davis Company.

Szlachter, B. N., et al. Feb. 1982. Relaxin in normal and pathogenic pregnancy. *Obstet. Gynecol.* 59:167.

Tamez, E. G. 1981. Familism, machismo, and childbearing practices among Mexican Americans. *J. Psychiatr. Nurs.* 19:21.

Worthington, B. S., et al. 1977. *Nutrition in pregnancy and lactation.* St. Louis: The C. V. Mosby Co.

Additional Readings

Anderson, R.; Lewis, S. Z.; Giachello, A. L., et al. 1981. Access to medical care among the Hispanic population of Southwestern United States. *J. Health Soc. Behav.* 22:78.

Ascher, B. May/June 1978. Maternal anxiety in pregnancy and fetal homeostasis. *J. Obstet. Gynecol. Neonatal Nurs.* 7:18.

Bash, D. M. Sept./Oct. 1980. Jewish religious practices related to childbearing. *J. Nurse Midwifery* 25:39.

Bullough, V. L., and Bullough, B. 1982. *Health care of the other Americans.* New York: Appleton-Century-Crofts.

Caplan, G. 1975. Psychological aspects of maternity care. *Am. J. Public Health.* 47:25.

DeGracia, R. T. 1979. Cultural influences on Filipino patients. *Am. J. Nurs.* 79:1412.

Ebrahim, G. J. 1980. Cross-cultural aspects of pregnancy and breast feeding. *Proc. Nutrition. Soc.* 39:13.

Friedman, M. M. 1981. *Family nursing: theory and assessment.* New York: Appleton-Century-Crofts.

Griffith, S. Nov./Dec. 1976. Pregnancy as an event with crisis potential for marital partners: summary of a study of interpersonal needs. *J. Obstet. Gynecol. Neonatal Nurs.* 5:35.

Horn, B. M. Nov. 1981. Cultural concepts and postpartal care. *Nurs. Health Care.* 2:516.

Kosasa, T. S., et al. 1974. Clinical use of a solid-phase radioimmunoassay specific for human chorionic gonadotropin. *Am. J. Obstet. Gynecol.* 19:6.

Marrs, R. P., and Mishell, D. R. 1980. Placental trophic hormones. *Clin. Obstet. Gynecol.* 23:721.

Press, I. 1978. Urban folk medicine: a functional overview. *Am. Anthropol.* 80:71.

Primeaux, M. Jan. 1977. Caring for the American Indian patient. *Am. J. Nurs.* 77:91.

Tyson, J. E. 1980. Changing role of placental lactogen and prolactin in human gestation. *Clin. Obstet. Gynecol.* 23:737.

ANTEPARTAL NURSING ASSESSMENT

■ CHAPTER CONTENTS

CLIENT HISTORY
    Definition of Terms
    Client Profile
    Obtaining Data
    Prenatal High-Risk Screening

INITIAL PHYSICAL ASSESSMENT

DETERMINATION OF DELIVERY DATE
    Nägele's Rule
    Uterine Size
    Ultrasound

INITIAL PSYCHOLOGIC ASSESSMENT

SUBSEQUENT PHYSICAL ASSESSMENT

SUBSEQUENT PSYCHOLOGIC ASSESSMENT

ROLE OF THE NURSE

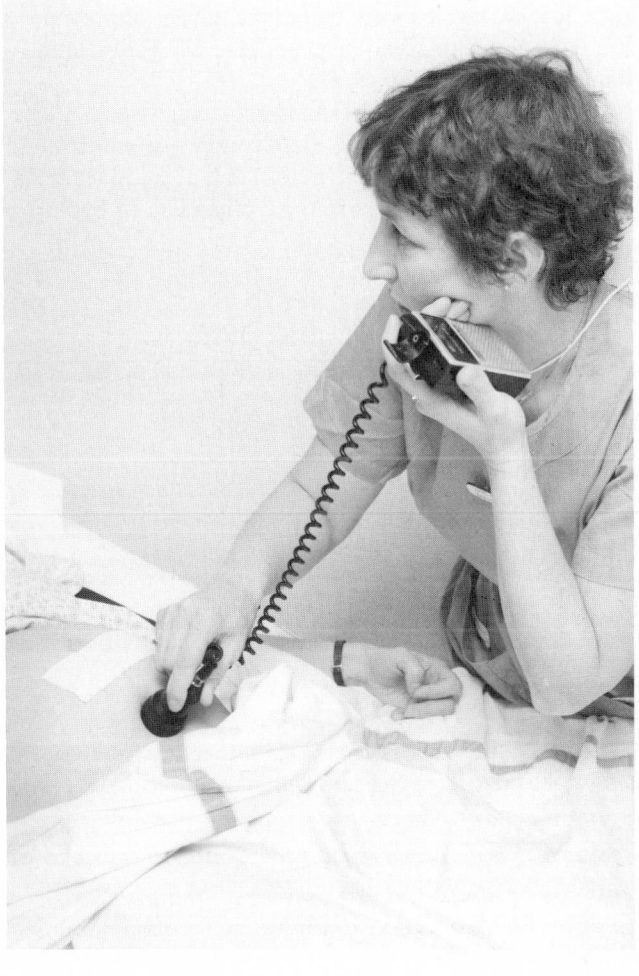

- Identify the essential components of a prenatal history.

- Explain the common obstetric terminology found in the history of a maternity client.

- Identify factors related to the father's health that should be recorded on the prenatal record.

- Describe the normal physiologic changes one would expect to find when performing a physical assessment on a pregnant woman.

- Explain how a woman's attitude toward childbearing can affect the course of her pregnancy.

The course of a pregnancy depends on a number of factors, including prepregnancy health of the woman, presence of disease states, emotional status, and past health care. Ideally, medical care before the advent of pregnancy has been adequate, and antenatal care will be a continuation of that established care.

If optimum maternal health is to be maintained, a thorough history and physical examination are essential to identify problem areas. The history and physical examination may be done by a nurse, by a physician, or by both.

CLIENT HISTORY

Definition of Terms

The following terms are used in the obstetric history of maternity clients:

Gestation: Weeks of gestation refers to the number of weeks since the first day of the last menstrual period (LMP).

Abortion: Delivery that occurs prior to the end of 20 weeks' gestation.

Preterm or premature labor: Labor that occurs after 20 weeks but before the completion of 37 weeks of gestation (pregnancy).

Postterm labor: Labor that occurs after 42 weeks of gestation.

Gravida: Any pregnancy, regardless of duration, including present pregnancy.

Primigravida: A woman who is pregnant for the first time.

Multigravida: A woman who is in her second or any subsequent pregnancy.

Para: Delivery after 20 weeks of gestation (pregnancy) regardless of whether the fetus is born alive or dead.

Nullipara: A woman who has not had a delivery at more than 20 weeks' gestation.

Primipara: A woman who has had one delivery at more than 20 weeks' gestation, regardless of whether the infant is born alive or dead.

Multipara: A woman who has had two or more deliveries at more than 20 weeks' gestation.

Stillbirth: A fetus born dead after 20 weeks of gestation.

The terms *gravida* and *para* refer to pregnancies, not to the fetus.

The following examples illustrate how these terms are applied in clinical situations:

1. Jean Smith has one child born at 38 weeks and is pregnant for the second time. At her initial prenatal visit, the nurse indicates her obstetric history as "gravida II para I ab 0." Jean Smith's present pregnancy terminates at 16 weeks' gestation. She is now "gravida II para I ab I."

2. Mrs. Alexander is pregnant for the fourth time. She has twins born at 35 weeks at home. She lost one pregnancy at 10 weeks' gestation and delivered another infant stillborn at term. At her prenatal assessment the nurse records Mrs. Alexander's obstetric history as "gravida IV para II ab I." Note that twins are considered as one pregnancy and delivery.

Because of the confusion that may result from this system when a multiple pregnancy occurs, a more detailed approach is used in some settings. Using the detailed system, gravida keeps the same meaning, while that of para is altered somewhat to focus on the number of infants born rather than the number of deliveries. A useful acronym for remembering the system is TPAL.

First digit, **T**—number of *term* infants born; that is, the number of infants born at 37 weeks' gestation or beyond.

Second digit, **P**—number of *preterm* infants born; that is, the number of infants born before 37 weeks' gestation.

Third digit, **A**—number of pregnancies ending in either spontaneous or therapeutic *abortion*.

Fourth digit, **L**—number of currently *living* children.

Using this approach, Jean Smith (described in the first example) would initially have been classified as "gravida 2 para 1001." Following her abortion she would be "gravida 2 para 1011." Mrs. Alexander would be described as "gravida 4 para 1212."

Client Profile

The history is essentially a screening tool that identifies the factors that may detrimentally affect the course of a pregnancy. Thus, for optimal prenatal care, the following information should be obtained for each maternity client at the first prenatal assessment:

1. Current pregnancy
   a. First day of last normal menstrual period
   b. Presence of cramping, bleeding, or spotting since last period
   c. Woman's attitude toward pregnancy (is this pregnancy planned?)
   d. Results of pregnancy tests, if they have been done
2. Past pregnancies
   a Number of pregnancies
   b. Number of abortions, spontaneous or induced
   c. Number of living children
   d. History of preceding pregnancies—length of pregnancy, complications (antepartal, intrapartal, postpartal), length of labor
   e. Perinatal status of previous children—birth weights, general development, complications, feeding patterns
   f. Blood type and Rh factor (if negative—medication after delivery for immunization)
   g. Prenatal education classes
3. Gynecologic history
   a. Previous infections—vaginal, cervical, sexually transmitted
   b. Previous surgery
   c. Age of menarche
   d. Regularity, frequency, and duration of menstrual flow
   e. History of dysmenorrhea
   f. Contraceptive history (if birth control pills were used, did pregnancy immediately follow cessation of pills? If not, how long after?)
4. Current medical history
   a. Weight
   b. Blood type and Rh factor, if known
   c. Any medications presently being taken (including nonprescription medications) or taken since the onset of pregnancy
   d. Alcohol and tobacco intake
   e. Illicit drug use and/or abuse
   f. Drug allergies

   g. Potential teratogenic insults to this pregnancy (such as viral infections, medications, x-ray examinations, surgery)
   h. Presence of disease conditions (such as diabetes, hypertension, cardiovascular disease, renal problems)
   i. Record of immunizations (especially rubella)
   j. Presence of any abnormal symptoms
5. Past medical history
   a. Childhood diseases
   b. Past treatment for any disease condition
   c. Surgical procedures
   d. Presence of bleeding disorders or tendencies (has she received blood transfusions?)
6. Family medical history
   a. Presence of diabetes, cardiovascular disease, hypertension, hematologic disorders, preeclampsia-eclampsia
   b. Occurrence of multiple births
   c. History of congenital diseases or deformities
   d. Occurrence of cesarean deliveries
7. Partner's history
   a. Presence of genetic conditions or diseases
   b. Age
   c. Significant health problems
   d. Previous or present alcohol intake, drug use
   e. Blood type and Rh factor
8. Personal information
   a. Age
   b. Educational level
   c. Previous or present use of drugs, alcohol, and cigarettes
   d. Cultural patterns that could influence pregnancy (such as dietary practices or self-medication)
   e. Acceptance of pregnancy
   f. Race or ethnic group (to identify need for prenatal genetic screening or counseling)
   g. Religion (for example, Jehovah's Witnesses—refusal of blood transfusions)
   h. Stability of living conditions
   i. Economic level
   j. Housing
   k. Any history of emotional or physical deprivation (herself or children)
   l. History of emotional problems
   m. Support systems
   n. Overuse or underutilization of health care system

Obtaining Data

A questionnaire like the one shown in Figure 10–1 is used in many instances to obtain information. The woman should be able to complete the questionnaire in a quiet place with a minimum of distractions.

Name _____   Age _____

Address _____   Home Telephone _____

What was the last year of schooling completed? _____

How old were you when your menstrual periods started? _____

How many days does a normal period last? _____

How many days are there between periods? _____

Do you have cramping with your periods? yes__no__

Is the pain: minimal _____

            moderate _____

            severe _____

What was the date of your last normal menstrual period? _____

Have you had bleeding or spotting
since your last menstrual period? yes__no__

Have you been on birth control pills? yes__no__

   If yes, when did you stop taking them? _____

How many previous pregnancies have you had? _____

How many living children do you have? _____

Have you had any abortions or stillbirths? yes__no__

   If yes, how many? _____

Were any of your previous babies born prematurely? yes__no__

List the birth weight of all previous children.

1. _____   3. _____

2. _____   4. _____

Did any of your children have problems immediately after birth?
yes__no__

   If yes, check the problems that occurred:

   Respiratory _____   Feeding _____

   Jaundice _____   Heart _____

   Bleeding _____

Did you have any problems with:

   previous pregnancies? yes__no__

      If yes, what was the problem? _____

   previous labors? yes__no__

      If yes, what was the problem? _____

previous postpartal periods: yes__no__

   If yes, what was the problem? _____

Are you Rh negative: yes__no__

Did you receive RhoGam after each pregnancy? yes__no__

What is your present weight? _____

Are you presently taking any prescripton or nonprescription drugs?
yes__no__

   If yes, please list medications:

1. _____   3. _____

2. _____   4. _____

Do you smoke? yes__no__

   If yes, how many cigarettes per day? _____

How much alcohol do you consume each day? _____

   each week? _____

If you have had any of the following diseases,
place a check beside it.

____	Chickenpox	____	High blood pressure
____	Mumps	____	Heart disease
____	Measles (3 day)	____	Respiratory disease
____	Measles (2 week)	____	Kidney disease
____	Asthma	____	Frequent bladder infections

If any of the following diseases is present in your family,
place a check beside the item.

____	Diabetes	____	Preeclampsia-eclampsia
____	Cardiovascular disease	____	Multiple pregnancies
____	High blood pressure	____	Congenital disorder
____	Breast cancer		

The following questions pertain to the father of this child.

What is the father's age? _____

Does he take prescription or nonprescription drugs? yes__no__

   If yes, please list the medications:

1. _____   3. _____

2. _____   4. _____

What is his alcohol intake each day? _____

   each week? _____

FIGURE 10–1 Sample prenatal questionnaire.

Further information may be elicited by direct interview. A quiet setting where privacy is assured creates a comfortable environment for the interview process. During the interview, the pregnant woman can expand or clarify her responses to the questionnaire. In addition, the initial interview offers the nurse the opportunity to begin establishing rapport with the client. This beginning dialogue sets the stage for a relationship in which the client feels comfortable asking questions of and expressing concerns to the nurse about her pregnancy, and the nurse can be an active educator/counselor to facilitate the client's understanding of her pregnancy, its influences on her, and how she influences her health care.

The expectant father should be encouraged to attend the initial and subsequent prenatal assessments. He may be able to contribute information to the history. In addition, the interview process may provide him with the opportunity to ask questions and express concerns that may be of particular importance to him.

Prenatal High-Risk Screening

A highly significant part of the prenatal assessment is the screening for high-risk factors. Risk factors are any findings that have been shown to have a negative effect on pregnancy outcome, either for the woman or her unborn child.

Many risk factors can be identified during the initial prenatal assessment; other conditions predisposing to maternal or fetal compromise may be detected by subsequent examinations. The nurse must be aware of these high-risk factors and their implications for a successful completion of pregnancy. It is important that high-risk pregnancies be identified early so that appropriate interventions can be instituted immediately.

All high-risk factors do not threaten the pregnancy to the same degree. To determine the possible effect of certain variables on the pregnancy, centers that provide prenatal care have devised various scoring tools. These scoring tools can be used to collect data and to identify the woman who needs to be observed more closely during the pregnancy course.

Some agencies use a risk scoring sheet, which is initiated at the first visit and then becomes a permanent part of the client's record. Information may be updated throughout the pregnancy as necessary. It is always possible that a pregnancy may begin as low risk and convert to high risk because of complications.

Table 10–1 identifies the major risk factors currently recognized. The table describes maternal and fetal/neonatal implications should the risk be present in the pregnancy. In addition to the factors listed, the perinatal health team also needs to evaluate such psychosocial factors as ethnic background; occupation, education; financial status; environment, including living arrangements and location; and the client's concept of health and that of her family or significant others, which might influence her attitude toward seeking health care.

INITIAL PHYSICAL ASSESSMENT

After a complete history is obtained, the woman is prepared for a thorough physical examination. The physical examination begins with assessment of vital signs, then proceeds to a complete examination of her body. The pelvic examination is performed last.

Before the examination, the woman should provide a clean voided urine specimen. After emptying her bladder, she is asked to disrobe and is given a sheet or some other protective covering. The woman who has emptied her bladder will be more comfortable during the pelvic examination, and the examiner will be able to palpate the abdominal organs more easily.

The physical examination is facilitated when the woman is at ease and comfortable.

Increasing numbers of nurses, as a result of the content of their basic education programs or their own expanding skills through physical assessment or practitioner courses, are prepared to perform physical examinations. The nurse who has not yet fully developed specific assessment skills assesses the woman's vital signs, explains the procedures to allay apprehensions, positions her for examination, and assists the examiner as necessary.

Each nurse is responsible for operating at the expected standard for someone with that individual nurse's skill and knowledge base. The following situation demonstrates this expectation.

Margo Cole is being seen in the clinic at 28 weeks' gestation. She began prenatal care at 12 weeks and her pregnancy to date has been uneventful. Pam Forbes graduated from her nursing program 9 months ago without having received any formal classes in physical assessment. Pam is doing the initial routine assessments for Margo and observes that Margo's weight gain has been excessive. When checking the vital signs she notes a significant increase in Margo's blood pressure. At this point Pam should be considering the possibility that Margo may be developing preeclampsia. Pam would continue her assessment by using a dipstick to check the urine for the presence of protein, query Margo about any recent problems with swelling, and do at least an initial check for any edema. Pam is not expected to diagnose the condition, but her charting should reflect her findings in a logical manner so that the clinician will be alerted, an in-depth assessment will be made, and treatment initiated if necessary.

The accompanying Initial Prenatal Physical Assessment Guide may be used by the nurse who is performing the initial prenatal physical examination (see Chapter 9 for *(Text continues on p. 236.)*

Table 10-1 Prenatal High-Risk Factors

Factor	Maternal implication	Fetal/neonatal implication
Social-personal		
Low income level	Poor antenatal care Poor nutrition ↑risk of preeclampsia	Low birth weight Intrauterine growth retardation (IUGR)
Poor diet	Inadequate nutrition ↑risk anemia ↑risk preeclampsia	Fetal malnutrition Prematurity
Living at high altitude	↑hemoglobin	Prematurity IUGR
Multiparity > 3	↑risk antepartum/postpartum hemorrhage	Anemia Fetal death
Weight < 100 lb	Poor nutrition Cephalopelvic dysproportion Prolonged labor	IUGR Hypoxia associated with difficult labor and delivery
Weight > 200 lb	↑risk hypertension ↑risk cephalopelvic dysproportion	↓fetal nutrition
Age < 16	Poor nutrition Poor antenatal care ↑risk preeclampsia ↑risk cephalopelvic dysproportion	Low birth weight ↑fetal wastage
Age > 35	↑risk preeclampsia ↑risk cesarean delivery	↑risk congenital anomalies ↑chromosomal aberrations
Smoking — one pack/day or more	↑risk hypertension ↑risk cancer	↓placental perfusion →↓O_2 and nutrients available Low birth weight IUGR Preterm birth
Use of addicting drugs	↑risk poor nutrition ↑risk of infection with IV drugs	↑risk congenital anomalies ↑risk low birth weight Neonatal withdrawal Lower serum bilirubin
Excessive alcohol consumption	↑risk poor nutrition Possible hepatic effects with long-term consumption	↑risk fetal alcohol syndrome
Preexisting medical disorders		
Diabetes mellitus	↑risk preeclampsia, hypertension Episodes of hypoglycemia and hyperglycemia ↑risk cesarean delivery	Low birth weight Macrosomia Neonatal hypoglycemia ↑risk congenital anomalies ↑risk respiratory distress syndrome
Cardiac disease	Cardiac decompensation Further strain on mother's body ↑maternal death rate	↑risk fetal wastage ↑perinatal mortality
Anemia:* hemoglobin < 9 g/dL (white) < 29% hematocrit (white) < 8.2 g/dL hemoglobin (black) < 26% hematocrit (black)	Iron deficiency anemia Low energy level Decreased oxygen carrying capacity	Fetal death Prematurity Low birth weight
Hypertension	↑vasospasm ↑risk CNS irritability →convulsions ↑risk CVA ↑risk renal damage	↓placental perfusion →low birth weight Preterm birth

Table 10–1   Prenatal High-Risk Factors Cont'd

Factor	Maternal implication	Fetal/neonatal implication
Thyroid disorder hypothyroidism	↑infertility ↓BMR, goiter, myxedema	↑spontaneous abortion ↑risk congenital goiter Mental retardation →cretinism ↑incidence congenital anomalies
hyperthyroidism	↑risk postpartum hemorrhage ↑risk preeclampsia Danger of thyroid storm	↑incidence preterm birth ↑tendency to thyrotoxicosis
Renal disease (moderate to severe)	↑risk renal failure	↑risk IUGR ↑risk preterm delivery
Obstetric considerations *Previous pregnancy* Stillborn	↑emotional/psychologic distress	↑risk IUGR ↑risk preterm delivery
Habitual abortion	↑emotional/psychologic distress ↑possibility diagnostic work-up	↑risk abortion
Cesarean delivery	↑probability repeat cesarean delivery	↑risk preterm birth ↑risk respiratory distress
Rh or blood group sensitization	↑financial expenditure for testing	Hydrops fetalis Icterus gravis Neonatal anemia Kernicterus Hypoglycemia
Current pregnancy Rubella (first trimester)		Congenital heart disease Cataracts Nerve deafness Bone lesions Prolonged virus shedding
Rubella (second trimester)		Hepatitis Thrombocytopenia
Cytomegalovirus		IUGR Encephalopathy
Herpesvirus type 2	Severe discomfort	Neonatal herpesvirus type 2 2° hepatitis with jaundice Neurologic abnormalities
Syphilis	↑incidence abortion	↑fetal wastage Congenital syphilis
Abruptio placenta and placenta previa	↑risk hemorrhage Bed rest Extended hospitalization	Fetal/neonatal anemia Intrauterine hemorrhage ↑fetal wastage
Preeclampsia/eclampsia	See hypertension	↓placental perfusion →low birth weight
Multiple gestation	↑risk postpartum hemorrhage	↑risk preterm birth ↑risk fetal demise

Elevated hematocrit*
  > 41% (white)
  > 38% (black)
	Increased viscosity of blood	Fetal death rate 5 times normal rate

*Data from Garn, S. M., et al. April 1981. Maternal hematologic levels and pregnancy outcomes. *Seminars in Perinatology* 5:155.

INITIAL PRENATAL PHYSICAL ASSESSMENT GUIDE

Assess	Normal findings	Alterations and possible causes*	Nursing responses to data†
Vital signs			
Blood pressure (BP)	90-140/60-90	High BP (essential hypertension, renal disease, pregestational hypertension, apprehension or anxiety associated with pregnancy diagnosis, exam, or other crises)	BP > 150/90 requires immediate consideration. Establish client's BP. Refer to physician if necessary. Assess patient's knowledge about high BP. Counsel on self and medical management.
Pulse	60-90/min Rate may increase 10 beats/min during pregnancy	Increased pulse rate (excitement or anxiety, cardiac disorders)	Count for one full minute. Note irregularities.
Respiration	16-24/min (or pulse rate divided by four) Pregnancy may induce a degree of hyperventilation; thoracic breathing predominant	Marked tachypnea or abnormal patterns	Assess for respiratory disease.
Temperature	36.2-37.6C (98-99.6F)	Elevated temperature (infection)	Assess for infection process or disease state if temperature is elevated. Refer to physician.
Weight	Depends on body build	Weight < 100 lb or >200 lb Rapid, sudden weight gain (preeclampsia-eclampsia)	Evaluate need for nutritional counseling. Obtain information on eating habits, cooking practices, foods regularly eaten, income limitations, need for food supplements, pica and other abnormal food habits. Note initial weight to establish baseline for weight gain throughout pregnancy.
Skin			
Color	Consistent with racial background; pink nail beds	Pallor (anemia) Bronze, yellow (hepatic disease, other causes of jaundice) Bluish, reddish, mottled Dusky appearance or pallor of palms and nail beds in dark-skinned patients (anemia)	The following lab tests should be performed: CBC, bilirubin level, urinalysis, and BUN. If abnormal, refer to physician.
Condition	Absence of edema Slight edema of extremities normal during pregnancy	Edema (preeclampsia) Rashes, dermatitis (allergic response)	Counsel on relief measures for slight edema. Initiate preeclampsia assessment. Refer to physician

*Possible causes of alterations are placed in parentheses.
†This column provides guidelines for further assessment and initial nursing interventions.

INITIAL PRENATAL PHYSICAL ASSESSMENT GUIDE Cont'd

Assess	Normal findings	Alterations and possible causes*	Nursing responses to data†
Lesions	Absence of lesions	Ulceration (varicose veins, decreased circulation)	Further assess circulatory status. Refer to physician, if lesion severe.
	Spider nevi common in pregnancy	Petechiae, multiple bruises, ecchymosis (hemorrhagic disorders)	Evaluate for bleeding or clotting disorder.
	Moles	Change in size or color	Refer to physician.
Texture	Moderately smooth	Dryness, roughness (dry skin)	Thyroid function tests should be performed.
		Scaliness, broken skin (hypothyroidism, vitamin A deficiency)	Determine usual daily vitamin A intake. Counsel about sources and methods of obtaining necessary vitamin A. If necessary, refer to physician.
Turgor — pinch skin	Skin is elastic and returns to normal shape after pinching	Skin maintains pinched or ``tent shape'' (dehydration)	Assess for other symptoms of dehydration. Identify ways to control fluid loss and replace necessary fluids. Refer to physician if severe.
Pigmentation	Café-au-lait spots	Six or more (Albright's syndrome or neurofibromatosis)	Consult with physician.
	Pigmentation changes of pregnancy include linea nigra, striae gravidarum, chloasma, spider nevi		Assure client that these are normal manifestations of pregnancy and explain the physiologic basis for the changes.
Hair Distribution	Even over entire body	Hirsutism, alopecia (Cushing's syndrome, hypothyroidism)	Assess for presence of other symptoms of Cushing's syndrome and hypothyroidism. Refer to physician.
Texture	Consistent with racial background	Brittleness, dryness (hypothyroidism, nutritional deficiency)	Evaluate nutritional status. Initiate appropriate dietary education. Evaluate thyroid function.
Head Size, movement, general appearance	Size appropriate to body; symmetrical; easily supported and moves with smooth control; facial symmetry	Lesions (skin disorders); observable vascularity; drooping of musculature (muscle or nerve disorder); edema; involuntary movement	Do expanded assessment of neurologic function. Refer to physician.
Temporal artery	Able to palpate temporal artery without discomfort to patient	Bounding, hard nodules; sensitivity to pressure (high or low carotid pressure)	Assess other pulses. Refer to physician.

*Possible causes of alterations are placed in parentheses.
†This column provides guidelines for further assessment and initial nursing interventions.

INITIAL PRENATAL PHYSICAL ASSESSMENT GUIDE Cont'd

Assess	Normal findings	Alterations and possible causes*	Nursing responses to data†
Scalp	Normal pattern	Scaliness, excess oiliness, nits or mites (head lice)	Evaluate hygiene. Institute programs to improve hygiene as needed and carry out medical treatment.
		Lumps or tenderness (infection)	Examine for local infection; if none found, refer to physician.
Neck			
Nodes	Small, mobile, nontender nodes	Tender, hard, fixed, or prominent nodes (infection, malignancy)	Examine for local infection. Refer to physician.
Trachea	Trachea should be in midline of neck; larynx, trachea, and thyroid rise with swallowing	Deviation to one side or the other; tension on one side or decreased expansion on one side	Chest x-ray examination should be done to identify normal or abnormal lung expansion. Refer to physician if deviation present.
Thyroid	Small, smooth lateral lobes palpable on either side of trachea; slight hyperplasia by third month of pregnancy	Enlargement or nodule tenderness (hyperthyroidism)	Listen over thyroid for bruits, which may indicate hyperthyroidism. Question client about dietary habits (iodine intake). Ascertain history of thyroid problems. Refer to physician.
Major vessels	Easily palpable, good pulse in carotid	Absence or diminished pulses (cardiovascular disease)	Refer to physician.
	Jugular veins	Not distended, nonpalpable (low cardiac output)	Assess level of distention with client at 45-degree angle. Refer to physician.
Eyes			
Near vision	Able to read print at about 18-in. distance	Any deviation from this standard	Refer to physician, for further evaluation.
Conjunctiva	Salmon-colored	Pale or infected	The following lab tests should be done: CBC, bilirubin level.
Sclera	White with a few small blood vessels	Localized and/or general hemorrhage; lesions; jaundice; increased vascularity; excess tearing; thick, purulent discharge; opacity of lens; scars; thick pearlike covering over pupil	Refer to physician, for further evaluation.
Eyelids	Smooth; move easily and close completely; when open, expose pupils equally; lashes full from inner to outer canthus; normal blinking	Exophthalmus (hypothyroidism), loss of elasticity, inflammation, purulent discharge, edema, ptosis, loss of lashes, accentuated or diminished blinking, nystagmus	Thyroid function tests (T_3–T_4) should be performed. Refer to physician.

*Possible causes of alterations are placed in parentheses.
†This column provides guidelines for further assessment and initial nursing interventions.

INITIAL PRENATAL PHYSICAL ASSESSMENT GUIDE Cont'd

Assess	Normal findings	Alterations and possible causes*	Nursing responses to data†
Pupils	Round and equal; respond briskly to light	Constantly constricted or dilated, abnormal in shape, unresponsive to light	Evaluate for associated ptosis and facial muscle weakness. Refer to physician.
Ears			
External auricle	Size, position, and shape within normal limit for head size	Absence, deformity, lesions, swelling, discharge, foreign bodies	Evaluate for associated problems. Refer to physician.
Inner ear — pull pinna and tilt away; use otoscope to examine tympanic membrane; check hearing	Cerumen Tympanic membrane flat, intact, pearly gray	Bulging, inflammation, tears Exaggerated sound; bulging membrane, reddened membrane (infection); poor perception of sound, no ability to hear	Refer to physician, for further evaluation.
Jaw			
Temporomandibular joint	Smooth, voluntary opening and closing, full range of motion	Partial movement, pain or tenderness, crepitation, dislocation	Refer to physician, for further evaluation.
Nose			
Patency and symmetry	Partial or fully open, normal contour	Closure or deformity (deviated septum), inflammation, bleeding, discharge, polyps, swelling, rhinitis, folliculitis	Refer to physician for deformities that are bothersome. Treat inflammation or bleeding.
Character of mucosa	Redder than oral mucosa		
Olfactory ability — ask patient to identify familiar smell (food, perfume); tests adequacy of first cranial nerve	In pregnancy, nasal mucosa is edematous in response to increased estrogen, resulting in nasal stuffiness and nosebleeds	Olfactory loss (first cranial nerve deficit)	Counsel client about possible relief measures for nasal stuffiness and epistaxis. Refer to physician for olfactory loss.
Head movement			
Place hand on jaw and try to return head to midline while patient holds head firmly in lateral position	Able to move head from side to side Resists movement back to midline	Examiner able to return head to midline (weakness of sternocleidomastoid — possible eleventh nerve problem)	Refer for neurologic evaluation.
Ask patient to shrug while examiner tries to prevent shoulders from rising	Equality of strength; able to raise shoulders	Unable to elevate shoulders under added pressure (weakness of sternocleidomastoid and trapezius muscles)	Refer for further neurologic evaluation.

*Possible causes of alterations are placed in parentheses.
†This column provides guidelines for further assessment and initial nursing interventions.

INITIAL PRENATAL PHYSICAL ASSESSMENT GUIDE Cont'd

Assess	Normal findings	Alterations and possible causes*	Nursing responses to data†
Sinuses			
Palpate frontal and maxillary sinuses	Smooth; normal body temperature	Tenderness; increased temperature; swelling (infection, inflammation)	Assess for other signs of allergy or infection.
Mouth			
Lips	Even border; pink mucous membrane, free of scaling, lesions; symmetrical shape and opening	Broken areas with mucocutaneous junction swelling, lesions (herpes simplex; benign or malignant lesions)	Discuss comfort measures for herpes. Refer to the physician for questionable lesions.
Tongue	Full mobility in mouth; pink color Moderate distribution of papillae over entire tongue Papillae moderately rough	Too large or thick; protruding from oral cavity; smooth; fissured lesions; geographically "hairy"; deviation of tongue from midline	Assess for signs of acromegaly, hypothyroidism, vitamin B_{12} deficiency. Reassure client that some of these signs appear with age.
Buccal mucosa, palate, pharynx	Pink, unobstructed, moist mucosa; minimal or absent swelling in tonsillar area; hard palate intact	Canker sore; white, curdy patches (thrush) Redness of pharynx; enlarged tonsil and uvula; white patches or gray membrane over throat	Refer if bony tumor not along midline. Culture for thrush and treat. Assess for infections. Counsel regarding seeking prompt health supervision for all infections or colds.
		Deviation of uvula plus soft palate fails to rise when patient says "ah" (tenth nerve paralysis)	Refer to physician for further neurologic evaluation.
Gums	May note hypertrophy of gingival papillae because of estrogen	Edema, inflammation (infection); pale (anemia)	Assess hematocrit for anemia. Counsel regarding dental hygiene habits. Refer to physician or dentist if necessary.
Chest and lungs			
Chest	Symmetrical, elliptical, smaller anteroposterior (A-P) than transverse diameter	Increased A-P diameter, funnel chest, pigeon chest (emphysema; asthma, chronic obstructive pulmonary disease, COPD)	Evaluate for emphysema, asthma, pulmonary disease (COPD).
Ribs	Slope downward from nipple line	More horizontal (COPD) Angular bumps	Evaluate for COPD. Evaluate for fractures. Consult physician.
		Rachitic rosary (vitamin C deficiency)	Consult nutritionist.
	No retraction or bulging of intercostal spaces (ICS) during inspiration or expiration; symmetrical expansion Tactile fremitus	ICS retractions with inspiration, bulging with expiration; unequal expansion (respiratory disease) Tachypnea, hyperpnea, Cheyne-Stokes respirations (respiratory disease)	Do thorough initial assessment. Refer to physician.

Refer to physician. |

*Possible causes of alterations are placed in parentheses.
†This column provides guidelines for further assessment and initial nursing interventions.

INITIAL PRENATAL PHYSICAL ASSESSMENT GUIDE Cont'd

Assess	Normal findings	Alterations and possible causes*	Nursing responses to data†
Percussion of posterior lungs	Bilateral symmetry in tone	Flatness of percussion, which may be affected by chest wall thickness	Evaluate for pleural effusions, consolidations, or tumor.
	Low-pitched resonance of moderate intensity	High diaphragm (atelectasis or paralysis), pleural effusion	Refer to physician.
Auscultation (see Procedure 10-1)	Upper lobes: bronchovesicular sounds above sternum and scapulas; equal expiratory and inspiratory phases	Abnormal if heard over any other area of chest	Refer to physician.
	Remainder of chest: vesicular breath sounds heard; inspiratory phase longer (3:1)	Rales, rhonchi, wheezes; pleural friction rub; absence of breath sounds; bronchophony, egophony; whispered pectoriloquy	Refer to physician.
Breasts	Supple; symmetry in size and contour; darker pigmentation of nipple and areola; may have supernumerary nipples, usually 5–6 cm below normal nipple line	"Pigskin" or orange-peel appearance; nipple retractions; swelling, hardness (carcinoma); redness, heat, tenderness, cracked or fissured nipple (infection)	Encourage monthly breast checks. Instruct client how to examine own breasts (Procedure 10-2). Refer to physician.
	Axillary nodes unpalpable or pellet size	Tenderness, enlargement, hard node; may be visible bump (infection); carcinoma	Refer to physician if evidence of inflammation.
	Pregnancy changes: 1. Size increase noted primarily in first 20 weeks 2. Become nodular 3. Tingling sensation may be felt during first and third trimester; woman may report feeling of heaviness 4. Pigmentation of nipples and areolas darkens 5. Superficial veins dilate and become more prominent 6. Striae seen in multiparas 7. Tubercles of Montgomery enlarge 8. Colostrum may be present after twelfth week 9. Secondary areola appears at 20 weeks, characterized by series of washed-out spots surrounding primary areola 10. Breasts less firm, old striae may be present in multiparas		Discuss normalcy of changes and their meaning with the client. Teach and/or institute appropriate relief measures (see Chapter 11). Encourage use of supportive brassiere.

*Possible causes of alterations are placed in parentheses.
†This column provides guidelines for further assessment and initial nursing interventions.

INITIAL PRENATAL PHYSICAL ASSESSMENT GUIDE Cont'd

Assess	Normal findings	Alterations and possible causes*	Nursing responses to data†
Heart (see Procedure 10-3)			
Size and placement	Lies in thoracic cavity within mediastinum; upper border lies behind upper portion of sternum; lower border lies at level of third left costal cartilage close to sternum	Enlargement (cardiac disease)	Complete initial cardiac assessment. Refer to physician.
Point of maximal intensity (PMI) or apical pulse	PMI 1–2 cm in diameter and located 7–9 cm left of midsternal point in the fourth or fifth intercostal space (May be further left of midsternal line during pregnancy)	Diffuse PMI located farther than 9 cm left of midsternal point (left ventricular hypertrophy or dilatation)	Assess other cardiac findings. Refer to physician, if indicated.
	Thrills not present Palpitation may occur in pregnancy due to sympathetic nervous system disturbance	Thrills, palpable vibrations that resemble a cat's purr, are associated with cardiac defects; thrusting of chest wall felt during palpation (cardiac disease)	Refer to physician.
Rate and rhythm	Normal rate and rhythm	Gross irregularity or skipped beats	Refer to physician. Twelve lead EKG may be part of cardiac evaluation process to screen for abnormalities of rhythm or electrical conduction.
	Rhythm may vary slightly with respirations	Three heart sounds or gallop rhythm may signal presence of decompensation or carditis	
Sounds	Normal heart sounds	Extra or prolonged sounds may signify valvular disease	Assure client of normalcy of short systolic murmurs in pregnancy. Refer to physician for abnormal sounds.
	No murmurs present (Short systolic murmurs that ↑ in held expiration are normal during pregnancy)	Murmur (obstruction to cardiac blood flow)	
Abdomen			
General appearance	Skin clear with exception of whitish silver striae of multiparas	Purple striae (Cushing's syndrome)	Assess for presence of other symptoms of Cushing's syndrome.
	Fine venous network	Dilated veins (vena cava obstruction)	
	Peristalsis may be visible in very thin women	Increased peristaltic waves (intestinal obstruction)	Refer to physician.
	Aortic pulsation may be visible in epigastrium	Increased pulsation (aortic aneurysm)	
	Pubic hair limited to pubic area	Hair distribution extending to umbilicus (bilateral polycystic ovary, Cushing's ovary, ovarian tumor)	

*Possible causes of alterations are placed in parentheses.
†This column provides guidelines for further assessment and initial nursing interventions.

INITIAL PRENATAL PHYSICAL ASSESSMENT GUIDE Cont'd

Assess	Normal findings	Alterations and possible causes*	Nursing responses to data†
	Umbilicus deeply indented early in pregnancy and more shallow as pregnancy progresses; at end of pregnancy, level with surface or may protrude slightly	Exudate or bleeding from umbilicus (infection, fistula) Herniation or bulging	Evaluate for infection.
Auscultation	Bowel sounds 5–34/min	Hyperactivity (hyperperistalsis)	Discuss dietary habits. Evaluate for stress-related factors. Refer to physician if indicated.
Palpation	Abdomen nontender and relaxed, especially during expiration	Muscle guarding (anxiety, acute tenderness); tenderness, mass (ectopic pregnancy, inflammation, carcinoma)	Evaluate client anxiety level. Refer to physician, if indicated.
	Diastasis of the rectus muscles late in pregnancy	Excessive separation of muscles	Assure client of normalcy of diastasis. Provide initial information about appropriate postpartum exercises.
	Liver nonpalpable	Rebound tenderness (peritoneal inflammation) Liver palpable below right costal margin, tender and/or nodules (suggest malignancy)	Refer to physician.
	Absence of pain	Pains in any abdominal quadrants; tenderness above inguinal ligaments (salpingitis)	Refer to physician for evaluation of specific cause.
Size	Flat or rotund abdomen Progressive increase in size of uterus due to pregnancy 10–12 weeks: fundus slightly above symphysis pubis 16 weeks: fundus halfway between symphysis and umbilicus	Size of uterus inconsistent with length of gestation (IUGR, multiple pregnancy, fetal demise, hydatidiform mole)	Reassess menstrual history regarding pregnancy dating. Evaluate increase in size using McDonald's method (p. 237). Use ultrasound to establish diagnosis.
	20–22 weeks: fundus at umbilicus 28 weeks: fundus three finger-breadths above umbilicus 36 weeks: fundus just below ensiform cartilage		
Fetal heartbeats	120–160 beats/min May be heard with Doptone at 10–12 weeks' gestation May be heard with fetoscope at 17–20 weeks	Failure to hear fetal heartbeat after 17–20 weeks (fetal demise, hydatidiform mole)	Refer to physician. Administer pregnancy tests. Use ultrasound to establish diagnosis.

*Possible causes of alterations are placed in parentheses.
†This column provides guidelines for further assessment and initial nursing interventions.

INITIAL PRENATAL PHYSICAL ASSESSMENT GUIDE Cont'd

Assess	Normal findings	Alterations and possible causes*	Nursing responses to data[†]
Fetal movement	Not felt prior to 20 weeks' gestation by examiner	Failure to feel fetal movements after 20 weeks' gestation (fetal demise, hydatidiform mole)	Refer to physician for evaluation of fetal status.
Ballottement	During fourth to fifth month, fetus rises and then rebounds to original position when uterus is tapped sharply	Failure to ascertain ballottement	Refer to physician for evaluation of fetal status.
Extremities Arms and hands	Hands warm, may be slightly moist; full range of motion; strong grip; good palpable pulses	Hands cold, stiff, tender; enlargement or deflation of phalanges; deviation of ulna or radius; presence of nodules (arthritis)	Evaluate for other symptoms of vascular disease or arthritis. Refer to physician if these are found or if data are questionable.
	In late pregnancy, may have some edema of hands	Marked edema (preeclampsia)	Initiate follow-up if client mentions that her rings feel tight.
Nails	Pink nail beds, nail base angle 160°, nail base firm	Clubbing (hypoxia); spoon nails (iron-deficiency anemia)	Evaluate for anemia or heart disease.
Legs	Toes pink; femoral, popliteal, posterior tibial, and dorsalis pedis pulses palpable	Unpalpable or diminished pulses (arterial insufficiency); pallor on elevation, cool temperature, skin atrophic and shiny, ulcerations, brown pigmentation around ankles (venous insufficiency, varicose veins)	Discuss prevention and self-treatment measures for varicose veins. Refer to physician if indicated.
Musculoskeletal system	Full range of motion	Limitation or deviation of joints Swollen, tender, hot joints and subcutaneous nodules (rheumatoid arthritis) Bony enlargement of joints (osteoarthritis) Knock knees, bowlegs, painful swelling of metatarsophalangeal joint (gout)	Determine which joints are involved. Refer to physician.
Spine Curvature	Normal spinal curves: concave cervical, convex thoracic, concave lumbar	Abnormal spinal curves: flatness, kyphosis, lordosis	Refer to physician for assessment of cephalopelvic disproportion. May have implications for administration of spinal anesthesia.
	In pregnancy, dorsal and lumbar spinal curve may be accentuated	Backache	See p. 258 for relief measures.
	Shoulders and iliac crests should be even	Uneven shoulders and iliac crests (scoliosis)	Refer very young clients to a physician. Discuss back stretching exercises with older clients.

*Possible causes of alterations are placed in parentheses.
[†]This column provides guidelines for further assessment and initial nursing interventions.

INITIAL PRENATAL PHYSICAL ASSESSMENT GUIDE Cont'd

Assess	Normal findings	Alterations and possible causes*	Nursing responses to data†
Vertebras	In straight vertical line Absence of tenderness	Curvature (kyphosis, scoliosis) Tenderness lateral to spine on flexion-extension or pressure	Refer to physician.
		Costovertebral angle tenderness (kidney infection or disease)	Obtain urinalysis. Refer to physician.
	Able to do straight leg raises without back pain	Back pain (disc disease)	Refer to physician.
	During advanced pregnancy, hypermotility of pelvic joints and accentuation of dorsal and lumbar curvature	Separation of symphysis, synchondrosis	
Reflexes	Reflexes normal and symmetrical	Hyperactivity, clonus (preeclampsia) Asymmetrical, diminished (cerebral or spinal nerve damage)	Evaluate for preeclampsia and cerebral or spinal nerve damage. (See Chapter 12 for specific nursing interventions.)
Pelvic area (see Procedure 10–4) External female genitals	Mons pubis covered with hair in shape of inverted triangle; labia majora symmetrical, not adherent or enlarged; vulva appears pink and moist	Lesions, hematomas, cellulitis, varicosities, urethral caruncle, inflammation of Bartholin's gland	Explain pelvic examination procedure (Procedure 10–4). Encourage woman to minimize her discomfort by relaxing her hips. Provide privacy.
	Small clitoris not exceeding 2 cm in length and 1 cm in width	Clitoral hypertrophy (masculinization)	
	In multiparas, labia majora loose and pigmented	Vulva inflamed, white patches present on mucosa and cervix (carcinoma)	
Urinary meatus	Urinary and vaginal orifices visible and appropriately located	Single meatus for urethra and vagina (fistula) Fistulous opening	Refer to physician.
		Urethral irritation and/or discharge (urethritis, foreign body)	Obtain smear, urinalysis. Refer to physician.
Vagina	Pink or dark pink in color	Grayish white patches (carcinoma)	Refer to physician.
	No bulging into vagina when patient strains	Bulging into vagina from upper wall (cystocele) Bulging into vagina from posterior wall (rectocele)	

*Possible causes of alterations are placed in parentheses.
†This column provides guidelines for further assessment and initial nursing interventions.

INITIAL PRENATAL PHYSICAL ASSESSMENT GUIDE Cont'd

Assess	Normal findings	Alterations and possible causes*	Nursing responses to data[†]
	Vaginal discharge odorless, nonirritating, thin or mucoid, clear or cloudy	Discharge associated with vaginal infections: 1. Monilial infection: thick, white, curdy 2. Trichomonal infection: profuse, watery, gray or green, frothy, with odor 3. Gardnerella vaginalis (hemophilus vaginalis): malodorous, gray. 4. Gonorrhea: green-yellow discharge, inflamed cervix and vulva	Obtain vaginal smear (Figures 10-2 and 10-3). See p. 355 for management of infections. Provide understandable verbal and written instructions to facilitate safe and effective treatment. Treat sexual partner if indicated.
	In multipara, vaginal folds smooth and flattened, entire vaginal canal widened; may have old episiotomy scar		
Cervix (Figure 10-4)	Pink color; os closed except in multiparas, in whom os admits fingertip	Eversion, reddish erosion, nabothian or retention cysts, cervical polyp; granular area that bleeds (carcinoma of cervix) Red spots on and around cervix (trichomonas vaginitis) Presence of string or plastic tip from cervix (IUD in uterus)	Provide client with a hand mirror and identify genital structures for her. Encourage her to view her cervix. Refer to physician if indicated. Advise client of potential serious risks of leaving an IUD in place during pregnancy. Refer to physician for removal.
	Pregnancy changes: 1-4 weeks' gestation: enlargement in anteroposterior diameter 4-6 weeks' gestation: softening of cervix (Goodell's sign) and cervicouterine junction (Ladin's sign); softening of isthmus of uterus (Hegar's sign); cervix takes on bluish coloring (Chadwick's sign) 8 weeks' gestation: uterus globular in shape and anteflexed against bladder 8-12 weeks' gestation: vagina and cervix appear bluish violet in color (Chadwick's sign)	Inability to elicit Goodell's sign (inflammatory conditions and carcinomas)	Refer to physician.
Uterus	Pear-shaped Located at upper end of vagina	Retroversion, retroflexion Prolapse	Discuss appropriate individualized exercises and need for rest. Refer to physician if indicated.

*Possible causes of alterations are placed in parentheses.
[†]This column provides guidelines for further assessment and initial nursing interventions.

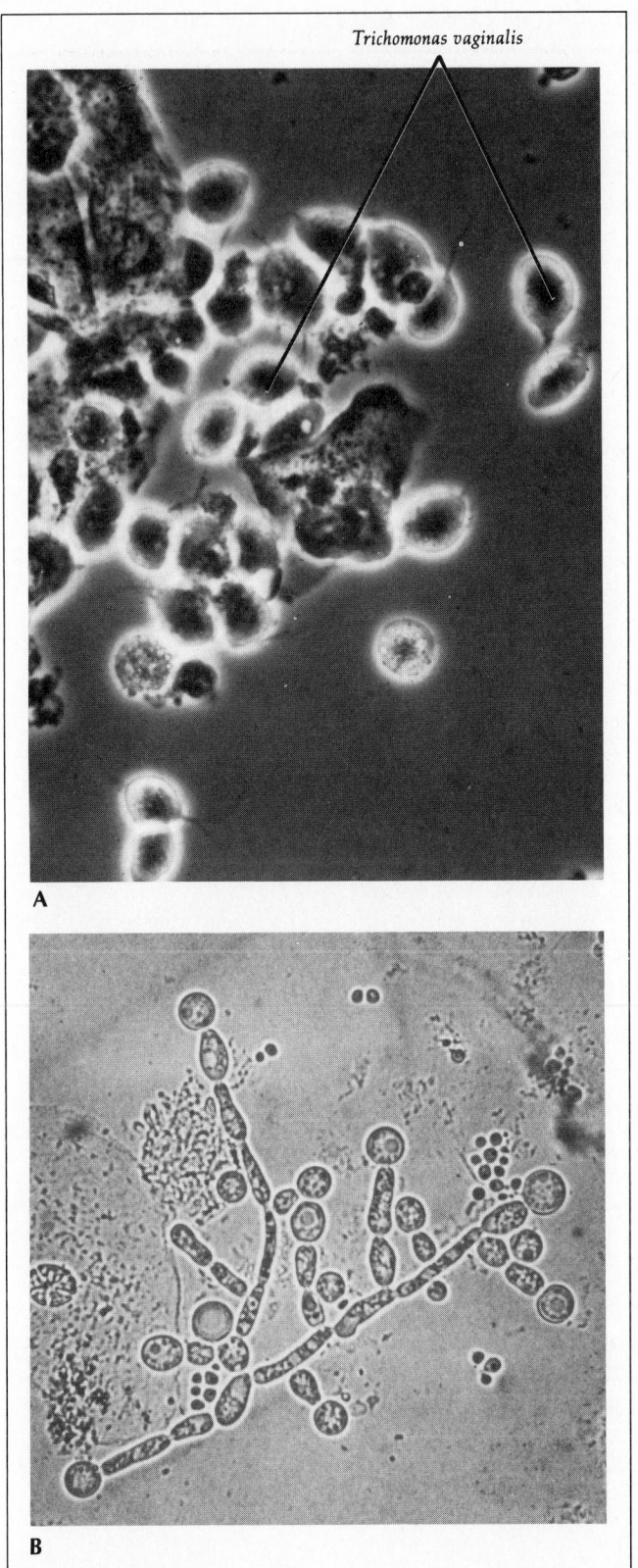

Trichomonas vaginalis

A

B

FIGURE 10–2 Microscopic appearance of microorganisms found in the vagina. **A,** *Trichomonas vaginalis.* **B,** The hyphae and spores of *Candida albicans.* (Courtesy of Tortora et al. 1982. *Microbiology.* Menlo Park, Calif.: Benjamin/Cummings Publishing Co.)

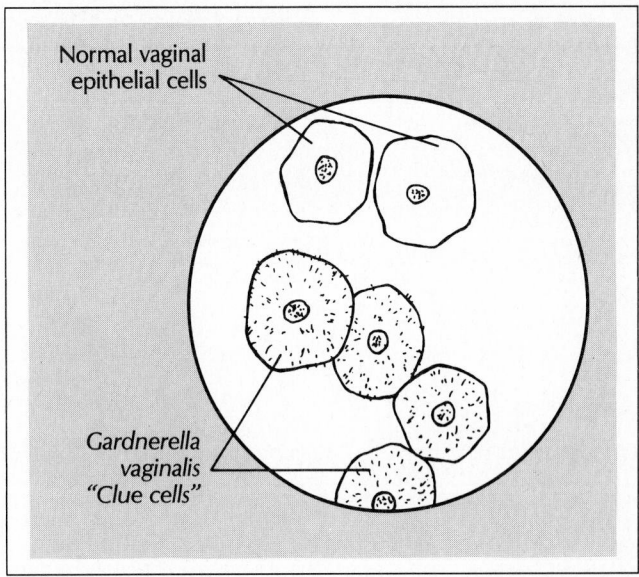

Normal vaginal
epithelial cells

*Gardnerella
vaginalis*
"Clue cells"

FIGURE 10–3 Depiction of the "clue cells" characteristically seen in *Gardnerella vaginalis.*

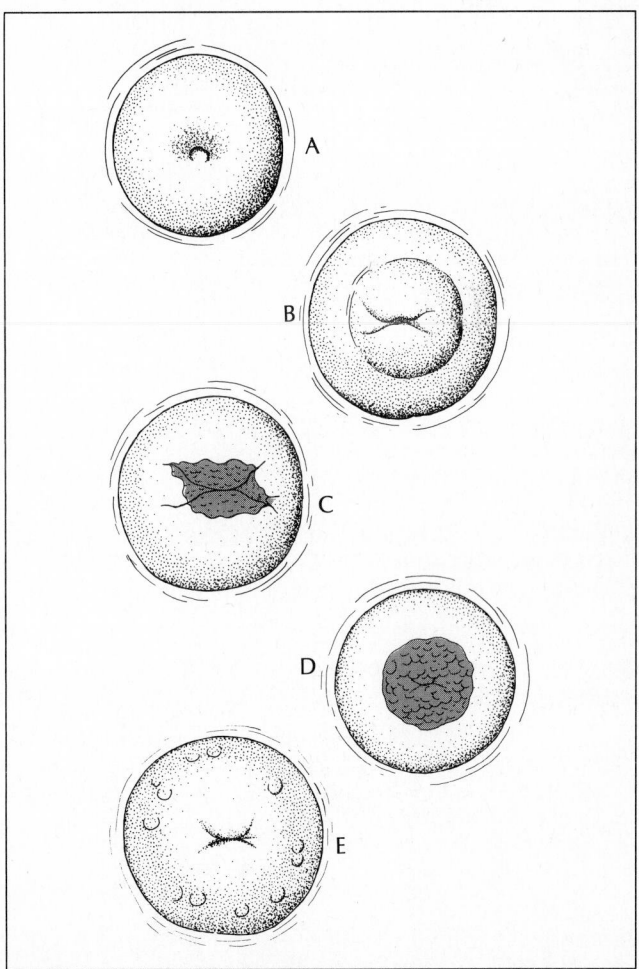

A

B

C

D

E

FIGURE 10–4 Common appearance of cervix on vaginal exam. **A,** Healthy nulliparous cervix. **B,** Lacerated multigravidous cervix. **C,** Everted cervix. **D,** Eroded cervix. **E,** Nabothian cysts.

INITIAL PRENATAL PHYSICAL ASSESSMENT GUIDE Cont'd

Assess	Normal findings	Alterations and possible causes*	Nursing responses to data†
	Mobile within pelvis	Fixed (pelvic inflammatory disease)	Refer to physician.
	Smooth surface	Nodular surface (fibromas)	
Ovaries	Small, walnut-shaped, nontender	Pain on movement of cervix (pelvic inflammatory disease) Enlarged or nodular ovaries (cyst, tumor, tubal pregnancy, corpus luteum of pregnancy)	Evaluate adnexal areas. Refer to physician.
Pelvic measurements	Internal measurements: 1. Diagonal conjugate 12.5 cm	Measurement below normal	Vaginal delivery may not be possible if deviations are present. Consider possibility of cesarean delivery. Determine CPD by radiological examination and ultrasound.
	2. Obstetric conjugate estimated by subtracting 1.5–2 cm from diagonal conjugate	Disproportion of pubic arch	
	3. Inclination of sacrum	Abnormal curvature of sacrum	
	4. Motility of coccyx External measurements: intertuberosity diameter >8 cm	Fixed or malposition of coccyx	
Anus and rectum Inspect sacrococcygeal and perianal area	No lumps, rashes, excoriation, tenderness	Hemorrhoids, rectal prolapse Nodular lesion (carcinoma)	Counsel about appropriate prevention and relief measures. Refer to physician for further evaluation.
	Cervix may be felt through rectal wall	Pilonidal cyst or sinus, anorectal fistula, anal fissure, rectal polyps, internal or external hemorrhoids	Counsel about appropriate relief measures (see Chapter 11).
	Stool negative for obvious or occult blood Symmetrical buttocks	Stool positive for blood (intestinal bleeding)	Refer to physician.
Laboratory evaluation Hematologic tests Hemoglobin	12–16 g/dL	<12 g/dL (anemia)	Hemoglobin <12 g/dL requires iron supplementation and nutritional counseling.
	Women residing in high altitude may have higher levels of hemoglobin		

*Possible causes of alterations are placed in parentheses.
†This column provides guidelines for further assessment and initial nursing interventions.

INITIAL PRENATAL PHYSICAL ASSESSMENT GUIDE Cont'd

Assess	Normal findings	Alterations and possible causes*	Nursing responses to data†
ABO and Rh typing	Normal distribution of blood types (Table 10-2) (p. 236)	Rh negative	If Rh negative, check for presence of anti-Rh antibodies. Check partner's blood type. If partner is Rh positive, discuss with client the need for antibody titers during pregnancy, management during the intrapartal period, and possible candidacy for RhoGAM.
Complete blood count (CBC)			
Hematocrit	38%–47%	Anemia or blood dyscrasias	Perform WBC and Schilling differential cell count.
Red blood cells (RBC)	4.2–5.4 million/μL		
White blood cells (WBC)	4500–11,000/μL	Presence of infection; may be elevated in pregnancy and with labor.	Evaluate for other signs of infection.
Differential			
Neutrophils	40%–60%		
Bands	up to 5%		
Eosinophils	1%–3%		
Basophils	up to 1%		
Lymphocytes	20%–40%		
Monocytes	4%–8%		
Syphilis tests—STS (serologic test for syphilis); complement fixation test; VDRL (Venereal Disease Research Laboratory); flocculation test	Nonreactive	Positive reaction STS tests may have 25%–45% incidence of biologic false positive results; false results may occur in individuals who have acute viral or bacterial infections, hypersensitivity reactions, recent vaccination, collagen disease, malaria, or tuberculosis	Positive results may be confirmed with the FTA-ABS tests (fluorescent treponemal antibody absorption tests). All tests for syphilis give positive results in the secondary stage of the disease; antibiotic tests may cause negative test results.
Gonorrhea culture	Negative	Positive	Refer for treatment.
Urinalysis			
Color	Pale golden yellow color	Orange, red, brown hues (porphyria, hemoglobinuria, urobilinuria, or bilirubinemia, treatment with phenazopyridine)	Assess for deviations. Porphyria may be indicated if urine becomes burgundy red on exposure to light.
Specific gravity	1.015–1.025	<1.015 (renal tubular dysfunction); >1.025 (ADH deficiency)	Refer to physician.
pH	4.6–8.0	Alkaline urine (metabolic alkalemia, *Proteus* infections, old specimen)	

*Possible causes of alterations are placed in parentheses.
†This column provides guidelines for further assessment and initial nursing interventions.

INITIAL PRENATAL PHYSICAL ASSESSMENT GUIDE Cont'd

Assess	Normal findings	Alterations and possible causes*	Nursing responses to data†
Glucose	Negative (small amount of glycosuria may occur in pregnancy)	Glycosuria (low renal threshold for glucose, diabetes mellitus, Cushing's disease, pheochromocytoma)	Assess blood glucose. Test urine for ketones.
Protein	Negative	Proteinuria (urine specimen contaminated with vaginal secretions, strenuous physical exercise, fever, kidney disease, postrenal infection, preeclampsia)	Repeat urinalysis. Instruct client in collection technique. If second specimen positive, do further assessment.
Red blood cells	Negative	Blood in urine (calculi, cystitis, glomerulonephritis, neoplasm)	Refer to physician.
White blood cells	Negative	Presence of white blood cells (infection in genitourinary tract)	Assess for other signs of infection. Refer to physician if indicated.
Casts	Negative	Presence of casts (nephrotic syndrome)	
Rubella titer	Hemagglutination-inhibition test (HAI) >1:10 indicates woman is immune	HAI titer <1:10	Immunization will be given within 6 weeks after delivery. Instruct client whose titers are <1:10 to avoid children who have rubella.
Antibody screen	Negative	Positive	For positive results, further testing should be done to identify specific antibodies. In addition, antibody titers may be done during pregnancy.
Sickle cell screen for black Americans	Negative	Positive; test results would include a description of cells	Refer to physician.
Papanicolaou (Pap) test	Negative‡	Test results that show atypical cells‡	Refer to physician. Discuss the meaning of the various classes with the client and importance of follow-up.
Chest x-ray	Clear	Infiltrate (pulmonary lesions, tuberculosis)	Provide lead shield for abdomen while film is taken. Note: Current trend is to avoid x-ray exposure to growing fetus. Chest x-ray is not routinely done. If tuberculosis is suspected, PPD is performed. Chest x-ray examination would be indicated for positive PPD.

*Possible causes of alterations are placed in parentheses.
†This column provides guidelines for further assessment and initial nursing interventions.
‡The current trend is to report Pap test results as follows:
1. Negative
2. Atypical (this finding would describe the cells)
Some clinicians may still use Class I to Class V terminology, with Class I being negative and Class V cancer in situ. It is important to know the scoring system used by the laboratory doing the test.

Procedure 10-1   Auscultation of Chest

Objective	Nursing action	Rationale
Assess quality and intensity of breath sounds	Place diaphragm of the stethoscope on client's chest and listen for breath sounds. Instruct her to breathe in and out through her mouth. Note: Be observant for signs of hyperventilation. First listen to apexes or upper lobes of lungs, comparing one side with other. Progress systematically downward from apexes to posterior, lateral, and anterior chest, always comparing both sides. Allow two to three breaths in each area (Figure 10-5). Evaluate sounds as to pitch, intensity, quality, and relative duration of inspiratory phases.

Listen for adventitious or abnormal breath sounds. | Vesicular breath sounds can be heard over most of the lung area. Bronchovesicular breath sounds can be heard near main stem bronchi.

Bronchial or tubular breath sounds can be heard over trachea.

Absent or decreased breath sounds can occur in bronchial obstruction, emphysema, or shallow breathing. Increased breath sounds or change in pitch can occur in conditions causing lung tissue consolidation. Rales are noncontinuous sounds most frequently heard on inspiration. They are produced by moisture in tracheobronchial tree. Rhonchi and wheezes are continuous sounds and may be present on inspiration and expiration but usually are more prominent on expiration. They are produced when air flows across narrowed air passages. Friction rubs are grating or crackling sounds usually heard on inspiration and expiration. They are produced when pleura is inflamed. |

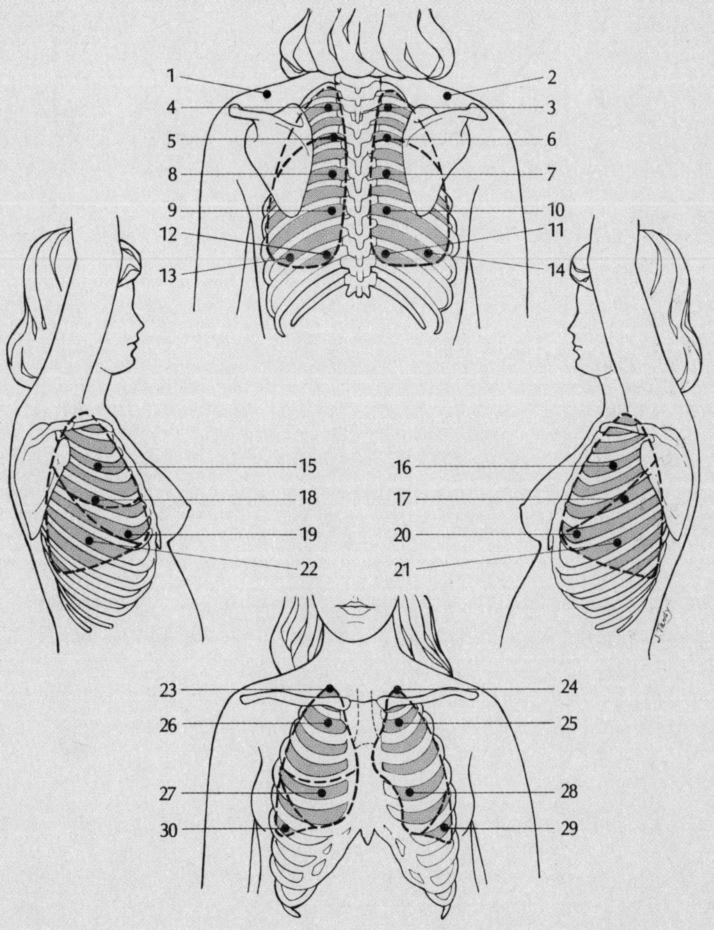

FIGURE 10-5 Suggested sequence for auscultation of the chest.

Procedure 10-2   Breast Self-Examination

Objective	Nursing action	Rationale
Provide instruction	Instruct woman as follows: 1. Lie down. Put one hand behind your head. With the other hand, fingers flattened, gently feel your breast. Press lightly (Figure 10-6,A). Now examine the other breast.	Over 74,000 American women develop breast cancer every year. About half die within 5 years. Experience shows that 95% of breast cancers are found by women themselves. When women discover lumps in their breasts at a very early stage, surgery can save 70%-80% of proven cancer cases.*
	2. Figure 10-6,B shows you how to check each breast. Begin as you see in C and follow the arrows, feeling gently for a lump or thickening. Remember to feel all parts of each breast.	
	3. Now repeat the same procedure sitting up, with the hand still behind your head (Figure 10-6,C).	
	Instruct woman to perform breast self-examination on monthly basis.	Monthly assessment will increase opportunity to identify breast changes. Nonpregnant women should check breasts at end of menstrual period.

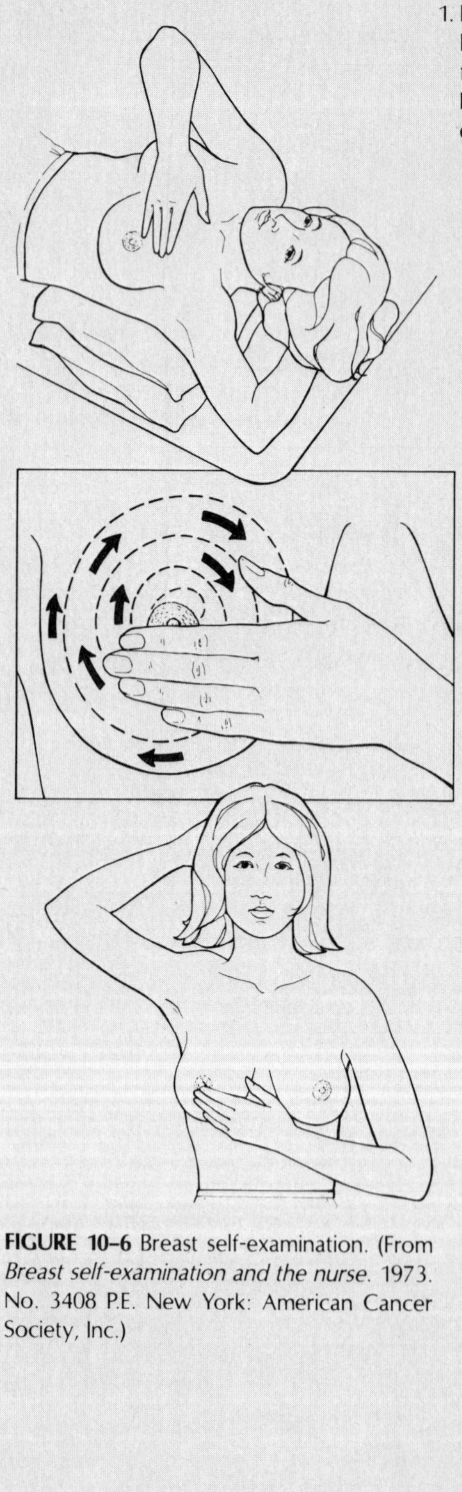

FIGURE 10-6 Breast self-examination. (From *Breast self-examination and the nurse.* 1973. No. 3408 P.E. New York: American Cancer Society, Inc.)

*From American Cancer Society. 1973. *Breast self-examination and the nurse.* No. 3408 PE.

Procedure 10–3   Cardiac Examination

Objective	Nursing action	Rationale
Provide optimal positioning for assessment	In quiet, comfortably warm room, have woman remove all clothing from upper torso. Place client in supine semi-Fowler's position with upper body elevated 30–40 degrees.	Client privacy is provided. Quiet warm room decreases shivering and subsequent muscular noises.
Assess chest to ascertain heart size and position	Percuss chest.	Determine adequacy of cardiac and respiratory systems (enlargement or displacement of the heart).
Determine the apex beat or PMI	Standing to right of woman, use fingertips and palmar aspect of right hand to palpate first over apex toward axilla and lower rib margin. PMI is usually located at fifth intercostal space 7–9 cm left of midsternal border, and is 1–2 cm in diameter. Optimal position is supine.	Malposition may indicate enlargement or abnormal placement of the heart.
Assess for presence of thrills	Palpate precordium at listening areas of heart.	Thrills are palpable vibrations that resemble cat's purr and are associated with cardiac defects.
Determine rate and rhythm	Auscultate with stethoscope (normal rate 60–100 beats/min). Palpate radial pulse; it should be simultaneous with the apical.	Rhythm may vary slightly with respirations. Deviations are gross irregularities or skipped beats.
Evaluate heart sounds	Auscultate during normal respiration, in deep expiration, and when client is holding her breath. Auscultate in same manner with woman on left side and then with her sitting up and slightly forward. Auscultate with stethoscope for normal sounds, abnormal sounds, and extra sounds at the four listening areas (Figure 10–7): 1. Apical or mitral area: left midclavicular line at fifth ICS. 2. Tricuspid or xiphoid area: lower left sternal border at fourth ICS. 3. Aortic area: second right ICS at the right sternal border. 4. Pulmonic area: second to third left interspace near left sternal border. Lightly place bell of stethoscope on chest for low-frequency sounds; firmly place stethoscope diaphragm against chest for high sounds. Listen for frequency (pitch), intensity (loudness), duration, and timing during cardiac cycle.	Auscultation with client in various positions allows detection of normal heart sound, low-frequency diastolic sounds, high-pitched diastolic murmurs of aortic or pulmonic valve insufficiency, and medium-pitched, harsh, systolic murmurs.

Procedure 10-3   Cardiac Examination Cont'd

Objective	Nursing action	Rationale
	Listen for first heart sound (S₁) at second right or left ICS. Use diaphragm of stethoscope.	S_2 in this area. S_1 may sound slightly split. Extra sound in right ICS may signify aortic valvular disease. Extra or prolonged sounds in left ICS space may indicate pulmonic valvular disease.
	Listen at heart apex in fifth left ICS.	S_1 louder than S_2; S_2 may sound split on inspiration.
	Use bell of stethoscope to listen for extra or abnormal heart sounds.	S_3 immediately follows S_2 and corresponds to syllable rhythm in "Kentucky." Physiologic third heart sound may be present in children. In older woman, third heart sound is pathologic. Fourth heart sound may immediately precede S_1, and heart rhythm is similar to syllable rhythm in "Tennessee."
	Listen for presence of murmurs. Determine location, timing, and duration.	Harsh blowing or rumbling sounds may radiate along flow of blood downstream from source and may be of continuous duration.

FIGURE 10-7 Auscultation of heart sounds.

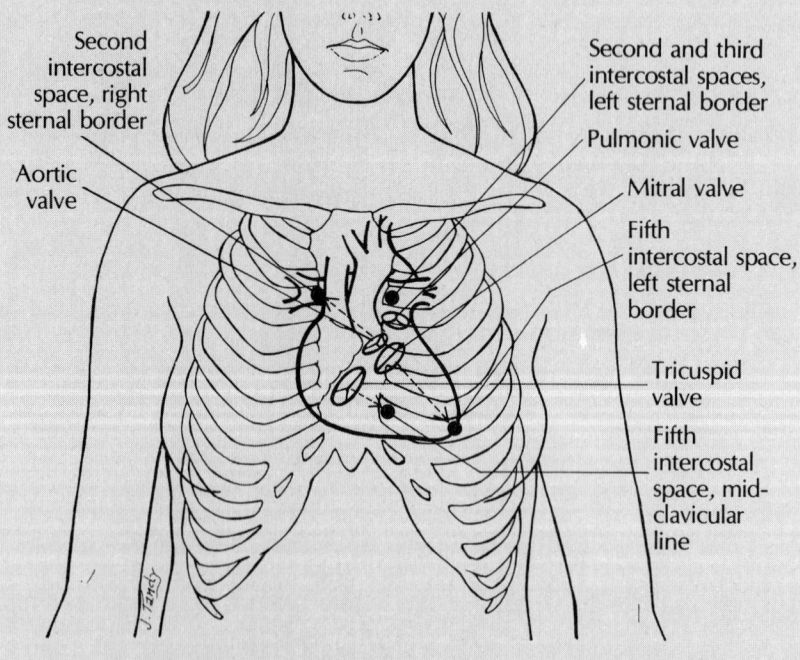

Second intercostal space, right sternal border

Aortic valve

Second and third intercostal spaces, left sternal border

Pulmonic valve

Mitral valve

Fifth intercostal space, left sternal border

Tricuspid valve

Fifth intercostal space, mid-clavicular line

Procedure 10–4 Assisting with Pelvic Examination

Objective	Nursing action	Rationale
Prepare client	Explain procedure.	Explanation of procedure decreases anxiety.
	Instruct client to empty her bladder and to remove clothing below waist. She may be encouraged to keep her shoes on and may be given a disposable drape to hold in front of herself.	Comfort is promoted during internal examination. She may feel more comfortable with shoes on rather than supporting her weight with bare heels against cold stirrups.
	Position client in lithotomy position with thighs flexed and adducted. Place her feet in stirrups. Buttocks should extend slightly beyond end of examining table (Figure 10–8).	
	Drape client with a sheet, leaving flap so perineum can be exposed.	
Ensure smooth accomplishment of procedure	Prepare and arrange following equipment so that they are easily accessible:	Examination is facilitated.
	1. Various-sized vaginal specula, warmed prior to insertion.	Warmed speculum assists in lubrication and facilitates initial insertion when culture and smears are to be taken; many standard lubricants cannot be utilized.
	2. Glove.	
	3. Lubricant.	
	4. Pelvimeter.	
	5. Materials for Pap smear and gonorrhea culture.	
	6. Good light source.	
Provide support to client as physician or nurse practitioner carries out examination	Explain each part of examination as it is performed: inspection of external genitals, vagina, and cervix; bimanual examination of internal organs.	Relaxation is promoted.
	Instruct client to relax and breathe slowly.	
	Advise client when speculum is to be inserted and ask her to bear down.	When speculum is inserted, woman may feel intravaginal pressure. Bearing down helps open vaginal orifice and relax perineal muscles.
	Lubricate examiner's finger well prior to bimanual examination.	
Provide client comfort at end of examination	Assist client to sitting position.	Supine position may create postural hypotension.
	Provide tissues to wipe lubricant from perineum.	Upon assuming sitting position, vaginal secretions along with lubricant may be discharged.
	Provide privacy for client to dress.	Comfort and sense of privacy is promoted.

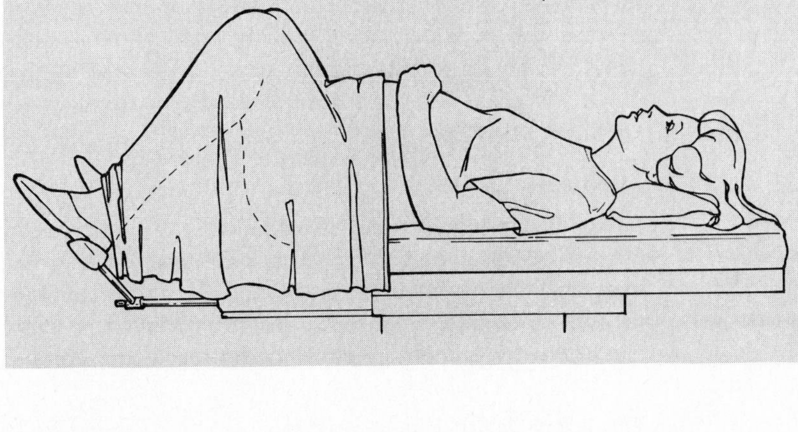

FIGURE 10–8 Woman in lithotomy position and draped for a pelvic examination.

Table 10–2   Normal Distribution of Blood Types According to Race (in percent)*

Blood group	Whites	Blacks	American Indians	Orientals
O	45	49	79	40
A	40	27	16	28
B	11	20	4	27
AB	4	4	1	5
Rh-positive	60	72	86	95
Rh-negative	40	28	14	5

*From Miller, W. 1977. *Technical manual of American Association of Blood Banks*. Washington, D.C.: The Association.

a discussion of the diagnosis of pregnancy). The assessment guide is detailed so that maternity nurses using it will be able to utilize the information pertinent to them in their role, at their level of expertise, and based on the practices and policies of each agency.

Thoroughness and a systematic procedure are the most important considerations when performing a physical exam. To facilitate completeness, the assessment guide is organized into four columns: area to be assessed, normal findings, alterations and possible causes of the alterations, and nursing response to data. The nurse should be aware that certain organs and systems are assessed concurrently with other systems.

Nursing interventions based on assessment of the normal physiologic and psychologic changes associated with pregnancy, and client teaching and counseling needs that have been mutually agreed upon are discussed in more detail in Chapter 11.

DETERMINATION OF DELIVERY DATE

Nägele's Rule

The delivery date, or estimated date of confinement (EDC), can be determined in a number of different ways. The most common method is Nägele's rule. To utilize this method, take the first day of the last menstrual period (LMP), subtract 3 months, and add 7 days. For example:

First day of LMP	November 21
Subtract 3 months	− 3 months
	August 21
Add 7 days	+ 7 days
EDC	August 28

A simpler method is to change the months to numerical terms:

November 21 becomes	11—21
Subtract 3 months	− 3
	8—21
Add 7 days	+ 7
EDC	August 28

If a woman with a history of menses every 28 days remembers her LMP and was not taking oral contraceptives prior to becoming pregnant, Nägele's rule may be a fairly accurate determiner of her predicted delivery date. However, if her cycle is irregular or 35–40 days in length, the time of ovulation may be delayed by several days. If she has been on oral contraceptives, ovulation may be delayed several weeks following her last menses. Ovulation usually occurs 14 days before the onset of the next menses, not 14 days after the previous menses.

Uterine Size

PHYSICAL EXAMINATION

When a woman is examined in the first 10–12 weeks of her pregnancy and the nurse practitioner or physician thinks that her uterine size is compatible with her menstrual history, uterine size may be the single most important clinical method for dating her pregnancy. In many cases, however, women do not seek obstetric attention until well into their second trimester, when it becomes much more difficult to evaluate specific uterine size. In the case of the obese woman, it is most difficult to determine uterine size early in a pregnancy.

FUNDAL HEIGHT

Fundal height may be used as an indicator of uterine size, although this is at best only accurate within about 4 weeks and cannot be used late in pregnancy. A centimeter tape measure is used to measure the distance abdominally from the top of the symphysis pubis to the top of the uterine fundus (McDonald's method). Fundal height usually correlates with gestational age until the third trimester, when fetal weights vary considerably. Thus at 26 weeks' gestation, fundal height is probably about 26 cm. At 20 weeks' gestation, the fundus is about 20 cm and at the level of the umbilicus in an average female.

McDonald's rule may also be used to measure fundal height in the second and third trimesters. Place the tape measure at the notch of the symphysis pubis and measure up over the fundus (Figure 10–9). Calculation is done as follows:

Height of fundus (in centimeters) × 2/7 =
Duration of pregnancy in lunar months
  Example: 28 cm × 2/7 = 8 lunar months
Height of fundus (in centimeters) × 8/7 =
Duration of pregnancy in weeks
  Example: 28 cm × 8/7 = 32 weeks

If the woman is very tall or very short, fundal height will differ.

Measurements of fundal height from month to month and week to week may give indications of intrauterine growth retardation (IUGR) if there is a lag in progression, or indications of the presence of twins or hydramnios if there is a sudden increase in height. Unfortunately, this method of dating a pregnancy can be quite inaccurate in obese women, in women with uterine fibroids, and in mothers who develop hydramnios.

QUICKENING

Fetal movements felt by the mother may give some indications that the fetus is nearing 20 weeks' gestation. However, quickening may be experienced between 16 and 22 weeks' gestation, so this is not a completely accurate method. One can begin to listen for a fetal heartbeat weekly after the woman experiences quickening and can use this indication to assist documentation for a delivery date.

FETAL HEARTBEAT

The fetal heartbeat can be detected as early as week 16 and almost always by 19 or 20 weeks of gestation with an ordinary fetoscope. In the case of twins or the obese woman, it may be later than this before the fetal heartbeat can be detected. Fetal heartbeat may be detected with the ultrasonic Doppler device (Figure 10–10) as early as 8 weeks (Leopold and Asher, 1974) although the average is 10–12 weeks' gestation.

Ultrasound

In the first trimester, ultrasound scanning can detect a gestational sac as early as 5–6 weeks after the LMP, fetal heart activity by 9–10 weeks and occasionally earlier, and fetal breathing movement by 11 weeks of pregnancy.

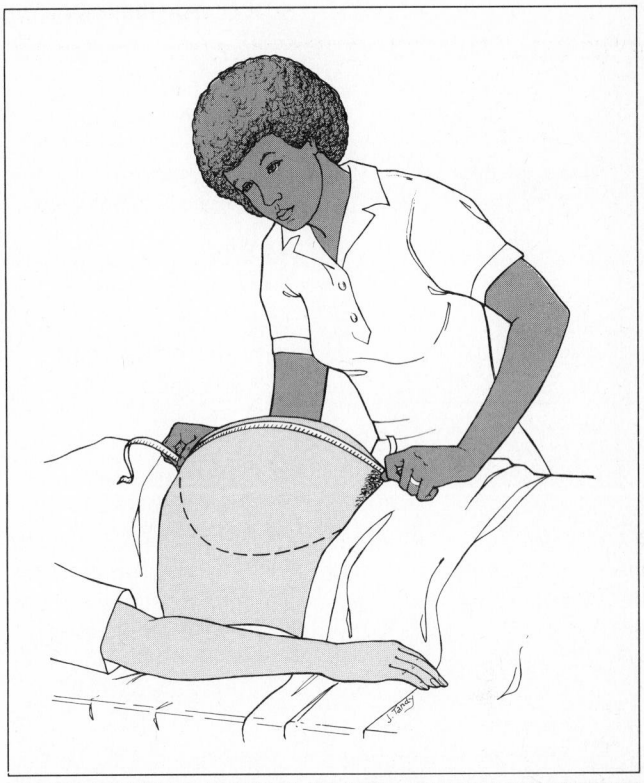

FIGURE 10–9 Use of McDonald's method to measure fundal height.

Crown-to-rump measurements can be made for assessment of fetal age until the fetal head can be defined. Biparietal diameter measurements can be made by approximately 12–13 weeks, and are more accurate earlier in pregnancy when less biologic variation occurs.

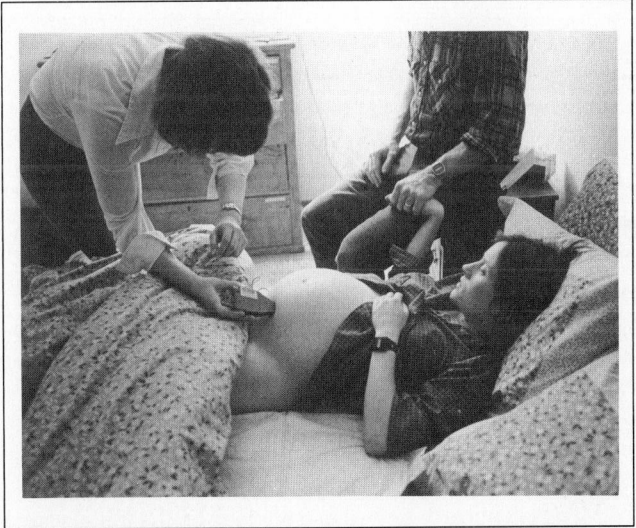

FIGURE 10–10 Listening to fetal heartbeat with Doppler device.

INITIAL PSYCHOLOGIC ASSESSMENT GUIDE

Assess	Normal findings	Alterations and possible causes*	Nursing responses to data†
Psychologic status	Excitement and/or apprehension; ambivalence	Marked anxiety (fear of pregnancy diagnosis, fear of medical facility)	Establish lines of communication. Active listening is useful. Establish trusting relationship. Encourage woman to take active part in her care.
		Apathy Display of anger with pregnancy diagnosis	Establish communication and begin counseling. Use active listening techniques.
Educational needs	May have questions about pregnancy or may need time to adjust to reality of pregnancy		Establish educational, supporting environment that can be expanded throughout pregnancy.
Support systems	Can identify at least two or three individuals with whom woman is emotionally intimate (partner, parent, sibling, friend, etc.)	Isolated (no telephone, unlisted number); cannot name a neighbor or friend whom she can call upon in an emergency; does not perceive parents as part of her support system	Institute support system through community groups. Develop trusting relationship with health care professionals.
Economic status	Source of income is stable and sufficient to meet basic needs of daily living and medical needs	Limited prenatal care Poor physical health Limited utilization of health care system Unstable economic status	Discuss available resources for health maintenance and delivery. Institute appropriate referral for meeting expanding family's needs — food stamps, etc.
Stability of living conditions	Adequate, stable housing for expanding family's needs	Crowded living conditions Questionable supportive environment for newborn	Refer to appropriate community agency. Work with family on self-help ways to improve situation.

* Possible causes of alterations are placed in parentheses.
† This column provides guidelines for further assessment and initial nursing interventions.

INITIAL PSYCHOLOGIC ASSESSMENT

At the initial visit the woman may be most concerned with the diagnosis of pregnancy. However, during this visit she (and her partner, if he is present) is also evaluating the health team that she has chosen. The establishment of the nurse–client relationship will enable the woman to better evaluate the health team and also provides the nurse with a basis for an atmosphere that is conducive to interviewing, support, and education. A psychologic assessment is difficult to obtain if the client does not feel free to talk.

Many clients are excited and anxious on the initial visit. Because of this, the initial psychologic assessment is general and the goal is to set the foundation for a trusting nurse–client relationship.

SUBSEQUENT PHYSICAL ASSESSMENT

The recommended frequency of prenatal visits is as follows:

• Monthly for the first 32 weeks of gestation.
• Every 2 weeks to week 36.
• After week 36, every week until delivery.

The accompanying Subsequent Physical Assessment Guide provides a systematic approach to the regular physical examinations that the pregnant woman should undergo for optimal prenatal care.

SUBSEQUENT PHYSICAL ASSESSMENT GUIDE

Assess	Normal findings	Alterations and possible causes*	Nursing responses to data[†]
Vital signs			
Temperature	36.2–37.6C (98–99.6F)	Elevated temperature (infection)	Evaluate for signs of infection. Refer to physician.
Pulse	60–90/min Rate may increase 10 beats/min during pregnancy	Increased pulse rate (anxiety, cardiac disorders)	Note irregularities. Evaluate anxiety and stress.
Respiration	16–24/min	Marked tachypnea or abnormal patterns (respiratory disease)	Refer to physician.
Blood pressure	90–140/60–90 (falls in second trimester)	>140/90 (preeclampsia)	Assess for edema, proteinuria, hyperreflexia. Refer to physician. Schedule appointments more frequently.
Weight gain	First trimester: 2–4 lb Second trimester: 11 lb Third trimester: 11 lb	Excessive weight gain (excessive caloric intake, edema, preeclampsia)	Discuss appropriate weight gain. Provide nutritional counseling. Assess for presence of edema.
Edema	Small amount of dependent edema, especially in last weeks of pregnancy	Edema in hands, face, legs, feet (preeclampsia)	Identify any correlation between edema and activities, blood pressure or proteinuria. Refer to physician if indicated.
Uterine size	See Initial Physical Assessment Guide for normal changes during pregnancy	Unusually rapid growth (multiple gestation, hydatidiform mole, hydramnios, miscalculation of EDC)	Evaluate fetal status. Determine height of fundus using McDonald's rule (p. 237). Use diagnostic ultrasound.
Fetal heartbeat	120–160/min Funic souffle	Absence of fetal heartbeat after 20 weeks of gestation (maternal obesity, fetal demise)	Evaluate fetal status.
Laboratory evaluation			
Hemoglobin	12–16 g/dL Pseudoanemia of pregnancy	<12g/dL (anemia)	Provide nutritional counseling. Hemoglobin may be repeated at 7 months' gestation. Women of Mediterranean heritage need a close check on hemoglobin because of possibility of thalassemia.
Antibody screen	Negative	Positive	Refer for further testing to identify specific antibodies. Titers may be indicated.
Urinalysis	See Initial Physical Assessment Guide (pp. 229–230) for normal findings	See Initial Physical Assessment Guide (pp. 229–230) for deviations	Repeat urinalysis at 7 months' gestation.

SUBSEQUENT PHYSICAL ASSESSMENT GUIDE Cont'd

Assess	Normal findings	Alterations and possible causes*	Nursing responses to data†
Protein	Negative	Proteinuria, albuminuria (contamination by vaginal discharge, urinary tract infection, preeclampsia)	Obtain dipstick urine sample. Refer to physician if deviations are present.
Glucose	Negative Note: Glycosuria may be present due to physiologic alterations in glomerular filtration rate and renal threshold	Persistent glycosuria (diabetes mellitus)	Refer to physician.
Danger signs of pregnancy	Client knows to report following danger signs immediately:	Lack of information	Provide appropriate teaching.
	1. Sudden gush of fluid from vagina	Premature rupture of membranes	Encourage women to report danger signs.
	2. Vaginal bleeding	Placenta abruptio, previa Lesions of cervix or vagina "Bloody show"	Refer to physician immediately for evaluation.
	3. Abdominal pain	Premature labor, placenta abruptio	
	4. Temperature above 38.3C (101F) and chills	Infection	
	5. Dizziness, blurring of vision, double vision, spots before eyes	Hypertension, preeclampsia	
	6. Persistent vomiting	Hyperemesis gravidarum	
	7. Severe headache	Hypertension, preeclampsia	
	8. Edema of hands, face, legs, and feet	Preeclampsia	
	9. Muscular irritability, convulsions	Preeclampsia, eclampsia	
	10. Epigastric pain	Preeclampsia — ischemia in major abdominal vessels	
	11. Oligouria	Renal impairment, decreased fluid intake	
	12. Dysuria	Urinary tract infection	
	13. Absence of fetal movement	Maternal medication, obesity, fetal death	

* Possible causes of alterations are placed in parentheses.
† This column provides guidelines for further assessment and initial nursing interventions.

SUBSEQUENT PSYCHOLOGIC ASSESSMENT

Periodic prenatal examinations offer the nurse an opportunity to assess the maternity client's psychologic needs and emotional status. If the woman's partner attends the prenatal visits, his needs and concerns can also be identified.

The interchange between the nurse and client will be facilitated if it takes place in a friendly, trusting environment. Provide time for the client to ask questions and to air concerns. If the nurse provides the time and demonstrates genuine interest, the client will feel more at ease bringing up questions that she may believe are silly or concerns that she has been afraid to verbalize.

During the subsequent psychologic assessments, a client may manifest dysfunctional behavior patterns such as the following:

- Increasing anxiety
- Inability to establish communication
- Inappropriate responses or actions
- Denial of pregnancy
- Inability to cope with stress

- Failure to acknowledge quickening
- Failure to plan and prepare for the baby (for example, living arrangements, clothing, feeding methods)

If the client appears to have these or other critical psychologic problems, the nurse should refer her to the appropriate professionals.

The accompanying Subsequent Psychologic Assessment Guide provides a model for the psychologic evaluation of both the pregnant client and the expectant father.

SUBSEQUENT PSYCHOLOGIC ASSESSMENT GUIDE

Assess	Normal findings	Alterations and possible causes*	Nursing responses to data†
Expectant mother Psychologic status	Pregnancy changes: First trimester: incorporates idea of pregnancy; may feel ambivalent, especially if she must give up desired role; usually looks for signs of verification of pregnancy, such as increase in abdominal size, fetal movement, etc. Second trimester: baby becomes more real to woman as abdominal size increases and she feels movement; she begins to turn inward, becoming more introspective Third trimester: begins to think of baby as separate being; may feel restless and may feel that time of labor will never come; remains self-centered and concentrates on preparing place for baby	Increasing stress and anxiety Inability to establish communication; inability to accept pregnancy; inappropriate response or actions; denial of pregnancy; inability to cope	Encourage woman to take an active part in her care. Establish lines of communication. Establish a trusting relationship. Counsel as necessary. Refer to appropriate professional as needed.
Educational needs: self-care measures and knowledge	Knowledge about following: Breast care Hygiene Rest Exercise Nutrition Relief measures for common discomforts of pregnancy	Inadequate information	Teach and/or institute appropriate relief measures (see Chapter 11).
Sexual activity	Client knows how pregnancy affects sexual activity	Lack of information about effects of pregnancy and/or alternate positions during sexual intercourse	Provide counseling.

*Possible causes of alterations are placed in parentheses.
†This column provides guidelines for further assessment and initial nursing interventions.

SUBSEQUENT PSYCHOLOGIC ASSESSMENT GUIDE Cont'd

Assess	Normal findings	Alterations and possible causes*	Nursing responses to data†
Preparation for parenting	In last few weeks of pregnancy, couple has prepared equipment, clothing, and place for baby	Lack of preparation (denial, failure to adjust to baby, unwanted child)	Counsel. If lack of preparation is due to inadequacy of information, provide information (see Chapter 11).
Preparation for childbirth	Client aware of following: 1. Prepared childbirth techniques 2. Normal processes and changes during childbirth		If couple chooses particular technique, refer to classes (see Chapter 11 for description of childbirth preparation techniques). Encourage prenatal class attendance. Educate woman during visits based on current physical status. Provide reading list for more specific information.
	3. Problems that may occur as a result of drug and alcohol use and of smoking	Continued abuse of drugs and alcohol; denial of possible effect on self and baby	Review danger signs that were presented on initial visit.
	Woman has met other physician and/or nurse-midwife who may be attending her delivery in the absence of primary physician and/or nurse-midwife	Introduction of new individual at delivery may increase stress and anxiety for patient and partner	Introduce woman to all members of group practice.
Impending labor	Client knows signs of impending labor: 1. Uterine contractions that increase in frequency, duration, intensity 2. Bloody show 3. Expulsion of mucous plug 4. Rupture of membranes	Lack of information	Provide appropriate teaching, stressing importance of seeking appropriate medical assistance.
Expectant father Psychologic status	First trimester: may express excitement over confirmation of pregnancy and of his virility; concerns move toward providing for financial needs; energetic; may identify with some discomforts of pregnancy and may even exhibit symptoms	Increasing stress and anxiety Inability to establish communication Inability to accept pregnancy diagnosis Withdrawal of support Abandonment of the mother	Encourage expectant father to come to prenatal visits. Establish lines of communication. Establish trusting relationship.
	Second trimester: may feel more confident and be less concerned with financial matters; may have concerns about wife's changing size and shape, her increasing introspection		Counsel. Let expectant father know that it is normal for him to experience these feelings.

*Possible causes of alterations are placed in parentheses.
†This column provides guidelines for further assessment and initial nursing interventions.

SUBSEQUENT PSYCHOLOGIC ASSESSMENT GUIDE Cont'd

Assess	Normal findings	Alterations and possible causes*	Nursing responses to data[†]
	Third trimester: may have feelings of rivalry with fetus, especially during sexual activity; may make changes in his physical appearance and exhibit more interest in himself; may become more energetic; fantasizes about child but usually imagines older child; fears of mutilation and death of woman and child arise		Include expectant father in pregnancy activities as he desires. Provide education, information, and support. Increasing number of expectant fathers are demonstrating desire to be involved in many or all aspects of prenatal care, education, and preparation.

*Possible causes of alterations are placed in parentheses.
[†] This column provides guidelines for further assessment and initial nursing interventions.

ROLE OF THE NURSE

As pregnancy is increasingly viewed as a normal physiologic process and not a disease condition, the nurse is assuming a more important role in prenatal clinics and obstetricians' offices. It is often the nurse who develops the initial client rapport and with whom the client identifies. This facilitates prenatal counseling and education. A nurse who is also a certified nurse-midwife may be the primary caregiver during an uncomplicated pregnancy. A nurse who is a nurse practitioner may be sharing this role with a physician. An office nurse may complement the physician's role by added assessments while focusing on the counseling and psychologic aspects of pregnancy.

With each antepartal visit, an environment of comfort and open communication should be established. The nurse should convey an attitude of concern for the client as an individual and an availability to listen and discuss the woman's concerns and desires. This rapport can be initiated as the nurse evaluates the vital signs and weight of the client. A supportive atmosphere coupled with the guidelines found in the subsequent physical and psychological assessments will enable the nurse to identify needed areas of education and counseling.

SUMMARY

Assessment of psychologic, social, cultural, and physical data forms the framework of specific medical and nursing interventions throughout a woman's pregnancy. The nurse must have a thorough understanding of the normal physical changes that occur during pregnancy so that deviations can be recognized and treated in an appropriate manner.

References

Leopold, G. R., and Asher, W. M. 1974. Ultrasound in obstetrics and gynecology. *Radio. Clin. North Am.* 12:127.

Garn, S. M., et al. April 1981. Maternal hematologic levels and pregnancy outcomes. *Seminars in Perinatology.* 5:155.

Miller, W., ed. 1977. *Technical manual of American Association of Blood Banks.* Washington, D. C.: The Association.

Additional Readings

Danforth, D., ed. 1982. *Obstetrics and gynecology.* 4th ed. Philadelphia: Harper & Row.

Malasanos, L., et al. 1981. *Health assessment.* 2nd ed. St. Louis: The C. V. Mosby Co.

Varney, H. 1980. *Nurse-midwifery.* Boston: Blackwell Scientific Pub., Inc.

■ 11 ■

THE EXPECTANT FAMILY: NEEDS AND CARE

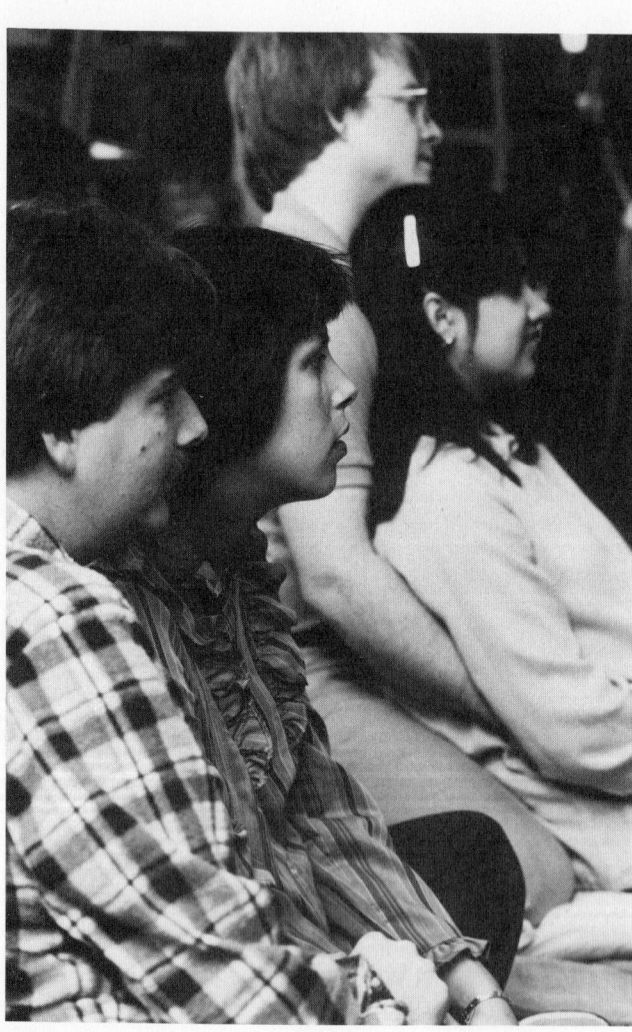

■ **CHAPTER CONTENTS**

PREGNANCY AND THE EXPECTANT FAMILY
Pregnancy as a Crisis
Pregnancy as a Developmental Stage

THE EXPECTANT FAMILY'S RESPONSES TO PREGNANCY
The Mother
The Father
Siblings
Grandparents

COMMON DISCOMFORTS OF PREGNANCY
First Trimester
Second and Third Trimesters
Nursing Responsibilities

COMMON CONCERNS DURING PREGNANCY
Breast Care
Clothing
Bathing
Employment
Travel
Activity and Rest
Exercises
Sexual Activity
Dental Care
Immunizations

Teratogenic Substances

Medications

Smoking

Alcohol

NUTRITION

Maternal Weight Gain

Nutritional Requirements

Vegetarianism

Factors Influencing Nutrition

Nursing Responsibilities

ANTEPARTAL NURSING MANAGEMENT

Assessment: Establishing the Data Base

Interventions

Classes for Family Members during Pregnancy

SELECTED METHODS OF CHILDBIRTH PREPARATION

Read Method

Psychoprophylactic (Lamaze) Method

Bradley Method

Hypnosis

PREPARING THE ADOLESCENT FOR CHILDBIRTH AND CHILDREARING

Physical Changes of Adolescence

Psychosocial Effects of Adolescence

The Pregnant Adolescent

The Adolescent Father

Parents' Reactions to Adolescent Pregnancy

Nursing Management of the Pregnant Adolescent

Prenatal Education for the Adolescent

■ OBJECTIVES

- Identify a family's responses to pregnancy and the appropriate nursing interventions.

- Identify the common discomforts occurring during pregnancy, their possible causes, and appropriate nursing interventions to alleviate the discomforts.

- Discuss the main areas of prenatal care requiring nursing assessment and instruction.

- Identify some of the concerns that the expectant couple may have regarding sexual activity.

- Compare nutritional needs during pregnancy and lactation with normal requirements.

- Identify the special dietary needs of pregnant women of various ethnic backgrounds.

- Identify socioeconomic and cultural influences on pregnancy and prenatal practices.

- Explain how the general nutrition of the woman before pregnancy affects the development of the infant.

- Describe the areas of assessment utilized in establishing a data base for the expectant family.

- Discuss nursing interventions for the family during pregnancy.

- Describe communication skills that parents may use to enhance family well-being.

- Compare and contrast methods of childbirth preparation.

- Determine differences between nursing management for adolescent childbirth and adult childbirth.

The body of the pregnant woman undergoes tremendous changes. These changes precipitate a number of physical discomforts that require intervention by the nurse who is managing the client's prenatal care. Generally, the nurse will find it sufficient to educate the client about self-care measures that promote relief of these annoying and possibly painful conditions. However, occasionally other nursing actions are required, depending on the severity of the problem or the ability of the woman to assume responsibility for her own care.

Pregnancy also precipitates a number of questions and concerns from the woman and her family regarding hygiene, possible changes in life-style, and nutrition. The nurse often assumes the roles of teacher and counselor for families who need information about pregnancy or who are having difficulty understanding how to adjust their lives to this event.

This chapter focuses on the family's response to pregnancy and on the common discomforts and concerns arising during pregnancy. It discusses hygiene and relief measures and examines the dynamics and significance of proper nutrition.

The chapter then considers various aspects of antepartal nursing management. This begins with the establishment of an appropriate data base, then explores cultural considerations, anticipatory guidance that is indicated and even considers some basic communication skills. Content is also presented on various types of childbirth preparation classes.

A discussion of antepartal needs and care would not be complete without considering the pregnant adolescent. This is done in depth in this chapter and then highlighted throughout the remainder of the book.

PREGNANCY AND THE EXPECTANT FAMILY

Pregnancy as Crisis

Pregnancy is a crisis in a family's life and therefore is accompanied by stress and anxiety, whether or not the pregnancy is desired. *Crisis* can be defined as any naturally occurring turning point (courtship, pregnancy, parenthood, death, or loss of a loved one) that necessitates intrapersonal and interpersonal changes and reorganization. *Stress* is any stimulus that evokes the affective responses of anxiety. Stress disrupts the individual's usual behavior, affect, and attitude and results in anxiety. *Anxiety* is a free-floating, poorly defined apprehensiveness about a vague threat of loss. The loss or threat of loss may be physical (body integrity), psychosocial (established relationships), or economic.

Pregnancy can be considered a maturational crisis, since it is a common event in the normal growth and development of the family. During a crisis, the individual or family is in disequilibrium. Egos weaken, usual defense mechanisms lose their effectiveness, unresolved material from the past reappears, and intrapersonal and interpersonal relationships shift. The period of disequilibrium and disorganization is characterized by abortive attempts to solve the perceived problems. If the crisis is unresolved, it will result in maladaptive behaviors in one or more family members, and possible disintegration of the family. Families who are able to resolve a maturational crisis successfully will return to normal functioning and can even strengthen the bonds in the family relationship (see Chapter 30).

Crisis and its potential for successful resolution are affected by the individual or family's (a) present level of organization or disorganization; (b) past experiences of success or failure with crisis, stress, and anxiety; (c) established coping patterns, productive or unproductive; and (d) availability and effectiveness of resources.

Pregnancy, whether it terminates in elective or spontaneous abortion or in a term infant, is a turning point in a couple's life. Pregnancy confirms one's biologic capabilities to reproduce, and it is evidence of one's participation in sexual activity and as such is an affirmation of one's sexuality. For beginning families, pregnancy is the transition period from childlessness to parenthood. If the pregnancy terminates in the birth of a child, the couple enters a new stage of their life together, one characterized by irreversibility and awesome responsibilities.

The expectant couple may be unaware of the physical, emotional, and cognitive state peculiar to pregnancy. The couple may anticipate no problem from such a normal event as pregnancy and therefore may be confused and distressed by the feelings and behaviors commonly associated with childbearing.

If the expectant woman is married or has a stable partner, she no longer is only a mate but also must assume the role of mother. Her partner will soon be a father. Career goals and mobility may be thwarted for one or both partners. Each partner begins to see the other in a different light. Their relationship takes on a different meaning to them and within the larger family and community. Their life-style changes. Role reorientation and re-identification are inevitable with each additional pregnancy and child. The set routines, family dynamics, and interactions are altered again with each pregnancy and require readjustment and realignment.

Even if a pregnant woman, by design or circumstance, is without a stable partner but plans to keep the baby or place it for adoption, her need for changes in role identity, for psychobiologic maturation, and for self-actualization still remains. The woman is no longer a separate individual. She must now consider the needs of another being who is totally dependent on her, at least during the pregnancy.

Decisions regarding financial matters also need to be made at this time. Will the woman work during the pregnancy and return to work after the baby is born? If she chooses to return to work, how soon after the birth of the child will she return? Many men have strong feelings about being the provider and caretaker of the family. Decisions may also need to be made about the division of tasks within in the home. If the woman expects to share household and child-care tasks with the man but he believes that women take care of home and children and men provide the income, conflicts will inevitably arise. When these differences are discussed openly, needs are identified, and solutions are agreed upon, the newly forming family moves toward meeting the needs of its members.

Colman and Colman (1972) undertook a comprehensive study of parents' reactions to pregnancy and found that, although it is a time of crisis, pregnancy can be a rewarding experience, especially if the couple has formed a trusting alliance and are sincere in their desire to share in every aspect of the experience. However, a weak relationship is often in greater jeopardy during pregnancy, especially if the man is forced to become involved in childbirth education classes and to be the woman's coach during labor and her supporter in the delivery room.

The couple must face the realities of labor and delivery before parenthood can be realized. Many nonparents have little idea what labor entails. Frequently, their information is based on experiences related to them by family members or friends, and these tales are often fraught with myths and exaggerations. Classes in prepared childbirth can help them overcome much of this lack of information or misinformation (see the discussion on specific methods of childbirth preparation later in this chapter).

Labor is threatening in many respects. Pain, disfigurement, disruption of bodily function, and even death are potential threats for the woman. The man faces the potential disfigurement of his wife, impairment of her health, or her death. Both fear that the baby may be ill or disfigured. The expectant couple is subject to anxiety during this period, and no one can reassure them about the outcome.

Colman and Colman (1972) describe a wide range of expected and normal reactions during pregnancy. Some are physical, others are basically emotional, and they often overlap. Colman and Colman observed that couples go through similar feelings and reactions during pregnancy whether it is their first, second, or third pregnancy, with a wide range of possible reactions. These reactions parallel the developmental tasks discussed in the next section, and the extremes of reactions may indicate the degree to which the task is accomplished. Both partners' possible reactions to the pregnancy are given in Table 11–1.

Pregnancy as a Developmental Stage

As discussed in Chapter 3, Duvall (1977) views the period of pregnancy and childbirth as a developmental stage in the expanding family that parallels the individual's psychosocial developmental tasks. Pregnancy can be a period of support or conflict for the couple, depending on the amount of adjustment each is willing to assume to maintain the family's equilibrium.

Three tasks are usually complementary and not likely to cause conflict:

1. The couple plans for the first child's arrival together, collecting information on how to be a mother and a father.
2. Each continues to participate in some separate activities with friends or family members. This may cause some conflict if the partners become too divergent in their activities unless an effort is made to limit these types of associations.
3. As time passes the man assumes the role of breadwinner and the woman assumes the role of homemaker. She prepares for the birth with layette and nursery organization, and the man becomes more overtly concerned with the financial responsibilities.

Each member of the expectant family must adjust to the experience of pregnancy and its implications. The psychologic integrity and growth of the family depends on the resolution of certain conflicts and acceptance of changes within the family structure as well as within each individual.

THE EXPECTANT FAMILY'S RESPONSES TO PREGNANCY

The Mother

The pregnant woman undertakes several psychologic tasks during pregnancy to establish a foundation for a healthy, mutually gratifying relationship with her infant.

1. *Acceptance of pregnancy.* She must resolve any ambivalence about pregnancy and eventually accept the embryo-fetus as part of herself; that is, she must establish bonds of attachment. Failure in this task may result in lack of responsiveness or in a sense of detachment or estrangement after giving birth.
2. *Acceptance of termination of pregnancy.* Toward the end of pregnancy, the woman prepares herself psychologically for physical separation from the fetus. Quickening during the second trimester has a dual effect: it helps the mother form bonds of attachment and helps her perceive the fetus as a separate individual. The discomforts of late pregnancy, mounting tension over impending labor, and eagerness to know the sex and appearance of the baby assist her in relinquishing intimacy with the fetus. Baby showers and gifts of baby clothes and equipment also help her acknowledge the separateness (and smallness) of the coming baby.
3. *Acceptance of mother role.* Rubin (1967) describes three phases of establishing one's identity with the

Table 11–1   Parental Reactions to Pregnancy

First trimester		Second trimester Cont'd	
Mother's reactions	**Father's reactions**	**Mother's reactions**	**Father's reactions**
Informs father secretively or openly	Differ according to age, parity, desire for child, economic stability	Remains regressive and introspective; all problems with authority figures projected onto partner; may become angry as if lack of interest is sign of weakness in him	If he can cope, will give her extra attention she needs; if he cannot cope, will develop a new time-consuming interest outside of home
Feels ambivalent toward pregnancy; anxious about labor and responsibility of child	Acceptance of pregnant woman's attitude or complete rejection and lack of communication		
Is aware of physical changes; daydreams of possible miscarriage	Is aware of his own sexual feelings; may develop more or less sexual arousal	Continues to deal with feelings as a mother and looks for furniture as something concrete	May develop a creative feeling and a "closeness to nature"
Develops special feelings for, renewed interest in mother, with formation of own mother identity	Accepts, rejects, or resents mother-in-law	May have other extreme of anxiety and wait until ninth month to look for furniture and clothes for baby	May become involved in pregnancy and buy or make furniture
	May develop new hobby outside of family as sign of stress		
Second trimester		**Third trimester**	
Mother's reactions	**Father's reactions**	**Mother's reactions**	**Father's reactions**
Feels movement and is aware of fetus and incorporates it into herself	Feels for movement of baby, listens to heartbeat, or remains aloof, with no physical contact	Experiences more anxiety and tension, with physical awkwardness	Adapts to alternative methods of sexual contact
Dreams that partner will be killed, telephones him often for reassurance	May have fears and fantasies about himself being pregnant; may become uneasy with this feminine aspect in himself	Feels much discomfort and insomnia from physical condition	Becomes concerned over financial responsibility
		Prepares for delivery, assembles layette, picks out names	May show new sense of tenderness and concern; treats partner like doll
Experiences more distinct physical changes; sexual desires may increase or decrease	May react negatively if partner is too demanding; may become jealous of physician and of his/her importance to partner and her pregnancy	Dreams often about misplacing baby or not being able to deliver it; fears birth of deformed baby	Daydreams about child as if older and not newborn; dreams of losing partner
		Feels ecstasy and excitement; has spurt of energy during last month	Renewed sexual attraction to partner
			Feels he is ultimately responsible for whatever happens

mother role: (a) rejection, (b) fantasizing oneself in the role, and (c) actively seeking information and role models. This self-concept as mother begins with the first pregnancy for most women. The self-concept expands with actual experience as a mother and continues to grow throughout subsequent childbearing and childrearing. Occasionally a woman never identifies with the mother role but instead plays the role of babysitter or older sister. For many women, the nurse is a role model. The way the nurse interacts with the baby and nur-

tures the mother's self-esteem and self-confidence can influence the mother's responsiveness to her baby and view of herself.

4. *Resolution of fears about childbirth.* During pregnancy, primitive emotional material reemerges, including fantasies about childbirth. Some women do not resolve their fantasies; instead, they suppress their fears and refrain from preparing for labor. These women want to "leave it all up to the doctor" and often request "something to put me out completely." For these women,

childbirth may be psychologically traumatic. Other women attempt to master their fears through various methods: psychoprophylactic preparation, reading, or classes.

5. *Bonding*. The attachment of a woman to her child and her binding commitment to nurture the child begin during pregnancy. Thus the maternal response may be influenced to some extent by the positiveness or negativeness of a woman's pregnancy. The maternal response and attachment are discussed in greater detail in Chapter 28.

The Father

For the expectant father, pregnancy is a psychologically stressful time because he, too, is facing the transition from nonparent to parent or from parent of one or more to parent of two or more.

Expectant fathers experience many of the same feelings and conflicts experienced by expectant mothers when the pregnancy has been confirmed. Contradictory feelings may occur when men first become aware of the pregnancy. For example, with most men, there is an initial source of pride in their virility implicit with fertilization whether the pregnancy was planned or not. At the same time, feelings of ambivalence are prevalent. The extent of ambivalence depends on multiple factors, such as whether the pregnancy was planned, his relationship with his partner, previous experiences with pregnancy, his age, and economic stability.

FIRST TRIMESTER

After the initial excitement of the announcement of the pregnancy to friends and relatives, and their congratulations, an expectant father may begin to feel left out of the pregnancy. He is also often confused by his partner's mood changes and perhaps bewildered by his responses to her changing body. He may resent the attention given to the woman and the need to change their relationship as she experiences fatigue and a decreased interest in sex. Many questions begin to haunt him at this time. A worry he will have throughout the pregnancy is the expense of having a baby. In addition, he is concerned about what kind of father he will be and may become involved with many memories regarding his own father.

Some expectant fathers experience *mitleiden* and develop symptoms similar to those of the pregnant woman: weight gain, nausea, and various aches and pains. The exact significance of this phenomenon is unknown. It may be a means for the man to identify with his partner and the pregnancy.

SECOND TRIMESTER

The father's role in the pregnancy is still vague in the second trimester, but his involvement can be facilitated by his watching and feeling fetal movement. Many women report that their partner kisses them on their abdomen more in pregnancy than at any other time. Both may find this sexually arousing and, during the second trimester especially, it can be a facilitator in increasing sexual activity. Some couples fantasize that the unborn baby is thus bringing them closer together (Bittman and Zalk, 1978).

It is helpful if the father, as well as the mother, has the opportunity to hear the fetal heartbeat; however, that would involve a visit to the physician's office. It takes a very confident expectant father to withstand the stares of women in the obstetrician's office, which has traditionally been a woman's domain. Not all physicians are comfortable in including fathers as part of the prenatal visit, although involvement of fathers in antepartal care is increasing.

As with expectant mothers, the expectant father needs to confront and resolve some of his own conflicts about the fathering he experienced. He will need to gradually sort out those behaviors in his own fathering that he wants to imitate and those he does not want to be part of his fathering behaviors. This process usually occurs gradually as the pregnancy progresses.

The middle trimester has been described by some authors as "quietly tumultuous" months for men. They feel that some men may avoid feeling fetal movement initially because of the envy they experience in not being able to carry the pregnancy, a not-so-uncommon feeling but one that is rarely expressed (Bittman and Zalk, 1978). Others believe men respond with mixed feelings to palpation of fetal movement—excitement is experienced but so is increased concern about the well-being of the fetus (Colman and Colman, 1972).

The woman's appearance begins to change at this time too, and men react differently to the physical change. For some it may have the effect of decreasing their sexual interest, and for others, it may have the opposite effect. A multitude of emotions are experienced by both partners, and thus, it continues to be an important time for them to communicate and accept each other's feelings and concerns. In situations in which the expectant mother's demands dominate the relationship, the expectant father's resentment may increase to the point that he is spending more time at work, involved in a hobby, or with his friends. The behavior is even more likely if the expectant father did not want the pregnancy and/or if the relationship was not a good one prior to the pregnancy.

THIRD TRIMESTER

If the couple have communicated effectively their concerns and feelings to one another and grown in their relationship, the third trimester becomes a special and rewarding time. A more clearly defined role evolves at this time for the expectant father, and it becomes more obvious how the couple can prepare together for the coming event. They may become involved in childbirth education classes, and more concrete preparations for the arrival of the baby begin, such as shopping for cribs, car seats, and other equipment. In contrast, if the expectant father has developed a detached attitude about the pregnancy prior to this time, it is unlikely he will become a willing participant even though his role becomes more obvious.

Concerns and fears may recur. Many men are afraid of hurting the unborn baby during intercourse. Some feel uncomfortable with fetal activity that occurs during foreplay or after intercourse, which may make it seem that the unborn baby was an observer. The father may also begin to have anxiety and fantasies about what could happen to his partner and the unborn baby during labor and delivery, and feels a great sense of responsibility. The questions asked earlier in pregnancy emerge again. What kind of parents will he and his partner be? Will he really be able to help his partner in labor? Can they afford to have a baby? Is his job really stable?

COUVADE

For centuries, primitive societies recognized the crisis potential of childbearing and prescribed behaviors and imposed taboos related to pregnancy, birth, and new parenthood. The term *couvade* refers to the observance of certain rituals and taboos by the male to signify the transition to fatherhood. Acting out these socially acceptable and patterned behaviors establishes the man's new identity for himself and others. Some taboos restrict his actions. For example, he may be forbidden to eat certain foods, to kill certain animals, or to carry certain weapons prior to and immediately after the birth. Perhaps these societies recognized a potential threat to the woman and unborn child if the energy from some of his aroused feeling was not rechanneled.

With couvade, the father plays an active and vital role during the woman's labor. In one culture, the father is expected to cry out and writhe in apparent agony while he is attended by several people and ceremoniously "delivered" of a pile of stones between his legs. His cries draw the attention of any lurking harmful spirits. Meanwhile the woman delivers quietly, alone or with one attendant, some distance away and safe from the harmful spirits.

The father's participation in the couvade affirms his psychosocial and biophysical relationship to the woman and child. Recent trends in this country toward a more active role of the father during pregnancy and childbirth may be a couvade in embryonic stage.

Siblings

It is commonly recognized that the introduction of a new baby into the family unit is usually the beginning of sibling rivalry. Sibling rivalry results from children's fear of change in the security of their relationships with their parents. Some of the behaviors demonstrating feelings of sib-

ling rivalry may even be directed toward the mother during the pregnancy as she experiences more fatigue and less patience with her toddler. Parents' early recognition in pregnancy of the potential effects of this new relationship and initiation of constructive steps at this time to decrease negative aspects of the interaction help minimize the problems of sibling rivalry.

For many expectant parents, concern for the newborn is coupled with concern for the needs of any older children at home. Many parents begin to prepare for introducing the new baby before its birth.

Preparation for the young child begins several weeks prior to the anticipated birth and is designed according to the age and experience of the child. Because they do not have a clear concept of time, young children should not be told too early about the pregnancy. When the toddler is told, he or she may expect the baby in the next hour, or within a day or two. From the toddler's point of view, "several weeks" is an extremely long time. The mother may let the child feel the baby moving in her uterus, explaining that this is "a special place where babies grow." (Many parents need to be reminded to use the word *uterus* rather than *stomach,* because *stomach* connotes something being eaten and something that can be vomited. Thus some children develop a dread of eating or defecating or become afraid when they see their mother vomiting.) The child can assist in unpacking the baby's clothes and putting them in drawers or in preparing the nursery room or area. The child will probably be interested in trying on the clothes, lying in the crib, and trying out other baby items.

If the child is ready for toilet training, it is most effectively done several months before or after the baby's arrival. Parents should know that the older, toilet-trained child may regress to wetting or soiling because he or she sees the new baby getting attention for such behavior. Any move from crib to bed or from one room to another should precede the baby's birth. The older, weaned child may want to drink from a bottle again after the new baby comes. Lack of knowledge of these common occurrences can be frustrating to the new mother and can compound the stress that she feels during the early postpartum days.

During the pregnancy, if possible, the older child should be introduced to a new baby for short periods to get an idea of what a new baby is like. This introduction dispels fantasies that the new arrival will be big enough to be a playmate.

Pregnant women may also find that bringing their children to a prenatal visit may be helpful after they have been told about the expected baby. The children are encouraged to become involved in prenatal care and to ask any quesions they may have. They are also given the opportunity to hear the baby's heartbeat, either with a stethoscope or with the Doppler. This helps make the baby more real to them (Figure 11-1).

The school-age child should be involved in the pregnancy with the pregnancy viewed as a family affair. Thus the child is not excluded from the experience. Teaching about the pregnancy should be based on the child's level of understanding and interest. Overeager parents may have a tendency to go into lengthier and more in-depth responses than the child is interested in. Some children voice more curiosity than others. Books at their level of understanding can be made available in the family areas of the home. Involvement in family discussions, attendance at sibling preparation classes, encouragement of the child to feel fetal movement, and an opportunity to listen to the fetal heart are some activities that supplement the learning process and help make the school-age child feel a part of the pregnancy, and not isolated from it.

The older child may appear to have a sophisticated knowledge base, but it may be intermingled with many misconceptions. One 36-year-old multipara related that when her 14-year-old son was told about her pregnancy, he was concerned about her age and a need for an amniocentesis. He had learned about the association of increased incidence of genetic disease with increased age in his science class at school, and was concerned about the fetus. In contrast, however, he was very naive about childbirth itself.

Even after the birth, siblings need to feel that they are part of the family affair. Changes in hospital regulations allowing siblings to visit their mother and the new baby facilitate this process. On arrival at home, siblings can share in "showing off" the new baby.

Preparation of siblings for the arrival of a new baby is essential in minimizing sibling rivalry. Other critical factors, however, are equally important. These include the amount of parental attention focused on the new arrival, amount of parental attention given the older child after the new arrival, and parental reinforcement of regressive and/or aggressive behavior.

Grandparents

The first relatives told about a pregnancy are usually the grandparents. Although relationships with parents can be very complex, this period in a family's life most often promotes a closer relationship between the expectant couple and their parents. The expectant mother may find she is increasing contact with her mother, and anticipates finding the support she needs from the relationship. The expectant father may find he is doing the same with both of his parents. But how are the expectant grandparents responding to the pregnancy? Usually they become increasingly supportive of the expectant couple, even if disapproval of the couple's marriage and/or other conflicts were previously present.

Grandparents may be unsure about the amount of involvement they are "allowed" during the pregnancy and childbearing process. Most want to be helpful; thus, some

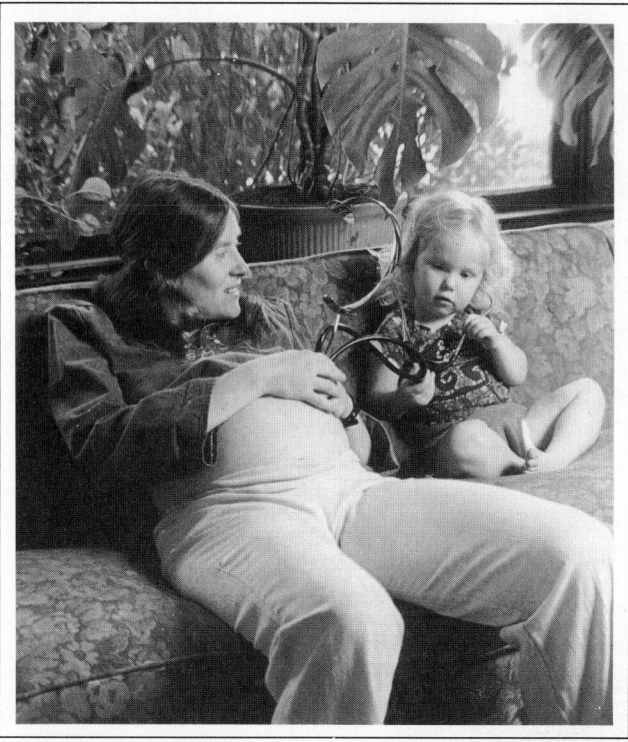

FIGURE 11-1 Children respond positively when they hear the heartbeat of their sibling-to-be.

may bestow advice and/or gifts unsparingly. Since grandparenting can occur over a wide span of years, people's response to this role can vary considerably. For some, this new role may occur at a relatively young age, and the connotation of aging that accompanies the role may affect their response to the pregnancy. The younger grandparent, therefore, may be active in her or his own life through work and other activities, and may not demonstrate as much interest as the young couple would like.

It can be difficult for even sensitive grandparents to know how much involvement the couple may want. The mood changes of the expectant mother, as well as other complex factors in the relationship, cause her to ask for advice and the next moment turn away. Expectant couples want to feel in control of their new situation, which may be initially difficult in their changing roles. Grandparents find that this factor, as well as changing roles in their own life (for example, retirement, financial concerns, menopause of the expectant grandmother, death of a friend), may contribute to conflicts in the changing family structure. Some parents of expectant couples may already be grandparents and have already developed their own style of grandparenting, which will be an important factor in how they respond to the pregnancy.

Childbearing and childrearing practices are very different for today's childbearing couple. It helps family cohesiveness for young couples to share with interested grandparents what today's practices are and why they feel they are effective. At the same time, it is important for young couples to listen to any differences expectant grandparents want to explain. When grandparents give advice, it helps to remember that they care. When their recommendations seem effective, it is significant to grandparents that young couples do listen.

In some situations, young couples feel they are receiving more advice than they can tolerate. Too often they perceive parents' suggestions as criticizing their ability to prepare adequately for the childbearing process, and later as criticism of their care of the newborn. The advice may not be difficult to deal with during the pregnancy, but becomes a different situation if a grandparent plans to help in the home after the arrival of the newborn. It then becomes essential for the young couple to discuss the problem and agree on a plan of action. The role of the helping grandparents when the new baby is brought home needs to be clarified prior to the event to ensure a comfortable situation for all.

COMMON DISCOMFORTS OF PREGNANCY

Common discomforts of pregnancy are often referred to as minor discomforts by health care professionals. These discomforts, however, are not minor to the pregnant woman. A woman whose fourth pregnancy is aggravating her varicose veins and whose pendulous abdomen is creating severe backache will be quite uncomfortable. Varicose veins can even predispose her to complications if she does not use preventive methods that also promote relief. The primigravida who is unaware that the dizziness she is experiencing is common in pregnancy may suffer considerable anxiety.

The discomforts of pregnancy are a result of physiologic and anatomic changes. These changes are fairly specific to each of the three trimesters (Figure 11–2).

Some preexisting problems, such as hemorrhoids and varicose veins, are aggravated during pregnancy. These discomforts worsen with enlargement of the gravid uterus; thus they may appear in the second trimester and become intensified in the third trimester. For women who do not have these preexisting conditions, the second trimester of pregnancy may be a relatively comfortable time. The discomforts caused by the enlarging uterus do not affect them until the last trimester or even until the last month.

Table 11–2 identifies the common discomforts of pregnancy, influencing factors, and appropriate interventions.

First Trimester

NAUSEA AND VOMITING

Nausea and vomiting are early symptoms in pregnancy, with some form of nausea occurring in the majority of pregnant women. This symptom appears sometime after the first missed menstrual period and usually ceases by the fourth missed menstrual period. Some women develop only an aversion to specific foods, many experience nausea upon arising in the morning, and others experience nausea throughout the day. Vomiting does not occur in the majority of these women.

Various theories attempt to explain the etiologic factors of nausea and vomiting in early pregnancy, but the specific cause is not known. A common theory attributes the nausea to hormonal changes related to hCG levels in the body. The initial presence of serum gonadotropin occurs at the same time that nausea and vomiting commence, and the gradual cessation of nausea and vomiting occurs as the reaction to serum gonadotropin subsides.

Another theory suggests that changes in carbohydrate metabolism may create a slight decrease in blood glucose levels in early pregnancy. Nausea may occur as the result of the sensations of intense hunger. Emotional factors and fatigue are considered by many authorities to have a role in the experience of nausea and vomiting (Pritchard and MacDonald, 1980.)

Interventions. Treatment of nausea and vomiting is not always successful, but symptoms can be reduced. The nurse must assess when the nausea and/or vomiting occurs to be helpful in suggesting methods of relief. For some women, nausea may be relieved simply by avoiding the odor of certain foods or other conditions that precipitate the problem. If nausea occurs most frequently during early morning, the woman can be encouraged to try various simple remedies such as eating dry crackers or toast before slowly arising. In general it is usually helpful to eat small but frequent meals and to avoid greasy and highly seasoned foods. Some women find unusual remedies that they claim to be helpful. If these remedies are not harmful to their pregnancy, they should be encouraged to continue using them.

Generally, nausea and vomiting cease by the fourth month of pregnancy. If they do not, hyperemesis gravidarum (a complication of pregnancy discussed in Chapter 12) may develop. For women suffering extreme nausea and vomiting in the first trimester, antiemetics may be ordered by the physician; however, antiemetics should be avoided if at all possible during this time because of possible teratogenic effects on embryo development.

NASAL STUFFINESS AND EPISTAXIS

Once pregnancy is well established, elevated estrogen levels may produce edema of the nasal mucosa resulting in nasal stuffiness, nasal discharge, and obstruction. Epistaxis may also result. Cool air vaporizers may be helpful, although the problem is often unresponsive to treatment. Women experiencing these problems find it difficult to sleep and may resort to nasal sprays and decongestants to relieve the problem. Such interventions can exaggerate the nasal stuffiness and create other discomforts. In addition,

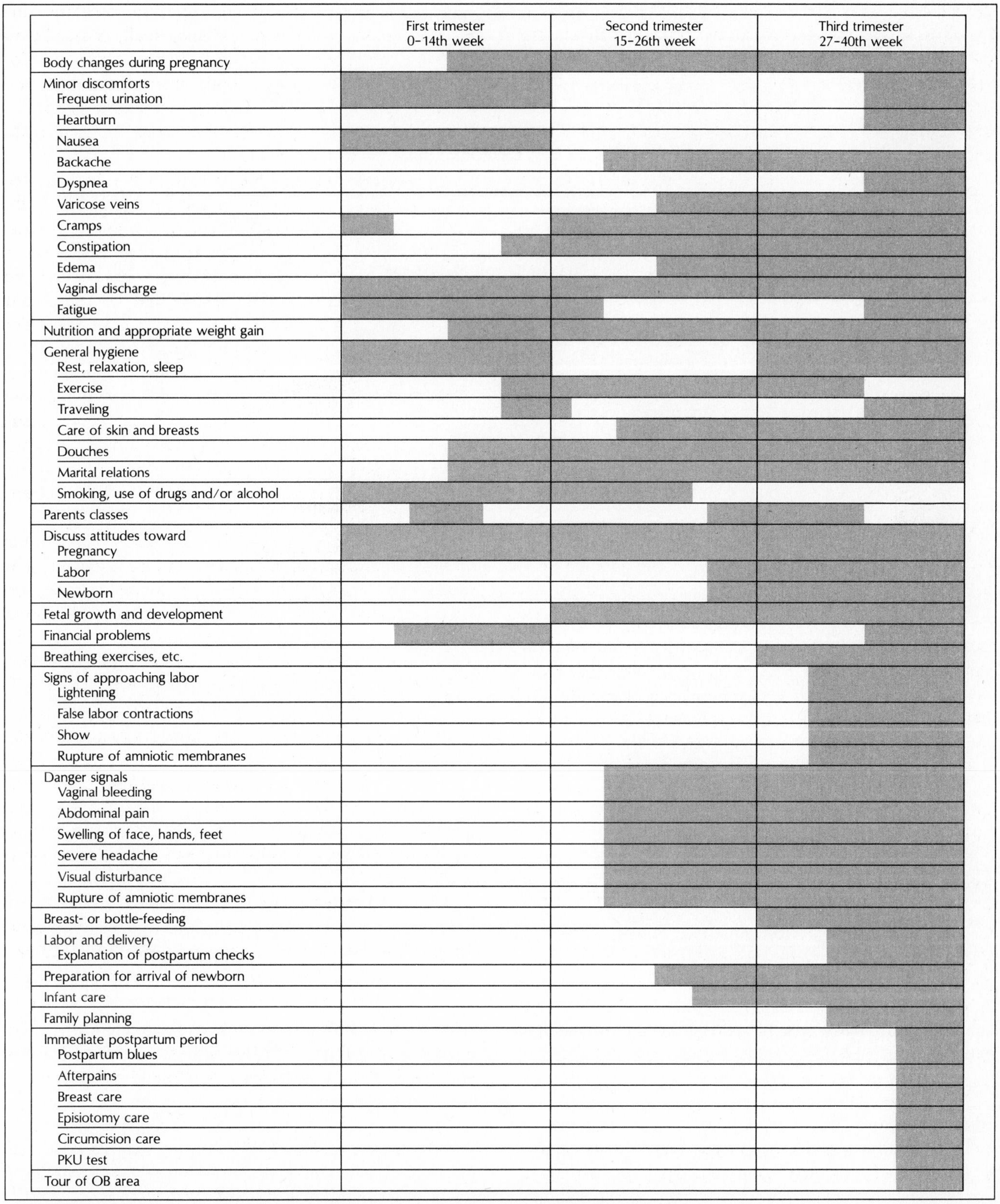

	First trimester 0–14th week	Second trimester 15–26th week	Third trimester 27–40th week
Body changes during pregnancy			
Minor discomforts Frequent urination			
Heartburn			
Nausea			
Backache			
Dyspnea			
Varicose veins			
Cramps			
Constipation			
Edema			
Vaginal discharge			
Fatigue			
Nutrition and appropriate weight gain			
General hygiene Rest, relaxation, sleep			
Exercise			
Traveling			
Care of skin and breasts			
Douches			
Marital relations			
Smoking, use of drugs and/or alcohol			
Parents classes			
Discuss attitudes toward Pregnancy			
Labor			
Newborn			
Fetal growth and development			
Financial problems			
Breathing exercises, etc.			
Signs of approaching labor Lightening			
False labor contractions			
Show			
Rupture of amniotic membranes			
Danger signals Vaginal bleeding			
Abdominal pain			
Swelling of face, hands, feet			
Severe headache			
Visual disturbance			
Rupture of amniotic membranes			
Breast- or bottle-feeding			
Labor and delivery Explanation of postpartum checks			
Preparation for arrival of newborn			
Infant care			
Family planning			
Immediate postpartum period Postpartum blues			
Afterpains			
Breast care			
Episiotomy care			
Circumcision care			
PKU test			
Tour of OB area			

FIGURE 11-2 Timetable for discomforts, concerns, and changes during pregnancy. This bar graph demonstrates the approximate times during pregnancy when a woman will experience concerns or need information in each category. From this data a plan for teaching is made to present the information prior to her need, enabling the woman to better understand and be prepared for her experience. (From *Maternity nursing today*, 2nd ed., by Clausen, J. © 1977 McGraw-Hill, Inc. Used with permission of McGraw-Hill Book Co.)

Table 11–2   Common Discomforts of Pregnancy

Discomfort	Influencing factors	Interventions
First trimester		
Nausea and vomiting	Increased levels of hCG Changes in carbohydrate metabolism Emotional factors Fatigue	Avoid odors or causative factors Dry crackers or toast before arising in morning Small but frequent meals Avoid greasy or highly seasoned foods Dry meals with fluids between meals Carbonated beverages
Urinary frequency	Pressure of uterus on bladder in both first and third trimester	Important to void when urge is felt Increase fluid intake during the day Decrease fluid intake *only* in the evening to decrease nocturia
Breast tenderness	Increased levels of estrogen and progesterone	Well-fitting supportive bra (described on p. 260)
Increased vaginal discharge	Hyperplasia of vaginal mucosa and increased production of mucus by the endocervical glands due to the increase in estrogen levels	Cleanliness, daily bathing Avoid douching, nylon underpants and panty hose; cotton underpants are more absorbent; powder can be used to maintain dryness if not allowed to cake
Nasal stuffiness and epistaxis	Elevated estrogen levels	May be unresponsive but cool air vaporizers may help; avoid use of nasal sprays and decongestants
Ptyalism	Specific causative factors unknown	Astringent mouthwashes, chewing gum, or sucking hard candy
Second and third trimester		
Heartburn (pyrosis)	Increased production of progesterone; decreasing gastrointestinal motility and increasing relaxation of cardiac sphincter; displacement of stomach by enlarging uterus; thus regurgitation of acidic gastric contents into esophagus	Small and more frequent meals Low sodium antacids Avoid overeating, fatty and fried foods, lying down after eating, and sodium bicarbonate
Ankle edema	Prolonged standing or sitting Increased levels of sodium due to hormonal influences Circulatory congestion of lower extremities Increased capillary permeability Varicose veins	Frequent dorsiflexion of feet when prolonged sitting or standing occurs Elevate legs when sitting or resting Avoid tight garters or restrictive bands around the legs

the use of any medications in pregnancy should be avoided if possible.

PTYALISM

Ptyalism is a rare discomfort of pregnancy in which excessive, often bitter saliva is produced. Causal theories are vague, and effective treatments are limited. Astringent mouthwashes, chewing gum, or sucking on hard candy may minimize the problem of ptyalism.

URINARY FREQUENCY AND URGENCY

One of the most common discomforts in pregnancy is frequency and urgency of urination. It occurs early in pregnancy because of the pressure of the enlarging uterus on the bladder. This condition subsides for a while when the uterus moves out of the pelvic area into the abdominal cavity, around the twelfth week. Although the glomerular filtration rate increases in pregnancy, it does not cause a significant increase in urine output. Frequency recurs in the last trimester as the enlarging uterus begins to press on the bladder again. Coughing or sneezing in the last month may even cause leakage of urine.

As long as other symptoms of urinary tract infection do not appear, frequency and urgency of urination are considered normal during the first and third trimesters.

Interventions. There are no methods of decreasing the frequency and urgency of urination in pregnancy. Fluid intake should never be decreased in attempts to prevent

Table 11–2 Common Discomforts of Pregnancy Cont'd

Discomfort	Influencing factors	Interventions
Varicose veins	Venous congestion in the lower veins which increases with pregnancy Hereditary factors (weakening of walls of veins, faulty valves) Increased age and weight gain	Frequent elevation of legs Supportive hose Avoid crossing legs at the knees, standing for long periods, garters, and hosiery with constricting bands
Hemorrhoids	Constipation (see following discussion) Increased pressure from gravid uterus on hemorrhoidal veins.	Avoid constipation Ice packs, topical ointments, anesthetic agents, warm soaks, or sitz baths; gentle reinsertion into rectum as necessary
Constipation	Increased levels of progesterone cause general bowel sluggishness Pressure of enlarging uterus on intestine Iron supplements Diet, lack of exercise, and decreased fluids	Increase fluid intake, fiber in the diet, exercise Develop regular bowel habits Stool softeners as recommended by physician
Backache	Increased curvature of the lumbosacral vertebras as the uterus enlarges Increased levels of hormones cause softening of cartilage in body joints Fatigue Poor body mechanics	Proper body mechanics Use of the pelvic tilt exercise Comfortable working heights Avoid wearing high-heeled shoes Avoid lifting heavy loads Avoid fatigue
Leg cramps	Imbalance of calcium/phosphorus ratio Increased pressure of uterus on nerves Fatigue Poor circulation to lower extremities Pointing the toes	Dorsiflexion of feet in order to stretch affected muscle Evaluation of diet Heat to affected muscles
Faintness	Postural hypotension Sudden change of position causing venous pooling in dependent veins Standing for long periods in warm area Anemia	Arise slowly from resting position Avoid prolonged standing in warm or stuffy environments Evaluation of hematocrit/hemoglobin
Dyspnea	Decreased vital capacity from pressure of enlarging uterus on the diaphragm	Proper posture when sitting and standing At night sleep propped up with pillows for relief if problem occurs

frequency. Tightening of the pubococcygeus muscle, known as *Kegel's exercises* (discussed on p. 263) can help maintain good perineal muscle tone. The function of the pubococcygeus muscle is to support internal organs and control voiding. The leaking of urine during pregnancy is usually limited only to pregnancy, unless there is excessive relaxation of the muscles. The muscle tone is believed to gradually weaken with each pregnancy, and bladder problems can occur when multigravidas are older if perineal muscle tone is not maintained.

BREAST TENDERNESS

Sensitivity of the breast occurs early and continues throughout the pregnancy. Increased levels of estrogen and progesterone play large roles in the soreness and tingling sensation felt in the breast and in the increased sensitivity of the nipples.

Interventions. A well-fitting supportive brassiere gives the most relief for this discomfort. The qualities of a proper supportive brassiere are discussed in the section on breast care (p. 260).

INCREASED VAGINAL DISCHARGE

Increased vaginal discharge (leukorrhea) is common in pregnancy. The discharge is usually whitish, consisting of mucus and exfoliated vaginal epithelial cells. It occurs as the result of hyperplasia of vaginal mucosa and increased production of mucus by the endocervical glands. In addition, an accompanying reduction in the acidity of the secretions allows organisms to grow more easily.

Interventions. Cleanliness is important in preventing excoriation and vaginal infections. Daily bathing should be adequate, and douching should not be necessary in pregnancy if vaginal infections do not occur. Nylon underpants and pantyhose retain heat and moisture in the genital area; thus absorbent cotton underpants should be worn to help prevent problems. Bath powder is also helpful in maintaining dryness and promoting comfort. The pregnant woman should be encouraged to report any change in vaginal discharge and any irritation in the perineal area. These changes frequently indicate vaginal infections (Chapter 12).

Second and Third Trimesters

It is more difficult to classify discomforts as specifically occurring in the second or third trimester, since many problems are due to individual variations in women, such as number of previously existing conditions. The symptoms discussed in this section usually do not appear until the third trimester in primigravidas but do occur earlier with each succeeding pregnancy.

HEARTBURN (PYROSIS)

Heartburn is the regurgitation of acidic gastric contents into the esophagus. It creates a burning or irritating sensation in the esophagus and radiates upward, sometimes leaving a bad taste in the mouth. It can occur anytime in pregnancy but is most common in the second half. Heartburn appears to be primarily a result of the displacement of the stomach by the enlarging uterus. The increased production of progesterone in pregnancy, decreases in gastrointestinal motility, and relaxation of the cardiac sphincter also contribute to heartburn.

Interventions. Activities that aggravate heartburn are overeating, ingesting fatty and fried foods, and lying down soon after eating. These situations should therefore be avoided. The woman should be encouraged to eat smaller and more frequent meals to accommodate the decreased size of her stomach. Antacids such as aluminum hydroxide, magnesium trisilicate, and magnesium hydroxide (Amphojel, Gelusil, and Maalox) can be recommended. However, common household remedies containing sodium bicarbonate (baking soda) should never be used for heartburn during pregnancy because of potential electrolyte imbalance.

ANKLE EDEMA

Most women experience ankle edema in the last part of their pregnancy because of the increasing difficulty of venous return from the lower extremities. Prolonged standing or sitting and warm weather increase the edema. It is also associated with varicose veins. Ankle edema becomes a concern only when accompanied by hypertension or proteinuria or when the edema is not postural in origin.

Interventions. The aggravating conditions just mentioned should be avoided. If the woman has to sit or stand for long periods, frequent dorsiflexion of her feet will help contract muscles, thereby squeezing the fluid back into circulation. Tight garters or other restrictive bands around the leg should not be worn. During rest periods, the woman should elevate her legs and hips as described in the following section on varicose veins.

VARICOSE VEINS

Varicose veins are a result of weakening of the walls of veins or faulty functioning of the valves. Some people have an inherited weakness in these walls. Poor circulation in the lower extremities predisposes to varicose veins in the legs and thighs. With poor circulation, the valves of the veins prevent the blood from going downward, and stasis of the blood exerts pressure, with gradual weakening of the walls, resulting in varicosities. In other instances, faulty functioning of the valves results in pooling of blood in the lower extremities with concomitant pressure on the vein walls. Occupations requiring prolonged standing or sitting contribute to congestion of blood in the lower extremities.

Pregnancy plays a significant role in creating conditions that cause varicose veins. The weight of the gravid uterus in the pelvis aggravates the development of varicosities in the legs and pelvic area by preventing good venous return. Most women who do not have other predisposing factors can avoid the development of varicose veins in pregnancy with good preventive measures. Some women, however, experience obvious changes in the veins of their legs. Increased maternal age, excessive weight gain, a large fetus, and multiple pregnancy can all contribute to the problem.

Women with varicosities in their legs experience aching and tiredness in the lower extremities, with the discomfort increasing throughout the day. They frequently become discouraged by the discoloration in the veins of their legs and by obvious blemishes. Prevention or relief of the discomfort occurs when good venous return from the lower extremities is restored.

Interventions. Preventive and relief measures include frequent elevation of the legs. One important habit that the pregnant woman can develop is always elevating her legs when she sits down. A more effective method to promote venous return is to lie on her back on the floor or bed with her legs resting at a right angle against the wall (Figure 11–3).

A pregnant woman should not sit for long periods of time or cross her legs at the knees, because of the pressure on her veins. She should not wear garters or hosiery with constricting bands. She should also avoid standing for long periods of time. However, supportive hose or elastic stockings may be extremely helpful, depending on the amount of discomfort. Supportive hose should be put on upon rising in the morning and should be cleansed daily with soap and warm water to help retain their elasticity.

Treatment of varicose veins by the injection method or by surgery is not recommended during pregnancy. The woman should be aware that treatment may be needed after pregnancy because the problem will be aggravated by a succeeding pregnancy.

Phlebothrombosis and thrombophlebitis are possible complications of varicose veins, but they usually do not occur in a healthy pregnant woman. If these complications occur, the cause is often a local injury.

Vulvar varicosities may also be a problem in pregnancy, although they are less common. Varicosities in the vulva and perineum cause aching and a sense of heaviness in these areas. Support in this area promotes relief. Elevation of only the legs aggravates vulval varicosities by creating stasis of blood in the pelvic area. Therefore, it is important that the pelvic area also be elevated to promote venous drainage into the trunk of the body. More than one firm pillow under the hips may be needed to accomplish this elevation. Near the end of pregnancy, this position may be extremely awkward; the woman may best relieve uterine pressure on the pelvic veins by resting on her side.

HEMORRHOIDS

Hemorrhoids are varicosities of the veins around the lower end of the rectum and anus. In the nonpregnant state, hemorrhoids are usually caused by the straining that occurs with constipation. When a woman becomes pregnant, the gravid uterus creates pressure on the veins and thus interferes with venous circulation. As the pregnancy progresses and the fetus grows, greater pressure on the veins and displacement of intestines occur, increasing the problem of constipation and often resulting in hemorrhoids.

Some women may not be aware of hemorrhoids in pregnancy until the second stage of labor, when the hemorrhoids appear as they push. Hemorrhoids that occur in pregnancy or at delivery usually subside, and they become asymptomatic after the early postpartal period.

Women who have hemorrhoids prior to pregnancy probably experience more difficulties with them during pregnancy because of the aggravating conditions just discussed.

Symptoms of hemorrhoids include itching, swelling, and pain, as well as hemorrhoidal bleeding. Internal hemorrhoids are located above the anal sphincter and are responsible for bleeding, usually with defecation. They are not usually painful unless they protrude from the anus. External hemorrhoids are located outside the anal sphincter. They are not usually the source of bleeding or pain; however, thrombosis of these hemorrhoids can occur, and in that case they become extremely painful. The thrombosis may resolve itself in 24 hours, or it can be treated in the physician's office by incising and evacuating the blood clot.

Interventions. Relief can be found by gently reinserting the hemorrhoid. Reinsertion is aided by gravity; therefore, reinsertion is more successful if the woman lies on her side or in the knee-chest position. She places some lubricant on her finger and presses against the hemorrhoids, pushing them inside. She holds them in place for 1–2 minutes and then gently withdraws her finger. The anal sphincter should then hold them inside the rectum. The woman will find it especially helpful if she can then maintain a side-lying position for a time, so this method is best done before bed or prior to a daily rest period.

Avoidance of constipation is an important factor in preventing and/or relieving the discomfort of hemorrhoids. Relief measures for existing hemorrhoid symptoms include ice packs, use of topical ointments and anesthetic agents, and warm soaks.

CONSTIPATION

Conditions in pregnancy that predispose the woman to constipation include general bowel sluggishness caused by increased progesterone and steroid metabolism; displace-

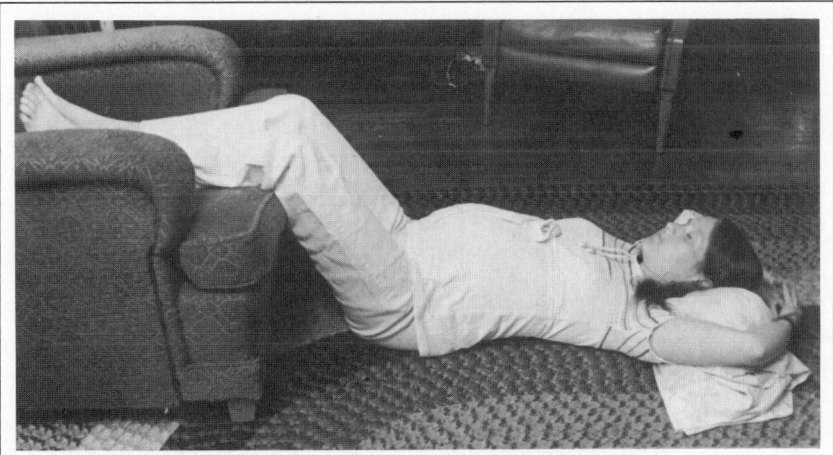

FIGURE 11-3 Swelling and discomfort from varicosities can be decreased by lying down with the legs elevated.

ment of the intestines, which increases with the growth of the fetus; and oral iron supplements, which may be needed by the pregnant woman.

Interventions. Increased fluid intake, adequate roughage or bulk in the diet, daily bowel habits, and adequate daily exercise can often maintain good bowel function in women who have not had previous problems. Women who try to develop these daily habits during pregnancy will be prepared to maintain good bowel function after delivery; meanwhile, they may need to use mild laxatives, stool softeners, and suppositories as recommended by their physician. The nurse should help women with constipation to develop good daily bowel habits and to avoid becoming dependent on laxatives during pregnancy, a habit that may continue after delivery.

BACKACHE

Many pregnant women experience backache. As the uterus enlarges, increased curvature of the lumbosacral vertebras occurs. Circulating steroid hormones cause a softening and relaxation of pelvic joints; thus the growing uterus stretch-

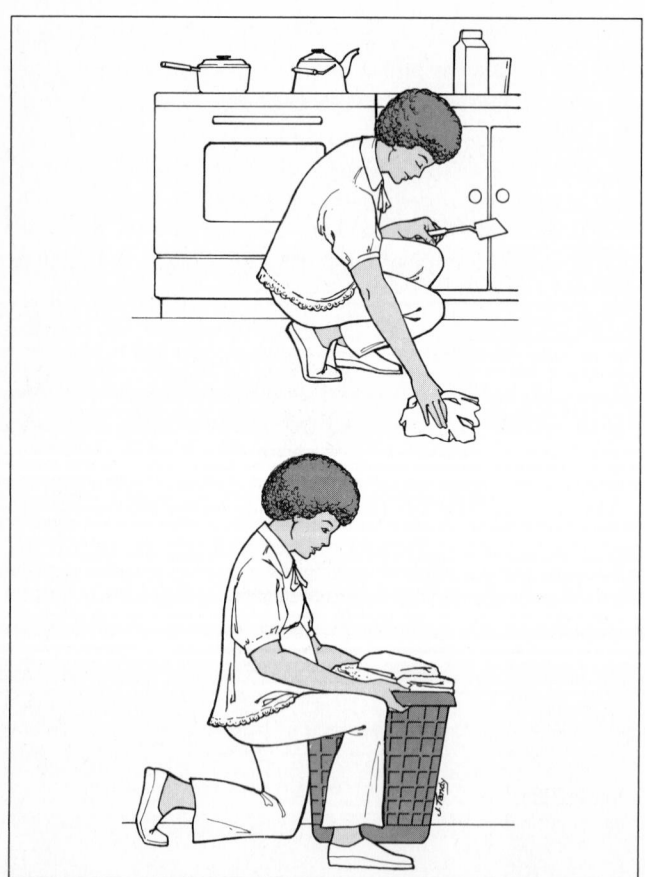

FIGURE 11–4 Proper body mechanics must be used by the pregnant woman when picking up objects from floor level or when lifting objects.

es the abdominal muscles, and the increasing weight creates a gradual tilt of the anterior portion of the pelvis. As the anterior portion of the pelvis tilts downward, the spinal curvature increases. If the woman does not learn how to correct this curvature, the strain on the muscles and ligaments will cause backache.

Interventions. An exercise called the *pelvic tilt* can help restore proper body alignment. As the anterior pelvis is tilted upward, the curvature of the back is automatically decreased, relieving much of the discomfort. If proper body alignment is maintained throughout pregnancy, backaches can be relieved or even prevented. See discussion on exercises, p. 262.

The application of proper body mechanics throughout pregnancy, in conjunction with proper posture, is also important. The pregnant woman should not curve her back by bending over to lift or pick up items from the floor. The strain is felt in the muscles of the back. Instead, leg muscles should be used to do the work. The woman can keep her back straight by bending her knees to lower her body into the squatting position (Figure 11–4). Her feet should be placed 12–18 in. apart to maintain body balance. When lifting heavy objects such as a child, she should place one foot slightly in front of the other, keeping it flat on the floor, and lower herself to the other knee. The object is held close to her body for lifting. This same principle of keeping the back straight and bending the knees applies when the woman sits down or gets out of a chair.

Work heights that require constant bending of the back can contribute to backache and therefore should be adjusted as necessary. Women who do not experience backache in pregnancy may become aware of it later as they bend to change a newborn's diaper.

A pendulous abdomen contributes to backache by increasing the curvature of the spine. The use of a good supportive maternity girdle is discussed in the section on clothing, as is the role of high-heeled shoes in increasing the lumbosacral curvature (p. 261).

LEG CRAMPS

Leg cramps are painful muscle spasms in the gastrocnemius muscles. They occur most frequently at night after the woman has gone to bed but may occur at other times. Extension of the foot can often cause leg cramps, so the pregnant woman should be warned not to do so while doing exercises for childbirth preparation or when she is resting.

Leg cramps are seen more frequently in women who consume large quantities of dairy products and may be caused by an imbalance of the calcium/phosphorus ratio of the body. Milk and cheese contain larger amounts of phosporous than calcium and the phosporous level of the blood increases when they are ingested. A decline in tissue calcium levels often accompanies elevated phosphorus levels and may result in muscle spasm. Spasms may be alleviated or avoided by decreasing the amount of dairy products consumed and by adding supplementary calcium to the diet (Aladjem, 1980).

Leg cramps are more common in the third trimester because of increased weight of the uterus on the nerves supplying the lower extremities. Fatigue and poor circulation in the lower extremities contribute to this problem.

Interventions. Immediate relief of the muscle spasm is achieved by stretching the muscle. This is most effectively done with the woman lying on her back and another person pressing the woman's knee down to straighten her leg while pushing her foot toward her leg (Figure 11–5). Foot flexion techniques, massage, and warm packs can be used to alleviate discomfort from leg cramps.

The physician may recommend that the woman drink no more than a pint of milk daily and take calcium lactate, or the physician may suggest a quart of milk daily and prescribe aluminum hydroxide gel. Aluminum hydroxide gel stops the action of phosphorus on calcium by absorbing the phosphorus and eliminating it directly through the intestinal tract. The treatment recommendations depend on the frequency of the leg cramps.

When planning a treatment regimen, one must be careful not to totally exclude milk from the woman's diet, because it is an excellent source of other essential nutrients.

FAINTNESS

Faintness is experienced by many pregnant women, especially in warm, crowded areas. The cause of faintness is a combination of changes in the blood volume and postural hypotension due to venous pooling of blood in the dependent veins. Sudden change of position or standing for prolonged periods can cause this sensation, and fainting can occur.

Interventions. If faintness is experienced from prolonged standing or from being in a warm, crowded room, the woman should lower her body to a sitting position, with her head lowered between her legs. If this procedure does not help, the woman should be assisted to an area where she can lie down and get fresh air. When arising from a resting position, she should move slowly.

SHORTNESS OF BREATH

Shortness of breath occurs as the uterus rises into the abdomen and causes pressure on the diaphragm. This problem worsens in the last trimester as the enlarged uterus presses directly on the diaphragm, decreasing vital capacity. When lightening occurs in the last few weeks of pregnancy in the primigravida, the fetus and uterus move down in the pelvis, engagement occurs, and the woman experiences considerable relief. Because the multigravida does not usually experience lightening until labor, shortness of breath will continue throughout her pregnancy.

Interventions. During the day, relief can be found by sitting straight in a chair and by using proper posture when standing. If distress is great at night, the woman can sleep propped up in bed, with several pillows behind her head and shoulders.

Nursing Responsibilities

As described in this chapter, there is a fairly predictable pattern of concerns specific to the different trimesters of pregnancy. The health care of the maternity client with these discomforts and concerns becomes more effective with the use of problem-oriented medical records (POMR) (Chapter 2).

A basic responsibility of the nurse caring for the pregnant woman is to continually assess and anticipate the presence of discomforts. The nurse should be aware of appropriate interventions and should be able to evaluate the effectiveness of the relief measures used by the woman. If these methods are not effective, the nurse must determine why they are not helpful. Is it a result of inaccurate assessment of the source of discomfort or of incomplete client education? The woman may not be using the self-care measures correctly, or the plan may include ineffective or inappropriate relief measures for this individual. After the situation is reevaluated, nursing interventions can be changed as necessary.

The major goal of prenatal care is maintenance of the intrauterine pregnancy. A related problem is the woman's

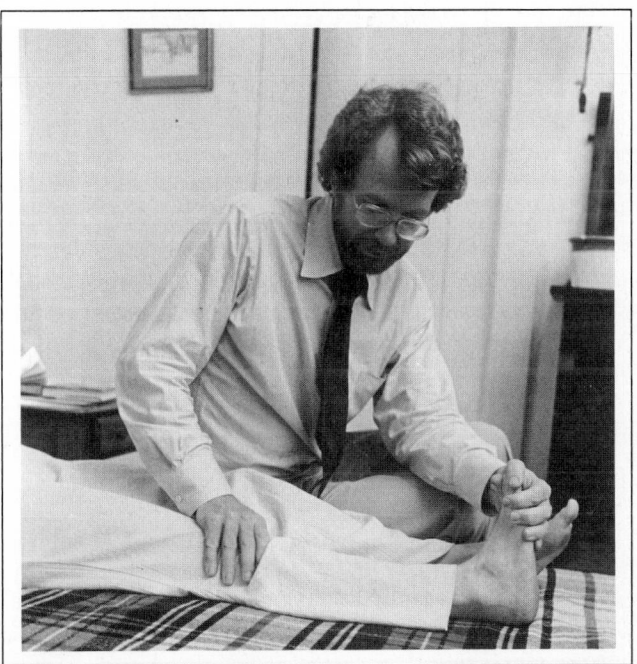

FIGURE 11–5 The expectant father can help relieve the woman's painful leg cramps by dorsiflexing the foot while holding her knee flat.

reactions to the changes in her body and life-style she undergoes because of her pregnancy.

The following SOAP narrative note is an example of this nursing process. (For explanation of SOAP, review Chapter 2.) Mrs. B., gravida II para I, is 7 months pregnant. Her daughter is 18 months old.

Problem: Backache.

Subjective: "My back is really starting to bother me now. I can hardly pick up Sarah any more. I don't know what I'll do!"

Objective: Her posture exaggerates the curvature of her spine. She walks with her hand on the middle of her back as she enters the room.

Assessment: Back discomfort is causing increased distress for Mrs. B. She needs information about the relationship of her changing shape and body alignment and has to use good body mechanics when lifting her daughter.

Plan: Focus on educational needs in this area.

1. Explain causes of backache during pregnancy.
2. Teach use of leg muscles when lifting.
3. Discuss ways of limiting amount of lifting required.
4. Teach pelvic tilt exercises to be done three times day.
5. If other measures do not provide enough comfort, discuss the helpfulness of a good supportive girdle.

COMMON CONCERNS DURING PREGNANCY

Breast Care

Whether the pregnant woman plans to bottle- or breast-feed her infant, proper support of the breasts is important to promote comfort, retain breast shape, and prevent back strain, particularly if the breasts become large and pendulous. The sensitivity of the breasts in pregnancy is also relieved by good support.

Because there is no voluntary muscle tissue in the breasts, loss of shape will occur if the woman does not wear a supportive brassiere. Many people falsely believe that sagging breasts are a result of breast-feeding. Breasts do become heavier when nursing, but it is the lack of proper support that causes tissues to sag.

A well-fitting supportive brassiere has the following basic qualities:

1. Straps are wide and do not stretch (elastic straps soon begin to lose their support with the weight of the breasts and constant washing).
2. All breast tissue fits comfortably into the bra cup.

3. The brassiere has tucks or other devices to expand its size with the enlarging chest circumference.
4. The nipple line is supported approximately midway between elbow and shoulder. At the same time, the brassiere is not pulled up in the back by the weight of the breasts.

Cleanliness of breasts is important, especially as the woman begins to produce colostrum. Colostrum, which can form crusts on the nipples, should be softened with the use of an ointment such as Massé cream and then removed with warm water. If a woman is planning to breast-feed, she should not use soap on the nipples because of its drying effect, which can lead to cracking of the skin.

Preparation of the breasts for breast-feeding is meant to help toughen the nipples and to prevent their dryness and cracking when the baby begins to nurse. After a daily bath, the woman should use a rough towel to dry the nipples, but the rubbing should not be allowed to cause soreness or irritation. The nipple can then be rolled by grasping it between thumb and forefinger and gently rolling it for a short time each day. Again, the nipple should not be irritated by this process. Woman who have sensitive skin, such as those with red hair, can benefit considerably from this preparation.

Nipple-rolling is more difficult with flat or inverted nipples, but women with these kinds of nipples still find this measure helpful in preparing their breasts for breast-feeding. Inverted nipples are relatively uncommon but do make breast-feeding difficult and sometimes too frustrating. Breast shields designed specifically for correcting inverted nipples can be worn during pregnancy. The shields appear to be the only measure that really helps if nipples are inverted. The mother will need to be committed to breast-feeding to succeed if she has truly inverted nipples. For further discussion of inverted nipples see Chapter 27.

Oral stimulation of the nipple by the woman's partner during sex play is also an excellent technique for toughening the nipple for breast-feeding. If a couple enjoys this, they should be encouraged to continue throughout the pregnancy.

Clothing

Clothing in pregnancy can be an important factor in how the woman feels about herself and her appearance. Maternity clothes, however, can be expensive, and are worn for a relatively short period of time. The maternity clothes that were worn during a first pregnancy may not be seasonally appropriate for the next pregnancy. Women who can afford the maternity clothes they want and those who can sew can dress stylishly. However, for women in lower socioeconomic levels, the expense is a problem. Possible solutions include buying used clothing and trading or exchanging maternity clothes with friends or relatives.

Clothing affects a woman's general comfort in pregnancy. Clothing should be loose and nonconstricting for both general comfort and the prevention of some of the specific discomforts of pregnancy. For example, restricting bands around the waist can be uncomfortable; those around the lower extremities, such as garters, can interfere with venous circulation and predispose to varicose veins or aggravate existing ones.

Maternity girdles are not considered necessary for most pregnant women, but some women who are accustomed to wearing girdles may feel more comfortable in continuing this practice during pregnancy. It is important for them to be aware that the girdle is for support and not for constriction of the abdomen. Women who have large, pendulous abdomens benefit considerably from a well-fitting supportive girdle. Without this support, the pendulous abdomen increases the curvature of the back and is a source of backache and general discomfort. Tight leg bands on girdles should be avoided.

High-heeled shoes aggravate back discomfort by increasing the curvature of the back and should not be worn if the woman experiences backache or problems with balance. Shoes should fit properly and should feel comfortable.

Bathing

With the increase of perspiration and mucoid vaginal discharge that occurs in pregnancy, daily bathing is important. Bathtub bathing was once a controversial subject because of a concern about water entering the vagina and causing infection. This controversy no longer exists. The only time the pregnant woman is advised not to bathe in a bathtub is in the presence of ruptured membranes or vaginal bleeding. However, caution is needed, since balance becomes a problem in pregnancy. Rubber mats in the tub and use of hand grips are important safety measures.

Some pregnant women have had difficulty getting out of the bathtub without assistance. This predicament seems to occur when extremely warm water is used or in hot weather in the latter part of pregnancy.

Employment

Fetotoxic hazards in the environment, overfatigue, excessive physical strain, and medical or obstetric complications are the major deterrents to employment during pregnancy. Employment involving balance should be terminated during the last half of pregnancy to protect the mother.

Fetotoxic hazards in the environment are always a concern to the expectant couple. If the pregnant woman or the woman contemplating pregnancy is working in industry, she should contact her company physician or nurse about possible hazards in her work environment. Some industrial products, such as turpentine and lead paint (which are also occasionally found in the home), are considered toxic substances during pregnancy.

Many women continue working during pregnancy because their income is necessary for the family or because their career is personally satisfying and important to them. Others may feel a need to work throughout pregnancy to help prevent boredom, which often occurs in the transition from being employed to being at home.

Travel

Pregnant women often have many questions about the effects of travel on them and on their fetus. If medical or obstetric complications are not present, there are no restrictions on travel. Travel does not harm the fetus or mother, although it can increase the discomforts of pregnancy and the possibility of accidents.

Travel by automobile can be especially fatiguing, aggravating many of the discomforts of pregnancy. The pregnant woman needs frequent opportunities to get out of the car and walk. A good pattern to follow is to stop every 2 hours and walk around for approximately 10 minutes. Seat belts should be worn low, under the abdomen, and should not fit tight. Although these restraints can cause internal damage in the event of an accident, statistics demonstrate that within the general population, greater mortality occurs as a result of ejection from the car. Thus seat belts and shoulder straps are recommended for the pregnant woman (Crosby and Costiloe, 1971).

As pregnancy progresses, flying or travel by train is recommended for long-distance traveling. The availability of medical care at one's destination also becomes an important factor for the near-term pregnant woman who is traveling.

Activity and Rest

Normal participation in exercise can continue throughout pregnancy. The woman should check with her physician about strenuous sports in which she is skilled, such as skiing, diving, and horseback riding. In general, however, the woman is no longer discouraged from those sports in which she has some skill if she has a healthy pregnancy. Pregnancy, however, is not the appropriate time to learn new strenuous sports because of the general strain and discomfort created. Safety is also a factor as it is for anyone learning a new sport, especially when it is complicated by the increased awkwardness that often occurs with the enlarging abdomen. Walking is an excellent exercise for pregnant women and is recommended as a daily outdoor exercise.

Exercise plays a role in prevention of constipation, in body conditioning, and in mental hygiene. However, an important rule to follow, especially during pregnancy, is not to overdo.

Adequate rest in pregnancy is important for both physical and emotional health. The pregnant woman experiences an increased need for sleep throughout her pregnancy, particularly in the first and last trimesters, when she tires easily. She will find that she has less resilience throughout pregnancy when she does not get adequate rest.

Eight hours of sleep is essential for many women, but individuals have varying needs. Time to rest during the day is also important. Finding this time may be difficult for mothers of small children and for women who work. The nurse can help the expectant mother examine her daily schedule and develop a realistic plan for short periods of rest and relaxation.

Sleeping becomes more difficult during the last trimester of pregnancy with the enlarging abdomen, increased micturition, and activity of the fetus. It becomes difficult for the pregnant woman to find a comfortable position. Figure 11–6 shows a position most pregnant women find helpful. Various methods of progressive relaxation of the mind and muscles similar to exercises taught in prepared childbirth classes can be helpful in preparing the woman for sleep. The most simple technique involves the gradual contraction and relaxation of muscle groups, beginning with flexion of the feet and moving upward to the top of the head.

Exercises

Exercises utilized for body conditioning in pregnancy are referred to as prenatal exercises. These exercises, however, can be used effectively by anyone and are not specific to pregnancy. In pregnancy they help strengthen muscle tone in preparation for delivery and promote more rapid restoration of muscle tone after delivery. Those women who are concerned about permanent change in body image as a result of the childbearing process will find that physical changes in pregnancy can be reduced considerably by faithfully practicing prescribed body conditioning exercises early in the prenatal period, as well as during the puerperium.

A great variety of body conditioning exercises are taught, but only a few will be discussed here. The pelvic tilt, or pelvic rocking, an important exercise in preventing and/or reducing back strain, also strengthens abdominal muscle tone.

The pregnant woman can learn the pelvic tilt in the following manner. While lying on her back, she puts her feet flat on the floor with her knees in the air to help prevent further strain and discomfort (Figure 11–7). She relieves the curvature in her back by pushing the raised area toward the hard surface. She or her partner can place hands under her back to feel the change in body alignment. It is then easier to apply the pelvic tilt when she is standing with her back against a wall and to maintain this body alignment throughout the day. The pelvic tilt includes the simultaneous movements of tightening the buttocks and abdominal muscles and "tucking under" the buttocks. The exercise can be performed on hands and knees and used while sitting in a chair.

The woman may start at 10 to 20 repetitions three times daily and increase *as tolerated* to 50 repetitions three times per day.

ABDOMINAL MUSCULATURE

The most basic exercise to increase abdominal muscle tone is tightening abdominal muscles in synchronization with respirations. It can be done in any position, but initially may be best learned lying supine. With knees flexed and feet flat on the floor, the woman expands her abdomen as

FIGURE 11–6 Position for relaxation and rest as pregnancy progresses.

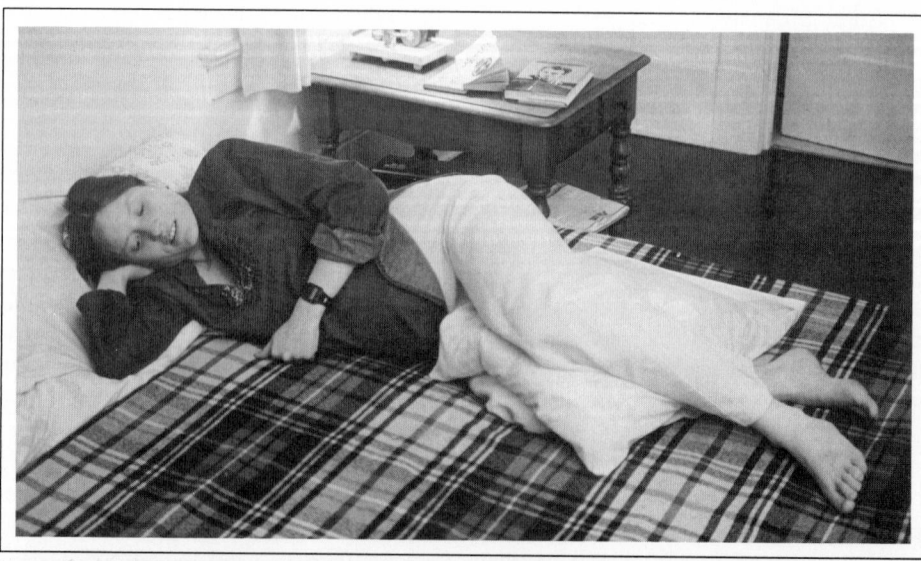

she slowly takes a deep breath. As she slowly exhales, she gradually pulls in her abdominal muscles until they are fully contracted. She relaxes for a few seconds, and then continues to repeat the exercise.

Partial sit-ups are exercises to strengthen abdominal muscle tone and are done according to individual comfort levels. When doing a partial sit-up, the woman would be lying on the floor as described above. It is imperative that this exercise be done with the knees flexed and the feet flat on the floor to avoid undue strain on the lower back. Her arms are outstretched toward her knees as she slowly pulls her head and shoulders off the floor to a comfortable level (if she has poor abdominal muscle tone, it may not be very far). She then slowly returns to the starting position, takes a deep breath, and repeats the exercise. To strengthen the oblique abdominal muscles, she repeats the process, only this time reaches one arm to one side of her knees, slowly returns to the floor, takes a deep breath, and then reaches to the opposite side.

These exercises can be done approximately five times in a sequence, with the sequence being repeated at other times during the day as desired. It is important that the exercises be done slowly, and muscle strain and overtiring be prevented.

PERINEAL MUSCULATURE

Perineal muscle tightening, also referred to as Kegel's exercises, is taught in all major types of childbirth education classes for the purpose of strengthening the pubococcygeus muscle and increasing its elasticity (Figure 11–8). The specific muscle group to be activated can be felt by

the woman when she stops her stream of urine when voiding. Continued practice of Kegel's exercises during voiding should be discouraged because it has been associated with urinary stasis and potential urinary tract infection. An effective practice method recommended by childbirth educators is for the woman to think of her perineal muscles as an elevator on the first floor of a structure, and to gradually contract to the third or fourth floor where she holds it for a few seconds, and then gradually relaxes the area (Fenlon et al., 1979). Contracting of the buttocks and thighs should not occur if the exercise is properly done.

Kegel's exercises can be done at almost any time. Women use certain clues for remembering to do them, such as each time they are stopped by a traffic signal or during each television commercial. Others do Kegel's exercises while waiting in a check-out line or talking on the telephone. It should be done whenever the woman thinks of it during the day.

TAILOR SITTING

The pregnant woman should assume a cross-legged sitting position whenever possible (Figure 11–9). The tailor sit stretches the muscles of the inner thighs in preparation for labor and delivery.

Sexual Activity

As a result of the physiologic, anatomic, and emotional changes of pregnancy, the couple usually has many questions and concerns about sexual activity during pregnancy. These questions most commonly relate to concerns about

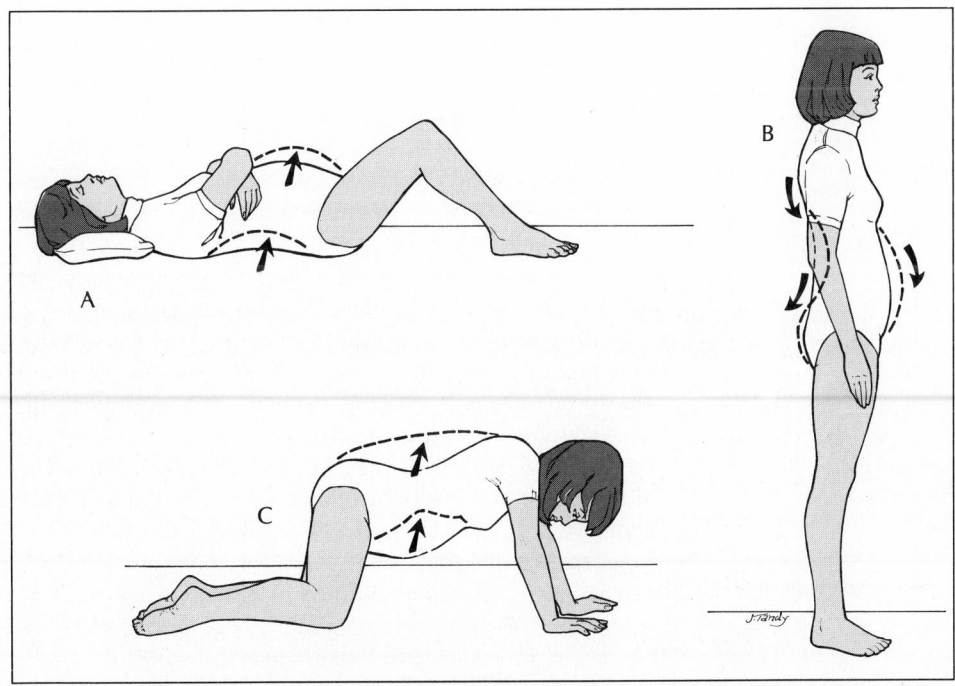

FIGURE 11–7 Pelvic tilt exercise relieves exaggerated lumbosacral curvature of pregnancy. This exercise may be done in three ways: **A,** lying supine; **B,** standing; **C,** on hands and knees.

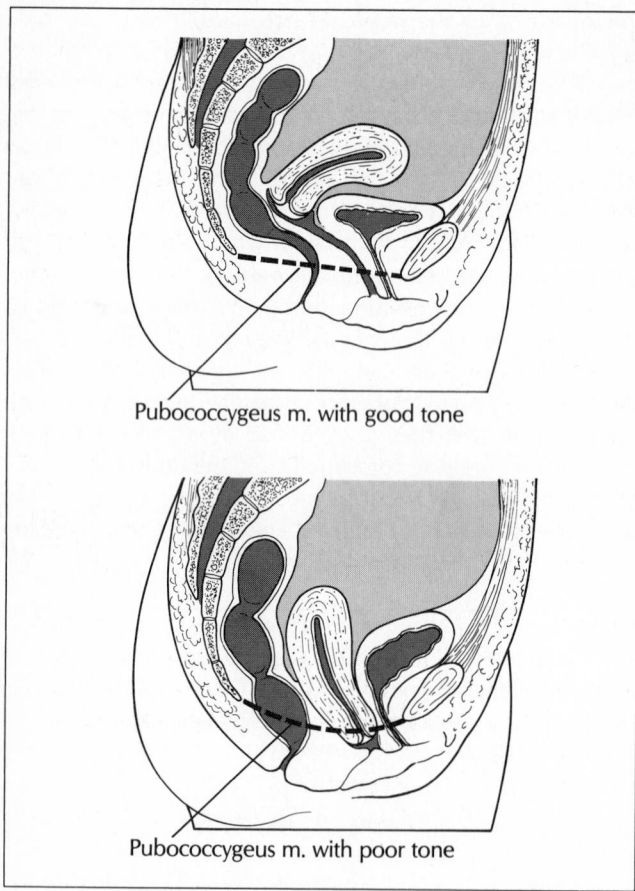

Pubococcygeus m. with good tone

Pubococcygeus m. with poor tone

FIGURE 11–8 Kegel's exercises. The woman learns to tighten the pubococcygeus muscle, which improves support to the pelvic organs.

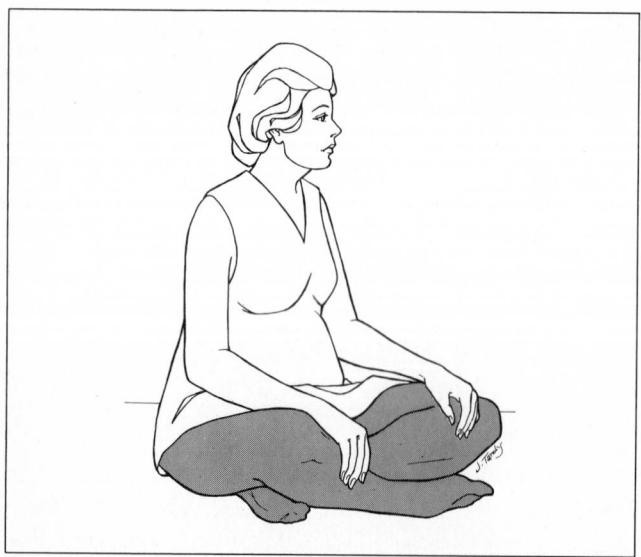

FIGURE 11–9 Tailor sit. The pregnant woman sits on the floor in cross-legged style. This exercise aids in stretching the adductor muscles of the legs.

injuring the baby or the woman and about changes in sexual desire of the couple.

In the past, only minimal information on this subject could be found in medical and nursing textbooks and in literature for expectant couples. Generally, couples were warned to refrain from intercourse in the last 6–8 weeks of pregnancy and to continue their abstinence for another period of time after the baby was born. It was thought that abstaining from sexual activity would help prevent discomfort for the pregnant woman and, theoretically, prevent infection, premature rupture of the membranes, and premature labor. In practice, however, these fears seem to be unfounded. With the growing amount of research about sexual response in the general population, reliable information is being gathered concerning the sexual activity of expectant couples. In a healthy pregnancy without complications there is no valid reason to prohibit coital and noncoital sexual behavior for the pregnant woman and her partner (Alouf and Barglow, 1981; Lion, 1982). Valid obstetric contraindications to coitus in pregnancy are limited only to pregnancies in which bleeding complications are present, membranes are ruptured, or there are other complications that may lead to premature delivery.

The expectant mother experiences many changes in sexual desire and response; they seem to be related to the various discomforts that occur during pregnancy. In the first trimester, many women experience loss of desire for sexual intercourse, which is probably related to the degree of fatigue or nausea and vomiting they are experiencing. For women who develop breast tenderness, any fondling of the breasts may no longer be desirable. To prevent discomfort, it may be necessary to use coital positions in which there is no direct pressure on the pregnant woman's breasts.

Probably the optimum time for sexual activity during pregnancy is in the second trimester. The excessive fatigue, nausea, and vomiting have subsided, and with the vascular congestion of the pelvis, the woman may experience greater sexual satisfaction than she experienced prior to pregnancy.

Interest in coitus usually begins to decrease again around the third trimester, as the woman's abdomen begins to protrude prominently. She is more uncomfortable in general, and fatigue occurs frequently. In addition, shortness of breath, painful ligaments, urinary frequency, and decreased mobility all affect sexual interest and activity (Swanson, 1980). If they are not already being used, alternative coital positions other than the traditional male superior position will have to be considered. Other positions are side-by-side, female superior, and rear-entry. Alternatives to intercourse, such as mutual masturbation, may be considered. It is important, however, that the couple feel comfortable with their chosen alternatives.

The pregnant woman may be alarmed by the orgasmic

changes that may occur in the last trimester. Instead of the rhythmic contractions of orgasm, she may experience a contraction lasting up to one minute, which may be followed by cramps and backache (Zalor, 1976). Masturbation often creates a more intense contraction than occurs with intercourse (Masters and Johnson, 1966). There is no evidence, however, that these contractions cause premature labor in the large majority of pregnant women (Solberg et al., 1973).

There have been reports in the literature of maternal deaths from air embolism caused by forceful blowing of air into the vagina during orogenital sex play (Aronson and Nelson, 1967; Fatteh et al., 1973).

Sexual activity does not have to include intercourse. Many of the nurturing and sexual needs of the pregnant woman can be satisfied by cuddling, kissing, and being held by her partner. The warm, sensual feelings that are present during these activities can be an end in themselves. Increased use of masturbation, however, may be important for her partner.

The sexual needs of men during their partner's pregnancy have not been studied. Their sexual desires, however, are also affected by many factors in pregnancy, such as their previous relationship with their partner, acceptance of the pregnancy, attitudes toward their partner's change of appearance, and concern about hurting the expectant mother or baby.

It is important for the expectant couple to be aware of their changing sexual desires, the normality of these changes, and the importance of communicating these changes to each other so that they can make nurturing adaptations. The nurse has an important role in helping the expectant couple facilitate this process. Currently a sexual health assessment is considered an integral part of prenatal care. Thus it is essential that nurses feel comfortable about their own sexuality and be well informed about the subject. In counseling expectant couples, an accepting and nonjudgmental attitude is important. The couple must feel free to express concerns about sexual activity, and the nurse must be able to respond and give anticipatory guidance in a comfortable manner.

Occasionally a woman initiates discussion about her sexual concerns, especially if she feels that she has good rapport with the nurse. More often the nurse must introduce the matter.

A statement such as "Many couples experience changes in sexual desire in pregnancy" can initiate the discussion. This generalization can be followed by an exploration of the couple's personal experience (Green, 1975). The nurse can ask a question such as "What kind of changes have you experienced?" rather than "Have you experienced any changes?"

The presence of both partners during sexual counseling is most effective in fostering communication between them.

Dental Care

Proper dental hygiene is important in pregnancy. In spite of such discomforts as nausea and vomiting, possible ptyalism, and heartburn, regular oral hygiene must not be neglected. The hyperemia of pregnancy, however, may cause conditions that discourage the woman from taking proper care of her teeth. These conditions are hypertrophy and tenderness of the gums and susceptibility to pain associated with her teeth.

Many people believe that the fetus derives its calcium from the woman's teeth to aid in the development of its tooth and skeletal structure. This is not true. The calcium in the woman's teeth cannot be altered. The calcium and phosphorus required by the fetus are obtained from the pregnant woman's diet.

The pregnant woman is encouraged to have a dental checkup early in her pregnancy. Women who neglect to obtain dental care prior to pregnancy become aware of dental problems during this time and thus may associate these problems with pregnancy. General dental repair and extractions can be done during pregnancy, preferably under local anesthetic. Dental x-ray examinations and extensive dental work should be delayed when possible until after delivery. Dental care needed during pregnancy requires consultation between the dentist and the maternal health care professional.

Immunizations

All women of childbearing age need to be fully aware of the risks of receiving specific immunizations if pregnancy is possible. Expectant women, especially those who intend to travel throughout the world, should be aware of the immunizations that are contraindicated during pregnancy. In addition, it is important that expectant women clearly understand the recommendations that are made regarding immunizations at certain times, as when influenza epidemics occur.

Immunizations with attenuated live viruses should not be given in pregnancy because of the teratogenic effect of the live viruses on the developing embryo. Vaccinations using killed viruses can be used. Recommendations for immunizations during pregnancy are given in Table 11–3.

Teratogenic Substances

Teratogenic factors are substances that adversely affect the normal growth and development of the fetus in utero. Most of the effects of these substances are immediately recognizable at birth as gross anatomical abnormalities. Some abnormalities that are related to teratogenic causes might not be identified for years. A well-known example is the development of cervical cancer in adolescent females whose mothers took diethylstilbestrol (DES) during pregnancy.

Suspected teratogenic substances are multiple. The use of x rays in the first trimester of pregnancy is associated with increased incidence of congenital abnormalities and, thus, contraindicated during that period. Controversy surrounds the use of radiology at other times in pregnancy as having a potential association with childhood leukemia (Swartz and Reichling, 1978).

Some environmental factors are also suspected as being teratogenic, but due to the complexities of the environment, causal relationships are difficult to demonstrate. Nevertheless, some definitive research has been done. For example, studies conducted on pesticides resulted in some pesticides being withdrawn from the market as a potential causative factor of increased spontaneous abortion in areas where their use was widespread. In contrast, insecticide levels have been found in maternal and fetal circulatory systems without associated teratogenic problems (Hayes, 1981c). Moreover, expectant women who live in high altitude areas have been found to have an increased incidence of small-for-gestational-age babies.

Table 11–3 Recommendations of American College of Obstetricians and Gynecologists for Specific Immunizations during Pregnancy*

Immunizations	Notes
Tetanus-diphtheria	Give if no primary series, or no booster in 10 years
Poliomyelitis	Not recommended routinely for adults but mandatory in epidemics
Mumps	Contraindicated
Rubella	Contraindicated
Influenza	Evaluate pregnant women for immunization according to criteria applied to other persons
Typhoid	Recommended if traveling in endemic region
Smallpox	No need; smallpox has been eradicated
Yellow fever	Immunize before travel to high risk area; risk of yellow fever to mother and fetus greater than risk from immunization
Cholera	Only to meet travel requirements
Rabies	Same as nonpregnant
Hepatitis-A	After exposure or before travel in developing countries

*From Pritchard, J. A., and MacDonald, P. 1980. *Williams obstetrics.* 16th ed. New York: Appleton-Century-Crofts, p. 321.

During pregnancy, women need to have a realistic perspective of potential environmental hazards. Those factors which are suspected as a hazard to the general population should obviously be avoided if possible. The expectant woman must remember that factors present in the environment for lengthy periods of time, such as pollution, have not resulted in epidemics of newborn defects.

Much research is being conducted on medications, alcohol, and smoking, and their roles as teratogenic substances. This information is discussed in the following sections.

Medications

The prevalent use of medication in pregnancy is of great concern. Studies have demonstrated that the average pregnant woman takes many more medications than commonly believed, including over-the-counter drugs as well as prescription drugs. Medications sold over the counter may be as dangerous as prescription drugs. Studies involving aspirin demonstrate that it induces a degree of platelet dysfunction in the fetus. Salicylates are associated with increased incidence of anemia, hemorrhage, prolonged gestation, and a variety of malformations. Offsetting these studies, however, was a large research project with data demonstrating that there was not an increased risk for malformations (Hayes, 1981c).

A major difficulty, even for women who attempt to eliminate all medication in pregnancy, involves ingestion of potential teratogenic medications for therapeutic purposes before pregnancy is diagnosed. It can be a problem for any woman, but especially for those with irregular menstrual cycles or for those who, because of great faith in their method of contraception, do not anticipate pregnancy. Although it is generally felt that the process of teratogenesis does not occur until the eleventh or twelfth day after fertilization, this leaves enough time for damage to be done before a woman's first missed menstrual period—given a regular cycle and nonexpectations of a pregnancy (Hayes, 1981a). Table 11–4 identifies possible effects of selected drugs on the fetus or neonate.

As previously indicated, the greatest concern for gross structural defects in the fetus is during the first trimester when organogenesis is occurring. Innumerable factors determine if a fetus in utero will have gross structural defects when the mother has taken a known teratogenic substance in this period. The medication dosage and timing of ingestion correlated with the specific period of organogenesis is critical, as well as other factors about the substance and a variety of individual metabolic and circulatory factors in the mother, placenta, and fetus.

Although the first trimester is the critical period for teratogenesis, some medications are known to have teratogenic effect when ingested in the second and third trimesters. Two examples of prescription drugs include tetracycline and sulfonamides. Tetracycline taken in late pregnancy is commonly associated with staining of teeth in children and has been shown to retard limb growth in premature infants; thus, it is felt ingestion should be avoided in pregnancy. Sulfonamides in the last few weeks of pregnancy are known to compete with bilirubin attachment of protein-binding sites, resulting in the occurrence of jaundice in the newborn and occasional kernicterus (Hayes, 1981c).

Other medications are known to affect the fetus in much the same way that an adult is affected by an overdosage. For example, the use of anticoagulants to treat thromboembolism in the mother can interfere with clotting factors in the fetus. However, this risk is lessened by frequent monitoring of prothrombin time in the mother, accompanied by appropriate changes in dosages of the anticoagulants. Heparin does not cross the placenta, so it is safer for the fetus than warfarin (Coumadin) and other anticoagulants. Moreover, warfarin is associated with multiple congenital anomalies when taken in early pregnancy (Rao and Arulappu, 1981).

Many women in pregnancy need medication for definitive therapeutic purposes such as the treatment of infections, allergies, or multiple other pathologic processes. In these situations, the problem can be extremely complex. Known teratogenic agents are not prescribed and usually can be replaced by medications considered safe. Reliable data about how innumerable medications affect a fetus and availability of information are lacking. The most commonly available drug reference is the *Physicians Desk Reference (PDR)*. A survey was conducted concerning statements about drugs in the *PDR*, their known effect on the fetus in utero, and recommendations for use in the pregnant woman. The findings demonstrated that no statements whatsoever were included in regard to use during pregnancy for 65.9% of the drugs. With the other 34.1% of the drugs, the statements that mentioned pregnancy were associated with lists of vitamins and/or mineral supplements that should be safe, medications that specifically do not have data available regarding their use in pregnancy, and statements saying medications were either safe, contraindicated and/or associated with teratogenesis (Hayes, 1981b). It must be remembered that the *PDR* is not all-inclusive, particularly for over-the-counter medications.

Caution should be the watchword when caring for pregnant women who have been taking medications. Although some studies demonstrate conclusive results, many cases are isolated, and the woman should not be unduly alarmed. When a pregnant woman asks about the harmful effects of medication in pregnancy, it is important to find out *why* she is asking before listing examples. It is essential that the pregnant woman check with her physician about medications that she was taking when pregnancy occurred and about any nonprescription drugs that she is contemplating using. A good rule to follow is that the advantage of

Table 11–4 Possible Effects of Selected Drugs on Fetus and Neonate*

Maternal drug	Effect on fetus and neonate
Alcohol	Cardiac anomalies, growth retardation, potential teratogenic effect
Antibiotics	
Amphotericin B (Fungizone)	Multiple anomalies, abortion
Kanamycin	Hearing loss
Tetracycline	Inhibition of bone growth in prematures, staining of deciduous teeth
Streptomycin	Hearing deficit and eighth cranial nerve damage
Chemotherapeutic agents	
Amethopterin (methotrexate)	Anomalies, retardation
Aminopterin	Anomalies, retardation
Chlorambucil (Leukeran)	Anomalies, retardation
Cyclophosphamide (Cytoxan)	Anomalies
Mitomycin C (Mutamycin)	Anomalies, abortion
Endocrine agents	
Androgens	Masculinization
Estrogens	Feminization, late-onset malignancy in females
Iodine	Congenital hypothyroidism
Methimazole (Tapazole)	Goiter, mental retardation
Progestins, oral	Masculinization, advanced bone age
Tolbutamide (Orinase)	Teratogenic effect
Hematologic agents	
Vitamin K (excessive)	Hyperbilirubinemia
Warfarin (Coumarin)	Malformations, CNS and eye abnormalities, perinatal hemorrhage
Sedatives-tranquilizers	
Phenothiazine	Hyperbilirubinemia
Promethazine (Phenergan)	Decreased platelet count
Others	
Drugs to control epilepsy	Low level of coagulatory factors II, VII, IX, X
Quinine	Deafness, thrombocytopenia
Salicylate (excessive)	Bleeding, low birth weight

*Modified from Overbach, A. M. 1974. Drugs used with neonates and during prenancy, III. Drugs that may cause fetal damage or cross into beast milk. *RN.* 37(12):39; and O'Brien, T. E., and Balmer, J. A. March 1981. Drugs and the human fetus. *U.S. Pharmacist.*

using a particular medication must outweigh the risks. Any medication with possible teratogenic effects must be avoided.

Smoking

Many studies in the last several years have shown that infants of mothers who smoke have a lower birth weight than infants of mothers who do not smoke. In addition, many studies have found that the intrauterine growth retardation (IUGR) increases as the number of cigarettes increases; the IUGR was minimal or eliminated when smokers stopped smoking early in the pregnancy (Naeye, 1981).

The specific mechanism of smoking's effect on fetuses is not known, but various theories have been proposed. Many authorities theorize that passage of carbon monoxide through the placenta produces intrauterine hypoxia. The carbon monoxide blood levels are increased in smoking women and cross the placental barrier. The carbon monoxide attaches to hemoglobin before oxygen does, thus decreasing perfusion of oxygen to fetal tissues (Longo, 1977). Others suggest that the nicotine in tobacco has a direct effect on the fetus through its vasoconstrictive actions and/or indirect action by impairment of placental perfusion (Haworth et al., 1980).

The third and most controversial theory attempts to correlate a relationship of decreased maternal weight gain in pregnancy with cigarette smoking as the cause of IUGR. A study by Davies and associates in 1976 investigated the various effects of cigarette smoking in the latter half of pregnancy on maternal weight gain and fetal growth. They studied 1159 mother–infant pairs and found that pregnant women who did not smoke gained significantly more weight than women who were heavy smokers (15 cigarettes/day), with an intermediate weight gain by light-to-moderate smokers (1–14 cigarettes/day). The size of the infants varied similarly. Infants born to nonsmokers were larger than those born to heavy smokers. Drawing on their study, Davies and colleagues suggested that increasing weight gain in smoking mothers might help to prevent the harmful effects of smoking on fetal growth.

Since that study, however, multiple studies have been done to contradict its findings. For example, one study was done with 8193 women in which an attempt was made to eliminate all major contributing factors of IUGR other than cigarette smoking (Naeye, 1981). The results of this study demonstrated that the newborns of women who smoked throughout pregnancy did experience IUGR independent of the mothers' pregravid weight and their total weight gain in pregnancy. Another study looked at average daily dietary intakes as well as total weight gain, and found that newborns of smoking mothers were significantly smaller than newborns of nonsmoking mothers, but pregnancy weight and dietary intake were equivalent in both groups (Haworth et al., 1980).

Hundreds of chemical compounds are found in tobacco smoke. It may be some time before the mechanisms actually causing IUGR are known. Studies are demonstrating, however, that any decrease in smoking during pregnancy will result in better fetal outcome. Pregnancy may be a difficult time for a woman to stop smoking, but she should be encouraged to reduce the number of cigarettes she smokes daily. The need to protect her unborn baby can increase her motivation.

Alcohol

Recognition of alcohol as a teratogenic substance in pregnancy was initially reported in the medical literature in 1968 (Lemoine et al., 1968). At that time, newborns with a specific combination of characteristics became associated with the common factor of heavy alcohol consumption by their mothers during the pregnancy. Since that time, much research has been done to validate this association. (Chapter 12 discusses this subject in detail.)

Further research has since been completed focusing on the amount of alcohol consumption in pregnancy that increases the risk of the *fetal alcohol syndrome* (FAS) in the fetus. Most of the research demonstrates that heavy consumption of alcohol in pregnancy increases the risk of FAS, but the effect of moderate consumption of alcohol in pregnancy is still not clear. Although moderate consumption may not produce FAS, some research has indicated increased association with altered growth, abnormal neurobehavioral development, and spontaneous abortion (Sokol, 1981). General conclusions are that the risk of teratogenic effects increases proportionally with increase in average daily intake of alcohol (Hanson et al., 1978). Pregnant women who have an occasional drink should not be unduly alarmed about the effect it will have on the fetus.

Studies also note that once women are aware of the pregnancy, most decrease their alcohol consumption because of concern for the fetus. The alcohol consumption immediately after conception and prior to the awareness of the pregnancy may be of greatest concern. Not only is this a critical period, but the problem is doubly critical as alcohol consumption and abuse are rapidly increasing among women in the childbearing age. Some feel the occasional binge, in which the woman becomes highly intoxicated, can be as harmful as heavy daily consumption, particularly if binges occur during the critical periods of organogenesis. Alcohol should always be considered foremost as a drug and not just as a beverage. Alcohol passes the placental barrier within minutes after consumption, with the potential alcohol blood levels in the fetus becoming equivalent to maternal alcohol blood levels.

Increased research is needed to determine the results of alcohol consumption in various stages of pregnancy. Some congenital anomalies are obviously a result of substance abuse during organogenesis. Awareness of the critical period of rapid development of brain cells in the fetus during the last trimester has created concerns of the effect of alcohol consumption during this period. Decreased consumption of alcohol in midpregnancy is associated with fewer incidents of growth retardation.

Some believe that maternal malnutrition in conjunction with chronic alcoholism is the cause of the growth retardation. Other research has demonstrated, however, that no significant difference in the nutritional status exists among pregnant women who were categorized according to amount of alcohol consumed (Ouellette et al., 1977). It has been found that alcohol interferes with the passage of amino acids across the placental barrier, thus interfering with availability of nutritious elements to the fetus; therefore, the nutrition and alcohol factors may play important roles (Lin and Maddatu, 1980).

Assessment of a woman's alcoholic intake should be a chief part of each woman's medical history, with questions asked in a direct and nonjudgmental manner. All women should be counseled about the role of alcohol in pregnancy. When pregnant women become aware of the risk of alcohol to their fetus, most usually attempt to modify their alcoholic consumption. If heavy consumption is involved, these women should be referred early to an alcoholic treatment program. Since the drug disulfiram (Antabuse), often used in conjunction with alcohol treatment, is suspected as a teratogenic agent, counselors in these programs need to be aware of a woman's pregnancy.

NUTRITION

Pregnancy is affected not only by the nutritional intake of the woman during pregnancy but also by her nutritional status prior to the pregnancy. Good nutrition is the result of proper eating for a lifetime, not just during pregnancy. The age of the mother is also an important factor. An expectant teenager has the additional needs of pregnancy superimposed on her needs for continued growth. This situation presents a double dilemma, since nutritional intake tends to be deficient during teenage years.

Another factor is the parity of a woman. The mother's nutritional needs and pregnancy outcome are influenced by the number of pregnancies she has had and the interval between them.

The effects of the expectant mother's nutritional status on the fetus have been demonstrated by animal studies. Such experiments have shown that nutritional deficiencies may cause smaller litters, increased malformations, and smaller offspring. Nutrition and many other factors are interrelated; more evidence points to the role of prenatal nutrition in infant well-being (Committee on Maternal Nutrition, 1970).

Conditions that occurred in several European countries during World War II, as well as experiments conduct-

ed during that period, led to identification of dietary factors which were recognized as affecting the outcome of pregnancy (Committee on Maternal Nutrition, 1970):

- the nutritional status of the woman prior to pregnancy
- the severity of the deficiency and its duration
- the time of gestation during which the deficiency occurs

As a result of the work of researchers such as Winick (1968, 1977) the effects of nutrient deficiency on cell and organ growth can be measured. Because the DNA content of mammalian cells remains a constant factor, the cell size and cell number of various organs can be estimated. Two formulas are used to obtain the information needed:

$$1. \quad \frac{\text{Amount of DNA in tissue}}{\text{Amount of DNA per cell (6.22ng)}} = \begin{array}{l}\text{Number of}\\\text{cells in organ}\\\text{or tissue}\end{array}$$

$$2. \quad \frac{\text{Amount of protein in tissue sample}}{\text{Total DNA of sample}} = \text{Cell size}$$

Nutritional effects on growth during the prenatal period and early development have been measured using these formulas.

The result is the theory that growth occurs in three overlapping stages: (a) growth by increase in cell number, (b) growth by increases in cell number and cell size, and (c) growth by increase in cell size alone. It is now thought that nutritional problems that interfere with cell division may have permanent consequences; but if the nutritional insult occurs when cells are mainly enlarging, the changes are reversible when normal nutrition occurs. These concepts are of supreme importance when related to brain development. A deficiency of vital nutrients does interfere with neuronal division, and its effects may continue into the neonatal period for about 2½ years, until myelination and other aspects of brain development are complete.

Growth of fetal and maternal tissues requires increased quantities of essential dietary components. Table 11–5 compares the recommended dietary allowances (RDA) of the National Academy of Sciences for nonpregnant females with those for pregnant and lactating teenage and adult women.

Most of the recommended nutrients can be obtained by eating a well-balanced diet each day. The basic food groups and recommended amounts during pregnancy and lactation are presented in Table 11–6.

Maternal Weight Gain

A relationship exists between maternal weight gain and infant birth weight. A weight gain of 11–13.6 kg (25–30 lb) is recommended, with the average being 12 kg (26 lb). The optimal weight gain depends on the height and bone structure of the individual and also on the prepregnant nutritional state.

The optimum pattern of weight gain during pregnancy consists of a gain of 1–2 kg (2–4 lb) in the first trimester followed by a relatively linear rate of gain averaging 0.4 kg (slightly less than a pound) per week throughout the last two trimesters. The pattern of gain is more important than the total amount. Sudden sharp increases in weight after the twentieth week of pregnancy may indicate excessive water retention and should be evaluated.

There are special concerns for weight gain in the obese woman. Pregnancy is not a time for dieting, and severe weight restriction with women in pregnancy can result in maternal ketosis, a threat to fetal well-being. Although obesity is a complex problem, pregnancy is a practical time to evaluate quality of diet in the obese woman. Studies of maternal obesity in pregnancy demonstrate that large babies are common even though pregnancy-induced hypertension (PIH) is the most common complication. Recent studies also indicate that obesity in pregnancy does not increase the need for operative delivery as once believed (Edwards et al., 1978; Colandra et al., 1981).

Women who are 10% or more below their recommended weight prior to conception also have special dietary concerns in pregnancy. Research has demonstrated that these women have a higher incidence of low-birth-weight (LBW) infants than women who are at a normal weight and have gained the same amount of weight during

their pregnancy (Edwards et al., 1978). Inadequate weight gain in pregnancy for both underweight and normal weight women, however, increases the risk of delivering LBW babies for both groups.

Research conducted by Naeye (1979) emphasizes the importance of individualizing optimal weight for each woman from conception. Naeye demonstrates that optimal weight gain needs to be based on the woman's body build (classified as overweight, underweight, or normal weight for height), rather than an average weight suggested for all women. He found that for the best outcome of pregnancy, the optimum weight gain for grossly overweight women was 16 lb; for women with normal prepregnancy weight, 20 lb; and for underweight women, 30 lb.

Nutritional Requirements

CALORIES

Calorie (cal) is a term used to designate that amount of heat required to raise the temperature of 1 g of water 1C. The *kilocalorie* (kcal) is equivalent to 1000 cal and is the unit used to express the energy value of food.

An extra daily caloric allowance of about 300 cal above the individual requirement, or a total of 2300–2400 calories per day, throughout pregnancy is considered adequate for most women. This does not take into consideration such factors as physical activity.

Table 11–5 Recommended Dietary Allowances for Women 15–40 Years of Age*

Nutrient	Nonpregnant (15–18 years)	(19–22 years)	(23–40 years)	Pregnant	Lactating
Energy, calories	2100	2100	2000	+300	+500
Protein (g)	46	44	44	+30	+20
Vitamin A (µg RE)	800	800	800	+200	+400
Vitamin D (µg)	10	7.5	5	+5	+5
Vitamin E (IU)	8	8	8	+2	+3
Ascorbic acid (mg)	60	60	60	+20	+40
Folacin (µg)	400	400	400	+400	+100
Niacin (mg)	14	14	13	+2	+5
Riboflavin (mg)	1.3	1.3	1.2	+0.3	+0.5
Thiamine (mg)	1.1	1.1	1.0	+0.4	+0.5
Vitamin B$_6$ (mg)	2.0	2.0	2.0	+0.6	+0.5
Vitamin B$_{12}$ (µg)	3.0	3.0	3.0	+1.0	+1.0
Calcium (mg)	1200	800	800	+400	+400
Phosphorus (mg)	1200	800	800	+400	+400
Iodine (µg)	150	150	150	+25	+50
Iron (mg)	18	18	18	†	†
Magnesium (mg)	300	300	300	+150	+150
Zinc (mg)	15	15	15	+5	+10

*From *Recommended dietary allowances.* 9th ed. 1980. Washington D.C.: Committee on Dietary Allowances Food and Nutrition Board, National Academy of Sciences, National Research Council.
†This iron requirement cannot be met by ordinary diets. Therefore, the use of 30–60 mg supplemental iron is recommended.

Table 11–6   Daily Food Plan for Pregnancy and Lactation*

Food group	Nutrients provided	Food source	Recommended daily amount during pregnancy	Recommended daily amount during lactation
Dairy products	Protein; riboflavin; vitamins A, D, and others; calcium; phosphorus; zinc; magnesium	Milk — whole, 2%, skim, dry, buttermilk Cheeses — hard, semisoft, cottage Yogurt — plain, low-fat Soybean milk — canned, dry	3–4 eight-ounce cups; used plain or with flavoring, in shakes, soups, puddings, custards, cocoa Calcium in 1 c milk equivalent to 1½ c cottage cheese, 1½ oz hard or semisoft cheese, 1 c yogurt, 1½ c ice cream (high in fat and sugar)	4–5 eight-ounce cups; equivalent amount of cheeses, yogurts, etc.
Meat group	Protein; iron; thiamine, niacin, and other vitamins; minerals	Beef, pork, veal, lamb, poultry, animal organ meats, fish, eggs; legumes, nuts, seeds, peanut butter, grains in proper vegetarian combination (vitamin B$_{12}$ supplement needed)	2 servings (1 serving = 3–4 oz) Combination in amounts necessary for same nutrient equivalent (varies greatly)	2½ servings
Grain products, whole grain or enriched	B vitamins; iron; whole grain also has zinc, magnesium, and other trace elements; provides fiber	Breads and bread products such as cornbread, muffins, waffles, hot cakes, biscuits, dumplings; cereals; pastas; rice	4–5 servings daily: 1 serving = 1 slice bread, ¾ c or 1 oz dry cereal, ½ c rice or pasta	5 servings
Fruits and fruit juices	Vitamins A and C; minerals; raw fruits for roughage	Citrus fruits and juices, melons, berries, all other fruits and juices	3–4 servings (1 serving for vitamin C): 1 serving = 1 medium fruit, ½–1 c fruit, 4 oz orange or grapefruit juice	Same as for pregnancy
Vegetables and vegetable juices	Vitamins A and C; minerals; provides roughage	Leafy green vegetables; deep yellow or orange vegetables such as carrots, sweet potatoes, squash, tomatoes; green vegetables such as peas, green beans, broccoli; other vegetables such as beets, cabbage, potatoes, corn, lima beans	3–4 servings (1 or 2 servings should be raw; 1 serving of dark green or deep yellow vegetable for vitamin A): 1 serving = ½–1 c vegetable, 2 tomatoes, 1 medium potato	Same as for pregnancy, except 1–2 servings of foods that provide vitamin A

*The pregnant woman should eat regularly, three meals a day, with nutritious snacks of fruits, cheese, milk, or other foods between meals if desired. (More frequent but smaller meals are also recommended.)
One should diet only under the guidance of one's primary health care provider.
Four to six glasses (8 oz) of water and a total of eight to ten cups (8 oz) total fluid should be consumed daily. Water is an essential nutrient.
An occasional alcoholic drink is permissible, but the expectant woman should avoid frequent or heavy drinking.

Table 11–6   Daily Food Plan for Pregnancy and Lactation* Cont'd

Food group	Nutrients provided	Food source	Recommended daily amount during pregnancy	Recommended daily amount during lactation
Fats	Vitamins A and D; linoleic acid	Butter, cream cheese, fortified table spreads; cream, whipped cream, whipped toppings; avocado, mayonnaise, oil, nuts	As desired in moderation (high in calories): 1 serving = 1 tbsp butter or enriched margarine	Same as for pregnancy
Sugar and sweets		Sugar, brown sugar, honey, molasses	Occasionally, if desired, but not recommended	Same as for pregnancy
Desserts		Nutritious desserts such as puddings, custards, fruit whips, and crisps; other rich, sweet desserts and pastries	Occasionally, if desired (high in calories)	Same as for pregnancy
Beverages		Coffee, decaffeinated beverages, tea, bouillon, carbonated drinks	As desired, in moderation	Same as for pregnancy
Miscellaneous		Iodized salt, herbs, spices, condiments	As desired	Same as for pregnancy

*The pregnant woman should eat regularly, three meals a day, with nutritious snacks of fruits, cheese, milk, or other foods between meals if desired. (More frequent but smaller meals are also recommended.)
One should diet only under the guidance of one's primary health care provider.
Four to six glasses (8 oz) of water and a total of eight to ten cups (8 oz) total fluid should be consumed daily. Water is an essential nutrient.
An occasional alcoholic drink is permissible, but the expectant woman should avoid frequent or heavy drinking.

PROTEIN

Protein supplies the amino acids (nitrogen) required for the growth and maintenance of tissue and other physiologic functions. Protein also contributes to the body's overall energy metabolism. In the absence of the preferred energy source, carbohydrate, about 58% of total dietary protein may become available as glucose and is oxidized as such to yield energy. The protein requirement for the pregnant woman is at least 74–76 g/day.

An important source of protein is milk, which provides approximately half the protein in the diet. A quart of whole milk supplies 32 g of protein, whereas the same quantity of skim or 2% low-fat milk yields 40 g.

Milk can be incorporated into the diet in a variety of ways, including soups, puddings, custards, sauces, and yogurt. Beverages such as hot chocolate and milk-and-fruit drinks can also be included, but they are high in calories. Various kinds of hard and soft cheese and cottage cheese are excellent protein sources, although cream cheese is categorized as a fat source only.

Protein equivalents for a cup of milk are 1 cup of yogurt, 1½ ounces of hard or semisoft cheese, ¼ cup (2 ounces) of cottage cheese, or 1½ cups of ice cream (which also contains more fat and calories).

In cases of allergy to milk (lactose intolerance) or for women who practice vegetarianism, dried or canned soy-base milk may be acceptable. It can be used in food preparation or as a beverage. Tofu, or soybean curd, may be used to replace cottage cheese. Goat's milk and goat's milk cheese sometimes may be tolerated by those who are allergic to cow's milk. Frequently, milk in cooked form is readily tolerated. Commercial coffee creamers have little or no nutritional value and must not replace milk in the diet. (See p. 281 for discussion of lactose intolerance.)

Individuals who have difficulty drinking milk or who are vegetarians sometimes prepare a high-protein drink made from a mixture of ingredients. A quart of this drink prepared in the morning can be used between meals throughout the day and is an easy way to increase protein intake. Ingredients may vary but generally include 3 cups of milk (cow, goat, or soy), ½ cup dry nonfat milk powder (cow or soy), 2 tbsp wheat germ, 2 tbsp brewer's yeast or protein powders, fruit, and vanilla (eggs are optional). These ingredients are mixed together and stored in a covered container in the refrigerator.

Meat, poultry, fish, eggs, and legumes are also good sources of protein. Small amounts of complete animal protein can be combined with partially complete plant protein for an excellent, well-utilized supply of protein. Several examples of complementary proteins are eggs and toast, tuna and rice, cereal and milk, spaghetti with meat sauce, macaroni and cheese, or a peanut butter sandwich.

FAT

Fats serve as valuable sources of energy for the body. The fat content of the maternal diet is associated with calorie level and linoleic acid intake. Linoleic acid is an essential nutrient found mainly in plant sources.

Research in the past decade has greatly increased our understanding of lipid and lipoprotein metabolism at all ages. This knowledge may eventually be used to normalize the cholesterol metabolism of the fetus and infant, thereby controlling these factors for a lifetime.

A high cholesterol level is the most common hyperlipidemia found in the perinatal state. It can be modified in the infant by changing dietary cholesterol and saturated fat. Commercial formulas with modified lipid content are now available for those concerned about dietary fat control in infant feeding (Tsang and Glueck, 1975).

It is difficult to determine the amount of maternal cholesterol being transferred to the fetus through the placenta. Fetal plasma levels do not correlate with maternal levels. The fetus does synthesize cholesterol, mainly in its liver and adrenals and in the placenta. The fetal brain synthesizes its own cholesterol, using primarily glucose, whereas the other sites use both glucose and acetate for cholesterol production.

Cholesterol content of umbilical cord blood is usually lower than adult levels. The lipoprotein content and composition may also be different (Tsang and Glueck, 1975).

CARBOHYDRATES

Carbohydrates provide protective substances and bulk as well as energy. Carbohydrates contribute to the total need for calories. If the total caloric intake is not adequate, the body uses protein for energy. Protein then becomes unavailable for growth needs. In addition, protein breakdown leads to acidosis. Ketosis can be a problem, especially in diabetic women, due to glycosuria, reduced alkaline reserves, and lipidemia. Intermittent glycosuria is not uncommon during pregnancy.

Carbohydrate needs increase, especially during the last two trimesters, as do the caloric needs for optimal weight gain and growth of the fetus, placenta, and other related maternal tissues. Productive carbohydrates can be found in milk, fruits, vegetables, and whole-grain cereals and breads.

MINERALS

The absorption of minerals improves during pregnancy, and mineral allowances are increased to allow for the growth of new tissue.

Calcium and phosphorus. Calcium and phosphorus are involved in energy and cell production and in acid-base buffering. Calcium is absorbed and utilized more efficiently during pregnancy, so the woman may store more than needed. Some calcium and phosphorus are required early in pregnancy, but most of the fetus's bone calcification occurs during the last 2–3 months. Teeth first begin to form at about the eighth week of gestation and are formed by birth. The 6-year molars begin to calcify just before birth. This means that calcium is particularly important as a structural element. At term, the fetus contains about 28 g of calcium.

If the pregnant woman's reserves of calcium are low, she should increase her calcium intake early in pregnancy. The minimum daily requirement of calcium for the pregnant adult woman is 1200 mg.

A diet that includes 3–4 cups of milk or an equivalent alternate and is nutritionally adequate for pregnancy will provide sufficient calcium and phosphorus. Frequently, the dietary intake of phosphorus exceeds the calcium intake. An excess of phosphorus can be avoided by limiting milk to 1 pint and meat to one serving daily and by ensuring that magnesium intake is adequate to effect proper utilization of calcium. Sources of calcium are listed in nutrition textbooks. Phosphorus is readily supplied through calcium- and protein-rich foods, especially milk, eggs, and meat.

Iodine. Inorganic iodine is excreted in the urine during pregnancy. Enlargement of the thyroid gland may occur if iodine is not replaced by adequate dietary intake or additional supplement.

The iodine allowance of 175 μg/day can be met by using iodized salt. When sodium is restricted, the physician may prescribe an iodine supplement.

Sodium. The sodium ion is essential for proper metabolism. Sodium intake in the form of salt is never entirely curtailed during pregnancy, even when hypertension or preeclampsia–eclampsia is present. It is recommended that food be seasoned to taste during cooking. Salty foods such as potato chips, ham, sausages, and sodium-based seasonings can be eliminated to avoid excessive intake.

Zinc. Zinc was added to the National Academy of Sciences' list of recommended dietary allowances in 1974, when it was recognized as a nutrient factor affecting growth. The RDA in pregnancy is 20 mg. Sources include milk, liver, shellfish, and wheat bran.

Magnesium. Magnesium is essential for cellular metabolism and structural growth. The RDA for pregnancy is 450 mg. Sources include milk, whole grains, beet greens, nuts, legumes, and tea.

Iron. Normal red blood cell formation is dependent on

adequate intake of several nutrients, including essential amino acids, vitamins B_6 and B_{12}, folic acid, ascorbic acid, and other vitamins and minerals, such as iron, copper, and zinc. If any one of these nutrients is missing from the diet, various types of anemia can result. Anemia is probably the most common problem in pregnancy, because nutritional anemia occurs frequently in nonpregnant women and the risk of anemia is increased by normal physiologic changes of pregnancy.

Anemia is generally defined as a decrease in the oxygen-carrying capacity of the blood. It results in a significant reduction in hemoglobin per decaliter of blood, in the volume of packed red cells per decaliter of blood (hematocrit), or in the number of erythrocytes per milliliter of blood.

The normal hematocrit in the nonpregnant woman is 38%–47%. In pregnancy the level may drop as low as 34%, even in the presence of adequate nutrition. This condition is called the *physiologic anemia of pregnancy* and is a result of increased plasma volume, which dilutes the hemoglobin and causes a drop in hemoglobin level between 24 and 32 weeks' gestation. After 20 weeks, the fetus requires extra iron stores, which further contributes to the symptoms of anemia.

Anemia in pregnancy is mainly caused by low iron stores, low nutrient intake, and increased needs. It is essential that the iron requirements balance the iron intake. This is a problem in nonpregnant women and even more so in pregnant ones. Total iron requirement for a single pregnancy varies from 750–900 mg, with the average being 800 mg (Kitay and Harbart, 1975). The iron cost of pregnancy is as follows:

Extra iron used in		
Products of conception	370	mg
Maternal blood increase	+290	mg
	660	mg
Less iron saved by cessation		
of menses	−120	mg
Total	540	mg

The Committee on Maternal Nutrition (1970) recommends that a simple iron salt such as ferrous gluconate, ferrous fumarate, or ferrous sulfate be given in amounts of 30–60 mg daily during the second and third trimesters of pregnancy. Supplements may not be given during the first trimester because of rapid changes that are occurring in the developing embryo. Ingesting more than 200 mg/day does not improve hematologic response significantly and may contribute to constipation.

By careful selection of foods high in iron, the daily iron intake can be increased considerably. Good sources of iron include liver and green leafy vegetables. Cereals are highly fortified with iron. Check the labels of various cereals to determine the approximate quantity of iron added. It should be noted that nonmeat sources of iron need an en-

hancing factor such as vitamin C to improve their absorption.

(See Chapter 12 for more information on anemia as a complication of pregnancy.)

VITAMINS

Everyone knows about the need for vitamins, but few have a thorough understanding of what they are and how they function in the body. Essentially, vitamins are organic substances that are necessary for life and growth. They are found in small amounts in specific foods and generally cannot be synthesized by the body.

Vitamins are grouped according to solubility. Those vitamins that dissolve in fat are A, D, E, and K; those soluble in water include vitamin C and the B complex. An adequate intake of all vitamins is essential during pregnancy; however, several are required in larger amounts to fulfill specific needs.

□ *FAT-SOLUBLE VITAMINS* The fat-soluble vitamins A, D, E, and K are stored in the liver and thus are available should the dietary intake become inadequate. The major complication related to these vitamins is not deficiency but toxicity due to overdose. Unlike water-soluble vitamins, excess amounts of A, D, E, and K are not excreted in the urine. Toxic symptoms include nausea, gastrointestinal upset, dryness and cracking of skin, and loss of hair.

Vitamin A. Vitamin A is involved in the growth of epithelial cells, which line the entire gastrointestinal tract and which compose the skin. Vitamin A plays a role in the metabolism of carbohydrates and fats. In the absence of A, the body loses its ability to synthesize glycogen, and the manner in which the body handles cholesterol is also affected. The protective layer of tissue surrounding nerve fibers does not form properly if vitamin A is lacking.

Probably the best-known function of vitamin A is its effect on vision in dim light. The components of the light-sensitive color pigments in the eye recombine in the dark to form visual purple, which depends on a constant supply of vitamin A in its alcohol form, retinol. In this manner, vitamin A prevents night blindness. Vitamin A is associated with the formation and development of healthy eyes in the fetus.

If maternal stores of vitamin A are adequate, the overall effects of pregnancy on the woman's vitamin A requirements are not very remarkable. The blood serum level of vitamin A decreases slightly in early pregnancy, rises in late pregnancy, and falls before onset of labor.

Both vitamin A (retinol) and its precursor, carotene, cross the placenta. Levels of vitamin A in the fetus are somewhat less than maternal values. The RDA for vitamin A during pregnancy is increased to 5000 IU (international units) from 4000 IU to allow for fetal storage of the vitamin.

Excessive intake of preformed vitamin A in large doses is toxic to both children and adults. Careful monitoring should be provided for those who regularly ingest more than 2000 retinol equivalents (6700 IU) of preformed vitamin A. The carotenes are not harmful if taken in excess but cause yellow skin; the discoloration disappears when intake is reduced. There are indications that excessive intake of vitamin A in the fetus can cause bone malformation, cleft palate, possible renal anomalies, jaundice, and skeletal pain.

Rich plant sources of vitamin A include deep green and yellow vegetables; animal sources include liver, liver oil, kidney, egg yolk, cream, butter, and fortified margarine.

Vitamin D. Vitamin D is best known for its role in the absorption and utilization of calcium and phosphorus in skeletal development. Calcium metabolism is a complex process involving ionized and protein-bound calcium, inorganic phosphorus, vitamin D, parathyroid hormone, and calcitonin. In the serum, calcium and phosphorus tend to have a reciprocal relationship. Approximately half of the total serum calcium is protein-bound and half is ionized. More than 98% of the calcium and 85% of the phosphorus exist as hydroxyapatite, a calcium phosphate salt, in bone. Calcium ions in the bone and serum are in a state of flux in relationship to each other, and this dynamic condition is regulated by parathyroid hormone and calcitonin. A form of vitamin D, D_3 (hydroxycholecalciferol), is responsible for intestinal transport of calcium and for parathyroid hormone-induced bone resorption.

To supply fetal needs for the development of skeletal tissue, the RDA for the second half of pregnancy is 400 IU of vitamin D. A deficiency of vitamin D results in rickets, a condition caused by improper calcification of the bones. It is treated with relatively large doses of vitamin D under a physician's direction.

Main food sources of vitamin D include fortified milk, margarine, butter, liver, and egg yolk. A quart of milk in the daily diet provides the 400 IU needed during pregnancy.

Excessive intake of vitamin D is not usually a result of food ingestion but of high-potency vitamin preparations. Overdoses during pregnancy can cause hypercalcemia or high blood calcium levels due to withdrawal of calcium from the skeletal tissue. Continued overdose can also causes hypercalcemia and eventually death, especially in young children. Symptoms of toxicity are excessive thirst, loss of appetite, vomiting, weight loss, high irritability, and high blood calcium levels.

Vitamin E. The major function of vitamin E, or tocopherol, in the body lies in its role as an antioxidant. This substance will take on oxygen, thus preventing another substance from undergoing chemical change. For example, vitamin E helps spare vitamin A by preventing its oxidation in the intestinal tract and in the tissues. It decreases the oxidation of polyunsaturated fats, thus helping to retain the flexibility and health of the cell membrane. In protecting the cell membrane, vitamin E affects the health of

all cells in the body. Its role during pregnancy is not known.

Vitamin E is also involved in certain enzymatic and metabolic reactions. It is an essential nutrient for the synthesis of nucleic acids required in the formation of red blood cells in the bone marrow. Vitamin E has also been found to be beneficial in treating certain types of muscular pain and intermittent claudication, in surface healing of wounds and burns, and in protecting lung tissue from the damaging effects of smog. Another well-established use for vitamin E is in the treatment of hemolytic anemia of infants. The newborn's need for vitamin E has been widely recognized, and human milk provides adequate vitamin E, whereas cow's milk is lower in E content. These functions may help explain the abundant claims and cures attributed to vitamin E, many of which have not been scientifically proved.

Deficiency symptoms of vitamin E are related to long-term inability to absorb fats. In humans, malabsorption problems exist in cases of cystic fibrosis, liver cirrhosis, postgastrectomy, obstructive jaundice, pancreatic problems, and sprue.

The recommended intake of vitamin E is increased from 8 IU for nonpregnant females to 15 IU for pregnant women. The vitamin E requirement varies with the polyunsaturated fat content of the diet. Vitamin E is widely distributed in foodstuffs, especially vegetable fats and oils, whole grains, greens, and eggs.

Vitamin E oil has been used by pregnant women externally on abdominal skin to facilitate stretching of the skin and possibly to alleviate permanent stretch marks. It is questionable whether taking high doses of vitamin E internally will accomplish this goal or will satisfy any other claims related to reproduction or virility.

Vitamin K. Vitamin K, or menadione as used synthetically in medicine, is an essential factor for the synthesis of prothrombin; its function is thus related to normal blood clotting. Synthesis occurs in the intestinal tract by the *Escherichia coli* bacteria normally inhabiting the large intestine. These organisms generally provide adequate vitamin K. Newborn infants, having a sterile intestinal tract and receiving sterile feeding, lack vitamin K. Thus a dose of menadione is often given the newborn as a protective measure.

Intake of vitamin K is usually adequate in a well-balanced prenatal diet; an increased requirement has not been identified. Secondary problems may arise if an illness is present that results in malabsorption of fats or if antibiotics are used for an extended period, which would inhibit vitamin K synthesis.

□ *WATER-SOLUBLE VITAMINS* Since water-soluble vitamins are excreted in the urine, only small amounts are stored, and so there is little protection from dietary inadequacies. It is therefore essential that adequate amounts be eaten daily. During pregnancy, the water-soluble vitamins are decreased in maternal serum levels, whereas high concentrations are found in the fetus.

Vitamin C. The requirement for ascorbic acid (vitamin C) is increased in pregnancy from 60–80 mg. The major function of vitamin C lies in the formation and development of connective tissue and the vascular system. Ascorbic acid is essential to the formation of collagen, an intercellular cementlike substance. Collagen may be thought of as the cement that holds cells together, just as mortar holds bricks together. If the collagen begins to disintegrate due to lack of ascorbic acid, cell functioning is disturbed and cell structure breaks down, resulting in muscular weakness, capillary hemorrhage, and eventual death. These are symptoms of scurvy, the disease related to vitamin C deficiency. Infants fed diets consisting mainly of cow's milk become deficient in vitamin C, and they constitute the main population group that develops scorbutic symptoms (Food and Nutrition Board, 1980).

Maternal plasma levels of vitamin C progressively decline throughout pregnancy, with values at term being about half those at midpregnancy. It appears that ascorbic acid concentrates in the placenta; thus levels in the fetus are 50% or more above maternal values.

There are no recognized effects of ascorbic acid deficiency on the outcome of pregnancy. However, the use of extremely high ascorbic acid supplements (up to 5 g daily) in pregnancy is questionable. No specific complications of fetal hypervitaminosis C have been found, but the possibility exists that fetal metabolism could be adversely affected by an oxidizing agent such as ascorbic acid. The infant accustomed to a high maternal intake of ascorbic acid during the entire gestational period will suffer from an acute deficiency state that could be harmful when the maternal supply is stopped at birth.

A nutritious diet for pregnancy should meet the body's needs for vitamin C without additional supplementation. Common food sources of vitamin C include citrus fruit, tomatoes, cantaloupe, strawberries, potatoes, broccoli, and other leafy greens. Ascorbic acid is readily destroyed by oxidation. Therefore, care must be taken in the storage and preparation of foods containing vitamin C.

B vitamins. The B vitamins—which include thiamine (B$_1$), riboflavin (B$_2$), niacin, folic acid, pantothenic acid, vitamin B$_6$, and vitamin B$_{12}$—serve as vital coenzyme factors in many reactions, such as cell respiration, glucose oxidation, and energy metabolism. The quantities needed, therefore, invariably increase as caloric intake increases to meet the increased metabolic and growth needs of pregnancy.

The *thiamine* requirement for pregnancy increases somewhat from the prepregnant level of 1.1 mg to 1.5 mg. Sources include pork, liver, milk, potatoes, enriched breads, and cereals.

Riboflavin allowances are possibly related to protein allowances, energy intake, and metabolic body size. Vita-

min B$_2$ deficiency is manifested by cheilosis and other skin lesions. During pregnancy, women may excrete less riboflavin and still require more, because of increased energy and protein needs. An additional 0.3 mg/day is recommended. Sources include milk, liver, eggs, enriched breads, and cereals.

An increase of 2 mg daily in *niacin* intake is recommended during pregnancy and 5 mg during lactation, although no information on the niacin requirements of pregnant and nursing women is available. Sources of niacin include meat, fish, poultry, liver, whole grains, enriched breads, cereals, and peanuts.

Folic acid is directly related to the outcome of pregnancy and to maternal and fetal health. Folic acid deficiency is associated with several complications of pregnancy and can cause fetal damage. About 40 years ago, it was noted that pregnant women with macrocytic anemia often responded to treatment with autolyzed yeast or crude liver extract but failed to respond to the purified liver extract used in treatment of addisonian pernicious anemia. Later it was learned that these women were victims of folate deficiency and that the yeast and crude liver extracts contained folic acid (Committee on Maternal Nutrition, 1970).

Megaloblastic anemia due to folate deficiency is rarely found in the United States, but those caring for pregnant women must be aware that it does occur. When no iron deficiency exists, a series of changes characterizes overt megaloblastic anemia. Anemia and megaloblastic erythropoiesis do not develop until about the twentieth week (Herbert, 1962).

Folate deficiency can occur in the absence of overt anemia. Various studies have shown folate deficiency to be associated with abruptio placentae, abortion, fetal malformation, and other late bleeding conditions (Committee on Maternal Nutrition, 1970). It has been further pointed out that severe maternal folate deficiency may have other unrecognized effects on the fetus and newborn. Hemorrhagic anemia in the newborn infant is attributed to folate deficiency.

One researcher suggests that folate deficiency causes irreversible damage to the products of conception—embryo and trophoblast—very early in pregnancy (Committee on Maternal Nutrition, 1970). He urges that folic acid supplementation begin no later than onset of pregnancy and preferably before.

Normal serum folic acid levels in pregnancy should range from 3–15 mg/mL; a value less than 3 mg/mL constitutes acute deficiency. Serum folate depends on absorption and ingestion of folic acid; thus, if the level is low in pregnancy, a folate deficiency may exist. The erythrocyte folate level is perhaps a better indicator of folate nutrition, but it is a late indicator of the anemia present (Kitay and Harbart, 1975). If no other complications are present, folic acid therapy brings immediate response. The stage of pregnancy or puerperium is important in determining the dosage. Prenatally an intake of 400 μg (0.4 mg) daily by mouth may induce remission. Postnatally a routine nutritious diet generally provides adequate folate to alleviate symptoms; however, it is wise to give additional folate therapy to build up stores and promote rapid hematologic changes. Iron supplementation is also recommended, since iron is an essential factor in hemoglobin formation. The latest revision of the RDA recommends 800 μg (0.8 mg) for all dietary sources during pregnancy. Pure sources of folacin are effective in less than a fourth of this amount.

Folic acid and iron are the only nutritional supplements generally recommended during the course of pregnancy. The increased need for other vitamins and minerals can be met with an adequate diet.

The best food sources of folates are green leafy vegetables, kidney, liver, food yeasts, and peanuts. As indicated by the list of food sources in Table 11–7, many foods contain small amounts of folic acid. In a well-planned diet, folate intake should be adequate. Note that cow's milk contains a small amount of folic acid, but goat's milk contains none. Therefore, infants and children who are given goat's milk must receive a folate supplement to prevent a deficiency. Adults can generally receive adequate folate from other food sources.

Dietary intake of folic acid can be altered by preparation methods. Since folic acid is a water-soluble nutrient, care must be taken in the cooking process. Loss of the vitamin from vegetables and meats can be considerable when cooked in large amounts of water.

No allowance has been set for *pantothenic acid* in pregnancy. On the basis of some studies, it may be advisable to supplement the diet with 5–10 mg of pantothenic acid daily. Sources include liver, egg yolk, yeast, and whole-grain cereals and breads.

Vitamin B₆ (pyridoxine) has long been associated biochemically with pregnancy. The classic test for B_6 nutrition is xanthinuric acid excretion following a tryptophan test load. The excretion of xanthinuric acid increases progressively throughout pregnancy until term, when levels may be 10 to 15 times those found in nonpregnant women. Also, blood levels of B_6 fall during gestation to about one-fourth the amounts found in nonpregnant women or during early pregnancy. The B_6 levels in the fetus are greater than those in the pregnant woman.

It is believed that these changes are due to metabolic adjustment during pregnancy rather than to B_6 deficiency. Rose and Braidman (1971) suggest that estrogenic stimulation of corticosteroid and the resultant increase in trypto-

Table 11–7   Folic Acid Content of Selected Foods*

Food	Amount	Folic acid (μg)	Food	Amount	Folic acid (μg)
Yeast, torula	1 tbsp	240.0	Snap beans, green, fresh	3½ oz	27.5
Beef liver, cooked	2 oz	167.6	Peas, green, fresh	3½ oz	25.0
Yeast, brewer's	1 tbsp	161.8	Cauliflower buds, fresh	1 c	22.2
Cowpeas, cooked	½ c	140.5	Shredded wheat cereal	1 biscuit	16.5
Pork liver, cooked	2 oz	126.0	Wheat flakes cereal	1 c	16.4
Asparagus, fresh	3½ oz	109.0	Figs, fresh	3 small	16.0
Wheat germ	1 oz	91.5	Blackberries, fresh	⅔ c	13.7
Spinach	3½ oz	75.0	Sweet potatoes, fresh	½ medium	12.0
Soybeans, cooked	½ c	71.7	Walnut halves, raw	8–15	11.5
Wheat bran	1 oz	58.5	Oysters, canned	3½ oz	11.3
Kidney beans, cooked	½ c	57.6	Pork (ham)	3½ oz	10.6
Broccoli, fresh	⅔ c	53.5	Filberts, raw	10–12	10.0
Brussels sprouts, fresh	3½ oz	49.0	Banana, fresh	1 medium	9.7
Whole-wheat flour	1 c	45.6	Cantaloupe, diced, fresh	⅔ c	9.0
Garbanzos, cooked	½ c	40.0	Cottage cheese	1 oz	8.8
Wheat bran cereal	1 c	35.0	White flour	1 c	8.8
Beans, lima, fresh	3½ oz	34.0	Peanut butter	1 tbsp	8.5
Asparagus, green, fresh	3½ oz	32.4	Blueberries, fresh	⅔ c	8.0
Cabbage, fine shreds	1 c	32.3	Turkey	3½ oz	7.5
Chocolate	1 oz	28.1	Celery, diced, fresh	1 c	7.0
Corn, fresh	3½ oz	28.0	Potatoes, peeled	1 medium	6.8
			Raspberries, fresh	¾ c	5.0

*Modified from Hardinga, M. G., and Crooks, H. N. 1961. Lesser known vitamins in food. *J. Am. Diet. Assoc.* 38:240.

Suggested Menus for Adequate Prenatal Vegetarian Diets—Day 1

Meal pattern	Mixed diet	Lacto-ovovegetarian	Lacto-vegetarian	Seventh-Day Adventist	Vegan
Breakfast					
Fruit	¾ c orange juice	Same as mixed diet	Same as mixed diet	Same as lacto-ovovegetarian	¾ c orange juice
Grains	½ c granola, 1 slice whole wheat toast				1 c granola, 1 slice whole grain toast
Meat group	1 scrambled egg with cheese		1 oz cheese melted over toast (no egg)		
Fat	1 tsp butter				1 tsp sesame butter
Milk	½ c milk				1 c soy milk
Midmorning					
Milk	1 c hot chocolate	Same	Same	Same	1 c protein drink*
Lunch					
Meat group/vegetable	1 c lentil chowder† (made with ground beef)	1 c lentil chowder† (no ground beef)	1 c lentil chowder† (no ground beef)	1 c lentil chowder† (made with vegeburger)‡	1½ c lentil chowder† (1 tbs torula yeast, wheat germ added)
Grains	1 corn muffin	Same	Same	Same	2 corn muffins§
Fat	1 tsp butter, honey				2 tsp margarine, honey
Fruit/dessert	½ peach, ½ c cottage cheese salad				½ peach, ½ c tofu salad
Tea	1 c tea				
Midafternoon					
Milk	¾ c vanilla pudding	Same	Same	Same	1 c pudding (soy milk)
Fruit	¼ c sliced banana				½ banana
Grain	1 graham cracker				1 graham cracker with peanut butter

phan oxygenase are responsible. Later in pregnancy, a true deficiency state may occur due to increased fetal uptake combined with the changes induced by hormones (Pitkin, 1975).

The RDA for vitamin B$_6$ during pregnancy is 2.6 mg, an increase of 0.6 mg over the allowance for nonpregnant women. Since pyridoxine is associated with amino acid metabolism, a higher-than-average protein intake requires increased pyridoxine intake. Generally, meeting the slightly increased need is possible from dietary sources, which include wheat germ, yeast, fish, liver, pork, potatoes, and lentils.

Vitamin B$_{12}$, or cobalamin, is the cobalt-containing vitamin and is found in animal sources only. Rarely is B$_{12}$ defi-

ciency found in women of reproductive age. Vegetarians are known to develop a deficiency, however, so it is essential that their dietary intake be supplemented with this vitamin. Occasionally vitamin B$_{12}$ levels decrease during pregnancy but increase again after delivery. The RDA during pregnancy is 4 μg/day.

Vitamin B$_{12}$ is absorbed either by simple diffusion or by a specific mechanism involving the intrinsic factor, which is a glycoprotein secreted by the parietal cells of the stomach. The intrinsic factor acts as a carrier for the vitamin in its passage to the ileum and ileal mucosal cells (Food and Nutrition Board, 1980).

A deficiency in vitamin B$_{12}$ may occur when there is difficulty related to absorption. Pernicious anemia results

Suggested Menus for Adequate Prenatal Vegetarian Diets—Day 1 Cont'd

Meal pattern	Mixed diet	Lacto-ovovegetarian	Lacto-vegetarian	Seventh-Day Adventist	Vegan
Dinner					
Meat group/ vegetable	¾ c meat sauce (onion, celery, carrot, tomato, mushroom in sauce), parmesan cheese	¾ c tomato sauce (same vegetables as in mixed diet), ¼ c cheese	Same as lacto-ovovegetarian	Same as lacto-ovovegetarian (add vegeburger‡ to tomato sauce)	Same as lacto-ovovegetarian (use tofu instead of cheese)
Grains	¾ c spaghetti, bread	1 c whole wheat spaghetti, 1 slice French bread	Same as lacto-ovovegetarian		
Vegetable	Mixed vegetable salad	Mixed vegetable salad with ¼ c sprouts, ½ egg, ½ oz cheese, ¼ c kidney beans added	(No egg in salad)		(Add tofu; no egg in salad)
Fat	Oil-vinegar dressing, ½ tsp butter	Same as mixed diet			1 tsp margarine
Fruit	Fresh pear or baked pear half				
Tea	1 c tea				
Bedtime					
Milk	1 c milk	Same	Same	Same	
Meat group/ vegetable	2 tsp peanut butter in celery or on wheat crackers				1 c protein drink*
Grain					Corn muffin§

* Protein drink recipe is given on p. 272. Use soy milk instead of cow or goat milk. Do not use eggs.
† Lentil chowder is made from lentils, celery, carrots, potatoes, onion, and tomatoes.
‡ Vegeburger is made from meat analogs.
§ Wheat germ and soy flour are added to corn muffin mixture.

when the body is unable to absorb cobalamin. Infertility is a complication when this type of anemia is present.

Vegetarianism

Vegetarianism is the dietetic choice of many persons. Some are vegetarians for religious reasons (Seventh-Day Adventists); others believe that this practice leads to a healthier body and mind.

There are several types of vegetarians. *Lacto-ovovegetarians* include milk, dairy products, and eggs in their diet. Occasionally fish, poultry, and liver are allowed. *Lactovegetarians* include dairy products but no eggs in their diets.

Vegans are considered "pure" vegetarians; they will not eat any food from animal sources.

Whether the family is currently practicing vegetarianism or is considering it as an alternative, during pregnancy it is vital that the expectant woman eat the proper combination of foods to obtain adequate nutrients. An adequate pure vegetarian diet contains protein from unrefined grains (brown rice and whole wheat), legumes (beans, split peas, lentils), nuts in large quantities, and a variety of cooked and fresh vegetables and fruits. Complete protein may be obtained by eating any of the following food combinations at the same meal: legumes and whole-grain cereals, nuts and whole-grain cereals, or nuts and legumes. Seeds may be used in the vegetarian diet if the quantity is large

Suggested Menus for Adequate Prenatal Vegetarian Diets—Day 2

Meal pattern	Mixed diet	Lacto-ovovegetarian	Lacto-vegetarian	Seventh-Day Adventist	Vegan
Breakfast					
Fruit	½ c applesauce	Same	Same	Same	Same
Grains	¾ c oatmeal, 1 slice whole grain toast				
Meat group	2 tbsp peanut butter, 1 tsp honey				
Milk	½ c milk				
Midmorning					
Fruit	1 medium orange	Same	Same	Same	Same
Lunch					
Meat group	Sandwich: ½ c tuna or egg salad, 2 tsp mayonnaise, 2 slices whole grain bread,	(½ c egg salad)	(2 oz cheese)	(½ c egg salad)	½ c tofu in mixed vegetable scramble, 2 tbsp wheat germ, 2 slices whole grain bread, 2 tbsp sesame butter, honey
Fat		Same	Same	Same	
Grains					
Vegetables	¼ c alfalfa sprouts, lettuce				
Fruit/dessert	Small banana				1 medium banana
Milk	1 c cream of tomato soup; ½ c milk				Cream of tomato soup; ½ c soy milk
Midafternoon					
Milk	½ c yogurt	Same	Same	Same	1 c soy yogurt
Fruit	½ c fruit				½ c fruit
Grain	2 tbsp wheat germ				2 tbsp wheat germ

enough. Because proteins are less concentrated in plant tissue than in animal tissue, it is necessary for vegetarians to eat larger quantities of food to meet body needs.

Sample vegetarian menus that meet the requirements of good prenatal nutrition are given on pp. 278–281.

For those families interested in altering their dietary habits, Register and Sonnenberg (1973) provide practical suggestions in the use of the vegetarian diet. They recommend the following principles in changing from a nonvegetarian to a lacto-ovovegetarian diet:

1. Decrease all empty-calorie foods as much as possible.

2. Increase the intake of the basic food groups to provide sufficient calories.

3. Use an increased amount of legumes, nuts, and possibly meat analogs (food products derived from soy and wheat) to replace meat.

4. Increase the intake of whole-grain products that supply protein, B vitamins, and iron to the diet.

5. Increase the intake of dairy products, using nonfat and low-fat milk, cottage cheese, cheeses, and other foods, to provide additional protein and vitamin B_{12}.

For changing from a lacto-ovovegetarian diet to a pure vegetarian diet, Register and Sonnenberg (1973) have additional recommendations:

1. Maintain an adequate calorie intake so that the body will not burn protein for caloric needs.

2. Increase the intake of foods that contain nutrients such as calcium and riboflavin, which are supplied in significant amounts by the milk group. Other sources of these nutrients include fortified soybean milk preparations; leafy green vegetables; legumes, especially soybeans; nuts, particularly almonds; and dried fruits.

Suggested Menus for Adequate Prenatal Vegetarian Diets—Day 2 Cont'd

Meal pattern	Mixed diet	Lacto-ovovegetarian	Lacto-vegetarian	Seventh-Day Adventist	Vegan
Dinner					
Meat group	3 oz baked chicken	1 c bean and cheese enchilada casserole	Same as lacto-ovovegetarian	Same as lacto-ovovegetarian	1 c bean and tofu enchilada casserole
Grain	½ c brown rice pilaf, bran muffin	1 c brown rice pilaf, bran muffin			1 c brown rice pilaf, bran muffin
Vegetables	½ c broccoli, tossed green salad with tomato	¾ c broccoli, tossed green salad with tomato			¾ c broccoli, tossed green salad with tomato
Fat	Russian dressing Butter	Cheese dressing Butter			French dressing Margarine
Fruit/dessert	Peach crisp	Peach crisp (with wheat germ and sunflower seeds)			Peach crisp (with wheat germ and sunflower seeds)
Milk	1 c milk	1 c milk			Soya hot chocolate
Bedtime					
Milk	1 c hot chocolate	Same	Same	Same	1 c hot soya/carob beverage
Meat group	1 oz cheese				Peanut butter (2 tbsp)
Grain	Rye-Krisp				Sesame crackers

3. Supplement the diet with vitamin B_{12}, since there is no practical plant source.

Factors Influencing Nutrition

Armed with knowledge of nutritional needs and food sources for these nutrients, the nurse may educate the maternity client so that nutritional adequacy can be maintained or instituted during pregnancy. In addition to the recommended diet, other factors need to be considered. What is the age, life-style, and culture of the pregnant woman? What food beliefs and habits does she have? What a person eats is determined by availability, economics, and symbolism. These factors and others will influence the expectant mother's acceptance of the nurse's intervention.

LACTOSE INTOLERANCE

"In the United States, over two thirds of blacks, Mexican Americans, American Indians, Ashkenazic Jews, and Orientals are lactose intolerant" (Rosenberg, 1977). More than 50% of this population may exhibit the intolerance with the consumption of milk (Bayless et al., 1975). Symptoms may include abdominal distention, discomfort, nausea, vomiting, loose stools, or cramps.

In counseling pregnant women who might be intolerant of milk and milk products, the nurse should be aware that even one glass of milk can produce symptoms (Bayless et al., 1975). One study found that Vietnamese adults preferred to drink canned milk with sucrose (Anh et al., 1977). The sucrose with the milk seemed to decrease the likelihood of symptoms. Possible milk alternatives such as custards, milk with sugar, milk with Ovaltine, and green leafy vegetables may assure an adequate intake of calcium (Campbell and Chang, 1973).

PICA

Pica is the eating of substances that are not ordinarily considered edible or to have nutritive value. Most women who practice pica in pregnancy eat such substances only during that time. The reasons given by many of these women are usually associated with relief of various discomforts of pregnancy or beliefs related to producing a beautiful baby (Curda, 1977).

Pica is most commonly found in poverty-stricken areas, where diets tend to be inadequate, but may also be found in other socioeconomic levels. The substances most commonly ingested in this country are dirt, clay, starch, and freezer frost. Iron-deficiency anemia is the most common concern in pica. Studies indicate that ingestion of

Table 11-8   Food Practices of Various Ethnic and Religious Groups

Cultural group	Staple foods	Prohibitions or foods not used	Food preparation
Jewish Orthodox	Meat: Forequarter of cattle, sheep, goat, deer Poultry: chicken, pheasant, turkey, goose, duck Dairy products	No blood may be eaten in any form Combining milk and meat at meal not allowed; milk and cheese may be eaten before meal, but must not be eaten for 6 hours after meal containing meat	Animal slaughter must follow certain rules, including minimal pain to animal and maximal blood drainage Two sets of dishes are used: one for meat, one for milk meals
	Fish with fins and scales No restrictions on cereals, fruits, or vegetables	No shellfish or eels	
Mexican American	Main vegetables: corn (source of calcium) and chili peppers (source of vitamin C); pinto beans or calice beans; potatoes Coffee and eggs Grain products: corn is basic grain; tortillas from enriched flour made daily	Milk rarely used	Chief cooking fat is lard Usually beans are served with every meal
Chinese	Rice is staple grain and used at most meals Traditional beverage is green tea Most meats are used, but in limited amounts Fruits are usually eaten fresh	Milk and cheese rarely used Meat considered difficult to chew, so may be eliminated from child's diet	Foods are kept short time and are cooked quickly at high temperature so that natural flavors are enhanced and texture and color are maintained Chief cooking fat is lard or peanut oil
Japanese	Seafood (raw fish) eaten frequently Most meats; large variety of vegetables and fresh fruits Rice is staple grain, but corn and oats also used	Milk and cheese rarely used	Chief cooking fat is soybean oil

laundry starch contributes to iron deficiency not because of the number of calories it provides without the presence of iron but rather because of actual interference with iron absorption (Talkington et al., 1970). The same study reported that ingestion of large amounts of clay did not interfere with the absorption of iron. However, a study by Minich and colleagues (1969) reports significant impairment of iron absorption with clays from three specific regions. Other problems with pica have been reported, including severe hypokalemia and intestinal obstruction (Curda, 1977). The ingestion of starch may be associated with excessive weight gain.

It is important that nurses be aware of pica and its implications for the woman and fetus. Assessment for the practice of pica is an important part of a nutritional history. Nurses may detect this practice as they help determine appropriate and effective relief measures for discomforts the woman is experiencing. Reeducation of the expectant woman is important in helping her to decrease or eliminate this practice.

FOOD MYTHS

The relationship of food to pregnancy is reflected in some common beliefs or sayings. Nurses frequently hear that the pregnant woman must eat for two or that the fetus takes from the mother all the nutrients it needs. The practice of

Suggested Menus for Adequate Prenatal Diet for Various Cultural Groups—Day 1*

Meal	Caucasian	Chicano[†]	Southern U.S.	Oriental[†]	Jewish	Italian[†]
Breakfast	Peaches Oatmeal/milk Toast with peanut butter Milk	Peaches Oatmeal/milk Corn tortilla Refried beans Milk	Peaches Oatmeal/milk Cornbread with molasses Milk	Peaches Steamed rice/ milk (soy) Rice cracker Tea	Peaches Oatmeal/milk Bagel with unsalted butter Milk	Peaches Oatmeal/milk Bread with butter Cheese Coffee/milk
Midmorning	Fruit/juice	Fruit/juice	Fruit	Fruit	Fruit	Fruit/juice
Lunch	Cheese omelet and vegetables Whole grain muffin with butter Lettuce and tomato salad Raw apple Milk	1 fried egg Refried beans with cheese Corn tortilla Fresh tomato and chilis Banana Milk	1 fried egg Black-eyed peas and salt pork Cornbread with molasses Turnip greens Ice cream	Miso soup Chinese omelet (with bean sprouts, pepper, green onion, mushroom) and fried rice Spinach Tea	Cheese omelet Brown rice Lettuce and tomato salad Honey cookie Milk	Cheese omelet Zucchini, green salad Grapes/cheese Milk
Midafternoon	Fruit Cottage cheese	Fruit Cottage cheese	Fruit	Fruit Tofu	Fruit	Fruit Cheese
Dinner	Roast beef and gravy Whole grain roll with butter Parsley, carrots, cabbage slaw Banana cream pie Tea	Refried beans with cheese Fried macaroni Tortilla Carrots, steamed tomato, chilis Corn pudding Milk	Beef stew with vegetables (carrots, greens) Dumplings Steamed potato, cabbage slaw Corn pudding	Beef strips with pan-fried vegetables Brown rice, steamed Milk custard	Beef stew with vegetables Barley pilaf Cooked cabbage Unsalted butter Coffeecake Fruit/juice	Spaghetti and meatballs with tomato sauce Italian bread with butter Sauteed eggplant, cabbage, salad Fruit Coffee/milk
Bedtime	Milk Wheat crackers 1 oz cheese	Milk Tortilla with beans Cheese	Milk Corn pudding	Ice cream	Ice cream	Ice cream

* Modified from American Dietetic Association. *Cultural food patterns in the U.S.A.*
† Encourage use of milk, since it is not ordinarily included in diets of members of these cultural groups.

pica, for example, has roots in myth. Common beliefs regarding pica include (a) that laundry starch will make the newborn lighter in color, and (b) that the baby will "slide out" more easily during delivery (Curda, 1977).

CULTURAL, ETHNIC, AND RELIGIOUS INFLUENCES

Cultural, ethnic, and occasionally religious background determines one's experiences with food and influences food preferences and habits. People of different nationalities are accustomed to eating different foods because of the kinds of foodstuffs available in their countries of origin. The way food is prepared varies, depending on the customs and traditions of the particular ethnic and cultural group. In addition, the laws of certain religions prescribe particular foods, prohibit others, and direct the preparation and serving of meals.

In each culture, certain foods have symbolic significance. Generally, these symbolic foods are related to major life experiences such as birth, death, or developmental milestones. (General food practices of different cultural and ethnic groups are presented in Table 11-8. Sample daily menus for differing cultural groups that meet minimal nutritional requirements during pregnancy are presented on p. 283.)

For example, Navajo Indian women believe that eating raisins will cause brown spots on the mother or baby. Many black Americans believe that craving one food excessively can cause the baby to be "marked"; some say a birthmark's shape can be correlated with the shape of the food the mother craved during pregnancy. This belief is also held by some Mexican American women. Also, milk consumption is considered by some Mexican Americans to make their babies too big, thereby creating difficult deliveries.

The traditional Chinese classify food as either hot or cold, and these classifications are related to the balance of forces for good health. Since childbirth is considered a cold condition, it must be treated with hot foods, such as chicken, squash, and broccoli. Vietnamese women believe that eat-

Suggested Menus for Adequate Prenatal Diet for Various Cultural Groups—Day 2*

Meal	Caucasian	Chicano†	Southern U.S.	Oriental†	Jewish	Italian†
Breakfast	Orange juice Pancakes with butter/syrup Sausage Milk	Tortilla Scrambled egg with beans and cheese Milk	Melon or fruit in season Cornmeal grits with molasses Biscuit with cream gravy Milk	Steamed millet Rice cracker Tofu Tea	Orange juice Potato pancakes with unsalted butter Fried eggs Milk	Orange Farina/milk Whole grain bread with butter Coffee/milk
Midmorning	Fruit juice	Melon or orange	Fruit juice	Fruit Egg drop soup	Fruit/cheese Chicken noodle soup	Fruit/cheese
Lunch	Cheese on toasted whole wheat bread Vegetable soup Raw carrots, pickles Pineapple Milk	Bean and cheese enchilada Tomato, chilis Fruit Milk	Cheese on whole wheat bread Mustard greens, tomato wedges Buttermilk	Tofu with steamed brown rice and vegetables Cooked greens	Cottage cheese blintzes with fresh whipped butter Broccoli, tomatoes Milk	Cheese on whole wheat bread Minestrone soup Green salad Fruit Coffee/milk
Midafternoon	Milk and fruit shake	Apple or banana	Fruit	Ice cream	Ice cream	Ice cream
Dinner	Baked chicken Biscuit with butter Sweet potato Broccoli Fruit salad Sponge cake Beverage	Stewed chicken Tortilla Sweet potato Spinach, raw carrots Juice	Ham hocks with rice and tomato, onion, and okra Cornbread with molasses Sweet potato, collards Buttermilk	Pork with fried rice and vegetables Broccoli, raw green salad Rice custard pudding Tea	Green cabbage with ground lamb stuffing Rye bread with unsalted butter Sweet potato, broccoli, raw green pepper, cucumber, pickles Fruit juice	Chicken tettrazini (with pasta) Whole grain Italian bread with butter Broccoli, green salad Grapes/cheese Coffee/milk
Bedtime	Milk Crackers with peanut butter Banana	Milk Cheese Tortilla with beans	Biscuit with peanut butter Fruit	Rice crackers Cheese Fruit	Pumpernickel bread Cheese Fruit	Cheese Fruit

*Modified from American Dietetic Association. *Cultural food patterns in the U.S.A.*
† Encourage use of milk, since it is not ordinarily included in diets of members of these cultural groups.

ing "unclean foods" such as beef, dog, and snake during pregnancy will cause the baby to be born an imbecile. Cabbage is also avoided because it is believed to produce flatulence that might bring on false labor (Clark, 1978).

PSYCHOSOCIAL FACTORS

Food is frequently considered a symbol of friendliness, warmth, and social acceptance. Sharing one's table with others has been practiced for centuries. Food has also been symbolic of motherliness; that is, taking care of the family and feeding them well is a part of the traditional mothering role. The mother influences her children's likes and dislikes by what she prepares and by her attitude about foods. Certain foods are assigned positive and negative values as reflected by such statements as "Milk helps one grow" and "Coffee stunts one's growth."

Some foods and food-related practices are associated with status. Some foods are prepared "just for company." Other foods are served only on specific occasions—for example, holidays such as Thanksgiving.

Socioeconomic factors. One's socioeconomic level may be a determinant of one's nutritional status. Poverty-level families are unable to afford the same types of food that higher-income families can. Thus, pregnant women with low incomes frequently are at risk for poor nutrition.

Education also plays a role in one's nutritional status, since one's educational level is frequently related to one's economic status.

Psychologic factors. Nutritional well-being can be directly affected by a person's emotional state. For example, one psychologic disorder, anorexia nervosa, which occurs primarily in adolescent girls, is manifested chiefly by self-inflicted starvation, resulting in malnutrition and ultimately death if not treated. Loss of appetite is also a common symptom of serious depression.

The expectant woman's attitudes and feelings about her pregnancy will certainly have an influence on her nutritional status. The woman who is depressed or who regards this event as unwanted and unwelcome may manifest these feelings by loss of appetite or by improper food practices, such as overindulgence in sweets or alcohol.

Nursing Responsibilities

The important components of and influences on a nutritionally balanced diet for the pregnant woman have been thoroughly discussed. Each person's view of nutrition and of its relationship to the pregnancy depends on previous teaching and dietary habits. A complete diet history and assessment of nutritional status must be made by the health care team to facilitate planning an optimal diet with each woman. During the data-gathering process, the nurse has an opportunity to discuss important aspects of nutrition in the context of the family's needs and life-style.

The nutritional questionnaire (Figure 11–10) can be used by the client and nurse to record the data base from which the plan of nursing interventions can be developed to fit the woman's individual needs. The sample questionnaire has been filled in to demonstrate this problem-oriented process.

Assessment of nutritional status is begun by the nurse as the questionnaire is completed. According to the format of problem-oriented medical records, the formulation of a partial problem list and initial plans follows the assessment. Following is an example of the process of POMR:

Assessment:

- Weight gain of 10 lbs during the first 2 months of pregnancy
- Limited information about present nutritional needs
- Limited budget, has obtained food stamps

Problem list (partial):

1. Limited nutritional information
2. Low intake of calcium and iron.
3. Excessive weight gain and empty calories.
4. Limited food budget.

Initial plans (partial):

Problem 1. Limited nutritional information.

   a. Review basic food groups and requirements.
   b. Compare present intake with recommended diet for the pregnant young adult.
   c. Recommend in-depth diet counseling if required.

Problem 2. Low intake of calcium and iron.

   a. Plan additional 3–4 cups of milk in daily intake.
   b. Encourage eating of foods high in iron. If this is not realistic (dislikes liver and spinach), investigate use of iron supplement.

ANTEPARTAL NURSING MANAGEMENT

Assessment: Establishing the Data Base

During the initial contact with the expectant mother or couple, the nurse elicits an explicit client profile (p. 211): the family's environment, life-style, habits, and relationships; sources and adequacy of income; race and/or culture; client's temperament and usual way of coping with stressful situations; an average day; and impact of the pregnancy on self, family, and significant others. At subsequent visits the nurse may ask her what *mother* means to her, what she thinks an average day with the baby will be like, and what she expects from the father. The father can be asked similar questions about his expectations for fatherhood and for his partner as a mother.

Many nonparents are not prepared for the sleep and feeding patterns of newborns. They have not thought about their feelings about the inevitable crying of the newborn and what they will do when the baby cries. Many couples are surprised to discover the sometimes extreme discrepancy between the partner's view of parenthood and expectation of the other. Guided discussion of these topics allows parents-to-be to attack problems, to arrive at compromises, and to appreciate each other's uniqueness.

Personal habits relevant to pregnancy include patterns of diet, sleep, and sexual activity; exercise; hobbies; and use of drugs (alcohol, tobacco, caffeine, and others). A past health history, describing the type and kind of therapies and responses to illness, adds significantly to the data base. The family history reveals the woman's placement within a family tree and her social relationship to its members. While taking the family history, the nurse can inquire about the geographic and social distance from family members, the frequency of visits, and the expected assistance from family members during pregnancy and after delivery.

The data base is completed with a description of body functioning, a complete physical examination, and laboratory values (see Chapter 10).

From the health assessment, the nurse develops an initial plan for interventions during the couple's preparation for childbearing and childrearing. The plan anticipates the need for information, guidance, and physical care. Interventions are timed to coincide with the woman's (couple's) readiness and needs.

FIGURE 11–10 Sample nutritional questionnaire used in nursing management of a pregnant client.

NUTRITIONAL QUESTIONNAIRE

Name Susan Longmont　　　　　　　Date 1-16-84

Age 20

Ethnic group white middle class

Religion Protestant

Gravida 1　　　　Para 0　　　　EDC 8-7-84

Age of youngest child? NA

Birth weights of previous children? NA

Usual nonpregnant weight 115　　Present weight 125

Weight gain during last pregnancy? NA

Vitamin supplements? none

Current medications? aspirin for headache

Do you smoke? yes　　How much per day? 1–1½ packs

Eating patterns:

1. How many meals per day? 2 when 12:30 pm　6:30 pm
2. How many snacks per day? 3 when 10:30 am　4:00 pm　10:00 pm
3. What other foods are important to your usual diet? chocolate and candy bars
4. Amount per day 4 bars/week
5. Do you have any different food preferences now? no
6. Do you eat nonfoods such as:

		Amount
laundry starch	no	NA
ice	yes	10 cubes/day
other (name)	no	NA

7. What foods do you dislike or do not eat? spinach and dried beans
8. For added information complete a typical daily intake (24 hour recall is suggested).

Interventions

Any crisis situation makes the involved parties more vulnerable but also more amenable to intervention. Through physical and psychosocial closeness to the woman or couple and with a detailed health assessment, the nurse is in a good position to intervene therapeutically. Well-paced interventions reassure prospective parents and validate their feelings and thoughts.

Two primary functions of the nurse caring for the pregnant family are (a) to support the family unit and (b) to provide prenatal education. If these tasks are performed well, family members may gain greater problem-solving ability, self-esteem, self-confidence, feelings of self-worth, and ability to participate in health care. In addition, parents who feel good about themselves have a sounder foundation on which to build meaningful relationships with their children.

SUPPORT OF FAMILY UNIT

The problems and concerns of the pregnant woman, the relief of her discomforts, and maintenance of her physical health receive much attention. However, her well-being also depends on the well-being of those she is closest to. Thus the nurse must meet the needs of the woman's family to maintain the integrity of the family unit.

Do you have special problems in food preparation such as:

1. Physical disability   yes _____   no _✔_   Explain _____

2. Cooking appliances   yes _____   no _✔_   Explain _____

3. Refrigeration of food   yes _____   no _✔_   Explain _____

Who does the meal planning? _I do._____ shopping? _We both do.____

cooking? _I do most of the time but my husband likes to help._____

Are there transportation problems? _We have only one car but we go in the evening._

_____

Financial situation: _My husband is working and going to school._____

_I am not working.____ Foodstamps _yes_____ w/c _no_____

Do you have any previous nutritional problems? _No. I have never paid much attention

to food before, but now I have a lot of questions._____

Are there any problems with this pregnancy? Nausea _Yes, in the morning.____

Constipation _No_____ Other _NA_____

Assessment by the nurse following the completion of the questionnaire.

Basic estimated nutrient and caloric value of typical daily intake.

Please circle one of the following:

	low	adequate	high
Protein intake was	low	(adequate)	high
Caloric intake was	low	adequate	(high)
Calcium intake was	(low)	adequate	high
Iron intake was	(low)	adequate	high
Vitamin C intake was	low	(adequate)	high

□ *PARTNER* Anticipatory guidance of the expectant father is a necessary part of any plan of care. He may need information about the anatomic, physiologic, and emotional changes that occur during pregnancy and postpartum, the couple's sexuality and sexual response, and possible reactions that he may experience. He may wish to express his feelings about breast- versus bottle-feeding, the sex of the child, and other topics. If it is culturally and personally acceptable to him, the nurse refers the couple to expectant parents' classes for further information and support from other couples.

The nurse ascertains the father's intended degree of participation during labor and delivery and assesses his knowledge of coaching and comfort measures and his preparation for the sights, sounds, and smells he may experience. If the couple prefers that his participation be minimal or restricted, the nurse supports their decision. With this type of consideration and collaboration, the father is less apt to develop feelings of alienation, helplessness, and guilt during the intrapartal period. Thus the relationship between the couple may be strengthened and his self-esteem raised. He is then better able to provide physical and emotional support to his partner during the birthing process.

□ *SIBLINGS* The nurse incorporates in the plan for prenatal care a discussion about the negative feelings that older

Table 11–9   Activities or Rituals During Pregnancy

Culture	Activity	Cultural meaning or belief	Nursing intervention
Mexican American	Certain clothing is worn (muneco-cord worn beneath the breasts and knotted over the umbilicus, Brown, 1976)	Ensures a safe delivery	If practice does not cause any danger, do not interfere with it
	Use of spearmint or sassafras tea or benedictine (Brown, 1976)	Eases morning sickness	Assess use of herbs and determine safety of their use
	Use of cathartics during the last month of pregnancy (Brown, 1976)	Ensures a good delivery of a healthy boy	Assess use of cathartics Provide teaching about dangers of the practice and explore other culturally acceptable means of resolving constipation (high fiber foods)
Black American	Use of self-medication for many discomforts of pregnancy is common (Epsom salts, castor oil for constipation; herbs for nausea and vomiting; vinegar and baking soda for heartburn) (Carrington, 1978)	Improves health and builds resistance	Assess use of self-medication; discourage those practices that may present problems
American Indian (selected examples)	*Navajo* Meets with the medicine man 2 months prior to delivery (Farris, 1976) Exercise is important during pregnancy; woman is also taught to concentrate on good thoughts and to be joyful (Farris, 1976)	Prayers are said to ensure safe delivery and healthy baby "Body movement is said to produce efficiency and promote joy" (Sevcovic, 1979, p. 39)	Encourage the use of support systems
	Muckeshoot Indians Keep busy and walk a lot (Horn, 1982)	The baby will be born earlier, and the labor and delivery will be easier	
	Tonawanda Seneca Eat sparingly and exercise freely (Evaneshko, 1982)	Delivery will be easier	Assess nutritional patterns and provide teaching if needed
Vietnamese	Consume ginseng tea Woman is expected to carry on conversations and counsel fetus (Hollingsworth et al., 1980)	Believed to give strength	Assess use and be certain it is not taken to the exclusion of necessary nutrients

children may have. Parents may be distressed to see an older child become aggressive toward the newborn. Parents who are unprepared for the older child's feelings of anger, jealousy, and rejection may respond inappropriately in their confusion and surprise. The nurse stresses that open communication between parents and children (or act-

ing out feelings with a doll if the child is too young to verbalize) helps the children to master their feelings and may prevent them from hurting the newest sibling when they are unsupervised. Children may feel less neglected and more secure if they know that their parents are willing to help with their anger and aggressiveness.

Table 11–10 Proscribed Activities

Culture	Activity	Rationale
Mexican American	Pregnant woman should not look at the full moon (Brown, 1976)	It will cripple or deform the unborn child
	She should not hang laundry or reach high	This will cause knots in the umbilical cord
	Baby showers should not be planned until delivery time (Kay, 1978)	Earlier would invite bad luck or the ''evil eye''
	The woman should not allow herself to quarrel or express anger (Kay, 1978)	Consequences are spontaneous abortion, premature labor, or knots in the cord
Black American	Avoid any emotional fright (Carrington, 1978)	Baby will have a birthmark
	Avoid reaching up	The umbilical cord may wrap around the baby's neck
American Indian (selected examples)	*Navajo* Rug weaving is forbidden; carrying and lifting also avoided (Sevcovic, 1979)	Puts unnatural strain on the body
	Avoid funerals or looking at dead animals (Sevcovic, 1979)	Exposes the baby to the realm of the dead and may cause later illness to the baby
	Laguna Pueblo Do not sew with a bone or a needle (Farris, 1978)	This will have an unkind effect on the baby
Vietnamese	Do not attend weddings or funerals (Hollingsworth et al., 1980)	Bad luck for the newlyweds; the baby may cry

CULTURAL CONSIDERATIONS IN PREGNANCY

Specific actions during pregnancy are often determined by cultural beliefs. Certain rituals and activities are often prescribed while others are forbidden. Some beliefs, which are passed down from generation to generation, may be called "old wives' tales." At one time these beliefs certainly had some meaning, but with the passing of time the meanings have often been lost. Certain beliefs may seem superstitious. Other beliefs have definite meanings that are retained. Tables 11–9 and 11–10 present prescribed and proscribed activities that are still seen within certain cultures. The tables are not meant to be all-inclusive; they offer a few examples of cultural activities important during the prenatal period.

In working with clients of another culture, it is constructive for the health professional to be as open as possible to other beliefs. If certain activities are not harmful, there is no need to impose one's beliefs and practices upon another culture. If the activities are harmful, it would be best to consult or work with someone within the culture or someone aware of cultural beliefs and values to help modify a client's behavior. Some questions to guide nursing care during this phase are:

• What are the client's beliefs regarding diet?

• What activities should be done during pregnancy?
• What activities should not be done?
• How is morning sickness managed?
• Are other remedies used during this time?
• Who provides support and instruction within the culture?
• Are other healers active within the culture?

ANTICIPATORY GUIDANCE FOR THE PUERPERIUM

In addition to recognizing individual family needs, issues that could be potential sources of stress in the puerperium need to be discussed by the expectant couple. If compromises can be negotiated in pregnancy about predictable crises in the early postpartum period, conflict will be decreased considerably. Some issues to be resolved prior to the puerperium could include: the question of sharing of infant and household chores; help in the first few days; a realistically adjusted budget if the mother has been working; options for babysitting to decrease restrictions on the mother's as well as couple's freedom; if and/or when the woman will return to work after the baby's birth; and how to deal with sibling rivalry and regressive behaviors.

Resolution of these issues varies for each couple. For

example, some young couples have relatives in the community who will do babysitting for them. Many others are isolated from family members and find it economically difficult to hire babysitters. Exchanging babysitting chores with other couples can be an excellent solution. Couples who have developed friendships through prenatal classes learn about one another's views on infant care, and can establish future babysitting exchanges even when they are new to the community.

It is valuable for professionals who come in contact with childbearing couples to help them assess potential areas of stress in the puerperium. If couples are able to comfortably agree on the issues prior to the early postpartum period, their adjustment will come about with much greater ease and stability than if these issues have not been confronted and resolved.

TEACHING COMMUNICATION SKILLS

The nurse's role may be expanded to teaching parents specific communication skills that enhance family well-being. Whether this is the first child or not, learning and using these skills will strengthen family relationships. In addition, these communication skills directly benefit the nurse–client relationship.

The communication skills described in this section are based on the work of Gordon (1970), who formulated an easily understood and practical adaptation of well-established psychotherapeutic techniques. Three of the skills he described that enhance rapport are active listening, sending I-messages, and resolving conflicts through the "no-lose" method.

□ *ACTIVE LISTENING* Active listening is a well-tested technique for helping a person with a problem. The listener simply feeds back to the sender his or her understanding of the meaning and of the feelings underlying the sender's statement.

Active listening requires certain underlying attitudes, including (a) wanting to be helpful to the other person, (b) genuinely being able to accept the other's feelings, and (c) having a deep feeling of trust in someone's capacity to handle emotions and to work through them to find solutions to problems.

One significant application of active listening in the maternity clinical setting is in deescalation of the woman's concern about her health or the couple's worries about the well-being of the fetus. Active listening can give the worried couple relief as well as a sense that their concern is being taken seriously.

As in any consulting relationship, the nurse must allow the client to decide about the usefulness of the advice— that is, whether to "buy" the consultation. Also, the nurse must realize that repeated attempts to convert another to the nurse's viewpoint, once it has been fully explained, only increase the client's defensiveness and the likelihood that he or she will ignore the advice. These considerations

are also applicable to advice giving within the family situation.

□ *SENDING I-MESSAGES* The second communication skill described by Gordon is the ability to send I-messages. An I-message lets the sender tell another person how one feels about behavior that one finds unacceptable. An I-message has three components: (a) a nonblameful description of the behavior of the other person, (b) a statement of the concrete and tangible effect of that behavior on the sender, and (c) a statement of the sender's feelings about the behavior.

Nurses have many opportunities for using I-messages to communicate their needs to clients. I-messages allow nurses to express their feelings yet cause clients minimal embarrassment, guilt, or shame. This type of communication enlists the client's willingness to initiate behavior out of consideration for the nurse's needs. I-messages such as the following may be sent from nurses to clients: "I am concerned when you don't take your medication. It makes me afraid you'll have a relapse and the work done so far will be wasted." This nonblameful yet clear way for nurses to identify their needs generates minimal resistance, so that the client remains willing to modify behavior.

□ *NO-LOSE PROBLEM SOLVING* Many solutions to conflicts involve the imposition of one party's will on the other. For example, the parent "wins" at the expense of the child's needs, or the child "wins" at the expense of the parent's needs. In either case, the loser inevitably feels resentful of the winner, and the relationship is damaged. The no-lose method of problem solving is designed to make both parties "winners."

The first step is to identify the needs of each person, with full use of active listening and I-messages. Both persons then search for a solution that is acceptable to each. They offer possible solutions, evaluate them, and eventually make a decision on a final solution that satisfies both. No compromise is required after the solution has been selected, because both parties have already accepted it. No power is required to force compliance, because neither is resisting the decision.

Conflicts between nurses and their clients are inevitable, as they are in all human relationships. Authoritarian nurses who impose their solutions on clients without reference to the clients' needs will find that they have resentful and resistant clients who are less likely to adhere to the professional advice. Permissive nurses who yield to their clients often suffer through missed appointments, late payment for services, or incomplete medical histories; as a result, they feel abused and resentful of the time and energy spent with that client. The no-lose problem-solving process gives nurses, couples, and parents the tools they need to avoid authoritarian or permissive responses to conflict and ensures that everyone's needs are met.

The maternity encounter is not the only or even necessarily the best place to teach and acquire effective communication. Courses for couples that focus on these skills are probably more effective educational vehicles. However, because support for parents is often scarce, the maternity setting may provide an opportunity to reinforce the learning of these skills.

Classes for Family Members during Pregnancy

PRENATAL EDUCATION

Antepartal educational programs vary in their goals, content, leadership techniques, and method of teaching. Content of the classes is generally dictated by the goals. For example, the goals of some classes are to prepare the couple for childbirth, and therefore discomforts of pregnancy and care of the newborn may not be included. Other classes may be oriented only to pregnancy and not prepare the woman for labor and delivery. Special classes are also available for couples who know that the expectant mother will be having a cesarean delivery. Nurses should be aware of these variations and the goals of the couple before directing couples to specific classes.

□ ONE-TO-ONE TEACHING Teaching on an individual basis occurs when the client needs it. Anticipatory guidance is also a positive part of teaching, and its effective use is based on the nurse's knowledge of the maternity cycle, assessment of its effect on the woman and other family members, and judgment of how this knowledge should be applied to probable or existing needs. Anticipatory guidance is relevant in discussion of such topics as care of breasts in pregnancy, sexual activity, and preparation for labor and delivery.

Nurses' teaching skills improve as they become more aware of the needs of expectant families and as they broaden their base of knowledge. A continuous evaluation of the effectiveness of one's teaching is essential in developing these skills.

□ GROUP TEACHING Group discussion is an appropriate and worthwhile teaching method, and it allows for optimum use of the nursing process. The nursing process basically involves the continuous assessment of client needs through various methods of data collection, intervention determined by the nurse's interpretation of the needs and by knowledge and skills, and evaluation of how well the nursing intervention has met the client's needs. In group teaching, however, the nurse assesses the needs of the group instead of the needs of an individual. Knowledge of group skills thus becomes essential.

Auerbach (1968), a leader in the field of parent education, has listed nine basic assumptions about parent group education:

1. Parents can learn.
2. Parents want to learn.
3. Parents learn best what they are interested in learning.
4. Learning is most significant when the subject matter is closely related to the parents' own immediate experience.
5. Parents can learn best when they are free to create their own response to a situation.
6. Parent group education is as much an emotional experience as it is an intellectual one.
7. Parents can learn from one another.
8. Parent group education provides the basis for a remaking of experience.
9. Each parent learns in his own way.*

Other factors facilitate group teaching. Groups should contain no more than 20 members when couples are involved (fewer if only mothers are in the group). An informal and friendly environment must be maintained. The members must attend consistently, and other activities should be encouraged in order to increase cohesiveness of the group. Large classes whose members sit in rows listening to didactic presentations by the nurse lose their effectiveness. Even when a short period is allowed for questions at the end of the lecture, only a few group members are able to participate. This traditional approach cannot provide for continuous identification of members' learning needs.

Helping the group to set an agenda at the initial session of a series of classes is one way of assessing members' needs. The individuals in the group must first become comfortable with each other so that there is a general sharing of concerns, questions, and information. Various techniques can be used to help the group members become familiar with one another. For example, the group can be divided into subgroups of two or three couples. Each subgroup is asked to list specific questions or concerns they would like discussed in the series of classes and to rank them in the order of interest. The subgroups are given a limited amount of time in which to accomplish their task. This method also stimulates much exchange of personal information.

Anticipatory guidance is necessary if discussion of important areas of content is not requested by group members; the leader can check with the group to determine whether it is an area of interest to them. Time must also be allotted for helping the group to plan how the agenda will be utilized, perhaps by grouping topics into general areas of focus, and letting the group determine the sequence in which these areas will be discussed.

Nursing intervention takes many forms in group discussion and frequently overlaps with assessment and evaluation as specific interests and concerns are clarified. The

*From Auerbach, A. 1968. *Parents learn through discussion: principles and practice of parent group education.* New York: John Wiley & Sons, Inc.

nurse may need to draw other members into the discussion or to clarify information. However, most prenatal classes are not purely discussion groups but include films, tours of maternity wards, demonstrations, and lengthy explanations. In classes concerned with selected methods of childbirth preparation, many group members have read extensively on the subject and can contribute considerably to the discussion, whereas other members may know nothing about it and thus require more explanations and demonstrations by the nurse. In situations where group members know little about the method, a more structured approach to discussion and exercises may be useful.

Evaluation of the effectiveness of the teaching–learning process is also continuous, but it is the most nebulous aspect. Checking each individual's performance after demonstration of an exercise is the most concrete way to evaluate learning. Evaluating members' changes in attitude or misconceptions is more difficult. A general evaluation of the series may be conducted in the last class, or evaluation forms can be given to members to return by mail at a later date.

Some excellent books have been written giving specific directions on how to establish classes and how to be an effective group leader. Although initially the traditional didactic method is easiest to use, as a nurse begins to apply the nursing process in practice, skills gradually develop and the nurse becomes an effective leader in group discussion.

PREPARED SIBLING PROGRAMS

Many hospitals now endorse children's visiting hours on maternity wards. Children's visitation on maternity wards is felt to reduce problems of separation anxiety in young children when mothers are hospitalized for the labor–delivery and postpartum experience. In addition, classes are being sponsored by these hospitals and/or various community groups to prepare children for what to expect in their visits and to make them more comfortable in the hospital setting before their mother's hospitalization. Another purpose of many of these classes is to facilitate the parents' preparation of children for the introduction of a new baby into the family.

Usually only one class is involved, and the youngest age accepted is 3 years old. Children are brought to the hospital by a parent, but parents are not included in the class unless a child will not participate without them. Most instructors believe that it is difficult to focus on the children when accompanying parents are asking their own questions. On the other hand, instructors of the classes want the children to feel positive about the hospital environment, so would not force a child to attend without a parent.

The classes usually involve a tour of the maternity ward where the children will be visiting their mothers. Chil-

dren can relate to such items as television sets, electric beds, and telephones the mothers will use to call them. Footstools at the nursery window allow youngsters of all sizes and ages to see the new babies. Most tours involve a visit to a birthing room, but not to delivery rooms. After the tour, the children are provided an opportunity to see and/or hear more about what happens to the parents and newborn in the hospital, how babies are born, and what babies are like. They are also offered an opportunity to discuss their feelings about having a new baby in the family. Discussion sessions may be divided into two age groups, if ages of the children attending vary greatly.

At the completion of the class, parents are usually provided with additional resources about how to prepare their children for a baby in the family. Some programs have special certificates for the children who attended, refreshments with their parents, and/or gift packets with articles similar to what new mothers receive (lotion, diapers for the new baby).

An increasing number of hospitals allow attendance of siblings at birth in birthing room settings. These hospitals usually require the siblings to attend special classes to prepare them for this experience. In addition, a sibling-support person who is trusted by the child is expected to accompany the child so that he or she can be present without distracting the mother. A grandparent often fills this role.

Classes that prepare children for attendance at birth are limited and do vary. It is important that such children be familiar with what to expect during the labor and delivery process: how the parents will act, especially the sounds and faces the mother may make, the messiness and blood, equipment, and how the baby will look and act at birth. In addition, parents are encouraged to involve the child early in the pregnancy, including taking the child on a prenatal visit to see the birth attendant and listen to the fetal heart beat. Most advocates feel the child also needs to be comfortable with seeing the mother without clothes prior to seeing her during labor and delivery.

CLASSES FOR GRANDPARENTS

For many years, hospital regulations have prevented grandparents of the newborn from having much contact until mother and baby arrive home. Those regulations are beginning to change considerably, and health professionals are beginning to recognize the important role of grandparents with the arrival of a newborn and the potential influence they have on the childbearing family. In addition to more open and extended visiting hours within the hospital environment, some communities are establishing classes for grandparents. The major purpose of these classes is twofold: to increase grandparents' awareness of the changes that have occurred in approaches to childbearing and childcare, and to increase grandparents' awareness of their feelings and the potential areas of conflict.

SELECTED METHODS OF CHILDBIRTH PREPARATION

Various methods of childbirth preparation are taught in North America. General antepartal classes cover various aspects of the maternity cycle and care of the newborn. Some classes, however, are more specifically oriented to preparation for labor and delivery, are labeled with a name indicating a theory of reduction of pain in childbirth, and are accompanied by specific exercises to accomplish this task. The three most common methods of this type are the Read (natural childbirth), the Lamaze (psychoprophylactic), and the Bradley (partner-coached childbirth). Hypnosis is also discussed here because it is sometimes used to help the expectant mother reduce or even eliminate pain in labor and delivery.

The programs in prepared childbirth have some similarities. All have an educational component to help eliminate fear. The classes vary in the breadth and depth of their coverage of various subjects related to the maternity cycle, but all prepare the participants in what to expect during labor and delivery and in methods of relaxation. Except for hypnosis, these methods also teach exercises to condition muscles and breathing patterns used in labor. The greatest differences among the methods are in the theories of why they work and in the relaxation techniques and breathing patterns that are taught.

The advantages of these methods of childbirth preparation are several. The most important is that a healthier baby may be produced because of the reduced need for analgesics and anesthetics. Another advantage is the satisfaction of the couples for whom childbirth becomes a shared and profound emotional experience. In addition, proponents of each method claim that it shortens the labor process, which has been clinically validated.

All maternity nurses must know how these methods differ, so that they will be able to support the couple in their chosen method. It is important that the nurse assess the couple's emotional resources and their expectations for the birth experience, so that the nurse can more effectively help them achieve their goals.

Read Method

Dr. Grantly Dick-Read (1959) was an English physician and a pioneer in the childbirth preparation movement. After observing many women in labor and assisting them in delivery, he developed a theory of preparation for childbirth. In 1933 his first book was published, entitled *Natural Childbirth*. It created considerable furor among physicians in his country.

Dick-Read called his method *natural childbirth* because he felt the process of labor and delivery was originally a natural process. He believed that pain experienced during this time was mental in origin, stating that "theoretically nature made no provision for parturition to be painful." Most women experience pain because of the culturally induced fear that they associate with childbirth. Thus his preparation method is centered around the fear-tension-pain syndrome: If the fear of childbirth is removed, tension will be reduced and pain will be minimized. Dick-Read believed that fear of childbirth could be removed by education. In his classes, women were taught what to expect in labor and delivery and to understand the process. Achievement of relaxation was also important. Additional exercises included conditioning of muscles that would be used in childbirth and others directed to the control of respiration during contractions. His program of physical preparation was further developed with the assistance of Helen Heardman (1961), a physiotherapist who was a proponent of this method.

Classes teaching the Read method follow a basic pattern. Part of the class time is devoted to the educational component and the other part to demonstration and practice of exercises.

Relaxation is an important part of the Read method. The woman is taught to use passive relaxation methods, such as progressive contraction and relaxation of muscle groups from her head to her toes, which may result in her falling asleep. She is encouraged to use this technique in labor to help her sleep or nap between contractions. If she is not able to sleep, at least she can relax her muscles.

The pattern of respiration utilized in labor is basically abdominal breathing. The woman concentrates on forcing the abdominal muscles to rise. When she begins the class, she probably takes several breaths per minute, but she is gradually taught to take one breath per minute, with a 30-second inhalation and 30-second exhalation. This pattern of breathing lifts the abdominal muscles as the uterus rises forward with a contraction. Proponents of this method suggest the pressure of the abdominal muscles on the contracting uterus increases pain. The woman is encouraged to practice her breathing in various positions and while involved in various activities. She begins the breathing technique with the first contraction in labor. Laboring women utilizing the Read method should not be interrupted in the middle of a contraction while doing their breathing.

An effective "pushing" position is also taught, but pushing is not done until the second stage of labor when it is needed. Body conditioning exercises condition the appropriate muscles. Panting is also taught to prevent pushing when it is not necessary.

Dick-Read emphasized the importance of a supportive environment throughout labor and delivery. He believed that a major source of discomfort for a woman during labor was the suggestion of pain, which "emanates from doctors, nurses, and relatives who believe in pain" (Dick-

Read, 1959). Proponents of all prepared childbirth methods believe that this type of environment still exists in many institutions and is a major source of discomfort.

Dick-Read believed husbands should be educated because of their influence on their wives but that husbands should not be with their wives during labor if they were not helpful to them. He emphasized that analgesia and anesthesia were available for women using his method of natural childbirth but implied throughout his book that a woman is either improperly prepared or remiss in her duty as a mother if she requests them.

Psychoprophylactic (Lamaze) Method

The terms *psychoprophylactic* and *Lamaze* are used interchangeably. *Psychoprophylactic* means "mind prevention," and Dr. Fernand Lamaze, a French obstetrician, was the first person to introduce this method of childbirth preparation to the Western world. Psychoprophylaxis actually originated in Russia and is based on Pavlov's research with conditioned reflexes. Pavlov found that the cortical centers of the brain can respond to only one set of signals at a time and that they accept only the strongest signal; the weaker signals are inhibited. Pavlov's research also demonstrated that verbal representation of a stimulus can create a response. When the real stimulus is substituted, the conditioned response continues to be produced. This theory was successfully applied to preparation for childbirth by Russian physicians.

Lamaze first became familiar with the psychoprophylaxis method when attending a conference in Russia. He introduced the method in France in 1951, adding innovations of his own. It was popularized soon after in this country through Marjorie Karmel's book *Thank You, Dr. Lamaze* (1965). The method was called "painless childbirth" and thus received much resistance from the medical profession in this country because it was believed that women inevitably experience pain in childbirth. Also, with the growing development of many analgesic and anesthetizing agents, it did not seem necessary to condition women for childbirth.

Proponents of the method gradually organized and in 1960 formed a nonprofit group called the American Society for Prophylaxis in Obstetrics. Two of the founders were Marjorie Karmel and Elizabeth Bing, a physical therapist who had also written about childbirth preparation using this method (Bing, 1967). This organization helped establish many programs throughout the country and has become one of the most popular methods of childbirth education.

The two components of Lamaze classes involve education and training. Couples are taught about childbirth and are trained to do specific exercises. Instructors teaching the method in this country have modified many of the original exercises, but the basic theory of conditioned reflex remains the same. Women are taught to substitute favorable conditioned responses for unfavorable ones. Rather than restlessness and loss of control in labor, the woman learns to respond to contractions with conditioned relaxation of the uninvolved muscles and a learned respiratory pattern. Exercises taught in these classes include proper body mechanics and body conditioning, breathing techniques for labor, and relaxation.

Some of the body conditioning exercises are similar to those taught in other childbirth preparation classes, such as the pelvic tilt, pelvic rock, and Kegel's exercise. Other exercises strengthen the abdominal muscles for the expulsive phase of labor. The method of relaxing uninvolved muscle groups (neuromuscular control), however, is unique and is a pattern of active relaxation, which is in contrast to the Read method of passive relaxation. The woman is taught to become familiar with the sensation of contraction and relaxation of the voluntary muscle groups throughout her body. She then learns to contract a specific muscle group and relax the rest of her body. This process of isolating the action of one group of voluntary muscles from the rest of the body is called *neuromuscular disassociation* and is basic to the psychoprophylaxis method of prepared childbirth. This exercise conditions the woman to separate the voluntary muscles of her body from uterine activity by relaxation of uninvolved muscles while the uterus contracts.

The breathing patterns utilized in the Lamaze method are also different from other methods. Chest breathing patterns vary according to the phase of labor; breathing becomes progressively more shallow. (See Chapter 16 for the various levels of breathing.) Proponents of this method believe that the variety of chest breathing patterns helps keep the pressure of the diaphragm off the contracting uterus. The patterns of breathing taught in different classes do vary. Occasionally the woman is taught to use one pattern until it is no longer effective rather than in conjunction with the phases of labor.

Another major modification in the Lamaze method involves the goals of expectant couples. Lamaze and his supporters implied that, if the childbirth experience was to be successful (painless with no anesthetic), specific criteria must be adhered to. Couples using this method are now encouraged to set their own goals for success. Lamaze childbirth education in this country supplies them with the tools to assist them in accomplishing these goals. The couple is encouraged to discuss their goals with the obstetrician and maternity nursing personnel in labor and delivery. When the nursing staff are aware of what the couple hopes to accomplish and of the resources they have available, they will be able to support them more effectively in their endeavors.

In France, *monitrices* are specially trained to assist the woman in labor and delivery. In this country, the partner has become the specially trained individual. In the United States, the Lamaze method no longer means childbirth without anesthetics or pain. The couple's training, how- ever, helps the woman to reduce pain and even to elimi- nate the need for anesthetics. More important, the woman is prepared to be an active participant and to be in control of her experience.

Bradley Method

The Bradley method, frequently referred to as partner- or husband-coached natural childbirth, is basically Read's method with the important introduction of the partner or support person, who plays a vital role in coaching the woman throughout pregnancy in preparation for labor and delivery.

In his writings and talks, Bradley compares his method of natural childbirth to the natural instincts in animals. Af- ter observing that animals do not suffer pain during the birthing process, he suggests that their birthing behaviors can be adapted by women to alleviate their suffering. Brad- ley lists environmental characteristics sought by birthing animals and their natural habits that he feels are necessary to achieve natural childbirth: darkness, solitude, quiet, physical comfort, physical relaxation, controlled breathing, and the appearance of sleep (Bradley, 1981). The exer- cises used to accomplish the relaxation and controlled breathing are basically those used in the Read method. A book titled *Exercises for True Natural Childbirth* (1975) gives more explicit instructions on how to do these exer- cises. The book was written by Rhonda Hartman, a nurse who was an early advocate of this method and who worked with Bradley in teaching and promoting it.

Bradley's goal is to help women achieve an unmedi- cated pregnancy, labor, and delivery. Proponents of his method have established the American Academy of Hus- band-Coached Childbirth for certifying teachers in his method. The teachers are usually individuals who have used the method successfully.

Hypnosis

The use of hypnosis in childbirth is not as common as the other methods of preparation just discussed. It does not include active exercising and is not always taught in a group situation. However, hypnosis is similar to the other methods in that it reduces fear of childbirth by telling the woman what to expect, produces relaxation, and reduces or eliminates pain.

The basic technique of hypnosis used in obstetrics is known as the *hypnoreflexogenous method,* first described in the Western hemisphere by Santiago Roig-Garcia (1961). The method is a combination of hypnosis and con- ditioned reflexes. Proponents believe that if a woman's re- sponse to labor has been verbally conditioned through posthypnotic suggestion, only rarely does the woman need enter a hypnotic state during labor.

During the hypnotic sessions, hypnosis is used to mod- ify the woman's existing perceptions of labor and delivery to eliminate fear and anxiety and to perceive contractions as a painless sensation. In addition, a low excitability level of the cortex occurs with hypnosis and posthypnotic sug- gestion. Proponents of this method feel that they are pre- paring the woman for a normal physiologic process, not a surgical procedure. Specific techniques of producing anes- thesia and analgesia are not taught but are believed to be by-products of the method (Werner et al., 1982). Roig- Garcia (1961) describes the woman prepared hypnotically as managing the labor and delivery process "in a state of vigilance and wakefulness without the presence of a pain component."

Practitioners of the hypnoreflexogenous method pre- pare their clients for the recovery period as well as for labor and delivery. Posthypnotic suggestions to facilitate elimination, breast-feeding, and other postpartum activi- ties are incorporated successfully into the training ses- sions.

Hypnotists in obstetrics often use a modification of the hypnoreflexogenous method and add the concept of "glove anesthesia." When the client is able to reach a me- dium or complete trance, the hypnotist describes the pro- cess of anesthetizing the woman's hand from the wrist to her fingertips. The hypnotist describes the tingling sensa- tions the client will experience and the eventual numbness of her hand. When the subject is able to achieve the numb- ness in her hand, she can transfer this anesthesia to other parts of her body by suggestion and touch. Throughout these suggestions, the woman's experience in labor and delivery is described in a positive manner, and the hypno- tist attempts to prepare her for her experience on a step- by-step basis to prevent any element of surprise. By the last session, autohypnosis may be accomplished by the cli- ent (Tinterow, 1972). Posthypnotic suggestions are uti- lized automatically in labor, with the numbness from the abdominal area to the knees being achieved rapidly, inside and out. During labor, the woman is never unconscious and can carry out such activities as voiding. She should be disturbed as infrequently as possible and spoken to softly; discomfort should never be suggested.

The sessions just described are time-consuming be- cause they are often done on a one-to-one basis. The ob- stetrician is frequently the hypnotist and begins prepara- tion of the woman around the fifth or sixth month of pregnancy. Six to eight sessions may be incorporated as part of the woman's prenatal visits.

The utilization of the hypnoreflexogenous method without the additional introduction of "glove anesthesia" seems to be the most common method of hypnosis now used in obstetrics, probably because it can be taught in group sessions in less time.

It should be noted that one group of researchers be- lieve that their experience has demonstrated that only a small percentage of the population (20%–40%) was capable of achieving successful hypnoanesthesia when women were prepared specifically for a surgical process rather than "incorporating psychological concepts of natural childbirth" (Werner et al., 1982).

These researchers describe women who used the hypnoreflexogenous method to completely block out the discomfort of labor, although they were aware of the hardening sensation of the uterus. Those who were unable to block the discomfort totally experienced discomfort at the level of the sacrum, similar to that experienced with menstrual periods. Once the cervix was completely dilated, these women all became aware of the urge to bear down. Their posthypnotic suggestions were also helpful in preparing them for suturing of episiotomies, although some needed to enter a true hypnotic state for the procedure (Werner et al., 1982).

Much controversy has surrounded the use of hypnosis, perhaps because the mechanism of hypnosis is only vaguely understood. Trance also seems to connote mysticism and lack of control. Proponents of hypnosis, however, say that the subject does not follow through on suggestions that she ordinarily would not do anyway. There is no physical danger to the woman and baby, especially with the reduction or elimination of medications in labor and delivery.

The greatest disadvantage of hypnosis to the couple is that the man is usually not involved. In addition, some are concerned about the risk of producing psychosis in a woman who has emotional disorder. Others feel that this would be impossible (Tinterow, 1972).

PREPARING THE ADOLESCENT FOR CHILDBIRTH AND CHILDREARING

Pregnancy for the adolescent is a crisis situation, as it is for the adult. The adolescent, however, has a number of factors complicating her pregnancy and outcome. Immature physical development, incomplete tasks of adolescence, uncertain support systems, and unfinished education all combine to place the young woman at risk during childbearing and childrearing.

The teenage pregnancy rate has continued to increase during the last decade, with at least one in ten young women becoming pregnant each year (Guttmacher, 1981). Although contraceptive use has increased among adolescents, it has not kept pace with the increasing incidence of sexual activity.

Many factors contribute to the increase of adolescent pregnancy. Both the age of menarche and the age of first sexual intercourse are declining, contributing to earlier pregnancy exposure. Sex is advertised in every aspect of the media, making it more visible than ever before. Marriage is being delayed until later years, and cohabitation is

more acceptable and more widely practiced than 20 or even 10 years ago.

Many pregnant adolescents are continuing school, usually with their classmates, thus increasing their visibility in the community. Twenty years ago these young women were expelled from school and generally "disappeared" for 9 months. Fewer young women are choosing to legitimate their newborns by marriage, and more of them are choosing to keep their newborns rather than relinquish them.

Even though the incidence of adolescent pregnancy has increased, the birth rate is declining. This is partially because of the availability of legal abortion services. Nevertheless, adolescents are becoming pregnant in greater numbers. The physiologic, psychologic, and sociologic consequences must be addressed by the health care profession.

Physical Changes of Adolescence

The physical changes of pubescence are covered in Chapter 5. The effects of the hypothalamic–pituitary–ovarian axis should be reviewed to comprehend why the young woman is at risk for complications during childbearing.

Menarche occurs in adolescents about 1 year earlier than it did 50 years ago, the average age being just under 13 years (Nelson et al., 1979). The major physical changes of puberty include a height spurt, weight change, and the appearance of secondary sex characteristics. Some researchers hypothesize that a critical weight of 47–48 kg (104–106 lb) may trigger a change in metabolism to initiate menarche, although this concept has been challenged (Nelson, 1978).

The first menstrual cycles are irregular and usually anovulatory. The hypothalamic–pituitary–ovarian axis takes up to 5 years to complete maturation (Lemarchand-Beraud et al., 1982). Long bone growth is also incomplete until well after menarche.

Nutritional status is an important determinant of menarche. Undernourished girls tend to have a later menarche. Anemia can be a problem for adolescents, especially during the growth spurt that precedes menarche.

Psychosocial Effects of Adolescence

The period of adolescence is both agony and ecstasy. The agony lies in dealing with body changes, social and family relationship changes; the ecstasy lies in new discoveries, independence, and responsibilities. The almost schizophrenic struggle to become an adult while needing the security of childhood creates a turbulent era for the entire family.

Erikson (1963) has described the psychosocial development of the individual as occurring in eight stages. The stage of puberty-adolescence relates to resolution of identity versus role confusion. Developmental tasks of the adolescent have been described by many writers. Mercer (1979) has enumerated six tasks that include:

- acceptance and achievement of comfort with body image
- determination and internalization of sexual identity and role
- development of a personal value system
- preparation for productive citizenship
- achievement of independence from parents
- development of an adult identity

These tasks are overwhelming in their nature for many adolescents; the guidance, nurturing, and support offered by the family and community play a large part in determining successful integration.

Adolescent rebellion is a means by which young people work at accomplishing these tasks. Rebellion permits them to make the transition to adult social roles. In the same way that the toddler attempts independence from mother, the adolescent who rebels against parental and school authority is trying to make independent decisions. The widespread rebellion of the late 1960s exemplifies this struggle by young people.

The young adolescent (under age 14) still sees authority in parents; the middle adolescent relies on the peer group for authority and decision making. Middle adolescence is the critical time for challenging: experimenting with drugs, alcohol, and sex are avenues of rebellion. Older adolescents are more at ease with their individuality and decision making. The experiences of middle adolescence assist them in completing their developmental tasks. Understanding each adolescent's stage of psychosocial development will help the nurse in caring for a pregnant teen.

Cognitive development is another crucial change of adolescence. Young people move from concrete and egocentric thinking of childhood to abstract conceptualization (Piaget, 1972). The ability of the young adolescent to see herself in the future or forsee the consequences of her behavior is minimal. She perceives her focus of control as external; that is, that her destiny is controlled by others, parents, and school authorities. As she matures, learns to solve problems, to conceptualize, and to make decisions, she will gradually see herself as having control. The ability to see the consequences of her behavior results.

The Pregnant Adolescent

The psychoanalytic rationales for adolescent pregnancy have received major attention in the literature. The motivating phenomenon may be an acting out of oedipal conflicts of adolescence, using the pregnancy to maintain infantile dependence on the young woman's own mother. If the young woman's mother has been an inconsistent nurturer, the daughter may enter adolescence with deficits in her sense of time, reality testing, and her ability to handle frustration; thus, she has difficulty dealing with her developmental tasks (Spain, 1980).

Deficits in ego functioning have been cited as reasons for sexually acting out. Young women with poor ego integrity have little sense of self-worth and some hopelessness regarding their future. Other psychologic rationales include: unstable family relationships; needing someone to love; competition with the adolescent's mother; punishment of the adolescent's father and/or mother; emancipation from an undesirable home situation; and an attention-getting vehicle. Pregnancy may be a young woman's form of delinquency because this is one area that parents cannot control.

Another school of thought suggests that pregnancy is a result of unmotivated accidents. The adolescent who is as yet incapable of thinking abstractly is unable to perceive the consequences of her sexual activity. She has sex infrequently, often not planning to have it, and therefore does not consider contraception. She may have guilt feelings surrounding sex and may not be able to admit she is sexually active. She is incapable of understanding how pregnancy will affect her future. Rationale may include comments such as, "I'm too young to get pregnant," "I don't have intercourse often enough," or "It was the safe time of the month." Most young people have no idea of when they ovulate and how they conceive.

PHYSIOLOGIC RISKS OF THE PREGNANT ADOLESCENT

Previous research demonstrated that adolescents were more at risk than older women for a myriad of problems during pregnancy. New studies that control for age, race, socioeconomic status, and prenatal care show that adolescents over age 15 years and who receive early, thorough prenatal care have no greater risk than women over age 20 years. It is the young adolescent (under age 14) who remains at high risk for premature births; low-birth-weight (LBW) infants; pregnancy-induced hypertension (PIH) and its sequelae, cephalopelvic disproportion (CPD); and iron deficiency anemia (Carey et al., 1981). In this age group, prenatal care is the critical factor that most influences pregnancy outcome.

Pregnancy-induced hypertension represents the most prevalent medical complication in adolescents; the incidence of PIH is higher in teens than among older women. The etiology of PIH remains unclear, but hypotheses point to uterine ischemia, nutritional factors, and immunologic variances that appear to affect adolescents. There may be a suboptimal development of the uterine vasculature in the very young adolescent that predisposes them to PIH (Chesley, 1978).

Iron deficiency anemia is a problem in all pregnant women. The adolescent who begins her pregnancy already anemic, however, is at increased risk and must be followed closely as well as carefully counseled regarding her nutrition during pregnancy.

Table 11–11   Developmental Tasks of Adolescence and Their Implications During Pregnancy

Developmental tasks of adolescence (Mercer, 1979)	Impact on pregnant adolescent	Nursing implications
Acceptance and comfort with body image	Must learn to deal with changing body: enlarging breasts and abdomen, striae, chloasma, weight gain; she may not have yet incorporated the changes of puberty	Assist the client in determining what the changes of puberty meant to her; how she feels about the changes of pregnancy Help her think of ways in which she can feel good about herself
	May be reticent about wearing maternity clothes	Assess at what point in the pregnancy she begins to wear maternity clothes; ask why if she is not wearing them at the appropriate time
	May try fad diets or eat junk food, due to peer pressure and the slender image society has of women; does not want to get fat	Nutrition counseling will be in order for every adolescent Emphasize that pregnant women do not diet, she can lose the weight later; give exercises for pregnant women
	Must learn to cope with looking different from her peers	Elicit feelings about how she is coping with this; support from friends, family
Determination and internalization of sexual role and identity	May not be able to perceive of herself as a sexual being (pregnancy confers overt sexuality)	Elicit feelings about sexuality
	Must learn to incorporate the concept of becoming a mother	What does motherhood mean to the client?
	Must cope with possible changes in relationships with friends, boyfriend, and family	How does she see relationships changing? How is she dealing with this?
	May see her role as solely procreator, other opportunities for development of other female roles may be temporarily abandoned	What other roles does she see for herself now? In 5 years?
Development of a personal value system	Must cope with and adjust to the fact that she became pregnant; is this in conflict with her self ideal of chastity?	Discuss her feelings of conflict, if any: Is she living up to her expectations and how can she do so?
	Adjust to premature motherhood and the inherent responsibilities	Explore the value the client places on becoming a mother and having children How does she see her relationship with her newborn, now and 5 years from now?
	Incorporate problem-solving skills and decision-making skills	Explore values regarding career, school, marriage Reality test: ``Tell me how you see a typical day with a 2-month-old infant?''
Preparation for productive citizenship	Adjust to interruption of school May see school as unnecessary, or postpone indefinitely	Explore provisions for school while pregnant: when can she return? Refer to Social Service; discuss importance of education regarding her career and future
	Incorporate career goals with parenting; she may not consider working important	Discuss future economic consolidation Assist problem solving in this area

Table 11–11 Developmental Tasks of Adolescence and Their Implications During Pregnancy Cont'd

Developmental tasks of adolescence (Mercer, 1979)	Impact on pregnant adolescent	Nursing implications
Achievement of independence from parents	Cope with realities of pregnancy, and dependence on family (or someone) for financial help	Elicit what changes she perceives and how she feels about them Discuss the reality of her situation (reality testing is constructive) How can she adjust? How can she plan independence? Living at home may be out of the question; she may end up on welfare Check her home and family situation often during the pregnancy
	Adjust to need for financial assistance until she can earn her own living	What role will the father of the child play? If she does not live at home, who will support her?
Development of an adult identity	Learn to accept the responsibilities of adulthood and parenthood Learn to accept the responsibilities for her actions Learn to plan for her future	Encourage prenatal classes, parenting classes Discuss prenatal care and the effects on her pregnancy Explore options through all of the above

Teenagers between 15 and 19 years old have the second highest incidence of sexually transmitted diseases in the United States. The impact of herpesvirus and gonorrhea during a pregnancy increases the dangers greatly. Other problems seen in adolescents are cigarette smoking and drug use. The damage may be already done to the fetus by smoking or drug use by the time pregnancy is confirmed in young women.

PSYCHOLOGIC RISK OF PREGNANCY

The most profound psychologic risk to the pregnant adolescent is the interruption in completing her developmental tasks. Add to this the tasks of pregnancy and the young woman has an overwhelming amount of psychologic work to do, the completion of which will affect her own and her newborn's future.

The successful achievement of developmental tasks in the various life stages preclude completion of the next set of tasks. Unless one is able to complete the tasks of adolescence and incorporate an adult identity, the adult tasks will be difficult to attain. These tasks are building blocks to maturation and to positive self-growth.

Table 11–11 lists adolescent developmental tasks (as identified by Mercer), the impact on the pregnant adolescent, and nursing implications. Tasks of pregnancy are included in Table 11–12.

Through the nursing process, the nurse should assist the client in meeting these tasks during prenatal visits. An interdisciplinary approach, utilizing the social worker, nu-

tritional counselor, and school counselor will benefit the client.

SOCIOLOGIC RISK

The adolescent pregnancy not only affects the adolescent but society as well. The syndrome of failure (Waters, 1969) describes the sequence of events that the adolescent is at risk for, the brunt of which society must carry. This syndrome includes:

- failure to fulfill the functions of adolescence
- failure to remain in school
- failure to limit family size
- failure to establish stable families
- failure to be self-supporting
- failure to have healthy infants

The frustration of being forced into adult roles before one has completed adolescent developmental tasks causes a negative cascade of events that affects the adolescent's entire life.

Several studies have demonstrated that the majority of young women who become pregnant drop out of school and never complete their education (Furstenberg, 1976; Moore and Waite, 1977; Card and Wise, 1978). With the advent of programs for pregnant adolescents and adolescent mothers, it is hoped that this problem will be alleviated in the next decade. Much effort will need to be expended, however, to break this element of the failure

Table 11-12   Tasks of Pregnancy and the Adolescent

Task	Impact on adolescent	Nursing implications
Acceptance of pregnancy	May deny until well into pregnancy, thus having no alternative but to carry pregnancy	Counsel or refer for counseling regarding whether she will keep or relinquish her newborn Discuss importance of early prenatal care
	May have difficulty bonding with fetus which may carry over to unresponsiveness to newborn	Elicit feelings about pregnancy (see Table 11-11, developmental task I)
Acceptance of termination of pregnancy	Toward end of pregnancy may focus on "wanting it to be over"; may have trouble individuating fetus	Elicit why she has these feelings Assist with coping mechanisms Discuss preferred sex, names, showers, and readiness for newborn's arrival
Acceptance of mother role	May not perceive of newborn as being her own, especially if client's mother will be caring for the newborn; may think of newborn as a doll or sister	Discuss plans for newborn, include client's mother as indicated Elicit client's perception of motherhood (see Table 11-11, developmental task II) Discuss dreams, role playing, fantasies that she experiences Does she know any new mothers? Encourage prenatal classes
Resolution of fears about childbirth	May focus on labor and delivery as mutilating to her body	Encourage attendance at prenatal classes, childbirth education Offer literature or references for reading
	May not see childbirth education as necessary for coping and learning	Elicit expectations, knowledge and fears about childbirth Discuss analgesia, labor process, offer tour of facilities
	May have fantasies, dreams or nightmares about childbirth	Reinforce that fantasies or dreams are normal Encourage support person to attend classes with client
Bonding	May feel ambivalent about pregnancy and motherhood	Assess all parameters of feelings about pregnancy in other developmental tasks and tasks of pregnancy (Table 11-11) Refer for counseling if there is any sign of maladjustment to pregnancy

cycle. Lack of education reduces the quality of jobs available to these young women. Adolescent husbands also tend to obtain less prestigious careers, earn less income, and have less job satisfaction than male counterparts who marry at an older age. Although adolescent women are more immediately affected because of pregnancy, the young men they marry are also at risk.

Failure to limit family size is another element of the syndrome. The younger the adolescent at her first pregnancy, the more likely she is to become pregnant again while an adolescent. These young adolescents frequently fail to remain in school, neglect to use contraception, and do not remain in contact with the father of their child.

Repeat pregnancies during adolescence are also problematic due to the increased mortality and morbidity of the neonate. Psychosocial responsibilities escalate as the adolescent has to raise more children. These young women frequently fail to establish a stable family. Their family structure tends to be matricentric and monoparental, often the same family structure that the adolescent was raised in. If such women do marry, their divorce rate is the highest of any other age group in the United States. Certainly situations of poverty aggravate this problem.

Failure to be self-supporting logically follows lack of education and lost career goals. Many of these young women end up on welfare.

Finally, adolescents are at risk for having unhealthy newborns.

Both the adolescent and society pay for the results of teenage pregnancy. Rising medical costs as a result of increased morbidity and mortality of mother and neonate are assured, as are increased costs to the taxpayer for welfare. The long-term social costs of adolescent childbearing can be staggering.

The Adolescent Father

Historically, the unwed adolescent father has been met with less than supportive services. He has been characterized as the "putative" father in the literature on adolescent pregnancy. His stresses, concerns, and needs have been ignored by society. Research in this area is scant.

The fathers are usually within 3–4 years in age of the young woman. The couple is usually from similar socioeconomic backgrounds and have similar education. Many are involved in meaningful relationships. Frequently, the fathers are involved in the decision making regarding abortion or adoption. Recent literature confirms that many fathers are very involved in the pregnancy and in the childrearing, whether or not the fathers live with their children.

Psychologic and sociologic risks to the adolescent father are in many ways similar to the young woman's risks. Card and Wise (1978) found that the adolescent fathers achieve less formal education than older fathers and they enter the labor force earlier (with less education). Eleven years after high school graduation, adolescent fathers had more blue-collar jobs than did young men who postponed fathering. Although incomes were similar, those who had been adolescent fathers had less chance for job advancement. Logically, they would never attain the same financial security as their counterparts who had more education.

This same study also found that adolescent fathers married at a younger age and had larger families than the older fathers did. The divorce rate of adolescent fathers is two to four times greater than that of couples who postpone childbearing and marriage. Less formal education, earlier marriages, and large families all combine to create a financial disaster, which may be a factor in the high divorce rate.

Psychologically the young man's own maturation will be altered. His developmental tasks will be interrupted as he faces fatherhood. Because he is not mature, his level of cognitive development and decision-making skills will influence whether he remains supportive or flees the situation. Certainly, he will be more vulnerable to emotional stressors than will an adult man.

The stresses of pregnancy on the adolescent male come from many sources. He faces negative reactions from people in his environment, including his own family and the family of the young woman. Feelings of anger, shame, and disappointment will be aimed at him. Although both young people were involved in the act of intercourse, the young man is usually considered the guilty party. He will feel isolated and alone, and if the young woman's parents refuse to allow him to see her, his sole support may be gone.

Another source of stress arises from actual and perceived changes in his life. His educational and career goals may be threatened as he anticipates marriage or quitting school to support the young woman and his forthcoming child. His relationship with his peers may be altered as well.

A third stressor will be his concerns regarding the health of the young woman and the fetus. He may be quite protective, yet may not understand the physical and psychologic changes of pregnancy.

The adolescent father faces a serious situation, which may be overwhelming for him. The unresolved stress may lead to a severe crisis, manifested by abnormal adaptive behavior, marked depression, somatic symptoms, sexually deviant behavior, or even acute psychosis.

The implications for the health care team are important. Even if the couple has severed their relationship, the father should be sought to assess how he is coping and to offer him counseling. It may take assertive steps to find him as he may fear recrimination, legal or otherwise. He may not understand why he needs to come to the clinic and the nurse must let him know that the staff would like to help him, too.

If the couple is still together, the father should be told that his participation is important, that he is an excellent support person for the young woman, and that he is welcome to attend clinic and classes. Many clinics interview the couple routinely on the first prenatal visit.

The young man will need education regarding pregnancy, childbirth, childcare, and parenting. Some clinics have couples attend classes together, others offer "father" classes. In the area of parenting, men need to learn rates of growth and development so they understand their newborn's potential and do not become frustrated and dissatisfied with the child's behavior.

As part of his counseling, the nurse should assess the young man's stressors, his support systems, his plans for involvement in the pregnancy and childrearing, his future plans, and his health care needs. He should be referred to social services for an opportunity to be counseled regarding his educational and vocational future. When the father is involved in the pregnancy, the young mother feels less deserted, more confident in her decision making, and better able to discuss her future.

Parents' Reactions to Adolescent Pregnancy

Perhaps the first, most intense crisis of the pregnant adolescent is telling her parents that she is pregnant. The young woman may not talk about her pregnancy until it is obvious. Her mother is usually the first to find out and often attempts to protect the young woman's father from discovering his daughter is pregnant. Little research is available on the reactions of these fathers, however.

Parents' initial reactions to the news are usually shock, anger, shame, guilt, and sorrow. The angry mother may accompany her daughter to the clinic. The nurse must assess the disharmony that is occurring and explain the process of adaptation that follows.

The stereotype of the poor family accepting the pregnant daughter and her newborn unequivocally is not true. Studies of poor black families found that the mother was often angry and disappointed. These mothers had high aspirations, hoping that their daughters would fare better in life than they had.

Mothers frequently feel guilty about their daughters' pregnancies. They wonder what they have done wrong and feel they have been inadequate in their role as a parent. They are also angry because they are concerned about themselves. Just as their children are growing up and they see a new sense of freedom coming, they now have the responsibility of helping their daughters deal with a crisis. They may also feel angry at "being made a grandmother," perhaps at a young age. Once these reactions are dealt with, the atmosphere begins to return to normal. The mother becomes involved in decision making regarding abortion, adoption, marriage, and dealing with the father-to-be and his family. Family input in these matters is important in the adolescent's decision making. If the pregnant adolescent is encouraged by her family to carry and keep the newborn, she is unlikely to disregard her family's wishes and seek an abortion. On the other hand, if the adolescent is not allowed to remain at home because of her pregnancy, she is more likely to seek abortion or relinquish her newborn.

As the pregnancy progresses the mother begins to take on the grandmother role. She may begin to buy presents for the newborn and plan for the future. She may participate in prenatal care and classes and can be an excellent support system for her daughter. She should be encouraged to participate if the mother–daughter relationship is positive. The mother should be updated on obstetrical practice to clarify any misconceptions she might have. During labor and delivery, the mother will be a key figure for her daughter. Drawing on her own experience, she can offer reassurance and instill confidence in the adolescent.

The last stages of a mother's acceptance occur after her daughter's child is born. As the mother attempts to integrate her role of grandmother, an initial blurring of roles occurs. The grandmother now sees her daughter as a mother, and the daughter begins to identify herself as a mother. Role confusion may develop and sometimes continues for years—the grandmother may essentially do all the mothering and caretaking activities for the newborn,

while the daughter remains only a daughter and becomes a sibling of her newborn. Until the daughter is able to internalize her role as mother, the grandmother will be unable to completely identify as a grandmother.

This new role development is clouded by the adolescent's struggle to complete her tasks of adolescence. The wise mother will gently encourage a balance between helping her daughter parent and allowing her to complete the tasks of adolescence. As her daughter becomes more confident in the role of parent, the grandmother can gradually encourage more independence for the daughter.

Nursing Management of the Pregnant Adolescent

Early and thorough prenatal care is the strongest and most critical determinant for reducing morbidity and mortality for the adolescent and her newborn. This point cannot be overemphasized. The nurse must understand the special needs of the adolescent to successfully meet this challenge. The major objectives in the prenatal care of the pregnant adolescent are to:

- assure quality health care to eliminate complications of pregnancy
- develop a trusting relationship with the client
- assist the client in increasing her self-esteem
- assist the adolescent in her decision-making and problem-solving skills so that she may proceed with her developmental tasks and begin to assume responsibility for her life as well as her newborn's life

ASSESSMENT: ESTABLISHING THE DATA BASE

Within any one age group, the maturational level varies from one individual to another. Adolescent life-styles and support systems vary tremendously. It is imperative that the interdisciplinary health team have information regarding the expectant adolescents' feelings and perceptions about themselves, their sexuality, and the coming baby; their knowledge of, attitude toward, and anticipated ability to physically care for and financially support the infant; and their maturational level and needs.

The nurse must establish a data base to plan her interventions for the adolescent mother-to-be. The following information is necessary:

Family and personal history. Family diseases such as diabetes, cardiovascular diseases, epilepsy, blood dyscrasia, hereditary diseases, congenital anomalies, tuberculosis, mental illness; multiple pregnancies; cultural influences; relationship within family and with significant others; previous sexual experience and sex education; self-concept and family support; and coping methods.

Medical history. The adolescent's general health; past or current heart disease, diabetes mellitus, epilepsy, rheumatic fever, childhood diseases, blood dyscrasia, tuberculosis, urinary tract disease, drug sensitivity, allergies; immunization; recent viral diseases; and exposure to drugs or pollutants.

Menstrual history. Onset of menses, regularity and duration of menses, and any problems with menses.

Obstetric history. Number of pregnancies, interrupted pregnancies, abortions, premature deliveries, viable births; health status of any living children; neonatal complications and/or stillbirths; previous pregnancy complications; experience with contraceptive methods.

NURSING RESPONSIBILITIES

In addition to completing the prenatal assessment described in Chapter 10, the nurse must be attentive to the special problems of adolescents. The first visit to the clinic or office will be fraught with extreme anxiety on the part of the young woman. Not only will she be nervous because of her situation, but this may well be her first exposure to the health care system since childhood. Making this first experience as positive as possible will encourage her compliance in returning for follow-up care as well as ensure a favorable attitude toward the importance of health care for both her and her newborn.

Developing a trusting relationship with the pregnant client is critical to compliance. Honesty and respect for the individual young woman and a caring attitude promote self-esteem. A verbal contract at the first visit will enable the client to begin to take responsibility for health and care during pregnancy. As a role model the nurse's attitudes about self-health and responsibility affect the adolescent's maturation process.

An overview of what the client will experience over the prenatal course, along with thorough explanations and rationale for each procedure as it occurs, will foster the client's understanding and give her some measure of control. Actively involving the young woman in her care will give her a sense of participation and responsibility in her health care (Figure 11–11).

Depending on how young the adolescent is, this may be her first pelvic examination, a frightening experience for any woman. A thorough explanation of the procedure and technique is a must. Gentle and thoughtful examination technique will put the client at ease. A mirror is helpful in allowing the client to see her cervix, educating her about her anatomy, and giving her a part in the exam. If she is extremely anxious, she may even take part in speculum insertion; she should be told to insert it as she does a tampon.

Clinical pelvimetry is an essential tool in determining spacial capacity as a predictor for CPD. If the client is nervous and uncomfortable during the first pelvic exam, the pelvimetry may be deferred until the next visit, since it tends to be an uncomfortable procedure.

Baseline weight and blood pressure measurements will be valuable in assessing weight gain and predisposition to

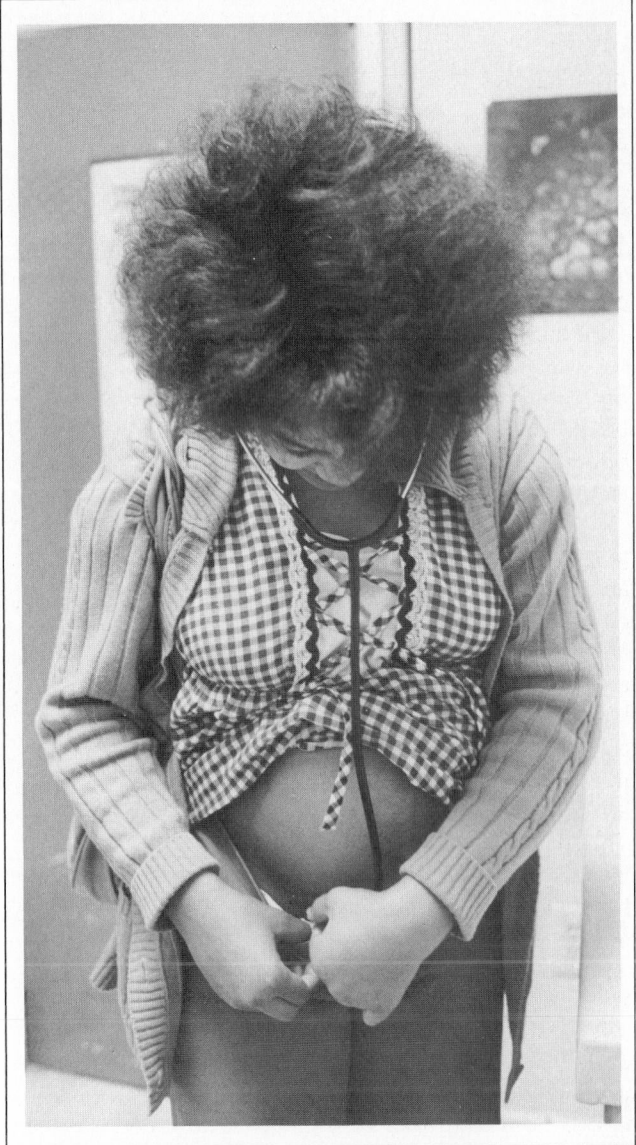

FIGURE 11–11 The nurse provides this young mother with an opportunity to listen to her baby's heartbeat. (© Suzanne Arms.)

PIH. The client may be encouraged to take part in her care by measuring and recording her weight. The nurse may use this time as an opportunity for assisting the young woman in problem solving: "Have I gained too much or too little weight?" "What influence does my diet have on my weight?" "How can I change my eating habits?"

Another way to introduce the subject of nutrition is during measurement of baseline and subsequent hemoglobin and hematocrit values. Since the adolescent is at risk for anemia, she will need education regarding the importance of iron in her diet.

The nurse must keep in mind that adolescents may fear laboratory tests, which can evoke early childhood

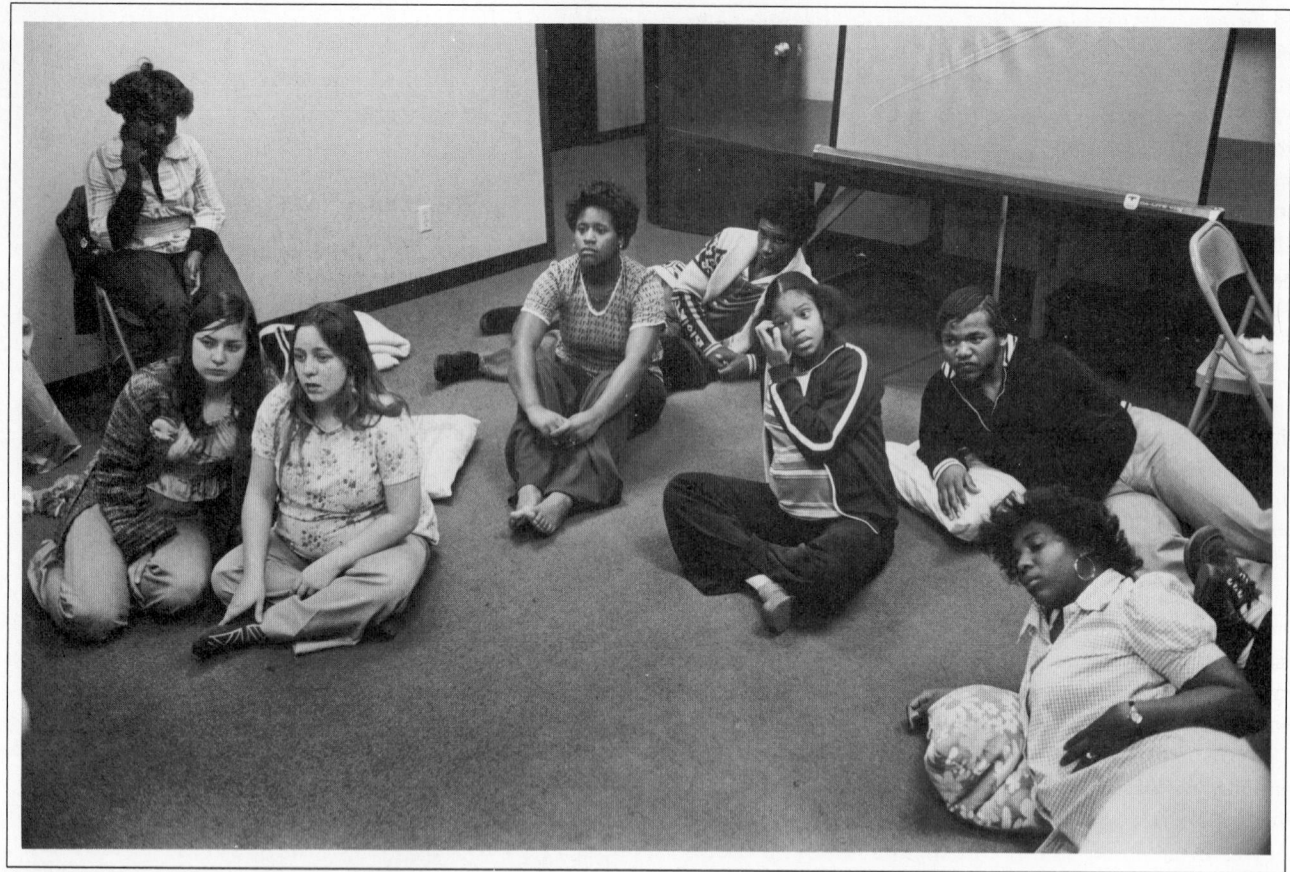

FIGURE 11-12 Prenatal classes may be designed especially for adolescents. (© Suzanne Arms.)

memories of being "stuck" with needles or hurt. Explanations help ease nerves and coordination of services will avoid multiple venous punctures.

A nutritional consultation is indicated for all adolescents. Group classes are helpful because peer pressure is strong among this age group.

PIH represents the most prevalent medical complication of pregnant adolescents. The criteria of blood pressure readings of 140/90 mm Hg are not acceptable as the determinant of PIH in adolescents. Women aged 14–20 years without evidence of high blood pressure usually have diastolic readings between 50 and 66 mm Hg. Gradual increases from the prepregnant diastolic readings, along with excessive weight gain, must be evaluated as precursors to PIH. This is one reason why early prenatal care is vital to management of the adolescent.

As mentioned earlier, adolescents have an increased incidence of sexually transmitted diseases. The initial prenatal examination should include a gonoccocal culture and wet prep for *Candida, Trichomonas,* and *Gardnerella.* Tests for syphilis should also be done. Education about sexually transmitted disease is important, as is careful ob-

servation of herpetic lesions or other symptoms throughout the client's pregnancy.

Substance abuse should be discussed with adolescents. It is important to review the risks associated with the use of cigarettes, caffeine, drugs, and alcohol with the young woman. She should be aware of the effects of these substances on her development as well as the development of the fetus.

Adolescents tend to be egocentric, and even the realization that their health and habits affect the fetus may not be regarded as important by them. It is often helpful to emphasize the effects of these practices on the client herself. Because of their immature cognitive development, the nurse must assist young women in problem solving and help them begin to visualize themselves in the future and imagine what the consequences of their actions might be. This can be accomplished by various introspective techniques. In addition, the nurse must understand that the developmental tasks of pregnancy must be met by the adolescent in addition to the stage-related developmental tasks she is already coping with. Table 11–12 identifies the tasks of pregnancy and their impact on the adolescent.

Ongoing parameters of care should include the same assessments that the older client receives. Special attention should be paid to evaluating fetal growth by measurement of fundal height, fetal heart tones, quickening, and fetal movement. The corresponding dates of auscultating fetal heart tones with the date of last menstrual period and quickening can be helpful in determining correct estimations of delivery time. If there is a question of size–date discrepancy by 2 cm either way, an ultrasound is warranted to establish fetal age so that instances of IUGR may be diagnosed and treated early.

The nurse must assess the family situation during the first prenatal visit. She should find out the level of involvement the adolescent desires from each of her family members. A sensitive approach to daughter and mother relationships helps motivate their communication. If the mother and daughter agree, the mother should be included in the client's care. Encouraging the mother to become part of the maternity team, grandmother crisis support groups, and counseling aids the mother in adapting to her role and in supporting her daughter.

The nurse should also help the mother assess her daughter's needs and assist her in meeting them. Some adolescents become more dependent during pregnancy, and some become more independent. The mother can ease and encourage her daughter's self-growth by understanding how to respond and to best support the adolescent.

Prenatal Education for the Adolescent

Many models can be referred to in establishing programs for prenatal education. Ideally, these programs should include the clinic and the school system. The clinic can benefit the adolescent by offering workshops on prenatal education, parenting skills, and childbirth classes. Schools are taking a larger role in making available special classes for adolescents in these same areas while providing academic classes.

The clinic can provide rap sessions in the waiting room, pamphlets to read, and films to view. Giving the clients something to do while they wait for their appointments may encourage them to return and also may help them learn. Decorating the clinic with attractive educational posters and creating an informal atmosphere establishes an environment where adolescents feel free to interact with professionals.

Adolescents respond more readily to classes that meet their needs; therefore classes that interest them will increase attendance (Figure 11–12). Concerns specific to their bodily changes, the effects of pregnancy, and what labor and delivery will be like have all been listed by adolescents as important areas. They also indicated interest in parenting skills. The subject of parenting is best brought up after delivery when the young woman is actually facing motherhood.

Areas that might be included in prenatal classes are anatomy and physiology, sex education, exercises for pregnancy and postpartum, contraception, labor and delivery, and growth and development of the fetus. Adolescents may want to participate in the teaching of these classes and should be encouraged to do so. Peer support and friendships can blossom among these young women, helping them all to mature.

The school has been cited by many adolescents as a preferred agency for education during pregnancy and early parenting. School systems are currently attempting to meet this need in a variety of ways. The most effective method appears to be mainstreaming the pregnant adolescent in academic classes with her peers and adding classes appropriate to her needs during pregnancy and early parenting. This is an ideal way to keep the adolescent in school, while assisting her in learning the skills she needs to cope with childbearing and rearing. She also will receive vocational guidance, which will be most beneficial to her future.

SUMMARY

The nurse needs comprehensive knowledge of the physiologic and psychologic aspects of pregnancy to effectively counsel the pregnant woman and her family about hygiene, relief measures for discomforts of pregnancy, and nutrition. The nurse must also be aware of possible family disequilibrium that may be associated with the crisis of pregnancy.

Those involved must adjust to changed roles and responsibilities, altered body image, fears related to the unborn child, and fears about labor and delivery.

In providing prenatal education to families, information should also be provided about the labor and delivery process and various methods of childbirth preparation. Families may benefit by learning communication skills, which will provide them with a means of dealing with their problems. These skills can also be integrated into their parenting methods.

The pregnant adolescent requires special attention

from the nurse. The young woman is at physical, psychologic, and sociologic risk because of her incomplete development. The expectant adolescent couple must be prepared to assume the role of father and mother before they are independent from their own parents.

If the expectant family is properly prepared for childbirth, this experience can be one of growth and development for all members. The nurse has a crucial role in ensuring that the family receives the opportunity to make the event a positive experience.

Resource Groups

American Society for Psychoprophylaxis in Obstetrics, 1523 L Street, NW, Washington, DC 20005. Provides information about the Lamaze method.

American Academy of Husband-Coached Childbirth, P.O. Box 5224, Sherman Oaks, CA 91403. Provides information about the Bradley method.

International Childbirth Education Association (ICEA), P.O. Box 20048, Minneapolis, MN 55420.

Maternity Center Association, 48 East 93rd Street, New York, NY 10028.

References

Aladjem, S. 1980. *Obstetrical practice.* St. Louis: The C. V. Mosby Company.

Alouf, F. E., and Barglow, P. 1981. Sexual counseling for the pregnant and postpartum patient. In *Gynecology and obstetrics,* vol. 2, ed. J. J. Sciarra et al. Hagerstown, Md.: Harper & Row.

Anh, N. T.; Thuc, T. K.; and Welsh, J. D. 1977. Lactose malabsorption in adult Vietnamese. *Am. J. Clin. Nutrition.* 30:468.

Aronson, M. E., and Nelson, P. K. 1967. Fatal air embolism in pregnancy resulting from an unusual sex act. *Obstet. Gynecol.* 30:127.

Auerbach, A. 1968. *Parents learn through discussion: principles and practice of parent group education.* New York: John Wiley & Sons, Inc.

Bayless, T. M., et al. 1975. Lactose and milk intolerance: clinical implications. *N. Engl. J. Med.* 292:1156.

Bing, E. 1967. *Six practical lessons for an easier childbirth.* New York: Bantam Books, Inc.

Bittman, S., and Zalk, S. R. 1978. *Expectant fathers.* New York: Hawthorne Books, Inc.

Bradley, R. A. 1981. *Husband-coached childbirth.* 3rd ed. New York: Harper & Row.

Brown, M. S. Sept./Oct. 1976. A cross-cultural look at pregnancy, labor, and delivery. *J. Obstet. Gynecol. Nurs.* 5:35.

Campbell, T., and Chang, B. April 1973. Health care of the Chinese in America. *Nurs. Outlook* 21:245.

Card, J. J., and Wise, L. L. July/Aug. 1978. Teenage mothers and teenage fathers: the impact of early childbearing on the parent's personal and professional lives. *Fam. Plan. Persp.* 10:199.

Carey, W. B., et al. Jan. 1981. Adolescent age and obstetric risk. *Seminars Perinatol.* 5:9.

Carrington, B. W. 1978. The Afro American. In *Culture childbearing health professionals,* ed. A. L. Clark. Philadelphia: F. A. Davis Company.

Chesley, L. C. 1978. *Hypertensive disorders in pregnancy.* New York: Appleton-Century-Crofts.

Clark, A. L., ed. 1978. *Culture childbearing health professionals.* Philadelphia: F. A. Davis Co.

Clausen, J. P., et al. 1977. *Maternity nursing today.* 2nd ed. New York: McGraw-Hill Book Co.

Colandra, C.; Abell, D. A.; and Beischer, N. A. 1981. Maternal obesity in pregnancy. *Obstet. Gynecol.* 57:8.

Colman, A. D., and Colman, L. 1972. *Pregnancy: the psychological experience.* New York: Herder & Herder.

Committee on Maternal Nutrition. 1970. *Maternal nutrition and the course of pregnancy: summary report.* Washington, D.C.: Food and Nutrition Board, National Academy of Sciences, National Research Council.

Crosby, W. M., and Costiloe, P. J. 1971. Safety of lapbelt restraint for pregnant victims of automobile collisions. *N. Engl. J. Med.* 284:632.

Curda, L. R. Spring 1977. What about pica? *J. Nurse-Midwifery.* 23:8.

Davies, D. P., et al. 1976. Cigarette smoking in pregnancy associated with weight gain and fetal growth. *Lancet.* 1:385.

Dick-Read, G. 1959. *Childbirth without fear.* 2nd ed. New York: Harper & Row.

Duvall, E. 1977. *Family development.* 5th ed. Philadelphia: J. B. Lippincott Co.

Edwards, L. E., et al. 1978. Pregnancy in the massively obese: course, outcome and obesity prognosis of the infant. *Am. J. Obstet. Gynecol.* 131:479.

Erikson, E. 1963. *Childhood and society.* 2nd ed. New York: W. W. Norton & Co., Inc.

Evaneshko, V. 1982. Tonawanda Seneca childbearing culture. In *Anthropology of human birth* ed. M. A. Kay. Philadelphia: F. A. Davis Company.

Farris, L. S. March/April, 1976. Approaches to caring for the American Indian maternity patient. *Am. J. Maternal Child Nurs.* 1:81.

————. 1978. The American Indian. In *Culture childbearing health professionals,* ed. A. L. Clark. Philadelphia: F. A. Davis Company.

Fatteh, A., et al. 1973. Fatal air embolism in pregnancy resulting from orogenital sex play. *Forensic Sci.* 2:247.

Fenlon, A.; McPherson, E.; and Dorchak, L. 1979. *Getting ready for childbirth.* Englewood Cliffs, N. J.: Prentice-Hall.

Food and Nutrition Board. 1980. *Recommended dietary allowances.* Washington, D. C.: National Academy of Sciences, National Research Council.

Furstenberg, F. July/Aug. 1976. The social consequences of teenage parenthood. *Fam. Plan. Persp.* 8:148.

Gordon T. 1970. *Parent effectiveness training.* New York: Peter W. Wyden, Publisher.

Green, R., ed. 1975. *Human sexuality: health practitioner's text.* Baltimore: Williams & Wilkins Co.

The Alan Guttmacher Institute. 1981. *Teen pregnancy: the problem that hasn't gone away.* New York, NY 10010.

Hanson, J. W.; Streissgrith, A. P.; and Smith, D. W. 1978. The effects of moderate alcohol consumption during pregnancy on fetal growth and morphogenesis. *J. Pediatr.* 92:457.

Hardinga, M. G., and Crooks, H. N. 1961. Lesser known vitamins in food. *J. Am. Diet Assn.* 38:240.

Hartman, R. 1975. *Exercises for true natural childbirth.* New York: Harper & Row.

Haworth, J. C., et al. July 1980. Fetal growth retardation in cigarette smoking mothers is not due to decreased maternal food intake. *Am. J. Obstet. Gynecol.* 137:719.

Hayes, D. June 1981a. Teratogenesis: a review of the basic principles with a discussion of selected agents. Part I. *Drug Intell. Clin. Pharm.* 15:444.

———. July/Aug. 1981b. Teratogenesis: a review of the basic principles with a discussion of selected agents. Part II. *Drug Intell. Clin. Pharm.* 15:542.

———. Sept. 1981c. Teratogenesis: a review of the basic principles with a discussion of selected agents. Part III. *Drug Intell. Clin. Pharm.* 15:639.

Heardman, H. 1961. *A way to natural childbirth: a manual for physiotherapists and parents to be.* Edinburgh: E. & S. Rivingsterne.

Herbert, V. 1962. Experimental nutritional folate deficiency in man. *Trans. Assoc. Am. Physicians.* 70:307.

Hollingsworth, A. O.; Brown, L. P.; and Brooten, D. A. November 1980. The refugees and childbearing: what to expect. *RN* 43:45.

Horn, B. M. 1982. Northwest coast Indians: the Muckleshoot. In *Anthropology of human birth,* ed. M. A. Kay. Philadelphia: F. A. Davis Company.

Karmel, M. 1965. *Thank you, Dr. Lamaze.* New York: Doubleday & Co., Inc.

Kay, M. A. 1978. The Mexican American. In *Culture childbearing health professionals,* ed. A. L. Clark. Philadelphia: F. A. Davis Company.

Kitay, D. Z., and Harbart, R. A. Sept. 1975. Iron and folic acid deficiency in pregnancy. *Clin. Perinatol.* 2:255.

Lemarchand-Beraud, T., et al. Feb. 1982. Maturation of the hypothalamo-pituitary-ovarian àxis in adolescent girls. *J. Clin. Endocrinol. Metabol.* 54:241.

Lemoine, P., et al. 1968. Children of alcoholic parents, observed anomalies (127 cases). *Quest Med.* 21:476.

Lin, G. W. J., and Maddatu, A. P. 1980. Effects of ethanol feeding during pregnancy on maternal-fetal transfer of a-aminosobutyric acid in the rat (abstract). *Alcoholism: Clin. Exp. Res.* 4:222.

Lion, E. M., ed. 1982. *Human sexuality in nursing process.* New York: John Wiley & Sons.

Longo, L. D. 1977. The biological effect of carbon monoxide on the pregnant woman, fetus and newborn infant. *Am. J. Obstet. Gynecol.* 129:69.

Masters, W. H., and Johnson, V. E. 1966. *Human sexual response.* Boston: Little, Brown & Co.

Mercer, R. 1979. *Perspectives on adolescent health care.* New York: J. B. Lippincott.

Minich, V., et al. 1969. Pica in Turkey: effect of clay upon iron absorption. *Am. J. Clin. Nutr.* 21:73.

Moore, K., and Waite, L. Sept./Oct. 1977. Early childbearing and educational attainment. *Fam. Plan. Perspect.* 9:220.

Naeye, R. L. Jan. 1981. Influence of maternal cigarette smoking during pregnancy on fetal and childhood growth. *Obstet. Gynecol.* 57(1):18.

———. Sept. 1979. Weight gain and the outcome of pregnancy. *Am. J. Obstet. Gynecol.* 135:3.

Nelson, R. M. 1978. Physiologic correlates of puberty. *Clin. Obstet. Gynecol.* 21:1137.

Nelson, W. E.; Vaughan, V. C.; and McKay, R. J., eds. 1979. *Textbook of pediatrics.* Philadelphia: W. B. Saunders.

O'Brien, T. E., and Balmer, J. A. March 1981. Drugs and the human fetus. *U.S. Pharmacist:* p. 44.

Ouellette, E. M., et al. 1977. Adverse effects on offspring of maternal alcohol abuse during pregnancy. *N. Eng. J. Med.* 297:528.

Overbach, A. M. 1974. Drugs used with neonates and during pregnancy. III. Drugs that may cause fetal damage or cross into breast milk. *RN* 37(12):39.

Piaget, J. 1972. Intellectual evolution of adolescence to adulthood. *Human Development.* 15:1.

Pitkin, R. M. Sept. 1975. Vitamins and minerals in pregnancy. *Clin. Perinatol.* 2:221.

Pritchard, J. A., and MacDonald, P. 1980. *Williams obstetrics.* 16th ed. New York: Appleton-Century-Crofts.

Rao, J. M., and Arulappu, R. 1981. Drug use in pregnancy: how to avoid problems. *Drugs* 22:409.

Register, U. D., and Sonnenberg, L. M. 1973. The vegetarian diet. *J. Am. Diet. Assoc.* 62:253.

Roig-Garcia, S. July 1961. The hypnoreflexogenous method: a new procedure in obstetrical psychoanalgesia. *Am. J. Clin. Hypnosis* 4:1.

Rose, D. P., and Braidman, I. P. 1971. Excretion of tryptophan metabolites as affected by pregnancy, contraceptive steroids and steroid hormones. *Am. J. Clin. Nutr.* 24:673.

Rosenberg, F. H. May 1977. Lactose intolerance. *Am. J. Nurs.* 77:823.

Rubin, R. 1967. Attainment of the maternal role. I. Processes. *Nurs. Res.* 16:272.

Sevcovic, L. 1979. Traditions of pregnancy which influence maternity care of the Navajo people. In *Transcultural nursing,* ed. M. Leininger. New York: Masson Publishing USA, Inc.

Sokol, R. J. 1981. Alcohol and abnormal outcomes of pregnancy. *Can. Med. Assoc. J.* 125(2):141.

Solberg, D. A., et al. 1973. Sexual behavior in pregnancy. *N. Engl. J. Med.* 288:1098.

Spain, J. 1980. Psychological aspects of contraceptive use in teenage girls. In *Psychological aspects of pregnancy, birthing and bonding,* ed. B. L. Blum. New York: Human Sciences Press.

Swanson, J. 1980. The marital sexual relationship during pregnancy. *J. Obstet. Gynecol. Neonatal Nurs.* 9(5):267.

Swartz, H. M. and Reichling, B. A. 1978. Hazards of radiation exposure for pregnant women. *J.A.M.A.* 239(18):1907.

Talkington, K., et al. 1970. Effect of ingestion of starch and some clays on iron absorption. *Am. J. Obstet. Gynecol.* 108:267.

Tinterow, M. M. 1972. Techniques of hypnosis. In *Obstetric analgesia and anesthetics,* ed. J. J. Bonica. Philadelphia: F. A. Davis Co.

Tsang, R. C., and Glueck, C. J. Sept. 1975. Perinatal cholesterol metabolism. *Clin. Perinatol.* 2:275.

Waters, J. L. June 1969. Pregnancy in young adolescents: a syndrome of failure. *South. Med. J.* 62:655.

Werner, M. E., et al. Jan. 1982. An argument for the revival of hypnosis in obstetrics. *Am. J. Clin. Hypnosis.* 24:149.

Winick, M. 1968. Changes in nucleic acid and protein content of the human brain growth. *Pediatr. Res.* 2:352.

————. April 12, 1977. *Maternal and Infant Nutrition Seminar.* Portland, Ore.

Zalor, M. K. May/June 1976. Sexual counseling for pregnant couples. *MCN* 1:176.

Additional Readings

Ashley, M. J. 1981. Alcohol use during pregnancy: a challenge for the '80's. *Can. Med. Assoc. J.* 125(2):141.

Baldwin, W. Jan. 1981. Adolescent pregnancy and childbearing: an overview. *Semin. Perinatol.* 5:1.

Blum, R. W., and Goldhagen, J. May 1981. Teenage pregnancy in perspective. *Clin. Pediatr.* 20:335.

Earls, F., and Siegel, B. July 1980. Percocious fathers. *Am. J. Orthopsychiatry.* 50:469.

Hott, J. R. 1976. The crisis of expectant fatherhood. *Am. J. Nurs.* 76:1436.

Jimenez, M. H., and Newton, N. Sept. 1979. Activity and work during pregnancy and the postpartum period: a cross-cultural study of 202 societies. *Am. J. Obstet. Gynecol.* 135:171.

Lamb, G. S., and Lipkin, M., Jr. 1982. Somatic symptoms of expectant fathers. *MCN* 7:110.

Leader, A.; Wong, K. H.; and Deitel, M. 1981. Maternal nutrition in pregnancy. Part I: a review. *Can. Med. Assoc. J.* 125:545.

Luke, B.; Hawkins, M. M.; and Petrie, R. H. 1981. Influence of smoking, weight gain and pregravid weight for height on intra-uterine growth. *A. J. Clin. Nutrition.* 34(7):1410.

McKay, S. R. 1980. Smoking during the childbearing year. *MCN* 5(1):46.

May, K. A. March/April 1978. Active involvement of expectant fathers in pregnancy: Some further considerations. *J. Obstet. Gynecol. Neonatal Nurs.* 7:7.

Meyer, M. B. 1978. How does maternal smoking affect birth weight and maternal weight gain? *Am. J. Obstet. Gynecol.* 131:888.

Olson, M. L. 1981. Fitting grandparents into new families. *MCN* 6:419.

Rosett, H. L.; Weiner, L.; and Edelin, K. C. 1981. Strategies for prevention of fetal alcohol effects. *Obstet. Gynecol.* 57:1.

Zellman, G. L. Jan./Feb. 1982. Public school programs for adolescent pregnancy and parenthood. *Fam. Plan. Perspect.* 14:15.

■ 12 ■

COMPLICATIONS OF PREGNANCY

■ CHAPTER CONTENTS

PREGESTATIONAL MEDICAL DISORDERS
    Cardiac Disease
    Diabetes Mellitus
    Thyroid Dysfunction
    Other Medical Conditions and Pregnancy

MEDICAL DISORDERS ASSOCIATED WITH PREGNANCY
    Hyperemesis Gravidarum
    Bleeding Disorders
    Incompetent Cervix

HYPERTENSIVE DISORDERS IN PREGNANCY
    Pregnancy-Induced Hypertension (Preeclampsia and Eclampsia)
    Chronic Hypertensive Disease

RH SENSITIZATION
    Fetal–Neonatal Implications
    Nursing Management

SURGICAL PROCEDURES DURING PREGNANCY
    Appendicitis
    Cholecystitis and Cholelithiasis
    Carcinoma of the Breast
    Carcinoma of the Cervix

ACCIDENTS AND TRAUMA

INFECTIONS
    Urinary Tract Infections
    Sexually Transmitted Diseases
    Vaginal Infections
    TORCH

DRUG USE AND ABUSE
    Drug Addiction
    Alcoholism

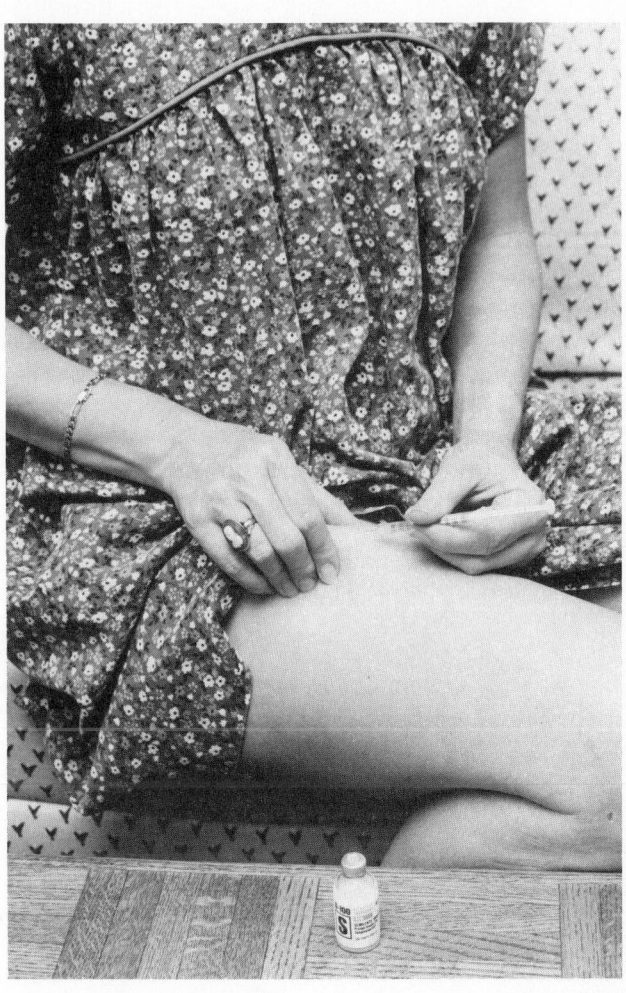

■ OBJECTIVES

- Discuss the effects of preexisting medical conditions on pregnancy.

- Differentiate the bleeding problems associated with pregnancy.

- Describe the development and course of hypertensive disorders associated with pregnancy.

- Explain the cause and prevention of Rh hemolytic disease of the newborn.

- Describe effects of surgical procedures on pregnancy, and how pregnancy may complicate diagnosis.

- Discuss some common infections that may be contracted during pregnancy or may coexist with pregnancy.

- Discuss possible teratogenic effects of infections and drugs.

- Discuss drug use and abuse during pregnancy.

Pregnancy puts stress on the healthy female biologically, physiologically, and psychologically. In the presence of certain factors, pregnancy may become a life-threatening event. It is therefore imperative that prenatal care be aimed toward specific identification, assessment, and management of the high-risk client.

In this chapter, the discussion focuses on pregestational medical disorders and specific disorders that are unique to the pregnant condition. The possible effects of these disruptions on the outcome of pregnancy are examined. In addition, infectious processes that may influence maternal and fetal well-being are described.

PREGESTATIONAL MEDICAL DISORDERS

Cardiac Disease

Heart disease is estimated to occur in 1%–2% of pregnancies (Danforth, 1982). Rheumatic heart disease formerly accounted for the great majority of cases, but recently congenital heart disease has become the leading cause of heart disease associated with pregnancy (Pritchard and MacDonald, 1980). This is due in part to newer surgical techniques enabling girls with congenital heart defects to live to childbearing age. It is also due to the fact that treatment of rheumatic fever with antibiotic therapy has reduced the incidence of valvular damage from rheumatic fever. Other less common causes of heart disease in pregnancy are syphilis; arteriosclerosis; coronary occlusion; and renal, pulmonary, and thyroid disorders.

The majority of expectant women with cardiac disease are able to complete a pregnancy successfully. Although heart disease remains the major nonobstetric cause of maternal death (Leman et al., 1981), statistics demonstrate a progressive decline in maternal mortality with this condition to an incidence in recent years of less than 1%. This significant reduction has evolved as a result of a better understanding of cardiovascular adaptation in pregnancy, more intensive prepregnancy and prenatal assessment and management, and a general improvement in the care of all cardiac clients.

The normal cardiovascular system during pregnancy exhibits several changes. Beginning early in the course of gestation, heart rate, cardiac output, and total blood volume increase. Cardiac output is increased by 40% and thus affects the increased heart rate. The blood volume begins to increase during the first trimester; the average blood volume increases by 40%, plateaus after 30 weeks' gestation, and shows little change during the last part of pregnancy (Burrow and Ferris, 1982).

The normal heart has adequate cardiac reserve to adjust to the increased demands of pregnancy with little difficulty. The client with cardiac disease has decreased cardiac reserve because her heart already has a higher work load. In the case of rheumatic endocarditis the mitral, aortic, or tricuspid valves may be involved, with mitral stenosis the most common lesion. Recurrent acute inflammation from bouts of rheumatic fever causes scar tissue formation on the valves. The scarring results in either stenosis (failure to open completely) or regurgitation due to failure to close completely, or a combination of both effects. Stenosis causes a decrease in blood flow through the valve, and therefore causes an increase in work load on the heart chamber just before the stenotic valve. A regurgitant (incompetent) valve allows blood to leak through when it is closed. Leaking increases the work load on the heart chambers on either side of the diseased valve.

With congenital heart disease the exact pathology depends on the specific defect in the septa, valves, or conduction system. Congenital defects commonly seen in pregnant women include atrial septal defect, ventricular septal defect, patent ductus arteriosis, pulmonary stenosis, and coarctation of the aorta. When surgical repair can be accomplished with no remaining evidence of organic heart disease, pregnancy may be undertaken with confidence. In such cases antibiotic prophylaxis is recommended to prevent subacute bacterial endocarditis at the time of delivery

(Noller, 1981b). When congenital heart disease is associated with cyanosis, whether the defect was originally uncorrected or whether the correction failed to relieve the cyanosis, the woman should be counseled to avoid pregnancy because the risk to her and the fetus would be high.

Eisenmenger's syndrome is a rare heart disease with poor prognosis. Pulmonary hypertension that accompanies the disease is due to a high pulmonary vascular resistance associated with right-to-left or bidirectional shunting through a large communication between the two circulations. Eisenmenger's syndrome is included here because the highest incidence of mortality of any isolated maternal cardiac defect results from this condition. Maternal mortality ranges from 30%–70% while fetal mortality exceeds 40% (Burrow and Ferris, 1982).

Regardless of the exact cause of the cardiac disease, whether of rheumatic or congenital origin, the same general signs and symptoms tend to appear. When cardiac reserve is strained, the heart compensates to increase its output by (a) ventricular dilatation, (b) ventricular hypertrophy, and (c) tachycardia. When these three mechanisms succeed in maintaining adequate blood flow to tissues without symptoms and in the presence of pathologic changes, the heart is in a state of compensation. Decompensation occurs when the heart, despite these mechanisms, is unable to cope with the work demands put upon it and must expend most of its reserve. At this point, symptoms develop with physical activity because the heart is unable to maintain adequate circulation. The most typical first sign of reduced cardiac reserve is a decreased tolerance for activity (Luckman and Sorenson, 1981).

CLASSIFICATION

To further clarify the severity of cardiac disease in pregnancy, the following classification of functional capacity has been standardized by the Criteria Committee of the New York Heart Association, Inc. (1955):

- Class I. No limitation of physical activity. Ordinary physical activity causes no discomfort; patients do not have anginal pain.
- Class II. Slight limitation of physical activity. Ordinary physical activity causes fatigue, dyspnea, palpitation, or anginal pain.
- Class III. Moderate to marked limitation of physical activity. During less than ordinary physical activity, patients experience excessive fatigue, dyspnea, palpitation, or anginal pain.
- Class IV. Unable to carry on any physical activity without experiencing discomforts. Even at rest, they experience symptoms of cardiac insufficiency or anginal pain.

Clients in classes I and II usually experience a normal pregnancy and have few complications, whereas those in classes III and IV are at risk for more severe complications.

CLINICAL MANIFESTATIONS

Clinical signs and symptoms that the pregnant woman with impending cardiac decompensation exhibits include:

- coughs (frequent, with or without hemoptysis)
- dyspnea (progressive, upon exertion)
- edema (progressive, generalized, including extremities, face, eyelids)
- heart murmurs (heard on auscultation)
- palpitations
- rales (auscultated in lung bases)

These progressive symptoms are indicative of congestive heart failure, the heart's signal of its decreased ability to meet the demands of pregnancy. It should be noted that this cycle is *progressive*, because some of these same behaviors are seen to a minor degree in a pregnancy without cardiac involvement.

Careful monitoring of these clients during the prenatal period is essential. If such symptoms appear, prompt medical actions are required to correct the cardiac status. Until cardiac function is improved, no obstetric manipulation should be attempted, because even the slightest stimulus might lead to cardiac failure.

FETAL–NEONATAL IMPLICATIONS

Infant mortality increases if maternal cardiac decompensation occurs. Uterine congestion, hypoxia, and elevation of carbon dioxide content of the blood not only compromise the fetus and decrease fetal weight gain but also frequently give rise to premature labor and delivery. The respiratory and metabolic acidosis suffered in utero as a result of suboptimal oxygenation of the fetus leads to cellular damage and predisposes the traumatized fetus to intrauterine fetal distress once labor begins. Moreover, oxygen transport and exchange are further reduced. Therefore, optimal fetal outcome can only be achieved through prevention of maternal cardiac decompensation.

The neonate who has suffered hypoxia in utero and during birth is at risk during the neonatal period, particularly if born prematurely. Favorable prognosis for the newborn of the cardiac client is based on maintenance of normal respiratory and metabolic functioning as determined by observation and laboratory testing. (See Chapter 25 for discussion of the nursing and medical care of the newborn with respiratory compromise.)

INTERVENTIONS

The primary goal of nursing care is to preserve the cardiac reserve function of the pregnant client. To do this it is necessary to maintain a balance between cardiac reserve and cardiac work load. Specific goals for nursing management are as follows:

1. Assess the stress of pregnancy on the heart's functional capacity.
   a. Compare the client's vital signs of pulse and respiration to the normal values expected during pregnancy.
   b. Establish activity level of client, including rest, and assess any changes in vital signs that may occur.
   c. Identify in order of priority the problems indicating cardiac decompensation (for example, dyspnea, cough, edema, pulse irregularity, rales in lung bases).
   d. Assess for other factors that would increase strain on the heart: anemia, infection, fear and anxiety, lack of support system, insufficient household help.
2. Support the woman's adaptive coping mechanisms to deal with stress.
   a. Teach the woman and her partner symptoms of cardiac decompensation and reasons for the need to decrease activity if symptoms occur.
   b. Reinforce physician's instructions, explaining the reason for each instruction.
   c. Allow ample time for the client to ask questions and encourage her to comment on her pregnancy and its progress.
   d. Answer the client's questions as fully as possible and in terms that she can understand.
   e. Carefully explain all nursing actions to the woman.
   f. Identify and utilize significant others, such as partner, mother, or friend, to give physical and psychologic support.
3. Identify the severity of the disease process.
   a. Note cardiac classification of the client.
   b. Identify problems in order of priority based on nursing diagnosis and client input.

Nursing management of the pregnant woman with cardiac disease involves varying tasks in the antepartal, intrapartal, and postpartal periods.

□ *ANTEPARTAL PERIOD* The following nursing actions are based on the physiologic and psychosocial needs of the pregnant cardiac client. All these actions are essential for any pregnant woman with cardiac disease, but the priority of nursing actions varies, depending on the severity of the disease process.

Adequate nutrition. A diet should be instituted that is high in iron, protein, and essential nutrients to meet the increased demands of pregnancy for increased blood volume and oxygen. However, sodium and calorie intake should be minimized.

Promotion of rest. Eight to ten hours of sleep are essential, with frequent daily rest periods. The nurse must assist the woman to understand the absolute necessity for this rest.

Protection from infection. It is vitally important to protect the heart from the additional stress of upper respiratory infections, which could lead to cardiac failure due to overload of the heart's reserve capacity.

Drug therapy. Besides the iron and vitamin supplements prescribed during pregnancy, the cardiac client may need additional drug therapy to maintain health. If the woman develops coagulation problems, the anticoagulant heparin may be used. Heparin offers the greatest safety to the fetus because it does not cross the placenta. The thiazide diuretics and furosemide (Lasix) may be used to treat congestive heart failure if it develops. Digitalis glycosides and common antiarrhythmic drugs may be used to treat cardiac failure and arrhythmias. These agents do cross the placenta but have no reported teratogenic effect. Penicillin prophylaxis to protect against infection, if not contraindicated by allergy, is encouraged.

Restriction of activity. Decreased exertion reduces fatigue, thereby promoting adequate ventilation and preservation of cardiac reserves.

Continuous monitoring of pregnancy. One or two prenatal visits per week for assessment of cardiac status are encouraged, especially between weeks 28 and 30 when the blood volume reaches maximum amounts.

Psychologic support. The client and her family are provided with information concerning her condition and management. This will increase their understanding and decrease anxiety. The nurse can counsel them regarding their preparation for childbirth, offer them encouragement to boost their morale, and put them in contact with self-help or support groups for high-risk pregnancies.

It is the aim of nursing to support the implementation of this care in the home. However, hospitalization may become necessary. The pregnant cardiac client is most prone to cardiac decompensation between weeks 28 and 32 of gestation. At that time the cardiac work load is highest. Careful assessment of the client's status is necessary to ensure safe culmination of pregnancy.

□ *INTRAPARTAL PERIOD* During labor and delivery, tremendous stress is normally exerted on the woman and the unborn fetus. This stress could be fatal to the fetus of a woman with cardiac disease because of the possible decreased oxygen and blood supply to it. It is therefore essential that the intrapartal management of a cardiac patient be aimed at reducing the amount of physical exertion and accompanying fatigue. Nursing actions include the following:

Continuous monitoring. Routine labor signs should be observed. Monitor fetal heart tones and contractions (see Chapter 15). Assess vital signs frequently, particularly if the pulse rate is 100/min or greater, and respirations are 25/min or greater, to determine whether there is progressive tachycardia or hyperventilation.

Assessment of pulmonary function. Dyspnea, coughing, and rales at the lung bases should be noted.

Proper positioning. To assure cardiac emptying and proper oxygenation, the semi-Fowler's and side-lying positions, with head and shoulders elevated, are recommended.

Supportive therapies. Supportive measures include use of prophylactic antibiotics, oxygen by mask if any pulmonary embarrassment such as dyspnea occurs, diuretics to decrease fluid retention, sedatives for rest and reduction of anxiety, analgesics with tranquilizers to potentiate action and reduce pain, and digitalis if signs of cardiac decompensation occur (listed on p. 311).

Assistance during delivery. Delivery by low torceps is the safest method, using a regional or local anesthetic to maintain controlled vaginal delivery, thereby reducing the stress of pushing and decreasing possible trauma to the newborn. The goal of nursing actions is to minimize the duration of the second stage of labor by encouraging and supporting relaxation. Cesarean delivery should be performed only if fetal or obstetric indications are present and not on the basis of heart disease alone.

Psychologic support. The nurse should remain with the patient to support and encourage her. The nurse should keep the patient and her family informed of labor progress and management plans, collaborating with them to fulfill their wishes for the birth experience as much as possible. The nurse needs to maintain an atmosphere of calm to lessen anxiety of the woman and her family.

□ *POSTPARTAL PERIOD* The postdelivery period is a most significant time for the cardiac patient. The rapid fluid shift resulting from the physiologic readaptation process means cardiac output and blood volume increase as the extravascular fluid is returned to the bloodstream for excretion.

After delivery, the intraabdominal pressure is reduced significantly, venous pressure is reduced, the splanchnic vessels engorge, and blood flow to the heart increases. The extravascular fluid moves into the bloodstream. This mobilization of fluid can place a great strain on the heart if excess interstitial fluid is present. Such stress on the heart could lead to cardiac decompensation, especially during the first 48 hours postpartum or as late as the sixth postnatal day. Continued nursing care includes the following actions:

1. *Assessment of postdelivery heart status.* The patient remains in the hospital for at least one week to allow for rest and recovery of cardiac function.

2. *Proper positioning.* The semi-Fowler's and side-lying positions, with elevation of head and shoulders, assist respiratory and cardiac function.

3. *Planning of activity schedule.* Based on nursing assessment of the patient's cardiac status as indicated by pulse and respirations, she begins a gradual and progressive activity program:

    a. Bed rest with nurse performing grooming, hygiene, and nutritional measures. As cardiac status improves, the woman may increase her performance of these activities of daily living.

    b. Progressive ambulation as tolerated. Assess pulse and respirations of patient before and after exercise to evaluate tolerance.

    c. Use of diet, administration of stool softeners, and mild local anesthetic to episiotomy site to facilitate bowel movement and urination without stress or strain.

4. *Psychologic support.* Encourage maternal–infant bonding process by providing frequent opportunities to see and hold newborn.

5. *Education and assistance of mother in newborn care.* For the first few days, as determined by cardiac status, the nurse will provide care for the newborn. This is best done at the mother's bedside to increase her contact with her newborn and to provide teaching opportunities. If the mother's cardiac condition is class I or class II, she may breast-feed her baby in bed. The nurse can assist her to a comfortable side-lying position with her head moderately elevated or to a semi-Fowler's position. The nurse should position the newborn at the breast and be available to burp the baby and reposition it at the other breast.

    The advisability of breast-feeding for the class III or class IV cardiac patient must be evaluated carefully. In many cases, because of the excessive fatigue factor and because the mother may be taking several medications that pass into the breast milk, breast-feeding may not be appropriate.

6. *Preparation for discharge.* The patient will need education, referrals, and support for her care and that of her newborn.

    a. Determine whether there are significant others to assist the mother at home in caring for self and neonate. Refer her to community homemaking services if needed.

    b. An activity schedule that is gradual and progressive and appropriate to patient's needs and home environment should be planned with the patient.

    c. Information regarding sexual relations and contraception should be given as appropriate.

Diabetes Mellitus

Another major complication of the maternity cycle is diabetes mellitus, an endocrine disorder of carbohydrate metabolism that results from inadequate production or utilization of insulin. It is characterized by hyperglycemia and glycosuria.

Insulin is a powerful hypoglycemic agent, normally produced by the β cells of the islets of Langerhans in the pancreas. It lowers blood glucose levels by enabling the glucose to move from the blood into muscle and adipose tissue cells. With inadequate amounts of insulin, the glucose cannot enter the cells but remains outside. The body cells become energy-depleted while the blood glucose level remains elevated. Fats and proteins in the body tissues are oxidized by the cells as a source of energy. This results in wasting of fat and muscle tissue of the body, negative nitrogen balance due to protein breakdown, and ketosis due to fat metabolism. The strong osmotic force of the glucose concentration in the blood pulls water from the cells into the blood, which results in cellular dehydration. The high level of glucose in the blood eventually spills over into the urine, producing glycosuria. Osmotic pressure of the glucose in the urine prevents reabsorption of water into the kidney tubules, causing extracellular dehydration.

These pathologic developments cause the four cardinal signs and symptoms of diabetes mellitus:

- Polyuria (frequent urination) results because water is not reabsorbed by the renal tubules due to the osmotic activity of glucose.
- Polydipsia (excessive thirst) is caused by dehydration from polyuria.
- Weight loss (seen in insulin-dependent diabetes, also called type I diabetes) is due to the use of fat and muscle tissue for energy.
- Polyphagia (excessive hunger) is caused by tissue loss and a state of starvation, which results from the inability of the cells to utilize the blood glucose.

Diagnosis of diabetes is based on the presence of clinical symptoms and laboratory tests showing elevated glucose levels in the blood and urine.

Diabetes mellitus disrupts approximately 1 in 300 pregnancies (Moore et al., 1981). Prior to the discovery of insulin in 1921, maternal mortality reported by Williams was 30%, and fetal mortality was 65% (Hellman and Pritchard, 1971). Since that time the management of the diabetic maternity patient has evolved into an interspecialty team approach, including medical internist, obstetrician, nutritionist, nurse, perinatologist, and pediatrician. This approach has been adopted to decrease maternal and

fetal risk of death in a pregnancy complicated by diabetes mellitus.

The overall changes in metabolism during pregnancy are profound in the healthy nondiabetic woman, but her physiologic tolerance for carbohydrate remains normal. This balance in the endocrine system is achieved in the following way. The increased activity of the maternal pancreatic islets results in the increased production of insulin. This is counterbalanced by the placenta's increased production of the hormone human placental lactogen (hPL), also called human chorionic somatomammotropin (hCS), which diminishes the effectiveness of maternal insulin. The hPL is secreted primarily in the third trimester and increases tenfold over the last 20 weeks of gestation. In addition, the elevated levels of progesterone and estrogens may help block insulin action (Burrow and Ferris, 1982).

Insulin requirements of pregnant women increase because of the insulin antagonism and altered insulin utilization that exists during pregnancy. A rise in the glomerular filtration rate in the kidneys in conjunction with decreased tubular glucose reabsorption results in glycosuria. A decrease in the normal fasting blood glucose occurs in pregnancy, but free fatty acids and ketones are increased. In summary, the delicate system of checks and balances that exists between glucose production and glucose utilization is stressed by the growing fetus, who derives energy from glucose taken solely from maternal stores. This stress is referred to as the *diabetogenic effect* of pregnancy. Thus any preexisting disruption in carbohydrate metabolism is augmented by pregnancy, and any diabetic potential may precipitate *gestational diabetes,* which is defined as diabetes diagnosed during pregnancy.

CLASSIFICATION OF DIABETES MELLITUS

States of altered carbohydrate metabolism have been classified several different ways. Table 12–1 shows the current accepted classification, a result of the 1979 report of a special committee of the National Institutes of Health (National Diabetes Data Group, 1979). This classification contains three main categories: diabetes mellitus (DM), impaired glucose tolerance (IGT), and gestational diabetes (GDM). The DM group is subdivided into three types:

1. *Type I or insulin-dependent diabetes mellitus (IDDM).* Type I formerly was called juvenile-onset diabetes, ketosis-prone diabetes, or unstable or brittle diabetes. Insulin-dependent diabetes can occur at any age but is usually seen in young persons. Little or no insulin is produced by the pancreas in type I diabetes.

2. *Type II or noninsulin-dependent diabetes mellitus (NIDDM).* Type II has been called maturity-onset diabetes, but has been described in children. Persons with type II diabetes are nonketosis-prone. Type II is further subdivided into obese and nonobese groups. Ideally, the type II disease is controlled by diet alone.

Table 12–1   Classification of Diabetes Mellitus (DM) and Other Categories of Glucose Intolerance*

1. Diabetes mellitus
   a. Type I, insulin-dependent (IDDM)
   b. Type II, noninsulin-dependent (NIDDM)
      (1) Nonobese NIDDM
      (2) Obese NIDDM
   c. Secondary diabetes
2. Impaired glucose tolerance (IGT)
3. Gestational diabetes (GDM)

* From National Diabetes Data Group of National Institutes of Health, 1979.

3. *Secondary diabetes.* The third type of diabetes is called secondary diabetes because it arises from another condition such as pancreatic disease (for example, pancreatitis or cystic fibrosis), hormonal disorder (for example, acromegaly or Cushing's syndrome), drug-induced conditions (for example, from steroids or birth control pills), or insulin-receptor abnormalities.

Impaired glucose tolerance (IGT) applies to persons whose fasting plasma glucose level is normal or only slightly elevated (140 mg/dL) but whose glucose tolerance tests show abnormal values. These persons are asymptomatic. IGT was formerly called chemical diabetes, borderline diabetes, or latent diabetes. Many persons in this group return to normal glucose tolerance spontaneously, but 1%–5% go on to develop overt diabetes each year (Price and Wilson, 1982).

Gestational diabetes mellitus (GDM) is diabetes that has its onset or is first diagnosed during pregnancy. Except for showing an impaired tolerance to glucose, the woman may remain asymptomatic or may have a mild form of the disease. Diagnosis of GDM is very important, however, because even mild diabetes causes increased risk for perinatal morbidity and mortality. After pregnancy women with GDM need to be reclassified as either type I, type II, IGT, or previously IGT, as determined by postpartal testing. Most women will revert to normal and can be reclassified as "previously IGT."

Table 12–2 shows White's classification of diabetes in pregnancy. This classification is still used in many agencies.

INFLUENCE OF PREGNANCY ON DIABETES

Pregnancy can affect diabetes in the following ways:

1. Diabetic control
   a. Change in insulin requirements
      (1) Frequently a decrease in insulin need occurs during the first trimester. Levels of hPL, an insulin antagonist, are low and use of glucose and glycogen by the woman and developing fetus is increased.
      (2) Insulin requirements begin to rise in the second trimester and may double or quadruple by the end of pregnancy as a result of placental maturation and hPL production.
      (3) Increased energy needs during labor may require increased insulin to balance intravenous glucose.
      (4) Usually an abrupt decrease in insulin requirement occurs after the birth of the placenta and loss of hPL in maternal circulation.
   b. Decreased renal threshold
   c. Dietary fluctuations due to nausea, vomiting, and cravings

   d. Increased risk of ketoacidosis, insulin shock, and coma
2. Possible accelerations of vascular disease
   a. Hypertension: increase in blood pressure of greater than 30 mm Hg systolic and 15 mm Hg diastolic
   b. Nephropathy: renal impairment
   c. Retinopathy

The primary concern is control of circulating blood glucose levels, which can be affected by severity of the diabetic disease state, emotional condition, and activity level. Awareness of the specific behaviors and stressors is vital to appropriate planning and subsequent implementation of nursing care.

INFLUENCE OF DIABETES MELLITUS ON PREGNANCY OUTCOME

The course of the pregnancy in a woman with diabetes mellitus is characterized by an increased incidence of maternal, fetal, and neonatal complications. The longer the woman has been diabetic, the higher the risk to the health of the fetus and the woman, especially if control of the diabetes has been poor in the years preceding pregnancy.

The most important complication is fetal mortality, which occurs at the rate of 10%–20%, or three to six times that for the general population. In contrast, maternal mortality is negligible.

Table 12–2 Classification of Diabetes in Pregnancy*

Class	Description
A	Gestational or chemical diabetes (abnormal glucose tolerance test)
B	Overt diabetes Onset after age 20 Duration less than 10 years No vascular involvement
C	Overt diabetes Onset before age 20 Duration 10 to 20 years No vascular involvement
D	Overt diabetes Onset before age 10 Duration more than 20 years Vascular involvement Benign retinopathy Leg calcification
E	Calcified pelvic vessels (this classification is not generally employed in current practice)
F	Diabetic renal impairment
R	Malignant retinopathy (proliferative)

* From White, P. 1965. Pregnancy and diabetes: medical aspects. *Med. Clin. North Am.* 49:1016.

The following sections discuss maternal, fetal, and neonatal problems caused by diabetes mellitus.

MATERNAL IMPLICATIONS

Hydramnios, or an increase in the volume of amniotic fluid, occurs in 6%–25% of pregnant diabetics (Burrow and Ferris, 1982). The exact mechanism causing the increase is unknown, although osmotic pressure, hypersecretion of amniotic fluid, and diuresis due to fetal hyperglycemia are suspected (Haynes, 1969). Premature rupture of membranes and onset of labor may be a problem, but only occasionally does this pose a threat. Amniocentesis may be utilized to decrease fluid volume; however, this procedure predisposes the diabetic client to potential infection, possible initiation of premature labor, possible premature separation of the placenta due to manipulation, and hemorrhage due to placental laceration.

Hypertensive disorders of pregnancy occur in about 12%–13% of diabetics and may be due to vascular changes resulting from the diabetes (Burrow and Ferris, 1982).

Ketoacidosis in the pregnant diabetic deserves special consideration. Hyperglycemia due to insufficient amounts of insulin can lead to a state of ketoacidosis as a result of the increase in ketone bodies (which are mildly acidic) in the blood released in metabolism of fatty acids. Ketosis develops slowly but can eventually lead to coma in the woman. The risk of fetal death is increased to 50% or higher if ketoacidosis is not promptly treated (Burrow and Ferris, 1982) because the fetal enzyme systems cease functioning in an acidotic environment. In pregnancy, particularly in the presence of prolonged vomiting, carbohydrate deficiency may lead to ketosis as fat cells are metabolized for energy needs. Measurement of blood glucose levels will easily differentiate starvation ketosis (a hypoglycemic state treated with glucose solution) from diabetic ketoacidosis (a hyperglycemic state treated with insulin).

The pregnant diabetic is also at risk for dystocia caused by cephalopelvic disproportion due to macrosomia (an LGA fetus). Anemia may develop as a result of vascular involvement and of nausea and vomiting caused by hormonal changes. Infections of the urinary tract, particularly monilial vaginitis, commonly develop because of glycosuria. The client should not be allowed to go past term because of the increased incidence of intrauterine fetal death. Because of fetal macrosomia, induction of labor is often not successful; then cesarean delivery is performed.

FETAL–NEONATAL IMPLICATIONS

The incidence of stillbirths increases markedly with gestations carried beyond 36 weeks. In some instances, these intrauterine deaths can be attributed to poor diabetic control and acidosis. Careful control of the pregnant woman's diabetes significantly reduces the incidence of mortality and morbidity in the neonate, especially morbidity associated with hypoglycemia (Guthrie and Guthrie, 1982). However, even in the well-controlled diabetic, fetal jeopardy remains a significant problem.

Previously, the primary cause of death for infants of diabetic mothers was RDS because these infants were almost always delivered early to avoid the possibility of intrauterine fetal death. Neonatal mortality was between 4% and 10%. With the widespread use of amniotic fluid analysis to determine fetal pulmonary maturity (see Chapter 13), the appropriate time for delivery is determined more carefully, and mortality has dropped to between 1% and 5%. At present, congenital anomalies are the leading cause of fetal–neonatal mortality in diabetic pregnancy. Birth defects may be the cause of perinatal loss in 20%–50% of the cases. These defects frequently involve the nervous system, heart, and skeletal system. Because organogenesis occurs in these three systems prior to 7 weeks' gestation, it seems that to further reduce mortality strict diabetic control must exist prior to conception (Burrow and Ferris, 1982).

Characteristically, infants of type I diabetic mothers (or classes A, B, and C) are LGA as a result of the high maternal levels of blood glucose, from which the fetus derives its glucose. These elevated levels provide a relentless stimulus to the fetal islets of Langerhans to produce insulin. The sustained fetal hyperinsulinism and hyperglycemia ultimately lead to excessive growth and deposition of fat. After birth the umbilical cord is severed, and thus the generous maternal blood glucose supply is eliminated. However, continued islet cell hyperactivity leads to excessive insulin levels and depleted blood glucose (hypoglycemia) in 2–4 hours. See Chapter 24 for discussion of the management of the infant of a diabetic mother.

Infants of mothers with more advanced diabetes, on the other hand, may demonstrate IUGR. This occurs because vascular changes in the diabetic woman decrease the efficiency of placental profusion and the infant is not as well sustained in utero.

TESTS FOR DIABETES MELLITUS

The pregnant woman's urine should be tested for glucose at every prenatal visit. Further testing for diabetes mellitus should be done if she has (a) glycosuria; (b) the cardinal symptoms of diabetes (polyuria, polydipsia, polyphagia, and weight loss); (c) obesity; (d) a family history of diabetes; or (e) an obstetric history that includes an LGA neonate weighing 4000 g or more at birth, hydramnios, unexplained stillbirth, neonatal death, or congenital anomalies.

□ *URINE TESTING* Glycosuria is not diagnostic of diabetes mellitus, but presence of glycosuria is indication for glucose tolerance testing. In the nonpregnant adult, glucose is not generally spilled into the urine until blood sugar level is 180 mg/dL or greater, making false-negative results possible. In the presence of pregnancy the renal threshold is lower, and glucose may spill into the urine when blood glucose levels are 130 mg/dL.

Tes-Tape and Dextrostix are methods of choice in urine testing. They are specific for glucose and do not show positive readings in the presence of lactose or fructose. Single-specimen urine tests are used in routine screening each antenatal visit.

A 24-hour urine test is sometimes ordered to measure the amount of glucose lost in a 24-hour period. The woman is instructed to discard the first morning voiding and then save all further voidings for 24 hours, including the first voiding the next morning. The urine should be kept refrigerated in a large container and taken to the laboratory promptly as soon as the collection is completed.

Urine tests are sometimes done in the insulin-dependent diabetic to determine insulin dosage. In this situation the glucose level in freshly produced urine is needed. Therefore, the client is asked to void one half-hour prior to the test to empty her bladder of old urine, then drink a glass of water, and void again. The second voided specimen is tested. The current trend is toward blood glucose measurements rather than urine testing for more accurate insulin determination, particularly with the availability of home blood glucose monitoring devices such as glucometers or dextrometers.

Urine is also tested for ketones. Acetest is specific for acetone, and Ketostix is specific for acetoacetic acid, the first by-product of fat oxidation. Both are simple tests for detecting ketones in the urine and are usually done routinely for type I (ketosis-prone) diabetes.

□ **BLOOD TESTS**

1. A fasting plasma glucose (FPG) test, commonly called a fasting blood sugar (FBS) test, is done to determine the amount of glucose that remains in the blood after a period of fasting. FPG testing should be used infrequently during pregnancy to avoid hypoglycemia and possible harm to the fetus.
   Preparation: No food and no liquids except water are allowed for 12 hours prior to the test (usually 8:00 PM to 8:00 AM).
   Method: Blood is drawn by venipuncture and sent to the laboratory.
   Results: The normal range is 80–120 mg/dL serum. Levels greater than 140 mg/dL on two occasions are indicative of diabetes mellitus.*

2. Two-hour postprandial (after meal) testing is a more sensitive test than FPG but is not considered totally diagnostic of diabetes.

*Guide used by the Diabetes Education Center, St. Louis Park Medical Center, Minneapolis, MN, prepared from *Classification of DM and other categories of glucose intolerance* from the National Diabetes Data Group, NIH, 1980.

Preparation: A high-carbohydrate diet is eaten for 2–3 days prior to the test. The individual then fasts (except for water) from midnight to breakfast. A high-carbohydrate breakfast or a glucose load of 100 g glucose is then consumed.
Method: Exactly 2 hours after the meal or glucose load, a single blood specimen is drawn by venipuncture and sent to the lab.
Results: The normal blood glucose level is less than 145 mg/dL 2 hours postprandial. A blood glucose level greater than 145 mg/dL is indicative of diabetes.

3. Oral glucose tolerance test (OGTT) is the most sensitive (with IGTT, discussed next) method for detecting diabetes mellitus or impaired glucose tolerance. It should not be used if the FPG is over 200 mg/dL. OGTT measures response to a measured amount of glucose.
   Preparation: For 3 days prior to the test the client eats a high-carbohydrate diet. Weight, fasting blood levels, and urine specimens are obtained the morning of the test.
   Method: 100 g* of glucose is given orally in lemon juice. Blood and urine samples are obtained at ½, 1, 1½, 2, and 3 hours after the glucose administration. No medications, smoking, or caffeine are permitted during the test. Light activity is recommended.
   Results: The following are normal levels for plasma glucose:

   Hours after glucose administration†
1 hour	185 mg/dL
1½ hours	160 mg/dL
2 hours	140 mg/dL
3 hours	120 mg/dL

   By 3 hours and thereafter the results should be less than 120 mg/dL. Mildly elevated values after glucose is administered with a normal blood glucose value at the initial time (fasting) is diagnosed as impaired glucose tolerance. According to the new National Institutes of Health interpretation of the test, fasting venous plasma glucose levels over 140 mg/dL and any value during the test over 200 mg/dL constitutes diabetes mellitus (Guthrie and Guthrie, 1982).

4. Intravenous glucose tolerance test (IGTT) is the preferred test in pregnancy, since glucose absorption from the intestinal tract may vary and alter findings of OGTT.
   Preparation: Same as for OGTT.
   Method: Same as for OGTT except instead of oral glucose, 50 mL of 50% glucose in sterile water is administered intravenously over a 4-minute period.

†Criteria established by Fahans and Conn, reported in Guthrie and Guthrie, 1982.

Results: It is normal for the 2-hour plasma glucose level to be no higher than the fasting level at the beginning of the test.

INTERVENTIONS

The major goals of nursing care are (a) to maintain a physiologic equilibrium of insulin production and glucose utilization during pregnancy and (b) to deliver an optimally healthy mother and neonate. To achieve these goals, good prenatal care must be of top priority, utilizing the previously discussed team approach. Antepartal nursing care of the diabetic woman is based on the previously identified nursing care principles and on the following principles:

- Thorough clinical assessment of disease process and client information
- Instruction and support
- Dietary regulation
- Urine and blood testing for glucose levels
- Establishment of insulin requirements
- Evaluation of fetoplacental functioning
- Assessment of fetal maturity

These principles are discussed in the next sections.

□ **ASSESSMENT OF DISEASE PROCESS AND CLIENT INFORMATION** Whether diabetes (usually type I) has been diagnosed before pregnancy occurs, or the diagnosis is made during pregnancy (GDM), careful assessment of the disease process and the client's understanding of diabetes is important. Thorough physical examination including assessment for vascular complications of the disease, any signs of infectious conditions, and urine and blood testing for glucose are essential on the first antenatal visit. Follow-up visits are usually scheduled twice a month during the first two trimesters and once a week during the last trimester. Assessment is also needed to yield information about the woman's ability to cope with the combined stress of pregnancy and diabetes, and her ability to follow a recommended regimen of care. Determination of the client's knowledge about diabetes and self-care is needed before formulating a teaching plan.

□ **INSTRUCTION AND SUPPORT** The nurse provides encouragement and information to the pregnant client with diabetes. Because diabetes mellitus is new to the woman with GDM, she may require a great deal more teaching than the woman whose diabetes is well established. There are few, if any, other disease entities in which management and outcome are as dependent on the client's understanding and ability to provide self-care. However, when diabetes is first diagnosed, the client's normal reaction may be disbelief or the question, "Why me?" The nurse needs to recognize this reaction and allow time for adjustment. The client may not be immediately ready for much teaching on the subject. A reaction often appears shortly after the teaching begins, namely, the client's fear that there is too much to cope with and that she is not up to it. Reassurances, time, support of family members, and sometimes a support group are helpful in this situation.

Teaching must be individualized and must include the partner or support person, who can provide better support when he or she understands the disease process and is prepared to deal with complications such as hypoglycemia or hyperglycemia (Table 12–3). Because a couple must learn such a significant amount of information in a relatively short time, it is important not to overload them with new information during any single session. Teaching sessions should be well planned and tailored to their needs. Repetition and review are often necessary, and visual aids, demonstrations, and written material are useful. In addition to the basic information presented to diabetic clients, the nurse must be prepared to teach about or discuss with the couple several other areas of concern.

Insulin administration. The nurse helps the couple learn to administer insulin. It must be understood that the daily responsibility for the injections must be the woman's, but the support person can help in emergency situations.

Dietary management. In the team approach to diabetes management, a dietitian usually works with the client to help plan meals within her calorie allotment. The diet plans should match the client's life-style and culture. Exchange lists for meal planning can be obtained from the American Diabetes Association. Another system called "Points in Nutrition" is available from the National Education Center in Kansas City, Kansas. Special cookbooks are also available and can be a great help to the diabetic.

Cesarean birth. Chances for a cesarean birth are increased if the pregnant woman is diabetic. This possibility should be anticipated—enrollment in cesarean birth preparation classes may be suggested. Many hospitals offer classes, and information is available through organizations such as Cesarean/Support Education and Concern (C/Sec., Inc.); Cesarean Birth Council; or the Cesarean Association for Research, Education, Support and Satisfaction in Birthing (CARESS). The couple may prefer simply to discuss cesarean birth with the nurse and their obstetrician and read some books on the topic.

Breast-feeding. The presence of diabetes is not a contraindication for breast-feeding, but lactation does affect the control of diabetes. Blood glucose levels may be lower because glucose is transferred from serum to breast to be converted to lactose, and energy is expended in milk production. Therefore calorie needs increase during lactation, and insulin must be adjusted accordingly. Lactose in the urine is normal during lactation. Thus, the urine should be tested with a diagnostic method specific for glucose.

Sexual functioning. Limited and conflicting evidence is available on whether diabetes decreases a woman's libido or orgasmic response. However, it can be assumed that if good control of diabetes is maintained, the chance of adverse effects is diminished.

Contraception. Low-dose oral contraceptives have

Table 12–3   Comparison of Hypoglycemia and Hyperglycemia*

	Hypoglycemia	Hyperglycemia
Causes	Too much insulin Too little food Increased exercise without increased food	Too little insulin Too much food (especially carbohydrate) Emotional stress Infection
Onset	Usually sudden (minutes to half-hour)	Slow (days)
Symptoms in general order of appearance	Nervousness Shakiness Weakness Hunger Sweaty Cool clammy skin Pallor Blurred or double vision Headache Disorientation Shallow respirations Irritability Convulsions Coma	Polyuria Polydipsia Dry mouth Increased appetite Tiredness Nausea Hot flushed skin Abdominal cramps Abdominal rigidity Rapid deep breathing Acetone breath Paralysis Headache Soft eyeballs Drowsiness Oliguria or anuria Depressed reflexes Stupor Coma
Laboratory findings: Urine	Glucose – negative Acetone – usually negative	Glucose – positive Acetone – positive
Blood	Glucose – 60 mg/dL or lower Acetone – negative	Glucose – ± 250 mg/dL Acetone – usually positive

Treatment: See Nursing Care Plan for Diabetes Mellitus

Other comas: Hyperosmolar coma is most often seen in persons over 60 years of age with type II diabetes. Lactic acidosis coma occurs in advanced stages of diabetes, especially in persons with uremia, arteriosclerotic heart disease, pneumonia, acute pancreatitis, chronic alcoholism, and bacterial infection.

* Adapted from Guthrie and Guthrie, 1982.

minimal effect on blood glucose levels, but oral contraceptives do increase the risk of vascular complications. For short-term use in diabetic women with no vascular involvement, the low-dose oral contraceptives may be used.

Intrauterine devices should be used only by women with well-controlled diabetes. Risk increases if infection or perforation develops.

Mechanical devices offer the lowest health risk to the diabetic woman. A diaphragm that is well fitted and used with spermicidal foam or jelly is very reliable. Reliability achieves almost 100% if the man also uses a condom.

If the couple is certain that they want no more children, vasectomy for the male may be the method of choice. Tubal ligation in the diabetic female carries slightly more risk than in the nondiabetic female.

Smoking. Smoking is contraindicated for both pregnancy and diabetes. Harmful effects on the maternal vascular system and the developing fetus result from smoking.

Travel. Insulin can be kept at room temperature while traveling. Small travel kits are available for carrying insulin, syringes, and glucagon. These items should always be carried on the person rather than in luggage in a baggage compartment. An identification bracelet or necklace stating that the person is diabetic should be worn. Meals can be arranged with airlines and exchange lists carried. The woman should learn to say "diabetes" in a few foreign languages. She should check with her physician for any instructions, prescriptions, or advice before leaving.

Support groups. Many communities have diabetes support groups or education classes, which can be most helpful to clients with newly diagnosed diabetes. Learning that others have faced a similar situation and hearing how they managed are great aids in trying to cope with a chronic disease.

Hospitalization. Hospitalization may become necessary during the pregnancy to evaluate blood glucose levels and adjust insulin requirements. Tests to determine fetal well-being also may be indicated. If the disease becomes uncontrolled, hospitalization is required.

□ *DIETARY REGULATION* Recommended daily food intake should be 30–35 kcal/kg, 150–200 g of carbohydrates, 125 g of protein, and 60–80 g of fat. The carbohydrates ingested should be primarily complex starches rather than concentrated sweets (Burrow and Ferris, 1982). The goal is to increase caloric intake with sufficient insulin to force glucose into the cells. Meals and snacks must be distributed to coincide with peaks in insulin activity. This is especially important when multiple doses of insulin are used. A regimen of three meals and three to four snacks per day, equally spaced, is best.

□ *URINARY AND BLOOD GLUCOSE DETERMINATIONS* The nurse should be aware of the correlation between urine glucose results and blood glucose levels. The blood glucose ideally should be maintained at 60–90 mg/dL after fasting and less than 120 mg/dL 2 hours after meals (Skyler et al., 1981). Fractional urine testing for glucose and acetone levels is done four times a day as needed. With highly motivated clients, if circumstances permit, home blood glucose monitoring at least four times daily is the most desirable approach. In the presence of control, optimal fetal outcome is enhanced, and the risk of ketoacidosis with subsequent fetal demise or retarded fetal growth is minimized.

Recently, a method of determining long-term diabetic control, measuring hemoglobin A_{1c}, (Hb A_{1c}) levels, has gained widespread clinical usage. When plasma glucose levels are increased, hemoglobin A_O is converted to Hb A_{1c}. This reaction is non-enzymatic and essentially irreversible. Because it is a relatively slow process, the Hb A_{1c} levels give a picture of the average serum glucose concentrations during the preceding 60 days. Lower levels occur with better control. It is interesting to note that although the levels are not predictive of malformation, the incidence of congenitally malformed infants is increased in women with high Hb A_{1c} levels in early pregnancy (Jovanovic and Peterson, 1982).

□ *ESTABLISHMENT OF INSULIN REQUIREMENTS* It has generally been held that women with gestational diabetes (White's class A) could be managed without insulin therapy. Dietary carbohydrate restriction has been considered adequate. Evidence is increasing, however, that insulin therapy begun early and continued through pregnancy improves fetal outcome (Guthrie and Guthrie, 1982). For these women, a low-dosage mixture of regular- and intermediate-acting (NPH or Lente) insulin given twice a day seems the best management. Oral hypoglycemics are contraindicated in pregnancy because of possible teratogenic effects.

Women with type I diabetes (White's classes B through F) are most often controlled with multiple insulin injections (Guthrie and Guthrie, 1982). Various combinations of regular- and intermediate-acting insulin are used. A common regimen is to give two-thirds of the total dose (NPH) in the morning before breakfast, divided as one part regular to two parts NPH, and one-third in the evening, divided half and half (Moore et al, 1981). The very long-acting insulin (Ultralente) may be taken instead each morning, with regular insulin before each meal. With multiple-injection therapy, tighter control can be achieved and more flexibility allowed in the timing and amount of foods than with single-injection therapy. Insulin dosage may be determined by finger-stick home blood-glucose monitoring. Hospitalization may be needed for achieving control and establishing insulin requirements, as mentioned earlier.

Medical technology may soon be able to provide long-acting insulin pumps for insertion into the pregnant diabetic. This would allow continuous subcutaneous infusion of insulin to approximate more closely the body's normal functioning.

□ *EVALUATION OF FETOPLACENTAL FUNCTIONING* Assessment of fetal well-being is essential. It is performed throughout the prenatal course, utilizing such clinical and chemical techniques as: (a) monitoring serum estriol levels, (b) monitoring insulin requirements (failure to require increased insulin dosages after first trimester or sudden drop in requirement should lead to doubt about placental functioning), (c) using ultrasonography to assess fetal growth, (d) measuring fundal height, and (e) administering nonstress and contraction-stress tests, begun at 30–32 weeks' gestation and performed at least once a week.

□ *ASSESSMENT OF FETAL MATURITY* Fetal lung maturity may be confirmed by obtaining a sample of amniotic fluid by amniocentesis and then determining the lecithin/sphingomyelin (L/S) ratio (see p. 385). Caution must be used in evaluating L/S ratio results since they may be falsely elevated in the diabetic woman.

An L/S ratio as high as 3:1 may be needed to indicate fetal lung maturity in the pregnant diabetic, compared with a ratio of 2:1 in the nondiabetic. A more accurate test to determine fetal lung maturity is that for phosphatidylglycerol (PG), a surfactant that is a precursor of lecithin. Most hospital laboratories are not set up to evaluate PG, and it may be necessary to refer the mother to a tertiary care center for the test. Acetone precipitable fraction and phosphatidylinositol (PI) values are other tests of fetal lung maturity. An acetone precipitable fraction greater than 50%, a small amount of PI, and a prominent amount of PG together with an L/S ratio greater than 2:1 reflect fetal lung maturity (Shields and Resnik, 1979).

LABOR

In the last 8–10 weeks of pregnancy the woman and fetus are monitored closely, usually on an ambulatory-care basis. If the fetal or maternal condition warrants it, the woman may be hospitalized the last few weeks for more careful observation. The woman whose blood glucose level remains within acceptable limits, whose estriol levels are rising, and whose fetus has a reactive nonstress test is doing well and can probably continue to term and deliver spontaneously. If intrauterine conditions threaten fetal survival, labor may be induced by oxytocin if the cervix is ready, or cesarean delivery may be needed.

Before allowing spontaneous or induced labor, pelvic adequacy is ascertained by careful clinical pelvimetry, as fetal macrosomia and maternal CPD are not uncommon in a diabetic pregnancy. The maternal blood glucose level is monitored closely during labor, every half-hour in some institutions, with the goal of maintaining the level between 60–100 mg/dL (Moore et al., 1981). Intravenous fluids and nutrients are provided. The daily doses of intermediate- or long-acting insulin are omitted, and hyperglycemia is prevented by doses of short-acting (regular) insulin, or insulin is added to the intravenous infusion of glucose and regulated by an infusion pump. It has been found that insulin clings to the plastic intravenous bag and tubing. To ensure that the client receives the desired dose, the intravenous tubing needs to be flushed with insulin before the prescribed amount is added to the intravenous bag of dextrose and water. The intravenous insulin is discontinued with completion of the third stage of labor.

If labor is being induced, intravenous oxytocin must also be monitored carefully. Its use is safest when regulated by an infusion pump. Vital signs are measured every 15 minutes, more often if they are depressed or elevated. Temperature is measured every 4 hours if membranes are intact, every 2 hours if ruptured. The woman is encouraged to labor on her side or any other safe comfortable position (even ambulatory if conditions allow) but not on her back because a supine position impairs circulation to the fetus.

The fetus is also observed closely during labor. Continuous electronic fetal monitoring provides the best information about baseline fetal heart rate, beat-to-beat variability, maternal contractions, and fetal response to maternal contractions.

The same principles of providing physical comfort, support, reassurance, information about progress, and explanation of all procedures that are needed by all women in labor are also needed by the diabetic woman and her support person. The nurse needs to collaborate with the couple to plan care that meets their realistic expectations for the childbirth experience.

POSTPARTUM

Postpartally the maternal insulin requirements fall significantly. This occurs because the levels of hPL, progesterone, and estrogen fall after placental separation and their anti-insulin effect ceases, resulting in decreased blood glucose levels. The diabetic mother may require no insulin for the first 24 hours or only one-fourth to one-half of her previous dose. Then, reestablishment of insulin needs based on blood sugar testing is necessary. Diet and exercise levels must also be redetermined.

Diabetic control and the establishment of parent–child relationships in light of neonatal needs are the priorities of this period. If her newborn must be cared for in a special care nursery, the mother needs support and information about the neonate's condition. Every effort must be made to provide as much contact as possible between the parents and their newborn. The decision to breast-feed should be supported for the woman who chooses this method.

In summary, a diabetic pregnancy demands thorough assessment, planning, and follow-up nursing care. The nursing assessment considers the biologic, psychologic, and sociologic needs of the woman and her family. Planning necessitates a coordinated team approach to assure optimal outcome, and follow-up care requires the nurse to have knowledge, understanding, and patience to implement and evaluate the required therapies successfully (see the accompanying Nursing Care Plan).

Thyroid Dysfunction

The thyroid gland is affected by the metabolic and hormonal changes that occur in pregnancy. However, thyroid dysfunction is not a common complication of pregnancy. The behaviors that result from pregnancy mimic those of the hyperthyroid state: increased metabolic rate, increased protein-bound iodine values, and increased ^{131}I intake. Evidence has shown that hypothyroid women ovulate irregularly, or, if pregnancy is achieved, their maintenance of the gravid state is difficult. It appears that infertility and high fetal mortality are characteristic of the hypothyroid state. In hyperthyroid women, there is no convincing evidence to support fertility impairment; however, there is a slight increase in neonatal mortality and a significant increase in the frequency of delivery of small-for-gestational-age (SGA) infants.

HYPERTHYROIDISM (THYROTOXICOSIS)

Hyperthyroidism is present in about 2 per 1000 pregnancies (Burrow and Ferris, 1982). Diagnosis of hyperthyroidism during pregnancy is difficult because of normal gesta-

NURSING CARE PLAN
Diabetes Mellitus in Prenatal, Intrapartal, and Postpartal Periods

CLIENT DATA BASE

Nursing history

1. Complete assessment: client and family
2. Identification of client's predisposition to diabetes
   a. Recurrent preeclampsia-eclampsia
   b. Previous LGA infants (≥4000 g)
   c. Hydramnios
   d. Unexplained fetal death
   e. Obesity
   f. Family history of diabetes

Physical examination

1. Length of gestation
2. Complaints of thirst and hunger
3. Recurrent monilial vaginitis
4. Frequent urination beyond first trimester and prior to third trimester
5. Fundal height greater than expectation for gestation
6. Obesity

Laboratory evaluation

1. Fasting plasma glucose (FPG)
2. 2-hour postprandial GTT
3. 3-hour IGTT or OGTT
4. Urine test for glucose
5. 24-hour urinary estriol

NURSING PRIORITIES

1. Observe for signs of hypoglycemia, hyperglycemia, preeclampsia
2. Test blood or urine daily for glucose
3. Dietary and insulin regulation as needed
4. Assess client and family needs for referral
5. Assess knowledge level of client relative to disease
6. During labor, monitor labor, amount and color of amniotic fluid, maternal and fetal status

CLIENT/FAMILY EDUCATION FOCUS

1. Discuss importance of strict dietary control, maintenance of appropriate blood glucose levels, adequate insulin coverage, and regular prenatal care for successful pregnancy outcome
2. Review signs and symptoms of hypoglycemia and hyperglycemia and the actions the client or her family should initiate if they appear
3. Provide appropriate literature about diabetes in pregnancy and refer the client/family to available resource and support groups

Note for diagnosis: 2 hr pp of 140 mg/dL is indicative of diabetes mellitus and a level of 110–140 mg/dL is suggestive of subclinical diabetes. May be confirmed with IGTT.

Problem	Nursing interventions and actions	Rationale
Dietary regulation	Maintain strict diet: 1. 30–35 kcal/kg 2. 150–200 g carbohydrate 3. 125 g protein 4. 60–80 g fat to provide approximately 35% of fetal stores 5. Sodium intake may be restricted	Maintain ideal weight in first trimester and average gain in last two trimesters (no more than 3–3.5 lb/month)
Insulin needs	Assess insulin needs: 1. Check lab results of FPG and 2-hour postprandial 2. Test urine four times daily using Tes-Tape or Dextrostix 3. Teach client use of home blood glucose monitoring device. Determine amount of insulin based on sliding scale. 4. Administer regular insulin or NPH or Lente insulin, or combination, as ordered	Sufficient insulin must be present to enable proper carbohydrate metabolism to take place; pregnancy requires a marked increase in circulating insulin to maintain normal blood glucose Fasting glucose level tends to be lower than nonpregnant value Effectiveness of insulin may be reduced by presence of hPL Insulin requirements fluctuate widely during pregnancy because of factors mentioned in text and because of lowered glucose tolerance, especially in second half of pregnancy, and fluctuate during intrapartal period because of depletion of glycogen stores during labor;

NURSING CARE PLAN Cont'd
Diabetes Mellitus in Prenatal, Intrapartal, and Postpartal Periods

Problem	Nursing interventions and actions	Rationale
		fluctuations during puerperium are a result of involuntary process; in addition, conversion of blood glucose into lactose during lactation may cause marked changes in glucose tolerance and/or hypoglycemia
Hypoglycemia	1. Teach client early signs of hypoglycemia and treatment	Self-care at home is a preventive measure so hypoglycemia will not become serious
	2. Observe for signs of hypoglycemia (see Table 12–3)	Correction of hypoglycemia and maintenance of controlled state provide optimal fetal health
	3. Treat within minutes of onset	Rapid treatment of hypoglycemia is essential to prevent brain damage as the brain requires glucose to function (skeletal and heart muscles can derive energy from ketones and free fatty acids)
	a. Obtain immediate blood samples for testing	Provides baseline information on glucose levels
	b. If client is alert give half a glass of orange juice or other liquid containing sugar; notify physician	Liquids are absorbed from the GI tract faster than solids; 10 g of glucose, which will reverse most hypoglycemic reactions, is the amount found in one-half glass orange juice, 2 tsp sugar or 1 or 2 hard candies
	c. If client is not alert enough to swallow give 1 mg glucagon subcutaneously or intramuscularly; notify physician	Glucagon triggers the conversion of glycogen stored in the liver to glucose
	d. If client is in labor with intravenous lines in place, 10–20 mL of 50% dextrose may be given IV Standing order should be available; notify physician	
Hyperglycemia	1. Teach client early signs of hyperglycemia and treatment	Client can recognize signs and administer self-treatment Client can also report any symptoms that may occur
	2. Observe for signs of hyperglycemia (see Table 12–3); administer treatment; notify physician	Administer insulin to restore body's normal metabolism of carbohydrate, protein, and fat
	a. Obtain frequent measurement of blood and urine glucose; measure urine acetone	Need to establish a baseline and to determine additional insulin dosage and prevent overtreatment; urine acetone indicates development of ketoacidosis
	b. Administer prescribed amount regular insulin subcutaneously or intravenously, or combination of routes	Regular insulin used because it acts immediately and is of short duration
	c. Replace fluids IV, orally, or both	Fluids are depleted in the process of ketoacidosis; hypotension can result from decreased blood volume due to dehydration
	d. Measure intake and output	Polyuria is an early sign of hyperglycemia; oliguria develops with hypotension and decreased bloodflow to kidneys
	e. Observe for symptoms of circulatory collapse; monitor BP and pulse	Circulatory collapse can result from hypotension
Preeclampsia	Observe and report any signs of preeclampsia (see discussion p. 336)	Preeclampsia is more prevalent in the pregnant woman with diabetes

NURSING CARE PLAN Cont'd
Diabetes Mellitus in Prenatal, Intrapartal, and Postpartal Periods

Problem	Nursing interventions and actions	Rationale
Vaginitis	Observe for symptoms of burning, itching, and leukorrhea; obtain vaginal smear; treat with prescription based on the causative organism and gestation	Vaginitis is more common in the woman with diabetes; treatment is specific to the organism
Urinary tract infections (UTI)	Observe for symptoms of frequency, urgency, and burning on urination; low back pain with kidney involvement	Incidence of UTI is increased in diabetes, possibly because the existence of glycosuria provides rich medium for bacterial growth
	Obtain urine specimen for culture and sensitivity	
	Administer prescribed antibiotics	Antibiotic prescribed is specific to causative organism
	Encourage fluids; measure intake and output	Increased fluid intake promotes urinary removal of organisms
Inadequate rest	Instruct client to rest frequently during day in lateral position	Lateral position has favorable influence on uteroplacental circulation and diminishes myometrial tone
Fear and lack of knowledge	Support and encourage client and partner:	By decreasing fear, the client will be more effective as a member of the antepartal-intrapartal health team
	1. Explain procedures	
	2. Allow them to ask questions	
	3. Assess their level of knowledge of childbirth and utilize this to teach about what is happening	
	4. Involve partner as much as possible	
	5. Utilize breathing and relaxation techniques to minimize amount of medication needed, especially if gestation is 36 or 37 weeks, to decrease fetal narcosis. For more detailed information, see Nursing Care Plan on labor and delivery, Chapter 16.	Fetal narcosis should be avoided
	6. Administer analgesics as needed in labor	
Compromise of fetoplacental status	Periodic assessments:	Continued slow rise of estriol indicates adequate functioning of maternal system, placental function, and fetal status, because estriol and creatinine require interplay of all three systems
	1. Level of plasma and/or urine estriol	
	2. Creatinine clearance	
	3. Regular assessment of fetal size	Assess fetal growth
	4. Ultrasonographs	Evaluate fetal size
	5. L/S ratio, or phosphatidylglycerol or phosphatidylinositol levels	2:1 ratio usually indicates fetal lung maturity sufficient to sustain infant in extauterine environment. In one-third of insulin-dependent women, L/S ratio fails to show a terminal rise; others show early excessive rise.
	6. NST or CST	
Size of fetus	Assessments:	Increased circulating glucose leads to increased deposition of fatty tissue in fetus
	1. Ultrasonographs	
	2. Measuring fundal height	Indicates uterine size, not necessarily size of fetus
Frequent hospitalization	Orient patient to surroundings and routines:	Admit prenatally to assess diabetic status
	1. Provide support	Admit if there are signs of incipient preeclampsia or infection
	2. Promote rest	Admit for most of third trimester if patient has microvascular disease, so that rest can be maintained and patient can be closely supervised

NURSING CARE PLAN Cont'd
Diabetes Mellitus in Prenatal, Intrapartal, and Postpartal Periods

Problem	Nursing interventions and actions	Rationale
Hydramnios	Assess size of uterus Assess signs of distress from hydramnios: 1. Respiratory distress 2. Stasis of fluid in legs	Diabetic clients are more prone to hydramnios, and it may develop rapidly
	Slow removal of amniotic fluid by transabdominal amniotomy may be done	Remove fluid slowly to prevent abruptio placentae and amniotic fluid embolus
Labor	Admit to unit: 1. Perform routine admission (see Nursing Care Plan on labor and delivery, Chapter 16) 2. Assess size of fetus and capacity of pelvis: ultrasonograph, x-ray pelvimetry 3. Administer IV fluids to maintain hydration and glucose to avoid depleting glycogen stores 4. Assess insulin needs by frequent blood glucose monitoring 5. Check urine acetone every hour 6. Continuously monitor fetal status 7. Alleviate induction concerns (see Nursing Care Plan on induction, Chapter 19)	Induction of labor at about 37 weeks, once fetal lung maturity is ascertained, may be recommended to ensure safe fetal outcome. Macrosomia is often associated with diabetes Increased exertion during labor alters insulin needs Ketonuria indicates increased need for insulin

Postpartum

Insulin needs	Assess insulin needs by blood glucose; client may not require insulin for first 24 hours after delivery	Removal of hPL from circulation permits more efficient utilization of insulin
Parent–infant bonding	Provide parents with frequent opportunities for contact with their newborn especially if in special care nursery Encourage rooming-in if newborn's condition permits Support breast-feeding if it is mother's chosen feeding method	Increased fears for the newborn's health may impede bonding
Postpartum hemorrhage	Frequently assess for vaginal bleeding and fundal firmness; massage to stimulate contraction if boggy; monitor BP and pulse	Higher incidence of postpartal hemorrhage in women with diabetes, due to overdistended uterus if LGA infant or hydramnios present

NURSING CARE EVALUATION

Client's diabetes will be controlled

Client will consume needed calories and nutrients

Client will have sufficient insulin to maintain control

Fetoplacental status will be monitored to avoid complications

Client education will be enhanced and client questions will be answered

NURSING DIAGNOSIS*	SUPPORTING DATA
1. Alteration in nutrition related to impaired carbohydrate metabolism	Symptoms of hypoglycemia or hyperglycemia (see Table 12–3) Glycosuria
2. Potential alteration in fetal health maintenance	Maternal hypoglycemia or hyperglycemia Abnormal findings in assessment of fetal size and status
3. Knowledge deficit about the effects of diabetes mellitus on pregnancy and pregnancy outcome	Expressed concerns or questions about specific aspects of diabetes during pregnancy

*These are a few examples of nursing diagnoses that may be appropriate for a person with this condition. It is not an inclusive list and must be individualized for each woman.

tional changes. Symptoms that are indicative include (a) a resting pulse rate greater than 100 beats/min, without slowing during Valsalva's maneuver; (b) muscle wasting, particularly of the quadriceps; (c) separation of the distal nail from its nail bed; (d) enlarged thyroid gland; (e) fine tremor of extended fingers; (f) exophthalmos with lid-lag in some cases; and (g) sweating. Serum thyroxine levels are not accurate determinants because of the influence of pregnancy.

With hyperthyroidism the incidence of premature delivery, postpartum hemorrhage, and possibly preeclampsia is increased. The major complication for both the hyperthyroid woman and the fetus is that of thyroid storm. This rare but frightening occurrence presents a clinical picture of extremely high fever, tachycardia, severe dehydration, sweating, and possible heart failure. In addition, mental function may be erratic. Prompt medical and nursing intervention include hospitalization and appropriate pharmacologic agents to reduce presenting behaviors and to achieve control. Thyroid storm most commonly occurs in pregnant women in whom the diagnosis of hyperthyroidism has been missed. It is therefore imperative that a thorough nursing prenatal assessment include careful history taking and close observation of the woman's physiologic and physical behaviors that may be indicative of increased thyroid function, as well as nervousness, heat sensitivity, fatigue, diarrhea, and insomnia.

□ *FETAL-NEONATAL IMPLICATIONS* Hyperthyroidism in newborns is even more uncommon than in the woman. It is seen more often in male neonates, which is contrary to the general trend of hyperthyroid dysfunction. Neonates born to mothers with this complication should have serum thyroxine (T_4) determinations done at birth and should be observed carefully during the first two weeks of life for signs of hyperthyroidism. Breast-feeding is generally contraindicated for women taking antithyroid medication because it is excreted in the milk.

□ *INTERVENTIONS* Treatment of hyperthyroidism involves a choice between drug therapy and surgical intervention. These alternatives must be weighed in view of gestational age and thyroid function. A variety of drugs can be used to control the overactivity of the sympathetic nervous system, to block the uptake of iodine by the thyroid gland, or to inhibit the production of the thyroid hormone. The drug of choice is the thyroid inhibitor propylthiouracil. These drugs do cross the placenta and interfere with fetal thyroid function. Overtreatment of the woman with hyperthyroid drugs may result in fetal hypothyroidism, fetal goiter, and deficient development, especially of the central nervous system. Therefore, the client is given the lowest possible dose. The goal is to maintain serum thyroxine in the high normal range.

If drug therapy is not effective, surgical resection of part of the thyroid gland is indicated. In the pregnant woman, the most favorable time would be after the first trimes-

ter to decrease the risk of spontaneous abortion. The size, friability, and vascularization of the thyroid gland must be reduced prior to surgery with concurrent administration of propylthiouracil and iodine (Lugol's solution or SSKI).

HYPOTHYROIDISM

Hypothyroidism in its extreme form is usually accompanied by amenorrhea and anovulation, with resultant sterility. It is rare, only one-tenth as common as hyperthyroidism (Danforth, 1982). However, a less severe deficiency is compatible with conception, although abortion is not uncommon. Generally, diagnosis is made based on the results of laboratory findings of free serum thyroxine concentrations, which are estimated by calculation of the free thyroxine index. Determination of radioactive iodine uptake is contraindicated during pregnancy because the substance is readily taken up by the fetal thyroid.

Additional supportive data include suggestive medical history and physical signs, such as a decreased basal metabolic rate, a firm diffuse goiter (enlarged thyroid gland), fatigability, cold intolerance, myxedema, constipation, dry skin, headache, and delayed deep tendon reflexes.

In pregnancy, relative iodine deficiency may be induced by increased renal iodide clearance and increased hormonogenesis.

□ *FETAL-NEONATAL IMPLICATIONS* The newborn of a hypothyroid mother has a slightly increased risk of being born with congenital goiter or with true cretinism. There are also reports of an increased risk for development of congenital anomalies (Danforth, 1982). If the neonate has hypothyroidism, there is increased risk of hyperbilirubinemia. To detect hypothyroidism in the neonate, newborns are now routinely screened for serum thyroxine levels.

□ *INTERVENTIONS* As soon as diagnosis is confirmed, treatment should begin to decrease the possibility of fetal mortality. Fetal health is monitored by ultrasonographic measurement of the biparietal diameter and fetal femur length at midgestation and again after 32 weeks. Weekly nonstress tests are important after 35 weeks of gestation. Replacement thyroid therapy is apparently needed to sustain normal growth and development of the fetus. Replacement doses are prescribed, and the free thyroxine index is used to monitor the adequacy of medication. Iodine administration is desirable as a means of reducing the risk of cretinism in the newborn. Early abortions from multiple causes often exhibit low levels of protein-bound iodine. However, thyroid medication should not be used prophylactically in the hope of reducing fetal death.

Other Medical Conditions and Pregnancy

ANEMIA

Anemias in pregnancy may be due specifically to the pregnancy, or they may exist coincidentally with the pregnancy. Iron deficiency anemia and megaloblastic anemia may be caused by the pregnancy. A rare category, refractory anemia, is any anemia for which no cause is found, and which does not respond to treatment but is immediately improved by delivery. There are many nonpregnancy-induced anemias, acquired or hereditary, some of which may be exacerbated by pregnancy.

□ *IRON DEFICIENCY ANEMIA* Anemia is the most common medical complication of pregnancy and 77% of anemias in pregnancy are of the iron deficiency type (Burrow and Ferris, 1982).

A pregnant woman needs at least an extra 1000 mg of iron intake during the pregnancy to compensate for the 300–400 mg of iron transferred to the fetus; 500 mg for the increased red blood cell mass in her own increased circulating blood volume; another 100 mg for the placenta; and 180–200 mg for the normal blood loss at delivery (Danforth, 1982). Approximately 200 mg of iron will be conserved due to the functional amenorrhea of pregnancy, but many women begin pregnancy in a slightly anemic state. The greatest need for increased iron intake is in the second half of pregnancy. When the iron needs of pregnancy are not met, hemoglobin (Hgb) falls below 11 g/dL. Serum ferritin levels, indicating iron stores, are below 12 μg/L. In pregnancy mild anemia can rapidly become more severe; therefore it needs immediate treatment.

Maternal implications. The woman with iron deficiency anemia is more susceptible to infection, tires easily, has an increased chance of postpartal hemorrhage, and tolerates poorly even minimal blood loss during delivery. If the anemia is severe (Hgb less than 6 g/dL), cardiac failure may ensue.

Fetal–neonatal implications. Abortion and prematurity rates are increased, and the neonate may be dysmature. With severe anemia the incidence of stillbirth and SGA neonates is increased. Fetal iron stores are not significantly impaired. The fetus may be hypoxic during labor due to impaired uteroplacental oxygenation (Danforth, 1982).

Interventions. Iron supplements are essential during pregnancy because dietary sources alone cannot meet the extra gestational requirements. Usually oral doses of a ferrous salt, for example, ferrous sulfate, 300 mg (60 mg of elemental iron) taken two to three times daily with meals (together with 1 mg of folic acid to prevent megaloblastic anemia) are adequate to restore hemoglobin to 12 g/dL. With a twin pregnancy a larger dose is needed. (The woman should be reminded to keep iron tablets out of reach of children.) If a large dose of iron causes vomiting and diarrhea or the anemia is discovered late in pregnancy, parenteral iron, for example, an iron dextran complex (Imferon), may be needed.

□ *MEGALOBLASTIC ANEMIA* Increased folic acid metabolism during pregnancy can rapidly result in folic acid deficiency. Folic acid is needed for DNA synthesis necessary for the normal division of red blood cell precursors. In its absence, the precursor cells fail to divide, mature abnor-

mally, and become enlarged red blood cells but are fewer in number. Bone marrow biopsy may be necessary to establish the diagnosis.

Megaloblastic anemia is associated with malnutrition and may affect 2% of pregnant women in the United States. It can develop rapidly, often occurring late in pregnancy. Hemoglobin levels as low as 3–5 g/dL are not uncommon (Danforth, 1982).

Interventions. Treatment consists of taking 1 mg of folic acid daily. The nurse can help the pregnant client avoid megaloblastic anemia by teaching her food sources of folic acid and cooking methods for preserving folic acid. The best sources are leafy green vegetables, red meats, fish, poultry, and legumes. Up to 50%–90% of folic acid can be lost with cooking in large volumes of water. Microwave cooking destroys more folic acid than conventional cooking.

□ *SICKLE CELL ANEMIA* Sickle cell anemia is a recessive autosomal disease. The individual must inherit the trait (HbS) from both parents (in other words, the person is homozygous for the trait). The sickle cell trait is carried by 8% of American blacks, who are usually asymptomatic. Carriers are heterozygous, with one normal HbA gene and one HbS gene. The anemia itself is present in about 0.7% blacks in the United States (Danforth, 1982).

The abnormal red blood cells are sickle or crescent shaped. A polypeptide chain in the hemoglobin protein is altered in that the amino acid valine is substituted for glutamic acid. This single substitution, which has been located in the sixth position of the β chain, out of 509 amino acids on four possible chains, causes the anemia. The result of this substitution is low solubility of the hemoglobin in the presence of decreased oxygenation. The red blood cells become distorted, rigid, and interlocked with one another, which causes vascular obstruction in the capillaries. This is called *sickling*, and varies in frequency of occurrence by the amount of the S hemoglobin in the red blood cells (with levels below 40% there is seldom a crisis) and other hemoglobin factors. Low oxygen pressure as in high temperature, dehydration, infection, or acidosis may precipitate a crisis. A hemolytic crisis may occur with profound anemia, jaundice, and high temperature, or a painful crisis may occur with capillary thrombosis and infarction in various organs.

Maternal implications. The client with sickle cell anemia usually relates a history of frequent illnesses and recurrent abdominal and joint pains, and is found to be extremely anemic. The client may appear undernourished and have long, thin extremities. Ulcers on ankles or jaundiced sclerae are often present. Pregnancy may aggravate the anemia and bring on more frequent crises. The chance of developing preeclampsia increases to a one in three risk. Risk of urinary tract infection, pneumonia, congestive heart failure, and pulmonary infarction is also increased. Mortality is about 1% (McPhee and Bell, 1981).

Fetal–neonatal implications. Abortion, fetal death, and prematurity lead to a perinatal death rate of about 50% (Danforth, 1982). IUGR is also a characteristic finding in neonates of sickle cell anemic women.

Interventions. Because no specific antisickling agent has been found, the goal of treatment is to reduce the anemia and decrease the chance of infection or a sickle cell crisis. Good nutrition and inclusion of folic acid supplements are essential. Increased hydration, good hygiene practices, and the avoidance of people with infections should be emphasized by the nurse. Small daily transfusions of packed cells may be necessary during a hemolytic crisis, and maternal exchange transfusions also help improve maternal condition. Bed rest may decrease the chance of premature birth. During labor, oxygen supplementation should be used continuously, and additional blood should be available as blood loss during delivery is poorly tolerated. When both parents are known to carry the trait, genetic counseling is indicated so that they can understand the risks associated with the disease and make decisions regarding future pregnancies accordingly.

Table 12–4 describes some less commonly seen medical conditions that may be found in women of childbearing age. The table briefly identifies the maternal and fetal–neonatal implications of each disease.

MEDICAL DISORDERS ASSOCIATED WITH PREGNANCY

Disruptive conditions that arise during the gestational period are the result of many high-risk factors, such as age, blood type, socioeconomic status, parity, psychologic well-being, and predisposing chronic illnesses (see Chapter 10). The major thrust of prenatal nursing care should be toward screening clients for these complications and toward supportive therapies that will facilitate optimal health for mother and fetus.

Hyperemesis Gravidarum

Hyperemesis gravidarum is pernicious vomiting during pregnancy. In its early stages, it may be difficult to diagnose because initially vomiting does not occur after each feeding. However, true hyperemesis progresses to a point at which the woman not only vomits everything she swallows but retches between meals.

The cause of hyperemesis during pregnancy is still debatable but probably is related to trophoblastic activity and gonadotropin production and is stimulated or exaggerated by psychologic factors. Incidence varies in different geographic locations in the United States and has declined in recent decades, but on the average hyperemesis appears in approximately 3.5 cases per 1000 deliveries (Mannor, 1981).

The pathology of hyperemesis in extreme cases begins with dehydration. This leads to fluid–electrolyte imbalance, and alkalosis from the loss of hydrochloric acid. More prolonged vomiting can result in loss of predominantly alkaline intestinal juices and occurrence of acidosis. Hypovolemia from dehydration leads to hypotension and increased pulse rate, with increased hematocrit and blood urea nitrogen levels and decreased urine output. Severe potassium loss (hypokalemia) interferes with the ability of the kidneys to concentrate urine, and disrupts cardiac functioning. Starvation causes severe protein and vitamin deficiencies. Characteristic symptoms include jaundice and hemorrhage due to deficiencies of vitamin C and B-complex vitamins and bleeding from mucosal areas due to hypothrombinemia.

Fetal or embryonic death may result, and the woman may suffer irreversible metabolic changes or death.

The differential diagnosis may involve infectious diseases such as encephalitis or viral hepatitis, intestinal obstruction, hydatidiform mole, or peptic ulcer.

It is imperative that diagnosis be made so that necessary therapy may be started. In severe cases, hospitalization is required. The objectives of nursing management include control of vomiting, correction of dehydration, restoration of electrolyte balance, and maintenance of adequate nutrition.

INTERVENTIONS

Initially, the patient with hyperemesis gravidarum is given nothing orally, with administration of intravenous fluids of at least 3000 mL in the first 24 hours. This therapy provides fluid, glucose, vitamin (B-complex, C, A, and D), and electrolyte replacement. Desired urine output is 1000 mL/24 hours. Intake and output are measured. Oral hygiene is especially important as the mouth is very dry and may be irritated from the vomitus. Use of barbiturates and antiemetics may be helpful in controlling nausea and vomiting, but is controversial because of possible teratogenic effects.

Usually in 48 hours the woman's condition improves sufficiently to begin oral feedings. Six small dry feedings followed by clear liquids is one treatment of choice. Another method is 1 oz of water offered each hour, followed as tolerated by clear, then nourishing liquids, progressing on succeeding days to low-fat soft and general diets.

Nursing care should be supportive and directed at maintaining a relaxed, quiet environment. Because emotional factors have been found to play a major role in this condition, psychotherapy is recommended. With proper treatment, prognosis is favorable.

Bleeding Disorders

During the first and second trimesters of pregnancy, the major cause of bleeding is abortion. This is defined as the termination of a pregnancy prior to 28 weeks of gestation or prior to viability of the fetus. Abortions are either *spontaneous*, occurring naturally with no artificial means, or *induced,* occurring as a result of artificial or mechanical interruption (see Chapter 6 for discussion of induced abortion). *Miscarriage* is a lay term applied to abortion.

Other complications that can cause bleeding in the first half of pregnancy are ectopic pregnancy (1 of every 200 pregnancies) and hydatidiform mole (1 of every 2000 pregnancies). In the second half of pregnancy, particularly in the third trimester, bleeding may develop that may be fatal to woman and fetus. Two major causes of bleeding at this time are placenta previa (1 of every 200 pregnancies) and abruptio placentae (1 of every 50 to 270 pregnancies) (Bernstine, 1981).

GENERAL PRINCIPLES OF NURSING INTERVENTION

All bleeding during pregnancy should be carefully evaluated. Therefore, antepartal teaching regarding bleeding as a warning sign should be stressed. It is often the nurse's responsibility to make the initial assessment of bleeding. In general, the following nursing measures should be implemented for pregnant patients being treated for bleeding disorders:

- Constant monitoring of vital signs of blood pressure and pulse is imperative
- Observe patient for behaviors indicative of shock, such as pallor, clammy skin, perspiration, dyspnea, or restlessness
- Count pads to assess amount of bleeding over a given time period; any tissue or clots expelled should be saved
- If pregnancy is of 20 weeks' gestation or beyond, assess fetal heart tones
- Prepare for intravenous therapy
- Prepare equipment for examination
- Have oxygen therapy available
- Collect and organize all data, including antepartal history, onset of bleeding episode, laboratory studies (hemoglobin, hematocrit, and hormonal assays)
- Assess coping mechanisms of patient in crisis. Give emotional support to enhance her coping abilities by continuous, sustained presence, by clear explanation of procedures, and by communicating her status to her family. Most important, prepare the patient for possible fetal loss. Assess her expressions of anger, denial, silence, guilt, depression, or self-blame.

SPONTANEOUS ABORTION

Many pregnancies are lost in the first trimester as a result of spontaneous abortion. Statistics are inaccurate, because some women may have aborted but were unaware that they were pregnant during the early weeks of gestation (through week 8). The bleeding is seen as a heavy menstrual period.

Approximately 82% of spontaneous abortions occur in the first trimester, with only 18% in the second. The over-

all figures range from 15%–20% of all pregnancies, according to the National Center for Health Statistics cited in Borg and Lasker (1981).

□ *ETIOLOGY* When a spontaneous abortion occurs, the woman and her family must search for a cause so that they may plan knowledgeably for future family expansion. However, even with current technology and medical advances, a direct cause cannot always be determined. The genetic findings for a couple may include the following (Danforth, 1982):

1. Chromosomal structure and number are normal in both partners, but abnormal offspring can result sporadically and unpredictably.
2. One member of couple is a carrier of a balanced translocation. Repeated abortion may result.

The most common causes of spontaneous abortion are related to abnormal development of the embryo or fetus. The abnormal development may be due to drugs or genetic makeup, faulty implantation due to abnormalities of the female generative tract, placental abnormalities, chronic maternal diseases, and endocrine imbalances.

Most spontaneous abortions appear to be related to imperfections in sperm or ova or to effects of teratogenic drugs, as discussed later in this chapter. Abnormalities of the woman's generative tract may be a result of organ imperfections, such as an undeveloped uterus, double uterus, or adhesions of the adnexa as a result of pelvic inflammatory disease. Abortion may also result from uterine fibroid tumors (leiomyoma). Sometimes abortion occurs in midpregnancy as a result of an incompetent cervix. The weakened cervix is unable to remain closed and painlessly dilates, the membranes rupture, and the products of conception are expelled. This is often the cause of second trimester habitual abortion.

Maternal infections, if left untreated, can emit toxins that stimulate abortion. Endocrine imbalances, particularly a reduction in progesterone and estrogen in early pregnancy, can retard the normal growth of the endometrial lining of the uterus. In later pregnancy, a decrease in hCG produced by the placenta can cause loss of pregnancy. Maternal malnutrition has also been implicated in abortion. Other chronic maternal diseases affecting embryonic and fetal growth include essential hypertensive vascular diseases, ABO incompatibility, chronic nephritis, and in the second trimester, syphilis. It is commonly believed that psychic trauma and accidents are the primary causes of abortion, but statistics do not generally support this belief.

□ *CLASSIFICATION* Spontaneous abortions are subdivided into the following categories so that they can be differentiated clinically (Table 12–5):

1. *Threatened abortion.* The fetus is jeopardized by unexplained bleeding, cramping, and backache. Bleeding may persist for days. The cervix is closed. It may be

Table 12–4   Less Common Medical Conditions and Pregnancy

Condition	Brief description	Maternal implications	Fetal/neonatal implications
Multiple sclerosis	Neurologic disorder characterized by destruction of the myelin sheath of nerve fibers	Although the disease is not altered by pregnancy, fatigue may bring on relapses; the woman must have adequate rest	No known effect
	The condition occurs primarily in young adults and, although marked by periods of remission, progresses to marked physical disability in 10–20 years	Uterine contraction strength is not diminished but since sensation frequently is lessened, labor may be almost painless	
		The woman should carefully consider decision to have a child because of the increased burden child care would place on her	
Myasthenia gravis	Neurologic disease commonly seen in young adult females, characterized by progressive weakening of the muscles of the face and upper torso; prior to the discovery of the effectiveness of treatment with anticholinesterase drugs such as neostigmine, the death rate was extremely high	Pregnancy has no predictable effect; exacerbations may occur equally in all three trimesters

Because adequate rest is important, the pregnant client should plan for extra help with child care | No known associated fetal anomalies with the disease or medication

Infants may be SGA

Myasthenia attacks may occur in the newborn during the first month but they respond well to medication; infants usually have normal muscle tone within 3–8 weeks |
| Systemic lupus erythematosus (SLE) | Chronic autoimmune collagen disease, characterized by exacerbations and remissions; symptoms range from characteristic rash to inflammation and pain in joints to fever, nephritis, depression, cranial nerve disorders, and peripheral neuropathies | Mild cases—little risk to mother or fetus

Severe cases—because of extra burden on the kidneys, therapeutic abortion may be indicated

Woman must be careful to avoid fatigue, infection, strong sunlight, and so on

Acute postpartum exacerbation is common and often severe | Increased incidence of spontaneous abortion, stillbirth, prematurity, and SGA neonates

Rarely, the neonate shows manifestations of the disease which respond to steroids and disappear within 3 months |

followed by partial or complete expulsion of pregnancy (Figure 12–1).

2. *Imminent abortion.* Bleeding and cramping increase. The internal cervical os dilates. Membranes may rupture. The term *inevitable abortion* applies.

3. *Complete abortion.* All the products of conception are expelled.

4. *Incomplete abortion.* Part of the products of conception

are retained, most often the placenta. The internal cervical os is dilated and will admit one finger.

5. *Missed abortion.* The fetus dies in utero but is not expelled. Uterine growth ceases, breast changes regress, and the woman may report a brownish vaginal discharge. The cervix is closed. Diagnosis is made based on history, pelvic examination, a negative pregnancy test, and may be confirmed by ultrasound if necessary.

Table 12–4   Less Common Medical Conditions and Pregnancy Cont'd

Condition	Brief description	Maternal implications	Fetal/neonatal implications
		Prophylactic treatment beginning a few weeks prior to delivery is recommended (Noller, 1981a)	
Epilepsy	Chronic disorder characterized by seizures; may be idiopathic or secondary to other conditions such as head injury, metabolic and nutritional disorders such as PKU or vitamin B_6 deficiency, encephalitis, neoplasms, or circulatory interferences	Seizure frequency often increases during pregnancy, with slightly higher incidence of hyperemesis gravidarum, preeclampsia, and vaginal hemorrhage A woman who has been seizure-free for a year should be withdrawn from medication prior to conception; a woman who requires medication has a 90% chance of having a normal child; women who seek advice after the first trimester should be maintained on their medication	Slightly higher incidence of congenital anomalies and perinatal mortality Certain anticonvulsant medications have teratogenic effects
Maternal phenylketonuria (PKU)	Inherited recessive single-gene anomaly (see Chapter 26)	Proper diet is mandatory prior to conception and during pregnancy; the woman should be counseled that her children will either inherit the disease or be carriers depending on the zygosity of the father for the disease	Limited data on the offspring of treated parents; if serum phenylaline levels are normal, excellent chance offspring will be normal In untreated women, increased incidence of mental retardation, congenital heart defects, and other problems
Tuberculosis (TB)	Infection caused by *Mycobacterium tuberculosis;* inflammatory process causes destruction of lung tissue, increased sputum, and coughing; found primarily among persons with poverty and malnutrition and among refugees from countries where TB is prevalent	If TB inactive due to prior treatment, relapse rate no greater than for nonpregnant women Mild cases—medication, extra rest, and limited contact with others recommended Serious cases—if pulmonary surgery such as pneumonectomy or lobectomy are indicated, they are usually tolerated by the fetus	If maternal TB is inactive, mother may breast-feed and care for her infant If TB is active, neonate should not have direct contact with mother until she is noninfectious

If the fetus is retained beyond 6 weeks, fetal autolysis results in the release of thromboplastin and disseminated intravascular coagulation (DIC) may develop.

6. *Habitual abortion.* Abortion occurs consecutively in three or more pregnancies.

□ *DIAGNOSIS* A primary consideration in the differential diagnosis of a bleeding condition is to determine whether vaginal bleeding is related to spontaneous abortion or due to other factors. One of the more reliable indices of evaluation is the presence of pelvic cramping and backache. These symptoms are usually absent in bleeding caused by polyps, ruptured cervical blood vessels, or cervical erosion.

Laboratory evaluations do not provide much help in establishing a diagnosis. If blood loss has been significant, the hemoglobin level will be lowered. Results of pregnancy

Table 12-5   Classification of Spontaneous Abortion (First and Second Trimesters)

Category	Signs and symptoms	Products of conception
Threatened	Vaginal bleeding, cramping, backache	May be partially or totally expelled
Imminent	Vaginal bleeding, cramping, backache, cervical dilatation	Will be partially or totally expelled
Complete	Same as imminent abortion	Totally expelled
Incomplete	Same as imminent abortion	Partially expelled
Missed	Weight loss, decrease in breast size, continued amenorrhea	Remain in utero
Habitual	Loss of three or more successive pregnancies	

tests are not particularly helpful, because they may remain positive for as long as two weeks after fetal death.

□ **INTERVENTIONS** The therapy prescribed for the pregnant woman with bleeding is restriction of activities, bed rest, abstinence from coitus, and perhaps sedation. If bleeding persists and abortion is imminent or incomplete, the patient is hospitalized, intravenous therapy or blood transfusions may be utilized to replace fluid, and dilatation and curettage or suction evacuation is performed to remove the remainder of the products of conception. If the woman is Rh-negative and not sensitized, Rh_o (d) immune globulin (RhoGAM) is given within 72 hours.

In missed abortions, the products of conception eventually are expelled spontaneously. If this does not occur within 1 month to 6 weeks after fetal death, hospitalization is necessary. Suction evacuation or dilatation and curettage is done if the pregnancy is in the first trimester. Beyond 12 weeks' gestation, induction of labor by intravenous oxytocin and prostaglandins may be used to expel the dead fetus.

Habitual abortion can be extremely distressing to the couple desiring a child. For a woman who has already lost a fetus in a previous pregnancy, the crucial time is the month corresponding to the time of the previous abortion. She may become more upset and fearful at that time (Weil,

FIGURE 12-1 Types of spontaneous abortion. **A,** Threatened abortion. **B,** Imminent abortion. **C,** Complete abortion. **D,** Incomplete abortion.

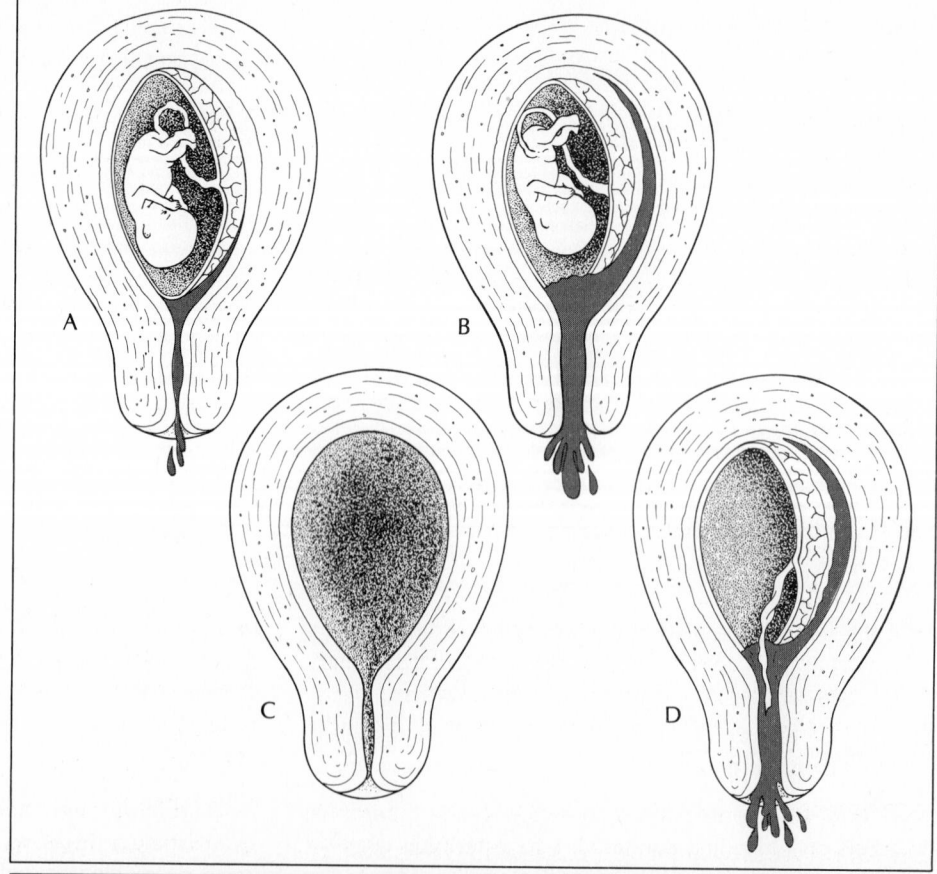

1981). Chances for carrying the next pregnancy to term after one spontaneous abortion are as good as they are for the general population. Chances of successful pregnancy decrease with each succeeding abortion, however. Defective embryo is usually the cause and may be of genetic origin. Bicornuate and septate uterus have been implicated, as have thyroid and nutritional deficiencies. If the cause can be determined, specific therapy can often be implemented to correct it, for example, thyroxine and nutritional supplements or surgery to correct uterine malformation. If an incompetent cervix is the cause of habitual abortion, it can usually be corrected by a surgical procedure (see p. 336), and the woman usually has a successful pregnancy.

The physical pain of the cramps and the amount of bleeding may be more severe than a couple anticipates, even when they are prepared for the possibility of an abortion. Nurses need to be aware that couples feel unprepared for their first experience of spontaneous abortion (Borg and Lasker, 1981). Nurses should offer support in dealing with the physical experience.

Providing emotional support is an important task for nurses caring for women who have aborted. Feelings of shock or disbelief are normal at first. Couples who approached the pregnancy with feelings of joy and a sense of expectancy now feel grief, sadness, and possibly anger. For those who were perhaps less than joyful or even negative about their pregnancy, there may be guilt and blame. The woman may harbor negative feelings about herself, ranging from lowered self-esteem, resulting from a belief that she is lacking or abnormal in some way, to a notion that the abortion may be a punishment for some wrongdoing.

The nurse can offer invaluable psychologic support to the woman and her family by encouraging them to verbalize their feelings, by allowing them the privacy to grieve, and by sympathetically listening to their concerns about this pregnancy and future ones. The nurse can aid in decreasing any feelings of guilt or blame by supplying the woman and her family with information regarding the causes of spontaneous abortion and possibly referring them to other health care professionals for additional help, such as a genetic counselor if there is a history of habitual abortions.

The nurse assesses the responses of the woman and her family to this crisis and evaluates their coping mechanisms and ability to comfort each other. If these are inadequate the family should be referred for additional help. The grieving period following a spontaneous abortion usually lasts 6–24 months (Borg and Lasker, 1981). Many couples can be helped during this period by an organization or support group established for parents who have lost a fetus or newborn.

ECTOPIC PREGNANCY

Ectopic pregnancy is an implantation of the blastocyst in a site other than the endometrial lining of the uterine cavity. It may result from a number of different causes, including tubal damage caused by pelvic inflammatory disease, previous pelvic or tubal surgery, hormonal factors that may impede ovum transport and thus mechanically stops the forward motion of the egg in the fallopian tube, tubal atony or spasms, and blighted conceptus. The actual pathogenesis occurs when such conditions are present and the fertilized ovum is prevented or slowed in its progress down the tube.

The most common type is a tubal pregnancy, in which implantation occurs in a fallopian tube. Other less common types of ectopic pregnancy are abdominal and cervical (Figure 12–2).

Incidence of ectopic pregnancy in the United States ranges from 1 in 80 to 1 in 200 live births (Danforth, 1982).

Initially the normal symptoms of pregnancy may be present, specifically amenorrhea, breast tenderness, and nausea. The hormone hCG is present in the blood and urine. As time passes the woman may experience spotting or irregular bleeding, lower abdominal pain, and faintness. As the pregnancy progresses, the chorionic villi grow into the wall of the tube or site of implantation and a blood supply is established. Thus bleeding occurs when the tube ruptures, causing the characteristic symptoms of sharp pain, syncope, and referred shoulder pain as the abdomen fills with blood.

In many instances, however, the symptoms are less obvious. One-fourth of ectopic pregnancies may involve uterine enlargement (Aladjem, 1980). Physical examination usually reveals adnexal tenderness; an adnexal mass is palpable in approximately one-half of the cases (Danforth, 1982).

If internal hemorrhage is profuse, the woman rapidly develops signs of hypovolemic shock. More commonly the bleeding is slow (chronic), and the abdomen gradually becomes rigid and very tender. If bleeding into the pelvic cavity has been extensive, vaginal examination causes extreme pain and a mass of blood may be palpated in the cul-de-sac of Douglas.

Laboratory tests may reveal low hemoglobin and hematocrit levels and rising leukocyte levels. The hCG titers are lower than in intrauterine pregnancy.

The following procedures are utilized in establishing the diagnosis:

- A careful assessment of menstrual history, particularly the LMP, should be undertaken

- Careful pelvic exam should be performed to identify any abnormal pelvic masses

- Laparoscopy may reveal an extrauterine pregnancy and is especially helpful in the event of an unruptured tubal pregnancy

- Culdoscopy may reveal clotted blood, possibly including an aborted conceptus

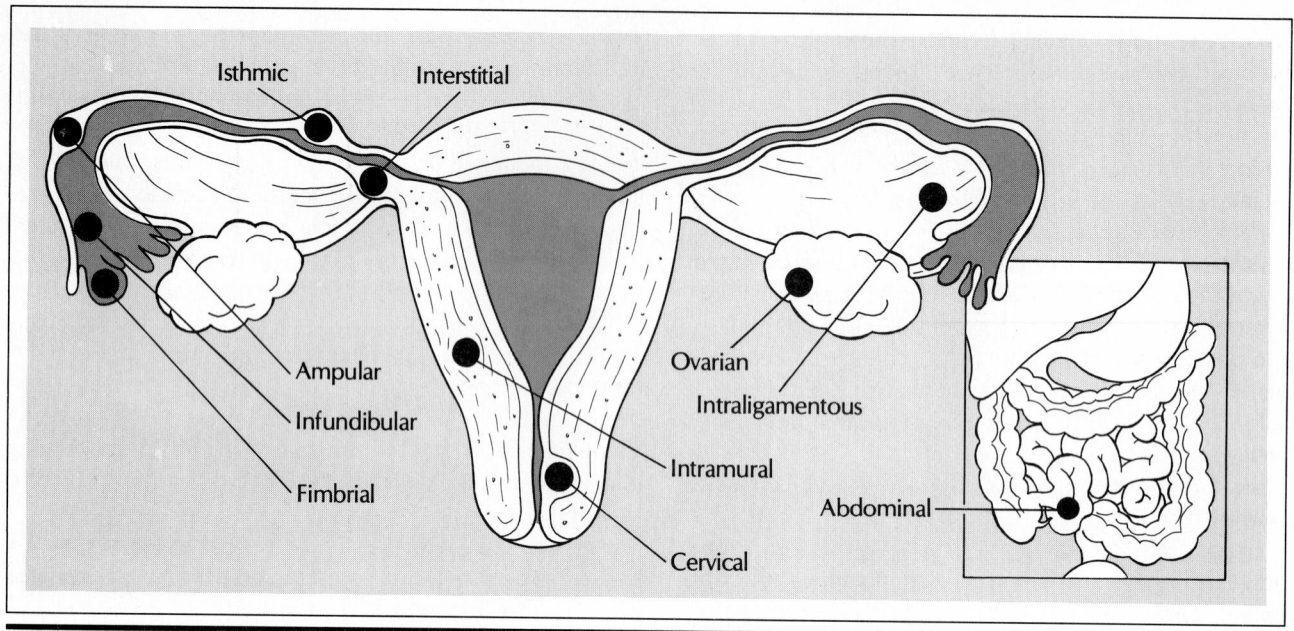

FIGURE 12–2 Various implantation sites in ectopic pregnancy.

- Laparotomy will give a confirmed diagnosis and allow opportunity for immediate treatment

- Ultrasound may be useful in identifying a gestational sac in an unruptured tubal pregnancy, but its most common value is in confirming an intrauterine pregnancy and ruling out an ectopic one

It is important to differentiate an ectopic pregnancy from other disorders with similar clinical presenting pictures. Consideration must be given to possible uterine abortion, ruptured corpus luteum cyst, appendicitis, salpingitis, torsion of the ovary, ovarian cysts, and urinary tract infection.

□ *INTERVENTIONS* Once the diagnosis of ectopic pregnancy has been made, surgical intervention is initiated. Intravenous therapy and blood transfusion are utilized to replace fluid loss. The affected tube and sometimes the ovary are removed surgically. If massive infection is found, a complete removal of uterus, tubes, and ovaries may be necessary. However, every effort is made to leave a normal tube, ovary, and uterus so that childbearing may be a future possibility. If childbearing is a consideration and the woman's contralateral tube has been damaged, salpingostomy (incision into tube to remove pregnancy) may be done. The risk of a subsequent tubal pregnancy is 10%–20% (Danforth, 1982). During surgery, the most important risk to be considered is potential hemorrhage. Bleeding must be controlled, and replacement therapy should be on hand. Blood transfusions may be necessary to allay shock. The Rh-negative nonsensitized woman is given $Rh_0(D)$ immune globulin.

The client and her family will need emotional support during this difficult time. Their feelings and responses to this crisis will probably be similar to those that occur in cases of spontaneous abortion. As a result, similar nursing actions are required for these patients (see p. 332).

HYDATIDIFORM MOLE

Hydatidiform mole is a gestational trophoblastic disease characterized by proliferation of the trophoblastic epithelium and the formation of numerous clear, avascular vesicles derived from the chorionic villi (Danforth, 1982). These vesicles are distended with fluid and form characteristic grapelike clusters. Usually no embryo is present. The cause is unknown (Figure 12–3).

The incidence of hydatidiform mole is 1 in 1500 pregnancies in the United States, but it occurs much more frequently in other countries. For instance, Taiwan has an incidence of 1 in 125, while in Mexico the incidence is 1 in 200 pregnancies. In addition, women who are older than 45 years have more than ten times greater risk of developing hydatidiform mole than women aged 20–40 years (Pritchard and MacDonald, 1980).

Initially the clinical picture is similar to that of pregnancy. Toward the end of the first trimester, however, characteristic signs begin to appear. One of the classic symptoms is vaginal bleeding. The blood may be bright red or brownish ("prune juice") and may last a short time or occur intermittently for weeks. Because of the bleeding, anemia is frequently seen. Uterine size in advance of the length of gestation may occur due to the rapid proliferation of the trophoblastic cells. Because serum hCG levels are significantly higher than would be seen in a normal pregnancy, severe nausea and vomiting are present. Symptoms of PIH prior to 24 weeks' gestation are strongly suggestive of a molar pregnancy. No fetal heart tones are heard, nor can fetal movement be discerned by abdominal palpation.

Clinical results of sonography reveal no fetal skeleton and often show a characteristic molar pattern. However, since similar patterns have been produced by uterine fibroids, a tangential section of a normal placenta, and even by pregnancies with multiple fetuses, the ultrasound should be repeated in 1–2 weeks and carefully evaluated in conjunction with the patient history (Pritchard and MacDonald, 1980).

□ *INTERVENTIONS* In some instances the woman may pass some of the grapelike clusters, and the mole spontaneously aborts. In most instances, however, therapy begins with complete emptying of the uterine cavity by suction curettage, followed by sharp curettage for any remaining fragments. Because of the potential for hemorrhage and the blood previously lost, whole blood should be available and further bleeding controlled with oxytocin. In women of high parity the malignancy rate is approximately 15% and in women over age 40 years the malignancy rate is 35%; consequently, hysterectomy may be appropriate (Danforth, 1982).

Nursing measures must include support for the woman/couple now no longer pregnant. (See Nursing Interventions for Spontaneous Abortion.) Additional counseling regarding future pregnancies may be necessary in light of the fact that a few of these women develop recurring moles or choriocarcinoma, a rare but highly malignant form of cancer for which survival rates of greater than one year are uncommon.

The patient treated for hydatidiform mole should receive follow-up therapy for a year. This consists of weekly measurement of serum hCG levels until they have been negative for 3 weeks; then monthly for 6 months, followed by every 2 months for the next 6 months. Pregnancy is to be avoided for a year because the elevated hCG levels associated with pregnancy would cause confusion as to whether choriocarcinoma had developed. Previously, contraception was accomplished with birth control pills; however, oral contraceptives may delay the fall in hCG levels after evacuation of the mole and thus are being more carefully evaluated (Pritchard and MacDonald, 1980).

Continued high or rising hCG titers are abnormal. If this occurs dilatation and curettage are performed, and tissue is examined. If malignant cells are found, chemotherapy for choriocarcinoma is started, using either methotrexate or dactinomycin. If therapy is ineffective, the choriocarcinoma has a tendency to metastasize rapidly.

If, after a year of supervisory therapy, the hCG serum titers are within normal limits, a couple may be assured that subsequent normal pregnancy can be anticipated with low probability of recurrent hydatidiform mole.

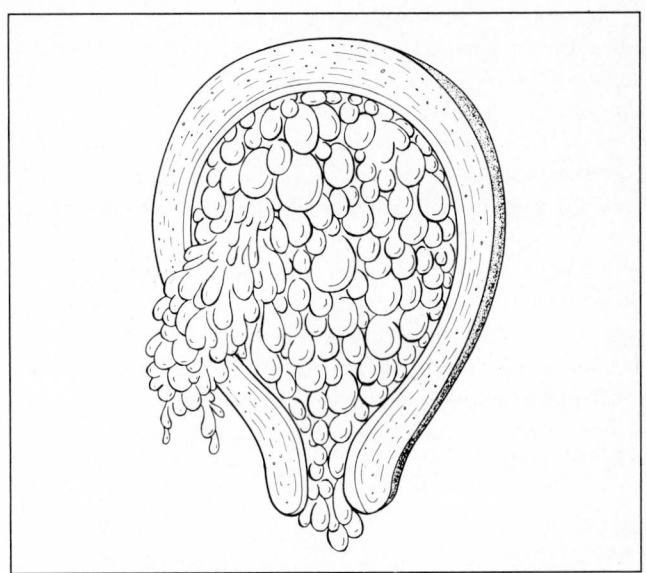

FIGURE 12–3 Hydatidiform mole.

PLACENTA PREVIA

In placenta previa, the placenta is improperly implanted in the lower uterine segment, perhaps on a portion of the lower segment or over the internal os. As the lower uterine segment contracts and the cervix dilates in the later weeks of pregnancy, the placental villi are torn from the uterine wall, thus exposing the uterine sinuses at the placental site. Bleeding begins, but because its amount depends on the number of sinuses exposed, initially it may be either scanty or profuse. The classic symptom is painless vaginal bleeding usually occurring after 20 weeks' gestation. See Chapter 18 for an in-depth discussion of placenta previa.

ABRUPTIO PLACENTAE

Abruptio placentae is the premature separation of the placenta from the uterine wall. It occurs prior to delivery and usually during the labor process. See Chapter 18 for an in-depth description of abruptio placentae.

Incompetent Cervix

Cervical incompetence is associated with repeated second trimester abortions. A possible cause is previous cervical trauma associated with dilatation and curettage, conization, or cauterization or cervical lacerations with previous deliveries (Pritchard and MacDonald, 1980).

Diagnosis is established by eliciting a positive history of repeated, relatively painless and bloodless second trimester abortions. Serial pelvic exams early in the second trimester reveal progressive effacement and dilatation of the cervix and bulging of the membranes through the cervical os.

Incompetent cervix is managed surgically with a Shirodkar-Barter operation (cerclage), or a modification of it by McDonald, which reinforces the weakened cervix by encircling it at the level of the internal os with suture material. A purse-string suture is placed in the cervix between 14 and 18 weeks of gestation. The procedure should not be done if any of the following conditions exist: the diagnosis is in doubt, membranes are ruptured, vaginal bleeding and cramping exists, or the cervix is dilated beyond 3 cm. Some advocate surgical repair of the cervix prior to repeat pregnancy. Once the suture is in place, a cesarean delivery may be planned (to prevent repeating the procedure in subsequent pregnancies), or the suture may be released at term and vaginal delivery permitted. Success rate for carrying the pregnancy to term is approximately 80%.

HYPERTENSIVE DISORDERS IN PREGNANCY

Pregnancy-Induced Hypertension (Preeclampsia and Eclampsia)

Pregnancy-induced hypertension (PIH) is a broad term for a specific category of hypertensive disorder that includes preeclampsia and eclampsia as categories (Willis, 1982). The former term *toxemia of pregnancy* was based on the theory that a toxin produced in the pregnant woman's body caused the hypertension, edema, and proteinuria associated with the disease. This theory has been abandoned, and the term is no longer appropriate.

PIH is characterized by the development of hypertension, excessive weight gain caused by fluid retention resulting in edema, and proteinuria. PIH is seen most often in the last 10 weeks of gestation, during labor, or in the first 12–48 hours after delivery.

The only cure for preeclampsia is termination of the pregnancy. Eclampsia is manifested by development of convulsions and coma in a woman with preeclampsia. If prompt and intensive antepartal care is given to pregnant women, eclampsia may be prevented.

INCIDENCE

PIH occurs in 5%–7% of all pregnancies. For teenagers, young primigravidas, and women of low income the risk of developing PIH is 10%–30% (Gant and Worley, 1980) and for women with chronic hypertension the chances are 25%–35%. Approximately one-third of women who have had PIH will develop it in a subsequent pregnancy. The incidence also increases with advanced maternal age. Because of improved antepartal care, preeclampsia cases have declined considerably in recent years. Eclampsia develops in approximately 5% of women with preeclampsia. With early diagnosis and careful management of the pre-

eclamptic state, the incidence of eclampsia is being reduced to a rarity in the United States. PIH remains, however, the third leading cause of maternal death in the United States.

ETIOLOGY

The cause of PIH is unknown. Many factors are believed to play a role in it. Predisposing factors to the development of PIH include diabetes mellitus, hypertension, renal disease, malnutrition (especially low protein diet), obesity, hydatidiform mole, multiple pregnancy, hydramnios, previous diagnosis of PIH, and a familial tendency to PIH. Women who develop PIH have an increased responsiveness to the vasopressor angiotensin II weeks before any clinical evidence of the disease appears. Women with chronic hypertension who later develop superimposed PIH show this same increased responsiveness (Worley et al., 1979). Circulating angiotensin II levels and plasma renin activity are lower in women with preeclampsia (Willis, 1982).

The cause of edema with PIH is unknown. It is usually the first symptom to appear, although PIH can occur without edema. Hypovolemia results from the plasma volume lost to the interstitial tissue. The role of hypovolemia in the etiology of PIH is controversial. Research indicates that decreased intravascular volume may cause the uterus to release a pressor substance. Others believe that the vasoconstriction precedes the blood volume decrease (Gant and Worley, 1980).

A recent, rather startling finding by Lueck et al. (1983) further clouds the issue of etiology in PIH. They observed multiple forms of a wormlike organism they tentatively named *Hydatoxi lualba* in the blood of women with preeclampsia-eclampsia and women with trophoblastic disease. They also located the organism in the umbilical cord blood of infants born to women with preeclampsia-eclampsia and in contact smears made from the placentas of women with this condition. In a related study Aladjem et al. (1983) were able to induce a preeclampsia-eclampsia-like syndrome in pregnant beagles by inoculating them intraperitoneally with a concentrate developed from the placentas of women with preeclampsia-eclampsia and hydatidiform mole containing the *H. lualba* organism. The researchers state that they recognize the need for confirmation of their findings by other investigators, but the possible implications should such confirmation be made are staggering.

NORMAL PHYSIOLOGY AND PATHOPHYSIOLOGY OF PIH

The vasoconstriction and hypovolemia of PIH are in contrast to the physiologic changes in a normal pregnancy (Figure 12–4). Normally blood volume increases 30%–50% during pregnancy, peripheral vascular resistance decreases, and pregnancy-induced arterial dilatation occurs. The increased blood volume is necessary to perfuse the placenta and the increased tissue mass of uterus and

(Text continues on p. 340.)

NURSING CARE PLAN
Preeclampsia-Eclampsia (PIH)

PATIENT DATA BASE

Nursing history

1. Complete assessment: patient and family
2. Identification of patient's predisposition to preeclampsia-eclampsia
   a. Primigravida
   b. Presence of diabetes mellitus
   c. Multiple pregnancy
   d. Hydramnios
   e. Hydatidiform mole
   f. Preexisting vascular or renal disease
   g. Adolescent or "elderly" gravida

Physical examination

1. Blood pressure — if possible compare with baseline
2. Observe for edema — note weight gain > 1 kg/wk
3. Patient's weight — obtain weekly weight gain if possible
4. Evaluate for hyperreflexia
5. Assess presence of visual disturbances, headache, drowsiness, epigastric pain

Laboratory evaluation

1. Urine for urinary protein: 1 g protein/24 hr = 1-2+; 5 g protein/24 hr = 3-4+
2. Hematocrit: Elevation of hematocrit implies hemoconcentration, which occurs as fluid leaves the intravascular space and enters the extravascular space
3. BUN: Not usually elevated except in patients with cardiovascular renal disease
4. Blood uric acid appears to correlate well with the severity of the preeclampsia-eclampsia (Note: thiazide diuretics can cause significant increases in uric acid levels)

NURSING PRIORITIES

1. Carefully monitor patient's vital signs, urinary output, hyperreflexia
2. Evaluate fetal status
3. Provide support to patient and family
4. Observe for signs of worsening condition:
   a. Increase in BP
   b. Decrease in hourly urine output ≤ 30 mL/hr
   c. Increased drowsiness
   d. Increased hyperreflexia
   e. Development of severe headache
   f. Visual disturbances
   g. Epigastric pain
   h. Convulsion

CLIENT/FAMILY EDUCATIONAL FOCUS

1. Discuss significance of PIH for the health of the woman and her fetus
2. Explain treatment modalities and their rationale
3. Explore possible long-term implications of PIH, such as need for frequent rest, the possible need to stop working if the woman is employed, and the possibility of hospitalization
4. Provide opportunities to discuss questions and individual concerns of the woman and her family

NURSING CARE PLAN Cont'd
Preeclampsia-Eclampsia (PIH)

Problem	Nursing interventions and actions	Rationale
Water retention	Weigh patient daily; gain of 1 kg/wk or more in second trimester or ½ kg/wk or more in third trimester is suggestive of PIH	Weight gain and evidence of edema are due to sodium and water retention
	Assess edema (Danforth, 1982) + (1 +) Minimal; slight edema of pedal and pretibial areas + + (2 +) Marked edema of lower extremities + + + (3 +) Edema of hands, face, lower abdominal wall, and sacrum + + + + (4 +) Anasarca with ascites	Decreased renal plasma flow and glomerular filtration contribute to retention; actual mechanisms are not clear
	Maintain patient on bed rest	Bed rest produces an increase in GFR
	Maintain normal salt intake (4–6 g/24 hr)	Normal salt intake is now advised, but excessive salt intake may cause the condition to become more severe
Hypertension	Assess BP every 1–4 hr, using same arm, with patient in same position	Blood pressure can fluctuate hourly; BP increases as a result of increased peripheral resistance due to peripheral vasoconstriction and arteriolar spasm Diastolic pressure is a better indicator of severity of condition
Proteinuria	Obtain clean voided urine specimen	Urine contaminated with vaginal discharge or red cells may test positive for protein
	Test urine for proteinuria, hourly and/or daily	Helps evaluate severity and progression of preeclampsia Proteinuria results from swelling of the endothelium of the glomerular capillaries Escape of protein is enhanced by vasospasm in afferent arterioles
Decreased urine output	Insert indwelling catheter	Catheter facilitates hourly urine assessment Renal plasma flow and glomerular filtration are decreased
	Determine hourly urine output; notify physician if urine output ≤ 30 mL/hr	Increasing oliguria signifies a worsening condition
Inadequate protein intake	Provide adequate protein: 1.5 g/kg/24 hr for incipient and mild preeclampsia	Plasma proteins affect movement of intravascular and extravascular fluids
	Patients with severe preeclampsia will be NPO ("nothing by mouth")	
Hyperreflexia	Assess knee, ankle, and biceps reflexes	Assessing reflexes helps determine level of muscle and nerve irritability
	Promote bed rest; allow patient to rest quietly in a darkened, quiet room Limit visitors	Rest reduces external stimuli
	Administer sedation as ordered (diazepam or phenobarbital orally or IM)	Sedation is frequently ordered
	Administer magnesium sulfate per physician order: 1. IM dose: 5–10 g of 50% solution every 4–6 hours	Magnesium sulfate is cerebral depressant; it also reduces neuromuscular irritability and causes vasodilatation and drop in BP Therapeutic blood level is 6–8 mg/dL

NURSING CARE PLAN Cont'd
Preeclampsia-Eclampsia (PIH)

Problem	Nursing interventions and actions	Rationale
	2. IV dose: 20 mL of 10% solution or as continuous infusion at a rate of 1 g/hr	
	Before administering subsequent doses of magnesium sulfate, check reflexes (knee, ankle, biceps)	Knee jerk disappears when magnesium sulfate blood levels are > 10 mg/dL
		Toxic signs and symptoms develop with increased blood levels; respiratory arrest can be associated with blood levels of 12–15 mg/dL
	Check respirations and measure urine output	Cardiac arrest can occur if blood levels are 15 mg/dL
	Do not give magnesium sulfate if:	
	1. Reflexes are absent	
	2. Respirations are < 14–16/min	
	3. <100 mL urine output in past 4 hours	Kidneys are only route for excretion of magnesium sulfate
	Have calcium gluconate available	Calcium gluconate is antidote for magnesium sulfate
Convulsions	Provide supportive care during convulsion:	
	1. Place tongue blade or airway in patient's mouth, if can be done without force	Acts to maintain airway and to prevent patient from biting tongue
	2. Suction nasopharynx as necessary	Removes mucus and secretions
	3. Administer oxygen	Promotes oxygenation
	4. Note type of seizure and length of time it lasts	
	After seizure, assess for uterine contractions	Precipitous labor may start during seizures
	Assess fetal status	Continuous fetal monitoring is necessary to identify fetal stress
	Maintain seizure precautions:	
	1. Quiet, darkened room	Quiet reduces stimuli
	2. Have emergency equipment available—O_2, suction, padded tongue blade	
	3. Pad side rails	Padding protects patient
Increased fetal morbidity and mortality	Assess fetal status; monitor fetal heart tones every 4 hours if patient has mild eclampsia	Evaluates fetal status
	Patient with severe preeclampsia-eclampsia requires continuous fetal monitoring	
Increased risk of abruptio placentae	Assess for signs of abruptio placenate:	40%–60% of women with abruptio placentae have preeclampsia; in patients with severe preeclampsia-eclampsia, abruption occurs in 10%–15% of the cases (Danforth, 1982)
	1. Vaginal bleeding	
	2. Uterine tenderness	
	3. Change in fetal activity	
	4. Change in fetal heart rate	
	5. Sustained abdominal pain	

NURSING CARE EVALUATION

Infant delivered	Woman independent in activities of daily living
Blood pressure within normal range	Mother able to care for infant
Absence of protein in urine	Mother understands and can verbalize course of condition, diet and medication instructions, infant care, and symptoms to report to physician (Davidson et al., 1977)
Symptoms of preeclampsia-eclampsia resolved or controlled	

NURSING CARE PLAN Cont'd
Preeclampsia-Eclampsia (PIH)

NURSING DIAGNOSIS*	SUPPORTING DATA
1. Fluid volume excess related to sodium and water retention	Daily weight gain Peripheral edema Hypertension Ascites Anasarca
2. Potential fluid volume deficit (intravascular) related to protein loss	Proteinuria Oliguria
3. Potential for maternal injury	Convulsions, abruptio placentae
4. Knowledge deficit about the condition and its treatment	Expressed concerns or questions about the effects of preeclampsia-eclampsia (PIH)

*These are a few examples of nursing diagnoses that may be appropriate for a person with this condition. It is not an inclusive list and must be individualized for each woman.

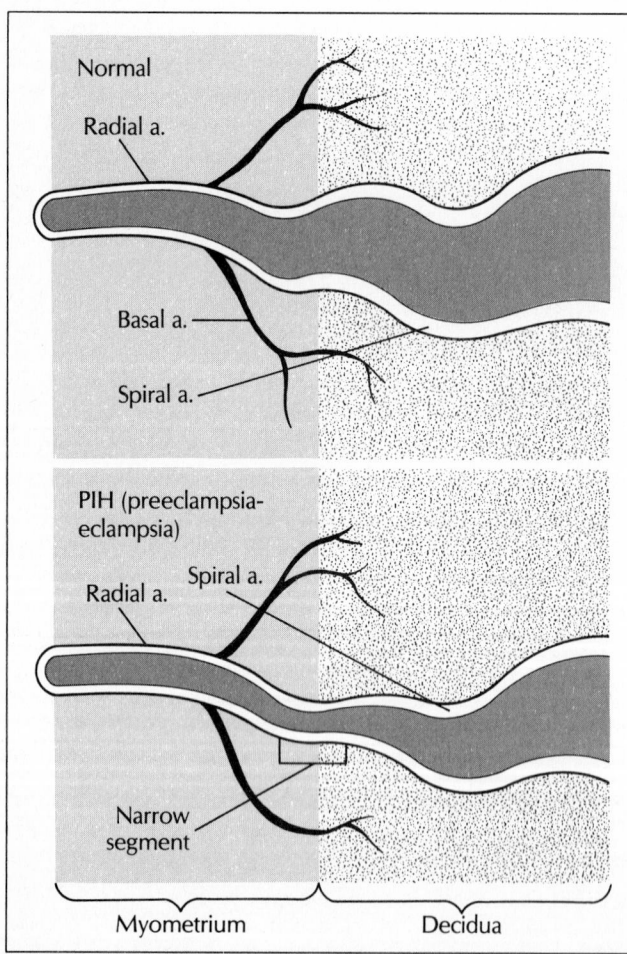

FIGURE 12–4 In normal pregnancy the passive quality of the spiral arteries permits increased blood flow to the placenta. In preeclampsia vasoconstriction of the myometrial segment of the spiral arteries occurs.

breasts. The higher blood volume also helps protect the fetus from impaired circulation due to maternal supine position, and it compensates for blood loss during delivery. The lowered peripheral vascular resistance results in slightly lower blood pressure from the middle of the first trimester through the second trimester, slowly returning to the woman's normal blood pressure during the third trimester.

The cause of normal hypervolemia of pregnancy is not clear. Increase in plasma renin levels stimulates secretion of aldosterone, which aids in reabsorption of sodium. Sodium retention increases total body water levels, a normal finding in pregnancy. Angiotensin II also stimulates production of aldosterone and is a potent vasopressor. Normally in pregnancy the smooth muscles of the blood vessels do not contract in response to the vasopressor. The glomerular filtration rate (GFR), which normally increases up to 50% in pregnancy, is reduced in PIH, although not to a rate as low as the prepregnant rate. Normally, during pregnancy creatinine, urea, and uric acid are cleared more quickly due to increased GFR, which results in lower serum and increased urine levels of these chemicals.

In PIH the reverse is true. Increased serum levels of uric acid are associated with poor fetal outcome. In addition serum proteins (albumin and globulin) are lost to the urine due to renal glomerular lesion or renal vascular spasm. Sodium reabsorption remains high and water is retained. Decreased urinary output (oliguria) results from decreased renal blood flow and decreased GFR.

Changes in clotting factors have been associated with PIH. Fibrinolytic activity normally is decreased during pregnancy but increases immediately after delivery. In some women with PIH, fibrinolytic activity remains low even 24 hours postpartum (Condie, 1976). Decreased platelet count, chronic intravascular coagulation, and fibrin deposits in small blood vessels leading to microangiopathic hemolytic anemia have all been described in connection with PIH. Controversy exists about the exact relation of these findings to the disease.

Effects of PIH on the CNS cause blurred vision, scotomata (blind spots), headache, and hyperreflexia. Vasospasm of the retina account for the visual changes. Headaches are usually frontal and occipital and may be constant. Vasospasm of the cerebral vessels is also responsible for the headaches. Pathophysiology of CNS hyperactivity is uncertain. Cerebral edema is usually cited as a causative factor. Hyperreflexia may be due to increased intracellular sodium and decreased intracellular potassium levels. Convulsions may result from vasoconstriction and cerebral ischemia (Chesley, 1978).

CLINICAL MANIFESTATIONS

Mild preeclampsia. Preeclampsia may be mild or severe. Women with mild preeclampsia may exhibit an almost asymptomatic pregnancy. Little or no peripheral edema may be evident following bed rest. Their blood pressure may be 140/90 or more, or about 30 mm Hg above their baseline systolic pressure and 15 mm Hg above their baseline diastolic pressure. The elevated blood pressure is noted on two separate readings at least 6 hours apart. This is an important consideration, because a young woman who may normally manifest a blood pressure of 90/60 would be hypertensive at 120/80, which is a marked increase above her baseline norm. Therefore, an essential part of the nursing assessment is to obtain a baseline blood pressure in early pregnancy. Urine testing may show a +1 or +2 albumin in a clean midstream specimen, and a 24-hour collection may contain 500 mg or more of protein. Proteinuria is a late development, the last of the three cardinal signs of preeclampsia to appear.

Severe preeclampsia. Severe preeclampsia may develop suddenly. Edema becomes generalized and readily apparent in face, hands, sacral area, lower extremities, and the abdominal wall. Edema is assessed on a 1+ to 4+ scale (see p. 338). Edema is also characterized by an excessive weight gain of more than 0.9 kg (2 lb) over a period of a couple of days to a week. Blood pressure is 160/100 or higher, a dipstick albumin measurement is +3 to +4, and the 24-hour urine protein is greater than 5 g. Hematocrit, blood urea nitrogen (BUN), serum creatinine, and uric acid levels are elevated. Other characteristic symptoms are frontal headaches, blurred vision, scotomata, nausea, vomiting, irritability, hyperreflexia, cerebral disturbances, oliguria (less than 400 mL of urine in 24 hours), pulmonary edema or cyanosis, and finally, epigastric pain. The epigastric pain is often the sign of impending convulsion (eclampsia) and is thought to be caused by increased vascular engorgement of the liver.

Eclampsia. The grand mal seizure of eclampsia may be preceded by an elevated temperature as high as 38.4C

(101.0F), or the temperature may remain normal. If the temperature spikes as high as 39.4C–40.0C (103F–104F), it is a very serious sign. The seizure begins with facial twitching. The woman's eyes usually are wide open and staring, with dilated pupils. The convulsion has three phases. The first phase is a tonic phase. All the woman's muscles contract, her back arches, arms and legs stiffen, and her jaw snaps shut, sometimes causing her to bite her tongue. Her respirations cease due to thoracic muscles held in contraction, and she becomes cyanotic. The tonic phase lasts 15–20 seconds, then the woman enters the clonic phase. Alternating forceful contraction and relaxation of all muscles causes the woman to thrash about wildly. She may remain apneic, or inhale and exhale irregularly as thoracic muscles contract and relax. Saliva and blood collected in her mouth may foam out. She remains cyanotic. Incontinence of urine and feces may occur. After about a minute the convulsive movements gradually cease and she slips into the third phase, a motionless coma which may last for less than an hour or for several hours. Respirations increase up to 50/min, and may be noisy and forceful. If the woman is not treated, the coma phase may be quite brief, and convulsions may recur in a few minutes.

Some women experience only one convulsion, especially if it occurs late in labor or during the postpartal period. Others may have from two to twenty or more. Unless they occur extremely frequently, the woman often regains consciousness between convulsions.

FETAL–NEONATAL IMPLICATIONS

Infants of women with hypertension during pregnancy tend to be SGA. The cause is related specifically to maternal vasospasm and hypovolemia, which result in fetal hypoxia and malnutrition. Decrease in fetal weight gain associated with maternal hypertension was found in one study to be more pronounced when the women were thin and had low pregnancy weight gains (Naeye, 1981). In addition, the neonate may be premature because of the necessity for early delivery.

Perinatal mortality associated with preeclampsia is approximately 10%, and that associated with eclampsia is 20%. When preeclampsia is superimposed on hypertensive vascular disease, the perinatal mortality may be higher.

At the time of delivery, the neonate may be oversedated because of medications administered to the woman, and may also have hypermagnesemia due to treatment of the woman with large doses of magnesium sulfate.

Fetal Assessment. Tests to evaluate fetal status are done more frequently as a pregnant woman's PIH progresses. Monitoring fetal well-being is essential to achieving a safe outcome for the fetus. The following tests are used:

• Fetal movement

• Nonstress test

- Ultrasonography for serial determination of growth
- Contraction stress test
- Estriol and creatinine determinations
- Amniocentesis to determine fetal lung maturity

These tests are described in detail in Chapter 13.

INTERVENTIONS—MILD PREECLAMPSIA

Blood pressure. The client's baseline blood pressure and number of weeks of gestation must be determined early in prenatal care. Arterial blood pressure varies with position, being highest when the client is sitting, intermediate when she is supine, and lowest when she is in the left lateral recumbent position. Therefore it is important that the client be in the same position each visit when the blood pressure is measured. For accuracy the cuff must be the proper size, the same arm should be used for comparison, and the blood pressure reading should be taken at approximately the same time of day. Both phases IV and V of Korotkoff's sounds (muffling and disappearance) should be recorded, because phase V is very low in many pregnant women.

Blood pressure is taken and recorded each antepartal visit. If the blood pressure rises or even if the normal slight decrease in blood pressure expected between 8 and 28 weeks of pregnancy is not manifest, the client should be followed more closely.

Roll-over test. Between 28 and 32 weeks of gestation the roll-over test may be used for selected primigravidas thought to be at risk for PIH. The client lies in the left lateral recumbent position for 15–20 minutes while her blood pressure stabilizes (evidenced by two successive readings of the same diastolic pressure). Then the woman is turned to the supine position, and her blood pressure is taken immediately and again in 5 minutes.

If the diastolic pressure rises 20 mm Hg or more in the supine position, it is considered a strong indication that the client will develop PIH. However, the roll-over test is no longer done as routinely as it once was, because it has not proven to have reliable predictive value, and because of the time involved in taking the test.

Diet and diuretics. Weight restriction, low-salt diet, and diuretics are no longer recommended in managing PIH. Low maternal weight gain is detrimental to the fetus. Sodium restriction and diuretics may worsen the situation, because the body fluid lost decreases blood volume further and thereby decreases placental perfusion. Exceptions may be made if there is preexisting cardiac or renal disease.

Women with mild preeclampsia or women at risk for PIH are advised to follow a high-protein diet to replace proteins lost in the urine. Salt intake should be moderate (2.5–7.0 g/day). Since many Americans consume a high-sodium diet, this would mean avoiding foods such as potato chips, bacon, luncheon meats, hot dogs, pork rind, pret-zels, peanuts, and the like. Salt intake should not be restricted below 2–4 g (Willis and Sharp, 1982). Fluid intake of 6 to 8 glasses of water per day is recommended. Pushing fluids or restricting fluid intake has not been found advantageous.

Lateral recumbent position. Bed rest in the left lateral recumbent position has been found to be beneficial to women with PIH. The supine position compresses both the inferior vena cava and the aorta, diminishing blood supply to the gravid uterus. Renal arteries are also compressed in the supine position, decreasing blood flow to the kidneys. In the erect position the heavy uterus puts pressure on the iliac veins, pooling blood in the legs, which decreases central blood volume and uterine and renal supply. In some women, the right lateral recumbent position applies pressure on the inferior vena cava and on the right ureter. In the left lateral recumbent position, however, renal plasma flow, GFR, and placental perfusion are increased. Bed rest orders need not be complete, but if the condition worsens the amount of time spent in bed must increase. Drastic reduction in physical activity is beneficial (Gant and Worley, 1980).

Support and teaching. Four major areas of concern exist for a woman with a high-risk pregnancy (Weil, 1981). The first is fear of losing the fetus. Sex relations are another concern: she and her partner may be afraid to have intercourse for fear it might harm the baby. They may feel resentment because of this fear. A third worry concerns finances—health insurance does not always cover all the tests, the prolonged hospitalization and so on that may be associated with complications during pregnancy. Finally, the woman's partner may not understand her need for bed rest and may become resentful or feel neglected. The couple's normal social life is interrupted. The woman may become depressed or resentful about being left alone or may feel bored. She may resist having to ask people to do simple things for her. If she has small children she will have difficulty providing for their care. The woman who does not have children may worry that she never will.

The nurse should identify and discuss each of these areas with the couple. It is necessary to explain to them the reasons for bed rest. A woman with mild preeclampsia may feel very well and be unable to see the need for resting even a few hours a day. The nurse can refer them to many community resources such as homemaking services, a support group for the partner, or a hot-line. Arrangements may be made for the partner to attend childbirth classes if both are not able to, or a nurse may be found to teach the classes privately. In addition, the woman needs to know which symptoms are significant and should be reported at once. Usually the woman with mild preeclampsia is seen every 2 weeks, but she may need to come in earlier if symptoms indicate the condition is progressing. She must understand her diet plan, which must match her culture, finances, and life-style.

INTERVENTIONS—SEVERE PREECLAMPSIA

If the preeclampsia progresses to the severe stage, hospitalization is essential. The goal of care is to prevent convulsions by decreasing blood pressure and establishing adequate renal function, and to continue pregnancy until the fetus is mature. If the pregnancy is 36 weeks' gestation or more and fetal lung maturity is confirmed, labor is induced. If labor is unsuccessful, delivery is by cesarean birth. When the pregnancy is less than 36 weeks' gestation or when L/S ratio indicates immaturity, interventions are aimed at alleviating maternal symptoms to allow the fetus to mature.

□ ASSESSMENT

Blood pressure. Blood pressure should be determined every 2–4 hours, more frequently if indicated by medication or other changes in patient status.

Temperature. Temperature should be determined every 4 hours; every 2 hours if elevated.

Pulse and respirations. Respiration and pulse rates should be determined along with blood pressure.

Fetal heart rate. The fetal heart rate should be determined with the blood pressure or monitored continuously with the electronic fetal monitor if the situation indicates.

Urinary output. Every voiding should be measured. Frequently, the patient will have an indwelling catheter. In this case, hourly urine output can be assessed. Output should be 700 mL or greater in 24 hours or at least 30 mL per hour.

Urine protein. Urinary protein is determined hourly if an indwelling catheter is in place or with each voiding. Readings of 3+ or 4+ indicate loss of 5 g or more of protein in 24 hours.

Urine specific gravity. Specific gravity of the urine should be determined hourly or with each voiding. Readings over 1.040 correlate with oliguria and proteinuria.

Edema. The face (especially eyelids and cheekbone area), fingers, hands, arms (ulnar surface and wrist), legs (tibial surface), ankles, feet, and sacral area are inspected and palpated for edema. The degree of pitting is determined by pressing over bony areas.

Weight. The patient is weighed daily at the same time, wearing the same robe or gown and slippers. Weighing may be omitted if the woman is to maintain strict bed rest.

Pulmonary edema. The patient is observed for coughing. The lungs are auscultated for moist respirations.

Deep tendon reflexes. The patient is assessed for evidence of hyperreflexia in the brachial, wrist, patellar, or Achilles tendons (Table 12–6). The patellar reflex is the easiest to assess. Clonus should also be assessed by vigorously dorsiflexing the foot while the knee is held in a fixed position. Normally no clonus is present. If it is present, it is measured as 1–4 beats and is recorded as such.

Placental separation. The patient should be assessed hourly for vaginal bleeding and/or uterine rigidity.

Table 12–6 Deep Tendon Reflex Rating Scale

Rating	Assessment
4+	Hyperactive; very brisk, jerky or clonic response; abnormal
3+	Brisker than average; may not be abnormal
2+	Average response; normal
1+	Diminished response; low normal
0	No response; abnormal

Headache. The patient should be questioned about the existence and location of any headache.

Visual disturbance. The patient should be questioned about any visual blurring or changes, or scotomata. The results of the daily fundoscopic exam should be recorded on the chart.

Laboratory blood tests. Daily tests of hematocrit to measure hemoconcentration; blood urea nitrogen, creatinine, and uric acid levels to assess kidney function; serum estriol determinations to assess fetal status; clotting studies for any indication of thrombocytopenia or DIC, and electrolyte levels for deficiencies are all indicated.

Level of consciousness. The patient is observed for alertness, mood changes, and any signs of impending convulsion or coma.

Emotional response and level of understanding. The patient's emotional response should be carefully assessed, so that support and teaching can be planned accordingly.

□ THERAPY

Bed rest. Bed rest must be complete. Stimuli that may bring on a convulsion should be reduced. The client should be placed in a private room in a quiet location but where she can be watched closely. Visitors should be limited to close family or main support persons. The woman should maintain the left lateral recumbent position most of the time, with side rails up for her protection. She should not receive phone calls because the phone ringing may be too jarring.

Diet. A high-protein, moderate-sodium diet is given as long as the client is alert and has no nausea or indication of impending convulsion.

Fluid and electrolyte replacement. The goal of fluid intake is to achieve a balance between correcting hypovolemia and preventing circulatory overload. Fluid intake may be oral or supplemented with intravenous therapy. Intravenous fluids may be started "to keep lines open" in case they are needed for drug therapy even when oral intake is adequate. The amount of fluid intake should be 1000 mL plus the amount of urinary output of the previous 24 hours (Cavanagh and Knuppel, 1981). Criteria vary for determining appropriate fluid intake. Electrolytes are replaced as indicated by daily serum electrolyte levels.

Medication. A sedative, such as diazepam (Valium) or phenobarbitol is sometimes given to encourage resting quietly in bed.

Antihypertensives. The drug of choice is the vasodilator hydralazine (Apresoline) (Gant and Worley, 1980). It effectively lowers blood pressure without adverse fetal effects. Hydralazine generally is given when the diastolic pressure is higher than 110 mm Hg. It may be administered either by slow intravenous push or drip methods. Hydralazine produces tachycardia; therefore the patient's pulse must be monitored with the blood pressure when the client is receiving hydralazine. Measure blood pressure every 2–3 minutes after the initial dose, and every 5–10 minutes thereafter. The diastolic pressure reading is maintained at 90–100 mm Hg to ensure adequate uteroplacental flow. The fetal heart tones are monitored continuously during hydralazine therapy. Hydralazine is not intended for long-term use.

Anticonvulsants. Magnesium sulfate ($MgSO_4$) is the treatment of choice for convulsions. Its CNS-depressant action reduces possibility of convulsion. Blood levels of $MgSO_4$ should be maintained between 4.0 and 7.5 mg/dL. Excessive blood levels should be avoided because at 10 mg/dL deep tendon reflexes fade, at 15 mg/dL respiratory paralysis and/or cardiac arrest occurs. (See Drug Guide for magnesium sulfate.)

Teaching and support. The development of severe preeclampsia is a cause for increased concern to the patient and her family. Increased stress can elevate blood pressure. A nursing goal is to decrease anxiety and provide an atmosphere of confidence and calm. The patient and her partner's most immediate concerns usually are about the prognosis for herself and the fetus. The nurse can offer honest and hopeful information. She can explain the plan of therapy and the reasons for procedures to the extent that the woman or her partner are interested. Understanding the reason for a procedure such as complete bed rest increases compliance. The nurse should keep the couple informed of the fetal status. Eye contact, voice, and manner can show that the nurse cares and can encourage them to express feelings and ask questions. The woman might worry or feel guilty, thinking that she may have brought on the preeclampsia. Concerns about family at home or financial concerns and questions about the length of her hospital stay may also be expressed. The nurse provides as much information as possible and seeks other sources of information or aid for the family as needed. Nurses can offer to contact a minister or hospital chaplain for additional support.

INTERVENTIONS—ECLAMPSIA

The occurrence of a convulsion is frightening to any family members who may be present, although the woman will not be able to recall it when she becomes conscious. Therefore, offering explanations to the family member while caring for the patient, and to the woman herself later, is essential.

When the tonic phase of the contraction begins, the woman should be turned to her side if she is not already in that position to aid circulation to the placenta. Her head should be turned face down to allow saliva to drain from her mouth. Attempting to insert a padded tongue blade has been questioned, but if it can be done without force, injury may be prevented to the patient's mouth. The side rails should be padded, or a pillow put between the woman and each side rail.

After 15–20 seconds the clonic phase starts. When the thrashing subsides, intensive monitoring and therapy begin. An oral airway is inserted, the woman's nasopharynx is suctioned, and oxygen administration is begun by nasal catheter. Fetal heart tones are monitored continuously. Maternal vital signs are monitored every 5 minutes until they are stable, then every 15 minutes. Magnesium sulfate is given intravenously. Diazepam is also used by some clinicians, but because of the depressant effect on the fetus, it should not be given when delivery is expected within an hour or two.

The lungs are auscultated for pulmonary edema. The woman is watched for circulatory and renal failure and for signs of cerebral hemorrhage. Furosemide (Lasix) may be given for pulmonary edema, digitalis for circulatory failure. Urinary output is monitored. The patient is observed for signs of placental separation, first evidenced by decreasing fetal heart rate. She should be checked every 15 minutes for vaginal bleeding, which may or may not be present with abruptio placentae. The abdomen is palpated for uterine rigidity. While she is still unconscious, the patient should be observed for onset of labor. Convulsions increase uterine irritability and labor may ensue. While the woman is comatose, she is kept on her side with the side rails up.

Invasive hemodynamic monitoring may be instituted, either central venous pressure (CVP) or pulmonary artery wedge pressure (PAWP) using a Swan-Ganz catheter. Both these procedures carry risk to the client and the decision to use them should be made judiciously.

When the patient's vital signs have stabilized, urinary output is good, and the maternal and fetal hypoxic and acidotic state alleviated, delivery of the fetus should be considered. Delivery is the only known cure for PIH. If the neonate will be preterm, it may be necessary to transfer the patient to a perinatal center for delivery. The woman and her partner deserve careful explanation about the status of the fetus and the woman, and the treatment they are receiving. Plans for delivery and further treatment must be discussed with them.

LABOR AND DELIVERY

The plan of care for the woman with PIH in labor depends on both maternal and fetal condition. The patient may

DRUG GUIDE Magnesium Sulfate (MgSO₄)

OVERVIEW OF OBSTETRIC ACTION

MgSO₄ acts as a CNS depressant by decreasing the quantity of acetylcholine released by motor nerve impulses and thereby blocking neuromuscular transmission. This action reduces the possibility of convulsion; this is why MgSO₄ is used in the treatment of preeclampsia. Because magnesium sulfate secondarily relaxes smooth muscle it may decrease the blood pressure, although it is not considered an antihypertensive, and may also decrease the frequency and intensity of uterine contractions.

ROUTE, DOSAGE, FREQUENCY

MgSO₄ may be given intramuscularly (IM) or intravenously (IV).

IV: The intravenous route allows for immediate onset of action and avoids the discomfort associated with IM administration. It must be given by an infusion pump for accurate dosage.
Loading dose
250 mL D₅W (5% dextrose in water) with 4 g MgSO₄ is administered over 20 minutes.
Maintenance dose
Based on serum magnesium levels and deep tendon reflexes, 1–3 g/hr is administered (Berkowitz et al., 1981).

IM: Initial loading dose involves 10 g in 50% solution divided into two injections and administered into each buttock (deep IM) in conjunction with the 4 g IV loading dose just described.
Maintenance dose
5 g every 4 hours in 50% solution is administered if deep tendon reflexes, respirations, and urine output are satisfactory. This route is very painful and avoided whenever possible.

Maternal contraindications

Extreme care is necessary in administration to women with impaired renal function because the drug is eliminated by the kidneys and toxic magnesium levels may develop.

Maternal side effects

Sweating, flushing, depression or absence of reflexes, hypothermia, muscle weakness, oliguria, confusion, circulatory collapse, and respiratory paralysis are all possible side effects. Rapid administration of large doses may cause cardiac arrest.

Effects on fetus/neonate

The drug readily crosses the placenta. Hypermagnesia in the newborn may have contributed to low Apgar scores and symptoms of lethargy, hypotonia, and weakness (Berkowitz et al., 1981).

NURSING CONSIDERATIONS

1. Monitor blood pressure continuously with IV administration and every 15 minutes with IM administration.

2. Monitor respirations closely. If the rate is less than 14–16/min, magnesium toxicity may be developing and further assessments are indicated.

3. Assess knee jerk (patellar tendon reflex) for evidence of diminished or absent reflexes.

4. Determine urinary output. Output less than 30 mL/hr may result in the accumulation of toxic levels of magnesium.

5. If the respirations or urinary output fall below specified levels or if the reflexes are diminished or absent, no further magnesium should be administered until these factors return to normal.

6. The antagonist of magnesium sulfate is calcium. Consequently an ampule of calcium gluconate should be available at the bedside. The usual dose is 10 mL of a 10% solution given IV over a period of about 3 minutes.

7. IM administration of MgSO₄ is painful and irritating. Therefore it is given deep into the gluteal muscle with 1% procaine to reduce the pain. The dose is divided between both buttocks and given Z-track with a long needle (Wheeler and Jones, 1981) or by circular rotation with the area massaged well afterwards.

8. Monitor fetal heart tones continuously with IV administration.

9. Continue MgSO₄ infusion for approximately 24 hours after delivery as prophylaxis against postpartum seizures.

have mild or severe preeclampsia, may become eclamptic during labor, or may have been eclamptic prior to the onset of labor. Therefore, careful monitoring of blood pressure and checking for edema and protein-urea levels are necessary for all women in labor. The prenatal record should be obtained so that current blood pressure readings may be compared with the baseline reading. If PIH was previously diagnosed, the labor may be induced by intravenous oxytocin when there is evidence of fetal maturity and cervical readiness. In very severe cases, cesarean delivery may be necessary regardless of fetal maturity.

A family member should be encouraged to stay with the woman as long as possible throughout labor and delivery. This is especially needed if the woman has been transferred to a high-risk center from another facility. The patient in labor and the family member or support person should be oriented to the new surroundings and kept informed of progress and plan of care. The woman should be cared for by the same nurses throughout her hospital stay.

The laboring woman with PIH must receive all the care and precautions needed for normal labor as well as those required for managing PIH. The patient may receive both intravenous oxytocin and MgSO₄ simultaneously. The woman in labor who develops a blood pressure higher than 160/110 may be given MgSO₄ intravenously (see Interventions—Severe Preeclampsia, p. 343). Because MgSO₄ has depressant action on smooth muscle, uterine contractions may diminish and labor may be augmented with oxytocin. Another method of inducing labor in the woman with PIH is to administer oxytocin intravenously and then during the course of labor give intravenous MgSO₄. Equipment and intravenous lines for both fluids must be checked frequently to ensure that they are being administered at the proper rate. Infusion pumps should be used to guarantee accuracy. Bottles and tubing must be labeled carefully. In addition, Barocca C, a yellow dye, may be added to the bottle or bag containing oxytocin (Kelly and Mongiello, 1982b). The yellow color will decrease the chance of confusion between the two bottles and fluid lines.

The woman with PIH in labor is kept in the left lateral recumbent position for most of labor, turning to right side only when needed. As mentioned earlier, the aorta and inferior vena cava are compressed when the woman is in the supine position.

Both woman and fetus are monitored carefully throughout labor. Signs of progressing labor are noted. In addition, the nurse must be alert for indications of worsening PIH, placental separation, pulmonary edema, circulatory renal failure, and fetal distress; all are more likely in a woman with PIH than in the normotensive client.

During the second stage of labor the woman is encouraged to push while lying on her side. If she is unable to do so comfortably or effectively, she can be helped to a semi-sitting position for pushing and to resume the lateral posi-

tion between each contraction. Delivery in Sims's or semi-sitting position should be considered. If lithotomy position is elected, a wedge should be placed under the right buttock to displace the uterus. If delivery is by cesarean birth due to fetal distress, a wedge under the woman's right buttock is indicated (Kelly and Mongiello, 1982a). During labor, oxygen is administered to the woman as indicated by fetal response to contractions.

Administration of anesthesia and analgesia during labor and delivery of the hypertensive client is an area of controversy. Pritchard and MacDonald (1980) recommend meperidine (Demerol) for labor. They and others recommend pudendal block rather than epidural anesthesia for delivery, because an epidural has hypotensive effects that may further decrease placental perfusion. A pediatrician and/or anesthesiologist must be available to care for the neonate on delivery. They must be aware of all amounts and times of medication the woman has received during labor.

POSTPARTUM

The woman with PIH usually improves rapidly after delivery, although seizures can still occur during the first 48 hours postpartum. For this reason, when the hypertension is severe the patient may continue to receive hydralazine or magnesium sulfate postpartally.

The amount of vaginal bleeding should be noted carefully. Because the woman with PIH is hypovolemic, even normal blood loss can be serious. The eclamptic patient is likely to lose twice as much blood as the normotensive patient. Rising pulse rate and falling urine output are indications of excessive blood loss. The uterus should be palpated frequently and massaged when needed to keep it contracted.

Blood pressure and pulse are checked every 4 hours for 48 hours. Hematocrit may be measured daily. The woman is instructed to report any headache or visual disturbance. No ergot products are given, as they are hypertensive. Intake and output recordings are continued for 48 hours postpartum. Increased urinary output within 48 hours after delivery is a highly favorable sign. With the diuresis, edema recedes and blood pressure returns to normal.

Postpartal depression can develop after the long ordeal of the difficult pregnancy. Family members are urged to visit, and as much mother–infant contact as possible should be allowed. There may be fears about a future pregnancy. The couple needs information about the chance of PIH occurring again. They also should be given family planning information. It is recommended that they delay the next pregnancy at least 2 years. Oral contraceptives generally have been contraindicated due to their potential hypertensive effect, although conflicting data exist. Pritchard and MacDonald (1980) believe the low-dose estrogen pill may be used, if the client is given careful follow-up care.

Chronic Hypertensive Disease

Chronic hypertension exists when the blood pressure is 140/90 or higher before pregnancy, or a blood pressure of 140/90 or higher develops before the twentieth week of gestation and/or persists indefinitely following delivery (Gant and Worley, 1980). The cause of chronic hypertension has not been determined.

Chronic hypertensive clients who have been taking antihypertensive medication or diuretics prior to pregnancy usually continue the medication during pregnancy at the lowest effective dose. There is some indication that the woman has less chance of developing preeclampsia if she continues to take hydralazine (Apresoline) or methyldopa (Aldomet) (Welt et al., 1981). If the hypertension develops early in pregnancy with no other indication of preeclampsia, controversy exists about whether antihypertensive medication is needed. Hydralazine or methyldopa or a combination of the two are usually the agents given (Willis and Sharp, 1982). The client is watched carefully for the development of edema or proteinuria.

Chronic hypertension of long standing is usually associated with vascular changes such as arteriosclerosis, retinal hemorrhage, and renal disease. These conditions are seen most commonly in the older pregnant woman. *Chronic hypertensive vascular disease* is the name given to these changes.

Chronic hypertension with superimposed preeclampsia. Preeclampsia may develop in a woman previously found to have chronic hypertension. When elevations of systolic blood pressure 30 mm Hg or of diastolic blood pressure 15–20 mm Hg above the baseline are discovered on two occasions at least 6 hours apart, proteinuria develops, or edema occurs in the upper half of the body (Gant and Worley, 1980), the woman needs close monitoring and careful management. Her condition often progresses quickly to eclampsia, sometimes before 30 weeks of pregnancy.

Late or transient hypertension. Late hypertension, as defined by Gant and Worley (1980), exists when transient elevation of blood pressure occurs during labor or in the early postpartal period, returning to normal within 10 days postpartum.

RH SENSITIZATION

Rh sensitization results from an antigen-antibody immunologic reaction within the body. Sensitization most commonly occurs when an Rh-negative woman carries an Rh-positive fetus, either to term or terminated by spontaneous or induced abortion. It can also occur if an Rh-negative nonpreg-

nant woman receives an Rh-positive blood transfusion.

The red blood cells from the fetus invade the maternal circulation, thereby stimulating the production of Rh antibodies. Because this usually occurs at delivery, the first offspring is not affected. However, in a subsequent pregnancy Rh antibodies cross the placenta and enter the fetal circulation, causing severe hemolysis. The destruction of fetal red blood cells causing anemia in the fetus is proportional to the extent of maternal sensitization (Figure 12–5).

Several forms of Rh antigen exist. The factors implicated in pathogenesis, in order of antigenic potential, are D, C, E, c, e, and, hypothetically, d (d has never been demonstrated but is thought to exist). There are many genetic combinations (genotypes) possible, such as CDE, cDe, Cde, and so forth. The D antigen is most significant clinically in that it provides the strongest stimulus to antibody formation in Rh-negative people. Therefore, individuals who are homozygous for the D antigen (DD) or heterozygous (Dd) are Rh-positive; those whose genotype is dd are Rh-negative. Despite the antigenicity of the D factor, only 10% of pregnancies with Rh-positive fetuses result in immunization of Rh-negative women, even after five pregnancies. This phenomenon has been attributed to a rapid lysis of fetal cells entering the maternal bloodstream.

Approximately 85% of white, 95% of black, and 99% of Oriental populations are Rh-positive (Danforth, 1982). The incidence of hemolytic disease from Rh sensitization is about three times as high among whites as among blacks and is rarely seen in Orientals.

Fetal–Neonatal Implications

Each year 10,000 infants in the United States die of Rh hemolytic disease (Danforth, 1982). If treatment is not initiated, the anemia resulting from this disorder can cause marked fetal edema, called *hydrops fetalis*. Congestive heart failure may result, as well as marked jaundice (called *icterus gravis*) which can lead to neurologic damage (kernicterus). This severe hemolytic syndrome is known as *erythroblastosis fetalis*.

The possibility also exists that an Rh-negative female fetus carried by an Rh-positive mother may become sensitized in utero. This female would not demonstrate signs of hemolytic disease, but since she would be sensitized before even becoming pregnant she would have a positive indirect Coomb's test when receiving prenatal care with her first Rh-positive fetus.

Nursing Management

MATERNAL AND PATERNAL SCREENING

At the first prenatal visit (a) a history is taken of previous sensitization, abortions, blood transfusions, or children

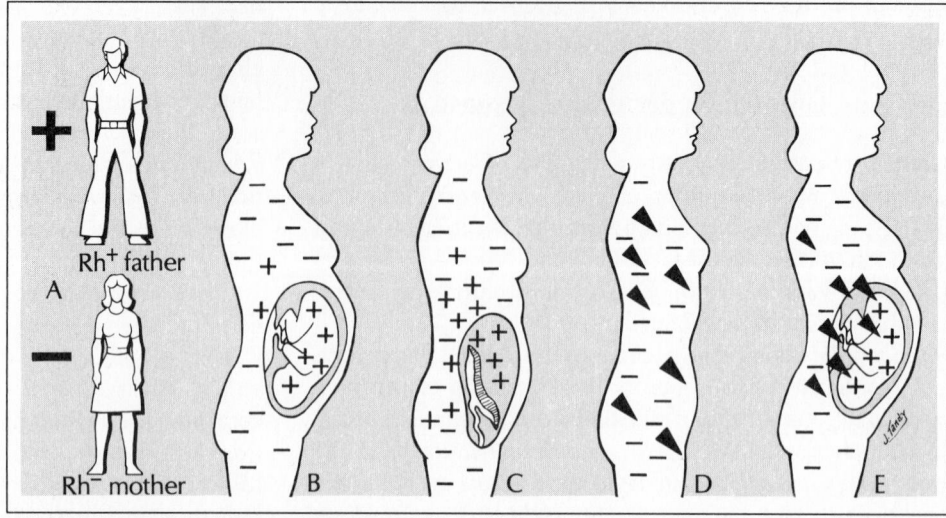

FIGURE 12–5 Rh isoimmunization sequence. **A,** Rh-positive father and Rh-negative mother. **B,** Pregnancy with Rh-positive fetus. Some Rh-positive blood enters the mother's blood. **C,** As placenta separates, further inoculation of mother by Rh-positive blood. **D,** Mother sensitized to Rh-positive blood; anti-Rh-positive antibodies are formed. **E,** With subsequent pregnancies with Rh-positive fetus, Rh-positive red blood cells are attacked by the anti-Rh-positive maternal antibodies causing hemolysis of red blood cells in the fetus.

who developed jaundice or anemia during the neonatal period; (b) maternal blood type (ABO) and Rh factor are determined and a routine Rh antibody screen is done; and (c) presence of other medical complications such as diabetes, infections, or hypertension are identified.

If the woman is Rh-negative (dd), the father of the unborn child is asked to come into the clinic or physician's office to be assessed for his Rh factor and blood type. If he is homozygous for Rh-positive (DD), all his offspring will be Rh-positive. If he is heterozygous (Dd), 50% of his offspring can be Rh-negative and 50% heterozygous for Rh-positive. If the father is Rh-negative, all their children will be Rh-negative, and no Rh incompatibility with the mother will occur. If the father is Rh-positive or the mother is known to have previously carried an Rh-positive fetus, further testing and careful management are needed.

PRENATAL ASSESSMENT AND INTERVENTIONS

Goals for prenatal management include identification and treatment for maternal conditions that predispose to hemolytic disease, identification and evaluation of the Rh-sensitized woman, coordinated obstetric–pediatric efforts for prenatal and/or postnatal treatment for the seriously affected neonate, and prevention of Rh sensitization if none is present.

When screening has identified the Rh-negative woman who may be pregnant with an Rh-positive fetus, an indirect Coombs' test or antibody screen is done to determine if the woman is sensitized (has developed isoimmunity) to the Rh antigen. The indirect Coombs' test measures the amount of antibodies in the maternal blood. A specimen of maternal blood is diluted to specific concentrations. Rh-positive red blood cells are added to the maternal blood sample. It the woman's serum contains antibodies, the Rh-positive red blood cells will agglutinate (clump) when rabbit immune antiglobulin is added. The titer (the amount or level of antibodies) is determined by the dilution at which the Rh-positive red blood cells clumped.

Titers should be determined monthly during the first and second trimesters, biweekly during the third trimester, and the week before the due date. If the test shows a maternal antibody titer of 1:16 or greater early in pregnancy, a Delta optical density (ΔOD) analysis of the amniotic fluid is performed at 26 weeks. If the titer is 1:16 or less late in pregnancy, delivery at 38 weeks or spontaneous labor at term can be anticipated.

Negative antibody titers can consistently identify the fetus *not* at risk. However, the titers cannot reliably point out the fetus in danger, because the level of the titer does not correlate with the severity of the disease. For instance, in a severely sensitized woman, antibody titers may be moderately high and remain at the same level although the fetus is being more and more severely affected. Conversely, a woman sensitized by previous Rh-positive fetuses may show a high fixed antibody titer during a pregnancy in which the fetus is Rh-negative (Danforth, 1982).

The most valuable indicator of fetal status is the ΔOD analysis. Amniotic fluid, obtained by transabdominal amniocentesis, is separated from its cellular components by centrifuge. The amount of pigment from the degradation of red blood cells can be measured when in solution in amniotic fluid. The fluid is subjected to spectrophotometric studies to determine the severity of the fetal hemolytic process and the obstetric–pediatric management.

If the spectrophotometric readings are in zone I (A) ΔOD at 450 nm, a normal or mildly anemic neonate may be anticipated and delivery at term may be permitted. Prognosis for this newborn is good, but phototherapy or exchange transfusion may be necessary A reading in zone II (B) ΔOD at 450 nm indicates a moderately anemic fetus who may be hydropic or stillborn if delivered at term. Once the fetus reaches viability, induced vaginal or cesarean delivery is indicated. A fair prognosis and possible need for exchange transfusion can be anticipated. Readings within zone III (C) ΔOD at 450 nm indicate a severely affected fetus who may require intrauterine transfusion every 1–2 weeks between weeks 26 and 32 until viability is reached, followed by delivery, usually cesarean. Neonatal exchange transfusion is anticipated. Prognosis is guarded.

PRENATAL INTERVENTIONS

Two primary interventions are available to the physician to aid the fetus whose blood cells are being destroyed by maternal antibodies: early delivery of the fetus and intrauterine transfusion, both of which carry risks. Ideally, delivery should be delayed until fetal maturity is confirmed at about 36–37 weeks. This is possible for most pregnancies with spectrophotometric readings in zones I and II (A and B). Only fetuses with a prognosis of death before 32 weeks as indicated by the ΔOD 450 nm amniotic readings should be given intrauterine transfusion (Pritchard and MacDonald, 1980). This procedure should be done before hydrops develops because the red blood cells injected into the fetal peritoneal cavity will be absorbed more slowly by the hydropic fetus. However, if ascites has already developed, the feus should still be transfused since it has a better chance of survival with the transfusion than without it (Bowman, 1981).

□ *INTRAUTERINE TRANSFUSION* Intrauterine transfusion is done to correct the anemia produced by the red blood cell hemolysis (see Procedure 12–1). If intrauterine transfusion is considered, the location of the placenta and fetal position are determined by ultrasound, an amniocentesis is done, and 30 mL of radiopaque dye is injected into the amniotic fluid. The fetus swallows the fluid containing the dye, making it possible to visualize the fetal gastrointestinal tract with fluoroscopy. The woman is admitted to the hospital, sedated, and taken to the x-ray department the day after the dye is injected.

With the woman under local anesthesia and using fluoroscopy a plastic catheter threaded through an 18 cm, 17-gauge Touhy needle is introduced through the abdomen into the intrauterine space and into the fetal peritoneal cavity. About 100 mL of packed red blood cells is selected for transfusion according to the following criteria: the specimen must be less than 24 hours old (blood over 24 hours old has lost the enzyme 2,3-diphosphoglycerase, which is necessary before oxygen can be released from the red blood cells into the tissues), type O, Rh-negative, and cross-matched against the mother's serum (Danforth, 1982).The blood is transfused into the fetus. Diaphragmatic lymphatics absorb the red blood cells into fetal circulation within a week after transfusion. Repeat transfusions can be scheduled every 7 days to 3 weeks until the fetus is sufficiently mature to tolerate delivery.

About 50%–60% of transfused nonhydropic fetuses survive. The procedure is hazardous to the fetus, resulting in mortality in 6% of cases. Direct trauma to the fetus with the needles and catheter is possible. Maternal complications are few; those that occur are usually due to bleeding or infection. The neonate is usually delivered about the thirty-fourth week. In general, premature neonates are more susceptible to damage from hemolytic disease, often require exchange transfusion, and require intensive nursery care.

POSTPARTAL INTERVENTIONS

The goals of postpartal care are to prevent sensitization in the as-yet-unsensitized pregnant woman and to treat the isoimmune hemolytic disease in the neonate.

□ *TREATMENT OF THE MOTHER* The Rh-negative mother who has no titer (indirect Coombs' negative, nonsensitized) and who has delivered an Rh-positive fetus (direct Coombs' negative) is given an intramuscular injection of 1 mL or 300 mg of anti-Rh_0 (D) gamma globulin such as RhoGAM within 72 hours so that she does not have time to produce antibodies to fetal cells that entered her bloodstream when the placenta separated. The anti-Rh_0 (D) gamma globulin works to destroy the fetus cells in the maternal circulation before sensitization occurs, thereby blocking maternal antibody production.

The normal dose of RhoGAM should suppress the immune response to approximately 30 mL whole Rh-positive blood. However, if a larger fetomaternal bleed may have occurred, a Kleihauer-Betke test can be performed and, based on the results, the dose of RhoGAM can be increased as necessary (Aladjem, 1980). Administration of RhoGAM provides temporary passive immunity to the mother, which prevents the development of permanent active immunity (antibody formation).

Procedure 12-1   Intrauterine Transfusion
Intrauterine transfusion is done only between 23 and 32 weeks of gestation. Amniocentesis is done
24 hours prior to admission, and radiopaque dye is instilled into the amniotic cavity.

Objective	Nursing action	Rationale
Prepare patient	Explain procedure	
Maintain patient comfort	Administer medications as ordered: 1. Morphine sulfate 10 mg 2. Sodium phenobarbital 90 mg 3. Promethazine 25 mg	Promotes relaxation and decreases discomfort
Prepare skin	Cleanse abdomen with 10-min Betadine scrub	Decreases possibility of infection
Transport	Transport patient to x-ray unit via stretcher	Use of stretcher promotes patient comfort and helps maintain cleansed abdomen
Locate fetal gastrointestinal system	Under sterile technique, physician inserts 17-gauge Touhy needle into fetal peritoneal cavity; catheter is threaded through needle and needle is removed; 5-10 mL radiopaque dye is inserted	Television fluoroscopy is utilized to visualize peritoneal cavity Checks placement of catheter in peritoneal cavity
Perform intrauterine transfusion	Fresh O Rh-negative blood is infused through catheter, and catheter is removed	Infuse 50 mL in fetus of 24 weeks' gestation; repeat every 7-21 days until a total of 350 mL is given or fetal maturity is assured
Monitor vital signs	Assess BP every 10-15 min, pulse and respirations every 2-15 min Assess fetal heart tones every 10-15 min with fetoscope or continuously if using electronic monitoring equipment	Assists in identification of transfusion reactions or other problems

When the woman is Rh-negative and not sensitized and the father is Rh-positive or unknown, RhoGAM is also given after each abortion, ectopic pregnancy, or amniocentesis. By the eleventh week of fetal life, the D-antigen is often present and can stimulate maternal isoimmunization, which would jeopardize the next Rh-positive fetus. Rho-GAM is not given to the neonate or the father. It is not effective for and should not be administered to a previously sensitized woman. However, sometimes after delivery or an abortion, the results of the blood test do not clearly show whether the mother is already sensitized to the Rh antigen or not. In such cases, the Rh_0 immunoglobulin should be given as it will cause no harm.

Pritchard and MacDonald (1980) state that 1.8% of Rh-negative women will develop isoimmunization during pregnancy with an Rh-positive fetus, rather than after delivery as is normally expected. Therefore, they advocate that a single intramuscular dose of 300 mg of Rh_0 immuno-globulin be administered to all Rh_0-negative nonimmunized women at 28 to 32 weeks' gestation and again within 72 hours after delivery.

When administering RhoGAM, the nurse must follow the instructions on the packet of RhoGAM carefully. The used packet containing the vial of drug cross-matched to the woman's serum is returned to the pharmacy, where it is saved. The woman is observed for possible symptoms of blood transfusion reaction.

Occasionally, the coating of maternal antibodies on fetal cells may block an accurate typing of cord blood; that is, an Rh-positive fetus may be erroneously typed as Rh-negative. Consequently, the RhoGAM will not be given, and the woman may become sensitized.

Rh sensitization and the resultant hemolytic disease of the newborn are less common today because of the development of RhoGAM. See Chapter 25 for treatment of the neonate.

SURGICAL PROCEDURES
DURING PREGNANCY

Surgery can generally be undertaken during pregnancy without affecting the course of the pregnancy or causing harm to the fetus. Trauma and diseases that require surgical treatment occur with about the same frequency in pregnant and nonpregnant women. They are age-related: disease occurs more frequently in the older adult while injury or accident occurs more often in the younger person and therefore is seen more often in pregnancy.

Although general preoperative and postoperative care is similar for gravid and nongravid women, special considerations must be kept in mind whenever the surgical client is pregnant. The early second trimester is the best time to operate because there is less risk of causing spontaneous abortion or early labor, and the uterus is not so large as to impinge on the abdominal field.

The preoperative chest radiograph and electrocardiogram, which are routine for persons over age 40, should be done on the same basis for the pregnant woman. If a chest radiograph is done, the fetus should be shielded from the radiation. Because of decreased intestinal motility and decreased free gastric acid secretion during pregnancy, stomach emptying time is delayed, which increases risk of vomiting during induction of anesthesia and during the postoperative period. Therefore, a nasogastric tube is recommended prior to major surgery. An indwelling urinary catheter prevents bladder distention, decreases risk of injury to the bladder, and promotes ease of monitoring output. Support stockings during and after surgery help prevent venous stasis and the development of thrombophlebitis. Fetal heart tones must be monitored before, during, and after surgery.

Pregnancy causes increased secretions of the respiratory tract and engorgement of the nasal mucous membrane, often making breathing through the nose difficult. Because of this pregnant women often need an endotracheal tube or tracheostomy for respiratory support during surgery.

Maternal hypoxia must be guarded against during surgery as uterine circulation will be decreased and reduced fetal oxygenation results very quickly.

Surgery should never be performed with the gravid woman in a flat supine position. A wedge must be placed under the right hip to tilt the uterus off major blood vessels, during both surgery and the recovery period.

No evidence exists that local or general anesthetics given to the expectant woman produce any congenital defects (Iffy and Kaminetzky, 1981), although increased incidence of spontaneous abortion and congenital anomalies has been reported in pregnancies of anesthesiologists and operating room staff. Spinal or epidural anesthesia may produce hypotension and respiratory apnea in the pregnant woman. The frequency and degree of the hypotension increase with higher anesthetic levels. This can be guarded against with preanesthetic infusion of 900–1000 mL of fluid.

Blood loss during surgery must be monitored carefully. Measurement of fetal heart tones gives the best indication of blood loss. Because of the normal increased blood volume of pregnancy, uterine blood flow may be reduced significantly before the maternal blood pressure begins to fall. Fluid replacement should be done with balanced electrolyte solution, and whole blood if needed.

Appendicitis

Nonobstetric abdominal emergencies occur in about 1 out of 1000 pregnancies. Of these, appendicitis is the most common. Symptoms are abdominal pain, diffuse and cramplike. It may become localized, usually over the area of the appendix. As pregnancy advances, the point of maximum tenderness tends to be higher as the cecum is displaced upward and toward the right. Sometimes the client may continue to locate her pain at McBurney's point even when the appendix is higher. Temperature may be elevated to 37.8–39C (100–102.2F), although not at the onset of pain. The woman may experience nausea and vomiting. Rebound tenderness and muscle guarding are present with appendicitis early in pregnancy, but they are less obvious in the last trimester.

Diagnosis may be difficult because abdominal palpation is hindered by the enlarged uterus, organs are displaced, and the leukocyte count is normally slightly elevated in pregnancy. In early pregnancy ectopic pregnancy must be considered. Other conditions to be ruled out are pyelonephritis, gallbladder disease, round ligament pain, false labor, adnexal and uterine pathology, and acute gastritis. If diagnosis is in doubt, a celiotomy or laparotomy must be performed. A few cases of acute appendicitis subside spontaneously. Most do not, and maternal and fetal mortality are high if treatment is delayed; they are low if surgery is prompt. With adequate hydration and broad-spectrum antibiotics the client should do well after surgery. If the appendix has ruptured, a drain must be placed in the incision.

Cholecystitis and Cholelithiasis

Incidence of gallbladder disease during pregnancy is comparable for similar-age nonpregnant women. Medical therapy is preferable to surgical intervention during pregnancy, unless attacks recur or the symptoms become acute.

Pain is usually in the upper right quadrant, radiating to the back and scapula. Nausea and vomiting are often severe. High temperature and jaundice may occur. In late pregnancy gallbladder disease is more difficult to diagnose.

It must be differentiated from hiatal hernia, appendicitis, acute intestinal obstruction, and pyelonephritis. If the client becomes jaundiced due to an obstructed bile duct, hepatitis must be considered in the differential diagnosis. Diagnosis is aided by ultrasound, which can visualize the gallbladder and any stones. If the attacks are mild, the client will be treated with analgesics, intravenous medication, nasogastric suction, and a low-fat diet. In early pregnancy, surgery may be deferred until the second trimester, although if the attack is severe, surgery must be done without delay.

Carcinoma of the Breast

The development of breast cancer during pregnancy is rare, but the normal hypertrophy of the pregnant woman's breast makes it easier for a beginning malignancy to be missed on palpation. During lactation, too, a malignancy may go unrecognized, or an inflammatory cancer be mistaken for acute mastitis.

Breast cancer may spread more rapidly during pregnancy (Danforth, 1982). It is thought this is due to increased vascularity of the breast during pregnancy. However, prognosis and 5-year survival rates are the same as for the nonpregnant woman, based on the stage of cancer when diagnosed. Mastectomy is the treatment of choice and can be performed without harm to the fetus. Radiation therapy can be damaging to the fetus, particularly in the first trimester, and cytotoxic agents have been associated with abortion, stillbirth, fetal anomalies, and premature labor. Therapeutic abortion does not alter the growth rate of the cancer.

After delivery, the woman is usually advised against becoming pregnant for at least 2 years. Because oral contraceptives are prohibited postmastectomy (Jochimsen et al., 1981), the client should be provided with mechanical contraceptives. Close supervision is needed, with possible follow-up treatment for the cancer.

Carcinoma of the Cervix

One in every 100 to 200 pregnant women is discovered to have cancer in situ on careful examination. When cancer is confirmed, usually by colposcopy and biopsy, treatment depends on the stage of the cancer and duration of the pregnancy. An in situ carcinoma is observed carefully during pregnancy, but treatment usually can be delayed until delivery and involution of the uterus. Treatment is by cervical conization with endocervical curettage to check for further lesions. Cryosurgery, laser surgery, or hysterectomy may be performed. Survival rates are excellent.

An invasive cervical cancer must be treated immediately. If the fetus is viable it is delivered by cesarean birth before treatment. Stage I invasive cervical carcinoma is treated by radical hysterectomy, while radiation therapy is indicated for more extensive invasive carcinoma. A fetus in first or early second trimester will usually abort spontaneously after radiation therapy begins, or may be removed by hysterotomy. Five-year survival rates depend on the stage of the cancer and are the same as for nonpregnant women.

ACCIDENTS AND TRAUMA

Accidents and injury are not uncommon during pregnancy. Fortunately, most accidents produce minor injuries and the outcome of the pregnancy is seldom affected. Late in pregnancy the woman has less balance and coordination, and may fall. Her protruding abdomen is vulnerable to a variety of minor injuries. The fetus is usually well protected by the amniotic fluid which distributes the force of a blow equally in all directions, and by the muscle layers of the uterus and abdominal wall. In early pregnancy, while the uterus is still in the pelvis it is shielded from blows by the surrounding pelvic organs, muscles, and bony structures.

Nevertheless, major trauma can happen to the pregnant woman, and some types of injuries have increased in frequency. Because travel during pregnancy is more common today, the woman is exposed to greater risk of accident than in previous years. Injuries from automobile accidents have become a major cause of nonobstetric maternal death. In conjunction, fetal death as a result of automobile-accident trauma may also occur. Seat belts have been known to injure the fetal head by sudden forceful pressure to the lower uterine segment. Despite this, lap and shoulder restraints are strongly recommended. The risk is greater without them because the mother could be fatally injured. Maternal mortality most often occurs from head trauma or hemorrhage. Unless the fetus is of more than 28 weeks' gestation and can be removed from the uterus within 20 minutes of maternal death it cannot be expected to survive. Uterine rupture may result from strong deceleration forces, with or without seat belts. Traumatic separation of the placenta can occur; it results in a high rate of fetal mortality. Premature labor is another serious hazard to the fetus, often following rupture of membranes during an accident. Premature labor can ensue even if the woman is not injured.

Maternal fractures, even of the pelvis, are tolerated well. However, ruptured bladder, retroperitoneal hemorrhage, and shock are complications one must be on guard for with a fractured pelvis.

Stab or gunshot wounds are another possible source of major trauma to the pregnant woman. Fetal or placental injury occurs in 89% of gunshot wounds to the abdomen, with a 66% perinatal mortality (Taylor and Slate, 1981). Stab wounds tend to cause less damage than bullet wounds.

Treatment of major injuries during pregnancy focuses initially on life-saving measures for the woman. Specifically, such measures include: establishing an airway, controlling external bleeding, and administering intravenous fluid to alleviate shock. The patient must be kept on her left side to avoid further hypotension. Fetal heart tones are monitored. Exploratory surgery is necessary following abdominal trauma to determine the extent of injuries. If the fetus is near term and the uterus has been damaged, cesarean delivery is performed. If the fetus is still immature, the uterus can often be repaired, and the pregnancy continues until term.

INFECTIONS

A major factor predisposing to risk in pregnancy is the presence of maternal infection, whether contracted prior to conception or during the gestational period. Frequently, abortion is the result of a severe maternal infection. If the pregnancy is carried to term in the presence of infection, the risk of fetal and maternal morbidity and mortality increases. In many instances of fetal risk due to infection, the woman presents few or no signs or symptoms. Therefore, it is essential to maternal and fetal health that diagnosis and treatment be prompt. Therapy must be based on an awareness of possible fetal effects as well as a desire for maternal well-being.

Urinary Tract Infections

Urinary tract infections affect 2%–10% of pregnant women. Stasis of urine, compression of ureters (especially the right ureter), decreased bactericidal capabilities of leukocytes in the urine, and vesicoureteral reflux (backward urine flow) make the pregnant woman more susceptible to urinary tract infection.

Asymptomatic bacteruria (bacteria in the urine actively multiplying without accompanying clinical symptoms) has been reported widely. Its incidence is estimated to be 4.0%–6.9% in all pregnant women, with higher rates for lower socioeconomic groups. The incidence increases with age and parity (Burrow and Ferris, 1982). *Escherichia coli* is usually the causative agent.

A woman who has had a urinary tract infection is more susceptible to a recurrent infection, either in the same or subsequent pregnancies. With acute urinary tract infection, especially with high temperatures, amniotic fluid infection may develop and a growth-retarded placenta may result. Increased risk of premature labor exists if the infection occurs near term.

A clean urine specimen should be obtained for culture from all pregnant women on their first antepartal visit. If bacteria are found in the urine, antibiotic therapy is begun even though the client may be asymptomatic. The woman is instructed to drink 3–4 liters of fluid per day. A follow-up urine culture is obtained a week after treatment is completed and every 1 or 2 months thereafter during pregnancy.

LOWER URINARY TRACT INFECTION

Cystitis is usually accompanied by a temperature of 38.4C (101F) or lower, frequency and urgency of urination with burning when voiding. Oral sulfonamides, particularly sulfisoxazole, are generally effective. These should only be used in early pregnancy, however, since they interfere with protein binding of bilirubin in the fetus. Use in the last few weeks of pregnancy can lead to neonatal hyperbilirubinemia and kernicterus. Other drugs that are usually effective and apparently safe for the fetus are ampicillin and nitrofurantoin (Furadantin). Nitrofurantoin crosses the placenta, but no harm to the fetus has been demonstrated. The tetracycline group is contraindicated because they cause retardation of bone growth and staining of fetal teeth.

The nurse should make sure the client is aware of good hygiene practices, since most bacteria enter through the urethra after having spread from the anal area. The nurse should also reinforce instructions or answer questions regarding the prescribed antibiotic, the amount of liquids to take, and the reasons for these treatments. Cystitis usually responds rapidly to treatment, but follow-up urinary cultures are important.

UPPER URINARY TRACT INFECTION

Acute pyelonephritis has a sudden onset with chills, high temperature of 39.6–40.6C (103–105F), and flank pain (either unilateral or bilateral). The right side is almost always involved because the large bulk of intestines to the left pushes the uterus to the right, putting pressure on the right ureter and kidney. Nausea, vomiting, and general malaise may ensue. With accompanying cystitis, frequency, urgency, and burning with urination may be experienced.

Edema of the renal parenchyma or ureteritis with blockage and swelling of the ureter may lead to temporary suppression of urinary output, which would be accompanied by severe colicky pain, vomiting, dehydration, and ileus of the large bowel.

The patient is hospitalized and started on intravenous antibiotic therapy as soon as an acute upper urinary tract infection is diagnosed by symptoms and urine culture. In the case of obstructed pyelonephritis, a blood culture is necessary. The client is kept in bed, lying on her left side. After a sensitivity report, the antibiotic may be changed to one more specific for the infecting organism. Ampicillin or nitrofurantoin, or one of these in combination with a sulfonamide, is commonly prescribed. If signs of urinary obstruction occur or continue, the ureter may be catherized to establish adequate drainage.

With appropriate drug therapy, the patient's temperature should return to normal. The pain subsides and the urine shows no bacteria within 2–3 days. Follow-up urinary cultures are needed to assure that the infection has been eliminated completely.

Sexually Transmitted Diseases

Sexually transmitted diseases (STDs), also called *venereal diseases,* are a group of infectious disorders contracted primarily through intimate sexual contact, oral or genital, with another person. The most common STDs are syphilis, gonorrhea, herpes simplex, chlamydia infections, cytomegalovirus infection, trichomonas vaginalis, monilial vulvovaginitis, and condyloma accuminata. There are several other relatively rare STDs. Cytomegalovirus and herpes simplex are discussed with the TORCH group; trichomonas and monilial infections are discussed under vaginal infections.

SYPHILIS

Syphilis is a chronic infection caused by a spirochete, *Treponema pallidum.* Syphilis can be acquired congenitally through transplacental inoculation, and can result from maternal exposure to infected exudate during sexual contact, or from contact with open wounds or infected blood. The incubation period is 10–60 days, and even though no symptoms or lesions are noted during this time, the client's blood contains spirochetes and is infectious.

Syphilis is divided into early and late stages. During the early stage (primary), a chancre appears at the site where the *Treponema pallidum* organism entered the body. Symptoms include slight fever, loss of weight, and malaise. The chancre persists for about 4 weeks and then disappears. In 6 weeks to 6 months, secondary symptoms appear. Skin eruptions called *condylomata* (not to be confused with condylomata accuminata), which resemble wartlike plaques, may appear on the vulva. Other secondary symptoms are acute arthritis, enlargement of the liver and spleen, iritis, and a chronic sore throat with hoarseness. When infected in utero, the newborn will exhibit secondary stage symptoms of syphilis.

The incidence of syphilis declined after discovery of penicillin, but since 1958 the incidence has been increasing. As a result of the increased incidence and the significant morbidity and mortality to the fetus in utero that this disease causes, serologic testing of every pregnant woman is recommended, and required by some state laws, at initial prenatal screening and is repeated in the third trimester.

The VDRL (Venereal Disease Research Laboratory) test and other nontreponemal antibody tests used in screening for syphilis can give false-negative results in the early incubating weeks of the disease. False-positive results can occur with many infectious diseases. If the clinical symptoms do not support the serologic findings, further testing may be done with a treponemal antibody test. In the pregnant client treatment with penicillin should begin after the first positive test rather than waiting for further testing.

□ *FETAL-NEONATAL IMPLICATIONS* One of the following outcomes can occur in the presence of untreated maternal syphilis: (a) second trimester abortion, (b) a stillborn infant at term, (c) a congenitally infected infant born prematurely or at term, or (d) an uninfected live infant. The clinical manifestations and treatment of the syphilitic newborn are discussed in Chapter 25.

□ *INTERVENTIONS* If testing of maternal serum is positive, treatment should be started immediately. It has been demonstrated that, in pregnancies treated before 18 weeks' gestation, the likelihood of fetal infection is almost nonexistent. If treatment is given later in pregnancy, congenital syphilis may have already developed.

For women with syphilis of less than a year's duration, 2.4 million units of benzathine penicillin G intramuscularly or 4.8 million units of procaine penicillin G are divided into three doses given 3 days apart. If syphilis is of long (more than a year) duration, these drugs are given but in total dosages of 6–9 million units intramuscularly in divided doses. Should the woman be allergic to penicillin, erythromycin can be given. Maternal serologic testing may remain positive for 8 months, and the newborn may have a positive test for 3 months.

GONORRHEA

Gonorrhea is an infection caused by the bacteria *Neisseria gonorrhoeae.* The expectant woman can be screened for this infection during her prenatal examination by means of a cervical culture. Many women with positive smears are asymptomatic. A chronic infection is usually found in the urethra, Skene's and Bartholin's glands, and the cervix. The infection generally remains localized to those areas until rupture of the membranes, at which time it can spread upward, causing endometritis, salpingitis, oophoritis, and pelvic peritonitis.

In acute gonorrheal infections in a gravid woman, the vulvar area and urethra are acutely inflamed. The discharge from the vagina is greenish yellow, and her vulva may be covered with a grayish exudate or condylomata. The cervix is often swollen and eroded and may secrete a foul smelling discharge in which the gonococci are present.

□ *FETAL-NEONATAL IMPLICATIONS* There are no congenital anomalies associated with gonorrhea. However, if untreated, morbidity in the fetus and neonate can result from ascending infectious gonorrhea during prolonged rupture of membranes or as a result of a vaginal delivery through an infected birth canal. The fetus is also at risk for prematurity because an acute gonorrheal infection may predispose to premature labor. For the fetus delivered through an infected birth canal, the result is a gonococcal eye infection known as *ophthalmia neonatorum*. Infections of the stomach, external ear canal, oropharynx, and anus can also occur. See Chapter 25 for further discussion on gonorrheal infection of the newborn and its treatment.

□ *INTERVENTIONS* Therapy consists of antibiotic treatment with aqueous procaine penicillin G given intramuscularly to the infected woman. A total dosage of 4.8 million units is administered, with 2.4 million units injected into each buttock. If the client is allergic to penicillin, kanamycin or erythromycin may be utilized. Additional treatment using twice the initial dose may be required if the cultures remain positive 7–14 days after completion of treatment. All sexual partners must also be treated or the woman may become reinfected.

If the woman has a positive culture at the time of labor, a cesarean delivery may be done to decrease the chances of the fetus contracting the infection in the birth canal.

CHLAMYDIAL INFECTIONS

Nongonococcal urethritis (NGU) is becoming one of the most common STDs in the United States. *Chlamydia trachomatis* has been established as the causative agent in 40%–50% of nongonococcal urethritis cases. *Chlamydia* may cause a concurrent infection in 30%–60% of the cases of gonococcal urethritis in males (Rafferty, 1981).

Chlamydial infection has been difficult to identify in women but has been found in cases of cervicitis and pelvic inflammatory disease. All women whose sexual partners have NGU should be treated. Most women who harbor *Chlamydia* are asymptomatic. The concerns in pregnancy are the possibilities of ophthalmia neonatorum (which persists despite treatment with silver nitrate) and newborn chlamydial pneumonia. The pneumonia may be primary or secondary to chlamydial conjunctivitis. It is speculated (Noller, 1981c) that a number of the pneumonias of newborns, currently considered viral, may in fact be due to the chlamydial organism.

The specific treatment for chlamydial infections is tetracycline. Tetracycline ophthalmic ointment is given to the infant for 3–5 weeks or until cultures are negative. Oral tetracycline is given to the mother following delivery. If chlamydial infection is discovered in the pregnant woman, or if a woman is sensitive to tetracycline, erythromycin is given instead. Ilotycin ophthalmic ointment, an erythromycin preparation, is also effective for the infant.

CONDYLOMATA ACCUMINATA

Condylomata accuminata are genital warts. They are common, and during pregnancy their growth is accelerated. The warts are caused by a virus similar to the one that causes skin warts. The virus usually is transmitted through sexual contact. The incubation period following exposure appears to be 2–3 weeks. The warts may be present on the vulva, vagina, and cervix. Evidence exists that the virus may be transmitted to the fetus during birth and cause development of laryngeal papillomas. This possibility is still under investigation, but if a causal relationship is found, care must be taken to clear all maternal lesions before delivery (Noller, 1981c).

All large areas of genital warts should be biopsied for neoplasia. The specimen label must indicate that the client is pregnant because increased cellular growth activity is normal for pregnancy.

The drug commonly used for treatment is topically applied podophyllin, which is thought to be teratogenic and in large doses has been associated with fetal death. During pregnancy the treatment of choice is hot cauterization or carbon dioxide laser. When there are only a few lesions, they may disappear spontaneously during the puerperium, or small doses of podophyllin may be applied postpartum.

Vaginal Infections

MONILIAL (YEAST) INFECTION

Monilial vaginitis is usually caused by the fungus *Candida albicans*, which normally is found in the intestinal tract. It can, however, invade the vagina, causing infection. Monilial infection is present in about 20% of pregnant women. It is commonly seen at term in women with poorly controlled diabetes (the organism thrives in a carbohydrate-rich environment) and in those on antibiotic or steroid therapy (these drugs reduce the numbers of Döderlein's bacilli, which are normally present flora). Diagnosis is made on the basis of a speculum exam, which reveals thick, white, tenacious cheeselike patches adhering to the pale, dry, and sometimes bluish vaginal mucosa. Additional symptoms include thick vaginal discharge, itching, dysuria, and dyspareunia.

□ *FETAL-NEONATAL IMPLICATIONS* If the monilial infection is not cured prior to delivery, the fetus may contract thrush by direct contact with the organism in the birth canal. The infection can also be contracted from contaminated hands, feeding equipment or breast, and bedding. Therefore, scrupulous cleanliness must be maintained. In most cases, the neonate does not display severe discomfort; however, some newborns have demonstrated difficulty in swallowing. Care of the neonate who has contracted this infection is discussed in Chapter 25.

□ *INTERVENTIONS* Treatment for monilial vaginitis involves the following nursing, medical, and self-care actions:

1. Explanation of proper wiping technique (front to back) following elimination.
2. Prescription of drug therapy.
   a. Miconazole or clotrimazole cream, applied to vulva and vaginal mucosa four times a day for a week.
   b. Insertion of nystatin (Mycostatin) vaginal suppositories, 0.5 g twice daily for 7–14 days.
3. Gentle bathing of vulva with weak sodium bicarbonate solution to relieve discomfort of pruritus. If topical treatment is being used, this should be done prior to, rather than after application of the medication.

4. Because *Candida* may be harbored in the folds of skin of the penis, it is important to treat the sexual partner to prevent recurrence of the vaginitis in the woman. Topical miconazole has usually been effective in eliminating the yeast infection from the male.

5. If miconazole cream is being used by both partners, sexual intercourse is permitted and may assure the spread of the cream throughout the vagina. With other methods of treatment, abstinence is recommended until both partners are cured.

TRICHOMONAS INFECTION

The parasite *Trichomonas vaginalis* causes a type of vaginitis common in both pregnant and nonpregnant women. It is often asymptomatic. The *Trichomonas* protozoan thrives in an alkaline environment. In the male, *Trichomonas* is found in the urogenital tract and may cause a urethritis, but most infected males are asymptomatic. The parasite is transmitted through sexual intercourse; therefore the male partner should be treated along with the woman.

Symptoms of *Trichomonas* infection include foamy, foul-smelling whitish or greenish-gray leukorrhea, itching and irritation of the vulva, dyspareunia, classic strawberry appearance of vagina and cervix, and urinary frequency and dysuria. There may also be excoriation and edema of the vulva. Some women are asymptomatic.

□ *INTERVENTIONS* Treatment consists of 2 g of metronidazol (Flagyl), taken orally immediately or 250 mg taken orally three times a day for 7 days. However, research has identified metronidazol as a possible teratogenic drug not recommended for use during the first half of pregnancy, although controversy exists about whether fetotoxicity actually occurs. Metronidazole may also be taken as a vaginal suppository. Intercourse should be avoided until both partners are cured.

At present there is no other treatment for *Trichomonas* infection. Symptoms may be relieved by vaginal irrigation with a comfortably warm, weak (15 mL, or 1 Tbsp, to 1 L) vinegar solution. However, during pregnancy, douching is generally contraindicated because it entails risk of air embolism due to the greatly increased vascularity of the genital tract (Kuczynski, 1980). If douching is recommended, a bulb-type syringe should never be used, as fatalities have occurred. The woman should be instructed to:

1. Empty her bladder and wash her hands carefully.

2. Assume a reclining position in a bathtub or on a toilet.

3. Cleanse the vulva by allowing the solution to flow out the nozzle and over the vulva and between the labia (this will also lubricate the nozzle).

4. With the douche bag only 6 inches (15 cm) above the vagina so that the water pressure is very low, gently insert the nozzle directing the tip backwards and downward 2–3 inches.

5. Rotate the nozzle while holding the labia together so the vagina fills and the solution reaches all surfaces.

6. Sit up and lean forward to complete emptying of vagina. Pat area dry. Clean equipment and wash hands again.

OTHER VAGINAL INFECTIONS

In the healthy woman, many flora normally inhabit the vagina, some of which are potentially pathogenic. As a result of antibiotics use, tissue trauma or, more often, unknown causes, vaginitis may develop from endogenous organisms. This occurrence is referred to as "nonspecific vaginitis." It may be caused by more than one type of bacteria: *Escherichia coli*, *streptococci*, and *staphylococci* often have been implicated. The *Hemophilus vaginalis* organism (also termed *Gardnerella vaginalis*) has been found in more than 90% of nonspecific vaginal infections, along with an increased concentration of anaerobic bacteria. Burning, pruritus, redness, and edema are characteristic symptoms. The characteristic "clue cell" is seen on the vaginal smear.

Various antibiotics are used in the treatment. It can be sexually transmitted; therefore both partners must be treated to prevent recurrence. A weak vinegar douche may provide relief (see Interventions for *Trichomonas*). Beta-lactose suppositories may enhance growth of Döderlein's bacilli to restore normal flora. Metronidazole (Flagyl) is used to treat severe cases, especially in nonpregnant women.

LISTERIAL INFECTION

Listeria monocytogenes bacteria have been recognized as a cause of perinatal infection since 1936. In recent years it has been recognized and reported more frequently in pregnant women, and it is suspected that many more cases go unreported. Although the bacteria are cultured from the vagina, the infection causes a systemic rather than a vaginal infection and may produce severe fetal–neonatal consequences. The infection in pregnant women is relatively rare, but early detection can save the life of the fetus; therefore it deserves mention here.

Transmission. How the infection is acquired by adults is unknown. The bacteria has been found in birds and mammals, including domestic and farm animals. It has been isolated in contaminated food and unpasturized milk, and is found in soil and fecal material. The bacteria are known to cross the placenta, but whether they also reached the fetus by an ascending infection from the vagina is not known. Listeriosis is diagnosed by isolating the causative organism in secretions or infected tissues or by identifying specific antibodies in the blood.

Maternal implications. Symptoms of listerial infection are similar to flu and often mistaken for it. The woman may have malaise, fever, chills, diarrhea, and back pain. Since she does not feel seriously ill, she usually does not report it. It is thought that the infection may frequently be asymptomatic or have only minor symptoms. The possibility exists that *L. monocytogenes* may be a cause of habitual abortion. Women experiencing habitual abortion should be assessed for the organism and treated if necessary (Danforth, 1982.)

Fetal–neonatal implications. If *L. monocytogenes* is contracted early in pregnancy, it can cause spontaneous abortion. If contracted between the seventeenth and twenty-eighth weeks it can cause fetal death or premature birth of an acutely ill neonate who dies hours later. Late in pregnancy the fetus may be born with congenital listeriosis (Gerrano, 1980).

Neonates with congenital listeriosis are characterized by prematurity, meconium staining, apnea at birth, flaccidity, papular erythematous skin rash, small lesions in the posterior pharynx, hepatosplenomegaly, and poor feeding. Mortality risk is high but varies with prematurity. Late-onset listeriosis, up to 4 weeks after delivery, usually results in meningitis. The neonate is usually full term, and the mortality is lower than for congenital listeriosis, but hydrocephalus and mental retardation may develop.

Interventions. Pregnant women can be instructed to practice thorough hand-washing after contact with animals and to notify their care providers whenever they have a flulike illness so that a vaginal culture can be taken.

Ampicillin in combination with an aminoglycoside should be started immediately after the diagnosis is made (Gerrano, 1980). Investigation has shown neonates of mothers treated with antibiotics have a survival rate of 71%, whereas the survival rate of neonates whose mothers were not treated is only 29% (Zervoudakis and Cederqvist, 1977).

The neonate with congenital listeriosis should be isolated and given antibiotic therapy and respiratory support. Scrupulous hand-washing should be used to prevent the spread of the infection. If it is cultured in the mother's lochia or urine, she may be given antibiotic therapy to prevent transmission. Careful hygiene and hand-washing are essential for the mother.

Because the infection often is not recognized before birth, the parents may have to deal unexpectedly with the crisis of an ill or dying neonate. Support for their grief is necessary. Prognosis for future pregnancies is good since the infection is uncommon. Vaginal and rectal cultures are taken periodically in subsequent pregnancies. They could be done prior to conception for the client's peace of mind.

TORCH

The TORCH group of infectious diseases are those identified as causing serious harm to the embryo-fetus. These are: toxoplasmosis (*TO*), rubella (*R*), cytomegalovirus (*C*), and herpesvirus type 2 (*H*). Some sources identify the (*O*) as other infections. The TORCH identification assists health team members to assess quickly the potential risk to each woman in pregnancy.

The importance of understanding what these infections are and identifying risk factors cannot be overemphasized—not only in light of maternal morbidity and mortality but also because of the serious effects on the fetus when the infection crosses the placenta. Exposure of the woman during the first 12 weeks of gestation may cause developmental anomalies. The three major viral infections are caused by rubella, cytomegalovirus, and herpesvirus type 2. Toxoplasmosis is a protozoal infection.

TOXOPLASMOSIS

Toxoplasmosis is caused by the protozoan *Toxoplasma gondii*. It is innocuous in adults, but when contracted in pregnancy, it is transmitted to the fetus in half the cases (Danforth, 1982). The pregnant woman may contract the organism by eating raw or poorly cooked meat or by contact with the feces of infected animals. In the United States the most common carrier is the cat, which transmits the infection by way of its feces. It is therefore strongly recommended that pregnant women avoid cat litter boxes.

The incubation period for the disease is 10 days. The woman with acute toxoplasmosis may be asymptomatic, or she may develop myalgia, malaise, rash, splenomegaly, and posterior cervical lymphadenopathy. Symptoms usually disappear in a few days or weeks. Diagnosis can be made by doing serologic tests, such as the Sabin-Feldman dye test. If diagnosis can be established by physical findings, history, and positive serologic results, the woman may be treated with sulfadiazine and pyrimethamine, which are administered for one month. Spiramycin (not yet available in the United States) has been shown to decrease fetal infections by 50% (Danforth, 1982). If toxoplasmosis is diagnosed before 20 weeks of gestation, therapeutic abortion should be considered because damage to the fetus is more severe than if the disease is acquired later.

The incidence of abortion, stillbirths, neonatal deaths, and severe congenital anomalies is increased in the affected fetus and neonate. In very mild cases, retinochoroiditis may be the only recognizable damage and it and other manifestations may not appear until adolescence or young adulthood. Severe neonatal disorders associated with congenital infection are neurologic abnormalities such as convulsions, coma, hypotonia, microcephaly, or hydrocephalus. Other conditions seen in the infant are chorioretinitis, ecchymosis, hepatosplenomegaly, intracranial calcifications, jaundice, microphthalmia, and pallor (anemia).

RUBELLA

The effects of rubella are no more severe, nor are there greater complications, in pregnant women than in non-pregnant women of comparable age. But the effects of this infection on the fetus and neonate are great, because rubella causes a chronic infection that begins in the first trimester of pregnancy and may persist for months after birth.

Estimates say that approximately 10%–20% of all pregnant women are susceptible to rubella. The only accurate method of screening is by performing a serology test, the test for hemagglutination inhibition (HAI). The presence of a 1:16 HAI titer or greater is evidence of immunity. A titer less than 1:8 indicates susceptibility, and repeat testing should be done to determine later infection. A fourfold rise in serum HAI titer or a high value initially indicates recent infection and the possibility of damage to the fetus.

□ *FETAL-NEONATAL IMPLICATIONS* The period of greatest risk for the teratogenic effects of rubella on the fetus is during the first trimester. If infection occurs between the third and seventh week of pregnancy, damage usually results in death. In the second month, 25% of affected fetuses may have serious defects, and if infection occurs in the third month, 15% of fetuses are affected. If infection occurs early in the second trimester, the resultant fetal effect is most often permanent hearing impairment.

Clinical signs of congenital infection are congenital heart disease, IUGR, and cataracts. Cardiac involvements most often seen are patent ductus arteriosis and narrowing of peripheral pulmonary arteries. Cataracts may be unilateral or bilateral and may be present at birth or develop in the neonatal period. A petechial rash is seen in some infants, and hepatosplenomegaly and hyperbilirubinemia are frequently seen. Other abnormalities may become evident in infancy, such as mental retardation or cerebral palsy. Diagnosis in the neonate can be conclusively made in the presence of these conditions and with an elevated rubella IgM antibody titer at birth.

Frequently, in women who had rubella during pregnancy, an infant is born with active viral infection. This is called the *extended rubella syndrome*. It is typified by one or more of the following disorders: cardiac maldevelopment, encephalitis, hepatosplenomegaly, jaundice, ocular abnormalities, pneumonitis, and thrombocytopenia or purpura. A tendency toward the development of leukemia in childhood has been noted. Thus, infected newborns often die early in infancy. Others survive longer, and isolation of newborns with active viral infection is mandatory; the active rubella has been cultured for as long as 1–1½ years after birth.

□ *INTERVENTIONS* The best therapy for rubella is prevention. Live attenuated vaccine is available and should be given to all children. It is recommended that women of childbearing age be tested for immunity and vaccinated if susceptible and if it is established that they are not pregnant. Health counseling in high school and in premarital clinic visits can emphasize the importance of screening prior to planning a pregnancy. Pregnant women are not vaccinated, although the initial concerns about the teratogenic potential of attenuated rubella virus vaccines has not been

confirmed (Mann et al., 1981). It is considered safe for newly vaccinated children to have contact with pregnant women.

If a woman who is pregnant becomes infected during the first trimester, therapeutic abortion is an alternative. Nursing support and understanding are vital at this time because such a decision may initiate a crisis for a couple who have planned for this pregnancy. They need objective data to understand the possible effects on their unborn fetus and the prognosis for the offspring.

CYTOMEGALOVIRUS

Cytomegalovirus (CMV) belongs to the herpesvirus group and causes both congenital and acquired infections referred to as *cytomegalic inclusion disease* (CID). The significance of this virus in pregnancy is related to its ability to be transmitted by asymptomatic women across the placenta to the fetus or by the cervical route during delivery.

CID is probably the most prevalent infection in the TORCH group. Nearly half of adults have antibodies for the virus. The virus can be found in urine, saliva, cervical mucus, semen, and breast milk. It can be passed between humans by any close contact such as kissing, breast-feeding, and sexual intercourse. Asymptomatic CMV infection is particularly common in children and gravid women. It is a chronic, persistent infection in that the individual may shed the virus continually over many years. The cervix can harbor the virus and an ascending infection can develop after delivery. Rarely, following placental infection the virus may stay in the uterus and infect fetuses of subsequent pregnancies. While the virus is usually innocuous in adults and children, it may be fatal to the fetus.

The cytomegalovirus is the most frequent agent of viral infection in the human fetus (Charles, 1981). It infects 0.5%–2.0% of neonates. The great majority of these infections are subclinical at birth, but about 10% later develop manifestations. Subclinical infections in the newborn are capable of producing mental retardation and auditory deficits, sometimes not recognized for several months, or learning disabilities not seen until childhood. CMV may be the most common cause of mental retardation.

Accurate diagnosis in the pregnant woman depends on the presence of CMV in the urine, a rise in IgM levels, and identification of the CMV antibodies within the serum IgM fraction. At present, none of the antiviral drugs has been effective in preventing CMV or in treating the congenital disease in the neonate.

For the fetus, this infection can result in extensive intrauterine tissue damage that is incompatible with life, in survival with brain damage, or in survival with no damage at all.

The infected neonate is often SGA and hypoplastic. The principal tissues and organs affected are the blood, brain, and liver. However, virtually all organs are potentially at risk. Hemolysis leads to anemia and hyperbilirubinemia. Thrombocytopenia, with subsequent petechiae and ecchymosis, often occurs. Another commonly seen effect is hepatosplenomegaly. Encephalitis, with signs ranging from lethargy to hypoactivity and convulsions, may occur. Cerebral palsy may develop. Microcephaly may be present at delivery, and chorioretinitis is apparent in 10%–20% of infants displaying symptoms of CMV.

HERPESVIRUS TYPE 2

Herpesvirus hominis (HVH) type 2, which causes the disease herpes simplex, affects the cervix, vagina, and external genitals and can be transmitted through sexual contact. Herpesvirus hominis type 1 is responsible for lip lesions (cold sores) and skin lesions, which are usually found above the umbilicus. Primary lesions of HVH-2 (herpes genitalis) consist of multiple vesicles involving the vulva, vagina, and cervix. Couples engaging in oral sex may develop HVH-2 lesions of the lips and mouth. Conversely, genital lesions caused by HVH-1 are sometimes seen.

Genital herpes is the second most common STD with evidence that it soon may be the first. The incubation period is 2–20 days after exposure, with an average of 6 days (Himell, 1981). The active infection lasts 3 weeks. Symptoms include genital irritation and itching; vaginal and urethral discharge, which may be copious and foul-smelling; enlarged tender lymph nodes in the inguinal area; and dysuria. The viral lesions begin as reddened papules. These become itchy pustular vesicles that break and form painful wet ulcers, which then dry and develop crusts. The ulcers are tiny (1–4 mm), usually occurring in clusters. They heal in 2–6 weeks without scarring (although sometimes with depigmentation) unless secondary bacterial infection develops in them. The initial herpes symptoms peak in 10–14 days and are usually gone in 3 weeks, although viral shedding may continue for 12 weeks or longer. If viremia is found with the initial infection, systemic symptoms of high temperature, malaise, liver involvement, meningitis, or encephalitis may occur (Himell, 1981).

After the initial symptomatic infection the woman may be free of lesions for weeks or months. The lesions usually recur several times a year at first and are almost always in the same locations as the original ones. Symptoms are usually less severe, the lesions last a shorter time, and the recurrences gradually become less frequent. The recurrent lesions shed virus for only about 2 weeks. Some individuals do not experience recurring infections. This clinical picture is typical, but some individuals have mild or even asymptomatic initial infections. Vaginal and cervical lesions are painless. Therefore a woman with no external lesions may have no symptoms except occasional vaginal discharge.

Genital herpes simplex with visible vescular lesions can be diagnosed by the characteristic clinical manifestations. If further diagnostic measures are needed, cultures are taken from active lesions. Serum may be analyzed for the presence of HVH-2 antibodies, but other antibodies, including HVH-1, may make the test invalid.

Control of the transmission of genital herpes simplex is difficult because viral shedding occurs in mild or asymptomatic cases, and may continue after lesions have healed. The woman with only internal lesions may not be aware of their presence and so passes on the infection.

Transmission of the HVH virus to the fetus almost always occurs after the membranes rupture, with ascendance of the virus from active lesions. It also occurs during vaginal delivery when the fetus comes in contact with genital lesions. Transplacental infection of the fetus is rare, apparently because the presence of circulating maternal antibodies to HVH-2 minimizes viremia (Noller, 1981c).

□ *FETAL-NEONATAL IMPLICATIONS* If active HVH infection occurs during the first trimester there is a 20%–50% rate of spontaneous abortion (Oleske and Minnetor, 1981), with associated chorioamnionitis. Infection after the twentieth week of gestation is related to increased incidence of premature birth but not to teratogenic defects. The premature infant is four times more susceptible to develop the infection after birth than is the full-term infant. The incidence of neonatal herpes in the United States is estimated at 1 in 3000 to 1 in 8000 live births, although there may be unrecognized cases (Oleske and Minnetor, 1981). By far the majority of perinatal infections are acquired during labor rather than earlier. Approximately 40%–50% of all infants who are born vaginally when active maternal genital lesions are present develop some form of HVH infection. The neonate can acquire the infection even if the mother is asymptomatic (Grossman et al., 1981).

The infected newborn is usually asymptomatic at birth but after an incubation period of 2–12 days develops symptoms of fever (or hypothermia), jaundice, seizures, and poor feeding. Approximately one-half of infected neonates develop the typical vesicular lesions confirming diagnosis. There is no definitive treatment. Some 50%–60% of the infants succumb to their infection. Half or more of the survivors have permanent visual damage and impaired psychomotor and intellectual development.

□ *INTERVENTIONS* Treatment is directed first toward relieving the woman's vulvar pain. Bacterial infections may be treated with cream containing sulfonamide. If the attack is severe, walking, sitting, and even wearing clothing may be painful. The client may be most comfortable in bed during the peak of the infection. Sitz baths twice a day may prevent secondary infection, and cotton underwear helps keep the genital area dry and promotes healing of the lesions (Himell, 1981).

When HVH-2 is suspected in the pregnant woman, amniocentesis can be performed to determine if there is fetal involvement. The amniotic fluid is tested for the presence of herpesvirus antibodies. If they are present, a cesarean delivery should not be performed; the presumably infected fetus should be delivered vaginally. Traditionally, if no infection is present on amniotic fluid analysis, a cesarean birth is indicated to protect the fetus from possible infection from the birth canal.

Recent studies of maternal viral cultures (Boehm et al., 1981; Grossman et al., 1981) have indicated that if the cultures show negative results, vaginal delivery may be permitted. The neonates in the studies were kept in isolation and did not develop clinically detectable evidence of infection.

HVH-2 virus has not been found in breast milk. Present experience shows that breast-feeding is acceptable if the mother scrubs and gowns to prevent any direct transfer of the virus.

A new drug, acyclovir (Zovirax), was approved by the FDA in 1982. It does not cure the infection or prevent recurrence. Acyclovir does reduce healing time of the initial attack and shortens the time that the live virus is in the lesions, thereby reducing the infectious period.

Nurses must be particularly concerned with client education for this fast-spreading disease. Clients must be informed of the association of genital herpes simplex with spontaneous abortion, neonatal mortality and morbidity, and the possibility of cesarean delivery. A client needs to inform her future health care providers of her infection. Clients also should know of the possible association of genital herpes with cervical cancer and the importance of a yearly Pap smear.

The woman who feels she acquired HVH-2 as a adolescent may be devastated as a mature young adult who wants to have a family. Clients may be helped by nursing counseling that allows expression of the anger, shame, and depression so often experienced by the herpes victim. Literature may be helpful and is available from Planned Parenthood and many public health agencies. The American Social Health Association has established the HELP program to provide information and the latest research results on genital herpes. The Association has a quarterly journal, *The Helper*, for nurses and herpes clients.

DRUG USE AND ABUSE

Indiscriminate drug use during pregnancy, particularly in the first trimester, may adversely affect the normal growth and development of the fetus. Originally it was thought that the placenta acted as a protective barrier to keep the drugs ingested by the woman from reaching the fetal system. This is not true. The degree to which a drug is passed to the fetus depends on the chemical properties of the drug, including molecular weight, and on whether it is administered alone or in combination with other drugs.

As discussed in Chapter 11, drugs adversely affecting fetal growth and development are called *teratogens*. They act on the developing organs to retard growth at crucial stages of organogenesis during the first trimester. Other drugs ingested by the expectant woman at other times dur-

ing the pregnancy may negatively influence the well-being of the fetus as well as produce critical problems in the neonate. Table 12–7 identifies common addictive drugs and their effects on the fetus and neonate. (Use of normal therapeutic drugs during pregnancy is discussed in Chapter 11.)

Drugs that are commonly misused include alcohol, amphetamines, barbiturates, hallucinogens, and heroin and other narcotics. Abuse of these drugs constitutes a major threat to the successful completion of pregnancy.

Drug Addiction

□ *MATERNAL IMPLICATIONS* Drug addiction has an adverse effect on the expectant woman. It affects her state of health, nutritional status, susceptibility to infection, and psychosocial condition. A majority of drug abusing pregnant women are malnourished and receive little or no antepartal care. Heroin-addicted pregnant women have two to six times the risk of PIH, malpresentation, third trimester bleeding, and puerperal morbidity (Pritchard and MacDonald, 1980). In addition, the risk of drug toxicity is present. In general, her psychologic and physiologic ability to handle the stress of pregnancy is severely reduced.

□ *FETAL-NEONATAL IMPLICATIONS* The fetus of a pregnant addict is at risk in the following ways:

1. The drug may cause chromosomal aberrations or may have a teratogenic effect on the fetus, resulting in congenital anomalies such as limb abnormalities.

2. The drug may induce physiologic and psychologic changes in the pregnant woman, resulting in placental dysfunction or fetal hypoxia or depression.

3. IUGR, increased rate of prematurity, and higher perinatal mortality are associated with maternal heroin addiction.

4. Symptoms of irritability, hyperactivity, hypertonia, sleep problems, and feeding difficulties may persist for 3–6 months in infants whose mothers are on low-dose methadone maintenance (Chasnoff et al., 1980).

5. About 50% of newborns of addicted mothers experience withdrawal symptoms severe enough to require treatment.

6. Taking a mixture of drugs may lead to maternal death and thus fetal death.

7. If the pregnant woman has periods of drug withdrawal, the fetus also appears to experience withdrawal as noted by increased fetal activity. Increased oxygen is needed by the fetus at these times. If the increased oxygen requirement is not met, for example, during labor, fetal distress with meconium-stained amniotic fluid will occur. Meconium aspiration is then a possibility.

The effects of drug abuse on the newborn are severe and include withdrawal behaviors, congenital malformations, and prematurity. Onset of withdrawal syndrome in

Table 12–7 Possible Effects of Selected Drugs of Abuse/Addiction on Fetus and Neonate

Maternal drug	Effect on fetus/neonate
I. Depressants	
A. Alcohol	Cardiac anomalies, IUGR, potential teratogenic effects, FAS
B. Narcotics	
1. Heroin	Withdrawal symptoms, convulsions, death, IUGR, respiratory alkalosis, hyperbilirubinemia
2. Methadone	Fetal distress, meconium aspiration; with abrupt termination of the drug, severe withdrawal symptoms, neonatal death
C. Barbiturates	Neonatal depression, increased anomalies; teratogenic effect(?); withdrawal symptoms, convulsions, hyperactivity, hyperreflexia, vasomotor instability
1. Phenobarbital	Bleeding (with excessive doses)
D. "T's and Blues" (combination of the following)	
1. Talwin (narcotic)	Safe for use in pregnancy; depresses respiration if taken close to time of birth
2. Amytal (barbiturate)	See barbiturates
E. Tranquilizers	
1. Phenothiazine derivatives	Withdrawal, extrapyramidal dysfunction, delayed respiratory onset, hyperbilirubinemia, hypotonia or hyperactivity, decreased platelet count
2. Diazepam (Valium)	Hypotonia, hypothermia, low Apgar score, respiratory depression, poor sucking reflex, possible cleft lip
F. Antianxiety drugs	
1. Lithium	Congenital anomalies; lethargy and cyanosis in the newborn
II. Stimulants	
A. Amphetamines	
1. Amphetamine sulfate (Benzedrine)	Generalized arthritis, learning disabilities, poor motor coordination, transposition of the great vessels, cleft palate
2. Dextroamphetamine sulfate (dexedrine sulfate)	Congenital heart defects, hyperbilirubinemia
B. Cocaine	Learning disabilities
C. Caffeine (more than 600 mg/day)	Spontaneous abortion, IUGR, increased incidence of cleft palate; other anomalies suspected
D. Nicotine (half to one pack cigarettes/day)	Increased rate of spontaneous abortion, increased incidence placental abruption, SGA, small head circumference, decreased length
III. Psychotropics	
A. PCP ("angel dust")	Flaccid appearance, poor head control, impaired neurologic development
B. LSD	Chromosomal breakage?
C. Marijuana	IUGR, potential impaired immunologic mechanisms

the addicted neonate may begin during the first 24–48 hours after birth (for example, for heroin) or be delayed several days (for example, for barbiturates) or up to 2–3 weeks (for example, for methadone). Symptoms of withdrawal from methadone may also occur earlier. Withdrawal symptoms in the neonate usually include tremors, agitation, sweating, and seizures. With heroin-addicted and methadone-maintained mothers, the level of drug abuse directly correlates with the severity of withdrawal behavior in the infant. Methadone withdrawal is generally more severe in doses above 20 mg/day. Barbiturates also cause a withdrawal syndrome in the neonate. The hallucinogens, such as LSD, are frequently taken in combination with other drugs, so it is difficult to determine the causative agents in many of the neonatal anomalies.

□ *INTERVENTIONS* Antepartal care of the pregnant addict

involves medical, socioeconomic, and legal considerations. The use of a team approach allows for the comprehensive management necessary to provide safe labor and delivery for woman and fetus. The essential components of care include the following:

1. Assess the client's general health status, with specific attention to skin abscesses and infections, as well as evaluation of other body systems.

2. Assess the client's obstetric condition. Determine whether a sexually transmitted disease is present. Estimate the length of gestation and approximate fetal size.

3. Assess drug use (type and amount) through urine testing. Clients are often unaware of actual amounts.

4. The management of heroin addiction includes the use of methadone, the current agent of choice in the treat-

ment or prevention of withdrawal symptoms. Dosage must be less than 20 mg/day to prevent severe withdrawal symptoms in the newborn. Hospitalization is necessary to initiate detoxification. "Cold turkey" withdrawal is not advisable during pregnancy because of potential risk to the fetus. Maintenance and support therapy are given during weekly prenatal visits.

Preparation for labor and delivery should be a part of the prenatal planning. Analgesic use should be avoided if possible, although it is not necessarily contraindicated. Relief of fear, tension, or discomfort may be achieved through nonnarcotic psychologic support and careful explanation of the labor process. Preferred methods of pain relief include the use of psychoprophylaxis and regional or local anesthetics such as pudendal block and local infiltration. These techniques are preferred to decrease further risk of additional fetal respiratory depression. Immediate intensive care should be available for the newborn who will probably be depressed, SGA, and premature. For care of the addicted newborn, see Chapter 25.

Alcoholism

MATERNAL IMPLICATIONS

Alcoholism has increased dramatically among women in the United States. The incidence is highest among women 20–40 years old; alcoholism is also seen in teenagers. Chronic abuse of alcohol can undermine maternal health by causing malnutrition, especially folic acid and thiamine deficiencies, bone marrow suppression, increased incidence of infections, and liver disease. As a result of alcohol dependency, withdrawal seizures may occur in the intrapartal period as early as 12–48 hours after cessation of drinking. Delirium tremens may occur in the postpartal period, and the neonate may suffer a withdrawal syndrome.

FETAL–NEONATAL IMPLICATIONS

Although concern for the effects of alcohol on the fetus has appeared in literature for centuries, only in the last decade

has fetal alcohol syndrome (FAS) been well documented. The syndrome has characteristic abnormalities, which vary in severity and combination. One of the most frequent findings is IUGR. FAS children typically do not catch up in growth after birth, and often remain "skinny kids." The newborn with FAS has characteristic facial abnormalities: short palpebral fissure, epicanthal folds, maxillary hyoplasia, micrognathia, long thin upper lip, and diminished or absent philtrum. In addition, there often are cardiac defects, limb and joint anomalies, and mental deficiency ranging from borderline to severe. The infant is usually irritable and hyperactive, has a high-pitched cry, and feeds poorly.

The FDA has recommended that pregnant women limit alcohol intake to no more than two drinks per day. FAS typically has been associated with the heavy drinker (five to six drinks per day). Recent research, however, has shown that far lesser amounts (only one to two drinks per day) may produce FAS (Danforth, 1982). Even as little as one drink per week may produce an SGA infant. The days surrounding implantation appear to be particularly critical. Thus, it is currently recommended that a woman should drink no alcohol for the month prior to conception (Danforth, 1982). It would be safest to also avoid alcohol completely for a month after conception and have only an occasional drink, preferably none at all, during pregnancy.

It is important that the nursing staff in the maternity unit be aware of the manifestations of alcohol abuse so that they can prepare for the client's special needs. The care regimen includes sedation to decrease irritability and tremors, seizure precautions, intravenous fluid therapy for hydration, and preparation for an addicted neonate. Although high doses of sedation and analgesics may be necessary for the woman, caution is advised because these can cause fetal depression.

Breast-feeding generally is not contraindicated, although alcohol is excreted in breast milk. Excessive alcohol consumption may intoxicate the infant and inhibit maternal let-down reflex. Discharge planning for the alcohol-addicted mother and newborn should be correlated with the social service department of the hospital.

SUMMARY

The diagnosis of high-risk pregnancy can be a shock to an expectant couple. The stress involved may lead to crisis unless appropriate nursing interventions are initiated.

A period of self-questioning follows the shock, during which the couple asks, "Did we make the right decision?" and "Have we done everything we should have to ensure a healthy pregnancy?" The self-doubt and guilt are even more pronounced if the pregnancy is unplanned. In this situation, the couple may feel they are being punished for

not initially wanting the pregnancy. Nursing care should be planned individually and in depth, depending on each couple's specific needs. The nursing assessment should include delineation of the factors that identify couples as high risk, identification of their level of understanding related to the specific disruption, evaluation of coping mechanisms utilized by the couple, and an awareness of the questions they need answered.

A crucial aspect of care will be the development of the nurse-client/family relationship. The trust and rapport that are established will be the supportive structure on which care is based. Specific nursing interventions include teaching and guidance related to necessary treatment and procedures; encouragement of communication among the couple, physician, and nurse; and support of the pregnant woman's self-esteem and body image. In addition, the nurse must support the physiologic function of the maternal–fetal unit as effectively as possible. Through these caring efforts, it is hoped that the high-risk pregnancy will result in a physiologically and psychologically healthy mother and child.

Resource Groups

Cesarean Association for Research, Education, Support and Satisfaction in Birthing (CARESS), Burbank, CA 91510.

Cesarean Birth Council, San Jose, CA 95101.

Cesarean/Support, Education and Concern (C/Sec., Inc), Dedham, MA 02026.

Epilepsy Foundation of America, 4351 Garden City Drive, Suite 406, Landover, MD 20785.

HELP Program, The American Social Health Association, P.O. Box 100, Palo Alto, CA 94302

References

Aladjem, S. 1980. *Obstetrical practice*. St. Louis: The C. V. Mosby Co.

Aladjem, S.; Lueck, J.; and Brewer, J. I. Jan. 1983. Experimental induction of a toxemia-like syndrome in the pregnant beagle. *Am. J. Obstet. Gynecol.* 145:27.

Berkowitz, R. L., Couston, D. R.; and Mochizuki, T. K. 1981. *Handbook for prescribing medications during pregnancy*. Boston: Little, Brown & Company.

Bernstine, R. S. 1981. Placenta abruptio. In *Principles and practice of obstetrics and perinatology*, ed. L. Iffy and H. A. Kaminetzky. New York: John Wiley & Sons.

Boehm, F. H., et al. 1981. Management of genital herpes simplex virus infection occurring during pregnancy. *Am. J. Obstet. Gynecol.* 141(7): 735.

Borg, S., and Lasker, J. 1981. *When pregnancy fails*. Boston: Beacon Press.

Bowman, J. M. 1981. Blood-group incompatabilities. In *Principles and practice of obstetrics and perinatology*, ed. L. Iffy and H. A. Kaminetzky. New York: John Wiley & Sons.

Burrow, G. N., and Ferris, G. F., 1982. *Medical complications during pregnancy*. 2nd ed. Philadelphia: W. B. Saunders Co.

Cavanagh, D., and Knuppel, R. A. 1981. Preeclampsia and eclampsia. In *Principles and practice of obstetrics and perinatology*, ed. L. Iffy and H. A. Kaminetzky. New York: John Wiley & Sons.

Charles, D. 1981. Cytomegalovirus infection. In *Principles and practice of obstetrics and perinatology*, ed. L. Iffy and H. A. Kaminetzky. New York: John Wiley & Sons.

Chasnoff, I. J., Hatcher, R.; and Burns, W. J. 1980. Early growth patterns of methadone-addicted infants. *Am. J. Dis. Child.* 134:1049.

Chesley, L. C. 1978. *Hypertensive disorders in pregnancy*. New York: Appleton-Century-Crofts.

Condie, R. G. 1976. Plasma fibrinolytic activity in pregnancy with particular reference to preeclampsia. *Aust. NZ Obstet. Gynecol.* 16:18.

Criteria Committee of the New York Heart Association, Inc. 1955. *Nomenclature and criteria for diagnosis of diseases of the heart and blood vessels*. 5th ed. New York: The Association.

Danforth, D. N., ed. 1982. *Obstetrics and gynecology*. 4th ed. Philadelphia: Harper & Row.

Davidson, S.V., et al. 1977. *Nursing care evaluation*. St. Louis: The C.V. Mosby Co.

Gant, N. F., and Worley, R. J. 1980. *Hypertension in pregnancy: concepts and management*. New York: Appleton-Century-Crofts.

Gerrano, S. 1980. Listerial infection: nursing care of mother and infant. *MCN* 5(6):390.

Grossman, J. H. III, et al. 1981. Management of genital herpes simplex virus infection during pregnancy. *Obstet. Gynecol.* 58(1):1.

Guthrie, D. W., and Guthrie, R. A. 1982. *Nursing management of diabetes mellitus*. 2nd ed. St. Louis: The C. V. Mosby Co.

Haynes, D. 1969. *Medical complications during pregnancy*. New York: McGraw-Hill Book Co.

Hellman, L. M., and Pritchard, J. A. 1971. *Williams obstetrics*. 14th ed. New York: Appleton-Century-Crofts.

Himell, K. 1981. Genital herpes: the need for counseling. *J. Obstet. Gynecol. Neonatal Nurs.* 10(6):446.

Iffy, L., and Kaminetzky, H. A., eds. 1981. *Principles and practice of obstetrics and perinatology*. New York: John Wiley & Sons.

Jochimsen, P., et al. April 1981. Pregnancy during adjuvant chemotherapy for breast cancer. *J.A.M.A.* 245:16.

Jovanovic, L., and Peterson, C.M. May/June 1982. Optimal insulin delivery for the pregnant diabetic patient. *Diabetes Care.* 5 (Suppl. 1):24.

Kelly, M. and Mongiello, R. 1982a. Maternal position and blood pressure during pregnancy and delivery. *Am. J. Nurs.* 82(5):809.

———. 1982b. Labor, delivery and postpartum. *Am. J. Nurs.* 82(5):813.

Kuczynski, H. J. March/April 1980. The pros and cons of douching: the nurse's role in counseling. *J. Obstet. Gynecol. Neonatal Nurs.* 9(2):90.

Leman, R. E., et al. 1981. Heart disease and pregnancy. *South. Med. J.* 74(8):944.

Luckman, J., and Sorenson, K. 1981. *Medical-surgical nursing: a psychophysiologic approach*, 2nd ed. Philadelphia: W. B. Saunders.

Lueck, J., et al. Jan. 1983. Observation of an organism found in patients with gestational trophoblastic disease and in patients with toxemia of pregnancy. *Am. J. Obstet. Gynecol.* 145:15.

Mann, J. M., et al. 1981. Assessing risk of rubella infection during pregnancy: a standardized approach. *J.A.M.A.* 245(16):1647.

Mannor, S. M. 1981. Hyperemesis gravidarum. In *Principles and practice of obstetrics and perinatology*, ed. L. Iffy and H. A. Kaminetzky. New York: John Wiley & Sons.

McPhee, S. J., and Bell, W. R. 1981. Anemia in pregnancy. In *Principles and practice of obstetrics and perinatology*, ed. L. Iffy and H. A. Kaminetzky. New York: John Wiley & Sons.

Moore, D. S.; Bingham, P. E.; and Kessling, O. 1981. Nursing care of the pregnant woman with diabetes mellitus. *J. Obstet. Gynecol. Neonatal Nurs.* 10(3):188.

Naeye, R. L. 1981. Maternal blood pressure and fetal growth. *Am. J. Obstet. Gynecol.* 141(7):780.

National Diabetes Data Group. 1979. *Classification of diabetes mellitus and other categories of glucose intolerance.* Washington, D.C.: National Institutes of Health.

Noller, K. L. 1981a. Autoimmune disorders in gestation. In *Principles and practice of obstetrics and perinatology*, ed. L. Iffy and H. A. Kaminetzky. New York: John Wiley & Sons.

————. 1981b. Heart disease in pregnancy. In *Principles and practice of obstetrics and perinatology*, ed. L. Iffy and H. A. Kaminetzky. New York: John Wiley & Sons.

————. 1981c. Sexually transmitted diseases in pregnancy. In *Principles and practice of obstetics and perinatology*, ed. L. Iffy and H. A. Kaminetzky. New York: John Wiley & Sons.

Oleske, S. M., and Minnetor, A. E. 1981. Herpes simplex infection during pregnancy. In *Principles and practice of obstetrics and perinatology*, ed. L. Iffy and H. A. Kaminetzky. New York: John Wiley & Sons.

Price, S. A., and Wilson, L. M. 1982. *Pathophysiology: clinical concepts of disease process*, 2nd ed. New York: McGraw-Hill Book Co.

Pritchard, J. A., and MacDonald, P. 1980. *Williams obstetrics*, 16th ed. New York: Appleton-Century-Crofts.

Rafferty, E. G. 1981. Chlamydial infections in women. *J. Obstet. Gynecol. Neonatal Nurs.* 10(4):299.

Shields, J., and Resnik, R. 1979. Fetal lung maturation and the antenatal use of glucocorticoids to prevent the respiratory distress syndrome. *Obstet. Gynecol. Surv.* 34:343.

Skyler, J.; Mintz, D.; and O'Sullivan, M. 1981. Management of diabetes and pregnancy. In *Diabetes mellitus*, vol. 5, ed. H. Rifken and P. Raskin. Bowie, Md: Robert J. Brady Co.

Taylor, H. W., and Slate, W. G. 1981. Trauma and diseases requiring surgery during pregnancy. In *Principles and practice of obstetrics and perinatology*, ed. L. Iffy and H. A. Kaminetzky. New York: John Wiley & Sons.

Weil, S. G. 1981. The unspoken needs of families during high-risk pregnancies. *Am. J. Nurs.* 81(11):2047.

Welt, S. I., et. al. 1981. Effects of prophylactic management and therapeutics in hypertensive disease in pregnancy: preliminary studies. *Obstet. Gynecol.* 57(5):557.

Wheeler, L., and Jones, M. B. 1981. Pregnancy-induced hypertension. *J. Obstet. Gynecol. Neonatal Nurs.* 10(3):212.

Willis, S. E. 1982. Hypertension in pregnancy: pathophysiology. *Am. J. Nurs.* 82(5):792.

Willis, S. E., and Sharp, E. S. 1982. Hypertension in pregnancy: prenatal detection and management. *Am. J. Nurs.* 82(5):798.

Worley, R. J., et al. Sept. 1979. Vascular responsiveness to pressor agents during human pregnancy. *J. Reprod. Med.* 23:115.

Zervoudakis, I. A., and Cederqvist, L. L. Oct. 1977. Effect of listeria monocytogenes septicemia during pregnancy on the offspring. *Am. J. Obstet. Gynecol.* 129:465.

Additional Readings

Ahlfars, K., et al. July 1981. Secondary maternal cytomegalovirus infection causing symptomatic congenital infections (letter). *N. Engl. J. Med.* 305(5):284.

Bartlet, D., and Davis, A. 1980. Recognizing fetal alcohol syndrome in the nursery. *J. Obstet. Gynecol. Neonatal Nurs.* 9:223.

Fisher, K. A., et al. July 1981. Hypertension in pregnancy: clinical-pathological correlations and remote prognosis. *Medicine* 60(4):267.

Floyd, C. C. 1981. Pregnancy after reproductive failure. *Am. J. Nurs.* 81(11):2050.

Foster, S. D. 1981. Magnesium sulfate: eclampsia management: effects on neonate. *MCN* 6(5):355.

Gilstrap, L. C., et al. 1981. Renal infection and pregnancy outcome. *Am. J. Obstet. Gynecol.* 141(6):709.

Harris, R. E., et al. 1981. Cystitis during pregnancy: a distinctive clinical entity. *Obstet. Gynecol.* 57(5):578.

Morrison, J. C., et al. Feb./March 1981. Management of the pregnant patient with cardiovascular disease. *C.V.P.* 9:17.

Shaywitz, S. E.; Caparulo, B. D.; and Hodgson, E. S. 1981. Development of language disability as a consequence of prenatal exposure to ethanol. *Pediatrics.* 68(6):850.

Ueland, K. 1980. Intrapartum management of the cardiac patient. *Clin. Perinatol.* 8(1):155.

Whitley, R. J., et al. 1980. The natural history of herpes simplex virus infection of mother and newborn. *Pediatrics* 66(4):489.

13

DIAGNOSTIC ASSESSMENT
OF FETAL STATUS

■ CHAPTER CONTENTS

ULTRASOUND
    Procedure
    Clinical Application

MATERNAL ASSESSMENT OF FETAL ACTIVITY

NONSTRESS TESTING
    Interpretation of NST
    Procedure
    Prognostic Value

CONTRACTION STRESS TEST
    Indications and Contraindications
    Procedure
    Clinical Application

ESTRIOL DETERMINATIONS
    Estriol Metabolism
    Patterns of Excretion
    Urinary Estriol Determinations
    Urinary versus Plasma (Serum)
    Estriol Determinations

HUMAN PLACENTAL LACTOGEN

AMNIOTIC FLUID ANALYSIS
    Amniocentesis
    Clinical Application
    Evaluation of Fetal Maturity
    Identification of Meconium Staining
    Antenatal Genetic Screening

AMNIOSCOPY

X-RAY EXAMINATION

FETOSCOPY

IMPLICATIONS OF PRENATAL TESTING FOR DELIVERY

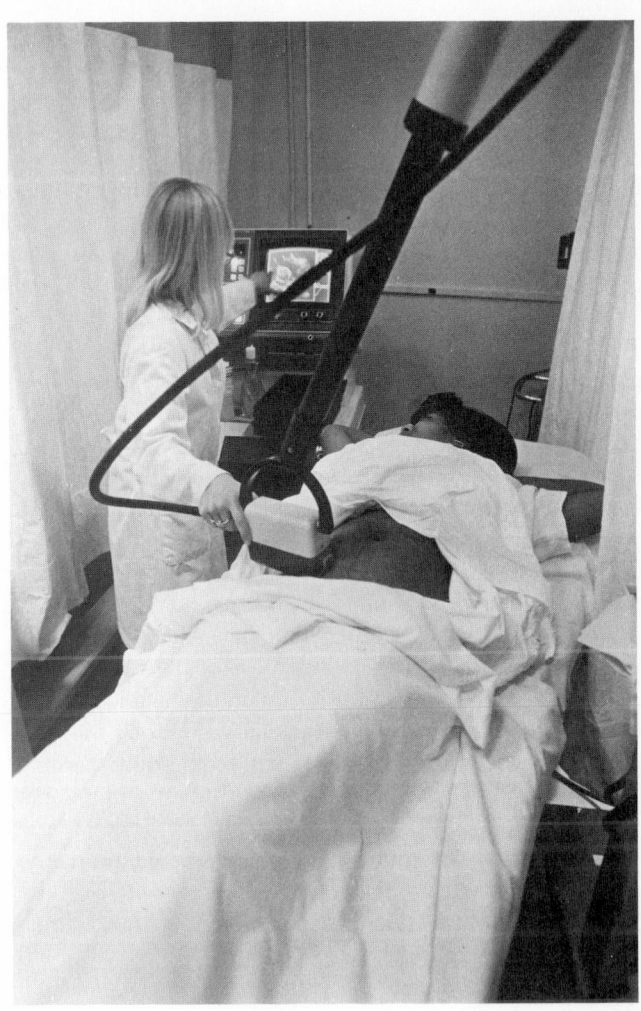

■ OBJECTIVES

- Compare the NST and the CST, giving indications, contraindications, and predictive value of each.

- Discuss the value of amniocentesis in relation to a positive CST.

- Outline the suggested protocol for monitoring a high-risk client with regard to NST–CST–L/S ratio–estriols.

- List indications for amniocentesis.

- Discuss the nurse's role in teaching the client the breast self-stimulation test.

- List indications for performing ultrasonic examination.

- Discuss the value of estriols and amniotic fluid analysis with regard to fetal well-being.

During the past 15–20 years, an increasing amount of interest has been focused on the problems of the high-risk pregnant woman, her management, and conditions that might affect her unborn child, because at-risk women and infants have a significantly greater chance of morbidity or mortality before or after delivery. Prematurity, congenital anomalies, mental retardation, cerebral palsy, and other conditions seem to be associated with the presence of certain factors during pregnancy or during delivery. Perinatal morbidity and mortality can be considerably reduced by early skillful diagnosis and appropriate, thorough, and highly intensive antepartal care of the pregnant woman. Thus, health care professionals are beginning to concentrate their efforts on identifying women who are at greater risk for developing problems that may affect their well-being and that of the fetus.

In an attempt to reduce perinatal mortality and morbidity, the field of perinatology has evolved. During the past decade, much knowledge has been acquired concerning the intrauterine environment of the fetus. Physicians, nurses, ultrasonographers, dieticians, social workers, and neonatologists are combining their efforts and expertise to contribute to the growing amount of information about the development of the fetus and the kinds of insult to which the fetus is susceptible.

A variety of tests of placental function and fetal well-being are of value in monitoring the health status of the fetus. These tests include diagnostic ultrasound, measurements of specific hormones and enzymes in maternal plasma and urine, amniocentesis for lung maturity studies, amnioscopy, and fetal stress tests. Some risk always exists with each procedure, so fetal morbidity and mortality should be considered before a particular procedure is done. Certainly not all high-risk pregnancies require the same procedures. One must be certain that the advantages outweigh potential risks and added expense. Each of these tests has its limitations in terms of diagnostic accuracy and applicability. No one test should be used to determine fetal status in the management of the high-risk client, but rather these tests should be used as adjuncts to good clinical judgment by the health care team.

Women who are considered to be at high risk and for whom the physician may order tests of placental function, fetal maturity, or fetal well-being include very young or older primigravidas and women with chronic hypertension, preeclampsia, diabetes mellitus, pregnancy beyond 42 weeks' gestation, Rh isoimmunization, previous unexplained stillborn or intrapartal loss, sickle cell hemoglobinopathies, suspected IUGR, maternal cyanotic heart disease, or other medical complications. (See Chapter 10 for further discussion of high-risk cases and Chapter 12 for descriptions of various conditions that may threaten the successful completion of pregnancy.)

ULTRASOUND

Valuable information concerning the fetus may be obtained from *pulsed-echo ultrasound*. Intermittent sound waves of extremely high frequency can be transmitted by means of an alternating current to a transducer, which is applied to the maternal abdomen. Ultrasonic sound waves are reflected off tissues of varying densities, and echoes return to the crystal and are changed to electrical signals. These signals are amplified and displayed on an oscilloscope or screen. The types of ultrasound are:

1. *A-mode (amplitude mode)*. Ultrasonic sound waves directed into the maternal abdomen are reflected back by maternal and fetal tissues and the fetal skull in A-mode ultrasound. The returning echoes are displayed on the oscilloscope as spikes. The height of the spikes varies according to the distance of reflecting tissues and/or structures, and is proportional to the amplitude of the returning echoes. A-mode has essentially been replaced by real-time ultrasound (see Figure 13–1,A).

2. *B-mode (brightness mode)*. In the B-mode ultrasound, the returning echoes are displayed on an oscilloscope as dots, and the brightness of the dots varies with the intensity of the reflected echoes. The dots coalesce to form a two-dimensional black and white static (fixed)

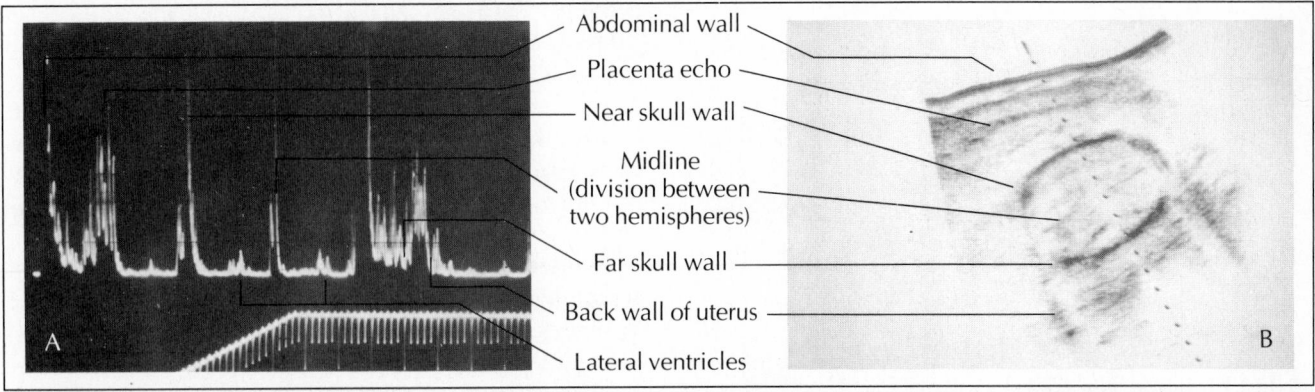

Abdominal wall
Placenta echo
Near skull wall
Midline
(division between
two hemispheres)
Far skull wall
Back wall of uterus
Lateral ventricles

A

B

FIGURE 13-1 Two methods of obtaining information about the fetus. Both scans are of the same fetus and were taken at the same time. The fetus is at 24 weeks' gestation. **A,** A-mode. Echo bounces off structures and is recorded as a spike. **B,** B-mode. The abdominal wall, internal structures, and fetal head can be visualized. The lateral ventricles cannot be visualized in the B-mode.

image of the scanned structure. Although gross structures can be identified, subtle tissue changes cannot be identified with the white on black image (Figure 13-1,B).

3. *Gray-scale ultrasound.* Gray-scale ultrasound provides for detection of a wide range of returning echoes (that is, strong echoes from the edges of structures and weaker echoes from inside the same structure). Through the use of many shades of gray (gray scale) the static or fixed image provides for visualization of the density of various internal structures (Figure 13-2).

4. *Real-time.* Real-time scanning utilizes gray scale and a continuous number of rapid fixed images produced by a transducer which are displayed on a small screen (similar to a television screen). Changes in tissue and/or structure position give the impression of motion because of the continuous rapid fixed images. In addition to visualizing motion, the operator may "freeze" an image on the screen and take a polaroid picture of the image for a permanent record. Real-time ultrasound is useful throughout pregnancy but is particularly helpful in late pregnancy for assessment of fetal breathing movements, cardiac activity, bladder function; fetal position; fetal abnormalities; multiple gestations; and location of the placenta. Additional advantages include the portability of the unit, and low cost to client.

The use of diagnostic ultrasound is advantageous because it is noninvasive and painless, allows the physician to study a client serially, is nonradiating to both woman and fetus with no known harmful effects to either, permits differentiation of soft tissue masses, and provides immediate information to the practitioner (Tamura and Sabbagha, 1981).

Procedure

Except for the instance of localizing the placenta for amniocentesis, the client is usually scanned with a full bladder. This enables the sonographer to assess other structures in relation to the bladder and in particular to determine the relationship of vagina and cervix to the bladder. This is

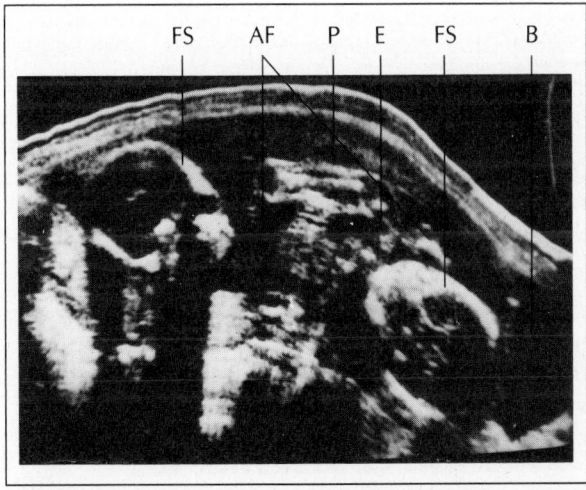

FS   AF   P   E   FS   B

FIGURE 13-2 Gray scale. Longitudinal scan demonstrating twin gestation, anterior placenta, fetal extremity. Both BPDs are at approximately 25-26 weeks' gestation. (AF = amniotic fluid; FS = fetal skull; E = extremity; B = woman's urinary bladder; P = placenta.) (Courtesy Section of Diagnostic Ultrasound, Department of Diagnostic Radiology, Kansas University Medical Center.)

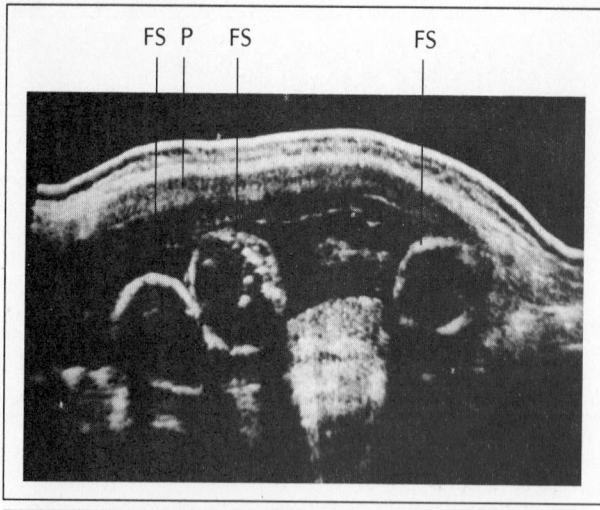

FIGURE 13-3 Transverse gray-scale scan demonstrating triplets. BPDs of all fetal skulls are at approximately 27 weeks' gestation. Anterior placenta (P) is shown. (Courtesy Section of Diagnostic Ultrasound, Department of Diagnostic Radiology, Kansas University Medical Center.)

particularly important in the case of vaginal bleeding in which a placenta previa is suspected. The cervical internal os is halfway between the sacral promontory and the base of the bladder. If the lower part of the placenta extends to the internal os, placenta previa is diagnosed. If the lower uterine segment cannot be visualized, the degree of previa cannot be ascertained. The client should be advised to drink one quart of water approximately 2 hours prior to the examination and to refrain from emptying her bladder.

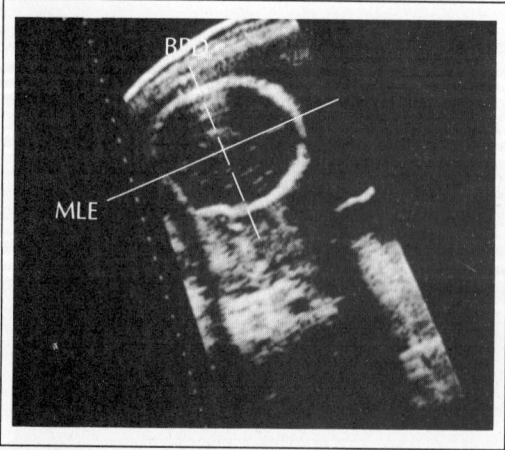

FIGURE 13-4 Transverse scan of 25-26 weeks' fetal skull. BPD is measured perpendicular to midline echo (MLE). (Courtesy Section of Diagnostic Ultrasound, Department of Diagnostic Radiology, Kansas University Medical Center.)

If the bladder is not sufficiently filled, she should be given three to four 8-oz glasses of water to drink. She may be rescanned 30-45 minutes later.

A sonogram requires 20-30 minutes and is uncomfortable to the woman only to the extent that she must lie flat on her back, a position most unphysiologic and uncomfortable for a pregnant woman. She may also experience discomfort due to distention of her bladder. Some women, particularly those near term with a large fetus, develop supine hypotension and experience nausea, vertigo, and lightheadedness due to compression of the abdominal aorta and inferior vena cava from pressure of the gravid uterus. This discomfort can be relieved by elevating the feet and turning the body to the lateral recumbent position. Mineral oil or transmission gel is generously spread over the maternal abdomen, and the sonographer slowly scans with a transducer longitudinally and transversely in sections across the abdomen to gain an entire picture of the contents of the uterus.

Clinical Application

Ultrasound is valuable for monitoring pregnancy in a variety of ways, including the following:

- Early identification of pregnancy
- Identification of multiple fetuses (Figure 13-3)
- Measurement of the biparietal diameter of the fetal head or fetal femur length to date pregnancy or to help identify IUGR (Figure 13-4)
- Detection of such fetal anomalies as hydrocephaly (Figure 13-5), microcephaly, anencephaly, ascites, myelomeningocele, and polycystic kidneys
- Detection of hydramnios (Figure 13-6) or oligohydramnios
- Placental localization for amniocentesis or determination of placenta previa
- Detection of intrauterine devices
- Detection of placental abnormalities
- Determination of fetal position and presentation
- Detection of fetal death
- Observation of fetal heart rate and respiration by real-time scanning
- Detection of incomplete or missed abortions and ectopic pregnancies
- Placental grading

EARLY PREGNANCY DETECTION

In managing the high-risk pregnant woman, it is of utmost importance to know the gestational age of the fetus to correlate data from all available tests. Pregnancy may be detected by diagnostic ultrasound as early as the fifth or sixth week following the LMP. A small collection of ringlike echoes may be seen within the uterus, and this is called the *gestational sac*. By the eighth week, stronger echoes representing the fetus may be seen along with the developing placenta. Fetal heart pulsations may be seen at 9–10 weeks. The placenta may be seen clearly at approximately 11–12 weeks' gestation, the fetal skull at 14 weeks' gestation in 95% of cases (Leopold and Asher, 1975), and the fetal thorax at about 16 weeks' gestation (Ragan, 1976).

The most accurate time for dating a pregnancy by diagnostic ultrasound is between 18–24 weeks' gestation with an accuracy of ±4½ days. A sonogram obtained during this time can be of great benefit in helping to date a pregnancy if confirmed by a second sonogram a few weeks later.

MEASUREMENT OF BIPARIETAL DIAMETER OF FETAL HEAD

By far the most important application of ultrasound is in the measurement of the biparietal diameter (BPD) of the fetal head. The BPD is the widest diameter of the fetal skull and is perpendicular to the fetal midline echo. This echo is apparently either the falx cerebri or the interhemispheric fissure of the fetus (McQuown, 1977). Measurement of the BPD provides the physician with a useful tool for following fetal development.

Tables correlating the BPD with fetal gestation vary from one institution to the next, undoubtedly because of socioeconomic and geographic factors inherent in the populations for which the tables were derived. Nevertheless, serial determinations on the same fetus using the same tables can be used as a gross measure of the progress of fetal development. If growth of the fetal head follows a normal curve as gestation advances, one can be assured that the fetus is growing at a normal rate. However, if the curve begins to flatten, the physician must be on the alert for IUGR of the fetus and must then consider this a high-risk case and evaluate the fetus by additional means, such as estriol determinations, nonstress tests, and possibly contraction stress tests.

Until about week 32, the fetal head grows about 3 mm/week (O'Sullivan, 1976) and thereafter at about 1.8 mm/week (Thompson et al., 1965; McQuown, 1977). One can obtain BPD measurements beginning in the thirteenth week of gestation. Detection of IUGR and an accurate prediction of fetal age can be most reliably achieved between 20 and 30 weeks of gestation, when the most rapid growth in the BPD occurs. After 40 weeks' gestation the BPD shows a growth of less than 1 mm/week; thus sonograms obtained at this point are not of value. Generally, the BPD measurement correlates closely with gestational age especially if serial determinations were obtained from early in the pregnancy. If only one determination is made late in pregnancy, the gestational age is less accurate (*see* Appendix C for evaluation of biparietal diameters).

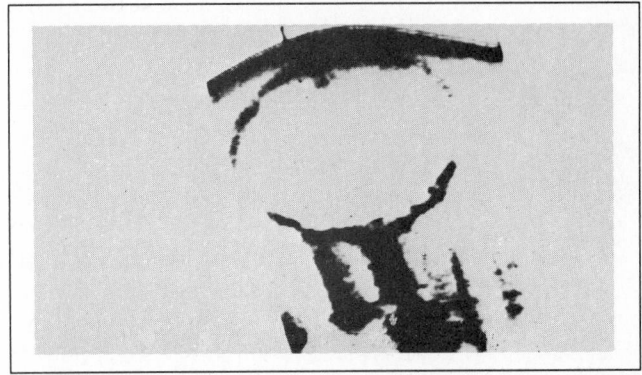

FIGURE 13–5 Hydrocephalic fetal skull at term. Note the minimal brain tissue in the bottom center. The large clear portion denotes fluid.

MEASUREMENT OF CROWN-TO-RUMP LENGTH

During the first trimester measurement of the crown-to-rump length (CRL) of the fetus is most useful. CRL is the longest length of the fetus (excluding the yolk sac). From approximately 6½ weeks the fetus grows in a linear fashion at about 1 cm/week up until week 14 (Gottesfeld, 1980). By 10–11 weeks, CRL and gestational sac diameters can be correlated with increased accuracy in gestational dating. Since the most common reason of unexpected enlargement of the uterus is for the client to be "off dates," the CRL and BPD correlation may be used to correct such an error after appearance of the fetal BPD at 12 to 13 weeks (Gottesfeld, 1980). Following the first trimes-

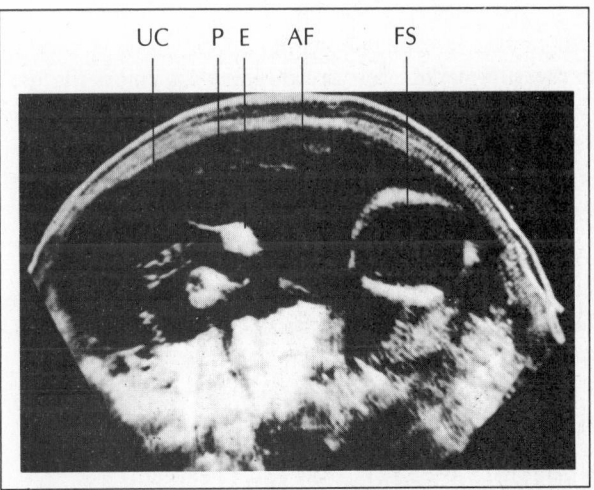

FIGURE 13–6 Transverse scan demonstrating fetal skull (FS), anterior placenta (P), extremities (E), umbilical cord (UC), and marked hydramnios (AF = amniotic fluid). (Courtesy Section of Diagnostic Ultrasound, Department of Radiology, Kansas University Medical Center.)

ter when differentiation of fetal head and trunk begins, the CRL is of limited value and the use of various other measurements for gestational dating and growth becomes important.

MEASUREMENT OF FEMUR LENGTH

Femur length is being investigated by many as an alternative means of assessing gestational age. Hohler and Quetal (1981) demonstrated in their study that from 23–40 weeks' gestation there is a constant linear relationship between the growth of the BPD and that of the fetal femur. They suggest that if the FL to BPD ratio is above normal limits it may be due to overestimation of femur length; underestimation of BPD; malposition of the fetal head making measurement difficult; or the existence of microcephaly. They believe that femur length may possibly be used as an alternative to measuring BPD with regard to assessing gestational age in normal pregnancies after 22 weeks.

To be truly accurate, femur growth rate charts should be developed by each institution with regard to the population served. Factors such as altitude and race would obviously have an effect upon standards found in any given population.

ABDOMINAL MEASUREMENTS

Measurement of the abdominal circumference (measurement at the level of the umbilical cord) provides data to aid in the detection of abnormal growth patterns. In IUGR, fetal abdominal girth ceases to grow due to the depletion of glycogen in the fetal liver and also to diminished accumulation of subcutaneous tissue overlying the fetal abdomen. Since different authors have reported differences in abdominal circumference measurements, for optimum accuracy each institution should develop its own standards for its particular client population. Abdominal circumference measurements alone are meaningless unless the gestational age of the fetus has been defined by CRL or serial BPDs. It appears to be most useful between 34–36 weeks' gestation in differentiating those normal fetuses from those at risk for IUGR.

HEAD-TO-ABDOMEN RATIOS

Head-to-abdomen ratios have also been utilized. The ratio normally approaches 1:0 at 35–36 weeks' gestation (Bree and Mariona, 1980); prior to this the ratio is greater than one. This measurement may be helpful in diagnosing IUGR.

DETECTION OF FETAL ABNORMALITIES

Only gross abnormalities of the fetus are readily detectable by sonography at present. The two major abnormalities are anencephaly and hydrocephaly. In general, when the BPD is more than 10.8 cm (McQuown, 1977), hydrocephaly should be suspected. Normally there is a 1:1 ratio

between the BPD and the measurement of the fetal thorax. If the chest is 5 mm or more smaller than the head size, one should suspect hydrocephaly. Anencephaly may be assumed if the fetal skull cannot be visualized after 14 weeks' gestation. Frequently, hydramnios is seen with this condition, and the trunk is able to be well visualized. Occasionally meningomyelocele may be detected, as can hydrops and ascites in the erythroblastotic infant. Hydramnios is easily identifiable by the large areas of echo-free spaces.

FETAL GROWTH DETERMINATION

As mentioned earlier, ultrasound provides the physician with a means of monitoring fetal growth. If the BPD of the fetal head is more than two standard deviations less than the mean for that particular gestational age, IUGR is suspected.

Intrauterine growth retardation is classified as symmetrical (primary) or asymmetrical (secondary). In symmetrical IUGR, all organs are reduced in size with equal reduction in body weight and head size. This growth retardation is noted in the first half of the second trimester. Symmetrically growth-retarded infants rarely experience asphyxia and labor is tolerated as it is in a normal pregnancy.

Asymmetrical IUGR is characterized by sparing of the head and brain but there is a resultant reduction in body size, apparently caused by a compromise in the uteroplacental blood flow. This type of IUGR comprises the majority of cases and is usually not evident prior to the third trimester. Fetuses with secondary IUGR are particularly at risk for perinatal asphyxia, pulmonary hemorrhage, hypocalcemia, and hypoglycemia in the neonatal period (Bree and Mariona, 1980). Birth weight will be reduced to the tenth percentile, whereas cephalic size may be between the ninety-fifth and fifteenth percentile.

Causes of IUGR may be the result of a single or combination of placental, maternal, or fetal problems, or may result without any apparent cause noticed antenatally. These infants are gestationally "mature," not premature, and are also termed SGA infants.

After prematurity, IUGR is the greatest cause of perinatal mortality. Between 3%–7% of all pregnancies are complicated by IUGR. Growth-retarded infants have a fivefold increase in perinatal asphyxia and an eightfold higher perinatal mortality rate than normal infants (Hobbins, 1982).

The earlier the gestational age is accurately assessed, the better one is able to predict IUGR. If one suspects a growth-retarded fetus, serial sonograms should be done from the twentieth to thirtieth week. The IUGR infant shows abnormal BPD growth, whereas the normal infant demonstrates a normal growth curve. A fetus with a BPD that is small for its gestational age which appears to grow normally is probably one with inaccurate dates. On the other hand, a fetus with a small BPD for its gestational age which does not show a normal weekly growth curve may be assessed to have growth retardation; this fetus should be further assessed with other means of antenatal surveillance. By performing serial cephalometry, the type of IUGR may be closely assessed, and fetuses can be evaluated further with abdominal-chest measurements, nonstress and contraction stress tests, and estriol levels to ascertain fetal status. Obviously, it becomes mandatory with a high-risk fetus to evaluate these other parameters to determine the optimal timing of delivery prior to onset of severe hypoxia or intrauterine death.

The question of when to deliver growth-retarded infants is still undecided. Some physicians, in light of pulmonary maturity, effect delivery of these infants by 37–38 weeks' gestation in hope of preventing long-term CNS deficits. Others choose to wait until other assessment parameters exhibit fetal jeopardy (for example, a positive contraction stress test, decreasing estriol levels, and so on).

FETAL BREATHING MOVEMENTS

Fetal breathing movements detected by A-scan and B-mode techniques have been studied over the last decade. With improved resolution using newer real-time equipment, evaluation of fetal breathing is now being suggested as a measure of fetal health. Episodic breathing movements have been reported by Patrick et al. (1978a). Manning (1977) reports observing fetal breathing movements as early as the eleventh week of gestation. After 36 weeks of gestation, the breathing movements are thought to be similar to those of the term neonate.

Three types of patterns of fetal breathing movements have been observed. The first pattern is the most common and is characterized by rapid initial movements, with a gradual decline in number. This pattern is associated with generalized fetal movements before and after the pattern is observed. The second pattern is characterized by rapid breathing movements interspersed with slower movements. Fetal movements occur less frequently. The third pattern is the least frequent in occurrence and consists of isolated fast breathing movements, which occur at the rate of 10–15/min. This pattern is not usually accompanied by fetal movements (Manning, 1977).

Patrick and associates (1978b) observed three additional patterns of fetal breathing, which are similar at 30–31, 34–35, and 38–39 weeks' gestation:

1. Significant increase in the amount of time fetuses spend breathing in the second and third hours following maternal meal.

2. Circadian rhythm in fetal breathing (increased time spent in breathing during the middle of the night during maternal sleep).

3. Episodes of fetal breathing plus gross body movements occurring for periods of 20–60 minutes out of every 1–1½ hours of observed time.

Natale (1981) in a study of more than 2000 hours of observation (more than 120 normal human fetuses) during the last 10 weeks of pregnancy found the longest period of apnea to be 65 minutes at 30–31 weeks of gestation, 105 minutes at 34–35 weeks, and 120 minutes at 38–39 weeks. Natale concluded that fetal apneic episodes of up to two hours are normal. Increased breathing 60 minutes after the peak in maternal plasma glucose concentrations was also noted. The fetal breathing remained elevated during the second and third hours following the oral ingestion of 50 g of glucose. Following administration of 25 g of intravenous glucose there was a 45–60 minute lag between the peak in maternal plasma glucose concentrations and the peak in fetal breathing activity.

It is not known why fetal breathing increases after an increase in maternal glucose concentration. Natale (1981) suggests that since glucose is utilized by the brain as a source of energy and the end-product of aerobic oxidation of glucose is carbon dioxide and water, it might be possible that an excess of carbon dioxide produced by increased glucose oxidation might stimulate the chemosensitive areas of the brain stem and produce increased fetal breathing activity. This would explain the 45–60 minute lag between peaks in maternal plasma glucose concentration and fetal breathing activity. Natale noted that fetal breathing was seen in 97% of the cases during the second and third hours following oral ingestion of 50 g of glucose at 32–34 weeks' gestation. Increased breathing was noted between 30 and 60 minutes following administration of 25 g of glucose given by intravenous bolus.

Richardson and associates (1979) noted that fetal breathing stopped with the onset of the active phase of labor, but that periodic increases in heart rate variability continued to occur, suggesting that in labor fetal breathing is a poor indication of fetal health and has little relationship to changes in fetal heart rate variability.

Certain drugs affect breathing. Meperidine and methyldopa seem to increase the incidence of fetal apnea. An increase in breathing has been noted to occur following administration of terbutaline sulfate, a bronchodilator (Boddy et al., 1974). A-scan imaging has demonstrated that fetal death is preceded by patterns of prolonged apnea or gasping and apnea (Tamura and Manning, 1981).

LOCALIZATION OF PLACENTA

Ultrasound is valuable in localizing the placenta for amniocentesis and in detecting placenta previa. Placentas appear to be located on the anterior surface of the uterine wall in approximately 40% of the cases (Ragan, 1976), and in some instances the placenta may cover the entire anterior uterine surface. By visualizing its location, the physician can avoid puncturing the placenta during amniocentesis. Ultrasound can also be used to locate a pool of amniotic fluid, thereby showing the physician exactly where and how deep to insert the needle for amniocentesis.

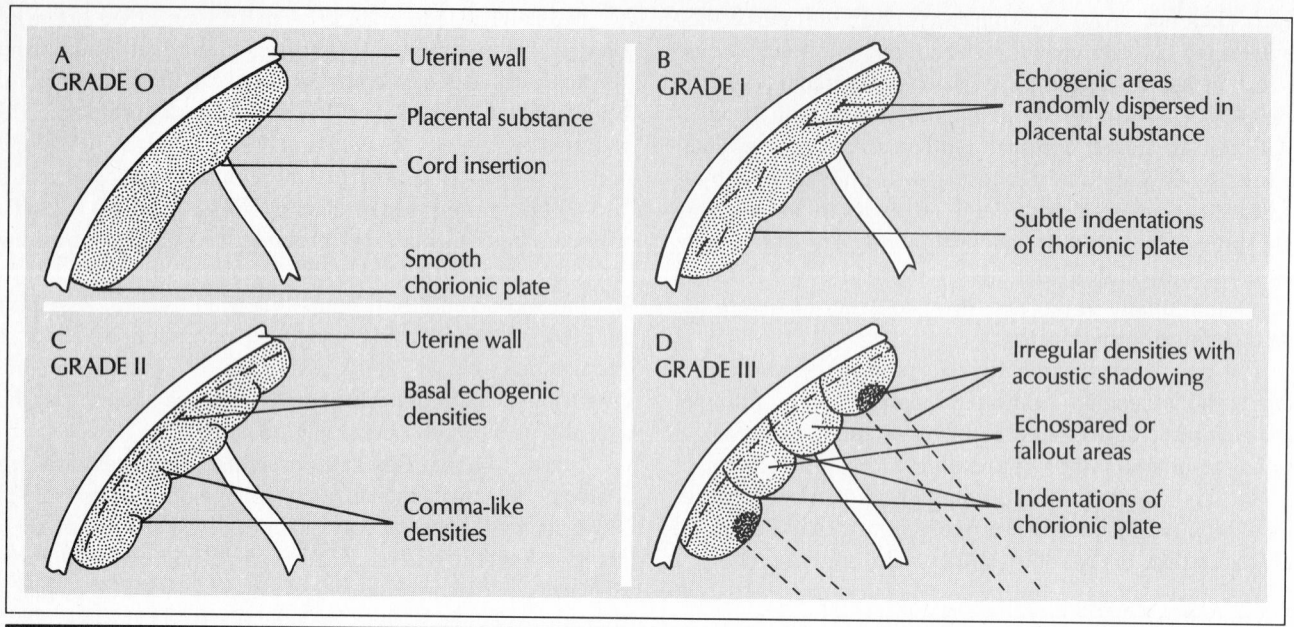

FIGURE 13–7 A, Diagram showing the ultrasonic appearance of a grade 0 placenta. **B,** Diagram showing the ultrasonic appearance of a grade I placenta. **C,** Diagram showing the ultrasonic appearance of a grade II placenta. **D,** Diagram showing the ultrasonic appearance of grade III placenta. (From Grannum, P. A. T.; Berkowitz, R. L.; and Hobbins, J. C. 1979. The ultrasonic changes in the maturing placenta and their relation to fetal pulmonic maturity. *Am. J. Obstet. Gynecol.* 133:916.)

PLACENTAL GRADING

Placental grading (grades 0–III) is based on morphologic changes in the basal and chorionic plates and the intervening placental substance. Placental maturational changes may be noted as early as 12 weeks' gestation (grade 0) with increasing changes (grades I–III) visualized by ultrasound until term. Figure 13–7 diagrams these changes in grade as described by Grannum, Berkowitz, and Hobbins (1979). The authors note that any given placenta may contain more than one grade and that the most mature grade should be used when total assessment is made. The grade is described according to the degree of calcification, although at present the reason for the calcification and its relationship to pulmonary maturity is not clear (Spirit and Kagan, 1980).

Grade III placentas appear to be correlated with L/S ratios greater than 2:1, indicating fetal lung maturity. In their research, Grannum and coworkers (1979) noted that when correlating ultrasonic maturational changes with mature L/S ratios, the L/S ratio was 2:1 or greater in 100% of their cases with grade III placentas and in 88% with grade II placentas.

Placental grading has been used as a possible means of determining fetal pulmonary maturity in high-risk pregnancies, such as those complicated by hypertension, diabetes, and Rh isoimmunization, in which amniocentesis would be difficult or hazardous to perform. The grading should only be used as an adjunct, though, since it has been reported that even with grade III placentas, an immature (less than 2:1) L/S ratio can be found in complicated pregnancies (Quinlan and Cruz, 1982).

RISKS OF ULTRASOUND

Much has been documented regarding the effects of X rays on the fetus during the first 8 weeks of gestation. As yet, no clinical studies demonstrate teratogenic effects due to diagnostic ultrasound. The consensus is that ultrasound is a safe procedure. Detailed controlled clinical studies and long-term evaluation of fetuses in utero are now in progress.

MATERNAL ASSESSMENT OF FETAL ACTIVITY

Maternal assessment of fetal activity has been advocated by many clinicians as a sign of fetal status. Counting of fetal movements by the client presently is being utilized during the third trimester as a screening test. It can be performed by the woman at her convenience without any expense. Many factors affect fetal reactivity, such as sound, drugs, cigarette smoking, sleep states of the fetus, blood glucose levels, and time of day. The expectant mother's perception of fetal movements and accuracy in documentation may also be influenced by many factors, so this may not be a reliable indicator of fetal status with some women. Fetuses have demonstrated stretching, rolling, and limb movements as seen on ultrasound, many of which are not gross movements and are not felt by the client. Most women are aware, however, when the activity of their fetus changes drastically and will report this if they have been told to be cognizant of it. Some clinicians have clients use fetal movement records (FMR) or a fetal activity diary (FAD). By keeping a written record of movements at particular time intervals during the day, the woman is made more aware of her fetus's activity.

The number of fetal movements required for reassurance is controversial and warrants further investigation. Freeman and Garite (1981) report that two or more movements in an hour are reassuring, while fewer than two should be reported to the clinician for evaluation with a nonstress test.

Clients should be reassured that there are fetal rest–sleep states during which minimal or no movement may occur. In a study by Patrick and coworkers (1982) it was noted that there were periods of up to 75 minutes in which gross fetal movements were totally absent. Other investigators have found similar results in their observations. Even though fetal movements may be a sign of fetal well-being, episodic absence of movement is characteristic of normal fetuses. Clients need to be reassured of this.

NONSTRESS TESTING

Much has been written about nonstress testing (NST), or fetal heart rate (FHR) acceleration determinations, as a predictor of fetal well-being (Trierweiler et al., 1976; Schifrin 1977). NST has become a widely accepted method of evaluating fetal status. Accelerations of the FHR imply an intact central and autonomic nervous system which is not being affected by intrauterine hypoxia. It has been demonstrated that those infants who sustain a negative contraction stress test (discussed later) generally exhibit accelerations of FHR (this is termed a reactive NST). Thus the NST may be used as a preliminary screening test for the contraction stress test.

The NST involves observation of baseline variability of the FHR and acceleration of FHR with fetal movement. Even though increased variability cannot be completely evaluated with an external fetal monitor, a loss of variability is significant. Loss of variability is usually seen in prematurity, fetal sleep, and after the administration of certain drugs to the client (such as barbiturates and magnesium sulfate). However, it must be emphasized that loss of variability may also result from an hypoxic condition occurring in the fetus.

Interpretation of NST

Reactive test. A reactive NST shows at least two accelerations of FHR with fetal movements, of 15 bpm, lasting 15 seconds or more, over 20 minutes (Figure 13–8).

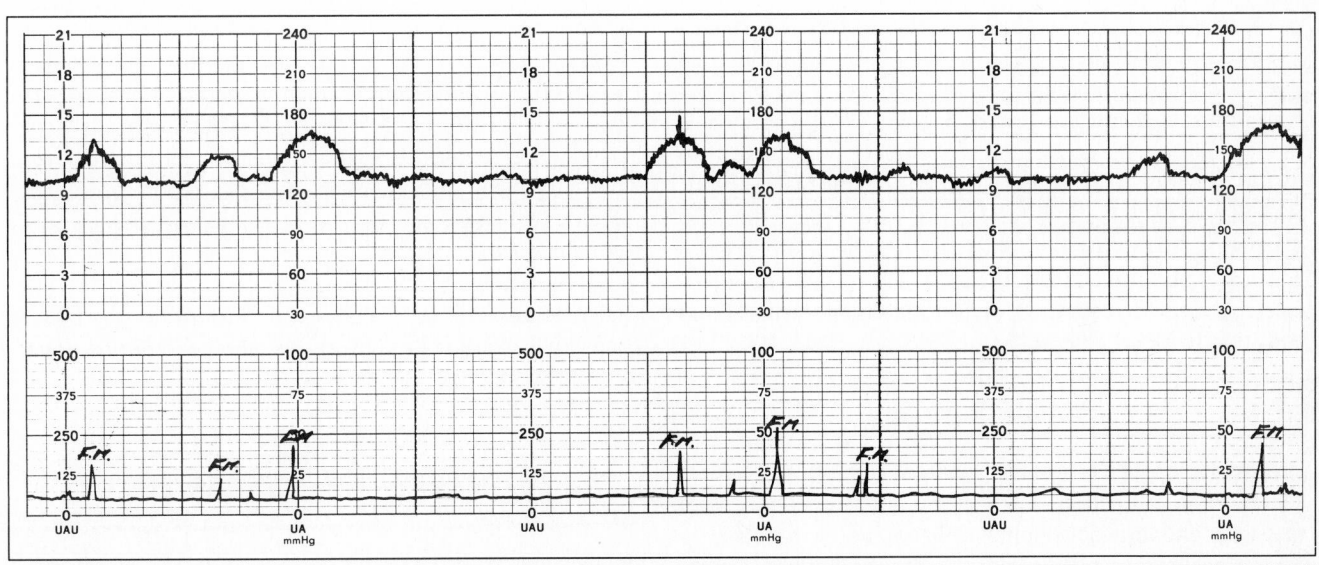

FIGURE 13–8 Example of a reactive nonstress test (NST). Accelerations of 15 beats/min, lasting 15 seconds with each fetal movement (FM). *(Top of strip = fetal heart rate; bottom of strip = uterine activity tracing.)*

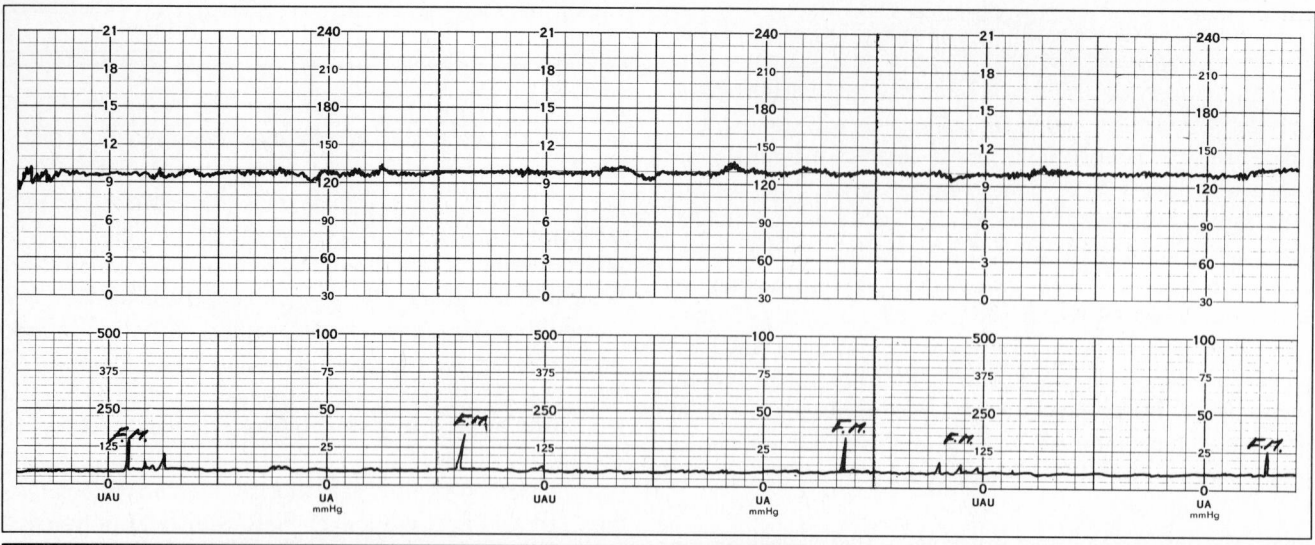

FIGURE 13-9 Example of a nonreactive NST. There are no accelerations of FHR with fetal movement (FM). Baseline FHR = 130 beats/min; tracing of uterine activity is on the bottom of the strip.

Nonreactive test. In a nonreactive NST, the reactive criteria are not met (Figure 13-9).

Unsatisfactory test. An unsatisfactory NST yields uninterpretable registration of FHR or inadequate fetal activity.

Note that criteria for the NST appear to vary from one author to another. Some require two accelerations of the FHR in 20 minutes; others require two in 10 minutes.

Procedure

The client is placed in a semi-Fowler position and an electronic fetal monitor is applied (see discussion on p. 434).

Recordings of the FHR are obtained for approximately 30–40 minutes (minimum of 20 minutes). The client or nurse must activate the "mark button" on the electronic fetal monitor with each fetal movement. The nurse also makes notations regarding baseline activity of the FHR, and uterine activity. If no fetal movements occur after 30–40 minutes of observation, the client may be asked to eat a light meal and return for retesting. Fetal movements often increase due to distention of the maternal stomach and elevation in blood glucose.

Prognostic Value

Bishop (1981) has reported that acceleration of FHR seems to be a function of advancing gestational age, fetal maturity, and fetal development. Bishop notes that there is a high occurrence of false-positive results (that is, a nonreactive test) prior to 30 weeks' gestation. Since delivery is seldom indicated prior to this time, nonstress testing may not be justified before 30 weeks. The NST and the contraction stress test both have higher incidences of false-positive rather than false-negative results. Attainment of a reactive test appears to be indicative of fetal well-being, whereas nonreactive results do not necessarily indicate fetal jeopardy and therefore require further evaluation of fetal status by other parameters. The correlation between a reactive NST and a negative contraction stress test is high.

The high incidence of nonreactive NSTs appears to be dependent on many factors; therefore all nonreactive tests should be followed by additional testing. Some authors advocate rescheduling the NST again within the same 24 hours, while others suggest an immediate contraction stress test. When the NST is reactive, the test should be repeated in a week. Any change in maternal or fetal status (such as decreased fetal movement, falling estriols, vaginal bleeding, or deterioration of maternal condition) warrants more frequent testing. Many authors recommend twice-weekly testing for clients with prolonged pregnancy or diabetes (Figure 13-10).

The NST is useful because it is simple and relatively quick to perform, permits easy interpretation, is less expensive, has no contraindications, and need not be done in a hospital setting.

CONTRACTION STRESS TEST

Kubli et al. (1969) have suggested that placental function may be divided into two components: nutritive (or metabolic) and respiratory. Nutritive deficit may result in IUGR, producing infants who are small for gestational age. These

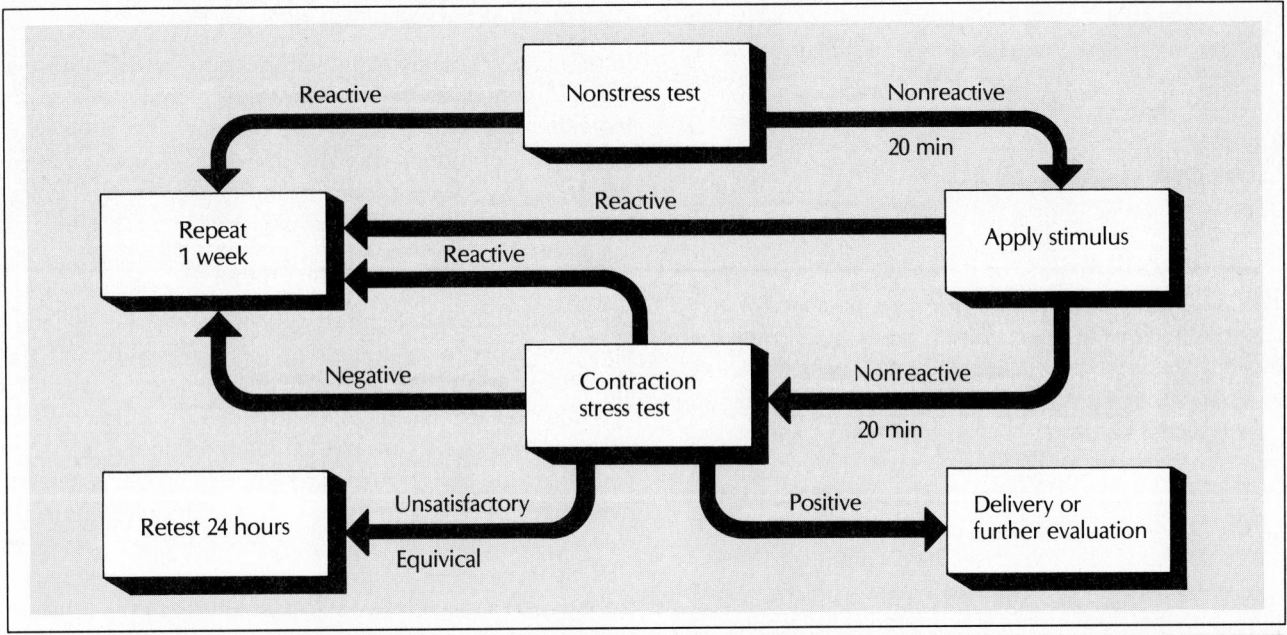

FIGURE 13–10 Flow chart indicating recommended management of nonstress test. (From Evertson, L. R.; Gauthier, R. J.; Schifrin, B. S.; et al. 1979. Antepartum fetal heart rate testing. I. Evolution of the non-stress test. *Am. J. Obstet. Gynecol.* 133(1):131.)

fetuses may be followed with serial sonograms, urinary and plasma estriol determinations, and clinical surveillance of fundal progression. The contraction stress test (CST) is a means of evaluating the respiratory function of the placenta and is most helpful in evaluating cases of chronic placental insufficiency and women whose estriol values may be abnormally low or difficult to interpret.

The CST is an external antenatal means of monitoring the respiratory reserve of the uterine–placental–fetal unit. It enables the health care team to identify the fetus at risk for intrauterine asphyxia by observing the response of the fetal heart rate to the stress of uterine contractions (spontaneous, oxytocin-induced) and to intervene if necessary. With an increase in intrauterine pressure during contractions, there is a transient reduction in blood flow to the intervillous space of the placenta and therefore decreased oxygen transport to the fetus. In most instances this reduction is well tolerated by a healthy fetus, but if there is insufficient placental reserve, fetal hypoxia, depression of the myocardium, and late decelerations of the FHR will occur as placental reserve is exceeded. In the intrapartal period, late decelerations of FHR have been associated with fetal metabolic acidosis (low fetal scalp pH), newborns with low Apgar scores, and, rarely, fetal intrapartal death (Weingold, 1975). Hon and Quilligan (1967) define *late decelerations* as decreases in the FHR that are uniform and have their onset late in the uterine contraction phase. Late decelerations have their onset at or just following the acme of the contraction and occur repetitively. (See Chapter 15 for further discussion of FHR patterns.)

Indications and Contraindications

The CST is indicated for pregnancies at risk for placental insufficiency or fetal compromise because of the following:

- IUGR
- Diabetes mellitus
- Heart disease
- Chronic hypertension
- Preeclampsia-eclampsia
- Sickle cell disease
- Suspected postmaturity (42 weeks' gestation)
- History of previous stillborn or intrapartal loss
- Rh sensitization with meconium-stained amniotic fluid
- Abnormal estriol excretion
- Hyperthyroidism
- Renal disease
- Nonreactive NST

Contraindications for the CST are as follows:

1. Third trimester bleeding (placenta previa or marginal abruptio placentae).
2. Previous classical cesarean delivery.
3. Instances in which the risk of possible premature labor outweighs the advantage of the CST.
   a. Premature rupture of the membranes.

b. Incompetent cervix or Shirodkar-Barter operation (cerclage—surgical procedure in which an incompetent cervix is encircled with suture to prevent it from dilating before the end of 40 weeks' gestation).

c. Multiple gestation.

Procedure

A necessary component of the CST is the presence of uterine contractions which occur three times in 10 minutes. The contractions may occur spontaneously (which is somewhat unusual), or they may be induced (stimulated) by utilizing oxytocin. The most common method of stimulating uterine contractions for a CST is through the use of intravenous administration of oxytocin (Pitocin). Consequently, the CST has been called oxytocin challenge test (OCT). Some facilities use the breast self-stimulation test (BSST). The development of this method is based on the knowledge that endogenous oxytocin is produced in response to stimulation of the breasts or nipples.

The CST is performed on an outpatient basis by qualified perinatal nurses well acquainted with fetal monitoring and the interpretation of various FHR patterns. Most agencies require the tests be administered in or near the labor and delivery unit, in case adverse reactions to oxytocin stimulation occur. The procedure, reasons for administering the test, equipment, and normal variations in monitoring that occur during the test should be clearly explained to the client prior to the test to alleviate apprehension. A consent form is signed. The client should empty her bladder prior to beginning the CST, because she may be confined to bed for 1½–2 hours.

During the test, the client assumes a semi-Fowler position to avoid supine hypotension. After the area of clearest fetoscopic heart tones is noted, the ultrasonic transducer (from the electronic fetal monitor) is placed on the client's abdomen so that the FHR may be accurately recorded on the monitoring strip. (See Chapter 15 for further discussion of fetal monitoring.) To record uterine contractions, the tocodynamometer (pressure transducer) is placed over the area of the uterine fundus. For the first 15 minutes the nurse records baseline measurements, including blood pressure, fetal activity, variations of the FHR during fetal movement, and spontaneous contractions. In addition, pertinent medical and obstetric information may be obtained from the client to aid in her further management.

After a 15-minute baseline recording, if three spontaneous contractions of good quality lasting 40–60 seconds have occurred in a 10-minute period, the results are evaluated and the test is concluded. If no contractions have occurred or if they are insufficient for interpretation, intravenous oxytocin solution is administered or breast stimulation is done.

CST WITH INTRAVENOUS OXYTOCIN

Intravenous 5% dextrose in normal saline or lactated Ringer's solution is infused in the client's hand or forearm (note: if client is diabetic, normal saline should be used). A piggy-back infusion of oxytocin in a similar solution is administered by means of a constant infusion pump to measure accurately the amount of oxytocin being infused.

BREAST SELF-STIMULATION TEST

Baseline data are obtained through assessment and continuous monitoring, as described for CST. In BSST, the breasts are stimulated by application of warm washcloths and then by manual nipple rolling of one nipple. When sufficient contraction criteria for interpreting the test have been met, the test is concluded. Continued assessment is maintained until contractions subside. The results are reviewed, recorded, and explained to the client. As with CST by intravenous oxytocin administration, breast stimulation is discontinued if late decelerations are repetitive or if they occur three times (Freeman, 1982).

Clinical Application

A CST is usually not done prior to 28 weeks' gestation because, in light of a positive test, delivery and extrauterine survival would be questionable, and sufficient research has not been done to determine whether the same test results apply to a fetus of this gestation.

CSTs are usually begun at approximately 32–34 weeks' gestation and are repeated at weekly intervals until the client delivers. Should the client's condition deteriorate, the CST should be repeated as soon as possible.

A *negative CST* (Table 13–1 and Figure 13–11) has high prognostic value in that it implies that placental support is adequate. If that is the case, the physician can avoid premature intervention and gain approximately one additional week of intrauterine life for the fetus (Freeman, 1975). A negative test also suggests that the fetus would be likely to tolerate the stress of labor should it ensue within the week (Schifrin et al., 1975).

A woman who exhibits a *positive CST* (Table 13–1 and Figure 13–12) may have a fetus whose placental reserves are compromised. In many instances there is minimal baseline variability of the FHR (a condition that is usually not seen with healthy fetuses). Most frequently, acceleration of the FHR with fetal movement is absent or diminished, representing inadequate autonomic nervous system control of the fetal heart rate. However, a positive CST does not appear to be as reliable an indicator of fetal status as a negative one (Freeman, 1975). False-positive results may occur due to maternal hypotension during the test, which produces late decelerations. Intravenous oxytocin-induced contractions may be more

Table 13-1   Interpretation of CST Results

CST	Findings	CST	Findings
Negative test	Three contractions of good quality in 10 min, lasting 40 or more sec, without late decelerations (Figure 13–11)	Hyperstimulation	Contractions closer than every 2 min or lasting more than 90 sec with late decelerations; healthy fetus may show decelerations during a prolonged contraction Repeat in 24 hr
	Contraction of good quality lasting more than 90 sec; hyperstimulation without late deceleration (Figure 13–13)	Suspicious test	Nonrepetitive late decelerations occurring with less than 50% of contractions Repeat in 24 hr
	Usually associated with good variability of the FHR and acceleration of FHR with fetal movement	Unsatisfactory test	Recording cannot be interpreted or contractions are inadequate, as a result of one or more of following factors:
Positive test	Occurrence of repetitive, persistent late decelerations with more than 50% of contractions; frequency of contractions need not be three in 10 min (Figure 13–12)		1. Obesity 2. Excessive maternal or fetal activity 3. Hydramnios 4. Fetal hiccups 5. Bowel sounds
	Usually associated with decreased variability and lack of acceleration of the FHR with fetal movement		Repeat in 24 hr (may need to wait one week if unable to obtain contractions)

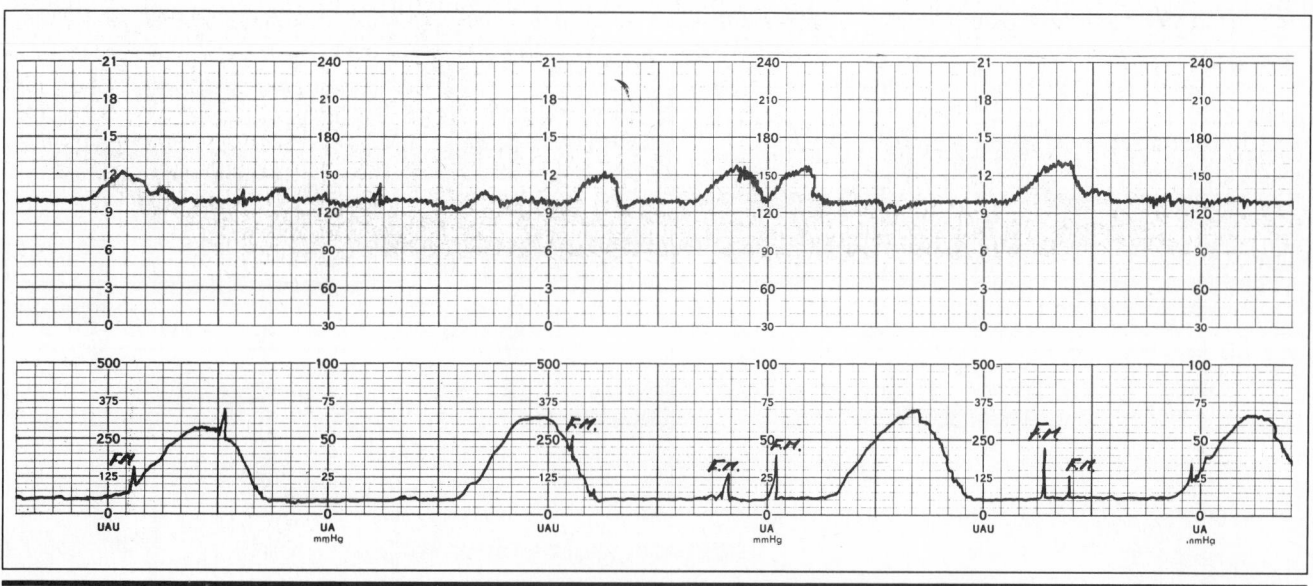

FIGURE 13–11 Example of a negative CST (and reactive NST). Baseline FHR = 130 with acceleration of FHR of at least 15 beats/min lasting 15 seconds with each fetal movement (FM). Uterine contractions recorded on bottom half of strip indicate three contractions in 8 minutes (with monitor paper speed at 3 cm/min).

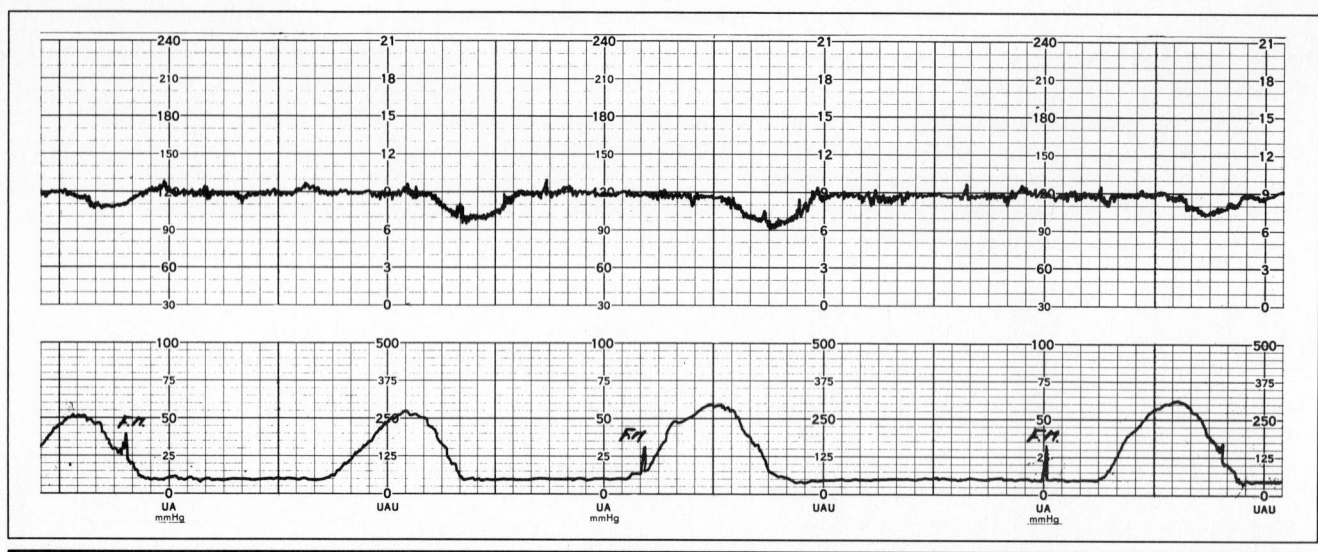

FIGURE 13-12 Example of a positive contraction stress test (CST). Repetitive late decelerations occur with each contraction. *Note:* There are no accelerations of FHR with three fetal movements (FM): Baseline FHR = 120 beats/min. Uterine contractions *(bottom half of strip)* occurred three times in 8 minutes.

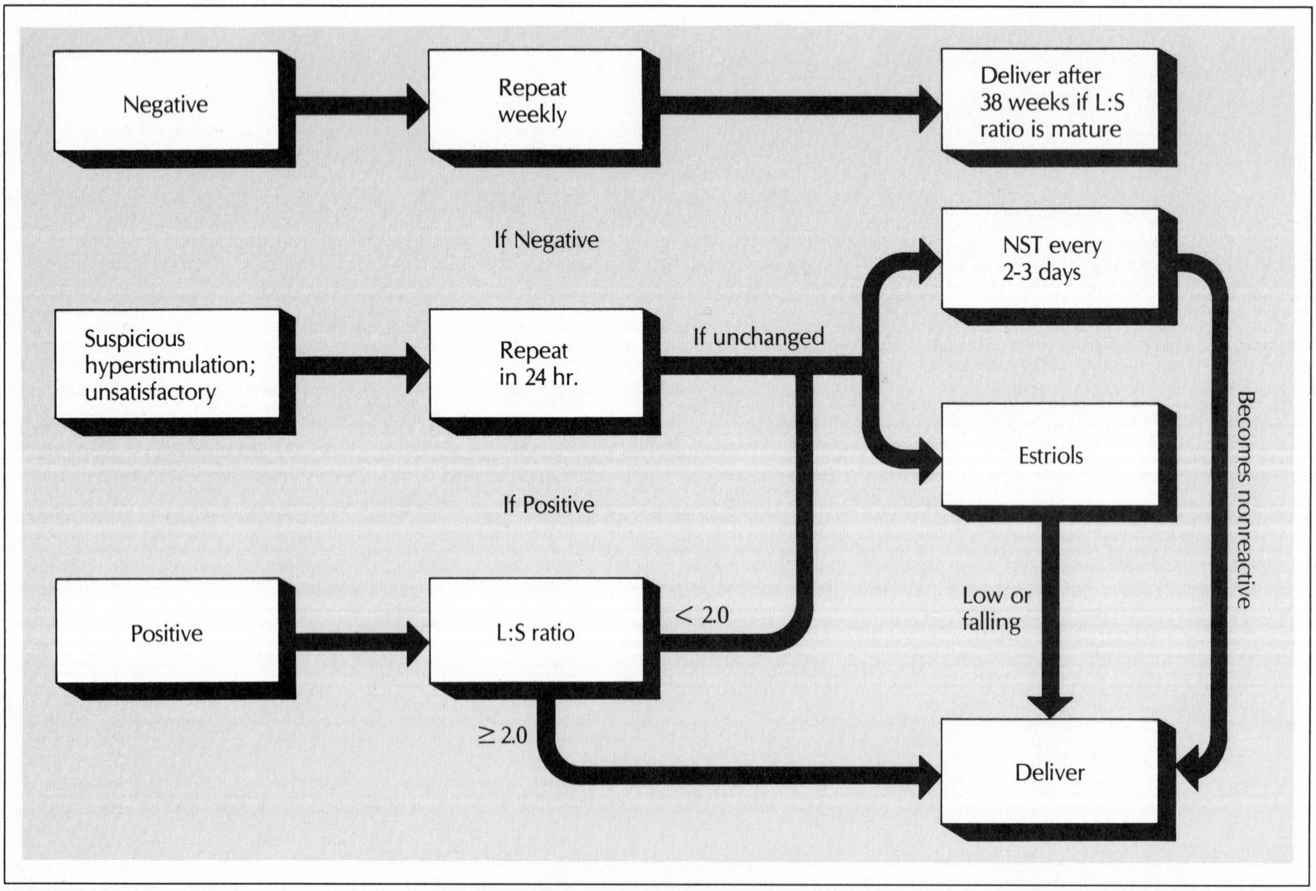

```
Negative ──────▶ Repeat ──────────────▶ Deliver after
                  weekly                   38 weeks if L:S
                                           ratio is mature

              If Negative                              NST every
                                                       2-3 days

Suspicious                                                          Becomes nonreactive
hyperstimulation; ──────▶ Repeat ──── If unchanged
unsatisfactory            in 24 hr.                     Estriols

              If Positive                          Low or
                                                   falling

Positive ──────▶ L:S ratio  < 2.0

                           ≥ 2.0                       Deliver
```

FIGURE 13-13 Flow chart indicating CST management protocol. (From Freeman, R. K., and Garite, T. J. 1981. *Fetal heart rate monitoring.* Baltimore: Williams & Wilkins, p. 166.)

stressful than would normally occur during labor as a result of hyperstimulation, which might not be detected with an external pressure transducer.

Clients with positive test results may be managed differently according to their specific situation. Other parameters of fetal status must be taken into consideration, and on the basis of all available data, the pregnancy may be allowed to continue or labor may be induced (Figure 13–13).

If the CST is positive, yet the fetus demonstrates acceleration of FHR with fetal movement (reactive NST), the CST may have false-positive results (about 50% of cases). Many of these clients will tolerate trial induction of labor (Huddleston, 1980).

If the CST is positive and there is no acceleration of FHR with fetal movement (nonreactive NST), the CST result appears to be ominous. It has been reported that loss of reactivity of the FHR is a late sign of fetal hypoxia, and this occurs earlier than appearance of late decelerations.

Delivery is usually considered if it has been determined that the fetus's lungs are mature. Whether the woman with a positive CST should have a cesarean delivery depends on how rapidly the fetus must be delivered to avoid possible fetal distress, on the adequacy of dilatation, on the softness and effacement of the cervix ("ripeness") at the time, and on the woman's condition.

ESTRIOL DETERMINATIONS

The amount of estrogen excreted in the urine of a pregnant woman has been used as an indicator of metabolic placental function and a predictor of fetal jeopardy in the management of the high-risk pregnancy. About 90% of the estrogen excreted in urine is in the form of *estriol*, and the presence of this hormone appears to be a reflection of the integrity of the maternal–fetal–placental unit. Estriol levels increase in both urine and blood as pregnancy goes to term, with significant amounts being produced in the third trimester. To maintain optimal estrogen metabolism, there must be a healthy fetus; a normally functioning, intact placenta; and a healthy mother. As the fetus grows and matures, estriol production increases; when growth becomes retarded, production levels off; and when there is fetal distress and the placenta has reached its limit, estriol production decreases. Serial estriol determinations are used in the obstetric management of high-risk clients with hypertension, preeclampsia, diabetes, renal disease, suspected placental insufficiency, IUGR, and postmaturity. Current opinion indicates the test is less reliable in clients with chronic hypertension and severe diabetes with renal changes.

Estriol Metabolism

Estrogen is produced by the placenta and depends on precursors received from both woman and fetus. There is a constant interplay between mother, fetus, and placenta, and all must be healthy and functioning well for estrogen production to be within normal limits.

Estrogen precursors from the mother and placenta (primarily cholesterol and pregnenolone) are transported across the placenta, synthesized by the fetal adrenal glands, and turned into dehydroepiandrosterone sulfate. Hydroxylation occurs in the fetal liver, and the androgens are then converted by the placenta to estriol and other estrogens and are excreted into the maternal circulation. Some of this material is returned to the fetus, and the remainder is conjugated with acids in the maternal liver and excreted by the kidneys.

Patterns of Excretion

Four patterns of estriol excretion are generally seen, as Figure 13–14 indicates (Green et al.,1969):

- *Pattern I.* All serial levels fall within the normal range and continue to rise until term.

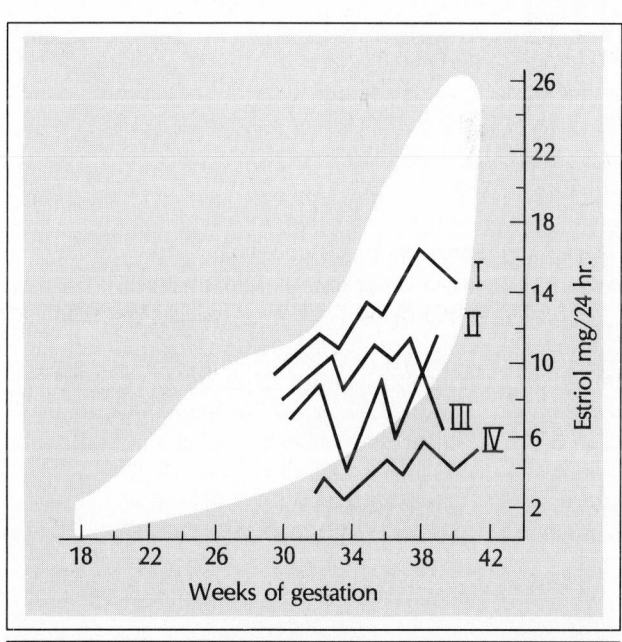

FIGURE 13–14 Estriol excretion patterns and the range of normal excretion *(light area)*. Excretion patterns I and II have critical levels of 12 mg/24 hr at term. Pattern III rises normally but falls before term. Pattern IV stays at low excretion levels. (From Green, J. W., et al. 1969. Correlation of estriol excretion patterns of pregnant women with subsequent development of their children. *Am. J. Obstet. Gynecol.* 105:730.)

- *Pattern II.* Levels are within subnormal range and yet rise so that the critical level of 12 mg is reached at term.
- *Pattern III.* Values are within the normal range but suddenly fall, either abruptly or gradually. This is an ominous pattern and is seen with fetal death due to a deterioration of the intrauterine environment.
- *Pattern IV.* Values are never within the normal range. Morbidity and mortality are high with this group. It is questionable whether this pregnancy should continue if fetal lungs are mature.

The range of normal values is broad, and various patterns are seen. A single 24-hour estriol measurement that falls in the normal range does not necessarily indicate fetal well-being, just as a single drop in production does not necessarily indicate fetal jeopardy. Of more significance than any specific value is the general trend in day-to-day or week-to-week values. Estriol production fluctuates daily, so one must be careful not to assume that the fetus is in jeopardy when in fact the fluctuation is normal. Generally, a drop of 50% or more from the previous mean level may signify fetal distress (Tulchinsky, 1975). Some clinicians may use a drop of greater than 40% occurring on two consecutive determinations as the significant change. Decreases of 30% may be due to laboratory variation or normal daily fluctuation. A fall in estriol is usually gradual, except in the case of diabetes, in which the drop may be more dramatic due to abrupt changes in glucose metabolism.

Estriol production reaches a plateau at about 40–41 weeks' gestation and decreases slowly thereafter. Thus, in the case of suspected postmaturity, if estriols are rising, the woman's estimated date for delivery may be incorrect. Urinary excretion of more than 30 mg/24 hr indicates absence of postmaturity, and therefore intervention may be delayed (Gobelsmann, 1977). If values are low but increasing, serial values indicate that the fetus is growing.

Decreasing estriol levels from previously low levels are a poor prognostic sign. Critical levels (lower limits than normal) of estriol excretion are 7 mg/24 hr at 30 weeks' gestation and 12 mg/24 hr at 40 weeks' gestation. A value of 4 mg/24 hr may indicate impending fetal death. Chronically low values may be indicative of IUGR. When low values are obtained, one must consider the following possibilities:

- Laboratory error
- Incomplete 24-hour urine collection
- Incorrect gestational age
- Drugs such as ampicillin, heroin, methadone, methenamine mandelate (Mandelamine), neomycin, or steroids
- Placental steroid sulfatase deficiency
- Chronic uteroplacental insufficiency
- Anencephaly or hydrocephaly
- Maternal pyelonephritis
- Maternal anemia
- Fetal congenital adrenal hypoplasia

Urinary Estriol Determinations

PROCEDURE

Clients must be given a clear explanation by the nurse or physician concerning the urinary collection procedure they must perform for estriol determination. The client must understand why all her urine must be saved, why it must be refrigerated, when to bring it to the laboratory, and what the results mean.

The client discards the first urinary specimen of the morning and then collects all urine in a clean container, which is kept refrigerated to prevent formation of bacteria and breakdown of estrogen products. The time that she first empties her bladder the first day is the time she should collect her final specimen the following morning. For example, if she first voids at 7 AM on Wednesday, the final specimen to be collected should be at 7 AM on Thursday. The client must be informed as to the time that she must bring the specimen to the laboratory so that it can be processed the same day to avoid delay in obtaining results. She should be told to report any incidence of forgetting to collect a particular voiding, because this will alter test results.

SERIAL DETERMINATIONS

In managing the high-risk client, it is necessary to obtain serial determinations. Estriol determinations are usually instituted at approximately 32–34 weeks' gestation and are collected no more than once or twice a week unless abnormal. Prior to 32 weeks' gestation, delivery is usually not contemplated due to immaturity of the fetus, although the physician may wish to begin to look at estriol excretion as early as 28 weeks in clients with chronic hypertension, preeclampsia, or fetal IUGR.

Estriol determinations may be indicated two to three times each week later in the pregnancy or even daily, as in the case of the diabetic nearing term, because there is a greater risk of missing a significant fall in estriol levels if only twice-weekly determinations are obtained. Estriols tend to fall more slowly in women with chronic hypertension, preeclampsia, and postmaturity. Therefore, twice-weekly determinations are usually sufficient.

Some authorities believe that normal levels begin to fall into an abnormal range about 72 hours before the death of the fetus actually occurs. An abrupt fall is an ominous sign of fetal distress, and until proven otherwise by other parameters, it suggests that the condition of the fetus is rapidly deteriorating.

Because of problems in collection, maternal renal disease, ingestion of medications by the woman, or other factors, estriol determinations should not be used as the sole determining factor in judging the status of the fetal–maternal–placental unit.

Urinary versus Plasma (Serum) Estriol Determinations

Urinary estriol determinations have been used longer than plasma determinations. For this reason, many institutions tend to rely more on urinary assays. Both seem to give the same type of information regarding the status of the maternal–fetal–placental unit, although values do vary. One must be aware of normal values within one's own laboratory. Generally, the plasma (serum) value is approximately one-third the total urine values.

Advantages of plasma over urinary estriol determinations include (a) ease of collection, (b) less difficulty in processing results, (c) less time needed to collect specimens, (d) less time needed to obtain results, (e) less expense, (f) fewer errors in collection, (g) possibility of obtaining two or more plasma samples for analysis in a single day.

Disadvantages of plasma collection are that (a) experience in using them has been limited and techniques are still in the stages of development and refinement, so they are done in only a few centers; (b) erroneously high plasma levels may be obtained with impaired renal clearance; and (c) considerable diurnal variation exists in plasma estriol levels.

Disadvantages of urinary collection include (a) errors in collection of urine (usually incomplete), (b) inconvenience of 24-hour collection, and (c) the amount of time needed to collect urine (24 hours) and to process results (6–8 hours). In addition, low values may be a result of impaired maternal renal function rather than fetal jeopardy.

HUMAN PLACENTAL LACTOGEN

Human placental lactogen (hPL) is a protein produced by the syncytiotrophoblast cells of the placenta in increasing amounts during the normal course of pregnancy, reaching a peak of about 7 μg/mL at term. It is measured by radioimmunoassay or hemagglutination inhibition methods utilizing maternal serum. Current opinion indicates mild enthusiasm for this test in clinical practice.

AMNIOTIC FLUID ANALYSIS

One of the most valuable studies available in the management of the pregnant woman is the analysis of the amniotic fluid, which is obtained by a technique known as *amniocentesis*. Examination of the fluid can provide information regarding the following:

- Degree to which Rh immunization has progressed
- Fetal lung maturity
- Presence of meconium, which may indicate fetal distress
- Chromosomal analysis (see Chapter 7 for further discussion)
- Detection of neural tube defects through α-fetoprotein analysis (see Chapter 7 for further discussion)

Amniocentesis

Amniotic fluid may be obtained by either transabdominal or suprapubic amniocentesis. The procedure is fairly simple, although complications do occur rarely (less than 1%). The fetus, umbilical cord, or placenta may be punctured inadvertently, causing injuries ranging from minor scratches of fetal parts to intrauterine hemorrhage, leading to fetal distress and intrauterine death. Placental perforation could result in hemorrhage from the fetal circulation, which could lead to fetal anemia or to increased sensitization of the Rh-negative mother. Intraamniotic infection and induction of premature labor are also hazards. Complications are rare, but the client does need to be informed of them. Generally, an operative permit is signed for this procedure.

PROCEDURE

Amniocentesis may be done on an outpatient basis but should be performed near a delivery suite should acute fetal distress be encountered. The client should empty her bladder prior to the amniocentesis so that the bladder is not entered instead of the uterus. Amniotic fluid and urine may look similar, and if there is a possibility that urine was obtained during a suprapubic tap, the fluid should be checked for pH and protein content with a dipstick. Amniotic fluid has a high protein content (Goldstein, 1977), which is not a normal finding in urine unless the woman has been spilling protein in her urine as a result of preeclampsia or renal disease.

The abdomen is scanned by ultrasound for placental and fetal location, and to locate an adequate pocket of fluid. The amniocentesis, or "tap," is done immediately, before the fetus has the opportunity to move. The needle insertion site is of the utmost importance, because the fetus, placenta, umbilical cord, bladder, and uterine arteries must all be avoided. The importance of locating the placenta cannot be stressed enough, especially in cases of Rh isoimmunization, in which trauma to the placenta increases fetal–maternal transfusion and worsens the immunization. In addition, if the placenta is anterior a suprapubic tap may be required to avoid puncturing the placenta. Except for very late in pregnancy, the fetal head may be displaced upward and the amniocentesis may be done suprapubical-

FIGURE 13-15 Amniocentesis. Woman is usually scanned by ultrasound to determine the placental site and to locate a pocket of amniotic fluid. As the needle is inserted, three levels of resistance are felt as the needle penetrates the skin, fascia, and uterine wall. When the needle is placed within the uterine cavity, amniotic fluid is withdrawn.

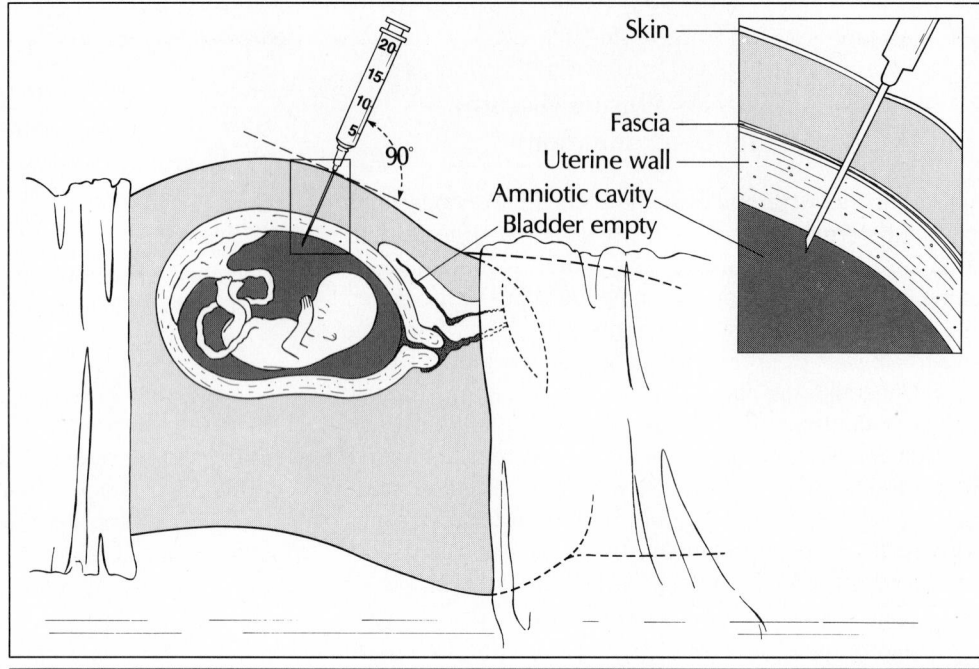

ly. If this is not feasible, it is usually done laterally (Figure 13-15). In the last few weeks of pregnancy, the fetus may occupy what appears to be all the available space in the uterus. There may be a decrease in the amount of available amniotic fluid. With the aid of ultrasound, fluid can usually be located, although in some cases it is impossible.

After the abdomen is scanned, the skin of the maternal abdomen is cleansed with an agent such as thimerosal (Merthiolate), Betadine, or hexachlorophene (pHisoHex). A local anesthetic such as lidocaine (1-2 mL of 1% solution) may be injected just under the skin to anesthetize the area. Many physicians choose not to do this, because they think it frequently causes more discomfort than inserting the spinal needle. A 3-6-inch or 22-gauge spinal needle is inserted into the uterine cavity. Generally, fluid immediately flows into the needle, which is attached to a syringe. From 15-20 mL of amniotic fluid is withdrawn, placed in test tubes covered with tape (to shield the fluid from light to prevent breakdown of bilirubin and other pigments), and sent to the laboratory for analysis. The needle is withdrawn, and the FHR is assessed for approximately 15 minutes. If the client's vital signs and the FHR are normal, she is allowed to leave.

If the amniotic fluid becomes contaminated with blood, the fluid should be centrifuged immediately. The client is observed closely for 30-40 minutes for alterations in the FHR. The blood should be tested to determine whether it is maternal or fetal by performing an Apt test. Some physicians routinely give Rh-negative women RhoGAM after amniocentesis, provided that they are not already sensitized at that time. If the amniotic fluid from these clients is contaminated with blood, the sample should be tested to

identify fetal cells. In this situation, a larger dose of immune globulin is required.

NURSING INTERVENTIONS

The nurse assists the physician during the amniocentesis. Nursing responsibilities are listed in Procedure 13-1. In addition, the nurse supports the client undergoing amniocentesis. Clients are usually apprehensive about what is about to happen as well as about the information that will be obtained by amniocentesis. The physician generally explains the procedure prior to the client's signing the consent form. As it is being performed, the client may need additional emotional support. She may become anxious during the procedure. In addition, the woman may become lightheaded, nauseated, and diaphoretic from lying on her back with a gravid uterus compressing the abdominal vessels. The nurse can provide support to the client by further clarifying the physician's instructions or explanations, by relieving the woman's physical discomfort when possible, and by responding verbally and physically to the client's need for reassurance.

Clinical Application

EVALUATION OF RH-SENSITIZED PREGNANCIES

The first studies of amniotic fluid were done in the early 1950s for the evaluation of bilirubin pigment in the amniotic fluid of Rh-sensitized mothers. By looking at the optical density of the fluid, the analyst could determine the degree to which the fetus was affected.

Bevis (1956) reported that, by analyzing amniotic fluid

Procedure 13-1   Amniocentesis

Objective	Nursing action	Rationale
Prepare client	Explain procedure Reassure client Have client sign consent form Have client empty bladder.	Anxiety will be decreased with information To indicate client's awareness of risks and consent to procedure To decrease risk of bladder perforation
Prepare equipment	Collect supplies: 3 mL syringe with 25-gauge needle Local anesthetic (1% procaine or 1% lidocaine) 3-6-inch 22-gauge spinal needle with stylet 10 mL syringe 20 mL syringe Three 10 mL test tubes with tops (amber-colored or covered with tape)	 Amniotic fluid must be shielded from light to prevent breakdown of bilirubin
Monitor vital signs	Obtain baseline data on maternal BP, pulse, respiration, and FHR Monitor every 15 minutes	Status of client and fetus is assessed
Locate fetus and placenta	Provide assistance as physician palpates for fetal position Assist with real-time ultrasound	 Real-time ultrasound is used to locate fetal parts and placental location. Amniocentesis is usually performed laterally on side of fetus opposite limbs to avoid puncture of cord; a suprapubic centesis is done if the placenta is anterior
Cleanse abdomen	Scrub abdomen with Betadine (or other cleansing agent)	Incidence of infection is decreased
Collect specimen of amniotic fluid	Obtain test tubes from physician; provide correct identification; send to lab with appropriate lab slips	
Reassess vital signs	Determine client's BP, pulse, respirations, and FHR; palpate fundus to assess fetal and uterine activity; monitor client with external fetal monitor for 20-30 minutes after amniocentesis Have client rest on left side	Fetus may have been inadvertently punctured Uterine contractions may ensue following procedure; treatment course should be determined to counteract any supine hypotension and to increase venous return and cardiac output
Complete client record	Record type of procedure done, date, time, name of physician performing test, client-fetal response, and disposition of specimen	Client records will be complete and current
Educate client	Reassure client; instruct her to report any of the following side effects: 1. Unusual fetal hyperactivity or lack of movement 2. Vaginal discharge—clear drainage or bleeding 3. Uterine contractions or abdominal pain 4. Fever or chills	Client will know how to recognize side effects or conditions that warrant further treatment

of the Rh-sensitized mother, valuable information could be gained concerning the progress of her pregnancy. Liley (1961) produced a graph that is now universally used in determining the severity of hemolytic disease in the fetus (Figure 13–16).

If a sensitized Rh-negative woman produces an incompatible Rh-positive fetus, antibodies cross the placenta and cause hemolytic anemia in the fetus. Concentrations of bilirubin and other breakdown products from destroyed red blood cells can be detected in amniotic fluid by spectrophotometry. By plotting their concentration or optical density at 450 mu on a Liley curve, the physician can ascertain the degree to which the fetus is affected and the need for intervention or intrauterine transfusion.

Liley categorized the degree of hemolytic disease into three zones. If the optical density falls in zone I (low zone) at 28–31 weeks' gestation, the fetus either will be unaffected or will have only mild hemolytic disease. Amniocentesis should be repeated in 2 or 3 weeks. When the optical

density falls in zone II (midzone), amniocentesis is repeated frequently so that the trend can be determined. The age of the fetus and the trend in optical density indicate the necessity for intrauterine transfusion or premature delivery. Optical densities falling in zone III (high zone) indicate that the fetus is severely affected and death is a possibility. The decision concerning delivery or intrauterine transfusion depends on the gestational age of the fetus. After about 32 or 33 weeks of gestation, early delivery and extrauterine treatment are probably preferred to performing intrauterine transfusion.

OPTICAL DENSITY

The measurement of optical density is a reflection of the amount of pigment bilirubin present in the amniotic fluid. Bilirubin may be found in amniotic fluid as early as the twelfth week of pregnancy, reaching its highest concentrations between 16–30 weeks' gestation (Leiker and Hensleigh, 1975). As pregnancy continues, the amount of bilirubin progressively decreases, finally disappearing near term.

The amount of bilirubin in amniotic fluid can be determined by a technique described by Liley (1961): evaluation of the optical density (ΔOD) at 450 mu. Although this method cannot be used as an absolute indicator of fetal maturity, many investigators agree that, once the optical density of amnitic fluid falls to zero, fetal maturity is almost assured. Conditions in which incresed values are found include anencephaly, intestinal obstruction, and sometimes deteriorating hydrops fetalis. Optical density cannot be used as an indication of fetal maturity in the Rh-sensitized woman.

Evaluation of Fetal Maturity

In managing the woman–fetus at risk, the physician is constantly faced with the possibility of having to deliver an infant prior to term and before the onset of labor. There are many indications for early termination of pregnancy, including repeat cesarean delivery, premature rupture of the membranes, diabetes, hypertensive conditions in the pregnant client, and placental insufficiency. Unfortunately, the most common cause of perinatal mortality is prematurity and complications arising from pulmonary immaturity (Leiker and Hensleigh, 1975); delivery of an infant with immature pulmonary function frequently results in RDS, also known as hyaline membrane disease (see Chapter 25).

Because gestational age, birth weight, and the rate of development of organ systems do not necessarily correspond, it may be necessary to determine the lung maturation of the fetus by amniotic fluid analysis, before elective delivery. Concentrations of certain substances in the amniotic fluid reflect the pulmonary condition of the fetus (see p. 385). In many cases, delivery of the infant can be delayed until the lungs show maturity.

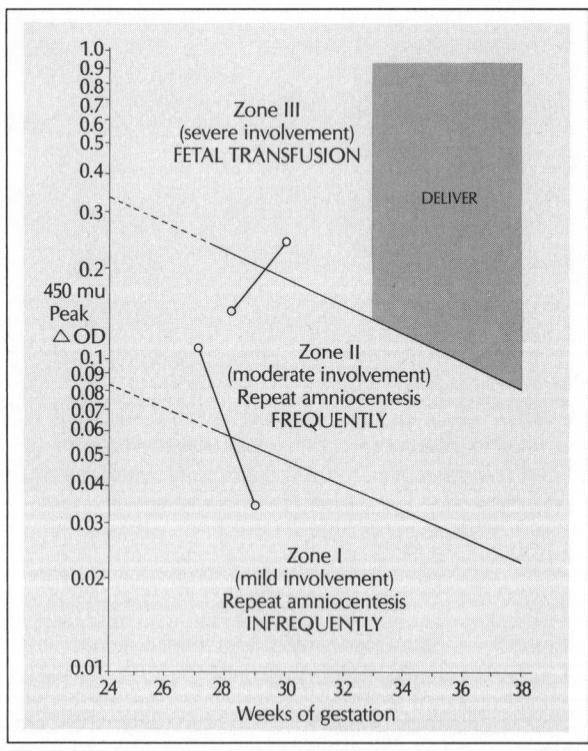

FIGURE 13–16 The density of amniotic fluid can be useful in determining the severity of erythroblastosis fetalis. There are three zones of optical density, which are correlated with the degree to which the fetus is affected by this condition. In this graph, management of the Rh-sensitized pregnancy is related to the condition of the fetus and gestational age. (Modified from Liley, A. W. 1961. Liquor amnii analysis in the management of the pregnancy complicated by rhesus sensitization. *Am. J. Obstet. Gynecol.* 32:1359.)

L/S RATIO

The alveoli of the lungs are lined by a substance called *surfactant*, which is composed of phospholipids. Surfactant lowers the surface tension of the alveoli during extrauterine respiratory exhalation. By lowering the alveolar surface tension, surfactant stabilizes the alveoli, and a certain amount of air always remains in the alveoli during expiration. When a newborn with mature pulmonary function takes its first breath, a tremendously high pressure is needed to open the lungs. Upon breathing out, the lungs do not collapse and about half the air in the alveoli is retained. An infant born too early in his or her development, when synthesis of surfactant is incomplete, is unable to maintain lung stability, resulting in underinflation of the lungs and development of RDS.

Fetal lung maturity can be ascertained by determining the ratio of two components of surfactant—lecithin and sphingomyelin. Early in pregnancy the sphingomyelin concentration in amniotic fluid is more than that of lecithin, resulting in a low *lecithin/sphingomyelin* (L/S) *ratio*. At about 30–32 weeks' gestation, the amounts of the two substances become equal. The concentration of lecithin begins to exceed that of sphingomyelin, rising abruptly at about 35 weeks' gestation (Gluck, 1975). Concurrently, sphingomyelin begins to decrease. Fetal maturity is attained when the L/S ratio is 2:1 or greater; that is, when the amount of lecithin found in the amniotic fluid is at least two times that of sphingomyelin (Figure 13–17).

RDS is associated with pulmonary immaturity; thus RDS does not develop in infants whose L/S ratio is 2:1 (except in diabetics).

Laboratories vary in their criteria and methods for determining L/S ratios. One must be aware of these differences when interpreting results.

Under certain conditions of stress, premature maturation of the fetal lungs may be seen. The lung seems to react in different ways to acute and chronic stress. Conditions in which one may see accelerated maturation of the lungs include premature rupture of the membranes, acute placental infarction, placental insufficiency, chronic abruptio placentae, renal hypertensive disease due to degenerative forms of diabetes, cardiovascular hypertensive disease, and severe chronic preeclampsia-eclampsia. In addition, the smaller of parabiotic twins may manifest lung maturity prematurely. Prolonged rupture of the membranes after 72 hours seems to have an acute effect on lung maturation, causing an abrupt rise in the L/S ratio (signifying lung maturity), independent of previous L/S ratios or gestational age (Richardson et al., 1974).

Delayed maturation is often seen in infants born to mothers with class A, B, and C diabetes, in those born to mothers with nonhypertensive glomerulonephritis or hydrops fetalis, and in the smaller of nonparabiotic twins (Gluck, 1975).

Should amniotic fluid be contaminated due to bloody tap, it has been suggested that fetal lung maturity be assessed by looking for phosphatidylglycerol, since it is not found in blood and L/S ratios may be inaccurate when fluid is so contaminated (Bustos et al., 1979).

LUNG PROFILE

As mentioned earlier, the most universally used assay in evaluating functional pulmonary maturity in the fetus is the L/S ratio. However, problems that may be incurred in this determination include:

- High false-negative rate
- Unpredictability of a value that is borderline
- Unpredictability of blood-contaminated specimens
- Occasional false-positive values associated with such conditions as Rh disease, diabetes, and severe birth asphyxia

Some of these difficulties have been overcome by utilizing a lung profile of amniotic fluid to evaluate fetal lung maturity, and by looking for the presence of lecithin (phosphatidylcholine) and phosphatidylglycerol (PG) which are reported to be the major phospholipids of surfactant (Hallman et al., 1976; Kulovich et al., 1979).

Lecithin accounts for approximately 80% of the total

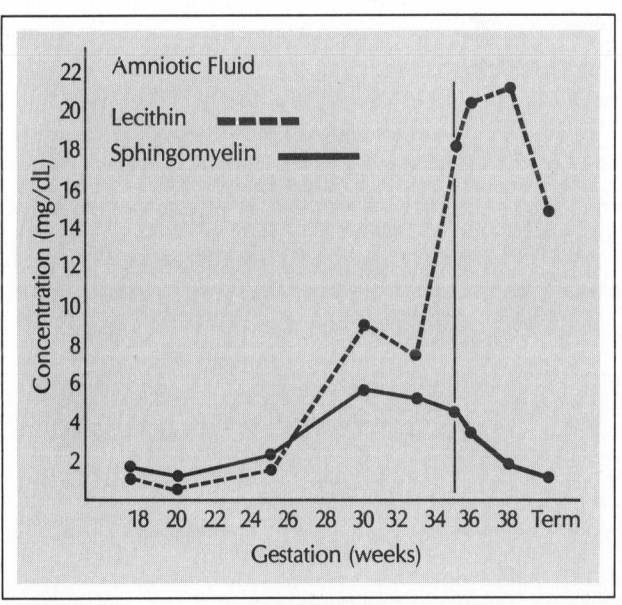

FIGURE 13–17 Mean concentrations in amniotic fluid of sphingomyelin and lecithin during gestation. The acute rise in lecithin at 35 weeks marks pulmonary maturity. (From Gluck, L., et al. 1971. Diagnosis of the respiratory distress syndrome by amniocentesis. *Am. J. Obstet. Gynecol.* 109:441.)

phospholipids in surfactant. Phosphatidylglycerol is the second most abundant phospholipid. Phosphatidylinositol (PI), as reported by Hallman et al. (1976), increases in amniotic fluid after 26–30 weeks of gestation, peaks at 36–37 weeks, and then decreases gradually, whereas phosphatidylglycerol, appearing after 35 weeks, continues to increase until term (Figure 13–18). In instances of diabetes, complicated by premature rupture of the membranes, or vascular disease, or severe preeclampsia-eclampsia, phosphatidylglycerol may be present before 35 weeks' gestation. It is helpful to know this fact, as early intervention in the event of lung maturation will lead to the best fetal outcome and prevention of RDS (Gabbe, 1982).

The incidence of RDS in infants delivered of diabetic mothers with L/S ratios of 2:1 or greater is significant. Although it has been reported that a delay in the appearance of phosphatidylglycerol in diabetic gestations may occur, the presence of additional phospholipid assists the physician in assessing the overall pulmonary status of the fetus in diabetic pregnancies (Cunningham et al., 1982). Kulovich et al. (1979) and Cunningham et al. (1982) reported delayed appearance of phosphatidylglycerol in the lung profile of class A diabetics until 37 weeks or later. Others have reported that it may begin to appear in the amniotic fluid of normal pregnancies between 35 and 37 weeks (Hallman et al., 1976; Kulovich et al., 1979). It appears that lung maturity can be confirmed in most pregnancies if phosphatidylglycerol is present in conjunction with an L/S ratio of 2:1.

The lung profile, developed by Gluck and associates, is a useful tool in the assessment of lung maturity in the fetus of the diabetic woman. This profile evaluates the relationship between not only lecithin and sphingomyelin, but also the presence of phosphatidylglycerol and phosphatidylinositol. It has been suggested that when the former is present in diabetic gestations and the L/S ratio is 2:1, one can be confident that respiratory distress will not occur in the neonate. Only the larger facilities are presently able to perform analysis of these two phospholipids, but it is hoped that this assay will be available some day for use with all diabetic pregnancies.

SHAKE TEST (FOAM STABILITY TEST)

Introduced by Clements et al. (1972), the shake test is a quick and inexpensive test for prediction of fetal lung maturity. It is based on the ability of surfactant in the amniotic fluid to form bubbles or foam in the presence of ethanol. The test requires 15–30 minutes. Exact amounts of 95% ethanol, isotonic saline, and amniotic fluid are shaken together for 15 seconds. The persistence of a complete ring of bubbles on the surface of the liquid after 15 minutes indicates a positive shake test, indicating lung maturity. There is an extremely high false-negative rate but a low false-positive rate. Factors that may account for false negativity include dirty glass test tubes and contamination of the reagents or amniotic fluid. The L/S ratio test is normally not done when the shake test is positive, because the shake test indicates fetal lung maturity. If the optical density and creatinine values do not correlate with the shake test finding, the L/S ratio should be obtained regardless of the shake test result.

The foam stability index (FSI) is a new, rapid test which is read by special spectrophotometry.

CREATININE LEVEL

Amniotic creatinine progressively increases as pregnancy advances. This may be due to excretion of fetal urine, reflecting fetal kidney function, or to muscle mass. The use of this value alone to assess maturity is not advisable, because a high creatinine value may be a reflection of muscle mass in a particular fetus and not necessarily indicate kidney maturity. For example, the macrosomic fetus of a diabetic woman may have high creatinine levels due to increased muscle mass, or the small, growth-retarded infant of the hypertensive may demonstrate a low level of creatinine due to decreased muscle mass; in these cases creatinine values can be misleading if used without other data. Nevertheless, when fetal growth (muscle mass) and kidney maturity are at odds, the creatinine is still more indicative

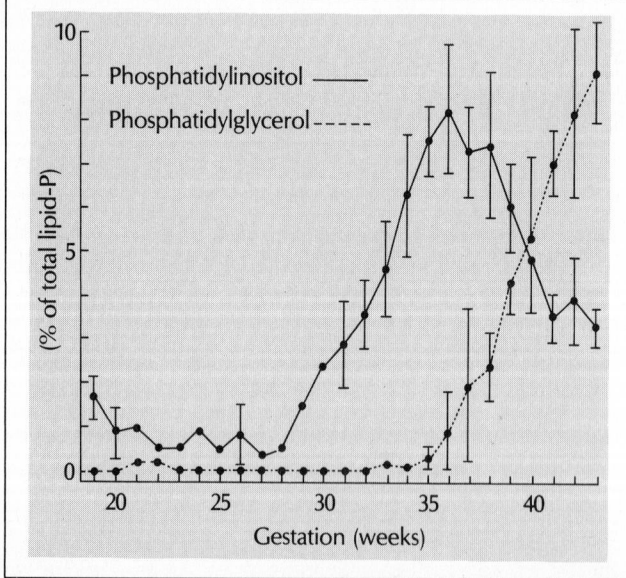

FIGURE 13–18 The content of phosphatidylinositol and phosphatidylglycerol in amniotic fluid during normal gestation. The phospholipids were quantified by measuring the phosphorus (P) content and expressed as percentages of total lipid phosphorus. Means ± standard deviations of three to five samples are shown for each point. (From Hallman, M., et al. 1976. Phosphatidylinositol and phosphatidylglycerol in amniotic fluid: indices of lung maturity. *Am. J. Obstet. Gynecol.* 125:616.)

of fetal kidney maturity. Creatinine levels of 2 mg/dL of amniotic fluid seem to correlate closely with a pregnancy of 37 weeks or more (Pitkin, 1975).

As long as the maternal serum creatinine is not elevated, measurement of creatinine level has a certain degree of reliability when used in conjunction with other maturity studies. An elevated maternal serum creatinine results in increased amniotic fluid levels. The woman's serum creatinine levels should be determined if the creatinine in the amniotic fluid is not what would normally be expected for a particular gestational age.

CYTOLOGIC EXAMINATION OF FETAL CELLS

One simple test of maturity, which can be done in the physician's office or at the bedside, is the staining of fetal fat cells in the amniotic fluid with Nile blue sulfate. The fetus sheds cells during its intrauterine life. In the last weeks of pregnancy the sebaceous glands gradually begin to function and cells are sloughed into the amniotic fluid. Sebaceous cells are different from other fetal cells in that they contain lipid globules. The number of these fat cells increases as the fetus matures, and the percentage of these cells present in the amniotic fluid gives an indication of gestational age. When the number of sebaceous cells (which stain orange with Nile blue sulfate) is less than 2%, there is a prematurity rate of about 85%. If more than 20% of the cells in the fluid stain orange, the infant will weigh at least 2500 g. Andrews (1970) states that, if 10% of the cells stain orange, the gestational age is 36 weeks in about 95% of cases. Others use 20% as the critical level of maturity.

Identification of Meconium Staining

Any episode of hypoxia in utero may result in an increased fetal peristalsis, relaxation of the anal sphincter, and passage of meconium into the amniotic fluid. The amniotic fluid is normally clear, but the presence of meconium makes the fluid greenish.

Meconium staining may also be observed when amniocentesis is done. After the membranes have ruptured, meconium staining may be observed in the drainage from the vagina.

Once meconium staining is identified, more assessments must be made to determine if the fetus is suffering ongoing episodes of hypoxia.

Antenatal Genetic Screening

Antenatal intrauterine diagnosis by amniocentesis of many disorders that may result in a seriously deformed or mentally deficient child is a major advance in the field of perinatology. Indications for genetic amniocentesis and management are discussed in Chapter 7.

AMNIOSCOPY

Visualization of the amniotic fluid through the membranes with an amnioscope is a technique employed to identify meconium staining of the fluid. In many institutions, evidence of meconium in the amniotic fluid is an indication for delivery. In other centers, additional evidence of fetal distress must be demonstrated before delivery is contemplated.

Before the amniotic membranes have ruptured, the meconium staining can be observed by amnioscopy. In this procedure, an amnioscope is placed in the vagina and against the fetal presenting part. The amniotic fluid can be visualized through the amniotic membranes.

Problems associated with amnioscopy include the possibility of inadvertently rupturing the membranes during the examination, an insufficiently dilated cervix through which to insert the amnioscope, intrauterine infection, and occasional difficulty in interpreting the color of the amniotic fluid. Amnioscopy may be a difficult procedure to perform if the woman is in active labor, because she may have difficulty maintaining proper position for the examination.

Amnioscopy is not widely practiced as a screening procedure for detection of meconium because of varying opinions regarding the clinical significance of meconium staining.

X-RAY EXAMINATION

Because of the increasing popularity and use of diagnostic ultrasound, x-ray examination is not employed as frequently as it was in the past. X-ray examination may be used to measure the diameters of the pelvis (pelvimetry) late in pregnancy or during labor. It can also give information regarding shape and size of the pelvis and the relationship of the baby's presentation, position, and station to the woman's pelvis. An x-ray examination may be performed when clinical pelvimetry is questionable, when abnormal presentation and position are evidenced, when labor is prolonged or arrested, or if abnormal development of the fetus is suspected.

Fetal body length and head diameters are almost impossible to measure, but it is possible to estimate fetal age by the appearance of ossification centers. By week 36 of pregnancy, the distal femoral epiphysis is present in approximately 80% or more of fetuses; there is evidence of the proximal tibial epiphysis in 70% to 75% of fetuses at term. The time of appearance of ossification centers seems to be affected by race and sex. The ability to demonstrate these ossification centers by x-ray examination confirms the duration of pregnancy, but their absence does not negate maturity.

Whenever a woman in labor must go to the x-ray department, it is imperative that a nurse accompany her with an emergency delivery pack. The client is often frightened and worried, because there is obviously something abnormal taking place. The nurse's presence can be reassuring to the woman because the nurse can handle the situation should delivery ensue in the x-ray room. Frequently, the woman is left alone by the x-ray technicians or attendants for short periods of time, and the presence of the nurse can be of much comfort to her. The nurse can also be of help in positioning the client for taking the films. The nurse should at all times be aware of the progress of labor and notify the physician immediately if delivery seems imminent.

FETOSCOPY

Fetoscopy, a technique for directly observing the fetus and obtaining a sample of fetal blood or skin, was discovered in 1972. Real-time ultrasound is utilized to visualize a pool of amniotic fluid in an effort to locate an area in which to insert a cannula and trocar. Following insertion, ultrasound is used to direct the endoscope to the desired part of the fetus for viewing and sampling. Skin biopsies may be obtained as well as blood samples. A 26-gauge needle is inserted into the umbilical cord under direct visualization while blood samples are withdrawn.

Many diagnoses, including short-limb dysplasias, spina bifida, and cleft lip and palate have been diagnosed by fetoscopy, but with the advent of ultrasound the need for fetoscopy has been obviated. It is still used to diagnose various skin malformations and diseases such as sickle cell anemia, β-thalassemia, hemophilia A, von Willebrand disease, and chronic granulomatous disease (Hobbins, 1982).

With fetoscopy, it is possible to obtain fetal blood during the second trimester and thus aid in intrauterine fetal exchange transfusion. There may be trauma to the fetus during peritoneal transfusion, but fetoscopy seems to eliminate or at least decrease this incidence. Since one is able to aspirate fetal blood and replace a siilar amount with donor blood, the incidence of cardiac overload could be decreased.

Only a few perinatal centers utilize this procedure due to risks involved which include fetal mortality (7.5%), vaginal leakage of amniotic fluid (7%), premature labor (10%), and infant mortality due to premature labor (2%) (Hobbins, 1982).

IMPLICATIONS OF PRENATAL TESTING FOR DELIVERY

Guidelines for prenatal testing in relation to timing of delivery for the high-risk woman are presented in Figures 13–10 and 13–13. It seems to be the general opinion that when both CST and estriol levels indicate fetal jeopardy, whether or not the fetus is mature it should be delivered. If either the CST or the estriol values indicate jeopardy and if lung maturity has been attained, the physician usually chooses to deliver the infant. If only one of the parameters of fetal health status signifies jeopardy and the fetus is immature, the fetus is usually not delivered immediately but rather observed closely and delivered when fetal lung maturity is reached or when further evidence of fetal jeopardy or deterioration of maternal or fetal condition is found.

SUMMARY

It is difficult to assess fetal status in many situations. Each woman must be treated individually in light of her specific circumstances. In addition, there is no one system of care intended for all high-risk clients. Clinical judgment by the attending physician, based on data obtained during the nursing assessment and coupled with appropriate tests of fetal well-being, will ultimately aid in deciding each pregnancy's outcome.

One of the most difficult problems in the management of the high-risk woman is timing of delivery. The physician must weigh the possible disadvantages of delivering a premature infant against the risk to that fetus of remaining in

the unhealthy, less than optimal intrauterine environment. For this reason, extremely intensive obstetric care and an accurate index of fetal well-being are essential for the management of pregnancies at risk.

The expert clinical judgment and care rendered by the attending physician and other highly specialized associates is of the greatest significance. The many studies and tests available to the woman at risk are used only as adjuncts to good clinical management. These tests are of little value if the client does not understand her condition and is unable to assume some of the responsibility for her own management and care. Generally, clients are willing to participate in their care, keep regular appointments, inform their physicians and caregivers about changes in their health status, and cooperate in necessary evaluation procedures. Unfortunately, the group of women in which maternal and infant mortality and morbidity are highest is also the group least motivated or able to cooperate in their health maintenance. These clients are frequently of low socioeconomic status, poorly educated, poorly nourished, and/or teenagers. Much time and effort is required to educate these women to ensure that they receive the best care and follow-up treatment.

The nurse is in a prime position to offer support and reassurance and to provide valuable input for the care of the high-risk client. Through the nurse's efforts, the flow of information to and from the client at risk can be maintained, thus ensuring optimal care for both her and her unborn child. In addition, the establishment of regionalized centers for high-risk pregnant clients, with specialized teams of workers and with electronic and biochemical monitoring of the fetus, will further enhance the potential for a successful childbirth experience.

References

Andrews, B. F. 1970. Amniotic fluid studies to determine maturity. *Pediatr. Clin. North Am.* 17:49.

Bevis, D. C. A. 1956. Blood pigments in haemolytic disease of the newborn. *J. Obstet. Gynaecol. Br. Emp.* 63:68.

Bishop, E. H. 1981. Fetal acceleration test. *Am. J. Obstet. Gynecol.* 141 (8):905.

Boddy, K., et al. 1974. Intrauterine fetal breathing movement. In *Modern perinatal medicine*, ed. L. Gluck. Chicago: Year Book Medical Publishers.

Bree, R. L., and Mariona, F. G. 1980. The role of ultrasound in the evaluation of normal and abnormal fetal growth. In *Seminars in ultrasound*, ed. H. W. Raymond, and W. J. Zwiebel. New York: Grune & Stratton.

Bustos, R., et al. 1979. Significance of phosphatidylglycerol in amniotic fluid in complicated pregnancies. *Am. J. Obstet. Gynecol.* 133 (8):903.

Clements, J. A., et al. 1972. Assessment of the risk of respiratory distress syndrome by a rapid test for surfactant in amniotic fluid. *N. Engl. J. Med.* 286:1077.

Cunningham, M. D., et al. 1982. Improved prediction of fetal lung maturity in diabetic pregnancies: A comparison of chromatographic methods. *Am. J. Obstet. Gynecol.* 142 (2):198.

Freeman, R. K. 1975. The use of the oxytocin challenge test for antepartum clinical evaluation of uteroplacental respiratory function. *Am. J. Obstet. Gynecol.* 121:487.

————. 1982. Stress testing: conceptual origin and current applications. Proceedings of sixth International Symposium on Perinatal Medicine, Corometrics Medical Systems, Inc. Las Vegas, Nevada.

Freeman, R. K., and Garite, T. J. 1981. *Fetal heart rate monitoring.* Baltimore: Williams & Wilkins.

Gabbe, S. G. 1982. Amniotic fluid indices of maturity. In *Protocols for high risk pregnancies,* ed. J. T. Queenan and J. C. Hobbins. Oradell, N.J.: Medical Economics Co., Inc.

Gluck, L., et al. 1971. Diagnosis of respiratory distress syndrome by amniocentesis. *Am. J. Obstet. Gynecol.* 109 (3):441.

————. 1975. Fetal maturity and amniotic fluid surfactant determinations. In *Management of the high-risk pregnancy,* ed. W. N. Spellacy. Baltimore: University Park Press.

Gobelsmann, U. April 1977. The clinical value of estriol determinations. From the proceedings of the second International Symposium on Perinatal Medicine. Las Vegas, Nevada.

Goldstein, A. I. 1977. Amniocentesis: indications, techniques, complications and alpha-fetoprotein. In *Advances in perinatal medicine,* ed. A. Goldstein. New York: Symposia Specialists, Stratton Intercontinental Medical Books Corp.

Gottesfeld, K. R. 1980. The use of ultrasound in the first trimester of pregnancy. In *Seminars in ultrasound,* ed. H. W. Raymond, and W. J. Zwiebel. New York: Grune & Stratton.

Grannum, P. A.; Berkowitz, R. L.; and Hobbins, J. C. 1979. The ultrasonic changes in the maturing placenta and their relation to fetal pulmonic maturity. *Am. J. Obstet. Gynecol.* 133 (8):915.

Green, J. W., et al. 1969. Correlation of estriol excretion patterns of pregnant women with subsequent development of their children. *Am. J. Obstet. Gynecol.* 105:730.

Hallman, M., et al. 1976. Phosphatidylinositol and phosphatidylglycerol in amniotic fluid: Indices of lung maturity. *Am. J. Obstet. Gynecol.* 125:616.

Hobbins, J. C. 1982. Fetoscopy. In *Protocols for high risk pregnancies,* ed. J. T. Queenan and J. E. Hobbins. Oradell, N.J.: Medical Economics Co., Inc.

Hohler, C. W., and Quetal, T. A. 1981. Comparisons of ultrasound femur length and biparietal diameter in late pregnancy. *Am. J. Obstet. Gynecol.* 141 (7):761.

Hon, E. H., and Quilligan, E. J. 1967. The classification of fetal heart rate. II. A revised working classification. *Conn. Med.* 31:781.

Huddleston, J. F. 1980. Stress and non-stress testing. In *Gynecology and obstetrics*, vol. 3, ed. J. J. Sciarri. Philadelphia: Harper & Row.

Kubli, E. W., et al. 1969. In *The feto-placental unit*, eds. Pecile and Finzi. Amsterdam: Excerpta Medica Foundation.

Kulovich, M. V., et al. 1979. The lung profile. I. Normal pregnancy. *Am. J. Obstet. Gynecol.* 135:57.

Leiker, J., and Hensleigh, P. 1975. Amniotic fluid analysis. *J. Kansas Med. Soc.* 76:159.

Leopold, G., and Asher, W. 1975. *Fundamentals of abdominal and pelvic ultrasonography.* Philadelphia: W. B. Saunders Co.

Liley, A. W. 1961. Liquor amnii analysis in the management of the pregnancy complicated by rhesus sensitization. *Am. J. Obstet. Gynecol.* 32:1359.

Manning, F. A. 1977. Fetal breathing movements. *Postgrad. Med.* 61:116.

McQuown, D. 1977. Ultrasound in pregnancy. In *Advances in perinatal medicine,* ed. A. Goldstein. New York: Symposia Specialists, Stratton Intercontinental Medical Books Corp.

Natale, R. 1981. Real-time ultrasound patterns of fetal activity. *Perinatol. Neonatol.* 5:47.

O'Sullivan, M. J. 1976. Acute and chronic fetal distress. *J. Reprod. Med.* 17:320.

Patrick, J. E., et al. 1978a. Human fetal breathing movements and gross fetal body movements at weeks 34–35 of gestation. *Am. J. Obstet. Gynecol.* 130:693.

Patrick, J.; Natale, R.; and Richardson, B. 1978b. Patterns of human fetal breathing at 34–35 weeks' gestational age. *Am. J. Obstet. Gynecol.* 132:507.

Patrick, J. E., et al. 1982. Patterns of gross fetal body movements over 24-hour observation intervals during the last 10 weeks of pregnancy. *Am. J. Obstet. Gynecol.* 142(4): 369.

Pitkin, R. M. 1975. Fetal maturity: nonlipid amniotic fluid assessment. In *Management of the high-risk pregnancy,* ed. W. N. Spellacy. Baltimore: University Park Press.

Quinlan, R. W., and Cruz, A. C. 1982. Ultrasonic placental grading and fetal pulmonary maturity. *Am. J. Obstet. Gynecol.* 142(1):111.

Ragan, W. 1976. Ultrasound in obstetrics. *Am. Fam. Physician.* 14(3):130.

Richardson, B.; Natale, R.; and Patrick, J. 1979. Human fetal breathing activity during induced labor at term. *Am. J. Obstet. Gynecol.* 133:247.

Richardson, C. J., et al. 1974. Acceleration of fetal lung maturation following prolonged rupture of the membranes. *Am. J. Obstet. Gynecol.* 118:1115.

Schifrin, B. S. April 1977. Antepartum fetal heart rate monitoring. From the proceedings of the second International Symposium on Perinatal Medicine. Las Vegas, Nevada.

Schifrin, B. S., et al. 1975. Contraction stress test for antepartum fetal evaluation. *Am. J. Obstet. Gynecol.* 45:436.

Spirit, B. A., and Kagan, E. H. 1980. Sonography of the placenta. In *Seminars in ultrasound,* ed. H. W. Raymond, and W. J. Zwiebel. New York: Grune & Stratton.

Tamura, R. K., and Manning, F. A. 1981. Fetal breathing movements. In *Gynecology and obstetrics,* vol. 3. ed., J. J. Sciarri, Philadelphia: Harper & Row.

Tamura, R. K., and Sabbagha, R. E. 1981. Assessment of fetal weight. In *Diagnostic ultrasound applied to obstetrics & gynecology,* ed. R. E. Sabbagha. Hagerstown, Md.: Harper & Row.

Thompson, H. E., et al. 1965. Fetal development as determined by ultrasonic pulse echo technique. *Am. J. Obstet. Gynecol.* 92:44.

Trierweiler, M. W., et al. 1976. Baseline fetal heart rate characteristics as an indicator of fetal status during the antepartum period. *Am. J. Obstet. Gynecol.* 125:623.

Tulchinsky, D. 1975. The value of estrogen assays in obstetric disease. In *Plasma hormone assays in evaluation of fetal well-being,* ed. A. Klopper. Edinburgh: Churchill Livingstone.

Weingold, A. B. 1975. Intrauterine growth retardation: obstetrical aspects. *J. Reprod. Med.* 14:244.

Additional Readings

Aladjem, S., and Brown, A. 1977. *Perinatal intensive care.* St. Louis: The C. V. Mosby Co.

Braly, P. B., and Freeman, R. K. 1977. The significance of fetal heart rate activity with a positive oxytocin challenge test. *Am. J. Obstet. Gynecol.* 50:689.

Fava, G. A., et al. 1982. Psychological reactions to amniocentesis: a controlled study. *Am. J. Obstet. Gynecol.* 143(5): 509.

Gelman, S. R., et al. 1980. Fetal movements and ultrasound: effect of maternal intravenous glucose administration. *Am. J. Obstet. Gynecol.* 137(4):459.

————. 1982. Fetal movements in response to sound stimulation. *Am. J. Obstet. Gynecol.* 143(4):484.

Hohler, C. W., and Quetal, T. A. 1982. Fetal femur length: equations for computer calculation of gestational age from ultrasound measurements. *Am. J. Obstet. Gynecol.* 143(4):479.

Littlefield, V., and Subert, G. Sept./Oct. 1978. The group approach to problem-solving for pregnant diabetic women. *MCN* 4:274.

Lubchenco, L. O., et al. 1963. Intrauterine growth as estimated from liveborn birth weights data at 24 to 42 weeks of gestation. *Pediatrics.* 32:793.

O'Brien, G. D., and Queenan, J. T. 1981. Growth of the ultrasound fetal femur length during normal pregnancy. *Am. J. Obstet. Gynecol.* 141:7.

Rayburn, W. F., et al. 1982. Conditions affecting non-stress test results. *Obstet. Gynecol.* 59(4):491.

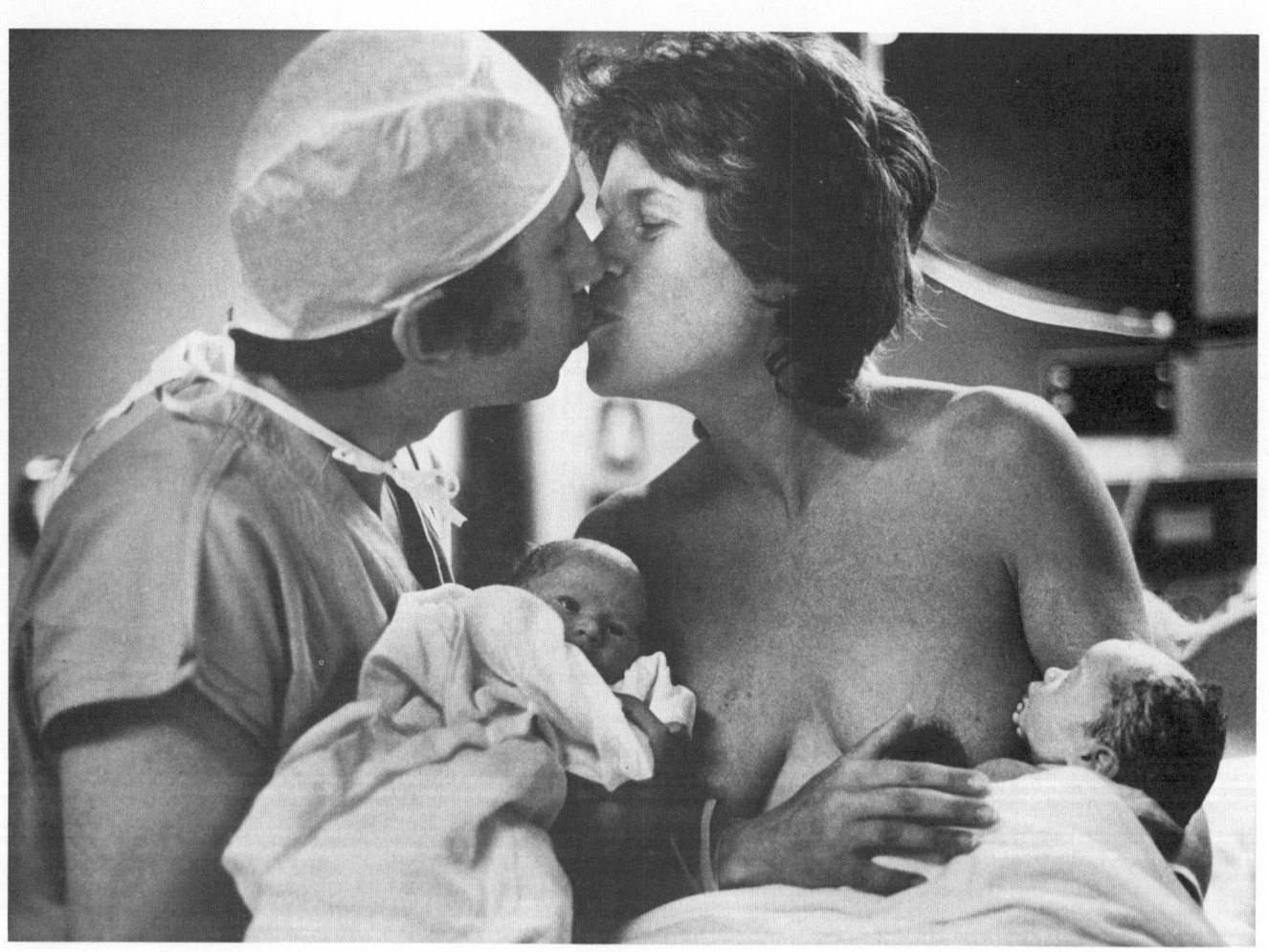

· IV ·

LABOR AND DELIVERY

Chapter 14 ■ Processes and Stages of Labor and Delivery

Chapter 15 ■ Intrapartal Nursing Assessment

Chapter 16 ■ The Family in Childbirth: Needs and Care

Chapter 17 ■ Obstetric Analgesia and Anesthesia

Chapter 18 ■ Complications of Labor and Delivery

Chapter 19 ■ Elective Obstetric Procedures

Chapter 20 ■ Birthing Options

PROCESSES AND STAGES OF LABOR AND DELIVERY

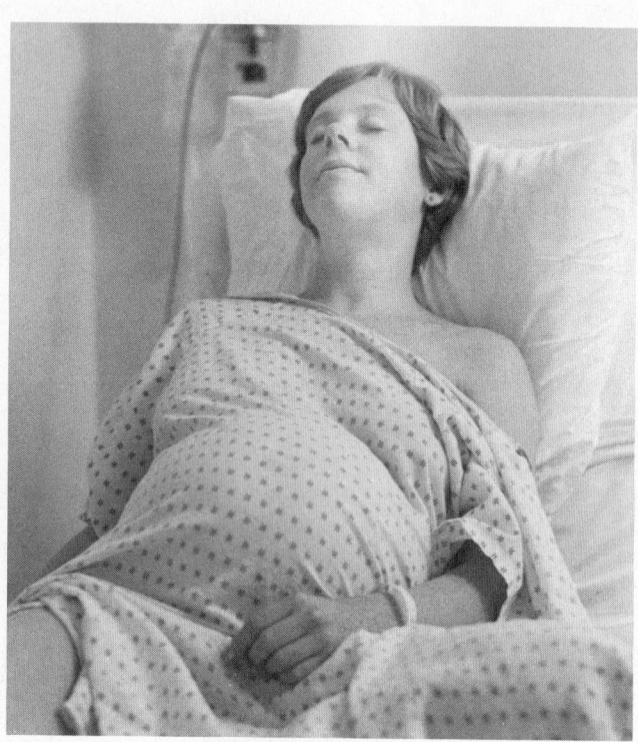

■ CHAPTER CONTENTS

CRITICAL FACTORS IN LABOR
    The Passage
    The Passenger
    The Powers
    The Psyche

PHYSIOLOGY OF LABOR
    Possible Causes of Labor Onset
    Biochemical Interaction
    Myometrial Activity
    Intraabdominal Pressure
    Musculature Changes of Pelvic Floor

MATERNAL SYSTEMIC RESPONSE TO LABOR
    Cardiovascular System
    Blood Pressure
    Fluid and Electrolyte Balance
    Gastrointestinal System
    Respiratory System
    Hemopoietic System
    Renal System
    Response to Pain

FETAL RESPONSE TO LABOR
    Biomechanical Changes
    Cardiac Changes
    Hemodynamic Changes
    Positional Changes

PREMONITORY SIGNS OF LABOR
    Lightening
    Braxton Hicks Contractions

Cervical Changes

Bloody Show

Rupture of Membranes

Sudden Burst of Energy

Other Signs

Differences Between True and False Labor

STAGES OF LABOR AND DELIVERY

First Stage

Second Stage

Third Stage

Fourth Stage

■ OBJECTIVES

- Discuss the significance of each type of pelvis to the birth process.

- Examine the factors that influence labor and the physiology of the mechanisms of labor.

- Describe the fetal positional changes that constitute the mechanisms of labor.

- Discuss the probable causes of labor onset and the premonitory signs of labor.

- Differentiate between false and true labor.

- Describe the physiologic and psychologic changes occurring in each of the stages of labor.

The process of labor and delivery is the culmination of the entire maternity cycle, and it marks the ultimate crisis to the childbearing woman, the fetus, and the family. The series of events by which the fetus, placenta, amniotic fluid, and fetal membranes (the products of conception) are expelled from the maternal body is appropriately called *labor* because this word implies an expenditure of energy to obtain a goal or product. The terms *childbirth, parturition,* and *confinement* have been used as synonyms for this process.

During the months of gestation, the fetus and the gravid woman prepare to accommodate themselves to each other during the birth process. The fetus progresses through various stages of growth and development, preparing for the independence of extrauterine life. The gravid woman undergoes various physiologic and psychologic adaptations during pregnancy that gradually prepare her for childbirth and the role of mother. For both woman and fetus the onset of labor marks a significant change in their relationship.

CRITICAL FACTORS IN LABOR

Four factors are of critical importance in planning individualized nursing care for the laboring woman: the passage, the passenger, the powers, and the psyche. The "four Ps," as they are commonly known, are defined as follows:

1. Passage
   a. Size of the pelvis (diameters of the pelvic inlet, midpelvis, and outlet)
   b. Type of pelvis, (gynecoid, anthropoid, platypelloid, or android)
   c. Ability of the cervix to dilate and efface and ability of the vaginal canal and introitus to distend
2. Passenger
   a. Fetal head (size and presence of molding)
   b. Fetal attitude (flexion or extension of the fetal body and extremities)
   c. Fetal lie
   d. Fetal presentation (the part of the fetal body entering the pelvis in a single or multiple pregnancy)
   e. Fetal position (relationship of the presenting part to the pelvis)
3. Powers
   a. The frequency, duration, and intensity of uterine contractions as the passenger is moved through the passage
   b. The duration of labor
4. Psyche
   a. Physical preparation for childbirth
   b. Sociocultural heritage
   c. Previous childbirth experience
   d. Support from significant others
   e. Emotional integrity

The progress of labor is critically dependent on the complementary relationship of these four factors. Abnormalities in the passage, the passenger, the powers, or the psyche can alter the outcome of labor and jeopardize both the gravid woman and the fetus (Nurses Association of the American College of Obstetricians and Gynecologists, 1974). Complications involving the four Ps are discussed in Chapter 18.

The Passage

In both males and females the pelvis provides support for the body weight and for the lower extremities. In the female, however, the pelvis must also adapt to the demands of childbearing (Pritchard and MacDonald, 1980). Because the process of labor essentially involves the accommodation of the fetus to the bony pelvis through which it must descend, the size and shape of the maternal pelvis must be assessed by the health care team.

The true pelvis, which forms the bony canal through which the baby must pass, is divided into three sections: the inlet, the pelvic cavity (midpelvis), and the outlet. These are described in detail in Chapter 4, as are the pelvic measurements that influence the childbirth outcome. The techniques used to determine these measurements are described in Chapter 15.

TYPES OF PELVES

Familiarity with the types of pelves contributes to the understanding of the mechanism of labor and of the relationship of passage, passenger, and powers during the intrapartal period. The Caldwell-Moloy classification of the types of pelves is based on pertinent characteristics of both male and female pelves (Caldwell and Moloy, 1933). Consideration is given to the size of the sacrosciatic notch, flaring of the pelvic brim, the shape of the inlet, and the relationship of the greatest anteroposterior diameter to the greatest transverse diameter.

The four classic types of pelves are *gynecoid, android, anthropoid,* and *platypelloid* (Figure 14–1). Mixed types of pelvic configurations occur more frequently than pure types.

Gynecoid pelvis. The normal female pelvis is the gynecoid type (see Figure 14–1). The inlet is rounded, with the anteroposterior diameter a little shorter than the transverse diameter. All the inlet diameters are at least adequate. The posterior segment is broad, deep, and roomy, and the anterior segment is well rounded. The gynecoid midpelvis has nonprominent ischial spines, straight and parallel side walls, and a wide, deep sacral curve. The sacrum is short and slopes backward. All of the midpelvic diameters are at least adequate. The gynecoid pelvic outlet has a wide and round pubic arch; the inferior pubic rami are short and concave. The anteroposterior diameter is long and the transverse diameter adequate. The capacity of the outlet is adequate. The bones are of medium structure and weight.

Approximately 50% of female pelves are classified as

gynecoid. The influence of a gynecoid pelvis on labor is favorable. Descent is facilitated and rapid because the fetal head usually engages in the transverse or oblique diameter with adequate flexion and engagement occurs at midpelvis. The occipital anterior position at delivery is common (Oxorn, 1980).

Android pelvis. The normal male type is the android pelvis (see Figure 14–1). The inlet is heart-shaped. The anteroposterior and transverse diameters are adequate for delivery, but the posterior sagittal diameter is too short and the anterior sagittal diameter is long. The posterior segment is shallow because the sacral promontory is indented, resulting in a reduced capacity. The anterior segment is narrow, and the forepelvis is sharply angled. The android midpelvis has prominent ischial spines, convergent side walls, and a long, heavy sacrum inclining forward. All the midpelvic diameters are reduced. The distance from the linea terminalis to the ischial tuberosities is long, yet the overall capacity of the midpelvis is reduced. The android outlet has a narrow, sharp, and deep pubic arch; the inferior pubic rami are straight and long. The anteroposterior diameter is short and the transverse diameter is narrow. The capacity of the outlet is reduced. The bones are of medium to heavy structure and weight.

Approximately 20% of female pelves are classified as android. The influence of an android pelvis on labor is not favorable. Descent into the pelvis is slow. The fetal head usually engages in the transverse or occipital posterior diameter in asynclitism with extreme molding. Arrest of labor is frequent, requiring difficult forceps manipulation (rotation and extraction), and the deep, narrow pubic arch may lead to extensive perineal lacerations. Cesarean delivery may be required.

Anthropoid pelvis. The anthropoid pelvis is often described as apelike (see Figure 14–1). The inlet is oval, with a long anteroposterior diameter and an adequate but rather short transverse diameter. Both the posterior and anterior segments are deep; the posterior sagittal diameter is extremely long, as is the anterior sagittal diameter. The anthropoid midpelvis has variable ischial spines, straight side walls, and a narrow and long sacrum that inclines backward. The midpelvic diameters are at least adequate, making its capacity adequate. The anthropoid outlet has a normal or moderately narrow pubic arch; the inferior pubic rami are long and narrow. The outlet capacity is adequate, and the bones are of medium weight and structure.

Approximately 25% of female pelves are classified as anthropoid. The influence of the anthropoid pelvis on labor is favorable. Usually the fetal head engages in the anteroposterior or oblique diameter in the occipital-posterior position. Labor and delivery progress well.

Platypelloid pelvis. The platypelloid type refers to the flat female pelvis (see Figure 14–1). The inlet is distinctly transverse oval, with a short anteroposterior and extremely short transverse diameter. The posterior sagittal and anterior sagittal diameters are short. Both the anterior and pos-

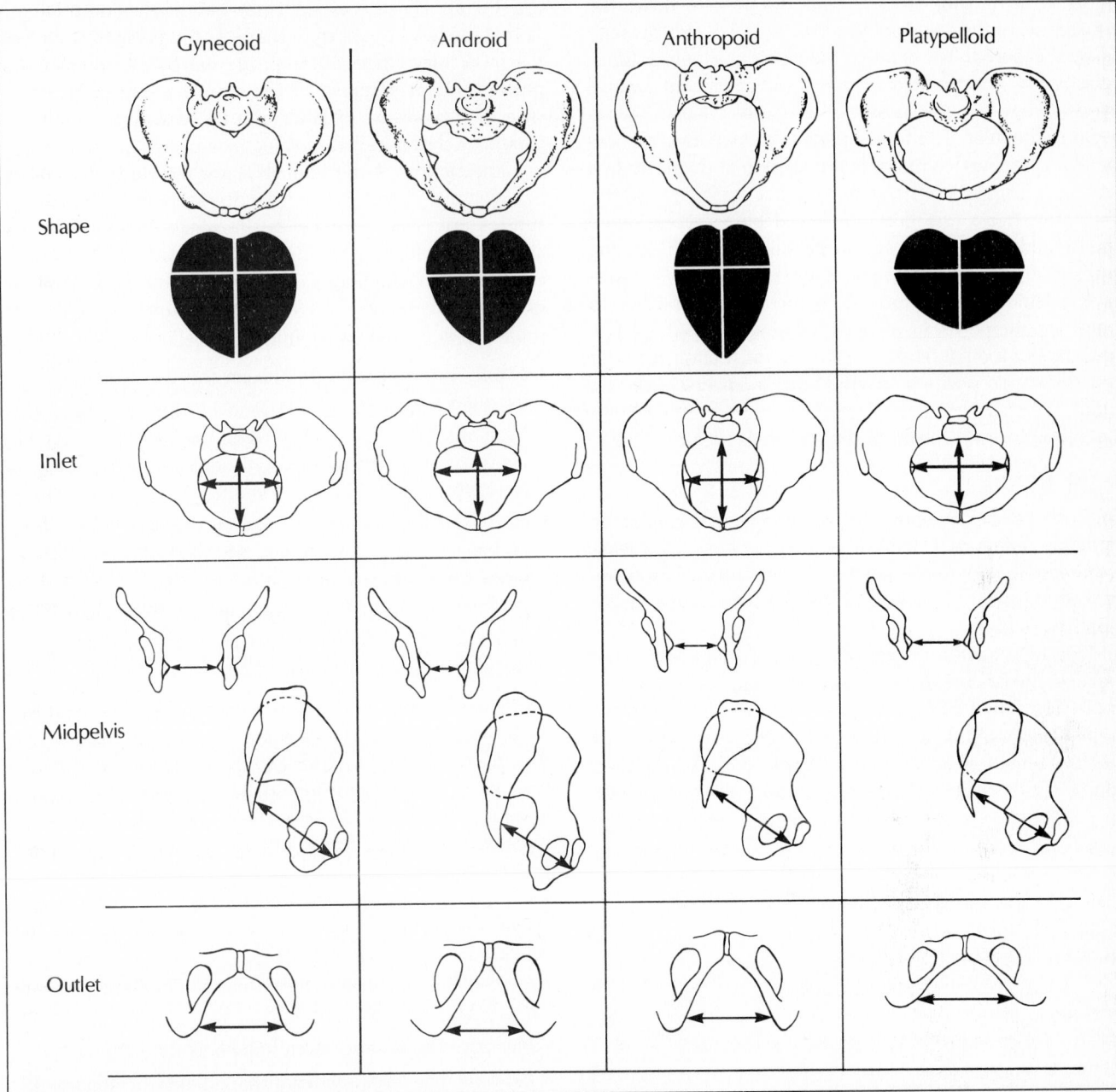

FIGURE 14–1 Comparison of Caldwell-Moloy pelvic types.

terior segments are shallow. The platypelloid midpelvis has variable ischial spines, parallel side walls, and a wide sacrum with a deep curve inward. Only the transverse diameter is adequate; thus the midpelvic capacity is reduced. The platypelloid outlet has an extremely wide pubic arch; the inferior pubic rami are straight and short. The transverse diameter is wide but the anteroposterior diameter is short. The outlet capacity is inadequate. The platypelloid bones are similar to the gynecoid type.

Only 5% of the female pelves are classified as platypelloid. The influence of the platypelloid pelvis on labor is not favorable. The fetal head usually engages in the transverse diameter with marked asynclitism. If the infant can transverse the inlet, it rotates at or below the spines, and delivery is rapid through the wide arch. But frequently there is delay of progress at the inlet, requiring a cesarean delivery.

The Passenger

The fetal passenger must accommodate itself to the maternal passage during labor. To pass through the relatively immobile pelvis, the fetus goes through a series of maneuvers to align its body.

which measurement is actually being reported. For example, the suboccipitobregmatic diameter notes the distance from the undersurface of the occiput to the center of the bregma, or anterior fontanelle. Fetal skull measurements are given in Figure 14–4.

Much can be learned from these diameters regarding the degree of extension or flexion of the fetal head. Extension of the head results in a larger diameter presenting than if the head is strongly flexed. Alterations in flexion of the fetal head can yield problems during the process of labor. The fetus endeavors to accommodate its most favorable head diameters to the limited measurements of the bony pelvis.

FETAL ATTITUDE

Fetal attitude, or habitus, refers to the relation of the fetal parts to one another. The normal attitude of the fetus, providing there is adequate amniotic fluid, is one of moderate flexion of the head and extremities on the abdomen and chest. This ovoid attitude has been called the *fetal position*. The back bows outward, the chin rests on the sternum, and the arms and thighs are flexed on the chest and abdomen. The fetus assumes various attitudes during the pregnancy, flexing and extending the arms, legs, and body. An extremely flexed and cramped attitude is maintained if the fetus has insufficient space in which to stretch, such as occurs in oligohydramnios (scant amniotic fluid) (Greenhill and Friedman, 1974).

Alterations in fetal attitude cause the fetus to present various diameters of the head to the maternal passage. With increased extension of the passenger's head, a larger diameter of the fetal skull must be accommodated by the pelvis. This alteration from a normal fetal attitude often contributes to a difficult labor. The fetus assumes a military attitude (chin up, shoulders back) when the head is moderately extended. Marked and excessive extension of the fetal head yield brow and face presentations.

FETAL LIE

Fetal lie refers to the relationship of the cephalocaudal axis of the fetus to the cephalocaudal axis of the pregnant woman. The passenger may assume either a transverse lie or a longitudinal lie. A *transverse lie* occurs when the long axis of the fetus is perpendicular to the woman's spine. The abdomen appears oval from left to right, with the buttocks of the fetus on one side and the head on the other. A *longitudinal lie* is assumed when the cephalocaudal axis of the fetus is parallel to the woman's spine. Depending on the fetal part entering the pelvis first, a longitudinal lie may either be a cephalic (head) or breech (buttocks) presentation.

FETAL PRESENTATION

Fetal presentation is determined by the body part of the passenger that enters the pelvic passageway first. This

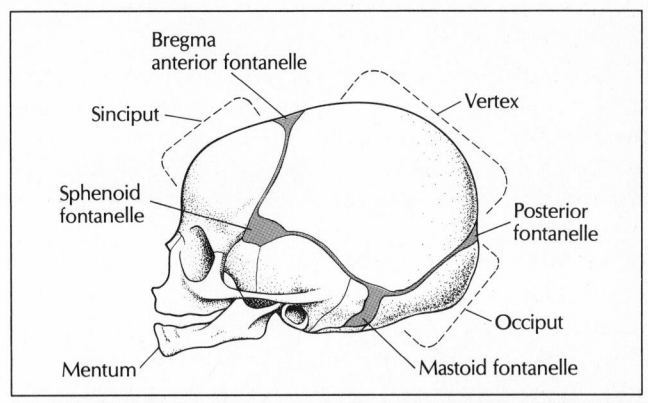

FIGURE 14–3 Lateral view of the fetal skull. The landmarks that have significance in obstetrics are identified.

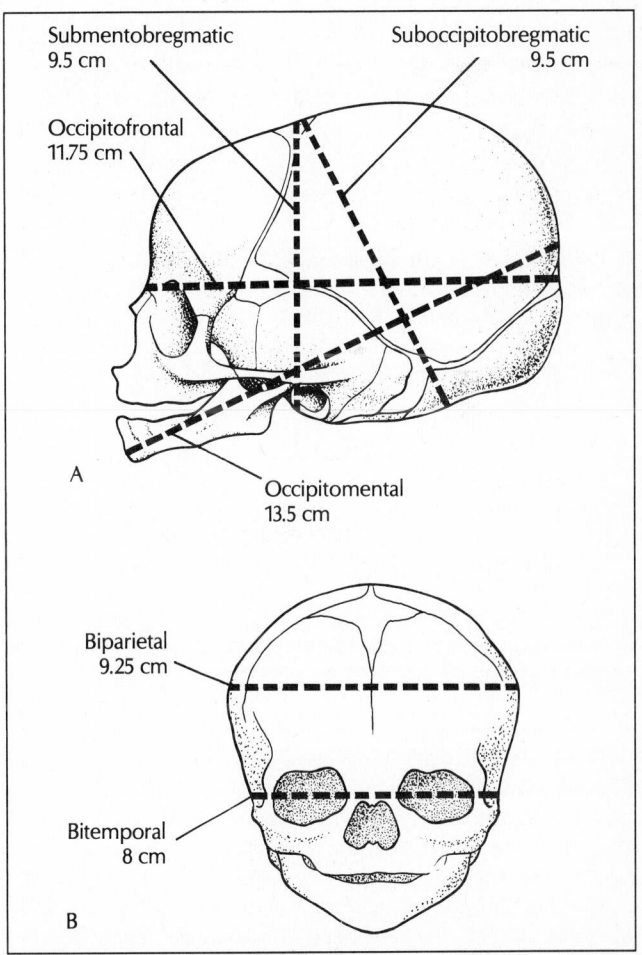

FIGURE 14–4 A, Anteroposterior diameters of the fetal skull. When the vertex of the fetus presents and the fetal head is flexed with the chin on the chest, the smallest anteroposterior diameter (suboccipitobregmatic) enters the birth canal. **B,** Transverse diameters of the fetal skull.

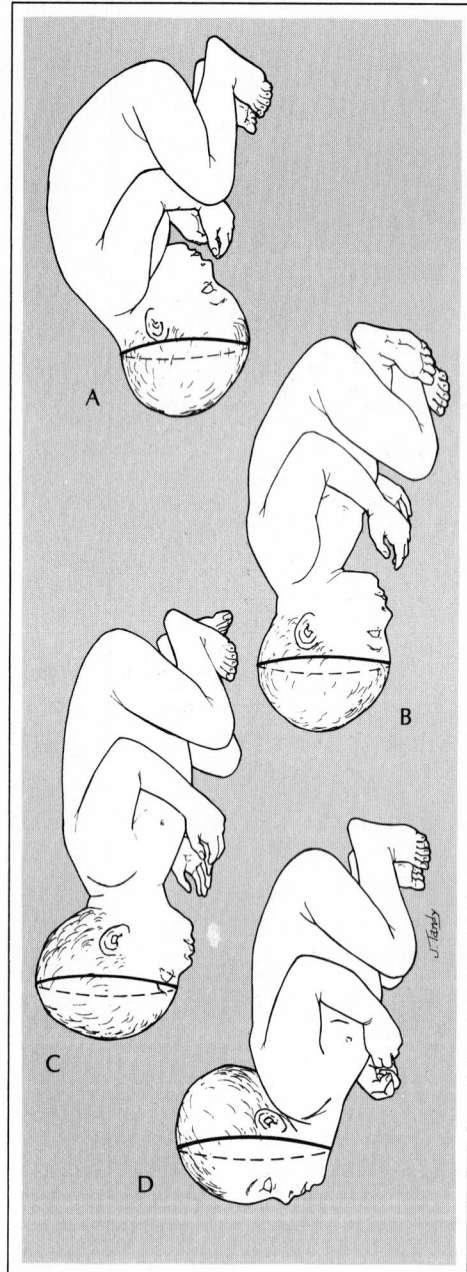

portion of the fetus is referred to as *presenting part*. Depending on the attitude of the fetal extremities to its body and the fetal lie, the presentation is either cephalic, breech, or shoulder.

□ *CEPHALIC PRESENTATIONS* The fetal head presents itself to the passage in approximately 95% of term deliveries (Danforth, 1982). The cephalic presentations are classified according to the degree of flexion or extension of the fetal head. Thus the fetal attitude becomes critical in determining the type of cephalic presentation in each case.

There are four types of cephalic presentation. *Vertex presentation*, in which the head is completely flexed on the chest, is the most common cephalic presentation; the smallest diameter of the passenger's head (suboccipitobregmatic) enters the passage in this presentation (Figure 14–5,A). *Military (median vertex) presentation* occurs when the fetal head is neither flexed nor extended and the occipitofrontal diameter is presented (Figure 14–5,B). A *brow presentation* is assumed when the fetal head is partially extended and the occipitomental diameter, the largest anteroposterior diameter, is presented to the maternal pelvis (Figure 14–5,C). The most extreme cephalic presentation is the *face presentation* in which the head is hyperextended (complete extension) and the submentobregmatic diameter presents to the maternal pelvis (Figure 14–5,D).

□ *BREECH PRESENTATIONS* Breech or pelvic presentations occur in 3% of term births. These presentations are classified according to the attitude of the passenger's hips and knees (see Figure 14–6 and Chapter 18, p. 554). A *complete breech* occurs when the fetal knees and hips are both flexed, placing the thighs on the abdomen and the calves on the posterior aspect of the thighs. On vaginal examination both buttocks and feet can be palpated. Flexion of the hips and extension of the knees changes a complete breech to a *frank breech*. This presentation causes the fetal legs to extend onto the abdomen and chest, presenting the buttocks alone to the pelvis. The buttocks and genitals are palpable on vaginal examination when the passenger assumes a frank breech presentation. A *footling breech* presentation occurs when there is extension both at the knees and at the hips. A *single footling breech* presentation occurs if only one foot is presenting; a *double footling breech* occurs if both feet enter the pelvis first. In all variations of the breech presentation the sacrum is the landmark to be noted. See Chapter 18 for further discussion of the implications of the breech presentations for labor and delivery.

□ *SHOULDER PRESENTATION* A shoulder presentation, usually referred to as a *transverse lie*, is assumed by the fetus when its cephalocaudal axis lies perpendicular to the maternal spine (see Chapter 18, p. 555). The fetus appears to lie crosswise in the uterus. Most frequently the shoulder is the presenting part in a transverse lie. In this case the acromion process of the scapula is the landmark to be noted. However, the fetal arm, back, abdomen, or side may present in a transverse lie. This presentation may

FIGURE 14–5 Cephalic presentations. **A,** Vertex presentation. Complete flexion of the head allows the suboccipitobregmatic diameter to present to the pelvis. **B,** Military (median vertex) presentation, with no flexion or extension. The occipitofrontal diameter presents to the pelvis. **C,** Brow presentation. The fetal head is in partial (halfway) extension. The occipitomental diameter, which is the largest diameter of the fetal head, presents to the pelvis. **D,** Face presentation. The fetal head is in complete extension and the submentobregmatic diameter presents to the pelvis.

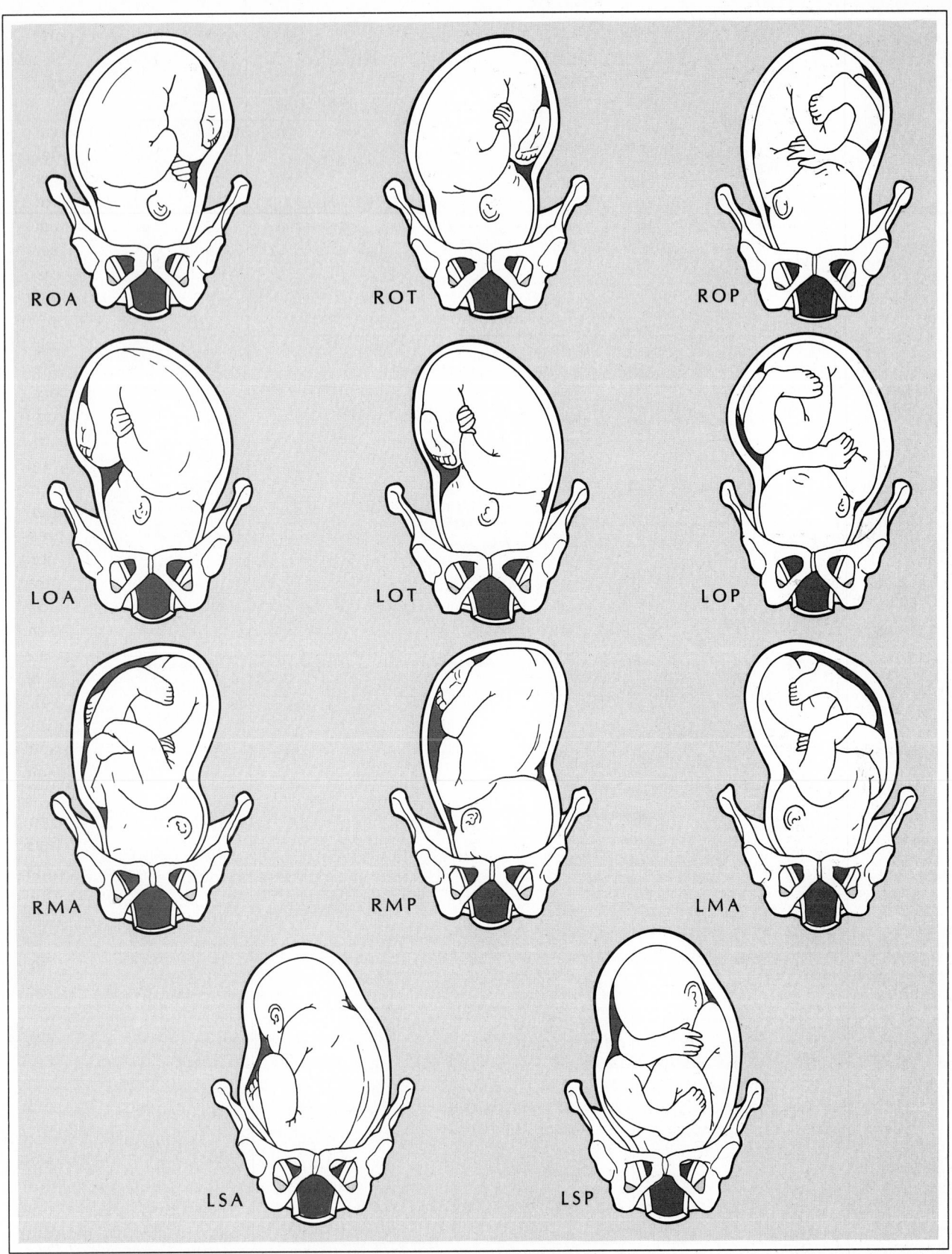

FIGURE 14–6 Categories of presentation. (Courtesy Ross Laboratories, Columbus, Ohio.)

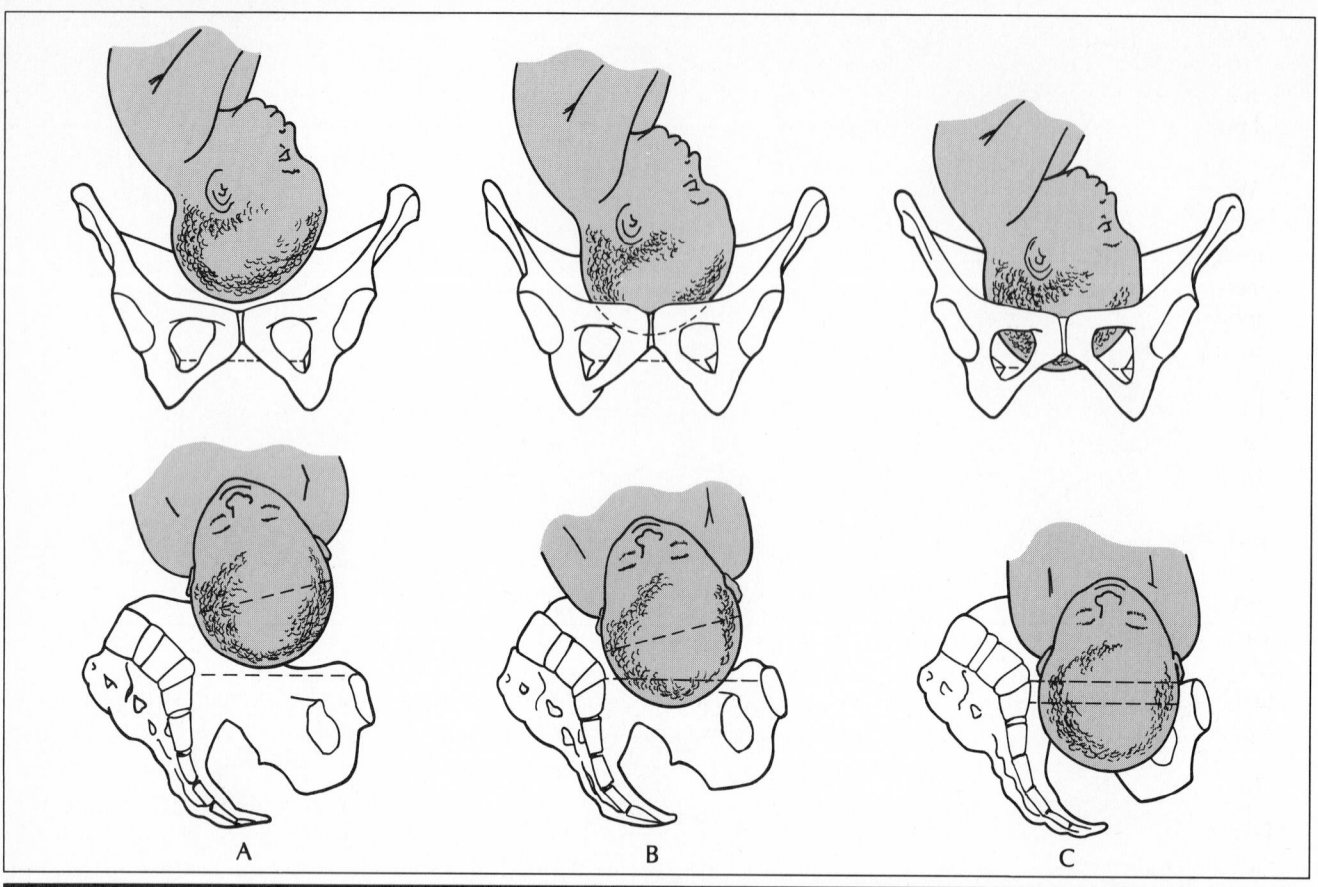

FIGURE 14–7 Process of engagement. **A,** Floating. **B,** Dipping. **C,** Engaged.

be caused by placenta previa (implantation of the placenta over the cervical os), small pelvic measurements, or excessive relaxation of the abdominal walls in women who have borne many children (grandmultiparas). Unless the fetus rotates during labor to a longitudinal lie, the delivery must be accomplished by cesarean birth. See Chapter 18 for further discussion of the transverse lie and other malpresentations, and their effects on the labor and delivery processes.

□ *FUNCTIONAL RELATIONSHIPS OF PRESENTING PART AND PASSAGE Engagement* of the presenting part takes place when the largest diameter of the presenting part reaches or passes through the pelvic inlet (Figure 14–7). The biparietal diameter is the largest dimension of the fetal skull to pass through the pelvis in a cephalic presentation. The intertrochanteric diameter is the largest to pass through the inlet in a breech presentation. Once the criteria for engagement have been met, the bony prominences of the presenting part are usually descending into the midpelvis (near the level of the ischial spines).

A vaginal examination determines whether engagement has occurred. In primigravidas, engagement usually occurs 2 weeks before term. Multiparas, however, may experience engagement several weeks before the onset of

labor or during the process of labor. If engagement has occurred, it means the adequacy of the pelvic inlet has been validated. Engagement does not suggest that the midpelvis and outlet are also adequate, however.

The presenting part is said to be *floating* (or ballottable) when it is freely movable above the inlet. When the presenting part begins to descend into the inlet, before engagement has truly occurred, it is said to be *dipping* into the pelvis.

Station refers to the relationship of the presenting part to an imaginary line drawn between the ischial spines of the maternal pelvis. In a normal pelvis, the ischial spines mark the narrowest diameter of the pelvis that the fetus must encounter. These spines are not sharp protrusions that harm the fetus but rather are blunted prominences at the midpelvis. The ischial spines as a landmark have been designated as zero station (Figure 14–8). If the presenting part is higher than the ischial spines, a negative number is assigned, noting centimeters above zero station. Station −5 is at the inlet, and station +4 is at the outlet; the presenting part can be visualized upon viewing the woman's perineum—delivery is imminent. During the process of labor, the presenting part should move progressively from the negative stations to the midpelvis at zero station and into the positive stations. Failure of the presenting part to descend in the presence of strong contractions may be due to disproportion between the maternal pelvis and fetal presenting part, or a short and/or entangled umbilical cord.

When both pelvic and fetal planes are parallel, the relationship is said to be *synclitic.* Thus in a cephalic presentation, engagement occurs in synclitism when the biparietal diameter of the fetal head is parallel to the sacrum and the symphysis pubis. Engagement in synclitism takes place when the uterus is perpendicular to the inlet, not retroflexed or anteflexed. Synclitic engagement also indicates that the pelvis is roomy.

Asynclitism indicates that the uterus is not perpendicular to the inlet and that the fetal head is not parallel to the planes of the pelvis. This usually occurs with small pelvic diameters or with weak abdominal musculature that allows the uterus to tilt anteriorly or posteriorly. When there is a large fetal head or small pelvic diameters, asynclitism facilitates engagement by allowing a smaller diameter of the fetal head to enter the pelvis. Persistent asynclitism may cause difficulties, however, preventing normal rotation of the head in the pelvis (Oxorn, 1980).

FETAL POSITION

Fetal position refers to the relationship of the landmark on the presenting fetal part to the front, sides, or back of the maternal pelvis. The landmark on the fetal presenting part is related to four imaginary quadrants of the pelvis: left anterior, right anterior, left posterior, and right posterior. These quadrants assist in designating whether the presenting part is directed toward the front, back, left, or right of the passage. The landmark chosen for cephalic presentations is the occiput in vertex presentations and the mentum in face presentations. Breech presentations use the sacrum as the designated landmark, and the acromion process on the scapula is noted in shoulder presentations. If the landmark is directed toward the center of the side of the pelvis, it is designated as a *transverse position,* rather than anterior or posterior.

Three notations are used to describe the fetal position:

1. Right (R) or left (L) side of the maternal pelvis.
2. The landmark of the fetal presenting part: occiput (O), mentum (M), sacrum (S), or acromion process (A).
3. Anterior (A), posterior (P), or transverse (T), depending on whether the landmark is in the front, back, or side of the pelvis.

Abbreviations are formed from these notations to assist the health care team in communicating the fetal position. Hence, when the fetal occiput is directed toward the back and to the left of the passage, the abbreviation used is LOP (left-occiput-posterior). The term *dorsal* (D) is used when denoting the fetal position in a transverse lie; it refers to the fetal back. Thus the abbreviation RADA indi-

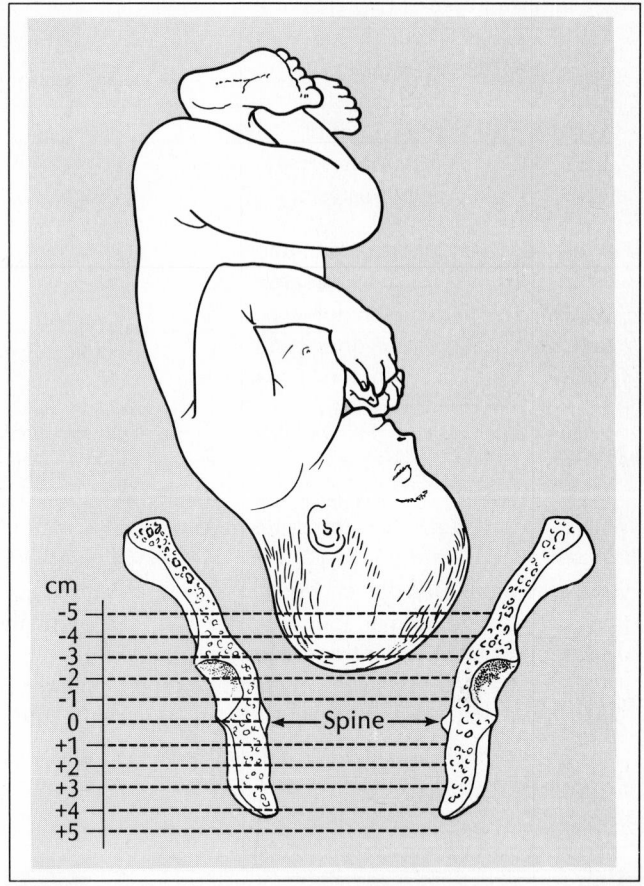

FIGURE 14–8 Measuring station of the fetal head while it is descending.

cates that the acromion process of the scapula is directed toward the woman's right and the passenger's back is anterior.

Following is a list of the positions for various fetal presentations, some of which are illustrated in Figure 14–6:

Positions in vertex presentation:
ROA	Right-occiput-anterior
ROT	Right-occiput-transverse
ROP	Right-occiput-posterior
LOA	Left-occiput-anterior
LOT	Left-occiput-transverse
LOP	Left-occiput-posterior

Positions in face presentation:
RMA	Right-mentum-anterior
RMT	Right-mentum-transverse
RMP	Right-mentum-posterior
LMA	Left-mentum-anterior
LMT	Left-mentum-transverse
LMP	Left-mentum-posterior

Positions in breech presentation:
RSA   Right-sacrum-anterior
RST   Right-sacrum-transverse
RSP   Right-sacrum-posterior
LSA   Left-sacrum-anterior
LST   Left-sacrum-transverse
LSP   Left-sacrum-posterior

Positions in shoulder presentation:
RADA   Right-acromion-dorsal-anterior
RADP   Right-acromion-dorsal-posterior
LADA   Left-acromion-dorsal-anterior
LADP   Left-acromion-dorsal-posterior

The fetal position influences labor and delivery. For example, posterior position causes a larger diameter of the fetal head to enter the pelvis than an anterior position. With a posterior position, pressure on the sacral nerves is increased, causing the laboring woman backache and pelvic pressure and perhaps encouraging her to bear down or push earlier than normal. (See Chapter 18 for an in-depth discussion of malpositions and their management.)

Assessment techniques to determine fetal position include inspection and palpation of the maternal abdomen, and vaginal examination (see Chapter 15 for further discussion of assessment of fetal position).

The Powers

Primary and secondary powers work complementarily to deliver the fetus, the fetal membranes, and the placenta from the uterus into the external environment. The primary power is uterine muscular contractions, which effect the changes of the first stage of labor—complete effacement and dilatation of the cervix. The second power is the use of abdominal muscles in pushing during the second stage of labor. The pushing adds to the primary power after full dilatation has occurred.

UTERINE RESPONSE

In labor, uterine contractions are rhythmical but intermittent, which allows for a period of uterine relaxation between contractions. This period of relaxation allows uterine muscles to rest and provides respite for the laboring woman. It also restores uteroplacental circulation, which is important to fetal oxygenation and adequate circulation in the uterine blood vessels.

Each contraction has three phases: (a) *increment,* the "building up" of the contraction (the longest phase); (b) *acme* or the peak of the contraction; and (c) *decrement* or the "letting up" of the contraction. When describing uterine contractions during labor, the terms frequency, duration, and intensity are used. *Frequency* refers to the period of time between the beginning of one contraction to the beginning of the next contraction.

The *duration* of each contraction is measured from the beginning of the increment to the completion of decrement (Figure 14–9). In beginning labor, the duration is about 30 seconds. As labor continues duration lengthens to an average of 60 seconds with a range of 45–90 seconds (Varney, 1980).

Intensity refers to the strength of the uterine contraction during acme. In most instances it is estimated by palpating the contraction but it may be measured directly through the use of an intrauterine catheter. When estimating intensity by palpation, the nurse determines whether it is mild, moderate, or strong by judging the amount of indentability of the uterine wall during the acme of a contraction. If the uterine wall can be indented easily, it is considered mild. Strong intensity would be achieved when the uterine wall cannot be indented. Moderate intensity falls between these two ranges. When intensity is measured by the use of an intrauterine catheter, the normal resting tonus (between contractions) averages 10 mm Hg of pressure. During acme the intensity ranges from 30–55 mm Hg of pressure (Cibils, 1981). (See discussion on stages of

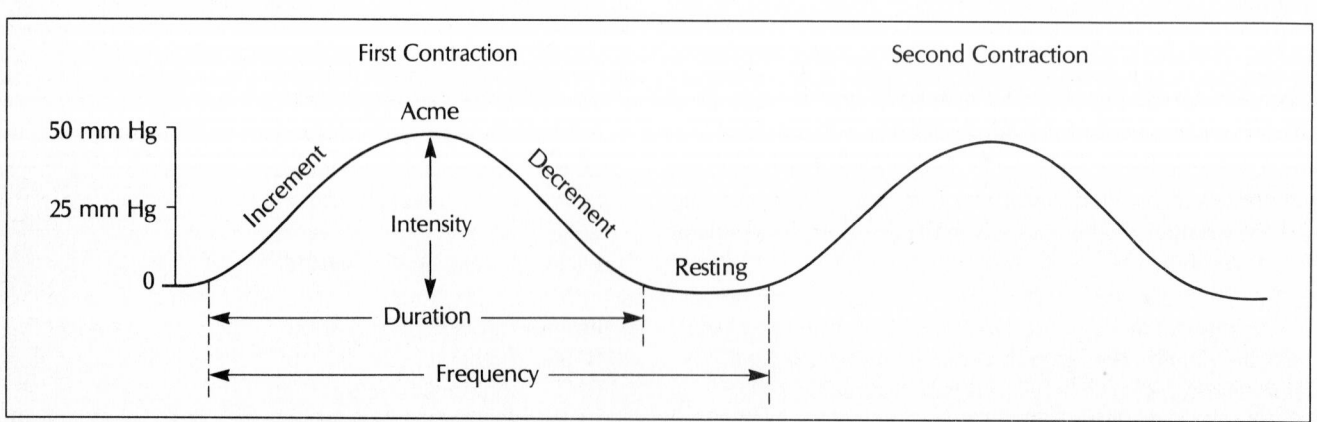

FIGURE 14–9 Characteristics of uterine contractions.

labor, p. 416; and Chapter 15 for further discussion of assessment techniques.)

At the beginning of labor, the contractions are usually mild, of short duration, and relatively infrequent. As labor progresses, the duration lengthens, the intensity increases, and the frequency is every 2–3 minutes. It is important to remember the contractions are involuntary and the laboring woman cannot control their duration, frequency, or intensity.

The Psyche

Colman and Colman (1971) describe labor as a journey into the unknown that is uncertain, irrevocable, and uncontrollable. The woman is uncertain about what her labor will be like: nulliparas face a totally new experience, and multiparas cannot be certain what each new labor will bring. The woman does not know whether she will live up to her expectations for herself in relation to her friends and relatives, whether she will be physically injured through laceration, episiotomy, or cesarean incision, or whether significant others will be as supportive as she imagines (Mercer, 1981). The woman faces an irrevocable event—the birth of a new family member—and, consequently, disruption of life-style, relationships, and self-image. Finally, the woman must deal with concerns about her loss of control of bodily functions, emotional responses to an unfamiliar situation, and reactions to the pain associated with labor.

Various factors influence a woman's reaction to the physical and emotional crisis of labor. Her accomplishment of the tasks of pregnancy, usual coping mechanisms in response to stressful life events, support system, and preparation for childbirth and cultural influences are all significant factors.

COPING MECHANISMS

Westbrook (1979) suggests that "the ways in which a person copes with an event is dependent on how the event is experienced as well as the coping skills the person has acquired." Therefore, coping mechanisms related to pregnancy are expected to be consistent with those typical of the individual and influenced by perception of the experience. Westbrook looked at three groups of new mothers by socioeconomic level (working, middle, and upper-middle class) in relation to positive and negative aspects of childbearing (that is, their perception of the experience) and coping mechanisms. Positive aspects of childbearing include enhancement of the woman's femininity, feelings of well-being, sense of value as a person, and feelings of maturity.

Negative aspects of childbearing include rejection of the pregnancy and/or infant; anticipation of problems during labor (fear, poor performance, lack of support); fear of physical harm to self during labor; physical discomfort of pregnancy; problems of infant care and worries about con-

flicting advice; the family's coping abilities, and the well-being of the infant.

Perceptions of the pregnancy, labor and delivery experience by women varied significantly by socioeconomic status in that coping mechanisms vary from class to class. Some typical coping strategies are confrontation, avoidance, optimism, seeking interpersonal help, fatalism, and control. Working-class women expressed positive attitudes toward childbearing, experiencing it as a satisfying and enhancing experience. On the other hand, they had negative attitudes toward labor compared with the middle-class and upper-middle class women. They complained of more physical discomfort and were, in general, more fearful of the physical processes of childbearing. These responses may reflect the perceptions of working-class women that they are less in control of events. It also suggests a greater use of fatalistic mechanisms and avoidance rather than confrontation (which is used more by middle-class and upper-middle class women) in coping strategies. The working-class women also had the lowest attendance at childbirth classes despite adequate time, availability, and transportation, further indicating their reliance on avoidance of these activities related to perceived uncontrollable stresses (in this case, the childbirth classes were intended to help them to deal with physical control of labor).

Coping mechanisms and stressors also affect the outcome of pregnancy. Women with high levels of anxiety have a significantly higher incidence of complications of pregnancy, such as preeclampsia, hemorrhage, fetal distress, forceps delivery, prolonged and precipitate labor (Crandon, 1978). This was also true for women with poor coping skills.

SUPPORT SYSTEMS

The childbearing experience has traditionally been a group endeavor centered around the laboring woman. Long recognized as a major developmental transition or crisis, childbirth has brought with it numerous rites of passage (Chaney, 1980). These rituals typically included both father and mother as well as significant members of the family and community. The role of the father has been often considered to have direct bearing on the outcome of the pregnancy (Heggenhougen, 1980).

In most developed Western countries relatively little attention has been paid to the role of the father and support systems in childbirth. Changes in practice by the medical profession have not related to the needs of the family during childbirth. Rather, the experience of the family has been forced to adapt to the needs of the caretakers. Only in the past decade has a significant thrust toward family-centered maternity care, and concern for the intrapartal needs of the family, been prevalent. As recently as the mid-1970s many hospitals continued to ban fathers from the labor rooms.

Current research and theory suggest the role of the

father and the family has both direct and indirect impact on the perception of the childbirth experience as a satisfying one on the part of the mother (Doering et al., 1980). The interaction between the laboring woman and her support persons may be observed throughout the stages of labor (Klein et al., 1981).

PREPARATION FOR CHILDBIRTH

Much attention has been focused on preparation during pregnancy as a way of increasing the woman's ability to cope during childbirth, decreasing her experienced stress, anxiety, and pain, and imparting satisfaction with the childbearing experience. Pain management has been "viewed as the primary factor in providing a good childbirth experience" (Humenick, 1981), although current research does not support this concept. Doering and Entwisle (1975) point out that preparation for childbirth does not necessarily lead to a decrease in pain. Physical and psychologic awareness of the childbearing experience, that is, maternal awareness without spinal or general anesthesia or heavy analgesia, leads to increased experiences of satisfaction in childbearing. Humenick (1981) further suggests that mastery, or control, of the childbearing experience is the key factor in perceived satisfaction. Humenick defines control as "continuing to be able to influence the decisions made, not surrendering all decisions and responsibilities to care providers, but rather maintaining a working alliance." In this respect childbirth education is helpful in increasing positive reactions to the birth experience in that it provides the laboring woman and her support persons with greater opportunities to control, or master, her labor experience.

Factors relating to control, although complex, support the mastery model. Factors that have the potential to be supportive include knowledge of the labor and delivery process, acquisition of skills to be used in coping with labor, ability to have influence in decisions, adequate and appropriate support from others, and adequate knowledge concerning alternatives. On the other hand, factors that may be potential stressors include fear and anxiety, excessive fatigue level, low pain tolerance, a sense of helplessness, loss of dignity, feelings of being abandoned or alone, and threats to the life or health of the woman and fetus (Humenick, 1981). Women whose coping mechanisms include avoidance and/or fatalism, who do not perceive themselves in control of their lives or the stresses in their lives, have greater anxieties regarding the actual birth experience (Westbrook, 1979). Women who attend childbirth preparation classes tend to need less medication during labor, are more aware, and perceive their experiences as more satisfying when compared with women who do not attend.

In the mastery model, pain is included among the numerous stressors of both positive and negative aspects of pregnancy and childbearing. Childbirth preparation education provides the opportunity to increase control and accomplish the psychologic tasks women set for themselves in labor, thereby facilitating a more positive birth experience.

PHYSIOLOGY OF LABOR

Possible Causes of Labor Onset

For some reason, usually at the appropriate time for the uterus and the fetus, the process of labor begins. Although medical researchers have been conducting numerous studies to determine the exact cause, it still remains a mystery. Some of the more widely accepted theories are discussed in the following sections.

OXYTOCIN STIMULATION THEORY

Oxytocin can be administered in minute quantities to a woman at term to initiate labor because the myometrium is increasingly sensitive to oxytocin prior to and during labor, perhaps due to stimulatory effects of circulating estrogen (Challis and Mitchell, 1981). However, convincing evidence is lacking to prove that maternal or fetal oxytocin initiates labor. Oxytocin does have an effect on the permeability of sodium in the myometrium and raises the intracellular calcium levels that are needed for muscle contraction (Huszar, 1981). During the second stage of labor, increased plasma levels of oxytocin may be found, which supports the theory that oxytocin helps maintain labor and aids involution (Takahashi and Burd, 1980; Challis and Mitchell, 1981).

PROGESTERONE WITHDRAWAL THEORY

Progesterone has been reported to inhibit the estrogen effect of increased contractility by raising the resting membrane potential in the myometrial cells. It may stabilize the myometrial membrane-bound pools of calcium, thereby limiting uterine contractility (Anderson, 1978). Although some researchers feel there is insufficient evidence to show that progesterone levels in the maternal blood supply fall before labor, others report that progesterone metabolism in the fetal membranes is marked by decreases near term. The decrease in progesterone metabolism may be due to a progesterone-binding protein, which is present near term in the chorion and amnion (Challis and Mitchell, 1981). The decrease may facilitate prostaglandin synthesis in the chorioamnion, which results in an increase in uterine contractility (Takahashi and Burd, 1980). Although no general agreement exists regarding a decrease in progesterone metabolism, many researchers support the theory that a rising estrogen and decreasing progesterone ratio is important in raising levels of uterine contractility (Huszar, 1981).

ESTROGEN STIMULATION THEORY

Estrogen causes irritability of the myometrium, perhaps through an increase in concentrations of actin and myosin (contractile proteins) and adenosine triphosphate (ATP), which is the energy source for contractions. In addition, estrogen may promote prostaglandin synthesis in the decidua and fetal membranes. This enhances myometrial muscle contraction. Once the muscle cell is irritable and contracts, the presence of estrogen also enhances the propagation of impulses over the uterine muscle (Takahashi and Burd, 1980).

FETAL CORTISOL THEORY

Liggins (1973) found that the removal of the fetal lamb's pituitary gland and adrenal cortex delays the onset of labor. Thus he has postulated that the fetus may play an important role in the initiation of labor. He also has reported premature labor in sheep that were infused with cortisol or ACTH. This phenomenon has not been confirmed in humans. Research continues; there is a possibility that cortisol affects the biochemistry of the fetal membrane (Takahashi and Burd, 1980).

FETAL MEMBRANE PHOSPHOLIPID–ARACHIDONIC ACID–PROSTAGLANDIN THEORY

According to the theory of fetal membrane phospholipid–arachidonic acid–prostaglandin interaction, estrogen promotes storage of esterified arachidonic acid in the fetal membranes. Withdrawal of progesterone activates phospholipase A_2, which is an enzymatic liberator. Phospholipase A_2 hydrolyzes phospholipids to liberate arachidonic acid in a nonesterified form. The arachidonic acid acts on prostaglandins E_2 or $F_{2\alpha}$ or both in the decidual membranes. Prostaglandin stimulates the smooth muscle to contract, especially in the myometrium. Prostaglandin is present in increased quantities in the blood and amniotic fluid just prior to and during labor. The exact relationship of prostaglandins to the initiation of labor has yet to be established (Challis and Mitchell, 1981; Huszar, 1981). Evidence is mounting that prostaglandin is a final step in the pathway toward initiation of labor (Takahashi and Burd, 1980).

DISTENTION THEORY

Distention theory was proposed after observations that multiple gestation and/or hydramnios conditions were associated with premature labor. Evidence exists that with increasing stretching of the uterus, there is an increase in the synthesis, myometrial concentration, and the release of $PGF_{2\alpha}$.

Biochemical Interaction

In the past, it was thought that the contraction wave of the uterus was controlled by pacemakers. Currently, it is sug-

gested that the myometrial cells participating in the pacemaker activity do not differ from surrounding cells, nor is the pacemaker activity limited to a specific site (Wolfs and Van Leeuwen, 1979). The contraction wave of the uterus begins in the fundus, which contains the greatest concentration of myometrial cells, and moves downward throughout the entire myometrium. Because the contraction wave moves quickly, the myometrium appears to contract as a unit. Myometrial contraction efficiency depends on four basic systems:

1. The contractile substances (actin and myosin)
2. A source of energy (ATP)
3. Cellular electrolyte exchange (calcium, sodium, and potassium)
4. Endocrine stimulus for conduction (oxytocin, $PGF_{2\alpha}$, and acetycholine)

Myometrium has both alpha-receptors, which stimulate uterine contractions, and beta-receptors, which have the opposite effect (Aladjem, 1980). Norepinephrine and epinephrine can stimulate the alpha- or beta-receptors. Which receptors they affect depends on the hormones that are present. If progesterone is present, norepinephrine and epinephrine stimulate the beta-receptors and the muscles remain quiet. If estrogen is present, norepinephrine and epinephrine stimulate the alpha-receptors and the muscle is excitable.

Myometrial Activity

Stretching of the cervix causes an increase in endogenous oxytocin, which increases myometrial activity. This is known as the *Ferguson reflex*. Pressures exerted by the contracting uterus vary from 20–60 mm Hg, with an average of 40 mm Hg.

In true labor the uterus divides into two portions. This division is known as the *physiologic retraction ring*. The upper portion, which is the contractile segment, becomes progressively thicker as labor advances. The lower portion, which includes the lower uterine segment and cervix, is passive. As labor continues, the lower uterine segment expands and thins out.

With each contraction the musculature of the upper uterine segment shortens and exerts a longitudinal traction on the cervix, causing effacement. *Effacement* is the taking up of the internal os and the cervical canal into the uterine side walls. The cervix changes progressively from a long, thick structure to a structure that is tissue-paper thin (Figure 14–10). In primigravidas, effacement usually precedes dilatation. This musculature remains shorter and thicker and does not return to its original length. This phenomenon is known as brachystasis. The space in the uterine cavity decreases as a result of brachystasis.

The uterus elongates with each contraction, decreas-

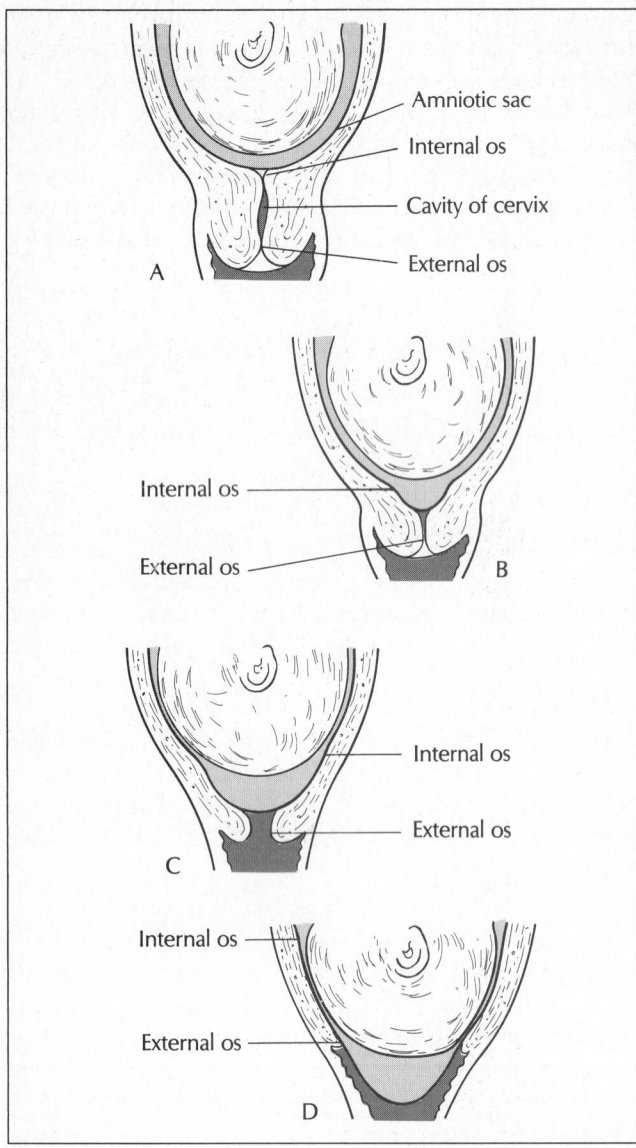

FIGURE 14-10 Effacement of the cervix in the primigravida. **A,** At the beginning of labor there is no cervical effacement or dilatation. **B,** Beginning cervical effacement. **C,** Cervix is about one-half effaced and slightly dilated. **D,** Complete effacement and dilatation.

ing the horizontal diameter. This elongation causes a straightening of the fetal body, pressing the upper pole against the fundus and thrusting the presenting part down toward the lower uterine segment and the cervix. The pressure exerted by the fetus is called the fetal axis pressure. As the uterus elongates, the longitudinal muscle fibers are pulled upward over the presenting part. This action, plus the hydrostatic pressure of the fetal membranes, causes cervical *dilatation*. The cervical os and cervical canal widen from less than a centimeter to approximately

10 cm, allowing delivery of the fetus. When the cervix is completely dilated and retracted up into the lower uterine segment, it can no longer be palpated.

The round ligament contracts with the uterus, pulling the fundus forward, thus aligning the fetus with the bony pelvis.

Intraabdominal Pressure

After the cervix is completely dilated, the maternal abdominal musculature contracts as the woman pushes. The pushing that the woman does aids in expulsion of the infant and the placenta after delivery. If the cervix is not completely dilated, bearing down can cause cervical edema, which retards dilatation, and can cause maternal exhaustion as a result of straining. Tearing and bruising will also result from bearing down upon an incompletely dilated cervix.

Musculature Changes in the Pelvic Floor

The levator ani muscle and fascia of the pelvic floor draw the rectum and vagina upward and forward with each contraction, along the curve of the pelvic floor. As the fetal head descends to the pelvic floor, the pressure of the presenting part causes the perineal structure that was once 5 cm in thickness to change to a structure of less than a centimeter, and a normal physiologic anesthesia is produced as a result of the decreased blood supply to the area. The anus everts, exposing the interior rectal wall as the fetal head descends forward (Pritchard and MacDonald, 1980).

MATERNAL SYSTEMIC RESPONSE TO LABOR

Cardiovascular System

A strong contraction greatly diminishes or completely stops the blood flow in the branches of the uterine artery which supplies the intervillous space. This leads to a redistribution of the blood flow to the peripheral circulation and an increase in peripheral resistance, resulting in an increase of the systolic and diastolic blood pressure and a slowing of the pulse rate. The amount of change in maternal blood pressure and pulse is also dependent on the maternal position. Supine hypotension has an occurrence rate of 10%–15%. When it occurs, it further taxes the cardiovascular system by decreasing venous return from the lower extremities (Cibils, 1981).

Cardiac output is increased by 10%–15% during rest periods between contractions in early labor and by 30%–

50% in the second stage (Albright, 1978). Additional increases and decreases in cardiac output mirror the changes in uterine pressure; that is, an increase in cardiac output as the contraction builds and peaks, and a slow return to precontraction cardiac output as the contraction diminishes.

There is an additional effect on hemodynamics during the bearing down efforts in the second stage. When the laboring woman holds her breath and pushes against a closed glottis (Valsalva maneuver), intrathoracic pressure rises. As intrathoracic pressure increases, the venous return is interrupted and leads to a rise in the venous pressure. In addition, the blood in the lungs is forced into the left atrium which leads to a transient increase in cardiac output, blood pressure, and pulse pressure, and bradycardia develops. As venous return to the lungs continues to be diminished as the breath continues to be held, a decrease in blood pressure, pulse pressure, and cardiac output occurs (Cibils, 1981).

When the next breath is taken (Valsalva maneuver is interrupted), the intrathoracic pressure is decreased. Venous return increases, which leads to refilling of the pulmonary bed and results in recovery of the cardiac output and stroke volume. This process is repeated with each pushing effort (Cibils, 1981).

Immediately after delivery, cardiac output peaks with an 80% increase over prelabor values, and then in the first 10 minutes decreases 20%–25%. Cardiac output further decreases 20%–25% in the first hour after delivery (Albright, 1978).

Blood Pressure

As a result of increased cardiac output, systolic blood pressure rises during uterine contractions. In the immediate postpartal period the arterial pressure remains essentially normal even though the cardiac output increases due to peripheral vasodilatation.

Supine hypotensive syndrome has been demonstrated radiographically in 90% of women at term. Although in clinical practice approximately 10%–15% of women demonstrate clinical symptoms (hypotension, tachycardia), some women may suffer supine hypotensive syndrome and remain asymptomatic due to compensatory mechanisms. These women are at risk because even though they are initially asymptomatic, placental perfusion is slowly compromised by arterial peripheral vasoconstriction (Albright, 1978).

Women with the highest risk of developing supine hypotensive syndrome are nulliparas with strong abdominal muscles and tightly drawn abdominal skin, gravidas with hydramnios and/or multiple pregnancy, and obese women. Other predisposing factors include hypovolemia, dehydration, hemorrhage, metabolic acidosis, administration of narcotics which results in vasodilation and inhibits compen-

satory mechanisms, and administration of regional anesthesia that results in sympathetic blockade.

Fluid and Electrolyte Balance

Diaphoresis and hyperventilation occur during labor, which alters electrolyte and fluid balance from insensible loss. The muscle activity elevates the body temperature, which increases sweating and evaporation from the skin. The rise in the respiratory rate as the woman responds to the work of labor increases the evaporative water volume, because each breath of air must be warmed to the body temperature and humidified (Dukes and Bowen, 1976). With the increased evaporative water volume, adequate hydration via parenteral fluids during labor becomes increasingly important.

Gastrointestinal System

During labor, additional reduction of gastric motility and absorption of solid food occurs. The gastric emptying time is further prolonged. It is not uncommon for a laboring woman to vomit stomach contents of food that was ingested up to 12 hours previously.

Respiratory System

Oxygen consumption, which increased approximately 20% during pregnancy, is further increased during labor. During the early first stage oxygen consumption increases 40%, with a further increase to 100% during the second stage.

Minute ventilation increases to 20–25 L/min (normal 10 L/min), and in the nonprepared and unmedicated client it may reach 35 L/min or more. This hyperventilation results in a rise in the maternal pH in early labor, followed by a return to normal toward the end of the first stage. If the first stage is prolonged, the maternal pH may become acidotic (Albright, 1978).

Hemopoietic System

Leukocyte levels may elevate to 25,000 or more during labor. Although the precise cause of the leukocytosis is unknown, it may be due to the strenuous exercise and stress response of labor (Pritchard and MacDonald, 1980). Plasma fibrinogen increases, and blood coagulation time decreases. Blood glucose levels may decrease, due to the increased activity of uterine and skeletal muscles (Varney, 1980).

Renal System

The base of the bladder is pushed forward and upward when engagement occurs. The pressure from the presenting part may lead to edema of the tissues due to impaired drainage of blood and lymph from the base of the bladder (Pritchard and MacDonald, 1980).

Approximately one-third to one-half of all laboring women have slight proteinuria of $1+$ as a result of muscle breakdown from exercise. An increase to $2+$ or above is indicative of pathology (Varney, 1980).

Response to Pain

THEORIES OF PAIN

Many theories of pain have evolved during the past century. The traditional theory of pain is known as the *specificity theory*. It proposes that a specific pain system carries messages from pain receptors in the body to a pain center in the brain. However, too many clinical facts are neglected in this model of a rigid, closed system. The amount and quality of pain experienced by an individual are modified by psychologic and environmental variables.

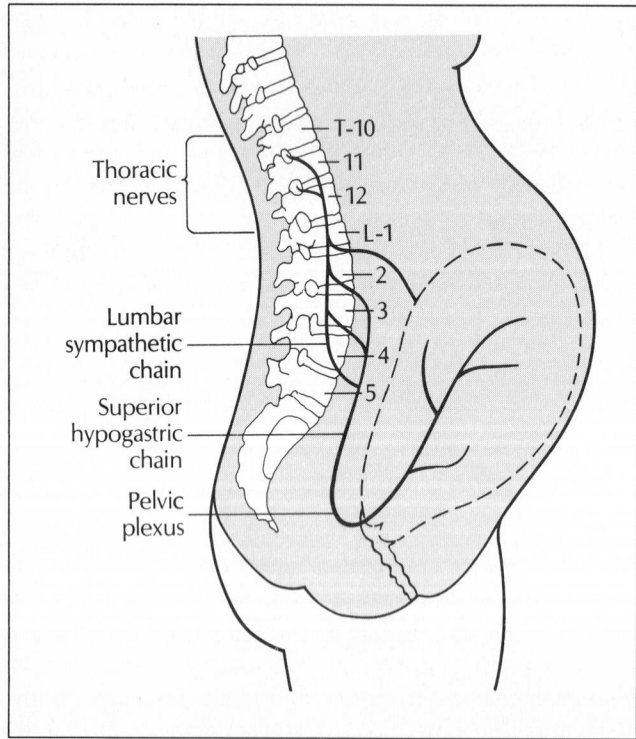

FIGURE 14–11 Pain pathway from uterus to spinal cord. Nerve impulses travel through the uterine plexus, pelvic plexus, inferior hypogastric plexus, middle and superior hypogastric plexus, and the lumbar sympathetic chain and enter the spinal cord through the twelfth, eleventh, and tenth thoracic nerves. (Modified from Bonica, J. J. 1972. *Principles and practice of obstetric analgesia and anesthesia.* Philadelphia: F. A. Davis Co., p. 492.)

The simplest form of response to stimuli is a protective mechanism, the withdrawal reflex that occurs in the sensorimotor arc. For example, when the hand is placed on a hot object, pain nerve fibers transmit impulses to the dorsal root of the spinal cord. Each impulse is transmitted through synapses to the ventral root and returns to the local muscles as a motor impulse causing a jerking movement away from the hot object. This reaction occurs before the sensory information is processed by the brain; the hand is lifted before pain is perceived. Even this simple mechanism does not occur in isolation. The individual is thrown off balance by the reflex action, and immediately the entire body moves to restore equilibrium. This type of reflex action occurs during an intramuscular injection—the person flinches as the skin is penetrated.

The *pattern theory* of pain attempts to incorporate the psychologic aspects of pain ignored by the specificity theory. The pattern theory proposes that particular networks or patterns of nerve impulses are produced by the summation of sensory input at the dorsal horn cells. Pain results when the total output of these cells exceeds a critical level as a result of excessive stimulation of receptors or of pathologic conditions that enhance the summation of impulses. The patterns of impulses travel over multiple pathways and enter widespread regions of the brain.

When the mechanisms suggested by the specificity and pattern theories are examined, valuable complementary concepts come to light. The *gate-control theory* proposed by Melzack (1973) has attempted to integrate all aspects of pain into a comprehensive theory. According to this view, pain results from activity in several interacting specialized neural systems.

The gate-control theory proposes that a mechanism in the dorsal horn of the spinal column, probably the substantia gelatinosa, serves as a valve or gate that increases or decreases the flow of nerve impulses from the periphery to the central nervous system. The uterus-to-spinal cord pain pathway along a single sensory tract is illustrated in Figure 14–11. The gate mechanism is influenced by the size of the transmitting fibers and by the nerve impulses that descend from the brain. Psychologic processes such as past experiences, attention, and emotion may influence pain perception and response by activating the gate mechanism. The gates may be opened or closed by central nervous system activities, such as anxiety or excitement, or through selective, localized activity (Melzack, 1973). The gate-control theory has two important implications for obstetrics: Pain may be controlled by tactile stimulation, and pain can be modified by "maximizing central control factors by means of special training in childbirth education, using suggestion, distraction and behavioral conditioning" (Clark and Affonso, 1979).

PAIN DURING LABOR

The pain associated with the first stage of labor is unique in that it accompanies a normal physiologic process. Even though perception of the pain of childbirth is greatly deter-mined by cultural patterning, there is a physiologic basis for discomfort during labor. Pain during the first stage of labor arises from (a) dilatation of the cervix, (b) hypoxia of the uterine muscle cells during contraction, (c) stretching of the lower uterine segment, and (d) pressure on adjacent structures. The primary source of pain is dilatation or stretching of the cervix. Nerve impulses travel through the uterine plexus, inferior hypogastric (pelvic) plexus, middle hypogastric plexus, superior hypogastric plexus, and the lumbar sympathetic and lower thoracic chain and enter the spinal cord through the posterior roots of the twelfth, elev-enth, and tenth thoracic and first lumbar nerves. As with other visceral pain, pain from the uterus is referred to the dermatomes supplied by the twelfth, eleventh, and tenth thoracic nerves. The areas of referred pain include the low-er abdominal wall and the areas over the lower lumbar region and the upper sacrum (Figure 14–12).

During the second stage of labor, discomfort is due to (a) hypoxia of the contracting uterine muscle cells, (b) dis-tention of the vagina and perineum, and (c) pressure on adjacent structures. The nerve impulses from the vagina and perineum are transmitted by way of the pudendal nerve plexus and enter the spinal cord through the posteri-or roots of the second, third, and fourth sacral nerves (Fig-ure 14–13).

Pain during the third stage results from uterine con-tractions and cervical dilatation as the placenta is expelled (Figure 14–14). The mechanism for the transmission of nerve impulses is the same as for the first stage of labor. This stage of labor is short, and the primary need for anes-thesia after this phase of the labor process is for episiot-omy repair.

FACTORS AFFECTING RESPONSE TO PAIN

Because pain is a total psychosomatic experience, many factors affect the individual's perception of pain impulses. All human societies have developed patterns of behavior for the maternal role during childbirth. Some psychologic and environmental influences particularly appropriate to labor are discussed here.

□ *CULTURAL BACKGROUND* Individuals tend to respond to painful stimuli in the way that is acceptable in their culture. It is important to realize the many varieties of response to pain to assess a client's need for assistance. The absence of crying and moaning does not necessarily mean that pain is absent, nor does the presence of crying and moaning necessarily mean that pain relief is desired at that moment. Some cultures believe it is natural to communicate the pain experience, no matter how mild. Members of some cultures stoically accept pain out of fear or because it is expected of them.

Cultural attitudes about childbirth itself may be a fac-tor in the reaction to pain. The San Blas Indians of Panama view childbirth as a shameful event that must be hidden from men and children. Labor is frequently prolonged and so painful that women lose consciousness (Newton, 1964). At the other extreme, the Navajo Indians of the southwest-ern United States view childbirth as an open social event. All who come to give support are invited to stay and eat (Lockett, 1939). The sensations of labor are not thought of as painful by Navajo women. In fact, the language has two words for labor, one meaning painful labor and the other meaning normal labor (McCammon, 1951). Acculturation has no doubt modified these attitudes since the original studies were done.

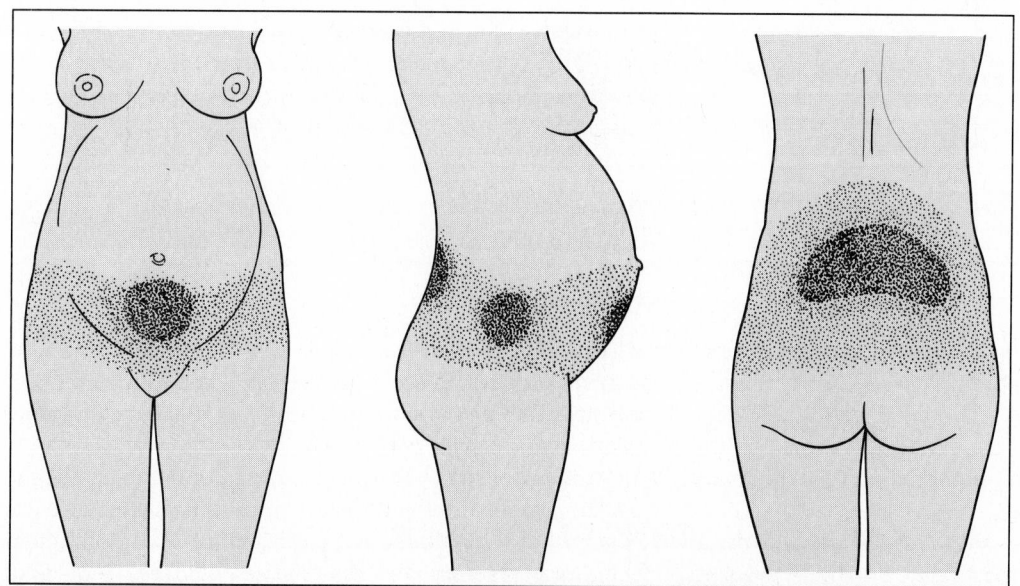

FIGURE 14–12 Area of ref-erence of labor pain dur-ing the first stage. Density of stippling indicates inten-sity of pain. (From Bonica, J. J. 1972. *Principles and practice of obstetric anal-gesia and anesthesia.* Phila-delphia: F. A. Davis Co., p. 108.)

FIGURE 14–13 Distribution of labor pain during the later phase of the first stage and early phase of the second stage. Cross-hatched areas indicate location of the most intense pain; dense stippling, moderate pain; and light stippling, mild pain. Note that the uterine contractions, which at this stage are very strong, produce intense pain. (From Bonica, J. J. 1972. *Principles and practice of obstetric analgesia and anesthesia.* Philadelphia: F. A. Davis Co., p. 109.)

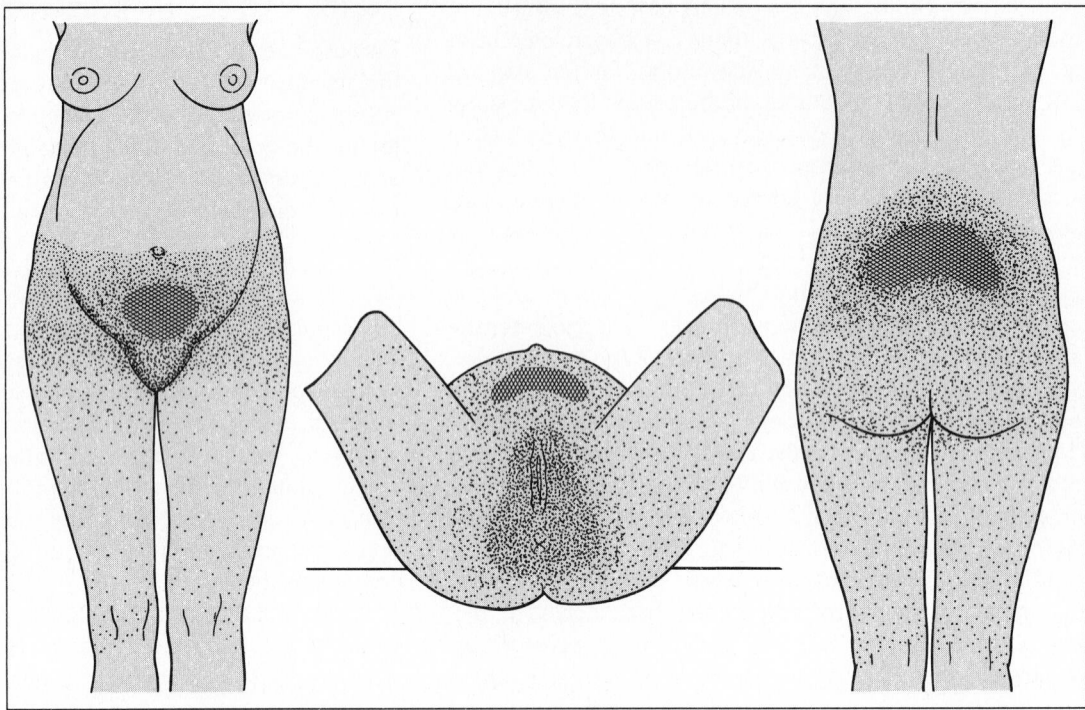

FIGURE 14–14 Distribution of labor pain during the later phase of the second stage and actual delivery. The perineal component is the primary cause of discomfort. Uterine contractions contribute much less. (From Bonica, J. J. 1972. *Principles and practice of obstetric analgesia and anesthesia.* Philadelphia: F. A. Davis Co., p. 109.)

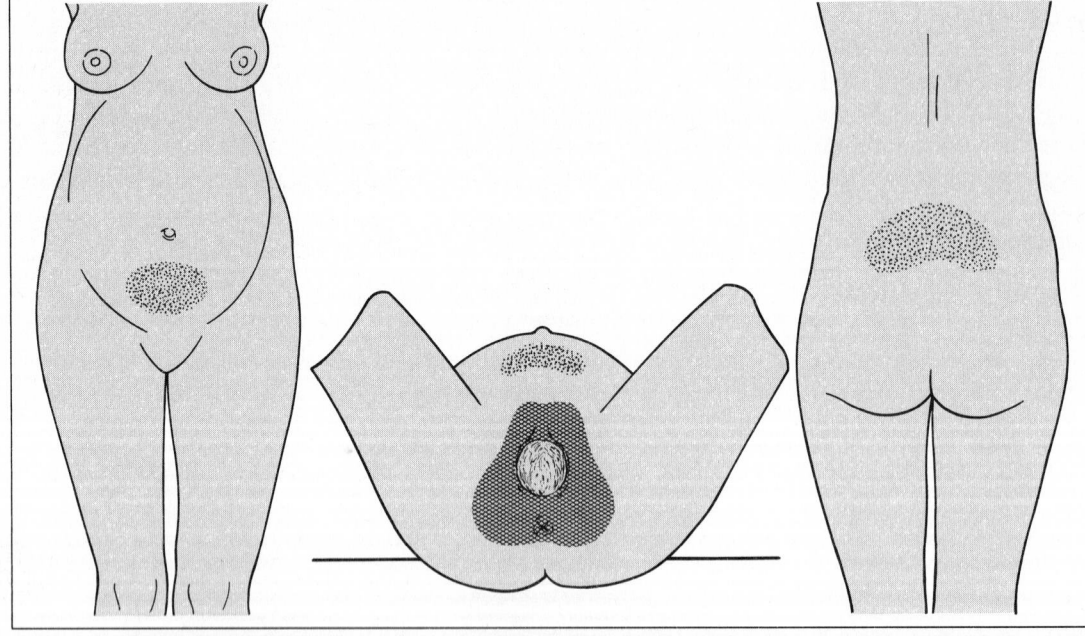

Among many in North America, interest in psychoprophylactic preparation and partner participation in childbirth has increased following a liberalized attitude toward sexuality and childbearing. The father's presence in the labor room has become an expected routine in many hospitals.

Many cultural groups in North America, such as those of Mexican, Arab, and Southeast Asian origin, believe that childbearing is an exclusively female experience. Women during childbirth do not want to share labor with their male partners but derive comfort from the support of female relatives and health personnel.

It is important, however, to avoid stereotyping clients because of their ethnic backgrounds since exposure to North American culture and expectations may modify the behavioral response to pain. Nurses who are providing support during labor must recognize that there are ways of reacting to pain, which are different from one's personal views of appropriate behavior. Nurses must be familiar with the cultural beliefs of those they are likely to assist during labor and use this knowledge along with assessment skills to verify the type of support that is needed.

□ *FATIGUE AND SLEEP DEPRIVATION* Exhaustion may be so great that a laboring woman's attention wanders from the physical stimuli of childbirth, or it may have the opposite effect, lowering the powers of resistance and self-control to produce an exaggerated response. Fatigue from sleep deprivation affects an individual's response to pain in several ways. The fatigued person has less energy and a decreased ability to use such usual strategies as distraction or imagination as coping mechanisms in dealing with pain. The fatigued woman in labor may choose a less demanding alternative, such as analgesia (McCaffery, 1972). This is a particularly important factor in laboring clients because prolonged prodromal labor may interfere with sleep. A woman may begin the active phase of labor in an exhausted state and have difficulty coping with the discomfort of frequent intense contractions.

□ *PERSONAL SIGNIFICANCE OF PAIN* The significance of pain is closely related to the woman's self-concept as well as to cultural expectations. She may view labor as a fearful event, one she has dreaded throughout pregnancy, or she may view it as the happiest event of her life. Pain may be interpreted by some women as punishment for perceived sins, such as engaging in premarital intercourse or feeling ambivalent toward the pregnancy. Others who have had psychoprophylactic preparation for childbirth may consider the pain a test of their ability to cope with a challenging event. If such women do not handle the pain of labor according to their expectations, they tend to experience a sense of failure, which threatens not only their self-concept but also their ability to mother. Consequently, it is vital that childbirth instructors and nurses stress to each woman that the reaction to childbirth is varied and individual. A woman should not feel a sense of failure if she requires analgesia to assist her in coping. The primary goal of psychoprophylactic preparation is not totally unmedicated childbirth but a childbirth experience that is satisfying to both father and mother.

□ *PREVIOUS EXPERIENCE* One's previous experience with pain affects one's ability to manage current and future pain. Particularly painful experiences can condition one to expect the same degree of pain in a similar situation. All persons, with very few exceptions, have experienced pain. It appears likely that those who have had more experience with pain are more sensitive to painful stimuli.

□ *ANXIETY* Anxiety related to pain must be approached on two levels, that associated with anticipation of pain and that associated with the presence of pain. While a moderate degree of anxiety about impending pain is necessary for the person to handle the pain experience, anxiety during the pain experience should be reduced as much as possible by nursing intervention. Anxiety during labor produces tension, which increases the intensity of the pain.

Anxieties unrelated to the pain can also intensify the pain experience. For many young women, admission for labor and delivery is their first hospitalization. Routine procedures, rules and regulations, equipment, and the general environment are unfamiliar and anxiety-provoking. For many women the spontaneous onset of labor has an element of surprise. Although the event is expected and even anticipated, few women are totally prepared for the actual onset of labor and hospitalization. Last-minute details must be completed. Arrangements for the care of other children have usually been made but now must actually be carried out. Having to leave young children for a few days is accompanied by varying degrees of anxiety for any mother.

Separation from loved ones is another major source of anxiety. Unfortunately, some institutions throughout the United States still do not allow husbands and significant others to be with the laboring woman during labor and delivery. One study of postoperative pain revealed that married persons seem to experience less pain than unmarried persons, possibly because of the emotional support given by the spouse (Bruegel, 1971). Of course, the implications of this study are not related solely to the married state, because many stable relationships are formed outside of marriage, but to the probability that the presence of the partner decreases anxiety. When anxiety is decreased by the support of a significant person, pain perception is decreased.

□ *ATTENTION AND DISTRACTION* Both attention and distraction have an influence on the perception of pain. When pain sensation is the focus of attention, the perceived intensity is greater. Preoccupation with an activity lessens pain perception. The classic example is the football player who is unaware of an injury until the game is over. Only then does he experience painful sensation from the injury.

A sensory stimulus can serve as a distraction because the person's attention is focused on the stimulus rather than the pain, for example, providing a client with a back rub. Cutaneous sensations are carried by large-diameter afferent fibers, which can inhibit the pain sensation carried by small-diameter fibers. This is a component of the gate-control theory of pain discussed earlier. Cutaneous stimulation to relieve pain may also be explained by the theory of extinction or perceptual dominance. It is possible that sensory input may extinguish pain or raise its threshold.

FETAL RESPONSE TO LABOR

In the presence of a normal fetus the mechanical and hemodynamic changes enforced by normal labor have no adverse fetal effect (Aladjem and Brown, 1974).

Biomechanical Changes

High pressures are exerted on the fetal head during contractions and to an even greater extent after rupture of the membranes. During labor's second stage, the pressures may rise as high as 200 mm Hg (Aladjem and Brown, 1974).

Cardiac Changes

Researchers have demonstrated that fetal heart rate decelerations can occur with intracranial pressures of 40–55 mm Hg. The currently accepted explanation for this is hypoxic depression of the CNS, which is under vagal control. The absence of these head compression decelerations in some women in labor is explained by the existence of a threshold that is more gradually reached in the presence of intact membranes and lack of maternal resistance. These changes are innocuous in the normal fetus (Aladjem and Brown, 1974).

Hemodynamic Changes

The adequate exchange of nutrients and gases to and from the fetal capillaries and the intervillous space depends on a number of factors, one of which is the fetal blood pressure. Fetal blood pressure serves as a protective mechanism for the normal fetus for the stresses of the anoxic period,

which are enforced by the contracting uterus during labor. The fetal and placental reserve is enough to see the fetus through these anoxic periods without adversity (Aladjem and Brown, 1974).

Positional Changes

So that the fetus can make the transition from intrauterine life to extrauterine life, the fetal head and body must adjust to the passage by certain positional changes, often called *cardinal movements* or *mechanisms of labor.* These changes are described in the order in which they occur (Figure 14–15).

Descent. Descent is thought to occur because of four forces: (a) pressure of the amniotic fluid, (b) direct pressure of the fundus on the breech, (c) contraction of the abdominal muscles, and (d) extension and straightening of the fetal body. The head enters the inlet in the occiput transverse or oblique position, because the pelvic inlet is widest from side to side. The sagittal suture is an equal distance from the maternal symphysis pubis and sacral promontory.

Flexion. Flexion occurs as the fetal head descends and meets resistance from the soft tissues of the pelvis, the musculature of the pelvic floor, and the cervix.

Internal rotation. The fetal head must rotate to fit the diameter of the pelvic cavity, which is widest in the anteroposterior diameter. As the occiput of the fetal head meets resistance from the levator ani muscles and their fascia,

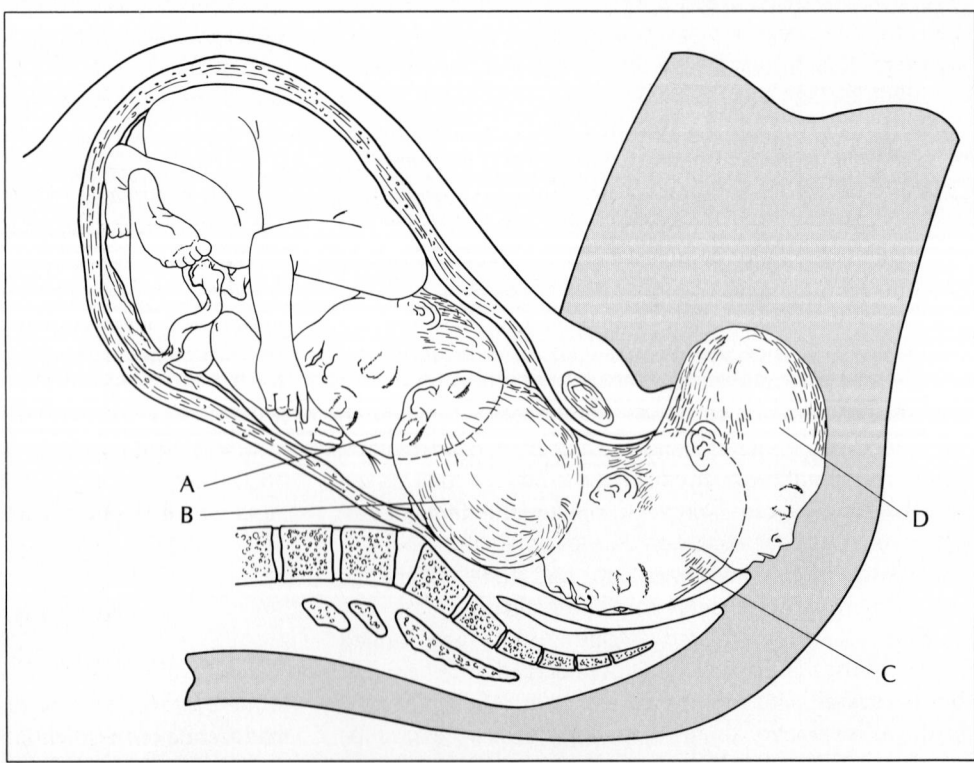

FIGURE 14–15 Mechanism of labor. **A,** Descent. **B,** Flexion. **C,** Internal rotation. **D,** Extension. (External rotation not shown.)

the occiput rotates from left to right and the sagittal suture aligns in the anteroposterior pelvic diameter.

Extension. The resistance of the pelvic floor and the mechanical movement of the vulva opening anteriorly and forward assist with extension of the fetal head as it passes under the symphysis pubis. With this positional change, the occiput, then brow and face, emerge from the introitus.

Restitution. The shoulders of the infant enter the pelvis obliquely and remain oblique when the head rotates to the anteroposterior diameter through internal rotation. Because of this rotation the neck becomes twisted. Once the head delivers and is free of pelvic resistance, the neck untwists, turning the head to one side (restitution), and aligns with the position of the back in the birth canal.

External rotation. As the shoulders rotate to the anteroposterior position in the pelvis, the head is turned farther to one side (external rotation).

Expulsion. After the external rotation and through expulsive efforts of the laboring woman, the anterior shoulder meets the under surface of the symphysis pubis, slips under it, and as lateral flexion of the shoulder and head occurs, the anterior shoulder is born before the posterior shoulder. The body follows quickly (Oxorn, 1980). The adaptations of the newborn to extrauterine life are discussed in Chapter 21.

PREMONITORY SIGNS OF LABOR

Most primigravidas and many multiparas experience signs and symptoms of impending labor.

Lightening

The majority of primigravidas experience the phenomenon of *lightening* before the onset of labor. This feeling occurs because the fetus begins to settle into the pelvic inlet. With its descent, the uterus moves downward, and the fundus no longer presses on the diaphragm.

The woman can breathe more easily after lightening. With increased downward pressure of the presenting part, however, the woman may notice leg cramps or pains due to pressure on the nerves that course through the obturator foramen in the pelvis, increased pelvic pressure, and increased venous stasis leading to dependent edema. Vaginal secretions increase due to congestion of the vaginal mucous membranes. In theory, primigravidas experience lightening because of increased intensity of Braxton Hicks contractions and the bracing action of abdominal muscles of good tone. Engagement then results. In one study, the mean interval between engagement and delivery in primigravidas was found to be 1.39 weeks (Weekes and Flynn, 1975).

Braxton Hicks Contractions

Prior to the onset of labor, Braxton Hicks contractions, the irregular, intermittent contractions that have been occurring throughout the pregnancy, may become uncomfortable. The pain seems to be in the abdomen and groin but may feel like the "drawing" sensations experienced by some with dysmenorrhea.

The contractions may occur for a few weeks, a few days, or just hours prior to the onset of true labor. False labor is uncomfortable and may be exhausting as the woman remains awake, wondering if "this is it." Since the contractions can be fairly regular, she has no way of knowing if they are the beginning of true labor. She may come to the hospital for a vaginal examination to determine if cervical dilatation is occurring. Frequent episodes of false labor and trips back and forth to the physician's office or hospital may frustrate or embarrass the woman, who feels that she should know when she is really in labor. Reassurance by nursing personnel can ease embarrassment.

Cervical Changes

For some time, the "ripening" (softening) of the cervix was thought to be caused by increasing intensity of Braxton Hicks contractions. Liggins (1978) suggests that softening of the cervix begins in the second half of pregnancy. Within a few days before the onset of labor, the cervix becomes even more soft and begins to efface and dilate slightly. The mechanism for this ripening is biochemical and is the result of changes in the connective tissue of the cervix. Research centers on the possible interplay of estrogen, progesterone, and prostaglandins as causative agents in the progressive cervical changes during pregnancy (Liggins, 1978).

Bloody Show

With softening and effacement of the cervix, the mucous plug (accumulated cervical secretions that have closed off the opening of the uterine cavity) is often expelled, resulting in a small amount of blood loss from the exposed cervical capillaries. The resulting pink-tinged secretions are called *bloody show.*

Bloody show is considered a sign of imminent labor, which usually begins within 24–48 hours. Sometimes vaginal examination with manipulation of the cervix may also result in a blood-tinged discharge, which may be confused with bloody show.

Rupture of Membranes

In approximately 12% of women, the amniotic membranes rupture before the onset of labor. This is called rupture of membranes (ROM). Labor usually begins within 24 hours for 80% of these women. When the membranes rupture, the open pathway into the uterus causes danger of infection. Frequently when labor does not begin within 12 hours after rupture of the membranes, it is induced if the gestation is near term (40 weeks).

When the membranes rupture, the amniotic fluid may be expelled in large amounts. Danger of the umbilical cord washing out with the fluid (prolapse of umbilical cord) results. Because of this threat and the possibility of infection, the woman is advised to notify her physician/nurse-midwife and proceed to the hospital. In some instances, the fluid is expelled in small amounts and may be confused with episodes of urinary incontinence associated with urinary urgency, coughing, or sneezing. The discharge may be checked to ascertain its source and to determine further action. After assessment the woman may feel embarrassed to find out she is having urinary incontinence. (See Chapter 15 for assessment techniques.)

Sudden Burst of Energy

Some women report a sudden surge of energy approximately 24–48 hours before labor. They may do their spring housecleaning or rearrange all the furniture (referred to as the "nesting instinct"). The nurse in prenatal teaching should warn prospective mothers not to overexert themselves at this time so that they will not be excessively tired at labor's onset. The cause of the energy spurt is unknown.

Other Signs

Additional premonitory signs may include a loss of weight of 1–3 pounds resulting from fluid loss and electrolyte shifts produced by changes in estrogen and progesterone levels, and increased backache and sacroiliac pressure from the influence of relaxin hormone on the pelvic joints. Some women report diarrhea, indigestion, or nausea and vomiting just prior to the onset of labor. The causes are unknown.

Differences Between True and False Labor

The contractions of true labor produce progressive dilatation and effacement of the cervix. They occur regularly and increase in frequency, duration, and intensity. The discomfort of true labor contractions usually starts in the back and radiates around to the abdomen, and is not relieved by ambulation (in fact, it may intensify).

The contractions of false labor do not produce *progressive* cervical effacement and dilatation. Classically, they are irregular and do not increase in frequency, duration, and intensity. The contractions may be perceived as a hardening or "balling up" without discomfort, or discomfort may occur mainly in the lower abdomen and groin. The discomfort may be relieved by ambulation and/or sedation (Table 14–1).

It is helpful for the woman to know the characteristics of true labor contractions as well as the premonitory signs of ensuing labor. However, sometimes the only way to accurately differentiate between true and false labor is by assessment of dilatation. The woman must feel free to come in for accurate assessment of labor and should never be allowed to feel foolish if it is false labor. The nurse must reassure the woman that false labor is common and that it often cannot be distinguished from true labor except by vaginal examination.

STAGES OF LABOR AND DELIVERY

There are three stages of labor. The first stage begins with the beginning of true labor and ends when the cervix is completely dilated at 10 cm. The second stage begins with complete dilatation and ends with the birth of the infant. The third stage begins with the expulsion of the infant and ends with the delivery of the placenta.

Some clinicians identify a fourth stage of labor. During this stage, which lasts 1–4 hours after delivery of the placenta, the uterus effectively contracts to control bleeding at the placental site (Pritchard and MacDonald, 1980).

Table 14-1 Comparison of True and False Labor

True labor	False labor
Contractions are at regular intervals	Contractions are irregular
Intervals between contractions gradually shorten	Usually no change
Increase in duration and intensity	Usually no change
Discomfort begins in back and radiates around to abdomen	Discomfort is usually in abdomen
Intensity usually increases with walking	Walking has no effect or lessens contractions
Progressive cervical dilatation and effacement	No change

The management of the laboring woman is discussed in Chapter 16.

First Stage

The first stage of labor is divided into the *latent* and the *active* phase. Friedman (1978) has further described and defined the active phase, according to cervical dilatation, as acceleration phase, phase of maximum slope, and deceleration phase. In addition, Friedman developed concepts based on the physiologic objectives of labor, calling them preparatory, dilatational, and pelvic divisions. The preparatory division includes the latent and acceleration phase, the dilatational division includes the phase of maximum slope, and the pelvic division commences with the deceleration phase. Each phase of labor is characterized by physical and psychological changes (Figure 14–16).

LATENT PHASE

The latent phase begins with the onset of regular contractions and is represented by a flat slope of cervical dilatation to about 3–4 cm. As the cervix begins to dilate, it also effaces, although little or no fetal descent is evident. The latent phase averages 8.6 hours but should not exceed 20 hours for nulliparas, and averages 5.3 hours but should not exceed 14 hours in multiparas.

Uterine contractions become established during the latent phase and increase in frequency, duration, and intensity. They may start as mild contractions lasting 15–30 seconds with a frequency of 15–30 minutes and progress to moderate ones lasting 30–40 seconds with a frequency of 5–7 minutes. They average 40 mm Hg during acme from a baseline tonus of 10 mm Hg.

In the early or latent phase of the first stage of labor, contractions are usually mild and the client feels able to cope. She may be relieved that labor has finally started and, while she may be anxious, is able to recognize and express those feelings of anxiety. She is often talkative and smiling and will be eager to talk about herself and answer questions. Excitement is high, and her mate or other support person are often as elated as the client.

ACTIVE PHASE

During the active phase, the cervix dilates from about 3–4 cm to 10 cm (complete dilatation), which marks the end of the first stage. Fetal descent is progressive.

The active period begins with the *acceleration phase* as cervical dilatation changes from a flat slope (as in the latent phase) to an upward curve. The *phase of maximum slope* covers the period of time when cervical dilatation progresses from approximately 3–4 cm to 8 cm. The cervical dilatation should be at least 1.2 cm/hr in nulliparas, and 1.5 cm/hr in multiparas (Friedman, 1978).

The *deceleration phase* is the last part of the active

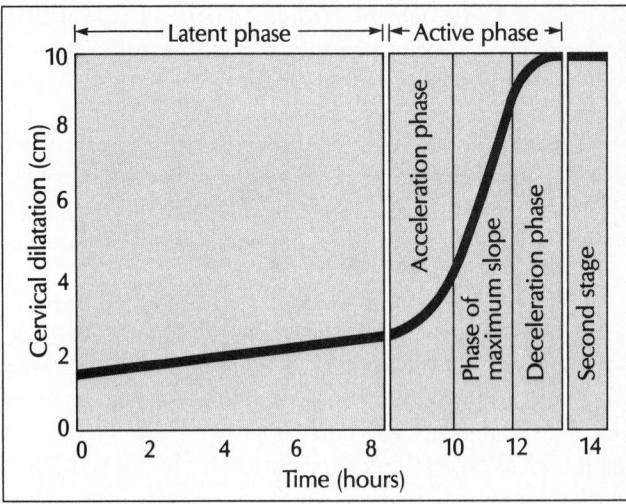

FIGURE 14–16 Composite of the average dilatation curve for nulliparous labor based on analysis of the data derived from the patterns traced by a large, nearly consecutive series of gravidas. The first stage is divided into a relatively flat latent phase and a rapidly progressive active phase. The active phase has three identifiable component parts — an acceleration phase, a linear phase of maximum slope, and a deceleration phase. (From Friedman, E. A. 1978. *Labor: clinical evaluation and management,* 2nd ed. New York: Appleton-Century-Crofts, p. 33, Figure 3.)

phase. The cervical dilatation slows as it progresses from 8–10 cm and the rate of fetal descent increases. The average rate of descent is at least 1 cm/hr in nulliparas, and 2.0 cm/hr in multiparas. The deceleration phase should not be longer than 3 hours for nulliparas and 1 hour for multiparas (Friedman, 1978). The deceleration phase may be referred to as *transition.*

During the active phase, contractions become more frequent, are longer in duration, and increase in intensity. By the end of the active phase, contraction frequency is usually every 2–3 minutes, with a duration averaging 60 seconds. The intensity is moderate or strong.

As the client enters the early active phase, her anxiety tends to increase as she senses the fairly constant intensification of contractions and pain. She begins to fear a loss of control, and may exhibit coping mechanisms to maintain control. A decreased ability to cope may be noted along with a sense of helplessness. Clients who have support persons available, particularly fathers, experience greater satisfaction and less anxiety throughout the birth process than those without these supports (Doering et al., 1980).

When the woman enters the active phase of the first stage, she may demonstrate significant anxiety. She becomes acutely aware of the increasing force and intensity of the contractions. She may become restless, frequently changing position. The most commonly expressed fear at this time is that of abandonment; it becomes crucial that the nurse be available as backup and relief for the support person. By the time the client enters the active phase, she is inner-directed and, often, tired. At the same time the support person may be feeling the need for a break, rest, or walk. The client should be reassured that she will not be left alone and should always be told where her support people are if they leave the room and where her nurse is should the client need her.

The woman may also have fears about tearing open or splitting apart with the force of the contractions (Kopp, 1971). Many clients experience a sensation of pressure so great with the peak of a contraction that it seems to them that their abdomens will burst open with the force. The client should be informed that this is a normal sensation and reassured that such bursting will not happen.

By the time the client reaches the deceleration phase (transition) she will most likely be withdrawn and inner-focused. She may increasingly doubt her ability to cope with her labor. The deceleration or transition phase is associated with increasing apprehension and irritability. The client does not want to be left alone but also does not want anyone to talk to or touch her. However, with the next contraction, she may ask for verbal and physical support. Other characteristics that may accompany this phase are hyperventilation as the woman increases her breathing rate, restlessness, difficulty understanding directions, a sense of bewilderment and anger at the contractions, statements that she "cannot take it anymore," requests for medication, hiccupping, belching, nausea, vomiting, beads of perspiration on upper lip, and increasing rectal pressure.

The woman in this phase is anxious to "get it over with" and is often terrified of being left alone. She may be amnesic and sleep between her now-frequent contractions. Her support persons may start to feel helpless and may turn to the nurse for increased participation as their efforts at alleviating the client's discomfort seem less effective.

As dilatation approaches completion, increased rectal pressure and uncontrollable desire to bear down, increased amount of bloody show, and rupture of membranes may result.

□ *AMNIOTIC MEMBRANES* At the beginning of labor the amniotic membranes bulge through the cervix in the shape of a cone. As labor progresses and dilatation occurs, the membranes assume the shape of a large watch crystal. They may rupture before labor or any time during labor. If the chorion ruptures and the amnion remains intact, the infant may deliver with the amnion covering its head. The child is then said to be born with a *caul*. Rupture of membranes (ROM) generally occurs at the height of an intense contraction with a gush of the fluid out the introitus. If this occurs in transition, then descent of the fetal head will follow.

Second Stage

The second stage of labor (also called the expulsive stage) begins with complete dilatation of the cervix (10 cm) and ends with delivery of the infant. It should be completed within an hour after the cervix becomes fully dilated for primigravidas (multiparas average 15 minutes). Contractions may be 60–90 seconds in duration, are strong in intensity, and have a frequency of 2–3 minutes. Descent of the fetal presenting part continues until it reaches the perineal floor.

As the fetal head descends, the woman has the urge to push because of pressure of the fetal head on the sacral and obturator nerves. As she pushes, intraabdominal pressure is exerted from contraction of the maternal abdominal musculature. As the fetal head continues its descent, the perineum begins to bulge, flatten, and move anteriorly. There may be a further increase in the amount of bloody show. The labia begin to part with each contraction. Between contractions the fetal head appears to recede. With succeeding contractions and maternal pushing effort, the fetal head descends further, and crowning (encircling of the fetal head by introitus) occurs, signifying that delivery is imminent (Danforth, 1982) (Figure 14–17).

The woman may feel a sense of relief that the delivery is near, and that she can now push. Some women feel a sense of control, which comes from being able to now have active involvement. Others (particularly those without childbirth preparation) may become frightened, and tend to fight each contraction and any attempt of others to persuade them to push with contractions. Such behavior may be frightening and disconcerting to her support persons. The client may feel she has lost control and become embarrassed and apologetic. The woman may demonstrate extreme irritability toward the staff or her supporters in an attempt to regain control over external forces against which she feels helpless. Some may feel acute and increasingly severe pain as the perineum distends. Usually, a psychoprophylactically prepared woman feels a sense of relief from the acute pain she felt during the transition phase.

SPONTANEOUS DELIVERY (VERTEX PRESENTATION)

As the head distends the vulva with each contraction, the perineum becomes extremely thin and the anus stretches and protrudes. With assistance from the physician or nurse-midwife, the head is delivered slowly under the symphysis pubis, with the face sliding over the perineum. (See Chapter 16 for medical and nursing interventions to facilitate the delivery process.) After delivery of the head, restitution and external rotation of the head occurs. When the anterior shoulder meets the under side of the symphysis pubis, gentle traction applied to the infant's head aids in delivery. The body then follows.

Delivery of infants in other than vertex presentations is discussed in Chapter 18.

Third Stage

PLACENTAL SEPARATION

After the infant is delivered, the uterus firmly contracts, diminishing its capacity and the surface area of placental attachment. The placenta begins to separate because of this decrease in surface area. As this separation occurs, bleeding results in the formation of a hematoma between the placental tissue and the remaining decidua. This hematoma accelerates the separation process. The membranes are the last to separate. They are peeled off the uterine wall as the placenta extrudes into the vagina.

Signs of placental separation usually appear around 5 minutes after delivery of the infant. These signs are (a) a globular-shaped uterus, (b) a rise of the fundus in the abdomen, (c) a sudden gush or trickle of blood, and (d) further protrusion of the umbilical cord out of the introitus.

PLACENTAL DELIVERY

When the signs of placental separation appear, the woman may bear down to aid in placental expulsion. If this fails and the clinician has ascertained that the fundus is firm, gentle traction may be applied to the cord while pressure is exerted on the fundus. The weight of the placenta as it is guided into the placental pan aids in the removal of the membranes from the uterine wall. Even though a placenta is not considered to be retained until after 30 minutes have elapsed from completion of the second stage of labor, Pritchard and MacDonald (1980) recommend manual removal if the placenta has not separated in 5 minutes after the birth to reduce the blood loss of the third stage. However, the danger of this method is the introduction of pathogens into the uterine cavity.

If the placenta separates from the inside to the outer margins, it is delivered with the fetal or shiny side presenting (Figure 14–18). This is known as the *Schultze mechanism* of placental delivery, or more commonly *shiny Schultze*. If the placenta separates from the outer margins inward, it will roll up and present sideways with the maternal surface delivering first. This is known as the *Duncan method* of placental delivery, and is commonly called *dirty Duncan* because the placental surface is rough-appearing.

Nursing and medical interventions during the third stage of labor are discussed in detail in Chapter 16.

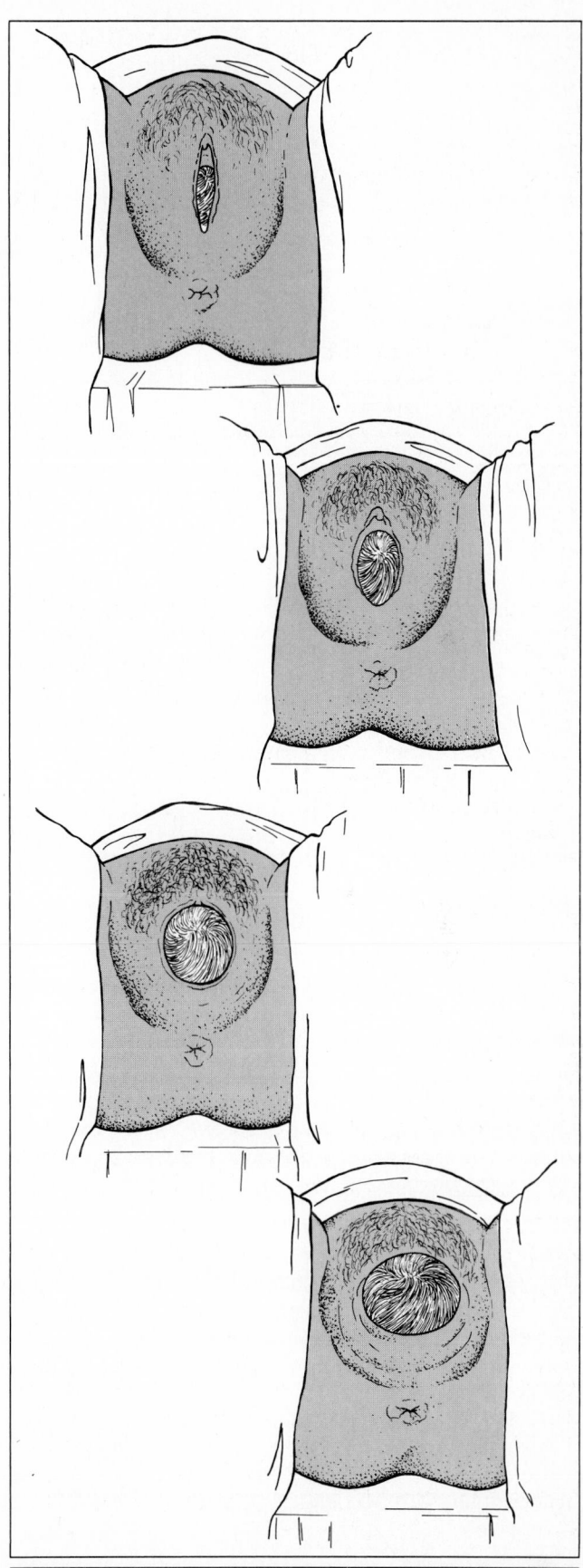

FIGURE 14–17 Progressive dilatation of the introitus during the second stage of labor.

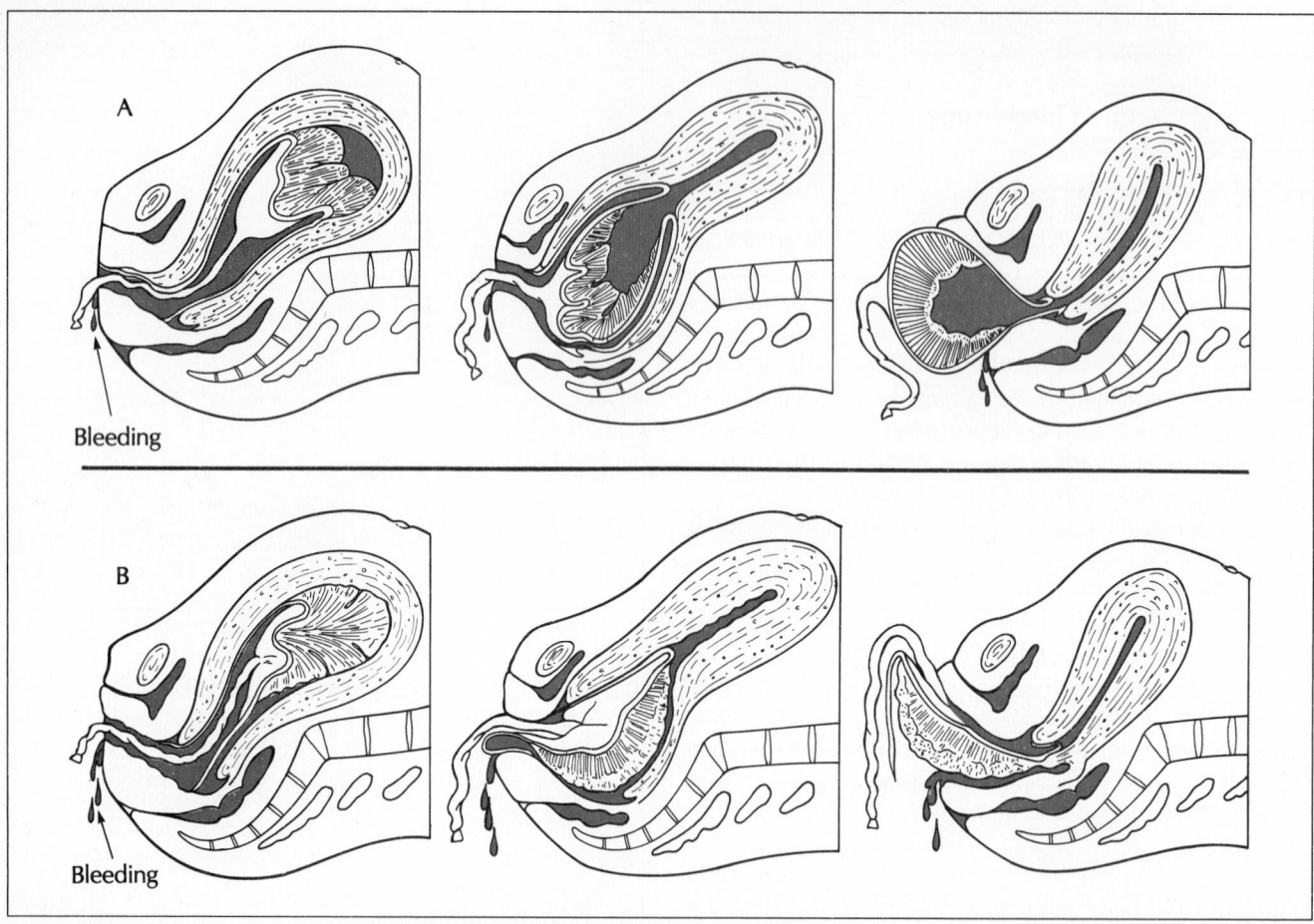

FIGURE 14–18 Placental separation and delivery. **A,** Schultze mechanism. **B,** Duncan mechanism.

Fourth Stage

The period of time from 1–4 hours after delivery, in which physiologic readjustment of the mother's body begins, is designated as the fourth stage of labor.

With the delivery, hemodynamic changes occur. Blood loss at delivery may be up to 500 mL. With this blood loss, and the lifting of the weight of the gravid uterus from surrounding vessels, blood is redistributed into venous beds. This results in a moderate drop in both systolic and diastolic blood pressure, increased pulse pressure, and moderate tachycardia (Cibils, 1981).

The cerebrospinal fluid pressure, which increased during labor, now drops with the delivery of the neonate and rapidly recovers normal values (Cibils, 1981).

The uterus remains contracted and is in the midline of the abdomen. The fundus is usually midway between the symphysis pubis and umbilicus. Its contracted state provides for constriction of the vessels at the placental implantation site. Immediately after delivery of the placenta, the cervix is patulous and thick.

Signs or symptoms of nausea and vomiting usually cease and the woman may be thirsty and hungry. She may experience a shaking chill, which is thought to be associated with the ending of the physical exertion of labor. It is not uncommon for the bladder to be hypotonic due to trauma during the second stage and/or the administration of anesthetics which may decrease sensations. Hypotonic bladder leads to urinary retention. Management of this stage is discussed in Chapter 16.

SUMMARY

The wonderful phenomenon of labor—the process of birth—is a period of transition for the pregnant woman, because it is the climax of her waiting. A competent maternity nurse must understand the physiologic and psychologic changes during normal labor and delivery to enable her to support and intervene appropriately.

References

Aladjem, S., and Brown, A. K. 1974. *Clinical perinatology.* St. Louis: The C. V. Mosby Co.

Aladjem, S. 1980. *Obstetric practice.* St. Louis: The C. V. Mosby Co.

Albright, G. A. 1978. *Anesthesia in obstetrics: maternal, fetal and neonatal aspects.* Menlo Park, Calif.: Addison-Wesley.

Anderson, N. C. July 1978. Physiologic basis of myometrial function. *Semin. Perinatol.* 2:211.

Bruegel, M. A. 1971. Relationships of post-operative anxiety to perceptions of postoperative pain. *Nurs. Res.* 20:26.

Bonica, J. J. 1960. *Mechanisms and pathways of pain in labor.* Chicago: Abbott Laboratories.

Caldwell, W. E., and Moloy, H. C. 1933. Anatomical variations in the female pelvis and their effect on labor with a suggested classification. *Am. J. Obstet. Gynecol.* 26:479.

Cibils, L. A. 1981. *Electronic fetal-neonatal monitoring.* Boston: PSG Inc.

Challis, J. R., and Mitchell, B. F. July 1981. Hormonal control of preterm and term parturition. *Semin. Perinatol.* 5:192.

Chaney, J. A. March/April 1980. Birthing in early America. *J. Nurs. Midwife.* 25:5.

Clark, A. L., and Affonso, D. D. 1979. *Childbearing: a nursing perspective.* Philadelphia: F. A. Davis Co.

Colman, A. D., and Colman, L. L. 1971. *Pregnancy: the psychological experience.* New York: Herder & Herder.

Crandon, A. J. 1978. Maternal anxiety and obstetric complications. *J. Psychosom. Res.* 23:109.

Danforth, D., ed. 1982. *Textbook of obstetrics and gynecology.* 4th ed. Philadelphia: Harper & Row.

Doering, S. G., and Entwisle, D. R. 1975. Preparation during pregnancy and ability to cope with labor and delivery. *Am. J. Orthopsych.* 45:825.

Doering, S. G. et al. March 1980. Modeling the quality of women's birth experience. *J. Health Social Behavior.* 21:12.

Dukes, J. H., and Bowen, J. C. 1976. Fluid and electrolytes: basic concepts and recent developments. *Contemp. OB/Gyn.* 8:173.

Friedman, E. A. 1978. *Labor: clinical evaluation and management.* 2nd ed. New York: Appleton-Century-Crofts.

Greenhill, J. P., and Friedman, E. A. 1974. *Biological principles and modern practice of obstetrics.* Philadelphia: W. B. Saunders Co.

Heggenhougen, H. K. Nov./Dec. 1980. Father and childbirth: an anthropological perspective. *J. Nurs. Midwife.* 25:21.

Humenick, S. S. Summer 1981. Mastery: the key to childbirth satisfaction? a review. *Birth Fam. J.* 8:79.

Huszar, G. July 1981. Biology and biochemistry of myometrial contractility and cervical maturation. *Semin. Perinatol.* 5:216.

Klein, R. P., et al. Fall 1981. A study of father and nurse support during labor. *Birth Fam. J.* 8:161.

Kopp, L. M. 1971. Ordeal or ideal—the second stage of labor. *Am. J. Nurs.* 71:1140.

Liggins, G. C. 1973. Fetal influences on myometrial contractility. *Clin. Obstet. Gynecol.* 16:148.

————. July 1978. Ripening of the cervix. *Semin. Perinatol.* 2:261.

Lockett, C. 1939. Midwives and childbirth among the Navajo. *Plateau (North Arizona Society of Science and Art)* 12:15.

McCaffery, M. 1972. *Nursing management of the patient with pain.* Philadelphia: J. B. Lippincott Co.

McCammon, C. S. 1951. Study of 475 pregnancies in American Indian women. *Am. J. Obstet. Gynecol.* 61:1159.

Melzack, R. 1973. *The puzzle of pain.* New York: Basic Books, Inc.

Mercer, R. A. March/April 1981. A theoretical framework for studying factors that impact on the maternal role. *Nurs. Res.* 30:73.

Newton, N. June 1964. Some aspects of primitive childbirth. *J.A.M.A.* 188:10.

Nurses Association of the American College of Obstetricians and Gynecologists (NAACOG). April 24, 1974. The four Ps. Postgraduate course. Las Vegas, Nevada.

Oxorn, H., 1980. *Human labor and birth.* New York: Appleton-Century-Crofts.

Pritchard, J., and MacDonald, P. C. 1980. *Williams obstetrics.* 15th ed. New York: Appleton-Century-Crofts.

Takahashi, K., and Burd, L. 1980. Initiation of labor. In *Gynecology and obstetrics,* ed. J. J. Sciarri, Philadelphia: Harper & Row.

Varney, H. 1980. *Nurse-midwifery.* Boston: Blackwell Scientific Publications, Inc.

Weekes, A. R., and Flynn, M. J. 1975. Engagement of fetal head in primigravidae and its relationship to duration of gestation and onset of labor. *Br. J. Obstet. Gynecol.* 82:7.

Westbrook, M. T. 1979. Socioeconomic differences in coping with childbearing. *Am. J. Comm. Psychol.* 7:397.

Wolfs, G. M., and van Leeuwen, M. 1979. Electromyographic observations on the human uterus during labor. *Acta Obstet. Gynecol. Scand.* (Suppl.) 90:1.

Additional Readings

Davis, J. A. June 1982. The place of birth. *Arch. Dis. Child.* 57:406.

Fullerton, J. D. T. March/April 1982. Choice of in-hospital or alternative birth environment as related to the concept of control. *J. Nurse Midwifery.* 27:17.

Garfield, R. E., et al. June 1981. Appearance of gap junctions in the myometrium of women during labor. *Am. J. Obstet. Gynecol.* 140:154.

Goodlin, R. C., et al. May 1982. Determinants of maternal temperature during labor. *Am. J. Obstet. Gynecol.* 143:97.

Griffith, S. May/June 1982. Childbearing and the concept of culture. *J. Obstet. Gynecol. Neonatal Nurs.* 11:181.

Huszar, G., et al. Jan. 1982. Biochemistry and pharmacology of the myometrium and labor: regulation at the cellular and molecular levels. *Am. J. Obstet. Gynecol.* 142:225.

Lavery, J. P., et al. July 1982. The effect of labor on the rheologic response of chorioamniotic membranes. *Obstet. Gynecol.* 60:87.

McKay, S. Summer 1982. Maternity care in China: report of a 1982 tour of Chinese medical facilities. *Birth.* 9:105.

Murata, Y. June 1982. Advances on the horizon. *Clin. in Perinatol.* 9:433.

Okita, J. R., et al. Feb. 1982. Initiation of human parturition. *Am. J. Obstet. Gynecol.* 142:432.

Richardson, P. Spring 1982. Significant relationships and their impact on childbearing: a review. *Maternal-Child Nurs. J.* 11:17.

Scott-Palmer, J., et al. 1981. Pain during childbirth and menstruation: a study of locus of control. *J. Psychosom. Res.* 25:151.

■ 15 ■

INTRAPARTAL NURSING ASSESSMENT

■ CHAPTER CONTENTS

MATERNAL ASSESSMENT

    History

    Intrapartal High-Risk Screening

    Intrapartal Physical Assessment

    Assessment of Pelvic Adequacy

    Intrapartal Psychologic Assessment

    Methods of Evaluating Labor Progress

FETAL ASSESSMENT

    Determination of Fetal Position and Presentation

    Evaluation of Fetal Status During Labor

    Fetal Heart Rate Patterns

    Value of Electronic Fetal Monitoring

    Psychologic Reactions to Electronic Monitoring

    Nursing Care and Responsibilities

    Additional Assessment Techniques

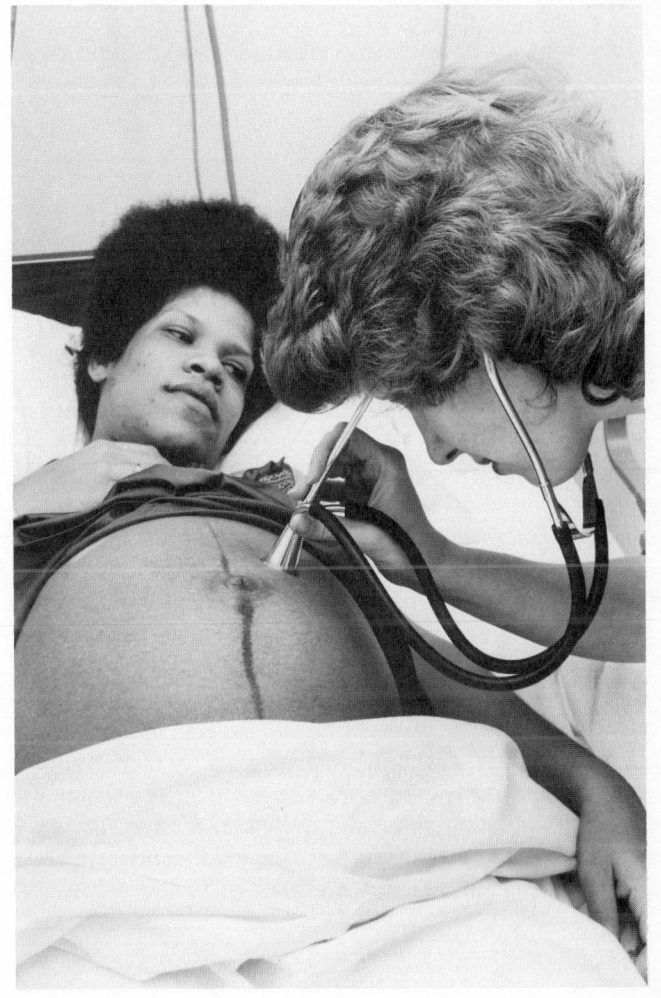

■ OBJECTIVES

- Discuss intrapartal physical and psychologic assessment.

- Identify the methods used to evaluate the progress of labor.

- Describe the procedure for performing Leopold's maneuvers and the information that may be obtained.

- Differentiate the various methods of electronic fetal monitoring giving advantages and disadvantages of each.

- Differentiate baseline and periodic changes and describe the appearance of each and their significance.

- Outline steps to be performed in the systematic evaluation of fetal heart rate tracings.

- Identify nonreassuring fetal heart rate patterns and nursing interventions that should be carried out in the management of fetal distress.

- Discuss the indications for fetal blood sampling and state related pH values.

- Discuss psychologic reactions to electronic fetal monitoring.

The physiologic changes that occur during the process of labor call for many adaptations of the mother and fetus. Assessment becomes more crucial because the changes are rapid and involve two individuals, mother and child, both of whom require frequent reevaluation and intervention.

Most labors are uncomplicated for the woman and fetus. However, the potential for risk is great because of the rapidity of the changes. Thus the nurse must be aware of factors that can change a normal labor to a high-risk one.

The number and efficacy of intrapartal assessment techniques have increased over the years. In the past, nurses assessed the laboring woman and fetus by palpation and auscultation. These methods gave the nurse only intermittent information about the woman and fetus. Uterine contractions were estimated to be mild, moderate, or strong, and judgments varied according to the palpating hand.

In the past, FHTs were auscultated between contractions and usually for only 15 seconds. The 15-second rate was multiplied by 4 for the rate per minute. The nurse who was wise enough to auscultate right after the end of a contraction could hear what is termed *late decelerations*. However, many nurses would listen through the deceleration period and record the best rate. Nurses could also ascertain tachycardia and bradycardia by auscultation.

Assessment of abnormal labor through FHTs is best accomplished by continuous monitoring. With the advent of electronic monitors, this is now possible. Electronic and other techniques to assess maternal and fetal status during labor are discussed in this chapter.

MATERNAL ASSESSMENT

History

A client history may be obtained in an abbreviated format when the woman is admitted to the labor and delivery area. Each agency has its own admission form but similar information is usually obtained. Relevant data include:

- Client's name and age

- Attending physician or certified nurse-midwife

- Personal data: blood type, Rh factor, results of serology testing, prepregnant and present weight, allergies to medications, foods, or substances

- History of previous illness, such as TB, heart disease, diabetes, convulsive disorders, thyroid disorders

- Problems in the prenatal course, for example, elevated blood pressure, bleeding problems, recurrent urinary tract infection

- Pregnancy data: gravida, para, abortions, neonatal deaths

- The method the woman has chosen for infant feeding

- Prenatal education class attendance

- Client requests regarding labor and delivery (for example, no enema, no analgesic or anesthetic, father in delivery room, and so on)

Table 15–1   Intrapartal High-Risk Factors

Factor	Maternal implication	Fetal/neonatal implication
Abnormal presentation	↑ Risk cesarean delivery ↑ Risk prolonged labor	Cesarean delivery Prematurity ↑ Risk congenital abnormality Neonatal physical trauma
Multiple gestation	↑ Uterine distention→ ↑ risk postpartum hemorrhage ↑ Risk premature labor	Low birth weight Prematurity Feto-fetal transfusion
Hydramnios	↑ Discomfort ↑ Distention	↑ Risk esophageal or other high alimentary tract atresias ↑ Risk CNS anomalies (myelocele)
Oligohydramnios	Maternal fear of ``dry birth''	↑ Risk congenital anomalies ↑ Risk renal lesions Postmaturity
Meconium staining of amniotic fluid	↑ Psychologic stress due to fear for fetus	Fetal asphyxia ↑ Risk meconium aspiration ↑ Risk pneumonia due to aspiration of meconium
Premature rupture of membranes (48 hours)	↑ Risk infection (amnionitis)	↑ Risk infection Prematurity
Premature labor	Fear for baby	Prematurity Respiratory distress syndrome Prolonged hospitalization
Induction-tetanic contractions	↑ Risk hypercontractility of uterus ↑ Risk uterine rupture	Prematurity if gestational age not assessed correctly Hypoxia
Abruptio placentae-placenta previa	Hemorrhage ↓ Uterine contractions after delivery	Fetal asphyxia Fetal exsanguination ↑ Perinatal mortality
Prolonged labor	Maternal exhaustion	Fetal asphyxia Intracranial birth injury
Precipitous labor (<3 hr)	Perineal lacerations	Tentorial tears Neonatal asphyxia
Prolapse of umbilical cord	↑ Fear for fetus	Fetal asphyxia
Fetal heart aberrations	↑ Fear for fetus	Tachycardia, acute asphyxic insult, bradycardia Chronic asphyxia Congenital heart disease
Uterine rupture	Hemorrhage Death	Fetal asphyxia Fetal hemorrhage Fetal death

Intrapartal High-Risk Screening

As part of the history and assessment, the nurse should consider intrapartal factors that may develop which would designate the client as high risk. Intrapartal high-risk factors are shown in Table 15–1. The table includes maternal and fetal or neonatal implications. The factors are pre-sented prior to the intrapartal physical assessment guide so that they can be kept in mind during the assessment.

Intrapartal Physical Assessment

A physical examination is included as part of the admission procedure and as part of the ongoing care of the client.

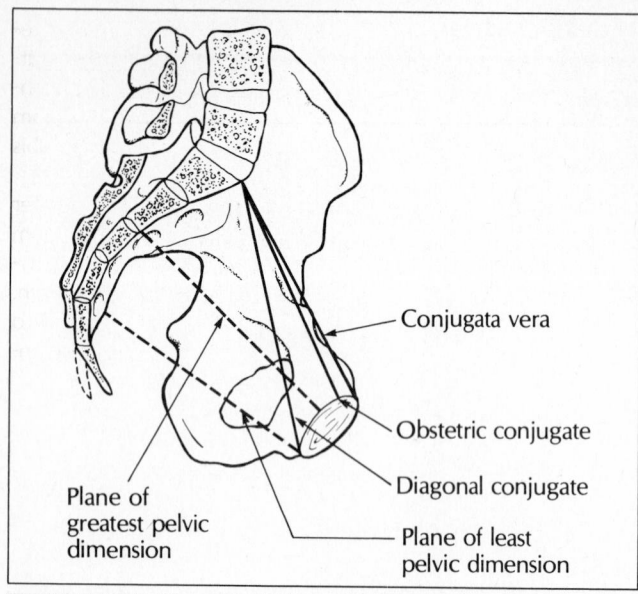

FIGURE 15–1 Anteroposterior diameters of the pelvic inlet and their relationship to the pelvic planes.

The assessment becomes the basis for initiating nursing interventions.

The intrapartal physical assessment is not as complete and thorough as the initial prenatal physical examination (Chapter 10), but it does involve assessment of some body systems and of the actual labor process. The accompanying Intrapartal Physical Assessment Guide provides a framework for the maternity nurse's examination of the laboring woman.

The guide includes assessments performed immediately upon admission and continued as an ongoing assessment. Others may be assessed only once. Critical admission assessments include vital signs, labor status, fetal status, and laboratory and psychologic evaluation. These assessments will be continued throughout the labor process. Assessments that are done only once as part of the admission data, if time permits, include evaluation of weight, breasts, lungs, and heart (in many institutions assessments of breasts, lungs, and heart are omitted).

Assessment of Pelvic Adequacy

The pelvis may be assessed by x-ray pelvimetry at the discretion of the obstetrician but should always be assessed vaginally. Nurses with special preparation may perform the vaginal assessment and interpret pelvimetry findings. This is sometimes referred to as *clinical pelvimetry.*

PELVIC INLET

The important anteroposterior diameters of the inlet for childbearing are the diagonal conjugate, the obstetric conjugate, and the true conjugate, or conjugata vera (Figure 15–1). Others are the transverse (13.5 cm) and the oblique diameters (12.5 cm).

The anteroposterior diameter of the pelvic inlet may be assessed by attempting to reach from the lower border of the symphysis pubis to the sacral promontory with the middle finger. The clinician should determine the length of the finger before attempting this. The diagonal conjugate can then be measured by marking the place where the proximal part of the hand makes contact with the pubis (Figure 15–2). Then the distance is measured (about 12.5 cm). The obstetric conjugate can be estimated by subtracting 1.5 from the length of the diagonal conjugate. At about 11 cm in length, it is the smallest and thus the most important anteroposterior diameter through which the fetus must pass. It is measured by x-ray examination from the sacral promontory to the upper inner point on the symphysis that extends farthest back into the pelvis. The true conjugate extends from the upper border of the symphysis pubis to the sacral promontory. It can be determined by subtracting 1.0 cm from the diagonal conjugate.

PELVIC CAVITY (MIDPELVIS)

Important midpelvic measurements include the plane of greatest dimension, or midplane (12.75 cm), and the planes of least dimension (anteroposterior diameter, 11.5–12.0 cm; posterior sagittal diameter, 4.5–5.0 cm; and transverse diameter, 10.5 cm). These latter diameters can be measured digitally.

Location of the sacrospinous ligament, a firm ridge of tissue, makes location of the ischial spines easier. When this ligament is located, the examiner should run the fingers along it laterally toward the anterior portion of the pelvis. The spines may range from a small firm bump like the knuckle of a finger (termed *not encroaching*) to a very prominent bone. The space between the ischial spines (transverse diameter) is estimated according to the prominence of the spines.

The sacrosciatic notch should admit two fingers. A wide notch means that the sacrum curves back posteriorly, giving the anteroposterior diameter of the midpelvis a greater length. A narrow notch indicates a decreased diameter. The width of the sacrosciatic notch is more accurately evaluated through x-ray examination but can be estimated through vaginal examination.

The length of the sacrospinous ligament is measured by tracing the ligament from its origin on the ischial spines to its insertion on the sacrum. It is usually 4 cm or two to three finger breadths long.

The capacity of the cavity can be assessed by sweeping the fingers down the side walls bilaterally to evaluate the shape of the pelvic side walls—whether convergent, divergent, or straight. The curvature, inclination, and hollowness of the sacrum help indicate the capacity of the posterior pelvis. It is estimated digitally by palpating the sacrococcygeal junction and by inching up toward the

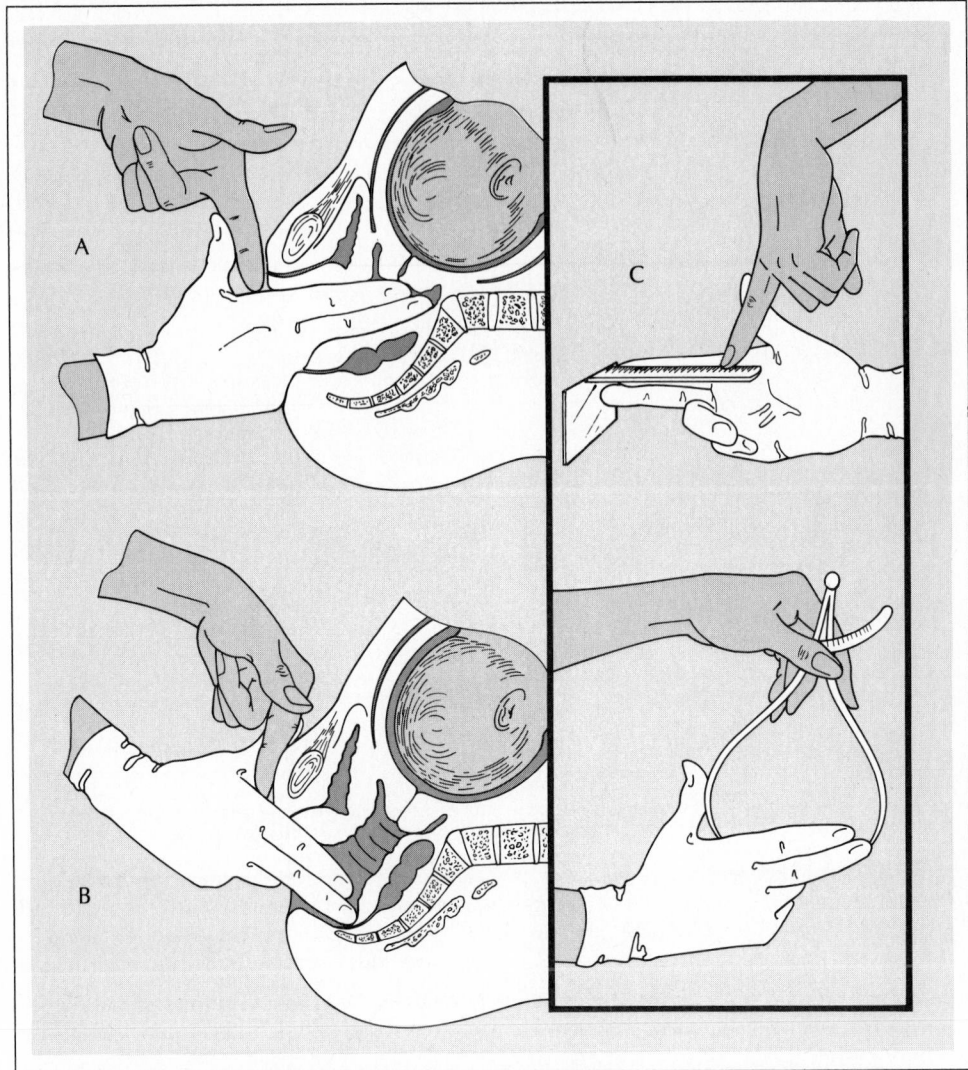

FIGURE 15-2 Manual measurement of inlet, midpelvis, and outlet. **A,** Estimation of diagonal conjugate, which extends from lower border of symphysis pubis to sacral promontory. **B,** Estimation of anteroposterior diameter of the outlet, which extends from the lower border of the symphysis pubis to the tip of the sacrum. **C,** Methods that may be used to check manual estimation of anteroposterior measurements.

promontory. The examiner then estimates the hollowness of the sacrum, which is normally hollow.

If the lumbar curve changes, it can increase or decrease the pelvic inclination and influence the progress of labor, because the fetus has to adapt itself to a curved path as well as to the different diameters of the true pelvis.

PELVIC OUTLET

The anatomic anteroposterior diameter of pelvic outlet, which is normally 9.5 cm, may be measured digitally (Figure 15-3, p. 433). The mobility of the coccyx is determined by pressing down on it with forefinger and middle finger during the initial vaginal exam. An immobile coccyx can decrease the diameter of the outlet. The obstetric anteroposterior diameter of the outlet is normally 11.5 cm.

The transverse diameter of the outlet is measured by placing the fist between the ischial tuberosities. Another method of measurement is to use the Thom's pelvimeter. The transverse diameter normally measures 8 cm.

The suprapubic angle is estimated by palpating the bony structure externally. It should be 85°–90°. The suprapubic angle is estimated by placing two fingers side by side at the border of the symphysis (Figure 15-4, p. 434). It is probably reduced if the examiner cannot separate his or her fingers.

The length and shape of the pubic rami affect the transverse diameter of the outlet. The pubic ramus is expected to be short and concave inward, as opposed to straight and long.

The height and inclination of the symphysis pubis are measured and the contour of the pubic arch is estimated. Excessively long or angulated bone structure shortens the diameter of the obstetric conjugate. Height can be deter-

(Text continues on p. 432.)

INTRAPARTAL PHYSICAL ASSESSMENT GUIDE: FIRST STAGE OF LABOR

Assess	Normal findings	Alterations and possible causes of alterations*	Nursing responses to data base†
Vital signs			
Blood pressure	90–140/60–90 or no more than 15–20 mm rise over baseline BP during early pregnancy	High blood pressure (essential hypertension, preeclampsia, renal disease, apprehension or anxiety) Low blood pressure (supine hypotension)	Evaluate history of preexisting disorders and check for presence of other signs of preeclampsia Turn woman to her side, and recheck blood pressure Do not assess during contractions. Implement measures to decrease anxiety and then reassess
Pulse	60–90 beats/min	Increased pulse rate (excitement or anxiety, cardiac disorders)	Evaluate cause. Reassess to see if rate continues. Report to physician
Respirations	16–24/min (or pulse rate divided by 4)	Marked tachypnea (respiratory disease) Hyperventilation (anxiety)	Assess between contractions. If marked tachypnea continues, assess for signs of respiratory disease Encourage slow breaths if client is hyperventilating
Temperature	36.2–37.6C (98F–99.6F)	Elevated temperature (infection, dehydration)	Assess for other signs of infection or dehydration
Weight	15–30 lb greater than prepregnant weight	Weight gain > 30 lb (fluid retention, obesity, large infant, hypertension of pregnancy)	Assess for signs of edema
Breasts	Slightly firm	Mass in any area of breasts (cysts, neoplasms)	Withhold hormones that prevent lactation from women who have breast masses or a history of problems or clients who plan to breast-feed
Lungs	Normal breath sounds (see irregular breath sounds, Procedure 10–1)	Rales, rhonchi, friction rub (infection)	Reassess; refer to physician
Heart	Normal heart sounds (see Procedure 10–3); grade II/VI systolic ejection murmur is normally found in pregnant women due to extra blood volume passing through heart valves	Murmurs	Refer to physician
Fundus	At 40 weeks' gestation, located just below xyphoid process	Uterine size not compatible with estimated delivery time (SGA, polyhydramnios, multiple pregnancy)	Reevaluate history regarding pregnancy dating. Refer to physician for additional assessment

* Possible causes of alterations are placed in parentheses.
† This column provides guidelines for further assessment and initial nursing interventions.

INTRAPARTAL PHYSICAL ASSESSMENT GUIDE Cont'd

Assess	Normal findings	Alterations and possible causes of alterations*	Nursing responses to data base†
Edema	Slight amount of dependent edema	Pitting edema of face, legs, abdomen (preeclampsia)	Check deep tendon reflexes for hyperactivity, check for clonus; refer to physician
Hydration	Normal skin turgor (see Prenatal Initial Physical Assessment Guide, Chapter 10)	Poor skin turgor (dehydration)	Assess skin turgor; refer to physician for deviations
Perineum	Tissues smooth, pink color (see Prenatal Initial Physical Assessment Guide, Chapter 10)	Varicose veins of vulva	Exercise care while doing a perineal prep. Note on client record need for follow-up in postpartal period. Reassess after delivery
	Clear mucus	Profuse, purulent drainage	Suspect gonorrhea. Report to physician. Initiate care to newborn's eyes. Notify neonatal nursing staff and pediatrician
	Presence of small amount of bloody show which gradually increases with further cervical dilatation	Hemorrhage	Assess BP and pulse, pallor, diaphoresis; report any marked changes
			(Note: Gaping of vagina and/or anus and bulging of perineum are suggestive signs of second stage of labor)
Energy status	Sufficient energy to complete the work of labor	Exhaustion, acetone in urine (deficiency in metabolism of glucose and/or fat, decreasing uterine activity in long labor)	Provide clear liquid with glucose content or hard candy in early labor. IV with dextrose in late labor. Dipstick urine. Assess quality of contractions. Refer to physician
Pelvic adequacy			
Inlet	Diagonal conjugate, 12.5 cm Obstetric conjugate, 11 cm True conjugate, 11.5 cm	Inadequate measurements	Determine fetal presentation, lie, and position. Inform physician if cephalopelvic disproportion is suspected
Cavity	Midplane, 12.45 cm Anteroposterior, 11.5–12 cm Posterior sagittal, 4.5–5 cm Transverse, 10.5 cm	Narrowed measurements	Assess engagement and fetal descent
Outlet	Bituberous width, 8 cm Mobile coccyx height <6 cm	Contractures, immobile coccyx	May need to explain and prepare client for a pelvimetry
Symphysis pubis	Mobile coccyx, height 6 cm Inclination: 85°–90°		May need to explain and prepare client for cesarean delivery

* Possible causes of alterations are placed in parentheses.
† This column provides guidelines for further assessment and initial nursing interventions.

INTRAPARTAL PHYSICAL ASSESSMENT GUIDE Cont'd

Assess	Normal findings	Alterations and possible causes of alterations*	Nursing responses to data base†
Labor status			
Uterine contractions	Regular pattern (Table 15-2 shows normal characteristics during first stage)	Failure to establish a regular pattern, prolonged latent phase Hypertonicity Hypotonicity	Evaluate whether client is in true labor. Ambulate if in early labor Evaluate client status and contractile pattern
Cervical dilatation	Progressive cervical dilatation from size of fingertip to 10 cm (Table 15-2 and Figures 15-5 and 15-6)	Rigidity of cervix (frequent cervical infections, scar tissue, failure of presenting part to descend)	Evaluate contractions, fetal engagement, position, and cervical dilatation. Inform client of progress
Cervical effacement	Progressive thinning of cervix (see Figure 15-5)	Failure to efface (rigidity of cervix, failure of presenting part to engage). Cervical edema (pushing effort by woman before cervix is fully dilated and effaced, trapped cervix)	Evaluate contractions, fetal engagement, and position Notify physician/nurse-midwife if cervix is becoming edematous. Work with client to prevent pushing until cervix completely dilated
Fetal descent	Progressive descent of fetal presenting part from station −5 to +4 (see Figure 15-8)	Failure of descent (abnormal fetal position or presentation, a macrosomic fetus, inadequate pelvic measurement)	Evaluate fetal position, presentation, and size Evaluate maternal pelvic measurements
Membranes	May rupture before or during labor	Rupture of membranes more than 12-24 hours before initiation of labor	Assess for ruptured membranes using Nitrazine test tape before doing vaginal exam Instruct clients with ruptured membranes to remain on bed rest, if presenting part is not engaged Keep vaginal exams to a minimum to prevent infection

	Findings on Nitrazine test tape:
	  Probably intact membranes
	    yellow pH 5.0
	    olive pH 5.5
	    olive green pH 6.0
	  Probably ruptured membranes
	    blue-green pH 6.5
	    blue-gray pH 7.0
	    deep blue pH 7.5
		False-positive results may be obtained if large amount of bloody show is present or if previous vaginal examination has been done using lubricant	Assess fluid for consistency, amount, odor. Assess FHR frequently. Assess fluid at regular intervals for presence of meconium staining

	Amniotic fluid clear, no odor	Greenish amniotic fluid (fetal distress)	Assess FHR. Do vaginal exam to evaluate for prolapsed cord. Apply fetal monitor for continuous data. Report to physician.

* Possible causes of alterations are placed in parentheses.

† This column provides guidelines for further assessment and initial nursing interventions.

INTRAPARTAL PHYSICAL ASSESSMENT GUIDE Cont'd

Assess	Normal findings	Alterations and possible causes of alterations*	Nursing responses to data base†
		Strong odor (amnionitis)	Take client's temperature and report to physician
Fetal status			
FHR	120–160 beats/min	<120 or >160 beats/min (fetal distress); abnormal patterns on fetal monitor: decreased variability, late decelerations, variable decelerations (p. 454)	Initiate interventions based on particular FHR pattern (p. 451)
Presentation	Cephalic, 97% Breech, 3%	Face or brow presentation	Report to physician. After presentation is confirmed as face or brow, client may be prepared for cesarean delivery
Assessment methods 1. Visualization of abdomen (p. 441) 2. Leopold's maneuvers (p. 441) 3. Vaginal examination (Procedure 15–1)		Transverse lie	Report to physician Prepare client for cesarean delivery
Position	LOA most common (Figure 15–9)	Persistent occipital-posterior position; transverse arrest	Carefully monitor maternal and fetal status
Activity	Fetal movement	Hyperactivity (may precede fetal hypoxia)	Carefully evaluate FHR. May apply fetal monitor.
		Complete lack of movement (fetal distress or fetal demise)	Carefully evaluate FHR. May apply fetal monitor
Laboratory evaluation			
Hematologic tests			
Hemoglobin	12–16 g/dL	<12 g (anemia, hemorrhage)	Evaluate woman for problems due to decreased oxygen-carrying capacity caused by lowered hemoglobin
CBC			
Hematocrit	38%–47%	Presence of infection or blood dyscrasias	Evaluate for other signs of infection or for petechia, bruising, or unusual bleeding
RBC	4.2–5.4 million/μL		
WBC	4,500–11,000/μL		
WBC differential			
Neutrophils	56%		
Bands	3%		
Eosinophils	2.7%		
Basophils	0.3%		
Lymphocytes	34%		
Monocytes	4%		
Serologic testing			
STS or VDRL test	Nonreactive	Positive reactive (see Chapter 10, Initial Prenatal Physical Assessment Guide)	For reactive test, notify newborn nursery and pediatrician

* Possible causes of alterations are placed in parentheses.
† This column provides guidelines for further assessment and initial nursing interventions.

INTRAPARTAL PHYSICAL ASSESSMENT GUIDE Cont'd

Assess	Normal findings	Alterations and possible causes of alterations*	Nursing responses to data base†
Urinalysis			
Glucose	Negative	Glycosuria (low renal threshold for glucose, diabetes mellitus)	Assess blood glucose. Test urine for ketones. Ketonuria and glycosuria require further assessment of blood sugars.‡
Ketones	Negative	Ketonuria (starvation ketosis)	
Proteins	Negative	Proteinuria (urine specimen contaminated with vaginal secretions, fever, kidney disease); proteinuria of 2+ or greater found in uncontaminated urine may be a sign of ensuing preeclampsia	Instruct client in collection technique. Incidence of contamination from vaginal discharge is common.
Red blood cells	Negative	Blood in urine (calculi, cystitis, glomerulonephritis, neoplasm)	Assess collection technique
White blood cells	Negative	Presence of white blood cells (infection in genitourinary tract)	Assess for signs of urinary tract infection
Casts	None	Presence of casts (nephrotic syndrome)	

* Possible causes of alterations are placed in parentheses.
† This column provides guidelines for further assessment and initial nursing interventions.
‡ Glycosuria should not be discounted. The presence of glycosuria necessitates follow-up.

mined by placing the index finger of the gloved hand up to the superior border of the symphysis. The examiner should measure the length of the first phalanx of the index finger (normally about 2.5 cm). Inclination may be determined by externally placing one finger on the top of the symphysis while the internal finger palpates the internal margin. An imaginary line is drawn between the fingers and the angle is estimated.

Table 15–2   Correlation of Cervical Dilatation and Uterine Activity During Phases of First Stage

	Latent phase	Active phase	Transition
Dilatation	0–3 cm	4–7 cm	7–10 cm
Contractions			
Frequency	Every 15–30 min	Every 3–5 min	Every 2–3 min
Duration	15–30 sec	30–60 sec	45–90 sec
Intensity	Mild	Moderate	Strong

A posterior inclination with the lower border of the pubis slanting inward decreases the anteroposterior diameter. The anteroposterior sagittal diameter is the most significant diameter of the outlet, as it is the shortest diameter through which the infant must pass. Estimating the contour of the pubic arch provides information on the width of the angle at which these bones come together. The pubic arch has obstetric importance; if it is narrow the infant's head may be pushed backward toward the coccyx, making extension of the head difficult. This condition is called *outlet dystocia*, and forceps (outlet) delivery is required. (See Chapter 19 for further discussion.) Fetal head injury or deep perineal laceration may occur.

In questionable situations some pelvic measurements should be determined by means other than digital methods, for example, by ultrasound or x-ray pelvimetry. X-ray pelvimetry reveals the shape and type of pelvis, the true internal measurements, the fetopelvic relationship, and the estimated fetal size (Oxorn, 1980).

X-ray evaluation is recommended in the following cases:

• During most dysfunctional labors, particularly if the physician is considering using oxytocin

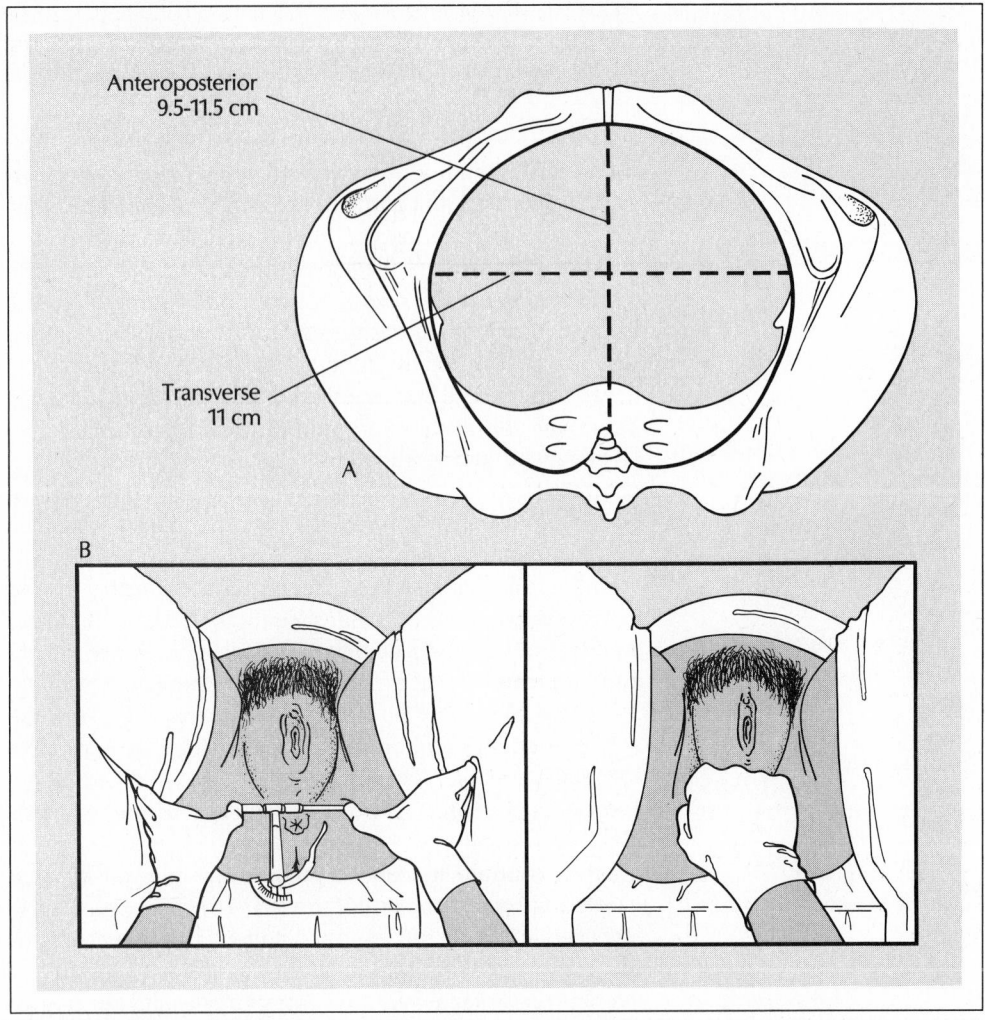

FIGURE 15–3 A, Diameters of the pelvic outlet. **B,** Measurement of the transverse diameter of the outlet. *Left,* use of Thom's pelvimeter; *right,* use of closed fist.

Anteroposterior
9.5–11.5 cm

Transverse
11 cm

A

B

- In women with abnormal clinical measurements if there is a question about pelvic adequacy after vaginal examination has been performed during early labor
- During a trial labor for contracted pelvis before a decision to administer oxytocin or to perform cesarean delivery is made
- In breech positions during labor at term or whenever an abnormal fetal position is suspected
- In clients who have had disease or injury involving the bony pelvis or hips
- In clients who have had difficult labors or large infants previously
- Whenever there is suggestive evidence of disproportion, such as a floating head during early labor in a primigravida*

*From Willson, J. R., and Carrington, E. 1979. *Obstetrics and gynecology.* 6th ed. St. Louis: The C. V. Mosby Co., p. 468.

Intrapartal Psychologic Assessment

Assessment of the laboring woman's psychologic status is an important part of the total assessment. The woman brings to labor previous ideas, knowledge, and fears. Assessment of her psychologic status enables the nurse to meet her informational and support needs. The nurse can support the woman and her partner, or in the absence of a partner, the nurse may become the support person. See the accompanying Intrapartal Psychologic Assessment Guide.

Methods of Evaluating Labor Progress

CONTRACTION ASSESSMENT

Uterine contractions may be assessed by palpation and/or continuous electronic monitoring.

Palpation. Contractions are assessed for frequency, duration, and intensity by placing one hand on the uterine

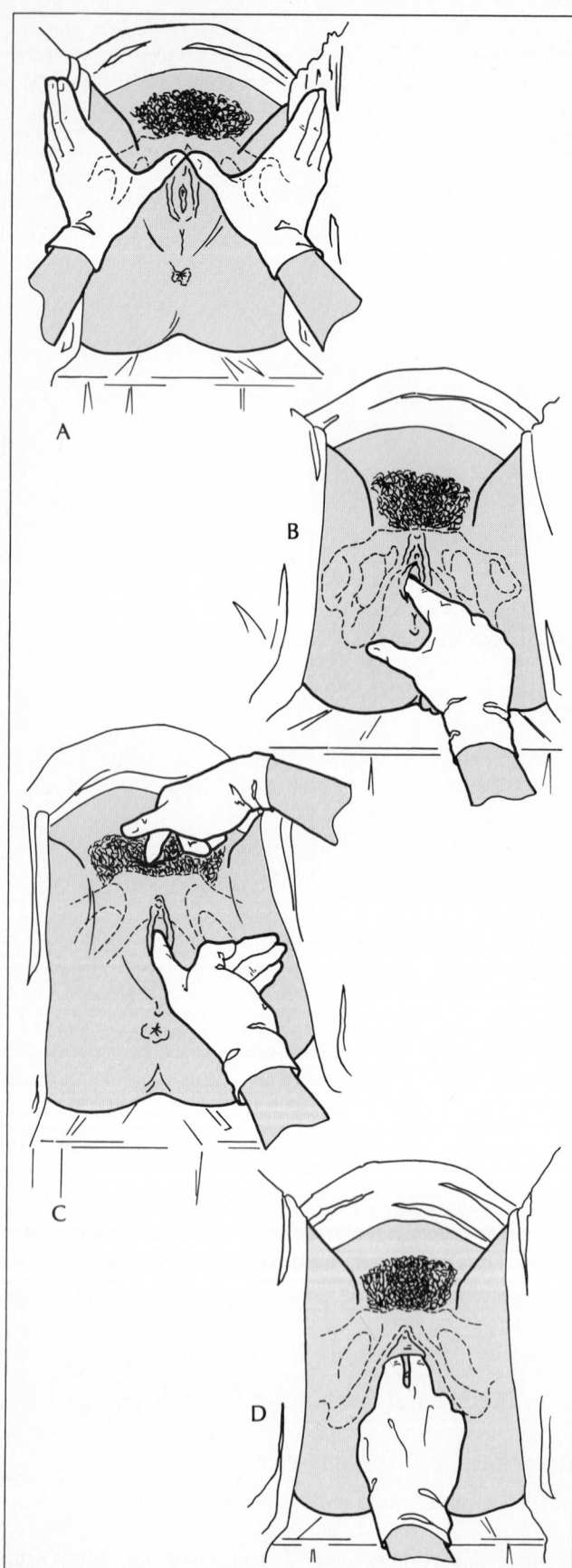

FIGURE 15–4 Evaluation of outlet. **A,** Estimation of subpubic angle. **B,** Estimation of length of pubic ramus. **C,** Estimation of depth and inclination of pubis. **D,** Estimation of contour of suprapubic angle.

fundus. The hand is kept relatively still as excessive movement may stimulate contractions or may cause discomfort. To determine duration the time is noted when tensing of the fundus is first felt (beginning of contraction) and again as relaxation occurs (end of contraction). During the acme of the contraction, intensity can be evaluated by estimating the indentability of the fundus. At least three successive contractions should be assessed to provide enough data to determine the contraction pattern. Since frequency is determined by noting the time from the beginning of one contraction to the beginning of the next, if contractions began at 7:00, 7:04, and 7:08, the frequency would be every 4 minutes.

Electronic monitoring. Electronic monitoring of the uterine contractions provides continuous data. In many agencies, it may be routinely done for all high-risk clients and all clients who are having oxytocin-induced labor.

External monitoring with tocodynamometer. An indirect method for monitoring uterine activity is by use of the tocodynamometer, which contains a flexible disk that responds to pressure. This disk is strapped to the woman's abdomen directly over the fundus, which is the area of greatest contractility, and it records the external tension exerted by contractions (Figure 15–10). The pressure is amplified and recorded on graph paper. The advantages to this method are that (a) it may be used prior to rupture of membranes antepartally and intrapartally and (b) it provides a continuous recording of the duration and frequency of contractions. The major disadvantage is that this method does not record the magnitude or intensity of a contraction. Another disadvantage to this method is that sometimes the strap bothers the woman, because it requires frequent readjustment as she changes position.

Internal monitoring of uterine pressure during labor is discussed on page p. 446.

CERVICAL ASSESSMENT

Cervical dilatation and effacement are evaluated directly by sterile vaginal examination (see Procedure 15–1, Intrapartal Vaginal Examination, p. 436). The vaginal examination can also provide information regarding membrane status, fetal position, and station of the presenting part.

EVALUATION OF LABOR PROGRESS

□ **FRIEDMAN GRAPH** Evaluation of the intensity, frequency, and duration of contractions does not present the entire birthing picture. Nurses can document labor progress objectively by using the Friedman graph, which evaluates uterine activity, cervical dilatation, and fetal descent.

(Text continues on p. 440.)

INTRAPARTAL PSYCHOLOGIC ASSESSMENT GUIDE

Assess	Normal findings	Alterations and possible causes of alterations*	Nursing response to data base[†]
Support system Physical intimacy of mother–father (or mother–support relationship)	Care-taking activities such as soothing conversation, touching	Limited physical contact or continual clinging together (may reflect normal pattern for this couple or their attempt to cope with this situation)	Encourage care-taking activities that appear to comfort the woman; encourage support to the woman; if support is limited, the nurse may take a more active role
	Support person stays in close proximity	Maintaining a distance from woman for prolonged periods (may be normal pattern for this couple or may indicate strained relationship, or anxiety with labor situation)	Encourage support person to stay close (if this seems appropriate)
Relationship of mother–father (or support person)	Involved interaction	Limited interaction (may reflect normal interaction pattern or strained relationship)	Support interactions; if interaction is limited, the nurse may provide more information and support
Anxiety	Some anxiety and apprehension is within normal limits	Rapid breathing, nervous tremors, frowning, grimacing or clenching of teeth, thrashing movements, crying, increased pulse and blood pressure (anxiety, apprehension)	Provide support and encouragement
Preparation for childbirth	Client has some information regarding process of normal labor and delivery	Insufficient information	Add to present information base
	Client has breathing and/or relaxation techniques to use during labor	No breathing or relaxation techniques (insufficient information)	Support breathing and relaxation techniques that client is using; provide information if needed
Response to labor	Latent phase: relaxed, excited, anxious for labor to be well established Active phase: becomes more intense, begins to tire Transitional phase: feels tired, may feel unable to cope, needs frequent coaching to maintain breathing patterns	Inability to cope with contractions (fear, anxiety, lack of education)	Provide support and encouragement; establish trusting relationship Provide support, coaching if needed
Coping mechanisms	Ability to cope with labor through utilization of support system, breathing, relaxation techniques	Marked anxiety, apprehension (insufficient coping mechanisms)	Support coping mechanisms if they are working for the client; provide information, and support if client is exhibiting anxiety or needs additional alternatives to present coping methods

* Possible causes of alterations are placed in parentheses.
[†] This column provides guidelines for further assessment and initial nursing interventions.

Procedure 15–1   Intrapartal Vaginal Examination

Objective	Nursing action	Rationale
Prepare client	Explain procedure, indications for carrying out procedure, and what information is being obtained Position client in lithotomy position with thighs flexed and abducted; instruct her to put heels of feet together Drape so that only the perineum is exposed Encourage her to relax her muscles and legs during procedure	Explanation of procedure decreases anxiety and increases relaxation of woman during procedure Prevents contamination of area during examination and provides for visualization of external labor progress signs Provides as much privacy as possible
Assemble and prepare equipment	Have following equipment easily accessible: • Sterile disposable gloves • Lubricant • Nitrazine tape test prior to first examination	Examination is facilitated and can be done quickly
Use aseptic technique during examination	If leakage of fluid has been noted or if client reports leakage of fluid, use Nitrazine test tape before doing vaginal exam; a single sterile glove may be used; the test tape is placed just inside the vagina (see p. 430 for Nitrazine results)	Nitrazine test tape registers a change in pH if amniotic fluid is present (unless a lubricant has already been used)
	Put on both gloves; using thumb and forefinger of left hand, spread labia widely, insert well-lubricated second and index fingers of right hand into vagina until they touch the cervix, without touching surrounding vulvar structures; in some labor and delivery units only one sterile glove is used for a vaginal exam	Avoid contaminating hand by contact with anus; positioning of hand with wrist straight and elbow tilted downward allows fingertips to point toward umbilicus and find cervix
Determine status of fetal membranes	Palpate for movable bulging sac through the cervix; observe for expression of amniotic fluid during exam; perform Nitrazine paper test first	If bag of waters is intact, it will feel like a bulge; if the membranes have ruptured, amniotic fluid may be expressed while performing the vaginal examination; determination of membrane integrity is important, as membranes can act as dilating wedge during labor and safeguard against ascending infection to fetus in utero
Determine status of labor progress during and after contractions	Carry out vaginal examination during and between contractions	Examination between contractions reveals degree of cervical dilatation and effacement when presenting part is not under pressure of contractions During a contraction, examination reveals information about the maximum amount of thinning, dilatation, and descent possible under influence of contractions
Identify degree of: 1. Cervical dilatation	Palpate for opening or what appears as a depression in the cervix with a surrounding circular ridge of tissue	Estimation of the diameter of the depression identifies degree of dilatation

Procedure 15–1   Intrapartal Vaginal Examination Cont'd

Objective	Nursing action	Rationale
	Estimate diameter of cervical opening in centimeters (0–10 cm) (Figures 15–5 and 15–6)	One finger is approximately 1.5–2 cm cervical dilatation
2. Cervical effacement	Palpate the thickness of the surrounding circular ridge of tissue; estimate degree of thinning in percentages	Degree of thinning determines the amount of lower uterine segment that has been taken up into the fundal area

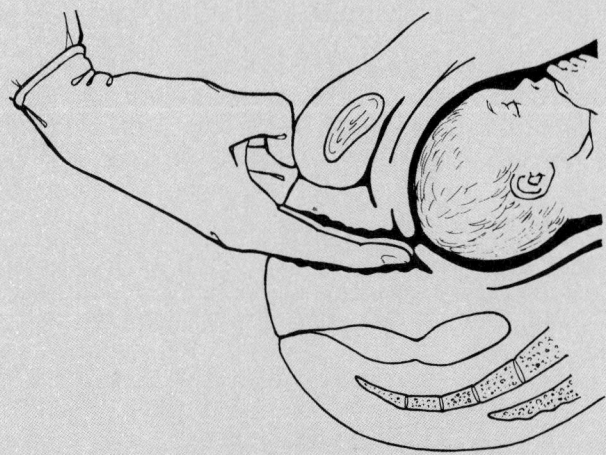

FIGURE 15–5 Vaginal palpation of cervical dilatation, effacement, amniotic membranes, and presenting part.

FIGURE 15–6 Cervical dilatation measurement tool.

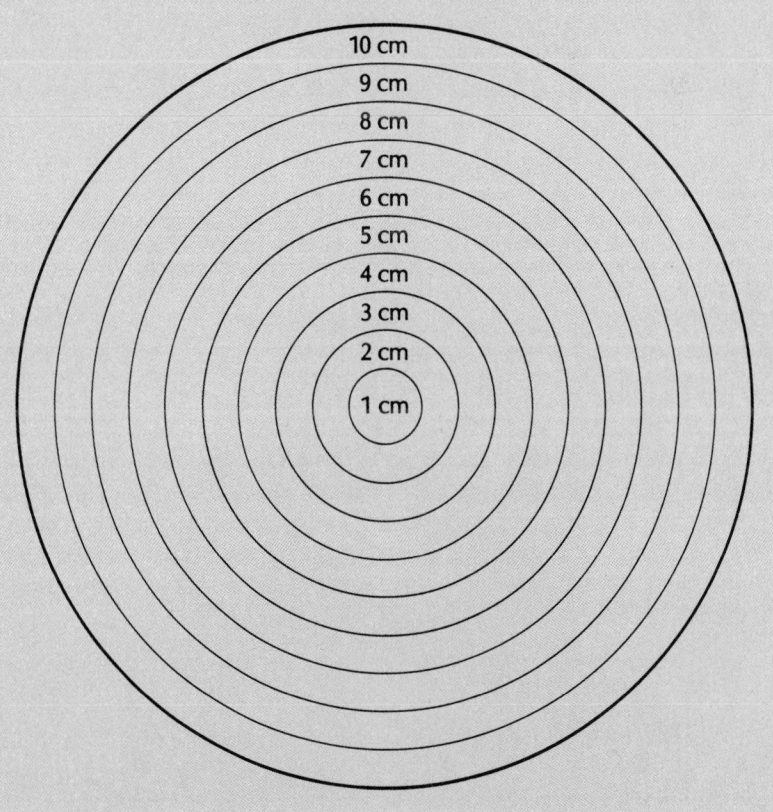

Procedure 15–1   Intrapartal Vaginal Examination Cont'd

Objective	Nursing action	Rationale
Determine presentation and position of presenting part	As cervix opens, palpate for presenting part and identify its relationship to the maternal pelvis (Figures 15–7 to 15–9) • In vertex presentation, palpate for sutures and fontanelles and relate the occiput to one of the four quadrants of the maternal pelvis • In face presentation, palpate facial features • In breech presentation, palpate buttocks and sacrum	Presenting part is easier to palpate through a dilated cervix, and differentiation of landmarks is easier Position is determined by relationship of occiput to quadrants of maternal pelvis Position is determined by relationship of sacrum to quadrants of maternal pelvis

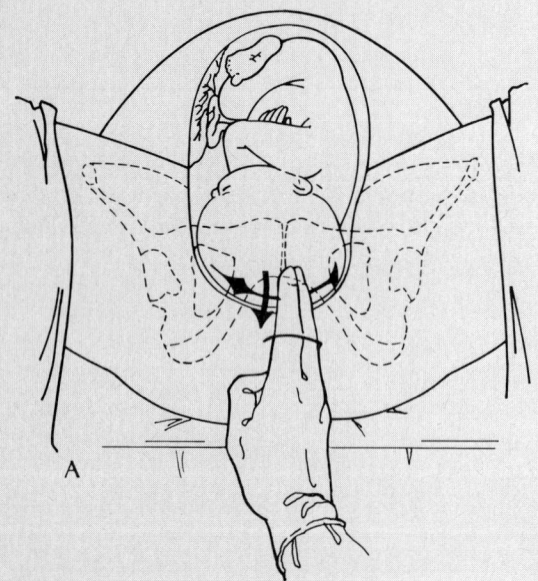

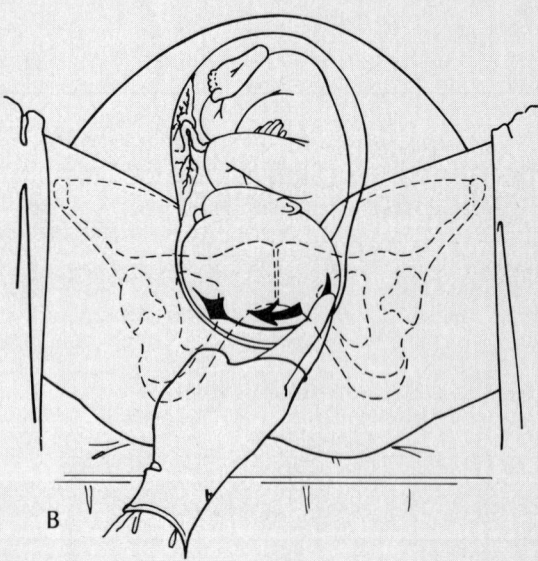

FIGURE 15–7 Assessment of fetal position and station. **A,** Palpate sagittal suture and assess station. **B,** Identify posterior fontanelle. **C,** Identify anterior fontanelle.

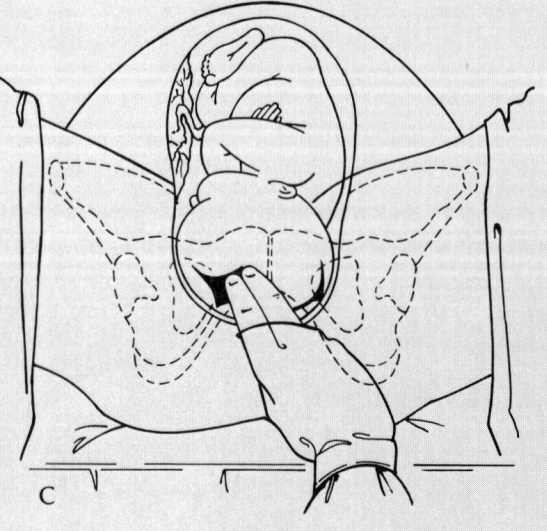

Procedure 15–1   Intrapartal Vaginal Examination Cont'd

Objective	Nursing action	Rationale

High head	Flexion and descent	Engaged	Deeply engaged	On pelvic floor and rotating	Rotation into A.P.
Pelvic brim					

Membranes intact	Sagittal suture in transverse diameter	Cervix dilating Head descending		Occiput rotating forward	Rim of cervix felt

FIGURE 15–8 *Top,* the fetal head progressing through the pelvis. *Bottom,* the changes that the nurse will detect on palpation of the occiput through the cervix while doing a vaginal examination. (From Myles, M. F. 1975. *Textbook for midwives.* Edinburgh: Churchill Livingstone, p. 246.)

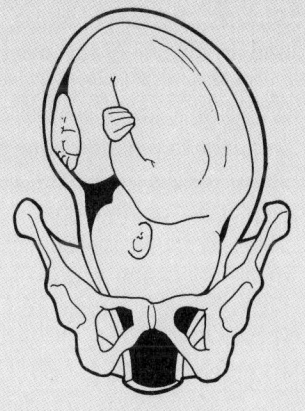

FIGURE 15–9 Palpation of presenting part in LOA position. Posterior fontanelle is in upper right.

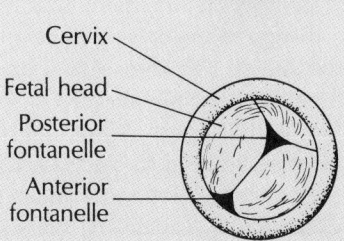

Cervix
Fetal head
Posterior fontanelle
Anterior fontanelle

Procedure 15-1   Intrapartal Vaginal Examination Cont'd

Objective	Nursing action	Rationale
Determine station and whether engagement has occurred	Locate lowest portion of presenting part, then palpate the side walls of the pelvis for the ischial spines; estimate in centimeters the relationship of the lowest portion of presenting part to the ischial spines (see Figures 15-7 and 15-8)	Identification of station provides information as to degree of descent and some information about adequacy of maternal pelvis Engagement occurs when the presenting part is at or below the level of the ischial spines
Inform client about progress in labor	Discuss with client findings of the vaginal examination and correlate them to her progress in labor	Assists the client in identifying progress and reinforces need for frequency of procedure Information is reassuring and supportive for client and family
Identify possible complications	Observe for bleeding (more than bloody show)	Bleeding is a contraindication for vaginal examination, because it might indicate placenta previa
	Observe for prolapse of umbilical cord into vaginal canal, or for evidence of fetal distress (which might suggest prolapse)	Indicates prolapsed cord

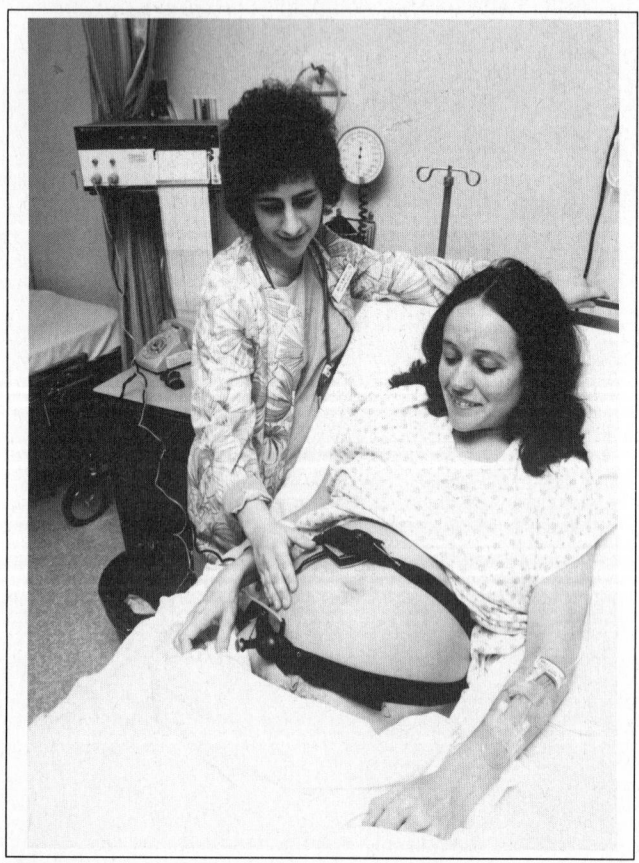

FIGURE 15-10 Client with external monitor applied.

To use the Friedman graph, one needs special graph paper and skill in determining cervical dilatation and fetal descent. The numbers at the bottom of the graph in Figure 15-11 are hours of labor from 1 to 16. Vertically, at the left, cervical dilatation is measured from 0 to 10 cm. The vertical line on the right indicates fetal station in centimeters, from −5 to +5 (Friedman, 1970). When one plots cervical dilatation and descent on the basic graph, a characteristic pattern emerges: an S curve represents dilatation and an inverse S curve represents descent.

When the laboring woman enters the hospital, she is asked at what time regular contractions began. A sterile vaginal examination determines cervical dilatation and the station of the presenting part of the fetus. This information is plotted on the graph. To determine the appropriate point to begin plotting data, the nurse must know how many hours the woman has been having regular contractions. In the example shown in Figure 15-11, on admission the cervix was dilated 2-3 cm after 4 hours of labor, and the station was −1. Later examinations are noted on the graph. When the client was in the eleventh hour of labor, the graph indicates that cervical dilatation was 8 cm and the station was zero. At 14 hours of labor, the graph indicates spontaneous delivery.

When utilizing the Friedman graph, the following method may be used to calculate the progress in centimeters of cervical dilatation per hour (or maximum slope of active dilatation). Divide the difference between two consecutive observations by the intervening time interval to obtain the value for the slope in centimeters per hour. For example, in the case illustrated in Figure 15–11, at 9½ hours of labor, the cervix is dilated 5 cm. At 11 hours of labor, the cervix is dilated 8 cm. The difference between these two observations is 3 cm. Divide the difference by the intervening time interval, which is 1½ hours: 3 cm ÷ 1½ = 2 cm/hr.

Evaluation of the woman's labor progress through use of the Friedman graph will assist in identifying normal or abnormal labor patterns.

FETAL ASSESSMENT

Determination of Fetal Position and Presentation

Fetal position is determined by a combination of factors, using various senses and technology. Assessment of the maternal abdomen for fetal position may be done by inspection, palpation, auscultation of fetal heart tones, determination of presenting part by vaginal examination and utilization of ultrasound.

INSPECTION

The nurse should observe the client's abdomen for size and shape. Attention should be given to the lie of the fetus by assessing whether the shape of the uterus projects up and down (longitudinal lie) or left and right, which indicates a transverse lie.

PALPATION

Use of Leopold's maneuvers provides a systematic evaluation of the maternal abdomen. Frequent practice with these maneuvers increases the proficiency of the examiner in determining fetal position by palpation. Difficulty may be encountered in performing these techniques on an obese client or on a client who has excessive amniotic fluid (hydramnios).

Leopold's maneuvers should be performed before listening to the fetal heart tones (FHTs). Auscultation of the FHTs is facilitated by locating the fetal back, because the sound of the heart tones is carried with more intensity through the fetal back and the uterine wall; it becomes diffused as it passes through the amniotic fluid.

Care should be taken to ensure the client's comfort during Leopold's maneuvers. The client should have recently emptied her bladder and should lie on her back with her abdomen uncovered. To aid in relaxation of the abdominal wall, the shoulders should be raised slightly on a pillow and the knees drawn up a little. The procedure should be completed between contractions. The examiner's hands should be warm (Figure 15–12).

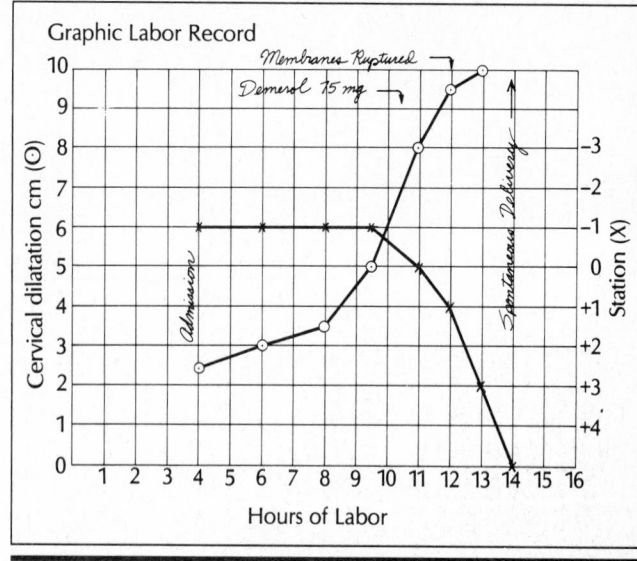

FIGURE 15–11 Example of charting labor progress on a Friedman graph. (Modified from Friedman, E. A. July 1970. An objective method of evaluating labor. *Hospital Practice.* 5 (7): 87.)

Consideration should be given to several questions while inspecting and palpating the maternal abdomen:

• Is the fetal lie longitudinal or transverse?
• What is in the fundus? Am I feeling buttocks or head?
• Where is the fetal back?
• Where are the small parts or extremities?
• What is in the inlet? Does it confirm what I found in the fundus?
• Is the presenting part engaged or floating?
• Is there fetal movement?
• How large is the fetus?
• Is there one fetus or more than one?
• Is fundal height proportionate to the estimated gestational age?

First maneuver. Facing the client, palpate the upper abdomen with both hands (Figure 15–12). What is the shape, size, consistency, and mobility of the form that is found? The fetal head is firm, hard, and round and moves independently of the trunk. The breech feels softer and symmetrical and has small bony prominences; it moves with the trunk.

Second maneuver. After ascertaining whether the head or the buttocks occupies the fundus, the nurse tries to determine the location of the fetal back and notes whether it is on the right or left side of the maternal abdomen. Still facing the client, the nurse palpates the abdomen with deep but gentle pressure, using her palms (Figure 15–12). The right hand should be steady while the left

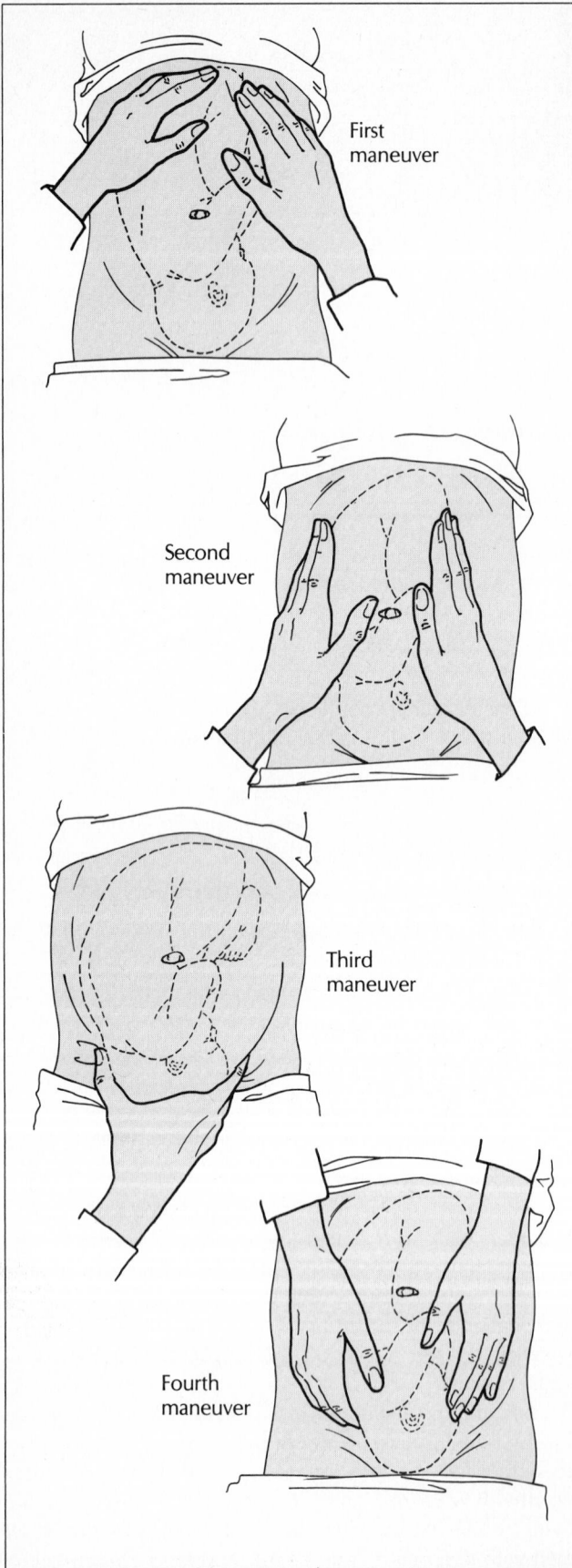

First maneuver

Second maneuver

Third maneuver

Fourth maneuver

FIGURE 15–12 Leopold's maneuvers for determination of fetal position and presentation.

hand explores the right side of the uterus. The maneuver is then repeated, probing with the right hand and steadying the uterus with the left hand. The fetal back should feel firm and smooth and should connect what was found in the fundus with a mass in the inlet. Once the back is located, the nurse validates the finding by palpating the fetal extremities (small knobs and protrusions) on the opposite uterine wall.

Third maneuver. Next the nurse should determine what fetal part is lying over the inlet by gently grasping the lower portion of the abdomen just above the symphysis pubis with the thumb and fingers of the right hand (Figure 15–12). This maneuver yields the opposite information from what was found in the fundus and validates the presenting part. If the head is presenting and is not engaged, it may be gently pushed back and forth.

Fourth maneuver. For this portion of the examination, the nurse faces the client's feet and attempts to locate the cephalic prominence or brow. Location of this landmark assists in assessing the descent of the presenting part into the pelvis. The fingers of both hands are moved gently down the sides of the uterus toward the pubis (Figure 15–12). The cephalic prominence (brow) is located on the side where there is greatest resistance to the descent of the fingers toward the pubis. It is located on the opposite side from the fetal back if the head is well flexed. However, when the fetal head is extended, the occiput is the first cephalic prominence felt, and it is located on the same side as the back. Therefore, when completing the fourth maneuver, if the first cephalic prominence palpated is on the same side as the back, the head is not flexed. If the first prominence found is opposite the back, the head is well flexed and a normal labor can be anticipated (Oxorn, 1980).

VAGINAL EXAMINATION AND ULTRASOUND

Additional assessment techniques to determine fetal position and presentation include vaginal examination and use of ultrasound if necessary. During the vaginal examination, the presenting part may be palpated if the cervix is dilated, and information about the position of the fetus and the degree of flexion of its head (in cephalic presentations) can be obtained.

X-ray examination is not usually advised to determine normal fetal presentations because of the potential risks to the fetus. For obese women or women in whom abdominal palpation is difficult, x-ray evaluation assists in identifying possible problem situations because x-ray film gives accurate information concerning position, presentation, flexion, and degree of descent of the fetal part.

Evaluation of Fetal Status During Labor

AUSCULTATION OF FHTS

The fetoscope has been the primary means of assessing the status of the fetus in utero since its development in 1917. It is still the primary means of antepartal surveillance, and in many hospitals it is the primary means for "normal" clients in labor.

The fetoscope is a subjective means of assessment, but used adjunctively with other means it can be most helpful. Instead of haphazardly searching over the client's abdomen for FHTs, the nurse should first perform Leopold's maneuvers. Not only will this indicate the general location for listening for FHTs, but it will aid in determining whether there are multiple fetuses and whether the fetus is in a transverse lie or breech presentation.

In cephalic presentation, FHTs are best heard in the lower quadrant of the maternal abdomen. In breech presentation they are heard at or above the level of the maternal umbilicus. In transverse lie, FHTs may be found just above or just below the umbilicus. As the presenting part descends and rotates through the pelvic structure during labor, the location of the FHTs tends to descend and move toward the midline. Clients may give a clue when they feel fetal kicking on one side of the abdomen. The fetal back is usually found on the opposite side of the kicking. FHTs may be heard most clearly at the fetal back (Figure 15–13).

The maternal abdomen is first palpated to determine fetal position. The FHTs are counted for 15 seconds and multiplied by 4 to obtain the number of beats per minute. The nurse should occasionally listen for one full minute through a contraction to detect any abnormal heart rate especially if tachycardia, bradycardia, or irregular beats are heard. It is advantageous to manipulate the fetus while listening for FHTs to determine whether the heart rate accelerates with fetal movement. This is thought to be a sign of fetal well-being. If the heart rate slows without any apparent movement, the nurse should listen for one full minute. The FHR should be auscultated every 30–60 minutes in early labor, every 15 minutes during active labor, and every 5 minutes during second stage of labor. If decelerations are noted, the client should be electronically monitored to rule out abnormalities in fetal heart rate.

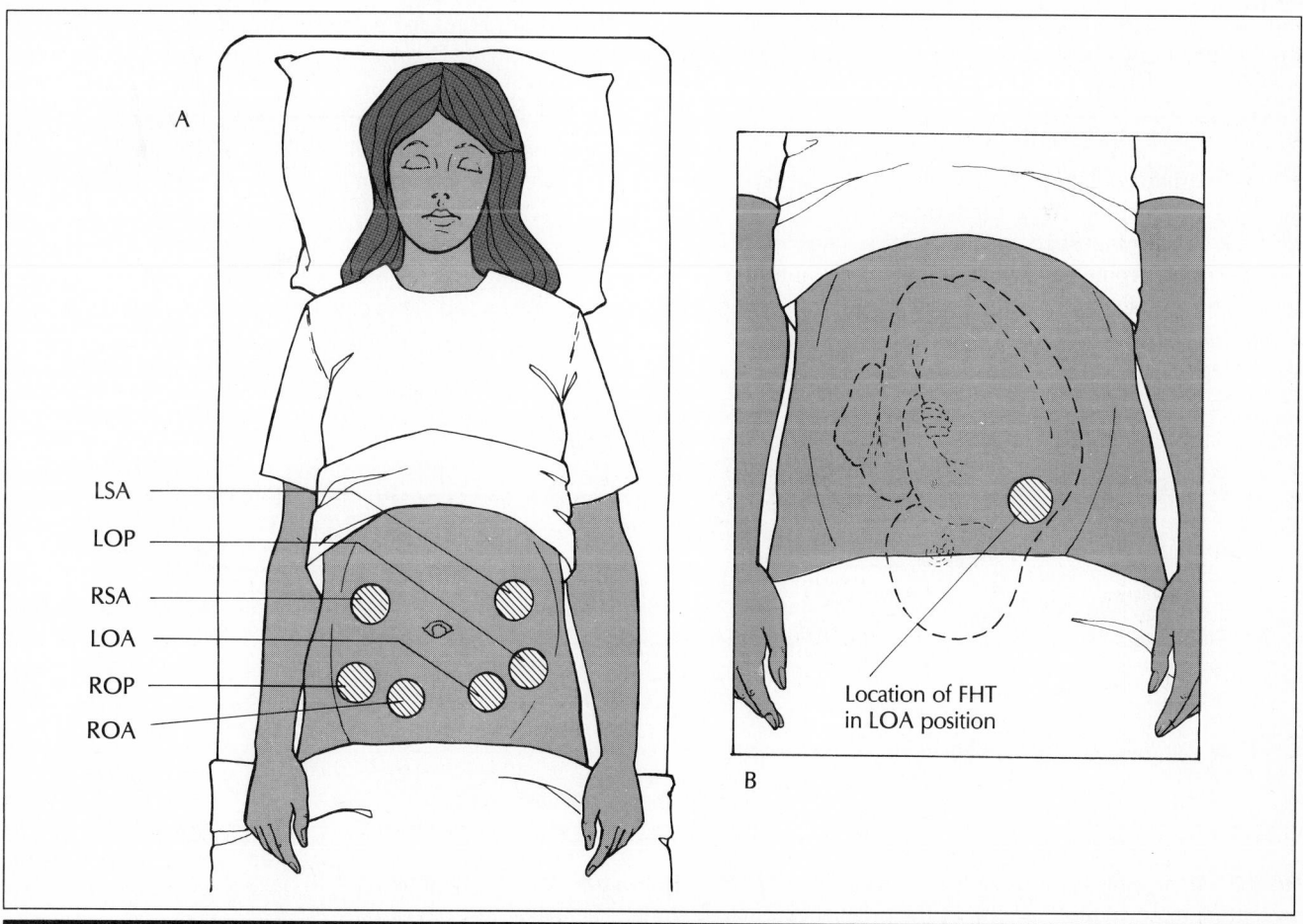

LSA
LOP
RSA
LOA
ROP
ROA

Location of FHT in LOA position

FIGURE 15–13 Location of FHR in relation to the more commonly seen fetal positions.

Only gross changes in FHR may be detected with the fetoscope; therefore subtle changes that occur in response to contractions may not be heard. It is difficult to hear the FHR during the peak of a contraction; by waiting until 30 seconds afterward (as was the custom for many years), abnormal responses are not detected, thereby missing early signs of fetal distress. Two significant problems with auscultation are (a) the inherent error that occurs in counting, and (b) the difference noted between instantaneous and average FHR. Instantaneous fetal monitoring is based on measurement of the time interval between successive FHR beats. Figure 15–14 demonstrates the differences noted when comparing instantaneous rates with those that are averaged by auscultation. One can see that accelerations and variable decelerations, which would be undetected by auscultatory means, are noted through use of fetal monitoring.

Periodic auscultation of the fetal heart with a fetoscope was thought to be an adequate method of assessment of fetal status during labor until about 1970, when electronic monitoring techniques were found to provide a more complete assessment of intrauterine fetal status. The electronic method enables the nurse or physician to be more assured of fetal well-being or to detect fetal distress by observing the continuous fetal heart rate and the periodic changes that occur during and after contractions of the uterus, and allows one to intervene if necessary.

ELECTRONIC MONITORING

There are two methods of assessing FHR during labor: indirect (external) and direct (internal). The indirect method may be accomplished by means of a fetoscope, fetal electrocardiography, and Doppler ultrasound (intermittent or continuous). Direct monitoring utilizes a scalp electrode and provides for continuous flow of FHR information.

Uterine contractions may be monitored externally by means of a tocodynamometer or internally through use of an intrauterine pressure catheter.

□ *INDICATIONS FOR ELECTRONIC FETAL MONITORING* Any client with previous history of medical or obstetric problems that might affect the status of labor or the health of the fetus should be monitored by continuous electronic fetal monitoring. Clients whose labor is being augmented or induced with oxytocin need close observation by this means because of the possibility of hyperstimulation. Some physicians advocate monitoring only those clients considered to be at risk or high risk, while many authorities in the field of perinatology feel the procedure is mandatory for all clients in labor. All abnormal fetal heart rates should be monitored.

Electronic monitoring provides information that is not readily available through auscultatory means. Advantages and disadvantages of methods of monitoring are outlined in Table 15–3.

□ *EXTERNAL MONITORING*
Fetal electrocardiography. Beat-to-beat FHR may be assessed by external fetal electrocardiographic monitoring. Three electrodes, placed appropriately on the maternal abdomen, pick up electrical fetal impulses of the QRS complex and are recorded by the monitor. Unfortunately, maternal QRS and P waves are also transmitted; therefore data from this method are more difficult to interpret. The maternal impulses are larger signals, however, and can usually be identified. This method is difficult to use because client movement may interfere with the electrical impulses transmitted and completely obliterate the fetal electrocardiographic signal. Another problem arises when maternal and fetal signals occur simultaneously and the tracing becomes difficult to interpret. Yet another difficulty results when maternal and fetal rates are similar or one is

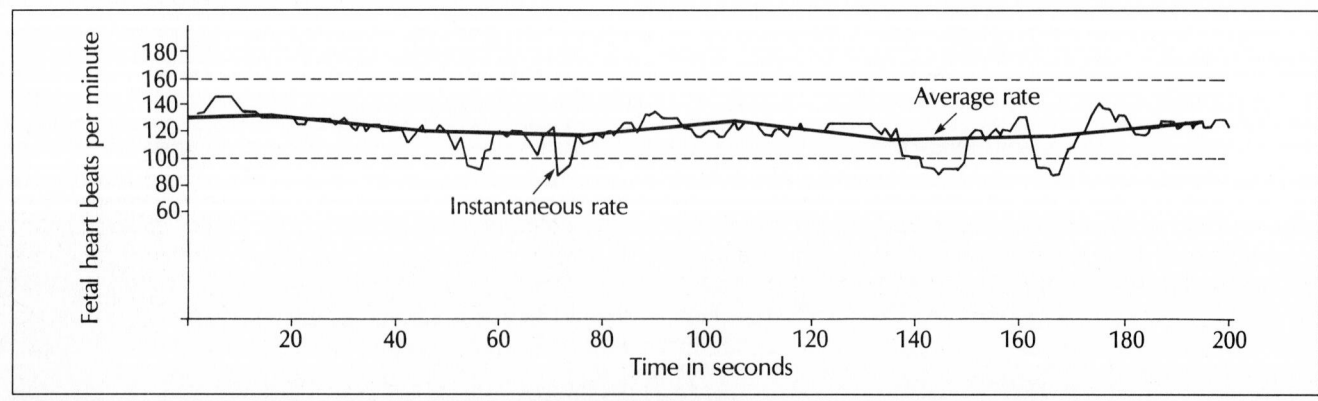

FIGURE 15–14 Comparison of instantaneous and average fetal heart rates. The average FHR illustrates a more constant rate, while the instantaneous rate illustrates the normal variation of the fetal heart rate. (From Hon, E. 1976. *An introduction to fetal heart rate monitoring.* 2nd ed. Los Angeles: University of Southern California School of Medicine, p. 9.)

Table 15-3 Advantages and Disadvantages of Various Monitoring Methods

Method	Advantages	Disadvantages
Fetoscope	Inexpensive Noninvasive Easy to use Easily transported	Intermittent information Gives no information regarding contractions Cannot assess variability or periodic changes in FHR Cannot hear FHT until 18 weeks' gestation
Doppler (pocket-sized ultrasound)	Inexpensive Noninvasive Easily transported Can hear FHT as early as 10–12 weeks	Gives no information regarding contractions Cannot assess variability Cannot assess variability or periodic changes in FHR unless severe Intermittent information
External monitoring	Continous information Noninvasive Uses: antepartal testing, and during labor Gives permanent record Can grossly assess contractions Can assess decreased variability and periodic changes Useful for client teaching	Equipment is expensive Subject to artifact Cannot assess variability unless decreased and then must confirm with internal monitoring Cannot quantitate contractions Belts uncomfortable to some clients Subject to double and half counting
Internal monitoring	Accurate, continuous information Gives fetal ECG Not subject to artifact Client more mobile in bed Can quantitate contractions Can assess variability Accurate assessment of periodic changes Useful for client teaching	Equipment is expensive Need personnel to interpret Requires 2–3 cm dilated cervix and ruptured membranes Requires knowledgeable personnel to apply equipment Client confined to bed or chair Slight increased risk of maternal or fetal infection Subject to double and half counting Invasive
Telemetry	Accurate, continuous information Client can be mobile (out of bed or in hall) Same other advantages of internal monitoring	Equipment is expensive Invasive Not widely used at the present time Same disadvantages of internal monitoring

half or double the other. In these cases of uniform patterns, it becomes impossible to measure true R-R intervals (Freeman and Garite, 1981). Electrocardiography has been utilized for antepartal stress testing, but has not been as successful as Doppler ultrasound for the client in labor.

Ultrasound. Ultrasound utilizes the Doppler principle. FHR may be monitored intermittently by use of a pocket-sized device or continuously by use of a fetal monitor. The external fetal monitor offers the advantage of a continuous flow of information, which is also visualized on an oscilloscope and recorded on graph paper. Prior to the placement of the ultrasonic transducer on the maternal abdomen, FHTs should be auscultated to determine the area of clearest sounds for optimal clarity of the tracing. A water-soluble gel is applied to the crystals of the underside of the transducer to aid in conduction of fetal heart sounds.

Continuous sound waves, which are emitted from the transmitting crystals, bounce off the beating heart or blood as it moves through the vessels in the cardiovascular system. The signals are then reflected back to receiving crystals and displayed on the oscilloscope and graph paper.

The transducer inadvertently may be directed toward a pulsating maternal vessel. In this case, the maternal signal will be noted rather than that of the fetal circulation. To avoid this, maternal pulse should be checked while using ultrasound.

Contractions can be monitored externally by use of a tocodynamometer (or "toco"), which is a pressure device

FIGURE 15–15 Tocodynamometer and ultrasonic technique to monitor maternal and fetal status during labor. (From Hon, E. 1972. *An introduction to fetal heart monitoring.* Los Angeles: University of California School of Medicine, p. 65.)

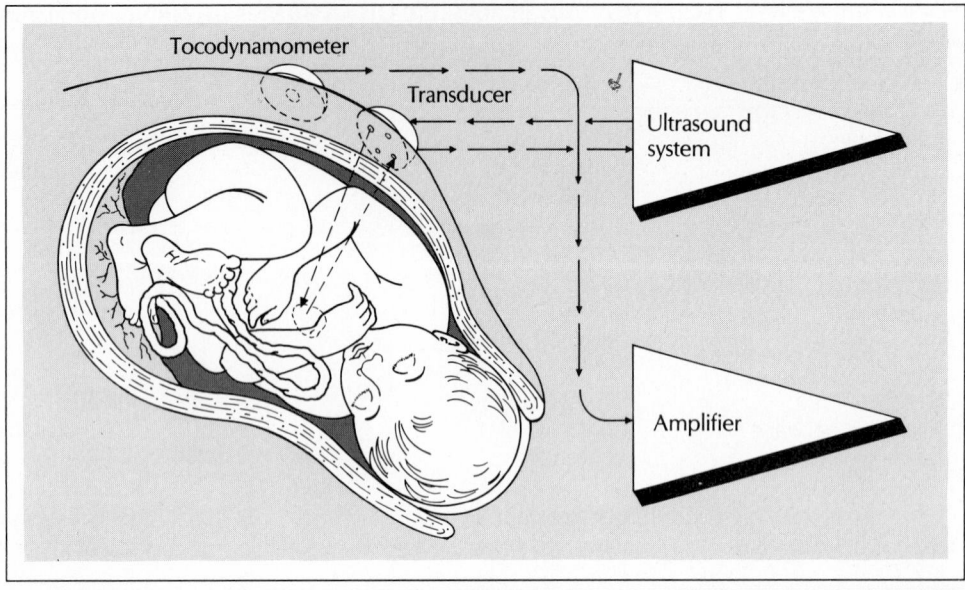

(Figure 15–15). As the uterine muscles contract, pressure is exerted against a projection on the underside of the "toco," which has been applied to the maternal abdomen by means of an elastic belt. The pressure creates an electrical signal that is transmitted to the monitor and recorded on the graph paper. Uterine contractions can be assessed for frequency but not for intensity. The intensity (which is displayed on the graph paper) is affected by how tightly the belt is applied around the maternal abdomen. When the belt is tight enough, one should be able to note the beginning of contractions on the monitor prior to or at the time the client begins to feel them. The client's most frequent complaint regarding fetal monitoring is the tightness of the belts, but if reasons are explained and belts frequently adjusted, most clients are more understanding and do not object.

Some disadvantages of external monitoring have been noted. In the case of a very obese client, an active fetus, or polyhydramnios, the FHR may be difficult to monitor by external means: the recording may look "scratchy" or "noisy," and data received will be incomprehensible (Figure 15–16). The external monitor is subject to artifact from extraneous noises such as maternal bowel sounds, fetal movement, maternal movement, and noises emitted from the monitor and in the labor room. This artifact may make it difficult to accurately assess variability of the FHR. When external monitoring is used, some mothers may feel compelled to lie quietly to avoid the need to readjust the belts.

External and internal monitoring are both subject to half and double counting of FHR (Figure 15–17). If the FHR is more than 180 beats/min, the monitor may divide the number in half (half count). For example, a FHR of 184 beats/min may be displayed as a rate of 92. Double counting may occur when the FHR is less than 70 beats/

min and the monitor doubles the rate. For example, a FHR of 60 may be displayed as a rate of 120. The nurse must be aware of this fact and periodically auscultate FHR to ascertain if the displayed rate is accurate.

□ **INTERNAL MONITORING** Internal monitoring is accomplished through use of an internal spiral electrode and an intrauterine pressure catheter (Figure 15–18). The cervix must be dilated at least 2 cm, the presenting fetal part accessible by vaginal examination, and the membranes ruptured. Even though it is not possible to apply the electrode and catheter under sterile conditions, this procedure should be performed as aseptically as possible. The vulva should be cleansed with Betadine (or other cleansing agent). A small electrode is attached to the fetal epidermis of the presenting part (scalp or buttocks). After determining fetal position by vaginal examinations, the examiner (physician or nurse) inserts the electrode, which is encased in a plastic guide, to the level of the internal cervical os and attaches it to the presenting part, being careful not to apply it to the face, suture lines, scrotum, or fontanelles. The electrode is rotated clockwise until it is attached to the presenting part and then disengaged from the guide tube. The guide tube is then removed and the end wires are connected to a leg plate that is attached to the woman's thigh. The cable from the leg plate is connected to the monitor.

The spiral electrode provides for an instantaneous and continuous recording of the FHR, demonstrating accurate baseline, periodic changes, and true baseline variability. The nurse must be aware that even though the FHR is recorded and appears to be that of the fetus, the monitor may actually be recording maternal heart rate. In the absence of a FHR, as in fetal death, the electrical signal picks up maternal heart rate (Figure 15–19). It is therefore criti-

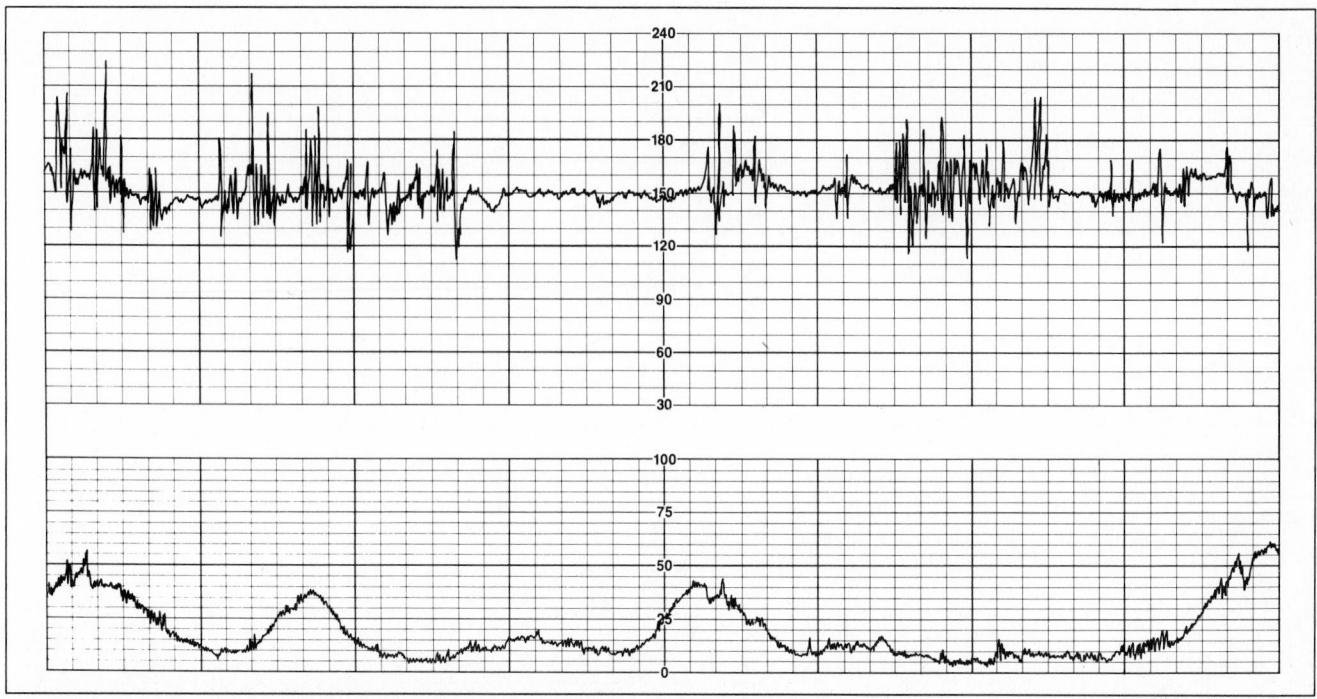

FIGURE 15–16 Noisy direct monitoring. (From Barden, T. F. 1976. *Selected pattern interpretations.* Slide No. 4. Wallingford, Conn.: Corometrics Medical Systems, Inc.)

cal that even with electronic monitoring the nurse must occasionally assess maternal pulse in relation to the FHR recording and question the client regarding movement of the fetus. On occasion the scalp electrode records a "scratchy" tracing and may contain many upward and downward deflections. In this case, the nurse should check to be certain it is properly attached to the presenting part.

Intensity of uterine contractions may be assessed by means of an intrauterine catheter (a small polyethylene tubing), inserted directly into the uterine cavity. The guide tube encasing the catheter is advanced as far as the internal cervical os and then the tubing is slowly threaded into the uterine cavity, usually in the area where fetal small parts are located. It is advanced only as far as the black marking indicated on the catheter, which should be visualized at the opening to the vaginal vault. The catheter and strain gauge are filled with sterile water (not saline as this will corrode the transducer). The gauge is then connected to the monitor. For measurement of accurate baseline resting tone of the uterus, the strain gauge should be adjusted to the height of the maternal xiphoid process. With the client in the supine position, this will approximate the level of the tip of the intrauterine catheter. By this means, a closed pressure system is maintained so that increases in intrauterine pressure with uterine contractions or hypertonus may be visualized.

In many institutions the intrauterine catheter is only utilized during oxytocin augmentation or induction, when

it is particularly important to quantitate the intensity and frequency of contractions to avoid hyperstimulation and possible uterine rupture due to overadministration of oxytocin. A slightly increased incidence of maternal infection (approximately 1%) may be noted following use of the intrauterine catheter, but this seems to be dependent on the duration of ruptured membranes and length of labor.

It is of particular importance that the nurse evaluate the client's labor status by means other than the fetal monitor. As with any type of technology, no machine is flawless and the monitor cannot fill the role of the nurse. One should never rely solely on data recorded by a machine. Technology is only useful as an adjunct to good nursing care. For example, the catheter often becomes clogged with vernix and therefore the recorded pressure is inaccurate. The catheter must be flushed occasionally to avoid this. All too often clients are in active labor with adequate contractions that are regarded as "poor quality" because the monitor was not functioning properly. The nurse routinely should palpate the intensity of the contractions and compare her assessment with that of data recorded by the monitor.

TELEMETRY

Fetal ECG and intrauterine pressure may be monitored through the use of telemetry. In telemetry a two-channel radio transmitter is placed into the vaginal vault, a pressure device placed in the uterus, and a scalp electrode

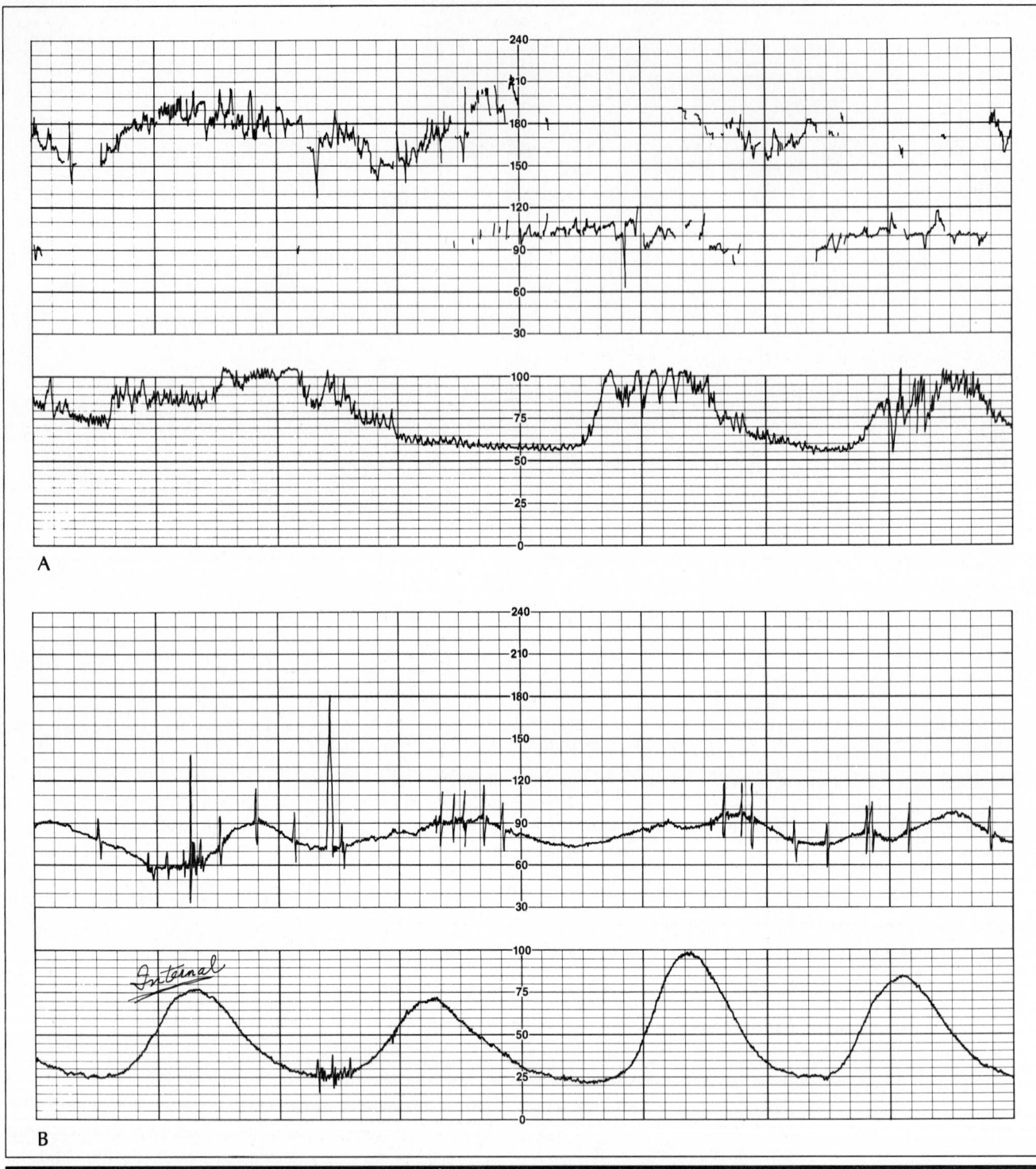

FIGURE 15–17 Incorrect tracing resulting from doubling. Fetal heart rate tracing in **A** was obtained using an indirect method (external monitor). Fetal heart rate tracing in **B** was obtained with direct method (internal device). (Modified from Paul, R. H., and Petrie, R. H. 1973. *Fetal intensive care: current concepts – monitoring records with self instruction.* Los Angeles: University of Southern California School of Medicine, Postgraduate Division, p. 21.)

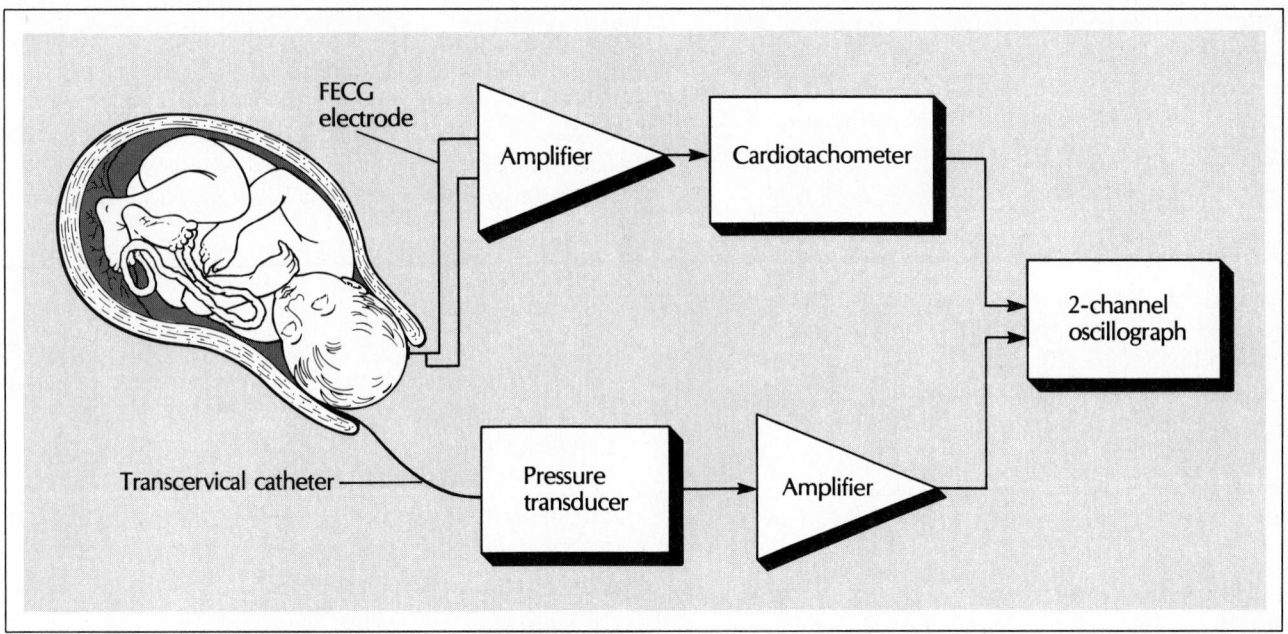

FIGURE 15–18 Direct monitoring of the fetus by scalp electrode. The pressure of the uterine contractions is being measured by transcervical catheter. (From Hon, E. 1976. *An introduction to fetal heart monitoring.* 2nd ed. Los Angeles: University of Southern California School of Medicine, p. 72.)

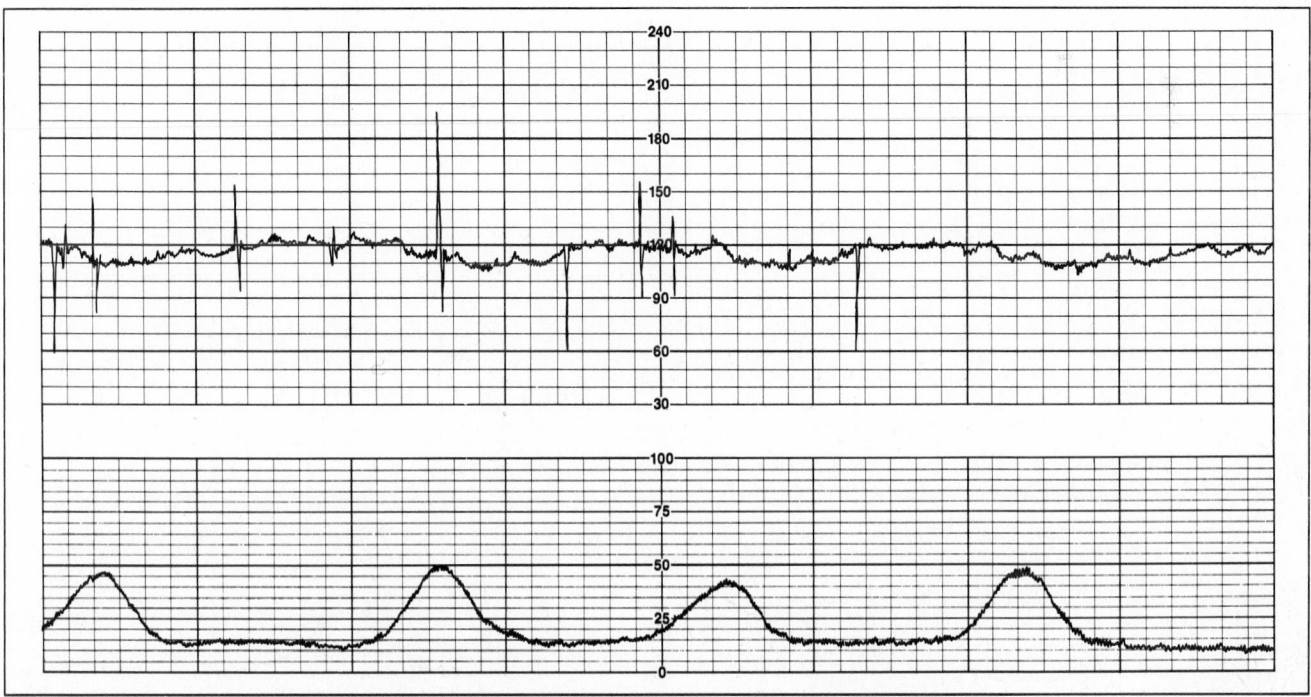

FIGURE 15–19 Erroneous fetal heart rate tracing. Fetal heart rate was actually the maternal heart rate. (Modified from Paul, R. H., and Petrie, R. H. 1973. *Fetal intensive care: current concepts — monitoring records with self instruction.* Los Angeles: University of Southern California School of Medicine, Postgraduate Division, p. 65.)

applied to the presenting fetal part. Information derived from these sources is relayed to a cardiotachometer at a central nursing station where data may be evaluated. The advantage of telemetry is that it permits the client to ambulate within a given distance from the monitor receiver.

Fetal Heart Rate Patterns

Fetal heart rate is evaluated by assessing both baseline and periodic changes. Normal FHR ranges from 120–160 beats/min (Figure 15–20). More important than FHR are the periodic changes that occur in response to the intermittent stress of uterine contractions. A sick fetus may have a normal heart rate, but demonstrate slight periodic changes indicative of intrauterine hypoxia. General principles of management of FHR patterns are presented in Table 15–4.

BASELINE RATE

The baseline refers to the average FHR observed during a 10-minute period of monitoring.

BASELINE CHANGES

Baseline changes in FHR are defined in terms of 10-minute periods of time. These changes are tachycardia, bradycardia, and beat-to-beat variability of the heart rate.

TACHYCARDIA

Tachycardia is defined as a rate of 160 beats/min or more for a 10-minute segment of time. Moderate tachycardia has rates of 160–179 beats/min. Severe tachycardia is defined as 180 beats/min or more. Although tachycardia may occur without apparent reason, possible causes include:

- Prematurity, which results in an immature autonomic nervous system

- Maternal fever, which results in an increase in sympathetic nervous system stimulation and an increase in the maternal metabolic rate, thus increasing the fetal oxygen demand

- Mild or chronic fetal hypoxemia, which results in an effort by the fetus to compensate for the oxygen deficit with increased sympathetic nervous system stimulation

- Fetal infection, which results in a fetal stress reaction to pathogens

- Fetal anemia

- Beta sympathomimetic drugs given to the pregnant woman

- Maternal anxiety, which causes maternal epinephrine to cross the placenta

- Fetal tachyarrhythmias

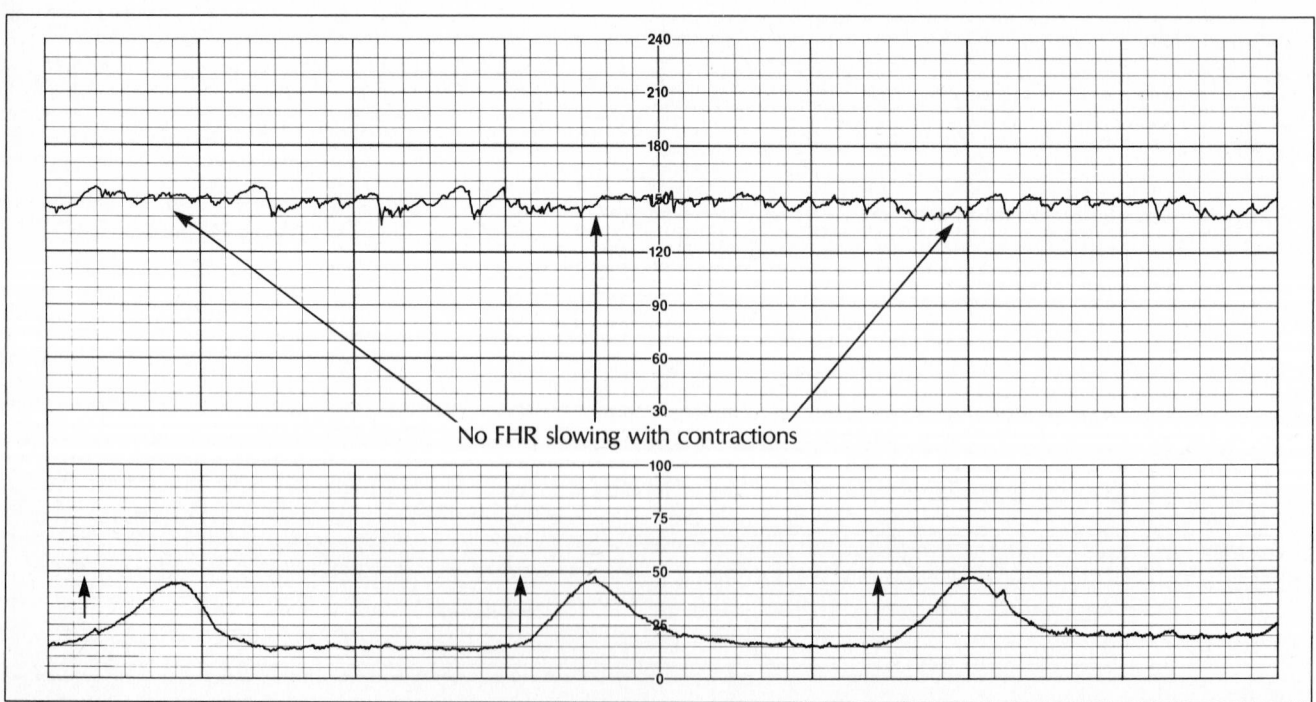

FIGURE 15–20 Normal fetal heart rate pattern utilizing internal monitoring. Note normal FHR, 140–158 beats/min, presence of long- and short-term variability, and absence of decelerations with adequate contractions.

Table 15–4   General Principles of Management of FHR Patterns

Pattern	Therapeutic intervention
Normal	Evaluate maternal vital signs
	Follow labor by means of vaginal examination at appropriate intervals
	Observe and assess quality of labor and FHR patterns
	Document data and assessment of findings
	Assure adequate hydration
	Change maternal position when indicated
	Decrease or discontinue oxytocin when indicated
	Administer oxygen when needed
	Maintain continual flow of communication
Tachycardia	Assess maternal temperature
	Reconfirm EDC
	Monitor for changes in FHR pattern
Bradycardia	Monitor for changes in FHR pattern
Early decelerations	Monitor for changes in FHR pattern
Variable decelerations	
Isolated or occasional	Monitor for changes in FHR pattern
Severe	Change maternal position to one in which FHR pattern is most improved
	Discontinue oxytocin if it is being administered
	Perform vaginal examination to assess for prolapsed cord or imminent delivery
	Administer 100% oxygen by tight face mask
	Monitor FHR continuously to assess current status and for further changes in FHR pattern
If variable decelerations are severe and uncorrectable and client is in	
Early labor	Cesarean delivery should be performed
Second stage labor	Vaginal delivery should be permitted unless baseline variability is decreasing or FHR is progressively rising, then cesarean delivery
Late decelerations occasional with good or increased variability	Monitor for further FHR changes
	Maintain client in side-lying position
	Maintain good hydration
	Discontinue oxytocin if being administered
	Administer oxygen
	Monitor maternal blood pressure and pulse for signs of hypotension
	Treat hypotension
Late decelerations persistent with good variability	Maintain side-lying position
	Administer oxygen
	Discontinue oxytocin if being administered
	Assess maternal blood pressure and pulse
	Begin intravenous fluids to maintain volume and hydration
	Assess labor progress
	Perform fetal blood sampling; if pH stays above 7.25, continue monitoring and resample; if pH shows downward trend (between 7.25 and 7.20) or is below 7.20, deliver by most expeditious means

- Maternal hypothyroidism
- Maternal drugs which inhibit the transmission of vagal response to the S-A node (such as atropine, hydroxyzine, phenothiazine)
- Excessive fetal activity

BRADYCARDIA

Fetal bradycardia is defined as a rate of less than 120 beats/min for a 10-minute segment of time. Mild bradycardia ranges from 100–119 beats/min and is considered benign. Moderate bradycardia is a fetal heart rate less than

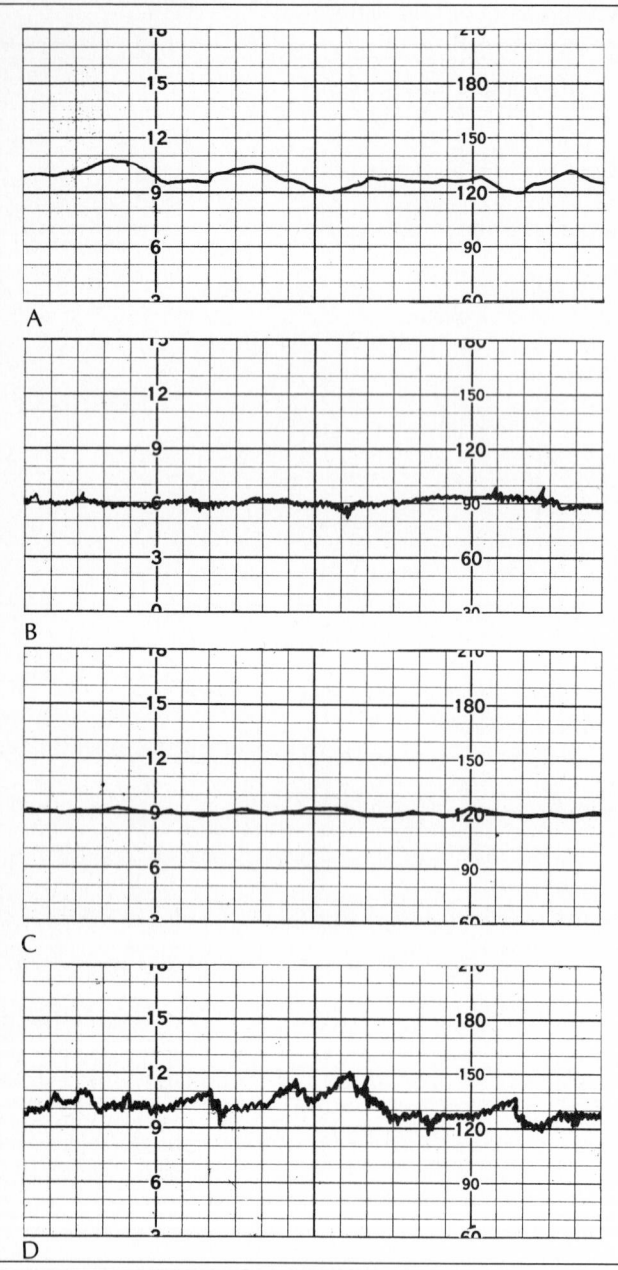

FIGURE 15–21 Long-term and short-term fetal heart rate variability. **A,** Long-term variability/no short-term variability. **B,** Short-term variability/no long-term variability. **C,** No long- or short-term variability. **D,** Long- and short-term variability.

100 beats/min. Severe bradycardia is an FHR less than 70 beats/min and is associated with a rapidly occurring fetal acidosis. Causes of fetal bradycardia include:

- Fetal hypoxia
- Fetal arrhythmias as seen with congenital heart block
- Drugs such as β-adrenergic (sympathetic) blocking agents (these include anesthetic agents used as paracervical and epidural blocks)
- Prolapse or prolonged compression of umbilical cord.

BASELINE VARIABILITY

One of the most important parameters of fetal well-being is noted in the *variability* of the FHR. This term refers to the irregularity of the FHR as noted on the graph paper. A healthy fetus normally demonstrates an irregular FHR baseline, which is caused by an interplay of the sympathetic and parasympathetic nervous systems. Variability refers to the interval between fetal heart beats. It consists of two components—long-range and short-range variability—both of significance in evaluating fetal status. Long-term variability refers to the larger rhythmic fluctuations that occur from two to six times per minute with a range of 5–15 beats/min. Long-term variability is increased by fetal movement and decreased when the fetus is in a sleep cycle. Short-term variability refers to beat-to-beat fluctuations in the baseline, which average 2–3 beats/min (Figures 15–21 and 15–22). Generally, long-term variability has been classified as follows (Hon, 1976):

No variability	0–2 beats/min
Minimal variability	3–5 beats/min
Average variability	6–10 beats/min
Moderate variability	11–25 beats/min
Marked variability	more than 25 beats/min

Rather than specifically count beats, it is probably only necessary to look at variability and classify it as minimal (or none), average, or marked. Fluctuations are due to the interplay of the parasympathetic and sympathetic components of the autonomic nervous system, as mentioned earlier. Therefore, when decreased variability is noted, one must suspect some compromise of these mechanisms. Decreasing fluctuations should be considered a warning sign of fetal jeopardy indicating that fetal reserve is being depleted. Increased variability has not been as well defined and the causes are unknown.

The nurse needs to keep in mind that true variability can only be evaluated by internal monitoring. The external monitor may demonstrate "normal" variability due to the presence of artifact, when in fact it is decreased. If variability appears to be decreased, this warrants application of an internal electrode. Decreased variability may be seen with the following conditions:

- Administration of hypnotics, analgesics, parasympathetic blocking agents, or magnesium sulfate to the mother
- Deep fetal sleep (in this case, decreased variability should not last longer than 15–20 minutes)
- Fetal congenital anomalies
- Parasympatholytics (phenothiazines, atropine) administered to client
- An immature fetus (less than 32 weeks' gestation)
- Fetal hypoxia and acidosis
- Fetal tachycardia
- Fetal anatomic brain damage

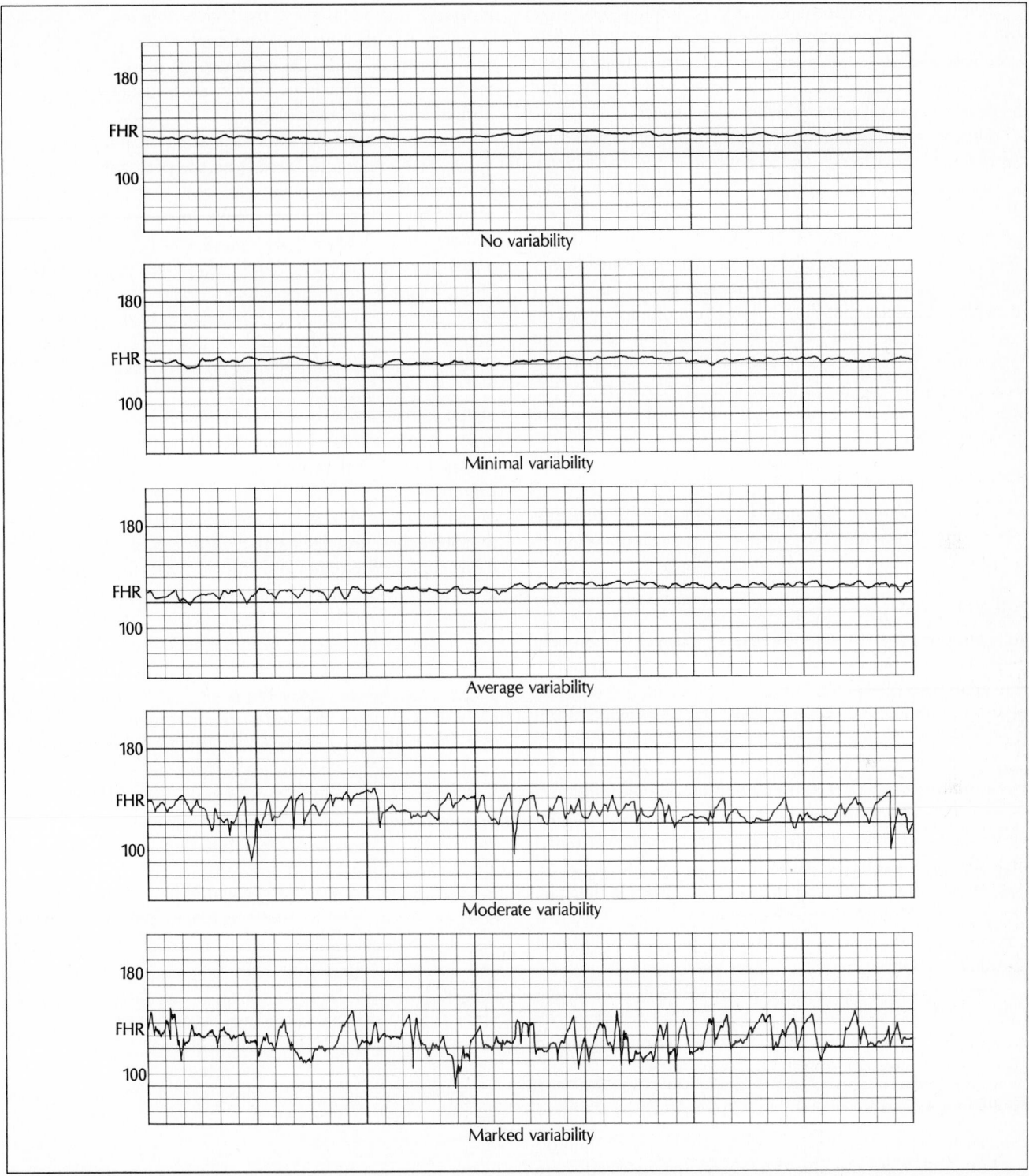

FIGURE 15-22 Types of variability. No variability = 0-2 beats/min; minimal variability = 3-5 beats/min; average variability = 6-10 beats/min; moderate variability = 11-25 beats/min; marked variability = more than 25 beats/min. (From Hon, E. 1976. *An introduction to fetal heart rate monitoring.* 2nd ed. Los Angeles: University of Southern California School of Medicine, p. 41.)

Stimuli such as maternal activity, abdominal palpation, and myometrial contractions may increase variability. Complete loss of variability may occur with complete heart block. If tachycardia accompanies loss of variability, fetal prognosis is usually poor (Boehn et al., 1978).

Druzen and colleagues (1979) noted that short-term variability tended to be due to actions of the parasympathetic nervous system, while long-term variability was due to actions of the sympathetic system. Modanlou and co-workers (1977) suggested that in the state of neonatal hypoxemia, short-term variability appeared to be reduced early with loss of long-term variability occurring later. Druzen et al. (1979) reported that the earliest effect of hypoxemia on variability appeared to be an increase in both short- and long-term variability. Severe and prolonged fetal hypoxia with accompanying acidemia results in diminished FHR variability, probably because of the effect of hypoxia and acidosis on the CNS.

PERIODIC CHANGES

Periodic changes are transient decelerations or accelerations of the FHR from the baseline. They usually occur in response to contractions and fetal movement.

ACCELERATIONS

Accelerations are transient increases in the FHR normally caused by fetal movement. As the fetus moves in utero, the heart rate increases similar to when adults exercise and their heart rate increases. When the fetus quiets down the heart rate returns to normal. Often acceleration accompanies contractions, usually due to fetal movement in response to pressure of the contracting uterine musculature. Accelerations of this type are thought to be a sign of fetal well-being and adequate oxygen reserve. Accelerations may also be caused by partial occlusion of the umbilical cord. In this instance a transient period of decreased placental return and fetal hypotension are seen, resulting in a baroreceptor response that increases the FHR (Freeman and Garite, 1981).

Accelerations may be periodic or sporadic and of uniform or variable shape (Krebs et al., 1982). Periodic accelerations occur in conjunction with contractions; sporadic accelerations may occur with fetal movement.

DECELERATIONS

Decelerations are periodic decreases in FHR from the normal baseline. Hon and Quilligan (1967) categorized them into three types, "early," "late," and "variable," according to when they occur in the contraction cycle and to their waveform (Figure 15–23). In their earlier work, Hon and Quilligan also referred to these deceleration patterns as Types I, II, and III.

□ *EARLY DECELERATIONS* Early decelerations are due to compression of the fetal head as it progresses down the birth canal. They have a uniform, smooth waveform that inversely mirrors that of the corresponding contraction. Beginning at the onset of the contraction and ending as the contraction ends, the nadir (lowest point) occurs at the peak of the contraction. The nadir is usually within the normal fetal heart rate range.

Generally early decelerations are benign and seen late in labor when the fetal head is on the perineum. Increased intracranial pressure results in local changes in cerebral blood flow, which in turn results in stimulation of vagal centers and produces a slowing of heart rate through the vagus nerve (Figure 15–24). If this pattern occurs early in labor, it may be due to head compression from cephalopelvic disproportion. A nurse must take great care in differentiating this type of deceleration from late decelerations: they look identical yet differ in time of onset.

Early decelerations are not associated with loss of variability, tachycardia, or other FHR changes, nor are they associated with fetal hypoxia, acidosis, or low Apgar scores. Early decelerations are viewed as a reassuring FHR pattern.

□ *LATE DECELERATIONS* Late decelerations are due to uteroplacental insufficiency as the result of decreased blood flow and oxygen transfer to the fetus through the intervillous space during uterine contractions causing hypoxemia (Figure 15–25). They have a smooth, uniform shape, which inversely mirrors the contraction (as do early decelerations), but are late in their onset. They begin at or within a few seconds after the peak of the contraction; the nadir is noted near the end of the contraction. They tend to occur with every contraction. When uteroplacental reserve is adequate, normally the fetus tolerates the transient stress of repetitive contractions. If fetal hypoxia occurs because of a decrease in uteroplacental blood flow (for example, from maternal hypotension or excessive uterine activity), late decelerations generally occur.

This pattern is always considered an ominous sign but does not necessarily require immediate delivery of the fetus. If late decelerations do not appear to be worsening and the variability of the FHR is good, delivery may be delayed although the fetus warrants constant observation. Should decelerations worsen or variability decrease, fetal blood sampling for pH determination is indicated to further evaluate acid-base status of the fetus.

Sometimes late decelerations are noted, which upon evaluation are found to be due to supine position of the laboring woman. In this case, decreased uterine blood flow to the fetus due to supine hypotension may be alleviated by raising the client's upper trunk or turning her to the side to displace pressure of the gravid uterus from the inferior vena cava. If the client is allowed to remain flat on her back, the fetus will continue to have decelerations due to oxygen compromise.

Late decelerations normally occur within the normal heart rate range (120–160 beats/min) and may be quite obvious or very subtle and almost indistinguishable. Some

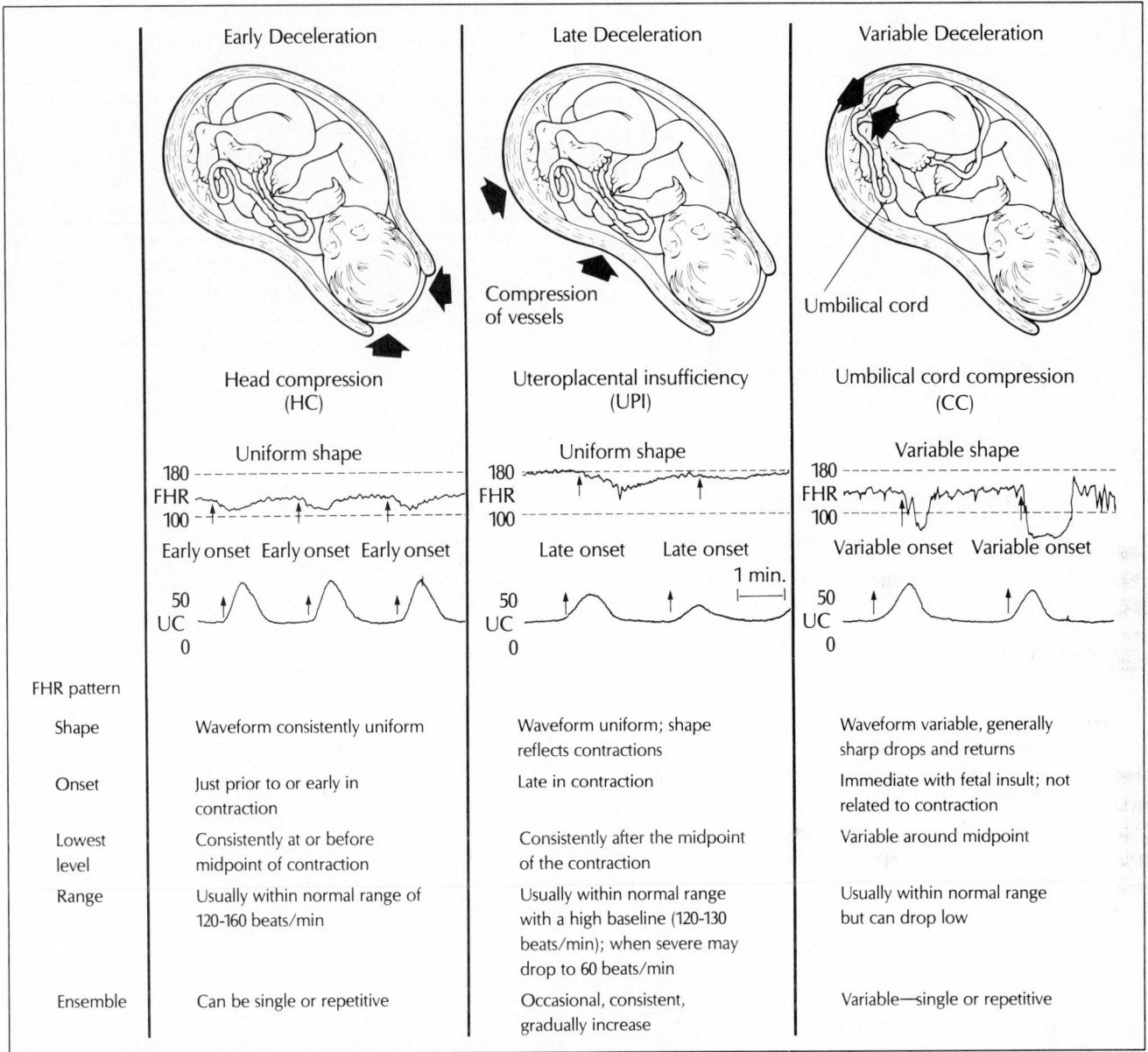

FIGURE 15–23 Types and characteristics of early, late, and variable decelerations. (From Hon, E. 1976. *An introduction to fetal heart rate monitoring.* 2nd ed. Los Angeles: University of Southern California School of Medicine, p. 29.)

fetuses at highest risk demonstrate a flat FHR baseline with late decelerations that are barely noticeable. It must be kept in mind that the depth of the deceleration does not indicate the severity of the insult.

Chronic uteroplacental insufficiency during pregnancy results in intrauterine growth retardation and if severe enough, antenatal death. When uteroplacental insufficiency is acute due to factors occurring during labor, fetal distress may ensue. If not properly treated intrapartal fetal death may occur.

□ **VARIABLE DECELERATIONS** Variable decelerations are appropriately named in that they vary in their onset, occurrence, and waveform. They are thought to be due to umbilical cord occlusion (which in essence cuts off the low resistance fetal placental circulation), and the resulting increase in peripheral resistance in the fetal circulation causes fetal hypertension. The fetal hypertension results in stimulation of the baroreceptors in the aortic arch and carotid sinuses. This results in an outflow from the parasympathetic system causing a sudden slowing effect on the

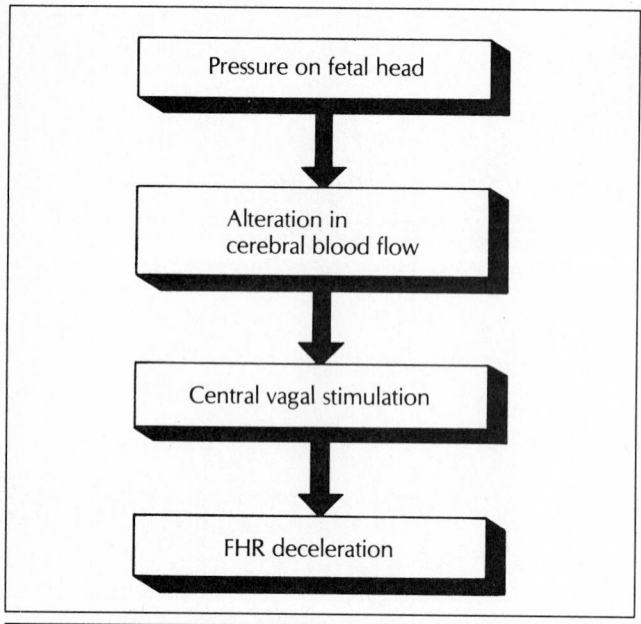

FIGURE 15–24 Mechanism of early deceleration (head compression). (Adapted from Freeman, R. K., and Garite, T. J. 1981. The physiologic basis of fetal monitoring. In *Fetal heart rate monitoring*. Baltimore: Williams & Wilkins, ch. 2, p. 13.)

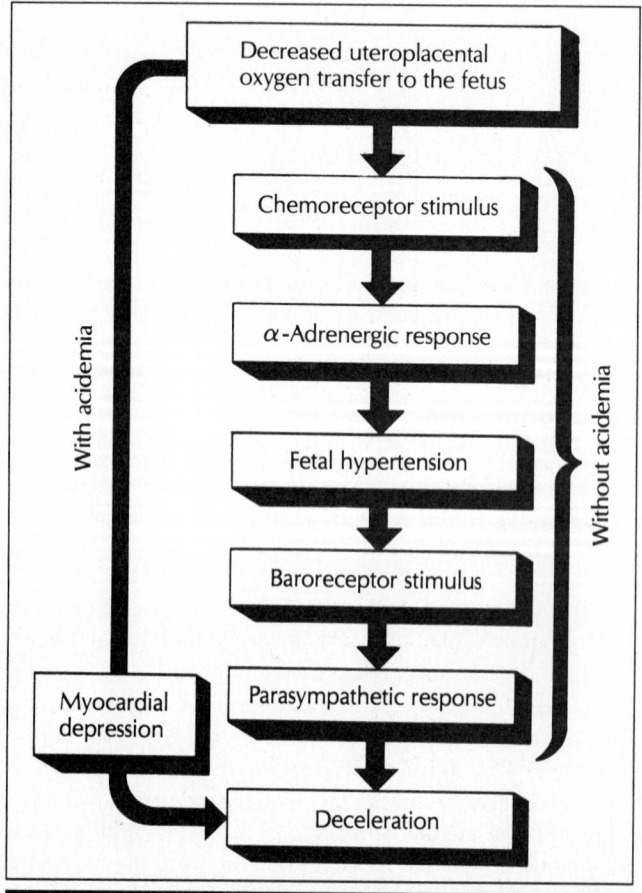

fetal atrial pacemaker (bradycardia) (Freeman and Garite, 1981). Either the fetus squeezes the cord or rolls over onto it, transient pressure is exerted on the cord from compression, or the cord is around the neck of the fetus. An occasional or isolated variable deceleration is usually benign. Variable decelerations that are repetitive and begin to worsen during the course of labor are of concern. Variable decelerations usually fall outside the normal FHR range and are classified as mild, moderate, and severe. They are acute in onset, vary in duration and intensity, and abruptly disappear when the insult of cord compression is relieved (Figure 15–26).

If decelerations are repetitive, one should suspect a nuchal cord or occult prolapse of the cord. If this pattern begins to be evident early in labor, the possibility arises of development of late decelerations due to repetitive stress causing uteroplacental insufficiency. In this instance, cesarean delivery might be warranted.

Decelerations that seem to deviate more from the baseline and lengthen are ominous and warrant further investigation. When they are prolonged and severe, a significant oxygen deficit develops from myocardial depression, resulting in hypoxemia and subsequent fetal metabolic acidosis (Freeman and Garite, 1981). If allowed to continue, fetal death may result.

With progressively worsening variable decelerations, an "overshoot" may occur. This is a blunt, smooth acceleration following the contraction and may be due to an attempt of the fetus to compensate for hypoxemia through sympathetic and adrenal mechanisms (Martin and Gingerich, 1976).

Variable decelerations are frequently seen toward the latter stages of labor when the membranes are ruptured, which decreases protection to the cord as the fetus descends down the birth canal. Variable decelerations usually do not warrant immediate delivery unless loss of variability and/or a rising baseline accompanies them. Often, repositioning the client corrects this type of pattern.

□ *MIXED PATTERNS/PROLONGED DECELERATIONS* It is possible to see a combination of periodic changes in FHR. This is probably the most confusing monitoring tracing. Prolonged decelerations (longer than 60–90 seconds) may occur with hypertonus associated with contractions, after administration of paracervical block or epidural anesthesia, and with sudden occult or frank prolapse of the umbilical cord. When decelerations happen following administration of regional anesthesia, the client should be turned on her side, evaluated for hypotension, and administered a

FIGURE 15–25 Mechanism of late deceleration. (From Freeman, R. K., and Garite, T. J. 1981. The physiologic basis of fetal monitoring. In *Fetal heart rate monitoring*. Baltimore: Williams & Wilkins, ch. 2, p. 15.)

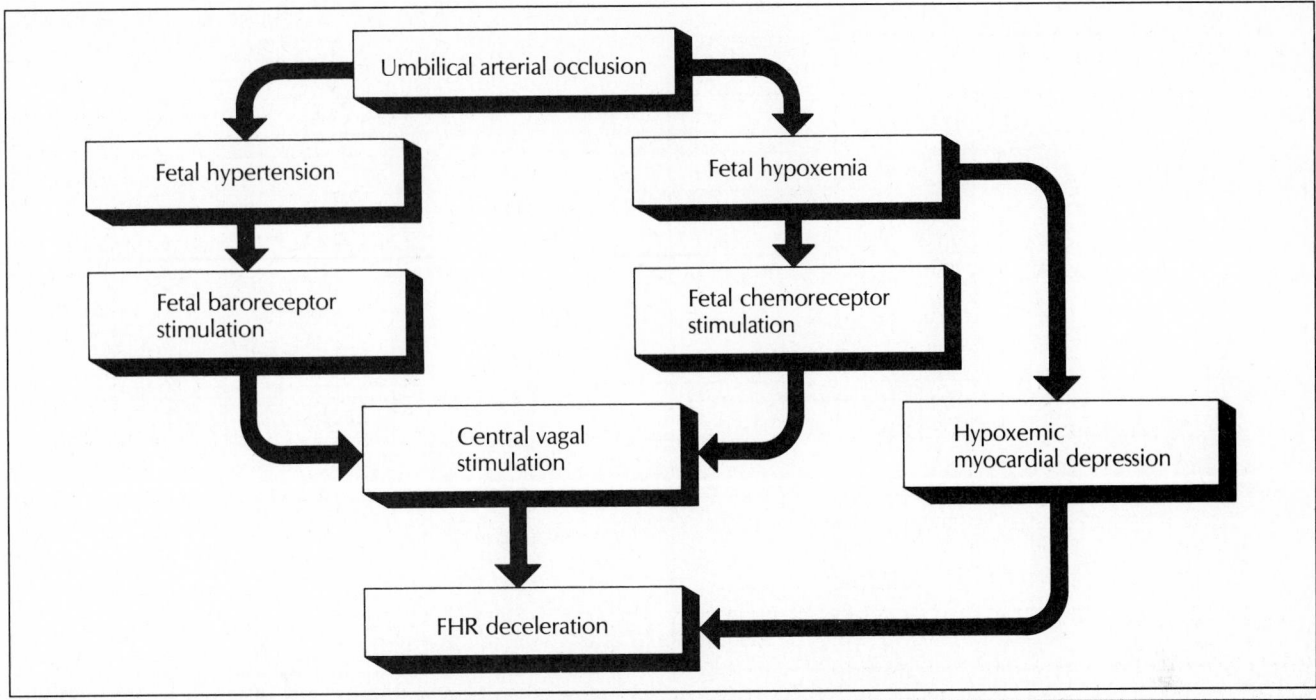

FIGURE 15–26 Mechanism of variable deceleration. (Adapted from Freeman, R. K., and Garite, T. J. 1981. The physiologic basis of fetal monitoring. In *Fetal heart rate monitoring.* Baltimore: Williams & Wilkins, ch. 2, p. 15.)

bolus of intravenous fluid (500–600 mL) to fill the dilated vascular space.

Mixed and unusual patterns and prolonged decelerations should be considered pathologic, especially if associated with loss of baseline variability. In cases of mixed deceleration patterns, further assessment by means of fetal blood sampling is indicated to evaluate acid-base status of the fetus.

□ *SINUSOIDAL PATTERNS* Occasionally an unusual pattern is seen that is referred to as sinusoidal. It is characterized by an undulant sinewave, which is equally distributed above and below the baseline. One sees long-term variability (5–15 beats/min) and an absence of short-term variability. The FHR baseline appears to "wander" or oscillate in a uniform pattern of 2–6 cycles per minute without specific accelerations during fetal activity. Fetal activity may be minimal or absent. The baseline FHR usually ranges from 110–150 beats/min (Figure 15–27).

Significant confusion regarding the definition and significance of the sinusoidal pattern exists, although the pattern seems to "imply severe fetal jeopardy and impending death" (Modanlou and Freeman, 1982). In a review of the literature of 41 sinusoidal patterns, Modanlou and Freeman noted that true sinusoidal heart rate was seen most frequently in the severely affected Rh-sensitized fetus and neonate or in fetuses compromised by severe anemia of a different origin. It was also noted in fetuses and neonates with perinatal asphyxia and/or CNS insult. In addition, they found that the only cases in which true sinusoidal patterns were seen without significant morbidity were in fetuses whose mothers had received alphaprodine (Nisentil) analgesia during labor. They support the hypothesis that the cause of sinusoidal heart rate may be due to tissue hypoxia of the cardiac center.

REASSURING AND NONREASSURING FHR PATTERNS

FHR patterns need to be assessed for evidence that shows whether they are reassuring or nonreassuring. Reassuring patterns include (Freeman, 1982):

1. No periodic changes
2. Early decelerations
3. Variable decelerations that do not exceed the following limits:
   a. Accelerations lasting less than 45 seconds
   b. Return to baseline is abrupt
   c. Baseline rate is not increasing
   d. Baseline variability is not decreasing
4. FHR accelerations
   a. With contractions
   b. With fetal movement

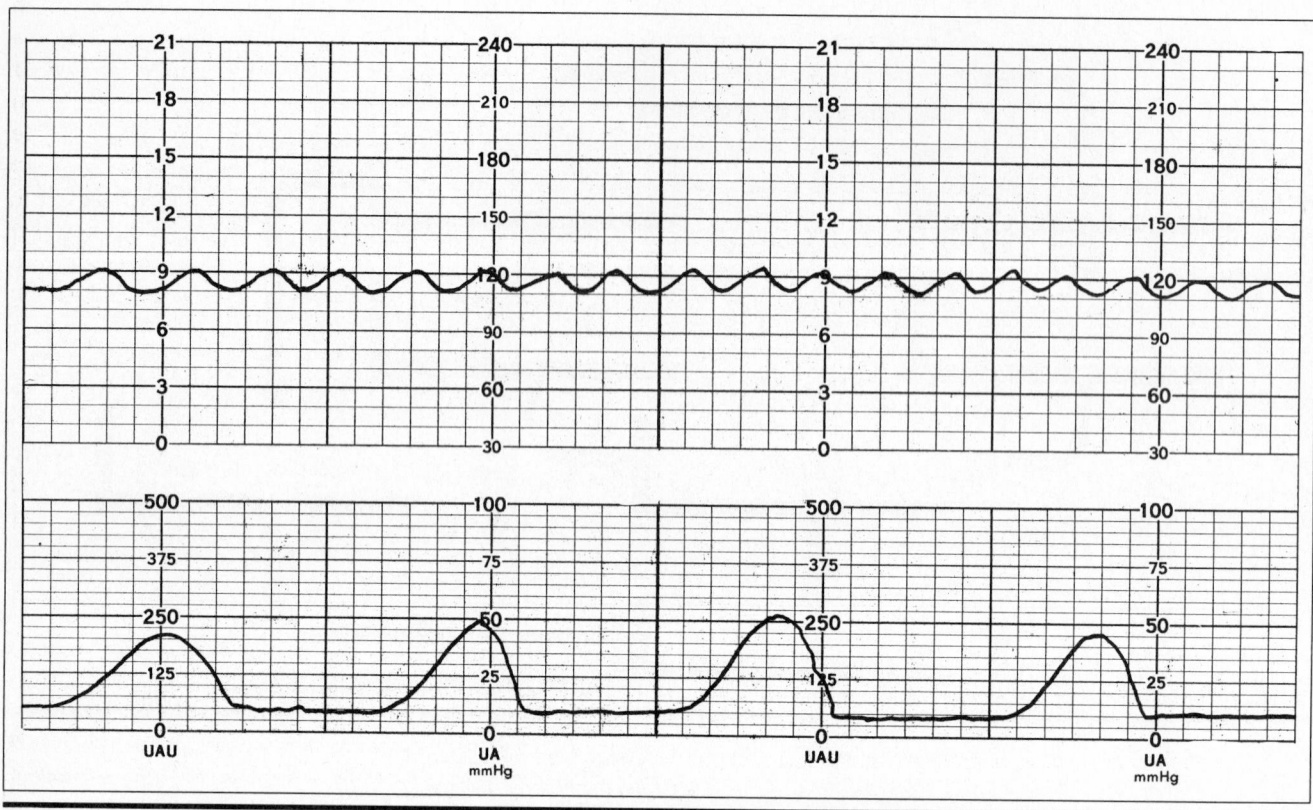

FIGURE 15–27 Fetal heart rate tracing demonstrating sinusoidal pattern. Note absence of short-term variability, and wandering baseline of the FHR.

Nonreassuring patterns include (Freeman, 1982):

1. Intermittent late deceleration with good FHR variability
2. Variable deceleration that exceeds the criteria (in reassuring patterns) with respect to duration and/or rate of return but still has good FHR variability and no rising baseline
3. Total loss of FHR variability with deceleration
4. Prolonged deceleration due to:
   a. Paracervical block
   b. Epidural block
   c. Supine hypotension
   d. Following vaginal examination or manipulation

Ominous FHR patterns include (Freeman, 1982):

1. Persistent, uncorrectable late decelerations with loss of FHR variability with or without fetal tachycardia
2. Variable decelerations accompanied by:
   a. Loss of FHR variability
   b. Fetal tachycardia
   c. Prolonged "overshoot"
   d. Blunted shapes
3. Sinusoidal FHR patterns

□ *PRETERMINAL PATTERNS* The preterminal fetus usually demonstrates an FHR pattern different from that of fetal distress. Most dying fetuses demonstrate tachycardia (al-

though not always) and loss of variability, and have a period of profound bradycardia just before death. Variable decelerations with rounded or "blunted" edges may be noted. The baseline may appear to "wander" or to be "fixed."

Often a preterminal fetus is severely damaged due to major congenital anomalies, making implications for delivery questionable. Cases of cesarean birth with delivery of neonates having severe fetal anomalies have been reported. Until more is known regarding preterminal patterns, it cannot be presumed that the fetus is unsalvageable.

Value of Electronic Fetal Monitoring

In spite of several years of experience with fetal monitoring, the benefits for neonatal outcome for the normal client are not yet conclusive. Certainly electronic monitoring has identified problems during labor that otherwise would have been undetected, and intervention has meant the survival of thousands of infants who might otherwise have died during labor. The standard of care in the United States has been moving toward monitoring all high-risk clients. In 1979 the Task Force of the National Institutes of Health recommended that electronic fetal monitors be considered in the management of high-risk clients "whenever the potential benefits of the technique exceed the known risks."

High-risk clients, who account for approximately 25% of the obstetric population, account for only about one-half of the perinatal morbidity and mortality. The remainder of the perinatal casualties come from the low-risk group (75% of the obstetric population) (Wilson and Schifrin, 1980). Obviously, classification of clients according to risk (low or high) prior to labor is not predictive of whether pregnancy outcome will be positive or not. Hobel et al. (1973) found that 23% of their clients who were low risk antepartally became high risk during labor. Furthermore, this group accounted for significantly higher morbidity and mortality than either the group who were high risk antepartally and low risk during labor, or low risk antepartally and low risk during labor. Moreover, low-risk clients demonstrated more problems during labor than did high-risk clients.

Significant reductions in infant and perinatal mortality are evident in past years. A large proportion of the lowered mortality has been attributed to the introduction of fetal monitoring.

Neutra and colleagues (1978), in examining data from 16,529 births over a 7-year period, found that the increased risk of neonatal death when not using electronic fetal monitoring rose 1.4 times, but that use of electronic fetal monitoring in the 26% of labors with obvious risk factors would avert 87% of the potentially preventable neonatal deaths. Their conclusion was that the major value of fetal monitoring is to identify either the unstressed normal fetus or the one in severe distress.

Haverkamp and associates (1979) compared the reliability and accuracy of fetoscopic auscultation by knowledgeable and competent clinical nurses with findings recorded by the electronic monitor. They found no differences in perinatal outcome with respect to Apgar scores or neonatal course. This study was small (483 high-risk clients), the women were all of low socioeconomic status, and all were categorized as high risk without allusion to specific problems. A 1:1 nurse/client ratio was maintained using strict criteria for assessment during labor.

Only four randomized controlled studies have compared auscultation to electronic fetal monitoring. Many clinicians feel these four studies are insufficient to support the monitoring of all laboring clients. Therefore, many conclude that in a well-screened population the value of electronic monitoring over careful auscultation is of little or no increased benefit. Yet others contend that electronic fetal monitoring gives an indication of normality, and they prefer to use it for that reason. It has been shown that the cesarean delivery rate increases with the use of electronic fetal monitoring; some feel this fact detracts from its value.

Unfortunately, electronic fetal monitoring is a better predictor of good outcome when patterns are reassuring than of poor fetal outcome when patterns are nonreassur-

ing. Schifrin and Dame (1973) reported a high correlation between reassuring FHR patterns and Apgar scores and a low correlation between nonreassuring patterns and Apgar scores. They found that less than one-half of clients with nonreassuring FHR patterns deliver infants with 5-minute Apgar scores below 7. The literature seems to indicate that FHR patterns are more predictive of abnormal conditions resulting in the fetus than are Apgar scores (Freeman and Garite, 1981). FHR patterns suggestive of fetal hypoxia and/or acidosis seem to correlate with depression of the infant at birth and with adverse outcomes in long-term (1-year) follow-up studies (Freeman and Garite, 1981).

Only one long-term follow-up study exists relating to long-term sequelae of monitored infants (Freeman and Garite, 1981). To accurately determine the value of electronic monitoring, more studies are necessary. Nevertheless, the mere fact that clients are monitored by such a detailed technology in conjunction with optimal nursing and medical assessment seems to assure greater surveillance during the stress of the intrapartal period.

Psychologic Reactions to Electronic Monitoring

The nurse plays an important role in providing information about fetal monitoring. Many clients have no knowledge of monitoring unless they have attended a prenatal class that dealt with this subject. Some women enter labor with preconceived negative ideas about this technology garnered from articles they have read in popular literature. Studies regarding reactions of women to intrapartal electronic fetal monitoring reveal that most women react positively to the monitor; those with negative feelings seem to be in the minority. A study by Dulock and Herron (1976) noted clients had a more positive attitude after delivery compared with predelivery attitudes. Starkman (1976) stated that the most positive aspect of her study was that clients with a previous history of intrapartal problems responded most favorably to the fetal monitor as a protector against disaster. Positive reactions expressed by clients in documented studies include feelings that the fetal monitor offered reassurance as a protector (as an extension of the obstetrician). It also acts as an aid in communication, an extension of the client (as a provider of information to the physician), an extension of the fetus (confirmation that the baby is "okay"), and a facilitator of involvement of the woman's partner in the labor experience. The clients appreciated the use of the monitor as a distraction or diversion during labor, and as an aid in mastery (for example, in Lamaze breathing).

Negative feelings about the monitor expressed by clients were resentment (more attention paid to fetal monitor by partner and staff); physical discomfort; decreased mobility; and frustration due to mechanical difficulties with the monitor. The women who had negative reactions felt the monitor was anxiety-producing (due to auditory information). They also experienced fear of injury to baby (Dulock and Herron, 1976; Starkman, 1976, 1977; Shields, 1978; Molfese et al., 1982).

Nurses should examine their own feelings about monitoring and give clients the opportunity to talk about feelings regarding use of it. Nurses have influence in modifying attitudes and providing information. The nurse's attitudes influence the type of nursing care provided. If nurses express negativism or lack of confidence in the equipment, they may not be able to incorporate this technology into their nursing assessment and therefore may give inadequate care and support to the client.

The emphasis in maternity nursing is directed toward meeting the physical, emotional, and psychosocial needs of the client with concern for the fetus. Through use of the monitor, maternal and fetal surveillance is enhanced. Yet the nurse must not lose sight of the client's needs and expend energies on overreliance on the monitor. The monitor only provides information for the nurse's evaluation of the client's status to provide the best care. Although technology should be appreciated for the additional information it offers, monitors do not care for clients; nurses do. In fact, because of the high standards of care needed when electronic fetal monitoring is used, most facilities find that additional staff is needed to properly educate clients and utilize this new technology.

Nursing Care and Responsibilities

Prior to application of the monitor, the nurse should fully explain to the client the reason for it and the information

Table 15–5   Evaluating FHR Tracings

I. *Stimulus*—uterine contractions
  A. Calibrate the system
  B. Baseline uterine resting tone
  C. Contractions
    1. Frequency
    2. Duration
    3. Intensity
II. *Response*—Fetal heart rate changes
  A. Calibrate the system
  B. Baseline changes
    1. FHR
    2. Amount of variability
  C. Periodic changes
    1. Accelerations
    2. Decelerations
      a. Uniform
        (1) Late
        (2) Early
      b. Nonuniform
        (1) Variable

that can be derived from its use. The nurse tells her how the monitor may be helpful in identifying the beginning of contractions and thus can aid in breathing during the various stages of labor. An explanation alleviates apprehensions about equipment that may be totally unfamiliar to the client. During labor it is advantageous to educate the client regarding possible application and use of the internal equipment as the physician may quickly decide to convert to this method while examining the client. Clients who are informed about the possibility of internal monitoring are better prepared if a quick decision must be made to apply electrode or catheter.

After the monitor is applied, basic information should be recorded on a label that is attached to the monitor strip. The data included are the date, client's name, physician, hospital number, age, gravida, para, EDC, membrane status, and maternal vital signs. As the monitor strip continues to run and care is provided, it is important that documentation of occurrences during labor be recorded not only in the medical record but also on the fetal monitoring tracing as well. The following information should be included on the tracing:

1. Vaginal examination (dilatation, effacement, station, and position)
2. Amniotomy
3. Maternal vital signs
4. Maternal position changes
5. Application of internal monitor
6. Medications
7. Oxygen information
8. Maternal behaviors (emesis, coughing, hiccups)
9. Fetal blood sampling

This information is helpful in later evaluation of a tracing. The tracing is considered to be a legal part of the client's medical record and is submissible in court. All pertinent information should be appropriately documented.

INTERPRETATION OF FHR TRACINGS

As in interpreting an ECG tracing, one needs a systematic approach in evaluating FHR tracings to avoid misinterpreting findings on the basis of inadequate or erroneous data. (See Table 15–5 for method of systematic evaluation.) Too often, nurses evaluate FHR changes without assessing other factors, such as contraction patterns, calibration of equipment, or baseline resting tone. Developing a systematic approach in evaluation allows the nurse to make a more accurate and rapid assessment, to have ease in communication of data to physicians and staff, and a systematic, universal language for documentation in the client's record.

In assessing tracings, the nurse should first identify the stimulus—the contractions. Before being able to differentiate between late and early decelerations, the nurse must assess the contraction pattern (frequency, duration, and intensity of contractions, and baseline resting tone). To do this, the monitoring system is calibrated to ensure it is functioning properly for optimal evaluation. If it is not, data may be misinterpreted. Contractions should be in evidence on the tracing at or even before the time the client actually feels them. If not, adjustments are needed. The fetal heart rate range occurring as a response to the stress of uterine contractions is noted. Again, the monitor should be calibrated. Often the internal electrode becomes displaced from the presenting part. In this case the tracing demonstrates much artifact, rendering interpretation impossible. It is difficult to differentiate between "noise" in the tracing and possible fetal cardiac arrhythmias or heart block. Baseline changes should be assessed: What is the FHR? Is it increasing? Is it decreasing? Is the variability increasing or decreasing?

Finally, the nurse looks at periodic changes. Are there accelerations with fetal movement? Are "blunted" accelerations following contractions? Are there decelerations? Late and early decelerations are uniform; variable decelerations are nonuniform. The timing of late decelerations is critical, so the monitor must be accurately adjusted to ensure that as much contraction as possible is being recorded by the monitor.

Only after thorough evaluation using a systematic approach to assessment can data obtained from electronic fetal monitoring be of benefit in predicting fetal outcome.

In many institutions it is not the nurse's perogative to diagnose specific types of decelerations, but adequate care cannot be given unless the nurse has sufficient knowledge about pattern interpretation. Unless a nurse is able to distinguish nonreassuring patterns from reassuring ones and can take responsibility for evaluating the status of labor, the nurse cannot be relied upon to detect impending problems. In some institutions the nursing professional is asked to be specific in documenting interpretation of FHR pattern. In other settings, the nurse simply describes the pattern without classifying it. No matter what the institution's policy is, nurses must be knowledgeable in the recognition of FHR patterns and accurate in communicating their assessment of fetal status to the physician.

Additional Assessment Techniques

MONITORING OF FETAL ACID-BASE STATUS

When nonreassuring or confusing FHR patterns are noted, it becomes necessary to seek additional information regarding the acid-base status of the fetus. This is accomplished by means of fetal blood sampling, which is usually done from the fetal scalp, but may be performed on the fetus in the breech position.

When oxygen perfusion to the fetus is compromised,

fetal hypoxia ensues and metabolism changes from aerobic to anaerobic, resulting in the production of lactic acid. This causes a state of acidosis and therefore a drop in the pH level. With fetal blood sampling, a higher correlation exists between low pH levels and low Apgar scores; with fetal monitoring, there is a high correlation between normal FHR patterns and high Apgar scores. This may be due to the fact that changes in fetal scalp blood pH occur only after significant anaerobic metabolism, whereas late decelerations may occur with early hypoxemia before the development of metabolic acidosis (Freeman and Garite, 1981). One must assess the risks of waiting against the risks of intervention by cesarean delivery to achieve higher Apgar scores.

Quilligan (1981) recommends scalp sampling under the following conditions: moderate and severe variable decelerations with good variability, mild and moderately severe variable decelerations with poor variability, or late decelerations. He recommends immediate cesarean delivery with severe late decelerations accompanied by poor variability. Freeman (1982) recommends the following indications (if one or more criteria are present) for fetal blood sampling:

1. Persistent uncorrectable late decelerations with good variability in a client who is expected to deliver in less than 2 hours.
2. Clients with confusing FHR patterns in which there are elements that could be considered ominous.
3. Clients with total loss of FHR variability but no deceleration pattern.

Fetal blood sampling requires that the membranes be ruptured, the cervix be at least 2–3 cm dilated, and that the presenting part not be above −2 station. Sampling is not done when patterns are ominous, and is contraindicated in acute emergencies and in cases of vaginal bleeding. In these instances, delivery by the most expeditious means is indicated.

FETAL BLOOD SAMPLING PROCEDURE

Equipment needed for fetal blood sampling is available in sterile disposable trays. Items needed are:

- Four or five 200 μL heparinized capillary tubes
- 2 mm blade on long handle
- Conical endoscope with light source
- Silicone spray or grease
- 10 to 15 sponges
- Long-handled sponge holder

Procedure. The client's vulva and perineum should be thoroughly cleansed with Betadine and sterile drapes arranged. A conical vaginal endoscope is inserted into the vagina and through the cervix to facilitate visualization of

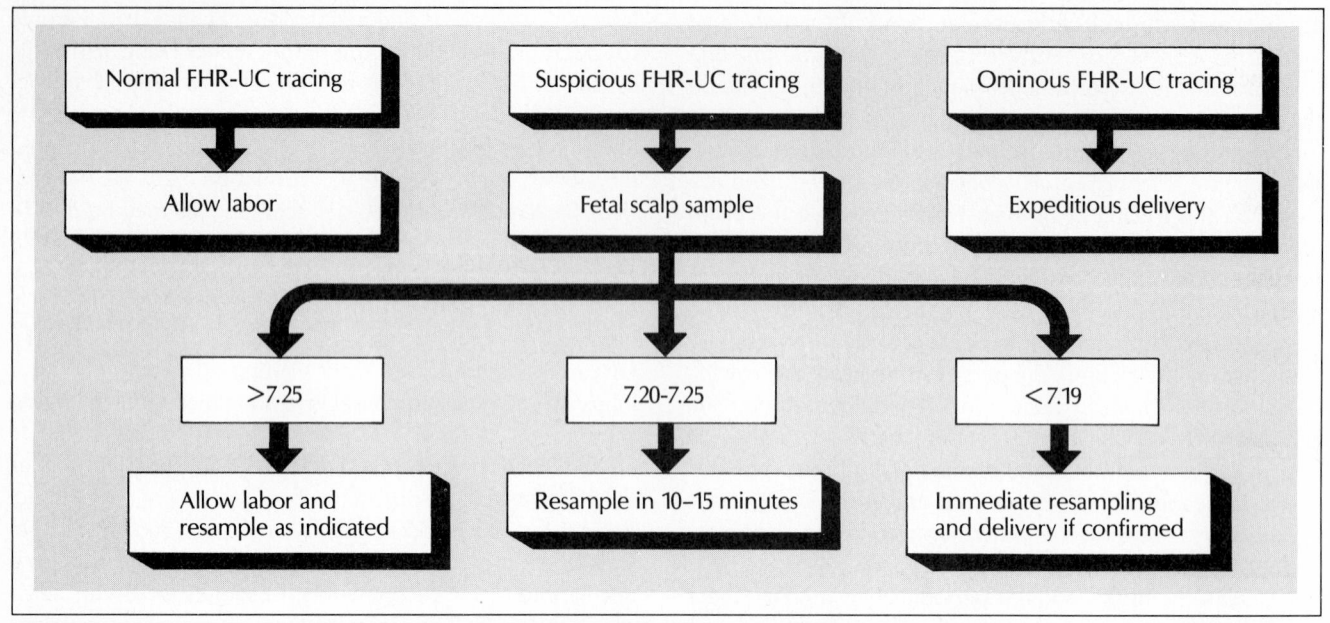

FIGURE 15–28 Guidelines for using fetal scalp pH. (From Monheit, A., and Cousins, L. Aug. 1981. When do you measure scalp blood pH? *Contemp. OB/GYN.* Med Econ. Co. Inc.)

the fetal site to be sampled. Working through the endoscope, the physician cleanses the site to remove vernix, blood, and amniotic fluid. Silicone spray is then applied to the site to provide a surface for the formation of a globule of blood. The site is punctured with a 2 × 2 mm microscalpel. A small amount of blood is then collected in a long heparinized glass capillary tube and immediately assessed for pH value. Approximately one-fourth tube of blood is needed for determining pH and three-fourths for evaluating complete blood gases (pH, P_{CO_2}, P_{O_2}, and base-deficit values). The clotting mechanism is compromised when pH is lowered; therefore oozing at the site may occur for a period of time. Loss of even minimal amounts of blood may be disastrous to the fetus. To avoid serious blood loss, pressure should be applied to the puncture site throughout two maternal contractions, then the site should be observed throughout a third contraction. After the procedure close observation for vaginal bleeding should be carried out to assure that what may appear to be heavy bloody show is not a fetal hemorrhage from the puncture site. Results of pH determination should be readily available in 10–15 minutes for this procedure to be effective.

Normal pH values during labor are at or above 7.25 pH, with 7.20–7.24 pH considered preacidotic. Values below 7.20 pH indicate serious acidosis (Petrie and Pollack, 1976). Freeman and Garite (1981) state the necessity of immediate resampling when the pH is 7.20–7.25 to confirm the value and to determine whether there is a trend toward acidosis. They recommend cesarean delivery when pH value is in the 7.20–7.25 range. Other authorities ad-

vocate waiting for the value to decrease to 7.20 pH or below before a cesarean (Monheit and Cousins, 1981). (Figure 15–28 shows guidelines for using fetal scalp pH.)

Kubli and coworkers (1969) demonstrated a correlation between the pH value of the fetal scalp and various FHR patterns. The more severe the heart rate pattern, the more likely the fetus is to be acidemic. Paul and Petrie (1973) evaluated late decelerations and found that FHR variability correlated even more with pH value than the severity of the late decelerations, resulting in both acidosis and decreased Apgar scores. Typically, one would want to know the fetal pH value if late or moderate variable decelerations were present, especially in conjunction with unexplained loss of short-term variability.

Although not clinically in use at present, it is possible to continuously monitor fetal pH by application of a pH electrode embedded into the fetal scalp tissue. This electrode does not measure fetal blood pH level per se, but rather the subcutaneous tissue pH level. In hypoxia, initially an increase in alpha-adrenergic activity occurs with accompanying fetal hypertension, causing acidosis to occur in peripheral tissue more rapidly than in the central circulation. Conversely, as hypoxia is corrected, a recovery lag of the pH value in the peripheral tissue may result (Freeman and Garite, 1981).

Considerable skill is required for both continuous and intermittent fetal blood sampling. As yet, even intermittent sampling is not widely utilized due to the difficulty of the procedure and the unavailability of laboratories to obtain immediate results.

The major difficulties associated with fetal blood sampling include (Freeman and Garite, 1981):

1. Difficult procedure
2. Intermittent data
3. Scalp or buttocks data may not reflect data from the central circulation
4. Risks of fetal bleeding and infection
5. Data influenced by maternal acid-base status
6. Data influenced by carbon dioxide retention

The more information available about FHR monitoring, the less need for performing fetal blood pH sampling. Only in instances in which FHR patterns are suggestive of high risk, or are uninterpretable or worsening, is this adjunctive procedure indicated. Fetal blood sampling may obviate unnecessary cesarean delivery. Fetal blood sampling and electronic fetal monitoring are complementary tools. They help provide the physician with the knowledge he or she needs to make appropriate decisions about intervention or nonintervention.

SUMMARY

Effective thorough assessment of two individuals (woman and fetus) during the intrapartal period requires a nurse to have an understanding of normal and abnormal physiology of labor, risk factors, optimal use of monitoring techniques, the development of specific assessment skills, and knowledge of intervention techniques. Professional nursing responsibilities require in-depth understanding of the nursing process and a commitment to participate as an integral part of the health care team.

References

Boehn, F. H.; Graben, A. L.; and Hicks, M. M. 1978. Coordinated metabolic and obstetric management of diabetic pregnancy. *South Med. J.* 71:37.

Druzen, M.; Ikenoye, T.; Murata, Y.; et al. March 1979. A possible mechanism for the increase in FHR variability following hypoxemia. Presented at the 26th annual meeting of Society for Gynecological Investigation. San Diego, Calif.

Dulock, H. L., and Herron, M. 1976. Women's responses to fetal monitoring. *J. Obstet. Gynecol. Neonatal Nurs.* (Suppl.) 5(5):68s.

Freeman, R. K., and Garite, T. J. 1981. *Fetal heart rate monitoring.* Baltimore: Williams & Wilkins.

Freeman, R. K. April 1982. Fetal distress: diagnosis and management. Presented at the sixth International Symposium on Perinatal Medicine. Las Vegas, Nevada.

Friedman, E. A. 1970. An objective method of evaluating labor. *Hosp. Pract.* 5:82.

Haverkamp, A. D.; Orleans, M.; Langendoerfer, S.; et al. 1979. A controlled trial of the differential effects of intrapartum fetal monitoring. *Am. J. Obstet. Gynecol.* 134:399.

Hobel, C. J.; Hyvaninen, M. A.; Okada, D. M.; et al. 1973. Prenatal and intrapartum high risk screening. *Am. J. Obstet. Gynecol.* 117:1.

Hon, E. H. 1976. *An introduction to fetal heart rate monitoring.* 2nd ed. Los Angeles, Calif.: Univ. Southern Calif. Sch. of Med.

Hon, E., and Quilligan, E. J. 1967. The classification of fetal heart rate: II. A revised working classification. *Conn. Med.* 31:779.

Krebs, H. B.; Petres, R. E.; Dunn, L. J.; and Smith, P. J. 1982. Intrapartum fetal heart rate monitoring. *Am. J. Obstet. Gynecol.* 142(3):297.

Kubli, E. W.; Hon, E. H.; Khazin, A. F.; et al. 1969. Observations on heart rate and pH in the human fetus during labor. *Am. J. Obstet. Gynecol.* 104:1190.

Martin, C. B., and Gingerich, B. 1976. Factors affecting the fetal heart rate: genesis of FHR patterns. *J. Obstet. Gynecol. Neonatal Nurs.* (Suppl.) 5(5):305.

Modanlou, H.; Freeman, R. K.; and Braly, P. 1977. A simple method of fetal and neonatal heart rate beat-to-beat variability quantitation. *Am. J. Obstet. Gynecol.* 127:861.

Modanlou, H. D., and Freeman, R. K. 1982. Sinusoidal fetal heart rate pattern: its definition and clinical significance. *Am. J. Obstet. Gynecol.* 142(8):1033.

Molfese, V.; Sunshine, P.; and Bennett, A. 1982. Reactions of women to intrapartum fetal monitoring. *Obstet. Gynecol.* 59(6):705.

Monheit, A., and Cousins, L. Aug. 1981. When do you measure scalp and blood pH? *Contemp. OB/GYN.,* Med. Econ. Co., Inc.

National Institutes of Health, Institute of Child Health and Human Development. March 1979. Task force on predictors of fetal distress (draft), consensus development conference on antenatal diagnosis. Working document for discussion. Bethesda, Maryland.

Neutra, R. R.; Rienberg, S. E.; and Griedman, E. A. 1978. The effect of fetal monitoring on neonatal death rates. *N. Engl. J. Med.* 299:324.

Oxorn, H. 1980. *Human labor and birth.* New York: Appleton-Century-Crofts.

Paul, R. H., and Petrie, R. H. 1973. *Fetal intensive care: current concepts.* Los Angeles, Calif.: Univ. Southern Calif. Sch. of Med.

Petrie, R., and Pollack, K. J. 1976. Intrapartum fetal biochemical monitoring by fetal blood sampling. *J. Obstet. Gynecol. Neonatal Nurs.* (Suppl.) 5(5):52s.

Quilligan, E. J. July 1981. Fetal bradycardia: watch or deliver? *Contemp. OB/GYN.* 18:127.

Schifrin, B. S., and Dame, L. 1973. Fetal heart rate pattern prediction of Apgar score. *J.A.M.A.* 219:322.

Shields, D. Dec. 1978. Maternal reactions to fetal monitoring. *Am. J. Nurs.* 78:2110.

Starkman, M. N. 1977. Fetal monitoring/psychological consequences & management recommendations. *Obstet. Gynecol.* 50(4):500.

Starkman, M. N. 1976. Psychological responses to the use of the fetal monitor during labor. *Psychosom. Med.* 38:269.

Willson, J. R., and Carrington, E. 1979. *Obstetrics and gynecology.* 6th ed. St. Louis: The C. V. Mosby Co.

Wilson, R. W., and Schifrin, B. S. 1980. Is any pregnancy low risk? *Obstet. Gynecol.* 55(5):653.

Additional Readings

Banta, H. D., and Thacker, S. B. 1979. Assessing the costs and benefits of electronic fetal monitoring. *OB/GYN Surv.* 34(8):627.

Butnarescu, G. F.; Tillotson, D. M.; and Villarreal, P. P. 1980. Assessment of reproductive risk. In *Perinatal nursing,* vol. 2. New York: John Wiley & Sons.

Cranston, C. S. 1980. Obstetrical nurses' attitudes toward fetal monitoring. *J. Obstet. Gynecol. Neonatal Nurs.* 9(6):344.

Hon, E. H.; Zannini, D.; and Quilligan, E. J. 1975. The neonatal value of fetal monitoring. *Am. J. Obstet. Gynecol.* 122(4):508.

McDonough, M.; Sheriff, D.; and Simmel, P. 1981. Parents' responses to fetal monitoring. *MCN* 6:32.

NAACOG Technical Bulletin. 1980. The nurses' role in electronic fetal monitoring. No. 7.

Perez, R. H. 1981. Fetal monitoring. In *Protocols for perinatal nursing practice.* St. Louis: The C. V. Mosby Co.

Tucker, S. M. 1978. Electronic monitoring. In *Fetal monitoring and fetal assessment in high-risk pregnancy.* St. Louis: The C. V. Mosby Co.

■ 16 ■

THE FAMILY IN CHILDBIRTH:
NEEDS AND CARE

■ CHAPTER CONTENTS

NURSING MANAGEMENT OF ADMISSION

NURSING MANAGEMENT OF LABOR
    Cultural Considerations
    The Adolescent During Labor and Delivery
    Management of Pain Relief
    Nursing Care Plan

MANAGEMENT OF SPONTANEOUS DELIVERY
    Birthing Room
    Delivery Room
    Nursing Interventions
    Physician/Nurse-Midwife Interventions

IMMEDIATE CARE OF THE NEWBORN
    Apgar Scoring System
    Care of Umbilical Cord
    Physical Assessment of Newborn by
    Delivery Room Nurse
    Newborn Identification Procedures

**MANAGEMENT OF THE THIRD AND FOURTH
STAGES OF LABOR**
    Third Stage
    Fourth Stage

FACILITATION OF ATTACHMENT

**DELIVERY IN LESS-THAN-IDEAL
CIRCUMSTANCES**
    Precipitous Delivery
    Out-of-Hospital Births

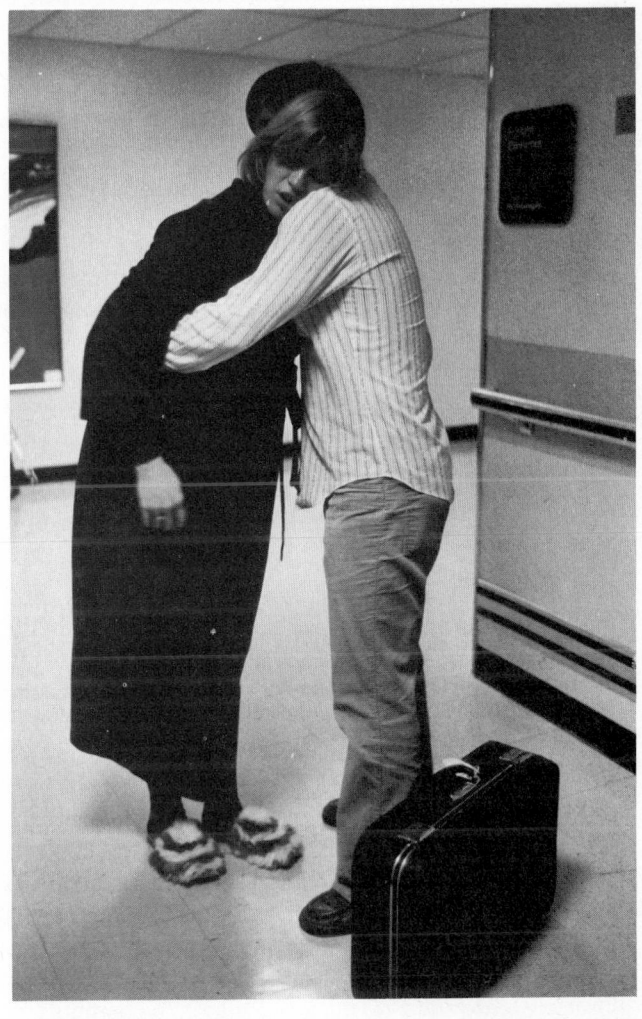

■ OBJECTIVES

- Identify the data base to be obtained and associated nursing care for the client during admission to the labor and delivery area.
- Discuss nursing interventions to meet the psychologic and physiologic needs of the client during each stage of labor and delivery.

- Identify the immediate needs of the newborn following delivery.
- Discuss immediate nursing care of the newborn.
- Discuss management of a delivery in less-than-optimal situations.

It is time for a child to be born. The waiting is over; labor has begun. The dreams and wishes of the past months fade as the expectant parents face the reality of the tasks of childbearing and childrearing that are ahead.

The couple is about to undergo one of the most meaningful and stressful events in their life together. The adequacy of their preparation for childbirth will receive its trial. The coping mechanisms and communication and support systems that they have established as a couple will be put to the test. In particular, the childbearing woman may feel that her psychologic and physical limits are about to be challenged.

The care rendered to all couples during labor and delivery can affect their feelings about this childbirth as well as future births. Nurses who can apply the concepts of the nursing process to their practice enhance the chances for each couple to have a positive childbearing experience.

The quality of nursing care received by the laboring couple depends on the accuracy of the nurse's assessment, diagnosis, and plan of care; skill in implementing that plan; and whether the outcomes of nursing interventions are desirable, expected, and positive. If the interventions are not successful, the nurse must evaluate the application of the nursing process and question whether the assessment and diagnosis were accurate, whether the objectives of the plan of care are realistic for that couple, and whether the interventions are appropriate for the identified problems.

Providing nursing care to the childbearing couple is challenging and rewarding. The nurse is participating in one of the most emotional experiences in life. Childbirth is usually joyous; sometimes it is a time of grief and sadness. In the event of complications, labor and delivery can be an extremely tense and stressful time for both the parents and the health care team. The needs of the childbearing couple in the event of crisis during or after labor and delivery are discussed in later chapters. In this chapter, however, the needs of the couple during normal labor and delivery are described, although normal delivery under less-than-ideal circumstances is also discussed.

NURSING MANAGEMENT OF ADMISSION

The client is instructed during her prenatal visits to come to the hospital if any of the following occur:

1. Rupture of amniotic membranes
2. Uterine contractions (nulliparas, 8–12 minutes apart; multiparas, 10–15 minutes apart)
3. Any vaginal bleeding

Early admission means less discomfort for the laboring woman when traveling to the hospital and more time to prepare for the delivery. Sometimes the labor is advanced and delivery is imminent but usually the client is in early labor at admission.

As the client enters the health care facility, she may be facing a number of unfamiliar procedures that health care providers tend to take for granted as routine practice. It is important to remember that all clients have the right to determine what happens to their bodies. *The client's informed consent should be obtained prior to any procedure that involves touching her body.* Informed consent requires that the client be given information about the procedure or care, its reasons, potential benefits and risks, and possible alternatives. To give informed consent, whether verbal or signed, the client should be considered a rational adult, and not under the influence of any medication that may affect her decision-making process. In most instances involving the nurse as the caregiver, the informed consent may be verbal. Each nurse needs to be aware of the requirements of the state and the individual hospital policies (Trandel-Korenchuk, 1982). (See Chapter 1 for additional discussion.)

The manner in which the client and her partner are greeted by the maternity nurse influences the course of the woman's hospital stay. It should be remembered that the sudden environmental change and sometimes impersonal technical aspects of the admission procedures can produce additional sources of stress. If she is greeted in a brusque, harried manner, she will be less likely to look to the nurse for support. A calm, pleasant manner is preferred when greeting the new admission. This calm manner indicates to the client that she is an important person and helps instill in the couple a sense of confidence in the staff's ability to provide quality care during this critical time.

Following the initial greeting, the client is taken into the labor room or birthing room. Some couples prefer to remain together during the admission process, and others prefer to have the partner wait outside. As the nurse helps the woman undress and get into a hospital gown, the nurse can begin conversing with her to establish the nursing data base. The experienced labor and delivery nurse can obtain essential information regarding the client and her pregnancy within a few minutes after admission, initiate any immediate interventions needed, and establish individualized priorities. The nurse is then able to make effective nursing decisions regarding intrapartal care: (a) Will a "prep" and/or enema be given? (b) Should ambulation or bed rest be encouraged? (c) Is more frequent monitoring needed? (d) What does the client want during her labor and delivery? (e) Is a support person available?

A major challenge for nurses is the formulation of realistic objectives for laboring women. Each woman has a different coping mechanism and support system. The single nullipara 14-year-old who has had no prenatal care and comes to the hospital alone does not bring the same coping mechanisms to the labor area as does the couple with a planned pregnancy who have attended prepared childbirth classes. The nurse may be the 14-year-old girl's support

system, whereas the nurse may be needed only minimally by the couple.

If indicated the client is assisted into bed. A side-lying or semi-Fowler's rather than supine position is most comfortable and avoids supine hypotensive syndrome (vena caval syndrome). When the pregnant woman assumes a supine position, the weight of the gravid uterus may cause partial occlusion of the vena cava (Figure 16–1). This occlusion results in shocklike symptoms as venous return to the heart is impaired, which produces hypotension, tachycardia, sweating, nausea and vomiting, and air hunger. Placental perfusion is also compromised. Recovery is immediate when the client is positioned on her side. The left side is favored because more pressure is then lifted from the vena cava, which is located slightly to the right of the midline. If recovery is not immediate, oxygen may be started by tight face mask, and intravenous fluids may be started. Occasionally a change in position to the other side is beneficial. The FHR should be closely monitored to assess fetal status.

Establishing rapport is a high priority and should be the first task. After the essential information is obtained from the client and her records, the nurse prepares to obtain appropriate objective data about vital signs, FHR, uterine activity, results of the sterile vaginal examination, and laboratory testing. (Chapter 15 considers intrapartal maternal assessment in depth.)

The nurse auscultates the FHR. (Detailed information on monitoring FHR is presented in Chapter 15.) The client's blood pressure, pulse, respiration, and oral temperature are determined. Contraction frequency, duration, and

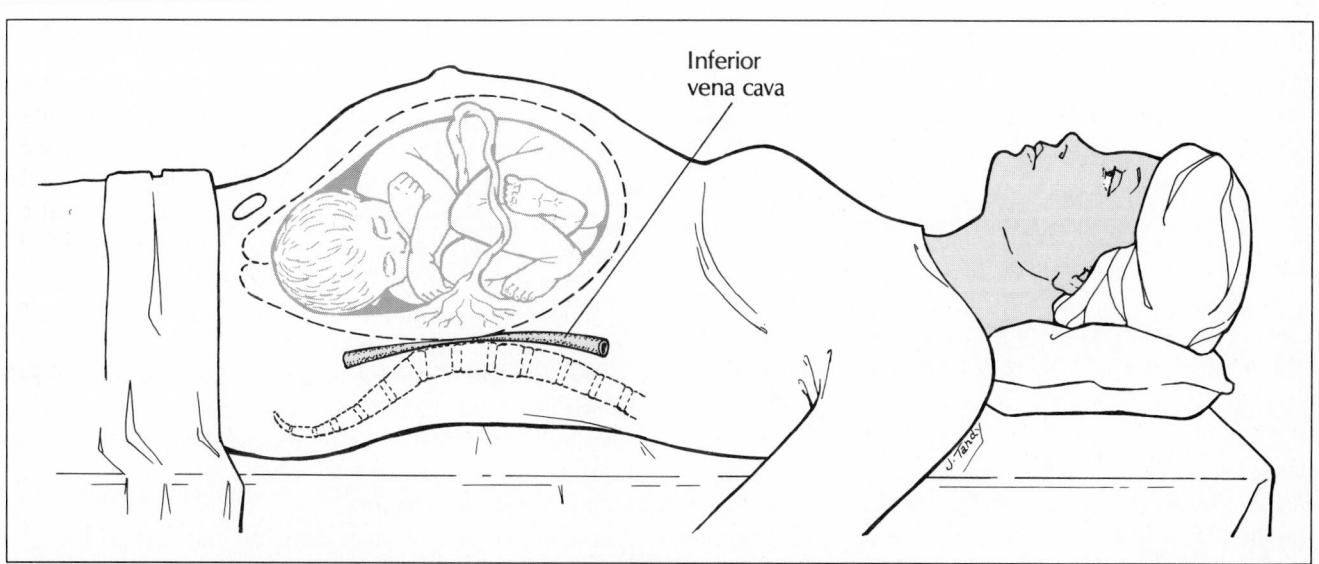

FIGURE 16–1 Venal caval syndrome. Gravid uterus compresses vena cava when the client is in a supine position. The blood flow returning to the heart is reduced, and maternal hypotension may result.

intensity are assessed; this may be done as other data are gathered. Before the sterile vaginal examination, the client should be informed about the procedure and its purpose. Afterward the nurse tells the client about the findings. It is important to remember that (a) if there are signs of advanced labor (frequent contractions, an urge to bear down, and so on), a vaginal examination must be done quickly, and (b) if there are signs of excessive bleeding or if the client reports episodes of bleeding in the last trimester, a vaginal examination should *not* be done.

Assessment of FHR, uterine contractions, and the results of the vaginal examination help determine whether the rest of the admission process can proceed at a more leisurely pace or whether additional interventions have higher priority. For example, auscultation of FHR of 110 beats/min necessitates the immediate application of a fetal monitor so that additional data may be obtained. The client's vital signs can be assessed after this is done.

After admission data are obtained, a clean-voided midstream urine specimen is collected. The client with intact membranes may walk to the bathroom. If the membranes are ruptured and the presenting part is not engaged, the woman is generally asked to remain in bed to avoid prolapse of the cord. Ambulation when membranes are ruptured may depend on client desires, clinician requests, or agency policy. The urine may be tested for the presence of protein, ketones, and glucose by using a dipstick before it is sent to the laboratory. This procedure is especially important if edema or elevated blood pressure is noted on admission. Proteinuria may be a sign of impending preeclampsia if it is 2+ or greater and not contaminated with blood or amniotic fluid. Ketonuria is a good index of starvation ketosis. Glycosuria is found frequently in pregnant women because of the increased glomerular filtration rate in the proximal tubules and the inability of these tubules to increase reabsorption of glucose. Although common, glycosuria should not be discounted. Researchers have demonstrated that 20% of pregnant women with glycosuria and with a strong family history of diabetes are class A, or latent, diabetics (Burrow and Ferris, 1982). Presence of glycosuria necessitates follow-up evaluation.

While the client is obtaining the urine specimen, the equipment for shaving the pubic area (referred to as the *prep*) and for the enema, if ordered, may be prepared. Many clinicians leave standing orders for prep measures and enema administration. Prep orders vary, but some believe that this form of skin preparation facilitates their work in the delivery room, makes perineal repair easier, and facilitates cleansing of the perineum in the postpartal period. The use of perineal preps is a controversial issue now. Many clients question the need for a prep and request that it be omitted. The nurse needs to ascertain the client's wishes in this matter. Clients who do not want a prep probably have discussed this with the physician/ nurse-midwife during the prenatal course. If a prep is to be

done, one of two types may be chosen: (a) *complete prep*, which is the removal of all pubic, perineal, and rectal hair; or (b) *mini prep*, which is the removal of perineal hair from the level of the clitoris, or lower edge of the vagina, downward to the rectum.

The nurse performing a prep washes hands and then positions the woman in the same manner as for a vaginal examination. A towel is placed under the client's buttocks. Lighting is adjusted so that the perineal area may be well visualized. The client is questioned about the presence of any moles or warts while the nurse is applying the soap solution with a gauze square or sponge provided in the prep set. The (right-handed) nurse holds the skin taut with the left hand, using a towel from the prep set or a single disposable glove to protect fingers, and shaves in short strokes, holding the razor in the right hand. The nurse works downward to the vagina. When the perineum has been shaved, the client is asked to turn to her left side and to assume the lateral Sims position. Again using the towel or disposable glove to protect the hand, the nurse pulls the upper buttock upward to expose the rectal area. After sudsing, the area around the rectum is shaved. The nurse must take care to prevent contaminants from the rectal area from entering the vaginal area.

The administration of an enema is also controversial. Proponents say the purposes of an enema are to: (a) evacuate the lower bowel so that labor will not be impeded; (b) stimulate uterine contractions; (c) avoid client embarrassment if bowel contents are expelled during pushing efforts; and (d) prevent contamination of the sterile field during delivery. Those who question the routine use of an enema on admission suggest that labor is impeded only by a severe bowel impaction, question whether labor is stimulated, and find that feces still may be expelled during pushing efforts. They also note that an enema may be an uncomfortable procedure.

After determining the client's wishes regarding an enema, the nurse notifies the clinician. The presence of some factors contraindicates the enema. They are vaginal bleeding, unengaged presenting part, rapid labor progress, and imminent delivery. These factors need to be identified. If an enema is to be given, the reasons and the procedure are explained to the client, and then the enema is administered while she is on her left side.

If the membranes are intact and labor is not far advanced, the client may expel the enema in the bathroom; otherwise she is positioned on the bedpan in bed. Raising the side rails on the bed will provide safety and facilitate self-positioning for comfort.

Before leaving the labor area, the nurse must be sure that the client knows how to operate the call system so that she can obtain help if she needs it. After the enema is expelled, the nurse monitors the FHR again to assess any changes. If the woman's partner has been out of the labor room, the couple is reunited as soon as possible.

In many hospitals, the admission process also includes signing a delivery permit, fingerprinting the pregnant woman for the infant records, and fastening an identification bracelet to the client's wrist.

Depending on how rapidly labor is progressing, the nurse notifies the clinician before or after completing the admission procedures. The report should include data concerning cervical dilatation and effacement, station, presenting part, status of the membranes, contraction pattern, FHR, any vital signs that are not in the normal range, the client's wishes, and her reaction to labor.

In addition to the physical labor admission procedures, laboratory tests are carried out. Hemoglobin and hematocrit values may be obtained to help determine the oxygen-carrying capacity of the circulatory system and the ability of the woman to withstand blood loss at delivery. Elevation of the hematocrit may indicate hemoconcentration of blood, which occurs with edema or dehydration, while a low hemoglobin, in the absence of other evidence of bleeding, suggests anemia. Blood may be typed and cross-matched if the client is in a high-risk category.

A serology test for syphilis is obtained if one has not been done in the last 3 months or if antepartal serology result was positive.

Nursing management of labor will be influenced by the physical, psychologic, and cultural data obtained during the admission process. An overview of some support measures the nurse may initiate are presented in Table 16–1. Detailed nursing actions are presented in Nursing Care Plan—Labor and Delivery, p.472.

NURSING MANAGEMENT OF LABOR

Cultural Considerations

Knowledge of specific values, customs, and practices of different cultures is as important in the labor phase as in the prenatal phase of the childbearing. Without this knowledge, a nurse is less likely to understand a client's behavior and may impose personal values and beliefs upon a client. As cultural sensitivity increases, so does the likelihood of providing high-quality care.

A culture often assigns certain superstitions, taboos, and beliefs regarding spirits around significant events such as the delivery of a child. This activity is often a mechanism for dealing with anxiety. For example, in a rural Cambodian home, a laboring woman often lies on a bed with a fire beneath it to drive away evil spirits (Hollingsworth et al., 1980). As soon as a baby is born to a Mexican American woman, she places her legs together to prevent air from entering the womb (Kay, 1978).

It is also common to prescribe certain activities for the relief of pain during childbirth. It is not uncommon for Southern U.S. white or black families to place a knife, razor, or ax under the bed to "cut the labor pains" (Murphee, 1968). During labor, the Laguna Pueblo Indian woman often holds onto a belt that has been blessed (Farris, 1978). In other tribes the medicine man may be called to give a special potion to the woman and to offer prayers for her. A badger claw is often given to a laboring Keresian Indian woman, since it is believed that badgers are good at "digging out" (Higgins and Wayland, 1981).

In looking at specific practices on position, food, and drink during labor, obvious differences between Western medicine and some cultures are apparent. In most non-European societies uninfluenced by Westernization, women assume an upright position in childbirth. Some traditional American Indian women give birth in upright positions. For example, the Pueblo woman gives birth on her knees and the Zuni woman kneels or squats while a midwife kneads her abdomen (Higgins and Wayland, 1981). In some tribes, certain teas made of juniper twigs may be given to relax the woman (Higgins and Wayland, 1981). In Southern black and white groups, three different teas are given "to keep the labor coming" and drinking of Coca Cola is encouraged (Murphee, 1968). Some of these beliefs may be encountered by maternity nurses today.

In working with clients from another culture, an awareness of historical beliefs and practices is helpful in understanding their behavior. In many cases, certain old practices are retained either in part or in full. An awareness of cultural values is also necessary, since specific behavior is often dictated by these traditional views. The three values that are especially important during labor are modesty, expression of pain, and the role of the father during labor and delivery. The following sections briefly describe some cultural differences in these areas.

MODESTY

Modesty is an important value for Oriental, Native American, and Mexican American women. Some Oriental women are not accustomed to male physicians and attendants and may prefer female physicians and attendants. For these three cultures pregnancy is often viewed as "female business" (Chung, 1977). Modesty is of great concern to these women, and exposure of as little of the client's body as possible is strongly recommended (Abril, 1977).

PAIN EXPRESSION

The role of culture in determining attitudes toward and reactions to pain was first explored by Zborowski (1952). His study was conducted with four groups: Jewish, Italian, Irish, and "Old Americans." Old Americans were defined as whites whose grandparents were born in the United States. Italian and Jewish cultures tended to be more emotional in their responses to pain than the Irish and Old Americans, who exhibited little emotional complaining, but reported on their pain instead.

Table 16–1   Normal Progress, Psychologic Characteristics, and Nursing Support During First and Second Stage of Labor

Phase	Cervical dilatation	Uterine contractions	Client response	Support measures
Stage 1 Latent phase	1–4 cm	Every 15–30 min, 15–30 sec duration Mild intensity	Usually happy, talkative, and eager to be in labor Exhibits need for independence by taking care of own bodily needs and seeking information	Get acquainted with client (and partner, if present) and ascertain her preparation and needs; initiate discharge planning; instruct her in breathing techniques if she has not had prenatal classes Orient family to equipment, monitors, procedures; allow client to participate in care Provide needed information
Active phase	4–7 cm	Every 3–5 min, 30–60 sec duration Moderate intensity	May experience feelings of helplessness; exhibits increased fatigue and may begin to feel restless and anxious as contractions become stronger; expresses fear of abandonment Becomes more dependent as she is less able to meet her needs	Encourage to maintain breathing patterns; provide quiet environment to reduce external stimuli and reassure Inform couple of labor progress Anticipate needs; allow client to assist in her care as she desires or is able to
Transition	8–10 cm	Every 2–3 min, 45–90 sec duration Strong intensity	Tires and may exhibit increased restlessness and irritability; may feel she cannot keep up with labor process and is out of control Physical discomforts Fear of being left alone May fear tearing open or splitting apart with contractions	Encourage client to rest between contractions; if she sleeps between contractions, wake her at increment of contraction so she can begin breathing pattern; this measure decreases feelings of being out of control Praise couple's efforts and inform them of progress Encourage continued participation of supports and provide support
Stage 2	Complete		May feel out of control; helpless; panicky	Gentle but firm directions to couple; maintain good eye contact with client; encourage inclusion and participation of support person

Differences in pain expression may also be seen among Orientals, blacks, and Mexican Americans. The laboring Oriental woman may not outwardly express pain for fear of shaming herself and her family (Hollingsworth et al., 1980). Orientals are anxious about losing face through one's behavior. Black women may also appear rather stoic in an effort to avoid showing weakness or calling undue attention to themselves (Carrington, 1978). Mexican American women, on the other hand, may be more expressive during labor. One way they may express pain and suffering is through groaning and moaning (Murillo-Rohde, 1979). Yet another behavior is for Mexican American women in labor to keep their mouths closed for fear of making the uterus rise. They are to yell only during exhalation (Kay, 1978).

Understanding pain behavior helps lead to an accurate assessment of the client's condition. Nonverbal communication becomes vital. In working with clients of another culture, language is often a barrier: if possible, an interpreter should be used. It is also important to be aware of communication differences, so that a nurse does not inadvertently indicate hostility, rejection, or lack of interest to a client.

In assessing clients' pain, it is beneficial for the nurse to assess personal views of physical and psychologic distress. One study of nurses in six different cultures found that nurses' beliefs regarding suffering reflected their cultural backgrounds (Davitz et al., 1976). For example, it was found that most Americans believe that Orientals feel less pain because their behavior does not appear to reflect pain. On the other hand, a nurse with a cultural background that dictates stoic behavior may have difficulty in understanding a client who has learned to freely express pain. An awareness of one's own values leads to a greater acceptance of another's behavior.

ROLE OF THE FATHER

In some cultures the husband or father attends the birth. In other groups the man is not present. In American Indian tribes, a midwife and female relatives traditionally assist the Indian woman giving birth. In the traditional Navajo tribe, all family members view the birth process (Farris, 1978). Oriental and Vietnamese fathers do not participate in childbirth since it is considered "women's work." Historically, black women provided emotional support to a woman during childbirth. Today many black women prefer to have their mothers present instead of the newborn's father (Carrington, 1978).

Who participates in the birth process is an important consideration for nurses. The participation of the father should not be assumed: his participation varies among cultures. A nurse's sensitivity to these different values alleviates unnecessary stress for the family. Nurses should be aware that fathers often do perform definite functions even though they may not participate in the actual childbirth. In this case they are still viewed as active participants. They may adhere to certain taboos, perform certain rituals, experience couvade, or even simulate labor (Heggenhougen, 1980).

The Adolescent During Labor and Delivery

The adolescent who has taken childbirth education classes is generally better prepared than the adolescent who has had no preparation. The prepared teenager usually better tolerates the labor experience. The nurse must keep in mind, however, that the younger the adolescent is, the less she may be able to actively participate in the process. Because of incomplete cognitive development, she may have less problem-solving capabilities. The younger teen may feel more threatened in terms of her ego-intactness and vulnerability to stress and discomfort.

The nurse becomes the primary advocate for the adolescent. The nursing support role varies depending on the client's own support system during labor. Not all young women in labor arrive with someone who will stay with her during childbirth. It is important for the nurse to establish a trusting relationship with the young client to assist her in maintaining control and understanding what is happening to her. Establishing rapport without recrimination for possible inappropriate behavior is essential. The adolescent who is given positive reinforcement for "work well done" will leave the experience with increased self-esteem, despite the emotional problems that may accompany her situation.

Each young woman in labor is different. The nurse must assess what each client brings to the experience. Nursing assessment asks the following questions:

- What are the client's attitudes and feelings about the pregnancy?
- Who will attend the birth and what is the person's relationship to the client?
- What does the client expect from the support person?
- What preparation has the client had for the experience?
- What are the client's expectations and fears regarding labor and delivery?
- How has her culture influenced her?
- What are her usual coping mechanisms?
- Does she plan to keep the newborn?

A verbal contract between nurse and client facilitates compliance and lets the adolescent know how the nurse will participate during the experience.

One of the greatest fears of any laboring woman is being left alone. The very young adolescent (under age 14) has fewer coping mechanisms and less experience to draw on than her older counterparts have. She needs to rely on the presence of someone at all times during labor. The very young adolescent may have unrealistic expectations of herself during labor. She will be more childlike and dependent than older teens and will require simple, concrete directions and explanations. During the transition phase she may become withdrawn and unable to express her need for nurturance. Measures to maintain her comfort and the nurse's touch and soothing encouragement help the client maintain control and meet her dependency needs.

During the second stage of labor, the young client may feel as if she is losing control and may reach out to those around her. This is her attempt to maintain ego-integrity. By remaining calm and being directive, the nurse helps the client to control feelings of helplessness.

The middle adolescent (age 14–17) often attempts to remain calm and unflinching during labor. This age group's coping behavior may be frustrating to the nursing staff because they appear aloof to nursing intervention and support. Although the nurse may not be able to break through

(Text continues on p. 482.)

NURSING CARE PLAN
Labor and Delivery

PATIENT DATA BASE

History

Client's name

Age of client

Obstetric history: gravida, para, abortions, fetal deaths, birth weight of previous children, complications during previous labors and deliveries

Estimated delivery date, calculated gestational age, and LMP (first day of last menstrual period)

Client and family medical history: health status of living children, medications taken during pregnancy, recent infections

Prenatal care: type and amount, any significant antepartal problems

Prenatal education: type of childbirth preparation

Pediatrician

Chosen method of infant feeding

Status of labor: when contractions began, when they became regular, quality of contractions; how client seems to be coping with contractions at this time

Status of membranes: intact, ruptured, time ruptured, fluid characteristics, amount of fluid

Time of last meal

Physical examination

(see Intrapartal Physical Assessment Guide, Chapter 15)

General appearance of client and partner (calm appearance or anxious)

Height and weight

Vital signs

Presence of edema

Abdomen and fundus (size and contour)

Hydration

Perineum

Uterine contractions

Nitrazine test

Vaginal examination: cervical dilatation and effacement, presentation and position of fetus, membranes

Fetal status (FHR)

Assessment of heart, lungs, and breasts may be done in some institutions

Laboratory evaluation

Hemoglobin

Hematocrit

CBC

Maternal blood type

Serologic tests

Urinalysis

NURSING PRIORITIES

1. Assess physical and psychologic status of client
2. Assess uterine contractile patterns
3. Assess status of fetus (FHR, position, presence of meconium, hyperactivity)
4. Assess labor progress
5. Prepare client for delivery
6. Support laboring client and coach (or partner) as needed

CLIENT/FAMILY EDUCATION FOCUS

1. Provide explanation of procedures as they are done
2. Discuss available options regarding labor and delivery
3. Provide opportunities to discuss individual questions and concerns of client and family

NURSING INTERVENTIONS

The interventions given here are based on common needs of laboring couples per stage of labor. Couples prepared in the psychoprophylactic method of childbirth are taught to begin the first concentrated breathing exercise when needed and to change to the next one only when the first one is not serving its purpose. Consequently, some couples may be able to use one or two breathing exercises throughout the entire labor experience. Although certain exercises are suggested with different labor phases, the couple need not use this particular breathing exercise if the need is not there. Similarly, nursing actions performed in one phase or stage of labor may need to be performed in other phases or throughout labor. The intervention depends on the problems identified with continued assessment.

Problem	Nursing interventions and actions	Rationale
FIRST STAGE		
Latent phase *Admission*	Greet couple warmly; orient couple to environment and admission procedures. Obtain history	Conveys acceptance, reduces anxiety, and establishes rapport Provides data base

NURSING CARE PLAN Cont'd
Labor and Delivery

Problem	Nursing interventions and actions	Rationale
	Assess maternal vital signs and FHR	Provides baseline values
	Notify physician or nurse-midwife of admission	
	Perform Intrapartal Physical Assessment (see Chapter 15)	
	Administer enema if ordered	Enema empties lower bowel; may stimulate uterine contractions, prevent contamination of sterile field during delivery, and facilitate descent of presenting part
	Perform perineal prep if ordered	Shaving of skin in pubic and perineal areas may facilitate perineal repair and cleansing of perineum in postpartal period
	Obtain urine specimen	Proteinuria of 2+ or more found in urine that is not contaminated with blood or amniotic fluid may be sign of ensuing preeclampsia
	Check FHR after woman expels enema	A change in fetal station may cause fetal distress if cord has progressed before presenting part
Physiologic maintenance	Assess vital signs:	Maternal vital signs provide information on state of dehydration, development of infection or maternal fetal complications
	1. Temperature every 4 hr unless >37.5C (99.6F), in which case check every 2 hr	
	2. Check BP, pulse, and respirations every hour; if BP >140/90, pulse >100, and/or respiration >22/min, notify physician	BP >140/90 requires more frequent reassessment and additional assessments of signs and symptoms of preeclampsia
Labor progress		
1. Dilatation	Begin charting on Friedman graph (see Figure 15-11)	Confirms normal or detects abnormal labor progression
a. Cervix 1–4 cm dilated		
b. Effacement occurring	Assess dilatation and effacement by vaginal examination	
2. Contractions	Assess contractions by palpation and/or electronic methods	
a. Becoming regular		
b. Frequency: every 15–30 min		
c. Duration: 15–30 sec		
d. Intensity: mild to moderate		
3. Bloody show and mucous plug	Ascertain presence of bloody show and passage of mucous plug	As labor begins, mucous plug is shed
		Beginning dilatation of cervix causes rupture of small capillaries in cervix, which results in blood-tinged mucus
Fetal status	Check FHR every 30–60 min as long as it remains between 120–160/min; if FHR is outside these parameters, continuous monitoring is recommended; at some time during early labor, attach external monitor for at least 15 min to assess fetal status; monitor may be removed and reapplied later or allowed to remain throughout labor, depending on findings	Evaluates fetal well-being, and provides information concerning fetal response to labor

NURSING CARE PLAN Cont'd
Labor and Delivery

Problem	Nursing interventions and actions	Rationale
	Palpate abdomen (Leopold's maneuvers, p. 441)	Determines fetal position
	Perform vaginal examination to assess degree of engagement of presenting part	Presenting part may be engaged in the nullipara and entering the inlet in the multipara
Activity	Encourage client to ambulate if desired unless any of following are present:	Ambulation may increase client comfort thereby reducing the need for analgesics; may be associated with shorter labors and may lower the incidence of FHR abnormalities (Flynn et al., 1978; McKay, 1980; Carr, 1980)
	1. Ruptured membranes	Prolapse of cord is possible
	2. Malpresentation and/or malposition of fetus	
	3. Vaginal bleeding	
	4. Advanced labor	Client may deliver suddenly
	5. Administration of analgesic agent	Client may feel dizzy or drowsy
	If the client cannot ambulate, encourage her to maintain a sitting position or a side-lying position; change positions frequently	The sitting position may promote client comfort; lateral side-lying position prevents supine hypotension syndrome and is associated with contractions of less frequency but greater intensity (McKay, 1980)
Discomfort (back or lower abdomen)	Assist in diversional activities — for example a conducted tour of facilities — if her membranes are intact and she can ambulate	Woman's attention is diverted away from her discomfort and contractions
		Tour familiarizes couple with the territory
	Assess couple's coping mechanisms for labor and answer their questions	Provides information; reduces fear of unknown; provides labor coping mechanism
	Anticipatory guidance may be needed for unprepared couple	
	Suggest to couple that they begin the following measures if needed:	Provides focus for attention and other busy work for the brain
	Effleurage	Stimulation eases abdominal discomfort
	Pelvic rocking or a back rub	Eases back discomfort
Sleep/rest	Encourage woman to relax	Reduces tension, conserves energy, and decreases discomfort
Sustenance	If clinician permits, woman may have clear liquids or ice chips	Provides energy and maintains hydration
	Do not give laboring woman solid foods	Gastrointestinal absorption is decreased during labor; client may vomit and aspirate gastric contents while under medication or anesthesia
Elimination	Encourage client to void every 2 hr or as needed	A full bladder can cause discomfort, impede descent of the fetus, and cause dysfunctional labor
	Check for bladder distention	Client may not have urge to void due to decreased tone of bladder from pressure from the presenting part

NURSING CARE PLAN Cont'd
Labor and Delivery

Problem	Nursing interventions and actions	Rationale
	If catherization is necessary, use small flexible catheter (no. 14 French) and lubricate well so it slides in easily; insert catheter between contractions, because during contraction fetal head presses down and makes insertion difficult and painful	Bladder trauma may predispose to post-partal urinary retention and cystitis
	Record intake and output	Evaluates hydration status
Care giving and receiving	Couple can usually manage during this phase of labor; nurse should periodically see if she can be of assistance	
	Provide privacy and prevent exposure by adequate draping during all procedures	Preserves modesty and demonstrates respect for individual
Psychologic maintenance	Listen and convey acceptance of behavior and attitudes	Couple usually is happy and relieved that this day has finally arrived; they may have some fear of the unknown and may anticipate problems
	Give correct information and support; inform couple of any procedures; answer any questions	
Active phase		
Physiologic maintenance	Assess vital signs: 1. Temperature every 4 hr unless >37.5C (99.6F), in which case check every 2 hr 2. BP, pulse, and respirations every hour	Evaluates maternal status
Labor progress	Chart data on Friedman graph	Provides objective means of assessing progress and detecting abnormal patterns

1. Dilatation
    a. Cervix 4-7 cm (active dilatation)
    b. Effacement complete (100%)
	Perform vaginal examination to assess dilatation and effacement	

	Encourage shallow chest breathing during examination (Lamaze — level 1)	Promotes relaxation

2. Contractions
    a. Regular
    b. Frequency: every 3-5 min
    c. Duration: 30-60 sec
    d. Intensity: moderate
	Assess contractions every 15 min	

3. Increase in bloody show and vaginal discharge	Change bed pads frequently	Promotes hygiene and comfort
	Wash perineum with warm water and dry the area	Keeps contaminants from reaching the vagina
Fetal status	Check FHR every 15 min by fetal monitor or by auscultation (immediately after contractions); count for at least 30 sec	Evaluates effect of active labor on fetus
Activity	Institute bed rest if client has been ambulatory up to this point, if she is tiring	Quality of contractions is better due to increased placental perfusion and increased O_2 transport to fetus; when client is on her back, uterus lies on vena cava and obstructs venous return from extremities; reduction of blood volume results in signs and symptoms of shock
	Assist coach in helping the woman into comfortable position (lateral position is recommended)	

NURSING CARE PLAN Cont'd
Labor and Delivery

Problem	Nursing interventions and actions	Rationale
	Observe for signs of vena caval syndrome, such as drop in BP; elevation of pulse; air hunger; pallor; moist, clammy skin; marked change in baseline FHR	
Discomfort 1. Feelings of pain increasing	Coach may suggest that client switch to another level of breathing (Lamaze—level 2) Offer pharmacologic support; if analgesic is administered: 1. Instruct client to remain in bed 2. Keep side rails up 3. Check maternal vital signs, FHTs, and fetal activity	Promotes safety; medication may make client dizzy and/or drowsy; client and/or fetus may respond poorly to medication
2. Backache	Administer or encourage coach to administer back rub (see Chapter 11)	Relieves discomfort
Sleep/rest	Provide environment conducive to relaxation (dim lights, decreased noise and activity in and out of room, soft music) Assist coach in identifying factors interrupting relaxation Offer to relieve labor coach	Relaxation enhances labor experience, conserves energy, and lessens pain Coach needs rest and sustenance
Sustenance	Provide ice chips Assess following parameters of hydration status: 1. Measure pulse and temperature for elevation 2. Check skin for dryness 3. Check client's lips for cracking and apply petroleum jelly or similar agent Intravenous electrolyte solution may be given at this time; monitor rate	Determines presence of dehydration and development of hypoglycemia; labor depletes the glycogen stores and thereby increases the chance of hypoglycemia Provides energy and prevents dehydration or corrects a dehydrated state
Elimination (bladder)	Continue to encourage woman to void every 2 hr; check for bladder distention	Prevents distention, discomfort, and trauma to bladder
Care giving and receiving 1. Dry mouth	Provide ice chips, mouth wash, glycerine swabs; assist her in brushing her teeth	Promotes comfort
2. Cracked lips	Apply petroleum jelly to lips	Promotes comfort
3. Vaginal discharges	Change linen and bed pads frequently Provide perineal care	Promotes hygiene and comfort and relieves discomforts from secretions
4. Diaphoresis	Sponge body and face	Relieves discomfort
Psychologic maintenance	Assure couple that efforts of labor are effective Provide information about labor progress	Couple becomes more serious and purposeful and less talkative; client is less receptive to instructions other than those given by her partner Decreases anxiety, because woman may begin to have fears or doubts about coping

NURSING CARE PLAN Cont'd
Labor and Delivery

Problem	Nursing interventions and actions	Rationale
	Avoid using words like *slow* when talking about progress	Connotations of the word *slow* can be discouraging
	Praise accomplishments of client and labor coach	Promotes confidence of laboring couple
Deceleration phase (Transition)	Continue graphic analysis of labor and physiologic parameters	Provides objective data about labor patterns
	Assess vital signs	
Labor progress	Continue graphic analysis	
1. Dilatation pattern	Assess by vaginal examination	
a. Cervix 8–10 cm		
b. Effacement complete (100%)	Multipara may be taken to delivery room at 8 cm cervical dilatation; nullipara may stay in labor room until dilatation is complete, fetus has descended, and there is perineal bulging	Tissues and muscles of birth canal in multipara are more relaxed, and birth process is more rapid; deceleration phase in multiparas lasts about 30 min
	Remain with couple	
2. Contractions	Assess each contraction	This is most active phase of first stage
a. Regular		
b. Frequency: every 2–3 min		
c. Duration: 45–90 sec		
d. Intensity: strong		
3. Heavy bloody show	Change bed pad and administer perineal care	Decreases chances of infection and provides comfort
4. Rupture of membranes	Monitor FHR immediately after membranes rupture (spontaneously or due to amniotomy)	Determines presence of prolapsed cord, which can occur with rupture of membranes if pelvic inlet is not occluded
	Inspect amniotic fluid for color, odor, amount, and consistency	To detect presence of meconium staining and infection
	Report and record observations	
	Perform vaginal examination, assessing dilatation, fetal position, and station	Rupture of membranes is usually sign of advanced progress
	Palpate for cord	Confirms absence of cord prolapse
	Dry perineum and change bed pad	Promotes comfort and good hygiene
Fetal status	Monitor fetal heart rate every 15 min or more frequently, especially in event of bradycardia or tachycardia; if bradycardia is noted immediately following contraction, apply fetal monitor to assess whether decelerations are present (see p. 454 for further discussion)	This is most active phase for fetus; uterus is contracting frequently, increasing anoxic periods for fetus
Discomfort		
1. Generalized discomfort	Coach should try variation of pant-blow breathing (Lamaze — Level 3)	Highly complex breathing pattern involves more mental concentration, thus decreasing pain reception at cerebral level
2. May have severe abdominal back pain or irritable abdomen	Apply firm pressure to lower abdomen and/or lower back	Alleviates some discomfort by producing counterpressure
	Apply heat to abdomen or back by using k-pad or hot water bottle	Warmth soothes muscle discomfort
	Palpate contractions lightly	

NURSING CARE PLAN Cont'd
Labor and Delivery

Problem	Nursing interventions and actions	Rationale
	Avoid pressure	
	Assist client to change position	
3. Trembling		May be due to very rapid labor
Sleep/rest	Assist coach in watching for tension and keeping woman relaxed	
	Encourage coach to awaken woman at beginning of contraction to begin her breathing exercises	Woman dozes between contractions and wakens at peak of contraction; breathing exercises provide focus of concentration, reducing perception of pain
Sustenance	Continue to observe for hypoglycemia	Deceleration phase of labor requires much energy
	Increase rate of parenteral fluids if signs of dehydration occur; due to great activity of this labor phase, client will probably not tolerate any quantity of oral intake	Fluid is lost by means of diaphoresis
	Offer sips or chips at frequent intervals	Breathing patterns tend to dry out the mouth
Elimination	Check for bladder distention	
Nausea and vomiting	Apply cold cloth to woman's throat	Helps alleviate nausea
	Elevate head of bed	
Care giving and receiving		
1. Diaphoresis (especially on upper lip and forehead)	Wash face; apply cool cloth to forehead	Promotes comfort
2. Hiccups, holding breath, urge to push	Check to see if complete dilatation has occurred; if it has not, urge woman to blow	Pushing on cervix that is not completely dilated results in cervical edema and increases danger of cervical lacerations and fetal head trauma; blowing exercise inhibits breath holding and pushing efforts
3. Leg tremors	Assure couple that this is normal and explain cause	Fetal head is pressing on nerves and blocks vessels to extremities
4. Muscle cramps in lower extremities	Place blankets over legs and feet	Circulation is diverted to uterus and upper body. Because of decreased circulation, extremities become cold.
	Extend client's leg and dorsiflex foot	Counteracts spasm, promoting relaxation
Hyperventilation	Encourage slow breathing, breathing with her if necessary	Hyperventilation increases loss of carbon dioxide and leads to respiratory alkalosis
	Client may breathe into paper bag	Woman may complain of tingling and numbness of lips, face, hands, and feet or may develop carpopedal spasms
Psychologic maintenance	Praise and encourage the laboring couple	
	Help them through one contraction at a time	Reinforces couple's ability to cope
	Convey an accepting, caring attitude	

NURSING CARE PLAN Cont'd
Labor and Delivery

Problem	Nursing interventions and actions	Rationale
	Coach (or nurse) should call woman by name, speak with firm, short commands, breathe with her, and maintain eye contact	Woman may become angry at nurse and labor coach, loss of control can occur
SECOND STAGE (EXPULSION PHASE)		
Physiologic maintenance	Assess vital signs	
Labor progress	Perform vaginal examination to assure complete dilatation (10 cm and 100% effaced)	
	Nullipara is taken to delivery room when perineal bulging is noted; after woman is in delivery room, check BP every 5–15 min and FHT after each contraction	Abdominal musculature contracts to assist with expulsion; the woman feels strong urge to push (similar to urge to defecate); anal eversion occurs, as does perineal bulging and flattening; introitus gradually opens wider with each contraction
	When client is taken to delivery room, provide scrub suit, boots, hat, and mask for partner if he is going into delivery room with her	
	Assess physiologic parameters of expulsion phase	
	Assist woman to a comfortable position for pushing	
	Elevate head of bed or delivery table 30°–60° or place pillows under head and torso; woman's legs should be spread slightly and knees slightly flexed (see Figure 16–5)	Facilitates expulsion; when woman's shoulders are raised, use of abdominal muscles is facilitated
	If woman's feet are to be placed in stirrups, lift both legs simultaneously to reduce muscle strain; feet should be supported with stirrups in low position with no pressure on popliteal area or calf of leg	Pressure on popliteal area or calf of leg may lead to thrombophlebitis
	Adjust handles so that client may pull back on them while pushing and so there is slight flexion of arm; at beginning of the contraction, the woman should be instructed to take two short breaths, holding third breath while leaning forward in a "C" position as she steadily bears down	Pushing adds the forces of intra-abdominal pressure to the existing intra-uterine pressure which moves the baby through the birth canal
	Encourage woman to exhale and inhale and repeat bearing-down effort until contraction ends	Providing intervals between the pushing effort minimizes the fall in maternal Po_2 and rise in Pco_2 (Nobel, 1981)
	Some women may prefer to exhale slightly during pushing efforts to avoid physiologic effects of Valsalva maneuver (see p. 409)	
	Encourage use of panting when pushing is undesirable	

NURSING CARE PLAN Cont'd
Labor and Delivery

Problem	Nursing interventions and actions	Rationale
Fetal status	Observe perineum for appearance of fetal vertex	Nullipara is transported to delivery room when vertex is visible at introitus without spreading labia
	Monitor FHR	Pressure is being exerted on fetal head with each expulsive effort
	Electronic monitoring device may be moved to delivery room with client to assess fetal response to efforts of delivery; if electronic monitoring device is not in use, auscultate FHR after each contraction	
Discomfort 1. May be decreasing 2. Stretching, burning sensations as infant moves into vagina and compresses perineal nerves	Praise pushing efforts; inform couple when head becomes visible (some delivery rooms have mirrors for couple to see infant emerge); provide cool wash cloth for forehead and face	Communicates success of couple's hard work Shows that client can work with forces of labor
Sleep/rest	Encourage woman to rest between contractions	Efforts of labor and delivery are exhausting
Psychologic maintenance	Praise and support couple	Woman feels relief that she can push; couple often feels satisfaction after each pushing effort
THIRD STAGE *Immediate postdelivery*	Note and record following: 1. Time of delivery of infant and position 2. Type of episiotomy and kind of suture used to repair incision 3. Analgesic or anesthetic agents used	Maintains correct delivery records Some anesthetics and blocking agents increase uterine relaxation, which may lead to hemorrhage
	4. Complications (excessive bleeding, uterine inertia, neonatal complications) Place newborn with parents as soon as possible	Complications may increase risk of hemorrhage or infection Early contact assists the attachment process
Delivery of placenta	Record delivery time and mechanism of placenta	Duncan delivery of placenta increases chance of incomplete separation, which in turn increases chance of hemorrhage due to retained placental fragments
	Administer and record oxytocic drugs Administer Deladumone or Ditate if woman is not breast-feeding Inspect intactness of placenta and check for irregularities of cord insertion Check maternal blood pressure and pulse Obtain cord blood	Increases uterine contractility Suppresses letdown of breast milk Duncan delivery of placenta increases chances of retention of placental tissue Assesses physiologic status If mother is Rh negative, send cord blood for direct Coombs' test; if mother is Rh positive, cord blood may be sent to laboratory to determine blood type and Rh

NURSING CARE PLAN Cont'd
Labor and Delivery

Problem	Nursing interventions and actions	Rationale
	Clinician does manual and visual examination of vagina to determine presence of lacerations	Prevents hemorrhage from undetected lacerations
FOURTH STAGE **First hour**	Assess vital signs:	Evaluates physiologic parameters for homeostatic adjustment
Physiologic maintenance	1. Temperature every hour; if it is not elevated, check every 4 hr 2. Check BP, pulse, and respirations every 15 min	Detects complications such as hemorrhage, hypovolemia, infection, and others
Assessment 1. Fundus	Check firmness and position of fundus every 15 min for the first hour—should be firm at midline at level of umbilicus or two finger-breadths below	Fundus must stay contracted to close off vessels at placental implantation site and to prevent hemorrhage
2. Perineum	Inspect perineum for redness, swelling, bruising, discharge, gaping, every 15 min for the first hour	Identifies excessive trauma that may hinder healing
3. Lochia	Check lochia for amount, color, presence of clots every 15 min for the first hour	Presence of clots may indicate retained placental fragments or uterine relaxation Saturation of more than one or two perineal pads in the first hour is considered excessive
4. Bladder	Palpate bladder for distention. Encourage client to void	Distended bladder can cause uterine atony and postpartal bleeding
Chilling	Cover woman with warmed blankets	Sudden release of intraabdominal pressure after emptying of uterus, reaction to fatigue, and exhaustion associated with stress of labor may cause chilling
Second to fourth hour **after delivery** *Physiologic and physical maintenance*	Perform previous assessment every 30 min as long as findings are within normal parameters	
	Give bed bath and prepare woman for transfer to postpartal unit; utilize time to assess learning needs with regard to self-care: massaging fundus, changing pads, perineal care after elimination	Promotes hygiene
Psychologic maintenance	Evaluate emotional status Provide quiet rest periods	

NURSING CARE EVALUATION

Client has had safe labor and delivery with no undue trauma or problems

Infant is delivered without undue trauma

Woman is transferred to postpartal unit when the following criteria are met:

1. Vital signs are stable

2. Uterus is firm, in the midline, and at the umbilicus

3. Lochia is moderate in amount

4. Bladder is not distended

NURSING CARE PLAN Cont'd
Labor and Delivery

Client understands self-care measures:

1. Massaging fundus and assessing its firmness
2. Changing pads
3. Care after elimination

NURSING DIAGNOSES*	SUPPORTING DATA
Knowledge deficit regarding normal labor and delivery process	Anxiety
	Frequently asks questions
	Expresses concern about what is to happen next
Alteration in comfort related to normal labor and delivery process	Grimacing with contractions
	Inability to maintain breathing patterns throughout contractions
	Anxiety
	Increased blood pressure and pulse

* These are a few examples of nursing diagnoses that may be appropriate for the laboring woman.
It is not an inclusive list and must be individualized for each woman.

the stoic barrier, the nurse needs to rise above frustration and realize that one's caregiving attitude will still affect the young woman, whether or not reciprocity exists. Many older adolescents who have participated in childbirth programs feel that they "know it all." The nurse's reinforcement in a nonjudgmental manner will help them "save face."

Older adolescents may be no more prepared for labor and delivery than younger counterparts. If she has not taken classes, she may require preparation and explanations. The older teenager's response to the stresses of labor, however, is similar to those of the adult woman.

The support person involved in the birthing process also needs the nurse's encouragement and support. The nurse must explain changes in a client's behavior and substantiate the client's wishes. Hospital rules that exclude people under age 16 may be waived to allow a young father-to-be to remain with the client. The nursing staff should reinforce young adolescents' feelings that they are wanted and important.

Even if the adolescent is planning to relinquish her newborn, she should be given the option of seeing and holding her newborn. She may be reluctant to do this at first, but it has been demonstrated that the grieving process after giving up a newborn is facilitated if the mother sees the infant. However, seeing or holding the newborn should be the client's choice.

The nurse should be alert to any physiologic complications of labor in the adolescent. A client's prenatal record is carefully reviewed for risks. Screening for PIH, CPD,

anemia, drugs ingested during pregnancy, sexually transmitted disease, and size–date discrepancies should be done. The use of the Friedman curve to plot the length of labor facilitates assessment of a prolonged stage I. It has been demonstrated that very anxious women may have prolonged labors due to increased adrenalin response. Cervical lacerations may occur during the birth due to a hypoplastic cervix in the young nulliparous client.

Any adolescent who has not had any prenatal care requires close observation during labor. Fetal monitoring is needed to establish fetal well-being. Adolescent women are at highest risk for pregnancy and labor complications and must be monitored intensively (Mercer, 1979).

Management of Pain Relief

One of the most important factors in determining a client's emotional reaction to labor and delivery is the support and encouragement she receives from hospital personnel in the labor and delivery unit.

A labor and delivery nurse is in the unique position of assisting during one of the most profound experiences of human existence. This nurse has the privilege of sharing in each couple's personal miracle. But it is sometimes difficult for the nurse, who may be admitting the seventh client toward the end of a busy shift, to share the enthusiasm and excitement of the expectant couple. Nurses who care for women in labor face a challenge. They must integrate sophisticated technical skills with sensitivity and an awareness of the influence of the nurses' attitude and behavior on the laboring woman's perceptions. A warm and supportive nurse helps set the stage for a satisfying childbirth experience.

ASSESSMENT

The first step in planning care for the client is assessment of factors that may contribute to discomfort in labor. Identification and validation of these factors provide a basis for nursing intervention that can decrease the degree of discomfort the woman experiences. Assessment of the pain experience has been categorized into eight possible types of behavioral response (McCaffery, 1972):

- Physiologic manifestations
- Body movement
- Facial expression
- Verbal statements
- Vocal behavior
- Physical contact
- Response to environment
- Patterns of handling pain

Many of these behaviors overlap in the total response to pain. The most frequent physiologic manifestations are increases in pulse, respiration, and blood pressure; dilated pupils; and an increase in muscle tension. In labor these reactions are transitory because of the intermittent nature of the pain. The increase in muscle tension is the most significant in labor because it may impede the progress of labor. Clients in labor are frequently seen voluntarily tightening skeletal muscles during a contraction and remaining motionless. Facial grimacing is also a common observation. Verbal statements relating to pain are generally reliable because requests for intervention usually mean that the woman has reached her tolerance level. Vocalization may take many forms during the first stage of labor. A grunting sound typically accompanies the bearing-down effort during the second stage of labor.

Some clients desire body contact during a contraction and may reach out to grasp the supporting person. As the intensity of the contractions increases with the progress of labor, the woman is less aware of the environment and may have difficulty hearing verbal instructions. The pattern of coping with labor contractions varies from the use of highly structured breathing techniques to loud vocalizations. Irritability and refusal of touch are common responses to the discomfort of the second stage of labor. The tense and frightened client is more likely to lose control during any stage of labor.

INTERVENTION

A decrease in the intensity of discomfort is one of the goals of nursing support during labor. (The total elimination of pain can only be accomplished with selected regional or general anesthetic techniques, which are discussed in Chapter 17.) Nursing measures used to decrease pain include:

- Ensuring general comfort
- Decreasing anxiety
- Providing information
- Using specific supportive relaxation techniques
- Administering pharmacologic agents as ordered by the physician

These measures are not mutually exclusive but are interrelated in the total management of care during labor.

□ *GENERAL COMFORT* General comfort measures are of utmost importance throughout labor. The client should be assisted to any position that she finds the most comfortable. A side-lying position is generally the most advantageous for the laboring woman. Care should be taken that all body parts are supported, with the joints slightly flexed. If the client is more comfortable on her back, the head of the bed should be elevated to relieve the pressure of the uterus on the vena cava. Back rubs and frequent change of position contribute to comfort and relaxation.

Fresh, smooth, dry bed linen promotes client comfort. Diaphoresis and the constant leaking of amniotic fluid contribute to discomfort. Changing the bed linen and gown of the woman who has intravenous fluidlines in place and is attached to the fetal monitor can be rather overwhelming to the beginning nurse and may be considered too much trouble by the experienced labor and delivery nurse, but the degree of effort required is far outweighed by the benefit to the laboring woman. To avoid having to change the bottom sheet following rupture of the membranes, the nurse may replace incontinent pads (chux) at frequent intervals. The perineal area should be kept as clean and dry as possible to prevent infection as well as to promote comfort.

Particular attention should be focused on the bladder. It should be kept as empty as possible. Even though the client is voiding, it is not unusual for urine to be retained because of the pressure of the fetal presenting part. A full bladder can be detected by palpation and percussion directly over the symphysis pubis. Some of the regional procedures for analgesia during labor contribute to the inability to void, and catheterization may be necessary. A full bladder adds to the discomfort during a contraction and may prolong labor by interfering with the descent of the fetus.

The client may experience dryness of the oral mucous membranes, as she is usually allowed no food or liquids by mouth. Even though the client may have intravenous fluids, the mouth still becomes dry. A lemon glycerine swab, popsicles, ice chips, or a wet 4 × 4 sponge may relieve the discomfort. Some prepared childbirth programs advise the client to bring lollipops to help combat the dryness that occurs with some of the breathing patterns. By relieving some of these minor discomforts the client is better able to use her coping mechanisms for dealing with pain.

□ *HANDLING ANXIETY* The anxiety experienced by women entering labor is related to a combination of factors inherent to the process. According to McCaffery (1972), anxiety is necessary during the anticipation of pain. She states that "during the anticipation of pain, pain relief is enhanced if the patient experiences a moderate amount of anxiety and this anxiety is channeled into methods of coping with pain." Note that she says moderate and not a high degree of anxiety and that the anxiety should be related only to the pain experience.

This concept can be correlated with the theory that a moderate degree of anxiety improves student performance on an examination whereas a high degree of anxiety decreases test performance. An excessive degree of anxiety interferes with one's ability to cope. Anxieties relating to other aspects of labor also inhibit coping mechanisms. One way to decrease anxiety that is not related to pain is to eliminate the unknown quality of labor by client teaching and by establishing a good rapport with the couple to preserve their personal integrity. In addition to being a good listener, it is important for the labor and delivery nurse to demonstrate genuine concern for the laboring woman. Remaining with the woman as much as possible conveys a caring attitude and dispels fears of abandonment. Praise for correct breathing, relaxation efforts, and pushing efforts not only provides positive reinforcement for repetition of the behavior but also decreases anxiety about the ability to cope with the process of labor.

□ *CLIENT TEACHING* Providing information about the nature of the discomfort that will occur during labor is important. Stressing the intermittent nature and maximum duration of the contractions can be most helpful. It is much easier to cope with pain when a period of complete relief is assured. Describing the type of discomfort and specific sensations that will occur as labor progresses helps the woman recognize these sensations as normal and expected when she does experience them.

Rectal pressure during the second stage may be interpreted as the need for a bowel movement. The instinctive response is to tighten muscles rather than bear down. A sensation of splitting apart also occurs in the latter part of the second stage, which tends to retard bearing-down efforts. If the woman expects these sensations and has been counseled that bearing down contributes to progress at this stage, she is more likely to listen to instructions and to make her best effort to control her responses. Descriptions of sensations should not be given unless the woman is also given instructions as to what she can do when the sensations occur. Some clients experience the urge to push during transition when the cervix is not fully dilated and effaced. This sensation can be controlled by panting, and instructions should be given prior to the time that panting is required.

A thorough explanation of procedures and equipment being used also decreases anxiety, thereby decreasing pain. Few women are prepared for the artificial rupturing of the membranes unless they have experienced it before. Assurance that it is no more uncomfortable than a vaginal examination decreases anxiety. Attachment to a fetal monitor can produce fear, because equipment of this type is associated with critically ill patients. Many labor and delivery units routinely monitor all women in labor. The beeps, clicks, and other strange noises should be explained, and a simplified explanation of the monitor strip should be given. The nurse can emphasize that the use of the monitor provides a more accurate way to assess the well-being of the fetus during the course of labor.

□ *SUPPORTIVE RELAXATION TECHNIQUES* Tense muscles increase resistance to the descent of the fetus and contribute to maternal fatigue. This fatigue increases pain perception and decreases the ability to cope with the pain experience. Comfort measures, massage, techniques for decreasing anxiety, and client teaching have been identified as contributing to relaxation. Other factors are adequate sleep and rest. The laboring woman needs to be encouraged to use the periods between contractions for rest and relaxation. A prolonged prodromal phase of labor may have prohibited sleeping. An aura of excitement naturally occurs with the onset of early labor, making it difficult to sleep although the contractions are mild and infrequent. An exhausted woman may be less enthusiastic about the delivery process and holding her newborn afterward.

Distraction is another specific method of increasing relaxation and coping with discomfort. During early labor, conversation or activities as light reading, bridge, or games such as Scrabble serve as distractors. One technique that is effective with moderate pain is to have the client concentrate on a pleasant experience she has had in the past. This requires a good imagination, but some women can close their eyes and recreate the pleasant experience. Another type of distraction is touch. Some women have the desire to touch another person during a painful experience, whereas others regard touching as an invasion of privacy or threat to their independence. When earlier assessment has not revealed this information about a client, nurses can make themselves available to the client who desires this support. One way to do this is by placing one's hand on the side rail of the bed within the client's reach. The person who needs touch will reach out for contact, and the nurse can pick up and follow through with this behavioral cue. Touch may be used to communicate to the client that dependency is allowed in stressful situations (Figure 16–2).

A specific type of cutaneous stimulation used prior to the transitional phase of labor is known as *abdominal effleurage* (Figure 16–3). Pain impulses are carried by small-

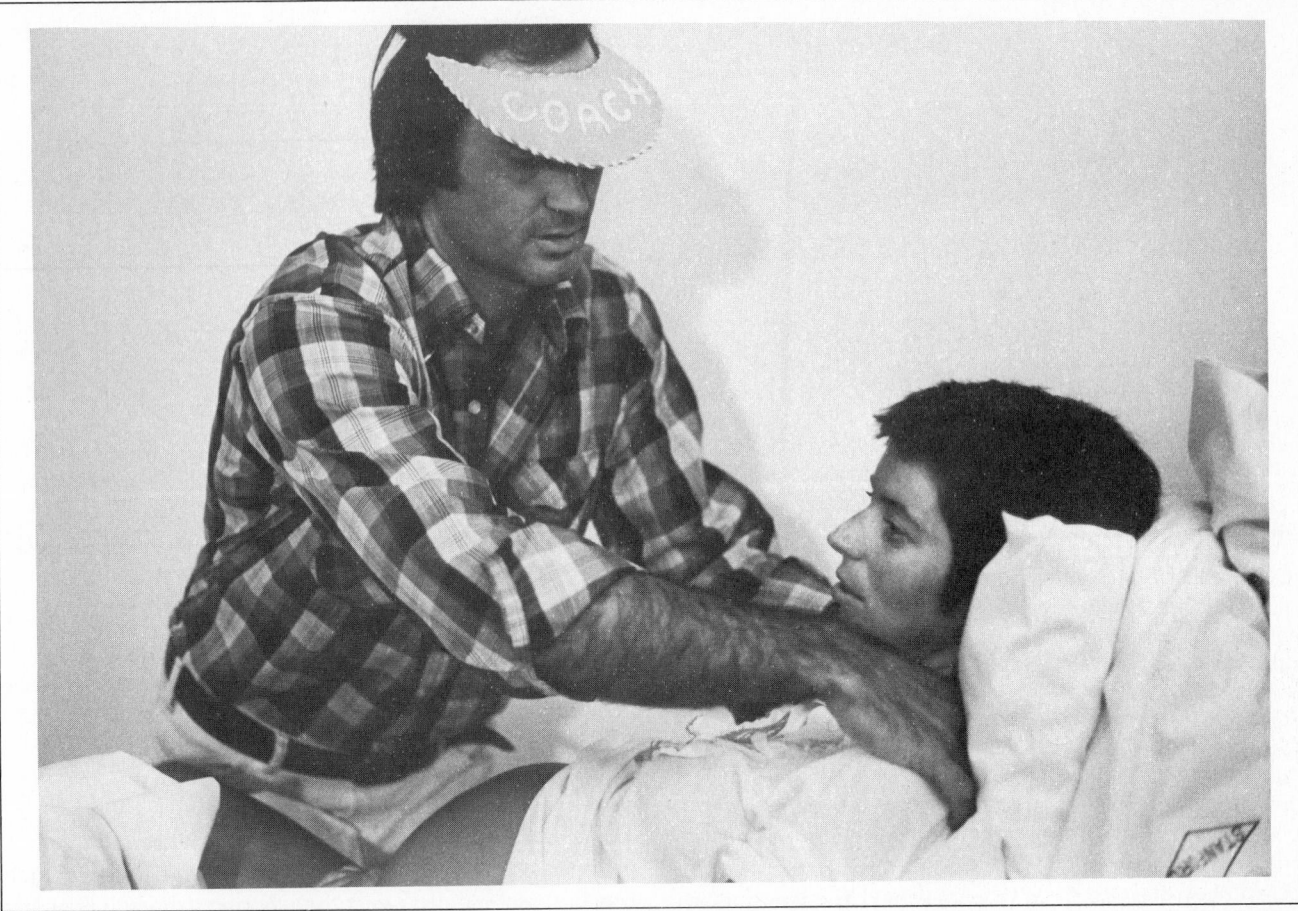

FIGURE 16–2 Woman's partner provides support and encouragement during labor. (© Suzanne Arms.)

diameter nerve fibers, and cutaneous sensations are carried by large-diameter nerve fibers. The theory is that the transmission of pain impulses is inhibited by the competing input from the large fibers. This light abdominal stroking is used in the Lamaze method of childbirth preparation. It is effective for mild to moderate pain but is not effective for intense pain. Deep pressure over the sacrum is more effective for relieving back pain.

In addition to the measures just described, the nurse can enhance the client's relaxation by providing encouragement and support for her controlled breathing techniques.

□ *CONTROLLED BREATHING* Controlled breathing may also be helpful to women during labor. Used correctly, it increases the client's pain threshold, permits relaxation, enhances the client's ability to cope with the uterine contractions, and allows the uterus to function more efficiently.

Lamaze breathing patterns utilize three patterns of chest breathing. The client begins with the first level breathing pattern and progresses to the second and third level as the contractions intensify. Each breathing pattern is preceded and ended with a deep cleansing breath, which consists of taking in a deep breath through the nose, and exhaling through the mouth (Figure 16–4).

First level (slow chest). The first breathing level is a slow and even chest breathing. The breath is taken in through the nose and exhaled out through the nose or mouth. The rate should be approximately 6 to 9 breaths per minute.

Second level (accelerated-decelerated). The second breathing pattern is useful when the contractions become more intense. It is more shallow and rapid and can be accelerated at the acme of the contraction and slowed as the contraction intensity decreases. The breath is taken in through the nose and exhaled out through the mouth.

Third level (pant-blow). The third breathing level is useful in the transition phase. The client takes more rapid

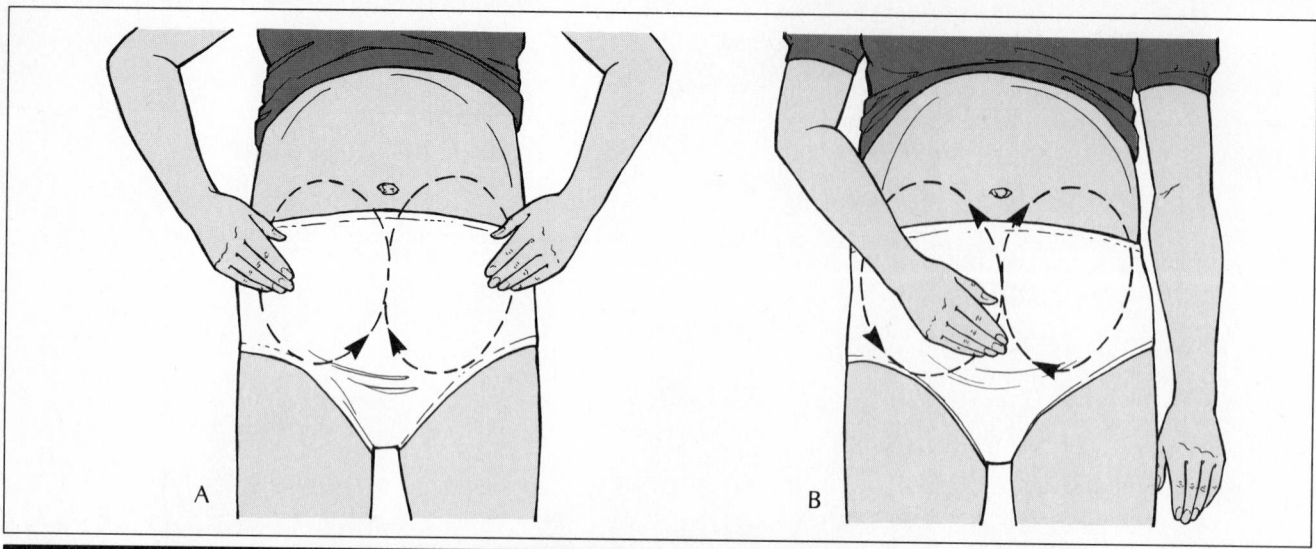

FIGURE 16-3 Effleurage is light stroking of the abdomen with the fingertips. **A,** Starting at the symphysis, the client lightly moves her fingertips up and around in a circular pattern. **B,** An alternate approach involves the use of one hand in a figure-eight pattern. This technique is used primarily in labor.

and shallow breaths throughout the contraction. The pattern is based on inhaling and exhaling through the mouth. After a cleansing breath, the mouth is held in a semismiling position and the breath is exhaled making a sound like "hee." After three of these "hee" breaths, the lips are slightly pursed as the next breath is exhaled making a "hoo" sound. This pattern (hee-hee-hee-hoo) is continued through the contraction and ended with a cleansing breath. During the "hee-hoo" breathing, the rate is kept at a shallow and rhythmic pace. If the mouth gets too dry, the tongue can be placed against the roof of the mouth (Fenlon et al., 1979).

Lamaze breathing is usually learned during prenatal classes and is practiced over a number of weeks before delivery. If the client has not learned Lamaze or another controlled breathing technique, it may be difficult to teach her quickly when she is admitted in active labor. In this instance, abdominal and pant-pant-blow breathing may be taught. Abdominal breathing consists of moving the abdominal wall upward as the breath is taken in and moving it downward as exhalation occurs. This method tends to lift the abdominal wall off the contracting uterus and thus may provide some relief of discomfort. The breathing is deep and rhythmical. As transition approaches, the client may feel the need to breathe more rapidly. To avoid hyperventilation, which may occur with deep abdominal breathing, the pant-pant-blow breathing pattern can be used.

As the client utilizes her breathing technique, the nurse can assess and support the interaction between the client and her coach or support person. In the absence of a coach, the nurse can assist the laboring woman by helping her identify the beginning of each contraction and encouraging her as she breathes through each contraction. Continued encouragement and support with each contraction throughout labor have immeasurable benefits. (See the Nursing Care Plan, p. 472, for additional comfort and support measures.)

Hyperventilation may occur when a client breathes very rapidly over a prolonged period of time. It results from an imbalance of oxygen and carbon dioxide (that is, too much carbon dioxide is exhaled, and too much oxygen remains in the body). The signs and symptoms of hyperventilation are tingling or numbness in tip of nose, lips, fingers, or toes; dizziness; spots before the eyes; or spasms of the hands or feet (carpal-pedal spasms). If hyperventilation occurs, the client should be encouraged to slow her breathing rate and to take more shallow breaths. With instruction and encouragement, many clients are able to change their breathing to rectify the problem. Encourage the client to relax and count out loud for her so she can pace her breathing during contractions. If the signs and symptoms continue or become more severe (that is, if they progress from numbness to spasms) the client can breathe into a paper surgical mask or a paper bag until symptoms abate (breathing into a mask or bag causes rebreathing of carbon dioxide). The nurse should remain with the client to give her reassurance.

Nursing Care Plan

The nurse continually assesses and supports maternal and fetal status throughout labor. The Nursing Care Plan for labor and delivery is based on the following factors:

- Physiologic maintenance patterns
- Labor progress (changes associated with parturition, such as dilatation and effacement, contractile patterns, bloody show, rupture of membranes)
- Fetal status patterns (physical responses of fetus to labor and fetal well-being)
- Activity state of client
- Discomforts of labor—patterns of sleep or rest (relaxation and amnesia-sleep)
- Sustenance (oral or parenteral intake and toleration of fluids)
- Elimination (all forms of output)
- Giving and receiving care (care the couple can perform for themselves or measures with which they need assistance)
- Psychologic maintenance patterns (progressive changes manifested during labor)

Many of the physical and psychologic changes that occur during labor and delivery are normal and predictable, and the outcome depends on the woman's internal system and the external support measures available to and used by the expectant couple. For example, the psychologic changes include manifestations of happiness, fear, anxiety, hostility, frustration, and success. As changes are exhibited, they should be identified and evaluated in terms of their normalcy, because occasionally deviations occur. Table 16–2 summarizes the immediate nursing action for physical problems that may occur. More specific intervention for deviations are detailed in Chapter 18.

MANAGEMENT OF SPONTANEOUS DELIVERY

Birthing Room

Couples often choose the birthing room for labor and delivery because of the more relaxed atmosphere maintained there. Consequently, preparation of the birthing room for delivery should be accomplished before the delivery is imminent. A delivery pack and instrument set can be placed on a small table close to the labor bed. Essentials for the immediate care of the newborn are prepared and emergency resuscitation equipment is available somewhere in the room. Often birthing rooms have a bed that may be adapt-

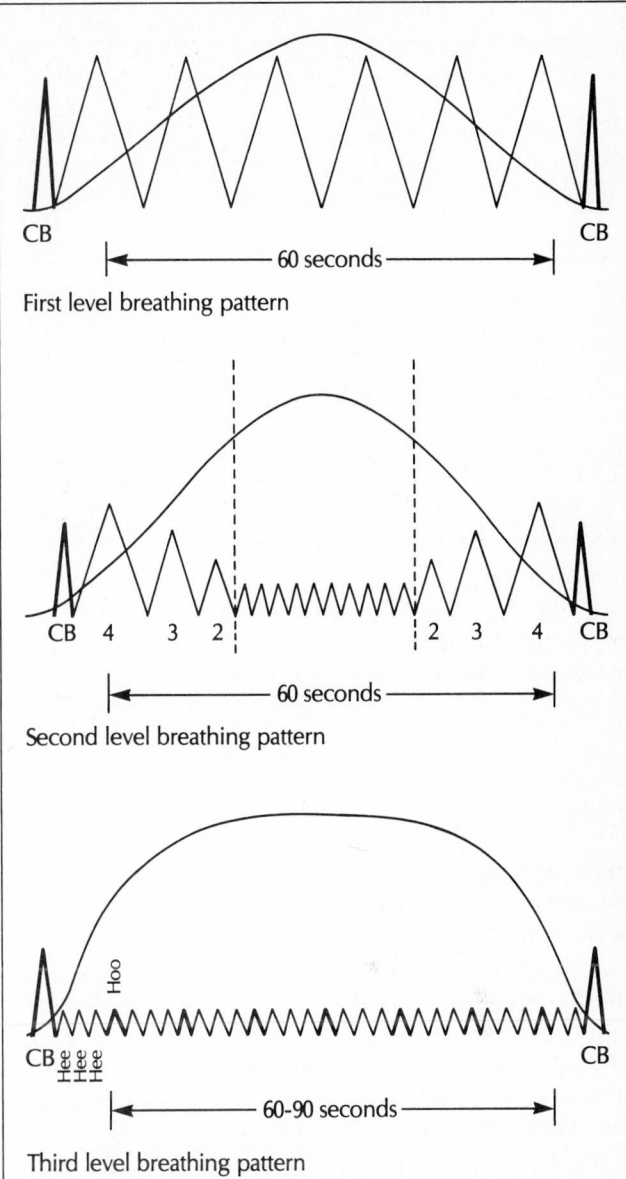

FIGURE 16–4 Lamaze breathing patterns. Each diagram represents a different breathing pattern. The curved line represents the uterine contraction. The peaked lines represent breaths that are taken during the contraction. Each breathing pattern begins and ends with a cleansing breath (CB). (From Fenlon, A., et al. 1979. *Getting ready for childbirth*. Englewood Cliffs, N.J.: Prentice-Hall, Inc.)

ed for delivery by removing a small section near the foot of it. Many of the same interventions described in the following section apply. After delivery, the newborn is placed with the mother or couple and their interaction is not interrupted.

Table 16–2 Deviations from Normal Labor Process Requiring Immediate Intervention

Problem	Immediate action	Problem	Immediate action
Client admitted with vaginal bleeding or history of painless vaginal bleeding	1. Do not perform vaginal examination 2. Assess FHR 3. Evaluate amount of blood loss 4. Evaluate labor pattern 5. Notify clinician immediately	Prolapse of umbilical cord	1. Relieve pressure on cord manually 2. Continuously monitor FHR; watch for changes in FHR pattern 3. Notify physician

Presence of greenish amniotic fluid	1. Continuously monitor FHR
	2. Evaluate dilatation status of cervix and determine whether umbilical cord is prolapsed
	3. Maintain client on complete bed rest
	4. Notify physician immediately
		Client admitted in advanced labor; delivery imminent	1. Proceed directly to delivery room
			2. Obtain necessary information:
			  a. Physician's name
			  b. Bleeding problems
			  c. Obstetric problems
			  d. FHR and maternal vital signs, if possible
			  e. Length of labor and last time she ate
			3. Direct ancillary personnel to telephone physician
			Do not leave client alone
			4. Provide support to couple

Absence of FHR and fetal movement	1. Notify physician 2. Provide emotional support to laboring couple (client has an idea that "something is wrong")		

Delivery Room

The instrument table, which is set up in advance, generally includes a linen pack containing a buttocks drape, two leg drapes, one abdominal drape, and several towels. Many delivery rooms are now using disposable linen packs. The delivery instruments can be sterilized in a large basin and are added to the table at the time it is set up. Equipment required in preparation for delivery varies somewhat from one hospital or agency to another.

The solution to be used for the perineal scrub is placed in a warm place so it will be warmed before using on the client. Some agencies use Betadine spray instead of a perineal scrub. Two gowns with towels, two pairs of gloves or more, and a sterile baby blanket should be added to the table when it is set up. Some delivery setups include a French catheter in a small basin. This may be wrapped separately and added if needed.

An instrument table is set up under sterile precautions, and it may be covered with sterile side sheets, labeled with the time and date, and initialed by the person who set it up. The table may be left for varying periods of time, depending on hospital/agency policy.

Most delivery rooms are equipped with a radiant-heated infant care unit, which is equipped with oxygen, suction, and an intermittent positive pressure breathing (IPPB) system that can be used with a mask or connected directly to an endotracheal tube. Before each delivery, this unit should be checked to make sure it is working and that a sterile area is available in which to place the infant. Two sterile towels are opened and placed in the unit for drying the newborn. If not left on continuously, the radiant heater is turned on at this time so that there will be a warm environment for the newborn.

It is suggested that the following equipment be available for neonatal care: a soft rubber ear bulb syringe for suctioning of the nose and mouth (this may be brought with the baby from the delivery table); a DeLee mucous suction trap; suction catheters (sizes 10, 12, and 14 French and sizes 8, 10, 12, and 14 French disposable plastic catheters with finger control); a laryngoscope with a working light; Miller size 0 premature and size 1 blade; and 2.5–4 mm or size 10, 12, and 14 endotracheal tubes with stylets for those clinicians who use them. A bag resuscitator should also be available if the heated unit does not have one (Korones, 1981).

Nursing Interventions

The nurse has responsibilities to four people in the delivery room: the woman, her partner/coach, the infant, and the clinician (physician or nurse-midwife).

The delivery is conducted under strict sterile precautions. Therefore, all those who enter the delivery room wear scrub apparel, caps, and masks and wash their hands. The mask is changed when it becomes damp because it does not provide an effective bacterial barrier when wet. The nurse assists the labor coach in donning the appropriate apparel for accompanying the woman to the delivery room.

Nursing duties include assisting with the transport of the woman to the delivery room and helping her onto the delivery table. During this time the nurse performs necessary tasks, continues an ongoing assessment, and provides appropriate comfort, support, and education to meet the specific needs as identified.

PREPARING THE WOMAN AND THE COACH FOR DELIVERY

□ *POSITIONING* The traditional lithotomy position for delivery enhances maintaining asepsis, assessing FHR, and performing episiotomy and repair. This position has the following disadvantages: (a) 3%–11% of clients develop supine hypotensive syndrome; (b) excessive pressure on legs results from stirrups; (c) aspiration from vomitus is more likely; (d) client may feel resentment at being forced to assume an ''embarrassing'' position; (e) tightening of the vagina and perineum as the thighs are flexed may increase the need for an episiotomy; (f) it may interfere with the frequency and intensity of contractions; and (g) the client works against gravity. The disadvantages noted may be eliminated if the client is positioned in a lithotomy posi-

tion with her back elevated at least 30–40° (McKay, 1981; Nobel, 1981).

In some agencies, the lateral Sims position is advocated for delivery. Although some medical procedures are more difficult to accomplish, this position is thought to be associated with the following advantages: (a) maternal hypotension is avoided; (b) contraction intensity remains unchanged; (c) there is no inhibition to push; (d) promotion of perineal and vaginal relaxation results in decreased need for episiotomy; and (e) it promotes client comfort (McKay, 1980).

The client may wish to assume a squatting position, and this may be encouraged in a birthing room setting but frowned on in a more traditional delivery room. The major advantage of squatting is the use of gravity to assist in delivery. Disadvantages of this position are difficulty in providing for client safety if she squats on a delivery table without side rails, and problems in assessing FHR. A squatting position also makes it more difficult for the clinician to control the birth process (McKay, 1980).

The position used for delivery is influenced by client and clinician desires and possibly by labor and delivery room protocols. If stirrups are used, they should be padded to alleviate pressure and both legs should be lifted simultaneously to avoid strain on abdominal and perineal muscles. The stirrups should be adjusted to fit the length of the

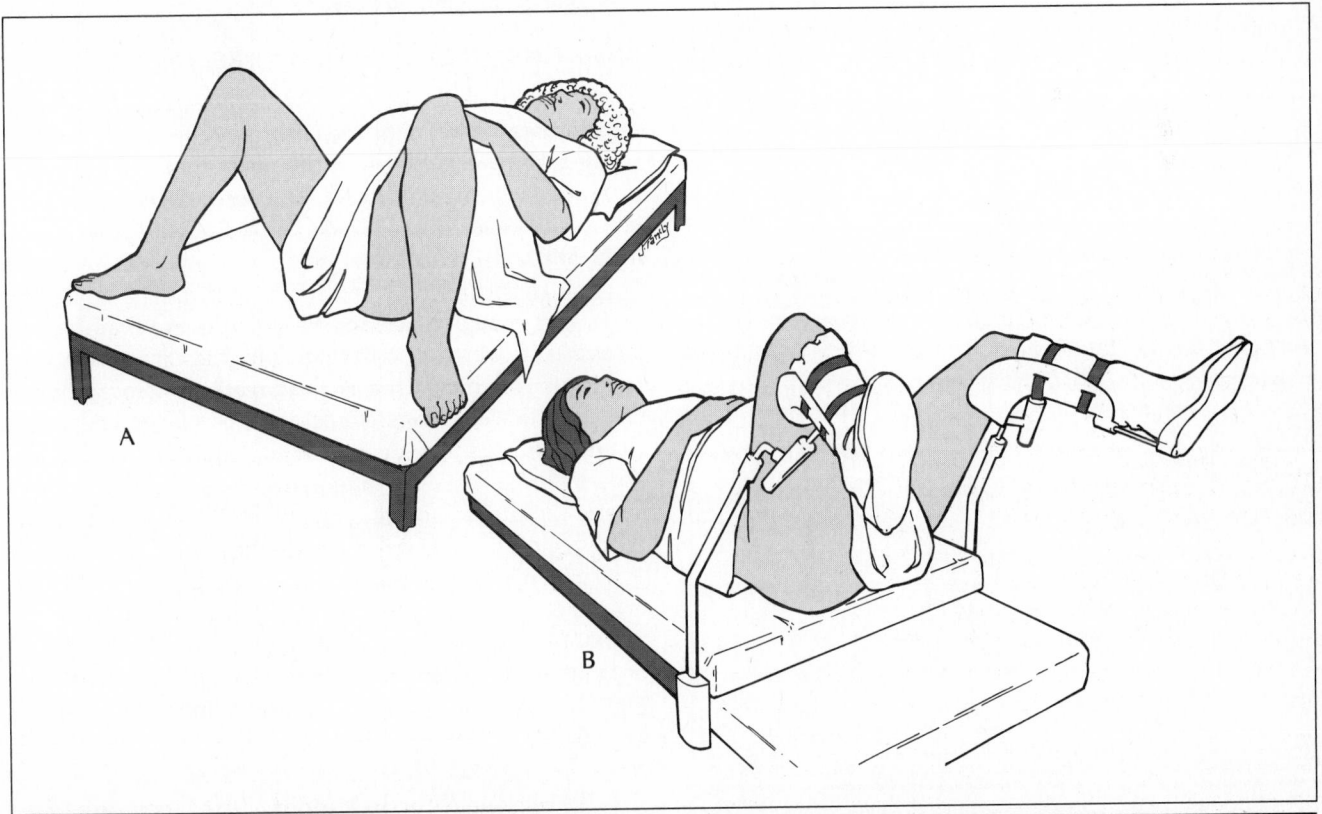

FIGURE 16–5 Examples of two positions of woman on the delivery table. **A,** Dorsal recumbent position. **B,** Lithotomy position.

woman's lower extremities (Figure 16–5). The feet are supported in the stirrup holders, and the height and angle of the stirrups are adjusted so there is no pressure on the popliteal or calf area of the woman's legs, which might cause discomfort and possible postpartal vascular problems. The expulsive efforts of the woman will be aided if the back of the delivery table is elevated about 30–60° and the handles on the delivery table are adjusted so she may pull back on them.

□ *CLEANSING THE PERINEUM* The woman's vulvar and perineal area is prepared in the following manner. A sterile prep tray containing two small basins with at least six large cotton balls in each cup should be set up. One cup contains a surgical scrub solution in sterile water, and the other cup contains sterile water. After thoroughly washing hands, the nurse dons sterile gloves and cleans the vulva and perineum with the scrub solution (Figure 16–6), then rinses with sterile water. Beginning with the mons, the area is scrubbed up to the lower abdomen. The second ball is used to scrub the inner groin and thigh of one leg, and the third cotton ball is used to scrub the other leg, moving outward to avoid carrying material from surrounding areas to the vaginal outlet. The last three cotton balls are used to scrub the labia and vestibule with one downward sweep each. The used cotton balls are then discarded.

The labor coach is provided a stool to sit on if desired. Both the woman and the coach are informed of procedures and progress and are supported throughout the delivery. Some delivery rooms come equipped with a mirror on the overhead light so that the couple may watch the delivery.

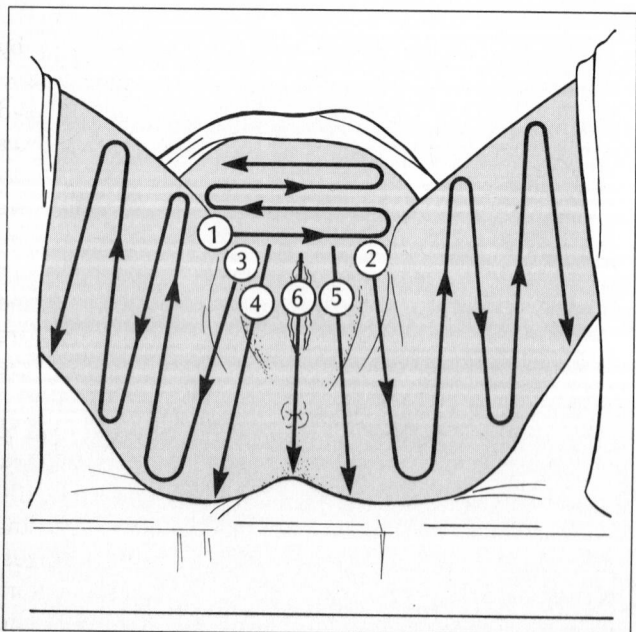

FIGURE 16–6 Cleansing the perineum prior to delivery. The nurse follows the numbered diagram, using a new cotton ball for each area.

The woman's blood pressure and the fetal heart rate are monitored between contractions, and contractions are palpated until delivery to assess status.

The nurse continues to assist the client in her pushing efforts. Traditionally, the Valsalva (closed glottis) method has been encouraged and the client is instructed to hold her breath for extended periods of time. (See p. 409 for discussion of maternal physiologic effects.) Currently, a modified Valsalva or exhalation breathing technique is suggested as an alternative to avoid the maternal and fetal effects associated with the Valsalva method. In the modified method, the client takes advantage of the spontaneous pushing effort that occurs after the cervix is completely dilatated. The client takes several deep breaths and then holds her breath for 5–6 seconds. Then, through slightly pursed lips, she exhales slowly every 5–6 seconds while continuing to hold her breath. Another breath is taken and the exhale breathing and pushing continues while the contraction is present (McKay, 1981) (Figure 16–7).

In spontaneous deliveries, the woman is encouraged to push until the fetal chin clears the perineum. The nurse instructs her to use her pattern of breathing until expulsion is complete. This procedure prevents a too-rapid delivery, which may traumatize or tear the maternal tissues. The head is often delivered between contractions, when control is easiest. Sometimes a gentle push from the woman is required for expulsion of the shoulders. Easy, gradual traction effects complete delivery of the infant.

ASSISTING THE PHYSICIAN/NURSE-MIDWIFE

The end third of the delivery table is retractable but should remain unretracted until the clinician is present so that a ready surface is available in the event that the infant arrives suddenly and unassisted. The nurse observes the perineum and keeps the clinician informed about the advancement of the delivery.

The clinician scrubs and dons a gown. The nurse ensures that enough gown and towel packs are available for all assistants who are scrubbing. After the clinician puts on sterile gloves, he or she is then ready to proceed with draping the client. One sterile drape is placed under the client's buttocks, one over each leg, and one over the abdomen. Some clinicians caution the client against touching any of the drapes so they remain sterile while others encourage her to reach up and touch the baby after delivery.

The nurse needs to anticipate the clinician's needs during the entire delivery and to obtain requested items such as extra sponges or sutures. A stool for the clinician to sit on is provided if desired. The overhead light is adjusted so that the maternal perineal area and introitus are well lighted.

Physician/Nurse-Midwife Interventions

When the fetal head has distended the perineum about 5 cm, the clinician may perform certain hand maneuvers to

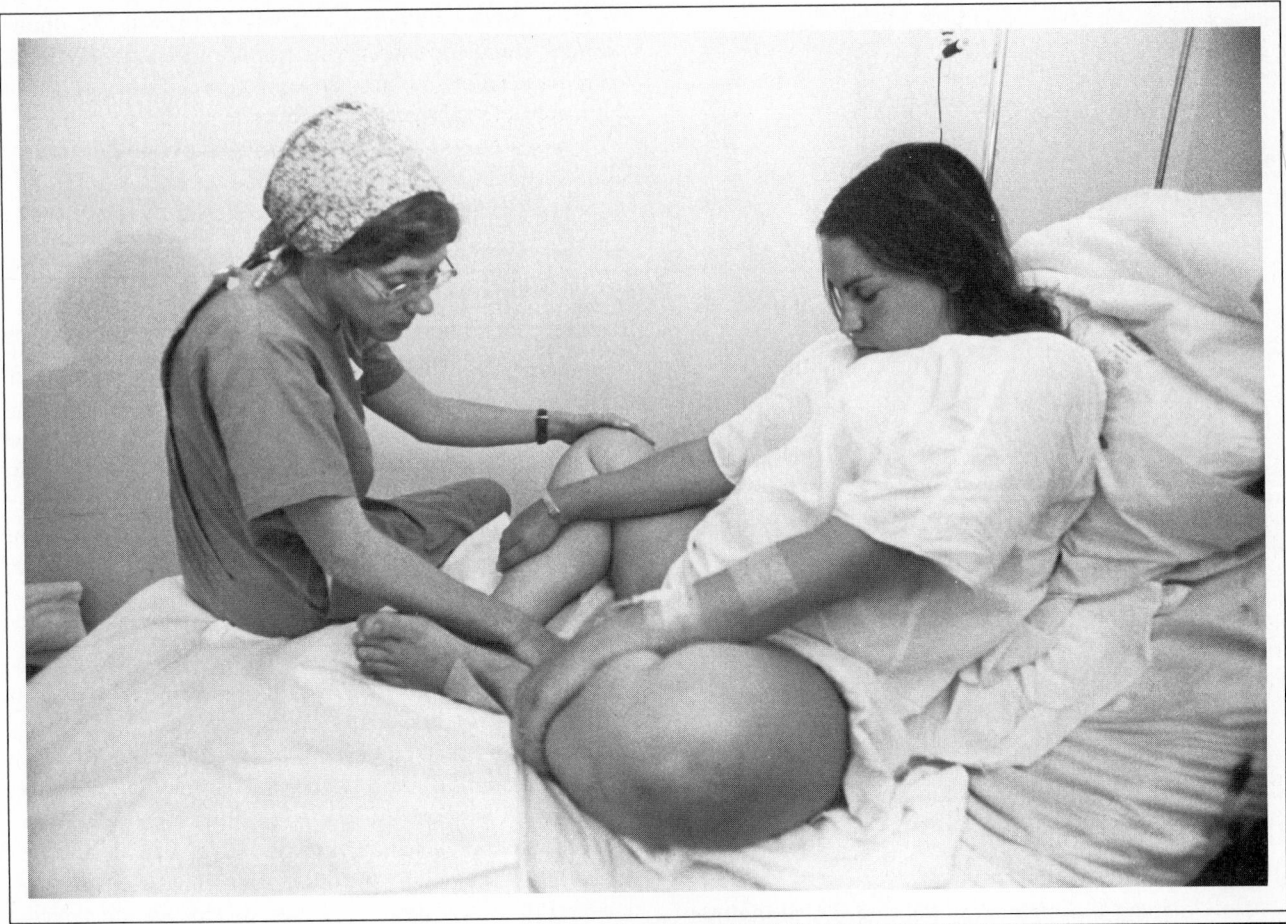

FIGURE 16–7 Nurse provides support during pushing efforts. (© Suzanne Arms.)

prevent undue trauma to the fetal head and maternal soft tissues. With a towel draped over one hand, the clinician applies pressure on the chin of the fetus through the maternal perineum. The other hand exerts gentle pressure on the occiput. This is the modified Ritgen maneuver (Figure 16–8). This maneuver permits the head to be delivered slowly under the symphysis pubis, with the face sliding successfully over the perineum. If tearing of the perineum is imminent, an episiotomy may be performed (see Chapter 19). After the infant's head is delivered, the clinician palpates the neck for the presence of a cord, which can be slipped over the fetal head if it is loose. If the cord is tight, it is double-clamped and cut.

Restitution and external rotation occur after the head is delivered. The only assistance needed during this time is support of the maternal perineum. While awaiting completion of external rotation, the clinician suctions the newborn's nose and mouth to remove mucus. When the newborn's shoulder appears at the symphysis pubis, the clinician may use both hands to grasp the newborn's head gently and pull downward for delivery of the anterior shoulder. Gentle upward traction facilitates delivery of the posterior shoulder.

Delivery of the newborn's body may be controlled by grasping the posterior shoulder with one hand, palm turned toward the perineum. The left hand may be used for this if the newborn is LOA. The right hand then follows along the infant's back, and the feet are grasped as they are delivered. The newborn's head is kept down and to the side as the newborn's feet, legs, and body are tucked under the clinician's left arm in a football hold. The clinician's right hand is then free for further care of the newborn and the newborn is securely held. The nose and mouth are suctioned with a bulb syringe, and respiratory passages are cleared.

There is considerable controversy about when to clamp and cut the cord. If the newborn is held at or below the introitus as cord clamping is delayed, as much as 50–100 mL of blood may be shifted from the placenta to the fetus. If the newborn is held 50–60 cm above the introitus, a negligible amount of blood is transferred to the newborn even after 3 minutes. The extra amount of blood added to the newborn's circulation may reduce the frequency of iron-deficiency anemia, which can occur later in infancy— or the circulatory overload may produce polycythemia and favor hyperbilirubinemia. Pritchard and MacDonald (1980)

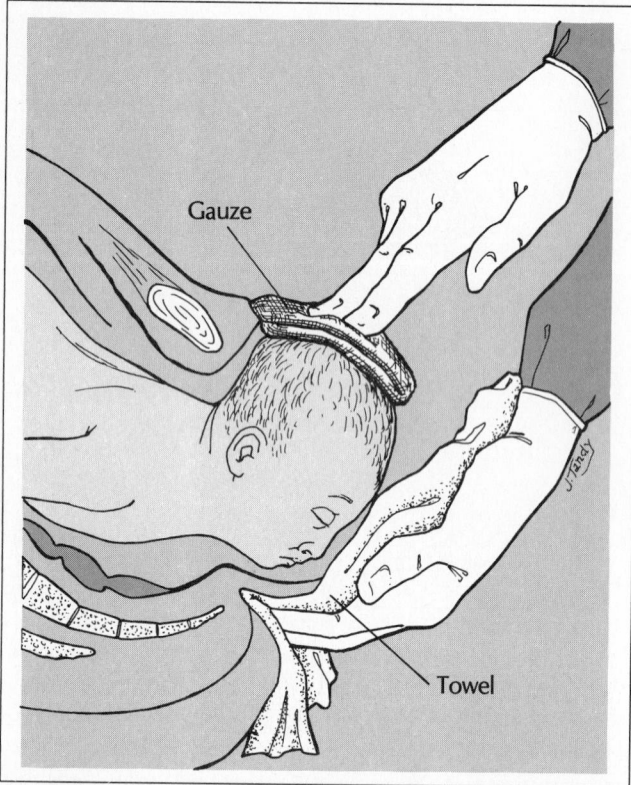

FIGURE 16–8 Delivery by modified Ritgen maneuver.

advocate clamping the cord after clearing the newborn's airway, which takes about 30 seconds. The newborn is not elevated above the introitus.

The cord is clamped with two Kelly clamps and cut between them. The clamp on the placental side is placed

Table 16–3   The Apgar Scoring System*

Sign	Score		
	0	1	2
Heart rate	Absent	Slow — below 100	Above 100
Respiratory effort	Absent	Slow — irregular	Good crying
Muscle tone	Flaccid	Some flexion of extremities	Active motion
Reflex irritability	None	Grimace	Vigorous cry
Color	Pale blue	Body pink, blue extremities	Completely pink

*From Apgar, V. Aug. 1966. The newborn (Apgar) scoring system, reflections and advice. *Pediatr. Clin. North Am.* 13:645.

on the mother's abdomen. A plastic cord clamp or umbilical tape may be applied on the newborn's cord about 2 cm from the newborn's abdomen, and then the Kelly clamp on the newborn's side may be removed.

Figures 16–9 to 16–16 on pp. 493 and 494 depict the labor and delivery experience of one family.

IMMEDIATE CARE OF THE NEWBORN

As soon as the newborn is delivered, the nurse notes on the delivery room record the time and sex and reports to the couple. If the mother is awake, she can be supported in a position to see the newborn. The clinician clears the newborn's airway and then clamps and cuts the cord. At this time the nurse approaches the instrument table and picks up a baby blanket by one corner, taking care not to contaminate the instrument table. The blanket is unfolded and draped over the nurse's arms and chest, again taking care not to contaminate the inner surface of the blanket. The clinician places the newborn on the blanket that covers the nurse's outstretched arms. The bulb syringe and any equipment that may be needed if the umbilical cord needs further attention are also handed to the nurse. As soon as the newborn is received, the nurse folds him toward her chest to maintain a secure hold and holds one leg through the blanket. The newborn is then placed in the radiant-heat unit and dried immediately. After drying, the newborn is placed on a clean, dry blanket and left uncovered under the radiant heat. Radiant heat warms the outer surface of objects; thus if the newborn is wrapped in blankets, the outer surface of the blanket is warmed instead of the newborn's skin. In some instances, the newborn is immediately given to the mother. Warmth can be maintained by placing warmed blankets over the newborn or providing skin-to-skin contact with the mother's chest. Personal wishes of the mother, clinician, or hospital policy and/or condition of the newborn may be the determining factor. The nurse needs to assure that warmth is maintained and that the airway is kept free from excessive mucus by frequent suctioning.

The newborn is placed in modified Trendelenburg position to facilitate drainage of mucus from the nasopharynx and trachea by gravity.

Apgar Scoring System

The Apgar scoring system (Table 16–3) was designed in 1952 by Dr. Virginia Apgar, an anesthesiologist. The purpose of this system is to evaluate the physical condition of the newborn at birth and the immediate need for resuscitation. The newborn is rated 1 minute after birth and again at 5 minutes and receives a total score ranging from 0 to 10 based on the following criteria:

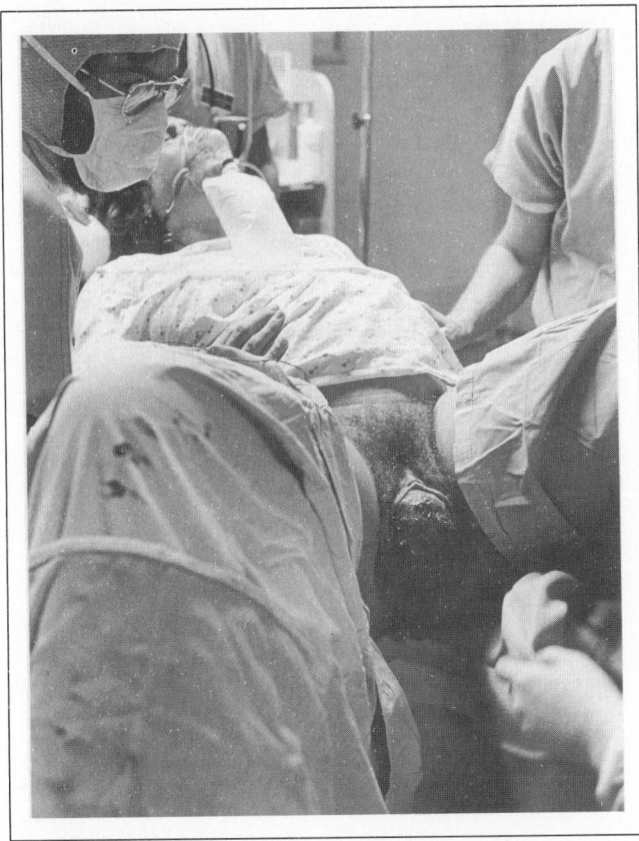

FIGURE 16-9 The fetal head is crowning. The father is by the mother's side. She is wearing an oxygen mask to facilitate her breathing.

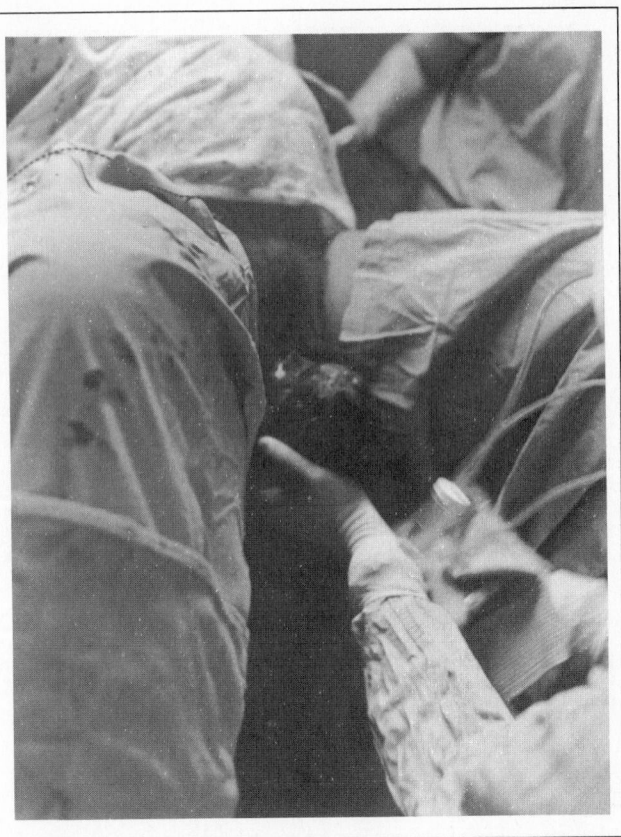

FIGURE 16-10 Note the clinician is controlling the delivery of the head by supporting the perineum.

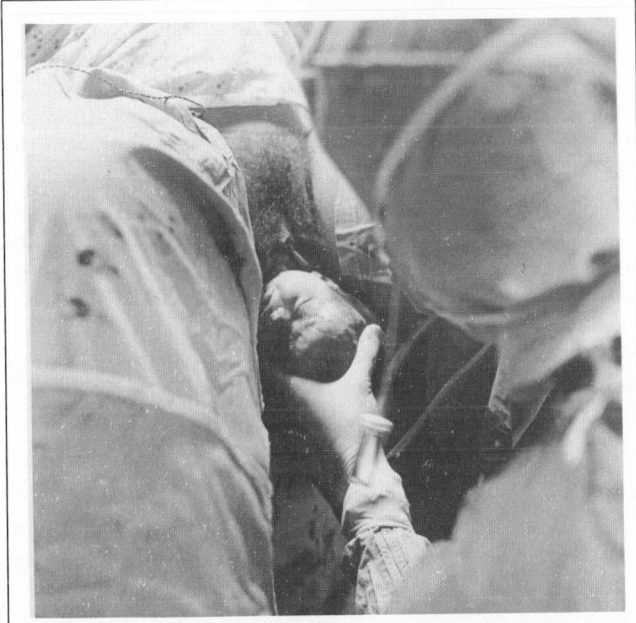

FIGURE 16-11 The head is delivered.

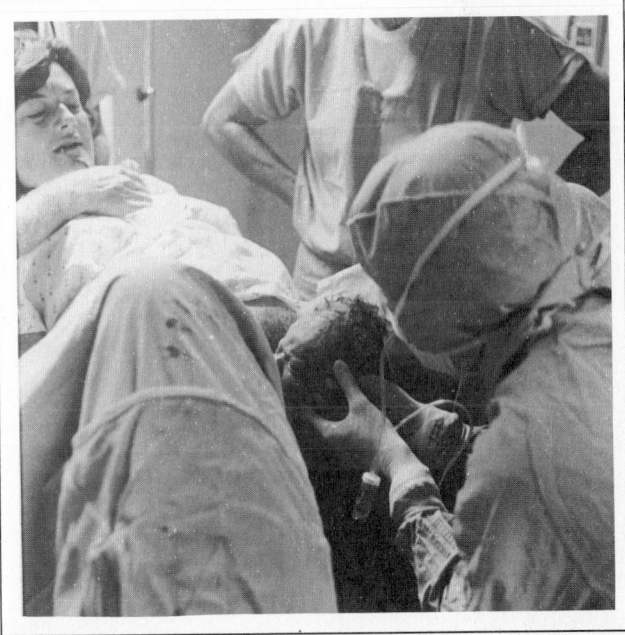

FIGURE 16-12 Note the molding of the infant's head. Restitution and external rotation have occurred.

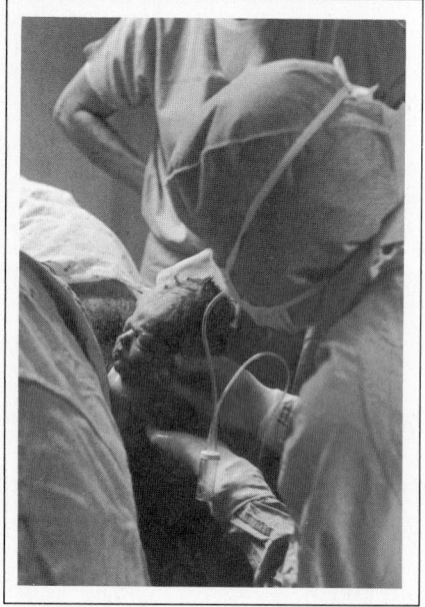
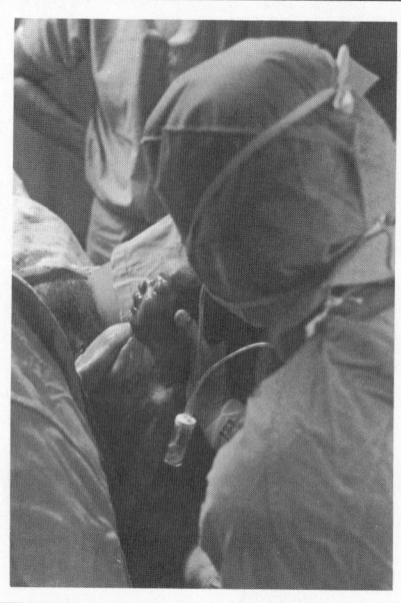
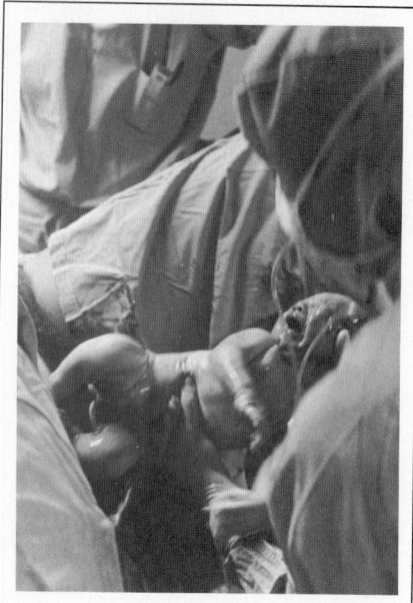

FIGURE 16–13 Delivery of the baby's shoulders.

FIGURE 16–14 Delivery of the baby's body.

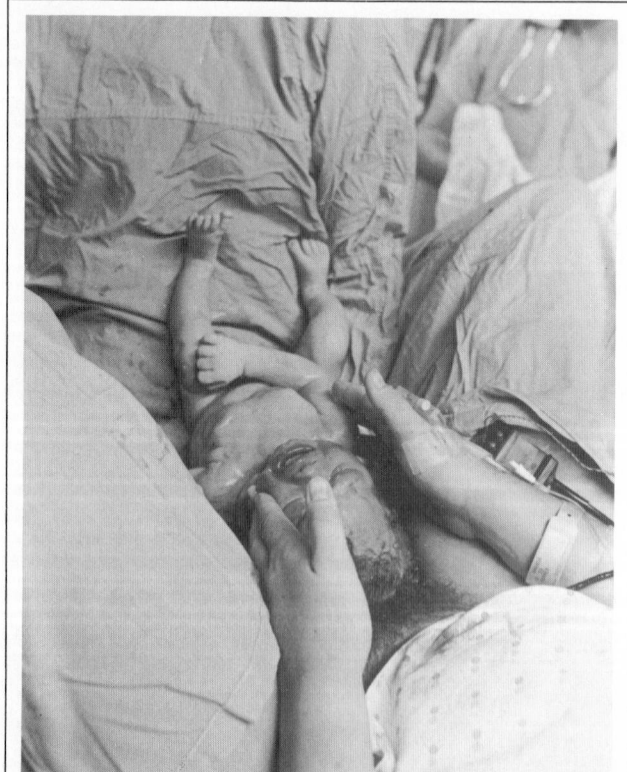

FIGURE 16–15 The infant rests between his mother's legs. Note that she is able to touch her baby immediately. The infant is held with his head lowered to facilitate drainage and to prevent aspiration of blood, amniotic fluid, and mucus.

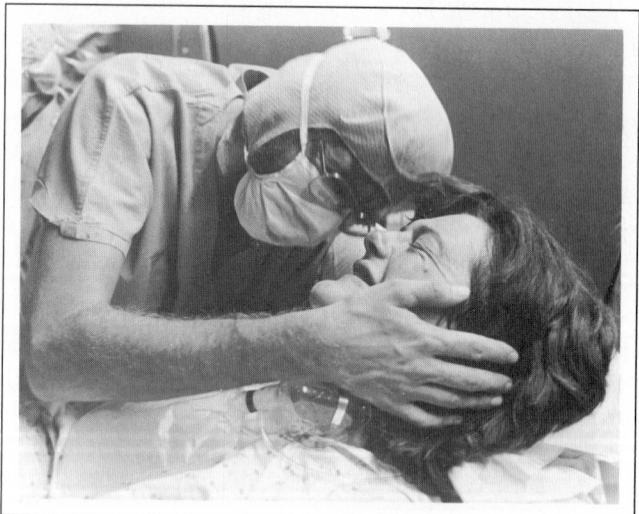

FIGURE 16–16 The new mother and father.

1. The *heart rate* is auscultated or palpated at the junction of the umbilical cord and skin. This is the most important assessment. A newborn heart rate of less than 100 beats/min indicates the need for immediate resuscitation.

2. The *respiratory effort* is the second most important Apgar assessment. Complete absence of respirations is termed *apnea*. A vigorous cry is indicative of good respirations.

3. The *muscle tone* is determined by evaluating the degree of flexion and resistance to straightening of the extremities. A normal newborn demonstrates flexion of the elbows and the hips, with the knees positioned up toward the abdomen.

4. The *reflex irritability* is evaluated by flicking the soles of the feet or by inserting a nasal catheter in the nose. A cry merits a full score of 2. A grimace is 1 point, and no response is 0.

5. The *color* is inspected for cyanosis and pallor. Generally, newborns have blue extremities, and the rest of the body is pink, which merits a score of 1. This condition is termed *acrocyanosis* and is present in 85% of normal newborns at 1 minute after birth. A completely pink newborn scores a 2 and a totally cyanotic, pale infant is scored 0.

A score of 8–10 indicates a newborn in good condition who requires only nasopharyngeal suctioning and perhaps some oxygen near the face. If the Apgar score is below 8, resuscitative measures may need to be instituted. See discussion in Chapter 25.

Care of Umbilical Cord

If the clinician has not placed a cord clamp (Hollister or Hesseltine, Figures 16–17 and 16–18) on the newborn's umbilical cord, it becomes the responsibility of the nurse to do so. Before applying the cord clamp, the nurse should examine the cut end for the presence of two arteries and one vein. The umbilical vein is the largest vessel, and the arteries are seen as smaller vessels. The number of vessels must be recorded on the delivery room and newborn records. The cord is clamped approximately ½–1 inch from the abdomen to allow room between the abdomen and clamp as the cord dries. The clamp must not catch any abdominal skin as this will cause necrosis of the tissue. The clamps are removed in the newborn nursery approximately 24 hours after the cord has dried.

Physical Assessment of Newborn by Delivery Room Nurse

An abbreviated systematic physical assessment is performed by the nurse in the delivery room to detect any

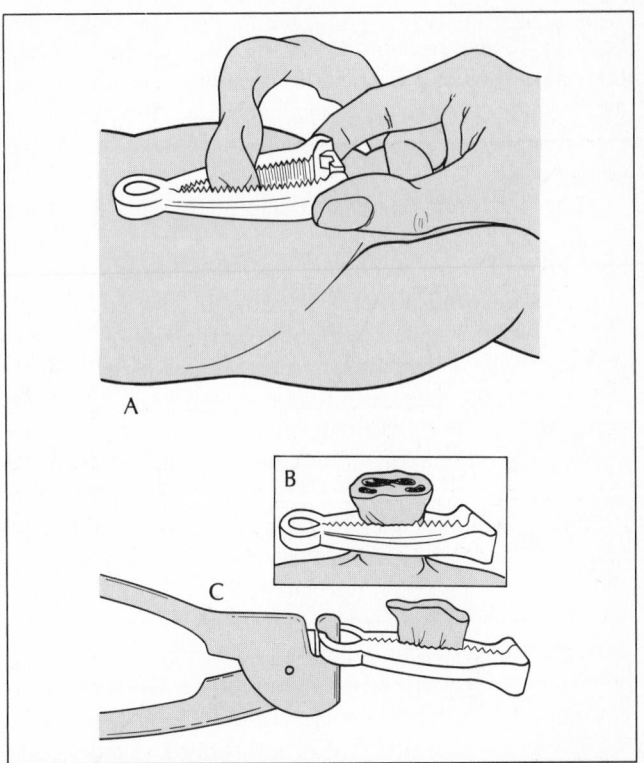

FIGURE 16–17 Hollister cord clamp. **A,** Clamp is positioned ½–1 inch from the abdomen and then secured. **B,** Cut cord. **C,** Plastic device for removing clamp after cord has dried.

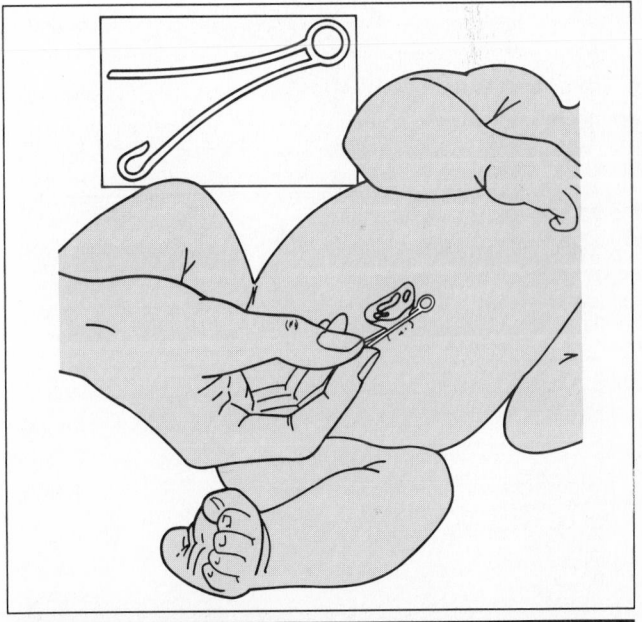

FIGURE 16–18 Hesseltine cord clamp is applied in a similar manner. Two clamps are often used to reduce the possibility of hemorrhage should one inadvertently open. When the cord has dried, the clamp may be removed manually.

abnormalities (Figure 16–19). First, the size of the newborn and the contour and size of the head in relationship to the rest of the body are noted. The newborn's posture and movements indicate tone and neurologic functioning. A flaccid or flexed upper extremity could mean a brachial plexus palsy.

The skin is inspected for discoloration, presence of vernix caseosa and lanugo, and evidence of trauma and desquamation. Vernix caseosa is a white, cheesy substance found normally on newborns. It is absorbed within 24 hours after delivery. Vernix is present in abundance on preterm infants and not at all on postterm newborns. A large quantity of fine hair (lanugo) is often seen on preterm newborns, especially on their shoulders, foreheads, backs, and cheeks. Desquamation of the skin is seen in postterm newborns.

Facial symmetry should be inspected. A one-sided cry may mean facial paralysis. A wide-eyed stare by an agitated newborn is a sign of intrauterine hypoxia.

The chest is inspected for retraction, grunting, or stridor, and the respiratory rate is counted before the newborn is disturbed. A normal rate is 30 to 40 respirations per minute.

The fontanelles and cranial sutures are palpated, and the fontanelles are measured if they appear excessively large. The widest point of the anterior fontanelle should be no greater than 5 cm. The posterior fontanelle should be no greater than 1 cm. Any molding or caput succedaneum

is noted. The hair is felt for texture. The eyes are gently opened and inspected for the presence and clarity of pupils. The nose is inspected for flaring, and the nares are checked for patency by introducing a catheter in each nostril. The mouth is palpated for intactness of the soft and hard palate, and the gums are inspected for the presence of membranous teeth, which must be removed because of the danger of aspiration. The location of the ears is checked by laying the finger at the edge of the eye and drawing an imaginary line back to the ears. The pinna should be located above the line. Ears set below the line are associated with congenital mental retardation and kidney problems. The pinna of the ears should be folded forward. They will stay folded or slowly return back in preterm newborns.

The newborn's neck is palpated bilaterally for size and presence of webbing. The clavicles are then palpated for intactness. Sometimes fractures occur in difficult deliveries. The breast tissue is measured for thickness, and any discharge is noted. Breast tissue that is 7 mm thick is seen in newborns over 39 weeks' gestation. About 4 mm is found in newborns who are of 37–38 weeks' gestation and 2 mm in newborns of less than 36 weeks' gestation. Any supernumerary nipples are noted.

The heart is auscultated for murmurs. About 90% of newborn murmurs are transient. The lungs are auscultated bilaterally for breath sounds. Absence of breath sounds on one side could mean a pneumothorax. Rales may be heard immediately after birth because of the presence of a small amount of fluid in the lungs, which will be absorbed. Ronchi indicate aspiration of oral secretions.

The newborn's abdomen is inspected for shape, size, contour, and abnormal pulsations. A pulsation around the epigastrium could indicate an enlarged heart. Distention could be a sign of congenital malformation. Localized flank enlargement is seen with enlarged kidneys. The edge of the liver is normally palpable below the right costal margin, and the tip of the spleen may also be palpated. The lower pole of each kidney may be felt abdominally 1 or 2 cm above the umbilicus. Anything below this level indicates enlargement. Distention of the bladder that occurs with obstructions may be palpated in the suprapubic region.

The genitals are inspected for sex verification, and any ambiguity is noted. Full rugation on the male scrotum indicates 39 weeks' gestation or more. Intermediate rugation is seen from 37–38 weeks. The scrotum is palpated for descended testes. Preterm newborns may have testes located in the inguinal canal. In female newborns, the clitoris is inspected for enlargement. Sometimes an enlarged clitoris may resemble a penis. The labia minora of preterm newborns are more prominent than the labia majora.

The anus is inspected for patency. If the newborn passes meconium or voids while in the delivery room, this is recorded on the delivery record and reported to the newborn nursery staff, because they are concerned about

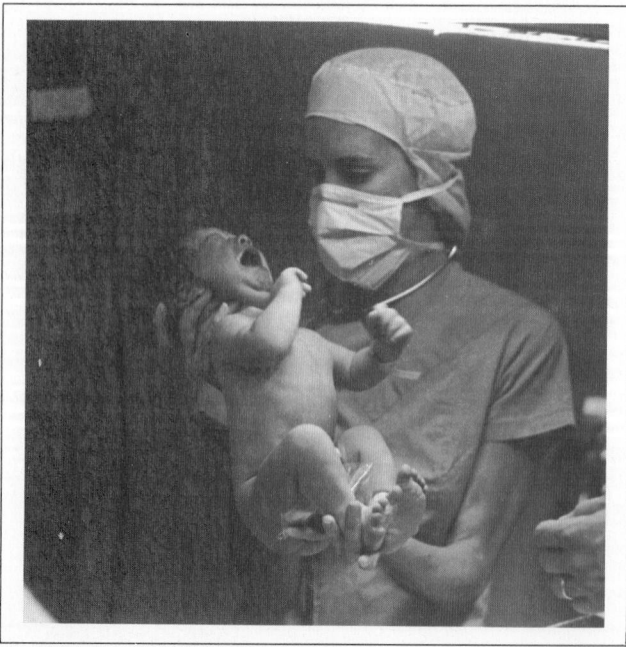

FIGURE 16–19 The delivery room nurse assesses the newborn. Notice the urine bag on the infant. (In most institutions, a urine collection is not done in the delivery room.)

the first voiding and defecation, which indicate normal system functioning.

The upper and lower extremities are inspected for the correct number of digits. Long fingernails are seen in the postterm newborn. To check for "hip click," which occurs with congenitally dislocated hips, the nurse flexes the legs at the knees and rotates them laterally. The soles of the feet are examined for creases. On newborns who are at 39 weeks of gestational age or more, the creases cover the entire foot. Creases on the anterior two-thirds of the feet are seen in newborns who are 37–38 weeks' gestation. In newborns less than 36 weeks, a single anterior transverse crease is found (Pritchard and MacDonald, 1980; Korones, 1981).

This brief examination reveals any gross abnormalities and permits a quick determination of gestational age. Most of this examination is accomplished by visual assessment. Further neurologic assessment and an in-depth physical examination are performed in the newborn nursery (see Chapter 22).

The newborn may be weighed and measured in the delivery room/birthing room or in the newborn nursery.

Newborn Identification Procedures

To assure that the parents are given the correct newborn, the mother and baby are tagged with identical bands or bracelets before the newborn is separated from the mother. One bracelet is applied to the mother's wrist, and two bracelets are applied to the newborn—one on each wrist, one on a wrist and one on an ankle, or one on each ankle. The bands must be applied snugly to prevent loss.

Most hospitals footprint the newborn and fingerprint the mother for further identification purposes. When preparing to footprint the newborn, the nurse wipes the soles of both the newborn's feet to remove any vernix caseosa, which interferes with the placement of ink on the foot creases.

See the accompanying Nursing Care Plan on the immediate care of the newborn.

MANAGEMENT OF THE THIRD AND FOURTH STAGES OF LABOR

Third Stage

After delivery, the clinician prepares for delivery of the placenta. As discussed in Chapter 14, the following signs suggest placental separation:

1. The uterus rises upward in the abdomen because the placenta settles downward into the lower uterine segment.

2. As the placenta proceeds downward, the umbilical cord lengthens.

3. A sudden trickle or spurt of blood appears.

4. The uterus changes from a discoid to a globular shape.

While waiting for these signs, the nurse palpates the uterus to check for ballooning of the uterus caused by uterine relaxation and subsequent bleeding into the uterine cavity.

After the placenta has separated, the client may be asked to bear down to facilitate delivery of the placenta. As discussed below, oxytocics are frequently given at the time of the delivery of the placenta. Oxytocin (Pitocin) 10 units may be given intravenously slowly along with methylergonovine maleate (Methergine) 0.2 mg intramuscularly. The nurse assesses and records maternal blood pressure before and after administration of oxytocics. The medications used vary with different clinicians. It is the nurse's responsibility to clearly understand and carry out the orders of the clinician and to record all medications on the delivery room record.

After the delivery of the placenta, the clinician inspects the placental membranes to make sure they are intact and that all cotyledons are present. This inspection is especially important with Duncan placentas. If there is a defect or a part missing from the placenta, a digital uterine examination is done. The vagina and cervix are inspected for lacerations, and any necessary repairs are made. The episiotomy may be repaired now if it has not been done previously. (See further discussion of episiotomy on p. 595). The fundus of the uterus is palpated; normal position is at the midline and below the umbilicus. If the fundus is displaced, it may be because of a full bladder or a collection of blood in the uterus. The uterus may be emptied of blood by grasping it anteriorly and posteriorly and squeezing.

The time of delivery of the placenta and the mechanism (Schultze or Duncan) is noted on the delivery record.

The uterine fundus is palpated at frequent intervals to ensure that it remains firmly contracted. The maternal blood pressure is monitored at 5- to 15-minute intervals to detect any untoward elevation, which may occur because of oxytocic drugs, or any decrease, which may be associated with excessive blood loss.

The client may be transferred to the recovery room after any active bleeding has subsided, the uterus is firm and well retracted, and maternal blood pressure and pulse are within normal limits.

USE OF OXYTOCICS

Clinicians advocate the use of oxytocic drugs (Pitocin, Syntocinon) to promote homeostasis through the stimulation of myometrial contractility after delivery. Each ampule of oxytocin contains 10 USP units/mL. The half-life of the compound is 3 minutes when given intravenously. Oxytocin should not be given by intravenous push in a large

NURSING CARE PLAN
Immediate Care of Newborn

PATIENT DATA BASE

History

Maternal prenatal history

Fetal status in utero (FHR, presence of meconium, hyperactivity)

Progress of labor and status of membranes

Type of delivery (spontaneous, forceps)

Physical examination

Estimation of newborn's status utilizing the Apgar scoring system at 1 and 5 min (score of 8–10: respirations present, cry strong, heart rate over 100, reflexes present, muscle tone good, and color dusky to pink)

Examination of cord for number of vessels, any hemorrhagic areas, and length

Complete short physical examination (see Neonatal Physical Assessment Guide, Chapter 22 for complete exam)

1. Sex of infant determined
2. No observable congenital anomalies

NURSING PRIORITIES

1. Establish a clear airway and adequate respiratory and cardiac effort
2. Stabilize temperature
3. Prevent infection
4. Identify newborn
5. Facilitate parent–newborn bonding

CLIENT/FAMILY EDUCATIONAL FOCUS

1. Discuss immediate care being given to the newborn
2. Provide opportunities to discuss individual questions and concerns of the client and family

Problem	Nursing interventions and actions	Rationale
Initial extrauterine adaptation	Determine and record Apgar score for infant at 1 and 5 min after birth If Apgar score is below 8 resuscitative efforts need to be instituted	Low Apgar score indicates need for possible resuscitative efforts
Respirations	Place infant in modified Trendelenburg position (lateral position)	Assists gravity drainage of mucus
	Gently suction nose and mouth with bulb syringe If respirations are depressed, suction with a DeLee catheter (Procedure 16–1); provide tactile stimulation; institute appropriate resuscitative measures as needed (see Chapter 25)	Vigorous suctioning that irritates the back of the throat can cause vagal stimulation which may lead to bradycardia; a DeLee catheter provides more efficient suctioning
	Administer O_2 by mask at 4–7 L/min if marked pallor or cyanosis is present	Provides additional O_2 and respiratory support
Temperature maintenance	Dry newborn thoroughly and place uncovered under radiant heat, or place on mother's chest and maintain skin-to-skin contact	Radiant heat works most efficiently on a dry surface; newborns remain naked so that radiant heat warms their skin surface
Protection from infection	Place clamp on umbilical cord using aseptic technique	Clamping cord also prevents bleeding Aseptic technique reduces chance of infection

NURSING CARE PLAN Cont'd
Immediate Care of Newborn

Problem	Nursing interventions and actions	Rationale
	Administer 1% silver nitrate solution in drops or place antibiotic ointment (Ilotycin) in newborn's eyes	Prevents ophthalmia neonatorum
Identification	Place two bracelets on infant (both wrists, both ankles, or one of each); NOTE: Newborn loses 5%–10% of birth weight, so bracelets must be snug	Assures identification
Congenital abnormalities	Assess for presence of malformations; observe and record number of vessels in cord	One artery in the umbilical cord is associated with genitourinary abnormalities
Bonding	Place newborn with mother and father as soon as possible	Facilitates formation of relationship between parents and child
	Encourage parents to unwrap and look at their newborn; assist mother with breast-feeding if she desires	
	Dim lights if possible so the newborn will readily open eyes	Establishment of eye contact is an important element in bonding process

NURSING CARE EVALUATION

Infant is delivered without undue trauma	Measures to prevent infections are instituted
Adequate respiratory effort is established	Identification of the newborn is accomplished
Neutral thermoregulation is provided	Attachment process is facilitated
	Any congenital abnormalities are noted

NURSING DIAGNOSIS*	SUPPORTING DATA
Potential impaired gas exchange	Excessive airway secretions
	Ineffective breathing patterns
	Total Apgar score of less than 8 (or individual score of 0 or 1 on respiratory effort)
	Pallor
	Cyanosis
	Flaccid
Potential for injury	Hypothermia
	Infection
	Birth trauma
Potential alteration in parenting	Lack of anticipated early parenting behaviors
	Birth trauma to newborn that necessitates separation of newborn from parents

*These are a few examples of nursing diagnoses that may be appropriate for a newborn. It is not an inclusive list and must be individualized for each newborn.

Procedure 16–1 DeLee Suction

Objective	Nursing action	Rationale
Clear secretions from newborn's nose and/or oropharynx	Tighten the lid on the suction collection bottle (Figure 16–20)	Avoids spillage of secretions and prevents air from leaking out of lid
	Place the whistle tip in your mouth; insert other end of tubing in newborn's nose or mouth for a distance of approximately 3-5 in.; provide suction by sucking on whistle tip	Provides suction / Clears nasopharynx / Gives gentle suction
	Continue suction as tube is removed	Avoids redepositing secretions in newborn's nasopharynx
	Continue reinserting tube and providing suction for as long as: 1. Secretions are being removed 2. Newborn continues to have depressed respirations 3. Movement of secretion can be heard with respiratory effort by ausculation of lungs	Facilitates removal of secretions / If meconium was present in amniotic fluid the baby may have swallowed some
	Occasionally the tube may be passed into the newborn's stomach to remove secretions or meconium that was swallowed before birth; if this action is needed, insert tube into newborn's mouth and then into the stomach	Secretions and/or meconium aspirate may be removed from newborn's stomach to decrease incidence of aspiration of stomach contents
	Provide suction and continue suction as tube is removed	

bolus because of the danger of maternal hypertension. It may be given intravenously or intramuscularly. Oxytocin may be added to 1000 mL of fluid and given intravenously over a period of hours.

The clinician may request that oxytocin (10 units) be given intramuscularly at the time of delivery of the anterior shoulder of the infant; some believe that this facilitates delivery of the placenta. Others question whether this method increases the incidence of neonatal hyperviscosity because an additional bolus of blood may be infused into the fetus when the uterus contracts (in response to oxytocin). At other times, oxytocin may be administered intramuscularly as the placenta delivers.

Oxytocin also has an antidiuretic effect. If given rapidly in an electrolyte-free solution, water intoxication could occur. Pritchard and MacDonald (1980) advocate the use of a solution that contains electrolytes coupled with an increase of the hormone's concentration rather than merely increasing the intravenous flow rate. See Drug Guides—Oxytocin, p. 590, and Methergine, p. 903.

CONTROLLING POSTPARTAL HEMORRHAGE

Ergonovine (Ergotrate) and methylergonovine (Methergine) are alkaloids derived from lysergic acid from the rye plant fungus. They may be given parenterally or orally and are used to control postpartal hemorrhage. Tetanic contractions are produced, with little tendency toward uterine relaxation. Transient but severe hypertension is a dangerous side effect with these drugs. For this reason they should not be given to clients with hypertensive problems or to clients who have received conduction anesthesia (Pritchard and MacDonald, 1980).

Fourth Stage

As soon as the placenta is delivered and the episiotomy or any vaginal lacerations are repaired, the delivery drapes may be removed. The nurse washes the perineum with gauze squares and sterile solution and dries the area with a sterile towel before placing the maternity pads. The client's legs are removed from the stirrups at the same time to avoid muscle strain. The legs may be bicycled to facilitate circulation return. The client is transferred to a recovery room bed, and the nurse helps her don a clean gown. The mother may feel cold and begin shivering. She can be covered with a warmed bath blanket, which may be covered by a second blanket. If the mother has not had a chance to hold her infant, she may do so before she is

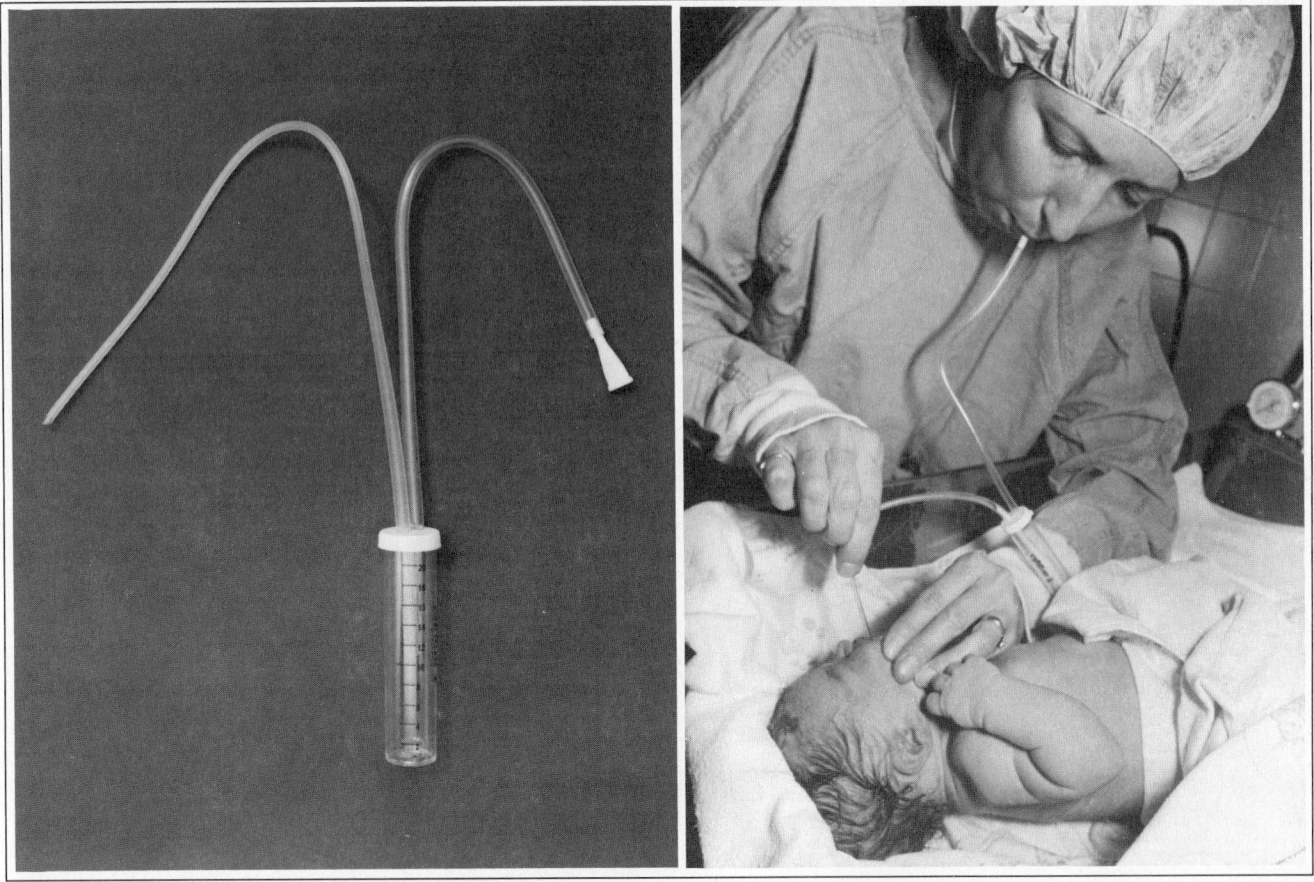

FIGURE 16–20 DeLee suction trap.

removed from the delivery room. The nurse ensures that the mother and father and newborn are provided with time to begin the attachment process. (See Chapter 28 for further discussion of attachment.)

The woman remains in the recovery room for a minimum of 1–2 hours; in some institutions she remains until she has voided for the first time. The recovery period requires close observation. The mother's oral temperature is taken once, unless it is elevated. Elevated temperature requires follow-up observation. Her blood pressure, pulse, respirations, consistency and position of fundus, and amount and character of vaginal flow are checked every 15 minutes for the first hour. Deviations from the normal ranges require more frequent checking. Blood pressure should return to the prelabor level, and pulse rate should be slightly lower than it was in labor. The return of the blood pressure is due to an increased volume of blood returning to the maternal circulation from the uteroplacental shunt. Baroreceptors cause a vagal response, which slows the pulse. A rise in the blood pressure may be a response to oxytocic drugs or may be caused by toxemia. Blood loss may be reflected by a lowered blood pressure and a rising pulse rate.

The fundus should be firm at the umbilicus or lower and in the midline. It should be palpated (Figure 16–21) but not massaged unless atonic. If it becomes boggy or appears to rise in the abdomen, the fundus should be massaged until firm; then with one hand supporting the uterus at the symphysis, the nurse should attempt to express retained clots. Overmassaging of the fundus causes an increased tendency toward uterine relaxation due to muscle exhaustion.

The nurse inspects the bloody vaginal discharge for amount and charts it as minimal, moderate, or heavy and with or without clots. This discharge, or *lochia rubra*, should be bright red. A soaked perineal pad contains approximately 100 mL of blood. If the perineal pad becomes soaked in a 15-minute period or if blood pools under the buttocks, continuous observation is necessary. Laceration of the vagina, cervix, or an unligated vessel in the episiotomy may be indicated by a continuous trickle of blood even though the fundus remains firm.

If the fundus rises and displaces to the right, the nurse palpates the bladder to determine whether it is distended. All measures should be taken to enable the mother to void. If she is unable to void, catheterization is necessary. Post-

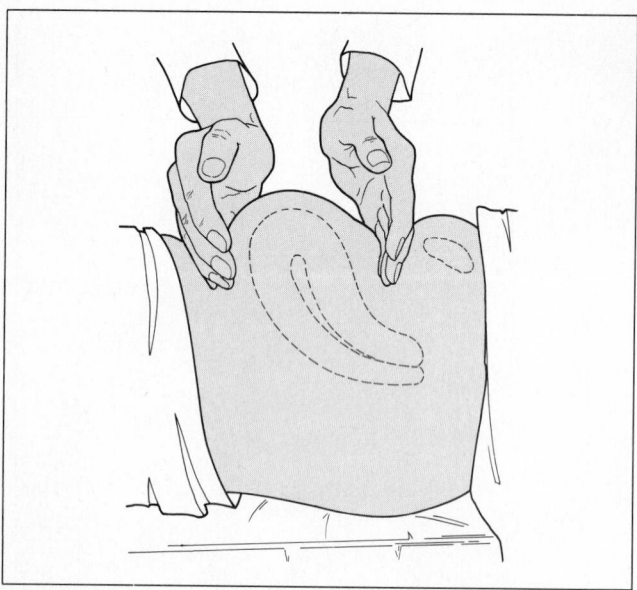

FIGURE 16–21 Suggested method of palpating the fundus of the uterus during the fourth stage. The left hand is placed just above the symphysis pubis, and gentle downward pressure is exerted. The right hand is cupped around the uterine fundus.

partal women have decreased sensations to void as a result of the decreased tone of the bladder as a result of the trauma imposed on the bladder and urethra during childbirth. The bladder fills rapidly as the body attempts to rid itself of the extra fluid volume returned from the uteroplacental circulation and of intravenous fluid that may have been received during labor and delivery. If the mother is unable to void, a warm towel placed across the lower abdomen or warm water poured over the perineum may help the urinary sphincter to relax and may thus facilitate voiding. A distended bladder can cause uterine atony and postpartal bleeding.

The perineum is inspected for edema and hematoma formation. With episiotomies, an ice pack often reduces swelling and alleviates discomfort.

The following conditions should be reported to the clinician: hypotension, tachycardia, uterine atony, excessive bleeding, or a temperature over 100F or 38C. The nurse should be aware that the blood pressure may not fall rapidly in the presence of dangerous bleeding in postpartal mothers because of the extra systemic volume. However, an increasing pulse rate may be noted before a decrease in blood pressure is detected. A normal blood pressure with the mother in the Fowler's position is a good confirmation of a normotensive woman.

Frequently women have tremors in the immediate postpartal period. It has been proposed that this shivering response is caused by a difference in internal and external body temperatures (higher temperature inside the body

than on the outside). Another theory proposes that the maternal organism is reacting to the fetal cells that have entered the maternal circulation at the placental site. A heated bath blanket placed next to the woman tends to alleviate the problem.

The couple may be tired, hungry, and thirsty. Some hospitals serve the couple a meal. The tired mother will probably drift off into a welcomed sleep. The father should also be encouraged to rest, because his role as one of the mother's major support systems is tiring physically and mentally.

After 2 hours or depending on agency policy, if the client's vital signs are stable with no bleeding, if her bladder is not distended, if her fundus is firm, and if her sensorium is fully reactive from any anesthetic agent that she may have received during delivery, the mother is usually transferred from the delivery unit to the postpartal floor.

FACILITATION OF ATTACHMENT

Dramatic evidence indicates that a sensitive period for attachment of mother and infant exists in the first few hours and even minutes after birth (Klaus and Kennell, 1982). Separation during this critical period not only delays attachment but may affect maternal and child behavior over a much longer period. At 1 month and 1 year after childbirth, mothers who were merely shown their infants after delivery and had them only briefly for 15- to 20-minute feeding periods demonstrated less eye contact and less soothing behavior during physical examination than did mothers who were allowed to hold their infants for an hour beginning 1–2 hours after delivery and for 5 hours on each of 3 succeeding days. The mothers with this extended contact asked twice as many questions about their children and used fewer commands at 2 years. The results of this and other research indicate that as soon as feasible the newborn needs to be united with his or her parents (Klaus and Kennell, 1982.)

Klaus and Kennell (1982) believe the bonding experience can be enhanced by at least 30–60 minutes of early contact in privacy. If this period of contact can occur during the first hour after birth, the newborn will be in the quiet state (state 4) and able to interact with parents by looking at them. Newborns also turn their heads in response to a spoken voice (see Chapter 21 for further discussion of newborn states).

The first parent–newborn contact may be brief (a few minutes) to be followed by a more extended period of time after uncomfortable procedures (delivery of the placenta and suturing of the episiotomy) are completed. When the newborn is returned to the mother, she can be assisted to begin breast-feeding if she so desires. Helping the mother change position on the delivery table to give her more room to hold the newborn, or assisting her to a sitting position may facilitate breast-feeding. Even if the newborn does not actively nurse, he or she can lick, taste, and smell the mother's skin. This activity by the newborn stimulates the maternal release of prolactin, which facilitates the onset of lactation.

Some nurses have found that darkening the delivery room by turning out most of the lights causes newborns to open their eyes and gaze around. This in turn enhances eye-to-eye contact with the parents. (Note: if the clinician needs a light source, the "spot light" can be left on.) Treatment of the newborn's eyes may also be delayed. Many parents who establish eye contact with the newborn are content to quietly gaze at their infant. Others may have more active involvement by touching and/or inspecting the newborn. Some mothers talk to their babies in a high-pitched voice, which seems to be soothing to newborns. Some couples verbally express amazement and pride when they see they have produced a beautiful, healthy baby. Their verbalization enhances feelings of accomplishment and ecstasy. Figure 16–22 shows a new parent establishing bonds with his newborn son.

Both parents need to be encouraged to do whatever they feel most comfortable in doing. Some parents prefer only limited contact with the newborn in the delivery room and instead desire private time together in a more quiet environment, such as the recovery room or postpartal area. In the current zest for providing immediate attachment opportunities, nursing personnel need to be aware of parents' wishes. The desire to delay interaction with the newborn does not necessarily imply a decreased ability of the parents to bond to their newborn (see Chapter 28 for further discussion of parent–newborn attachment).

DELIVERY IN LESS-THAN-IDEAL CIRCUMSTANCES

Emergency delivery occurs in a variety of physical settings and during a variety of climatic disturbances. The two areas that are addressed in this chapter are hospital births unattended by a clinician and unattended out-of-hospital births.

Precipitous Delivery

Occasionally labor progresses so rapidly that the maternity nurse is faced with the task of delivering the baby. This is called a *precipitous delivery*. The attending maternity nurse has the primary responsibility for providing a physically and psychologically safe experience for the woman and her baby.

A client whose physician or nurse-midwife is not present may feel disappointed, frightened, and abandoned, especially if she is not prepared through childbirth education. Fear is an inhibiting factor in birth rooms; therefore, the

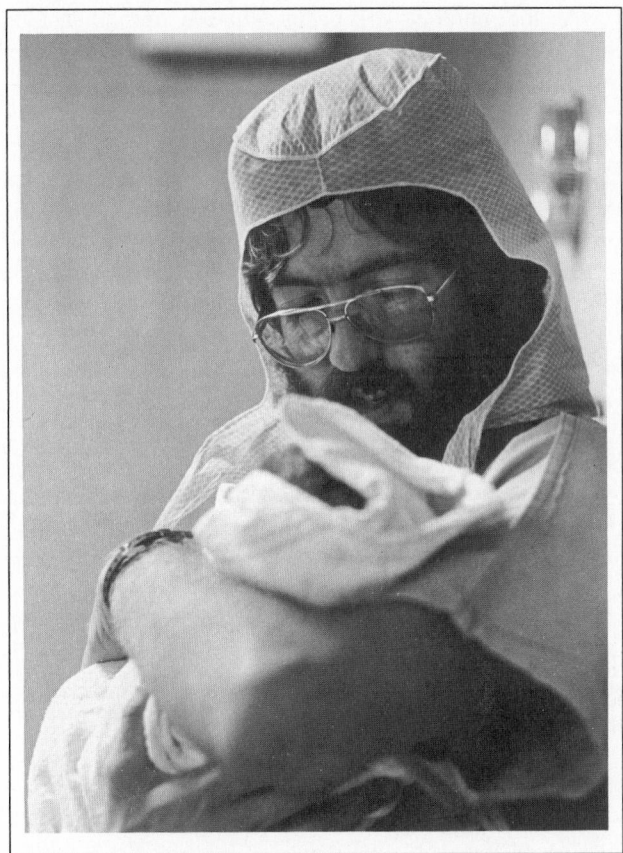

FIGURE 16–22 The father holds his son.

nurse can support the woman by keeping her informed about the labor progress and assuring the client that the nurse will stay with her. If delivery is imminent, the nurse must not leave the mother alone. Auxiliary personnel can be directed to contact the clinician and to retrieve the emergency delivery pack ("precip pack"). An emergency delivery pack should be readily accessible to the labor rooms. A typical pack contains the following items:

1. A small drape that can be placed under the client's buttocks to provide a sterile field.
2. Several 4 × 4 gauze pads for wiping off the newborn's face and removing secretions from the mouth.
3. A bulb syringe to be used to clear mucus from the newborn's mouth.
4. Two sterile clamps (Kelly or Rochester) to clamp the umbilical cord.
5. Sterile scissors to cut the umbilical cord.
6. A sterile umbilical cord clamp, either Hesseltine or Hollister.
7. A baby blanket to wrap the newborn in after delivery.
8. A package of sterile gloves.

As the materials are being gathered, the nurse must remain calm. The client is reassured by the composure of the nurse and feels that the nurse is competent.

DELIVERY OF INFANT IN VERTEX PRESENTATION

The nurse who manages a precipitous delivery in the hospital conducts it as follows. The client is encouraged to assume a comfortable position. If time permits, the nurse scrubs hands with soap and water and puts on sterile gloves. Sterile drapes are placed under the client's buttocks.

At all times during the delivery, the nurse gives clear instructions to the client, supports her efforts, and provides reassurance.

When the head crowns, the nurse instructs the client to pant, which decreases her urge to push. The nurse checks whether the amniotic sac is intact. If it is, the nurse tears the sac so the newborn will not breathe in amniotic fluid with the first breath.

The nurse may place an index finger inside the lower portion of the vagina and the thumb on the outer portion of the perineum and gently massage the area to aid in stretching of perineal tissues and to help prevent perineal lacerations. This is called "ironing the perineum."

With one hand, the nurse applies gentle pressure against the fetal head to prevent it from popping out rapidly. *The nurse does not hold the head back forcibly.* Rapid delivery of the head may result in tears in the woman's perineal tissues; in the fetus the rapid change in pressure within the fetal head may cause subdural or dural tears. The nurse supports the perineum with the other hand and allows the head to be delivered between contractions.

As the client continues to pant, the nurse inserts one or two fingers along the back of the fetal head to check for the umbilical cord. If the cord is around the neck, the nurse bends the fingers like a fish hook, grasps the cord, and pulls it over the baby's head. It is important to check that the cord is not wrapped around more than one time. If the cord is tightly looped and cannot be slipped over the baby's head, two clamps are placed on the cord, the cord is cut between the clamps, and the cord is unwound.

Immediately after delivery of the head, the mouth, throat, and nasal passages are suctioned. The nurse places one hand on each side of the head and exerts gentle downward traction until the anterior shoulder passes under the symphysis pubis. At this time, gentle upward pressure facilitates delivery of the posterior shoulder. The nurse then instructs the woman to push gently so that the rest of the body can be delivered quickly. The newborn must be supported as it emerges.

The newborn is held at the level of the uterus to facilitate blood flow through the umbilical cord. The nurse must be careful to avoid dropping the newborn, as the combination of amniotic fluid and vernix makes the newborn very slippery. The nose and mouth of the newborn are suctioned again, using a bulb syringe. The nurse then dries the newborn to prevent heat loss.

As soon as the nurse determines that the newborn's respirations are adequate, the infant can be placed on the mother's abdomen with the newborn's head slightly lower than the body to facilitate drainage of fluid and mucus. The weight of the newborn on her abdomen stimulates uterine contractions, which aid in placental separation. The umbilical cord should not be pulled.

The nurse is alert for signs of placental separation (slight gush of dark blood from the vagina, lengthening of the cord, or a change in uterine shape from discoid to globular). When these signs are present, the mother is instructed to push so that the placenta can be delivered. The nurse inspects the placenta to determine whether it is intact.

The nurse checks the firmness of the uterus. The fundus may be gently massaged to stimulate contractions and to decrease bleeding. Putting the newborn to breast also stimulates uterine contractions through release of oxytocin from the pituitary gland.

The umbilical cord may now be cut. Two sterile clamps are placed approximately 2–4 inches from the newborn's abdomen. The cord is cut between them with sterile scissors. A sterile cord clamp (Hollister or Hesseltine) can be placed adjacent to the clamp on the newborn's cord, between the clamp and the newborn's abdomen. The clamp *must not* be placed snugly against the abdomen, because the cord will dry and shrink.

The area under the mother's buttocks is cleaned, and her perineum is inspected for lacerations. Bleeding from lacerations may be controlled by pressing a clean perineal pad against the perineum and instructing the client to keep her thighs together.

□ *RECORD KEEPING* The following information is noted and placed on a delivery record:

1. Position of fetus at delivery.
2. Presence of cord around neck or shoulder (nuchal cord).
3. Time of delivery.
4. Apgar scores at 1 and 5 minutes after birth.
5. Sex of newborn.
6. Time of delivery of placenta.
7. Method of placental expulsion.
8. Appearance and intactness of placenta.
9. Mother's condition.
10. Any medications that were given to mother or newborn (per agency protocol).

□ *POSTDELIVERY INTERVENTIONS* If the physician arrives soon after delivery, the nurse assists him or her in the examination of the mother, newborn, and placenta. Other nursing interventions directed toward the newborn include the following:

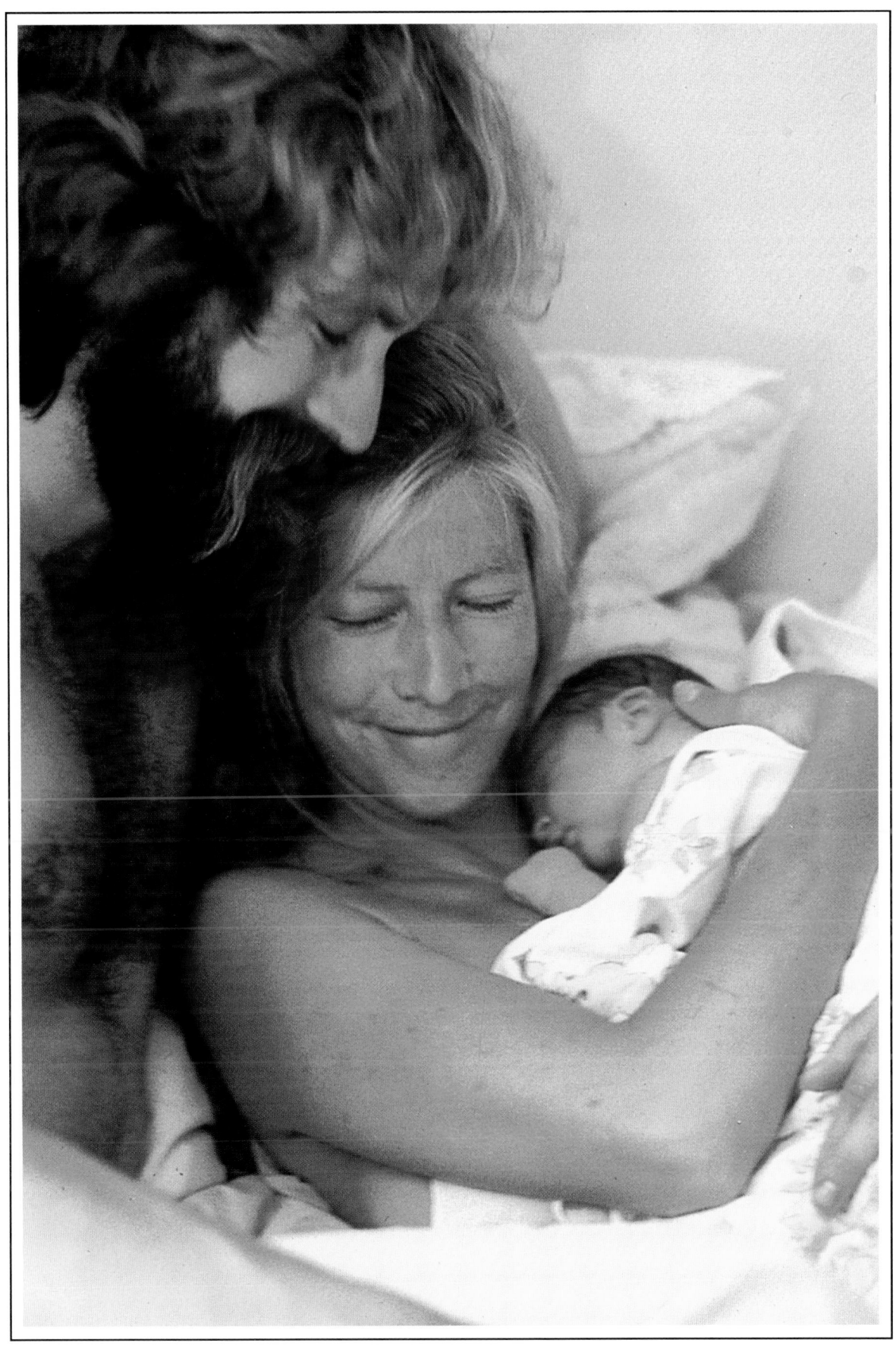

Plate I   Beginnings…

Plate II   Linea nigra

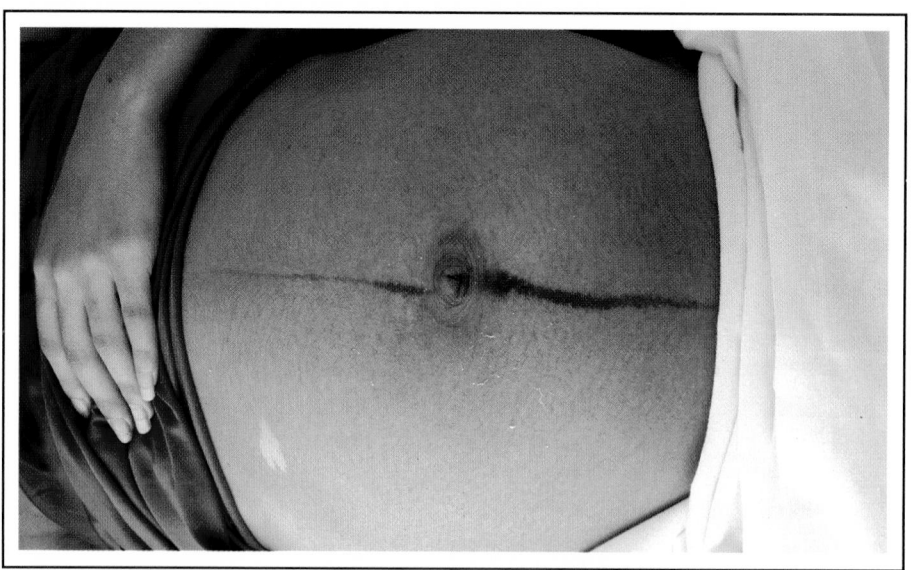

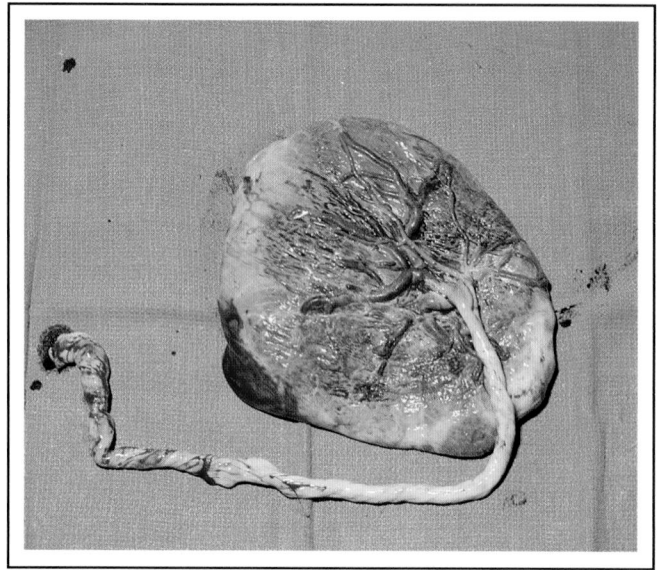

Plate III   Fetal side of placenta

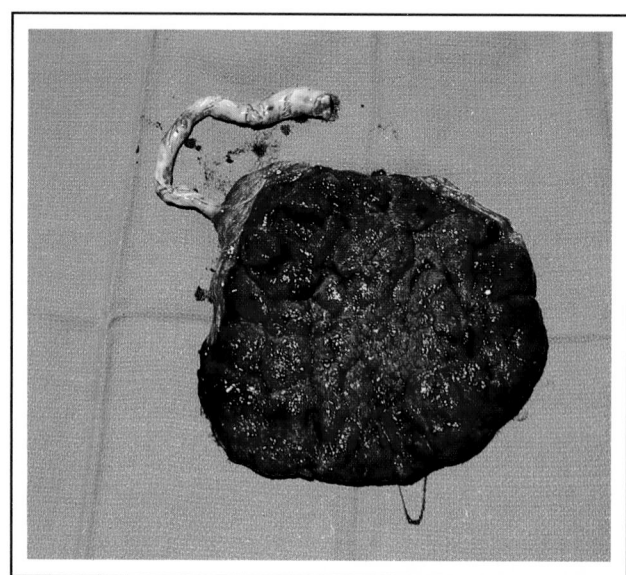

Plate IV   Maternal side of placenta

Plate V   Acrocyanosis

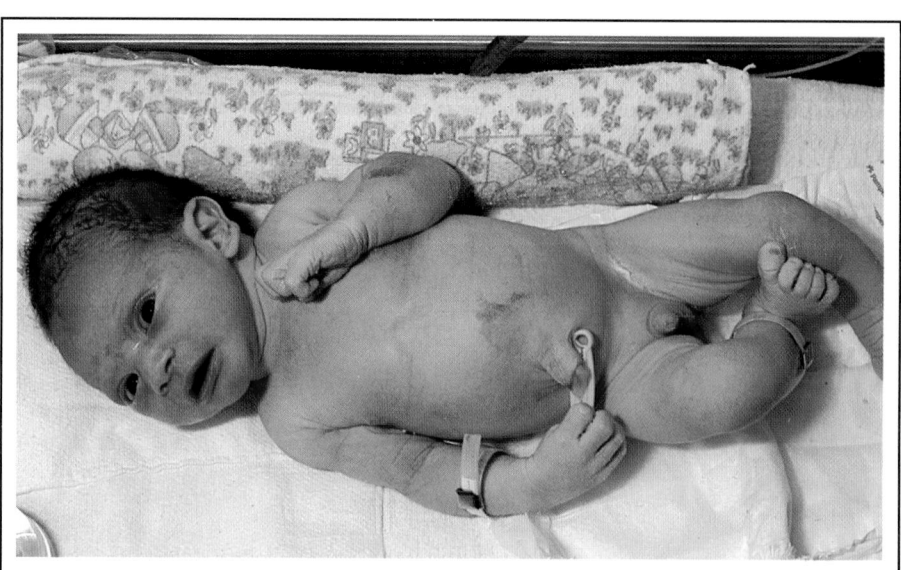

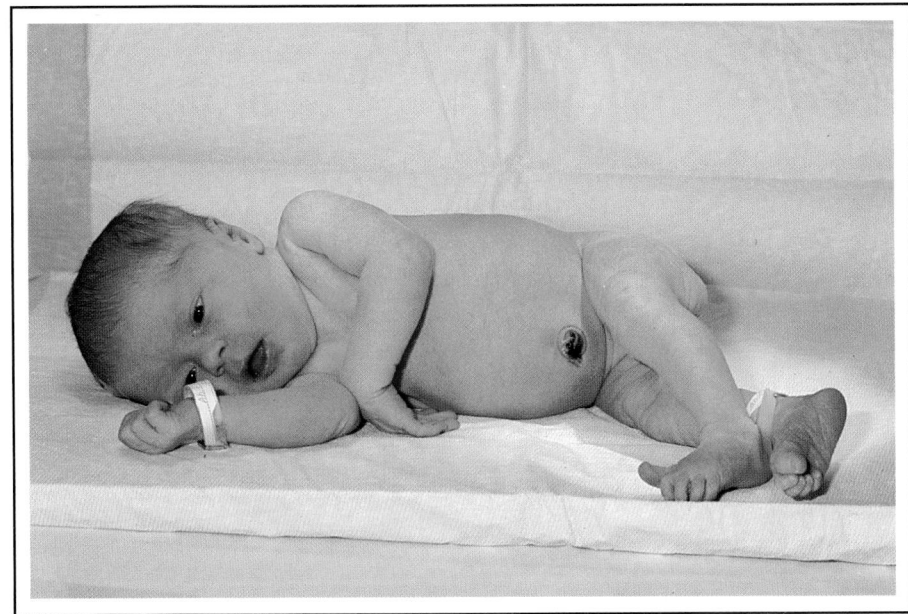

Plate VI   Normal newborn

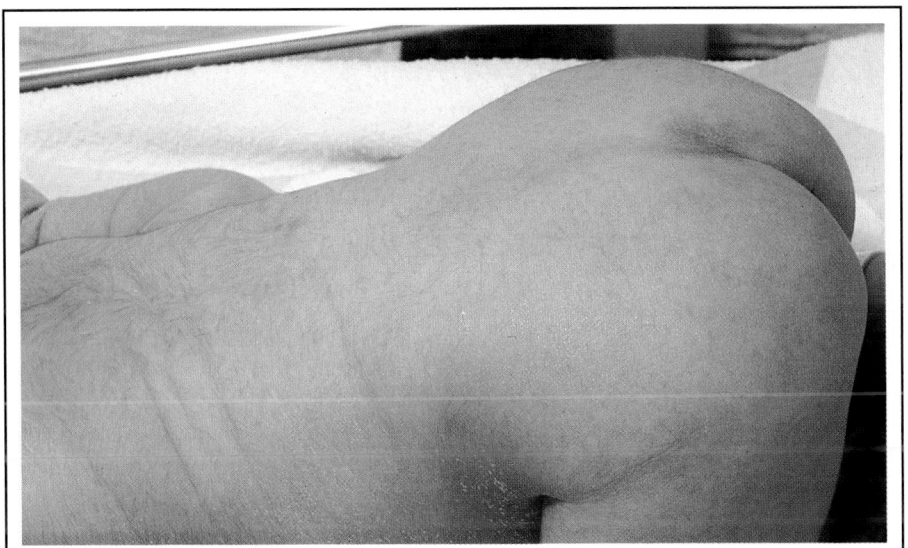

Plate VII   Mongolian spots

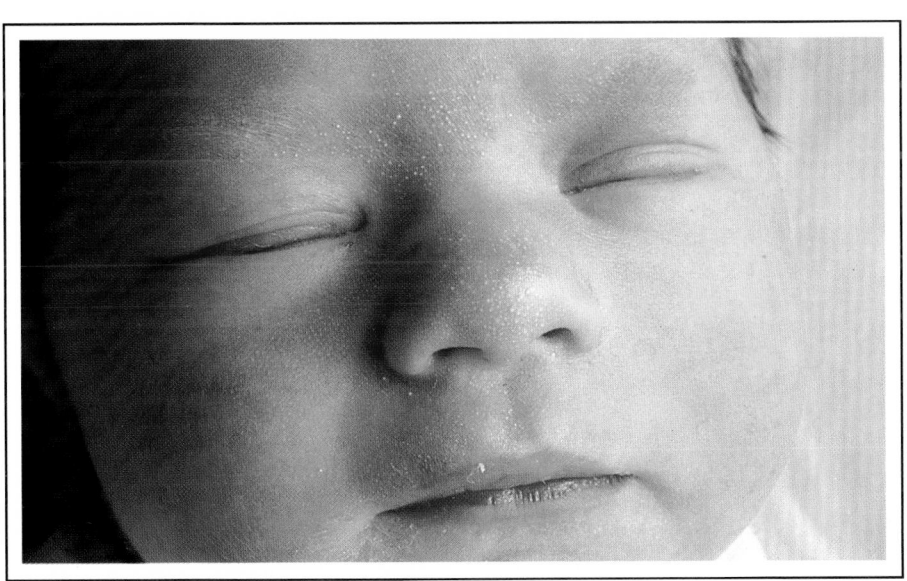

Plate VIII   Facial milia

Plate IX   Stork bites

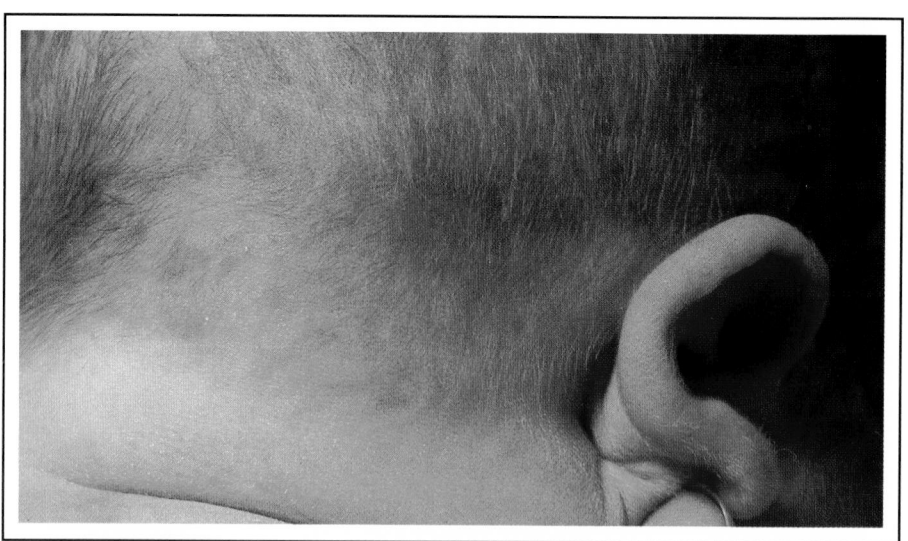

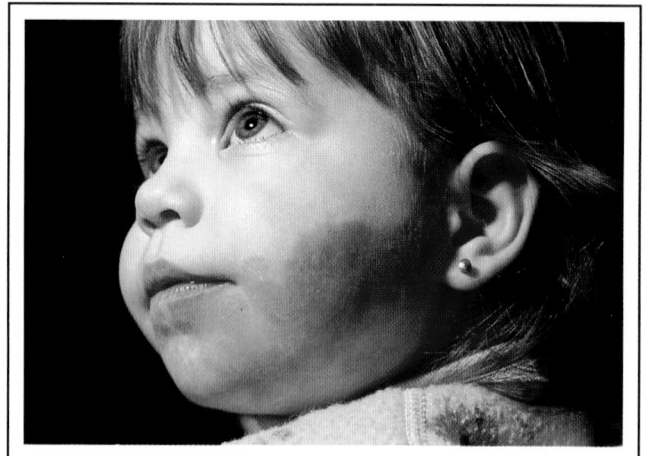

Plate X   Portwine stain

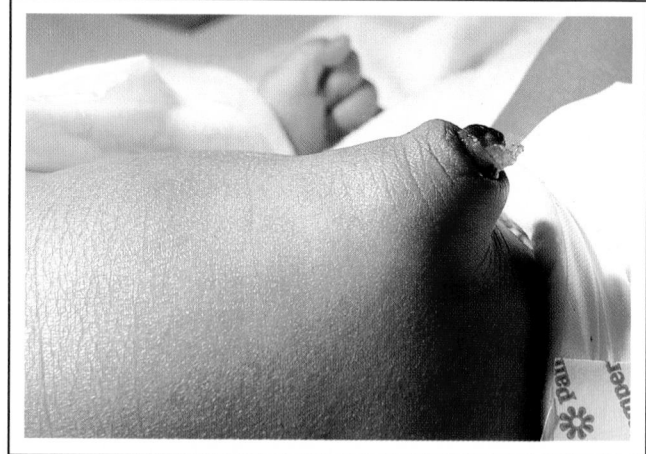

Plate XI   Umbilical hernia

Plate XII   Erythema toxicum

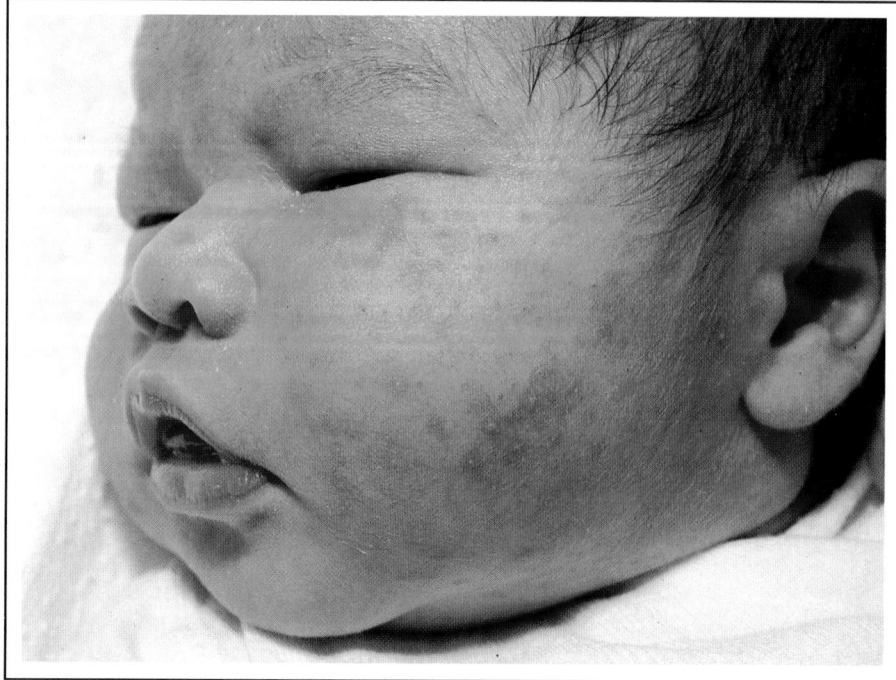

1. Keep the airway clear.
2. Maintain warmth.
3. Note and record a meconium stool or voiding.
4. Inspect the cord for the number of vessels and record this information.
5. Instill erythromycin (Ilotycin) or 1% silver nitrate or another appropriate prophylactic agent into the newborn's eyes.
6. Place identification bracelets on the newborn's wrists or ankles.
7. Transfer the newborn to the nursery.

If the newborn is premature, a careful evaluation of respiratory status should also be made.

Nursing interventions directed toward the mother are as follows:

1. Monitor vital signs every 5–15 minutes.
2. Assess firmness and position of uterus.
3. Evaluate amount of lochia and presence of clots.
4. Assess bladder fullness (a distended bladder can exert pressure on the uterus and increase the amount of bleeding).
5. Ensure her warmth.

Additional interventions include actions that enhance maternal–infant bonding. They include:

1. Encouraging the mother to look at and touch her baby.
2. Praising the mother for her accomplishments during labor and delivery.
3. If the mother desires, assisting her in assuming a position of comfort to breast-feed the infant.

The nurse should include the father in the bonding process. If he was present at the delivery, he should be praised for any support that he offered. If the father was not present, he is permitted to be with the mother and baby as soon as possible after the birth. He should be encouraged to hold and touch the baby.

If the physician's arrival is delayed or if the newborn is having respiratory distress, the newborn should be transported immediately to the nursery. *Be sure the newborn is properly identified before he or she leaves the delivery area.*

DELIVERY OF INFANT IN BREECH PRESENTATION

A significant factor in a breech delivery is that the smallest part of the fetus presents first; succeeding parts are progressively larger. The cervix is not as effectively dilated when the fetus is in breech presentation as when it is in the vertex position. Therefore, descent is usually slow and may not occur until the cervix is fully dilated and the membranes rupture.

The emergency delivery of an infant in breech position is conducted similarly to that of an infant in vertex presentation. However, when the breech crowns, the nurse instructs the woman to pant so that the part is delivered between contractions. The nurse supports the breech in both hands. The infant's body is lifted slightly upward for delivery of the posterior shoulder and arm. The newborn may then be lowered, and the anterior shoulder and arm will pass under the symphysis.

Flexion of the head occurs as with other presentations. It is important to maintain the flexion. The nape of the neck pivots under the symphysis, and the rest of the head is borne over the perineum by a movement of flexion.

The remaining delivery and postdelivery interventions for breech birth are described in the preceding section on precipitous delivery of an infant in vertex presentation.

Out-of-Hospital Births

Every woman who is in labor should be transported to a care facility as soon as possible. However, this is not always possible. Emergency deliveries may be necessary in various locations, such as in cars or out of doors. Home delivery is considered an emergency only if it is unexpected and unplanned.

If a hospital or birth center is not accessible and birth is imminent, the following are important considerations:

- Privacy for the delivering woman (or couple)
- A clean place to deliver
- Protection from infection
- Safeguard against hemorrhage

NURSING MANAGEMENT OF THE EXPECTANT MOTHER

The woman who is laboring under such unusual circumstances will need a great deal of psychologic support. The beautiful experience that she had planned is now impossible, and she may react with hostility, bitterness, and resentment. In addition, she may be extremely frightened and alarmed by the lack of equipment and skilled personnel. An attitude of calm and confidence helps both the nurse and the woman maintain control.

The nurse must communicate to the woman in labor that her needs are understood. In addition, the nurse must reassure the woman that the nurse will work with the woman (and her support persons) to provide the best experience under the circumstances.

Do not separate the mother from her partner or other persons whom she chooses to be present. However, the expectant mother should be screened from curious strangers, both for privacy and asepsis. The less exposure the mother and newborn have to strangers, the less chance they have of contracting infections. If the woman is inside a shelter, folding chairs or carts draped with blankets or coats make an efficient screen, as do sleeping bags tied to low-hanging branches of trees if one is outdoors. A private room is desirable if available. Women in labor take precedence over any other individual or group when it comes to the use of space and transportation.

A clean surface should be provided for the woman. Unread newspapers, clean towels, blankets, garment bags turned inside out, the inside of a coat, or even a shirt or pair of slacks turned inside out can be placed under the woman's hips to cover a floor, a carpet, or the ground.

If the room or car temperature can be regulated, a warm environment 26.7C–28.9C (80F–84F) degrees is preferred. Two roaring fires, one on each side of the woman, provide warmth if the delivery is outside.

If one is attending a birth in a shelter, one should obtain the following supplies if possible:

- Bulb syringe
- Cord clamp
- Scissors
- Basin
- Four bath blankets
- Four sheets
- Four towels
- Two pillows
- Two baby shirts
- A dozen diapers (cloth or disposable)
- Ophthalmic silver nitrate solution (to instill in newborn's eyes)
- Sterile water and eyedropper to rinse the newborn's eyes
- Two dozen peripads
- A sanitary belt

The delivery can proceed as described for an in-hospital precipitous delivery (p.503). Substitution may need to be made in equipment. Cord ties or new shoestrings may be used to tie the umbilical cord. A clean soft cloth may be used to wipe off the newborn's face and the inside of the mouth. A new razor or scissors (clean or boiled) may be used to cut the cord. If necessary, the cord may be left intact and the placenta may be wrapped in a blanket with the newborn. Care must be taken to keep the newborn and placenta close together so that no unnecessary traction is put on the umbilical cord.

NURSING MANAGEMENT OF THE NEWBORN

The care of the newborn under out-of-hospital circumstances is directed toward the same considerations as those born in a hospital or maternity center: protection from overstimulation, infection, and heat loss; adequate resuscitation; and facilitation of parent–infant bonding.

□ *PROTECTION FROM OVERSTIMULATION AND INFECTION* Loud music, very bright lights, and large numbers of extraneous personnel are usually not in evidence in hospitals, and they are contraindicated during any birth. Overstimulation can occur in the presence of a great deal of noise and activity. The chances of infection are increased by the number of people the newborn is exposed to.

At sites designated as shelters during natural disasters, such as schools or church basements, these forms of overstimulation are very much in evidence. Under these circumstances, the nurse attempts to provide the woman in labor a quiet, screened, and restricted area that has some soundproofing and indirect lighting. If this is not possible, the nurse should request that the noise level be lowered. If spotlights or lanterns are used, the newborn's eyes must be shielded, or the light should be adjusted so that it does not shine directly into the eyes. The number of people in the immediate area should be restricted to caregivers, the expectant mother's family, and other support persons she may choose.

□ *PROTECTION FROM HEAT LOSS* Protecting the newborn from heat loss without a radiant warmer is a challenge to the nurse attending the family under emergency conditions. Any of several methods may be available. If the environment is unheated, that is, below 27.8C (82F), the nurse dries the newborn thoroughly, especially the hair. The nurse instructs the mother to roll onto her side (even if the placenta has not separated) and places the newborn on its side against the mother, skin-to-skin, so they face each other. The mother and infant are then wrapped up together or covered by one of the following methods:

1. Wrap the pair with unused plastic food wrap. Do not cover the newborn's face.
2. Wrap them with a garment bag turned inside out. The newborn should be wrapped as if in a blanket, but the face must not be covered. If the temperature is very low, a cap should be fashioned for the newborn and taped or tied in place, because the majority of heat loss is from the head.
3. Place layers of unread newspapers over the mother and newborn. The nurse must ensure that the newborn's feet are well covered and that there are no gaps in the paper where the heat can be lost. It is better to provide too many newspapers than too few.
4. Drape the mother and newborn with clothing and cover with blankets, coats, and so on.

When the mother and newborn are wrapped together, the nurse need not disturb their ambient environment to check the temperature. The mother can check the newborn's body temperature by feeling the infant's stomach with the back of the fingers.

Even if the environment is warmer than 27.8C (82F), it is necessary to dry the newborn thoroughly and to protect from heat loss. Wrapping the newborn up with the mother in a blanket, coat, or other materials is recommended.

□ *ENSURING ADEQUATE RESUSCITATION* During an emergency situation outside of the hospital, resuscitation equipment may not be available. If the newborn is mildly depressed, institute the following measures:

1. Position the newborn on its side, with the head slightly lower than the trunk. This position facilitates drainage of mucus by gravity.
2. Wipe mucus from the newborn's face and mouth with a soft rag or your finger.
3. Keep the newborn dry and warm to avoid cold stress.
4. *Do not* hold the newborn by the ankles and slap the buttocks because these actions cause excessive stimulation of the newborn. *Do* rub the newborn's back and stimulate the bottom of the feet by stroking with your fingers.
5. If these measures are not effective and there is no respiratory effort, give mouth-to-mouth resuscitation.
6. Evaluate for the presence of a heartbeat by placing fingers over the sternum. If a heartbeat is absent, initiate cardiopulmonary massage.

FACILITATION OF PARENT-INFANT BONDING

The mother and father and newborn are encouraged to get to know each other. The nurse can point out the newborn's behavior and show the mother or couple how they can deal with this behavior. For example, if the newborn is looking at the mother's face, the nurse can encourage the mother to make eye-to-eye contact and to smile at the newborn. When the newborn puts fist or fingers in his or her mouth, the mother can offer to breast-feed. When the newborn no longer wants to nurse and shows signs of sleepiness, the mother can stroke the baby gently, hum, sing or rock the newborn. Give-and-take behavior by the mother or couple helps alleviate much of their fear that the delivery under these unusual circumstances has adversely affected their ability to make bonds with or take care of their baby.

SUMMARY

Labor and delivery can be a time of anxious or eager anticipation. The nurse must remember that the care rendered to the client and family at this time has an impact not only on the client's feelings about and reactions to this labor and delivery but also on future childbearing plans and expectations.

The nurse must be adept at intrapartal assessment; must be cognizant of the physiologic changes that are occurring and the wide range of emotional reactions to labor and delivery; and must incorporate these into the plan of care for meeting the needs of the childbearing couple.

The first hour after delivery is critical for both mother and newborn from both a physiologic and psychologic viewpoint. This period demands continued knowledgeable and caring nursing management.

References

Abril, Irene, F. May/June 1977. Mexican-American folk beliefs: how they affect health care. *Am. J. Mat. Child Nurs.* 2:168.

Apgar, V. Aug. 1966. The newborn (Apgar) scoring system: reflections and advice. *Pediatr. Clin. North Am.* 13:645.

Burrow, G. N., and Ferris, T. 1982. *Medical complications during pregnancy.* Philadelphia: W. B. Saunders Co.

Carr, K. C. Winter 1980. Obstetric practices which protect against neonatal morbidity: focus on maternal position in labor and birth. *Birth Fam. J.* 7:249.

Carrington, B. W. 1978. The Afro American. In *Culture childbearing health professionals,* ed. Ann L. Clark. Philadelphia: F. A. Davis Company.

Chung, J. J. March 1977. Understanding the Oriental maternity patient. *Nurs. Clin. North Am.* 12:67.

Davitz, L. J., et al. 1976. Suffering as viewed in six different cultures. *Am. J. Nurs.* 76:1296.

Farris, Lorene. 1978. The American Indian. In *Culture childbearing health professionals,* ed. Ann L. Clark. Philadelphia: F. A. Davis Company.

Fenlon, A., et al. 1979. *Getting ready for childbirth.* Englewood Cliffs, N. J.: Prentice-Hall, Inc.

Flynn, M., et al. 1978. Ambulation in labour. *Br. Med. J.* 2:591.

Higgins, P. G., and Wayland, J. R. Sept. 16, 1981. Labour and delivery in North America. *Nurs. Times* (Midwifery Suppl.):77.

Heggenhougen, H. K. Nov./Dec. 1980. Father and childbirth: an anthropological perspective. *J. Nurse Midwife.* 25:21.

Hollingsworth, A. O., et al. Nov. 1980. The refugees and childbearing: what to expect. *RN* 43:45.

Kay, M. A. 1978. The Mexican American. In *Culture child-bearing health professionals*, ed. Ann L. Clark. Philadelphia: F. A. Davis Company.

Klaus, M. H., and Kennell, J. H. 1982. *Parent–infant bonding*. St. Louis: The C. V. Mosby Co.

Korones, S. 1981. *High risk newborn infants: the basis for intensive nursing care*. 3rd ed. St. Louis: The C. V. Mosby Co.

McCaffery, M. 1972. *Nursing management of the patient with pain*. Philadelphia: J. B. Lippincott Company.

McKay, S. R. 1980. Maternal position during labor and birth: a reassessment. *J. Obstet. Gynecol. Neonatal Nurs.* 9:288.

—————. 1981. Second stage labor—has tradition replaced safety? *Am. J. Nurs.* 81:1061.

Mercer, R. 1979. *Perspectives on adolescent health care*. New York: J. B. Lippincott.

Murillo-Rohde, Ildaura. 1979. Cultural sensitivity in the care of the Hispanic patient. *Wash. State J. Nurs.* (Special Suppl.):25.

Murphee, Alice H. Sept. 1968. A functional analysis of southern folk beliefs concerning birth. *Am. J. Obstet. Gynecol.* 102:125.

Nobel, E. March/April 1981. Controversies in maternal effort during labor and delivery. *J. Nurse Midwife.* 26:13.

Pritchard, J., and MacDonald, P. C. 1980. *Williams obstetrics*. 16th ed. New York: Appleton-Century-Crofts.

Trandel-Korenchuk, D. M. 1982. Informed consent: client participation in childbirth decisions. *J. Obstet. Gynecol. Neonatal Nurs.* 11:379.

Zborowski, Mark. 1952. Cultural components in responses to pain. *J. Social Issues.* 8:16.

Additional Readings

Anderson, C. J. March/April 1981. Enhancing reciprocity between mother and neonate. *Nurs. Res.* 30:89.

Bramptom, B., et al. May/June 1981. Initial mothering patterns of low-income black primiparas. *J. Obstet. Gynecol. Neonatal Nurs.* 10:174.

Brown, M. S. Oct. 1976. A cross-cultural look at pregnancy, labor, and delivery. *J. Obstet. Gynecol. Neonatal Nurs.* 5:35.

Campbell, A., and Worthington, E. L. Jan./Feb. 1982. Teaching expectant fathers how to be better childbirth coaches. *Am. J. Mat. Child Nurs.* 7:28.

Colman, A. D., and Colman, L. L. 1971. *Pregnancy: the psychological experience*. New York: Herder & Herder.

Dean, P. G., et al. Jan./Feb. 1982. Making baby's acquaintance: a unique attachment strategy. *Am. J. Mat. Child Nurs.* 7:37.

Duignan, N. M., et al. 1975. Characteristics of normal labour in different racial groups. *Br. J. Obstet. Gynecol.* 82(8):593.

Dunn, D. M., and White, D. G. 1981. Interactions of mothers with their newborns in the first half-hour of life. *J. Adv. Nurs.* 6:271.

Elsherif, C., et al. March/April 1979. Coaching the coach. *J. Obstet. Gynecol. Neonatal Nurs.* 8:87.

Griffith, S. May/June 1982. Childbearing and the concept of culture. *J. Obstet. Gynecol. Neonatal Nurs.* 11:181.

Howley, C. May/June 1981. The older primipara: implications for nurses. *J. Obstet. Gynecol. Neonatal Nurs.* 10:182.

Worthington, E. L., et al. Jan./Feb. 1982. Which prepared-childbirth coping strategies are effective? *J. Obstet. Gynecol. Neonatal Nurs.* 11:45.

■ 17 ■

OBSTETRIC ANALGESIA AND ANESTHESIA

■ CHAPTER CONTENTS

METHODS OF PAIN RELIEF

    Systemic Drugs

    Regional Analgesia and Anesthesia

    Paracervical Block

    Peridural Block—Epidural and Caudal

    Subarachnoid Block (Spinal, Low Spinal, or Saddle Block)

    Pudendal Block

    Local Anesthesia

GENERAL ANESTHESIA

    Inhalation Anesthetics

    Intravenous Anesthetics

    Balanced Anesthesia

    Complications of General Anesthesia

    Medical Interventions for Acute Respiratory Obstruction

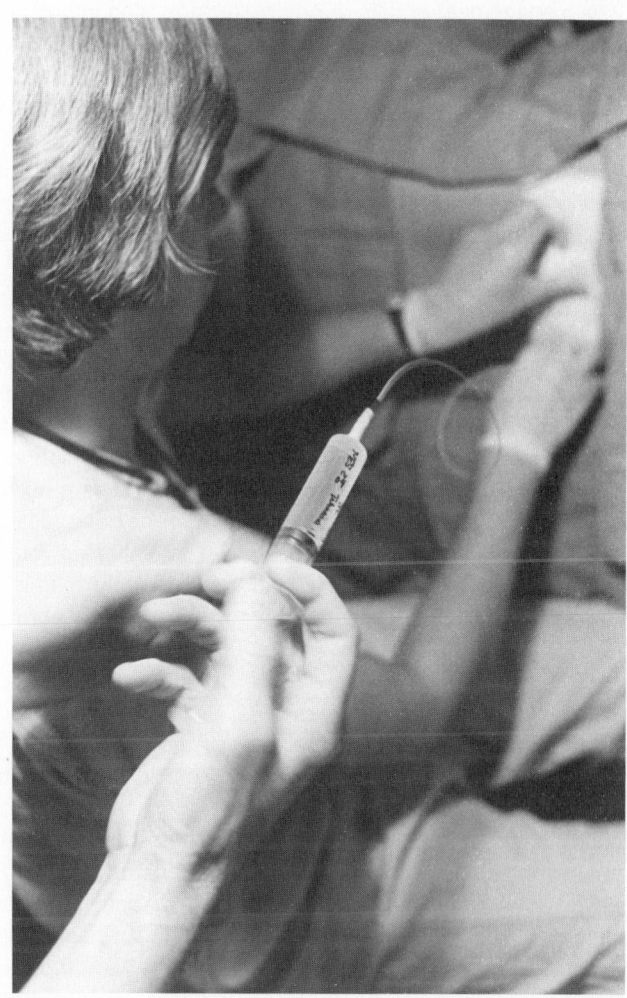

■ **OBJECTIVES**

- Describe the use of systemic drugs to promote pain relief during labor.

- Identify the major types of regional analgesia and anesthesia including area affected, advantages, disadvantages, technique, and nursing implications.

- Discuss the complications of regional anesthesia that may occur.

- Describe the major inhalation and intravenous anesthetics used to provide general anesthesia.

- Describe the major complications of general anesthesia.

The management of pain during parturition is an important aspect in the health care of the childbearing woman. The discomfort associated with labor and delivery has been a subject of concern throughout history. A woman's attitude toward childbirth and pain reflects her culture. During the early Greek, Roman, and Egyptian civilizations, the art of assisting women in childbirth was highly developed. Unfortunately, the practices from these cultures were displaced during the Dark Ages by ignorance and superstition.

It was not until the nineteenth century that health care for mothers and babies began to improve. One significant clinical advance was the introduction of anesthetic agents into obstetrics. Ether and chloroform were first used for labor and delivery in Great Britain by Sir James Simpson of the University of Glasgow. An outraged clergy claimed that the pain of childbirth was decreed by God as punishment for the fall from grace in the Garden of Eden. They cited the Bible (Genesis 3:16) as proof that women must suffer: "Unto the woman He said, I will greatly multiply thy sorrow and thy conception; in sorrow thou shalt bring forth children. . . ." In his defense of the practice, Simpson also used the Bible (Genesis 2:21) to propose that God used anesthesia for the creation of Eve: "And the Lord God caused a deep sleep to fall upon Adam. . . ."

The use of chloroform by Queen Victoria for the birth of her seventh child was the event that finally ended the controversy and sanctioned the use of anesthetic agents for childbearing. Since that time, many agents and techniques have been introduced. The goal of pain relief in childbirth is alleviation of discomfort in the woman while ensuring the safety of both mother and fetus. To date, no method or agent has been discovered that can meet all these criteria. The search for a safe, effective method of pain relief during labor and delivery thus continues in the twentieth century.

Theories of pain and factors affecting maternal response to the pain of childbearing are discussed in Chapter 14.

METHODS OF PAIN RELIEF

Reduction or relief of pain during labor is achieved by several different methods, including psychoprophylactic methods (which were discussed in Chapters 14 and 16) and systemic drugs and regional nerve blocks. This classification provides a convenient framework for exploring various alternatives for pain relief.

No method is mutually exclusive. The agents used for regional nerve blocks may enter general circulation and cause unwanted side effects. Systemic drugs such as meperidine (Demerol) or diazepam (Valium) may assist the tense psychoprophylactically prepared woman to regain control and to progress to a satisfying childbirth experience. Regional nerve blocks with analgesic doses of anesthetic agents administered during the course of labor are compatible with the goals of prepared childbirth.

Systemic Drugs

The goal of pharmacologic pain relief during labor is to provide maximal analgesia with minimal risk for the mother and fetus. Three factors must be considered in the use of analgesic agents: (a) the effects on the mother, (b) the effects on the contractions of labor, and (c) the effects on the fetus.

Maternal drug action is of primary importance because the well-being of the fetus depends on adequate functioning of the maternal cardiopulmonary system. Any alteration of function that disturbs the woman's homeostatic mechanism affects the fetal environment. Maintaining the maternal respiratory rate and blood pressure within normal range is thus of prime importance. The use of electronic fetal monitoring has provided a means of accurately assessing the effects of pharmacologic agents on uterine contractions. The Friedman labor curve provides a basis for determining the effects of drugs on the overall course of labor. (See Chapter 15 for discussion of the Friedman graph and electronic monitoring.)

All systemic drugs used for pain relief during labor cross the placental barrier by simple diffusion, with some agents crossing more readily than others. Drug action in the body depends on the rate at which the substance is metabolized by liver enzymes and excreted by the kidneys. The fetal liver enzymes and renal systems are inadequate to metabolize analgesic agents, so that high doses remain active in fetal circulation for a prolonged period of time. The fetal brain receives a greater amount of the cardiac output than the neonatal brain (Albright, 1978). The percentage of blood volume flowing to the brain is increased even further during intrauterine stress, so that the hypoxic fetus receives an even larger amount of a depressant drug. The blood–brain barrier is more permeable at the time of birth, a factor that also increases the amount of drug carried to the central nervous system.

Although systemic drugs affect the fetus, so do pain and stress experienced by the mother (Myers, 1975; Shnider and Levinson, 1979). Withholding medication from the tense and anxious client in labor may not accomplish the well-intentioned goal. A positive approach should be taken with the prepared couple so they understand that maternal discomfort and anxiety may have as much adverse effect on the fetus as a judicious amount of an analgesic agent.

Disagreement exists in the literature about the safest time for the administration of narcotics. In one study, peak depression of the fetus occurred during the second and third hour after intramuscular administration, with little or no effect during the first hour or after the fourth hour following injection (Shnider and Moya, 1964). Depressed newborns are reported to have a decrease in sucking effort, visual attentiveness, and overall activity for as long as four days after birth (Moore, 1972).

ADMINISTRATION OF ANALGESIC AGENTS

The optimal time for administering analgesia is determined after making a complete assessment of many factors. In general, an analgesic agent is administered to nulliparas when the cervix has dilated to 5–6 cm, and to multiparas when the cervix has reached 3–4 cm dilatation. This is only a generalization, however; the character of each labor must be taken into account. Analgesia given too early may prolong labor, and analgesia given too late is of no value to the client and may harm the fetus. In many institutions the nurse makes the decision as to when the analgesic ordered by the clinician is given. This decision is based on a complete assessment of the client as well as the progress of labor.

Currently, a minimal amount of an analgesic agent is given in labor. Oral analgesics are not used because of poor absorption and prolonged gastric-emptying time. The intramuscular and intravenous routes are more frequently utilized. When the prescribed route is intramuscular, a needle of sufficient length to penetrate the muscle is a necessity. One study revealed that blood levels of a drug were more than doubled when injected intramuscularly by physicians rather than by nurses. The physicians in the study used larger and longer needles, so that the agent entered the muscle rather than the subcutaneous fat (Dundee et al., 1974). When an agent is given intravenously, it should be administered no faster than 1 mL/min. Dilts (1981) recommends that all drugs be given intravenously because a smaller dose can be given, the onset of action can be more accurately predicted and the duration more accurate-

ly timed. It has been suggested that the intravenous injection be given with the onset of a contraction, when the blood flow to the uterus and the fetus is decreased. Whatever the route of administration, the power of suggestion on the part of the nurse greatly increases the effectiveness of the agent.

The general principles for administering analgesic drugs are as follows:

1. The client should be in an individual labor room.
2. The environment should be free from sensory stimuli, such as bright lights, noise, and irrelevant conversation, to allow the client to focus on the drug action.
3. An explanation of the effects of the medication should be given, including how long the effects will last and how the drug will make the client feel.
4. The client should be encouraged to empty her bladder prior to administration of the drug.
5. The baseline FHR and maternal vital signs should be recorded prior to administration.
6. The physician's written order should be checked, and the medication prepared and signed out on the narcotic or control sheet.
7. The client should be asked again if she is allergic to any medication and her arm band checked for identification.
8. The drug should be administered by the route ordered, using correct technique.
9. The side rails should be pulled up for client safety, and the reasons explained to the client.
10. The medication, dosage, time, route, and site of administration should be charted on the nurse's notes and on the monitor strip.
11. The FHR should be monitored to assess the effects of the medication on the fetus, and the client evaluated for the effectiveness of the analgesic agent.
12. The client should not be left alone. If no family member is present and it is necessary for the nurse to leave, the client should be given a short explanation and assurances that the nurse will return.

NARCOTIC ANALGESICS

□ *MORPHINE* Morphine, a CNS depressant, is thought to act on the corticothalamic pathways and the sensory areas of the brain. In addition to raising the pain perception threshold, morphine alters the reaction to pain. It has selected action on the medulla, depressing the respiratory and cough centers and stimulating the vomiting center. Morphine also is helpful in reducing increased cardiac output. It does not depress the myocardium.

Morphine is not often used in labor in most obstetrical units. When it is used, the common dosage is 10 mg intramuscularly or 1–2 mg in incremental intravenous doses. The peak effect following intravenous administration occurs in approximately 20 minutes. Peak effect after intramuscular injection occurs in the second hour and analgesia lasts for 4–6 hours. Fetal depression occurs about 2 hours after maternal intramuscular injection. Greater depression may occur with the morphine than with the use of meperidine: the fetal brain is more permeable to morphine (Albright, 1978).

□ *MEPERIDINE* Meperidine (Demerol) is frequently used for obstetric analgesia. This agent is almost as effective in relief of pain when compared to morphine. See Drug Guide—Meperidine (below) for further discussion.

NARCOTIC ANTAGONISTS

Narcotic antagonists counteract the respiratory depressant effects of the opiate-type narcotics. Levallorphan (Lorfan) is effective only against neonatal respiratory depression caused by narcotic analgesics. This antagonist acts by competing with narcotics in the respiratory center receptors and by displacing the narcotic molecules from the receptor sites. It is important to note that if the receptors are not occupied solely by narcotics, antagonist agents *produce* respiratory depression by occupying these sites. Therefore, this drug *increases* depression caused by barbiturates, tranquilizers, and other sedative drugs.

Levallorphan (Lorfan) 1.0 mg IV may be administered to the client 5–10 minutes before delivery to prevent respiratory depression of the newborn. The administration of this agent withdraws the analgesic effect of the narcotic and may result in an uncomfortable, uncooperative client.

Naloxone (Narcan) exhibits little pharmacologic activity in the absence of narcotics. Although it is an antagonist, it has little or no agonistic activity, and it can be used in cases of depressed newborns when a narcotic is thought to be involved. Neonatal depression will not be relieved if the depression is not due to narcosis, but depression will not be made worse. For neonatal dose, see Drug Guide—Narcan in Chapter 25.

DRUG GUIDE—MEPERIDINE HYDROCHLORIDE (DEMEROL)

OVERVIEW OF OBSTETRICAL ACTION

Meperidine hydrochloride is a narcotic analgesic that interferes with pain impulses at the subcortical level of the brain. In addition, it enhances analgesia by altering the physiologic response to pain, suppressing anxiety and apprehension, and creating a euphoric feeling. Meperidine hydrochloride is used during labor to provide analgesia. Peak analgesia occurs in 40–60 minutes with intramuscular and in 5–7 minutes with intravenous administration. Duration is 2–4 hours. Administration after labor has reached the active phase does not appear to delay labor or to decrease uterine contraction frequency or duration. Meperidine HCl crosses the placental barrier and appears in the fetus within 1–2 minutes after maternal intravenous injection (Morrison et al., 1982).

Route, dosage, frequency

IM: 50–100 mg every 3–4 hours
IV: 25–50 mg by slow intravenous push every 3–4 hours

Maternal contraindications

Hypersensitivity to meperidine, asthma
CNS depression
Respiratory depression
Fetal distress
Preterm labor if delivery is imminent
Hypotension
Respirations <12 per minute
Concurrent use with anticonvulsants may increase depressant effects

Maternal side effects

Respiratory depression
Nausea and vomiting, dry mouth

Drowsiness, dizziness, flushing
Transient hypotension
Bradycardia, palpitations
May precipitate or aggravate seizures in clients prone to convulsive activity (Giacoia and Yaffee, 1982)

Effect on fetus/neonate

Neonatal respiratory depression may occur if meperidine HCl is administered within 2–4 hours of delivery
Neonatal hypotonia, lethargy, interference of thermoregulatory response
Neurologic and behavioral alterations for up to 72 hours after delivery. Presence of meperidine in neonatal urine up to 3 days following delivery (Morrison et al., 1982)

NURSING CONSIDERATIONS

Assess client history, labor and fetal status, maternal blood pressure and respirations to identify contraindications to administration
Intramuscular doses should be injected deeply to avoid irritation to subcutaneous tissue
Intravenous doses should be diluted and administered slowly
Provide for client safety by instructing her to remain on bed rest, by keeping side rails up and placing call bell within reach
Evaluate effect of drug
Observe for maternal side effects
Observe newborn for respiratory depression, be prepared to initiate resuscitative measures and administer antagonist naloxone if needed

ATARACTICS

Ataractic drugs do not relieve pain but are reported to decrease apprehension and anxiety, to relieve nausea, and to potentiate the effects of narcotics. Agents frequently used in labor include promethazine (Phenergan), promazine (Sparine), hydroxyzine (Vistaril), and diazepam (Valium). Controversy still exists about the use of these drugs during labor. Many of the favorable reports are not from controlled studies. Evidence suggests that tranquilizers do not significantly affect the contractions of active labor.

The effects on the fetus are being questioned. The drugs may affect the attention span of the infant after delivery because these agents are poorly metabolized in the fetal and neonatal system. Many times, untoward fetal effects go unrecognized. Hypothermia and hypotonia in the newborn following intrapartal administration of diazepam (Valium) have been noted (Pritchard and MacDonald, 1980).

Ataractics may be given alone to reduce tension, or they may be combined with narcotics to potentiate the analgesic effect. In this case, the dosage of the narcotic is decreased by half. These agents may be given intramuscularly or intravenously. The peak action occurs within minutes when given intravenously and within 30–60 minutes when given intramuscularly.

SEDATIVES

Sedatives formerly played an important role in the pharmacologic management of labor. However, barbiturates have the disadvantage of producing restlessness in the presence of moderate to severe pain, and they readily cross the placental barrier, causing respiratory depression in the newborn.

The principal use of barbiturates in current obstetric practice is in false labor or in the early stages of prodromal labor. An oral dose of 100 mg of secobarbital (Seconal) or pentobarbital (Nembutal) promotes relaxation and allows the client to sleep a few hours. If the client is in false labor, the contractions usually stop. Women in prodromal labor enter the active phase of labor in a more relaxed and rested state.

There is no completely safe and satisfactory method of pain relief. When analgesia is used judiciously, however, it can be beneficial to the laboring woman and do little harm to the fetus. The woman who is free from fear and who has confidence in the medical and nursing personnel usually has a relatively comfortable first stage of labor and requires a minimum of medication. A positive attitude on the part of the professional nurse and the expectant parents is an essential part of pain relief.

Regional Analgesia and Anesthesia

Regional analgesia and anesthesia are achieved by injecting local anesthetic agents into an area that will bring the agent into direct contact with nervous tissue. Local agents stabilize the cell membrane, preventing initiation and transmission of nerve impulses. The methods most commonly utilized in obstetrics include paracervical block, peridural block (lumbar epidural and caudal), subarachnoid block (spinal for cesarean birth, low spinal for vaginal delivery—also known as *saddle block*), pudendal block, and local infiltration. The nerve blocks may be accomplished by a single injection or continuously by means of an indwelling plastic catheter. Regional techniques have gained widespread popularity in recent years and are particularly compatible with the goals of psychoprophylactic preparation for childbirth.

Although each technique has advantages and disadvantages, in general the advantages of a regional procedures are as follows:

1. Relief from discomfort is complete in the area blocked.
2. Depression of maternal vital signs rarely occurs.
3. Aspiration of gastric contents is virtually eliminated if no other adjunct sedation was administered.
4. Administration at the optimal time does not significantly alter the course of labor.
5. The woman remains alert and able to participate in the childbirth process.

The disadvantages include:

1. A high degree of skill is required for proper administration of most procedures.
2. Failures such as no effect or unilateral or incomplete anesthesia can occur even with experienced operators.
3. Side effects do occur with some techniques.
4. Systemic toxic reactions are more common than with agents used for general anesthesia.

Essential prerequisites for the administration of regional analgesia and anesthesia are knowledge of the anatomy and physiology of pertinent structures, techniques for administration, the pharmacology of local anesthetics, and potential complications. With the exception of nurse anesthetists and nurse-midwives, who may perform procedures for which they have been trained, nurses in the United States may *not* legally administer anesthetic agents. This admonition includes the reinjection of agents through indwelling catheters. However, the nurse must have an adequate knowledge of all aspects of regional anesthesia to provide client support and to give appropriate reinforcement of the administrator's explanation to the client. The nurse who has a thorough understanding of the techniques and agents can also provide more efficient assistance to the administrator. Client safety is increased when the nurse recognizes complications and immediately initiates appropriate intervention.

The relief of pain associated with the first stage of labor can be accomplished by blocking the sensory nerves sup-

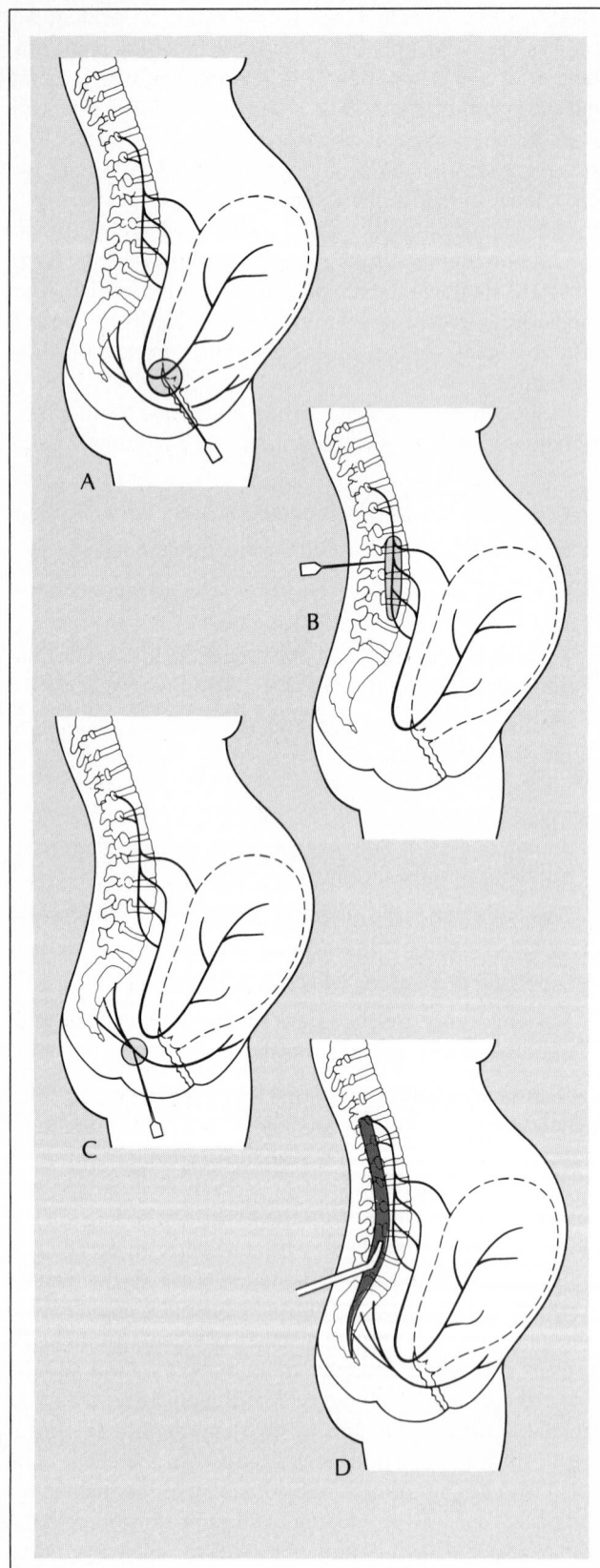

FIGURE 17–1 Schematic diagram showing pain pathways and sites of interruption. **A,** Paracervical block: relief of uterine pain only. **B,** Lumbar sympathetic block: relief of uterine pain only. **C,** Pudendal block: relief of perineal pain. **D,** Lumbar epidural block: dark area demonstrates peridural space and nerves affected, and white tube represents continuous plastic catheter. (From Bonica, J. J. 1972. *Principles and practice of obstetric analgesia and anesthesia.* Philadelphia: F. A. Davis Co., pp. 492, 512, 521, and 614.)

plying the uterus with the techniques of paracervical, lumbar sympathetic, and peridural (epidural and caudal) blocks. The relief of pain associated with the second stage and delivery can be alleviated with pudendal, peridural, (spinal, low spinal), and subarachnoid (saddle) blocks (Figure 17–1).

REGIONAL ANESTHETIC AGENTS

Two types of local anesthetic agents are currently available—the ester and amide types. The ester type includes procaine (Novocaine), chloroprocaine (Nesacaine), and tetracaine (Pontocaine). Esters are rapidly metabolized by plasma pseudocholinesterase; therefore, toxic maternal levels are not as likely to develop and placental transfer to the fetus is prevented. Amide types include lidocaine (Xylocaine), mepivacaine (Carbocaine), and bupivacaine (Marcaine). Amide types are more powerful and longer-acting agents. They readily cross the placenta, can be measured in the fetal circulation, and affect the fetus for a prolonged period of time.

Regional anesthetic agents block the conduction of nerve impulses from the periphery to the CNS. Although the mechanism of their action is not fully understood, it is thought that the agents do not allow sodium ions to enter the cell, thereby preventing depolarization. The neuronal membrane is stabilized in its resting state so that nerve impulses from the source of pain are not transmitted. Motor and sympathetic fibers of mixed spinal nerves may be blocked in the attempt to achieve loss of sensation. The types of peripheral nerve fibers are differentially sensitive to the agents. The smaller the fiber, the more sensitive it is to local anesthetics. It is possible to block the small C and A-Δ fibers, which conduct the sensations of pain, temperature, pressure and touch, without affecting the large, heavily myelinated A-α, A-β, and A-γ fibers, which continue to maintain muscle tone, position sense, and motor function (Bonica, 1972).

Absorption of local anesthetics depends primarily on the vascularity of the area of injection. The agents also contribute to increased blood flow by causing vasomotor paralysis. Higher concentration of drugs causes greater vasodilatation. Good maternal physical condition or a high metabolic rate aids absorption. Malnutrition, dehydration, electrolyte imbalance, and cardiovascular and pulmonary problems lower the threshold for toxic effects. The pH of

SUMMARY OF SIGNS AND SYMPTOMS OF SYSTEMIC TOXIC REACTIONS FROM LOCAL ANESTHETIC DRUGS*

Central nervous system effects
A. Stimulation of
  1. Cerebral cortex → excitement, disorientation, incoherent speech, convulsions
  2. Medulla
    a. Cardiovascular center → increased blood pressure and pulse
    b. Respiratory center → increased respiratory rate and/or variations in rhythm
    c. Vomiting center → nausea and/or vomiting
B. Depression of
  1. Cerebral cortex → unconsciousness
  2. Medulla
    a. Vasomotor → fall in blood pressure and rapid or absent pulse (syncope)
    b. Respiratory → variations in respiration and/or apnea

Peripheral effects
A. Cardiovascular (syncope)
  1. Heart → bradycardia, that is, depression from direct action of local anesthetic agent on myocardium
  2. Blood vessels → vasodilatation from direct action of local anesthetic agent on blood vessels

Allergic responses
A. Skin → urticaria, etc.
B. Respiration → depression ("clinical anaphylactic shock")
C. Circulation → depression ("clinical anaphylactic shock")

Miscellaneous reactions
A. Psychogenic
B. To other drugs, for example, vasoconstrictors

* From Moore, D. C. 1967. *Regional block,* 4th ed. Courtesy of Charles C. Thomas, Publisher, Springfield, Illinois.

tissues affects the rate of absorption, which has implications for fetal complications. The addition of vasoconstrictors such as epinephrine delays absorption and prolongs the anesthetic effect. Recent studies have demonstrated that epinephrine decreases uteroplacental blood flow, making it an undesirable additive in many situations. The breakdown of local anesthetics in the body is accomplished by the liver and plasma esterase, with the resulting substance being eliminated by the kidneys.

The weakest concentration and the smallest amount necessary to produce the desired results are advocated.

ADVERSE MATERNAL REACTIONS

Reactions to local anesthetic agents range from mild symptoms to cardiovascular collapse. The signs and symptoms of toxic reactions to local anesthetic agents are summarized in the box above. Mild reactions include palpitations, vertigo, tinnitus, apprehension, confusion, headache, and a metallic taste in the mouth. Moderate reactions include more severe degrees of mild symptoms plus nausea and vomiting, hypotension, and muscle twitching, which may progress to convulsions and loss of consciousness. The severe reactions are sudden loss of consciousness, coma, severe hypotension, bradycardia, respiratory depression, and cardiac arrest. Local toxic effects on tissues may also result with high concentrations of the agents. Anesthetic agents should not be used unless an intravenous line is in place.

Systemic toxic reactions most commonly occur with an excessive dose through too great a concentration or too large a volume. Accidental intravenous injection that suddenly increases the amount of the drug in maternal circulation results in depression of vasomotor, respiratory, and other medullary centers of the brain. It also depresses the heart and peripheral vascular bed. A massive intravascular dose can result in sudden circulatory collapse within 1 minute. Reactions to subcutaneous and extradural injection occur between 5 and 40 minutes. The short-acting agents can produce toxic reactions in 10–15 minutes (procaine), and the long-acting agents (mepivacaine), in 20–40 minutes. *It is imperative that the client be under close supervision by knowledgeable personnel throughout the time that the agent is being used.*

If epinephrine has been added to the anesthetic agent to prolong the anesthesia, it is necessary to differentiate between reaction to the anesthetic agent and to the epinephrine. Reaction to epinephrine is characterized by pallor, perspiration, a greater increase in blood pressure and pulse than occurs with reactions to anesthetic agents, and dyspnea.

Psychogenic reactions can occur, with symptoms similar to systemic toxic reactions. This phenomenon may occur as the procedure is begun and prior to the injection of the anesthetic agent. Regardless of the cause, the symptoms must be treated.

Allergic reactions to anesthetic agents may also occur.

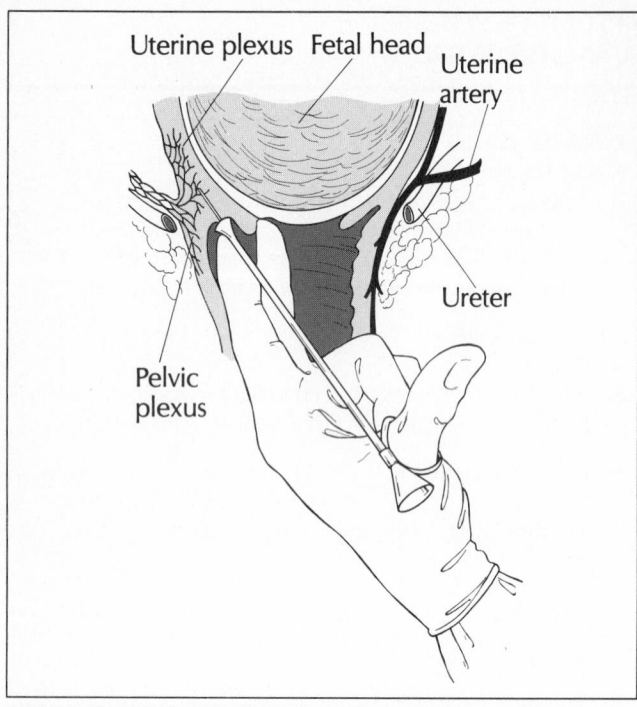

Uterine plexus   Fetal head   Uterine artery

Ureter

Pelvic plexus

FIGURE 17-2 Technique for paracervical block from needle in place at appropriate distance beyond guide. (From Bonica, J. J. 1972. *Principles and practice of obstetric analgesia and anesthesia.* Philadelphia: F. A. Davis Co., p. 515.)

The manifestations of the antigen-antibody reaction include urticaria, laryngeal edema, joint pain, swelling of the tongue, and bronchospasm. An antihistamine such as diphenhydramine (Benadryl) should be administered intravenously to treat allergic reaction (Bonica, 1972).

INTERVENTIONS

Treatment of systemic toxicity. In the treatment of mild toxicity, the administration of oxygen and intravenous injection of a short-acting barbiturate is advocated. Preparation must be made to treat convulsions or cardiovascular collapse. Specific interventions in the treatment of systemic toxicity are listed in the box on p. 515.

Treatment of convulsions. The best treatment for convulsions is administration of oxygen, administration of 40–60 mg of succinylcholine, and intubation (Bonica, 1972). This method is quick, and succinylcholine can be given intramuscularly if necessary. It does not depress maternal myocardial and medullary centers, nor does it depress the fetus. This treatment has an advantage over treatment with short-acting barbiturates such as thiopental or pentobarbital, which depress maternal myocardial and medullary centers as well as the fetus. Overdosage is also more frequent with the short-acting barbiturates.

Treatment of sudden cardiovascular collapse. In sudden collapse, assisted ventilation with 100% oxygen through

an endotracheal tube is indicated. The rate of intravenous fluids may be increased to support circulation. Vasopressors with inotropic action may be given, and in extreme cases, epinephrine and closed cardiac massage may be indicated.

Paracervical Block

The paracervical block is useful during the first stage of labor. It anesthetizes the inferior hypogastric plexus and ganglia to provide relief of pain from cervical dilatation but does not anesthetize the lower vagina or perineum. Indwelling catheters may be used for repeated injections. The woman should be in active labor and the cervix dilated 4–5 cm prior to injection. Uterine contractility may increase in frequency and in baseline uterine tone. The addition of epinephrine to the anesthetic agent is not recommended for this method because of its inhibitory effect on the myometrium. The agents advocated for this procedure are procaine (Novocaine) and tetracaine (Pontocaine). Lidocaine (Xylocaine), chloroprocaine (Nesacaine), and mepivacaine (Carbocaine) are also used. These ester types are better metabolized by the placenta with less transfer to the fetus.

The disadvantages of the paracervical block include the following: The vascularity of the area increases the possibility of rapid absorption, with resulting systemic toxic reaction. Hematomas may occur as a result of uterine vessel damage. Fetal bradycardia frequently follows paracervical block, with a reported incidence of 25%–85% (Pritchard and MacDonald, 1980).

The amide group of agents have the potential to produce direct fetal myocardial depression. The ECG of the fetus with bradycardia, in the absence of maternal hypotension or increase in uterine activity, resembles that of a conduction defect due to vagal stimulation instead of direct depression (Ettiger and McCant, 1976). Greiss et al. (1976) propose that the fetal bradycardia is caused by reduced placental blood flow associated with anesthetic drug action. Baxi et al. (1979) suggest the fetal heart rate changes are secondary to fetal hypoxia.

A paracervical block should not be used if evidence of placental insufficiency, fetal prematurity, or fetal distress exists (Albright, 1978).

TECHNIQUE

The proper method for administering a paracervical block is illustrated in Figure 17–2.

1. The client is placed in the dorsal recumbent position with knees flexed.
2. A 12.7–15.24 cm, 22-gauge needle is placed in a guide such as the Iowa trumpet, Kobak device, or Kohl's instrument, which allows the needle to extend 1–1½ cm beyond the tip.

3. The guide is placed in the lateral fornix of the vagina, and the needle is inserted through the vaginal mucosa.

4. Aspiration is done to make sure the needle is not in a blood vessel.

5. Between 5 and 10 mL of the anesthetic solution is injected.

6. The procedure is repeated on the opposite side.

7. If a continuous block is done, the plastic catheters are taped to the abdomen.

This technique provides adequate anesthesia until the woman reaches delivery, when another technique, such as pudendal block, becomes necessary.

NURSING IMPLICATIONS

As previously mentioned, fetal bradycardia is a problem with paracervical block. It is imperative to continuously monitor the FHR with electronic monitoring equipment. The fetal bradycardia usually occurs within 2–10 minutes following the paracervical block and lasts for 5–10 minutes. FHR baseline variability is diminished, and late decelerations may occur during the return of the preblock fetal heart rate pattern. At delivery, these neonates have normal Apgar scores if the FHR has been in the normal range for 30–50 minutes preceding delivery. During the bradycardic episode, the client should be in a side-lying position and receiving oxygen. Maternal hypotension, if present, should be treated with intravenous fluids. If fetal bradycardia persists for more than 10–15 minutes, fetal blood sampling may be done. Fetal bradycardia that continues for 30 minutes or longer may be due to fetal metabolic acidosis and immediate delivery should be considered (Albright, 1978).

Maternal complications following a paracervical block are rare, but the possibility of systemic toxic shock due to accidental injection into the maternal vascular system or unusually rapid absorption must always be kept in mind. Hematomas and infection at the site of the injections have been reported. Since paracervical block must be done in the lithotomy position, supine hypotensive syndrome may occur. Maternal blood pressure and pulse must be closely monitored for the first 15 minutes after injection or reinjection.

The duration of pain relief varies with the anesthetic agent used. When indwelling catheters have been left in place for reinjection, care must be taken to avoid dislodging the catheters when cleansing the perineum or examining the woman vaginally.

The bladder must also be constantly assessed because the anesthetized laboring woman may not be aware of the need to void. Stages of cervical dilatation must also be monitored because the paracervical technique blocks only the cervix and upper vagina. It is not sufficient for pain relief during delivery and episiotomy repair.

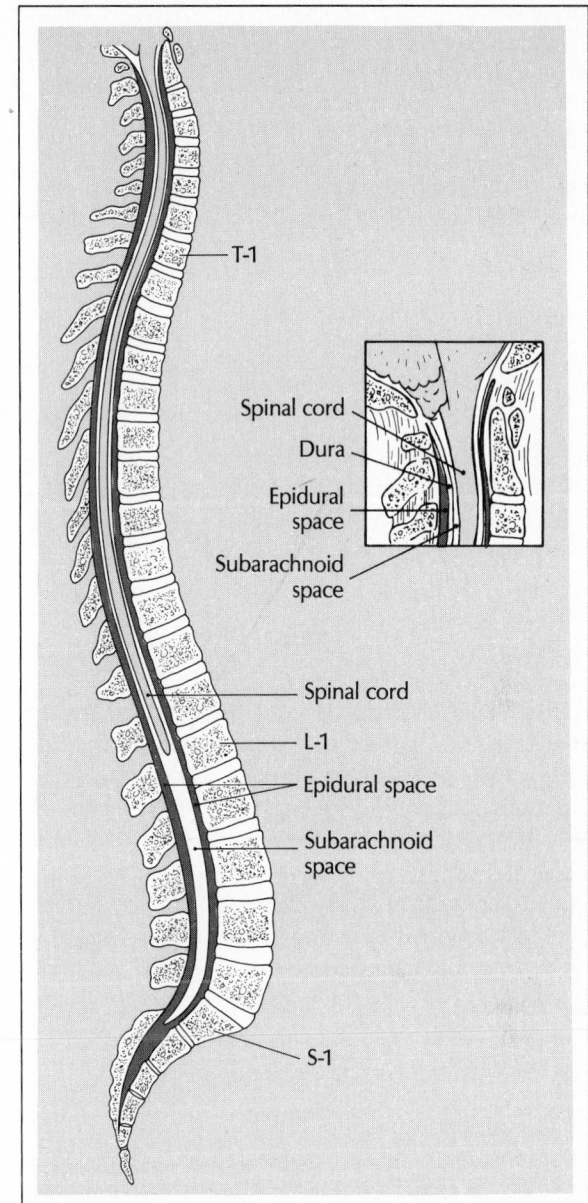

FIGURE 17–3 Epidural space.

Paracervical block should be used *only* in normal labor with an uncompromised fetus.

Peridural Block—Epidural and Caudal

Peridural anesthesia can provide pain relief throughout the entire course of labor. The peridural or *epidural space* is a potential space between the dura mater and the ligamentum flavum that extends from the base of the skull to the end of the sacral canal (Figure 17–3). It contains areolar tissue, fat, lymphatics, and the internal vertebral venous plexus. Access to the space may be through the lumbar or

FIGURE 17–4 Technique of epidural block. **A,** Proper position of insertion. **B,** Needle in the ligamentum flavum. **C,** Tip of needle in epidural space. **D,** Force of injection pushing dura away from tip of needle. (From Bonica, J. J. 1972. *Principles and practice of obstetric analgesia and anesthesia.* Philadelphia: F. A. Davis Co., p. 631.)

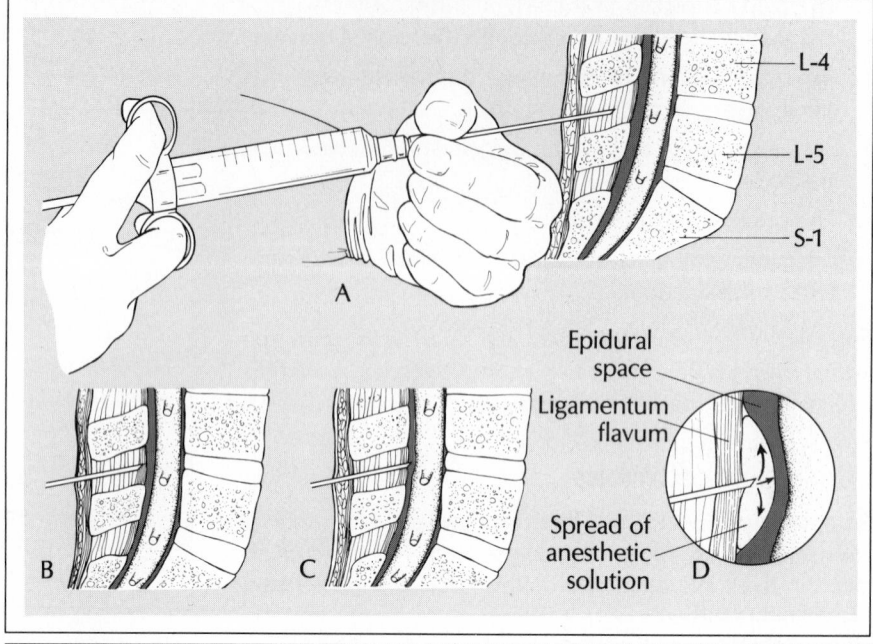

caudal area. The technique is most frequently used as a continuous block to provide analgesia and anesthesia from active labor through episiotomy repair. This method, particularly continuous lumbar epidural block, has become the obstetric anesthesia of choice in many areas of the United States.

Peridural anesthesia is advocated for premature labor and in the presence of maternal heart disease, hypertension, diabetes, and pulmonary disease (Greenhill and Friedman, 1974).

Disadvantages of peridural block are varied. Considerable skill is required for peridural techniques, and the incidence of success correlates highly with the skill and experience of the administrator. Pain relief is slower than with other methods, and a higher volume of anesthetic agent is required than for spinal anesthesia. Lumbar epidural block has a slight advantage over the caudal method in that anesthesia is more rapid and a smaller volume of anesthetic agent is necessary. Fewer bony abnormalities occur in the lumbar vertebras than in the sacrum. The administrator must guard against accidental perforation of the dura mater, particularly with the lumbar epidural method, and against the injection of an epidural dose into the spinal canal, with resultant high spinal anesthesia.

Perineal relaxation is another disadvantage; it interferes with internal fetal rotation. The incidence of persistent occipital-posterior and occipital-transverse positions increases. The woman may also find it difficult to bear down effectively. As a result, there is an increase in cesarean deliveries. Schifrin (1972) has reported that fetal heart rate patterns resembling uteroplacental insufficiency occur in about 25% of the cases who have peridural anesthesia during labor. These FHR patterns are related to maternal hypotension. The incidence of late deceleration increases

to 72% when maternal hypotension is present (Greenhill and Friedman, 1974). This condition is readily corrected by administering oxygen, turning the client on her left side, and increasing the flow rate of intravenous fluids.

Peridural anesthesia is contraindicated when hemorrhage is present or likely to occur, if there is local infection at the site of injection (such as a pilonidal cyst), and in the presence of central nervous system disease or any condition in which a convulsive seizure or hypotension might have serious effects (cardiac or pulmonary disease). It is also contraindicated when the client is unable to understand the implications and risks of the block or states she does not wish to have anesthesia.

TECHNIQUE FOR LUMBAR EPIDURAL BLOCK

The following steps must be taken in administering a lumbar epidural block:

1. The client is placed on her left side, shoulders parallel, with her legs slightly flexed. *The spinal column is not kept convex, as it is for a spinal block, because that position reduces the peridural space to a greater degree and stretches the dura mater, making it more susceptible to puncture.* (The epidural space is decreased during pregnancy because of venous engorgement. It is also smaller in obese and short individuals.)

2. The skin is prepared with an antiseptic agent.

3. A skin wheal is made to anesthetize the supraspinous and interspinous ligaments.

4. A short beveled 18-gauge needle with stylet is passed to the ligamentum flavum of the second, third, or fourth lumbar interspace (Figure 17–4). The ligamentum flavum is identified by its resistance to injection of saline or air. A rebound effect takes place.

5. Resistance disappears as the peridural space is entered.

6. Aspiration rules out penetration of a blood vessel.

7. A test dose of 2–3 mL of anesthetic agent is injected to make sure the dura mater has not been penetrated.

8. A test period of at least 5 minutes is allowed. During this time, vital signs and levels of anesthesia are checked to make sure that no untoward effects have occurred.

9. After checking again to make sure the dura mater has not been perforated, a single dose of 10–12 mL is injected to provide anesthesia for delivery.

TECHNIQUE FOR CONTINUOUS LUMBAR EPIDURAL BLOCK

The procedure for a continuous lumbar epidural block is the same as for a lumbar epidural block through step 5, after which the following steps are taken:

6. A plastic catheter is threaded 3–5 cm beyond the tip of the needle. Hyperesthetic response in the leg, hip, or back is sometimes elicited if the soft catheter touches a nerve in the peridural space. The needle is removed. (The plastic catheter is *never* pulled back through the needle. Risk of shearing plastic catheters must be kept in mind.)

7. The catheter is taped in place.

8. A test dose of 2–3 mL of anesthetic agent is injected.

9. An analgesic dose of 5–6 mL is given for relief of uterine pain during the first stage of labor. Additional injections are made through the catheter as necessary.

10. An anesthetic dose of 10–12 mL is given just prior to delivery, with the client sitting in an upright position.

Although other agents may be used for the epidural block, bupivacaine (Marcaine) is preferred because each injection produces analgesia for 2½–3 hours (Akamatsu and Bonica, 1974). Bupivacaine (Marcaine) and chloroprocaine (Nesacaine) produce good sensory analgesia with minimal motor blockade. A low concentration of the agent of choice is used to provide analgesia during labor, which avoids interference with fetal internal rotation due to paralysis of the perineal muscles. Reinforcing doses should be administered by the anesthesiologist before the anesthetic level has fallen considerably—otherwise tolerance to the agent and a reduction in the effectiveness of the block can occur. High concentrations are given for the "sitting dose" just prior to delivery to ensure good perineal relaxation.

□ *NURSING IMPLICATIONS* Continuous epidural analgesia may be initiated when active labor has been established. Relief of pain, anxiety, and apprehension results without interfering with the Ferguson reflex or rotation when a segmental block is done. A segmental block of the tenth and eleventh dermatomes is considered ideal for the first stage of labor. Contractions may be less intense for 10–20 minutes following injection, with gradual resumption of good-quality contractions.

In the absence of maternal hypotension, toxic reaction, or other maternal complications that interfere with uteroplacental transfer, the fetus is not likely to be affected during an epidural technique. Lavin and associates (1981) studied the effect on the FHR of the two most commonly used drugs for epidural anesthesia, bupivacaine (Marcaine) and chloroprocaine (Nesacaine). The results indicate that these agents have little effect on the fetal heart rate. Bupivacaine was associated with a slight increase in FHR variability. This study suggests that any change in the FHR should always be thoroughly investigated.

The most common maternal side effect of epidural anesthesia is hypotension. This is due to the sympathetic block and loss of peripheral resistance. Maternal blood pressure and pulse must be taken every 1–2 minutes after the injection for the first 15 minutes and every 10–15 minutes thereafter.

Systolic blood pressure below 100 mm Hg or a fall in systolic pressure greater than 30% of the baseline blood pressure requires treatment (Shnider and Levinson, 1979). Some clinicians attempt to avoid hypotension by preloading the woman with 500–1000 mL of lactated Ringer's solution. Treatment of the hypotension includes manual uterine displacement to the left, or maintaining a left side lying position, Trendelenburg position, increased rate of intravenous fluids, and oxygen by face mask. The nurse must be prepared to initiate these measures. (Ephedrine may be used to elevate the blood pressure if these actions are not effective.) The regimen for initial surveillance should be repeated each time the peridural catheter is reinjected with the agent.

Systemic toxic reaction can occur with epidural block as was described in the section on paracervical block. Since large quantities of anesthetic agent are used for epidural block, the likelihood of toxic reaction is higher than with some of the other regional procedures. The client should be engaged in conversation to permit evaluation of her sensorium. Total spinal anesthesia may result from accidental perforation of the dura mater or excessive spreading of the agent extradurally.

A distressing maternal problem is inadequate block, unilateral block, or block failure. Epidural anesthesia has a higher failure rate than spinal anesthesia, because the catheter must be properly placed for adequate analgesia to occur. A one-sided block is fairly common and can be overcome by having the client lie on the unanesthetized side and injecting more of the agent. A block may be effective except for a "spot" of pain in the inguinal or suprapubic area. Clark (1981) cites failure to block S_1 as the most likely cause. The sensitivity of the side of the foot to a pinprick demonstrates that S_1 is inadequately blocked, since this area is innervated by that nerve.

During epidural block the urge to void is diminished. The bladder must be checked carefully and the client encouraged to void at frequent intervals to obviate bladder distention. The client may also require more coaching during the second stage of labor since she cannot feel her contractions and does not experience the urge to push.

Headache (as occurs with spinal blocks) is *not* a side effect of epidural anesthesia, because the dura mater of the spinal canal has not been penetrated and there is no leakage of spinal fluid. Therefore, lying flat for a prescribed number of hours after delivery is not required. Ambulation should be delayed, however, until the effects of anesthesia have worn off. This may take several hours depending on the agent and the total dose used. Motor control of the legs is weak but not totally absent after delivery. Return of complete sensation and the ability to control the legs is essential before attempting ambulation. The woman must also be able to maintain blood pressure in a sitting or standing position. See Nursing Care Plan—Regional Anesthesia, next page, for further nursing actions.

TECHNIQUE FOR CAUDAL BLOCK

The caudal approach to the peridural space was formerly a popular procedure particularly when a catheter was used

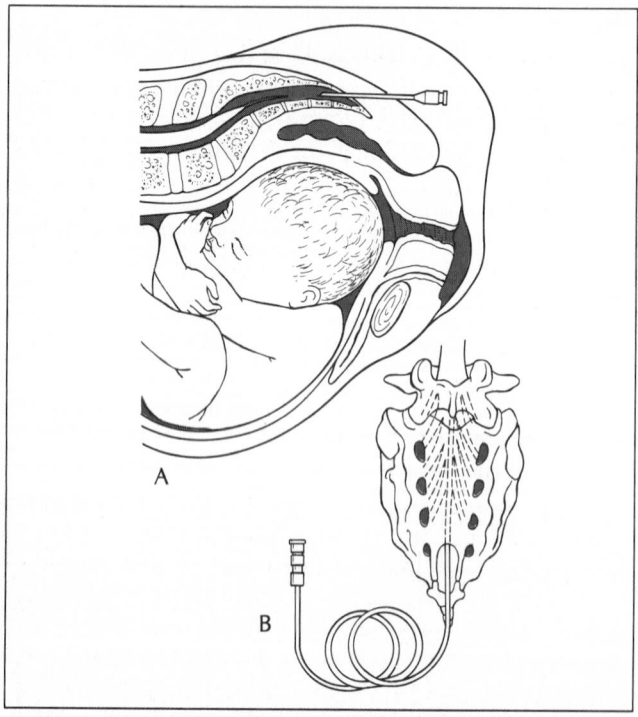

FIGURE 17–5 Caudal technique. **A,** Placement of needle in caudal canal. **B,** Plastic catheter in caudal canal. (From Regional anesthesia in obstetrics, Clinical Education Aid No. 17, Ross Laboratories, Columbus, Ohio.)

for administration of additional doses of anesthetic agent. At the lower end of the sacrum on the posterior surface of the fourth sacral vertebra is a U-shaped foramen covered by a thick layer of fibrous tissue that leads into the caudal portion of the peridural space.

The technique is as follows:

1. Although the knee-chest position makes the bony landmarks more prominent, it is most uncomfortable for the client. A lateral Sims position is better tolerated.

2. The skin is prepared with a suitable antibacterial agent.

3. A skin wheal is raised over the sacral hiatus and into the fascia.

4. An 18-gauge thin-walled stylet for a plastic catheter needle is passed through the skin at a 70° or 80° angle into the sacral hiatus until the sacrum is reached (Figure 17–5, *A*).

5. The needle hub is depressed toward the skin at a 35° or 40° angle and advanced into the sacral canal 2–3 cm.

6. Aspiration for blood or spinal fluid is done. If spinal fluid is obtained, the procedure should be discontinued at once. If blood is obtained, the needle is advanced for a short distance.

7. While palpating over the sacrum to detect crepitation from a needle that is improperly placed, 3 mL of air is rapidly injected. If major resistance to injection occurs, subperiosteal placement is indicated.

8. A test dose of 3 mL is given, and vital signs are monitored for at least 5 minutes. The level of hypoesthesia is also checked.

9. The agent is injected slowly into the caudal space for a single dose. A dose of 8–10 mL provides a low block affecting dermatomes S_1 to S_5; 20–30 mL sensitizes spinal nerves from T_{10} to S_5.

For continuous caudal block the procedure is the same, but once the needle is placed correctly, a plastic catheter is threaded through the needle and advanced 15 cm into the caudal space (see Figure 17–5, *B*). Initially 15–30 mL is given, with reinforcement doses every 45–90 minutes.

□ *NURSING IMPLICATIONS* A caudal block should be monitored in the same manner as an epidural block. With the caudal technique a larger volume of anesthetic solution is required so that the client must be watched closely for a toxic reaction. Relaxation of the anal sphincter and increased warmth of the extremities indicate proper placement of the catheter in the caudal canal. Vasodilatation may be detected by watching for increased redness of the large toe and the ball of the foot. Accidents unique to caudal block include perforation of the rectum and of the fetal scalp. The nursing measures given for epidural block apply to caudal block.

NURSING CARE PLAN
Regional Anesthesia

CLIENT DATA BASE

History

1. Maternal information
   a. Allergies to drugs (specifically anesthetic agents)
   b. Psychologic status
      (1) What type anesthesia does the client want and what kind will she accept?
      (2) Does the client understand the procedure?
      (3) What does she expect it to accomplish?
      (4) Is the client able to cope with the labor process and can she follow directions?
   c. Prenatal preparation and education
   d. Presence of other disease states, such as cardiovascular, pulmonary, and CNS disorders, and metabolic diseases
   e. Time of client's last meal
2. Fetal assessment
   a. Gestational age
   b. Status
   c. Stability of FHR

Physical examination

1. Determine whether site to be used for injection is free from infection

2. Determine whether hemorrhage is present or imminent
3. Evaluate blood pressure for evidence of hypotension
4. Note evidence of upper respiratory infection, which is a contraindication for general anesthesia

Laboratory evaluation

1. No specific tests required for woman
2. Fetal scalp samples may be obtained in presence of fetal distress

NURSING PRIORITIES

1. Maintain a safe environment for woman and fetus
2. Continuously monitor maternal status to recognize and to treat potential problems
3. Monitor fetal status
4. Promote thorough understanding of procedure through education of both parents

CLIENT/FAMILY EDUCATIONAL FOCUS

1. Discuss the purpose, expected effect, and possible side effects of anesthetic block
2. Discuss the procedure and the expected nursing care associated with the regional anesthesia
3. Provide opportunities to discuss questions and individual concerns of the woman and her family

Problem	Nursing interventions and actions	Rationale
Client's fear and anxiety	Thoroughly explain procedure, its effects, and its value to client and significant other	Regional anesthesia is frequently poorly understood and frightening for clients
	Provide an opportunity for questions and discussion	Thorough explanation during procedure ensures client cooperation
	Utilize charts and other teaching aids as necessary	
	Evaluate emotional significance of regional anesthesia to the client and intervene appropriately	
Adequate preparation for procedure	Have legal permits signed. Have client empty bladder	Regional anesthesia interferes with client's urge to void
	Begin intravenous fluids	Intravenous fluids maintain adequate hydration and provide systemic access in the event of untoward reactions or severe hypotension
		Clients receiving subarachnoid or peridural block are to be overhydrated for 5 min prior to the procedure
		Increased intravenous fluid intake decreases the possibility of maternal hypotension
	Position client correctly for procedure (see text for proper positioning for individual procedures)	

NURSING CARE PLAN Cont'd
Regional Anesthesia

Problem	Nursing interventions and actions	Rationale
	Assess maternal status: 1. Obtain baseline vital signs before any anesthetic agent is given 2. Monitor blood pressure every 5 min for 30 min following administration of anesthetic agent 3. Monitor pulse and respiration	Baseline reading allows more complete evaluation of maternal status Hypotension is a frequent complication of regional anesthesia Pulse may slow following spinal anesthesia due to decreased venous return, decreased venous pressure, and decreased right heart pressure Respiratory paralysis is a potential complication of regional anesthesia
	Assess fetal status: 1. Utilize fetal monitoring to establish a baseline reading of FHR and FHTs 2. Monitor FHR continuously	Maternal hypotension may interfere with fetal oxygenation and is evidenced by fetal bradycardia
	Observe, record, and report complications of anesthesia, including hypotension, fetal distress, respiratory paralysis, changes in uterine contractility, decrease in voluntary muscle effort, trauma to extremities, nausea and vomiting, loss of bladder tone, and spinal headache	
Hypotension	Observe, record, and report symptoms of hypotension, including systolic pressure <100 mg or a 25% fall in systolic pressure, apprehension, restlessness, dizziness, tinnitus, headache	
	Institute treatment measures: 1. Place client with head flat and foot of bed elevated	Gravity increases venous filling of the heart and the pulmonary blood volume; the result is an increase in stroke volume and cardiac output with a rise in blood pressure
	2. Increase IV fluid rate	Blood volume increases and circulation improves
	3. Administer O_2 by face mask	Oxygen content of circulating blood increases
	4. Administer vasopressors as ordered	Vasoconstriction occurs; vasopressors are not used in pregnant women unless absolutely necessary because they may further compromise the fetus
	Specific interventions for treatment of hypotension following peridural anesthesia: 1. Raise knee gatch on bed 2. Manually displace uterus laterally to left	Increases venous return (vena cava is usually to the right)
	3. Administer O_2 by face mask at 4–7 L/min	Face mask is method of choice, because woman in labor breathes through her mouth
	4. Increase rate of IV fluids.	

NURSING CARE PLAN Cont'd
Regional Anesthesia

Problem	Nursing interventions and actions	Rationale
	5. Keep client supine for 5–10 min following administration of block to allow drug to diffuse bilaterally; after 5–10 min position client on side	
	Specific interventions for hypotension following spinal anesthesia: 1. Administer O_2 by face mask at 4–7 L/min 2. Manually displace uterus to left 3. Increase rate of IV fluids 4. Place legs in stirrups	BP drops following spinal anesthesia, probably because of paralysis of the sympathetic vasoconstrictor fibers to blood vessels Increases venous return
Fetal distress	Observe, record, and report fetal bradycardia (FHR <120/min) and loss of beat-to-beat variability Institute treatment measures for maternal hypotension (Note: Paracervical blocks commonly cause a drop in FHTs for a short period of time)	Maternal hypotension causes decreased blood circulation to fetus and results in fetal hypoxia Amide group of anesthetic agents (bupivacaine, mepivacaine, and lidocaine) have potential to produce direct fetal myocardial depression; bradycardia may be caused by reduced placental blood flow
Respiratory paralysis and spinal blockade	Monitor respirations; if respiratory function is compromised, client exhibits restlessness, dizziness, drowsiness, dyspnea, and an inability to speak; lapse into unconsciousness, hypotension, and apnea quickly follows Immediate treatment includes following: 1. Support of ventilation 2. Increase in IV fluid rate 3. Preparation for cardiac resuscitation	Respiratory paralysis may occur with total spinal blockade and results from too concentrated a dose (for example, injected during a contraction) or too large a dose
Change in uterine contractility	Monitor uterine contractions manually or electronically; if uterine contractions cease, oxytocic agent may be administered	Anesthetic agents generally decrease uterine contractility (although increased contractility occasionally occurs); this decrease frequently prolongs labor for the client
Decrease in voluntary muscle effort	Monitor contractions; coordinate client's pushing effort with pressure of uterine contraction; delivery by forceps may be necessary	Loss of muscle control results in loss of ability to push Client does not have sensation of having contractions Pushing without contractions decreases effectiveness and tires the client
Trauma to extremities	Support extremity during movement Position legs securely so they cannot fall off stirrups or delivery table	Regional block anesthesia produces vasomotor paralysis

NURSING CARE PLAN Cont'd
Regional Anesthesia

Problem	Nursing interventions and actions	Rationale
	Move legs slowly	Sudden movement in client with vasomotor paralysis may precipitate hypotensive episode
Nausea and vomiting	Protect client from aspiration of vomitus	Nausea and vomiting may accompany hypotension and are related to hypoxia and excessive rise in BP following administration of vasopressor
	Move client slowly and gently	Nausea and vomiting are often related to sudden changes in position
Loss of bladder tone	Evaluate bladder distention	Regional anesthesia reduces feeling and control of sphincter muscles
	Insert Foley catheter if distention is present	Full bladder during second stage of labor increases chance of bladder trauma
Spinal headache	1. Preventive measures include: a. Use of small (25–26) gauge needle	Spinal headache is related to the leakage of spinal fluid; a small needle permits less fluid loss
	b. Maintenance of recumbent position for 6–12 hr following delivery	Headache, which commonly occurs when the client is upright, is related to decreased intracranial pressure
	c. Adequate hydration—IV fluids during labor and delivery, oral fluids following delivery 2. Administer analgesics as ordered 3. Use of ``blood patch'' for severe and incapacitating headache	Aids in fluid replacement

NURSING CARE EVALUATION

Client has not suffered injury

Client's BP, pulse, and respiration are within her normal limits

Fetus has not been compromised. FHTs remained fairly stable

Client understands type of regional block administered and possible side effects

NURSING DIAGNOSES*	SUPPORTING DATA
1. Anxiety and/or fear related to invasive, unfamiliar procedure	Lack of knowledge about regional anesthesia Preconceived notions, fears
2. Potential for maternal injury	Respiratory paralysis Maternal hypotension Decrease in voluntary muscle effort for bearing down Trauma to lower extremities Aspiration Loss of bladder tone Spinal headache

*These are a few examples of nursing diagnoses that may be appropriate for a woman receiving regional anesthesia. It is not an inclusive list and must be individualized for each woman.

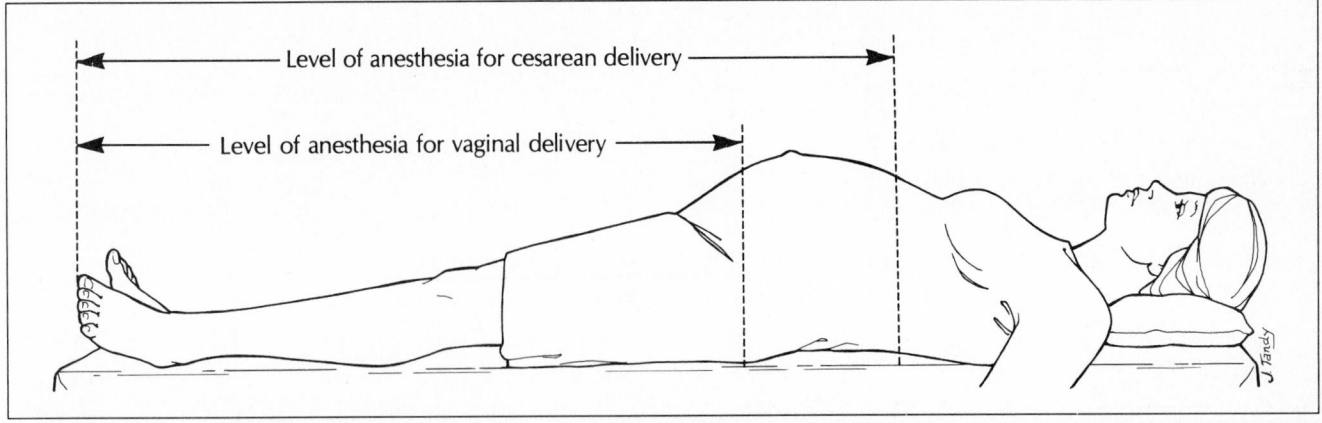

FIGURE 17-6 Levels of anesthesia for vaginal and cesarean deliveries. (From Regional anesthesia in obstetrics, Clinical Education Aid No. 17, Ross Laboratories, Columbus, Ohio.)

The caudal block method for peridural anesthesia has been largely replaced by lumbar epidural block. The epidural method is technically easier to perform, less painful for the client, more reliable, and requires a smaller amount of anesthetic agent.

Subarachnoid Block
(Spinal, Low Spinal, or Saddle Block)

In subarachnoid block, a local anesthetic agent is injected directly into the spinal fluid in the spinal canal to provide anesthesia for vaginal delivery and cesarean birth. For vaginal delivery, blockade to the T_{10} dermatome is usually effective, whereas cesarean delivery requires anesthesia to the T_8 dermatome (Figure 17-6). The term *saddle block* has been used to describe the subarachnoid block procedure used for vaginal delivery, but the term is incorrectly used in most cases because the area of the anesthesia is greater than the area anesthetized with a true saddle block (Pritchard and MacDonald, 1980). However, "saddle block" is a more acceptable term to the general public than "low spinal block."

The subarachnoid space is the fluid-filled area between the dura and the spinal cord. During pregnancy, the space decreases because of the distention of the epidural veins. Thus a specific dose of anesthetic produces a much higher level of anesthesia in the pregnant woman than in the nonpregnant woman. The procedure is usually done when the fetal head is on the perineum. Bearing down during the second stage of labor increases the anesthetic level to one higher than desired, so the injection must not be made while the woman is having a contraction.

When a low spinal block is properly administered, failure rate is low. The disadvantages include an extremely high incidence of maternal hypotension with resultant fetal hypoxia, maternal postspinal headaches, and maintenance of uterine tone, which makes intrauterine manipulation very difficult. Spinal anesthesia is contraindicated for clients with severe hypovolemia, regardless of the cause; central nervous system disease; infection over the site of puncture; and severe hypotension or hypertension. It is also contraindicated for clients who do not wish to have spinal procedures.

TECHNIQUE

The following steps are followed in administering a subarachnoid block:

1. The client is placed in a sitting position with feet supported on a stool.
2. Intravenous infusion should be checked for patency.
3. The client places her arms between her knees, bows her head, and arches her back to widen the intervertebral space.
4. Careful skin preparation is done, maintaining sterility.
5. A skin wheal is made over L_3 or L_4.
6. The double-needle technique is advocated (Figure 17-7). A 20- or 21-gauge needle, with stylet used as an introducer, is passed through the wheal into the interspinous ligament, ligamentum flavum, and epidural space.
7. A 25- or 26-gauge needle is inserted into the larger needle and advanced through the dura into the subarachnoid space.
8. Upon removal of the stylet, a drop of fluid can be seen in the hub of the needle if the spinal canal has been entered.
9. The appropriate amount of anesthetic agent (such as 4 mg of tetracaine (Pontocaine) for vaginal delivery and 8-10 mg for cesarean delivery) is injected slowly, and both needles are removed.

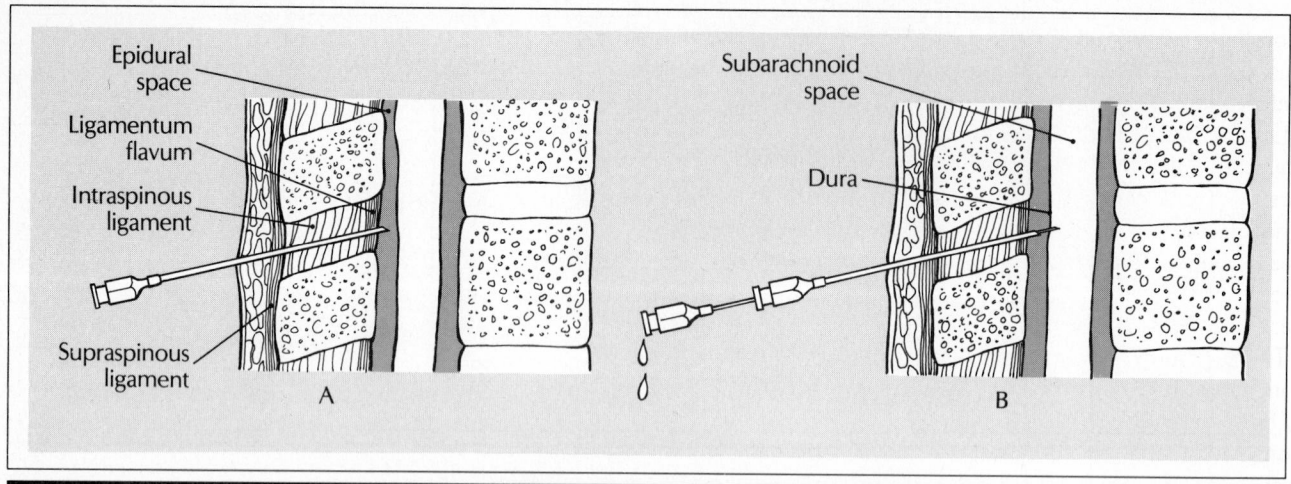

FIGURE 17–7 Double needle technique for spinal injection. **A,** Large needle in epidural space. **B,** 25–26 gauge needle in larger needle entering the spinal canal. (From Bonica, J. J. 1972. *Principles and practice of obstetric analgesia and anesthesia.* Philadelphia: F. A. Davis Co., p. 563.)

10. With hyperbaric solutions, the client remains sitting up for 45 seconds.

11. The client is placed on her back with a pillow under her head. Position changes can alter the dermatome level if done within 3–5 minutes. After 10 minutes, a position change will not affect the level of anesthesia.

12. Blood pressure, pulse, and respiration must be monitored every 1–2 minutes for the first 10 minutes then every 5–10 minutes.

NURSING IMPLICATIONS

The sitting position for the administration of spinal (subarachnoid block) anesthesia is preferred. Since the procedure is not done until the presenting part is on the perineum, sitting on the edge of the delivery table may be very difficult for the laboring woman. The nurse helps the client into a sitting position and provides encouragement and support during the procedure. The nurse informs the physician when a contraction is beginning so the anesthetic agent will not be injected at that time. After sitting upright for the prescribed number of minutes, a recumbent position is assumed and the legs are placed in stirrups. Monitoring of blood pressure begins immediately.

In the absence of maternal hypotension or toxic reaction there is no direct effect on the fetus with subarachnoid block. The amount of anesthetic used is too small to reach fetal circulation in a quantity that might cause fetal depression. A study by Caritis et al. (1980) compared the fetal acid-base balance and maternal blood pressure following spinal and epidural anesthesia. The observations suggest that infants delivered by cesarean birth with epidural anesthesia have higher blood pH levels and lower base deficit values in umbilical cord blood than infants delivered by cesarean birth with spinal anesthesia. Spinal anesthesia

was shown to be well tolerated by a healthy fetus when a fluid load in excess of 1000 mL preceded the injection. The extent to which the fetus is affected relates to the degree of maternal hypotension rather than a direct drug effect on the fetus. When maternal hypotension occurs, one is well advised to delay delivery for 4 or 5 minutes to allow the fetus to recover.

The most common serious maternal side effect of spinal (subarachnoid block) is hypotension. The incidence of hypotension is much higher for cesarean birth than for vaginal delivery because of the degree of sympathetic block (Clark, 1981). The importance of monitoring blood pressure and treatment of hypotension were addressed in the section on nursing implications following epidural block. The possibilities of total spinal anesthesia and toxic reaction must always be kept in mind.

As with other techniques that block pain sensation in the lower body, the laboring woman must be instructed when to bear down because she will not experience this urge. After delivery, the woman may not be able to move from the delivery table because of motor paralysis in her legs. Great care must be taken in the lifting technique to avoid injury to the woman's muscles and ligaments. Any sudden movement can precipitate a hypotensive episode.

The maternal complications of meningitis and arachnoiditis after spinal blocks have become rare with strict aseptic technique. Chemical irritation has been virtually eliminated with the use of single-dose disposable equipment.

Although much less serious than other complications, headache is an unpleasant aftermath of spinal anesthesia. Leakage of spinal fluid at the site of dural puncture is thought to be the cause. Several techniques have been suggested to decrease the possibility of headache. The use of a 25- or 26-gauge needle and avoidance of multiple perforations of the dura reduce the incidence. The incidence of spinal headache varies from about 70% after puncture with a 16-guage needle to only about 2% with a 25-gauge spinal needle (Shnider and Levinson, 1979). Hyperhydration and keeping the woman flat in bed for 6–12 hours after delivery have been recommended as preventive measures, but there is no evidence that these procedures are effective (Pritchard and MacDonald, 1980). Not all postpartal headaches in clients who had spinal anesthesia are a result of the procedure.

The postspinal block headache usually begins on the second postpartal day and lasts several days to a week. It may be of varying degrees of severity. The pain occurs or becomes worse when the client sits or stands and decreases or ceases when she lies down or flexes and extends her head.

Treatment consists primarily of bed rest, increased fluids, and analgesics for the mild or moderate forms. Severe and incapacitating headache has been treated successfully by a "blood patch" over the site of dural puncture. About 10 mL of blood is drawn from the client and immediately injected into the epidural space over the site of the perforation; the clot applies pressure and seals off the leak. In many cases, this procedure has dramatically relieved symptoms. The success rate ranges from 91%–100% (Abouleish et al., 1975).

Pudendal Block

The pudendal block technique provides perineal anesthesia for the latter part of the first stage, the second stage of labor, delivery, and episiotomy repair. An anesthetic agent is injected below the pudendal plexus, which arises from the anterior division of the second and third sacral nerves and the entire fourth sacral nerve. The pudendal nerve crosses the sacrosciatic notch and passes the tip of the ischial spine, where it divides into the perineal, dorsal, and inferior hemorrhoidal nerves. The perineal nerve, which is the largest branch of the pudendal plexus, supplies the skin of the vulvar area, the perineal muscles, and the urethral sphincter. The dorsal nerve supplies the clitoris, and the inferior hemorrhoidal nerve supplies the skin and muscles of the perianal region as well as the internal anal sphincter. Pudendal block provides relief of pain from perineal distention but does not relieve pain of uterine contractions.

Pudendal block is a relatively simple procedure but requires a thorough knowledge of pelvic anatomy to block the pudendal nerve adequately. A moderate dose of anesthetic agent (10 mL per side) has minimal effect on the woman and the course of labor. The urge to bear down during the second stage of labor may be eliminated, but the woman is able to do so with appropriate coaching. There is little effect on the uncompromised fetus unless overly rapid or intravascular injection occurs. The block

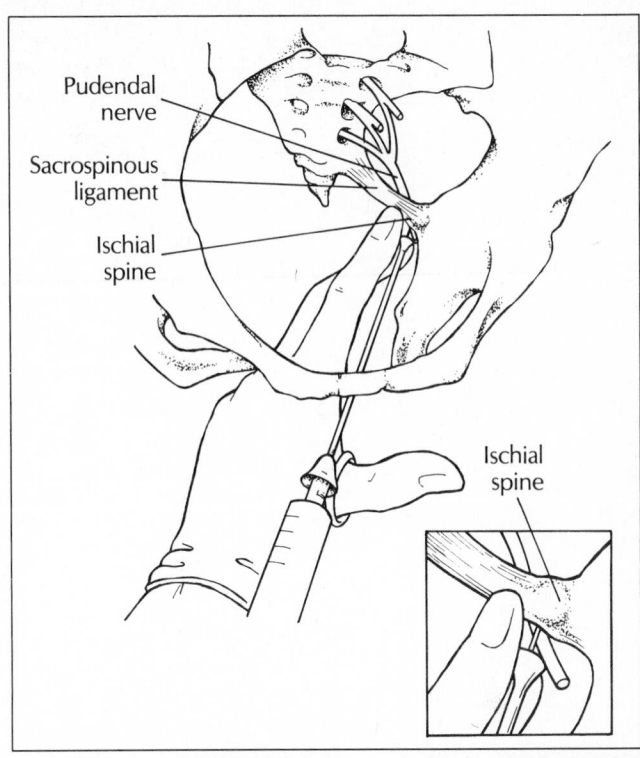

FIGURE 17–8 Technique for pudendal block. Inset shows needle extending beyond guide. (Modified from Bonica, J. J. 1972. *Principles and practice of obstetric analgesia and anesthesia*. Philadelphia: F. A. Davis Co., p. 495.)

may be done by a transvaginal or transperineal approach. Transvaginal injection is simpler, safer, and more direct, making it the procedure of choice.

TECHNIQUE

A pudendal block is administered as follows:

1. The client is placed in a lithotomy or dorsal recumbent position with the knees flexed.
2. A 12.7–15.24 cm, 22-gauge needle with guide is used to protect the vaginal wall and control needle depth.
3. The instrument is guided into the vagina until the ischial spine is reached (Figure 17–8).
4. The needle is advanced through the vaginal wall and, by the technique of individual operator preference, into the space where the pudendal nerve passes.
5. Following aspiration to make sure that the needle is not in a blood vessel, 3–5 mL of solution is injected.
6. The needle is advanced 1 cm more, aspiration is repeated, and another 3–5 mL of the agent is injected.
7. Injection of the agent into the pudendal nerve on the opposite side follows the same procedure.

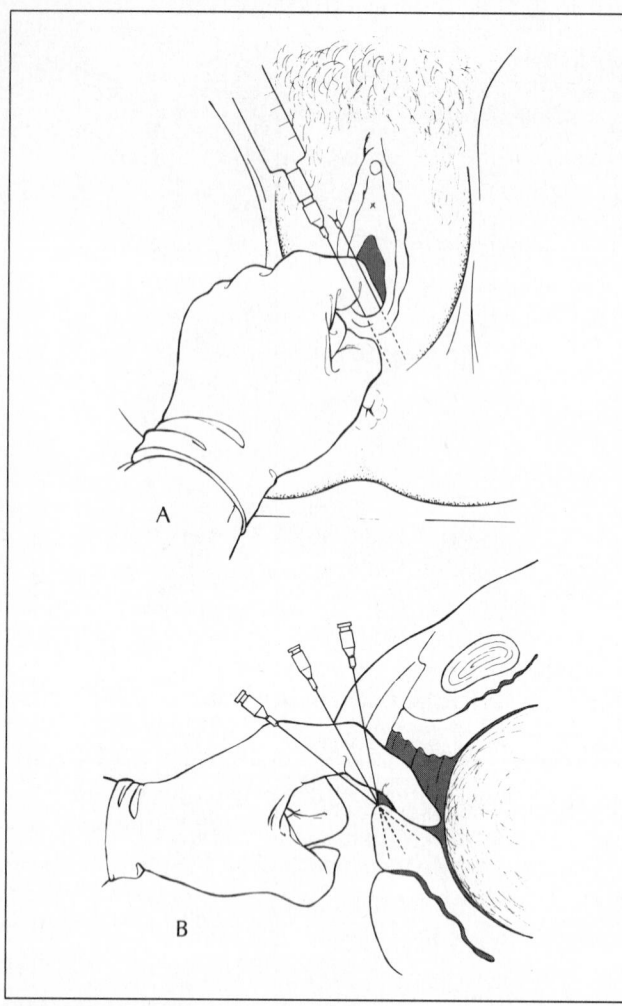

FIGURE 17–9 Local anesthesia. **A,** Technique of local infiltration for episiotomy and repair. **B,** Technique of local infiltration showing fan pattern for the fascial planes. (From Bonica, J. J. 1972. *Principles and practice of obstetric analgesia and anesthesia.* Philadelphia: F. A. Davis Co., p. 505.)

Local Anesthesia

Local anesthesia is accomplished by injection of an anesthetic agent into the intracutaneous, subcutaneous, and intramuscular areas of the perineum. It is generally used at the time of delivery for episiotomy repair and is especially useful for women delivering by psychoprophylactic methods of childbirth. The procedure is technically simple and is practically free from complications.

A disadvantage is that large amounts of solution must be used. Although any local anesthetic may be used, chloroprocaine (Nesacaine), lidocaine (Xylocaine), and mepivacaine (Carbocaine) are the agents of choice in local infiltration because of their capacity for diffusion.

TECHNIQUE

The technique of local anesthesia consists of injecting the agent with a long, sharp, beveled 22-gauge needle into the various fascial planes of the perineum (Figure 17–9). The procedure is deceptively simple; however, overdose may occur if the anesthetist does not wait for the anesthetic to take effect before injecting more solution. An excessive volume or concentration contributes to systemic toxic reactions and local toxic effects (Greenhill and Friedman, 1974). In the absence of maternal complications, there are no fetal effects when the procedure is done prior to delivery.

GENERAL ANESTHESIA

The goal of obstetric anesthesia is to provide maximal pain relief with minimal side effects to the woman and her fetus. Anesthetic techniques and drugs should be selected to meet their needs. Before the anesthetic procedure, intravenous fluids should be initiated so that access to the intravascular system is immediately available in case of emergency. Women who have had fluids withheld throughout the course of labor need an infusion for hydration and energy.

When used, general anesthesia is usually administered at the time of delivery, although some drugs serve as analgesic agents during labor. The method used to produce general anesthesia may be intravenous injection or inhalation.

No method or agent is without maternal and fetal hazards. All agents for general anesthesia cross the placental barrier and depress the nervous system of the fetus in varying degrees. Anesthetic deaths still remain a cause of maternal mortality in the United States, and half of the deaths are attributable to aspiration of vomitus during general anesthesia. Despite the maternal and fetal hazards, general anesthesia is still popular in much of North America.

Chloroprocaine (Nesacaine), which has a low toxicity, may be used if prompt but brief anesthesia is needed. Lidocaine (Xylocaine) has prompt effect and intermediate action. Other agents used are mepivacaine (Carbocaine) and bupivacaine (Marcaine). The possible maternal complications specific to pudendal block include broad ligament hematoma, perforation of the rectum, and trauma to the sciatic nerve. Pudendal block is frequently used in conjunction with paracervical block, or it may be the sole anesthetic technique used. It is compatible with the goals of psychoprophylactic preparation for childbirth. The transvaginal technique must be done before the fetal head has advanced too far in the birth canal. Demonstrable blood levels of anesthetic agents have been documented in the fetus but serious fetal complications are rare.

General anesthesia is indicated for a woman with certain obstetric complications. When hemorrhage or the threat of hemorrhage is present, general anesthesia may be the method of choice, because regional anesthesia with resulting sympathetic blockage and peripheral vasodilatation compounds the problem of hypovolemia. Any obstetric condition requiring uterine relaxation, such as delivery of the head in a breech presentation, internal version with the second twin, and tetanic contractions, is an indication for general anesthesia. Bonica (1972) states, "The potent inhalation anesthetics are the best uterine relaxants currently available because they act more rapidly and are better controlled than any other drugs." It is the procedure of choice in emergency cesarean section for fetal distress. General anesthesia is also used for clients with CNS disease and allergies to local anesthetic agents.

Many drugs have been used as obstetric anesthetic agents since chloroform was first used. Ether and nitrous oxide were first introduced in the eighteenth century for the relief of pain. Inhalation anesthetics depress the central nervous system in varying degrees, which correlate to the concentration of the agent in arterial blood entering cerebral circulation. By balancing the amount of a drug entering arterial circulation by way of the lung against the amount returning chemically intact to the lung by way of venous circulation, the anesthesiologist can control the concentration in the brain and keep the client at the level of anesthesia desired. Inhalation anesthetics are considered to be safer than intravenously administered drugs because the circulating concentrations can be more quickly and better controlled. Once injected, intravenous agents cannot be retrieved and must be metabolized by the body for excretion.

Nurses who care for anesthetized clients in the delivery and recovery rooms must be able to assess the client's level of anesthesia to provide appropriate intervention. Client's in stage I anesthesia respond to verbal orders even though sensorium is altered. It is important that only one person give commands. Otherwise, confusion results and the client cannot respond appropriately.

It must also be remembered that the client in stage II anesthesia is actually unconscious and unable to control behavior. The higher cortical centers are depressed by the anesthetic agent, releasing the lower motor and emotional centers from control. The client is not responsible for her actions at this level.

Inhalation Anesthetics

NITROUS OXIDE

Nitrous oxide is the oldest analgesic and anesthetic gaseous agent. It provides rapid and pleasant induction; it is nonirritating, nonexplosive, and inexpensive; and it provides less disturbance in physiologic functioning than any

other agent (Bonica, 1972). At a concentration of 40%, it produces excellent analgesia yet permits the laboring woman to cooperate. Little or no fetal depression occurs with this concentration. When used alone, there is no effect on the maternal respiratory center.

Nitrous oxide is generally used in combination with other agents for anesthesia. Although it is an excellent analgesic, nitrous oxide provides poor muscular relaxation. The main use of nitrous oxide is as an analgesic agent during the second stage of labor, as an induction agent or supplement to more potent inhalation anesthetics, and as a part of balanced anesthesia, discussed later in the chapter.

METHOXYFLURANE (PENTHRANE)

Of the more recent halogenated anesthetics, methoxyflurane is the most potent and the most widely used in obstetrics. Analgesic doses may be self-administered with an inhaler to provide pain relief during transition and the second stage of labor without significantly affecting the course of labor. Masks designed for self-administration should *never* be held over the client's face by nursing personnel, because the agent is not to be administered continuously.

Anesthetic doses provide smooth induction and emergence with minimal irritation of the tracheobronchial tree, although fetal depression occurs with high concentrations for a prolonged period of time. The addition of nitrous oxide and oxygen decreases the amount of methoxyflurane needed for effective anesthesia. When required for emergency conditions, a higher concentration can produce good uterine relaxation. One of its disadvantages, although enhancing its wide margin of safety, is the slow induction time. The emergence from anesthesia is also slow, and the client must be carefully supervised in the recovery room by nursing personnel.

HALOTHANE (FLUOTHANE)

Halothane, the vapor of a nonexplosive and nonflammable volatile liquid, is frequently used as a general anesthetic. Induction with this agent is smooth and rapid, safe and predictable. Halothane is nonirritating to the upper respiratory tract and causes little nausea or vomiting. It does cause depression of respiration and irritability of cardiac tissue resulting in arrhythmias. Only a moderate degree of muscle relaxation is produced. The agent increases blood flow to the uterus and does not contribute to uterine relaxation when used in low doses.

Intravenous Anesthetics

THIOPENTAL SODIUM (PENTOTHAL)

Thiopental sodium is an ultrashort-acting barbiturate that produces narcosis within 30 seconds after intravenous administration. Induction and emergence are smooth and pleasant, with little incidence of nausea and vomiting. The client goes from the first stage of anesthesia to the first plane of the third stage so rapidly that the clinical signs of the levels in between are difficult to detect. Barbiturates are nonirritating to the respiratory tract and are nonexplosive. They differ from the inhalation anesthetics in two major ways: (a) little or no analgesia occurs, and (b) the method of administration is less controllable.

Thiopental sodium is extremely irritating to tissues, and sloughing may result if infiltration occurs with high concentrations of the agent. Because of this effect, the integrity of the intravenous line must be checked prior to administration. The rapidity of action makes it valuable in convulsive states, particularly those that occur as side effects of local anesthetics. Maternal peak plasma concentration after injection may fall as much as 90% in 1 minute, so injection at the onset of a contraction prevents the fetus from receiving the transient high concentration of the agent. Hypotension, vasodilation and laryngospasm may occur and muscle relaxation is inadequate.

Thiopental sodium is rarely used alone, because the dosage required for anesthesia produces profound central nervous system depression. It is most frequently used for induction and as an adjunct to other more potent anesthetics. Significant neonatal depression does not occur with administration of single doses of less than 250 mg (Danforth, 1982).

KETAMINE (KETALAR, KETAJECT)

The intravenous agent ketamine is a dissociative anesthetic with amnesic and analgesic properties. It is a useful alternative to thiopental sodium for induction of general anesthesia and is most frequently used as a single-dose induction of general anesthesia.

Ketamine causes an increase in blood pressure and pulse and is the agent of choice for women who have bleeding complications and asthma. The agent should *never* be used in women with preeclampsia. Ketamine crosses the placental barrier within 60–90 seconds after injection, but causes little fetal depression with maternal doses of 0.5–1.0 mg/kg or less. Administration of higher doses is associated with neonatal respiratory depression and elevated bilirubin levels. The advantages of rapid action, retention of laryngeal and pharyngeal reflexes, elevation of blood pressure, and minimal respiratory depression make its use desirable.

Ketamine's disadvantages are a 10%–25% increase in maternal blood pressure and heart rate, transient apnea, and emergence reactions (Albright, 1978). The emergence reactions include dreamlike state, hallucinations, delirium, and confusion. By minimizing verbal, tactile, and visual stimulation, these reactions may be prevented. Use of ketamine may also induce amnesia about events surrounding delivery, which is unacceptable to many clients.

Balanced Anesthesia

A current trend in the management of a vaginal delivery requiring anesthetic or cesarean birth is the use of *balanced anesthesia*. The technique uses several different agents and routes of administration to produce the desired state of delivery or operative procedure. The fact that no single anesthetic agent is suitable for all people in all situations has led to the combined use of several agents and techniques for increased effectiveness and client safety. In this way, each agent is used for a specific purpose. Furthermore, because of the combined effect much smaller amounts of the agents can be given than if used alone.

An example of balanced anesthesia would be the use of an intravenous barbiturate (thiopental sodium) for sedation and rapid pleasant induction, then nitrous oxide and oxygen inhaled through a face mask for analgesia and anesthesia, followed by intravenous succinylcholine to produce muscle relaxation for intubation and better control of respiration, then a return to nitrous oxide and the face-mask inhalation of oxygen for maintenance. The purpose of balanced anesthesia is to obtain the maximum benefit from each agent and technique with a minimum of side effects for the client and newborn.

Complications of General Anesthesia

The primary dangers of general anesthesia are as follows:

FETAL DEPRESSION

Most general anesthetic agents reach the fetus in about 2 minutes. The depression in the fetus is directly proportional to the depth and duration of the anesthesia. The long-term significance of fetal depression in a normal delivery has not been determined. The poor fetal metabolism of general anesthetic agents is similar to that of analgesic agents administered during labor. General anesthesia is not advocated in cases in which the fetus is considered to be at high risk, particularly in premature delivery.

UTERINE RELAXATION

The majority of general anesthetic agents cause some degree of uterine relaxation, thereby increasing the incidence of cesarean and forceps delivery as well as postpartal uterine atony.

VOMITING AND ASPIRATION

Pregnancy results in decreased gastric motility and the onset of labor halts the process almost entirely. Food eaten hours earlier may still be in the stomach undigested. The nurse must ascertain when the laboring woman last ate and record this information on the client's chart and on her anesthesia record.

Even when food and fluids have been withheld, fasting gastric juice is highly acidic and can produce chemical pneumonitis if aspirated. Such pneumonitis is known as Mendelson's syndrome; the signs and symptoms are chest pain, respiratory embarrassment, cyanosis, fever, and tachycardia. It has become common procedure to administer an antacid during labor to neutralize the gastric contents. The usual dose is 30 mL of an antacid preparation 30–90 minutes before delivery. Gibbs and coworkers (1979) found that aspiration of an antacid also causes pulmonary damage. Whittington et al. (1979) reports two maternal deaths following aspiration of gastric contents even though the women had received antacid therapy during labor.

The result of a study by Detmer and colleagues (1979) suggests that cimetidine (Tagamet) may be more effective than antacid therapy in raising the pH level of gastric contents. However, Husemeyer and Davenport (1980), comparing the antacid effects of magnesium trisilicate and cimetidine found that the antacid was more effective in raising the pH level of gastric fluids in clients undergoing cesarean birth. There seems to be no final answer in the prevention of Mendelson's syndrome.

Vomiting and aspiration of undigested food or acidic gastric juice occurs most frequently during emergence from general anesthesia. Sellick's maneuver of applying cricoid pressure to compress the esophagus, thereby occluding the lumen to avoid regurgitation of stomach contents into the pharynx and trachea, is frequently practiced. Every nurse in the labor and delivery unit should be trained in the proper technique for applying cricoid pressure. All delivery room suites should have emergency equipment available to deal with complications such as aspiration.

Medical Interventions for Acute Respiratory Obstruction

The immediate medical treatment of acute respiratory obstruction includes the following measures:

1. Place the delivery table in a 30-degree head-down position, with the client on her right side.

2. Quickly suction pharynx and larynx or remove food with gauze-wrapped finger.

3. Perform laryngoscopy and endotracheal intubation. If the jaws cannot be forced open, succinylcholine may be given intravenously to facilitate removal of emesis and intubation. Cricoid pressure may be applied by the delivery room nurse.

4. Give 100% oxygen for pulmonary ventilation.

5. Perform bronchoscopy.

6. Tracheobronchial lavage is advocated by some, but this procedure remains controversial.

Follow-up care includes these measures:

1. *Broncholytic agents:* Aminophylline, 500 mg, slowly injected intravenously to produce bronchodilatation.

2. *Adrenocorticosteroids:* Cortisone, 100 mg, to decrease inflammatory response.

3. *Antibiotics:* Broad-spectrum agent to decrease secondary infection.

4. *Oxygen:* Intermittent positive pressure breathing (IPPB)

The use of a respirator and tracheostomy should *never* be delayed until the client is moribund. Should cardiac failure occur, it must be treated promptly and thoroughly (Bonica, 1972).

Obviously, the emergency interventions for aspiration just described constitute the recommended medical management of acute respiratory obstruction, but the *nursing* implications are very clear. Should aspiration occur, the labor and delivery room nurse should be prepared to act immediately by positioning the delivery table, turning the client on her right side, and initiating suction. The nurse may also be requested to apply cricoid pressure. During induction of and emergence from general anesthesia, the anesthesiologist must have an informed assistant able to provide help and give undivided attention if a crisis such as aspiration occurs.

SUMMARY

The complications that may occur during obstetric anesthesia are serious. Anyone who performs anesthetic procedures should be proficient in preventing, detecting, and managing all possible complications. Nursing personnel in labor and delivery suites must have a thorough understanding of anesthetic techniques, because nurses provide continual and direct care to clients and because the early detection of an incipient complication contributes to the success of medical management.

Psychoprophylactic preparation for childbirth has increased the use of regional anesthetic procedures for delivery and episiotomy repair, and this trend is increasing in popularity. The regional techniques are not without maternal and fetal hazards, however.

According to Bonica (1972), "High quality analgesic and anesthetic management requires observation of the five cardinal C's: Communication, Coordination, Cooperation, Courtesy, and (sometimes) Compromise by every member of the obstetric team." It is obvious that certain safeguards are required for the maximum protection of the woman and fetus. These include (a) continuing education in obstetric analgesia and anesthesia for clinicians and nurses; (b) better communication and cooperation among obstetricians, anesthesia personnel, nurses, and pediatricians; (c) establishment of department protocol for the administration of regional procedures, with input from all members of the obstetric team; and (d) the procurement of all equipment necessary to provide safe and effective obstetric anesthesia.

References

Abouleish, E.; de la Vega, S.; Blendingen, I., et al. 1975. Long-term follow-up of epidural blood patch. *Anesth. Analg.* 54:459.

Akamatsu, T. K., and Bonica, J. J. June 1974. Spinal and extradural analgesia-anesthesia for parturition. *Clin. Obstet. Gynecol.* 17:2.

Albright, G. A. 1978. *Anesthesia in obstetrics: maternal, fetal, neonatal aspects.* Menlo Park, Calif.: Addison-Wesley Publishing Co..

Baxi, L. V., et al. 1979. Human fetal oxygenation following paracervical block. *Am. J. Obstet. Gynecol.* 135:1109.

Bonica, J. J. 1972. *Principles and practice of obstetric analgesia and anesthesia.* Philadelphia: F. A. Davis Co.

Caritis, S. N., et al. 1980. Fetal acid base state following spinal or epidural anesthesia for cesarean section. *Obstet. Gynecol.* 56:610.

Clark, R. B. 1981. Conduction anesthesia. *Clin. Obstet. Gynecol.* 24:601.

Danforth, D., ed. 1982. *Obstetrics and gynecology.* 4th ed. New York: Harper & Row.

Detmer, M. D., et al. Sept. 1979. Prophylactic single-dose oral antacid therapy in the pre-operative period: a comparison of cimetidine and Maalox. *Anesthesiol.* 51:270.

Dilts, P. V. June 1981. Narcotic analgesia. *Clin. Obstet. Gynecol.* 24:597.

Dundee, J. W., et al. 1974. Plasma-diazepam levels following intramuscular injections by physicians and nurses. *Lancet* 2:1461.

Ettiger, B., and McCant, D. Sept./Oct. 1976. Effects of drugs on the fetal heart rate during labor. *J. Obstet. Gynecol. Nurs.* 5:3.

Giacoia, G. P., and Yaffe, S. 1982. Perinatal pharmacology. In *Gynecology and obstetrics*, vol. 3, ed. J. J. Sciarri. Philadelphia: Harper & Row.

Gibbs, C. P., et al. Nov. 1979. Antacid pulmonary aspiration in the dog. *Anesthesiol.* 51:380.

Greiss, F. C., et al. 1976. Effects of local anesthetic agents on the uterine vasculatures and myometrium. *Am. J. Obstet. Gynecol.* 124:8.

Greenhill, J. P., and Friedman, E. A. 1974. *Biological principles and modern practice of obstetrics.* Philadelphia: W. B. Saunders Co.

Husemeyer, R. P., and Davenport, H. T. 1980. Prophylaxis for Mendelson's syndrome before cesarean section: a comparison of cimetidine and magnesium trisilicate mixture regimes. *Br. J. Obstet. Gynecol.* 87:565.

Lavin, J. P., et al. 1981. The effects of bupivacaine and chloroprocaine as local anesthetics for epidural anesthesia on fetal heart rate monitoring parameters. *Am. J. Obstet. Gynecol.* 41:717.

Moore, D. C. 1967. *Regional block.* 4th ed. Springfield, Ill.: Charles C Thomas.

Moore, M. L. 1972. *The newborn and the nurse.* Philadelphia: W. B. Saunders Co.

Morrison, J. C., et al. 1982. Meperidine metabolism in the parturient. *Obstet. Gynecol.* 59:359.

Myers, R. E. 1975. Maternal psychological stress and fetal asphyxia: a study in the monkey. *Am. J. Obstet. Gynecol.* 122:47.

Pritchard, J. A., and MacDonald, P. C. 1980. *Williams obstetrics.* 16th ed. New York: Appleton-Century-Crofts.

Schifrin, B. S. 1972. Fetal heart rate patterns following epidural anaesthesia and oxytocin infusion during labour. *J. Obstet. Gynecol. Br. Commons.* 79:332.

Shnider, S. M., and Levinson, G. 1979. *Anesthesia for obstetrics.* Baltimore: Williams & Wilkins.

Shnider, S. M., and Moya, F. 1964. Effects of meperidine on the newborn infant. *Am. J. Obstet. Gynecol.* 36:1011.

Whittington, R. M.; Robinson, J. S.; and Thompson, J. M. Aug. 1979. Fatal aspiration (Mendelson's) syndrome despite antacids and cricoid pressure. *Lancet.* 2:228.

Additional Readings

Arnolds, C. W., et al. June 1981. Prepared childbirth. *Clin. Obstet. Gynecol.* 24:575.

Bean, C. A. 1974. *Methods of childbirth: a complete guide to childbirth classes and maternity care.* New York: Dolphin Books.

Block, C., et al. 1975. The effect of support of the husband and obstetrician on pain perception and control in childbirth. *Birth Family J.* 2:43.

Cogan, J. 1980. Effects of childbirth preparation. *Clin. Obstet. Gynecol.* 23:1

Davitz, L. J., and Davitz, J. R. 1980. *Nurses' response to patients' suffering.* New York: Springer Publishing Company.

Dimond, E. G. 1971. Acupuncture anesthesia: Western medicine and Chinese traditional medicine. *J.A.M.A.* 218:1558.

Horsley, J. A., and Crane, J. 1982. *Pain: deliberative nursing intervention.* New York: Grune & Stratton.

MacLaughlin, S. M., and Taubenheim, A. M. Jan./Feb. 1981. Epidural anesthesia for obstetric patients. *J. Obstet. Gynecol. Neonatal Nurs.* 10:9.

Samko, M. R., and Schoenfeld, L. S. 1975. Hypnotic susceptibility and the Lamaze childbirth experience. *Am. J. Obstet. Gynecol.* 121:631.

Veith, I. 1973. Acupuncture in traditional Chinese medicine—an historical review. *Calif. Med.* 118:70.

Wallis, L.; Shnider, S. M.; Palakniuk, R. J., et al. 1974. An evaluation of acupuncture analgesia in obstetrics. *Anesthesiol.* 41:596.

Willmuth, R., et al. 1978. Satisfaction with prepared childbirth and locus of control. *J. Obstet. Gynecol. Neonatal Nurs.* 7:33.

■ 18 ■

COMPLICATIONS OF LABOR AND DELIVERY

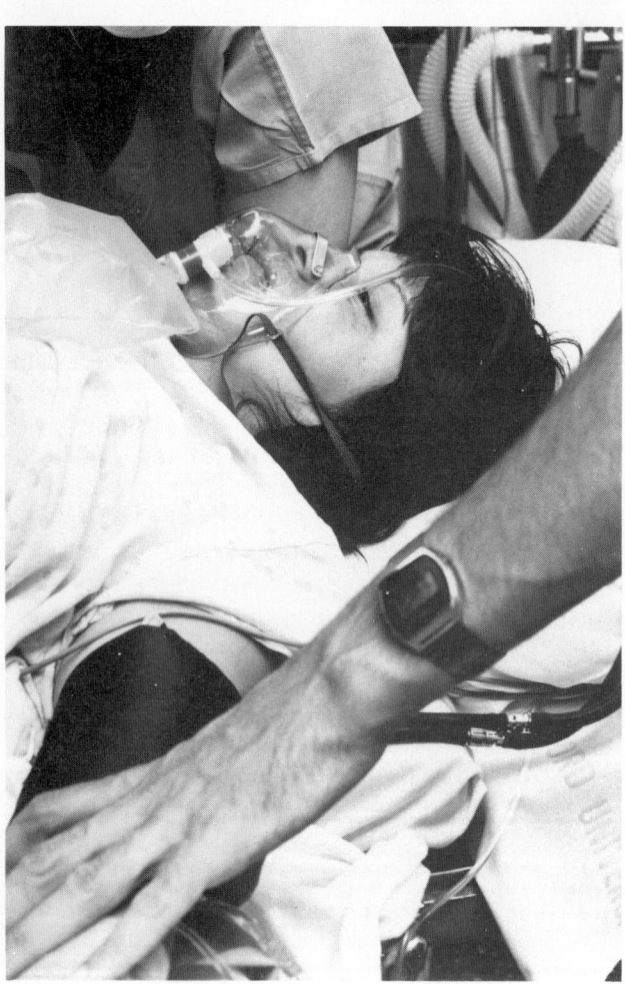

■ CHAPTER CONTENTS

COMPLICATIONS INVOLVING THE PSYCHE
    Interventions

COMPLICATIONS INVOLVING THE POWERS
    General Principles of Nursing Intervention
    Dysfunctional Labor Patterns
    Friedman's Classification of Dysfunctional Labor
    Dystocia Due to Uterine Rings
    Premature Rupture of Membranes
    Preterm Labor
    Ruptured Uterus

COMPLICATIONS INVOLVING THE PASSENGER
    Fetal Problems
    Developmental Abnormalities
    Multiple Pregnancies
    Fetal Distress
    Intrauterine Fetal Death (IUFD)
    Placental Problems
    Problems Associated with Umbilical Cord
    Problems Associated with Amniotic Fluid

COMPLICATIONS INVOLVING THE PASSAGE
    Contractures of the Inlet
    Contractures of the Midpelvis
    Contractures of the Outlet
    Implications of Pelvic Contractures

COMPLICATIONS OF THIRD AND FOURTH STAGES
    Postpartal Hemorrhage
    Inversion of Uterus
    Genital Tract Trauma

COMPLICATED CHILDBIRTH: EFFECTS ON THE FAMILY
    Nursing Management

■ OBJECTIVES

- Describe the psychologic factors that may contribute to complications during labor and delivery.

- Discuss dysfunctional labor patterns.

- Describe various types of fetal malposition and malpresentation and possible associated problems.

- Discuss abruptio placentae and placenta previa and associated bleeding problems.

- Discuss the nursing care that is indicated in the event of fetal distress.

- Discuss intrauterine fetal death including etiology, diagnosis, management, and the nurse's role in assisting the family.

- Discuss variations that may occur in the umbilical cord and insertion into the placenta.

- Discuss the implications of pelvic contractures on labor and delivery.

- Discuss complications of the third and fourth stages.

- Discuss the effects of complications in childbirth on the family.

The successful completion of the 40-week gestational period requires the harmonious functioning of four components: the passenger, passage, powers, and psyche. (These components are described in depth in Chapter 14.) Briefly, the passenger includes all the products of conception: the fetus, placenta, cord, membranes, and amniotic fluid. The passage comprises the vagina, introitus, and bony pelvis, and the powers are the myometrial forces of the contracting uterus. The psyche is the intellectual and emotional processes of the pregnant woman as influenced by heredity and environment and includes her feelings about pregnancy and motherhood. Disruptions in any of the four components may affect the others and cause *dystocia* (abnormal or difficult labor).

COMPLICATIONS INVOLVING THE PSYCHE

Stress, anxiety, and fear have a profound effect on the laboring woman. Erickson (1976) reported that the following complications can result in the woman's fear for herself and for her baby and in fear of dependency:

- Prolonged first stage of labor
- Prolonged second stage of labor
- Rotation of the infant's head
- Indicated low forceps
- Apgar scores of less than 5
- Apgar scores of 5 to 7

It was noted in this study that many of these factors are interrelated.

Stress produces neural and endocrine responses. The liver releases glucose to satisfy the body's increased energy needs. The bronchial tree dilates for increased oxygen intake, and the anterior pituitary is stimulated, which results in an increase in production of glucocorticoids and mineralocorticoids by the adrenal cortex. These hormones promote the retention of sodium and the excretion of potassium and also stimulate the posterior pituitary to release antidiuretic hormone for the conservation of water. The loss of potassium is postulated to assist in the reduction of myometrial activity. The reduction of glucose stores from stress and anxiety can drain the stores needed for the contracting uterus (Assali, 1972).

The sympathetic nervous system stimulates the adrenal medulla, resulting in the secretion of epinephrine, which increases the heart rate, cardiac output, and blood pressure. The sympathetic nervous system also stimulates the adrenals to release norepinephrine, which increases peripheral vasoconstriction and the blood flow to the vital organs. This physiologic reaction can adversely affect the contracting uterus. The uterus responds to α-excitatory and β-inhibitory effects of epinephrine. Through baroreceptor stimulation, epinephrine inhibits myometrial activity (β-receptors). Norepinephrine stimulates the α-excitatory receptors. The uterine musculature is then stimulated leading to uncoordinated or increased uterine activity (Reid et al., 1972; Lederman et al., 1977).

The anxiety, fear, and labor pain experienced by the laboring woman may produce a vicious cycle, resulting in increased fear and anxiety because of continued central pain perception. This leads to enhanced catecholamine release, which in turn increases physical distress and results in myometrial dysfunction. Ineffectual labor and myometrial dysfunction may occur, especially when epinephrine is the predominant substance released (Assali, 1972).

Nursing research supports the effectiveness of education in minimizing the stress accompanying the labor process. Timm (1979) in her experimental study evaluating prenatal education noted that pregnant women who attended prenatal classes required fewer medications during labor than women who were exposed to other structured programs during pregnancy. These findings were consistent regardless of age, race, or parity. Butane et al. (1980) identified pain and loss of control as the most unpleasant parts of labor according to 50 mothers' perceptions of their labor experiences. Generally, research findings indicate that women who participate in prenatal classes benefit by maintaining better control in labor, decreasing their use of ataractics and analgesics, manifesting more positive attitudes, and experiencing feelings of anticipation rather than trepidation (Lederman et al., 1979; Genest, 1981; Sasmor et al., 1981; Zacharias, 1981).

Interventions

Antepartal classes provide education about the developmental and psychologic changes that can be expected during childbirth. Couples learn coping mechanisms in the form of physical and emotional comfort measures, controlled breathing exercises, and relaxation techniques.

Unprepared couples can be taught many of these activities at the time of admission to the delivery room, especially if active labor has not begun. Information about the labor process, medical procedures, the environment, simple breathing exercises, and relaxation techniques can be given, thereby relieving some apprehension and fear. Even a woman in active labor who has had no prior preparation can achieve a good deal of relaxation from physical comfort measures, touch, constant attendance, therapeutic interaction, and possibly pharmacologic support.

If the laboring woman is suffering from complications such as those previously listed, the nurse should try to determine whether fear and stress are causative or contributing factors. Support measures can then be instituted to alleviate the psychologic distress, which will be helpful in relieving the physical distress.

COMPLICATIONS INVOLVING THE POWERS

The myometrial forces of the contracting uterus are dependent upon one or more contracting muscles stimulating the contraction of one or more adjacent muscles. The resulting wave of contractions then spreads for variable distances over the myometrium. The contractility of the uterus is affected by the following factors: (a) the energy source; (b) the ionic exchange of electrolytes; (c) the contractile proteins; and (d) the endocrine sources (Bonica, 1967; Danforth, 1982). See p. 406 for further discussion. These four factors must interact for effective labor to occur. Any disruption in the interaction of these factors may result in ineffective, dysfunctional labor.

Dysfunctional labor that causes a delay in the delivery of the newborn is due to problems with the mechanisms of parturition. Dysfunctional labor can have a profound effect on the woman as well as the fetus. Prolonged labor of over 24 hours' duration is associated with an increase in maternal and infant mortality, usually resulting from infection.

Fetal conditions associated with dysfunctional labor include fetal hypoxia and problems associated with cephalopelvic disproportion (CPD) between the maternal pelvis and fetus (such as bone fractures, internal hemorrhage, and neurologic changes resulting from compression). Friedman et al. (1977) conducted a study on the effects of dysfunctional labor on the fetus and newborn. They demonstrated a significant increase in perinatal mortality. At 8 months of age, a greater incidence of motor developmental abnormalities was seen in infants born to women who experienced dysfunctional labor. This finding was not verified when the children were 1 year of age.

General Principles of Nursing Intervention

The nurse can identify clients who have the potential for labor dysfunction by assessing the adequacy of their contractile system and by determining the source of any imbalance or disruption. Nursing interventions are directed toward restoring or maintaining the proper functioning and interactions of the physiologic components of labor as follows:

1. *Fluid-electrolyte imbalance and inadequate glucose level.* Exhaustion associated with prolonged labor can decrease the energy source, resulting in inadequate glucose replacement or diabetic hypoglycemia. Electrolyte imbalances may be caused by vomiting or profuse perspiration, both of which are common occurrences during labor. Intravenous fluids containing electrolytes and glucose are often recommended, because oral fluids are poorly tolerated in labor. The nurse can screen the maternal urine for ketones. Women with dehydration and ketosis exhibit an increase in pulse rate and temperature, a fruity odor of the breath, and a rise in the hematocrit. The diabetic client may need increased amounts of insulin for the utilization of the glucose.

2. *Imbalance in the contractile proteins.* This situation can occur in a number of medical disorders, such as anemia, PIH, and kidney disease. In preeclampsia and kidney disease, proteins are lost because of damage to the renal tubules from the disease processes. The nurse can help to lessen these potential problems through early prenatal counseling. Interventions may include dietary counseling, encouragement of adequate prenatal care, and early detection of problems. In addition, the nurse can encourage the expectant mother to rest in a lateral position to increase uterine and kidney perfusion.

3. *Endocrine imbalance.* Epinephrine-norepinephrine imbalances may result from anxiety, stress, fear, or pain.

Nursing interventions are aimed at relieving discomfort and at meeting the client's psychologic needs. Teaching appropriate breathing and relaxation techniques, administering analgesic or anesthetic agents, positioning the woman, and communicating clearly and sympathetically are helpful nursing measures that can reduce the woman's fears and discomfort.

In general, nursing actions are aimed toward resolving the physiologic imbalances that can affect the powers. However, the nurse must be able to identify the complications that result from these imbalances. In the following pages, specific conditions involving the powers are examined in terms of their effects on the woman and child, and specific nursing and medical interventions are described.

Dysfunctional Labor Patterns

In hypertonic labor patterns, ineffectual contractions of poor quality occur in the latent phase of labor. In hypotonic labor patterns, early labor is well established with effective contractions, but the active phase of labor becomes prolonged or halts. Either type of dysfunctional labor may result in prolonged labor, which has potentially serious implications for the woman and fetus.

HYPERTONIC LABOR PATTERNS

In hypertonic uterine motility, the resting tone of the myometrium rises more than 15 mm Hg and may rise as much as 50–85 mm Hg. The frequency of contractions is usually increased, whereas the intensity may be decreased (Figure 18–1). The number of fibers in the myometrium that are not contracting and are free to receive new impulses from the pacemakers is diminished, which results in an increased resting tone due to premature interruption of the refractory period (Pritchard and MacDonald, 1980).

Contractions are painful but ineffective in dilating and effacing the cervix, which may lead to a prolonged latent phase. Very anxious nulliparas at term or postterm are most commonly afflicted with hypertonic labor.

Maternal implications. Hypertonic labor patterns are extremely painful because of uterine muscle cell anoxia. There is an increase in uterine muscle tone but little cervical dilatation and effacement. Because hypertonic labor of-

ten occurs in the latent phase of labor, when dilatation may be no more than 2–3 cm, the woman may be accused of overreacting to her labor. She may be aware of the lack of progress and become anxious and discouraged. Women who have prepared for their labor and delivery may feel frustrated as their coping mechanisms are severely tested.

Fetal–neonatal implications. Fetal distress occurs early, because contractions interfere with the uteroplacental exchange. If this distress goes unidentified, the fetus may be lost. In any situation in which pressure on the fetal head is prolonged, cephalhematoma, caput succedaneum, or excessive molding may occur (Figure 18–2, p. 541). (See Chapter 21 for further discussion.)

Interventions. Management of hypertonic labor may include bed rest and sedation to promote relaxation and to reduce pain. Oxytocin is not administered to a woman suffering from hypertonic uterine activity because it is likely to accentuate the abnormal labor pattern (Pritchard and MacDonald, 1980). If the hypertonic pattern continues and develops into prolonged latent phase, the physician may use oxytocin infusion and/or amniotomy as treatment methods. These methods are only instituted after CPD and fetal malpresentation have been ruled out.

Nursing measures include identification and reporting of a dysfunctional labor pattern, provision of information to the laboring family, provision of an environment conducive to relaxation if sedation is ordered, and any supportive technique that the nurse can devise. The nurse may wish to try a change of position for the woman (lateral position may correct the hypertonic pattern), mouth care, effleurage, back rub, and change of linens. In addition, the labor coach may need assistance in helping the woman to cope.

Fluid imbalance must be prevented through adequate hydration. Urine ketones should be monitored hourly. The couple should be kept informed of labor progress.

Nursing measures in the event of fetal–neonatal distress are given in the Nursing Care Plan on p. 538.

HYPOTONIC LABOR PATTERNS

In hypotonic dysfunctional labor, uterine activity in early labor has been within normal limits, but then a hypotonic pattern consisting of infrequent uterine contractions of

(Text continues on p. 541)

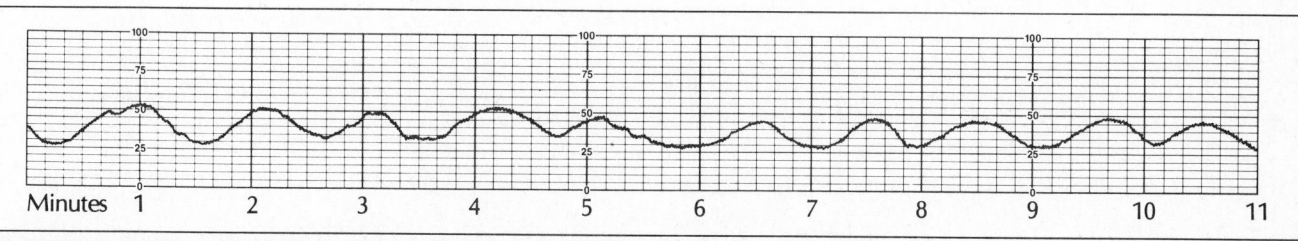

FIGURE 18–1 Hypertonic uterine motility.

NURSING CARE PLAN
Fetal Distress

CLIENT DATA BASE

History

Assess client for presence of predisposing factors:

1. Preexisting maternal diseases
2. Maternal hypotension, bleeding
3. Placental abnormalities

Physical examination

Asphyxia is suggested when one or more of the following are present:

1. FHR decelerations, decreased variability, tachycardia followed by bradycardia
2. Presence of meconium in amniotic fluid
3. Fetal scalp blood pH determination ≤ 7.20

Laboratory evaluation

Maternal hemoglobin and hematocrit

Urinalysis

NURSING PRIORITIES

1. Evaluate maternal and fetal status for variations requiring immediate intervention
2. Identify and correct interferences with transplacental gas exchange
3. Identify and report FHR decelerations and lack of baseline variability
4. In presence of fetal asphyxia, prepare woman for immediate delivery (either vaginally or by cesarean)

CLIENT/FAMILY EDUCATIONAL FOCUS

1. Discuss the problems that are occurring
2. Explain the treatment methods
3. Provide opportunities to discuss questions and individual concerns of the client and her family

Problem	Nursing interventions and actions	Rationale
Fetal asphyxia	Observe and record the signs of fetal asphyxia:	Fetal asphyxia implies hypoxia (reduction in P_{O_2}), hypercapnia (elevation of P_{CO_2}), and acidosis (lowering of blood pH) Anaerobic glycolysis (breakdown of glycogen) takes place in the presence of hypoxia, and the end product of this process is lactic acid, resulting in metabolic acidosis
	1. Presence of meconium in amniotic fluid	Fetal hypoxic episode leads to increased intestinal peristalsis and anal sphincter relaxation resulting in meconium release
	2. Decelerations in FHR	Vagal stimulation elicited through hypoxic brain tissues causes bradycardia
	3. Fetal hyperactivity	Fetus may initially become hyperactive in an attempt to increase circulation
	Initiate following interventions:	
	1. Administer O_2 to the client with tight face mask at 6–7 L/min, per physician order	Administration of O_2 may increase amount of oxygen available for transport to fetus Tight face mask is used because laboring woman tends to breathe through her mouth
	2. Change maternal position (lateral, left side preferred)	Changed maternal position may relieve compression of the maternal vena cava and the cord, thereby facilitating O_2 exchange

NURSING CARE PLAN Cont'd
Fetal Distress

Problem	Nursing interventions and actions	Rationale
	3. Prepare equipment for fetal blood sampling	Evaluate fetal acidotic state. Hypoxia causes increase in lactic acid and results in acidosis, which causes a drop in the pH of the fetal blood (normal pH is 7.25–7.30); other tests that may be done on fetal blood sample are O_2 pressure (normal 18–22 mm Hg), CO_2 pressure (normal 48–50 mm Hg), base deficit (normal 0–10 mg/L)
	4. Prepare patient for immediate delivery (may be vaginal or cesarean delivery)	
	5. Correct maternal hypotension if present: a. Administer IV fluids b. Assess any maternal bleeding; if present, replace circulatory fluids	Lowered maternal blood pressure or circulating blood volume affects O_2 exchange gradient of maternal–placental–fetal unit
	6. Decrease uterine contractions; if oxytocin is infusing, decrease infusion rate or discontinue oxytocin	Increased uterine tone decreases exchange at placental site and decreases fetal recovery time following contractions
Impaired blood flow through umbilical cord		
Cord compression	Observe and note variable decelerations of FHR If bradycardia lasts longer than 30 sec, change maternal position; if necessary, follow interventions listed under fetal asphyxia	Umbilical vessels may be partially or completely occluded by compression of the cord; cord may prolapse through cervix and vagina, or compression may occur when the cord is trapped between a fetal part and the bony pelvis; transient episodes of compression are reflected by variable decelerations (decelerations that are unrelated to uterine contractions)
Prolapsed cord	Evaluate for presence of predisposing factors: 1. Abnormalities in presentation: breech, shoulder, transverse lie 2. Rupture of membranes 3. Multiple gestation Observe for prolapse of the cord externally through vaginal introitus While doing vaginal exam, evaluate for presence of cord, which feels like rope and pulsates	Occult or obvious prolapse of the cord may cause complete depletion of fetal oxygen within 2½ min if compression is not relieved
	Institute emergency measures for prolapse of cord:	Emergency measures for a prolapsed cord are aimed at immediately relieving compression and reestablishing fetal–neonatal blood/oxygen circulation

NURSING CARE PLAN Cont'd
Fetal Distress

Problem	Nursing interventions and actions	Rationale
	1. Manually exert pressure on the presenting part; this must be done continuously, patient may be maintained in supine position, Trendelenburg, knee-chest position, or on her side with a pillow to elevate her hips 2. If occult prolapse is suspected, change maternal position to side-lying position 3. Notify physician immediately	
Impaired transplacental gas exchange	Assess woman for conditions that produce maternal hypoxia: 1. Severe pneumonia, maternal hypotension of any cause, congestive heart failure with diminished blood flow to maternal organs 2. Disturbed O_2 carrying ability of hemoglobin	Antepartal hypoxic insults influence the fetal response to labor and delivery by affecting O_2 exchange at placental site Severe maternal disorders, such as abruptio placentae, seriously jeopardize the fetus, but the effects may be more pronounced in a fetus who has had antepartal stress such as PIH, because O_2 exchange has been compromised and fetal reserve has decreased
	3. Low environmental oxygen tension at high altitudes, preeclampsia-eclampsia, apnea with convulsions, vena caval syndrome	Maternal hypoxia reduces O_2 tension in the blood that perfuses the placenta; fetal O_2 deprivation follows as the maternal–fetal Po_2 gradient is reduced or eliminated
	Assess client for placental problems (placenta previa, abruptio placentae) Maintain maternal blood pressure Maintain adequate maternal oxygenation by positioning (avoid supine position to prevent vena caval syndrome) and administration of O_2 as necessary	These maternal conditions reduce placental gas exchange by reducing surface area available for oxygen diffusion
	Replace circulating blood volume in presence of hemorrhage	Maternal blood loss may cause hypotension and impair perfusion of the intact portion of the placenta

NURSING CARE EVALUATION

Maternal conditions that produced maternal hypoxia are corrected or controlled	A live birth is accomplished with no signs of permanent damage from fetal asphyxia Maternal blood volume is restored

NURSING DIAGNOSES*	SUPPORTING DATA
1. Impaired fetal gas exchange related to prolapsed cord, cord compression, placental problems, or maternal hypoxia	Presence of meconium in amniotic fluid Decelerations in FHR Fetal hyperactivity
2. Fear related to knowledge of fetal distress	Anxiety Expressed concerns

* These are a few examples of nursing diagnoses that may be appropriate for this condition. It is not an inclusive list and must be individualized for each woman and fetus.

mild to moderate intensity and a marked slowing or arrest of cervical dilatation and fetal descent occurs. In this pattern the myometrial resting tone is below 8 mm Hg. Fewer than two to three contractions occur in a 10-minute period (Figure 18–3). Hypotonic labor may occur when uterine fibers are overstretched from twins, large singletons, hydramnios, and grandmultiparity. Hypotonic uterine motility also occurs when sedation such as meperidine (Demerol) is given in the latent phase of labor or in the presence of various degrees of CPD. It may also occur with bladder and bowel distention. Clinically, hypotonic uterine motility may occur in the latent or active phase but is most often seen in the active phase. It is painless and responds to oxytocin if conditions permit its use.

Maternal implications. If labor is prolonged, intrauterine infection can result, along with maternal exhaustion and psychologic stress. Any woman with a dysfunctional labor pattern is a candidate for postpartal hemorrhage, but the woman with hypotonic labor is especially threatened. If the hypotonic pattern persists, the uterus may be less likely to contract efficiently after delivery, which can lead to postpartal hemorrhage.

Fetal–neonatal implications. Fetal distress usually occurs late in hypotonic labor, and most often is due to ascending maternal pathogens (Paul and Petrie, 1973). Fetal tachycardia is observed on the electronic monitor or auscultated by the nurse. The newborn delivered of a mother with prolonged labor because of uterine hypotonia should be observed closely for signs of sepsis in the nursery.

Interventions. After CPD and fetal malpresentation have been ruled out, oxytocins may be given intravenously in a controlled intravenous infusion to improve the quality of uterine contractions. Intravenous fluid is also useful to maintain adequate hydration to prevent maternal exhaustion. Amniotomy may be done, and in some instances sedation may provide rest and promote relaxation for the laboring woman.

Nursing measures include assessment of contractions, and frequent monitoring of maternal vital signs and FHR. Maternal hydration may be assessed by maintaining intake and output records. The client should be encouraged to void every 2 hours, and her bladder should be checked for distention. Because her labor may be prolonged, the woman

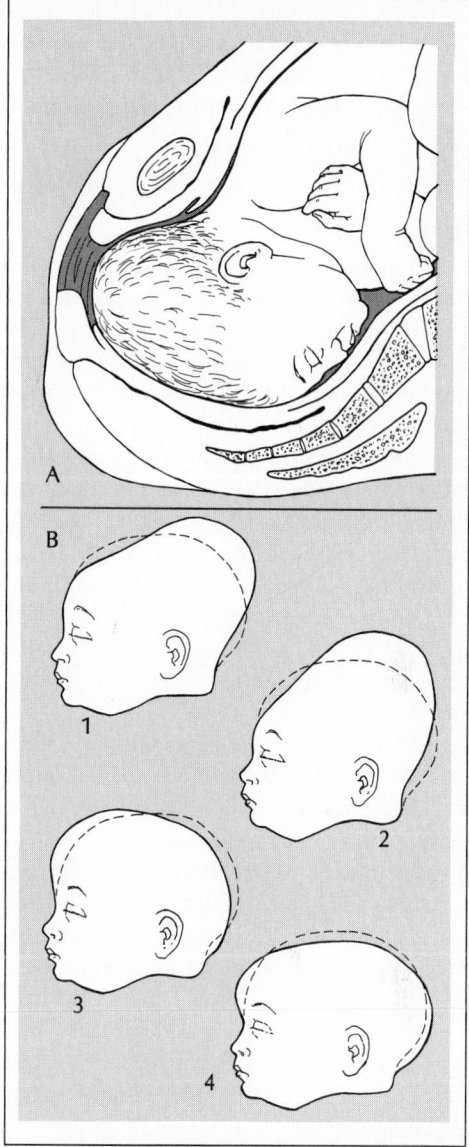

FIGURE 18–2 Effects of labor on fetal head. **A,** Caput succedaneum formation. The presenting portion of the scalp area is encircled by the cervix during labor, causing swelling of the soft tissue. **B,** Molding of fetal head in cephalic presentations: **1,** occiput anterior; **2,** occiput posterior; **3,** brow; **4,** face.

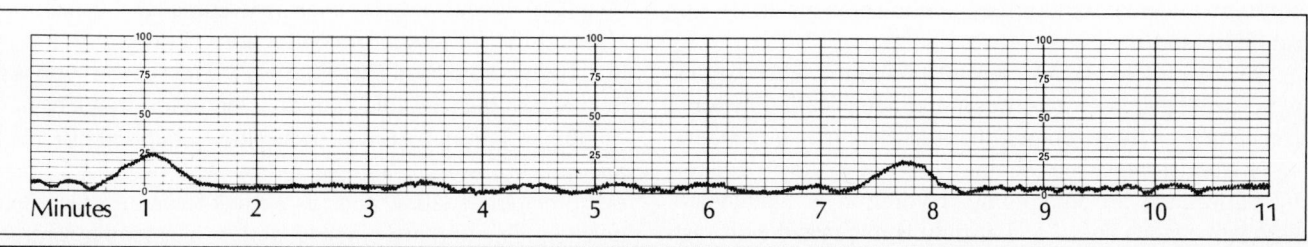

FIGURE 18–3 Hypotonic uterine motility.

must be observed for signs of infection (elevated temperature, chills, changes in characteristics of amniotic fluid). Vaginal examinations should be kept to a minimum. Nursing implications of oxytocin infusion are presented in Drug Guide—Oxytocin, p. 590.

PROLONGED LABOR

Labor lasting more than 24 hours is termed *prolonged labor*. In these cases usually the first stage is extended and the active and/or latent phase is prolonged. The cervix fails to dilate within a reasonable period of time. Early recognition and treatment are imperative to prevent maternal–fetal complications.

According to Oxorn (1980), the incidence of prolonged labor varies from 1%–7% and is most common in the nullipara. CPD, malpresentations, malpositions, labor dysfunction, and cervical dystocia are the principal causes. Other influencing factors are excessive use of analgesics, anesthetics, and sedatives in the latent phase of labor; premature rupture of the membranes in the presence of an uneffaced, closed cervix; and reduced pain tolerance associated with high anxiety.

Maternal implications. Prolonged labor usually has a deleterious effect on the woman. Intense but unproductive pain from labor contractions in the latent phase or a prolonged active phase is likely to result in maternal exhaustion and moderate to severe stress. In addition, she becomes a prime candidate for infection and hemorrhage from uterine atony, uterine rupture, or lacerations of the birth canal. An already stressful situation may be compounded by the necessity to deliver the fetus by forceps or cesarean birth. Support and encouragement become critical to assist the client and her partner in coping with the numerous potential and actual problems associated with prolonged labor.

Fetal–neonatal implications. Fetal distress may occur early or late in the labor depending on which phase of labor is prolonged. Uteroplacental perfusion may be impeded by the length of the labor, resulting in fetal asphyxia. Premature rupture of the membranes (PROM) increases the risk of infection for both fetus and neonate. Prolapse of the cord may occur after rupture of the membranes if the presenting part fails to descend and engage. Continuing pressure on the head or a delivery by forceps may cause soft tissue edema and bruising, and in some instances, cerebral trauma.

Interventions. Management of prolonged labor begins with identification of any causal and complicating factors. Depending on these factors, the treatment may be to stimulate labor through the administration of oxytocin and/or by performing an amniotomy. Hydration is maintained with intravenous fluids, and anxiety is minimized with rest and sedation. In the event of serious maternal–fetal distress, delivery is likely to be by forceps or cesarean birth.

Further discussion of the management of hypocontractility or hypercontractility patterns that may be precursors of prolonged labor is found on p. 537.

Nursing measures include monitoring maternal–fetus status. FHR patterns are assessed for any signs of distress, for example, subtle tachycardia followed by bradycardia, late decelerations, and decreasing variability. Amniotic fluid is observed for meconium staining and signs of infection. The nurse analyzes labor progress by collecting data on the pattern of the labor contractions, the degree of cervical dilatation and effacement, the stations of descent, and the fetal presentation. If the fetus is in a vertex presentation, the nurse may evaluate the amount of pressure on the fetal head by the presence or absence of a caput succedaneum and/or molding. Calculating fluid intake and output and checking urine for presence of ketones provide the nurse with information about the maternal hydration state. If the client is receiving oxytocin therapy, the nurse should implement appropriate nursing measures to ensure the safety of the woman and fetus. (For further information on the administration of oxytocin, refer to Chapter 19 and Drug Guide—Oxytocin, p. 590.)

Assisting the client and her partner to deal with the anxiety and frustration associated with a prolonged labor is another important nursing responsibility. The nurse offers support, encouragement, and information as appropriate. Comfort measures such as a change in position, oral hygiene, skin care, and cool washcloths to the forehead may help the woman relax. Encouraging the involvement of her partner in care of the client may further reduce anxiety.

Following delivery, the mother should be closely monitored for signs and symptoms of hemorrhage, shock, and infection. The fetus should be observed for signs of sepsis, cerebral trauma, and the appearance of cephalhematoma. Nursing actions for fetal distress are given on p. 538.

PRECIPITOUS LABOR

Precipitous labor is labor that lasts for less than 3 hours. The most common cause is the lack of resistance of the maternal tissues to the passage of the fetus (Oxorn, 1980). The other primary cause is intense uterine contractions of which there are two types (Figure 18–4). In the first type, uterine contractility increases in intensity and frequency. Myometrial contractions exert pressures of 50–70 mm Hg, and the frequency of contractions is greater than five in a 10-minute period (Assali, 1972). The second type is a myometrial tachysystole with only increased frequency.

Other factors that may contribute to hyperactive labor and delivery are (a) multiparity, (b) large pelvis, (c) previous precipitous labor, and (d) a small fetus in a favorable position. One or more of these factors, plus strong contractions, result in a rapid transit of the infant through the birth canal (Pritchard and MacDonald, 1980). In addition, hyper-

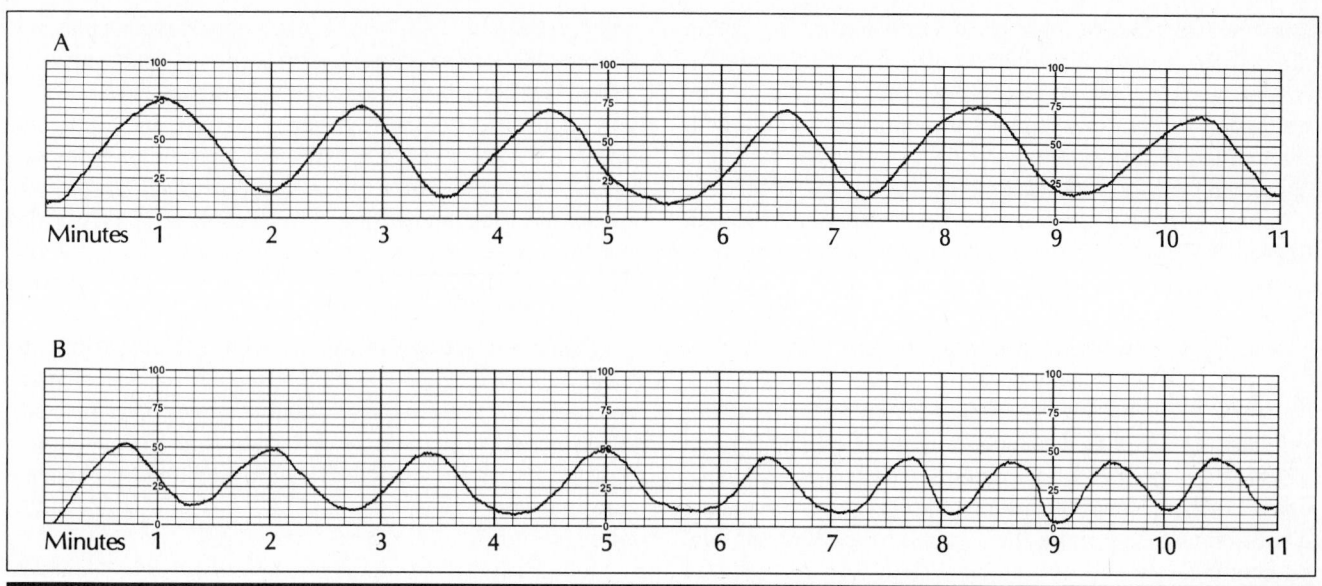

FIGURE 18–4 Patterns associated with precipitous labor. **A,** Hyperactive uterine contractility. **B,** Myometrial tachysystole.

active labor may be caused by oxytocin overdose, which can occur during induction of labor. In this case, dysfunctional labor is caused by medical error.

Precipitous labor and precipitous delivery are not the same. A precipitous delivery is an unexpected, sudden, and often unattended birth. See p. 503 for discussion of emergency delivery.

Maternal implications. If the cervix is effaced and the maternal soft tissues are not resistant to stretching, maternal complications may be few. However, if the cervix is not ripe (soft) and the maternal soft tissues are resistant, lacerations of the cervix, vagina, perineum, and periuretheral area may occur, because the tissues do not stretch adequately. There is also a possibility of uterine rupture. When resistance is present, amniotic fluid embolism may occur (p. 576). The woman is also at risk for postpartal hemorrhage due to expanded uterine fibers. In addition, she may experience a loss of control because of the rapidity of the labor process.

Fetal–neonatal implications. Decreased periods of uterine relaxation result in fetal hypoxia and hypercarbia. Clinically, an acidotic fetus demonstrates decreased beat-to-beat variability and eventually bradycardia. Vagal stimulation is elicited through hypoxic brain tissues, which causes the bradycardia. The same vagal stimulation causes an increase in intestinal motility, resulting in release of meconium in utero.

Any resistance of the maternal soft tissues to the fetal head, as can occur in precipitous labor, may cause cerebral trauma to the infant. If the birth is unattended and unassisted, the newborn infant may suffer from lack of care in the first few minutes of life. Suffocation and aspiration are possible complications (Paul and Petrie, 1973).

Interventions. During the intrapartal nursing assessment, the labor client who is at risk for hyperactive labor can be identified. The presence of any of the following factors may indicate potential problems:

- Previous history of rapid labor
- Accelerated cervical dilatation and fetal descent
- Uterine contractile patterns in which there is no uterine relaxation between contractions
- Pain that seems out of proportion to the contractions

If the client has a history of precipitous labor, she should be closely monitored, and an emergency delivery pack should be close at hand. The physician should be informed of any unusual findings on the Friedman graph. The nurse should be in constant attendance if at all possible. Comfort and rest may be promoted by assisting the woman to a comfortable position, providing a quiet environment, and administering sedatives as needed. Information and support are given before and after the delivery.

To avoid hyperstimulation of the uterus and possible precipitous labor during oxytocin administration, the nurse should be alert to the dangers of oxytocin overdosage (see Drug Guide—Oxytocin, p. 590). If the woman is receiving oxytocin, and an accelerated labor pattern develops, the oxytocin should be discontinued immediately and the client turned on her left side to improve uterine perfusion. Oxygen may be started to increase the available oxygen in the maternal circulating blood; this increases the amount available for exchange at the placental site.

General anesthetics and other drugs such as magnesium sulfate have been used in cases of hyperactive labor. The benefits and effectiveness of these agents are questionable. The ensuing delivery may be slowed by having the woman pant or blow with contractions. This method can be taught to the unprepared woman before active labor begins. It is also helpful for the nurse to breathe with the woman during this time. If delivery is imminent, the nurse can proceed with the emergency delivery procedure (Chapter 16). The nurse should *never* attempt to stop a delivery by holding the woman's legs together. This may cause trauma to the newborn's head.

Friedman's Classification of Dysfunctional Labor

Friedman (1978) has developed a method of defining and classifying abnormal labor patterns. His analysis of labor deals "with the relationship of cervical dilatation against elapsed time in labor and the comparable patterns of fetal descent with elapsed time as practical clinical tools for assessing individual labors" and for "detecting abnormali-

ties" (Friedman, 1978, p. 5). Four major classifications of abnormal labor patterns are (a) disorder of preparatory division of labor; (b) disorders of dilatational division of labor; (c) disorders of pelvic division of labor; and (d) precipitate labor disorders. Preparatory division includes the latent and acceleration phases. Dilatational division includes the maximum slope of dilatation. The pelvic division encompasses the deceleration phase, second stage, and phase of maximum slope of descent of the fetus (see Figure 14–16).

Abnormal labor patterns may occur in each major category. Table 18–1 lists the abnormal patterns and diagnostic criteria for each pattern. The first three categories (seven disorders) are based on the labor being prolonged or arrested in certain aspects. The fourth category concerns labor patterns that are too rapid in regard to cervical dilatation and/or fetal descent.

Friedman (1978) reports that the overall incidence of labor disorders is almost 8% and that nulliparas have labor

Table 18–1 Patterns of Abnormal Labor*

Pattern	Diagnostic criterion
Disorder of preparatory division of labor	
Prolonged latent phase	
Nulliparas	Latent phase duration of 20 hr or more
Multiparas	Latent phase duration of 14 hr or more
Disorders of dilatational division of labor	
Protracted active-phase dilatation	
Nulliparas	Maximum slope of dilatation of 1.2 cm/hr or less
Multiparas	Maximum slope of dilatation of 1.5 cm/hr or less
Protracted descent	
Nulliparas	Maximum slope of descent of 1.0 cm/hr or less
Multiparas	Maximum slope of descent of 2.0 cm/hr or less
Disorders of pelvic division of labor	
Prolonged deceleration phase	
Nulliparas	Deceleration phase duration of 3 hr or more
Multiparas	Deceleration phase duration of 1 hr or more
Secondary arrest of dilatation	Cessation of active-phase progression for 2 hr or more
Arrest of descent	Cessation of descent progression for 1 hr or more
Failure of descent	Lack of expected descent during deceleration phase and second stage
Precipitate labor disorders	
Precipitate dilatation	
Nulliparas	Maximum slope of dilatation of 5 cm/hr or more
Multiparas	Maximum slope of dilatation of 10 cm/hr or more
Precipitate descent	
Nulliparas	Maximum slope of descent of 5 cm/hr or more
Multiparas	Maximum slope of descent of 10 cm/hr or more

* From Friedman, E. A. 1978. *Labor: clinical evaluation and management.* 2nd ed. New York: Appleton-Century-Crofts.

problems six to nine times more often than multiparas. The most common disorders in nulliparas occur in arrest patterns (more than one-third) and prolonged latent phase (about one-third). Multiparas who have labor disorders are more likely to have prolonged latent phase (more than half), arrest disorders, and protraction disorders (the latter are fairly unusual).

When the labor pattern is plotted on a labor graph, objective data are available to identify a client's labor patterns as "normal" or "abnormal." Appropriate management techniques can then be implemented.

Dystocia Due to Uterine Rings

Retraction rings may be divided into two types: physiologic retraction rings and pathologic retraction rings. Pathologic retraction rings are further subdivided into Bandl rings and constriction rings. On the rare occasions when retraction rings are pathologic, immediate action is necessary to prevent serious maternal–fetal complications. Uterine retraction rings are described in the following two sections.

PHYSIOLOGIC RETRACTION RINGS

During the normal labor process, the upper uterine segment becomes thicker with each contraction and shorter as the volume of the contents decreases with the descent of the fetus. In turn, the musculature of the lower uterine segment is required to distend; it becomes thinner and

longer to accommodate the fetus. The boundary between these two segments, a ridge on the inner surface of the uterus, is known as a *physiologic retraction ring.*

PATHOLOGIC RETRACTION RINGS

A *pathologic retraction ring* is an extreme or exaggerated form of a physiologic retraction ring. It may occur as a result of obstructed labor. The most common type of pathologic retraction ring is the Bandl ring, which results from excessive retraction of the upper uterine segment and overdistention of the lower uterine segment (Figure 18–5). A Bandl ring often occurs as a result of obstructed labor; that is, when fetal descent is prevented by malposition of the fetus, CPD, or maternal tumors that block the downward movement of the fetus. The formation of a Bandl ring further obstructs labor as part of the fetus is above the ring and part is below the ring. As the ring rises with further uterine contractions, the lower uterine segment becomes even more distended and may rupture. Cesarean delivery is indicated since anesthetics and sedatives are usually ineffective in relaxing the ring (Oxorn, 1980).

A constriction ring forms when a localized ring of the myometrium becomes tetanic. The fetus or most of the fetus is located above the ring and cannot descend. The client experiences severe pain and her abdomen is extremely tender to palpation. Usually a constriction ring can be relaxed with general anesthesia or sedation, depending upon its intensity. Cesarean birth or forceps delivery is then performed.

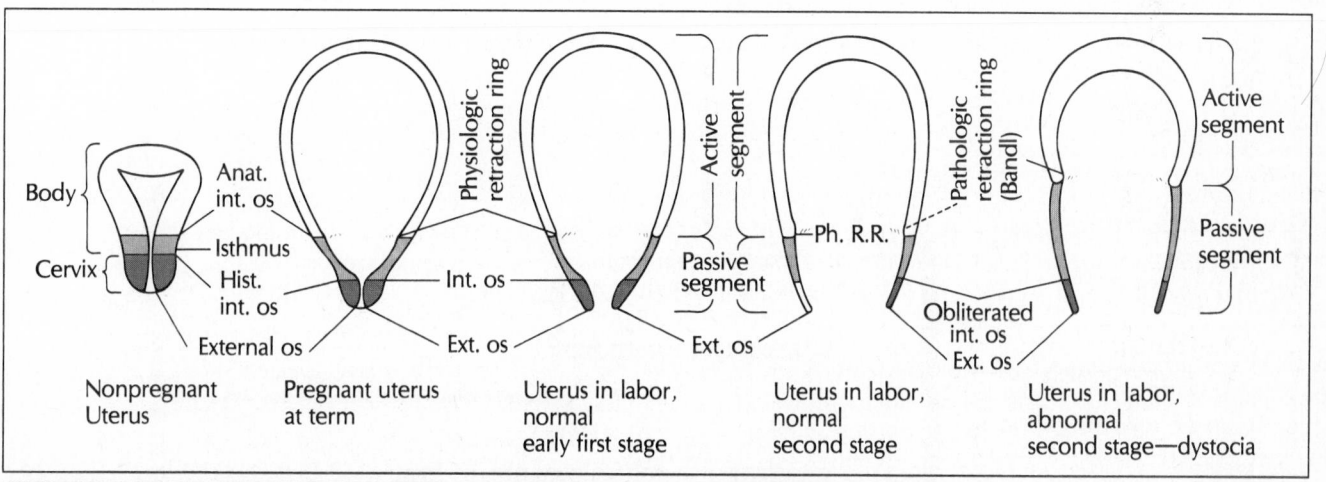

FIGURE 18–5 Sequence of development of the segments and rings in the pregnant uterus. Note comparison between the nonpregnant uterus, uterus at term, and uterus in labor. The passive lower segment of the uterine body is derived from the isthmus; the physiologic retraction ring develops at the junction of the upper and lower uterine segments. The pathologic retraction ring develops from the physiologic ring. Anat. Int. Os = anatomic internal os; Hist. Int. Os = histologic internal os; Ph. R. R. = physiologic retraction ring; E. O. = external os. (From Pritchard, J. A., and MacDonald, P. C. 1980. *Williams obstetrics.* 16th ed. New York: Appleton-Century-Crofts.)

Premature Rupture of Membranes

Premature rupture of the membranes is defined as the spontaneous rupture of the membranes 1 hour or more before the onset of labor (Oxorn, 1980). Although the etiology of PROM is not known, Benson (1977) indicates that irritating maternal secretions or bacteria may assist in the dissolution of the membranes. An incompetent cervix may be the cause of second-trimester PROM.

The incidence of PROM is approximately 10%–12% (Oxorn, 1980). Of these women, 80%–90% proceed into spontaneous labor within 48 hours, and 20% bear preterm neonates. In the presence of intrauterine infection or a large fetus, the latent phase of labor may be shortened. Conversely, the latent phase tends to be lengthened for nulliparas.

Maternal implications. The major maternal risks associated with PROM are ascending intrauterine infection and precipitation of a preterm labor. Either event represents a major stressor for the woman. If infection exists, induction of labor is necessary to evaluate the contents of the uterus. In the absence of infection, prolonged hospitalization may be indicated if the pregnancy is not at term (Figure 18–6).

Fetal–neonatal implications. Perinatal mortality from PROM is 5% overall and 30% for preterm neonates, because of the variety of complicating factors that may negatively affect the fetus or neonate (Oxorn, 1980). Infection is the leading cause of fetal–neonatal death. The most common site of infection is the respiratory tract. The preterm fetus is further jeopardized by the associated increased risks of malpresentation (especially breech) and prolapse of the cord. Chapter 24 contains additional information on the preterm neonate.

Interventions. Gestational age of the fetus and the presence or absence of maternal infections determine the management of PROM. After confirming with Nitrazine paper and a microscopic examination that the membranes have ruptured, the gestational age is calculated. Single or combination methods of calculation may be used, including the Nägele's rule, fundal height, ultrasound to measure the fetal BPD, and amniocentesis to identify lung maturity. If maternal signs and symptoms of infection are evident, antibiotic therapy (usually by intravenous infusion) is initiated immediately, and the fetus is delivered vaginally or by cesarean birth regardless of the gestational age. Upon admission to the nursery, the neonate is assessed for sepsis and

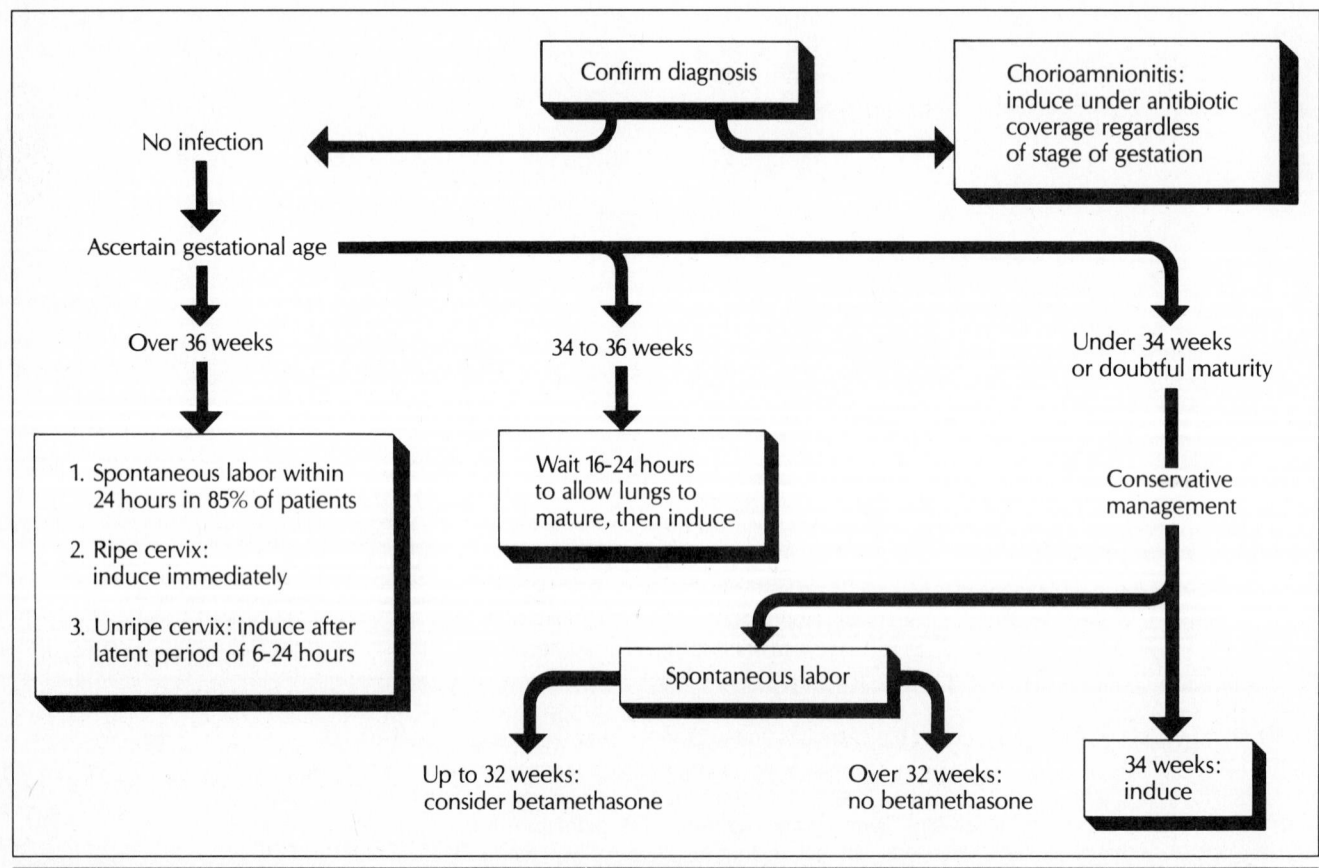

FIGURE 18–6 Premature rupture of membranes. (From Oxorn, H. 1980. *Human labor and birth.* 4th ed. New York: Appleton-Century-Crofts.)

DRUG GUIDE—BETAMETHASONE (CELESTONE SOLUPAN®)

OVERVIEW OF OBSTETRIC/FETAL ACTION

"Betamethasone is a glucocorticoid which acts to accelerate fetal lung maturation and prevent hyaline membrane disease by inhibiting cell mitosis, increasing cell differentiation, promoting selected enzymatic actions, and participating in the storage and secretion of surfactant" (Bishop, 1981). The best results are obtained when the fetus is between 30–32 weeks' gestation. However, some researchers have noted beneficial effects as early as 28 weeks and as late as 34 weeks. To obtain optimal results, delivery should be delayed for at least 24 hours after the end of treatment. If delivery does not occur, the effect of the drug disappears in about week. A female fetus seems more likely than a male to obtain the most prophylactic effect (Giacoia and Yaffe, 1982).

Route, dosage, frequency

Prenatal maternal intramuscular administration of 12 mg of betamethasone is given once a day for 2 days. Repeated treatment will be needed on a weekly basis until 34 weeks of gestation (unless delivery occurs).

Contraindications

Inability to delay birth for 48 hours

Adequate L:S ratio

Presence of a condition which necessitates immediate delivery (e.g., maternal bleeding)

Presence of maternal infection, diabetes mellitus, hypertension

Concomitant use of tocolytic agents may increase risk of maternal pulmonary edema (Bishop, 1981)

Gestational age greater than 34 weeks

Maternal side effects

Bishop (1981) reports that suspected maternal risks include (a) initiation of lactation; (b) increased risk of infection; (c) augmentation of placental insufficiency in hypertensive clients; (d) gastrointestinal bleeding; (e) inability to use estriol levels to assess fetal status; (f) pulmonary edema when used concurrently with tocolytics (such as ritodrine)

May cause NA^+ retention, K^+ loss, weight gain, edema, indigestion

Effects on fetus/neonate

Lowered cortisol levels between 1 and 8 days following delivery (Giacoia and Yaffe, 1982)

Possible suppression of aldosterone levels up to 2 weeks following delivery (Giacoia and Yaffe, 1982)

Hypoglycemia

NURSING CONSIDERATIONS

Assess client for presence of contraindications

Client education regarding possible side effects

Administer deep into gluteal muscle, avoid injection into deltoid (high incidence of local atrophy)

Periodic evaluation of BP, pulse, weight, and edema

Assess lab data for electrolytes

---

placed on antibiotics. Chapter 25 provides further information about the neonate with sepsis.

Management of PROM when maternal infection is not present may include induction of labor if gestation is more than 34 weeks (Oxorn, 1980). The induction may be delayed for 24 hours in the 34-to-36-week gestation. This delay is thought to permit elevation of maternal–fetal blood corticosteroids, thereby contributing to fetal lung maturity. If the gestation is less than 34 weeks, efforts are directed at maintaining the pregnancy. If the gestation is between 28 and 32 weeks and spontaneous labor is not present, the use of betamethasone (Celestone) may be considered. If labor is spontaneous and cervical dilatation is less than 4 cm, betamethasone (Celestone) may be given. The woman is given tocolytics in an attempt to delay the labor and delivery long enough to obtain the desired acceleration of fetal lung maturity. See Drug Guide—Betamethasone, above. Management of the preterm neonate is discussed in Chapter 24.

Nursing actions should focus on the woman, her partner, and the fetus. The time her membranes ruptured and the time of labor onset are recorded. The nurse observes the woman for signs and symptoms of infection by frequently monitoring her vital signs (especially temperature and pulse), describing the character of the amniotic fluid, and reporting elevated white blood counts (WBC) to the clinician. Uterine activity and fetal response to the labor are evaluated. Comfort measures may help promote rest and relaxation. Additionally, the nurse must ensure that hydration is maintained, particularly if the woman's temperature is elevated.

Providing psychologic support for the couple is not only essential but critical. The nurse may reduce anxiety by listening empathetically, relaying accurate information, and providing explanations of procedures. Preparing the couple for a cesarean birth, a preterm neonate, and the possibility of fetal or neonatal demise may be necessary.

Preterm Labor

Labor that occurs after 28 weeks but before 37 weeks of pregnancy is referred to as *preterm labor*. The causes may be fetal, maternal, or placental factors. Premature rupture of the membranes occurs in 20%–30% of the cases of preterm labor. In the other 70%–80% of cases, no known cause has been identified (Danforth, 1982). Maternal factors include cardiovascular or renal disease, diabetes, preeclampsia-eclampsia, abdominal surgery, a blow to the abdomen, uterine anomalies, cervical incompetence, and maternal infection (especially urinary tract infections). Fetal factors include multiple pregnancy, hydramnios, and fetal infection.

Maternal implications. In certain situations, such as preeclampsia-eclampsia, severe renal disease, or cardiovascular disease, continuation of the pregnancy would place the woman in jeopardy, and so no effort is made to prevent labor.

Maternal abdominal surgery is only performed when absolutely necessary and requires the awareness of the possibility that uterine manipulation or displacement may contribute to the early onset of labor.

The major implications for the client relate to psychologic stress factors related to her concern for her unborn child.

Fetal–neonatal implications. Mortality increases for neonates born before 37 weeks of gestation. Although the preterm infant is faced with many maturational deficiencies (fat storage, heat regulation, immaturity of organ systems), the most critical factor is the lack of development of the respiratory system—to the extent that life cannot be supported. If active labor can be delayed in the 34-to-36-week gestation for 16–24 hours, maternal–fetal blood corticosteroids elevate and contribute to fetal lung maturity (Oxorn, 1980). The acceleration of the maturation of the lungs occurs because of the stress-producing situation. In some instances, such as severe maternal diabetes or serious isoimmunization, continuation of the pregnancy may be more life-threatening to the fetus than the hazards of prematurity are. See Chapter 24 for in-depth consideration of the preterm neonate.

Interventions. Immediate diagnosis is necessary so that preterm labor can be stopped before it has advanced to a stage at which intervention will be ineffective. Labor is not interrupted if one or more of the following conditions are present:

- Active labor with cervical dilatation of 4 cm or more
- Presence of severe preeclampsia-eclampsia, which creates risk for the woman if the pregnancy continues
- Fetal complications (isoimmunization, gross anomalies)
- Ruptured membranes, which increase the risk of uterine infection (see exceptions, p. 547)
- Hemorrhage
- Fetal death

The drugs currently in use to arrest preterm labor are ritodrine (Yutopar), isoxsuprine (Vasodilan), and terbuta-

line sulfate (Brethine). Ritodrine, a β-mimetic agent, is currently FDA approved. See Drug Guide—Ritodrine, next page.

After labor ceases, additional ritodrine is given by the intramuscular or oral route in the amount of 10 mg every 2 hours during the first 24 hours. This dosage can be administered safely at a maximum of 120 mg in four to six divided doses over 24 hours. Ritodrine should be given to clients whose pregnancy is between 20 and 36 weeks' gestation and whose regular uterine contractions indicate progression into labor. The effectiveness or safety of the medication for use in labors in which the cervix has dilated more than 4 cm and effacement is more than 80% has not been documented (Foster, 1981).

Additional maternal effects include an elevation of maternal blood glucose and plasma insulin. Hyperglycemia may occur in women with abnormal carbohydrate metabolism, because of their inability to release more insulin, so the drug must be used with caution (Spellacy et al., 1978). Other maternal effects may include a slight lowering of serum iron resulting from the action of β-mimetics to activate hematopoiesis and also a decrease in serum potassium following treatment. This hypokalemia may "result from a displacement of the extracellular potassium into the intracellular space. This may be caused by beta-adrenergic induced release of insulin or/and pituitary vasopressin, which are both known to transport potassium ions into the cells" (Kauppila et al., 1978). See Drug Guide—Ritodrine, next page.

Isoxsuprine (Vasodilan), a β-mimetic compound, is given intravenously with a loading dose of 0.2–1.0 mg/min for about 24 hours. After preterm labor is arrested, isoxsuprine may be given orally. Side effects include hypotension and maternal and fetal tachycardia (Csapo and Herczeg, 1977). Brazy and Pupkin (1979) report fetal effects of isoxsuprine as increased incidence of hypotension, hypoglycemia, hypocalcemia, ileus, and death.

Terbutaline sulfate (Brethine), a selective $β_2$-receptor stimulator that is not FDA approved for use in preterm labor, may be given intravenously to arrest preterm labor. Treatment is initiated at 10 μg/min and may be increased by 5 μg/min to a maximum of 25 μg/min. When contractions cease, the effective infusion rate should be continued for 1 hour and then decreased by 5 μg/min until the lowest effective maintenance dose is reached. The infusion is continued for 8 hours. Subsequent treatment of 0.25 mg is given subcutaneously every 6 hours for 3 days, plus 5 mg orally three times a day. Maternal side effects include tachycardia (with little effect on the blood pressure), nervousness, tremor, and headache. Some researchers have indicated an additional side effect of pulmonary edema (Stubblefield, 1978). A mild fetal tachycardia may result. Neonatal hypoglycemia has also been noted (Epstein et al., 1979).

A new β-mimetic drug, Hexaprenaline (soon to be released for use), has fewer maternal side effects.

DRUG GUIDE—RITODRINE (YUTOPAR)

OVERVIEW OF OBSTETRIC ACTION

Ritodrine is a sympathomimetic β_2-adrenergic agonist. It exerts its effect on β_2-receptors which "are involved in glycogenolysis and relaxation of the smooth muscle of arterioles, the bronchi, and the uterus" (Lipshitz and Schneider, 1980). Ritodrine is FDA-approved for use in treatment of preterm labor.

Route, dosage, frequency

Add 150 mg of ritodrine to 500 mL IV fluid and administer as a piggy-back to a primary IV. Using an infusion pump, start infusion at 20 mL/hr. Rate may be increased by 10 mL/hr every 10 minutes until contractions cease. Maximum dosage is 70 mL/hr. When contractions cease, the infusion rate may be decreased by 10 mL/hr. The infusion may be maintained at a low rate for a period of hours to assure the contractions do not begin again. Before the intravenous infusion is discontinued, IM or PO administration is begun. Although protocols may differ in various clinical facilities, Foster (1981) reported that after labor ceases, ritodrine is administered by IM or PO route in the amount of 10 mg every 2 hours during the first 24 hours. This dosage can be administered safely to a maximum of 120 mg in four to six divided doses over 24 hours. The length of therapy varies.

Maternal contraindications

Preterm labor accompanied by cervical dilatation greater than 4 cm, chorioamniotitis, severe preeclampsia-eclampsia, severe bleeding, fetal death, significant IUGR contraindicate use of ritodrine, as do any of the following:

Hypovolemia, uncontrolled hypertension

Pulmonary hypertension

Cardiac disease, arrhythmias

Diabetes mellitus (use with caution)

Use with caution in clients receiving concurrent therapy with glucocorticoids

Gestation less than 20 weeks

Maternal side effects

Tachycardia, occasionally premature ventricular contractions (PVCs), increased stroke volume, increased systolic pressure, palpitations, tremors, nervousness, nausea and vomiting, headache, erythema

Decreased peripheral vascular resistance, which lowers diastolic pressure → widening of pulse pressure

Hyperglycemia

Metabolic acidosis

Hypokalemia (causes internal redistribution)

Pulmonary edema in clients treated concurrently with glucocorticoids, and who have fluid overload

Increased concentration of lactate and free fatty acids

Increase in plasma volume as indicated by decreases in hemoglobin, hematocrit, and serum albumin levels (Philipsen, 1981)

Effects on fetus/neonate

Fetal tachycardia

Increased serum glucose concentration

Fetal acidosis

Fetal hypoxia

Neonatal hypoglycemia, hypocalcemia

Neonatal paralytic ileus

Neonatal hypotension at birth

May decrease incidence of neonatal respiratory distress syndrome (Lipshitz, 1981)

NURSING CONSIDERATIONS

Assess client history and maternal and fetal status to determine contraindications to treatment with ritodrine

Explain procedure to client

Position woman in left lateral position to decrease incidence of hypotension and increase placental perfusion

Apply fetal monitor for continuous fetal and uterine contraction assessment

Assess contraction status, maternal blood pressure, pulse, and presence of maternal side effects prior to each increase in flow rate

Assess respiratory status for rate, rales, rhonchi

Assess fluid intake and output

Assess lab data on electrolytes

Have β-blocking agent available for emergency use

Notify physician if maternal pulse > 120 beats/min and/or FHR > 180 beats/min

If symptoms of side effects are severe, discontinue ritodrine infusion

Encourage patient to take PO dosages on time to provide adequate drug levels to assure continued uterine relaxation

At delivery assess newborn for side effects

Supportive treatment of the client in preterm labor consists of bed rest, monitoring vital signs (especially blood pressure and respirations), measuring intake and output, and continuous monitoring of FHR and uterine contractions. Placing the woman on her left side facilitates maternal–fetal circulation. Vaginal examinations are kept to a minimum.

An additional treatment may be recommended. Administration of glucocorticoids has an effect on the maturation of preterm lung membranes, and if given more than

24 hours before delivery, the incidence of respiratory distress syndrome may be reduced by 50% (Thornfeldt et al., 1978). Dexamethasone (Decadron) and/or betamethasone (Celestone) may be administered intramuscularly to the client and delivery is delayed at least 24 hours if possible. Oxorn (1980) recommends the use of betamethasone (Celestone) only when the period of gestation is less than 32 weeks. All specific fetal side effects are not known; the long-term effects of steroid treatment on the fetus still require investigation (Thornfeldt et al., 1978).

When labor cannot be arrested, a decision about type of delivery is made. Cesarean delivery is considered if fetal presentation is breech or transverse lie. If vaginal delivery is the method of choice, it is recommended that the amount of analgesics administered be kept to a minimum. Artificial rupture of membranes is usually deferred until the cervix is dilated at least 6 cm to reduce the possibility of cord prolapse. During the delivery, the fetal head is protected by the use of forceps and an episiotomy to reduce pressure. Qualified personnel who can assist the respiratory effort of the preterm infant should be present at delivery.

Emotional support for the woman and her partner during preterm labor and delivery is imperative. Common behavioral responses include feelings of anxiety and guilt about the possibility that the pregnancy will terminate early. With empathetic communication, the nurse can facilitate the expression of these feelings, thereby assisting the couple in the process of identifying and implementing coping mechanisms. The nurse also keeps the couple informed about the labor progress, the treatment regimen, and the status of the fetus so that their full cooperation can be elicited. In the event of imminent vaginal or cesarean delivery, the couple should be offered brief but ongoing explanations to prepare them for the actual birth process and the events following the birth.

Ruptured Uterus

A ruptured uterus is the tearing of previously intact uterine musculature or an old uterine scar after the period of fetal viability, as opposed to uterine perforation. The rupture may be through the three muscular layers of the uterus, which is termed a *complete rupture,* or through the endometrium and myometrium, which is called an *incomplete rupture.* The rupture can be caused by (a) a weakened cesarean scar, usually from a classic incision (Chapter 19); (b) obstetric trauma, such as may occur with any undue manipulation of the fetus at the time of delivery; (c) mismanagement of oxytocin induction or stimulation during labor; (d) obstructed labor; (e) congenital or acquired defects; or (f) external forces, such as trauma.

Signs and symptoms of a complete rupture include excruciating pain and cessation of contractions. Vaginal hemorrhage may appear, but bleeding is usually not profuse.

Massive intraperitoneal hemorrhage and hematomas of the broad ligament are hidden sources of bleeding and may account for the scant vaginal bleeding. Slight vaginal bleeding also may result from the bloodless dehiscence of the avascular cesarean delivery scar. The patient exhibits signs of shock, and the uterus can be palpated as a separate mass. An incomplete rupture may not be evident until after the birth of the baby, when maternal shock is profoundly out of proportion to the blood loss evident at the time of delivery.

The nurse should remember the warning signs of impending uterine rupture. The following may mean that the lower uterine segment is becoming acutely thin:

1. Restlessness and anxiety from severe pain and strong uterine contractions may occur.
2. No indication of labor progress is found by vaginal examination.
3. The lower uterine segment balloons out, simulating the appearance of a full bladder, and a pathologic retraction ring may be evident. This ring occurs when there is an abnormal division between the upper and lower uterine segments and is manifested by an indentation across the lower abdominal wall with acute tenderness above the symphysis.
4. On vaginal examination the cervix is found to stretch tautly around the presenting part, and a caput succedaneum may bulge out of the cervix into the vagina.

Maternal implications. If a ruptured uterus remains untreated, irreversible shock and death may occur. Occasionally, when a rupture goes undetected for a period of time, peritonitis results.

Fetal implications. In acute uterine rupture, the fetus extrudes into the abdominal cavity. The fetus, as it faces asphyxia, may become excessively active and exhibit bradycardia, which progresses to absence of heartbeat as it succumbs. All of this may take place within a few minutes.

Interventions. The nurse may be the one to identify the warning signs of impending rupture or maternal hemorrhage if rupture has occurred. In acute rupture, the nurse quickly mobilizes the staff for an emergency laparotomy. When the physiologic needs of the patient and the fetus are met, the nurse can focus on the emotional needs of the family. The family must have a clear understanding of the procedure and its implications for future childbearing. In addition, if fetal death has occurred, the couple should be given an opportunity to grieve and allowed to see their infant if they desire.

In the presence of a threatened rupture, cesarean delivery should be performed. If the rupture has already occurred, the abdomen is opened and the uterus removed. Some physicians repair a smooth tear if the bleeding is controllable. Greenhill and Friedman (1974) recommend sterilization if a hysterectomy is not done, because there is a danger of repeated rupture with subsequent pregnancies. Low incomplete ruptures or extension of cervical tears may be repaired through the vagina. Women who have ruptured uteruses are advised to have elective cesarean births with future pregnancies.

COMPLICATIONS INVOLVING THE PASSENGER

Complications involving the passenger include any abnormality of the fetus, placenta, umbilical cord, or amniotic fluid.

Fetal Problems

The progress of labor and delivery can be affected by the position and presentation of the fetus, fetal developmental abnormalities, and the presence of more than one fetus in the uterus.

MALPOSITIONS

□ *OCCIPUT-POSTERIOR POSITION* Persistent occiput-posterior position of the fetus is probably one of the most common complications encountered in obstetrics. Although this position may be normal in some races because of a genetically small transverse diameter of the midpelvis, it is considered a malposition because of the maternal and fetal difficulties that may result. It should be remembered that the fetus generally tries to accommodate to the passage it has to travel through. For a fetus in an occiput-posterior position to rotate to an occiput-anterior position, it must rotate 135 degrees (ROP to ROT to ROA to OA), and most fetuses accomplish this. But some do not, and in those cases labor progress may cease or the fetus may be delivered in a posterior position.

Signs and symptoms of a persistent occiput-posterior position are a dysfunctional labor pattern, a prolonged active phase, secondary arrest of dilatation or arrest of descent, and the complaint of intense back pain by the laboring woman. This back pain is caused by the fetal occiput compressing the sacral nerves. Further assessment may reveal a depression in the maternal abdomen above the symphysis. FHTs will be heard far laterally on the abdomen, and on vaginal examination one will find the wide diamond-shaped anterior fontanelle in the anterior portion of the pelvis. This fontanelle may be difficult to feel because of molding of the fetal head.

Interventions. According to Pritchard and MacDonald (1980), vaginal delivery is possible as follows:

1. Await spontaneous delivery.
2. Forceps delivery with the occiput directly posterior.
3. Forceps rotation of the occiput to the anterior position and delivery (Scanzoni's maneuver).

4. Manual rotation to the anterior position followed by forceps delivery.*

If the pelvis is roomy and the perineum is relaxed, as found in grandmultiparity, the fetus may have no particular problem delivering spontaneously in the occiput-posterior position. If, however, the perineum is rigid, the second stage of labor may be prolonged. A prolonged second stage is one that lasts over an hour in multiparas and 2 hours or more in nulliparas. One complication of the fetus delivering in the occiput-posterior position is the possibility of a third- or fourth-degree perineal laceration or extension of a midline episiotomy.

In the event of a prolonged second stage with arrest of descent due to occiput-posterior position, a midforceps or manual rotation may be done if no CPD is present. In cases of CPD, cesarean delivery is the treatment of choice.

In the past, a primary nursing intervention in cases of a persistent occiput-posterior fetal position has been the repositioning of the woman. The woman is turned from side to side; the force of gravity supposedly affects rotation. Whether the side position affects rotation is unknown; there is no documentation supporting this management. Turning the woman on her side does allow the labor coach the opportunity to administer counterpressure over the sacral area, which helps relieve the intense back pain experienced by the laboring woman. The modified knee-chest position tends to decrease some of the pressure on the sacral nerves, thereby decreasing discomfort. In addition, the side position increases uterine perfusion, which results in better labor and fetal oxygenation. The knee-chest position provides a downward slant to the vaginal canal, directing the fetal head down on descent.

□ *TRANSVERSE ARREST* In women with hypoactive labor or a diminished anteroposterior pelvic diameter (as seen with the platypelloid pelvis and diminished transverse diameter in the android pelvis), an incomplete rotation may occur, resulting in a transverse arrest. This may also result in arrest of descent and a prolonged second stage of labor. If the woman's labor is effective, spontaneous rotation may occur if she is allowed to continue to labor. If labor is poor and no CPD is present, the delivery may be accomplished by midforceps, manual rotation, or vacuum extractor. Occasionally the head is visible at the introitus even though the biparietal diameters have not entered the inlet. This situation is seen in cases of severe molding and caput formation. Cesarean delivery is the management of choice if the station is above +2 (Pritchard and MacDonald, 1980).

Maternal implications. Manipulation during delivery can cause maternal soft tissue damage. If the physician elects to deliver the patient when the fetus is in the occiput-posterior position, a mediolateral episiotomy may be per-

---

*From Pritchard, J. A., and MacDonald, P. C. 1980. *Williams obstetrics.* 16th ed. New York: Appleton-Century-Crofts, p. 818.

formed. Any prolonged pressure by the fetal head in one position may cause the woman later gynecologic problems, such as fistulas resulting from tissue anoxia. Postpartal hemorrhage may result from undetected lacerations or atony if the labor was hypoactive.

Fetal–neonatal implications. Unless a protraction or arrest disorder is present or an operative delivery is performed, fetal mortality is not increased with an occiput-posterior or transverse position, because most fetuses do rotate spontaneously. Perinatal and neonatal mortality also are not significantly increased when the second stage is longer than 3 hours in the absence of CPD (Cohen, 1977). Cerebral damage may be caused in cases of undetected CPD. The fetus should be observed in utero closely by the nurse, and at the time of delivery a pediatrician should be present if a midforceps delivery is anticipated.

Interventions. The nurse continues efforts to support and comfort the laboring woman. Continuous monitoring of contractions (character and frequency), amount of maternal discomfort, maternal vital signs, and fetal response to labor are important nursing interventions. The nurse

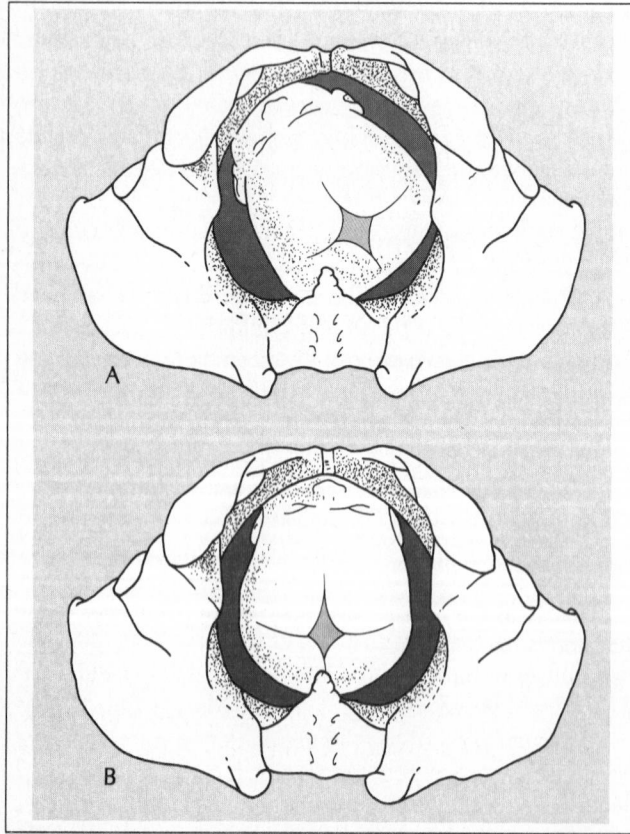

FIGURE 18–7 Left frontum anterior: LFrA. Labor: **A,** Descent, **B,** Internal rotation. (From Oxorn, H. 1980. *Human labor and birth.* 4th ed. New York: Appleton-Century-Crofts.)

notifies the physician in case of distress or dysfunctional labor.

The couple is prepared by the nurse for the extreme molding of the infant's head. The nurse remains alert for signs of postpartal hemorrhage.

MALPRESENTATIONS

Three vertex attitudes of the fetus are classified as abnormal presentations: the sinciput, brow, and face. The fetal body straightens out in these presentations from the classic fetal position to an S-shaped position. The sinciput presentation is probably the least problematic for the woman and fetus. In most cases, as soon as the head reaches the pelvic floor, flexion occurs and a vaginal delivery results.

In addition to the vertex malpresentation, the breech, shoulder (transverse lie), and compound presentations can cause significant difficulty during labor. These and the vertex presentations are discussed here.

□ **BROW PRESENTATION** The brow presentation occurs more often in the multipara than the nullipara and is thought to be due to lax abdominal and pelvic musculature. The largest diameter of the fetal head, the occipitomental, presents in this type of presentation. The nullipara whose fetus has a brow presentation commonly has a small infant. Upon descent into the inlet, the brow presentation frequently converts to an occiput position. Some brow presentations convert to face presentations. Leopold's maneuvers reveal a cephalic prominence on the same side as the fetal back. A brow presentation can be detected on vaginal examination by palpation of the diamond-shaped anterior fontanelle on one side and the orbital ridges and root of the nose on the other side (Figure 18–7).

Maternal implications. Delivery should be accomplished by cesarean birth in the presence of CPD or failure of the brow to convert to an occiput or face presentation. With a vaginal delivery, perineal lacerations are inevitable and may extend into the rectum or vaginal fornices.

Fetal–neonatal implications. Fetal mortality is increased due to injuries received during delivery and/or infection because of prolonged labor. The fetus should be observed closely during labor for signs of hypoxia as evidenced by late decelerations and bradycardia. Trauma during the birth process can include tentorial tears, cerebral and neck compression, and damage to the trachea and larynx.

Interventions. As long as dilatation and descent is occurring, active interference is not necessary. In the presence of labor problems but no CPD, a manual conversion may be attempted. Midforceps delivery in the presence of complete dilatation and fetal station at +2 is advocated by some medical experts. In the presence of failed conversions, CPD, or secondary arrest of labor, cesarean birth is the management of choice.

Nursing management of abnormal cephalic presentations includes close observation of the woman for labor aberrations and of the fetus for signs of distress. The nurse may need to explain the position to the laboring couple or to interpret what the physician has told them. The nurse should stay close at hand to reassure the couple, inform them of any changes, and assist them with labor-coping mechanisms.

At the time of delivery, adequate resuscitation equipment and pediatric assistance should be available.

In face and brow presentations, the appearance of the infant may be affected. The couple may need help in beginning the attachment process because of the infant's facial appearance. After the infant is inspected for gross abnormalities, the pediatrician and nurse can assure the couple that the facial edema and excessive molding are only temporary and will subside in 3 or 4 days.

□ *FACE PRESENTATION* Face presentation of the fetus occurs most frequently in multiparas, in preterm delivery, and in the presence of anencephaly. When performing Leopold's maneuvers, the nurse finds that the back of the fetus is difficult to outline, and a deep furrow can be palpated between the hard occiput and the fetal back (Figure 18–8). FHTs may be heard on the side where the fetal feet are palpated. It may be difficult to determine by vaginal examination whether a breech or face is presenting, especially if facial edema is already present. During the vaginal examination, palpation of the saddle of the nose and the gums should be attempted. When assessing engagement, the nurse must remember that the face has to be deep within the pelvis before the biparietal diameters have entered the inlet.

Maternal implications. The risks of CPD and prolonged labor are increased with face presentation. With any prolonged labor, the chance of infection is increased.

Fetal–neonatal implications. The fetus may develop caput succedaneum of the face during labor, and after delivery the edema gives the newborn a grotesque appearance. As with the brow presentation, the neck and internal structures may swell due to the trauma received during descent. Petechiae and ecchymoses are often seen in the superficial layers of the facial skin because of the birth trauma.

Interventions. If no CPD is present, if the chin (mentum) is anterior, and if the labor pattern is effective, the woman may deliver vaginally (Figure 18–9). Mentum posteriors can become wedged on the anterior surface of the sacrum (Figure 18–10). In this case as well as in the presence of cephalopelvic disproportion, cesarean birth is the management of choice.

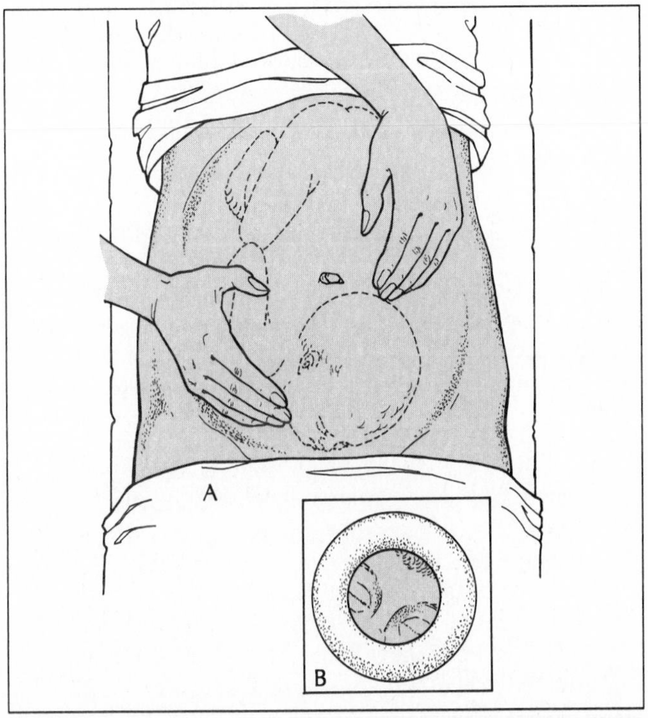

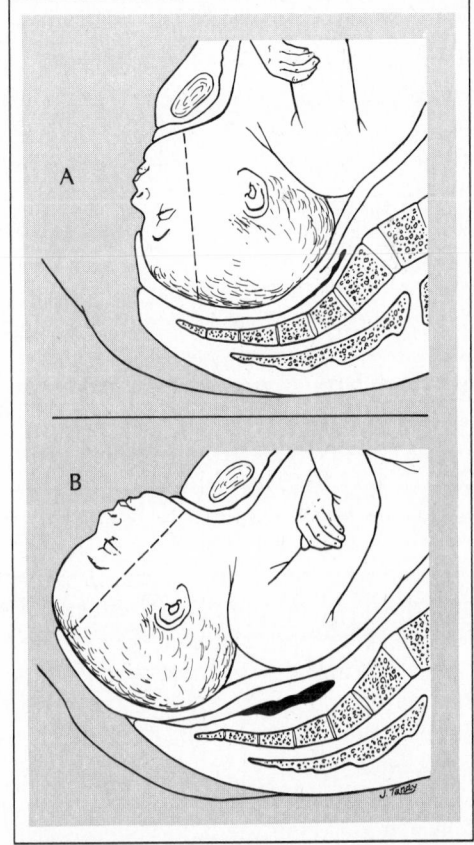

FIGURE 18–8 Face presentation. **A,** Palpation of the maternal abdomen with the fetus in RMP. **B,** Vaginal examination may permit palpation of facial features of the fetus.

FIGURE 18–9 Mechanism of birth in mentoanterior position. **A,** The submentobregmatic diameter at the outlet. **B,** The fetal head is born by movement of flexion.

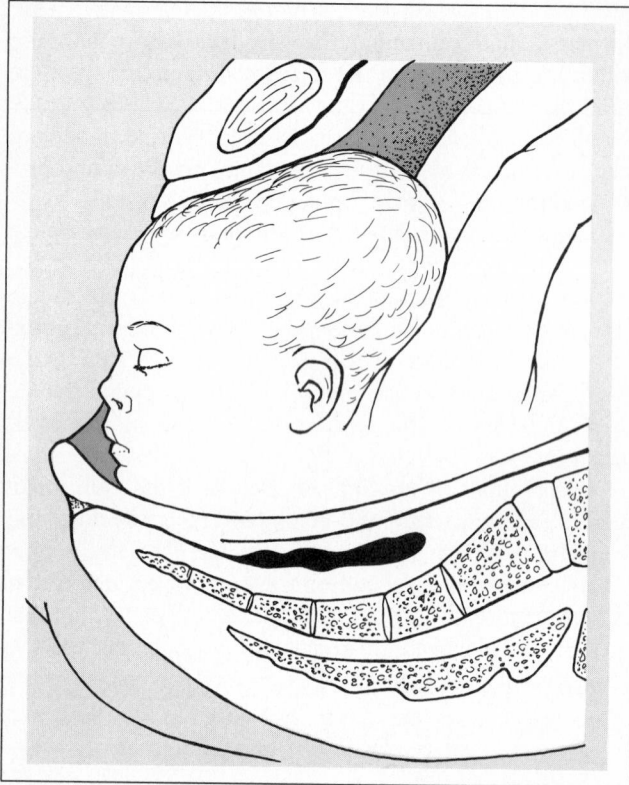

FIGURE 18–10 Mechanism of birth in mentoposterior position. Fetal head is unable to extend farther. The face becomes impacted.

Nursing interventions are the same as for brow presentation.

□ *BREECH PRESENTATIONS* The exact cause of breech presentation (Figure 18–11) is unknown. This malpresentation occurs in 3%–4% of all pregnancies and is associated with preterm birth, placenta previa, hydramnios, multiple pregnancies, grandmultiparity, fetal hydrocephaly, and fetal anencephaly. It has been postulated that in cases of preterm delivery, the fetus is small in relation to the overall size of the uterine cavity and has much room to move around. Consequently it may more easily assume any presentation. An incomplete breech, or footling, presentation prolongs labor because an effective dilating wedge is lacking. The most critical problem with a breech presentation is that the largest part of the infant (the head) delivers last. In the presence of fetomaternal disproportion, the pelvis is not really tried until it is virtually too late to salvage the fetus.

Frequently it is the nurse who first recognizes a breech presentation. On palpation the hard vertex is felt in the fundus and ballottement of the head can be done independently of the fetal body. The wider sacrum is palpated in the lower part of the abdomen. If the sacrum has not descended, on ballottement the entire fetal body will move. Furthermore, FHTs are usually auscultated above the um-

bilicus. Passage of meconium from compression of the infant's intestinal tract on descent is common.

There is a danger of prolapsed umbilical cord, especially in incomplete breeches, because space is available between the cervix and presenting part through which the cord can slip. If the infant is small and the membranes rupture, the danger is even greater. This is one reason why any woman admitted to the labor and delivery suite with a history of ruptured membranes should not be ambulated until a full assessment, including vaginal examination, is performed.

Maternal implications. Frequently a breech presentation necessitates cesarean delivery. The woman should have a clear understanding of the rationale for electing to deliver her child by this method.

In the event of vaginal delivery there is less maternal risk. The woman should, however, be carefully examined for lacerations or tears.

Fetal–neonatal implications. The incidence of perinatal mortality increases in breech presentations, especially in the multiparous woman and when oxytocin is used (Kochenour, 1977). (Nulliparous women may be at less risk because they may receive a more thorough evaluation than multiparous women.) Hyperextension of the fetal head can occur at the time of delivery if delivery is vaginal and can result in cervical cord injuries. Other fetal and neonatal dangers include the following (Korones, 1981):

1. Increased possibility of intracranial hemorrhage from a traumatic delivery of the head.

2. Spinal cord injuries caused by stretching and manipulation of the infant's body.

3. Hemorrhage into the fetal abdominal viscera, particularly the kidneys, liver, and spleen.

4. Brachial plexus palsy.

5. Fracture of the upper extremities.

Interventions. Cesarean delivery is being performed more in cases of breech presentation because of the increasing documentation of perinatal mortality and morbidity. Kochenour (1977) lists the following criteria for vaginal delivery:

> (1) The fetus should be presenting as a frank breech with an estimated fetal weight of less than 3500 grams, (2) the patient should have an adequate pelvis shown by x-ray pelvimetry, (3) a flat plate of the abdomen must exclude a hyperextended fetal head, (4) labor must progress normally and oxytocin should not be used for an arrested labor, (5) the second stage of labor should be less than one hour in duration, and (6) the patient should not be an elderly primigravida.*

*From Kochenour, N. 1977. The management of breech presentations. *PCC News.* 3(5):32.

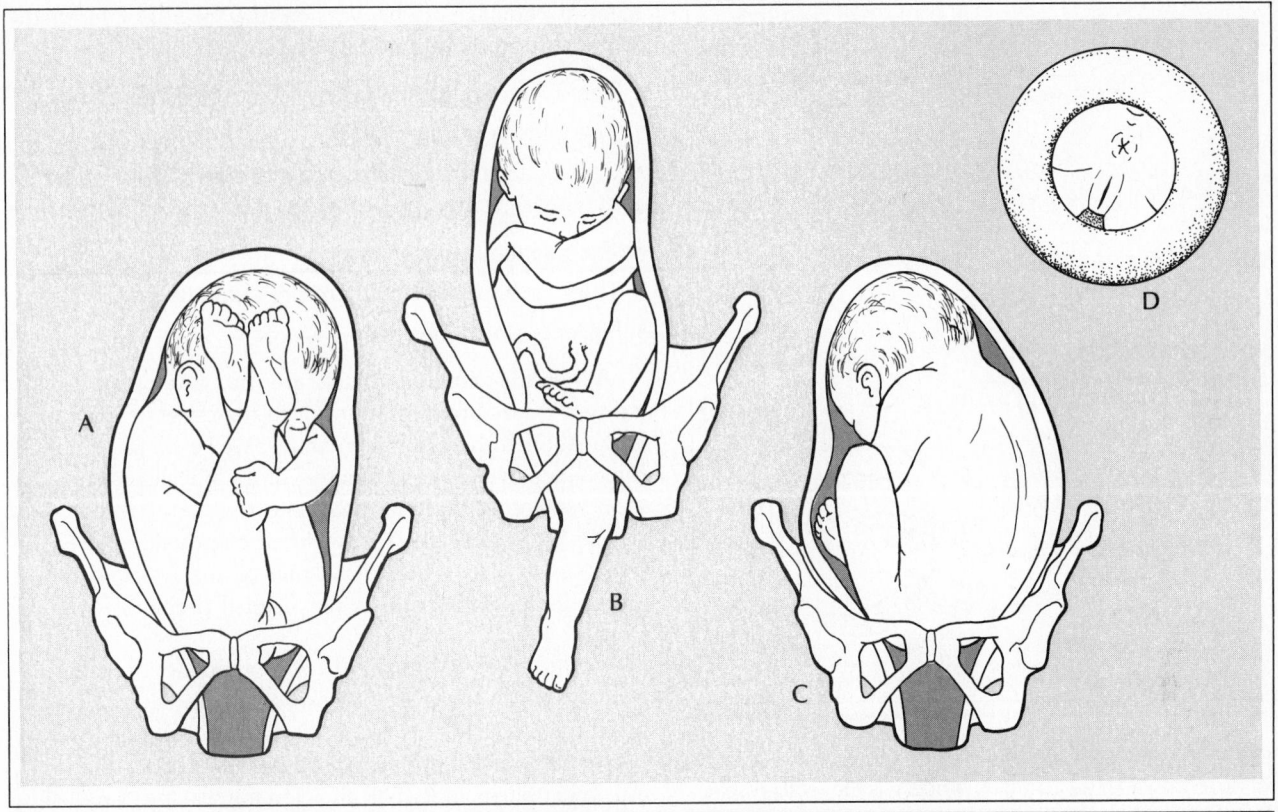

FIGURE 18–11 Breech presentation. **A,** Frank breech. **B,** Incomplete (footling) breech. **C,** Complete breech in LSA position. **D,** On vaginal examination, the nurse may feel the anal sphincter, which grips the nurse's finger. The tissue of the fetal buttocks feels soft.

Factors that contraindicate vaginal delivery are presence of prenatal complications, previous perinatal deaths, or birth trauma. There are two methods of delivering a breech fetus vaginally: partial breech extraction (assisted breech) and total breech extraction.

In the presence of strong uterine contractions, many breech deliveries may be accomplished spontaneously. As the force of the contractions and the woman's bearing-down efforts push the breech against the vulva, a generous episiotomy is made to give adequate room. As the infant is delivered, the physician supports the body and applies gentle downward traction. Flexion of the head is to be maintained. The shoulders emerge with continued pushing effort. The body is held slightly upward, and the head is delivered with the face directed back at the perineum.

In a number of breech presentations, more assistance is required to facilitate delivery. If there is any delay of proper flexion or descent of the head, it may be necessary to use forceps on the aftercoming head. The forceps commonly used are Piper forceps. An assistant (physician or nurse) holds the infant's body, which has been wrapped in a towel to provide handling ease. The physician's hands are then free to apply the Piper forceps and extract the head.

The nurse should include Piper forceps as a part of the delivery table setup. During the delivery process, the nurse may have to assist in the support of the infant's body if the physician elects to use forceps. The circulating nurse should monitor the FHR closely during the delivery.

Pediatric assistance should be available at the time of delivery. If meconium has been passed in utero, the pediatrician should examine the neonate for meconium aspiration.

□ *TRANSVERSE LIE (SHOULDER PRESENTATION)* A transverse lie occurs in approximately one in every 300 to 400 deliveries (Greenhill and Friedman, 1974). The infant's long axis lies across the woman's abdomen, and on inspection the contour of the maternal abdomen appears widest from side to side (Figure 18–12).

On palpation no fetal part is felt in the fundal portion of the uterus or above the symphysis. The head may be palpated on one side and the breech on the other. FHTs are usually auscultated just below the midline of the umbilicus. On vaginal examination, if a presenting part is palpated, it is the ridged thorax or possibly an arm that is compressed against the chest.

Maternal conditions associated with a transverse lie are grandmultiparity with lax uterine musculature; obstruc-

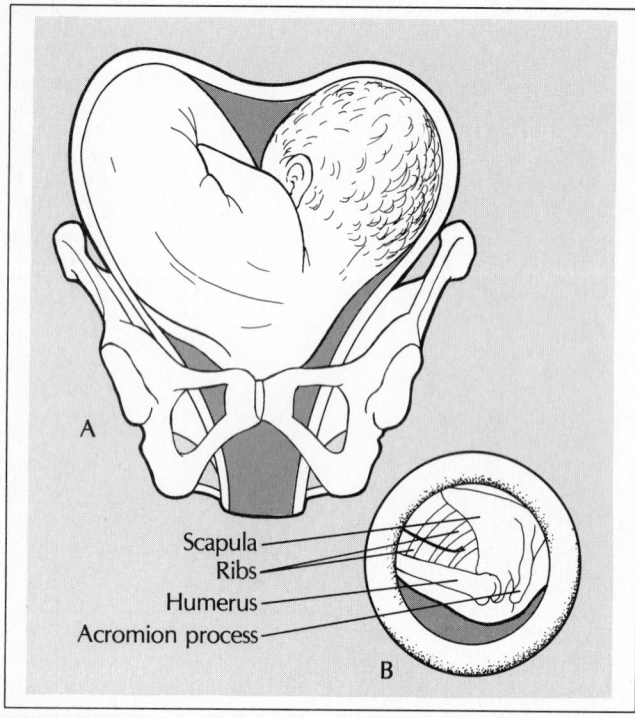

FIGURE 18–12 A, Shoulder presentation. **B,** On vaginal examination the nurse may feel the acromion process as the fetal presenting part.

tions such as bony dystocia, placenta previa, neoplasms, and fetal anomalies; hydramnios; and preterm labor. It is not uncommon in multiple gestations for one or more of the fetuses to be in a transverse lie. The nurse must be aware that careless vaginal examinations in the presence of unengagement may convert a dipping fetal head or breech presentation into a transverse lie. Also, premature amniotomy may assist a fetus that has not firmly entered the inlet into assuming this presentation.

Maternal implications. Labor can be dysfunctional in the presence of a transverse lie. Uterine rupture can occur. As in any case of prolonged labor, the woman is more prone to infection.

Fetal–neonatal implications. One danger of transverse lie is a prolapsed umbilical cord because there is nothing in the pelvic inlet to serve as a blocking agent. Prolapse of a fetal arm may also occur. If the woman is allowed to labor in the presence of a transverse lie, the fetus may succumb from asphyxia and trauma.

Interventions. The nurse can identify a transverse lie by inspection and palpation of the abdomen, by auscultation of FHTs in the midline of the abdomen (not conclusive), and by vaginal examination. The primary nursing actions are to assist in interpretation of the fetal presentation, to provide information and support to the couple, and to quickly prepare the woman for an operative delivery.

With a live fetus at term, cesarean delivery is the treat-

ment of choice. External version may be attempted if the following criteria are met:

- There is no indication for rapid termination of labor
- The fetus is highly movable
- Contractions are not strong and frequent
- There is no cephalopelvic disproportion
- The membranes are intact
- There is an adequate amount of amniotic fluid
- Placenta previa has been ruled out

When the required criteria are met, attempts at external version are appropriate prior to the onset of labor or in early labor. If the client is in active, well-established labor, the chance of success is minimal. If the physician succeeds in manipulating the fetal head into the maternal pelvis, it should be held in place for several contractions in an attempt to fix it in place. To eliminate the possible use of undue force, anesthesia is not used (Pritchard and MacDonald, 1980).

□ *COMPOUND PRESENTATION* A compound presentation is one in which there are two presenting parts. It can occur when the pelvic inlet is not totally occluded by the primary presenting part. If the prolapsed part is a hand, the delivery generally is not difficult. Sometimes the hand slips back and occasionally it is delivered alongside the head (Oxorn, 1980).

A compound presentation becomes a medical emergency when one of the presenting parts is the umbilical cord (see the discussion on prolapse of the umbilical cord on p. 574).

Developmental Abnormalities

MACROSOMIA

Fetal macrosomia occurs when a neonate weighs more than 4000 g at birth. This condition is more common among offspring of large parents and diabetic women and in cases of grandmultiparity and postmaturity.

Maternal implications. The pelvis that is adequate for an average-sized fetus may be disproportionately small for an oversized fetus. Distention of the uterus causes overstretching of the myometrial fibers, which may lead to dysfunctional labor and an increased incidence of postpartal hemorrhage. If the oversized fetus acts as an obstruction, the chance of uterine rupture during labor increases.

Fetal–neonatal implications. Fetal prognosis is guarded. If a macrosomic fetus is unsuspected and labor is allowed to continue in the presence of disproportion, the fetus can receive cerebral trauma from intermittent forceful contact with the maternal bony pelvis. During difficult operative procedures performed at the time of vaginal delivery, the fetus may become asphyxiated or receive neurologic damage from pressure exerted on its head.

Shoulder dystocia can occur if the shoulders become wedged between the sacrum and the pubic bone. During manual attempts to facilitate delivery, there is a danger of overstretching the fetal neck. If the cord has also been brought down into the bony pelvis and delivery is delayed, asphyxia from cord compression can occur.

Interventions. The maternal pelvis should be evaluated carefully if a large fetus is suspected. An estimation of fetal size can be made by palpating the crown-rump length of the fetus in utero, but the greatest errors in estimation occur on both ends of the spectrum—the macrosomic fetus and the very small fetus. Fundal height can give some clue. Ultrasound or x-ray pelvimetry may give further information about fetal size. Whenever the uterus appears excessively large, hydramnios, an oversized fetus, or multiple pregnancies must be considered as possible causes.

If shoulder dystocia occurs and delivery cannot be completed by various manual maneuvers, the physician may find it necessary to fracture the clavicles to save the neonate's life.

The nurse should monitor these labors closely for dysfunction, utilizing the Friedman graph. The fetal monitor is applied for continuous fetal evaluation. Early decelerations could mean disproportion at the bony inlet. Any sign of labor dysfunction or fetal distress should be reported to the physician.

The nurse inspects these neonates after delivery for skull fractures, cephalhematoma, and Erb's palsy and informs the nursery of any problems. If the nursery staff is aware of a difficult delivery, the newborn will be observed more closely for cerebral and neurologic damage.

Postpartally, the nurse checks the uterus for potential atony and the maternal vital signs for deviations suggestive of shock.

HYDROCEPHALY

In hydrocephaly 500–1500 mL of cerebrospinal fluid accumulates in the ventricles of the fetal brain. When this occurs before delivery, severe CPD results, because of the enlarged cranium of the fetus.

Abdominal palpation reveals the presence of a hard mass just above the symphysis; this is the unengaged head. If the presentation is breech, it is difficult on external palpation to discern between the breech and an enlarged head. A fetogram or sonogram is indicated in the presence of breech presentations to evaluate the cranium. Vaginal examination with a vertex presentation reveals wide suture lines and a globular cranium.

Maternal implications. Obstruction of labor can occur, and if the uterus is allowed to continue contracting without medical interference, uterine rupture can result.

Fetal–neonatal implications. Outlook for the fetus is poor. Frequently, other congenital malformations accompany this condition, such as spina bifida and myelomeningocele. The neonate is severely brain damaged and often succumbs during delivery or afterward in the nursery because of malformations and the presence of infection.

Interventions. Vaginal delivery cannot be accomplished without intervention. The treatment of choice is withdrawal of the cerebrospinal fluid, thus collapsing the fetal skull. If the fetus is in a cephalic presentation, this is accomplished by introduction of a 17-gauge needle into the ventricle after the cervix is 3 cm dilated. With a breech presentation, this may be accomplished with ultrasonic guidance to aid transabdominal craniocentesis. If cesarean delivery is performed, a transabdominal method of drainage is advocated to prevent excessive extension of the incision (Pritchard and MacDonald, 1980).

The nurse assists the physician with the procedures involved in the accomplishment of this delivery. The nurse also helps the couple to cope with this crisis and to deal with their grief.

OTHER FETAL MALFORMATIONS

Enlargement of various fetal parts could result in dystocia. These fetal problems include enlargement of fetal organs, such as a liver or distended bladder, and incomplete twinning, in which a partially developed twin is attached to the fetus. It is not uncommon for malpresentations and malpositions to accompany this type of gestation. Hydramnios (see p. 576) often accompanies the pregnancy that has a neurologically damaged fetus with defective swallowing.

Interventions. Cesarean birth is recommended to avoid a difficult vaginal delivery if a developmental problem is diagnosed early. Connected fetuses are often joined by movable tissue that can be manipulated without dismembering a fetus.

Nursing tasks fall in the realm of physical and emotional support of the laboring couple. Physical support includes physiologic maintenance of the woman's body functions during labor and assistance with comfort measures. Emotional support includes helping the couple with the grief process if there is a fetal loss. If the couple wishes to see the infant, the body should be made as attractive as possible. Cleaning the body of offensive odors and substances that cause disfigurement can be helpful. The infant can be wrapped in a blanket and presented to the couple with gentle, loving care. Empathetic nursing measures can make their acceptance and grief process easier.

Multiple Pregnancies

When two fetuses develop from the fertilization of one ovum, the twins are categorized as *monozygotic*. The twins are further classified as diamniotic, dichorionic, or monochorionic, depending on the period in which the division of the ovum occurs (Figure 8–22). Monozygotic twins are identical and thus the same sex.

Dizygotic twins result from the fertilization of two separate ova. They are diamniotic, dichorionic, and fraternal.

They may or may not be the same sex and are not identical. If the twins are of the same sex, the placenta is sent to the pathology laboratory for examination to determine whether they are monozygotic or dizygotic twins.

According to Pritchard and MacDonald (1980) the incidence of monozygotic twins is independent of race, heredity, age, parity, and fertility therapy. However, the incidence of dizygotic twinning is highly influenced by these factors.

IDENTIFICATION OF MULTIPLE GESTATIONS

When obtaining a maternal history, it is important to identify a family history of twinning. Equally important is a history of medication taken to enhance fertility. These facts should be noted on the antepartal record.

At each antepartal clinic visit, the nurse should measure the fundal height. With any growth, fetal movement, or heart tone auscultation out of proportion to gestational age by dates, twins should be suspected. During palpation, many small parts on all sides of the abdomen may be felt. If twins are suspected, the nurse should attempt to auscultate two separate heartbeats in different quadrants of the maternal abdomen. Use of the Doppler device may be helpful. Conclusive evidence of twins is found on sonography or x-ray examination.

Maternal implications. The increased incidence of PIH associated with multiple gestations is thought to result from an oversized uterus and increased amounts of placental hormones. Abortions are more common in multiple gestations, possibly because of genetic defects or poor placentation or implantation. Maternal anemia is more common, because the maternal system is nurturing more than one fetus. Third trimester bleeding from placenta previa occurs more frequently, as does hydramnios. Hydramnios may be due to increased renal perfusion from cross-vessel anastomosis of monozygotic twins. Placenta previa may be due to a decreased area of choice for implantation.

Complications during labor include (a) uterine dysfunction due to an overstretched myometrium, (b) abnormal fetal presentations, and (c) preterm labor. With rupture of membranes and hydramnios, abruptio placentae can occur. Danger of placental abruption after the delivery of the first twin also exists because of a decrease in the surface area of the uterus to which the placenta is still attached.

The woman pregnant with twins may experience more physical discomfort during her pregnancy, such as shortness of breath, dyspnea on exertion, backaches, and pedal edema, because of the oversized uterus.

Occasionally multiple pregnancies are not diagnosed until the time of delivery; this occurs most often in cases of preterm labor. If the family has physically, psychologically, and financially prepared for one baby, problems can arise when they are suddenly confronted with more than one child. In addition, infants of multiple pregnancies frequently require intensive care, and this may cause financial and emotional stress.

Fetal–neonatal implications. Fetal problems in the presence of multiple gestations are numerous. Labor is usually preterm. In addition, in the presence of monochorionic placentas with artery-to-artery anastomosis, fetoplacental circulation is compromised. One twin is overperfused and is born with polycythemia and hypervolemia and may have hypertension with an enlarged heart. This twin's amniotic sac exhibits hydramnios because of the increased renal perfusion and excessive voiding. The other twin has hypovolemia and exhibits IUGR. In the newborn period the neonate with increased perfusion has an increased chance of hyperbilirubinemia as the system tries to rid itself of the extra red blood cells. The other twin is anemic, with all the problems that SGA infants exhibit.

The cytoplasmic mass of all organs is diminished in multiple gestations, and the growth rate is decreased. Therefore, twins may suffer from intellectual and motor impairment.

The high rate of prematurity is associated with an increased incidence of respiratory distress syndrome (RDS). The incidence of fetal anomalies is also greater with twin gestations (Pritchard and MacDonald, 1980).

Interventions. Antepartally, the woman may need counseling about diet and daily activities. The nurse can help her plan meals to meet her increased needs. An increase of 300 calories or more over the recommended daily dietary allowance established by the Food and Nutrition Board of the National Research Council is advised for uncomplicated pregnancy (see Table 11–5). The daily intake of protein should be increased as much as 1.5 g/kg of body weight. Daily iron supplements of 60–80 mg and an additional 1 mg of folic acid are recommended.

Maternal hypertension is treated with bed rest in the lateral position to increase uterine and kidney perfusion. The nurse can help the woman schedule frequent periods of rest during the day. Family members or friends may be willing to care for the woman's other children periodically to allow her time to get rest. Back discomfort can be alleviated by pelvic rocking, good posture, and good body mechanics.

Occasionally in multiple pregnancies women exhibit nausea and vomiting past the first trimester. A diet consisting of dry, nongreasy foods may be helpful. Antiemetics may be necessary to provide relief. The woman is more prone to have a feeling of fullness after eating, and this may be alleviated by eating small but frequent meals.

In the event of fluid and electrolyte imbalance due to hypertension or hyperemesis, hospitalization may be necessary so that appropriate therapy may be instituted.

During labor, it is important to monitor both fetuses. An external electronic monitor can be applied to both fetuses, or if conditions permit, the internal monitor can be applied to the presenting twin and the external monitor can be applied to the other. The heart rate may be auscultated on different quadrants of the maternal abdomen, but continuous monitoring is more beneficial. Signs of distress should be reported immediately. The woman's labor should be plotted on the Friedman graph, and any sign of dysfunction should be reported to the clinician.

With twins, any combination of presentations and positions can occur (Figure 18–13). A fetogram assists in determining these presentations and positions.

Vaginal delivery is facilitated when the largest fetus is in vertex presentation and is the first to be born. However, in the event that the first fetus is in a breech position, the following can occur:

1. If the fetus is large, the head can be a problem to the bony pelvis.

2. If the fetus is small, its body can descend into the birth canal before complete dilatation has occurred.

3. The danger of a prolapsed cord exists.

If these problems are overcome, the delivery can proceed as any other breech delivery. Often real-time ultrasound is used in the delivery room to monitor position and heartbeat of the two infants.

The presentation, position, and lie of the second twin must be assessed quickly after the delivery of the first twin. If the breech or vertex is fixed in the pelvic inlet, the membranes may be ruptured and the woman allowed to labor under close supervision. The FHR of the second twin should be assessed closely. Occasionally diluted oxytocin is given if myometrial activity has not resumed within a 10-minute period.

Delivery in the presence of dysfunctional labor due to overstretched uterine fibers can be managed with cesarean birth or infusion of diluted oxytocin. Clinicians do not agree on the benefits and dangers of the two methods. Nor do they agree on the most beneficial type of analgesia and anesthesia to employ for the labor and delivery. In the presence of an unstable maternal circulatory system, as found with PIH, regional anesthetic agents such as epidurals or caudals can cause hypovolemic shock due to the blocking of the sympathetic nervous system. Large and continuous doses of narcotics can cause neonatal respiratory depression, especially if these infants are premature, as twins frequently are. Paracervical blocks have been known to cause transient fetal bradycardia. Pritchard and MacDonald (1980) advocate the use of the pudendal block at the time of delivery. Uterine relaxation can be obtained with halothane if internal podalic version for the second twin is required.

Cesarean delivery is advocated in the presence of fetal distress, previous cesarean birth, CPD, placenta previa, and sometimes severe pregnancy-induced hypertension. If the second twin is larger than the first and CPD exists, a cesarean delivery should be performed (Pritchard and MacDonald, 1980).

The nurse must prepare to receive two neonates instead of one. This means a duplication of everything, including the resuscitation equipment, radiant warmers, and

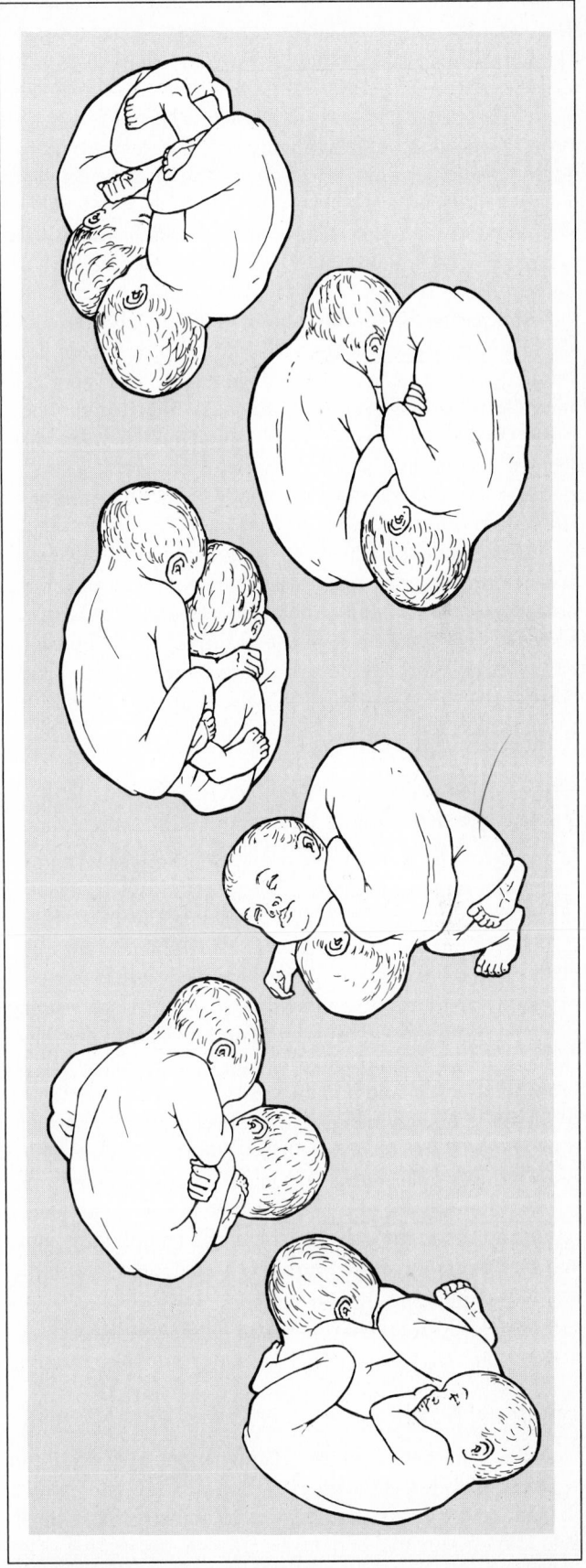

FIGURE 18–13 Types of twin presentations.

newborn identification papers and bracelets. Two staff members should be available for newborn resuscitation.

If twins are discovered at the time of delivery, the nurse must move quickly to prepare for the second newborn. The pediatric team may need to be notified at this time. While one nurse is monitoring the second twin in utero, the other nurse is caring for the already delivered newborn and preparing for the second. Special precautions should be observed to ensure correct identification of the neonates. The first born is usually tagged Baby A and the second, Baby B.

The matter of suppression of preterm labor is under debate. If the labor has been established, little can be done other than to proceed with the deliveries. The labor pattern and fetuses should be continuously monitored, whole blood prepared in case it is needed, and a functioning intravenous route established. Two scrubbed obstetricians, a pediatrician, and an anesthesiologist should be present at the time of preterm delivery.

After multiple deliveries, mothers are closely monitored for postpartal hemorrhage. In addition, the nurse determines the woman's or family's need for referral to social welfare agencies or public health clinics for follow-up care. The family may be unprepared financially and psychologically for the arrival of twins and thus at risk for further difficulties.

THREE OR MORE FETUSES

When three or more fetuses are present, maternal and fetal problems are potentiated. The more fetuses conceived, the smaller they tend to be at the time of delivery. Delivery of three or more fetuses is best accomplished by cesarean birth because of the risk of fetal insult due to decreased placental perfusion and hemorrhage from the separating placenta during the intrapartal period (Pritchard and MacDonald, 1980). Complicated obstetric maneuvers such as breech extraction and podalic version, the risk of prolapse of the cord, and an increase in fetal collision provide additional rationale for an abdominal delivery. Itzkowicz (1979) reviewed 59 triplet births and found that the majority delivered vaginally. He also noted that an abnormal presentation complicated the delivery of the second and third fetus and that mortality of the third fetus was double that of the first fetus. Depending on the maternal–fetal status, a cesarean birth may be in these neonates' best interests.

CONJOINED TWINS

Conjoined or Siamese twins occur when the division of the embryonic disk is incomplete. Labor dystocia is common. Vaginal delivery can be accomplished if the joining is pliable. When essential organs are shared, separation after delivery is usually not successful.

Fetal Distress

The most commonly observed initial signs of fetal distress include meconium-stained amniotic fluid (in a vertex presentation) and decelerations in FHR. Fetal scalp blood samples demonstrating a pH value of 7.20 or less provide a more sophisticated indication of fetal problems and are generally obtained when questions about fetal status arise. (For further discussion see p. 461.)

A variety of factors may contribute to fetal distress. The most common are related to cord compression, placental abnormalities, and preexisting maternal disease.

Maternal implications. Indications of fetal distress greatly increase the psychologic stress a laboring woman must face. The professional staff may become so involved in assessing fetal status and initiating corrective measures that they fail to give explanation and emotional support to the woman and her partner. It is imperative to provide full explanations of the problem and comfort to the couple. In many instances, if delivery is not imminent, the woman must undergo cesarean delivery. This operation may be a source of fear for the couple and of frustration, too, if they were committed to a shared, prepared delivery experience.

Fetal–neonatal implications. Prolonged fetal hypoxia may lead to mental retardation or cerebral palsy and ultimately to fetal demise.

Interventions. When evidence of possible fetal distress develops, initial interventions include changing the maternal position and administering oxygen by mask at 6–7 L/min. If fetal monitoring has not been used prior to this time, it is usually instituted. Fetal scalp blood samples are also taken. Probable cause is ascertained and further actions are based on a complete assessment of maternal–fetal status. The Nursing Care Plan on fetal distress (pp. 538–540) offers a framework for dealing with fetal distress caused by various conditions.

Intrauterine Fetal Death (IUFD)

Fetal death, often referred to as fetal demise, accounts for one-half of the perinatal mortality after the twentieth week of pregnancy. IUFD results from unknown causes or a number of physiologic maladaptions including preeclampsia-eclampsia, abruptio placentae, placenta previa, diabetes, infection, congenital anomalies, and isoimmune disease.

The cessation of fetal movement frequently is the first indication of fetal death. It is followed by a gradual decrease in the signs and symptoms of pregnancy. Fetal heart tones are absent and fetal movement is no longer palpable. Abdominal x-ray examination may reveal Spalding's sign, an overriding of the fetal cranial bones. In addition, maternal estriol levels fall. Diagnosis of IUFD is confirmed by absence of heart action on real-time ultrasonography.

In 75% of these cases, spontaneous labor begins within 2 weeks of the fetal death (Quilligan, 1980). Artificial rupture of the membranes is avoided because of the risk of introducing infection. If labor does not ensue, oxytocin or prostaglandins may be administered to induce labor.

Prolonged retention of the fetus may lead to the development of disseminated intravascular coagulation (DIC) (also referred to as *consumption coagulopathy*). After the release of thromboplastin from the degenerating fetal tissues into the maternal bloodstream, the extrinsic clotting system is activated, triggering the formation of multiple tiny blood clots. Subsequently, fibrinogen and factors V and VII are depleted, and the client begins to display symptomalogy of DIC. Fibrinogen levels begin a linear descent 3–4 weeks after the death of the fetus and continue to decrease without appropriate medical intervention. An in-depth discussion of DIC is found on p. 567.

The parents of a stillborn infant suffer a devastating experience, precipitating an intense emotional trauma. During the pregnancy, the couple has already begun the attachment process, which now must be terminated through the grieving process. The behaviors that couples exhibit while mourning may be associated with the five stages of grieving as described by Kübler-Ross (1969). Often the first stage is *denial* of the death of the fetus. Even as the initial birth attendant suspects fetal demise, the couple is hoping that a second opinion will be different. Some couples may not be convinced of the death until they view and hold the stillborn infant. The second stage is *anger*, resulting from the feelings of loss, loneliness, and perhaps guilt. The anger may be projected to significant others and health team members, or it may be omitted when the death of the fetus is sudden and unexpected. *Bargaining*, the third stage, may or may not be present depending upon the couple's preparation for the death of the fetus. If the death is unanticipated, the couple may have no time for bargaining. In the fourth stage, *depression* is evidenced by preoccupation, weeping, and withdrawal. Profound depression may necessitate psychiatric consultation. Physiologic postpartal depression appearing 24–48 hours after delivery may compound the depression of grief. The final stage is *acceptance*, which involves the process of resolution. This is a highly individualized process that may take months to complete.

The following nursing measures are recommended:

1. Listen to the couple; do not offer explanations. They require solace without minimizing the event.
2. Respond to denial with gentle, firm, and realistic statements.
3. Discuss with the couple the opportunity to see and hold the stillborn infant. Advocates of seeing the stillborn believe that viewing assists in dispelling denial and en-

ables the couple to progress to the next step in the grieving process. If they choose to see their stillborn infant, preparing the couple is absolutely essential. The nurse should describe what they will see by saying "the baby is cold," "the baby is blue," "the baby is bruised," or other appropriate statements. Some agencies routinely take a photo of the infant and let parents know it's available if they wish to have it.

4. Redirect the anger when possible rather than defending or avoiding the couple's hostile feelings.
5. Accept the weeping and depression. A couple may have intense feelings that they are unable to share with each other. Encourage them to talk together and allow emotions to flow freely.
6. Convey the message that time heals, but acknowledge that the memory is never completely obliterated.
7. Arrange for the woman to be assigned to a room that is away from new mothers and infants.
8. Prepare the couple for returning home. If there are siblings, each will progress through age-appropriate grieving. Provide the parents with information about normal mourning behaviors, both psychologic and physiologic.
9. Encourage the couple to consider participating in support groups for parents who have lost an infant. (See Chapter 30 for resource groups.)

Placental Problems

Maintenance of placental function is paramount to assure fetal well-being and continuance of the pregnancy. Because the placenta is so vascular, problems that develop are usually associated with maternal and possible fetal hemorrhage. Causes and sources of hemorrhage are reviewed in Table 18–2, and signs and symptoms of hemorrhage are presented in Table 18–3.

ABRUPTIO PLACENTAE

Abruptio placentae is the premature separation of the placenta from the uterine wall. Premature separation is considered a catastrophic event because of the severity of the hemorrhage that occurs. The incidence is about 1 in every 80 to 200 pregnancies (Pritchard and MacDonald, 1980). In 10% of the cases, the separation is severe, and fetal death or possibly maternal death occurs from hemorrhagic shock. In the other 90%, there is a less severe separation, and the results are not so serious. Increased risk of abruptio placentae occurs in women with a parity of five or more or who are over 30 years of age. Women with preeclampsia-eclampsia and renal or vascular disease are also at greater risk.

The cause of abruptio placentae is largely unknown. Theories have been proposed relating its occurrence to

Table 18–2   Causes and Sources of Hemorrhage

Causes and sources	Signs and symptoms
Antepartal period	
Abortion	Vaginal bleeding
	Intermittent uterine contractions
	Rupture of membranes
Placenta previa	Painless vaginal bleeding after seventh month
Abruptio placentae	
Partial	Vaginal bleeding; no increase in uterine pain
Severe	No vaginal bleeding
	Extreme tenderness of abdominal area
	Rigid, boardlike abdomen
	Increase in size of abdomen
Intrapartal period	
Placenta previa	Bright red vaginal bleeding
Abruptio placentae	Same signs and symptoms as listed above
Uterine atony in stage III	Bright red vaginal bleeding, ineffectual contractility
Postpartal period	
Uterine atony	Boggy uterus
	Dark vaginal bleeding
	Presence of clots
Retained placental fragments	Boggy uterus
	Dark vaginal bleeding
	Presence of clots
Lacerations of cervix or vagina	Firm uterus
	Bright red blood

decreased blood flow to the placenta through the sinuses during the last trimester. Excessive intrauterine pressure caused by hydramnios or multiple pregnancy may also be contributing factors.

□ **CLINICAL MANIFESTATIONS** Premature separation is subdivided into three types (Figure 18–14):

- *Covert (severe).* In this situation, the placenta separates centrally and the blood is trapped between the placenta and the uterine wall. Entrapment of the blood results in concealed bleeding.

- *Overt (partial).* In this case, the blood passes between the fetal membranes and the uterine wall and escapes vaginally. Thus the bleeding is revealed.

- *Placental prolapse.* Massive vaginal bleeding is seen in the presence of almost total separation.

The signs and symptoms of these three types of placental abruption are given in Table 18–4. In severe cases of covert abruptio placentae, a blood clot forms behind the placenta. With no place to escape, the blood invades the myometrial tissues between the muscle fibers. This occurrence accounts for the uterine irritability that is a significant sign of premature separation of the placenta. If hemorrhage continues, eventually the uterus turns entirely blue in color. After delivery of the neonate, the uterus contracts only with difficulty. This syndrome is known as a *Couvelaire uterus* and frequently necessitates hysterectomy.

As a result of the damage to the uterine wall and the retroplacental clotting with covert abruption, large amounts of thromboplastin are released into the maternal blood supply, which in turn triggers the development of DIC and the resultant hypofibrinogenemia. Fibrinogen levels, which are ordinarily elevated in pregnancy, may drop to incoagulable amounts within a matter of minutes as a

Table 18–3   Degree of Hemorrhage*

Severity	Signs and symptoms	Reduction in blood volume
Mild hemorrhage	Minimal tachycardia Slight decrease in BP Mild evidence of vasoconstriction, with cool hands and feet	15%–25% (750–1250 mL)
Moderate hemorrhage	Tachycardia (100–120 beats/min) Decrease in pulse pressure Systolic BP 90–100 mm Hg Restlessness, increased sweating, pallor, oliguria	25%–35% (1250–1750 mL)
Severe hemorrhage	Tachycardia > 120 beats/min Systolic BP decreased to 60 mm Hg and frequently unobtainable by cuff Mental stupor, extreme pallor, cold extremities, anuria	Up to 50% (2500 mL)

* Modified from Smith, I. I., and Weil, M. H. 1967. In *Diagnosis and treatment of shock*, eds. M. H. Weil and H. Shubin. Baltimore: Williams & Wilkins.

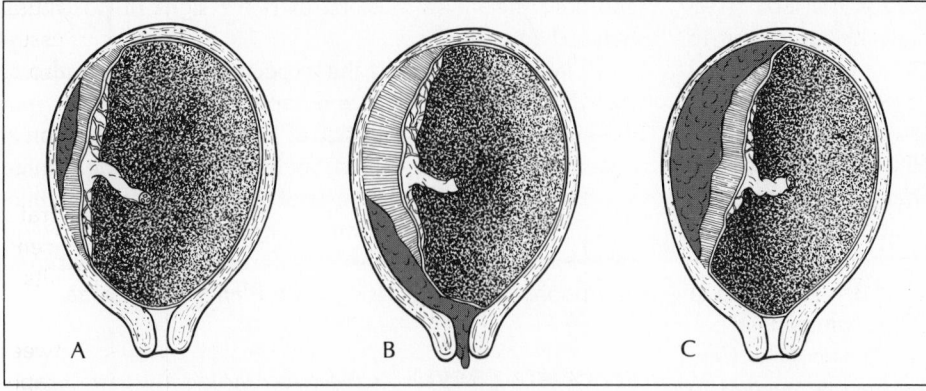

FIGURE 18-14 Abruptio placentae. **A,** Internal or concealed hemorrhage. **B,** External hemorrhage. **C,** Complete separation. (From Abnormalities of the placenta, Clinical Educational Aid no. 12, Ross Laboratories, Columbus, Ohio.)

result of rapidly developing premature separation of the placenta. Further information on DIC is found on p. 567.

Maternal implications. Maternal mortality is approximately 6%. Problems following delivery depend in large part on the severity of the intrapartal bleeding, coagulation defects (DIC), hypofibrinogenemia, and length of time between separation and delivery. Moderate to severe hemorrhage results in hemorrhagic shock, which ultimately may prove fatal to the mother if not reversed. In the postpartal period, mothers who have suffered this disorder are at risk for hemorrhage and renal failure due to shock, vascular spasm, intravascular clotting, or a combination of the three. Another cause of renal failure is incompatible emergency blood transfusion. Failure is directly proportional to the number of units transfused.

Fetal-neonatal implications. Perinatal mortality associated with premature separation of the placenta is about 15%. In severe cases in which separation is almost complete, infant mortality is 100%. In less severe separation, fetal outcome depends on the level of maturity. The most serious complications in the neonate arise from preterm labor, anemia, and hypoxia. If fetal hypoxia progresses unchecked, irreversible brain damage or fetal demise may result. With thorough assessment and prompt action on the part of the health team, fetal and maternal outcome can be optimized.

Interventions. Upon admission, the nursing assessment begins. Any sudden change in behavior, such as an aching pain in the abdomen, may signal the separation of the placenta during labor. Other important signs that should be noted include irritability of the uterus, faint or absent FHTs, fetal hyperactivity, meconium-stained amniotic fluid, increase in fundal height, any increase in bleeding, and symptoms of shock. Frequently, shock symptoms appear disproportionate to blood loss.

The psychologic aspects of the nursing care of this patient cannot be overestimated. Maternal apprehension increases as the clinical picture changes. Factual reassurance and an explanation of the procedures and what is happening are essential for the emotional well-being of the expectant couple. The nurse can reinforce positive aspects of the

woman's condition, such as normal FHTs, normal vital signs, and decreased evidence of bleeding.

If the separation is mild and gestation is near term, labor may be induced and the fetus delivered vaginally with as little trauma as possible. If the induction of labor by rupture of membranes and oxytocin infusion by pump does not initiate labor within 8 hours, a cesarean delivery is usually done. A longer delay would increase the risk of increased hemorrhage, with resulting hypofibrinogenemia. Supportive treatment to decrease risk of DIC includes typing and cross-matching for blood transfusions (at least three units), clotting mechanism evaluation, and intravenous fluids.

In cases of moderate to severe placental separation, a cesarean delivery is done after hypofibrinogenemia has been treated by intravenous infusion of cryoprecipitate or plasma. Vaginal delivery is impossible in the event of a Couvelaire uterus, because it would not contract properly

Table 18-4 Differential Signs and Symptoms of Abruptio Placentae

Covert (severe)	Overt (partial)	Placental prolapse
No overt bleeding from vagina	Vaginal bleeding	Massive vaginal bleeding
Rigid abdomen	Rigid abdomen	Rigid abdomen
Acute abdominal pain	Acute abdominal pain	Acute abdominal pain
Decreased blood pressure, increased pulse	Decreased blood pressure, increased pulse	Shock
Uteroplacental insufficiency	Uteroplacental insufficiency	Marked uteroplacental insufficiency

in labor. Cesarean delivery is necessary in the face of severe hemorrhage to allow an immediate hysterectomy to save both woman and fetus.

Medical and nursing management of complications of severe abruptio placentae is as follows. Hypovolemia is life-threatening and must be combated with whole blood. If the fetus is alive but in distress, emergency cesarean delivery is the method of choice. With a stillborn fetus, vaginal delivery is preferable unless shock from hemorrhage is uncontrollable. The hematocrit value should be maintained at 30%. Pritchard and MacDonald (1980) recommend a balanced salt solution of Ringer's lactate intravenously. Central venous pressure (CVP) monitoring may be needed to check fluid replacement. The nurse monitors fluid intake and output closely and accurately. Hourly recordings are suggested. Oliguria of less than 30 mL/hr should be reported to the physician. Intake may be increased or decreased depending on the output.

If a CVP line is inserted, elevations should be reported. The nurse should also look for signs of cough, rales, and shortness of breath, which might mean fluid overload and pulmonary edema.

Hourly bedside clotting times may be ordered and can be performed by the nurse. A stable clot that forms in less than 6 minutes indicates a good fibrinogen level. Blood that fails to clot within 30 minutes indicates a critically low clotting factor level. The time it takes the blood to clot plus retraction should be noted.

Measures should be taken to empty the uterus to prevent DIC from occurring. An amniotomy may be performed and oxytocin stimulation is advocated to hasten delivery. The nurse will find it difficult to palpate contractions because of the hypertonic state of the uterus. However, the woman may complain with regularity, which signals increased uterine tone. Progressive dilatation and effacement usually occur (Pritchard and MacDonald, 1980).

Postpartally the nurse should continue close monitoring of the mother's fluid intake and output and her vital signs. The uterus must be palpated frequently for atony. In addition, the nurse must be alert for signs of postpartal hemorrhage.

If lactation occurs at the expected time, it is evidence that the pituitary gland has escaped serious damage from ischemia and that the threat of Sheehan syndrome is reduced. The mother should be followed-up to determine whether menses returns. Tests of thyroid and adrenal function 4–6 months after delivery are part of proper follow-up care for patients who have suffered a severe placental abruption. (See the Nursing Care Plan for hemorrhage on p.569).

PLACENTA PREVIA

In placenta previa, the placenta is improperly implanted in the lower uterine segment. This implantation may be on a portion of the lower segment or over the internal os. As the lower uterine segment contracts and dilates in the later weeks of pregnancy, the placental villi are torn from the uterine wall, thus exposing the uterine sinuses at the placental site. Bleeding begins, but because its amount depends on the number of sinuses exposed, initially it may be either scanty or profuse.

The cause of placenta previa is unknown. Statistically it occurs in about 1 in every 167 deliveries with 20% being complete and is more common in multiparas (Pritchard and MacDonald, 1980). Women with a previous history of placenta previa as well as those who have undergone a low cervical cesarean delivery appear to be at greater risk for its occurrence.

The types of placenta previa are as follows (Figure 18–15):

• *Complete or total placenta previa.* The placenta totally covers the internal os.

• *Partial placenta previa.* A small portion of the placenta covers the internal os.

• *Low-lying or marginal placenta previa.* The placental edge is attached very close to but does not cover the internal os.

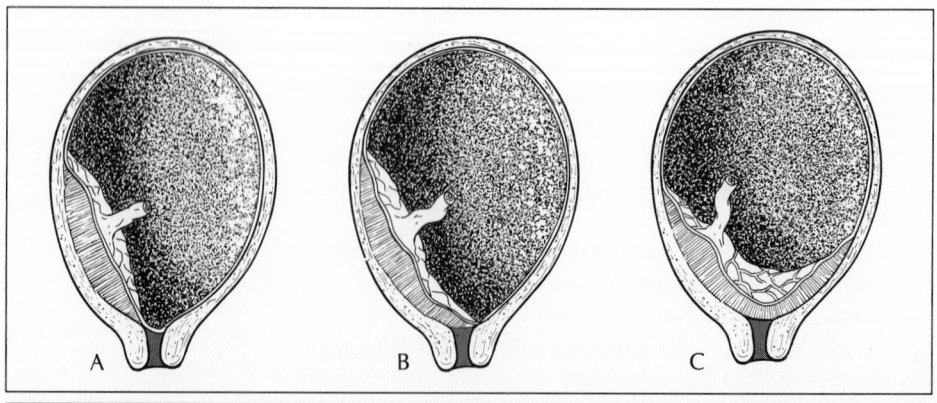

FIGURE 18–15 Placenta previa. **A,** Low placental implantation. **B,** Partial placenta previa. **C,** Total placenta previa. (From Abnormalities of the placenta, Clinical Educational Aid no. 12, Ross Laboratories, Columbus, Ohio.)

□ *CLINICAL MANIFESTATIONS* Painless, bright red vaginal bleeding is the best diagnostic sign of placenta previa. If this sign should develop during the last 3 months of a pregnancy, placenta previa should always be considered until ruled out by examination. Generally, the first bleeding episode is scanty. If no rectal or vaginal examinations are performed, it often subsides spontaneously. However, each subsequent hemorrhage is more profuse.

The uterus remains soft, and if labor begins, it relaxes fully between contractions. The FHR usually remains stable unless profuse hemorrhage and maternal shock occur. As a result of the placement of the placenta, the fetal presenting part is often unengaged, and transverse lie is common.

Diagnosis. Direct diagnosis of placenta previa can only be made by feeling the placenta inside the os. However, profuse bleeding can result from this examination, so it should only be performed under two specific circumstances: (a) when the pregnancy is beyond 37 weeks' gestation and the fetus is mature enough to be born, and (b) when recurring hemorrhages make it imperative that delivery take place immediately to save both the woman and the fetus. This examination, reserved for emergency situations, is called the *double setup procedure* (see Procedure 18–1), and it requires that everything be at hand to perform an immediate cesarean delivery should profuse bleeding ensue.

Indirect diagnosis is made by localizing the placenta

Procedure 18–1   Double Setup Examination

Objective	Nursing action	Rationale
Prepare patient	Explain procedure thoroughly. Consent form for a cesarean delivery is signed (in case it is needed)	Decreases anxiety. Informed consent is for legal purposes

Assemble and prepare equipment	Set up delivery room for a vaginal delivery:
	1. Assemble equipment on instrument table
	2. Warm infant crib
	3. Set out resuscitation equipment for newborn
	4. Obtain monitoring equipment:
	  a. Sphygmomanometer and stethoscope
	  b. Ultrasound fetal monitoring system or fetoscope
	Set up equipment for cesarean delivery if needed
		Sterile vaginal examination is done in the delivery room so that, if immediate delivery is required, a vaginal or cesarean delivery may be done

Position patient	Assist patient to delivery table; place legs in stirrups, raising both legs at same time	Reduces muscle strain
Maintain adequate fluids	If IV infusion has not already been started, begin one with a large-bore needle Administer fluids at a keep-open rate Administer oxygen and suction as needed	Patient is likely to develop excessive bleeding; IV is started so fluids may be administered quickly if needed
Assemble personnel	Required personnel include scrub nurse, circulating nurse, physician, physician's assistant, anesthesiologist, pediatrician, and nursery nurse	
Monitor procedure	Physician carefully performs vaginal examination; dependent on findings, interventions may be as follows: 1. Rupture of membranes 2. Vaginal delivery 3. Cesarean delivery	Method of treatment depends on presence and degree of placenta previa

FIGURE 18–16 Ultrasound of placenta previa.

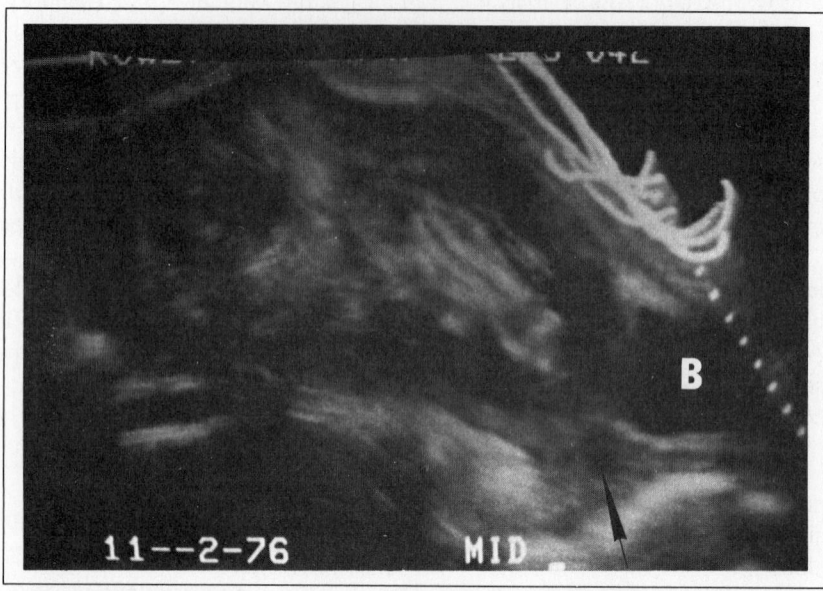

through tests that require no vaginal examination. The most commonly employed diagnostic test is the ultrasound scan (Figure 18–16).

Differential diagnosis. The differential diagnosis of cervical or uterine bleeding requires careful inspection and palpation. Suspicious areas should be biopsied. Partial separation of a normally implanted placenta may also exhibit painless bleeding, and a true placenta previa may not demonstrate overt bleeding until labor begins, thus confusing the diagnosis. Another important fact to note is that the causes of slight to moderate antepartal bleeding episodes in 20%–25% of patients are never accurately diagnosed.

Maternal implications. During the antepartal period, mild hemorrhage generally results in few, if any, maternal complications. A slight decrease in the hemoglobin and hematocrit levels may be apparent, and the woman may complain of fatigue.

The presence of placenta previa increases maternal risks in the postpartal period. Hemorrhage that may occur when the placental site is located in the lower uterine segment is a primary danger. This is the passive section of the uterus, and the contractility of this section of muscle fiber is poor. Uterine rupture could occur as a result of the weakening of the uterine musculature by the ingrowth of the placenta and the presence of its blood sinuses. Uterine infection from prolonged rupture of membranes, retained placental fragments, and possible anemia are also risks.

Fetal–neonatal implications. The prognosis for the fetus depends on the extent of placenta previa. Changes in the FHR and meconium staining of the amniotic fluid may be apparent. In a profuse bleeding episode, the fetus is compromised and does suffer some hypoxia. FHR monitoring is imperative on admission to the hospital, particu-

larly if a vaginal delivery is anticipated. This is important, because the presenting part of the fetus may obstruct the flow of blood from the placenta or umbilical cord. If fetal distress occurs, delivery is by cesarean birth.

After delivery of the neonate, blood sampling should be done to determine whether any newborn anemia has been caused by intrauterine bleeding episodes of the woman.

Interventions. Care of the patient with painless late gestational bleeding depends on (a) the week of gestation during which the first bleeding episode occurs and (b) the amount of bleeding. If the pregnancy is less than 37 weeks' gestation and if bleeding is scanty or has stopped, the placenta should be localized by indirect methods, such as real-time scanning. If placenta previa is ruled out, a vaginal examination may be performed with a speculum to assess the cause of bleeding (such as cervical lesions). If placenta previa is diagnosed, then *expectant management* is employed to delay delivery until about 37 weeks' gestation to allow the fetus to mature. Expectant management involves stringent regulation of nursing care as follows:

1. Bed rest with only bathroom privileges as long as the patient is not bleeding.
2. No rectal or vaginal exams.
3. Assessment of blood loss, pain, and uterine contractility.
4. Assessment of FHTs with external fetal monitor.
5. Monitoring of vital signs.
6. Complete laboratory evaluation: hemoglobin, hematocrit, Rh factor, and urinalysis.
7. Intravenous fluid (Ringer's lactate) with drip rate monitored.

8. Two units of cross-matched blood available for transfusion.

9. Communication with patient and family about what is happening and encouragement of their questions.

If frequent, recurrent, or profuse bleeding persists, a cesarean delivery is performed.

At 37 weeks, delivery is performed either by the vaginal route or by cesarean birth. This decision is based on knowledge of the degree of previa and of the feasibility of labor induction. The double setup examination provides this information (see Procedure 18–1). If the placenta does not cover the os, membranes are ruptured and a vaginal delivery is anticipated. If bleeding becomes profuse, a cesarean delivery is done.

Before a double setup procedure is performed, the laboring couple should be physiologically and psychologically prepared for possible surgery (Chapter 19). A whole-blood setup should be readied for intravenous infusion and a patent intravenous line established before any intrusive procedures are undertaken. The maternal vital signs should be monitored every 15 minutes in the absence of hemorrhage and every 5 minutes with active hemorrhage. The external tocodynamometer should be connected to the maternal abdomen to continuously monitor uterine activity.

The precautions of a double setup are taken because the vaginal examination can cause overt bleeding. The medical and nursing team scrub and prepare for surgery. The newborn nursery is alerted, and adequate infant resuscitation equipment is readied. An anesthesiologist is also present. The patient is prepared for a cesarean delivery in the usual manner. She is then taken to the delivery room (or operating room) and examined in the lithotomy position. A speculum examination confirms the presence or absence of placenta previa. If previa is found, a cesarean delivery is performed without delay. The fetus should be continuously monitored until the pregnancy is terminated.

The newborn's hemoglobin, cell volume, and erythrocyte count should be checked immediately and then monitored closely. The infant may require oxygen and administration of blood.

COMPLICATIONS ASSOCIATED WITH BLEEDING

Disseminated intravascular coagulation is an abnormal overstimulation of the coagulation process, secondary to an underlying disease. The coagulation process remains essentially the same, but certain medical conditions hasten and intensify the response to the point that hemorrhage may be life-threatening as coagulation factors are overconsumed.

Sepsis in the obstetric client may activate the intrinsic coagulation pathway because of damage to the endothelial cells. On the other hand, the extrinsic pathway is activated by the release of thromboplastin from damaged tissues in such conditions as abruptio placentae, toxemia, and retained products of conception. The normally high levels of tissue thromboplastin in the placenta and decidua of the uterus may contribute to the occurrence of DIC. Amniotic fluid released into the bloodstream from amniotic fluid emboli and intraamniotic saline infusions activates both pathways. With the initiation of the coagulation process, massive numbers of clots form rapidly. Fibrinogen becomes depleted as it is converted to fibrin. Platelets are entrapped in the clots, leading to a decrease in the number of platelets. The coagulation process also activates plasminogen conversion to plasmin, which can lyse fibrinogen (dissolve clots) and as the fibrin clots are destroyed, fibrin split products having an anticoagulant effect are released. Because of the elevated fibrin split products level, the decrease in the number of platelets, and the reduced fibrinogen level, the outcome is generalized bleeding. Ischemia of the organs follows from the vascular occlusion of the numerous fibrin thrombi. The multisite hemorrhages result in shock and potentially death (Figure 18–17).

The clinical manifestations of DIC begin subtly and become more overt with the severity of the disease. The signs and symptoms are indicators of degrees of bleeding ranging from generalized hemorrhage to minor generalized bleeding to localized bleeding in the form of purpura and petechiae. Confirmation of DIC is made with several blood tests. The prothrombin time (PT) test evaluates the extrinsic pathway in clotting. PT is prolonged in DIC. The intrinsic pathway is evaluated by testing the partial thromboplastin time, which is also prolonged in DIC. Platelets are decreased as are fibrinogen levels. Platelet counts below $50,000/\mu L$ result in spontaneous bleeding. Fibrinogen levels may be within normal ranges, but will be lower than the initial level. The number of fibrin split products is elevated. The frequency of testing depends upon the severity of the disease. Other more specific assays of the clotting factors may be recommended for the critically ill client (Talbert and Blatt, 1979).

DIC frequently can be resolved by correcting the underlying cause. In the obstetric client, terminating the pregnancy or treating the infection removes the causative factor.

Additional therapy is not required in moderate or low-grade DIC. In severe DIC, heparin therapy may be instituted. Although it is highly controversial, proponents of this treatment argue that the antithrombin activity of heparin neutralizes the free circulating thrombin to prevent the conversion of fibrinogen to fibrin and thus halts the coagulation process. The effectiveness of the medication is determined by the cessation of bleeding. Those who oppose the use of heparin feel it may potentiate hemorrhage.

Blood component therapy may also be necessary in severe DIC. Fresh frozen plasma and cryoprecipitate are given to increase the fibrinogen levels. The body's natural tendency to increase production of fibrinogen under stress

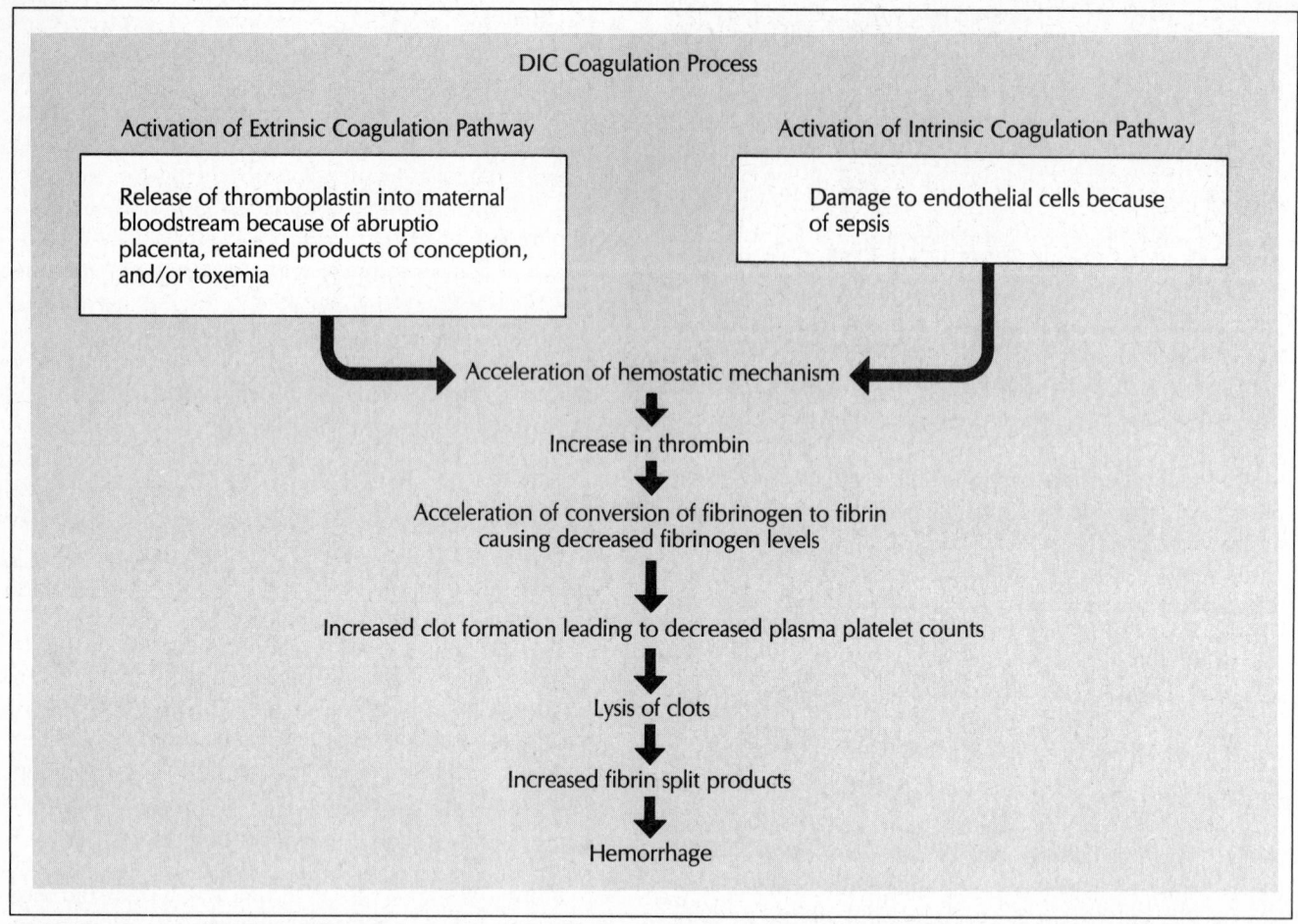

FIGURE 18–17 DIC coagulation process.

provides an additional source of fibrinogen. In the hemorrhaging client, platelets and other volume expanders may be administered.

The nurse should carefully observe for signs and symptoms of DIC in clients who are candidates for this complication. Bleeding from injection sites, epistaxis, bleeding gums, and the presence of purpura and petechiae on the skin may be signs of developing DIC. As appropriate, the nurse continues to monitor maternal–fetal status by checking vital signs, uterine activity, and FHR. In the event of a major blood loss, nursing measures are identified in the Nursing Care Plan on hemorrhage found on p. 569. Additional responsibilities of the nurse include monitoring the administration of heparin and blood products. Meeting the client's psychologic needs is another nursing priority: accurate, informative explanations should be offered frequently. A warm, understanding approach assists the client to cope with her anxiety and frustration (Jennings, 1979).

OTHER PLACENTAL PROBLEMS

Other problems of the placenta can be divided into those that are developmental and those that are degenerative.

Developmental problems of the placenta include placental lesions, placental succenturiata, circumvallate placenta, and battledore placenta. Degenerative changes include infarcts and placental calcification.

□ *PLACENTAL LESIONS* Angiomatous tumors, metastatic tumors, and cysts are classified as placental lesions. Cysts are the most common and occur in the chorionic membrane (Pritchard and MacDonald, 1980). About one-third of placental tumors are associated with maternal hydramnios. Maternal complications can result from hydramnios (see p. 576). Perinatal mortality is high because of the high rate of prematurity. These infants also have an increased incidence of metastatic lesions (Greenhill and Friedman, 1974).

□ *SUCCENTURIATE PLACENTA* In succenturiate placenta, one or more accessory lobes of fetal villi have developed on the placenta, with vascular connections of fetal origin (Figure 18–18,A, p. 574). Vessels from the major to the minor lobe(s) are supported only by the membranes, thus increasing the risk of the minor lobe being retained during the third stage of labor.

The gravest maternal danger is postpartal hemorrhage

(Text continues on p. 573.)

NURSING CARE PLAN
Hemorrhage

CLIENT DATA BASE

History

Identify factors predisposing to hemorrhage:

1. Presence of preeclampsia-eclampsia
2. Overdistention of the uterus
   a. Multiple pregnancy
   b. Hydramnios
3. Grandmultiparity
4. Advanced age
5. Uterine contractile problems
   a. Hypotonicity
   b. Hypertonicity
6. Painless vaginal bleeding after seventh month
7. Presence of hypertension
8. Presence of diabetes
9. History of previous hemorrhage or bleeding problems, blood coagulation defects, abortions
10. Retained placental fragments
11. Lacerations

Determine religious preference to establish whether client will permit a blood transfusion

Physical examination

Severe abdominal pain

Painless vaginal hemorrhage

Revealed or concealed bleeding (see Table 18-4)

Shock symptoms (decreased blood pressure, increased pulse, pallor)

Uterine tetany or uterine atony

Portwine amniotic fluid with abruptio placentae

Degree of hemorrhage (see Table 18-3)

Changes in FHR

Laboratory evaluation

Hemoglobin and hematocrit

Type and cross-match

Fibrinogen levels

NURSING PRIORITIES

1. If IV is not present, start one in large vein with large-bore plastic cannula
2. Evaluate blood loss (if possible, measure or weigh blood-soaked pads to facilitate adequate replacement)
3. Monitor vital signs, particularly pulse and BP
4. Measure urine output
5. Administer oxygen as necessary
6. Evaluate fetal status
7. Maintain fetal life-support mechanisms
8. Do not perform vaginal or rectal exam until placenta previa has been ruled out

CLIENT/FAMILY EDUCATIONAL FOCUS

1. Provide information regarding the cause of the hemorrhage
2. Discuss the assessment techniques and treatment associated with the hemorrhage
3. Provide opportunities for questions and individual concerns of the client and her family

Problem	Nursing interventions and actions	Rationale
Blood loss	Observe, record, and report blood loss	Hypovolemia causes decreased venous return to the heart and subsequent decrease in cardiac output; decreased cardiac output initiates sympathoadrenal response, which leads to increased peripheral resistance and tachycardia in an effort to maintain adequate tissue perfusion; decreased blood flow to kidney causes stimulation of juxtaglomerular apparatus to release hormones; this leads to retention of sodium ions and water (mechanism to increase blood volume) and increased reabsorption of water by distal tubules, which increases intravascular volume; cells do not receive sufficient O_2 or nutrients because of vasoconstriction of venules and arterioles (caused by increased catecholamines)

NURSING CARE PLAN Cont'd
Hemorrhage

Problem	Nursing interventions and actions	Rationale
	Assess patient experiencing decrease in blood volume using following parameters:	Release of catecholamines and cortisol during shock also stimulates release of fatty acids for energy production; as fatty acids are metabolized, there is increase in ketones; ketones are normally oxidized in the liver, but the hypoperfused liver cannot do this adequately, resulting in increase in metabolic acidosis
	1. Monitor rate and quality of respirations continuously	Initially respiratory rate increases as a result of sympathoadrenal stimulation, resulting in increased metabolic rate; pain and anxiety may cause hyperventilation
	2. Measure pulse rate	Increased pulse rate is an effect of increased epinephrine
	3. Assess pulse quality by direct palpation Determine pulse deficit by comparing apical-radial rates	Reflects circulatory status Thready pulse indicates vasoconstriction and reflects decreased cardiac output; peripheral pulses may be absent if vasoconstriction is intense Bounding pulse may indicate overload
	4. Compare present BP with patient's baseline BP; note pulse pressure	Hypotension indicates loss of large amount of circulatory fluid or lack of compensation in circulatory system As cardiac output decreases, there is usually a fall in pulse pressure Peripheral vasoconstriction may make accurate readings difficult
	5. Monitor urine output (decrease to less than 30 mL/hr is sign of shock): a. Insert Foley catheter b. Measure output hourly c. Measure specific gravity to determine concentration of urine	Vasoconstrictor effect of norepinephrine decreases blood flow to kidneys, which decreases glomerular filtration rate and the output of urine Inability to concentrate urine may indicate renal damage from vasoconstriction and decreased blood perfusion
	6. Assess skin for presence of following: a. Pallor and cyanosis: *Pallor* in brown-skinned persons appears yellowish-brown; black-skinned individuals appear ashen gray; generally pallor may be observed in mucous membranes, lips, and nail beds *Cyanosis* is assessed by inspecting lips, nail beds, conjunctiva, palms, and soles of feet at regular intervals; evaluate capillary refilling by pressing on nail bed and observing return of color; compare by testing your own nail bed b. Coldness	Skin reflects amount of vasoconstriction Pallor is determined by intensity of vasoconstriction Cyanosis occurs when the amount of unoxygenated hemoglobin in the blood is $\leq$ 5 g/dL blood Produced by slow blood flow

NURSING CARE PLAN Cont'd
Hemorrhage

Problem	Nursing interventions and actions	Rationale
	c. Clamminess	Caused by sympathetic stimulation of sweat glands
	Assess state of consciousness frequently	Diminished cerebral blood flow causes restlessness and anxiety; as shock progresses, state of consciousness decreases
	Measure CVP: Insert catheter into superior vena cava; intravenous fluid should run freely through catheter before measuring, and baseline zero mark should be marked on patient's chest; normal CVP is 5–10 cm H_2O	Provides estimation of volume of blood returning to heart and ability of both chambers in right heart to propel blood Low CVP indicates a decrease in the circulating volume of blood (hypovolemia)
	Assess amount of blood loss: 1. Count pads 2. Weigh pads and chux (1 g = 1 mL blood approximately) 3. Record amount of flow in a specific amount of time (for example, 50 mL bright red blood on pad in 20 min)	In obstetric patients, blood is replaced according to estimates of actual blood loss, rather than using parameters of increased and decreased BP
Reduction of hemoglobin	Position patient in supine position	Position keeps more blood volume available to vital centers
	Elevate right hip	Avoids pressure on vena cava
	Avoid Trendelenburg position	Trendelenburg position shifts heavy uterus against diaphragm and may compromise respiratory function
	Administer whole blood	Corrects reduced oxygen-carrying capacity
	Administer O_2 by face mask at 4–7 L/min	Woman in labor is mouth breather; using face mask assures better oxygen delivery
Hypovolemia	Relieve decreased blood pressure by administration of whole blood	Hypotension results from decreased blood volume
	While waiting for whole blood to be available, infuse isotonic fluids, plasma, plasma expanders, or serum albumin	Degree of hypovolemia may be assessed by CVP, hemoglobin, and hematocrit
Fluctuations in blood perfusion to vital organs	Monitor urine output hourly: 1. 50 mL/hr or more indicates safe renal perfusion 2. Less than 25 mL/hr indicates inadequate renal perfusion (tubular ischemia and necrosis can result) Monitor adequacy of fluid volume by evaluating CVP	Provides excellent measure of organ perfusion
Presence of hemorrhage	Observe for signs and symptoms of hemorrhage (see Tables 18–2 and 18–3)	Bleeding often stops as shock develops but resumes as circulation is restored
	If partial abruptio placentae is diagnosed, nurse and physician will: 1. Evaluate blood loss	

NURSING CARE PLAN Cont'd
Hemorrhage

Problem	Nursing interventions and actions	Rationale
	2. Assess uterine contractile pattern and tenderness 3. Monitor maternal vital signs 4. Assess fetal status 5. Assess cervical dilatation and effacement 6. Rule out placenta previa 7. Perform amniotomy and begin oxytocin infusion if labor does not start immediately or is ineffective	
	If severe abruptio placentae is diagnosed: 1. Perform same assessments as for partial abruptio placentae 2. Measure CVP 3. Replace blood loss 4. Effect immediate delivery 5. Observe for signs and symptoms of disseminated intravascular coagulation (DIC)	
	If uterine atony is diagnosed intrapartally, assess contractility of uterus and amount of vaginal bleeding; postpartally, massage uterus until firm and administer ergonovine intramuscularly or orally as ordered	Muscle fibers that have been overstretched or overused do not contract well; contraction of muscle fibers over open placental site is essential; slight relaxation of uterus muscle fibers leads to continuous oozing of blood
	If placental fragments have been retained, assess uterine contractility and vaginal flow	Interferes with contractility of uterus
	Massage uterus and scrape out uterine contents	Couvelaire uterus does not contract well because of presence of blood around muscle fibers
	If cervical or vaginal lacerations are found, they are repaired by the physician	
Fetal distress	Assess and monitor fetal heart rate (range 120–160 beats/min)	Hemorrhage from woman disrupts blood flow pattern to fetus, possibly compromising fetal status
	Observe for meconium in amniotic fluid	Hypoxia causes increased motility of fetal intestines and relaxation of abdominal muscles, with release of meconium into amniotic fluid
	Assist in obtaining fetal blood sample (pH < 7.2 indicates severe jeopardy)	
Fear	Instruct patient about procedures	Fear and anxiety affect release of catecholamines
	Remain calm	Increases patient's confidence

NURSING CARE PLAN Cont'd
Hemorrhage

Problem	Nursing interventions and actions	Rationale
Depletion of fibrinogen	Evaluate blood levels; at term, normal fibrinogen level is 375–700 mg/dL; critical level required to clot blood is 100 mg/dL Observe for signs and symptoms of DIC	Fibrinogen and fibrin are lost because of their accumulation in a retroplacental clot; further fibrinogen loss and additional coagulation failure may result from intravascular clotting and fibrinolysis
	Determine whether fetal demise is cause of fibrinogen depletion; conduct coagulation studies and measure fibrinogen levels; induce labor if patient is at risk	Dead fetus releases thromboplastin, which interferes with the clotting mechanism and lowers fibrinogen level
DIC	Monitor the administration of blood components as necessary (whole blood, platelets, cryoprecipitate, plasma)	Maintain the hematocrit value at 30% and above; elevate the platelet count and the fibrinogen levels
	Presence of hemorrhage—note previous interventions and rationale	
	Minimize anxiety with an empathetic approach and explanations	Increase client's feelings of security

NURSING CARE EVALUATION

Blood loss is corrected

Vital signs remain within normal range

Fetal heart tones are present and within normal range

NURSING DIAGNOSES*	SUPPORTING DATA
1. Decreased cardiac output related to hypovolemia and decreased venous return	Excessive bleeding or concealed bleeding Decreased blood pressure and/or changes in pulse pressure Increased pulse Pallor Cyanosis Decreased hematocrit value Decreased fibrinogen levels Decreased urine output Anxiety and/or restlessness Decreased CVP
2. Impaired gas exchange related to reduction of hemoglobin	Cyanosis Delayed capillary refill Dyspnea Generalized weakness
3. Fear related to hemorrhaging	Signs of anxiety and apprehension

* These are a few examples of nursing diagnoses that may be appropriate for a woman with this condition. It is not an inclusive list and must be individualized for each woman.

if this minor lobe is severed from the placenta and remains in the uterus. All placentas should be examined closely for intactness. If vessels appear to be severed at the margin of the placenta, the uterus should be explored for retained placental tissue. This condition usually is not diagnosed until after the delivery of the placenta (Pritchard and MacDonald, 1980). If the vascular connections rupture be-

tween the lobes, life-threatening fetal hemorrhage can result. At birth the infant should be inspected for pallor, cyanosis, retractions, tachypnea, tachycardia, and feeble pulse. The infant's cry will be weak and the muscle tone flaccid (Korones, 1981).

□ *CIRCUMVALLATE PLACENTA* In circumvallate placenta, the fetal surface of the placenta is exposed through a ring

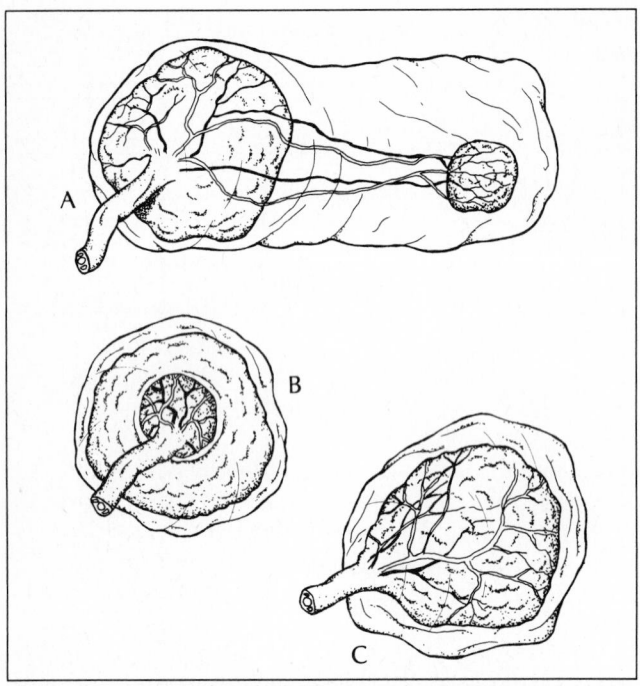

FIGURE 18–18 Placental variations. **A,** Succenturiate placenta. **B,** Circumvallate placenta. **C,** Battledore placenta. (From Abnormalities of the placenta, Clinical Educational Aid no. 12, Ross Laboratories, Columbus, Ohio.)

opening around the umbilical cord (Figure 18–18,*B*). The vessels descend from the cord and end at the margin of the ring instead of coursing through the entire surface area of the placenta. The ring is composed of a double fold of amnion and chorion with some degenerative decidua and fibrin between. The cause of this condition is unknown. Maternal–fetal problems include an increased incidence of late abortion or fetal death, antepartal hemorrhage, prematurity, and abnormal maternal bleeding during or following the third stage of labor, resulting from improper placental separation or shearing of membranes from the placenta.

□ *BATTLEDORE PLACENTA* In the case of battledore placenta, the umbilical cord is inserted at or near the placental margin (Figure 18–18,*C*). As a result, all fetal vessels transverse the placental surface in the same direction. The chances of preterm labor are high because of interference with fetal circulation and nutrition. Fetal distress or bleeding during labor is also likely because of cord compression or vessel rupture.

□ *PLACENTAL INFARCTS AND CALCIFICATIONS* In the aging process the placenta may develop infarcts and calcifications. They become significant if they cover a large enough area to interfere with the uterine–placental–fetal exchange. Altered exchange can also occur with certain maternal disease processes, such as hypertension. Infarcts are most often seen in cases of severe pregnancy-induced hypertension.

Problems Associated with Umbilical Cord

PROLAPSED UMBILICAL CORD

Conditions associated with a prolapsed cord include breech presentation, transverse lies, contracted inlets, small fetus, extra long cord, low-lying placenta, hydramnios, and twin gestations. Any time the inlet is not occluded and the membranes rupture, the cord can be washed down (Figure 18–19) into the birth canal in front of the presenting part.

Maternal implications. When predisposing factors to cord prolapse exist, the client should be considered high risk and should be monitored closely. If prolapse occurs prior to complete cervical dilatation, cesarean delivery is the treatment of choice.

Fetal–neonatal implications. Because with each contraction the umbilical cord becomes compressed between the maternal pelvis and the presenting part, fetal distress is common. If the cord ceases to pulsate, it is generally indicative of fetal demise.

Interventions. Bed rest is indicated for all laboring women with a history of ruptured membranes, until engagement with no cord prolapse has been documented. Furthermore, at the time of spontaneous rupture of membranes or amniotomy, the FHR should be auscultated for at least a full minute. During labor, if fetal bradycardia is detected on auscultation, the woman should be examined to rule out a cord prolapse. Electronic monitor tracings in the presence of cord prolapse show severe, moderate, or prolonged variable decelerations with baseline bradycardia. If these patterns are found, the nurse should examine the woman vaginally.

If a loop of cord is discovered, the gloved fingers are left in the vagina, and attempts are made to lift the fetal head off the cord to relieve the compression until the physician arrives. *This is a life-saving measure.*

The force of gravity can be employed to relieve the compression. The woman assumes the knee-chest position or the bed is adjusted to the Trendelenburg position and the patient should be transported to the delivery or operating room in this position. The nurse must remember that the cord may be occultly prolapsed with an actual loop extending into the vagina or lying alongside the presenting part. It may be pulsating strongly or so weakly that it is difficult to determine on palpation of the cord whether the fetus is alive. Greenhill and Friedman (1974) advocate that a Doppler device be used for auscultation before a fetal death is confirmed.

Occasionally a cord prolapses out the introitus. If this condition is identified in a home situation, some of the previously discussed life-saving actions can be implemented by the nurse. The lateral Sims position may be more feasible for the woman if the position is to be assumed for any extended period of time. The pelvis should be elevated on pillows. Compression on the cord can be relieved in the vagina as in the hospital situation, and wet dressings soaked in a mild salt solution should be wrapped around the protruding cord. The woman should be transported to the hospital immediately. If the cord is pale, limp, and obviously not pulsating, no action is necessary other than transport. At no time should attempts be made to replace the cord into the uterus, because this could cause devastating trauma to the cord and could greatly increase the possibility of intrauterine infection. Vaginal delivery (with or without forceps) is possible if the following criteria are met:

• Cervix is completely dilated
• A vertex is presenting at least at zero station
• Membranes are ruptured
• Pelvic measurements are adequate

If these conditions are not present, cesarean delivery is the method of choice. The woman is taken to the delivery room while the nurse vaginally relieves the pressure on the cord until the infant has been delivered. The medical and nursing team must work together quickly to facilitate delivery in this obstetric emergency.

UMBILICAL CORD ABNORMALITIES

Umbilical cord abnormalities include congenital absence of an umbilical artery, insertion variations, cord length variations, and knots and loops of the cord. Insertion variations include velamentous insertion and vasa previa, and cord length problems include long and short cords.

□ *CONGENITAL ABSENCE OF UMBILICAL ARTERY* Absence of an umbilical artery may have serious fetal implications. The incidence of all types of fetal anomalies is 25% with a "two-vessel" cord.

Immediately after the umbilical cord is cut, it should be inspected to determine whether the correct number of vessels is present. If an artery is absent, the nurse should examine the newborn more closely for anomalies and gestational age problems.

□ *VELAMENTOUS INSERTION* In a velamentous insertion condition, the vessels of the umbilical cord divide some distance from the placenta in the placental membranes (Figure 18–20).

Velamentous insertions occur more frequently in multiple gestations than in singletons. Other placental anomalies often accompany this condition, such as succenturiate placenta. If the vessels become torn during labor, fetal hemorrhage can occur and is signaled by FHR abnormalities accompanied by vaginal bleeding (Gabbe et al., 1977).

□ *VASA PREVIA* When the vessels of a velamentous insertion transverse the internal os and appear in front of the fetus, a vasa previa has occurred. Fetal hemorrhage with asphyxia is likely to result because the hemorrhage will

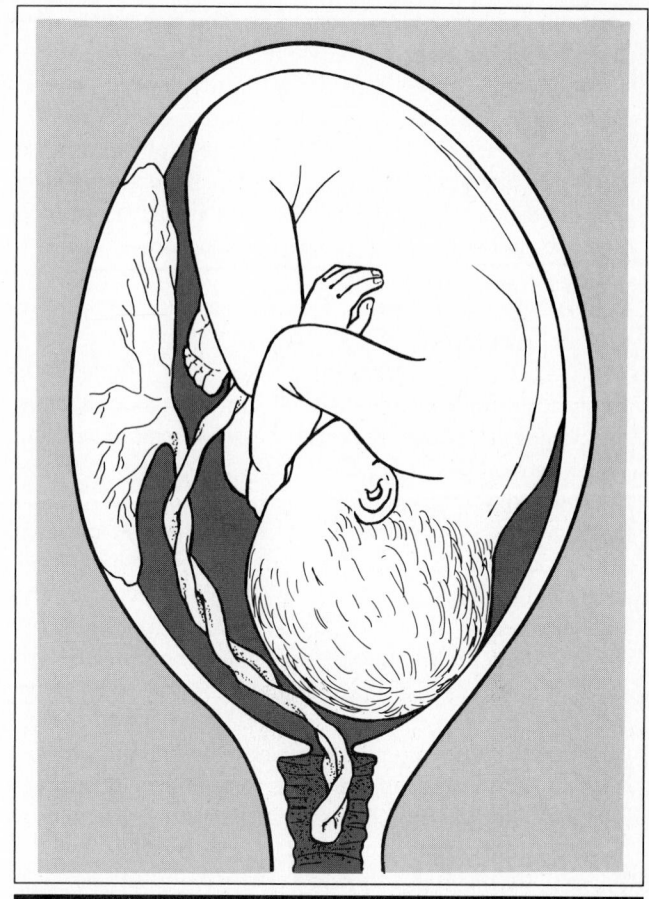

FIGURE 18–19 Prolapse of cord.

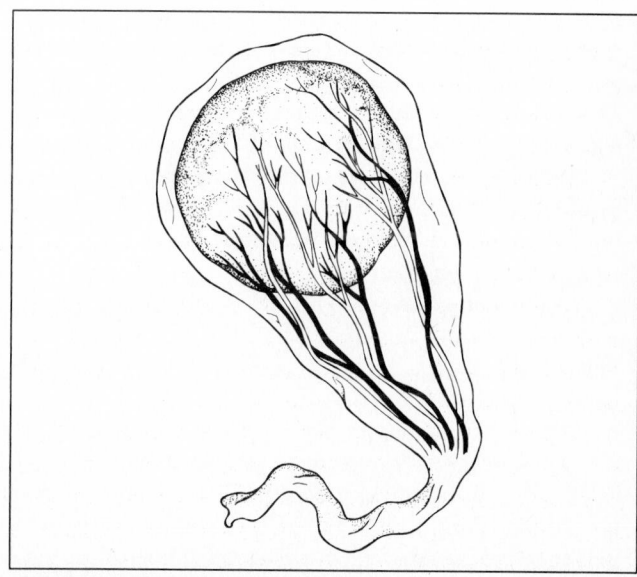

FIGURE 18–20 Placenta with a velamentous umbilical cord insertion.

increased in some cases of hydramnios, indicating that an increased functioning of the placental tissue may be contributory.

There are two types of hydramnios: chronic and acute. In the chronic type, the fluid volume gradually increases. Most cases are of this variety. In acute cases, the volume increases rapidly over a period of a few days.

Maternal implications. When the amount of amniotic fluid is over 3000 mL, the woman experiences shortness of breath and edema in the lower extremities from compression of the vena cava. If hydramnios is severe enough, she can experience intense pain. The acute form of hydramnios tends to be more severe. Milder forms of hydramnios occur more frequently and are associated with minimal symptoms. Hydramnios is associated with such maternal disorders as diabetes and Rh sensitization. As mentioned earlier, it may be found in multiple gestations.

Antepartally, if the amniotic fluid is removed too rapidly, abruptio placentae can result from a decreased attachment area. Because of these overstretched fibers, uterine dysfunction can occur intrapartally, and there is increased incidence of postpartal hemorrhage.

Fetal–neonatal implications. Fetal malformations and premature delivery are common with hydramnios; thus perinatal mortality is high. Prolapsed cord can occur when the membranes rupture, which adds a further complication for the fetus. The incidence of malpresentations is also increased.

Interventions. Hydramnios should be suspected when the fundal height increases out of proportion to the gestational age. As the amount of fluid increases, the nurse may have difficulty palpating the fetus and auscultating the FHTs. In the more severe cases, the maternal abdomen appears extremely tense and tight on inspection. On sonography, large spaces can be identified between the fetus and the uterine wall. Also at this time, an anencephalic infant or a dilated fetal stomach resulting from esophageal atresia may be identified, and multiple gestations may be confirmed. An x-ray fetogram will also show a radiolucent area of space and fetal skeletal defects if present.

If the accumulation of amniotic fluid has become severe enough to cause maternal dyspnea and pain, hospitalization and removal of the excessive fluid are required. This can be done vaginally or by amniocentesis. The dangers of performing the technique vaginally are prolapsed cord and the inability to remove the fluid slowly. If amniocentesis is performed, it should be done with the aid of sonography to prevent inadvertent damage to the fetus and placenta. The fluid should be removed slowly to prevent abruption (Pritchard and MacDonald, 1980).

When performing amniocentesis, it is vital to maintain sterile technique. The nurse can offer support to the couple by explaining the procedure to them. The nurse assists the clinician in interpreting sonographic or x-ray findings.

OLIGOHYDRAMNIOS

Oligohydramnios, in which the amount of amniotic fluid is severely reduced and concentrated, is a rare maternal finding. The exact cause of this condition is unknown. It is found in cases of postmaturity, with IUGR secondary to placental insufficiency, and in fetal conditions associated with renal and urinary malfunction. If oligohydramnios occurs in the first part of pregnancy, there is a danger of fetal adhesions (one part of the fetus may adhere to another part). Pulmonary hypoplasia has been found, theoretically due to lack of fluid inhaled in the terminal air sacs (Pritchard and MacDonald, 1980).

Maternal implications. Labor can be dysfunctional and can begin before term. It is usually extremely painful for the woman, and progress is protracted.

Fetal–neonatal implications. Fetal hypoxia may occur due to umbilical cord compression (Greenhill and Friedman, 1974). At birth these infants appear wrinkled and leathery, and serious skeletal deformities are often found (Pritchard and MacDonald, 1980).

COMPLICATIONS INVOLVING THE PASSAGE

The passage includes the maternal bony pelvis, beginning at the pelvic inlet and ending at the pelvic outlet, and the maternal soft tissues within these anatomic areas. A contracture in any of the described areas can result in CPD. Abnormal fetal presentations and positions occur in CPD as the fetus attempts to accommodate to its passage.

The gynecoid and anthropoid pelvic types usually are adequate for vertex delivery, but the android and platypelloid types predispose to CPD. Certain combinations of types also can result in pelvic diameters inadequate for vertex delivery. (See Chapter 14 for an in-depth description of the types of pelves and their implications for childbirth.)

Contractures of the Inlet

The pelvic inlet is contracted if the shortest anterior-posterior diameter is less than 10 cm or the greatest transverse diameter is less than 12 cm. The anterior-posterior diameter may be approximated by measuring the diagonal conjugate, which in the contracted inlet is less than 11.5 cm. Clinical and x-ray pelvimetry are used to determine the smallest anterior-posterior diameter through which the fetal head must pass. Sonography then can be utilized to measure the biparietal diameter of the fetal head, which averages 9.5–9.8 cm.

When both diameters are contracted, the incidence of difficult deliveries increases. The risks associated with inlet contractures are numerous. The course of labor tends to be prolonged with unsatisfactory dilatation of the cervix. Because the entire force of the labor contractions is exerted on the membranes, PROM may occur. The lack of fetal descent in the nullipara before the onset of labor may potentiate the risk of prolapse of the cord. In these cases, vertex presentations assume other presentations, such as face and shoulder. Pathologic retraction rings and uterine rupture may also develop. Perinatal mortality increases for the fetus. Excessive molding and skull fractures may lead to fetal intracranial hemorrhage. A large caput succedaneum may also form.

The management of inlet contractures begins with assessment of the size and presentation of the fetus, the pelvic configuration, uterine activity, cervical dilatation, and any problems during previous labors and deliveries. Based upon these findings, the decision is made to proceed with a trial labor or a cesarean delivery.

Contractures of the Midpelvis

Contractures of the midpelvis are more common than inlet contractures. The plane of the midpelvis is formed from the margin of the symphysis pubis through the ischial spines and touches the sacrum near the fourth or fifth vertebra. Although a satisfactory method of measuring the midpelvis manually does not exist, prominent spines, converging pelvic walls, or a narrow sacrosciatic notch can be ascertained on vaginal examination. Midpelvis contractures cause transverse arrest of the head, leading to potentially difficult midforceps delivery.

The treatment goal is to allow the natural forces of labor to push the biparietal diameter of the fetal head beyond the potential interspinous obstruction. Although forceps may be used, they cause difficulty because pulling on the head destroys flexion and the space is further diminished. A bulging perineum and crowning indicate that the obstruction has been passed.

Contractures of the Outlet

An interischial tuberous diameter of less than 8 cm constitutes an outlet contracture. Frequently, outlet and midpelvic contractures occur simultaneously. Whether vaginal delivery can occur depends on the woman's interischial tuberous diameter and the fetal posterosagittal diameter.

Implications of Pelvic Contractures

Maternal implications. Labor is prolonged and protracted in the presence of CPD, and premature rupture of membranes can result from the force of the unequally distributed contractions being exerted on the fetal membranes. In obstructed labor, uterine rupture can occur. With protracted descent, necrosis of maternal soft tissues can result from pressure exerted by the fetal head. Eventu-

ally necrosis can cause fistulas from the vagina to other nearby structures. Difficult forceps deliveries can also result in damage to maternal soft tissue.

Fetal–neonatal implications. If the membranes rupture and the fetal head has not entered the inlet, there is a grave danger of cord prolapse. Extreme molding of the fetal head can result in skull fracture or intracranial hemorrhage. Traumatic forceps deliveries can cause damage to the fetal skull and CNS.

Interventions. The adequacy of the maternal pelvis for a vaginal delivery should be assessed intrapartally as well as antepartally. During the intrapartal assessment, the size of the fetus and its presentation, position, and lie must also be considered. (See Chapter 15 for intrapartal assessment techniques.)

The nurse should suspect CPD when labor is prolonged, cervical dilatation and effacement are slow, and engagement of the presenting part is delayed. Contractions should be monitored continuously, and the labor progress should be charted on the Friedman graph. The fetus should also be monitored continuously.

If the physician is uncertain whether the infant will be delivered vaginally, a trial of labor may be given. The patient is allowed to labor to determine if the forces of the uterine contractions can overcome the actual or suspected disproportion. If contractions are not of adequate strength, the membranes are ruptured or oxytocin is administered to stimulate uterine activity. The trial of labor is allowed to continue only as long as dilatation and descent are progressive (Friedman and Sachtleben, 1976). The exact time limits (6–18 hours, rarely more than 24 hours) are based on the judgment of the physician. No fetal descent, ineffective contractions, and lack of progressive dilatation and effacement of the cervix are evidence of the failure of the trial of labor and cesarean delivery is done.

Nursing actions during the labor trial are the same as during any procedure in which oxytocin is being administered. The woman and fetus must be monitored continuously.

The couple may need support in coping with the stresses of this complicated labor. The nurse should keep the couple informed of what is happening and explain the procedures that are being utilized. This knowledge can reassure the couple that measures are being taken to resolve the problem.

COMPLICATIONS OF THIRD AND FOURTH STAGES

Postpartal Hemorrhage

Postpartal hemorrhage is defined as a loss of blood in excess of 500 mL in the first 24 hours following delivery.

Immediate postpartal hemorrhage is most commonly caused by uterine atony and lacerations of the vagina and cervix. In addition, retention of placental fragments may cause immediate or delayed postpartal hemorrhage.

UTERINE ATONY

Relaxation of the uterus (or insufficient contractions) following delivery can frequently be anticipated in the presence of (a) overdistention of the uterus that occurs with multiple fetuses, macrosomic fetus, or hydramnios; (b) dysfunctional labor that has already indicated the uterus is contracting in an other-than-normal pattern; (c) oxytocin stimulation or augmentation during labor; and (d) the use of anesthesia that produces uterine relaxation.

Hemorrhage from uterine atony may be slow and steady rather than sudden and massive. The blood may escape from the vagina or collect in the uterus. Because of the increased blood volume associated with pregnancy, changes in maternal blood pressure and pulse may not occur until blood loss has been significant.

After delivery of the placenta, the fundus should be palpated to assure that it is firm and well contracted. If it is not firm, vigorous massage should be instituted. Oxytocics (Pitocin, Methergine, or Ergotrate) may be given. If the bleeding persists, the physician undertakes bimanual uterine compression, which consists of using one gloved hand to massage the uterine fundus externally while the other gloved hand is inserted into the vagina and the closed fist is pressed against the uterus. With this procedure the uterus is compressed and massaged and hemorrhage from uterine atony can usually be controlled. If an intravenous line is not already infusing, one should be established with oxytocin (Pitocin) added at a rapid rate. Blood transfusions may be ordered. Oxygen at 4–7 L/min is given by face mask. The physician manually checks the uterine cavity for retained placental fragments and also inspects the cervix and vagina for lacerations. The combination of bimanual compression, oxytocics, and blood transfusion is usually effective in treating uterine atony. The fundus should be assessed frequently for the next few hours to see that it remains contracted.

RETAINED PLACENTA

Hemorrhage may occur after the delivery of the newborn but before delivery of the placenta. In this instance, the physician observes the firmness of the fundus and administers fundal massage if needed. When the placenta is ready to separate, expression (delivery) of the placenta is enhanced by massaging the fundus. If signs of placental separation have not occurred, the physician manually removes the placenta by inserting a gloved hand into the uterus and placing the fingers at the placental margin. Then the placenta is gently separated from the uterine wall. During this procedure, the other hand remains on the uterine fundus, externally. After delivery of the placenta, the consistency of the fundus is assessed. If it is boggy and bleeding contin-

ues, the same interventions instituted for uterine atony are performed.

RETAINED PLACENTAL FRAGMENTS

Hemorrhage from retained placental fragments is not usually a cause of immediate postpartal hemorrhage, but tends to be a major cause of later postpartal bleeding. To prevent this type of hemorrhage, the placenta should be inspected after delivery for evidence of missing pieces or cotyledons. The membranes should be inspected for absent sections or for vessels that traverse from the edge of the placenta outward along the membranes, which may indicate placenta succenturiate and a retained lobe. The uterine cavity may be checked for retained placental fragments or membranes.

PLACENTA ACCRETA

The chorionic villi attach directly to the myometrium of the uterus in placenta accreta. Two other types of placental adherence are placenta increta, in which the myometrium is invaded, and placenta percreta, in which the myometrium is penetrated. The adherence itself may be total, partial, or focal, depending on the amount of placental involvement.

The primary complication with placenta accreta is maternal hemorrhage. Breen and coworkers (1977) cite placenta previa, postpartal hemorrhage, and previous cesarean deliveries as being correlated with placental adherence. An abdominal hysterectomy may be the necessary treatment, depending on the amount and depth of involvement.

LACERATIONS

Lacerations of the cervix or vagina may be indicated when bright red vaginal bleeding persists in the presence of a well-contracted uterus. Shock that is out of proportion to blood loss may result from uterine laceration. Upper vaginal lacerations are most frequently in the posterior fornix. The physician inspects the lower aspects of the uterus, cervix, and vagina. If lacerations are found, they are sutured.

Inversion of Uterus

Uterine inversion occurs when the uterus turns inside out during the third stage of labor. This rare occurrence can be caused by a lax uterine wall coupled with undue tension on an umbilical cord when the placenta has not separated. Forceful pressure on the fundus with a dilated cervix and sudden emptying of the uterine contents may be contributing factors. Maternal bleeding with shock is rapid and profound. The fundus is absent from the abdominal cavity on palpation.

Interventions. The uterus must be replaced manually be grasping the vaginal mass, spreading the cervical ring with the fingers and thumb, and steadily forcing the fundus upward. The patient is often placed under deep anesthesia. Occasionally tocolytic agents are given (Oxorn, 1980).

Nursing interventions should be directed at management of shock. Volume replacement should be a priority. The nurse ascertains whether a vein is patent for intravenous infusion and initiates the collection of a blood sample for type and cross-matching. Blood pressure and pulse rate should be monitored every 5 minutes by the nurse until the anesthesiologist arrives and is ready to assume this duty.

Careful monitoring of the intake and output is vital. An indwelling catheter is usually inserted into the bladder after the uterus is replaced. Kidney function is a good indicator of adequate tissue perfusion and tissue damage from anoxia. The uterus should be assessed frequently to assure it remains contracted.

Genital Tract Trauma

HEMATOMA

The most common site of a genital tract hematoma is the lateral vaginal wall in the area of the ischial spines. If the hematoma is 3 cm or less and does not enlarge, it does not require therapy. A hematoma that continues to enlarge may allow enough blood loss to precipitate signs and symptoms of shock, sensations of intense internal pressure, and severe pain. In this instance, the hematoma should be drained, and the bleeding point located and ligated (Work, 1982).

First, nursing measures are directed toward further assessment when the patient complains of intense pressure and pain in the perineal or rectal area. The perineum should be inspected for bruising or areas of swelling. Maternal blood pressure and pulse are assessed.

Signs and symptoms of shock in the presence of a well-contracted uterus and no visible vaginal blood loss should alert the nurse to the possibility of hematoma. The hematoma may be palpated by gentle rectal exam, although this procedure may be quite uncomfortable for the patient. After alerting the physician, the nurse continues to monitor vital signs, and may initiate intravenous fluids if hypovolemic shock is developing.

PERINEAL LACERATIONS

A laceration of the perineal tissues may occur when there is excessive stretching of the perineal tissues or when there is an extension of the episiotomy. The laceration is repaired by suturing.

COMPLICATED CHILDBIRTH: EFFECTS ON THE FAMILY

A complicated pregnancy and difficult labor and delivery are crisis situations that can test the coping mechanisms of every individual involved. The family may respond to the crisis in relatively typical ways or may respond dysfunctionally.

During the antepartal period, the family may have ambivalent feelings toward a complicated pregnancy. Fear and anxiety about the woman's health and the health and welfare of the fetus may be exhibited as hostile behaviors and guilt feelings. The expectant mother may have feelings of inadequacy with regard to her womanhood and ability to reproduce (Cabela, 1977). The father may blame himself for impregnating his partner, or the family may accuse the health care team of poor management.

Simultaneously, the expectant parents, especially the woman, are emotionally investing themselves in the child. She perceives the child as part of herself. With birth, the child becomes a person in his or her own right and the process of attachment occurs.

When an infant is stillborn or dies following delivery, the couple must mourn and deal with the pain of detaching themselves. This process involves anger, guilt, pain, and sadness. However, because they have had little or no time to know the child as a person, the soothing part of the mourning process—"identification" built on memories, shared experiences, and mutual living—is absent (Furman, 1978).

Parents of an ill or deformed infant must not only resolve their feelings of guilt and grief, but they must also prepare themselves to care for that child. This couple may be unable to face the possibility that their infant may not survive. They may doubt their ability to properly care for the child. The costs of caring for the high-risk child are great, perhaps creating financial difficulties for the family. In addition, the emotional toll of caring for such a child may be extreme.

Nursing Management

The birth of an ill, abnormal, or stillborn infant presents the couple with the reality that they may have been fearing throughout pregnancy. It is imperative that the medical and nursing staff respond in supportive and sympathetic ways. Typically, however, health care personnel avoid eye contact and communication with the woman or family. Another common reaction on the part of the nursing staff is the use of cliches (Saylor, 1977). Comments such as "The poor thing is better off" of "You can have other children" are offered as comfort. However, the bereaved parents perceive the loss not only as the death of their child but also as a loss of a portion of themselves, and such comments by nursing personnel seem to negate the child's very existence.

When a malformed infant is born, powerful reactions, even among caregivers, are not unusual. Kennell (1978) points out that initially the staff may be fascinated to hear about and eager to see a malformed infant. Frequently, such a child is the focus of a great deal of staff attention in the nursery. After they have seen the newborn, they feel shock and sadness similar to that experienced by the parents. This reaction is especially common for those who have had little experience with congenital anomalies. Finally, in an effort to deal with their reactions, they have a tendency to wish to avoid the parents. In such instances it is frequently helpful to provide the staff with occasions to talk through their feelings so that they can be more supportive of the family in its grief. In some centers with intensive care nurseries, this practice has been formalized through regular staff meetings and has been of great benefit to staff and, indirectly, to families.

Basic actions the nurse can take to provide emotional support are often of real help to a family. When a labor is complicated or when the fetus has died, it is imperative that the client have consistent support and not be left alone. The partner should be encouraged to remain, and the nurse should also be present to observe the woman or couple and provide support. Thoughtful comfort measures such as ice chips, clean chux, and judicious use of analgesics also demonstrate caring attitudes (Kowalski and Osborn, 1977).

In the event of a stillborn delivery or infant death, the couple is given the opportunity to see and hold their child, regardless of condition or abnormality. They should not be forced, but if they are uncertain, the nurse can explain that fantasy is often worse than fact and that seeing the infant frequently facilitates the grieving process. The father must not make this decision for his partner. The couple should, of course, be prepared for what they will see. Simple explanations of the baby's appearance—including a description of color, skin, any abnormalities or bruises, and body temperature—will prepare them. The nurse should wipe off any blood or feces before showing the infant to the couple. At this time the nurse may tactfully point out attractive aspects of the infant's appearance so that he or she becomes more of an individual to the couple. Some agencies are even showing couples who so desire it infants stillborn before the age of viability and report positive results (Kowalski and Osborn, 1977).

When a malformed infant is born, the couple must deal with their mourning and with the future needs of their child. Kennell (1978) points out that whenever possible the parents and their infant should be kept together following delivery. Frequently, the newborn can be returned to the parents after a brief physical assessment in the nursery. The contact between the parents and infant may ultimately be a source of great satisfaction to the parents if successfully accomplished.

The decision to permit the siblings to view the dead newborn should be based on the child's age and personality. Adolescents may be offered a choice. Younger school-aged children are not helped by seeing the infant but may benefit by attending the funeral service. Some preschool children may benefit from attending the service with their parents, but they especially are *not* helped by seeing their dead sibling (Furman, 1978).

Any time a complication occurs during pregnancy, financial difficulties may occur, even in families that are not classified as low income. Financial strain may be embarrassing for the family, and they may be hesitant to voice their concerns. The nurse must be familiar with hospital, federal, and local resources in their community so that the caregivers can make them known to high-risk clients.

The parents of a child born with a disability require time to work through their feelings of grief. They then need and desire factual information about their child's disability, his or her special needs, and the care required. Using a collaborative approach, members of the health team can provide the necessary teaching and information. They can also refer the parents to community groups and resources that are directed toward providing financial assistance and helping the child develop to his fullest potential. Community groups also exist that provide support to the parents and can be a source of great comfort to them.

SUMMARY

Childbirth is traditionally viewed as normal, happy, and uneventful, and usually it is. However, a wide variety of complications may develop that represent a hazard to the woman and her unborn child. It is essential that the labor and delivery client be assessed carefully and provided with appropriate care to prevent problems when possible or to treat them to facilitate satisfactory outcome.

References

Assali, N. S. 1972. *Pathophysiology of gestation: maternal disorders.* New York: Academic Press.

Benson, R. C. 1977. *Handbook of obstetrics and gynecology.* Los Altos, Calif.: Lange Medical Publications.

Bishop, E. H. Nov. 1981. Acceleration of fetal pulmonary maturity. *Obstet. Gynecol.* (Suppl.) 58:48.

Bonica, J. J. 1967. *Principles and practices of obstetric analgesia and anesthesia.* Philadelphia: F. A. Davis Co.

Brazy, J. E., and Pupkin, M. J. 1979. Effects of maternal isoxsuprine administration on pre-term infants. *J. Pediatr.* 94:444.

Breen, J. L., et al. 1977. Placenta accreta, increta, and percreta: a survey of 40 cases. *Obstet. Gynecol.* 49:34.

Butane, P., et al. 1980. Mothers' perceptions of their labor experiences. *Mat. Child Nurs. J.* 9:73.

Cabela, B. 1977. Complications of childbearing: psychological and socioeconomic implications. In *Maternity nursing today,* eds. J. P. Clausen et al. New York: McGraw-Hill Book Co.

Cohen, W. 1977. Influence of the duration of second stage labor on perinatal outcome and puerperal morbidity. *Obstet. Gynecol.* 49:266.

Csapo, A. I., and Herczeg, J. Nov. 1977. Arrest of premature labor with isoxsuprine. *Am. J. Obstet. Gynecol.* 129:482.

Danforth, D., ed. 1982. *Obstetrics and gynecology.* 4th ed. Philadelphia: Harper & Row.

Epstein, M. F., et al. 1979. Neonatal hypoglycemia after beta-sympathomimetic tocolytic therapy. *J. Pediatr.* 94:449.

Erickson, M. 1976. The relationship between psychological variables and specific complications of pregnancy, labor and delivery. *J. Psychosom. Res.* 20:21.

Foster, S. D. 1981. Ritodrine for arrest of premature labor. *MCN.* 6:204.

Friedman, E. A. 1978. *Labor: clinical evaluation and management.* 2nd ed. New York: Appleton-Century-Crofts.

Friedman, E. A., and Sachtleben, M. R. 1976. Station of the fetal presenting part, VI. Arrest of descent in nulliparas. *Obstet. Gynecol.* 47:129.

Friedman, E. A., et al. 1977. Dysfunctional labor, XII. Long-term effects on infant. *Am. J. Obstet. Gynecol.* 127:779.

Furman, E. Winter 1978. The death of a newborn: care of the parents. *Birth Fam. J.* 5:214

Gabbe, S. G., et al. 1977. Fetal heart rate response to acute hemorrhage. *Obstet. Gynecol.* 49(2):247.

Genest, M. 1981. Preparation for childbirth—evidence for efficacy, a review. *J. Obstet. Gynecol. Neonat. Nurs.* 10:82.

Giacoia, G. P., and Yaffe, S. 1982. Perinatal pharmacology. In *Gynecology and obstetrics,* vol. 3, chapter 100, ed. J. J. Sciarri. Philadelphia: Harper & Row.

Greenhill, J. P., and Friedman, E. 1974. *Biological principles and modern practice of obstetrics.* Philadelphia: W. B. Saunders Co.

Itzkowicz, D. A. 1979. A survey of 59 triplet pregnancies. *Br. J. Obstet. Gynaecol.* 86:23.

Jennings, B. M. 1979. Improving your management of DIC. *Nursing 79.* 5:60.

Kauppila, A., et al. 1978. Effects of ritodrine and isoxsuprine with or without dexamethasone during late pregnancy. *Obstet. Gynecol.* 51(3):288.

Kennell, J. H. Winter 1978. Birth of a malformed baby: helping the family. *Birth Fam. J.* 5:219.

Kochenour, N. 1977. The management of breech presentations. *PCC News.* 3(5):32.

Korones, S. 1981. *The high risk newborn infant: the basis for intensive care.* St. Louis: The C. V. Mosby Co.

Kowalski, K., and Osborn, M. Jan./Feb. 1977. Helping mothers of stillborn infants to grieve. *Am. J. Mat. Child Nurs.* 2:29.

Kübler-Ross, E. 1969. *On death and dying.* New York: The Macmillan Co.

Lederman, R. P., et al. 1977. Endogenous plasma epinephrine and norepinephrine in last trimester pregnancy. *Am. J. Obstet. Gynecol.* 129:5.

Lederman, R. P., et al. 1979. Relationship of psychological factors in pregnancy to progress in labor. *Nurs. Research.* 28:94.

Lipshitz, J. July 1981. Beta-adrenergic agonists. *Seminars Perinatol.* 5:252.

Lipshitz, J., and Schneider, J. M. 1980. Inhibition of labor. In *Gynecology and obstetrics,* vol. 3, chapter 87, ed. J. J. Sciarri. Philadelphia: Harper & Row.

Oxorn, H. 1980. *Human birth and delivery.* 4th ed. New York: Appleton-Century-Crofts.

Paul, R. H., and Petrie, R. H. 1973. *Fetal intensive care: current concepts.* Los Angeles: University of Southern California School of Medicine.

Philipsen, T., et al. Sept. 1981. Pulmonary edema following ritodrine-saline infusion in premature labor. *Obstet. Gynecol.* 58:304.

Pritchard, J. A., and MacDonald, P. C. 1980. *Williams obstetrics.* 16th ed. New York: Appleton-Century-Crofts.

Quilligan, E. J. 1980. *Current therapy in obstetrics and gynecology.* Philadelphia: W. B. Saunders Co.

Reid, D. E., et al. 1972. *Principles and management of human reproduction.* Philadelphia: W. B. Saunders Co.

Sasmor, J. L., et al. 1981. Childbirth education in 1980. *J. Obstet. Gynecol. Neonat. Nurs.* 10:155.

Saylor, R. D. 1977. Nursing response to mothers of stillborn infants. *J. Obstet. Gynecol. Neonatal Nurs.* 6:39.

Spellacy, W. N., et al. July 1978. The acute effects of ritodrine infusion on maternal metabolism: measurements of levels of glucose, insulin, glucagon, triglycerides, cholesterol, placental lactogen and chorionic gonadotropin. *Am. J. Obstet. Gynecol.* 131(6):637.

Stubblefield, P. G. Oct. 1978. Pulmonary edema occurring after therapy with dexamethasone and terbutaline for premature labor: a case report. *Am. J. Obstet. Gynecol.* 132:341.

Talbert, L. M., and Blatt, P. M. 1979. Disseminated intravascular coagulation in obstetrics. *Clin. Obstet. Gynecol.* 22:4.

Thornfeldt, R. E., et al. May 1978. The effect of glucocorticoids on the maturation of premature lung membranes. *Am. J. Obstet. Gynecol.* 131:143.

Timm, M. M. 1979. Prenatal education evaluation. *Nurs. Research.* 28:338.

Work, B. A. Nov. 1982. Caring for genital tract birth trauma. *Contemp. Obstet. Gynecol.* 20:82.

Zacharias, J. F. 1981. Childbirth education classes: effects on attitudes toward childbirth in high risk indigent women. *J. Obstet. Gynecol. Neonat. Nurs.* 10:265.

Additional Readings

Berkowitz, R. L., et al. July 1978. The relationship between premature rupture of the membranes and the respiratory distress syndrome. *Am. J. Obstet. Gynecol.* 131:503.

Brodicks, K. 1965. *Patterns of shock: implications for nursing care.* New York: Macmillan Co.

Freeman, R. K. 1974. Management of acute fetal distress. In *A clinical approach to fetal monitoring.* San Leandro, Calif.: Berkeley BioEngineering, Inc.

————. 1974. Monitoring records from selected clinical cases. In *A clinical approach to fetal monitoring.* San Leandro, Calif.: Berkeley BioEngineering, Inc.

Friedman, E. A. 1974. *Management of difficult labor.* MedCom slide presentation.

Guyton, A. 1976. *Textbook of medical physiology.* Philadelphia: W. B. Saunders Co.

Klaus, M. H., and Fanaroff, A. A. 1973. *Care of the high risk neonate.* Philadelphia: W. B. Saunders Co.

Meissner, J. E. 1980. Predicting a patient's anxiety level during labor: a two part assessment tool. *Nurs. 80.* 10:50.

Miller, J. M., et al. Sept. 1978. Premature labor and premature rupture of the membranes. *Am. J. Obstet. Gynecol.* 132:1.

Ness, P. M., and Perkins, H. A. 1979. Cryoprecipitate as a reliable source of fibrinogen replacement. *J.A.M.A.* 241:1691.

Rayburn, W. F., et al. 1981. Umbilical cord length and intrapartum complications. *Obstet. Gynecol.* 57(4):450.

Rubin, R. 1961. Puerperal change. *Nurs. Outlook.* 9:753.

Young, B. K., et al. 1980. Intravenous dexamethasome for prevention of neonatal respiratory distress—a prospective controlled study. *Am. J. Obstet. Gynecol.* 138:203.

■ 19 ■

ELECTIVE OBSTETRIC PROCEDURES

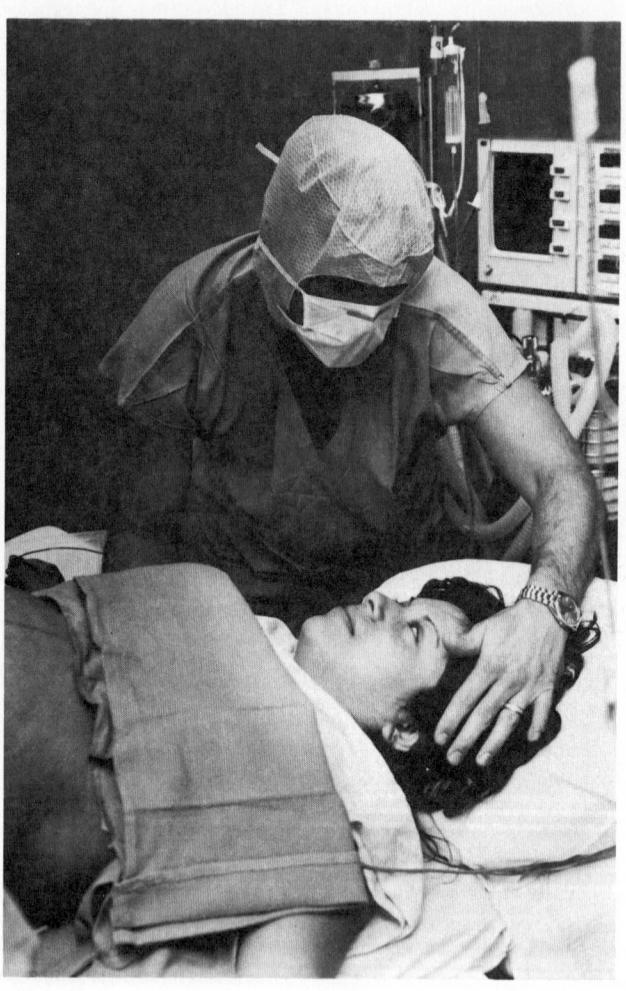

■ CHAPTER CONTENTS

VERSION

External or Cephalic Version

Internal or Podalic Version

Nursing Interventions

AMNIOTOMY

INDUCTION OF LABOR

Contraindications

Labor Readiness

Methods

Prostaglandin Administration

EPISIOTOMY

Nursing Interventions

FORCEPS DELIVERIES

Types of Forceps

Indications

Complications

Prerequisites for Forceps Application

Trial or Failed Forceps Delivery

VACUUM EXTRACTION

Nursing Interventions

CESAREAN BIRTH

Indications for Cesarean Delivery

Maternal Mortality and Morbidity

Types of Cesarean Deliveries

Uterine Incisions

Nursing Interventions for Family Having Cesarean Birth

Analgesia and Anesthesia

■ OBJECTIVES

- Describe the various methods for version and the nursing interventions for each method.

- Discuss the use of amniotomy in current maternity care.

- Compare methods for inducing labor, explaining their advantages and disadvantages.

- Describe the types of episiotomies performed, the rationale for each, and the associated nursing intervention.

- Describe the indications for forceps delivery and types of forceps that may be used.

- Discuss the use of vacuum extraction including indications, procedure, complications, and related nursing interventions.

- Explain the indications for cesarean birth, impact on the family unit, preparation and teaching needs, and associated nursing interventions.

The use of operative or other obstetric procedures has increased in recent years. More childbearing women are being identified as high risk, and the birth experience must be facilitated whenever possible in these cases to alleviate the possible dangers to the woman and infant. In addition, certain obstetric procedures are performed to accommodate the wishes of the expectant family or the physician.

Obstetric procedures discussed in this chapter are versions, amniotomy, induction of labor, episiotomy, forceps delivery, vacuum extraction, and cesarean birth.

VERSION

Version is the alteration of fetal position by abdominal or intrauterine manipulation to accomplish a more favorable fetal position for delivery. Three types of version are recognized. *External* or *cephalic version* (Figure 19–1) is externally accomplished; *podalic version* is an internal procedure; and *combined version* includes a simultaneous external and internal procedure.

External or Cephalic Version

The infant is rotated from a breech or transverse position to cephalic position by external abdominal manipulation. This version may be done before term and is more successful in multiparous women with lax abdominal walls.

The prerequisites for cephalic version are as follows (Pritchard and MacDonald, 1980; VanDorsten et al., 1981):

1. The presenting part must not be engaged.
2. The abdominal wall must be thin enough to permit accurate palpation.
3. The uterine wall must not be irritable.
4. There must be a sufficient quantity of amniotic fluid in the uterus, and the membranes must be intact. Oligo-

hydramnios or rupture of the membranes prevents adequate amniotic fluid from being present for unrestricted turning of the fetus.

Contraindications include the following:

1. Fetopelvic disproportion that would prevent a vaginal delivery.
2. Third-trimester bleeding.
3. Low implantation of the placenta.
4. Previous uterine surgery.

An external or cephalic version may be done with tocolysis (administration of ritodrine). With this method the woman receives intravenous ritodrine (Yutopar) to relax the uterus and under continuous fetal monitoring, the fetus is converted from breech to vertex presentation. The procedure is done at 37 weeks' gestation because most fetuses still in breech presentation at this time will not spontaneously convert. Proponents of this method cite a significant decrease in breech presentation at term (90% of fetuses converted remain in vertex presentation) and a resultant decrease in the number of cesarean deliveries (Fall and Nilsson, 1979; VanDorsten et al., 1981).

External or cephalic version under tocolysis is contraindicated in a woman with congenital or acquired heart disease, or thyroid dysfunction because of the risk of adverse effects of ritodrine (VanDorsten et al., 1981).

Internal or Podalic Version

Internal or podalic version is used to rotate a fetus in a vertex or transverse position to a breech position. The only indication for this is the delivery of the second twin (Pritchard and MacDonald, 1980). In this procedure, after the first twin is delivered the physician reaches up into the uterine cavity, grasps one or both feet of the second twin and draws them through the cervix.

The fetus, regardless of gestational size, is in danger during a podalic version. This emergency procedure should be utilized when prolapsed cord results in fetal dis-

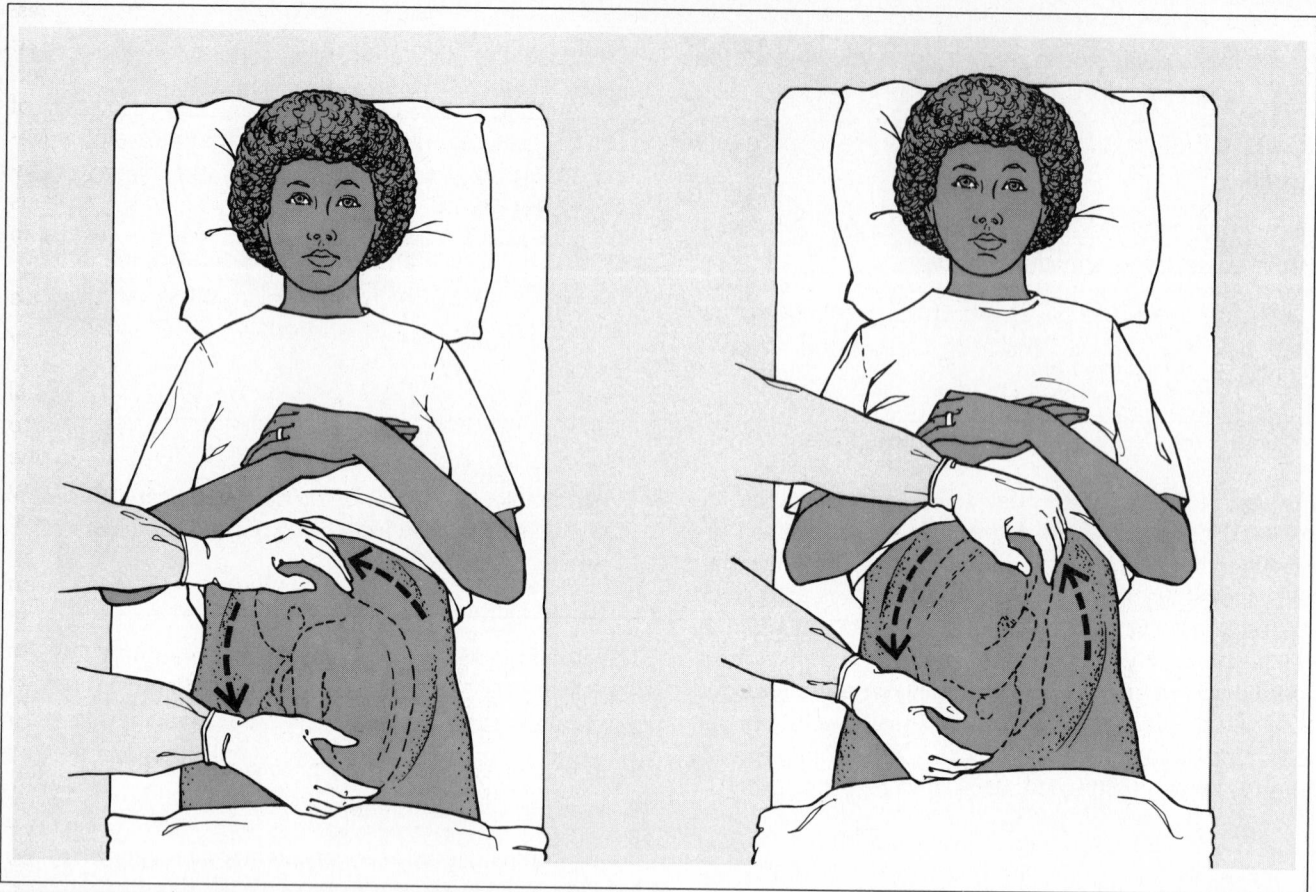

FIGURE 19–1 External version of fetus from breech to cephalic presentation.

tress, or when immediate delivery is required. If time permits, a planned cesarean birth is a more desirable procedure than podalic version.

During a podalic version there is a danger of uterine rupture in the presence of a stretched lower uterine segment. Prolapse of the umbilical cord may occur with a fully dilated cervix and an unengaged fetal part.

Nursing Interventions

Nursing care during an external version includes assessment of maternal blood pressure every 5 minutes and continuous monitoring of the fetus. These assessments should continue for 30 minutes after the version. For an internal version, the clinician may request an elbow-length version glove, which is worn over a regular sterile glove. After an internal version, the woman should be observed closely for hemorrhage because the intrauterine manipulation may cause trauma to the uterine musculature, thus preventing it from contracting properly (see Nursing Care Plan for hemorrhage in Chapter 18).

AMNIOTOMY

Amniotomy, the artificial rupturing of membranes, is probably the most common operative procedure in obstetrics. It may be done as a surgical method of labor induction or after active labor is established. In a study conducted by Martell et al. (1976), it was noted that 66% of all laboring women reach full dilatation with intact membranes. Of these women, 12% had intact membranes at the time of delivery. Martell et al. demonstrated that labor is shortened after an amniotomy if it is performed when the cervix is dilated 4–5 cm, probably because the hard fetal head comes in contact with the cervix and hastens cervical dilatation. However, Martell found that infants born following artificial rupture of the membranes at 4–5 cm cervical dilatation had a slightly lower pH and an increased incidence of early decelerations. These side effects could be deleterious in the case of a high-risk pregnancy, in which the fetus may already be compromised.

Before an amniotomy is performed, the fetus is assessed for presentation, position, and station. Unless the head is well engaged in the pelvis, most physicians do not advocate an amniotomy because of the danger of a prolapsed cord.

The nurse explains the procedure to the laboring woman, who is draped in preparation for a vaginal examination and whose perineum is prepared according to hospital procedure. The nurse may be asked to apply fundal pressure to move the presenting part down more firmly on the cervix. While performing a sterile vaginal examination, the physician introduces an amnihook (or other rupturing device) into the vagina. A small tear is made in the amniotic membrane. Following rupture of the membranes, amniotic fluid is allowed to escape. Opinion varies regarding how much fluid should escape. Proponents of slow escape suggest that slow escape of the amniotic fluid decreases the chance of prolapse of the umbilical cord or abruptio placentae that may occur with sudden reduction in uterine volume (Niswander, 1980). They stress that the amniotomy should be done between contractions if the presenting part is at a station of +1 or above (Danforth, 1982). Those favoring escape of a large amount of fluid believe it reduces uterine volume, which results in contraction of the myometrium and in turn in more effective contractions (Niswander, 1980).

Explanation of the sensations the laboring woman will feel helps decrease anxiety. She can expect to feel the draining of amniotic fluid onto her perineum but no increase in discomfort. It is imperative that the FHR be auscultated before and immediately after the procedure so that any changes from the previous FHR pattern can be noted. If changes are marked, the nurse should check for prolapse of the cord. The amniotic fluid should be inspected for amount, color, odor, and presence of meconium or blood. The perineal area is cleansed and dried after the procedure. There is now an open pathway for organisms to ascend into the uterus, so strict sterile precautions must be taken when doing vaginal examinations, the number of vaginal exams must be kept to a minimum, and the woman's temperature should be monitored every 2 hours.

INDUCTION OF LABOR

The American College of Obstetricians and Gynecologists defines *induction of labor* as the deliberate initiation of uterine contractions prior to their spontaneous onset (Hughes, 1972). The procedure may be either elective or medically indicated because of the presence of a maternal and/or fetal problem.

Elective induction is defined by the Food and Drug Administration as "the initiation of labor for the convenience of an individual with a term pregnancy who is free of medi-

cal indications." The practice of elective induction is questionable in some centers because of the associated maternal risks and the possibility of delivering a preterm infant. The client should be carefully evaluated for the presence of a medical condition that would contraindicate the procedure. Accurate gestational dating is essential. Elective induction may be indicated for a client who has had previous precipitous labors (lasting less than 3 hours) to avoid an unexpected out-of-the-hospital delivery.

Indicated induction may be considered in the presence of a preexisting maternal disease such as diabetes mellitus, chronic hypertensive vascular disease, and renal disease. Since these diseases are associated with possible placental insufficiency, fetoplacental function tests should be done to assist the physician in determining the need for and the timing of an induction. Additional tests for fetal maturity are necessary to determine the neonate's capacity for extrauterine survival.

Additional indications for medically indicated induction include severe preeclampsia-eclampsia, abruptio placentae, premature rupture of membranes, postterm pregnancy, severe fetal hemolytic disease, intrauterine growth retardation, and intrauterine fetal death (Niswander, 1980; Cibils, 1981).

Contraindications

All contraindications to spontaneous labor and vaginal delivery are contraindications to the induction of labor (Cibils, 1981).

Maternal contraindications are as follows:

- Previous uterine incision (cesarean birth, hysterotomy, myomectomy)
- Obstructions of the birth canal from soft tissue masses (myomas, fibroids, large cysts)
- Invasive carcinoma of the cervix
- Advanced maternal age
- Presence of herpesvirus type 2
- Cephalopelvic disproportion
- Placenta previa centrally located
- Grand multiparity (5 or more pregnancies)
- Overt uterine overdistension (hydramnios, multiple fetuses)
- Lack of client acceptance

Fetal contraindications are as follows:

- Severe fetal distress or abnormal results of contraction stress test
- Low birth weight or preterm fetus
- Abnormal fetal presentation (transverse, or possibly breech)

Before an induction is attempted, appropriate assessment must indicate that both client and fetus are ready for the onset of labor. This includes evaluation of fetal maturity and cervical readiness.

Labor Readiness

FETAL MATURITY

Early diagnosis of pregnancy with adequate recorded data during the early months of pregnancy is helpful in determining the expected date of delivery. External abdominal examination of the growing uterus also aids in determining fetal growth.

Amniotic fluid studies are beneficial in assessing fetal maturity. Serial ultrasound examinations are helpful, provided that the tests are performed early in the second trimester (20–22 weeks) and again prior to 38 weeks. It is difficult to estimate fetal age from one examination performed between 39 and 40 weeks' gestation. One needs to compare findings with those from earlier examinations. (See Chapter 13 for discussion of methods to assess fetal maturity.)

CERVICAL READINESS

The findings on vaginal examination will help determine whether cervical changes favorable for induction have occurred. Bishop (1964) developed a prelabor scoring system that has proved to be helpful in predicting the inducibility of patients (Table 19–1). Components evaluated are cervical dilatation, effacement, consistency, and position, as well as the station of the fetal presenting part. A score of 0, 1, 2, or 3 is given to each assessed characteristic. The higher the total score for all the criteria, the more likely it is that labor will ensue. The lower the total score, the higher the failure rate. A favorable cervix is the most important criterion for a successful induction.

The presence of a cervix that is anterior, soft, more than 50% effaced, and dilated at least 3 cm, with the fetal head at +1 station or lower is favorable for a successful induction (Danforth, 1982). (This is true even in the multipara.) In a study of 2000 birth inductions, Pakzad (1980) reports that if cervical maturity is disregarded, then a long induction will most likely develop.

A "ripe" cervix as an indicator for success is so widely accepted that several methods (including laminaria, catheters, and PG gel) to enhance ripening are being investigated (Jagoni et al., 1982).

Methods

The most frequently used methods of induction are amniotomy, intravenous oxytocin (Pitocin) infusion, or both.

AMNIOTOMY

The mechanism by which amniotomy stimulates labor is unknown. However, under favorable conditions, which include cervical readiness and position of the fetal head against the lower segment and dipping into the pelvis, about 80% of clients at term go into active labor within 24 hours after amniotomy (Cibils, 1981).

The advantages of amniotomy as a method of labor induction are as follows:

1. The contractions elicited are similar to those of spontaneous labor.
2. There is usually no risk of hypertonus or rupture of the uterus.
3. The client does not require close surveillance as in oxytocin infusion.
4. Fetal monitoring is facilitated because amniotomy does not interfere with the following:
   a. Scalp blood sampling for pH determinations.
   b. Scalp electrode application.
   c. Intrauterine catheter placement.
5. The color and composition of amniotic fluid can be evaluated.

Table 19–1   Prelabor Status Evaluation Scoring System*

| Factor | Assigned value | | | |
	0	1	2	3
Cervical dilatation	Closed	1–2 cm	3–4 cm	5 cm or more
Cervical effacement	0%–30%	40%–50%	60%–70%	80% or more
Fetal station	−3	−2	−1, 0	+1, or lower
Cervical consistency	Firm	Moderate	Soft	
Cervical position	Posterior	Midposition	Anterior	

*Modified from Bishop, E. H. 1964. Pelvic scoring for elective induction. *Obstet. Gynecol.* 24:266.

The following are disadvantages of amniotomy:

1. Once an amniotomy is done, delivery must occur regardless of subsequent findings that suggest delaying birth.
2. The danger of a prolapsed cord is increased.
3. There is a risk of infection from ascending organisms.
4. Compression and molding of the fetal head are increased.
5. Labor may not be successfully induced, resulting in cesarean delivery.

OXYTOCIN INFUSION

Intravenous administration is an effective method of initiating uterine contractions (inducing labor). Ten units of oxytocin (Pitocin) are added to 1 L of intravenous fluid (usually 5% dextrose in balanced salt solution—for example, 5% dextrose in lactated Ringer's). The resulting mixture will contain 10 mU of oxytocin per milliliter and the prescribed dose can be easily calculated. A second bottle of intravenous fluid is prepared and used to start and maintain the infusion. This avoids infusing a large dose of oxytocin as the line is begun and provides additional fluids while the oxytocin solution is being kept at a low infusion rate. After the infusion is started, the oxytocin solution is piggybacked to the primary tubing and the infusion is delivered with an infusion pump to ensure accuracy. The FDA recommends an initial dosage of 1–2 mU/min and further states the dosage "may be gradually increased in increments of no more than 1–2 mU/min until the patient experiences a contraction pattern similar to normal labor."

Many clinicians use a more aggressive approach, starting with 1–2 mU/min and increasing the amount in a stepwise manner to 4, 8, and 12 mU/min as needed for adequate contractions. Depending on the rate of infusion, maximum effect is reached in approximately 20–60 minutes; therefore it is advisable to increase the infusion rate at intervals of no less than every 20 minutes to a maximum rate of 20 mU/min (Pritchard and MacDonald, 1980; Cibils, 1981; Danforth, 1982). If the desired effects are not achieved with a dose of 20 mU/min, it is unlikely that higher doses will be successful, and they may increase the hazards to the woman and fetus (Danforth, 1982).

During administration, the goal is to achieve contractions every 2–3 minutes of good intensity, each of which lasts 40–50 seconds. The uterus should relax to normal baseline tone between contractions. In 75% of cases, the frequency of contractions increases steadily, and in 90% of cases the intensity increases as the oxytocin infusion rate is advanced in a stepwise manner until maximum uterine efficiency results. The tonus of the uterus is always affected (Cibils, 1981). If the infusion is further advanced after maximum efficiency is attained, the intensity diminishes,

tonus increases, and frequency remains high. There is a resultant decrease in the relaxation time between contractions, and tetanic (sustained) contractions may occur (Cibils, 1981).

Oxytocin induction is not without some associated risks. Rapid progression of infusion rates or continuance of a particular rate without adequate assessment of the uterine contractions may lead to hyperstimulation of the uterus, compromise of the fetus due to decreased placental perfusion, a rapid labor and delivery with the danger of cervical or perineal lacerations, or uterine rupture. Water intoxication may occur if large doses are given in electrolyte-free solution over a prolonged period of time (Cibils, 1981).

NURSING INTERVENTIONS

Constant observation and accurate assessments are mandatory to provide safe, optimal care for both woman and fetus. Baseline data (maternal temperature, pulse, respiration, blood pressure, and FHR) should be obtained before beginning the infusion. A fetal monitor is used to provide continuous data. Many institutions recommend obtaining a 15-minute recording before the infusion is started to obtain baseline data on uterine contractions and FHR. Before each advancement of the infusion rate, assessments of the following should be made: (a) maternal blood pressure, pulse; (b) rate and reactivity of the FHR tracing (any bradycardia or decelerations are noted); and (c) contraction status, frequency, intensity, duration, and resting tone between contractions. During the induction, assess urinary output to identify any problems with retention, fluid deficit, and possibility of the development of water intoxication. As contractions are established, vaginal examinations are done to evaluate cervical dilatation, effacement, and station. The frequency of vaginal examinations primarily depends on the number of pregnancies and on characteristics of contractions. For example, a mullipara with contractions every 5–7 minutes, each lasting 30 seconds, who does not perceive her contractions does not usually require a vaginal examination, but when her contractions are every 2–3 minutes, lasting 50–60 seconds with good intensity, a vaginal examination will be needed to evaluate her status. When evaluating the need for analgesia, a vaginal examination should be performed to avoid giving the medication too early and increasing the risk of prolonging labor, and to identify advanced dilatation and imminent delivery. The administration of analgesia within 2–4 hours before delivery may result in respiratory difficulties for the newborn. For additional information on nursing interventions, see Drug Guide—Oxytocin, p. 590, and Nursing Care Plan—Induction of Labor, p. 591.

Intravenous oxytocin may be given for augmentation of labor; see Drug Guide—Oxytocin for further discussion.

(Text continues on p. 595.)

DRUG GUIDE—OXYTOCIN (PITOCIN)

OVERVIEW OF OBSTETRIC ACTION

Oxytocin (Pitocin) exerts a selective stimulatory effect on the smooth muscle of the uterus and of the blood vessels. Oxytocin affects the myometrial cells of the uterus by increasing the excitability of the muscle cell, increasing the strength of the muscle contraction, and supporting propagation of the contraction (movement of the contraction from one myometrial cell to the next). Its effect on the uterine contraction depends on the dosage used and on the excitability of the myometrial cells. During the first half of gestation, little excitability of the myometrium occurs and the uterus is fairly resistant to the effects of oxytocin. However, from midgestation on, the uterus responds increasingly to exogenous intravenous oxytocin. When at term, cautious use of diluted oxytocin, administered intravenously, results in a slow rise of uterine activity. Depending on the rate of infusion, the maximum effect is achieved in 20–60 minutes. The half-life of exogenous circulating oxytocin is 3 minutes; half-life of uterine response is about 15 minutes (Cibils, 1981).

Oxytocin is used to induce labor at term and to augment uterine contractions in the first and second stages of labor. Oxytocin also may be used immediately after delivery to stimulate uterine contraction and thereby control uterine atony.

Oxytocin is not thought to cross the placenta because of its molecular weight and the presence of oxytocinase in the placenta (Giacoia and Yaffe, 1982). Oxytocin has an antidiuretic effect.

Route, dosage, frequency

For induction of labor: Add 10 units oxytocin (1 mL) to 1000 mL of intravenous solution. (The resulting concentration is 10 mU oxytocin per 1 mL of intravenous fluid.) Using an infusion pump, administer IV, starting at 0.5 mU/min and increasing the rate stepwise every 20 minutes until good contractions (every 2–3 minutes, each lasting 40–60 seconds) are achieved or to a maximum rate of 20 mU/minute (Cibils, 1981).

0.5 mU/min =	3 mL/hr	8	mU/min =	48 mL/hr
1.0 mU/min =	6 mL/hr	10	mU/min =	60 mL/hr
1.5 mU/min =	9 mL/hr	12	mU/min =	72 mL/hr
2 mU/min =	12 mL/hr	15	mU/min =	90 mL/hr
4 mU/min =	24 mL/hr	18	mU/min =	108 mL/hr
6 mU/min =	36 mL/hr	20	mU/min =	120 mL/hr

For augmentation of labor: Prepare and administer IV oxytocin as for labor induction. Increase rate until labor contractions are of good quality.

For administration after delivery of placenta: One dose of 10 units oxytocin (1 mL) is given intramuscularly or by slow intravenous push.

Maternal contraindications

Severe preeclampsia-eclampsia

Predisposition to uterine rupture (in nullipara over 35 years of age, paragravida 4 or more, overdistention of the uterus, previous major surgery of the cervix or uterus)

Cephalopelvic disproportion

Malpresentation or malposition of the fetus, cord prolapse

Preterm infant

Rigid, unripe cervix; total placenta previa

Presence of fetal distress

Maternal side effects

Hyperstimulation of the uterus results in hypercontractility, which in turn may cause the following:

   Abruptio placentae

   Impaired uterine blood flow → fetal hypoxia

   Rapid labor → cervical lacerations

   Rapid labor and delivery → lacerations of cervix, vagina, perineum, uterine atony, fetal trauma

   Uterine rupture

Water intoxication (nausea, vomiting, hypotension, tachycardia, cardiac arrhythmia) if oxytocin is given in electrolyte-free solution

Hypotension with rapid IV administration postpartum

Effect on fetus/neonate

Fetal effects are primarily associated with the presence of hypercontractility of the maternal uterus. Hypercontractility causes a decrease in the oxygen supply to the fetus, which is reflected by irregularities and/or decrease in FHR. Hyperbilirubinemia.

NURSING CONSIDERATIONS

Explain induction or augmentation procedure to client

Apply fetal monitor and obtain 15-minute tracing to assess FHR before starting IV oxytocin

For induction or augmentation of labor, start with primary IV and piggy-back secondary IV with oxytocin

Assure continuous fetal and uterine contraction monitoring

Assess FHR, maternal blood pressure, pulse, and uterine contraction frequency, duration, and resting tone before each increase in oxytocin infusion rate

Record all assessments and IV rate on monitor strip and on client's chart

Record all client activities (such as change of position, vomiting) and procedures done (amniotomy, sterile vaginal examination) and administration of analgesics on monitor strip to allow for interpretation and evaluation of tracing

Assess cervical dilatation as needed

Utilize nursing comfort measures

Discontinue IV oxytocin infusion and infuse primary solution when (a) fetal distress is noted (bradycardia, late or variable decelerations, meconium staining); (b) uterine contractions are more frequent than every 2 minutes; (c) sustained uterine contractions are seen; or (d) insufficient relaxation of the uterus between contraction or a steady increase in resting tone are noted; in addition to discontinuing IV oxytocin infusion, turn client to side, and if fetal distress is present, administer oxygen by tight face mask at 4–7 L/min; notify physician

NURSING CARE PLAN
Induction of Labor

CLIENT DATA BASE

History

Previous pregnancies

Present pregnancy course

Childbirth preparation

Estimated gestational age

See the Nursing Care Plan on labor and delivery, Chapter 16, for other information

Physical examination

1. Examination of pregnant uterus (Leopold's maneuvers to determine fetal size and position, p. 441)

2. Vaginal examination to evaluate cervical readiness

   a. Ripe cervix: feels soft to the examining finger, is located in a medial to anterior position, is more than 50% effaced, and is 2–3 cm dilated

   b. Unripe cervix: feels firm to the examining finger, is long and thick, perhaps in a posterior position, with little or no dilatation

3. Presence of contractions

4. Membranes intact or ruptured

5. Fetal size (Leopold's maneuvers, ultrasound)

6. Fetal readiness

7. CPD evaluation

8. Maternal vital signs and FHR before beginning induction

Laboratory evaluation

Fetal maturity tests (L/S ratio, creatinine concentrations, ultrasonography)

Maternal blood studies (CBC, hemoglobin, hematocrit, blood type, Rh factor)

Urinalysis

NURSING PRIORITIES

1. Monitor and evaluate status of mother and fetus continuously throughout the induction

2. Provide continuous physical and emotional support

3. Evaluate and monitor uterine response to induction

4. Evaluate and monitor fetal response to induction

5. Continuously evaluate client for complications associated with induction (abruptio placentae, fetal distress, any rise or decrease in maternal BP, hemorrhage, shock, uterine rupture, tetanic contractions)

CLIENT/FAMILY EDUCATIONAL FOCUS

1. Provide information regarding the induction procedure including action and side effects of medications, and expected action

2. Provide information regarding the fetal monitor, how it works, and the information that can be obtained from it

3. Provide opportunities for questions and individual concerns of the client and family

Problem	Nursing interventions and actions	Rationale
Client preparation	Assess client's feelings regarding induction Client may ask, "Will this work?" "How long will it take?" "Will it hurt more?"	Client may be apprehensive about what will happen, or feel a sense of failure that she cannot "go into labor by herself"
	Assess client's knowledge base regarding the induction process Provide needed information (for example, when the cervix is ripe, contractions should begin in 30–60 minutes); length of labor depends on a number of factors	After assessing knowledge base, appropriate information can be given to allay apprehension
	Assess knowledge of breathing techniques; if client does not have a method to use, teach breathing techniques before starting oxytocin infusion	Use of breathing techniques during contractions will help relaxation; although client may be apprehensive about induction, teaching a new breathing method will be easier before contractions are present
Changing client status Maternal vital signs	Assess maternal BP and pulse before beginning induction and then before each increase in infusion rate; do not advance infusion rate in presence of maternal hypertension or hypotension or radical changes in pulse rate	To establish baseline data and to assess client response to induction; client status may change rapidly

NURSING CARE PLAN Cont'd
Induction of Labor

Problem	Nursing interventions and actions	Rationale
Cervical dilatation	Evaluate cervical dilatation by vaginal examination with each oxytocin dosage increase after labor is established	When cervix responds by stretching or pulling, *do not* increase oxytocin dosage; overdosage may occur, causing rapid labor with possible cervical lacerations and fetal damage; when there is no change in the cervix, additional oxytocin is needed
Fetal status	Assess FHR by continuous electronic fetal monitoring. Obtain 15-minute tracing prior to beginning induction to evaluate fetal status; *do not* start infusion or advance rate (if induction has already begun) is FHR is not in range of 120–160 beats/min, if decelerations are present, or if variability decreases	Will provide continuous data regarding fetal response to induction
Contraction status	Apply monitor to obtain 15 minutes of tracing prior to starting induction	Establishes baseline data
	Assess contraction frequency, duration, and intensity prior to each increase in infusion rate	Evaluates uterine response to induction
	Do not increase rate of infusion if contractions are every 2–3 minutes, lasting 40–60 seconds, with moderate intensity	Desired effect has been obtained
	Discontinue oxytocin infusion if: 1. Contractions are more frequent than every 2 minutes 2. Contraction duration exceeds 75–90 seconds 3. Uterus does not relax between contractions	Uterus is being overstimulated and serious complications may develop for woman and fetus
Discomfort from contractions	Provide support to client as she uses breathing techniques	Contractions may build up more quickly with oxytocin induction
	Encourage use of effluerage, back rub, and other supportive measures (see Labor and Delivery Nursing Care Plan, p. 472)	Techniques help maintain relaxation and thereby decrease pain sensation
	Assess need for analgesia, obtain order and administer (as long as maternal BP, pulse, respiration and FHR are within normal range)	After labor is well established, analgesia may be given without delaying progress
Inadequate labor response	Increase oxytocin IV infusion rate every 20 minutes until adequate contractions are achieved; do *not* exceed an infusion rate of 20 mU/min	Uterine response to oxytocin may be individualized
	Check infusion pump to assure oxytocin is infusing; check whether pump is on, chamber refills and empties, level of fluid in IV bottle becomes lower; if problem is found, correct it and restart infusion at beginning dose	Oxytocin may not be infusing due to pump, mechanical, or human error
	Check piggy-back connection to primary tubing to assure solution is not leaking	

NURSING CARE PLAN Cont'd
Induction of Labor

Problem	Nursing interventions and actions	Rationale
Failed induction	Explain reasons, if known Provide support Discontinue oxytocin induction, continue to monitor maternal and fetal status until effects of oxytocin have subsided	Cervix may not have been ''ready'' (ripe) for induction; even though labor was not established, significant changes in the cervix may have occurred; oxytocin may have been improperly administered Failure of induction may increase client's personal feelings of failure or increase apprehension if delivery must be effected because of maternal and/or fetal problems
Hypotension	Position client on her side; encourage her to avoid supine position Monitor maternal BP and pulse and FHR every 15–20 minutes If client becomes hypotensive: 1. Keep her on her side, may change to other side 2. Discontinue oxytocin infusion 3. Increase rate of primary IV 4. Monitor FHR 5. Notify physican 6. Assess for cause of hypotension	To maintain optimal blood flow to uterus and placenta Woman is frequently on her back at beginning of induction while monitors are attached and IV is started; vena cava is obstructed, causing maternal hypotension, which may lead to fetal bradycardia; initial hypotension is secondary to peripheral vasodilation induced by oxytocin, which causes diminished blood supply to placenta and resultant decrease in O_2 supply to fetus Actions are directed toward improving blood flow and oxygenation of tissues
Infection	Use aseptic technique for starting and maintaining the IV	Asepsis reduces incidence of infection
	Maintain sterile technique when doing vaginal exams	Organisms may be introduced during vaginal examinations
	Assess client's temperature every 4 hours if membranes are intact, and every 2 hours if membranes are ruptured	Elevation of temperature may be associated with development of infection
	Assess IV site for redness, swelling when membranes are ruptured; assess amniotic fluid for odor and discoloration	May indicate local infection May be associated with chorioamnionitis
Water intoxication	Administer oxytocin in electrolyte solution	Oxytocin has slight antidiuretic effect, especially when administered in electrolyte-free solutions
	Assess and record fluid intake and output Monitor for nausea, vomiting, hypotension, tachycardia, cardiac arrhythmias	Provides information on hydration status These are signs and symptoms of water intoxication; they must be differentiated from other problems
Delivery of preterm infant	Correlate tests done to establish gestational age; calculate gestational age Notify pediatrician and nursery personnel if infant is preterm and induction must continue for medical reasons	Prematurity can occur due to incorrect evaluation of fetal age; specialized care may be needed
Tetanic contractions	Observe contraction frequency and duration. In presence of contractions lasting over 90 seconds: 1. Discontinue oxytocin infusion 2. Assess maternal status 3. Assess fetal status	Contractions lasting over 90 seconds with decreased resting tone may result in fetal hypoxia Ruptured uterus or abruptio placentae can result from drug-induced tumultuous labor

NURSING CARE PLAN Cont'd
Induction of Labor

Problem	Nursing interventions and actions	Rationale
Fetal hypoxia — asphyxia	Monitor FHR continuously (normal range is 120–160/min) In episodes of bradycardia (<120 beats/min) lasting for more than 30 sec, administer O_2 by face mask at 4–7 L/min Stop oxytocin infusion Position woman on left side if quick recovery of FHR does not occur	O_2 deficiency may occur over a long period of time; in cases of placental insufficiency or cord compression, compensated tachycardia may be evoked
	Carefully evaluate fetal tachycardia (>160/min) Sustained tachycardia may necessitate discontinuation of oxytocin infusion Assess for presence of meconium staining	Persistent fetal tachycardia causes more prominent O_2 deficiency (hypoxia) and CO_2 increase in fetal blood; vasoconstriction occurs, with increased fetal blood flow through coronary arteries, brain, and placenta; this increased demand on myocardial performance leads to cardiac decompensation if oxygen exchange is impaired and hypoxia continues Fetal hypoxia may also cause central vasomotor center to release adrenal catecholamines; at term, this enhances depolarization of cardiac pacemaker cells, which will result in direct bradycardia Bradycardia or subsequent reflex tachycardia temporarily remedies the O_2 deficiency
Rapid delivery	Assist with rapid delivery. Observe for: 1. Laceration of cervix and tissues in the birth canal 2. Fetal distress Evaluate postpartally: 1. Check mother for lacerations and contractility of fundus 2. Check neonate for birth injuries	Overstimulation or overdosage of oxytocin may occur as additional endogenous oxytocin is produced by maternal system Rapid delivery increases risk of cervical and soft tissue lacerations in birth canal Rapid labor and delivery may lead to uterine atony Pressure within fetal head changes rapidly with precipitous, rapid delivery; infant is prone to cerebral edema and hemorrhage

NURSING CARE EVALUATION

Normal sterile vaginal delivery is accomplished without complications (lacerations, precipitous delivery)

Postpartally the maternal fundus is firm; blood flow is moderate; blood pressure, pulse, and respirations are stable and within normal limits

Neonate's respirations, color, and temperature are within normal limits

Family bonding is begun by allowing interactions among mother, baby, and father in delivery room

NURSING CARE PLAN Cont'd
Induction of Labor

NURSING DIAGNOSES*	SUPPORTING DATA
1. Knowledge deficit related to induction procedure	Client unable to verbalize the purpose and procedure Expressed questions and concerns regarding the induction
2. Alteration in uterine blood flow related to hypertonic contractions	Contraction frequency of less than every 2 min and duration exceeding 60–90 sec Marked changes in FHR variability and rate Late decelerations
3. Alteration in fetal blood flow related to decreased uterine blood flow	Marked changes in FHR variability and rate Late decelerations Meconium staining of amniotic fluid Marked changes in fetal activity (hypo- or hyperactive)

*These are a few examples of nursing diagnoses that may be appropriate for a woman being induced. It is not an inclusive list and must be individualized for each woman.

Prostaglandin Administration

The use of prostaglandin $F_{2\alpha}$ (PGF$_{2\alpha}$) and prostaglandin E$_2$ (PGE$_2$) for induction is fairly routine in England, and is currently being studied for use in the United States.

In a comparison between intravenous infusion of PGF$_{2\alpha}$ and oxytocin, Baxie et al. (1980) reported that the use of either agent administered at low dose appeared to be equally satisfactory for induction of labor. Side effects of nausea and vomiting (which have been associated with PGF$_{2\alpha}$) were reported infrequently. One client receiving PGF$_{2\alpha}$ developed superficial phlebitis at the infusion site.

Intracervical application of PGE$_2$ gel has also been used for ripening the cervix and for induction of labor. In a study of 50 nulliparous clients with unfavorable cervical state, Ulmsten (1982) reported that 11 of 25 who received intracervical PGE$_2$ gel had successful induction of labor and delivered within 24 hours. The remaining 14 who received PGE$_2$ gel had significant improvement in cervical Bishop score. Two of the 25 who received a placebo gel delivered within 24 hours but the other 23 had no change in cervical Bishop score. In a subsequent open study, 54% had successful induction of labor, and the remaining undelivered clients had considerable ripening of the cervix, from a mean of 3.2 prior to treatment to 6.5 by 24 hours after treatment. No signs of gastrointestinal discomfort were observed.

Liggins (1978) notes that intravaginal PGE$_2$ gel is effective, free of side effects, and noninvasive. If excessive uterine activity occurs, the gel can be removed with minimal problems. Liggins states, "it seems not unlikely that future development of intravaginal administration of PG will replace amniotomy and oxytocin as the method of choice for induction of labor."

EPISIOTOMY

An *episiotomy* is a surgical incision of the perineal body extending downward from the vaginal orifice for obstetric purposes (Carter and Wolber, 1981). The purposes of an episiotomy are to minimize stretching of the perineal tissues and to decrease trauma to the fetal head during descent and delivery of the fetus.

The routine use of episiotomies is becoming an increasingly controversial issue. Various authors have found no evidence to support the reasons for episiotomies just listed (Cogan and Edmunds, 1977; Banta and Thacker, 1982). However, most medical textbooks still advocate the prophylactic use of this procedure.

The episiotomy is performed just before delivery, when the presenting part is beginning to crown, but before there is excessive stretching of the perineal tissues. The incision begins at the midline and may be extended down the midline through the perineal body, or it may extend at a 45-degree angle in a mediolateral direction to the right or left (Figure 19–2). A midline episiotomy is preferred if the perineum is of adequate length and no difficulty during delivery is anticipated, as the blood loss is less, the incision is easy to repair, and heals with less discomfort for the mother. The major disadvantage is that the midline incision may extend through the anal sphincter and rectum. In the presence of a short perineum or an anticipated difficult delivery, a mediolateral episiotomy provides more room and decreases the possibility of a traumatic extension into the rectum. The mediolateral episiotomy may be complicated by greater blood loss, a longer healing period, and more discomfort postpartally for the mother.

Coats et al. (1980) compared midline and mediolateral episiotomies. Their findings suggest that the pain experi-

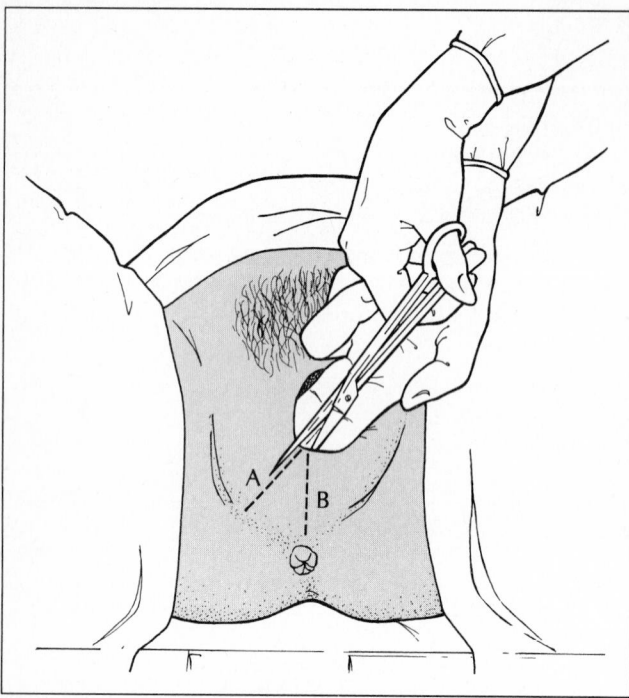

FIGURE 19–2 The two most common types of episiotomies are mediolateral **(A)** and midline **(B).**

enced after delivery was similar for both groups, although those with midline episiotomies began intercourse significantly earlier, which may indicate they had less discomfort. The group with midline episiotomies also had less bruising of the tissues and less scarring.

Less common types of episiotomies include lateral and complete perineotomy. The lateral episiotomy may be done when certain circumstances are present, such as posterior vulva and/or perineal lesions, making a midline or mediolateral episiotomy impractical. The advantages of a lateral episiotomy are essentially the same as a mediolateral incision. The major disadvantages, however, are the increased number of muscles involved and the difficulty of effecting adequate repair. A complete perineotomy may be done when traumatic or unexpected extension of a midline episiotomy is inevitable. The incision includes the distal midanterior rectal wall and the external rectal sphincter (Carter and Wolber, 1981). Although this procedure is usually reserved for those instances when there is an anticipated extension of a midline episiotomy, it may also be used intentionally in the presence of a large fetus, short perineum, or difficult presentation (Carter and Wolber, 1981). This type of episiotomy may also be referred to as an "episirectomy" or "episioprototomy."

Nursing Interventions

The episiotomy is usually performed with the client under a regional or light general anesthesia but may be per-

formed without anesthesia in emergency situations. (As crowning occurs, the distention of the tissues causes numbing.) Adequate anesthesia must be given for the repair.

Repair of the episiotomy (episiorrhaphy) is accomplished either during the period between delivery of the neonate and before delivery of the placenta or after the delivery of the placenta. Adequate lighting is necessary for clear visualization. The client needs to be supported during the repair as she may feel some pressure sensations. In the absence of adequate anesthesia, she may feel pain. Placing a hand on her shoulder, and talking with her can provide comfort and distraction from the repair process.

The type of episiotomy and type of suture used (usually chromic catgut 00 or 000) are recorded on the delivery record. This information should also be included in a report to the recovery room, so that adequate assessments can be made and relief measures can be instituted if necessary.

To alleviate pain and swelling after the repair, ice packs are beneficial for the first 8 hours. Hot sitz baths are recommended to increase the circulation to the area and to promote healing. The episiotomy site should be inspected every 15 minutes during the first hour after delivery and thereafter daily for redness, swelling, tenderness, and hematomas. Mild analgesic sprays and oral analgesics are ordered as needed. The mother will need instruction in perineal hygiene care and may need instructions about use of the analgesic spray. (See Chapter 27 for additional discussion of relief measures.)

FORCEPS DELIVERIES

Forceps may be used to provide traction, to rotate, or both. The forceps used in obstetrics have four parts: a blade, handle, shank, and lock. The blades are designated as right and left and are either fenestrated or solid. Most blades have a pelvic and cephalic curve and articulate at the lock. Fenestrated blades are lighter, grip the fetal head better, and are less likely to slip than solid blades.

There are two types of forceps deliveries. The delivery is termed *outlet forceps delivery* when the fetal head is visible on the perineum without spreading the labia. When the fetal head is higher than the level of the ischial spines, delivery is termed a *midforceps delivery*. The lower part of the fetal head must be at the level of the ischial spines and the biparietal diameter must have entered the inlet (engagement) to perform a midforceps delivery. Most midforceps deliveries are rotations of the fetus from an occiput-posterior or occiput-transverse position to an occiput-anterior position. *High forceps deliveries* (application of forceps before engagement of the fetal head) are no longer used because they are extremely dangerous for the woman and the fetus.

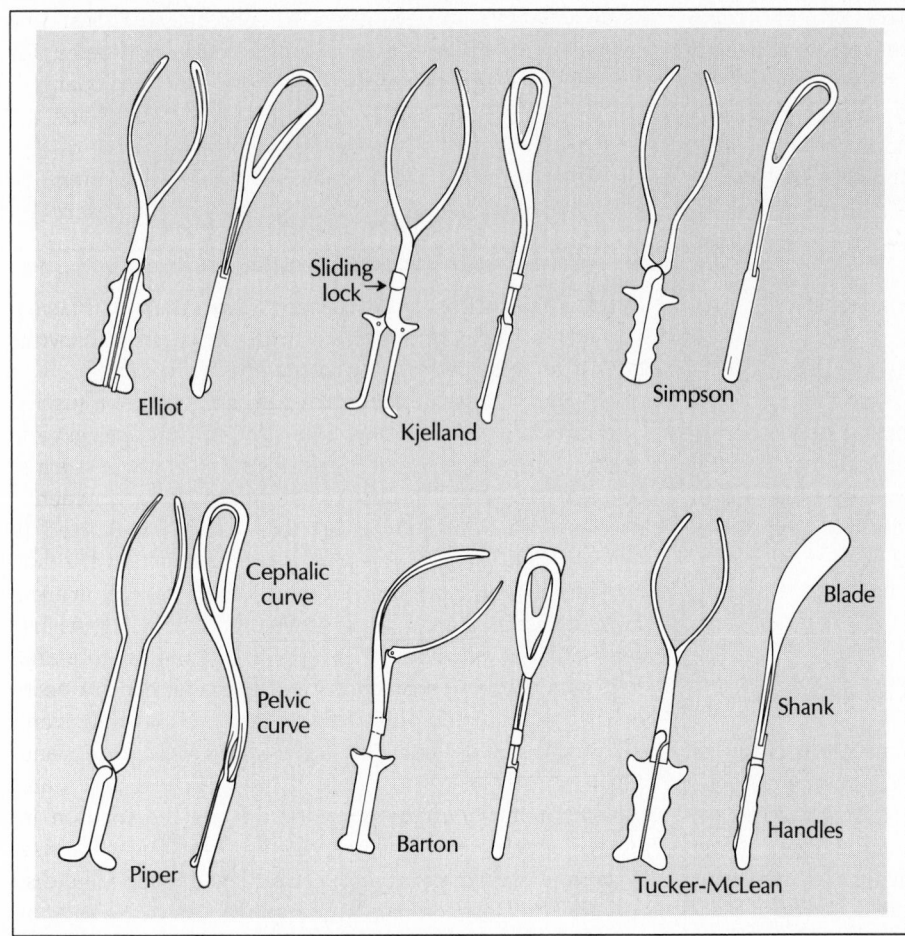

FIGURE 19–3 Forceps are composed of a blade, shank, and handle, and may have a cephalic and pelvic curve. (Note labels on Piper and Tucker-McLean forceps.) The blades may be fenestrated (open) or solid. The front and lateral views of these forceps illustrate differences in blades, open and closed shank, cephalic and pelvic curves.

Types of Forceps

The following forceps are depicted in Figure 19–3.

Simpson forceps are outlet forceps. They have a fenestrated blade and an English lock and are separated at the shanks to allow for cutting of the episiotomy after the application. These forceps can be used successfully on infants with well-molded heads.

Tucker-McLean forceps have a solid blade and closed shanks. They are also outlet forceps but may be used for midforceps rotations of fetuses in the occiput-posterior position. Due to the shape of the Tucker-McLean cephalic curve, they work well with premature infants with little molding.

The *Kjelland forceps* have a sliding lock with no pelvic curve. They are designed for occiput-posterior and occiput-transverse midforceps rotations.

The *Barton forceps* have one hinged blade and are used for midforceps rotation of the fetus from an occiput-transverse position to an occiput-anterior position.

Elliot forceps have a fenestrated blade and an English lock and are closed at the shanks. They are used as outlet forceps.

Piper forceps have long shanks that curve down. The handle is lower than the blades. The blades are fenestrated. The forceps are used for the aftercoming head of a fetus in a breech presentation.

Indications

Indications for the use of forceps include any condition that threatens the life of the woman or fetus. Maternal conditions include heart disease, acute pulmonary edema, intrapartal infection, or exhaustion. Fetal conditions include prolapsed cord, premature placental separation, and fetal distress. Forceps may be used electively to shorten the second stage of labor, sparing the woman the pushing effort, or when regional or general anesthesia has affected the woman's motor innervation and she cannot push effectively. They are advocated in preterm infant delivery (Pritchard and MacDonald, 1980), as discussed in Chapter 18.

Complications

Perinatal morbidity and mortality are increased with midforceps deliveries. Neonatal depression and birth trauma have been closely correlated with the use of midforceps, especially if a rotation is done (Friedman and Sachtleben, 1976). The incidence of postpartal hemorrhage is increased with midforceps deliveries if the second stage lasts over 3 hours. No such increase is found in cases in which operative techniques are not used but in which the second stage of labor is prolonged (Cohen, 1977). Friedman et al. (1977) also found a lower IQ score in children 3–4 years old who were delivered by midforceps compared with those delivered by low forceps or spontaneously.

Prerequisites for Forceps Application

Use of forceps requires complete dilatation of the cervix and knowledge of the exact position and station of the fetal head. The membranes must be ruptured to allow a firm grasp on the fetal head. The presentation must be vertex or face with the chin anterior, and the head must be engaged, preferably on the perineum. *Under no circumstances should there be any CPD.*

Trial or Failed Forceps Delivery

In a trial forceps procedure, the physician attempts to use forceps with the knowledge that there is a degree of CPD. If a good application cannot be obtained or if no descent occurs with the application, then cesarean delivery is the method of choice. A failed forceps procedure is an attempt to deliver with forceps without success (Pritchard and MacDonald, 1980).

NURSING INTERVENTIONS

It is the nurse's responsibility to provide the physician with the type of forceps requested. Frequently this request can be anticipated, as with outlet forceps or a premature delivery. The Piper forceps should always be available on the delivery table with a breech delivery in case they are needed.

The nurse can explain the procedure briefly to the woman if she is awake. With adequate regional anesthesia, the client should feel some pressure but no pain. Encourage her to maintain breathing techniques to prevent her from pushing during application of the forceps (Figure 19–4). The nurse monitors contractions and with each contraction the physician will provide traction as the client pushes. The FHR should be monitored continuously by the circulating nurse until the delivery. It is not uncommon to observe bradycardia as traction is being applied to the forceps. This bradycardia results from head compression and is transient in nature. With midforceps rotations, pediatric assistance may be needed. Adequate resuscitation equipment should be readied.

Occasionally the neonate will have a forceps bruise from the application. The parents should be informed about the presence of a bruise and told that it will disappear in a few days.

Neonates who have had a forceps delivery should be inspected for cerebral trauma and Erb's palsy if there was a difficult forceps extraction.

VACUUM EXTRACTION

Vacuum extraction is an obstetric procedure with widespread use throughout the world, although it has not gained as much popularity in the United States (Greis et al., 1981). The vacuum extractor is composed of a suction cup attached to a suction bottle (pump) by tubing. The suction cup, which comes in various sizes, is placed against the fetal occiput. The pump is used to create negative pressure (suction) and an artificial caput ("chignon") is formed. The vacuum pressure is begun slowly at 0.2 kg/cm^2 and then increased by intervals of 0.2 kg/cm^2 every 2 minutes until a maximum pressure of 0.8 kg/cm^2 is reached. The physician then applies traction in coordination with uterine contractions and the fetal head is delivered. The cup should not remain in place for longer than 20 minutes and "pull off" (slippage) should be avoided (Plauché, 1979).

The majority of physicians do not use the vacuum extractor until the cervix is fully dilated. The fetus should be in vertex presentation with a well-flexed head (Plauché, 1978). The most common indication for use of the vacuum extractor is prolongation of the first stage of labor. Other indications for its use include (a) fetal distress, (b) malpositions such as OP or OT, and (c) such maternal complications as cardiopulmonary disease, shock, pregnancy-induced hypertension, and abruptio placentae (Greis et al., 1981). Contraindications for use of the vacuum extractor include the presence of CPD, face, or breech presentation.

Major risks to the fetus with the use of the Malmström vacuum extractor reported by Plauché (1979) include possible tissue necrosis of the fetal scalp at the site of the cup attachment, and "cookie-cutter" avulsion of the fetal scalp associated with use of the cup to rotate the fetal position.

Greis et al. (1981) compared the vacuum extractor deliveries (Bird modification of the Malmström, and Neward lever hand-pump) with forceps deliveries. Use of the vacuum extractor was associated with a significantly lower incidence of severe birth canal damage and maternal bleeding. In addition, puerperal febrile morbidity was lowered. Neonatal complications included a high incidence of a "chignon" (which usually disappeared in a few hours), and increased incidence of cephalhematoma (24% with vacuum extractor versus 11% with forceps).

Currently, a soft silicone cup is being used in some centers. Advantages of this cup include greater pliability for ease in insertion into the vagina; better fit on the fetal head, which helps diffuse the extraction force; and reduced risk of cephalhematoma (Kappy, 1981).

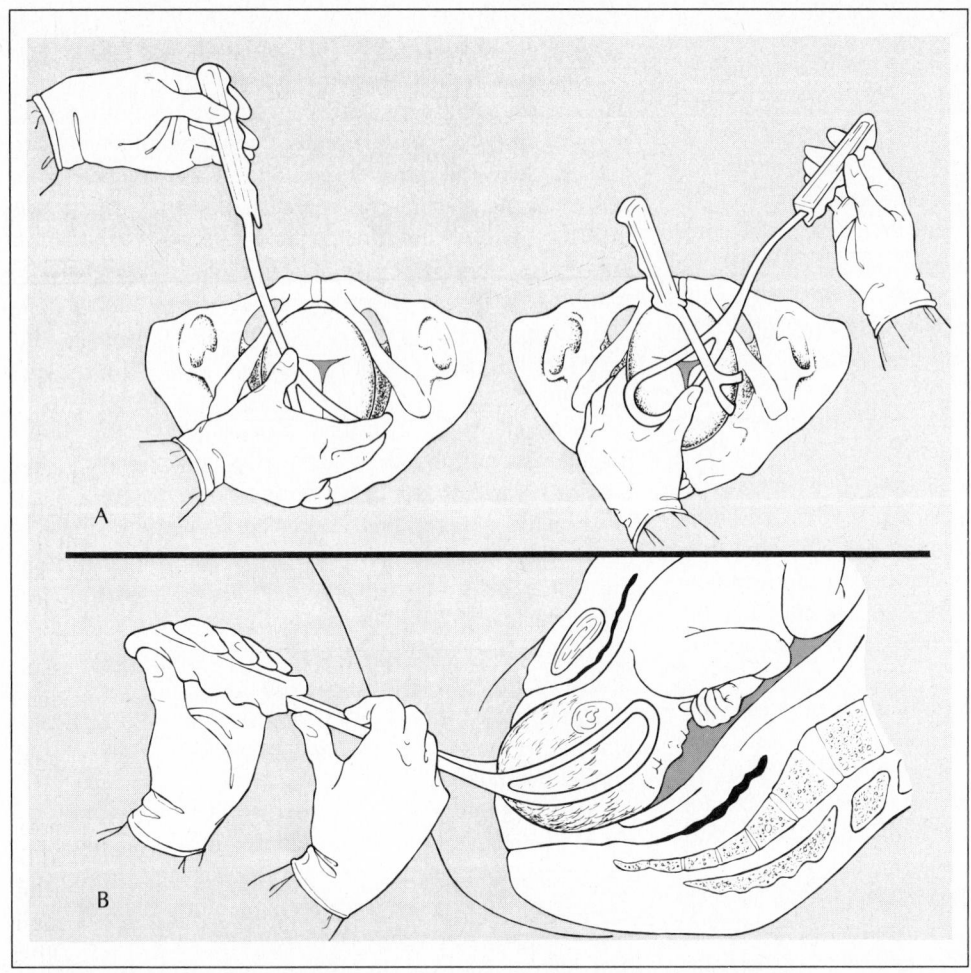

FIGURE 19–4 Application of forceps in occiput anterior (OA) position. **A,** The left blade is inserted along the left side wall of the pelvis, over the parietal bone. **B,** The right blade is inserted along the right side wall of the pelvis over the parietal bone. **C,** With correct placement of the blades, the handles lock easily. During contractions, traction is applied to the forceps in a downward and outward direction to follow the birth canal.

Nursing Interventions

The nurse may be responsible for gathering the equipment and providing the physician with the size of cup requested. Sterile tubing should be provided along with the cup. After the physician assembles the cup and tubing, he or she hands the distal end to the nurse to connect to the suction bottle. When the cup is applied to the fetal head, the nurse is directed to pump the suction.

The nurse should be ready to quickly release the suction in the event that the cup accidentally slips off during traction ("pull off") to prevent damage to the maternal tissues.

During the procedure, the client should be informed about what is happening. If adequate regional anesthesia has been administered, the woman feels only pressure during the procedure. The fetus should be auscultated every 5 minutes or more frequently, and proper infant resuscitation equipment should be readied if fetal problems are anticipated. The parents need to be informed that the caput (chignon) on the baby's head will disappear in a few hours.

Assessment of the newborn should include inspection and continued observation for cerebral trauma.

CESAREAN BIRTH

Cesarean birth is the delivery of the infant through an abdominal and uterine incision. The word *cesarean* is derived from the Latin word *caedere*, meaning "to cut." Cesarean birth is one of the oldest surgical procedures known to modern man. Until the twentieth century, cesarean delivery was primarily equated with an attempt to salvage the fetus of a dying woman. Today cesarean birth has become a common occurrence, with approximately one out of every six neonates being delivered by this method (NIH, 1980).

As a result of a nearly threefold increase in the incidence of cesarean births in the last decade, a National Institutes of Health (NIH) Consensus Development Conference was held in September 1980, to address issues concerning cesarean childbirth (National Institute of Child Health and Human Development, NIH Consensus Development, Statement on Cesarean Childbirth, The Cesarean Birth Task Force, 1980). Findings of the NIH Cesarean Birth Task Force will be discussed throughout this section.

Indications for Cesarean Delivery

Cesarean births are performed in cases of breech presentation, fetal distress, dysfunctional labor, and uteroplacental insufficiency from maternal disease conditions (Hibbard, 1976; Jones, 1976). The most commonly occurring indication for cesarean delivery is dystocia caused by CPD. Other indications for this procedure include prolapsed cord, placenta previa, abruptio placentae, IUGR, prolonged rupture of the membranes, genital herpes, prematurity, fetal distress and occasionally tumors blocking the vagina. Primary cesarean deliveries are increasingly done for breech presentations in nulliparas.

In the United States the incidence of cesarean birth has increased from 5.5% in 1970 to 15.2% in 1978 and 16% in 1980 (NIH, 1980). This trend is also evident in Canada. Factors that are thought to contribute to this increased rate are technologic advancements, social changes, changes in childbearing practices, increasing capability for infant survival, advances or changes in medical care, obstetric attitudes and practices, and the increasing percentage of complicated births.

Four diagnostic categories have had the greatest influence upon the increased incidence of cesarean birth. Dystocia (abnormal or difficult labor) accounted for 30% of the increase followed by repeat cesarean (25%–30%), breech presentation (10%–15%), and fetal distress (10%–15%) (NIH, 1980).

Technologic and medical advancements have altered the attitude toward cesarean birth from a "procedure of last resort" to an "alternative birth method." Technologic advancements include:

1. Refinements in surgical techniques for entry and closure of the uterus.
2. Monitoring of maternal and fetal physiology to identify pairs at risk from the forces of labor and vaginal delivery.
3. Developments in anesthesia enhancing maternal participation and comfort during delivery, as well as reducing depressant effects on the fetus.
4. Pharmacology and parental fluid therapy which decrease hazards of maternal hemorrhage and infection.

Social changes are associated with increasing numbers of cesarean deliveries. In conjunction with initiation of federal programs in the 1960s to promote maternal and child health, the socioeconomic disparity of women having cesarean births has decreased. A trend toward women receiving care from an obstetrician and delivering in larger hospitals is also evident. The increasing rate of cesareans in larger hospitals (greater than 1000 deliveries per year) has been higher than in smaller hospitals. Although there is no reliable data to support the claims, some speculate that the trend of third-party reimbursement and defensive

obstetrics to avoid malpractice lawsuits might also be contributing factors (NIH, 1980; Amirikia et al., 1981).

Changes in childbearing practices are also related to the increasing rate of cesarean deliveries. With the decreasing size of American families, the percentage of primigravida deliveries have increased. The incidence of cesarean births is nine times greater for the primigravida than the multigravida (Stichler and Affonso, 1980). An increasing number of women are choosing to have their children at a later age than a decade ago. Age is associated with a higher incidence of uterine inertia or dystocia, common conditions necessitating cesarean delivery (Boehm et al., 1981).

Although in 90% of all the primary cesarean births, the neonate weighs more than 2500 g, increasing numbers of cesareans are being done for low birth weight or preterm neonates (NIH, 1980). Some contend that this mode of delivery is more advantageous than subjecting the vulnerable preterm neonate to the stresses of a vaginal birth. It is difficult to assess the true effect of operative deliveries on neonatal mortality. Improved neonatal survival rates are also attributed to higher numbers of neonatal intensive care units, improvement in the specialty areas of maternal–fetal and neonatal medicine, and improved technology.

Changes in obstetric management have also resulted in the higher number of cesarean births. Improved antepartal monitoring, and electronic monitoring during labor for fetal distress are considered contributing factors. Also, attitudes have changed from vaginal delivery of the breech presentation and difficult forceps deliveries toward delivering these neonates by cesarean procedure.

Although the rationale for cesarean delivery is to improve pregnancy outcome, insufficient data exist regarding morbidity risk to the mother and neonate to support this claim. The NIH Consensus Development Statement on Cesarean Childbirth (1980) summarized the following data for cesarean birth outcomes:

Dystocia: No evidence that the infant greater than 2500 g had survival advantage.

Repeat cesarean: No mortality/morbidity data relative to risks or benefits to client or infant.

Breech: Insufficient data in terms of preferred method for all fetuses regardless of weight.

Fetal distress: No evidence relative to mortality risks associated with the method of delivery.

Whether pregnancy outcome is improved with cesarean birth remains an unanswered and controversial issue.

Electronic fetal monitoring to assess fetal distress has often been blamed for the increased cesarean birth rate. Some contend that fetal distress is diagnosed more often than it actually exists, resulting in unnecessary cesarean births. Yet, in controlled studies it has been found that in *experienced* hands a liberal use of fetal monitoring in low-

(Text continues on p. 605.)

NURSING CARE PLAN
Cesarean Birth

CLIENT DATA BASE

History

Previous pregnancies

Course of recovery from previous cesarean births

Present pregnancy course

Estimated gestational age

Childbirth preparation

Sensitivity to medications and anesthetic agents

Past bleeding problems

Physical examination

1. Fetal size, fetal status (FHR), and fetal maturity

2. Lung and cardiac status

3. Complete physical examination prior to administration of anesthetic

Laboratory evaluation

CBC

Hemoglobin and hematocrit

Type and cross-match for two units whole blood

Rh

Prothrombin time

VDRL

Urinalysis

NURSING PRIORITIES

1. Provide couple with factual information and support in preparation for their cesarean birth to enable them to make choices, feel in control, and minimize feelings of anxiety, loss, guilt, and helplessness

2. Support the couple's desires to participate in their birth experience within the constraints or options of the situation

3. Encourage couple to participate in the decision-making process for the cesarean birth experience and care during the preparatory, recovery, and postpartal periods

CLIENT/FAMILY EDUCATIONAL FOCUS

1. Maintain "birth-oriented" approach

2. Explain preparatory procedures and postoperative care measures

3. Provide opportunity for questions and concerns of the client and family.

Problem	Nursing interventions and actions	Rationale
Preparation for cesarean birth	Integrate cesarean birth information into childbirth preparation classes	Couples may deny the possibility of an unplanned cesarean birth Preparatory needs are basically the same for all couples anticipating childbirth Provides knowledge base, which will allow for adaptive coping responses should they deliver in either manner
	Emphasize the similarities between vaginal and cesarean delivery Minimize perceptions of "normal" versus "abnormal" birth	
	Provide factual information	Enables couples to make choices and participate in their birth experiences
	Encourage couple to discuss with obstetrician the approach and birth preferences in the event of a vaginal or cesarean birth	Opportunity to discuss needs and desires minimizes unrealistic expectations, disappointment and/or feelings of loss Promotes understanding of options, beliefs of birth attendant, and hospital policies Allows couple to do anticipatory problem solving and develop effective coping behaviors
Anticipated or repeat cesarean birth	Encourage expression of feelings	Enables couple to work through fears, ambivalent or unresolved feelings and grief associated with loss of vaginal birth
	Assess reaction to and interpretation of past cesarean birth experiences	Identifies need for information and opportunity to work through fears or unresolved feelings

NURSING CARE PLAN Cont'd
Cesarean Birth

Problem	Nursing interventions and actions	Rationale
	Encourage the development of mutual support by couples sharing their experiences and common concerns	Decreases sense of being "different" or "alone" by realizing that their fears and concerns are not unique and feelings of anger or guilt are normal
Previous negative cesarean birth experiences	Create a safe, nonthreatening environment for couples to work through unresolved negative feelings	Negative feelings may contribute to distortion of information, impede learning, and affect expectations of upcoming birth experience
	Encourage couples to identify events that would make this birth experience more positive	Allows for anticipatory problem solving, and enhances ability to meet goals and expectations for birth event
Independence and sense of confidence	Maximize the couple's opportunities to have choices and make decisions	Increases sense of control over one's body and experiences
Preparation for emergency cesarean	Avoid "last minute" approach	Avoids or minimizes reactions of anger, shock, resentment, panic, or crisis
	Keep couple informed as developments occur allowing for mutual decision making between the family and birth attendant, informing them of the facts, alternatives, and consequences of nonintervention	Gives couple control; helps them perceive their birth experience positively
Effective communication	Cover most salient points of what to anticipate: 1. What is going to happen to the woman's body and how it will feel 2. What and why specific procedures will be done 3. How to handle discomfort associated with procedures	Knowing what to expect increases coping capability
	Provide couple with brief period of privacy	Opportunity for them to pool their coping strengths to deal with the anxiety of the situation
	Inquire if couple has any questions about the decision	Opportunity for further clarification
	Prepare client in increments, giving information and rationale for each procedure	Crisis-altered cognitive grasp leads to information not being heard or misinterpreted
	Avoid silence	Often interpreted by the client as frightening and/or negative
	Employ eye contact and therapeutic touch	Conveys a feeling of caring and reality orientation
Postpartal visit by nurse attending birth	Describe the birth events, minute-by-minute, event-by-event	Fill in the "missing pieces" of the birth experience
	Encourage parents to tell story as many times as needed	Enables parents to psychologically integrate the birth experience and resolve negative feelings
Inclusion of father (or significant other) in birth	Support the presence of the father during intrapartal and postpartal periods if desired	Promotes family bonding, minimizes "missing pieces"; calming influence for the mother; shared experience

NURSING CARE PLAN Cont'd
Cesarean Birth

Problem	Nursing interventions and actions	Rationale
	Provide accurate, current information as developments occur	Reduces feelings of confusion, helplessness, and anxiety
	Serve as a support system for the father	
	Initiate father-infant contact immediately after delivery if infant stable	Promotes family bonding
	Allow parents and baby to be together in recovery room	
Recovery from surgery	Assess vital signs every 5 min until stable, then every 15 min for an hour, then every 30 min for 8 hours	Vital signs may vary in response to medications or anesthetic
Fluids and nutrition	Maintain intravenous infusion flow rate Check patency and inspect IV site for redness or swelling	IV fluids are maintained for 24-48 hours, or until bowel sounds are present; oxytocic agent is usually added to the IV infusion for a few hours after surgery to enhance contraction of uterine muscles
	Administer ice chips for first 24 hours, then advance diet as bowel sounds return	
Bladder drainage	Connect indwelling bladder catheter to dependent drainage. Catheter is usually removed 1-2 hours after IV fluids are discontinued	Enhances bladder emptying
	Measure urine output on first two voidings and check bladder for distention	Measuring urine provides information regarding adequate output and indicates whether the bladder is being emptied
Blood loss	Check hemoglobin and hematocrit a few hours after surgery and on first postoperative day	Identifies existence of anemia related to blood loss
Nausea and vomiting	Administer antiemetic as needed; check vital signs before administering	Establishes baseline vital signs; some antiemetics lower blood pressure
Pain	Administer pain medication as needed; assess vital signs before administering	Controls or alleviates pain at incision site and gas pains; establishes baseline vital signs, because pain medications may lower blood pressure
	Monitor maternal use if she is nursing	Many drugs taken by the mother are passed into the breast milk
	Place woman in comfortable position and splint incision when coughing or deep breathing	Provides support and relief of pain
Healing of incision	Inspect incision for redness, swelling, drainage, bruising, and separation of tissues	Healing of incision is facilitated when infection is absent; if signs of infection are present, antibiotic therapy is indicated
Bowel function	Auscultate bowel sounds	Bowel sounds are absent for 24-36 hours as a result of anesthetic and pain medication
	Progressive ambulation after 24 hours Discuss rationale for early ambulation and assist in the ambulation process	Ambulation enhances return of bowel function

NURSING CARE PLAN Cont'd
Cesarean Birth

Problem	Nursing interventions and actions	Rationale
	Offer positive reinforcement for all attempts and steps in ambulation process	
Pulmonary status	Turn patient and have her cough and deep breathe every 2 hours for 24 hours	Provides aeration of lungs and assists in preventing pulmonary complications
	Splint incision while she is coughing or deep breathing	Promotes comfort
Hemorrhage	Evaluate firmness and position of fundus	Monitor involution
	Palpate fundus after pain medication is administered to promote patient comfort	Palpation of fundus causes discomfort to the woman and is frequently neglected and therefore becomes increasingly important
	Fundus may be palpated from side of abdomen to avoid discomfort	Tenderness at incisional site
	Evaluate lochia	Lochia progresses from rubra to serosa to alba Increase in flow indicates inefficient contraction of uterus and/or subinvolution
Bonding	Enhance bonding by maintaining client comfort Provide information about the baby as soon as possible (such as sex, condition and normalcy) Provide early opportunities for parent-infant interaction	Interaction may be delayed because of recovery from anesthesia and discomfort in first few hours after delivery
	Discuss her feelings about the cesarean birth and her self-image as a mother	Feelings of failure associated with birthing experience can be generalized to ability to assume mothering role

NURSING CARE EVALUATION

No sign of infection is present	Client is discharged in good physical state
Involution proceeds normally	Education is provided for self-care and infant care

NURSING DIAGNOSES*	SUPPORTING DATA
1. Alteration in comfort: pain related to surgical procedure	Complaints of pain at incision site Gas pains
2. Potential alteration in bowel elimination	Absent or diminished bowel sounds Abdominal distention
3. Potential ineffective airway clearance	Reluctance to cough and deep breathe due to discomfort Rales, rhonchi Febrile
4. Potential alteration in parenting	Mother-infant bonding delayed Feelings of inadequacy, failure to have a "normal" birthing process
5. Knowledge deficit about postoperative course	Expressed concerns or questions about specific aspects of recovery from cesarean birth

*These are a few examples of nursing diagnoses that may be appropriate for a woman with this condition. It is not an inclusive list and must be individualized for each woman.

risk and high-risk clients does not cause a rise in the overall incidence of cesarean deliveries (Boehm et al., 1981). Electronic fetal monitoring does not necessarily raise the incidence of diagnosed fetal distress in a given population unless the population itself changes. The liberal attitude toward cesarean delivery for breech and other high-risk conditions has contributed more to its increased incidence than has electronic fetal monitoring.

Management of breech presentation has accounted for about 15% of the rise in the cesarean rate during the last 10 years. This trend was based on the increased incidence of neonatal morbidity and mortality thought to be secondary to vaginal delivery of a breech presentation. Subsequent studies have found that breech presentation is associated with both increased morbidity and mortality whether delivered by cesarean or vaginal route (Amirikia et al., 1981). Also, no improvement has been noted in perinatal mortality for breech presentation delivered by cesarean in contrast with vaginal delivery, other than in the fetus weighing 1000–1500 g (Mann and Gallant, 1979). When considering the route of delivery, fetal maturity, size, pelvic adequacy, presence of congenital anomalies, type of breech presentation, as well as the skill of the obstetrician must be considered.

A cesarean delivery is avoided if possible when the fetus is dead or too small to survive outside the uterus. The abdominal route increases maternal morbidity and mortality risks without any advantage for the fetus.

Maternal Mortality and Morbidity

Cesarean births have two to four times the maternal mortality of vaginal deliveries (NIH, 1980; Frigoletto et al., 1980; Amirikia et al., 1981). Mortality, although low (less than 0.02%), is most often due to anesthesia accidents and/or underlying medical conditions such as cardiac disease, renal disease, diabetes, or severe PIH.

Morbidity varies widely and depends upon the population assessed and the circumstances necessitating abdominal delivery. Major complications resulting from surgery include hemorrhage, blood clots, injury to the bladder or intestines and, most frequently, infection. The incidence of infection associated with cesarean delivery is five to ten times greater than with vaginal deliveries (Hawrylyshyn et al., 1981). The most common are endometritis and wound and urinary tract infections. Factors associated with increased risk for endometritis include onset and length of labor or rupture of the amniotic membranes prior to delivery. Hemostasis, increased operative time, blood loss, and trauma to the ovary are intraoperative factors that contribute to morbidity. The risk to the fetus of a traumatic vaginal delivery must be weighed against the risk of maternal morbidity.

Types of Cesarean Deliveries

The two most common types of cesarean deliveries are (a) the low-segment transverse or low cervical transverse, and (b) the classic.

The skin incision is either horizontal (Pfannenstiel or bikini) or vertical (classic) and is not indicative of the type of incision made into the uterus. With the horizontal skin incision, a transverse cut is made across the lowest and narrowest part of the abdomen. Since the incision is made just below the pubic hair line, it is almost invisible after healing. The limitations of this type of skin incision are that it does not allow for extension of the incision if needed, and it requires more time than the classic (vertical) incision. The classic (vertical) incision is made between the navel and the symphysis pubis. The incision can be made midline (most common) or paramedian (just off center) which allows for stronger scar formation. The type of skin incision is determined essentially by time factor or physician preference.

Uterine Incisions

The type of uterine incision is contingent upon the obstetric situation. The choice of incision affects whether the woman may have an opportunity for a subsequent vaginal delivery, along with risks for rupture of the uterine scar with a subsequent pregnancy.

The types of uterine incisions are low-segment transverse, classic, and low classic (Figure 19–5).

LOW-SEGMENT TRANSVERSE INCISION

Low-transverse method is the most common and most preferred for the following reasons:

1. The lower segment is the thinnest portion of the uterus. Therefore, an incision in this area results in a minimal blood loss.
2. The concentration of the contractile proteins actin and myosin is least in the lower uterine segment. Thus the chance of uterine rupture is decreased with subsequent pregnancies.
3. The chance of peritonitis is decreased.
4. There are fewer postoperative adhesions.

The limitations of the low-transverse incision are the following:

1. It takes longer to make and repair.
2. It is limited in size because of the presence of major blood vessels on either side of the uterus.

CLASSIC CESAREAN INCISION

The classic incision is used in the presence of adhesions from previous cesarean births, when the fetal position is the transverse lie, or with an anteriorly implanted placenta.

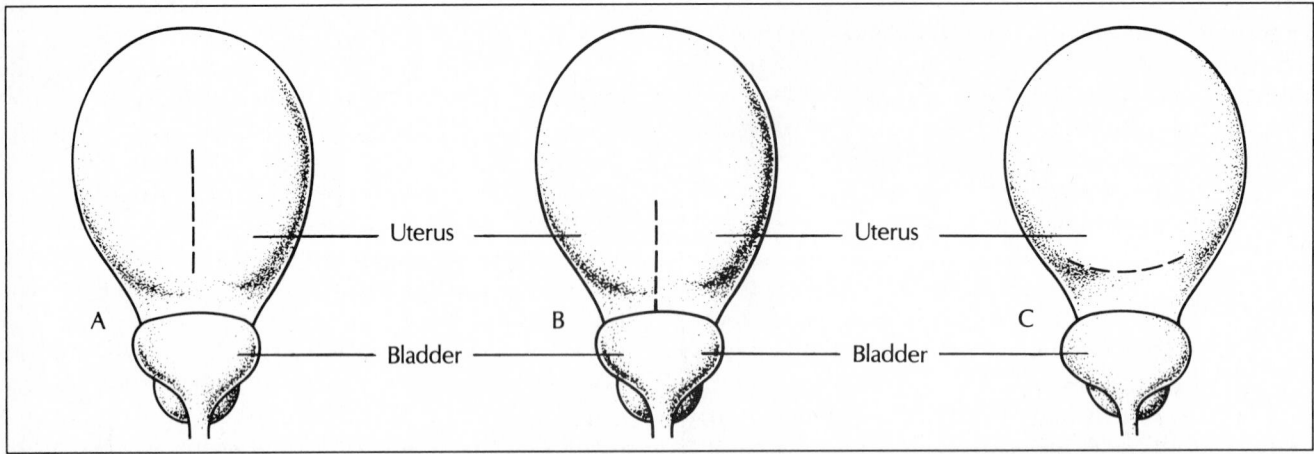

FIGURE 19–5 Types of uterine incisions for cesarean delivery **A,** Classic. **B,** Low classic. **C,** low uterine transverse.

Because large blood vessels in the myometrium are cut, there is more blood loss with this incision than with others and a slight increase in rupture of the uterine scar in subsequent labors.

LOW CLASSIC INCISION

The low classic (low flap vertical) incision is made into the lower uterine segment. Considered to be a compromise between the classic and transverse, it is as safe as a transverse, yet can be extended into a classic if necessary.

Elective Repeat Cesarean

In North America, elective repeat cesarean births are common following a primary cesarean. The dictum "once a cesarean always a cesarean" advocated by Cragin before the New York Medical Society in 1916 was based on the use of the classic uterine incision. The rationale for repeat cesarean was to avoid the risks of uterine rupture during labor. In 1974 more than 99% of women with previous cesareans were delivered by repeat cesarean in subsequent pregnancies, although contemporary practices involved the low-transverse incision in 99% of the cases (Lowe et al., 1976).

The trend is increasing to have a trial of labor and vaginal delivery after a primary cesarean in cases of nonrecurring indications (for example, cord accident, placenta previa, fetal distress). This trend has been influenced by client demand and a growing body of evidence suggesting that a properly conducted vaginal delivery after a cesarean poses less risk for maternal and neonatal mortality and morbidity than does a repeat cesarean (Lavin et al., 1982). In a review of the literature (1950–1980), Lavin and associates found that of those women allowed a trial of labor, 66.7% were successful in delivering vaginally. Successful vaginal delivery occurred in 74.2% of women with a nonrecurrent indication for their previous cesarean and in

33.3% of those whose indication for previous cesarean was CPD. Clients who had a prior vaginal delivery were more likely to deliver vaginally than those who did not (Lavin et al., 1982). Although a classic uterine scar increases the probability of uterine rupture, the precise increased risk cannot be accurately determined. The risks of uterine rupture (less than 1%) following a low-transverse incision in contrast to increased maternal and neonatal risks of a repeat surgical delivery are receiving renewed attention in obstetric management practices (Shy et al., 1981). This issue concerns not only client satisfaction and safety but is also related to health care costs.

A trial of labor should be attempted only when the chances for a vaginal delivery are positive. Precautions that should be taken to ensure a safe delivery include the following:

1. Contraindications for vaginal delivery (such as CPD, placenta previa, and abruptio placentae) ruled out.
2. Availability of medical records with complete information about the previous cesarean birth, course of delivery, and postoperative recovery.
3. Fully equipped medical center with full-time staff, operating room, and anesthesia readily available.
4. Readily available blood products.
5. Constant physician attendance during labor.
6. Following delivery of the neonate, the uterus should be explored to ascertain whether the uterine scar is intact.

Nursing Interventions for Family Having Cesarean Birth

PREPARATION FOR CESAREAN BIRTH

Cesarean birth is an alternative method of delivery. Since one out of every five or six deliveries is a cesarean, preparation for this possibility should be an integral part of every childbirth education curriculum. The attitude of the instructor in conveying factual information will affect the client's reaction to an unplanned cesarean birth. The instructor can emphasize the similarities between cesarean and vaginal births to minimize undertones of "normal" versus "abnormal" delivery (Affonso, 1981). This will diminish feelings of anger, loss, and grief.

All couples should be encouraged to discuss with their obstetrician what the approach would be in the event of a cesarean. They can also discuss their needs and desires as a couple under those circumstances. Their preferences may include the following:

- Participating in the choice of anesthetic
- Father (or significant other) being present during the procedures and/or delivery
- Father (or significant other) being present in the recovery or postpartum room
- Audio recording and/or taking pictures of the birth
- Delayed instillation of eye drops to promote eye contact between parent and infant in the first hours after delivery
- Physical contact or holding the newborn while on the delivery table and/or in the recovery room (if the mother cannot hold the newborn the father can hold the baby for her)
- Breast-feeding on the delivery table and/or in the recovery room

Information couples need about cesarean delivery are categorically the same as for vaginal birth. They include:

- Events in the preparatory phase
- Description or viewing of the delivery room
- Types of anesthesia
- Sensations that may be experienced
- Roles of significant others
- Interaction with neonate
- Immediate recovery phase
- Postpartal phase

The context in which this information is given should be "birth-oriented" rather than surgery-oriented.

PREPARATION FOR REPEAT CESAREAN BIRTH

When a couple is anticipating a cesarean birth, they have time to analyze and synthesize the information and to prepare for some of the specifics. Many hospitals or local groups (such as C-Sec Inc.) provide preparation classes for cesarean birth. The instructor should impart a feeling of normalcy and factual information, which will allow a couple to make choices and participate in their birth experience. Couples who have had previous negative experiences need an opportunity to describe what they felt contributed to these events. They should be encouraged to

identify what they would like to have altered and to list interventions that would make the experience more positive. Those who have had positive experiences need reassurance that their needs and desires will be met in the same manner. In addition, an opportunity should be given to discuss any fears or anxieties.

A specific concern of the client facing a repeat cesarean is "anticipation of the pain experience." She needs reassurance that subsequent cesareans are often less painful than the first. She will not experience the extreme fatigue that followed the primary cesarean if it was preceded by a long and/or strenuous labor. Giving this information will enable her to cope more effectively with stressful stimuli, including pain. The nurse can remind the client that she has already had experience with how to prevent, cope with, and alleviate painful stimuli.

PREPARATION FOR EMERGENCY CESAREAN DELIVERY

Usually a couple is prepared for an emergency cesarean by either the "last minute" or the "mutual decision" approach. All too frequently childbirth attendants wait until the last minute to inform the client of the need for a cesarean delivery under the guise of "sparing the couple undue anxiety." Ironically, the client's reaction to this delayed approach is not only excessive anxiety but also anger, shock, and resentment resulting in a state of crisis or panic (Affonso and Stichler, 1980). In contrast, the mutual decision approach between the birth attendants and the client keeps the family fully informed as developments occur. The clinician presents all the facts, suggests alternatives, and describes likely outcomes of nonintervention, allowing the expectant parents to participate in the decision making. The opportunity to make choices and have control over their birthing experience is the major factor influencing a couple's positive perception of the event (Affonso and Stichler, 1980).

The period preceding surgery must be used to its greatest advantage. The couple needs some time for privacy to assimilate the information given to them and to quickly pull together their strength to face this new crisis. It is imperative that caregivers utilize their most effective communication skills. Silence is often interpreted by the client as indicating danger for her and her fetus and/or caregiver anger resulting from her failure to perform (Affonso, 1981). The client may experience a sense of panic and/or fear. She may be confused and numb to instructions. It is essential for the attendant to address the salient points regarding what the couple may anticipate during the next few hours. Ask "What questions do you have about the decision?" This gives the couple an opportunity for further clarification. Prepare the client in increments, giving her information and the rationale for each procedure before commencing. In brief, before carrying out a procedure tell her (a) what you are going to do; (b) why you are going to do it; and (c) what sensations she may experience. This allows the client to be informed and to consent to the procedure. The client experiences a sense of control, and therefore less helplessness and powerlessness.

Often the phenomenon of memory lapse is more pronounced during crisis or panic states. "Missing pieces" are unremembered events or segments of time. Although not unique to cesarean birth this phenomenon contributes to a sense of loss or missing out for the woman. Her inability to remember may contribute to feelings of depression or anger. It is important for the delivery nurse to visit the client during the postpartal period to fill in the "missing pieces." Women, whether awake or asleep for the delivery, have confirmed the value of having the event relived for them minute-by-minute and event-by-event. This process is valuable because (a) it allows for reality orientation and correction of the client's misperceptions or misinformation; (b) it aids in psychologic integration of the birth event; and (c) it fosters the attachment process.

Preparation of the client for surgery involves more than the procedures of establishing intravenous lines and urinary catheter, or doing an abdominal prep. As discussed previously, good communication skills are very influential in helping the client stay in control. Therapeutic touch and eye contact do much to maintain reality orientation and control. These measures reduce anxiety for the client during the stressful preparatory period. All clients will experience some degree of anxiety and apprehension: behavioral manifestations of anxiety include withdrawal, crying, apologies, or inappropriate laughter. Increased heart rate, blood pressure, body temperature, dilated pupils, pallor and/or dry mouth are physiologic signs of anxiety. Anxiety also affects senses such as sight, hearing, as well as cognitive grasp. Severe anxiety often results in distortion of reality. The nurse should continually assess how the client is perceiving the event and coping with her apprehension.

If the cesarean delivery is scheduled and not an emergency, the nurse has ample time for preoperative teaching. The woman needs to practice her turning, coughing, and deep breathing. It is helpful if she is taught to splint her abdominal muscles when she coughs. The nurse should determine whether she wants to breast-feed or bottle-feed, so that medication to inhibit lactation can be sent to surgery if needed.

To prepare the woman for the surgery, she is given nothing by mouth, an abdominal and perineal prep is done (from below breasts to the pubic region), and an indwelling catheter is inserted to dependent drainage, to prevent bladder distention and obstructed delivery. An operative permit must be signed by the woman. At least two units of whole blood are readied for administration. An intravenous line is started, with an adequate size needle to permit blood administration, and preoperative medication is ordered. The pediatrician should be notified and adequate preparation made to receive the infant. The nurse should make sure that the infant warmer is functional and that appropriate resuscitation equipment is available. The circulating nurse assists in positioning the client on the operating table. Fetal heart rate should be ascertained before surgery and during preparation, since fetal hypoxia can result from supine maternal hypotension. The operating table may be adjusted so it slants slightly to one side. This helps relieve the pressure of the gravid uterus on the vena cava and lessens the incidence of supine maternal hypotension. The suction should be in working order, and the urine collection bag should be positioned under the operating table to ensure proper urinary drainage.

DELIVERY

There are conflicting opinions and policies about fathers in the delivery room during a cesarean birth. It is interesting that the reasons for excluding them are similar to those that excluded fathers from the vaginal birth environment. Examples of these opinions, which have since been proven to be invalid, include concerns about the father fainting, emotional trauma, increased risk of law suits or infection, and so on. The NIH Task Force on Cesarean Birth (1980), after considering this issue, concluded that "in spite of the widespread fears of adverse effects . . . there is no evidence of harm from fathers' participation." The American College of Obstetrics and Gynecology position statement states that they "cannot perceive strong medical indications or contraindications of the presence of fathers in the operating suite" (Affonso, 1981). In fact, it has been found the father's presence during the cesarean procedure leads to a more positive evaluation of the birth experience later by both the mother and father (Affonso, 1981). In addition, when the father was present for the delivery, the mother required less postpartal medication for pain, experienced less loneliness, and was less anxious about the baby's health.

When the father attends the cesarean birth he must scrub and wear the surgical gown and mask as do others in the operating suite. A stool can be placed beside the woman's head. The father can sit nearby to provide physical touch, visual contact, and verbal reassurance to his partner.

Other measures can be taken to promote the participation of the father who is not allowed or chooses not to be in the delivery room. They are:

1. Allowing the father to be near the delivery room where he can hear the newborn's first cry.

2. Encouraging the father to carry or accompany the infant to the nursery for the initial assessment.

3. Involving the father in postpartal care in the recovery room.

In addition to meeting the emotional and informational needs of the expectant parents, other nursing functions are carried out to assure physiologic support and safety of the woman and neonate. The nurse should stand by to connect the suction when the operating team is ready and should record the actual time the incision is made and the infant is delivered. An oxytocin preparation is administered intravenously just as the infant is born.

After delivery, the nurse assists the pediatrician with physiologic support of the neonate. After the infant's condition is stable, he or she should be shown to the woman if she is awake. Repeat administration of oxytocin during surgery may be necessary to control uterine bleeding. The circulating nurse assists with the application of the dressing to the incision and, with the aid of other staff, helps the woman back into bed.

Analgesia and Anesthesia

There is no perfect anesthesia for cesarean delivery. Each has its advantages, disadvantages, possible risks, and side effects. Goals for analgesia and anesthesia administration include safety, comfort, and emotional satisfaction for the client. Effects of analgesia and anesthesia upon the neonate vary. Different pharmacologic agents cross the placenta at different rates into the fetal bloodstream and are metabolized at varying rates. Other factors associated with the effects of drugs on the neonate include (a) dosage, (b) route of administration, (c) maternal metabolism, (d) health of fetus, and (e) length of time between administration of drug and delivery of the neonate. There are two classifications of anesthesia for cesarean delivery: general and conduction (spinal and epidural). See Chapter 17 for further discussion.

IMMEDIATE POSTPARTAL RECOVERY PERIOD

The postpartal recovery room must be equipped with suction and oxygen to adequately ensure a patent airway and to protect from respiratory obstruction resulting from secretions. The recovery room nurse should check the mother's vital signs every 5 minutes until they are stable, then every 15 minutes for an hour, then every 30 minutes until she is discharged to the postpartal floor. The nurse should remain with the woman until she is stable.

The dressing and perineal pad must be checked every 15 minutes for at least an hour, and the fundus should be gently palpated to determine whether it is remaining firm. The fundus may be palpated by placing a hand to support the incision. Intravenous oxytocin is usually administered to promote the contractility of the uterine musculature. If the client has been under general anesthesia, she should be positioned on her side to facilitate drainage of secretions, turned, and assisted with coughing and deep breathing every 2 hours for at least 24 hours. If she has received a spinal anesthetic, the level of anesthesia should be checked every 15 minutes until sensation has fully returned. It is important to monitor intake and output and to observe the urine for bloody tinge, which could mean surgical trauma to the bladder. The physician prescribes medication to relieve the mother's pain and nausea, and this should be administered as needed. Facilitation of parent–infant interaction following birth and postpartal care is discussed in Chapter 28.

SUMMARY

Elective and operative procedures are widely utilized in obstetrics. Amniotomy, the most common operative procedure, is performed to shorten labor. Labor can be induced when the fetus is mature and the cervix is ripe. Episiotomies reduce tearing of perineal tissues and promote their healing. Forceps were developed to assist in difficult delivery situations. Other alternatives to difficult deliveries include version procedures and cesarean birth. Operative obstetrics provides a means for health care practitioners to promote the safety, health, and comfort of the laboring woman and her fetus.

Resource Groups

Cesarean Birth Council International, P.O. Box 4331, Mountain View, CA 94040. Information, literature; parent advocacy.

Cesarean Connection, P.O. Box 11, West Mount, IL 60559. Clearinghouse for information and resources; newsletter.

C-Sec Incorporated, 66 Christopher Road, Waltham, MA 02154. Information, parent education groups for cesarean birth.

International Childbirth Education Association, Inc. Cesarean Birth Council, P.O. Box 20048, Minneapolis, MN 55420. Information, parent education regarding childbirth.

References

Affonso, D. D. 1981. *Impact of cesarean childbirth.* Philadelphia: F. A. Davis Co.

Affonso, D. D., and Stichler, J. F. March 1980. Cesarean birth: women's reactions. *Am. J. Nurs.* 80:468.

Amirikia, H., et al. May 1981. Cesarean section: a 15-year review of changing incidence, indications, and risks. *Am. J. Obstet. Gynecol.* 140:81.

Banta, D., and Thacker, S. B. Spring, 1982. The risks and benefits of episiotomy: A review. *Birth.* 9:25.

Baxie, L. V., et al. Jan. 1980. Induction of labor with low dose prostaglandin and oxytocin. *Am. J. Obstet. Gynecol.* 136:28.

Bishop, E. H. 1964. Pelvic scoring for elective inductions. *Obstet. Gynecol.* 24:266.

Boehm, F. H., et al. June 1981. The effect of electronic fetal monitoring on the incidence of cesarean section. *Am. J. Obstet. Gynecol.* 140:295.

Carter, F. B., and Wolber, P. G. 1981. Episiotomy. In *Gynecology and obstetrics,* vol. 2:1, chapter 67, ed. J. J. Sciarra. Hagerstown, Md.: Harper & Row.

Cibils, L. A. 1981. *Electronic fetal-maternal monitoring.* Boston: PSG Publishing Co.

Coats, P.M., et al. May 1980. A comparison between midline and mediolateral episiotomies. *Br. J. Obstet. Gynaecol.* 87:408.

Cogan, R., and Edmunds, E. P. 1977. The unkindest cut. *Contemp. OB/Gyn.* 9:55.

Cohen, W. 1977. Influence of the duration of second stage labor on perinatal outcome and puerperal morbidity. *Obstet. Gynecol.* 49:266.

Danforth, D. N., ed. 1982. *Obstetrics and gynecology.* 4th ed. Philadelphia: Harper & Row.

Department of Health, Education and Welfare. 1978. *Food and Drug Administration Bulletin.* New restrictions on oxytocin use, vol. 8. Oct/Nov. 1978.

Fall, O., and Nilsson, B. A. June 1979. External cephalic version in breech presentation under tocolysis. *Obstet. Gynecol.* 53:712.

Friedman, E., and Sachtleben, M. R. 1976. Station of the fetal presenting part. VI. Arrest of descent in nulliparas. *Obstet. Gynecol.* 47:129.

Friedman, E., et al. 1977. Dysfunctional labor. XII. Long-term effects on infant. *Am. J. Obstet. Gynecol.* 127:779.

Frigoletto, F. D., et al. April 1980. Maternal mortality rate associated with cesarean section: an appraisal. *Am. J. Obstet. Gynecol.* 136:969.

Giacoia, G. P. and Yaffe, S. 1982. Perinatal pharmacology. In *Gynecology and obstetrics,* vol. 3, chapter 100, ed. J. J. Sciarri. Philadelphia: Harper & Row.

Greis, J. B., et al. May 1981. Comparison of maternal and fetal effects of vaccum extraction with forceps or cesarean deliveries. *Obstet. Gynecol.* 57:571.

Hawrylyshyn, P. A., et al. Feb. 1981. Risk factors associated with infection following cesarean. *Am. J. Obstet. Gynecol.* 139:294.

Hibbard, L. 1976. Changing trends in cesarean sections. *Am. J. Obstet. Gynecol.* 75:798.

Hughes, E. C., ed., 1972. *Obstetrics-gynecology terminology.* Philadelphia: F. A. Davis Co.

Jagoni, N., et al. Jan. 1982. Role of the cervix in the induction of labor. *Obstet. Gynecol.* 59:21.

Jones, O. H. 1976. Cesarean section in present-day obstetrics. *Am. J. Obstet. Gynecol.* 76:798.

Kappy, K. A. Feb. 1981. Vacuum extractor. *Clinics in Perinatol.* 8:79.

Lavin, J. P., et al. Feb. 1982. Vaginal delivery in patients with prior cesarean section. *Obstet. Gynecol.* 59:135.

Liggins, G. C. July 1978. Ripening of the cervix. *Seminars in Perinatol.* 2:261.

Lowe, J., et al. Jan. 1976. Cesarean sections in U.S. PAS hospitals. *PAS reports.* 14:1.

Mann, L.I., and Gallant, J. Oct. 1979. Modern indications for cesarean section. *Am. J. Obstet. Gynecol.* 135:437.

Martell, M., et al. 1976. Blood acid-base balance at birth in neonates from labors with early and late rupture of membranes. *J. Pediatr.* 89:693.

Niswander, K. R. 1980. Induction of labor. In *Gynecology and obstetrics,* vol. 2, rev. ed. 1982. eds. J. J. Sciarra, and A. B. Gerbie. Hagerstown, Md.: Harper & Row.

NIH Cesarean Birth Task Force. 1980. National Institute of Child Development statement on cesarean childbirth. USDHHS, Building HHH, Rm 447F8, Washington, D. C. 20201.

Pakzad, K. G. Aug. 1980. Risks occurring in birth induction without considering cervix maturity. *J. Perinat. Med.* 8:27.

Plauché, W. C. Feb. 1978. Vacuum extraction: use in a community hospital setting. *Obstet. Gynecol.* 52:289.

————. June 1979. Fetal cranial injuries related to delivery with the Malmström vacuum extractor. *Obstet. Gynecol.* 53:750.

Pritchard, J. A., and MacDonald, P. C. 1980. *Williams obstetrics,* 16th ed. New York: Appleton-Century-Crofts.

Shy, K. K., et al. Jan. 1981. Evaluation of elective repeat cesarean section as a standard of care: an application of decision analysis. *Am. J. Obstet. Gynecol.* 139:123.

Stichler, J. F., and Affonso, D. D. March 1980. Cesarean birth. *Am. J. Nurs.* 80:466.

Ulmsten, U. March 1982. Intracervical application of prostaglandin gel for induction of term labor. *Obstet. Gynecol.* 59:336.

VanDorsten, J. P., et al. Oct. 1981. Randomized control trial of external cephalic version with tocolysis in late pregnancy. *Am. J. Obstet. Gynecol.* 141:417.

Additional Readings

Crowell, D. H., et al. Jan. 1980. Effects of induction of labor on the neurophysiologic functioning of newborn infants. *Am. J. Obstet. Gynecol.* 136:48.

Granat, M. 1976. Oxytocin contraindication in the presence of uterine scar. *Lancet.* 2:1411.

Luther, E. R., et al. June 1980. The effect of estrogen priming on induction of labor with prostaglandins. *Am. J. Obstet. Gynecol.* 137:351.

McNay, M. B., et al. 1977. Perinatal deaths: analysis by clinical cause to assess value of inductions of labour. *Br. Med. J.* 1:347.

Moolgasker, A. S., et al. Sept. 1979. A comparison of different methods of instrumental delivery based on electronic measurements of compression and traction. *Obstet. Gynecol.* 54:299.

O'Driscoll, K., and Geoghegan, F. April 1981. Haemorrhage in first born infants and delivery with obstetric forceps. *Br. J. Obstet. Gynaecol.* 88:577.

O'Herlihy, M. B., and MacDonald, M. B. 1979. Influence of preinduction prostaglandin E_2 vagina gel on cervical ripening and labor. *Obstet. Gynecol.* 54:708.

Sellers, S. M., et al. Jan. 1980. Release of prostaglandins past amniotomy is not mediated by oxytocin. *Br. J. Obstet. Gynaecol.* 87:43.

Sleiner, H., et al. Jan. 1979. Cervical ripening prior to induction of labor (intracervical applicaton of a PGE_2 viscous gel). *Prostaglandins.* 17:125.

Stewart, P. Jan. 1982. Spontaneous labor: when should the membranes be ruptured? *Br. J. Obstet. Gynaecol.* 89:39.

Stewart, P., et al. Mar. 1981. A comparison of oestradiol and prostaglandin E_2 for ripening the cervix. *Br. J. Obstet. Gynaecol.* 88:236.

Ulmsten, U., et al. Nov. 1979. Comparison of prostaglandin E_2 and intravenous oxytocin for induction of labor. *Obstet. Gynecol.* 54:581.

BIRTHING OPTIONS

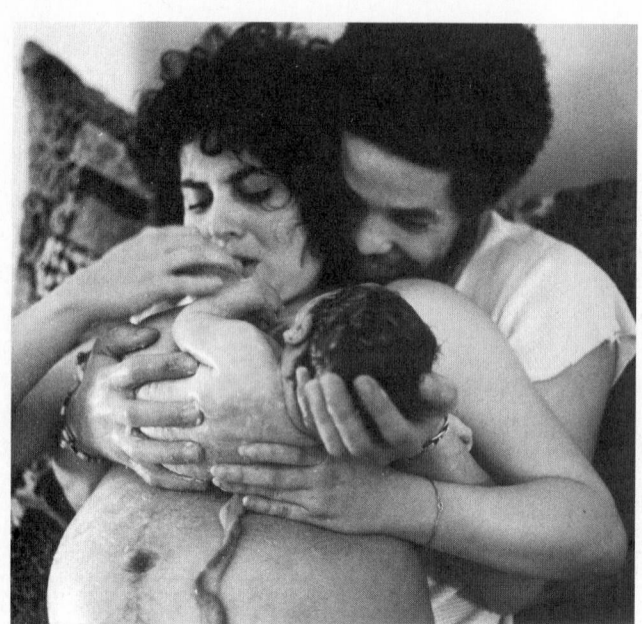

■ CHAPTER OUTLINE

BIRTHING OPTIONS
  Siblings at Birth
  Alternative Positions
  The Leboyer Method
  Birth Centers
  Early Discharge
  Home Births

■ OBJECTIVES

- Discuss sibling attendance at birth.

- Examine alternative birthing positions and settings for labor and delivery.

- Describe early discharge programs and subsequent postpartal assessment.

- Explore philosophy, preparation, and management of home birth.

BIRTHING OPTIONS

Maternal and neonatal death rates have fallen dramatically over the past 20 years, affording expectant parents what some would call the luxury of seeking joy and growth in the birth experience. Many couples no longer see birth as an isolated medical experience, but rather as a highly personal and significant life event and one over which they should have significant control (Burchell and Gunn, 1980). Consequently, the desires of expectant parents frequently include the following requests:

1. That labor and delivery be performed in a supportive, quiet, and relaxed environment.

2. That an enema and perineal shave not be given at admission.

3. That the father be allowed to participate as much as the couple desires.

4. That medications and treatments be administered only with the couple's permission and only after a complete explanation about their actions and possible side effects has been given.

5. That invasive fetal monitoring be avoided.

6. That forceps and anesthesia not be used unless medically indicated.

7. That the woman may labor and deliver in the same room and bed.

8. That an episiotomy not be performed.

9. That the baby be delivered in a dimly lighted room and gently handled.

10. That the parents be allowed maximal interaction with their child or that the infant be allowed to nurse immediately after delivery.

11. That the baby be allowed to remain with his or her parents.

12. That the labor and delivery be shared by persons significant to the couple.

Some hospitals are not equipped to meet some of these requests. Others refuse because they believe that certain procedures are necessary to maintain maternal and fetal well-being. Others refuse because of resistance to change to new ideas and methods. In any case, many ex-

pectant families are frustrated in their attempt to make decisions about the kind of childbearing experience they want. As a result, they are seeking alternate modes of maternity care and individuals who are more responsive to their desires.

Siblings at Birth

More couples are choosing to extend the "family-centered" concept beyond mother, father, and neonate by including their other children in the birth experience. Their desire is to emerge as a family in close touch with one another and to reclaim birth as a normal and significant life event. Many hospitals have yet to develop programs for postpartal sibling visitation, consequently having siblings attend a birth is often an even less available option. However, families who feel strongly that they want their children with them will probably do so even if they must create their own situation to carry out that choice.

Children less than 2 years of age generally have little interest in pregnancy or birth, but early preschool-age children are interested in babies and where they come from. Involvement in the pregnancy, preparations for the birth, and seeing the birth itself can help reduce these childrens' often unspoken fears and misconceptions. Their education and active involvement in the birth process helps children perceive themselves as being as important as the newborn and to see themselves as active rather than passive family members (Bliss, 1980). Involvement of siblings in the events surrounding birth also fosters the integration of the newborn into the family unit, with a resulting decrease in "normal" sibling rivalry. Early bonding and skin-to-skin contact between siblings are as valuable as they are between parent and newborn. Presence at the birth or at least frequent postpartal contact is also helpful in reducing the anger and anxiety elicited in toddlers and preschoolers by the separation from their mother.

The decision to have children present at birth is a very personal and individual one. Those who support this concept agree that some broad guidelines help maximize the experience for the entire family. It is generally accepted that children, like parents, benefit from some education prior to experiencing childbirth. This usually involves a combination of books, audiovisuals, models, parental discussion, formal education classes, and play experiences. Within the limits of their cognitive development, certain essential points should be covered. These include the anatomy and physiology of pregnancy, labor, and birth and some information about fetal development. It is important to tell them what they are likely to see or hear during the birth process. For example, they may be told:

- Labor is hard, intense work and mother will need to concentrate during her contractions. Between the contractions she may be able to talk and answer questions.

- The work of labor may be accompanied by sounds such as groaning and panting that the child has not heard before.

- Labor is uncomfortable and sometimes painful, but women's bodies are made in a special way to do this work without coming apart.

- Birth is generally very "wet"; this is to be expected and is okay.

Teaching children about the placenta and its delivery is also necessary, and information concerning the episiotomy and its repair is included when appropriate (Parma, 1979). Children as young as 3 years old can be given basic information tailored to meet their needs. Some practitioners recommend that children under 4 years old should be discouraged from attending birth because they are less likely to question what they do not understand and are more dependent on their mothers for emotional support (Leonard et al., 1979).

It is highly recommended that there be a support person or coach with the child whose sole responsibility is tending to the needs of the child. The support person should be well known to the child, warm, sensitive, flexible, knowledgeable about the birth process, and comfortable with sexuality and birth. They must be prepared to interpret what is happening as the child requires and intervene when necessary.

The child should be given the option of relating to the birth in whatever manner he or she chooses as long as it is not disruptive. Children should certainly understand that it is their own option to be there and that they may stay or leave the room as they choose. It may be helpful to elicit from the child exactly what he or she expects from the experience in order to best assist in meeting the child's goal.

Children vary in their responses, sometimes depending on the stage of labor and delivery. Leonard and colleagues (1979) found that in early labor children interacted more with their mother, asking questions, timing contractions, and engaging in tending, supportive interventions. In late labor, when the mother became less accessible most of the children withdrew somewhat and adopted more of an observer role. Whatever the child's coping style, it is intensified as labor progresses. During delivery some children chose to stand very close, while others preferred to distance themselves. Following delivery, the newborn was generally the center of attention and delivery of the placenta and any repairs frequently went unnoticed. Overall, no child showed any extreme distress and most seemed to notice maternal sounds more than any particular sight. At times they required some modulation of the intensity of the experience, which was usually accomplished by leaving the room.

Many agencies logically are concerned about neonatal infection when siblings are present. Parents are requested not to bring children who are obviously ill. Children are requested to perform an antiseptic scrub and put on a cover gown. In agencies that only allow sibling postpartal visits, infection has not been an issue.

In general, the presence of siblings at birth engenders feelings of interest and the desire to nurture "our" baby, as opposed to jealousy and rivalry directed at "mom's" baby. Instead of the mother mysteriously disappearing to the hospital, leaving the children at home, and returning with a demanding outsider, the family attending delivery together finds a new opportunity for closeness and growth through the sharing of the birth of a new member.

Alternative Positions

The upright posture for labor and delivery was considered normal in most societies until modern times. Squatting, kneeling, standing, and sitting were variously selected for birth by women. It has only been within the last two hundred years that the recumbent position has become more usual in the Western world. Its use in this century has been reinforced because of the convenience it offers in applying new technology. The lithotomy position has thus become the conventional manner in which North American women give birth in hospitals. In searching for alternative positions, consumers and professionals alike are refocusing on the practices of primitive cultures and midwives, where attention is on the comfort of the laboring woman rather than on the convenience of the birth attendant (Irwin, 1978) (Figure 20–1).

The traditional recumbent position for labor and lithotomy position for delivery provide for easier cleansing and visualization of the perineum, more convenient monitoring of FHR, easier handling of intravenous fluid therapy, and easier access for administering anesthesia and repairing the perineum (McKay, 1980). On the other hand, traditional positioning may also cause significant maternal hypotension due to the weight of the gravid uterus on the inferior vena cava and aorta. This drop in maternal blood pressure may have a marked influence on the development of fetal distress in labor. The dorsal recumbent position in labor also has been said to diminish the efficiency of uterine contractions, contribute to a loss of pelvic mobility, and

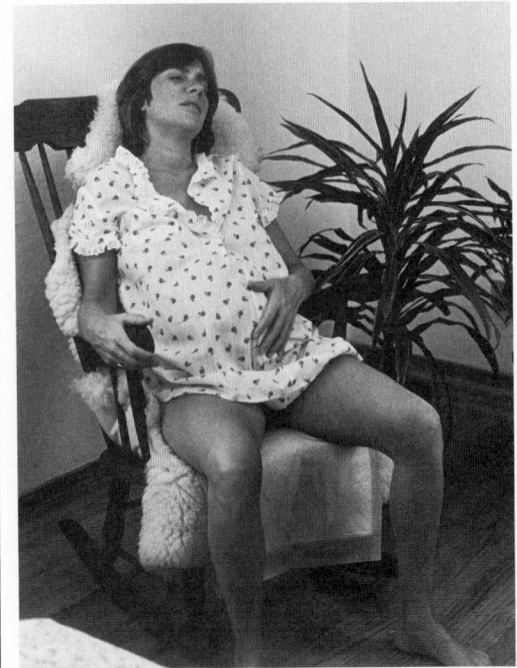

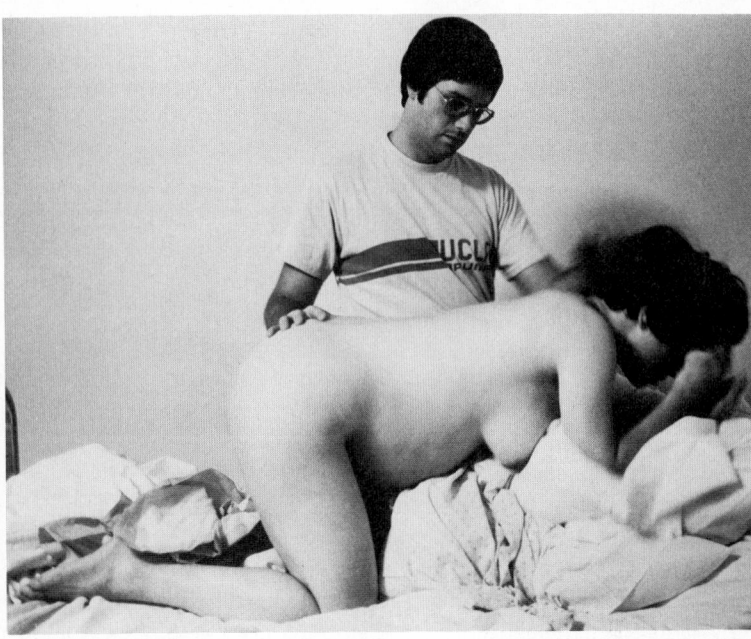

Figure 20–1 As long as no contraindications exist, the laboring woman is encouraged to choose a position of comfort. The nurse modifies her assessments and interventions as necessary. (© Suzanne Arms.)

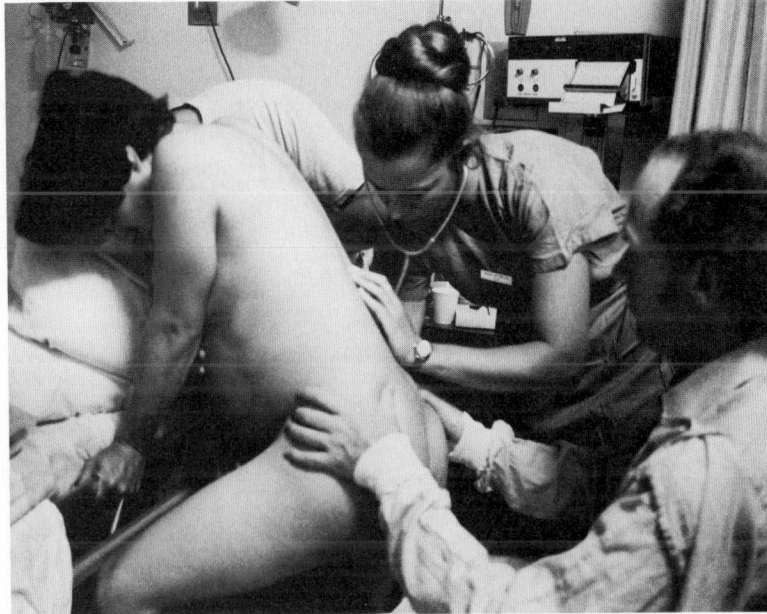

work against the forces of gravity, all culminating in a slower labor.

Proponents of more "natural" birth positions criticize the lithotomy position for its effects on maternal blood pressure, its attendant risks of thrombosis, emesis, and nerve lesions, and its high incidence of back pain. It has been shown that when the woman flexes her thighs the vagina tightens and narrows, contractions weaken and be-

come less regular, and increased force is required to give birth as the woman pushes "uphill." Consequently, episiotomies and forceps are required with disturbing frequency (McKay, 1980). Many women find the position not only unnatural, but also undignified and unnecessarily embarrassing. Without the aid of well-placed mirrors, the woman in the lithotomy position is visually and sometimes tactilely separated from her own birth experience.

An alternative position favored by some women and birth attendants is the left lateral Sims (Figure 20–2). In assuming this position for delivery, the woman lies on her left side with her left leg extended and her right knee drawn against her abdomen or flexed by her side. Those who favor this position find it increases overall comfort, does not compromise venous return from the lower extremities, and diminishes the chances of aspiration should vomiting occur. Women also perceive the lateral Sims as a more natural and comfortable position and less intrusive with no stirrups or overhead lights required. Birth attendants have found the position has a positive effect on the management of fetal shoulder dystocias. It also decreases the temptation to apply excess fundal pressure since the fundus is not as accessible. Fewer episiotomies are required in this position since the perineum tends to be more relaxed. Some data show the additional advantage of offering better control over precipitous deliveries (Irwin, 1978).

Critics of the lateral position cite the necessity of turning the woman on to her back to repair any episiotomy or lacerations, problems with difficult forceps deliveries, the inconvenience of adjusting standard obstetric drapes to the new position, and uncomfortable positioning for the birth attendant (Irwin, 1978). The position also offers no clear advantage in bringing the woman visually closer to the birth.

The squatting position is favored by some women primarily for the positive use it makes of gravity. Squatting is thought to facilitate the entrance of the presenting part into the pelvic inlet, thus hastening engagement. During the second stage of labor, squatting increases the size of the pelvic outlet and helps in the woman's bearing-down efforts. Some birth attendants object to this position because the perineum is relatively inaccessible and thus it is difficult for them to control the birth process. Squatting also increases the difficulty of administering analgesia, using instruments, and monitoring fetal status.

A semi-Fowler's position is advocated by some as an appropriate middle ground between the recumbent and upright positions. This position enhances the effectiveness of the abdominal muscle efforts while the client is pushing and thereby shortens the second stage of labor. By raising and supporting the torso, the woman is sometimes better able to view the birth process. At the same time, the birth attendant has access to the perineum. Many older delivery room tables are not capable of adjusting to a semi-Fowler's position, however.

The sitting position is becoming an option for more women with the increased availability of birthing chairs. The use of delivery chairs can be traced back to ancient Egyptian hieroglyphics and was broadly used in ancient Greek, Roman, and Incan civilizations. In the wake of the nineteenth-century battle against puerperal fever, birthing chairs began to vanish on hygienic grounds. Birthing chairs are being used again during the second stage of labor and are perceived by some women who use them as a positive way to actively participate in the birth process (Figure 20–3). The upright sitting position offers advantages similar to squatting and the semi-Fowler's position. It has been postulated that the weight of a term fetus is sufficient force in itself to supply much of what is needed to bring the newborn into the world. Proponents of the birth chair state that it makes possible spontaneous deliveries in births that would have required operative assistance in the recumbent

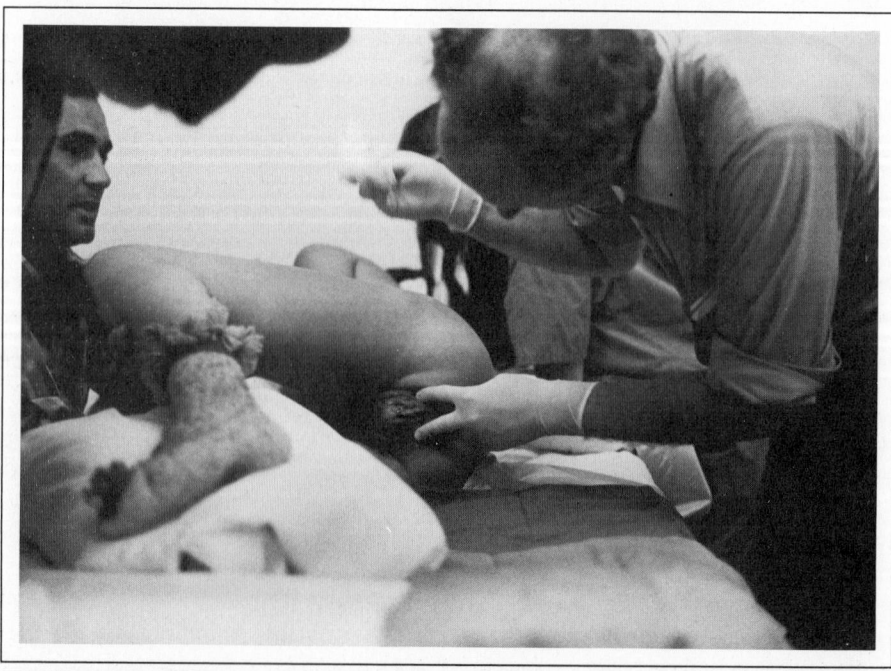

Figure 20–2 Side-lying delivery. Note that the woman's upper leg is supported by her partner. (© Suzanne Arms.)

position. Women experiencing severe back pain have found use of the chair can diminish or eliminate the pain. Birth attendants feel that a good working position can be easily achieved during deliveries in the birth chair. Other than the fact that it requires a change in birth attendants' approaches at delivery, the chief problem inhibiting widespread use of the birth chair has been the availability of reasonably priced, efficient chairs that meet hygienic requirements (Haukeland, 1981).

In reconsidering the many hazards that the recumbent position presents during the intrapartal period, as well as the advantages of the optional positions, convenience seems "... a very poor excuse for interfering with an event having such critical importance for the entire future of the child" (Dunn, 1976, p. 791).

The relative immobility imposed on women laboring in traditional settings is also being questioned. The ability to move about during labor seems important from both a physiologic and psychologic standpoint. Studies have shown that women allowed to ambulate during labor experience less discomfort, have shorter labors, require less frequent oxytocin augmentation, show a lower incidence of abnormal FHR patterns, and consequently achieve a greater sense of control and self-confidence in relation to their birth experience. Ambulation by laboring women has frequently been forbidden based on the presence of ruptured membranes or the necessity of monitoring FHR patterns. Some practitioners state that ruptured membranes should not be a contraindication to ambulation when the presenting part is well engaged. With the increased availability of telemetry, fetal monitoring need no longer interfere with maternal ambulation (McKay, 1980). Expectant couples, as well as some health care providers, are questioning why bedrest and restricted activity need to be prescribed for both preterm and term labor.

The Leboyer Method

In 1975 Leboyer introduced a birthing technique directed toward easing the newborn's transition to extrauterine life. In a conventional delivery the newborn is subjected to extreme changes in sensory input—bright lights, voices, suctioning, and being quickly dried and placed in blankets. Leboyer advocated a more soothing and tender approach to the handling of the newborn at delivery. The lights in the delivery room are dimmed, and the noise level, including talking, is kept to a minimum. As the newborn is delivered, the physician/nurse-midwife supports the infant by sliding a finger under each axilla, avoiding touching the head, to further reduce trauma. Suctioning is not done, and the newborn is placed on his or her stomach on the mother's bare abdomen. The mother is encouraged to gently stroke and touch the newborn in a massaging motion. Care is taken to keep the newborn's spine in a curved position similar to its position in utero. Clamping of the

umbilical cord is delayed until all pulsations have ceased out of respect for the innate rhythms of the new life. Leboyer (1976) believes that this delay helps the newborn's initial respiratory efforts as well as sheltering the newborn from anoxia at the time of birth. After the umbilical cord is clamped, the newborn is gently and slowly placed in a water bath that has been warmed to 98–99F. The newborn remains in the bath until he or she is completely relaxed. The warm water recreates the intrauterine environment in temperature and weightlessness. Following the bath the infant is carefully and gently dried and wrapped in layers of warm blankets. The head and hands are always left to move and play. The newborn is then placed on the side to assure minimal stress on the spine and maximum freedom of movement. The infant is left alone to quietly take in the new environment.

Critics of the Leboyer method have expressed concerns about several of the techniques involved. They question the ability of the birth attendant to quickly assess maternal and/or neonatal complications or calculate Apgar scores in

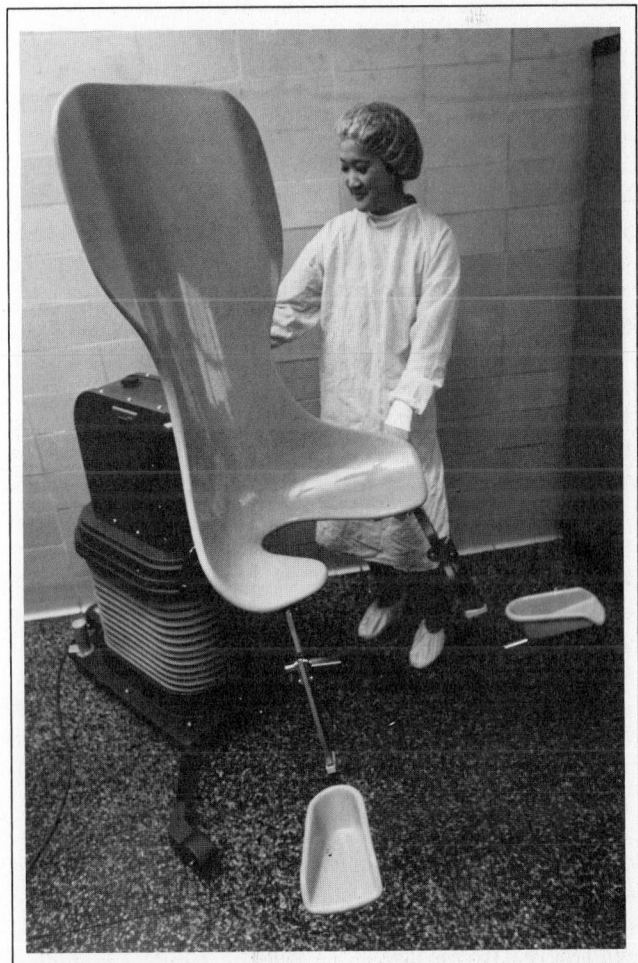

Figure 20–3 Birthing chair. Chair is contoured to provide optimum support. The chair can be tilted to various positions.

an environment of dim light. Traditional practitioners are concerned about the potentially high neonatal bilirubin levels associated with delayed cord clamping. Other critics fear an increase in neonatal skin infections from the skin-to-skin contact between mother and newborn, as well as from immersion in the water bath. Hypothermia related to the bath is also cited as a risk of the Leboyer method. On the other hand, proponents and couples themselves cite the advantages of the method as increased participation by the father in the birth process—particularly when he gives the bath—and the serenity of the birth experience (Crystle et al., 1980).

Birth Centers

Birth centers are maternity facilities located in a hospital or separate institution close to a health care agency. Factors playing a role in the evolution of the birth center concept include the women's movement, increased consumer demands for self-directed, family-centered maternity care, concern over the cost-effectiveness of applying highly technologic care to "normal" obstetrics, and recognition of a steadily increasing number of home births (Barton et al., 1980). Care in these alternative centers may be offered by various combinations of certified nurse-midwives, labor and delivery nurses, nurse practitioners, physicians, nonmedical assistants, public health nurses, and families themselves. Overall, birth centers require families to take more responsibility for the birth experience, while at the same time meeting their wishes for a more flexible and less costly way to give birth.

Birth centers strive for a warm, homelike atmosphere, with rooms similar to a typical bedroom at home. The room is generally furnished with a bed, in which the woman labors and delivers, comfortable chairs for the father and other relatives or friends, a cradle, and a private bath and/or shower. Some free-standing centers also have playrooms for siblings, kitchens where families may keep food or beverages, and other amenities. Most free-standing centers welcome children to whatever extent they choose to be involved, while hospital-based centers are somewhat more reluctant to allow total sibling participation.

Birth centers are generally equipped for emergencies with oxygen, suction, and resuscitation equipment. A system for rapid transport to more traditional settings is usually available.

In keeping with the concept of birth as a normal event, most birth center settings are set up for nurse-midwife management of labor and delivery rather than for obstetric technology and treatment. Therefore, these centers are not appropriate for high-risk deliveries. Couples intending to use the centers are screened during pregnancy for the following high-risk factors.

Social factors

- Fewer than three prenatal visits
- Nullipara older than 35 years of age
- Multipara older than 40 years of age

Preexisting maternal disease

- Chronic hypertension
- Renal, cardiac, or respiratory disease
- Diabetes
- Preeclampsia-eclampsia
- Anemia (hemoglobin less than 12 g/dL)

Previous pregnancy history

- Previous stillbirth, cesarean birth, or infant born with respiratory distress syndrome

Present pregnancy

- Preeclampsia-eclampsia
- Gestation less than 37 completed weeks or greater than 42 weeks
- Multiple pregnancy
- Abnormal fetal presentation
- Third-trimester bleeding or known placenta previa
- Multiparity greater than five
- Ruptured membranes for longer than 24 hours
- Estimated fetal weight of less than 5 lb or more than 9 lb
- Contracted pelvis or CPD
- Pelvic disease such as uterine malformations or active genital herpes

The presence of any one factor may not automatically exclude the woman from a birth room experience, but it does necessitate careful and continuous assessment. Generally, induction or conduction anesthesia is not used in birth centers.

Each center also has policies regarding various circumstances that would require the client to be transferred to a conventional labor and delivery setting. These may include, but are not limited to, the following:

- An increase in maternal temperature to over 100.4F (37.8C)
- A significant change in blood pressure
- Meconium staining
- Prolonged true labor
- Significant vaginal bleeding
- Prolonged second stage of labor (more than 2 hours for a nullipara and more than 1 hour for a multipara)
- The need for continuous fetal monitoring

The eligible couple is usually encouraged or in some instances required to attend prenatal classes. Some centers recommend as many as 10–12 weeks of preparatory education, and therefore require registration by approximately the twenty-second week of pregnancy. In some centers, a class that provides orientation to the birthing room is also required. Couples are encouraged to meet birthing room personnel and discuss the couple's desires and preferences for their birth experience.

The expectant mother is admitted to the birth center after labor has begun. She is encouraged to utilize breathing and relaxation techniques during the labor. She is supported and coached by those present. She may drink fluids as desired, but generally abstains from solid foods. The delivery occurs in the same room in which she has labored, eliminating the break in concentration and continuity required by changing rooms when delivery is imminent. The delivery itself is frequently unaccompanied by traditional obstetric procedures. Episiotomies are not routine, forceps are not used, and the woman may deliver in the position of her choice in many centers. After delivery, physical contact between the parents and newborn is encouraged. The mother may breast-feed immediately. Siblings and accompanying support persons are also encouraged to interact with the newborn as they choose.

In most instances rooming-in is immediate and healthy newborns and their families are never separated. The initial pediatric examination is conducted in the room with the family present. The mother and newborn are monitored for a minimum of 2–24 hours after delivery and then are discharged. In birthing centers in the hospital setting, some women may choose to forego early discharge and are transferred to the postpartal unit.

Home visits by birth center personnel are scheduled to occur within 24 hours of discharge and again 3 or 4 days after delivery. In some centers, weekly visits are made throughout the first 6 weeks after delivery. In others, the family is asked to return to the center on the sixth to seventh postpartal day and again at 5–6 weeks. The home visit provides an opportunity to see the family in their home setting, to make assessments of the mother and newborn, to answer questions, and to provide information and support. The accompanying Postpartal Home Visit Assessment Guide (p. 624) outlines the assessments that may be made. Detailed information on newborn and postpartal assessment is presented in Chapters 22 and 27.

Birth center deliveries are thought by many to provide a more natural and satisfying birth experience in a setting consistent with safe intrapartal and perinatal care. Birth centers offer a safe middle ground in the conventional hospital birth versus home birth furor. They are particularly useful for couples aware of the risks associated with out-of-hospital births and, at the same time, concerned with what they perceive as the risks of in-hospital birth. In most in-

stances, with proper screening and appropriate back-up care, no increased risk to women or newborns arises in birth centers.

CASE STUDY

Allison and Scott Jones are expecting their first child. During the pregnancy they have attended prenatal classes and have made special preparation in anticipation of using the birthing room at their local hospital. The pregnancy has proceeded without difficulty or problems.

When labor begins, they go to the hospital and are greeted by Marie Carlson, a nurse in the labor and delivery department. Ms. Carlson helps Allison and Scott get settled and completes the admission process. Allison is having contractions every 2–3 minutes lasting 45 seconds, and cervical dilatation is 5 cm. She is breathing with the contractions and is excited that the delivery day is at hand.

Ms. Carlson works to provide a comfortable, unhurried atmosphere. She is already acquainted with the Joneses because they have attended the prenatal classes that she teaches. She is familiar with their level of knowledge and will now work to support them as labor progresses. She notes that Allison and Scott are working well together in timing contractions and utilizing relaxation techniques and breathing methods. Ms. Carlson completes her physical assessment, then talks with the couple about the progress. Ms. Carlson leaves, letting the Joneses know she is available whenever they need her. She has found that parents who use the birthing room are well prepared and that she may not need to stay quite so close. She returns periodically to assess progress and to see how the Joneses are coping with the labor. As long as all is going well she allows the couple privacy. She has notified the physician/nurse-midwife of Allison's admission and labor status, who is now on the way to the hospital.

As Allison proceeds into transition, Ms. Carlson notes that the Joneses are needing more encouragement and support, so she stays in constant attendance. She assesses maternal, fetal, and labor status and keeps the Joneses informed of their progress.

Dr. J. G. Grey comes in to see the Joneses and stays close by because the labor is progressing rapidly. Toward the end of the transition, Ms. Carlson prepares the equipment to be used during delivery. She assists Allison in her pushing efforts when the cervix has completely dilated. During the delivery, she assists Allison, Scott, and Dr. Grey. The delivery is managed in the same unhurried manner. Ms. Carlson assesses the physical parameters and offers continuing support as Allison delivers a healthy-appearing baby girl. Ms. Carlson assesses the newborn quickly and then places her in her mother's arms.

The postdelivery recovery period is monitored closely so that any problems can be identified. Allison is recover-

(Text continues on p. 628.)

The following photographs were taken at a birth center. We wish to express our appreciation to the delivering couple for sharing their unique and moving childbirth experience.

There were two nurses and a physician in attendance. Unexpectedly the mother chose a standing delivery position, and the father helped support her body during the birth.

We do not advocate this particular delivery position. We do believe that every maternity nurse should be aware that there is no one "correct" way to have a baby. Each birth is special.

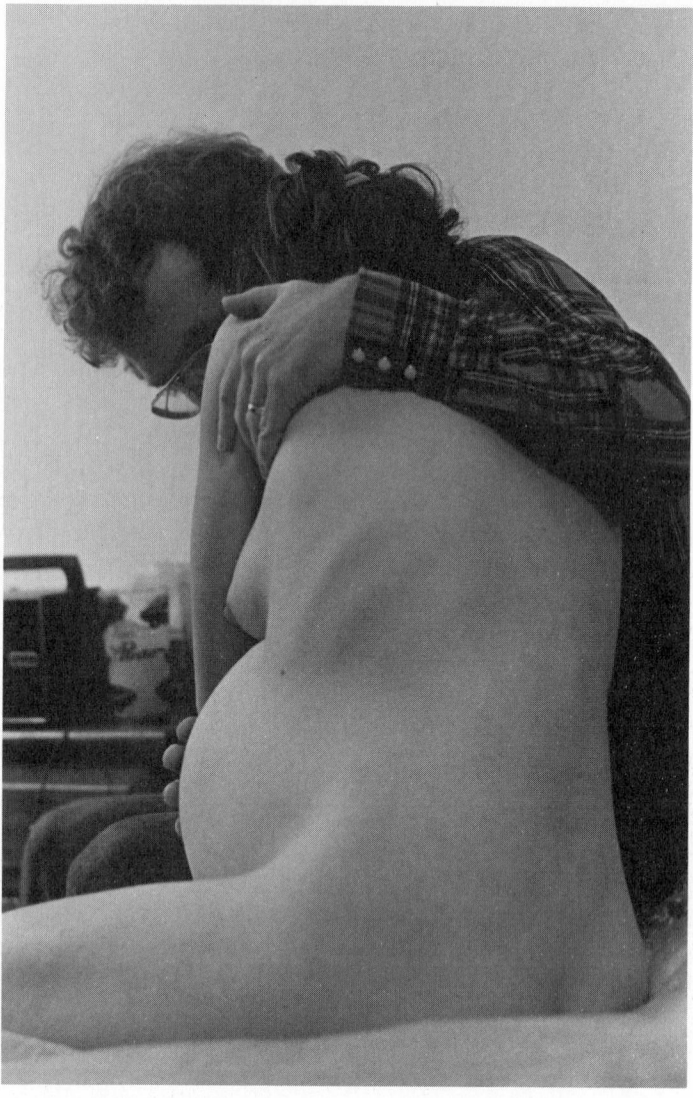

The woman is in labor. She has just taken a shower, and is now resting.

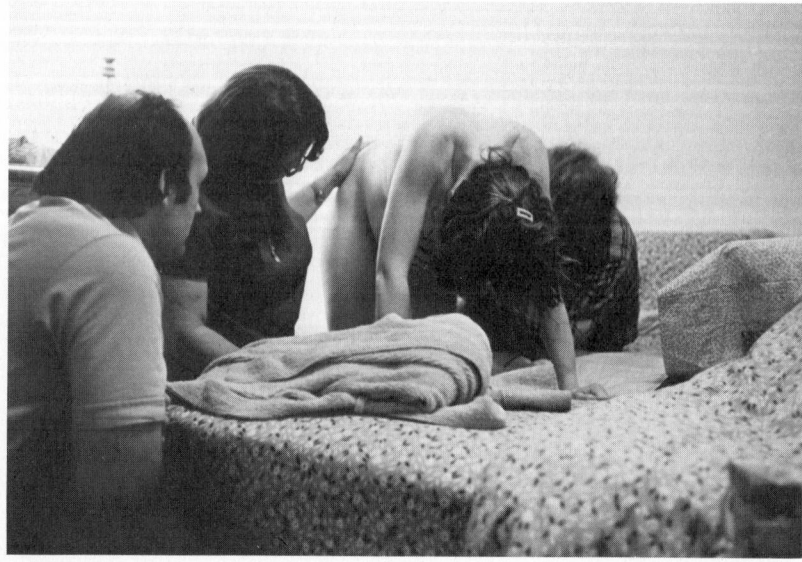

The woman walks around the room. Moments later she feels the urge to begin pushing. The nurse and her husband support her body as she begins to push.

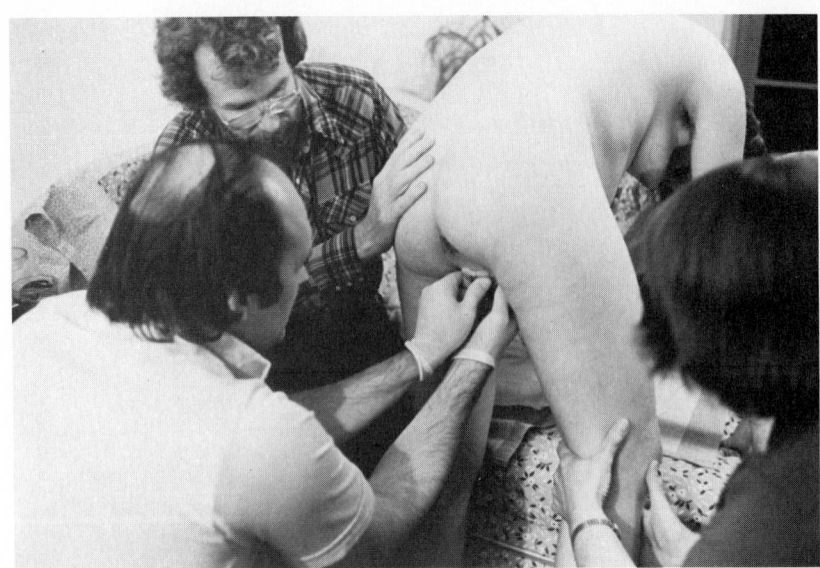

Within one minute the head has crowned, and rapid delivery ensues.

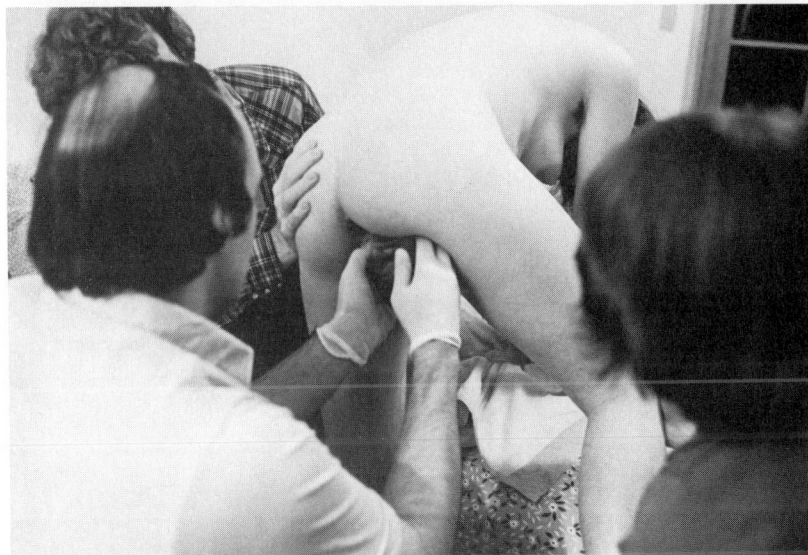

Delivery of the head is beginning.

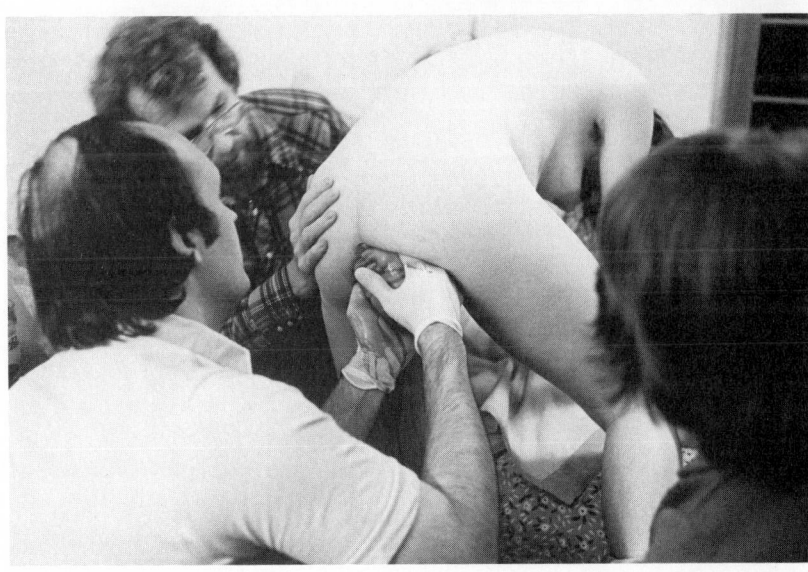

Complete delivery of the head.

External rotation and restitution have occurred.

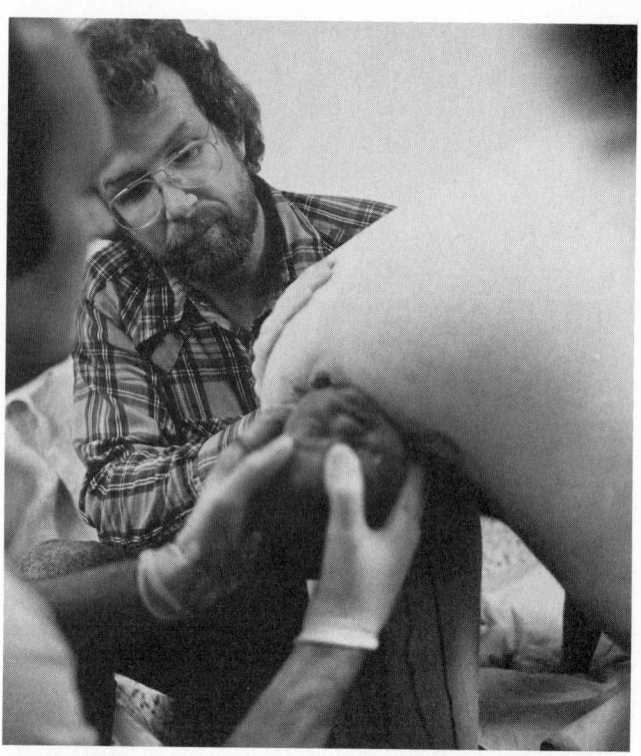

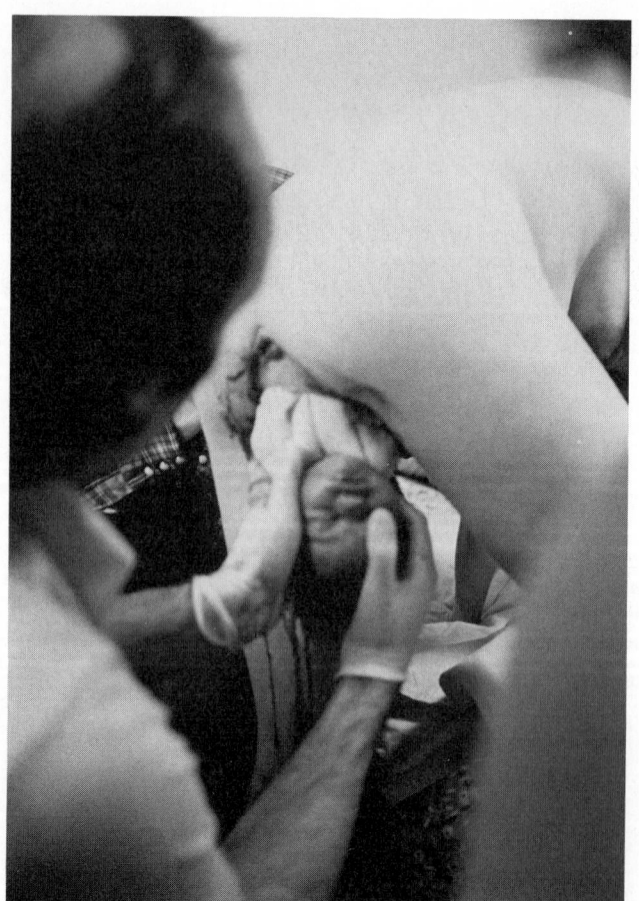

The mother pushes slightly to facilitate delivery of the infant's body.

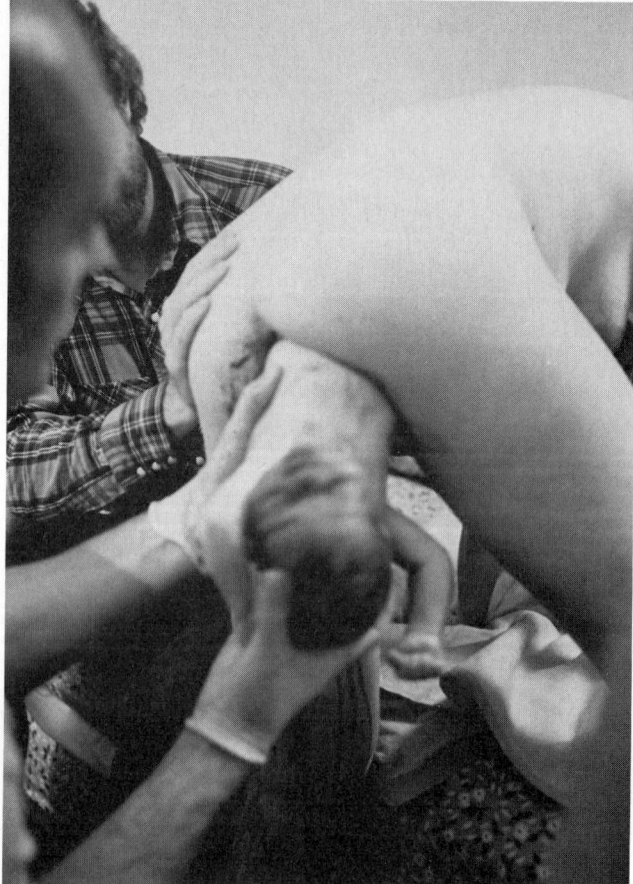

Delivery of the infant's body.

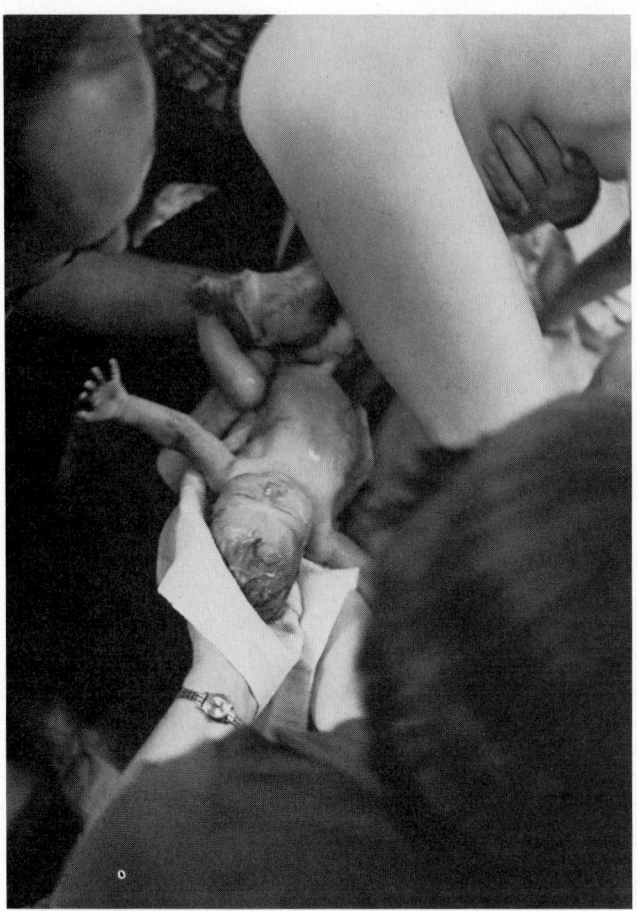

A little girl has been born. Note the nurse's position as she handles the newborn with a warm towel.

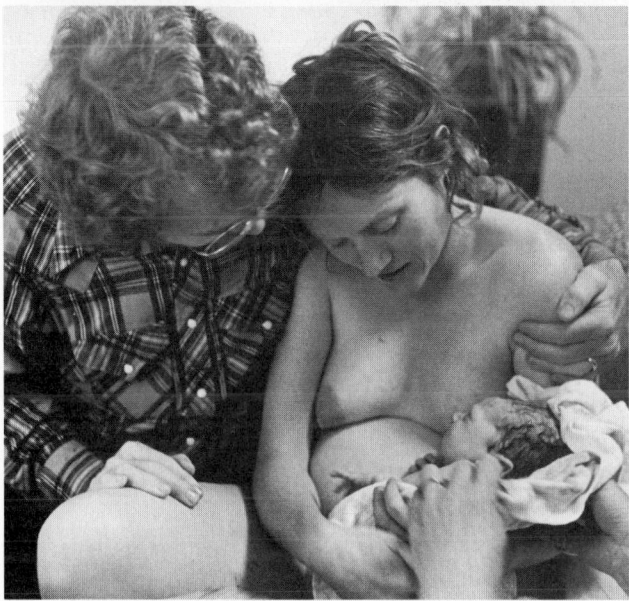

The nurse hands the baby to the mother. In this photograph the baby is two minutes old.

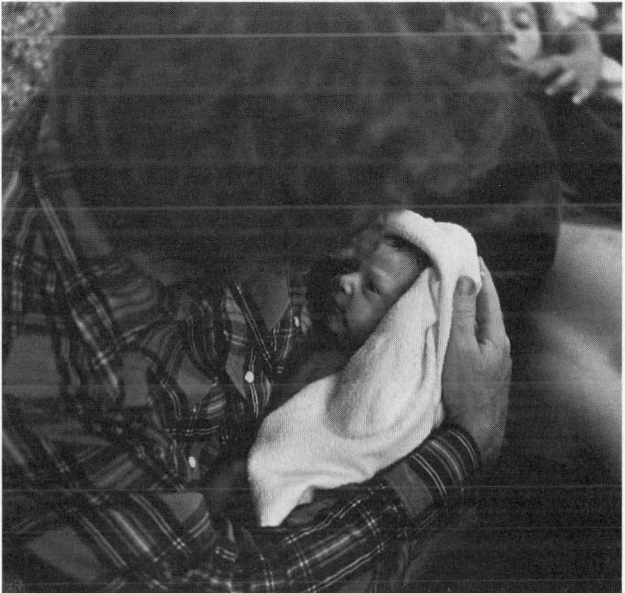

The father holds the baby five minutes after delivery. The nurse is standing behind the mother, covering her with warm blankets as the mother awaits delivery of the placenta.

POSTPARTAL HOME VISIT ASSESSMENT GUIDE
(24 hours after delivery)

Assess	Normal findings	Alterations and possible causes of alterations*	Nursing responses to data base†
Mother Vital signs	BP between 90/60 and 140/90 mm Hg	BP below 90/60 (reduction in blood volume)	For deviations in BP, refer to physician
		BP above 140/90 (hypertensive disorder)	If BP is elevated, assess patient for edema; obtain urinalysis for protein; may dipstick urine for protein
	Pulse 70–100	Pulse below 70 or above 100 (cardiac disorder)	Reevaluate pulse after a period of rest Report findings to physician
	Oral temperature 98–99F (36.6–37.1C)	Temperature above 100.4F (37.8C) (infectious process)	Assess for signs of infection; refer to physician
Breasts	Presence of colostrum, engorgement may be beginning	Absence of colostrum (inadequate letdown)	Assess mother's feeding practices; How long is newborn nursing? How often? Assess mother's fatigue level; assess newborn's activity level, rooting and sucking reflexes; assist mother during a feeding—this provides opportunity for assessment, encouragement, support, and teaching
	Nipples smooth, no evidence of cracking	Cracking of nipples (prolonged breast-feeding, unprepared nipples)	Assess mother's feeding practices; counsel her in cleansing of the breast and exposing the nipples to air
	Absence of localized swelling or redness	Localized swelling or redness (infectious process)	Instruct mother in breast massage; depending on severity of infection, mother may need to be counseled about alternate feeding methods and referred to physician/nurse-midwife
Fundus	Firm and in the midline	Boggy (inadequate uterine contractions) Out of midline (bladder distention)	Assist client in locating her fundus; encourage her to assess firmness and position twice a day, and to record results
	0–1 finger-breadths below the umbilicus	At or above umbilicus (inadequate uterine contractions)	Provide education regarding how and why to check the fundus and what actions to take if alterations are noted Assess lochia for amount and presence of clots Assess bladder for distention
	Progressive decrease in size	Subinvolution (inadequate contractions)	Assess lochia for amount and presence of clots Assess temperature

POSTPARTAL HOME VISIT ASSESSMENT GUIDE, Cont'd
(24 hours after delivery)

Assess	Normal findings	Alterations and possible causes of alterations*	Nursing responses to data base†
			Refer to physician/nurse-midwife if fundus remains boggy, if lochia is heavy, if voiding does not facilitate return of fundus to midline, if oral temperature is above 100.4F (37.8C)
Lochia	Lochia rubra for first 2–3 days; small clots	Excessive lochia—one pad saturated in 2 hours; large clots (inadequate uterine contractions, subinvolution, vaginal lacerations)	Assess fundus; if uterus is firm, assess for perineal laceration; if fundus boggy, provide massage; evaluate amount of lochia
	Odor similar to menstrual flow	Foul odor (infection)	If odor present, assess oral temperature and uterine tenderness; if boggy fundus, excessive lochia, foul odor, uterine tenderness, oral temperature above 100.4F remain, refer to physician
Episiotomy	Close approximation of skin edges; small amount of bruising	Separation of skin edges, excessive bruising, presence of indurated area at episiotomy site	Assess client's information regarding relief measures; provide education as necessary; if alterations are found, refer to physician
Bladder	No distention	Distention (loss of muscle tone, inability to empty bladder)	Implement interventions to assist voiding; if client unable to void, catheterization will be necessary; assess fluid intake, encourage adequate fluid intake
	Absence of frequency, urgency, and dysuria	Frequency, urgency, dysuria (bladder infection)	Assess temperature Refer to physician Assess fluid intake
Bowels	Bowel movement by third postpartal day	Constipation (inadequate fluid or nutritional intake; fear of pain when episiotomy is present)	Assess fluid and nutritional intake; encourage her to force fluids; stool softener may be needed; provide counseling and support if she indicates fear of defecation because of episiotomy
Fatigue level	Tired, exhausted after initial period of birth euphoria		Suggest alterations in home schedule to allow for periods of rest Encourage mother to rest while the newborn sleeps Counsel regarding gradual re-initiation of activity

POSTPARTAL HOME VISIT ASSESSMENT GUIDE, Cont'd
(24 hours after delivery)

Assess	Normal findings	Alterations and possible causes of alterations*	Nursing responses to data base†
			Discuss physical results of fatigue (reduced milk flow, problems establishing feeding, increased lochia) Explore family or support persons' availability to assume additional tasks
Psychologic well-being and adjustment	Emotional lability, feelings of pride or inadequacy with regard to labor and birth; transition through "taking-in" and "taking-hold" phases	Postpartal psychosis Inability of parents to assume new roles	Allow mother to review and discuss the birth Reassure client that she did well during labor and delivery Make references to positive features of the newborn and his or her response to the mother Provide positive reinforcement of mothering skills Reassure the client that her feelings at this time are normal Work with the mother as a consultant, allowing her to perform the mother skills Accept maternal passivity and dependency, making concrete suggestions for possible actions
	"Postpartum blues" Necessity to adjust to new roles and responsibilities	Marked postpartal depression	Explain the basis of "blues," reassuring the client they are common and temporary Permit the client to discuss and vent her feelings Assist the family and support persons in understanding and accommodating to the new mother's needs
Knowledge level	The woman understands normal postpartal changes and how to care for them Client has adequate knowledge of the following self-care measures: breast care, perineal care, sitz baths, fundal massage, adequate fluid intake, optimum nutrition, Kegel exercises The parents and other primary caregivers understand newborn care and newborn growth and development		Provide information based on individual need and learning readiness Focus on all the family members Reinforce previous knowledge Emphasize principles and encourage individual problem solving and application Provide anticipatory guidance regarding common newborn and family behaviors Discuss sibling rivalry and suggest approaches to reduce it

POSTPARTAL HOME VISIT ASSESSMENT GUIDE, Cont'd
(24 hours after delivery)

Assess	Normal findings	Alterations and possible causes of alterations*	Nursing responses to data base†
	The parents have realistic expectations of one another, the newborn, and other family members The siblings are adjusting to the newborn The parents have made plans for birth control		Include discussion of postpartal sexual feelings, resumption of sexual activity, and contraceptive alternatives
Newborn Vital signs	Axillary temperature 97–98F (36.1–36.6C)	Axillary temperature below 97F (36.1C) (inadequate temperature control, lack of subcutaneous fat)	Provide external means of warming newborn
	Apical pulse 110–160 beats/min	Apical pulse < 110 or > 160 (cardiac disorder)	Assess respirations and general color; refer to physician
	Respirations 30–60/min (count for one full minute)	Respirations above 60/min (respiratory problems)	Assess apical pulse, temperature, and general color; refer to physician
Skin color	Pinkish	Jaundice (hemolytic disease, physiologic jaundice)	Draw bilirubin; refer to physician
Umbilical cord	Dry	Moist, oozing, odor, exudate (infection); bleeding	Culture exudate; instruct mother in cleansing of cord and allowing exposure to air; refer to physician if needed
Feedings	6–8 per day	< 6 or > 8 (inadequate knowledge of feeding needs, disinterest of the newborn)	Assess mother's feeding practices and knowledge base; provide counseling Assess newborn's weight
Alertness	Awake for 1–4 hr per day	Excessive wakefulness or sleeping	Assess sleep habits, number and amount of feedings Counsel as necessary Instruct in expected newborn behavior
Baby care	Mother has adequate knowledge of the following baby care measures: bathing, feeding, sleeping habits, clothes, temperature (axillary, rectal), safety (home and car), quieting techniques	Inadequate knowledge	Assess knowledge base Provide counseling and information as needed
Attachment	Evidence of bonding with appropriate physical interactions: calling the newborn by name, feeding techniques established, newborn clean and well cared for	Poor infant hygiene, failure to gain weight, references to newborn using only pronouns or disparaging nicknames, lack of infant care supplies	Provide information and counseling

* This column provides guidelines for further assessment and initial nursing interventions.
† Possible causes of alterations are placed in parentheses.

ing without problems and is eager to learn more about her new daughter. Ms. Carlson talks to the Joneses to assess their level of knowledge and provides information that is needed. She does a physical assessment of the newborn and explains the findings to the Joneses. She assists Allison as she breast-feeds her baby for the first time. After the feeding, the nurse assists Scott in giving the baby her first bath. Ms. Carlson has found that the bath time provides opportunities to talk and share information.

During the recovery period, she provides quiet time for the new family to be together and get acquainted.

A few hours after delivery, Ms. Carlson assists the Joneses as they prepare for dismissal. She will be making a visit to the Joneses' home the next morning and then weekly, to assess the mother and newborn and to provide information and continued support.

Early Discharge

More hospitals are offering new mothers—whether they deliver in a conventional labor and delivery setting, a birthing room, or an in-hospital birth center—the option of early discharge. The concept generally includes any discharge occurring from 2–24 hours postpartally. Most institutions have written policies and criteria about the mother and the newborn for early discharge. Criteria for the mother may include any or all of the following:

- No antepartal or intrapartal complications
- A labor no longer than 30 hours for a primipara or 24 hours for a multipara
- An episiotomy or no greater than a third-degree laceration with no vaginal or cervical lacerations
- A spontaneous or low-forceps delivery
- Stable vital signs
- A firm uterine fundus
- Voiding without difficulty
- Ability to ambulate and provide care for herself and her newborn
- Help at home for 1–3 days
- Demonstrated understanding of home care instructions

Early discharge criteria for the neonate may include:

- Stable vital signs
- Normal physical examination
- An hematocrit level of 45%–65% and a Dextrostix result of greater than 45%
- At least one water feeding or two formula or breast-feedings

The desired practice is to follow up early discharges with home visits by labor and delivery, postpartum, or public health nurses. (See Postpartal Assessment Guide, p. 624.) The early discharge option offers both financial benefits, in terms of reducing the costs of obstetric care, as well as psychologic benefits by reuniting families in their homes more quickly. The most frequent neonatal problem requiring readmission to the hospital is hyperbilirubinemia. Research suggests readmission may be due to the high percentage of breast-feeding mothers who select this option, the trend toward late cord clamping in the birth experiences of this group, and the thorough assessments of nurses making home visits (Barton et al., 1980).

Home Births

Another alternative to the traditional hospital delivery is home birth. Couples who choose home birth are reported to share certain common attitudes and beliefs. In general, they believe that they hold primary responsibility for their own health, and as a group tend to define health and illness differently than the traditional medical establishment. Home birth couples frequently maintain strong beliefs regarding their rights and abilities to make their own birth choices. Couples choosing home births assume that the responsibility for the birth outcome is theirs; furthermore, they do not believe the hospital is necessarily the safest place to give birth, and see standard medical practice as frequently involving unnecessary trauma and intervention. Home birth couples are particularly desirous of responsibility and control and do not trust the conventional health delivery system to provide this. Confusing medical jargon, advanced technology that limits the laboring woman's activity, the necessity of adopting the dependent sick role, and the rigidity and loss of individualism associated with hospitalization are all factors in many couples' decisions to have a home birth (Bauwens and Anderson, 1978). Some immigrant women may feel that hospital routines and expectations will not allow them to conform to their cultural norms for childbearing behavior.

Therefore, in making the choice between home and hospital birth, medical risk is only one issue. Women and their families are also considering the social risks and benefits of birth location as well as acknowledging that their perceptions of medical risks do not always conform to the medical profession's definition of the same (McClain, 1981). Parents who have participated in home delivery find that it is a warm, close, loving experience for which they have responsibility and control. The newborn infant is immediately incorporated into the family, and the continuous contact between the newborn and the family facilitates the bonding process and establishment of a family unit. Siblings present during delivery are able to welcome the newborn into the family and are participants in an exciting and beautiful experience.

A home birth may be accompanied by unexpected complications, such as prolonged labor, malpresentation of the fetus, or bleeding problems. Adequate medical back-up care is an important part of a successful home birth. However, adequate medical back-up care is frequently unobtainable. Obstetricians as a group are particularly vocal opponents of home birth. Their opposition is often based on memories of serious emergencies they have witnessed at the time of birth. Therefore, home birth is usually seen by them as a regressive step in maternal–child care. Despite their opposition, the trend toward home births seems to be increasing rather than slowing. However, a side effect of physician opposition has been to make home births, when they do occur, even less safe. Couples planning a home birth may be refused physician-supervised prenatal care as well as birth attendance. Many physicians also refuse to act as back-up caregivers for the nurse-midwife attending a home birth. Hospital personnel in general also tend to oppose home birth. They may manifest this disapproval through punishing attitudes when couples unable to complete birth at home come to the hospital.

The safety of any home birth is maximized by thorough planning, careful prenatal care and screening, skilled physicians/nurse-midwives, and an organized and tested transport system to a facility where accepting caregivers are available. Because of marked disagreement about the home birth concept, conventional medicine has made many of these safety factors difficult to obtain (Zimmerman, 1980).

Home deliveries may be attended by a lay midwife, certified nurse-midwife (contingent upon the laws of respective states), or physician. Lay midwives rarely have an established educational program or state certification. Clients generally seek out any one particular midwife based on word-of-mouth recommendations from other women the midwife has attended. It has been suggested that lay midwives are responsible for much of the home birth movement. However, it is more likely that lay midwives are being actively sought by consumers to assist them in realizing their birth choice.

Certified nurse-midwives are well-educated, skilled practitioners, closely regulated by state nurse practice acts in terms of their scope of practice.

ASSESSMENT

Families who choose home birth should be screened and counseled extensively throughout the pregnancy. A number of different criteria must be met for a successful home birth experience. The following questions can be asked to determine the feasibility or desirability of home birth for a particular couple.

1. *Why does the couple desire a home birth?*
2. *Are they choosing home birth to challenge authority or to "get back" at the system?* The couple who perceives home birth as a political act may not have the pregnant woman's or the infant's best interest at heart. The couple may have had what they perceive as "bad" experiences with the health care system.

3. *What is the family's financial status?* The couple who chooses home birth for financial reasons may be at risk if their income is such that it precludes adequate nutrition and prenatal care.
4. *Is the woman able to adequately care for herself?* The woman who is unable to take proper care of herself because of psychologic or physical factors may not be in optimal condition to cope with the stresses of labor and delivery and therefore may be classified as high risk.

The expectant mother should undergo a thorough physical examination, including laboratory studies, to assess her health status. The amount of information and understanding about birth and related processes held by the family must also be evaluated so that counseling can be directed toward filling the gaps in their knowledge.

The presence of the following factors may preclude the possibility of home birth:

- Age under 16 years or over 40 years
- Weight under 100 lb or over 200 lb
- History of long labors
- Previous cesarean deliveries
- Previous intrapartal or postpartal bleeding problems
- Repeated miscarriages
- Previous Rh incompatibility
- Parity greater than five
- Malpresentation of fetus
- Previous delivery of preterm infant (under 38 weeks) or postmature infant (over 42 weeks)
- Presence of maternal disease (preeclampsia-eclampsia, diabetes, cardiac disease, respiratory disease, hydramnios, vaginal bleeding, herpesvirus type 2 infection)
- Psychologic risk factors
- Multiple pregnancy

If any of these high-risk factors are found during the assessment process, the family should be advised that home birth may not be in the woman's or infant's best interests.

ANTEPARTAL INTERVENTIONS

One of the most important prerequisites for a successful home birth is that the pregnant woman be in excellent health. The nurse can help the woman achieve this end by giving her and her family quality health care throughout the prenatal period. Education and counseling of the family are important aspects of this care, and these can be effectively accomplished through a series of childbirth classes. Classes begin in midpregnancy. It is emphasized throughout these classes that the expectant parents are ultimately responsible for the successful outcome of the planned home birth. The following subjects are stressed because they may affect the kind of birth and childrearing experiences the family has:

- Nutrition
- Exercise
- Breathing and relaxation techniques
- Normal physiologic changes during pregnancy
- Normal labor and delivery processes

The couple is encouraged to ask their physician for information about laboratory results, blood pressure, general physical condition of the expectant mother, and the status of the fetus (fetal heart rate). They are told to request information about possible complications and typical obstetric procedures. Nurses should encourage class members to cooperate with the physician and other members of the health care team should a hospital delivery become necessary.

Participants in these prenatal classes receive explanations about bonding and parenting. They are urged to read and study independently about the birth process as well as to participate in group learning experiences. In addition, couples are taught how to recognize problems that might need further attention.

In preparation for the home delivery the couple will need to have the following supplies available:

- Disposable underpads
- Sterilized cord tie and scissors
- Bulb syringe
- Four to six receiving blankets (to be warmed in the oven at 100F when labor begins so they will be warm for the newborn)
- Six towels
- Two sets of sheets
- Plastic sheet
- Sterile sheet (may be sterilized by placing in paper bag and putting it in the oven)
- Perineal pads and belt
- Large bowl for placenta and small bowl for scrub solutions
- Cotton balls and bottle of alcohol
- Betadine scrub solution

LABOR AND DELIVERY AT HOME

When labor begins, the nurse-midwife or physician is summoned to the home. She monitors the labor and provides support to the family. Maternal vital signs are monitored frequently, and FHR is assessed every 15 minutes. A vaginal examination is performed at the beginning of labor to ascertain position, presentation, dilatation, and effacement of the cervix, and this examination is repeated infrequently unless a problem arises.

The woman labors and delivers in whatever position she chooses. The pain she experiences is generally not seen as a negative aspect of the birth process. The woman may eat nourishing snacks while she is in labor, but usually restricts solids once true labor has started. Herbal and other natural teas are seen as particularly helpful by many women who select home birth. Women who deliver at home generally select a squatting, sitting, or standing position for the birth. A hands-on-knees position is recommended by many midwives in the event of a breech presentation. The second stage of labor may be prolonged compared with in-hospital birth, since much effort is made to "iron" the perineum and control the birth so neither episiotomies nor lacerations are an issue in a home birth. The third stage of labor may also be prolonged since oxytoxics are not routinely administered for home births. Just as with hospital births, the placenta is examined by the clinician for any abnormalities. The clinician may recommend to the couple that the placenta be kept at a cold temperature for 24 hours and taken to the hospital with the mother if there are postpartal bleeding problems.

Following delivery, which may be actively assisted by the father, couples usually prefer late cord clamping, immediate breast-feeding and unlimited contact between the infant, parents, siblings, and other significant people in attendance. Some couples report a renewed spirit of family, community, and celebration at home births.

The nurse-midwife remains with the family until maternal bleeding has stabilized, the mother has urinated, and the newborn baby has begun nursing. The nurse-midwife returns to the home 24 and 48 hours after delivery to check maternal bleeding and temperature and to assess the neonate's skin for jaundice. The nurse-midwife also assists the mother if she is having difficulty breast-feeding the infant. The attendant may frequently be called on to provide the family with information regarding the normal postpartal course and infant care and development. Nurse-midwives are usually available by telephone or during home visits to answer questions. The mother and newborn are examined by the physician/nurse-midwife 1 week and 6 weeks after birth.

INDICATIONS FOR HOSPITALIZATION

If a woman who has planned a home birth suddenly finds it necessary to seek hospital care, she is at risk both physiologically and psychologically. Either she, her fetus, or both are probably in distress if hospitalization was deemed necessary. Moreover, she is also vulnerable to disapproval, ridicule, and anger on the part of many hospital personnel. Her control over the birth process, which may have been a major factor in her decision to select home birth, is now almost totally gone. She must deal with her fears and concerns regarding the birth outcome, her guilt and responsibilities should the outcome be poor, and the unfamiliarity of her surroundings at this critical time.

Factors that may necessitate moving a planned home birth to the hospital include the following:

- Hard labor for longer than 8 hours without fetal descent
- The onset of true labor prior to 36 weeks' gestation
- Marked meconium staining
- An abnormal fetal heart rate or pattern
- Significant vaginal bleeding intrapartally or postpartally

The nurse who has initial contact with the family must be careful to remain nonjudgmental in attitudes or remarks. All care and procedures should be carefully explained with regard to what action is being done and its rationale. Care should be taken that any required procedure is not presented in a punitive way. Depending on the circumstances, it may be appropriate for the nurse to reassure the couple that their choice of birth location did not cause the current problem. Every effort should be made to give them any control and options possible in the new situation.

SUMMARY

Expectant parents are requesting and in some instances demanding options in what has been traditional maternity care. Many hospitals are now providing alternative birthing experiences through birthing centers and inclusion of Leboyer methods when requested. Other couples are choosing to forego any institutional contact, and opt to have their birth experience at home. The obstetric nurse needs to be informed of alternative birthing methods, their advantages and disadvantages. The role of assessment and teaching takes on an even more important aspect as contact with the client may be possible only over a short period of time.

With sound nursing and medical care, consumers of maternity care are probably best helped by making available to them a wide variety of birth options. In this way, society has its best chance of extending a satisfying and safe birth experience to every couple.

References

Barton, J., et al. 1980. Alternative birthing center: experience in a teaching obstetric service. *Am. J. Obstet. Gynecol.* 137:377.

Bauwens, E., and Anderson, S. 1978. Home births: a reaction to hospital environmental stressors. In *The anthropology of health*, ed. Eleanor Bauwens. St. Louis: The C. V. Mosby Co.

Bliss, J. 1980. New baby in the family. *Can. Nurse.* 76:42.

Burchell, R. C., and Gunn, J. 1980. The new birth experience. *J. Obstet. Gynecol. Neonat. Nurs.* 9:250.

Crystle, C. D., et al. 1980. The Leboyer method of delivery. An assessment of risk. *J. Repro. Med.* 25:267.

Dunn, P. M. 1976. Obstetric delivery today: for better or for worse? *Lancet* 1:790.

Haukeland, I. 1981. An alternative delivery position: new delivery chair developed and tested at Konigsberg Hospital. *Am. J. Obstet. Gynecol.* 141:115.

Irwin, H. W. 1978. Practical considerations for the routine application of left lateral Sims position for vaginal delivery. *Am. J. Obstet. Gynecol.* 131:129.

Leboyer, F. 1976. *Birth without violence.* New York: Alfred A. Knopf, Inc.

Leonard, C. H., et al. 1979. Preliminary observations on the behavior of children present at the birth of a sibling. *Pediatrics.* 64:950.

McClain, C. 1981. Women's choice of home or hospital birth. *J. Fam. Practice.* 12:1033.

McKay, S. R. 1980. Maternal position during labor and birth. A reassessment. *J. Obstet. Gynecol. Neonat. Nurs.* 9:288.

Parma, S. 1979. A family-centered event? Preparing the child for sharing in the experience of childbirth. *J. Nurse-Midwife.* 24:6.

Zimmerman, E. 1980. Home birth safety. *J. Obstet. Gynecol. Neonat. Nurs.* 9:191.

Additional Readings

Arms, S. 1975. *Immaculate deception.* Boston: Houghton Mifflin Co.

Brody, H., and Thompson, J. R. 1981. The maximum strategy in modern obstetrics. *J. Fam. Practice.* 12:977.

Enlien, M. 1975–1976. The family in labour. *Birth Fam. J.* 2:133.

Faison, J. B., et al. 1979. The childbearing center: an alternative birth setting. *Obstet. Gynecol.* 54:527.

Haire, D. 1972. *The cultural warping of childbirth.* Seattle, Wash.: International Childbirth Education Association.

Klaus, M. H., and Kennell, J. H. 1976. *Maternal–infant bonding: the impact of early separation or loss on family development.* St. Louis: The C. V. Mosby Co.

Lange, R. 1972. *The birth book.* Ben Lomond, Calif.: Genesis Press.

McKay, S. R. 1981. Second stage labor—has tradition replaced safety? *Am. J. Nurs.* 81:1016.

May, I. M. 1978. *Spiritual midwifery.* Summertown, Tenn.: The Book Publishing Company.

Ritche, C. A. 1976. Childbirth outside the hospital—the resurgence of home and clinic deliveries. *MCN.* 1:372.

Sumner, P. E., and Phillips, C. R. 1981. *Birthing rooms: concept and reality.* St. Louis: The C. V. Mosby Co.

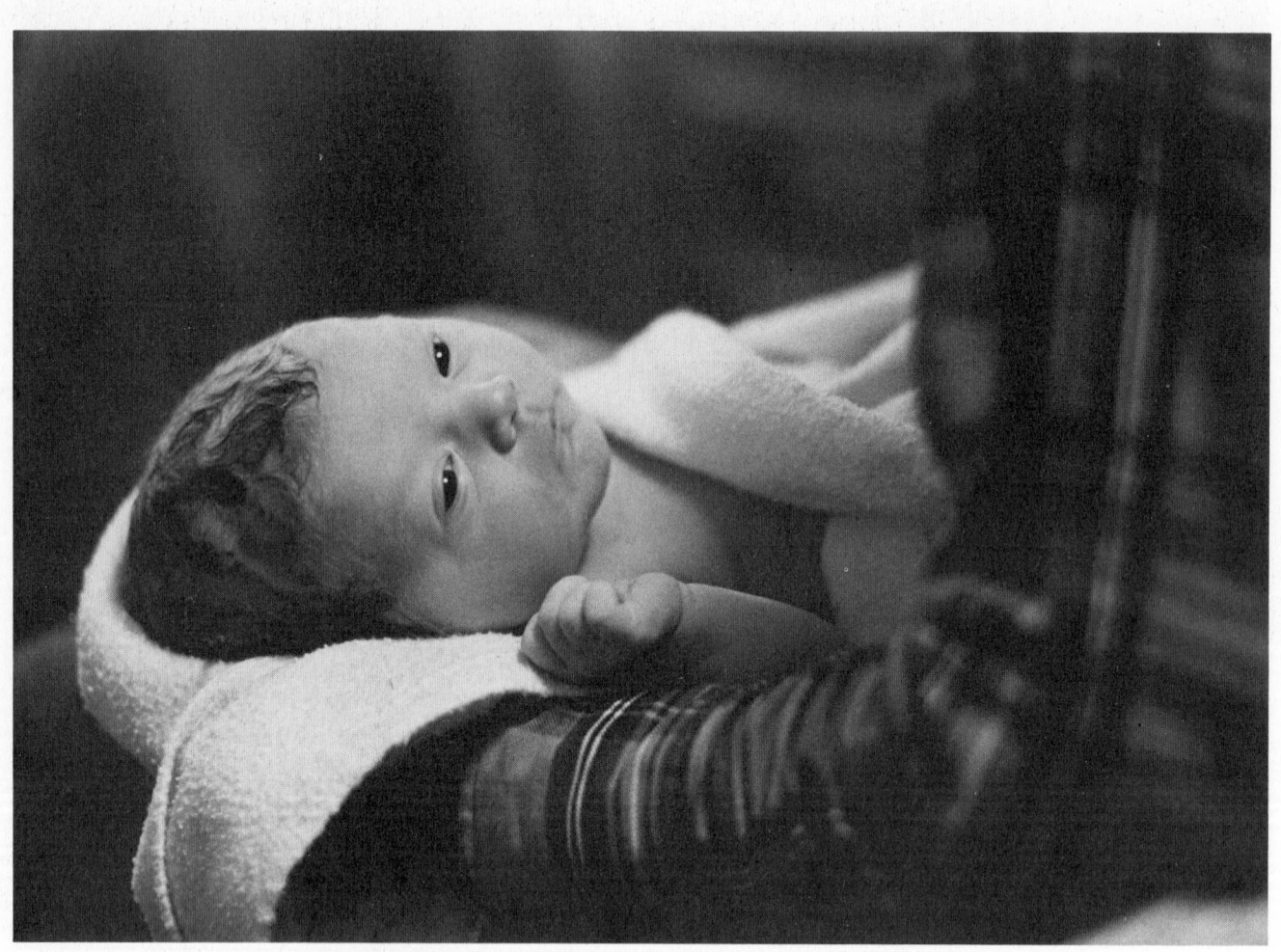

▪ V ▪

THE NEONATE

Chapter 21 ▪ Physiologic Responses
of the Newborn to
Birth

Chapter 22 ▪ Nursing Assessment of the Newborn

Chapter 23 ▪ The Normal Newborn: Needs and Care

Chapter 24 ▪ The High-Risk Newborn: Needs and Care

Chapter 25 ▪ Complications of the Neonate

Chapter 26 ▪ Congenital Anomalies

PHYSIOLOGIC RESPONSES
OF THE NEWBORN TO BIRTH

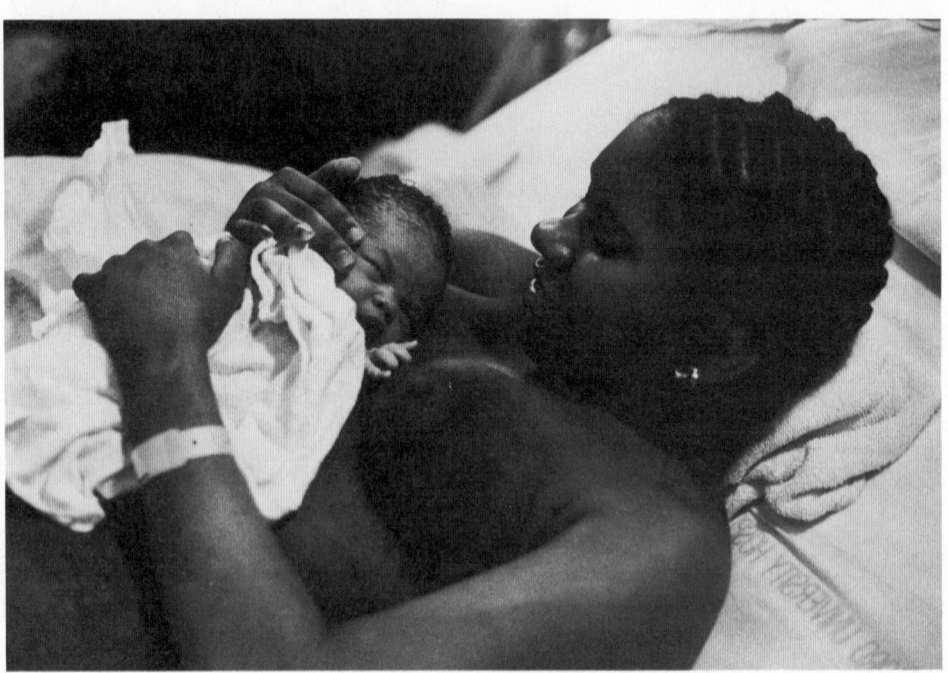

■ CHAPTER CONTENTS

RESPIRATORY ADAPTATIONS
    Initiation of Breathing
    Neonatal Pulmonary Physiology
    Characteristics of Neonatal Respiration

CARDIOVASCULAR ADAPTATIONS
    Embryology
    Fetal-Neonatal Transition Circulation
    Characteristics
    Oxygen Transport

HEMATOPOIETIC SYSTEM
    Neonatal Hematology

TEMPERATURE REGULATION
    Heat Loss
    Heat Production

HEPATIC ADAPTATION
    Iron Storage and Red Blood Cell Production
    Carbohydrate Metabolism
    Physiologic Jaundice—Icterus Neonatorum
    Coagulation

GASTROINTESTINAL ADAPTATION
    Functional Development
    Digestion of Carbohydrates
    Digestion of Proteins
    Digestion of Fats

GENITOURINARY ADAPTATION
    Kidney Development and Function
    Genital Development
IMMUNOLOGIC ADAPTATIONS

NEUROLOGIC AND SENSORY/PERCEPTUAL
FUNCTIONING
    Motor Activity
    Sensory Capacities of the Newborn
    States of the Newborn
    Neurologic Adaptations

■ OBJECTIVES

- Describe the physiologic changes of the transition from intrauterine to extrauterine life.

- Outline the cardiovascular and respiratory changes necessary to maintain neonatal ventilation and perfusion.

- Compare the adult, fetal, and neonatal hematopoietic systems.

- Describe nonshivering thermogenesis.

- Discuss the changing roles of the liver and gastrointestinal tract in the neonate.

- Determine the significance of the kidney in fluid and electrolyte balance in the neonate.

- Describe the immunologic response of the neonate.

- Describe the sensory/perceptual functioning of the newborn.

The neonatal period includes the time from birth through the twenty-eighth day of life. This period involves the adjustments from intrauterine to extrauterine life that the infant must make to effectively function as a unique individual. The nurse must be totally cognizant of a newborn's normal biopsychosocial adaptations to recognize deviations from it.

To begin life as an independent being, the neonate must first and foremost establish pulmonary ventilation in conjunction with marked circulatory changes. These radical and rapid alterations are crucial to the maintenance of life. In contrast, all other neonatal body systems can change their functions or establish themselves over a prolonged period of time.

RESPIRATORY ADAPTATIONS

The respiratory system is in a continuous state of development from fetal life to early childhood. During the first 20 weeks of gestation, growth of the primitive lung is limited to morphologic changes and to the differentiation of pulmonary, vascular, and lymphatic structures; biochemical activity is virtually nonexistent. At 20–24 weeks of fetal life, alveolar ducts begin to appear, followed by the generation of alveoli at 24–28 weeks. The alveolar epithelial cells then begin to differentiate into type I cells (structures necessary for gas exchange) and type II cells that contain lamellar bodies providing for the synthesis and storage of surfactant. *Surfactant* designates a group of surface-active phospholipids, of which lecithin is the most critical for alveolar stability. Biochemically, the synthesis of surfactant is initiated by the methylation pathway. Although this pathway is extremely vulnerable to hypoxia and acidosis, the lungs could be sufficiently mature to maintain extrauterine life by 26 weeks.

At 28–32 weeks of gestation, the number of type II cells further increases, and surfactant synthesis by the choline incorporation pathway begins. This shift is significant in that the choline pathway is less susceptible to acidosis and hypoxia, thus placing the preterm newborn in somewhat less jeopardy. Between the thirtieth and thirty-sixth week of fetal life, the lungs have functionally matured to allow more expansion, thereby increasing the newborn's ability to survive extrauterine life. Synthesis of surfactant and the resultant lung maturity may be accelerated between the thirty-fourth and thirty-sixth week, if the fetus resides in a high cortisol milieu (such as caused by PROM). At this time the lungs are structurally developed enough to permit maintenance of good lung expansion and adequate exchange of gases (Avery, 1981).

635

Initiation of Breathing

The ability of the neonate to breathe air immediately upon exposure to extrauterine life appears to be the consequence of weeks of intrauterine practice. In this respect, breathing can be perceived as a continuation of an intrauterine process as the lungs convert from a fluid to a gas medium. Fetal breathing movements (FBM)—chest wall movements of the fetus—can be detected by A and B scan ultrasound as early as 11 weeks of gestation. The pattern of FBM tends to be irregular and infrequent at 11 weeks, whereas a periodic pattern is established by 24 weeks, and a regular pattern at 34 weeks (Boddy, 1979). Marsal (1978) describes the following three types of FBM cycles occurring in the normal neonate:

1. Smooth, seesaw movements of the chest and abdomen (most frequent).
2. Periods of prolonged inspiration as if overcoming a large resistance.
3. Short interruptions in the course of inspiration.

The presence of FBM is associated with an intact CNS and as such is a reliable indicator of fetal well-being.

Absence of FBM may reflect normal periodic breathing or CNS depression. Fetal breathing pattern may be influenced by a variety of external and internal variables such as maternal exercise, smoking, infection, hypoglycemia, and hypoxia; the lasting effect on the fetus of each factor is not known (Manning and Feyerabend, 1976). At this time, deviations in FBM are unreliable predictors of fetal insult and do not dictate a poor prognosis unless validated by other indices of fetal status, such as the nonstress test (NST) and the contraction stress test (CST). The significance of FBM in establishing respiratory activity after birth and the impact on fetal well-being need to be further researched. Goldstein and Reid (1980) propose that FBM is essential for development of chest wall muscles (including the diaphragm) and to a lesser extent as a regulator of lung fluid volume and therefore of lung growth.

The initiation of extrauterine respiratory movement relies upon several chemical, thermal, sensory, physical, and mechanical stimuli that serve to provoke that vital first breath.

CHEMICAL STIMULI

An important chemical stimulator that contributes to the onset of breathing is transitory asphyxia of the fetus and newborn. The resultant elevation in Pco_2 and the decrease in pH and Po_2 are the natural outcome of normal vaginal delivery with cessation of placental gas exchange and umbilical cord pulsation and cutting. These changes, which are present in all newborns to some degree, stimulate the aortic and carotid chemoreceptors, initiating impulses that trigger the medulla's respiratory center. Although brief periods of asphyxia are a significant stimulator, prolonged asphyxia is abnormal.

THERMAL STIMULI

The significant decrease in ambient temperature after delivery (from 98.6F to 70–75F or 37C to 21–23.9C) is a significant thermal stimulus for initiation of breathing. As nerve endings in the skin are stimulated to transmit impulses to the medulla, the newborn responds with rhythmic respirations. Excessive cooling may result in profound depression and evidence of cold stress, but the normal temperature changes that occur are apparently within physiologic limits.

SENSORY AND PHYSICAL STIMULI

As the fetus is delivered from an environment characterized by sensory deprivation to one of sensory prominence, a number of physical and sensory influences appear to play a role in initiating respiration. They include the numerous tactile, auditory, and visual stimuli of birth. Historically, vigorous stimulation was provided by slapping the buttocks or heels of the newborn, but today greater emphasis is placed on gentle physical contact. Thoroughly drying the infant, for example, provides stimulation and ensures warmth in a far more comforting way.

MECHANICAL EVENTS

Fetal lungs continuously produce fluid during the latter half of intrauterine development. This secretion fills the lungs almost completely, expanding air spaces. Some of the fluid drains out of the lungs into the amniotic fluid and is soon swallowed by the fetus. The respiratory passages of a normal term fetus contain approximately 80–110 mL of fluid, which must be removed at the time of delivery to permit adequate movement of air. As the fetal chest is compressed through the birth canal during a normal delivery, approximately one-third of the fluid is squeezed out of the lungs because of increased intrathoracic pressure. The subsequent recoil of the chest wall after the birth of the newborn's trunk is thought to produce a small passive inspiration of air drawn into the lungs to replace the fluid that was squeezed out, thus overcoming the forces resisting the expansion of the lung. The fluid that has been left in the lungs is drawn back farther with each breath and is later absorbed into the bloodstream through the pulmonary capillaries and lymphatics. Some of the air is also forced into the proximal airways. An air–liquid interface (the surface boundary between these two components) is established in the smaller airways and alveoli. It is not known how quickly the remaining alveolar fluid is reabsorbed, but under normal circumstances it is reabsorbed after a few breaths or within the first hour after birth (Korones, 1981). Figure 21–1 summarizes the initiation of respiration.

Although the initial expiration should clear the airways of accumulated fluid and permit inspiration, it is wise to suction mucus and fluid from the newborn's mouth with a suction device (such as a DeLee or bulb syringe) as the

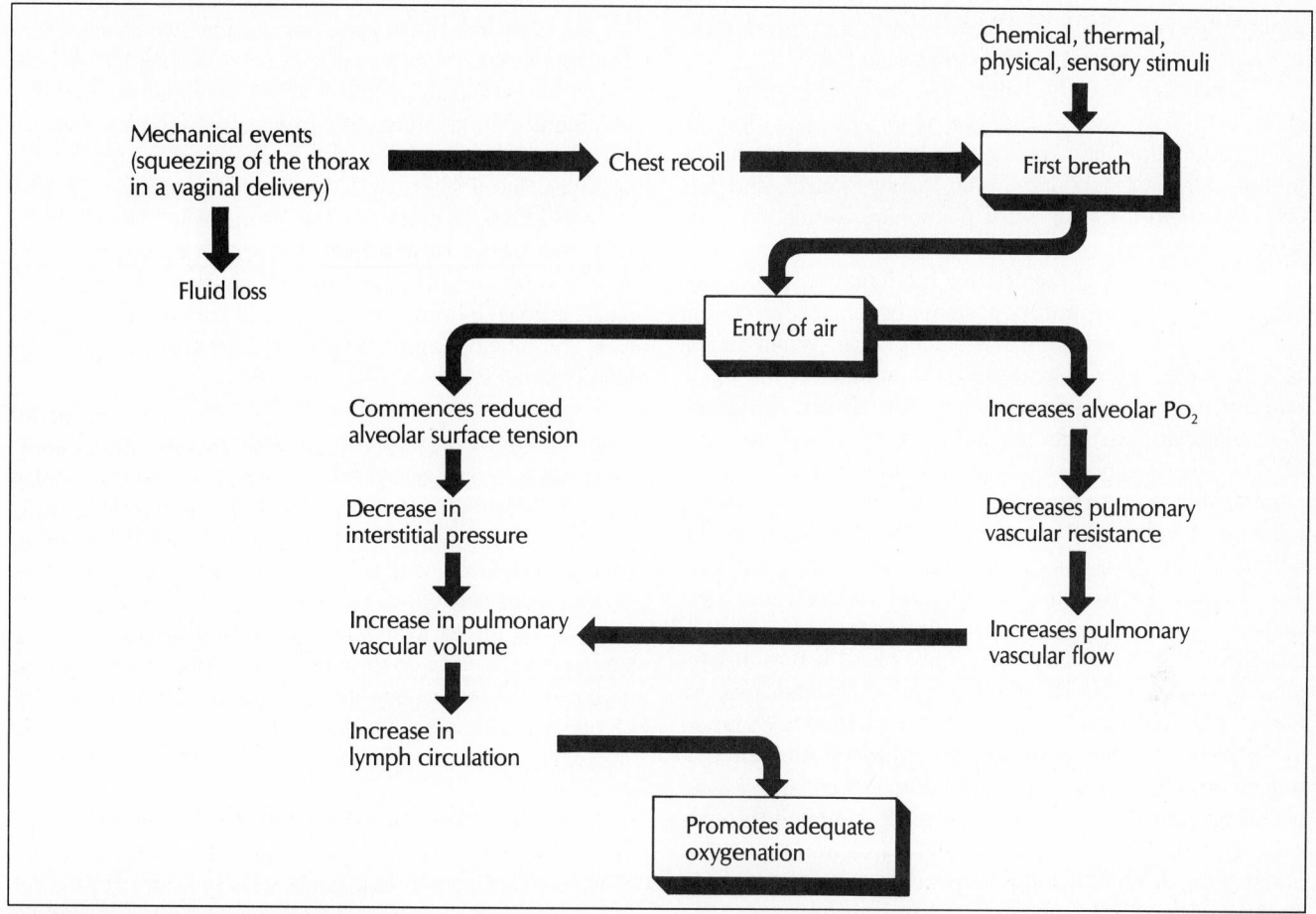

FIGURE 21-1 Initiation of respiration in the neonate.

head and shoulders are delivered and as the infant stabilizes (See Procedure 16–1 and Chapter 23).

Delay in clearing the lungs may result from (a) underdeveloped lymphatics, which decrease the rate at which the fluid is absorbed from the lungs, or (b) complications antenatally or during labor and delivery that interfere with adequate lung expansion and result in increased pulmonary vascular resistance and decreased blood flow. These complications may include inadequate compression of the chest wall in a very small neonate, the absence of chest wall compression in the neonate delivered by cesarean birth, or severe asphyxia at birth.

Spontaneous movements after birth also contribute to minute ventilation and influence the other physical and sensory factors. If the evacuation of pulmonary fluid is inhibited, bronchial obstruction with atelectasis may result.

Three major forces may oppose the initiation of respiratory activity: (a) surface tension in the alveoli, (b) the viscosity of pulmonary fluid within the respiratory tract, and (c) compliance of the lung. Because of surface tension within the alveoli, the small airways and alveoli would collapse between each inspiration were it not for the presence of surfactant, which reduces the cohesive force between the moist surfaces of the alveoli. Surfactant promotes lung expansion by preventing the alveoli from completely collapsing with each expiration and increases lung *compliance*, the ability of the lung to fill with air easily. When surfactant is decreased, compliance is also decreased and the pressure needed to expand the lungs with air increases. Resistive forces of the fluid-filled lung in conjunction with the small radii of the respiratory airways require the generation of pressures of 40–80 cm of water for the initial inflation of the lung. Generally, the first breath establishes a functional residual capacity (FRC) that is 30%–40% of the fully expanded lung volume. Residual air in the lungs after expiration alleviates the need for continuous high pressure for successive breaths. Indeed, the first breath of life may be the most difficult.

Neonatal Pulmonary Physiology

The first breath of life—the gasp in response to tactile, thermal, mechanical, and chemical changes associated with birth—initiates the serial opening of the alveoli. Thus begins the transition from a fluid-filled environment to an air-breathing existence, and from a dependent intrauterine existence to an independent extrauterine life.

To maintain life, the lungs must function immediately after birth. Two radical changes must take place for the lungs to function: first, pulmonary ventilation must be established through lung expansion following birth, and second, a marked increase in the pulmonary circulation must occur.

With the onset of respiration, the functions of the cardiovascular and respiratory systems become interrelated; hence the term *cardiopulmonary adaptation.* When air enters the lungs, the rise in alveolar Po_2 stimulates the relaxation of the pulmonary arteries, which in turn decreases the pulmonary vascular resistance. Simultaneously, lowered surface tension decreases interstitial pressure. Immediately, the vascular flow in the lung increases by 20%, followed by subsequent increases of 85% at 7 hours of life and 100% at 24 hours of life (Smith and Nelson, 1976). The greater blood volume contributes to the conversion from fetal circulation to neonatal circulation. After the establishment of pulmonary circulation, blood is well distributed throughout the lung, although the alveolae may or may not be fully ventilated. Increased shunting is common in the early neonatal period, largely through fetal circulation channels, the bronchial circulation, and collapsed alveoli. The bidirectional flow, or right-to-left shunting through the ductus arteriosus, may divert a significant amount of blood away from the lungs depending on the pressure changes of respiration, crying, and the cardiac cycle. For adequate oxygenation to occur, sufficient blood must be delivered by the heart to the lungs.

The function of the lung—to maintain oxygen and carbon dioxide exchange—is influenced by many factors. Chemical, pharmacologic, pulmonary reflex, pressoreceptor, and thermal factors influential in adult respiration regulation have not been as extensively evaluated in the neonate. The effect of chemical stimuli (Pco_2 and Po_2 concentrations) on newborn respirations has been studied, however. In response to hypercarbia (increased Pco_2), the newborn's respiratory rate increases to remove the retained CO_2. The consequences of hypoxia (decreased Po_2) as a ventilatory stimulus depend on temperature, hemoglobin content, and shunting of blood. The full-term neonate, however, tends to respond paradoxically by demonstrating brief hyperpnea, followed by respiratory depression. Cold stress accompanied by hypoxia results in immediate ventilatory depression.

From a physiologic standpoint, the movement of air into and out of the lungs (for oxygenation of the blood delivered by the heart) is accomplished by pressure differences, resistances to gas flow, and gaseous exchange. Pressure gradients within the respiratory system account for the flow of gas: (a) at inspiration there is decreased alveolar pressure, so that gas flows into the lungs; and (b) at expiration there is an increase in alveolar pressure, so that gas flows out of the lungs.

Gas flow into the lungs is opposed by two forces—lung compliance and airway resistance. Compliance is influenced by the elastic recoil of lung tissue and by anatomic variations. The anatomic differences between the neonate and the adult influence lung compliance. The infant has a relatively large heart and mediastinal structures that reduce available lung space. The protuberant abdomen further encroaches on the high diaphragm to decrease lung space. Anatomically, the neonatal chest is equipped with weak intercostal muscles, a rigid rib cage with horizontal ribs, and a high diaphragm that inhibits available space for lung expansion.

Impedance to ventilation is also offered by airway resistance, which depends on the radii, length, and number of airways as well as on lung compliance. A reduction in size of the airway, as in the anatomic size of an infant's airway as opposed to an adult airway, or continued retention of secretions within the airway will greatly increase resistance to gaseous flow.

Surface forces further affect lung compliance, as pressures are utilized to overcome surface-tension forces at the air-liquid interface of the alveoli. With respiration, the alveoli undergo changes: inspiration (the radius of the alveolus is greatest) and expiration (the radius of the alveolus is smaller).

The alveoli are lined with surfactant. This lining-layer functions to (a) lower surface tension as the radius of the alveolus is reduced in expiration (less pressure is required to hold the alveolus open); and (b) maintain alveolar stability by variance of the surface tension as the size of the alveolus changes.

The surfactant system develops systematically as gestation progresses. Recently, estimation of fetal pulmonary maturity by examination of amniotic fluid for phospholipids and lecithin/sphingomyelin ratio (L/S ratio) has become an accepted tool (see Chapter 13). The ratio of the surface-active phospholipids, lecithin, and sphingomyelin, is an indication of lung maturity.

These concentrations of lecithin and sphingomyelin are established in a definite changing relationship as pregnancy and gestation advance. In the immature fetal lung, the L/S ratio is less than 1:1; transitional ratios are about 1.5:1.0; and the mature ratio is greater than 2:1. Lecithin is produced via two major enzymatic pathways, the methyl-transferase system and the phosphocholine-transferase system (Figure 21–2). The methyl-transferase system is first detectable at 22–24 weeks' gestation, appears to contribute little to maturing surfactant, and increases gradually toward term. It is very susceptible to damage by acidosis, hypothermia, and hypoxia. The second enzymatic pathway, the phosphocholine-transferase system, demonstrates a peak in lecithin production at about 35 weeks' gestation, and lecithin levels rise rapidly toward term, paralleling late fetal lung development. It is a fairly stable system, relatively resistant to the insults of hypothermia. Clinically, the occurrence of the second pathway peak production closely corresponds with the marked decrease in incidence of idiopathic respiratory distress syndrome after 35 weeks of gestation. Production of sphingomyelin remains constant throughout gestation. The neonate delivered before the L/S ratio is 2:1 will have varying degrees of respiratory distress.

Although the L/S ratio continues to be used extensively in determining the fetal lung maturity, increasing recognition is being given to the presence of phosphatidylglycerol in the amniotic fluid (see discussion in Chapter 13). As a more mature component of the surfactant complex, its presence appears to ensure fetal lung maturity and reduces the incidence of false-positive L/S ratio readings, a common occurrence in the pregnant diabetic client.

Adequate oxygenation also depends on gaseous exchange at the cellular level. Within lung tissue this gas exchange depends on two principles. The first is diffusion, which is responsible for gas exchange between capillary blood and the alveoli and which depends on the substance (the gas and its pressure) crossing the membrane and the properties of the membrane (such as thickness and available surface area for exchange). The second is the ventilation/perfusion ratio within the alveolar space, which is necessary for adequate gaseous exchange. A delicate balance exists between blood flow (perfusion) and alveolar ventilation. Lung tissue that is ventilated poorly (decreased Po_2) promotes airway constriction. Alveolar ventilation is thus regulated to maintain constant alveolar and arterial carbon dioxide tension. A discussion of mechanisms affecting oxygen transport is found on p. 642–643.

Characteristics of Neonatal Respiration

Normal neonatal respiratory rate is 30–50 per minute. Respirations initially may be largely diaphragmatic, and have shallow and irregular depth and rhythm. Additionally, they are primarily abdominal and synchronous with the chest movement. Short periods of apnea are to be expected. When the breathing pattern is characterized by apnea lasting 5–15 seconds, *periodic breathing* is occurring. Periodic respiration is rarely associated with differences in skin color or heart rate changes, nor does it have prognostic significance. Tactile or other sensory stimulation increases the inspired oxygen and converts periodic breathing patterns to normal breathing patterns. Neonatal sleep states particularly influence respiratory patterns. With deep sleep, the pattern is reasonably regular. Periodic breathing occurs with rapid-eye-movement (REM) sleep, and grossly irregular breathing is evident with motor activity, sucking, and crying.

The neonate is an obligatory nose breather, and any obstruction will cause respiratory distress, so it is important to keep the throat and nose clear. If respirations drop below 30 or exceed 60 per minute when the infant is at rest, or if dyspnea or cyanosis occurs, the physician should

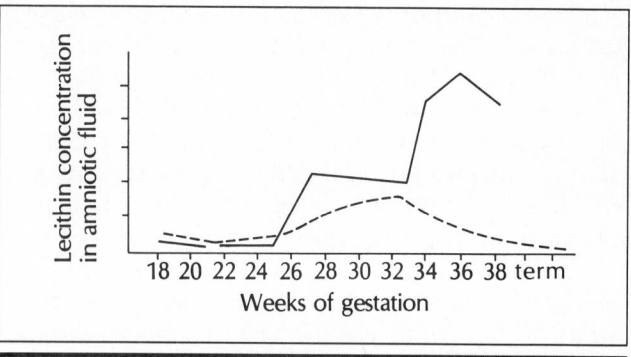

FIGURE 21–2 Development of lecithin in the fetal lung. The broken line represents the methylation pathway, and the solid line represents the phosphocholine transferase pathway. (From Gluck, L., and Kulovich, M. V. 1973. Fetal lung development. *Pediatr. Clin. North Am.* 20:373.)

be notified. (Some initial dyspnea or cyanosis may be normal.) Any increased use of the intercostal muscles may also indicate respiratory distress.

CARDIOVASCULAR ADAPTATIONS

Embryology

Early formation of the cardiovascular system is necessary, because the human ovum lacks sufficient yolk to provide nutrients for the rapidly growing embryo. On about the fifteenth to eighteenth day, a small cluster of cells, called the cardiogenic plate, can be identified. The cardiogenic plate is located at the cephalic end of the embryo in front of the tissue that will become the head. A small U-shaped cavity rapidly encircles the cardiogenic plate. The outer layer of this evolving structure will become the pericardium, the inner layer will develop into the myocardium and epicardium, and the remaining cells will migrate to form the endocardium. The head of the embryo grows forward as the pericardial cavity swings under, so that the early heart tissue becomes part of the developing thorax. Within the pericardial cavity, cells arrange themselves in long side-by-side strands. These strands develop into two thin-walled vessels that fuse together and form a single vessel that functions as a simple tubular heart. By the end of 21 days, this tubular heart has rhythmic contractions, forcing blood through primitive vessels in the developing embryo.

The tubular heart grows much more rapidly than the pericardial chamber within which it finds itself. As the tubular heart folds and doubles on itself, the venous end swings up toward the arterial end, and slight constrictions appear, dividing it into the primitive atrium and the primitive ventricle. As the heart continues to grow, complex rotation of the chambers occurs, until the ventricle becomes situated below the atrium. At the time, the embryo is 6 weeks old and one-half inch long, and its heart shows the general shape and markings that it will carry permanently (Toronto, 1972).

From 5–7 weeks, partitions are formed and a four-chambered heart is developed. First, masses of endocardial tissue, called *endocardial cushions,* grow together from the dorsal and ventral portions of the atrioventricular groove, forming the tricuspid and mitral valves and separating the atria from the ventricles. At the same time, a septum develops from the interventricular groove and grows toward the base of the heart, separating the right and left ventricles, but this septum is not completely developed until the eighth week. The distal cephalad ventricular septum divides the arterial end of the primitive tube, making two vessels out of one. One vessel becomes the aorta, which is connected to the ventricle. The other vessel is the pulmonary artery and is connected to the right ventricle.

A crescentic ridge appears on the dorsocephalic part of the atrium, forming a septum that rapidly grows toward the ventricle. Before it reaches the ventricle and closes completely, a new opening develops higher up in the septum. A second thin septum grows down and extends like a curtain over the aperture. This structure is called the *foramen ovale,* a unidirectional valve permitting blood to flow only from the right atrium into the left (Toronto, 1972).

The venous end of the primitive tube divides and separates, forming veins that empty into the atrium. These veins migrate and arrange themselves so that the superior vena cava, the inferior vena cava, and the coronary sinus empty into the right atrium and the pulmonary veins empty into the left atrium.

Fetal–Neonatal Transition Circulation

The lungs of the fetus do not function in utero; therefore, it is necessary to have a special circulatory system that will bypass most of the blood supply to the lungs. See Chapter 8 for a discussion of fetal circulation and Figure 8–13 for a pictorial presentation. At the time of birth, marked changes occur in the cardiovascular system. With the first breath of life and the cutting of the cord, the newborn begins the transition from intrauterine to extrauterine life.

During fetal life, blood with higher oxygen content is diverted to the heart and brain. Blood in the descending aorta is less oxygenated and supplies the kidney and intestinal tract. Limited amounts of blood, pumped from the right ventricle toward the lungs, enters the pulmonary vessels. In the fetus increased pulmonary resistance forces most of the blood through the ductus arteriosus into the descending aorta (Figure 8–13). Expansion of the lungs with the first breath decreases the pulmonary vascular resistance, as the clamping of the cord raises systemic vascular resistance and left atrial pressure. This physiologic mechanism marks the beginning of neonatal circulation and the integration of cardiopulmonary adaptation (Figure

21–3). Five major areas of change occur in cardiopulmonary adaptation.

1. *Increased aortic pressure and decreased venous pressure.* With severing of the cord, the placental vascular bed is eliminated and the intravascular space is reduced. Consequently, aortic blood pressure is increased. At the same time, separation from the placenta results in decreased blood return via the inferior vena cava, resulting in a small decrease in pressure within the venous circulation.

2. *Increased systemic pressure and decreased pulmonary artery pressure.* Pressure increases in the systemic circulation because severing the placenta produces greater systemic resistance. At the same time, adequate lung expansion produces increased pulmonary blood flow, while the increased blood Po_2 associated with initiation of respirations produces vasodilatation. The combination of increased pulmonary blood flow and vasodilatation results in decreased pulmonary artery resistance. With the opening of the vascular beds, the systemic vascular pressure decreases, causing perfusion of the other body systems.

3. *Closure of the foramen ovale.* Closure of the foramen ovale is a function of atrial pressures. In utero, pressure is greater in the right atrium, and the foramen ovale is open. Decreased pulmonary resistance and increased pulmonary blood flow result in increased pulmonary venous return into the left atrium, thereby increasing left atrial pressure slightly. The decreased pulmonary vascular resistance also causes a decrease in right atrial pressure. The pressure gradients are now reversed, left atrial pressure is greater, and the foramen ovale is functionally closed. Although the foramen ovale closes 1–2 hours after birth, a slight right-to-left shunting may occur in the early neonatal period. Any increase in pulmonary resistance may result in reopening of the foramen ovale, causing a right-to-left shunt. Permanent closure occurs within several months.

4. *Closure of the ductus arteriosus.* Initial elevation of the systemic vascular pressure above the pulmonary vascular pressure increases pulmonary blood flow by causing a reversal of the flow through the ductus arteriosus. Blood now flows from the aorta into the pulmonary artery. Furthermore, although the presence of oxygen causes the pulmonary arterioles to dilate, an increase in blood Po_2 triggers the opposite response in the ductus arteriosus—it constricts. If the lungs fail to expand or if Po_2 levels drop, the ductus remains patent. Fibrosis of the ductus occurs within 3 weeks, but functional closure is accomplished within 15 hours after birth.

5. *Closure of the ductus venosus.* Although the mechanism of initiating closure of the ductus venosus is not known, it appears to be related to mechanical pressure

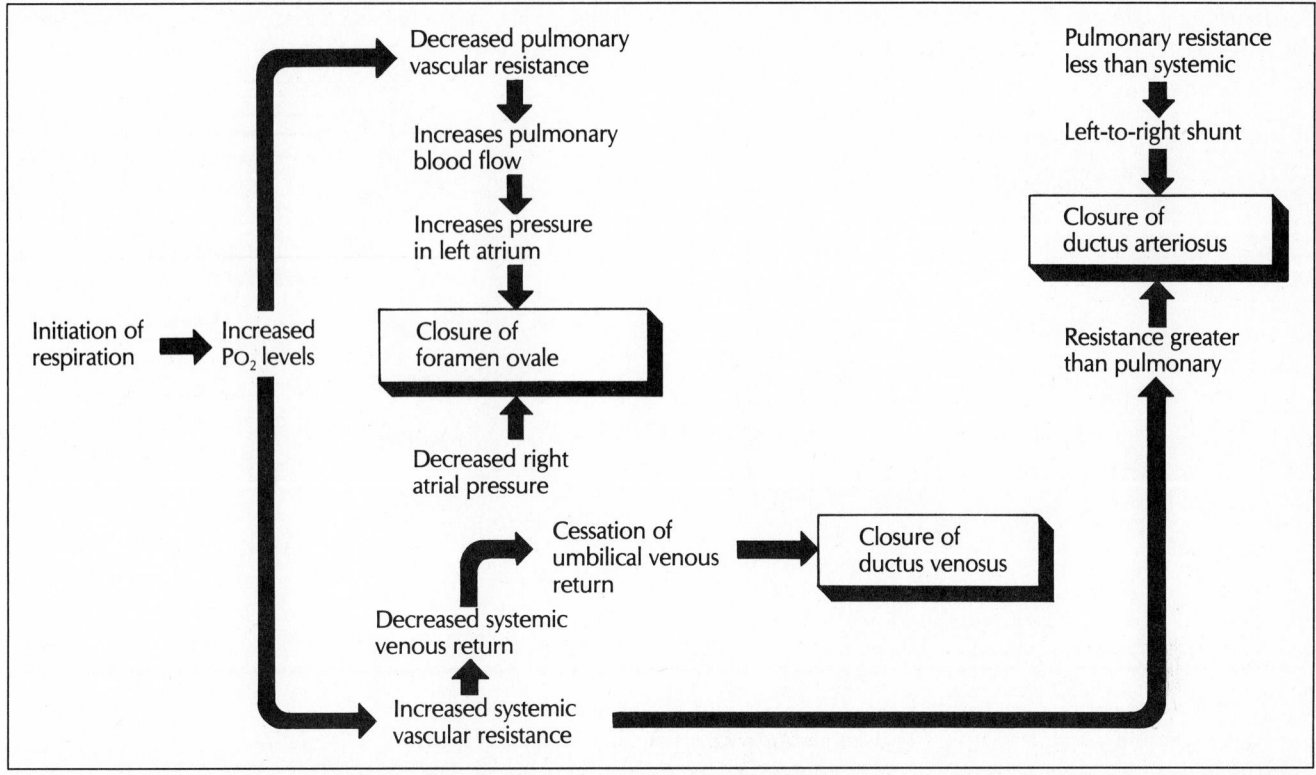

FIGURE 21-3 Transitional circulation — conversion from fetal to neonatal circulation.

changes after severing of the cord, redistribution of blood, and cardiac output. Closure of the bypass forces perfusion of the liver. Anatomic fibrosis occurs within 3–7 days (Korones, 1981) (Figure 21–4).

Characteristics

HEART RATE

Shortly after the first cry and the advent of cardiopulmonary circulation, the newborn heart rate accelerates to 175–180 beats/min. Thereafter the rate follows a fairly uniform course, decelerating to 115 beats/min at 4–6 hours of life, then rising and plateauing to approximately 120 beats/min at 12–24 hours of life (Smith and Nelson, 1976). The range of the heart rate in the full-term neonate is 70–90 beats/min while asleep and 120–150 while awake; it may be as high as 180 while crying. Apical pulse rates should be obtained by auscultation for a full minute, preferably when the neonate is asleep. Peripheral pulses should also be evaluated to detect any lags or unusual characteristics.

BLOOD PRESSURE

During the newborn period, the blood pressure tends to be the highest immediately after birth, and then descends to its lowest level about 3 hours of age. By 4–6 days of life, the blood pressure rises and plateaus at a level approximately the same as the initial level (Smith and Nelson, 1976). Blood pressure is particularly sensitive to the changes in blood volume that occur in the transition to neonatal circulation. Figure 21–5 describes this response (Smith and Nelson, 1976).

Blood pressure values during the first 12 hours of life vary with the birth weight. In the full-term resting neonate, the average blood pressure is 74/47 mm Hg and 64/39 mm Hg for the preterm newborn. Crying may cause an elevation of 20 mm Hg in both the systolic and diastolic blood pressure, thus accuracy is more likely in the quiet newborn. The measurement of blood pressure is best accomplished by using the Doppler technique or a 1–2 in. cuff and a stethoscope over the brachial artery.

HEART MURMURS

Murmurs are usually produced by turbulent blood flow. Murmurs may be heard when blood flows across an abnormal valve or across a stenosed valve, when there is an atrial septal or ventricular septal defect, or when there is increased flow across a normal valve. A transient murmur is often heard in newborns before the ductus arteriosus completely closes.

About 50%–60% of normal children have what are

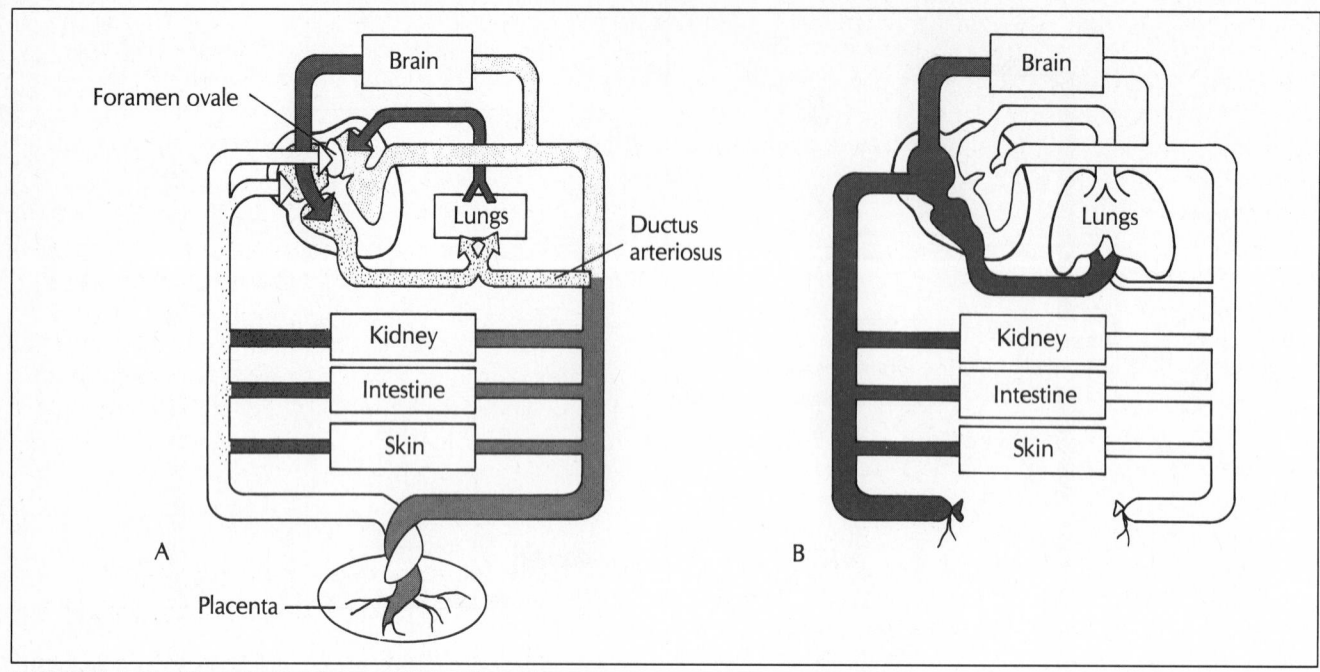

FIGURE 21-4 A, Schematic representation of fetal circulation. Oxygenated blood leaves the placenta by way of the umbilical vein (vessel without stippling). It flows into the portal sinus in the liver (not shown) and a variable portion of it perfuses the liver. **B,** Schematic representation of circulation in the normal newborn. After expansion of the lungs and ligation of the umbilical cord, pulmonary blood flow increases and left atrial and systemic arterial pressures rise while pulmonary arterial and right heart pressures fall. (From Avery, G. B. 1981. *Neonatology.* Philadelphia: J. B. Lippincott Co., pp. 184–185.)

called innocent or functional murmurs. In young children, a low-pitched, musical murmur heard just to the right of the apex of the heart is fairly common. There appears to be no structural or underlying reason for these murmurs. Func-

tional murmurs are always short in duration and midsystolic, never diastolic.

Occasionally, significant murmurs will be heard, including the murmur of a patent ductus arteriosus, the murmur of aortic or pulmonic stenosis, or the murmur of a small ventricular septal defect. See Chapter 26 for discussion of congenital heart defects.

CARDIAC OUTPUT

In the first 2 hours after birth when the ductus arteriosus remains mostly patent, about one-third of the ventricular output is returned to the pulmonary circulation. Minimal amounts of blood may also shunt from left to right through the foramen ovale. As a result, the left ventricle has a significantly greater volume load than the right ventricle. In the adult, right and left ventricular outputs are equal; in the neonate right ventricular output equals systemic blood flow, and left ventricular output equals pulmonary blood flow. Systemic blood volume and pulmonary blood volume are *not* equal in the neonate. The newborn's combined cardiac output (left and right ventricular) is greater per unit of body weight than in later childhood.

Oxygen Transport

The transportation of oxygen to the peripheral tissues is dependent upon the presence of hemoglobin found in the

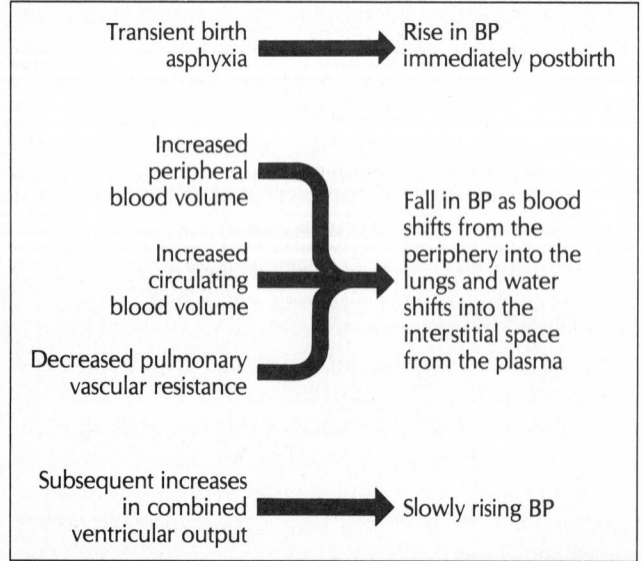

FIGURE 21-5 Response of BP to neonatal changes in blood volume.

erythrocyte. In the fetus and neonate, a variety of hemoglobins exist, the most significant being Hb F (fetal hemoglobin) and Hb A (adult hemoglobin). Approximately 70%–90% of hemoglobin in the fetus and neonate is of the fetal variety. Hb F and Hb A possess a reciprocal relationship; Hb F predominates during fetal life and the first few weeks postnatally, but is eventually replaced by Hb A. The greatest difference between Hb F and Hb A is related to the transport of oxygen.

The supply of oxygen to the tissues is regulated by several factors, including blood oxygen capacity, cardiac output, and hemoglobin–oxygen affinity (Schaeffer et al., 1977). Oxygen capacity is the maximum amount of hemoglobin and oxygen that can be bound and is directly affected by hemoglobin concentrations. One gram of hemoglobin is able to combine with 1.34 mL of oxygen. The actual amount of oxygen-bound hemoglobin divided by the oxygen capacity gives a percentage signifying *oxygen saturation*. Oxygen saturation, which is controlled by arterial oxygen tension (Pa_{O_2}) and hemoglobin–oxygen affinity usually has values between 96% and 98%. A significant reduction in the oxygen capacity results in an increased cardiac output to compensate for the decreased oxygen concentration of the hemoglobin.

Oxygen affinity, the amount of binding power between the hemoglobin and oxygen, affects the transfer of oxygen to the tissues. Increased affinity reduces oxygen delivery to the tissues, and decreased affinity results in more oxygen being released to the tissues. Hb F has a greater affinity for oxygen than Hb A; thus at any given oxygen tension, Hb F binds more oxygen and has a higher oxygen saturation than Hb A. However, fetal oxygen tension levels must be lower than in the adult for the fetal hemoglobin to release oxygen to the tissues. The reason for this difference is the presence of organic phosphates in the red blood cell.

Of the organic phosphates residing in the erythrocyte, 2,3 diphosphoglyceride (DPG) has been identified as being responsible for the release of oxygen to the tissues and for the dissimilarity in the oxygen affinity of Hb F and Hb A. The 2,3 DPG interacts with Hb A to decrease oxygen affinity and increase the availability of oxygen to the tissues. On the other hand, Hb F does not interact with 2,3 DPG to the same degree, thus hindering the freeing of oxygen to the tissues. Consequently, Hb F has greater oxygen affinity than Hb A.

The affinity of oxygen for hemoglobin is measured by the *oxygen dissociation curve*. The curve graphically demonstrates the relationship between Pa_{O_2} levels and the degree of oxygen saturation (Figure 21–6). The fetal curve is said to be shifted to the left when it is compared to the adult curve. Normally the fetal dissociation curve moves to the right as the increasing interaction between Hb A and 2,3 DPG facilitates the release of oxygen from the erythrocytes.

In the newborn the greater affinity of hemoglobin for oxygen in Hb F causes the shift to the left in the oxygen dissociation curve. More oxygen is bound to fetal hemoglobin, which increases the oxygen saturation compared with the adult, but less oxygen is available to the tissues at any partial pressure. This is advantageous for the fetus, who must maintain adequate oxygen uptake in the presence of very low oxygen tension (umbilical venous Po_2 cannot exceed the uterine venous Po_2) (Quilligan and Kretchmer, 1980). Because of this phenomenon, hypoxia in the neonate is particularly difficult to recognize because of the high concentration of oxygen in the blood. Clinical manifestations of cyanosis are lacking until low levels of oxygen are present. Shifts to the left in the curve also may be caused by alkalosis (increased pH) and hypothermia. Acidosis, hypercarbia, and hyperthermia may lead to shifts to the right in the oxygen dissociation curve.

HEMATOPOIETIC SYSTEM

Blood-forming tissues undergo dramatic developmental changes during fetal life to prepare for the transition to neonatal life. Early hematopoiesis occurs in the yolk sac. By the eighth to tenth week, the liver and spleen become the major sites for hematopoiesis, with the formation of normoblastic erythrocytes, platelets, and granulocytes. Bone marrow assumes the role of blood-forming organ around the eighteenth week of gestation. Bone marrow

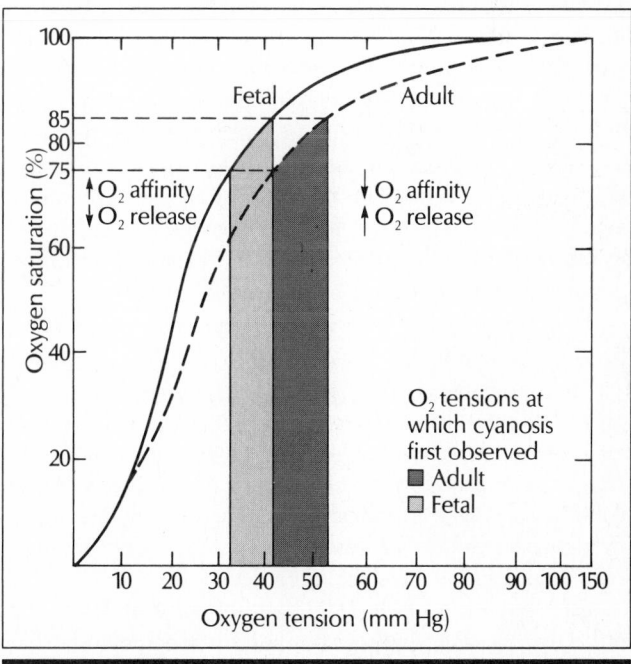

FIGURE 21–6 Fetal oxygen dissociation curve. (Modified from Klaus, M., and Fanaroff, A. A. 1973. *Care of the high-risk infant.* Philadelphia: W. B. Saunders Co., p. 122.)

initially produces more leukocytes but with the decline of liver hemopoietic function increasing numbers of red blood cells are formed. Fetal erythropoietin, which in part controls red blood cell production, is detectable in the last trimester of pregnancy. Its concentration in fetal blood and amniotic fluid increases with gestation. Fetal blood (umbilical vein) in utero is 50% oxygen saturated; this relative hypoxia causes increased amounts of erythropoietin to be secreted causing active erythropoiesis (an increase in nucleated red blood cells and reticulocytes). After birth, erythropoietin produced by the fetal liver normally may not be detectable until the kidney starts production, and erythroid activity recommences at 8–12 weeks postnatally.

Fetal red blood cell production is not significantly influenced by maternal erythropoiesis or maternal nutrition because iron, folate, and vitamin B_{12} are extracted by the fetus irrespective of maternal stores.

Fetal erythrocytes are larger than those present at birth but fewer in number. After birth, the red blood cell count gradually increases as cell size decreases. Neonatal red blood cells have a life span of 80–100 days, which is approximately two-thirds of an adult's red blood cell life span. In neonatal red blood cells, about 5% of the RBC's retain their nucleus.

Granular leukocytes, lymphocytes, monocytes, and megakaryocytes are first seen about the seventh week of gestation. During the first half of gestation, leukocytes are present in small numbers. Granular leukocytes differentiate into neutrophils, eosinophils, and basophils, which are present in the fetal circulating blood near the end of the first trimester. Granulocyte numbers increase in the last 2–3 months of fetal life. Lymphoblasts give rise to large and small lymphocytes in the lymph nodes at about 12 weeks' gestation. The thymus provides lymphoblasts to the lymph nodes and other lymphoid tissue, which then play a role in antibody formation. Lymphocytes attain two-thirds of the adult's value by 20 weeks' gestation and gradually continue to increase until term. Megakaryocytes appear in the liver and spleen as platelets at about 11 weeks' gestation and approach adult values by 30 weeks.

Hematologic values in the newborn are decidedly modified by several factors, which include (Smith and Nelson, 1976):

The site of the blood sample. Hemoglobin and hematocrit levels taken simultaneously are significantly higher in capillary blood than in venous blood. Sluggish peripheral blood flow creates red blood cell stasis, thereby increasing their concentration. Because of this, blood samples taken from venous blood sites are more accurate.

Delayed cord clamping and the normal shift of plasma to the extravascular spaces. Neonatal hemoglobin and hematocrit values are higher when a placental transfusion occurs postnatally. Placental vessels contain about 100 mL of blood at term, the majority of which can be transfused into the newborn by positioning the neonate below the level of the placenta and by late clamping of the cord. Blood volume increases by 40%–60% with late cord clamping (Korones, 1981). The increase is reflected by a rise in hemoglobin level and an increase in the hematocrit to 65% about 48 hours after birth (compared with 48% when the cord is clamped immediately). For greatest accuracy, the initial hemoglobin and hematocrit levels should be measured in the cord blood, although this is not a routine practice.

Gestational age. There appears to be a positive association between increasing gestational age, higher red blood cell numbers, and greater hemoglobin concentration. This means that the gestational age of the newborn influences the values.

Prenatal and/or perinatal hemorrhage. Occurrence of significant prenatal or perinatal bleeding decreases the hematocrit level and causes hypovolemia.

Neonatal Hematology

In the fetus, the hemoglobin and erythrocyte counts are high because of the nature of fetal circulation. In the first days of life hemoglobin concentration may rise by 1–2 g/dL above fetal levels as a result of placental transfusion, low oral fluid intake, and diminished extracellular fluid volume. By 1 week postnatally, peripheral hemoglobin is comparable to fetal blood counts. The hemoglobin level declines progressively thereafter (Hatch and Sumner, 1981), creating a phenomenon known as *physiologic anemia of infancy.*

A factor that influences the degree of physiologic anemia is the nutritional status of the neonate, because supplies of vitamin E, folic acid, and iron may be inadequate in the face of increased growth in the later part of the first year of life. Hemoglobin values fall, mainly from a decrease in red cell mass rather than from the dilutional effect of increasing plasma volume. Other contributing factors are that red cell survival is lower in neonates than in adults, and red cell production is less. Hemoglobin levels continue to decrease gradually during the first 3 months after birth, then begin to increase slowly as the infant grows to adulthood.

Leukocytosis is a normal finding because the trauma of birth stimulates increased production of neutrophils during the first week of life. Neutrophils then decrease to 35% of the total leukocyte count by 2 weeks of age. Eventually, lymphocytes become the predominant type of leukocyte and the total white blood count falls.

Blood volume of the term infant is estimated to be 80–85 mL/kg of body weight. The true amount of blood volume varies based on the amount of placental transfusion received. Normal blood values for the normal term infant are as follows:

Laboratory data	Normal range
Hemoglobin	15–20 g/dL
RBC	5.0–7.5 million/mm³

Hematocrit	43%–61%
WBC	10,000–30,000/mm³
Neutrophils	40%–80%
Eosinophils	2%–3%
Lymphocytes	30%–31%
Monocytes	6%–10%
Immature WBC	3%–10%
Platelets	100,000–280,000/mm³
Reticulocytes	3%–6%
Blood volume	78 mL/kg (early cord clamping)
	98.6 mL/kg (late cord clamping)
	82.3 mL/kg (third day after early cord clamping)
	92.6 mL/kg (third day after delayed cord clamping)

Knowledge of the concentrations of serum electrolytes is essential in monitoring the fluid and electrolyte status of the newborn. Table 21–1 depicts the blood chemistries of the normal newborn.

TEMPERATURE REGULATION

Temperature regulation is the maintenance of thermal balance by the dissipation of heat to the environment (heat loss) at a rate equal to the production of heat. Newborns are *homeothermic;* they attempt to stabilize their internal body temperatures within a narrow range in spite of significant temperature variations in their milieu.

Thermoregulation in the newborn is closely related to the rate of metabolism and oxygen consumption. Within a specific environmental range called the *thermal neutral zone* (TNZ), the rates of oxygen consumption and metabolism are minimal. Furthermore, within the limits of the TNZ, internal body temperature is maintained because of thermal balance. For an unclothed full-term neonate, the range of the TNZ is an ambient temperature of 32–34C (89.6–93.2F). The limits for an adult are 26–28C (78.8–82.4F). Thus, the normal newborn requires higher environmental temperatures to maintain a thermoneutral environment than does the adult. Establishment of a TNZ is affected by neonatal characteristics described in the following paragraphs.

The neonate has decreased thermal insulation and a thin epidermis, with blood vessels closer to the skin than an adult. Therefore, the circulating blood is influenced by changes in environmental temperature, and in turn influences the hypothalmic temperature-regulating center.

The flexed posture of the term infant decreases the surface area exposed to the environment, thereby reducing heat loss. Other neonatal characteristics such as size and age may also affect the establishing of a TNZ. Preterm SGA neonates require higher environmental temperatures to achieve a thermoneutral environment while a larger,

Table 21–1   Normal Blood Chemistry Values, Term Infants*

Determination	Sample source	Cord	1–12 hr	12–24 hr	24–48 hr	48–72 hr
Sodium, mmol/L	Capillary	147 (126–166)	143 (124–156)	145 (132–159)	148 (134–160)	149 (139–162)
Potassium, mmol/L		7.8 (5.6–12)	6.4 (5.3–7.3)	6.3 (5.3–8.9)	6.0 (5.2–7.3)	5.9 (5.0–7.7)
Chloride, mmol/L		103 (98–110)	100.7 (90–111)	103 (87–114)	102 (92–114)	103 (93–112)
Calcium, mg/dL		9.3 (8.2–11.1)	8.4 (7.3–9.2)	7.8 (6.9–9.4)	8.0 (6.1–9.9)	7.9 (5.9–9.7)
Phosphorus, mg/dL		5.6 (3.7–8.1)	6.1 (3.5–8.6)	5.7 (2.9–8.1)	5.9 (3.0–8.7)	5.8 (2.8–7.6)
Blood urea, mg/dL		29 (21–40)	27 (8–34)	33 (9–63)	32 (13–77)	31 (13–68)
Total protein, g/dL		6.1 (4.8–7.3)	6.6 (5.6–8.5)	6.6 (5.8–8.2)	6.9 (5.9–8.2)	7.2 (6.0–8.5)
Glucose, mg/dL		73 (45–96)	63 (40–97)	63 (42–104)	56 (30–91)	59 (40–90)
Lactic acid, mg/dL		19.5 (11–30)	14.6 (11–24)	14.0 (10–23)	14.3 (9–22)	13.5 (7–21)
Lactate, mmol/L		2.0–3.0	2.0			

*From Avery, G. B., ed. 1981. *Neonatology.* Philadelphia: J. B. Lippincott Co., p. 1175. Data from Acharya, P. T., and Payne, W. W. 1965. *Arch. Dis. Child.* 40:430 and Daniel, S. S., et al. 1966. *Pediatrics.* 37:942.

FIGURE 21-7 Thermal environment of newborn infants. Smaller infants have a higher neutral thermal environment. (Modified from Lubchenco, L. 1976. *The high-risk infant*. Philadelphia: W. B. Saunders Co., p. 133.)

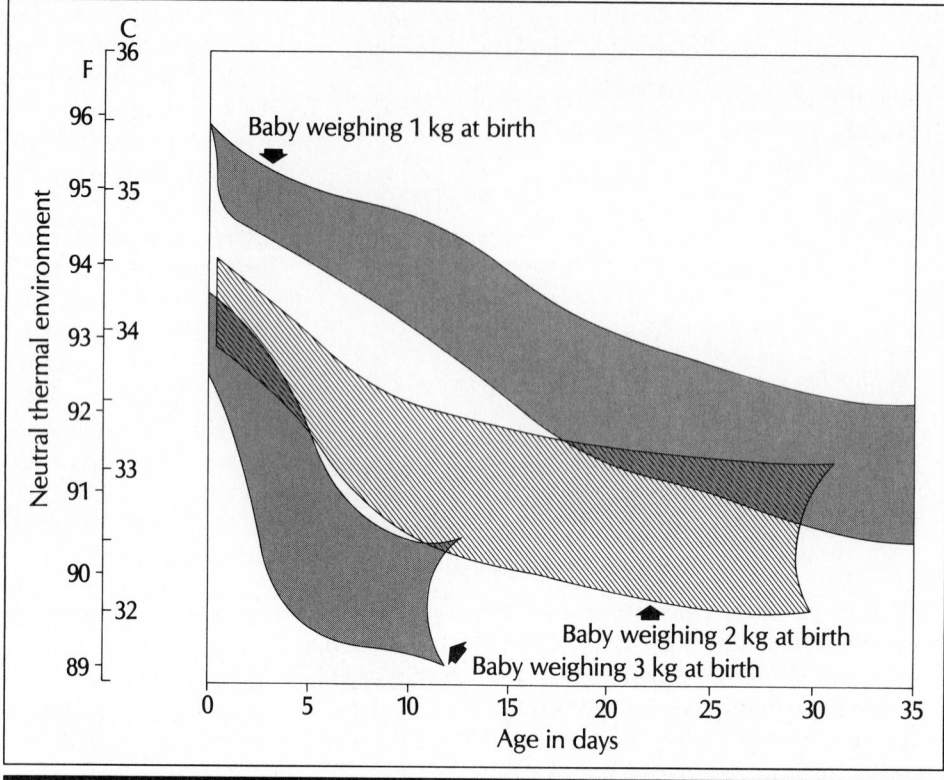

well-insulated newborn may be able to cope with lower environmental temperature. If the environmental temperature falls below the lower limits of the TNZ, the neonate responds with increased oxygen consumption and raised metabolism, which results in greater heat production. Prolonged exposure to the cold may result in depleted glycogen stores and acidosis. Oxygen consumption also increases with elevation, in the environmental temperature above the TNZ (Figure 21-7).

To accomplish thermal regulation, the neonate must possess a system of surface sensors to perceive temperature differences, a central control system (the hypothalamus), and a means to adjust heat production and heat loss (vasomotor control) (Avery, 1981). Vasomotor control facilitates the retention of heat through vasoconstriction and permits heat loss through vasodilatation.

Heat Loss

A newborn is at a distinct disadvantage in maintaining a normal temperature because of a larger body surface in relation to mass and a limited amount of insulating subcutaneous fat. With a body weight approximately 5% of the adult's and a body surface 15% of the adult's, the full-term newborn loses about four times the heat of an adult (Danforth, 1982). The neonate's poor thermal stability is primarily due to excessive heat loss rather than to impaired heat production.

Two major routes of heat loss are from the internal core of the body to the body surface, and from the external surface to the environment. Usually the core temperature is 0.5C higher than the skin temperature, providing for the continuous transfer or conduction of heat to the surface. The greater the difference in temperatures between core to skin, the more rapid the transfer. Heat loss from the body surface to the environment takes place by four avenues—convection, radiation, evaporation, and conduction.

Convection involves the loss of heat from the warm body surface to the cooler air currents. Heat loss by convection depends upon the temperature of the air and the velocity of the air flow. Air-conditioned rooms, oxygen by mask, and removal from an incubator for procedures without an overhead warmer as a heat source increase convective heat loss of the neonate. *Radiation* losses occur when heat transfers from the heated body surface to cooler surfaces and objects not in direct contact with the body. The walls of a room or of an incubator are potential causes of heat loss by radiation, even if the ambient temperature of the isolette is within the neutral thermal range for that infant. *Evaporation* is the loss of heat incurred when water is converted to a vapor. The newborn is particularly prone to lose heat by evaporation immediately after delivery when the infant is wet with amniotic fluid and during bath time. *Conduction* is the loss of heat to a cooler surface by direct skin contact. Chilled hands, cool scales, cold examination tables, and cold stethoscopes can cause the newborn to lose heat by conduction.

After birth, the highest losses of heat generally result from radiation and convection because of the newborn's large body surface compared with weight, and from thermal conduction because of the marked difference between core temperature and skin temperature. The neonate is able to respond to the cooler environmental temperature with adequate peripheral vasoconstriction, but this mechanism becomes less effective because of the minimal amount of fat insulation present, the large body surface, and ongoing thermal conduction. Because of these factors, minimizing heat loss of the newborn after delivery is imperative. Nursing measures for preventing hypothermia can be found in Chapter 25. Humidity, on the other hand, modifies heat loss by preventing evaporation.

Heat Production (Thermogenesis)

Upon being exposed to a cool environment, the neonate requires additional heat. Several sources of heat production, or *thermogenesis,* are available, including increased basal metabolic rate, muscular activity, and chemical thermogenesis (also referred to as *nonshivering thermogenesis*) mediated through the release of catecholamines (Schaeffer et al., 1977). Shivering, a form of muscular activity common in the cold adult, is rarely seen in the newborn, although it has been observed at ambient temperatures of 15C (59F) or less. If shivering does appear, it means the infant's metabolic rate has already doubled and the extra muscular activity does little to produce needed heat. Nonshivering thermogenesis (NST) is a particularly important mechanism of heat production unique to the newborn.

NST occurs when skin receptors perceive the environmental temperature changes and transmit sensations to the CNS, which in turn stimulates the sympathetic nervous system. Release of norepinephrine by the adrenal gland and at local nerve endings in the brown fat causes the metabolism of the triglycerides to fatty acids, thereby releasing heat to be distributed to the body. Brown fat is a major producer of heat for the cold-stressed neonate because of its greater heat production capacity.

Brown adipose tissue (BAT) or brown fat, the primary source of heat in the cold-stressed neonate, first appears in the fetus at about 26–30 weeks of gestation and continues to increase in supply until 2–5 weeks after the birth of a full-term neonate, unless it is depleted by cold stress. BAT is deposited in the midscapular area, around the neck, and in the axillas, with deeper placement around the trachea, esophagus, abdominal aorta, kidneys, and adrenal glands (Figure 21-8). It constitutes 2%–6% of the newborn's total body weight. This fat is called brown fat because of its dark color, which is due to its enriched blood supply, dense cellular content, and abundant nerve endings.

The structures of brown and white fat cells differ, as do

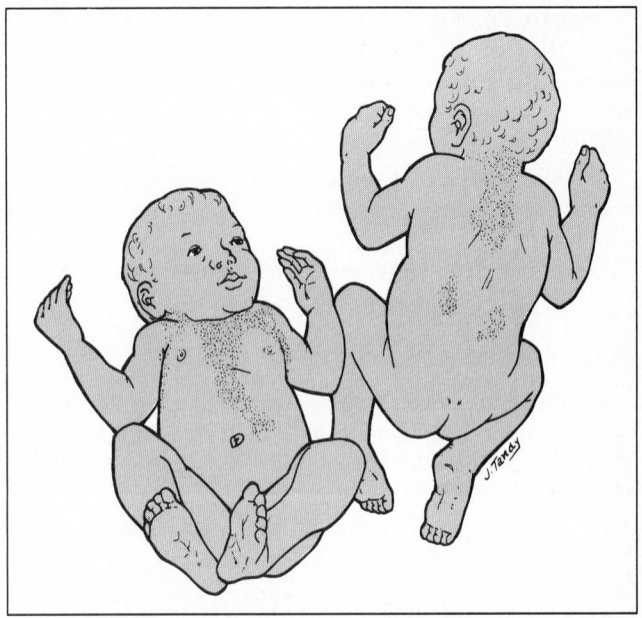

FIGURE 21–8 The distribution of brown adipose tissue (BAT) in the neonate. (Adapted from Davis, V. Nov./Dec. 1980. Structure and function of brown adipose tissue in the neonate. *J. Obstet. Gynecol. Neonat. Nurs.* 9:364.)

their functions. In brown fat, the large numbers of fat cells facilitate the rapidity with which triglycerides can be metabolized to produce heat. Energy is provided by the presence of glycogen and large numbers of mitochondria releasing adenosine triphosphate (ATP) for rapid metabolic turnover and production of heat. In addition, brown fat possesses a rich blood supply to enhance distribution of heat throughout the body, and a nerve supply for initiation of metabolic activity. This type of metabolism is specific to the newborn. The brown fat is metabolized and utilized within several weeks after birth (Korones, 1981).

After being exposed to cold, thermographic studies of newborns show an increase in the skin heat over the brown fat deposits in the neonate between 1 and 14 days of age. If the brown fat supply has been depleted, the metabolic response to cold will be limited or lacking. An increase in basal metabolism as a result of hypothermia results in an increase in oxygen consumption. A decrease in the environmental temperature of 2C (36F) is a drop sufficient to double the oxygen consumption of a term neonate (Schaeffer et al., 1977).

The normal term neonate is usually able to cope with the increase, but the preterm neonate may be unable to increase ventilation to the necessary level of oxygen consumption. As a consequence, maintaining an optimal thermal environment is an absolute necessity to prevent neonatal cold stress and the resulting metabolic physiologic responses. (See Chapter 25 for discussion of cold stress.)

Hypoxia and the effect of certain drugs (such as Demerol) may also prevent metabolism of brown fat. Demerol given to the laboring woman leads to a greater fall in the newborn's body temperature during the neonatal period. Reserpine given to experimental animals has been shown to diminish the body's stores of catecholamines, thereby interfering with heat conservation (Danforth, 1982). It is important to remember that neonatal hypothermia prolongs as well as potentiates the effects of many analgesic and anesthetic drugs in the neonate.

RESPONSE TO HEAT

Sweating is the usual initial response of the newborn to hyperthermia. The neonate has six times as many sweat glands as the adult, but their activity level is one-third that of the adult (Foster; Hey; and Katz, 1969). The glands have limited function until after the fourth week of extrauterine life. Dissipation of heat is accomplished by peripheral vasodilatation and augmentation of evaporation of insensible water loss. Oxygen consumption and metabolic rate also increase in response to hyperthermia.

HEPATIC ADAPTATION

The liver and gallbladder form at 4 weeks of fetal life. In the newborn, the liver is frequently palpable 2–3 cm below the right costal margin because it is relatively large and occupies about 40% of the abdominal cavity. The neonatal liver plays a significant role in iron storage, carbohydrate metabolism, conjugation of bilirubin, and coagulation.

Iron Storage and Red Blood Cell Production

In utero, the fetal liver stores iron for use in hemoglobin production during the early months of postnatal life and functions to varying degrees as a site of hematopoiesis beginning by the eighth week of gestation.

In the event that bone marrow activity is suppressed, the liver becomes more active to compensate for the decreased production of red blood cells. Neonatal iron stores are proportional to total body hemoglobin content and length of gestation. At birth, the term neonate has 270 mg of iron, and approximately 140–170 mg of this amount is in the hemoglobin (Schaeffer et al., 1977). If the mother's iron intake has been adequate, enough iron will be stored to last until the fifth month of neonatal life. At this time, foods containing iron or iron supplements must be given to prevent anemia in the infant.

Carbohydrate Metabolism

In the fetus the rate of glucose uptake by way of the umbilical circulation is closely related to the maternal blood glucose level. The concentration of glucose in fetal circulation is about one-fourth to one-third lower than in maternal blood (Korones, 1981). Glucose is the major source of energy in the fetus as indicated by increased fetal activity during the time of the most rapid rise in maternal glucose levels (Miller et al., 1978). Current studies indicate that amino acids, lactate, and perhaps free fatty acids and ketones are utilized for fuel (Crewell; Stys; and Battaglia, 1980).

Neonatal carbohydrate reserves are relatively low. One-third of this reserve is in the form of liver glycogen. Glucose is the main source of energy in the first few (4–6) hours after delivery. The blood glucose level falls rapidly and then stabilizes at values of 50–60 mg/dL for several days; by the third day postnatally, values increase to 60–70 mg/dL. Blood glucose levels are influenced by a balance between liver glucose output and peripheral uptake, body temperature, insulin concentration, and muscular activity. Hepatic glucose output is dependent on the following factors (Smith and Nelson, 1976): (a) adequate glycogen stores; (b) sufficient supplies of endogenous gluconeogenic substrate; (c) normally functioning hepatic gluconeogenic and glycogenolytic systems; and (d) a normal endocrine system for mediating these processes.

Glucose is stored as glycogen in the fetal liver starting at the ninth to tenth week of gestation (Korones, 1981). At term, neonatal glycogen stores are twice that of the adult. If the fetus or neonate experiences hypoxia, the glycogen stores are used and may be depleted to meet metabolic requirements. As stores of liver and muscle glycogen and blood glucose decrease, the neonate compensates by changing from a predominantly carbohydrate metabolism to fat metabolism. Energy is derived from fat and protein as well as from carbohydrates. The amount and availability of each of these "fuel substrates" is dependent upon constraints imposed by immature metabolic pathways (lack of specific enzymes or hormones) in the first few days of life.

Physiologic Jaundice—Icterus Neonatorum

The fetal liver begins to metabolize bilirubin at 12 weeks of gestation but this ability disappears by 36 weeks. The fetus does not conjugate bilirubin so that it can cross the placenta to be excreted. Physiologic jaundice, caused by accelerated lysis of fetal red blood cells, impaired conjugation of bilirubin, and increased bilirubin reabsorption from the intestinal tract does *not* have a pathologic basis, but rather is a normal biologic response of the newborn.

Schaeffer et al. (1977) describe five factors giving rise to physiologic jaundice, which may be due to interactions among the factors.

1. *Greater bilirubin loads to the liver.* In the neonate, the combination of an increased blood volume, largely due to delayed cord clamping, and accelerated lysis of the fetal red blood cell contributes to an increased bilirubin

level in the blood. The neonate has a shorter erythrocyte (RBC) life span (80–100 days instead of 120) and a proportionately larger amount of nonerythrocyte bilirubin formed than the adult. Therefore, newborns have two to three times greater production or breakdown of bilirubin.

Bilirubin values are further increased with reduced bowel motility, which enhances the reabsorption of bilirubin from the intestine via the enterohepatic pathway.

2. *Defective uptake of bilirubin from the plasma.* If the newborn does not ingest adequate calories, the formation of hepatic binding proteins diminishes, resulting in higher bilirubin levels.

3. *Defective conjugation of the bilirubin.* Decreased glucuronyl-transferase activity results in greater bilirubin values. (An in-depth discussion of the conjugation of bilirubin is found in Chapter 25.) The presence of the enzyme $3\alpha20\beta$ propregnandiol in breast milk is thought to further impede the conjugation of bilirubin.

4. *Defect in bilirubin excretion.* A congenital infection may cause impaired excretion. Delay in introduction of bacterial flora and decreased intestinal mobility can also delay excretion.

5. *Inadequate hepatic circulation.* Decreased oxygen supplies to the liver associated with neonatal hypoxia or congenital heart disease lead to a rise in the bilirubin level.

About 50% of full-term neonates and 80% of preterm neonates exhibit physiologic jaundice on about the second or third day after birth. The characteristic icteric (yellow) color results from increased levels of unconjugated bilirubin, which are a normal product of red blood cell hemolysis, and reflect a temporary inability of the body to eliminate bilirubin. The manifestations of physiologic jaundice appear *after* the first 24 hours postnatally. This differentiates physiologic jaundice from pathologic jaundice (Chapter 25), which is clinically evident at birth or within the first 24 hours of postnatal life. Serum levels of bilirubin are about 4–6 mg/dL before yellow coloration of the skin and sclera appears.

During the first week, unconjugated bilirubin levels in physiologic jaundice should not exceed 12 mg/dL in the full-term or preterm newborn (Avery, 1981). Peak bilirubin levels are reached between days 3 and 5 in the full-term infant and between days 5 and 6 in the preterm infant. These values are established for European and American newborns. Chinese, Japanese, Korean, and American Indian neonates have considerably higher bilirubin levels that persist for longer periods with no apparent ill effects (Gartner and Lee, 1977).

Nursery environment, including lighting, hinders the early detection of the degree and type of jaundice. Pink walls and artificial lights mask the beginning of jaundice in newborns. Daylight assists the observer in early recognition by eliminating distortions caused by artificial lights.

Nursery procedures are designed to decrease the probability of high bilirubin levels. These actions are as follows:

- The infant's body temperature is maintained at 97.6F (36.4C) or above, because chilling results in acidosis, which in turn decreases available serum albumin-binding sites, weakens albumin-binding powers, and causes elevated unconjugated bilirubin levels.

- Passage of stool is monitored for amount and type. Bilirubin is eliminated in the feces; inadequate stooling may result in reabsorption and recycling of bilirubin.

- Early feedings are encouraged to promote intestinal elimination and bacterial colonization, and to provide caloric intake necessary for formation of hepatic binding proteins.

If jaundice is suspected, the nurse can quickly assess the neonate's coloring by pressing his or her skin with a finger. As the blanching occurs, the nurse can observe the icterus (yellow coloring). If jaundice becomes apparent, nursing care is directed toward keeping the neonate well hydrated and promoting intestinal elimination. For specific nursing management and therapies, see the Nursing Care Plan on p. 831.

Physiologic jaundice may be very upsetting to parents; they require emotional support and thorough explanation of the condition. Necessary hospitalization of the newborn for a few additional days may be disturbing to parents. They should be encouraged to provide for the emotional needs of their newborn by continuing to feed, hold, and caress the infant. If the mother is discharged, the parents should be encouraged to return for feedings and feel free to telephone or visit whenever possible. In many instances, the mother, especially if she is breast-feeding, may elect to remain hospitalized with her infant; this decision should be supported.

BREAST-FEEDING JAUNDICE

Breast-feeding is implicated in prolonged jaundice in some newborns. The breast milk of some women is thought to contain an enzyme that inhibits glucuronyl transferase or to contain several times the normal breast milk concentration of certain free fatty acids, which are thought to inhibit the conjugation of bilirubin. The newborn's bilirubin level begins to rise about the fourth day after the mother's mature milk has come in. The level peaks at 2–3 weeks of age, and may reach 15–20 mg/dL. Interruption of nursing may be advised if bilirubin reaches 16–17 mg/dL (Avery, 1981). Within 48 hours after discontinuing breast-feeding, the neonate's serum bilirubin levels begin to fall and return to normal levels in 4–8 days.

Many physicians believe that breast-feeding may be resumed once other causes of jaundice have been ruled out, although the bilirubin concentrations rise to 1–3 mg/dL

(Avery, 1981) but do not reach previous high levels. Nursing mothers need encouragement and support in their desire to nurse their infants, assistance and instruction regarding pumping and expressing milk during the interrupted nursing period, and reassurance that nothing is wrong with their milk or mothering abilities.

Coagulation

The liver plays an important part in blood coagulation during fetal life and continues this function to some degree during the first few months following birth. Coagulation factors II, VII, IX, and X (synthesized in the liver) are activated under the influence of vitamin K and therefore are considered vitamin K-dependent. The absence of normal flora needed to synthesize vitamin K in the newborn gut results in low levels of vitamin K and creates a transient blood coagulation deficiency between the second and fifth day of life (Table 21–2). From a low point at about 2–3 days after birth, these coagulation factors rise slowly, but do not approach normal adult levels until 9 months of age or later. Increasing levels of these vitamin K-dependent factors indicate a response to dietary intake and bacterial colonization of the intestines. Although usually no clinical consequences arise, to combat the deficiency an injection of vitamin K (Aquamephyton) is given prophylactically on the day of birth. (Hemorrhagic disease of the newborn is discussed in more depth in Chapter 25.) Other coagulation factors having low cord blood levels are XI, XII, and XIII. Fibrinogen and factors V and VIII are near adult ranges (Buchanan, 1978).

Platelet counts at birth are in the same range as for adults, but neonates may manifest mild transient platelet-functioning defect. Neonatal platelets have less-than-normal levels of serotonin and are mildly deficient in adenine nucleotides, which alters the secondary platelet aggregation in the coagulation process. Phototherapy accentuates the platelet defect (Hatch and Sumner, 1981).

Prenatal maternal therapy with diphenylhydantoin (Dilantin) or phenobarbital (Luminal) causes abnormal clotting studies and neonatal bleeding in the first 24 hours after birth (Mountain et al., 1970). Infants born to mothers receiving coumadin (Warfarin) compounds may bleed because these agents cross the placenta and accentuate existing vitamin K-dependent factor deficiencies.

GASTROINTESTINAL ADAPTATION

During the first 4 weeks of gestation the intestine develops as a single tube, liver buds are evident, and the bile ducts and gallbladder begin to form. The intestine elongates at a rapid pace to form a loop that protrudes into the umbilical cord. For 6 weeks the small intestine grows and coils inside the cord until at 10 weeks it reenters the abdominal cavity. Meanwhile, the splanchic flexure, duodenum, and colon are held in place by the mesenteric bands. An abnormal exit or entrance of the intestine can result in such pathologies as an oomphalocele. Between the fifth and fortieth weeks, the intestine grows by a thousandfold. At term, it is about 240–300 cm in length, or about three to four times the crown-to-heel length of the neonate.

Differentiation and maturation of the structures necessary for digestion progress from the proximal to the distal

Table 21–2 Coagulation Factors and Test Values In Term and Preterm Infants*

	Normal	Term infant (cord blood)	Preterm infant (cord blood)
Fibrinogen (mg/dL)	200–400	200–250	200–250
Factor II (%)	50–150	40	25
Factor V (%)	75–125	90	60–75
Factor VII (%)	75–125	50	35
Factor VIII (%)	50–150	100	80–100
Factor IX (%)	50–150	25–40	25–40
Factor X (%)	50–150	50–60	25–40
Factor XI (%)	75–125	30–40	—
Factor XII (%)	75–125	50–100	50–100
Factor XIII (titer)	1:16	1:8	1:8
Partial thromboplastin time (sec)	30–50	70	80–90
Prothrombin time (sec)	10–12	12–18	14–20
Thrombin time (sec)	10–12	12–16	13–20

*From Avery, G. B., ed. 1981. *Neonatology*. Philadelphia: J. B. Lippincott Co., p. 570.

end of the system. By the seventh week of fetal life, villi begin to develop in the duodenum and jejunum. Microvilli become regular, with many mitochondria present below the villi. Development of the secretory and absorbing surfaces is greater than that of the supporting musculature. All glandular elements found in adult mucosa are present at birth, but the fetal structures are more shallow.

Enzymatic activity commences in the seventh to eighth week of gestation and progresses to maturity by 36–38 weeks of fetal life. Full maturity is achieved by this time, with the presence of enzymatic activity, and the ability to transport nutrients.

Functional Development

By birth, the neonate has experienced swallowing, gastric emptying, and intestinal propulsion. Swallowing by the fetus in utero is documented by the presence of lanugo and squamous cells in the meconium and the effectiveness with which the neonate completes the first feeding. In utero, swallowing is accompanied by gastric emptying and peristalsis of the fetal intestinal tract. By the end of gestation, in preparation for extrauterine life, peristalsis becomes much more active. Fetal peristalsis is also stimulated by anoxia, causing the expulsion of meconium into the amniotic fluid.

Air enters the stomach immediately after birth. The small intestine is filled within 2–12 hours and the large bowel within 24 hours. The salivary glands are immature at birth, and little saliva is manufactured until the infant is about 3 months old. The newborn's stomach has a capacity of about 50–60 mL. It empties intermittently, starting within a few minutes of the beginning of a feeding and completed between 2 and 4 hours after feeding. The newborn's gastric acidity is equal to an adult's but becomes less acidic in about a week and remains lower than that of adults for 2–3 months. The stomach secretes pepsinogen, which is necessary for protein digestion and production of hydrochloric acid. Both pepsinogen and hydrochloric acid are necessary for beginning the digestion of milk prior to its entrance into the small bowel. Digestion and absorption of nutrients are primarily functions of the small bowel, where pancreatic secretions digest starches and proteins. Bile secretions from the gallbladder through the bile duct aid in fat absorption, and duodenal secretions complete this complex process. The cardiac sphincter is immature, as is nervous control of the stomach, so some regurgitation may be noted in the neonatal period. Regurgitation of the first few feedings during the first day or two of life can usually be lessened by avoiding overfeeding and by burping the newborn well during and after the feeding.

When no other signs and symptoms are evident, vomiting is often self-limiting and ceases within the first few days of life. However, vomiting or continuous regurgitation should be observed closely. If the neonate has swallowed bloody or purulent amniotic fluid, lavage may be indicated to relieve the problem.

About 69% of normal term neonates pass meconium within 12 hours of life; 94% by 24 hours, and 99.8% within 48 hours (Schaeffer et al., 1977). Meconium is formed in utero from the amniotic fluid and its constituents, together with intestinal secretions and shed mucosal cells. It is recognized by its viscid, tarry, dark green appearance. Transitional (thin brown to green) stools consisting of part meconium and part fecal material are passed for the next day or two, after which the stools become entirely fecal. Generally, the stools of a breast-fed newborn are pale yellow (but may be pasty green); they are more liquid and more frequent than those of formula-fed neonates, whose are paler in color. Bowel movements are individualized but range from one every 2–3 days to as many as ten daily.

The term neonate has adequate intestinal and pancreatic enzymes to digest most simple carbohydrates, proteins, and fats.

Digestion of Carbohydrates

Those carbohydrates requiring digestion in the newborn are usually disaccharides (lactose, maltose, sucrose), which are split into monosaccharides (galactose, fructose, and glucose) by the enzymes of the intestinal mucosa. Lactose is the primary carbohydrate in the breast-feeding newborn and is generally easily digested and well absorbed. The only enzyme lacking is pancreatic amylase, which remains relatively deficient during the first few months of life. Therefore, newborns have trouble digesting starches (changing more complex carbohydrates into maltose).

Digestion of Proteins

Although proteins require more digestion than carbohydrates, they are well digested and absorbed from the neonatal intestine. Protein digestive enzymes have been present in the fetus from about midgestation. The proteolytic enzymes of the intestinal mucosa facilitate hydrolysis of protein while enterocytes transfer resultant amino acids to the blood.

Digestion of Fats

Fats are digested and absorbed less efficiently by the neonate than the child because of the minimal activity of the pancreatic enzyme lipase. The neonate excretes about 10%–20% of the dietary fat intake, compared with 10% for the adult. The fat in breast milk is absorbed more completely by the newborn than is the fat in cow's milk because it consists of more medium-chain triglycerides and breast milk contains lipase. (See Chapter 23 for a more detailed discussion of infant nutrition.)

Adequate digestion and absorption are essential for

neonatal growth and development. If optimal nutritional support is available, postnatal growth ideally should parallel intrauterine growth; that is, after 30 weeks of gestation, the fetus gains 30 g per day and adds 1.2 cm to body length daily. To gain weight at the intrauterine rate, the term neonate requires 120 calories per kilogram per day. Following birth, calorie intake is often insufficient for weight gain until the neonate is 5–10 days old. During this time there may be a weight loss of 5%–15%. Failure to lose weight when caloric intake is inadequate may indicate fluid retention. Shift of intracellular water to extracellular space and insensible water loss account for the 5%–15% weight loss.

GENITOURINARY ADAPTATION

Kidney Development and Function

By the fourth month of fetal life, the cortical and medullar portions of the kidney are differentiated. As growth continues, they migrate from the area of the fourth lumbar vertebra to the level of the first lumbar vertebra or the twelfth thoracic vertebra.

The newborn's kidneys are relatively large and may extend below the iliac crests; they are most easily palpable through the abdominal wall soon after birth. Because the infant pelvis is too small to contain it, the bladder is also an abdominal organ.

The physiologic features of the neonatal kidney include the following (Behrman, 1977):

1. The kidneys consist of a full complement of functioning nephrons.

2. The glomerular filtration rate of the kidneys is low, with the neonatal rate being 35 mL/min/1.73 m^2 body surface area, compared with the adult rate of 125 mL/min/1.73 m^2. Because of this physiologic inefficiency, the neonatal kidney is unable to dispose of water and solutes rapidly.

3. The juxtamedullary nephron is maturationally advanced and has the capacity to reabsorb Na$^+$ and H$^+$ and concentrate the urine.

4. A variable range of transport capacities is available as the nephron is highly developed functionally and anatomically.

In summary, the kidney is characterized by a low functional capacity with respect to a decreased rate of glomeruli flow, thus limiting its ability to relinquish fluids rapidly and efficiently. The limitation of tubular reabsorption can lead to inappropriate loss of substances present in the glomerular filtrate, such as amino acids and bicarbonate.

By 4 months of gestation, urine is found in the fetal bladder, and amniotic fluid analysis indicates that the fetus voids in utero. About 17% of newborns void at delivery, 92% by 24 hours, and 99% within 48 hours. A neonate who has not voided after 24 hours should be assessed for adequacy of fluid intake, bladder distention, restlessness, and symptoms of pain. The physician should be notified.

Unless edema is present, normal urinary output is often limited, and the voidings are scanty until fluid intake increases. (The fluid of edema is eliminated by the kidneys, so infants with edema have a much higher urinary output.) The first 2 days postnatally, the newborn voids two to six times daily; with a urine output of 30–60 mL per day. Subsequently, the neonate voids five to twenty-five times every 24 hours, with a volume of 30–50 mL/kg/24 hr. The initial bladder volume is 6–44 mL of urine.

Full-term neonates are not able to concentrate urine to the same extent as the adult. The maximum concentrating ability of the newborn is a specific gravity of 1.025. Feeding practices may affect the osmolarity of the urine. The inability of the neonate to further concentrate urine is due to the limited excretion of solutes in the growing newborn. The ability to fully concentrate urine is attained by about 3 months of age. Because the neonate's ability to handle excessive insensible fluid losses or restricted intake is strongly influenced by the limited ability to concentrate urine, the physiologic response to circumstances causing fluid loss is unpredictable.

Following the first voiding, the newborn's urine frequently appears cloudy (due to mucus content) and has a high specific gravity, which decreases as fluid intake increases. Occasionally pink stains ("brick dust spots") appear on the diaper. These are caused by urates and are innocuous. Blood may occasionally be observed on the diapers of female infants. This *pseudomenstruation* is related to the withdrawal of maternal hormones. Males may have bloody spotting from a circumcision. In the absence of apparent causes for bleeding, the physician should be notified. Normal urine during early infancy is straw-colored and almost odorless, although odor occurs when certain drugs are given or when infection is present.

The normal values of a urinalysis for a neonate include the following:

> Protein <5–10 mg/dL
>
> WBC < 2–3
>
> RBC 0
>
> Casts 0
>
> Bacteria 0

The concentration of bicarbonates (HCO$_3$) in the blood is controlled by the renal threshold. This mechanism permits the HCO$_3$ to remain in the blood only when the blood concentration is below a certain level. If the concentration rises above the renal threshold, the glomeruli-filtered

HCO_3 is reabsorbed and excreted in the urine. Therefore, because the renal threshold is low in the newborn, the HCO_3 concentration and buffering capacity are decreased, which may lead to acidosis and electrolyte imbalances.

Genital Development

In early fetal life, the gonad is bipotential in relation to sexual development (Figure 21–9). In the genetically determined male, the testes produce androgenic hormones, causing the distal wolffian duct to form the internal male genital tract, which includes the vas deferens, seminal vessels, and ejaculatory ducts. The hormones also promote growth of the genital tubercle and cause the fusion of the urogenital ridge. The testes secrete müllerian-inhibiting factor, which causes regression of the müllerian duct in the scrotum at term. The testes are usually present in the scrotum.

The sexually bipotential gonad under the influence of genetically female inducers develops ovaries. In response to maternal and placental estrogens, the paramesonephric duct (müllerian duct) develops into the uterine tubes and uterus. Since the male inducer substance is absent, the wolffian duct regresses. In the absence of androgens the undifferentiated external genitalia is stimulated by placental and maternal estrogens to differentiate into labia majora, labia minora, clitoris, and part of the vagina. A drop in estrogen after delivery causes involution of the female neonate's uterus in the first weeks of life, creating a mucoid vaginal discharge and some slight bleeding (pseudomenstruation).

The hyperestrogenism of pregnancy causes swelling of the breast tissue in both male and female newborns. Some neonates may secrete a discharge from the breast. In the past, this discharge was called "witch's milk."

IMMUNOLOGIC ADAPTATIONS

The cells that constitute the immune system appear early in fetal life, but usually are not *fully* activated until sometime after birth. Fetal albumin and globulin other than immunoglobulins are present throughout the last trimester of gestation.

The three major types of immunoglobulins—IgG, IgA, and IgM—are primarily involved in immunity. Of these three, only IgG crosses the placenta. The pregnant woman

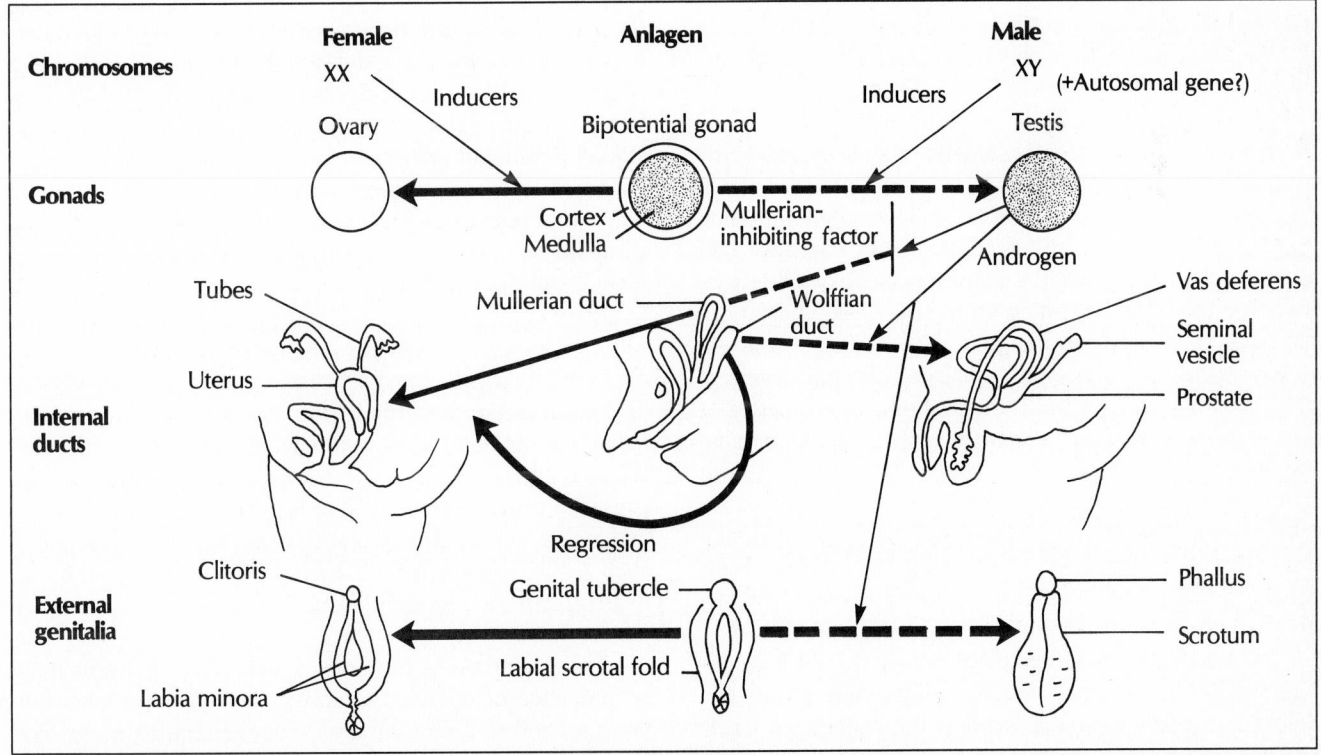

FIGURE 21–9 Normal sexual differentiation. Various inducers (*thin arrows*) are necessary for differentiation of the gonads and masculine development (*broken heavy arrows*). In the absence of these inducers, the differentiation is female (*solid heavy arrows*). (From Avery, G. B. 1981. *Neonatology*. Philadelphia: J. B. Lippincott Co., p. 1105.)

forms antibodies in response to illness or immunization. This process is called *active acquired immunity*. When IgG antibodies are transferred to the fetus in utero, *passive acquired immunity* results, because the fetus does not produce the antibodies itself.

The newborn possesses varying degrees of nonspecific and specific immunity. The nonspecific mechanism of opsonization, the process of coating invasive bacteria to ready them for ingestion by phagocytic cells, is impaired. Immunoglobulins (specific immunity) are a type of antibody secreted by the lymphocytes and plasma cells into the body fluids. The IgG level in newborns is 700–1300 mg/dL (Danforth, 1982). By 6 months of age, IgG levels vary from 200–1200 mg/dL. IgG is very active against bacterial toxins.

Because a transfer of maternal immunoglobin occurs primarily during the third trimester, preterm infants (especially those born prior to 34 weeks) may be more susceptible to infection. Infants receive immunity (if mother has specific antibodies) to tetanus, diphtheria, smallpox, measles, mumps, poliomyelitis, and a variety of other bacterial and viral diseases. The period of resistance varies: Immunity against common viral infections such as measles may last 4–8 months, whereas immunity to certain bacteria may disappear within 4–8 weeks.

The normal newborn does produce antibodies in response to an antigen, but not as effectively as an older child would. It is customary to begin immunization at 2 months of age, and then the infant develops actively acquired immunity.

IgM immunoglobulins are primarily antibodies to blood group antigens, gram negative enteric organisms, and some viruses in the expectant mother, although IgM production in the neonate occurs as part of the initial antigen–antibody response to practically all infectious agents. Because IgM does not normally cross the placenta, most or all is produced by the fetus beginning at 10–15 weeks' gestation. IgM levels in the newborn range from 0–30/dL in contrast to 10–90 mg/dL at 6 months of age. Elevated levels of IgM at birth (greater than 20 mg/dL) may be indicative of placental leaks or, more commonly, of antigenic stimulation in utero. Consequently, elevations suggest that the infant was exposed to an intrauterine infection such as rubella, syphilis, toxoplasmosis, herpesvirus, or cytomegalovirus. The lack of available maternal IgM in the newborn also accounts for the infant's increased susceptibility to gram negative enteric organisms such as *E. coli.*

The functions if IgA immunoglobulins are not fully understood, although they appear to provide protection mainly on secreting surfaces such as the respiratory tract, gastrointestinal tract, and eyes. Serum IgA does not cross the placenta and is not normally produced by the fetus in utero. Unlike the other immunoglobulins, IgA is not affected by gastric action. Colostrum, the forerunner of breast milk, is very high in secretory form of IgA. Consequently,

it may be of significance in providing some passive immunity to the infant of a breast-feeding mother.

Limited information is available on the remaining two immunoglobulins, IgE and IgD. IgE, which does not cross the placenta, contains skin-sensitizing reagins. IgD has no distinctive antibody function or activity and is found in minimal amounts in the cord blood.

NEUROLOGIC AND SENSORY/ PERCEPTUAL FUNCTIONING

The neonate responds to and interacts with the environment from the moment of birth in a predictable pattern of behavior that is somewhat shaped by the intrauterine experience. Brazelton (1975) found a positive association between newborn behavior and the nutritional status of the pregnant woman. Neonates with higher birth weight attended and responded to visual and auditory cues and exhibited more mature motor activity compared with low-birth-weight newborns.

Maternal environmental experiences also affect the fetus. If the fetal heart rate is monitored when a woman is smoking or being exposed to an auditory stimuli or emotional shocks, an increase in FHR is noted. Repetition of the stimuli leads to a decreased FHR response. Neonates exposed to intense noise during fetal life were significantly less reactive to loud sounds postnatally (Ando, 1970). The fetus is the recipient of a variety of external and internal stimuli that might influence neonatal behavior. The level of coping with these stressors may be displayed in neonatal behavioral responses varying from quietly dealing with the stimulation, to becoming overreactive and tense, to a combination of the two.

Motor Activity

The organization and the quality of the newborn's motor activity are influenced by a number of factors including the following (Brazelton, 1977): (a) sleep–wake states; (b) presence of environmental stimuli such as heat, light, cold, and noise; (c) conditions causing a chemical imbalance, such as hypoglycemia; (d) hydration status; (e) state of health; and (f) recovery from the stress of labor and delivery.

The performance of complex behavioral patterns may be reflective of neonatal integrity. The neonate who can bring a hand to a mouth may be demonstrating motor coordination as well as a self-quieting technique, thus increasing the complexity of the behavioral response. Neonates also possess complex organized defensive motor patterns as exhibited by the ability to approach and remove an obstruction, such as a cloth across the face.

Sensory Capacities of the Newborn

The newborn is able to process and respond to complex visual stimulation. For example, when a bright light is flashed into the neonate's eyes, the initial response is blinking, constriction of the pupil, and perhaps a slight startle reaction. However, with repeated stimulation, the newborn's response repertoire gradually diminishes and disappears; this is known as *habituation*. The capacity to ignore repetitious disturbing stimuli is a neonatal defense mechanism readily apparent in the noisy well-lighted nursery.

In addition to being able to disregard specific stimuli, the newborn has the ability to be alert to, to follow, and to fixate on complex visual stimuli that have a particular appeal and attractiveness to the neonate. The newborn prefers the human face and eyes and bright shiny objects. As the face or object is brought into the line of vision, the neonate responds with bright, wide eyes, still limbs, fixed staring. This intense visual involvement may last several minutes, during which time the neonate is able to follow the stimulus from side to side. Figures 21–10, 21–11, and 21–12 illustrate these responses. The newborn uses this sensory capacity to become familiar with family, friends, and surroundings (Figure 21–13).

AUDITORY CAPACITY

The newborn responds to auditory stimulation with a definite, organized behavior repertoire. The stimulus used to assess auditory response should be selected to match the state of the newborn. A rattle is appropriate for light sleep, a voice for an awake state, and a clap for deep sleep. As the neonate hears the sound, the cardiac rate rises, and a minimal startle reflex may be observed. If the sound is appealing, the newborn will become alert and search until the site of the auditory stimulus is located.

OLFACTORY CAPACITY

Neonates are able to distinguish their mother's breast pads from those of other mothers by 1 week postnatally (Brazelton, 1977). Apparently this phenomenon is related to the ability of the neonate to select by smell.

TASTE

The newborn responds differently to varying tastes. Sugar, for example, increases sucking. Sucking pattern variations also exist in newborns fed cow's milk or human breast milk (Brazelton, 1977). When breast-feeding, the neonate sucks in bursts with frequent regular pauses. The bottle-fed newborn tends to suck at a regular rate with infrequent pauses. The pauses in feeding may be used to interject social communication between the mother and neonate, whether at regular or irregular intervals.

TACTILE CAPACITY

The neonate is very sensitive to being touched, cuddled, and held. Often a mother's first response to an upset or crying newborn is touching or holding. Swaddling, a hand on the abdomen, or holding the arms to prevent a startle reflex are other methods that may soothe the newborn. The settled neonate is then able to attend to and interact with the environment.

SUCKING

When awake and hungry, the neonate displays rapid searching motions in response to the rooting reflex. Once feeding begins, the newborn establishes a sucking pattern according to the method of feeding. Finger sucking is not only present postnatally, but in utero. The neonate frequently uses sucking as a self-quieting activity, which assists in the development of self-regulation.

States of the Newborn

The state of consciousness of the neonate can be divided into two categories, the sleep state and the alert state (Prechtl and Beintema, 1964; Brazelton, 1977). Subcategories are identified under each major category.

SLEEP STATES

Sleep cycles in the neonate have been recognized and defined based on length of the time cycle. The length of the cycle is contingent upon the age of the neonate. At term, REM active sleep and quiet sleep occur in intervals of 45–50 minutes. REM is also present in both the first half and second half of quiet sleep. When viewed in percentages, about 45%–50% of the total sleep of the neonate is active sleep, 35%–45% is quiet (deep) sleep, and 10% of sleep is transitional between these two periods. It is hypothesized that REM sleep stimulates the growth of the neural system. Over a period of time, the neonate's sleep–wake patterns become diurnal; that is, the infant sleeps at night and stays awake during the day. (See Chapter 22 for in-depth discussion of assessment of neonatal states.)

1. *Deep or quiet sleep.* Deep sleep is characterized by closed eyes with no eye movements, regular even breathing, and jerky motion or startles at regular intervals. Behavioral responses to external stimuli are likely to be delayed. Startles are rapidly suppressed, and changes in state are not likely to occur.
2. *Active REM.* Irregular respirations, eyes closed with REM, irregular sucking motions, minimal activity, and irregular but smooth movement of the extremities can be observed in active REM sleep. Environmental and internal stimuli initiate a startle reaction and a change of state.

FIGURE 21-10 Fixation and intense interest in the human face. (From Schaeffer, A. J. et al. 1977. *Diseases of the newborn.* Philadelphia: W. B. Saunders Co., p. 42.)

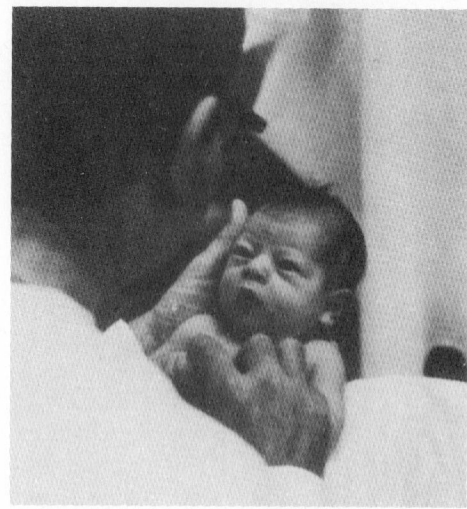

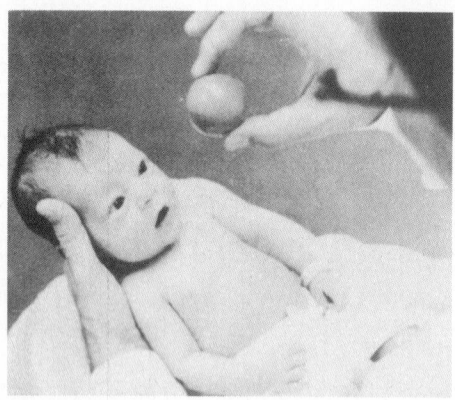

FIGURE 21-11 Following a red ball. (From Schaeffer, A. J. et al. 1977. *Diseases of the newborn.* Philadelphia: W. B. Saunders Co., p. 42.)

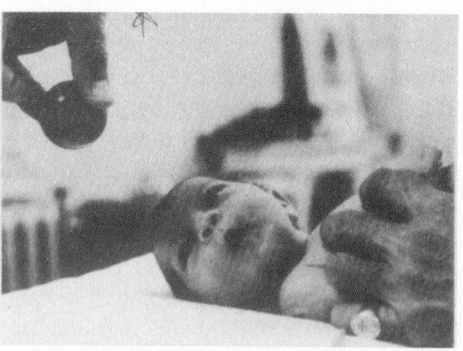

FIGURE 21-12 Head turning to follow. (From Schaeffer, A. J. et al. 1977. *Diseases of the newborn.* Philadelphia: W. B. Saunders Co., p. 42.)

FIGURE 21-13 Newborn's visual involvement and attentiveness to his mother. (© Suzanne Arms.)

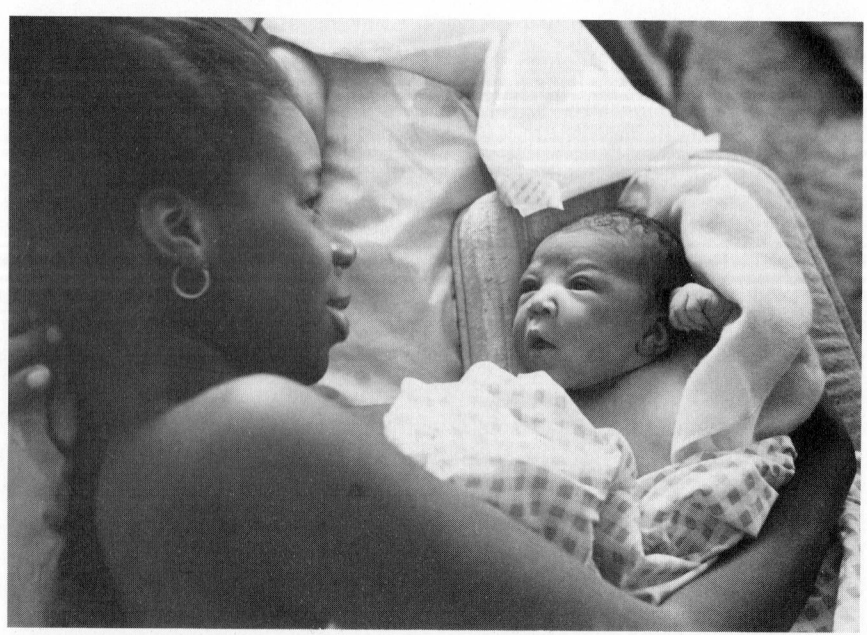

ALERT STATES

Waking states that last for varying amounts of time are influenced by fatigue, hunger, and other needs of the newborn. In the first 30–60 minutes after birth, many neonates display an alert state, characteristic of the first period of reactivity. About 12–18 hours after birth, the infant is again alert when the second period of reactivity occurs. A further description of these two periods of reactivity is found on p. 711. These periods of alert states tend to be short the first 2 days postnatally to allow the newborn to recover from the birth process. Subsequently, alert states are of choice or of necessity (Brazelton, 1977). Increasing choice of wakefulness by the neonate is indicative of a maturing capacity to achieve and maintain consciousness. Heat, cold, and hunger are but a few of the stimuli that can cause wakefulness by necessity. Once the disturbing stimuli are removed, sleep tends to recur.

The following are subcategories of the alert state (Brazelton, 1977):

1. *Drowsy or semidozing.* The behaviors common to the drowsy state are open or closed eyes, fluttering eyelids, semidozing appearance, and slow, regular movements of the extremities. Mild startles may be noted from time to time. Although the reaction to a sensory stimulus is delayed, a change of state often results.

2. *Wide awake.* In the wide awake state, the neonate is alert, follows, and fixates on attractive objects, faces, or auditory stimuli. Motor activity is minimal, and the response to external stimuli is delayed.

3. *Active awake.* The eyes are open and motor activity is quite intense with thrusting movements of the extremities in the active awake state. Environmental stimuli cause increase in startles or motor activity, but discrete reactions are difficult to distinguish because of generalized high activity level.

4. *Crying.* Intense crying is accompanied by jerky motor movements. Crying serves several purposes for the newborn. It may be used as a distraction from disturbing stimuli such as hunger and pain. Fussiness often allows the neonate to discharge energy and reorganize behavior. Most important, crying elicits an appropriate response of help from the parents.

Neurologic Adaptations

The formation and maturation of the nervous system is a complex process that is minimally, if at all, influenced by the actual birth process. Because many biochemical and histologic changes have yet to occur in the neonatal brain, the postnatal period is considered a time of risk to the development of the brain and nervous system. For the pattern of development, including intellect, to proceed, the maturation of the brain and associated nervous system needs to advance in an orderly, unhampered fashion.

The neurologic examination is used to determine the intactness of the neonatal nervous system (Chapter 22). It should begin with a period of observation, noting the general physical characteristics and behaviors of the newborn. Important behaviors to assess are the state of alertness, resting posture, cry, and quality of muscle tone and motor activity (Schaeffer et al., 1977).

Partially flexed extremities with the legs adducted to the abdomen is the usual position of the neonate. When awake, the newborn may exhibit purposeless, uncoordinated bilateral movements of the extremities. If these movements are absent, minimal, or obviously asymmetrical, neurologic dysfunction should be suspected. Eye movements are observable during the first few days of life. An alert neonate is able to fixate on faces and brightly colored objects. If a bright light shines in the newborn's eyes, the blinking response is elicited. The cry of the newborn should be lusty and vigorous. High-pitched cries, weak cries, or no cries are all causes for concern.

Muscle tone is evaluated with the head of the neonate in a neutral position as various parts of the body are passively moved. The newborn is somewhat hypertonic; that is, resistance to extending the elbow and knee joints is noted. Muscle tone should be symmetrical. Diminished muscle tone and flaccidity require further evaluation.

Specific deep tendon reflexes can be elicited in the neonate, but have limited value unless they are obviously asymmetrical. The knee jerk is brisk; a normal ankle clonus may involve three or four beats. Plantar flexion is present. Other reflexes, including the Moro, grasping, rooting, and sucking reflexes are characteristic of neurologic integrity.

SUMMARY

Birth propels the infant from a warm, weightless, fluid environment into a cold, dry, pressurized environment within a short time. Separation from the placenta requires that the infant assume responsibility for all major body functions. Immediate initiation of respiration and changes in the circulatory patterns are essential for extrauterine life. Within 24 hours after birth, the newborn's renal, gastrointestinal, hematologic, metabolic, and neurologic systems must function sufficiently for optimal progression to and maintenance of extrauterine life.

A basic understanding of these physiologic and neurobehavioral changes forms a foundation from which the nurse can more effectively assess (Chapter 22) and intervene (Chapter 23) to meet the health needs of the newborn and his or her family.

References

Ando, Y. 1970. Effects of intense noise during fetal life upon postnatal adaptability. *J. Acoust. Soc. Am.* 47:1128.

Avery, G. B. 1981. *Neonatology: pathophysiology and management of the newborn.* Philadelphia: J. B. Lippincott Company.

Behrman, R. E. 1977. *Neonatal–perinatal medicine.* St. Louis: The C .V. Mosby Co.

Boddy, K. 1979. Fetal breathing: its physiologic and clinical implications. *Hosp. Pract.* 14:89.

Brazelton, T. B. 1977. Neonatal behavior and its significance. In *Diseases of the newborn,* ed. A. J. Schaeffer, et al. Philadelphia: W. B. Saunders.

Brazelton, T. B. et al., 1975. Biomedical variables and neonatal performance of Guatemalan infants. Paper presented to American Academy of Cerebral Palsy, New Orleans.

Buchanan, G. R. 1978. Neonatal coagulation: normal physiology and pathophysiology. *Clin. Haematol.* 7:85.

Crewell, W. H.; Stys, S. J.; and Battaglia, F. C. 1980. Fetal pathophysiology. In *Fetal and maternal medicine,* ed. E. J. Quilligan, and N. Kretchmer. New York: John Wiley & Sons.

Danforth, D. H., ed. 1982. *Obstetrics and gynecology,* 4th ed. Philadelphia: Harper & Row.

Foster, K. G.; Hey, E. N.; and Katz, G. 1969. The response of the sweat glands of the newborn baby to thermal stimuli and to intradermal acetylcholine. *J. Physiol.* 203:13.

Gartner, L. M., and Lee, K. S. 1977. Jaundice and liver disease. In *Neonatal perinatal medicine,* ed. R. E. Behrman, St. Louis: The C. V. Mosby Co.

Goldstein, J. D., and Reid, L. M. 1980. Pulmonary hypoplasia resulting from phrenic nerve agenesis and diaphragmatic amyoplasia. *J. Pediat.* 97:282.

Hatch, D. J., and Sumner, E. 1981. *Neonatal anaesthesia.* Chicago: Year Book Medical Publishers.

Korones, S. B. 1981. *High risk newborn infants: the basis for intensive care nursing,* 3rd ed. St. Louis: The C. V. Mosby Co.

Manning, F. A., and Feyerabend, C. 1976. Cigarette smoking and fetal breathing movements. *Br. J. Obstet. Gynaec.* 83:262.

Marsal, K. 1978. Fetal breathing movements: characteristics and clinical significance. *Obstet. Gynecol.* 52:394.

Miller, F. C., et al. 1978. The effects of maternal blood sugar levels on fetal activity. *Obstet. Gynecol.* 52:662.

Mountain, D. R.; Hush, J.; and Gallus, A. S. 1970. Neonatal coagulation defect due to anticonvulsant drug treatment in pregnancy. *Lancet.* 1:265.

Prechtl, H. F. R., and Beintema, D. L. 1964. *The neurological examination of the full-term newborn infant.* London: Spastics Society International Medical Publications in association with William Heinemann Ltd.

Quilligan, E. J., and Kretchmer, N. 1980. *Fetal and maternal medicine.* New York: John Wiley & Sons.

Schaeffer, A. J., et al. 1977. *Diseases of the newborn.* Philadelphia: W. B. Saunders Company.

Smith, C. A., and Nelson, N. M. 1976. *The physiology of the newborn infant,* 4th ed. Springfield, Ill.: Charles C Thomas.

Toronto, A. F. 1972. *Structure and function of the heart.* Salt Lake City, Utah: Zion's Book Co.

Additional Readings

Avery, M. E.; Fletcher, B. D.; and Williams, R. G. 1981. *The lung and its disorders in the newborn infant,* 4th ed. Philadelphia: W. B. Saunders.

Brazelton, T. B. 1979. Behavioral competence of the newborn infant. *Sem. Perinatol.* 3:35.

Bryan, A. 1978. Control of respiration in the newborn. *Clin. Perinatol.* 5:293.

Gardner, S. 1978. The mother as an incubator . . . after delivery. *J. Obstet. Gynecol. Neonat. Nurs.* 8:174.

Gartner, L. M., and Lee, K. S. 1979. Effect of starvation and milk feeding on intestinal bilirubin absorption. *Gastroenterology* (abstract). 77:A13.

Gorski, P. A., et al. 1979. Stages of behavioral organization in the high risk neonate: theoretical and clinical considerations. *Sem. Perinatol.* 3:61.

Hallman, M. 1977. Absence of phosphatidylglycerol in respiratory distress syndrome in the newborn: a study of minor surfactant phospholipids in newborns. *Pediatr. Res.* 11:714.

Hill, S. T., et al. 1979. The effect of early parent–infant contact on newborn body temperature. *J. Obstet. Gynecol. Neonat. Nurs.* 8:287.

Hutton, N. J., et al. 1980. Urine collection in the neonate: effect of different methods on volume, specific gravity, and glucose. *J. Obstet. Gynecol. Neonat. Nurs.* 9:165.

Oehler, J. M. 1981. *Family-centered neonatal nursing care.* Philadelphia: J. B. Lippincott Company.

Parker, D., et al. 1981. Newborn behavioral assessment: research prediction, and clinical uses. . . . the Brazelton neonatal behavioral assessment scale. *Child Today.* 10 (4): 2.

Porth, C. M., et al. 1978. Temperature regulation in the newborn. *Am. J. Nurs.* 78:1691.

■ 22 ■

NURSING ASSESSMENT OF THE NEWBORN

■ CHAPTER CONTENTS

ESTIMATION OF GESTATIONAL AGE
Assessment of Physical Characteristics
Assessment of Neurologic Status

PHYSICAL EXAMINATION
General Appearance
Posture
Weight and Measurements
Temperature
Skin
Head
Face
Neck
Chest
Cry
Respiration
Heart
Abdomen
Genitals
Anus
Extremities
Back
Neurologic Status

NEONATAL PHYSICAL ASSESSMENT

NEONATAL BEHAVIORAL ASSESSMENT

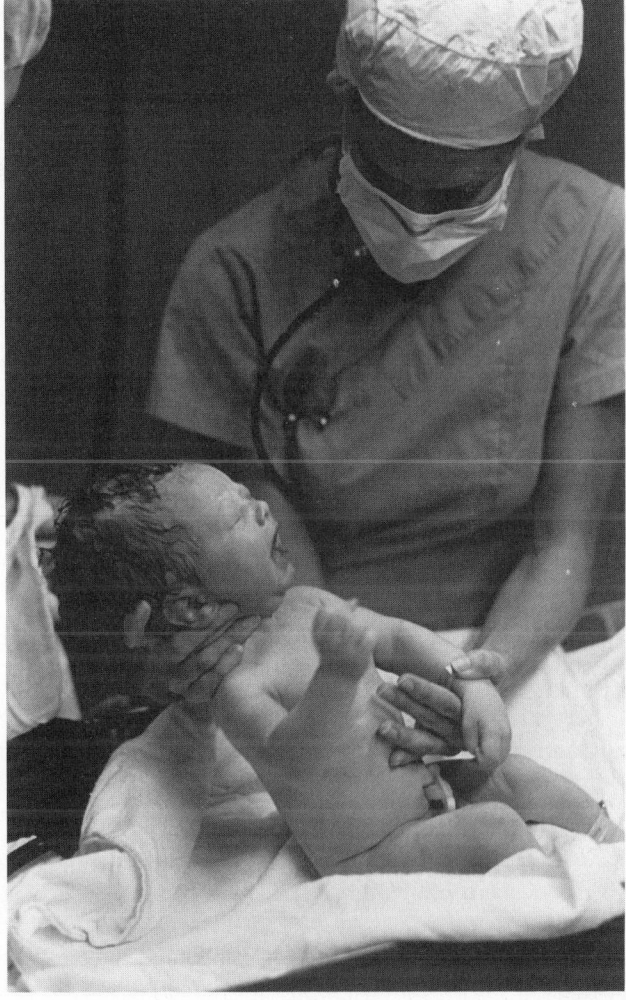

■ OBJECTIVES

- Describe the normal physical characteristics of the newborn.
- Identify the various methods of determining gestational age.

- Describe the neurologic and/or neuromuscular characteristics of the newborn and the reflexes that may be present at birth.
- Describe the components of the neonatal behavioral assessment.

The nurse is the only member of the health team who is a 24-hour observer of the neonate. In many hospitals a full-time medical staff is unavailable to provide constant medical care to the newborn. Because the pediatrician is present in the nursery for only a brief period of time, signs and symptoms of disease or injury of the newborn usually appear when the pediatrician is absent. Unlike the verbalizing adult client, the neonate communicates needs primarily by behavior. The nurse, through objective observations and evaluations, must be able to interpret this behavior into information about the neonate's condition and to respond with appropriate nursing interventions. This chapter focuses on the assessment of the neonate and on interpretations of the findings.

Assessment of the newborn is a continuous process designed to evaluate development and adjustments to extrauterine life. In the delivery room, the Apgar scoring procedure and careful observation of the neonate form the basis of assessment and are correlated with information such as:

- Maternal history
- Duration of labor
- Maternal analgesia and anesthesia
- Any complications of labor or delivery
- Apgar score
- Treatment instituted in the delivery room, in conjunction with determination of clinical gestational age
- Consideration of the classification of newborns by weight and gestational age and by neonatal mortality risk
- Physical examination of the newborn

Although an initial assessment of the newborn is done in the delivery room, the first thorough examination occurs in the nursery within 24 hours after delivery. When data from these various sources are incorporated with the findings of the assessment of the newborn in the nursery, a plan for nursing intervention is formulated.

The first 24 hours of life are significant because this period marks the critical transition from intrauterine to extrauterine life. Statistically, the risk of mortality and morbidity is high within this period. Nurses must establish the infant's gestational age and status on admission to the nursery so that careful attention can be given to age-related problems.

ESTIMATION OF GESTATIONAL AGE

Traditionally, the gestational age of a neonate was determined on the basis of the dates that the pregnant woman gave her physician about her last menstrual period. This method was accurate only 75%–85% of the time. Because of the problems that develop with the infant who is preterm or whose weight is inappropriate for gestational age, a more accurate system was developed to evaluate each newborn. Once learned, these observations can be made in a few minutes. Every neonatal nurse should be familiar with the methods for evaluating gestational age.

Clinical gestational age assessment tools have two components: external physical characteristics and neurologic and/or neuromuscular development evaluations. Physical characteristics include sole creases, amount of breast tissue, nature of the hair, cartilagenous development of the ear, testicular descent, and scrotal rugae or labial development. These objective clinical criteria are not influenced by labor and delivery nor do they change significantly within the first 24 hours after birth. During the first 24 hours of life, the newborn's nervous system is unstable during adjustment to extrauterine life; thus findings from neurologic evaluations that include reflexes or assessments dependent on the higher cortex centers may be less reliable during this period. Gestational assessment tools compensate for this problem by doing the scoring twice and averaging the two results or by delaying neurologic assessment until after 24 hours. If the neurologic component drastically deviates from the age generated by the external characteristics, the assessment is redone in 24 hours.

The neurologic components (excluding reflexes) can aid in assessing neonates of less than 34 weeks' gestation (Ballard et al., 1979). Between 26 and 34 weeks, neurologic changes are significant, whereas significant physical changes are less evident. The important neurologic changes consist of replacement of extensor tone by flexor tone progressing in a caudocephalad direction. Neurologic examination facilitates assessment of functional or physiologic maturation in addition to physical development. Of the current gestational assessment aids, Dubowitz and Dubowitz's tool (Figure 22–1, pp. 662–663) has been the most thoroughly documented and validated tool in clinical assessment of intrauterine growth alterations and preterm neonates (Robertson, 1979). This tool lists physical characteristics (Figure 22–1,A) and neuromuscular tone components (Figure 22–1,B) to be assessed upon admission to the nursery.

To calculate the gestational age, a score is given to each of the external physical characteristics and the neuromuscular components. Both scores are added, the total score is plotted on the graph (Figure 22–2, p. 664), and a corresponding gestational age is identified. A maximum score is 70, which corresponds with a gestational age of 43 weeks. For example, upon completing a gestational assessment of a 1-hour-old newborn, the nurse finds all the physical characteristics scored 3 each for a total of 27 and all neurologic assessments scored 3 each for a total neurologic score of 24. The physical characteristics score of 27 is combined with the neurologic score of 24 for a total score of 51. On the horizontal axis (total points), 51 is located and followed up the graph until reaching the diagonal intersecting line; the weeks of gestation is then read on the vertical line. Because all infants vary slightly in the development of physical characteristics and maturation of neurologic development, each of these areas will have some variance in score instead of all the physical characteristics having a score of 3 as in the example.

Two of the neuromuscular components cannot be assessed on very ill neonates or those on respirators—head lag and ventral suspension. The Dubowitz tool provides methods for scoring these two areas without changing the level of significance for the overall total tool (Dubowitz and Dubowitz, 1977).

Ballard's estimation of gestational age by maturity rating, a simplified version of the Dubowitz tool, has been reported as valid (Robertson, 1979). This tool deletes some of the neuromuscular tone assessments such as head lag, ventral suspension, and leg recoil. Ballard's tool is scored much like the Dubowitz method, with each physical and neuromuscular component given a value and the total score matched to a gestational age (Figure 22–3, pp. 665–666).

Both these tools lose validity when assessing neonates of less than 28 weeks' or over 43 weeks' gestation. An additional tool that is used is Brazie and Lubchenco's "Estimation of Gestational Age Chart" (Appendix D). Some nurseries use the physical characteristics component of this tool as an initial assessment for all neonates admitted to the nursery.

In carrying out gestational age assessments, the nurse should keep in mind that some maternal conditions cause metabolic alterations that affect certain gestational assessment components. Neonates of preeclamptic-eclamptic clients, who suffer some degree of oxygen deprivation during labor show a poor correlation with the criteria involving active muscle tone and edema. Neonates with RDS tend to be flaccid, edematous, and assume a "frogleg" posture—these characteristics affect the scoring of neuromuscular components. Maternal diabetes, although it appears to accelerate fetal growth, seems to retard maturation. Mater-

nal hypertensive states, which retard growth, seem to accelerate maturation. These factors warrant further study.

Assessment of Physical Characteristics

To accurately assess the neonate, one first evaluates characteristics that can be observed without disturbing the infant. As these observations are recorded on the chart, a pattern indicating gestational age quickly becomes apparent. Selected physical characteristics common to both the Dubowitz and Ballard assessment tools are presented here in the order in which they might be evaluated most effectively:

1. *Resting posture,* although a neuromuscular component, should be assessed as the infant lies undisturbed on a flat surface (Figure 22–4, p. 667).

2. *Skin* in the preterm neonate appears thin and transparent, with venules prominent over the abdomen early in gestation. As term approaches, the skin appears opaque because of increased deposition of subcutaneous tissue. Disappearance of protective vernix caseosa promotes skin desquamation.

3. *Lanugo,* a fine hair covering, decreases as gestational age increases. The amount of lanugo is greatest at 28–30 weeks and then disappears, first from the face, then from the trunk and extremities.

4. *Sole (plantar) creases* are reliable indicators of gestational age in the first 12 hours of life. After this, the skin of the foot begins drying, and creases appear. Development of sole creases is systematic, beginning at the anterior portion of the foot and, as gestation progresses, proceeding to the heel (Figure 22–5, p. 668). Plantar creases vary with race. Black infants' sole creases are less developed at term (Damoulaki-Sfakianaki et al., 1972).

5. *Breast tissue and areola* are palpated by application of the forefinger and middle finger to the breast area. Although Figure 22–6 (p. 669) utilizes the thumb and forefinger to improve visualization of the areola for purposes of this discussion, during actual assessment the nipple should not be grasped with thumb and forefinger, as skin and subcutaneous tissue will prevent accurate estimation of size. Traumatization of the breast tissue may also occur if this procedure is not done gently. As gestation progresses, the breast tissue mass and areola enlarge. However, a large breast tissue mass can occur as a result of conditions other than advanced gestational age. The infant of a diabetic mother tends to be LGA, and the accelerated development of breast tissue is a reflection of subcutaneous fat deposits. SGA term or postterm newborns may have utilized subcutaneous fat (which would have been deposited as breast tissue) to survive in utero; as a result, their lack of breast tissue may indicate a gestational age of 34–35

(Text continues on p. 668.)

FIGURE 22–1 Estimation of gestational age. **A,** External (superficial) criteria. **B,** Neurologic criteria. (From Dubowitz, L., and Dubowitz, V. 1977. *Gestational age of the newborn.* Menlo Park, Calif.: Addison-Wesley Publishing Co.)

EXTERNAL SIGN	SCORE				
	0	**1**	**2**	**3**	**4**
OEDEMA	Obvious oedema hands and feet; pitting over tibia	No obvious oedema hands and feet; pitting over tibia	No oedema		
SKIN TEXTURE	Very thin, gelatinous	Thin and smooth	Smooth; medium thickness. Rash or superficial peeling	Slight thickening. Superficial cracking and peeling esp. hands and feet	Thick and parchment-like; superficial or deep cracking
SKIN COLOUR (Infant not crying)	Dark red	Uniformly pink	Pale pink; variable over body	Pale. Only pink over ears, lips, palms or soles	
SKIN OPACITY (trunk)	Numerous veins and venules clearly seen, especially over abdomen	Veins and tributaries seen	A few large vessels clearly seen over abdomen	A few large vessels seen indistinctly over abdomen	No blood vessels seen
LANUGO (over back)	No lanugo	Abundant; long and thick over whole back	Hair thinning especially over lower back	Small amount of lanugo and bald areas	At least half of back devoid of lanugo
PLANTAR CREASES	No skin creases	Faint red marks over anterior half of sole	Definite red marks over more than anterior half; indentations over less than anterior third	Indentations over more than anterior third	Definite deep indentations over more than anterior third
NIPPLE FORMATION	Nipple barely visible; no areola	Nipple well defined; areola smooth and flat diameter <0.75 cm.	Areola stippled, edge not raised; diameter <0.75 cm.	Areola stippled, edge raised diameter >0.75 cm.	
BREAST SIZE	No breast tissue palpable	Breast tissue on one or both sides < 0.5 cm. diameter	Breast tissue both sides; one or both 0.5-1.0 cm.	Breast tissue both sides; one or both > 1 cm.	
EAR FORM	Pinna flat and shapeless, little or no incurving of edge	Incurving of part of edge of pinna	Partial incurving whole of upper pinna	Well-defined incurving whole of upper pinna	
EAR FIRMNESS	Pinna soft, easily folded, no recoil	Pinna soft, easily folded, slow recoil	Cartilage to edge of pinna, but soft in places, ready recoil	Pinna firm, cartilage to edge, instant recoil	
GENITALIA MALE	Neither testis in scrotum	At least one testis high in scrotum	At least one testis right down		
FEMALES (With hips half abducted)	Labia majora widely separated, labia minora protruding	Labia majora almost cover labia minora	Labia majora completely cover labia minora		

A

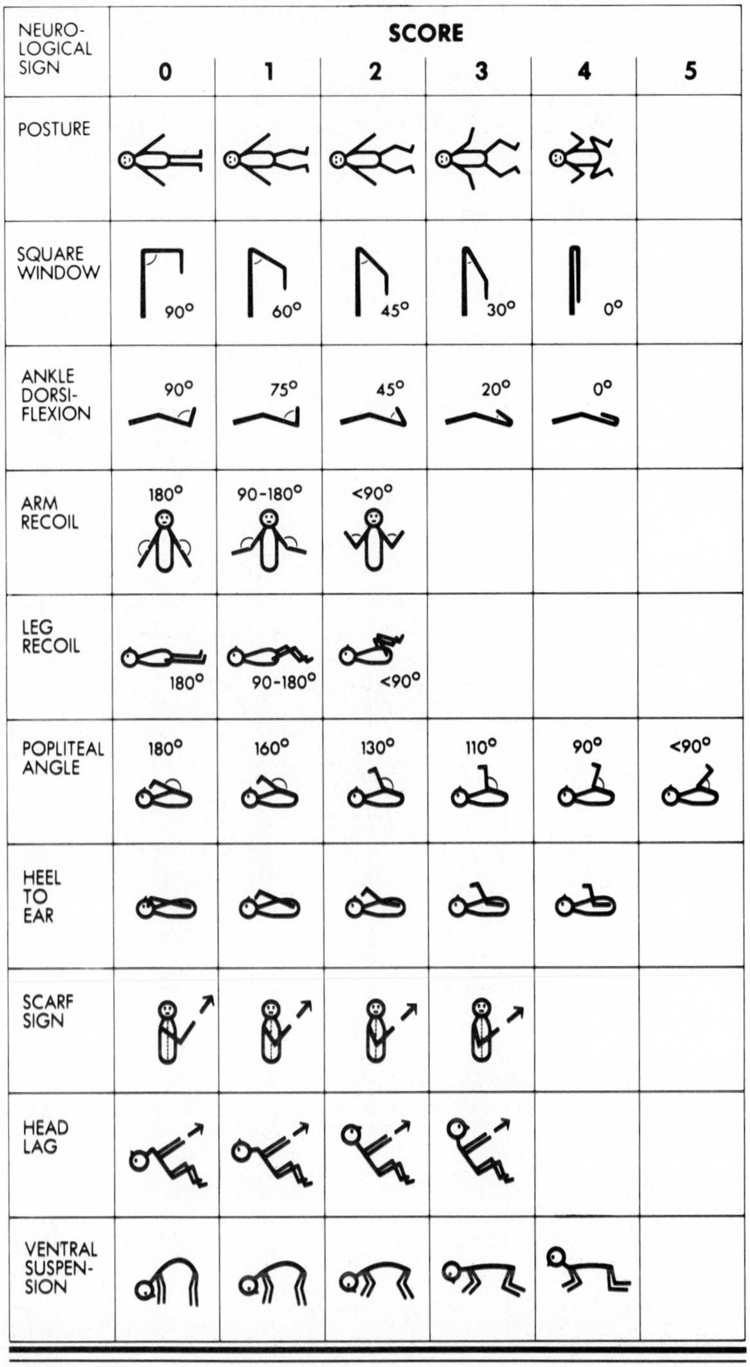

FIGURE 22-1 Continued.

NEURO-LOGICAL SIGN	SCORE					
	0	1	2	3	4	5
POSTURE						
SQUARE WINDOW	90°	60°	45°	30°	0°	
ANKLE DORSI-FLEXION	90°	75°	45°	20°	0°	
ARM RECOIL	180°	90–180°	<90°			
LEG RECOIL	180°	90–180°	<90°			
POPLITEAL ANGLE	180°	160°	130°	110°	90°	<90°
HEEL TO EAR						
SCARF SIGN						
HEAD LAG						
VENTRAL SUSPEN-SION						

B

FIGURE 22–2 Graph for reading gestational age from total score. (From Dubowitz, L., and Dubowitz, V. 1977. *Gestational age of the Newborn.* Menlo Park, Calif.: Addison-Wesley Publishing Co.)

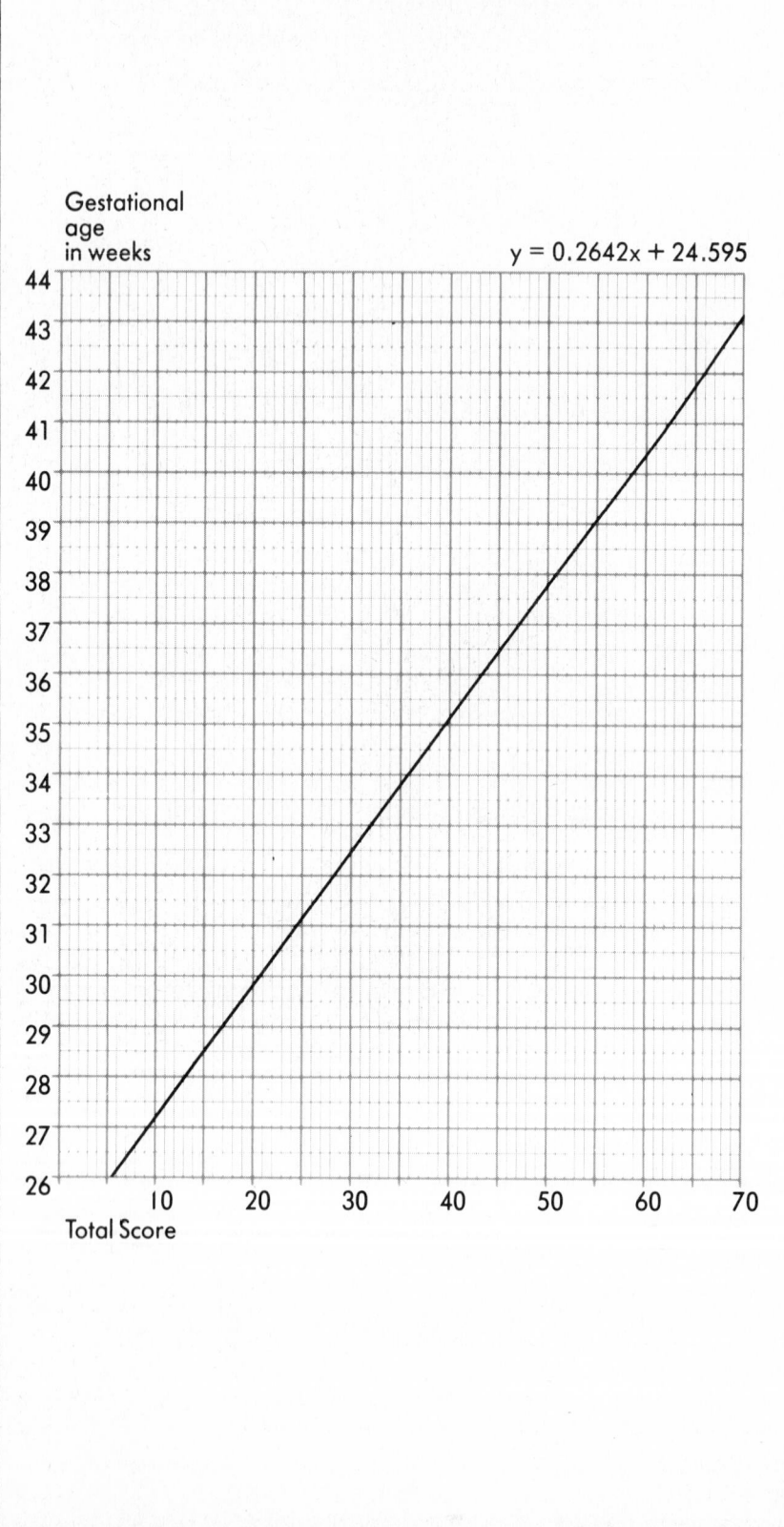

Estimation of Gestational Age
by Maturity Rating
Symbols: X=First exam   O=Second exam

Neuromuscular Maturity

	0	1	2	3	4	5
Posture						
Square window (wrist)	90°	60°	45°	30°	0°	
Arm recoil	180°		100°-180°	90°-100°	<90°	
Popliteal angle	180°	160°	130°	110°	90°	<90°
Scarf sign						
Heel to ear						

Gestation by dates _____ wks.

Birth date _____ Hour _____ am / pm

APGAR _____ 1 min _____ 5 min

Score	Wks
5	26
10	28
15	30
20	32
25	34
30	36
35	38
40	40
45	42
50	44

Physical Maturity

	0	1	2	3	4	5
Skin	gelatinous red, transparent	smooth pink, visible veins	superficial peeling and/or rash, few veins	cracking pale area, rare veins,	parchment, deep cracking, no vessels	leathery, cracked, wrinkled
Lanugo	none	abundant	thinning	bald areas	mostly bald	
Plantar creases	no crease	faint red marks	anterior transverse crease only	creases anter. 2/3	creases cover entire sole	
Breast	barely percept.	flat areola, no bud	stippled areola, 1-2 mm bud	raised areola, 3-4 mm bud	full areola, 5-10 mm bud	
Ear	binna flat, stays folded	sl. curved pinna, soft with slow recoil	well-curv. pinna, soft but ready recoil	formed and firm with instant recoil	thick cartilage, ear stiff	
Genitals (male)	scrotum empty, no rugae		testes decending, few rugae	testes down, good rugae	testes pendulous, deep rugae	
Genitals (female)	prominent clitoris and labia minora		majora and minora equally prominent	majora large, minora small	clitoris and minora completely covered	

Continued.

FIGURE 22–3 Newborn maturity rating and classification. (From Ballard, J. L., et al. 1977. A simplified assessment of gestational age. *Pediatr. Res.* 11:374. Figures adapted from Classification of the low-birth-weight infant by A. Y. Sweet in *Care of the high-risk infant* by M. H. Klaus and A. A. Fanaroff, W. B. Saunders Co, Philadelphia, 1977, p. 47.)

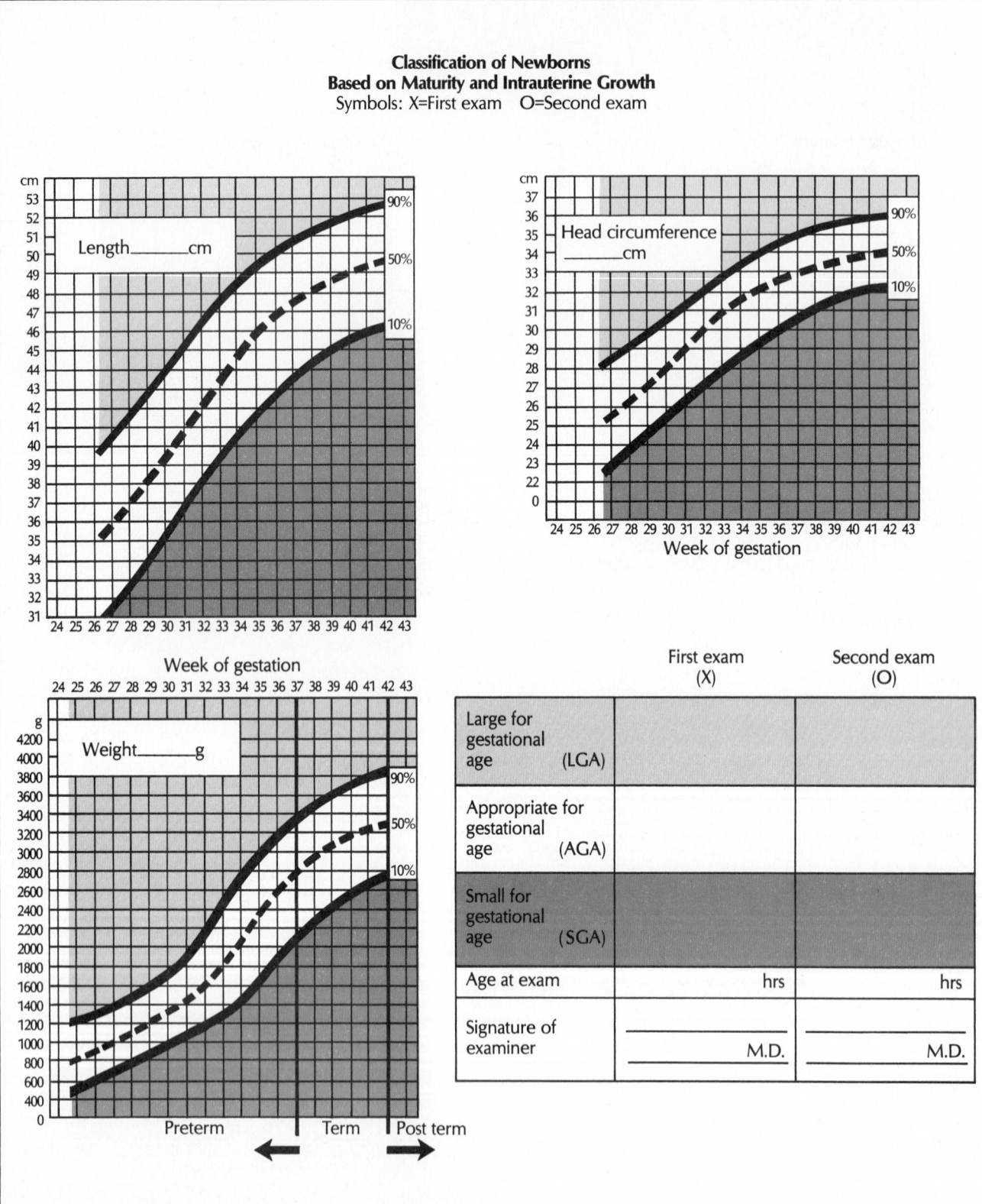

Classification of Newborns
Based on Maturity and Intrauterine Growth
Symbols: X=First exam   O=Second exam

	First exam (X)	Second exam (O)
Large for gestational age (LGA)		
Appropriate for gestational age (AGA)		
Small for gestational age (SGA)		
Age at exam	hrs	hrs
Signature of examiner	M.D.	M.D.

FIGURE 22–3 *Continued.*

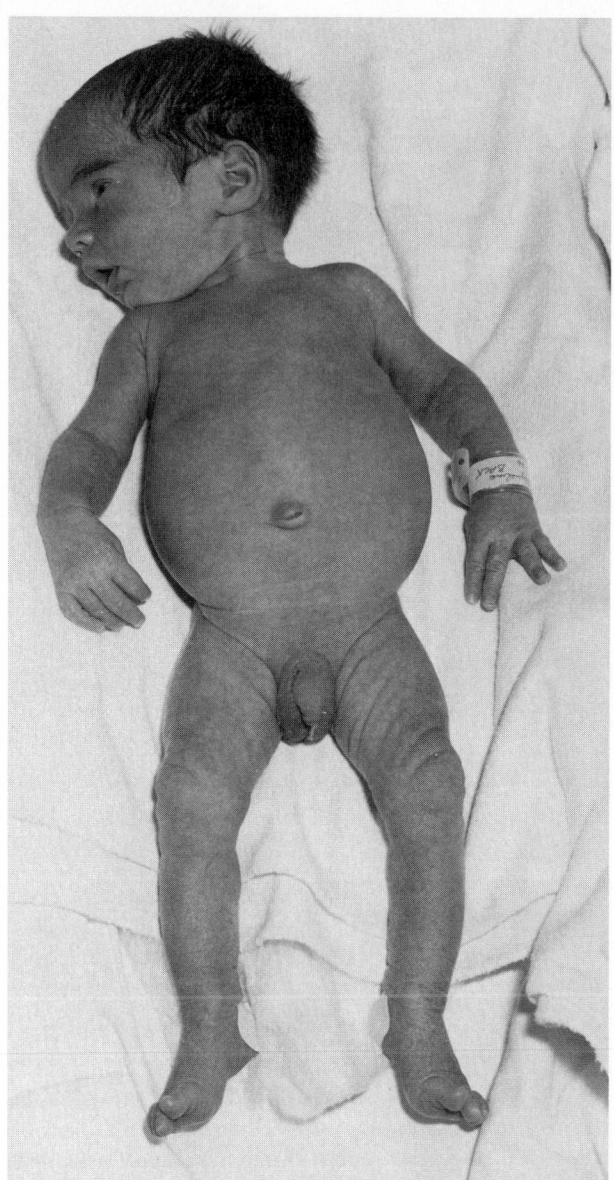

A

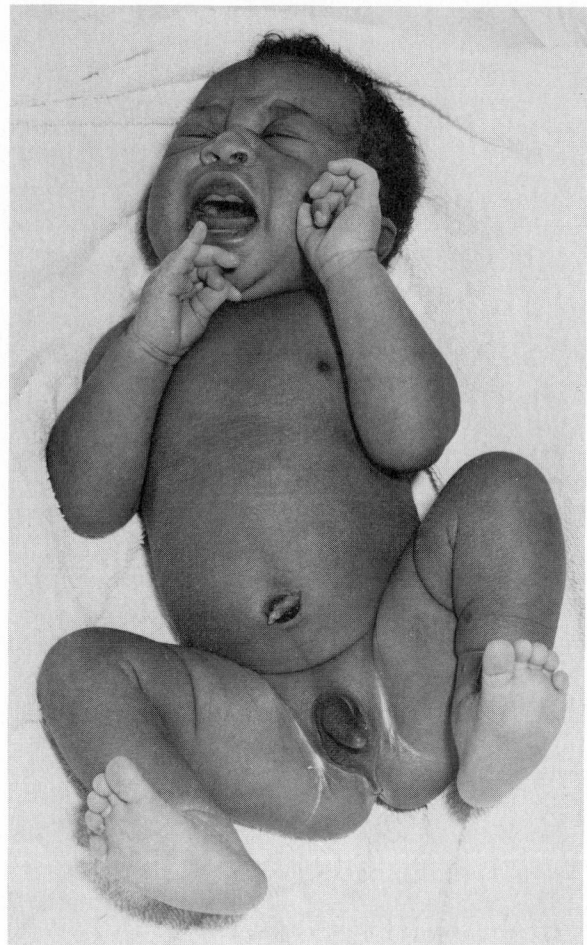

B

FIGURE 22–4 Resting posture. **A,** Infant exhibits beginning of flexion of the thigh. The gestational age is approximately 31 weeks. Note the extension of the upper extremities. **B,** Infant exhibits stronger flexion of the arms, hips, and thighs. The gestational age is approximately 35 weeks. **C,** The full-term infant exhibits hypertonic flexion of all extremities. (From Dubowitz, L., and Dubowitz, V. 1977. *Gestational age of the newborn.* Menlo Park, Calif.: Addison-Wesley Publishing Co.)

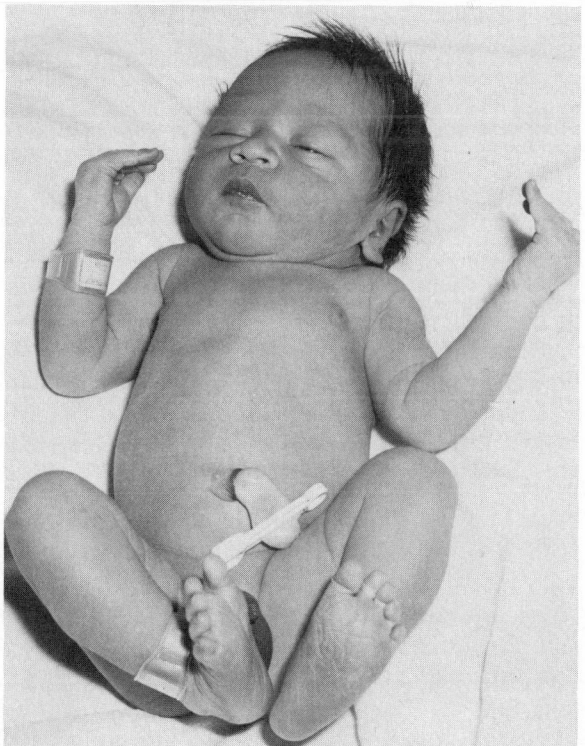

C

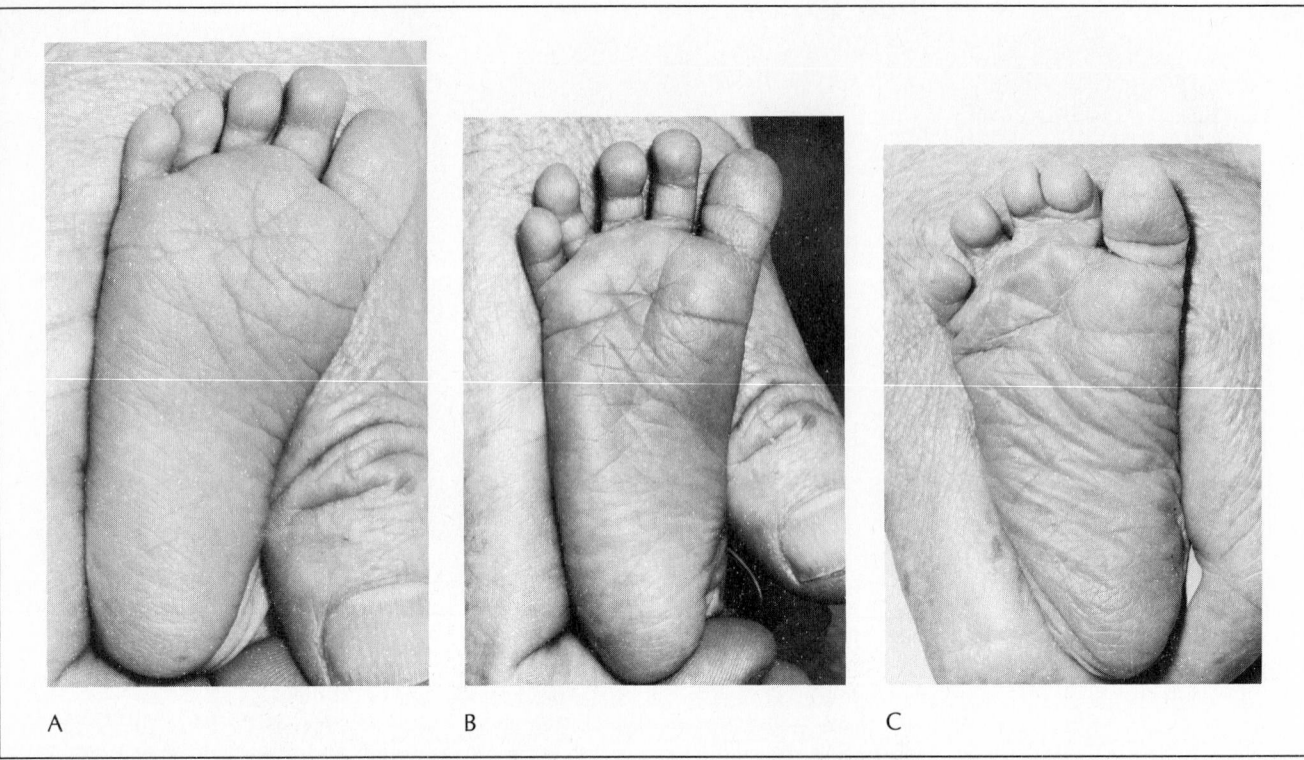

A   B   C

FIGURE 22–5 Sole creases. **A,** Infant has a few sole creases on the anterior portion of the foot. Note the slick heel. The gestational age is approximately 35 weeks. **B,** Infant has a deeper network of sole creases on the anterior two-thirds of the sole. Note the slick heel. The gestational age is approximately 37 weeks. **C,** The full-term infant has deep sole creases down to and including the heel. (From Dubowitz, L., and Dubowitz, V. 1977. *Gestational age of the newborn.* Menlo Park, Calif.: Addison-Wesley Publishing Co.)

weeks, even though other factors indicate a *term* or *postterm* neonate.

6. *Ear form and cartilage distribution* develop with gestational age. The deposition of cartilage gives the ear its shape and substance (Figure 22–7). An infant of less than 34 weeks' gestation has little cartilage deposition, so the ear folds over on itself and remains folded. By approximately 36 weeks' gestation, the pinna springs back slowly when folded. (This response is tested by holding the top and bottom of the pinna together with forefinger and thumb, then releasing the pinna and observing the response.) By term, the neonate's pinna is firm, stands away from the head, and springs back quickly from folding.

7. *Male genitals* are evaluated in terms of the size of the scrotal sac, the presence of rugae, and whether the testes have descended (Figure 22–8). Prior to 36 weeks the male has a small scrotum with few rugae, and the testes are palpable in the inguinal canal. By 36–38 weeks, the testes are found in the upper scrotum and rugae have developed over the anterior portion of the scrotum. By term the testes are generally located in the lower scrotum, which is pendulous and covered with rugae.

The appearance of the *female genitals* depends in part on subcutaneous fat deposition and therefore relates to fetal nutritional status. At 30–32 weeks' gestation, the clitoris is prominent, and the labia majora are small and widely separated. As gestational age increases, the labia majora increase in size. At 36–40 weeks, they nearly cover the clitoris. At 40 weeks and beyond, the labia majora cover the labia minora and clitoris (Figure 22–9).

The clitoris varies in size and occasionally is so large that it is difficult to identify the sex of the infant. This may be caused by adrenogenital syndrome, which causes excessive secretions of androgen and other hormones from the adrenals.

In the full-term female newborn some tissue may protrude from the floor of the vagina. This tissue, the hymenal tag, is a normal segment of the hymen and disappears in several weeks (Korones, 1981).

Other physical characteristics assessed by some gestational age scoring tools include the following:

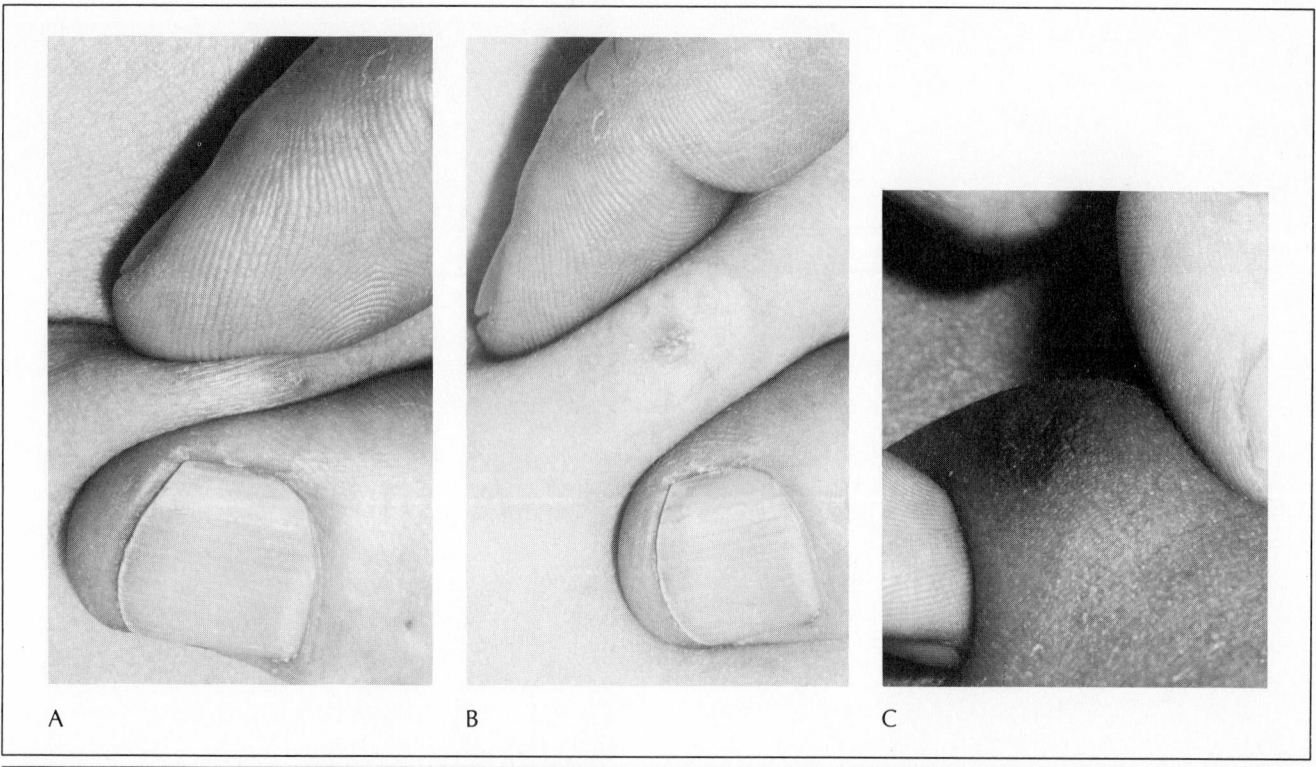

A   B   C

FIGURE 22–6 Breast tissue. **A,** Infant has a barely visible areola and nipple. No tissue is palpable. The gestational age is less than 33 weeks. **B,** Infant has a visible raised area. On palpation the area is 4 mm. The gestational age is 38 weeks. **C,** Infant has a 10 mm breast tissue area. The gestational age is 40–44 weeks. (From Dubowitz, L., and Dubowitz, V. 1977. *Gestational age of the newborn.* Menlo Park, Calif.: Addison-Wesley Publishing Co.)

1. *Vernix distribution* (and protection) decreases as term approaches. As a result, the preterm infant is covered with vernix, and the postterm infant has no vernix. After noting vernix distribution, the delivery room nurse dries the newborn to prevent evaporative heat loss. Thus vernix distribution is disturbed by the time the newborn enters the nursery. The delivery room nurse must communicate to the neonatal nurse the amount and areas of vernix coverage.

2. *Hair* of the preterm infant has the consistency of matted wool or fur and lies in bunches rather than in the silky, single strands of the term infant's hair.

3. *Skull firmness* increases as the infant matures. In a term neonate the bones are hard, and the sutures are not easily displaced. The clinician should not attempt to forceably displace the sutures.

4. *Nails* appear and cover the nail bed at about 20 weeks' gestation. Nails extending beyond the fingertips may be indicative of postterm neonate.

Assessment of Neurologic Status

The central nervous system of the human fetus matures at a fairly constant rate. Specific neurologic parameters cor-related to gestational age have been established. Tests have been designed to evaluate neurologic status as manifested by neuromuscular tone development. In the fetus, neuromuscular tone develops from the lower to the upper extremities. The neurologic evaluation requires more manipulation and disturbances than the physical evaluation of the neonate and therefore is difficult to administer if the newborn is ill and requires supportive therapies, which tend to immobilize the infant.

The neuromuscular evaluation (see Figure 22–1,*B*) is best performed when the infant has stabilized. The following characteristics are evaluated:

1. *Ankle dorsiflexion* is determined by flexing the ankle on the shin. The sole of the neonate's foot is pushed with the examiner's thumb while the fingers support the back of the neonate's leg. Then the angle formed between the foot and the interior leg is measured (Figure 22–10). This sign can be influenced by intrauterine position and congenital deformities.

2. The *square window sign* is elicited by flexing the neonate's hand toward the ventral forearm. The angle formed at the wrist is measured (Figure 22–11).

(Text continues on p. 672.)

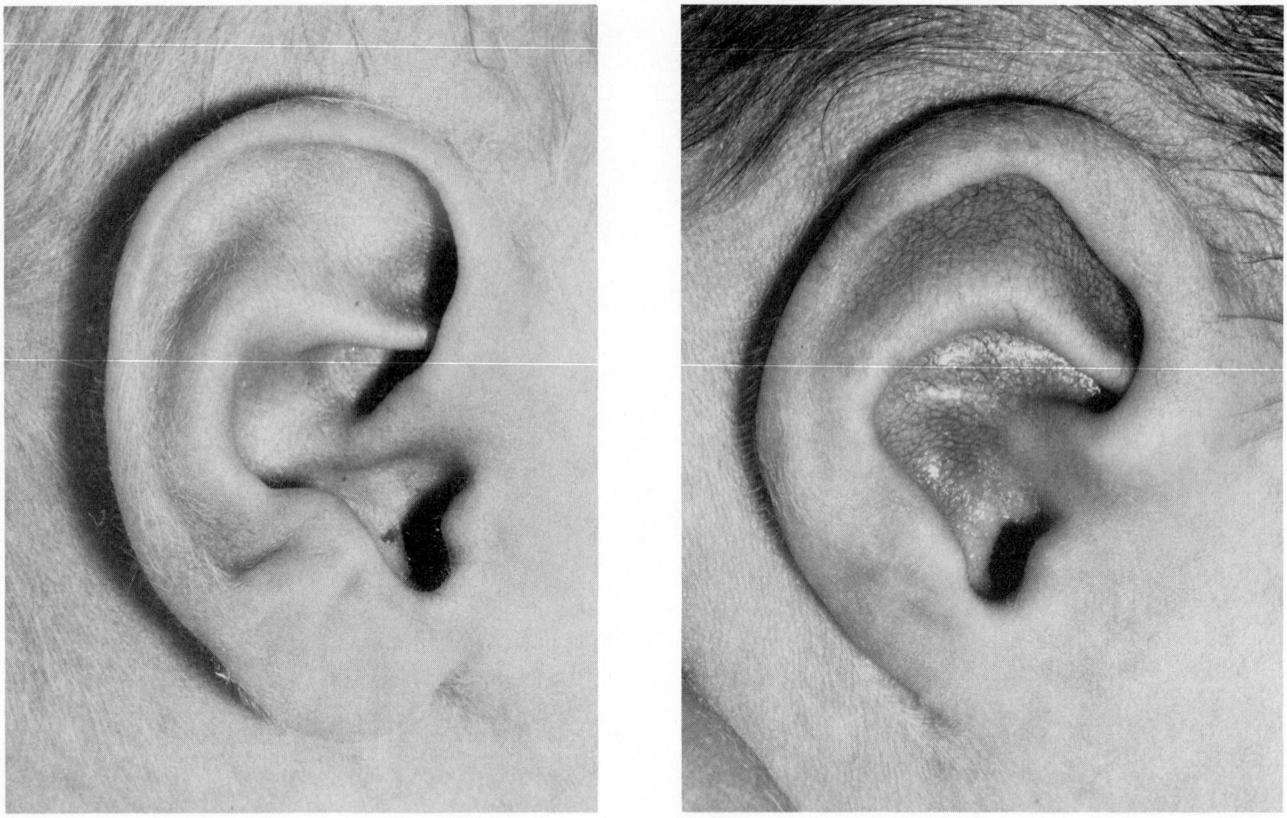

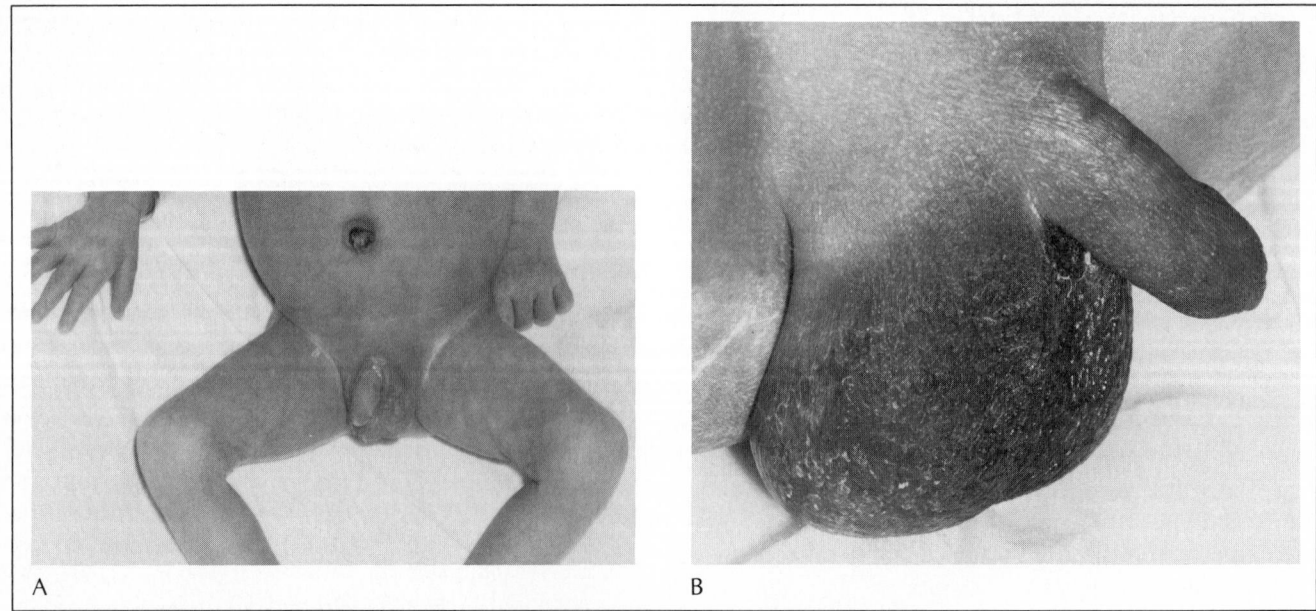

FIGURE 22–7 Ear form and cartilage. **A,** The ear of the infant at approximately 36 weeks' gestation shows incurving of the upper two-thirds of the pinna. **B,** Infant at term shows well-defined incurving of the entire pinna. (From Dubowitz, L., and Dubowitz, V. 1977. *Gestational age of the newborn*. Menlo Park, Calif.: Addison-Wesley Publishing Co.)

FIGURE 22–8 Male genitals. **A,** Preterm infant's testes are not within the scrotum. The scrotal surface has few rugae. **B,** Term infant's testes are generally fully descended. The entire surface of the scrotum is covered by rugae. (From Dubowitz, L., and Dubowitz, V. 1977. *Gestational age of the newborn*. Menlo Park, Calif.: Addison-Wesley Publishing Co.)

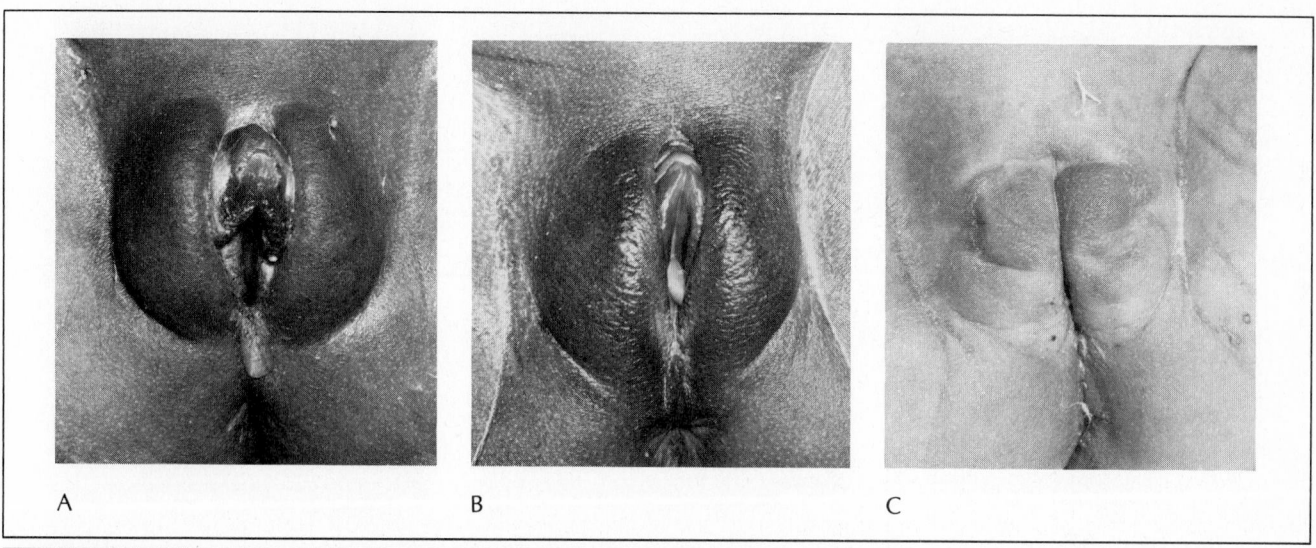

FIGURE 22–9 Female genitals. **A,** Infant has a prominent clitoris. The labia majora are widely separated, and the labia minora, viewed laterally, would protrude beyond the labia majora. The gestational age is 30–36 weeks. **B,** The clitoris is still visible; the labia minora are now covered by the larger labia majora. The gestational age is 36–40 weeks. **C,** The term infant has well-developed, large labia majora that cover both the clitoris and labia minora. (From Dubowitz, L., and Dubowitz, V. 1977. *Gestational age of the newborn*. Menlo Park, Calif.: Addison-Wesley Publishing Co.)

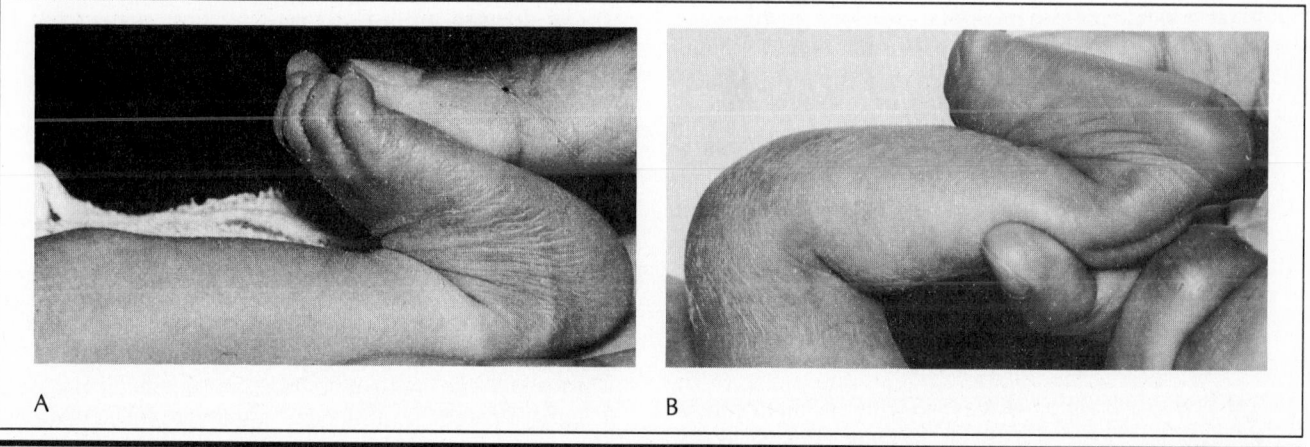

FIGURE 22–10 Ankle dorsiflexion. **A,** A 45° angle is indicative of 32–36 weeks' gestation. A 20° angle is indicative of 36–40 weeks' gestation. **B,** An angle of 0° is common at gestational age of 40 weeks or more. (From Dubowitz, L., and Dubowitz, V. 1977. *Gestational age of the newborn*. Menlo Park, Calif.: Addison-Wesley Publishing Co.)

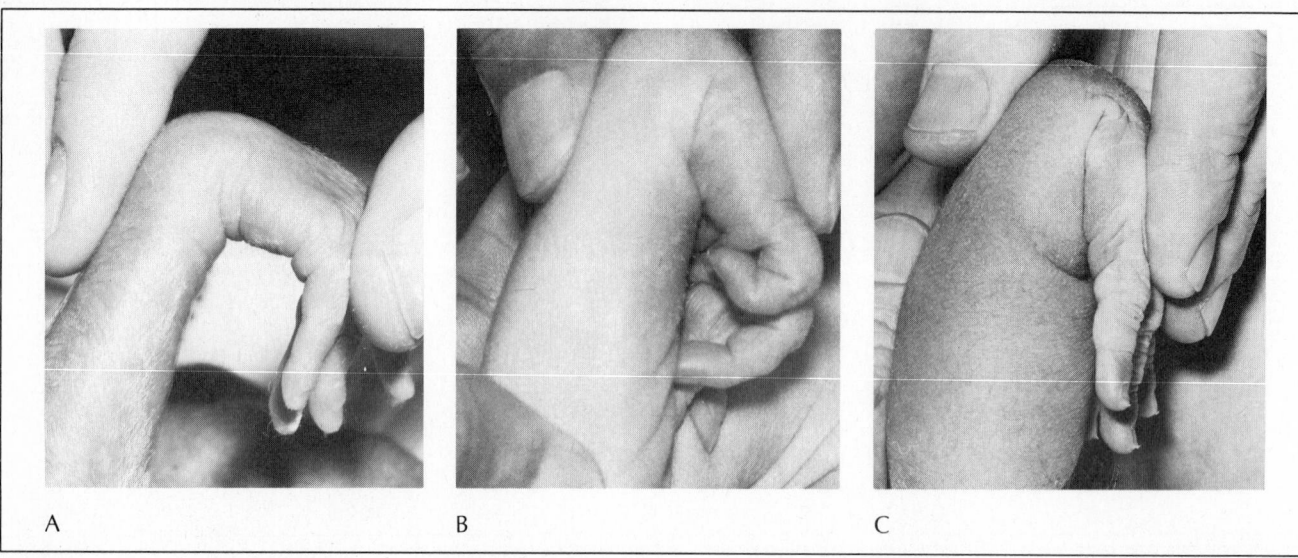

A   B   C

FIGURE 22–11 Square window sign. **A,** This angle is 90° and suggests an immature newborn of 28–32 weeks' gestation. **B,** A 30° angle is commonly found from 38–40 weeks' gestation. **C,** A 0° angle occurs from 40–42 weeks. (From Dubowitz, L. and Dubowitz, V. 1977. *Gestational age of the newborn.* Menlo Park, Calif.: Addison-Wesley Publishing Co.)

3. *Recoil* is a test of flexion development. About a 2-week delay occurs between the development of resting flexion and recoil (in the flexed position) in response to extension. Because flexion first develops in the lower extremities, recoil is first tested in the legs. The neonate is placed on his or her back on a flat surface. With a hand on the neonate's knees and while manipulating the hip joint, the nurse places the neonate's legs in flexion, then extends them parallel to each other and flat on the surface. The response to this maneuver is recoil of the neonate's legs. According to gestational age, they may not move or they may return slowly or quickly to the flexed position. Recoil in the upper extremities is tested by flexion at the elbow and extension of the arms at the neonate's side.

4. The *popliteal angle* is determined with the infant supine and flat. The thigh is flexed on the chest, and the examiner places an index finger behind the infant's ankle to extend the lower leg. The angle formed is then measured. Results vary from no resistance in the very immature infant to an 80° angle in the term infant.

5. The *heel-to-ear maneuver* is performed by placing the infant in a supine position and then gently drawing the foot toward the ear on the same side until resistance is felt. Both the popliteal angle and the proximity of foot to ear are assessed. In a very immature infant, the leg will remain straight and the foot will go to the ear or beyond.

Maneuvers involving the lower extremities of newborns who had frank breech presentation should be de-

layed to allow for resolution of flexor fatigue (Ballard et al., 1979).

6. The *scarf sign* is elicited by placing the neonate supine and drawing an arm across the chest toward the infant's opposite shoulder until resistance is met. The location of the elbow is then noted (Figure 22–12).

7. Head lag *(neck flexors)* is measured by pulling the neonate to a sitting position and noting the degree of head lag. Total lag is common in infants up to 34 weeks' gestation, whereas postmature infants (42 weeks) will hold their head in front of their body line.

8. Ventral suspension *(horizontal position)* is evaluated by holding the infant prone on the examiner's hand. The position of head and back and degree of flexion in the arms and legs are then noted. Some flexion of arms and legs indicates 36–38 weeks' gestation; fully flexed extremities, with head and back even, are characteristic of a term neonate.

9. *Major reflexes* such as sucking, rooting, grasping, Moro, tonic neck, and others are evaluated and scored.

A supplementary method of gestational age determination is evaluation of the vascular network over the ocular lens behind the cornea (Hittner et al., 1977).

Determination of gestational age and correlation with birth weight (Figure 22–13) enables the nurse to assess the infant more accurately and to anticipate possible physiologic problems. This information is then used in conjunction with a complete physical examination to determine priorities and to establish a plan of care appropriate to the individual infant.

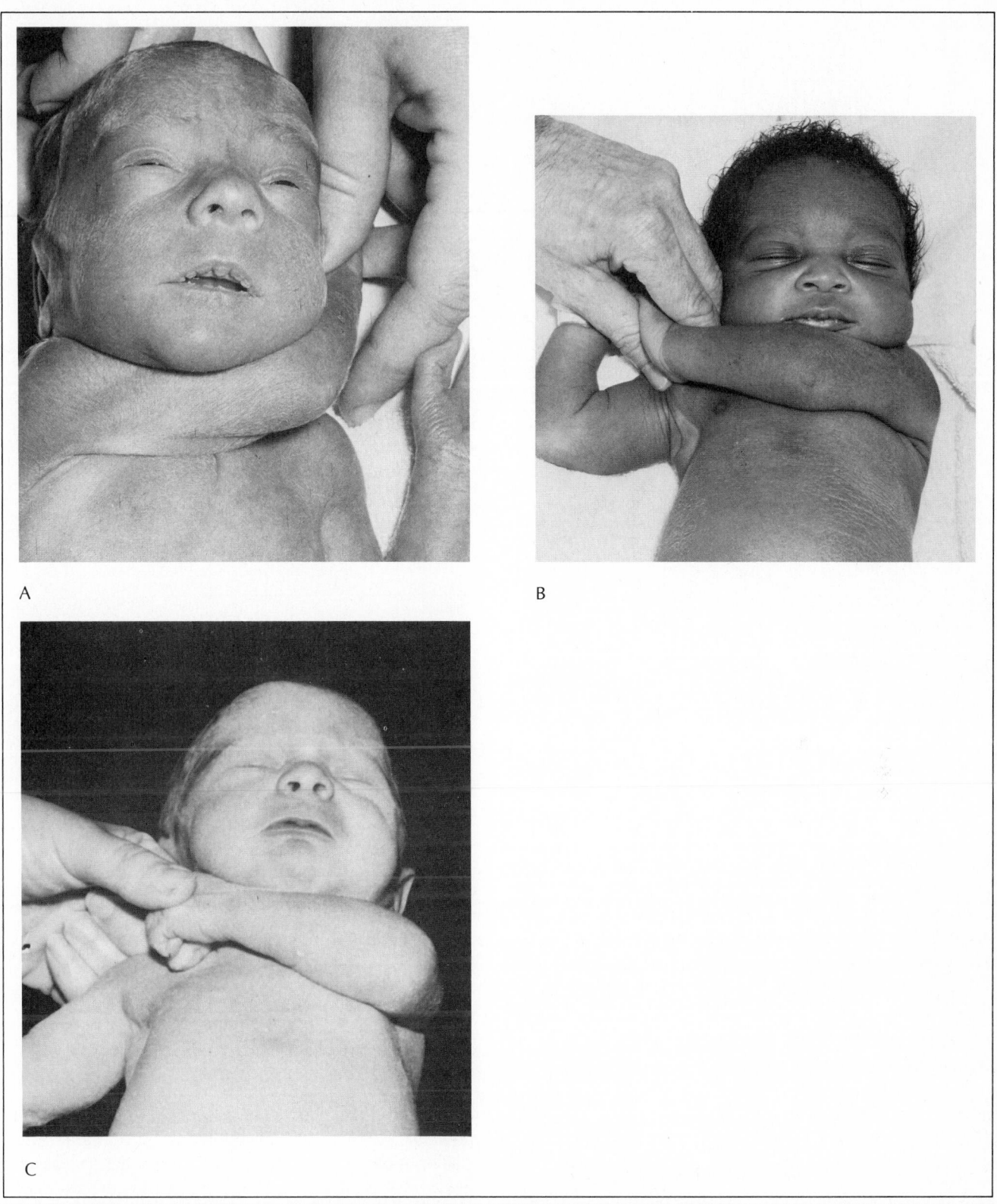

FIGURE 22–12 Scarf sign. **A,** No resistance is noted until after 30 weeks' gestation. The elbow can be readily moved past the midline. **B,** The elbow is at the midline at 36–40 weeks' gestation. **C,** Beyond 40 weeks' gestation, the elbow will not reach the midline. (From Dubowitz, L., and Dubowitz, V. 1977. *Gestational age of the newborn.* Menlo Park, Calif.: Addison-Wesley Publishing Co.)

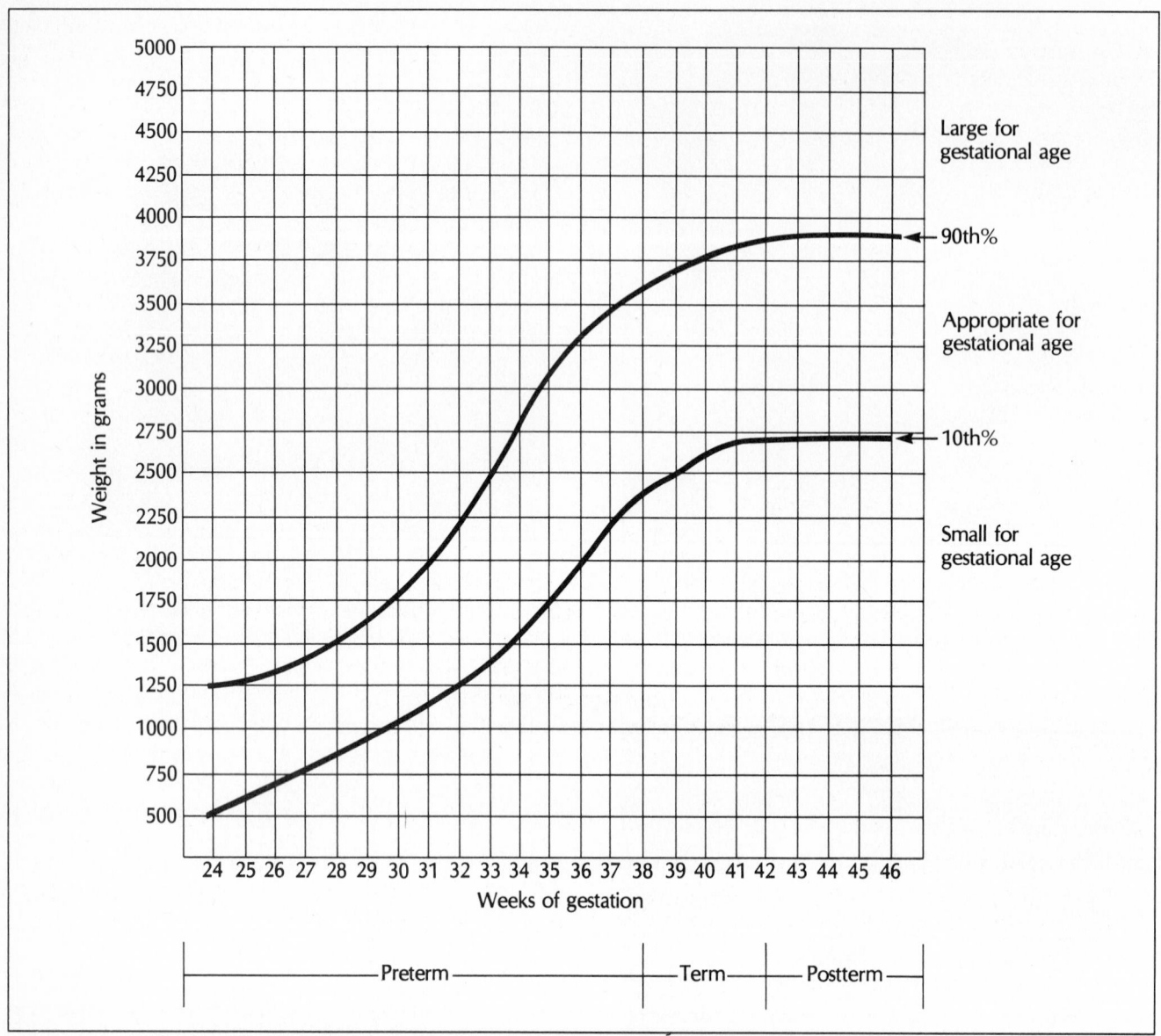

FIGURE 22–13 Classification of newborns by birth weight and gestational age. The newborn's birth weight and gestational age are plotted on the graph. The newborn is then classified as large for gestational age, appropriate for gestational age, or small for gestational age. (From Battaglia, F. C., and Lubchenco, L. O. 1967. A practical classification of newborn infants by weight and gestational age. *J. Pediatr.* 71:161.)

PHYSICAL EXAMINATION

After the initial determination of gestational age and related potential problems, a more detailed physical examination is conducted. The nurse should choose a warm, well-lighted area that is free of drafts. Completing a physical examination in the presence of the parents provides an opportunity to acquaint them with their unique newborn. The nurse should perform the examination systematically and record all findings. When assessing the physical and neurologic status of the newborn, the nurse should first consider general appearance and then proceed to specific areas.

General Appearance

The newborn's head is disproportionately large for the body. The center of the baby's body is the umbilicus rather than the symphysis pubis, as in the adult. The torso appears long and the extremities short. The flexed position that the neonate maintains contributes to the apparent shortness of the extremities. The hands are tightly clenched. The neck is short because the chin rests on the chest. Newborns have prominent abdomen, sloping shoulders, narrow hips, and rounded chest; they tend to stay in a flexed position similar to the one maintained in utero.

Posture

Although the newborn's posture is influenced by intrauterine position and type of delivery, a full-term newborn is usually flexed and will offer resistance when extremities are straightened. With a breech presentation, the feet are usually dorsiflexed and may take several weeks for the newborn to assume typical neonatal posture.

Weight and Measurements

The normal full-term white newborn has an average birth weight of 3405 g (7 lb, 8 oz), whereas black, Oriental, and American Indian newborns are usually somewhat smaller. Other factors that influence weight are age and size of parents, health of mother, and the interval between pregnancies. Half of all newborns weigh between 2950 g (6 lb, 8 oz) and 3515 g (7 lb, 12 oz). After the first week and for the first 6 months, the neonate's weight will increase about 227 g (8 oz) weekly.

Approximately 70%–75% of the neonate's body weight is water. During the initial newborn period (the first 3 or 4 days), there is a physiologic weight loss of about 5%–15% (depending on the size of the neonate) because of fluid shifts. Large babies may tend to lose more weight

because of greater fluid loss in proportion to birth weight. If weight loss is greater than expected, clinical reappraisal is indicated. Factors contributing to weight loss include small fluid intake resulting from delayed breast-feeding or a slow adjustment to the formula, increased loss of meconium, and urination. Weight loss may be marked in the presence of temperature elevation because of associated dehydration.

The length of the normal newborn is difficult to measure, because the legs are flexed and tensed. To measure length, infants should be flat on their backs with legs extended as much as possible. The average length is 49.4 cm (19.5 in.), with the range being 45.8–52.3 cm (18–20.5 in.). The newborn will grow approximately an inch a month for the next 6 months. This is the period of most rapid growth.

At birth the newborn's head is one-third the size of the adult head. The ratio of face to cranium is 1:8 in the infant and 1:2 in the adult. The circumference of the newborn's head is 33–35 cm (13–14 in.). For accurate measurement, the tape is placed over the most prominent part of the occiput and brought to just above the eyebrows (Figure 22–14,A). The circumference of the newborn's head is approximately 2 cm greater than the circumference of the newborn's chest at birth and will remain in this proportion for the next few months. (Factors that alter this measurement are discussed on p. 679.)

The chest is rounded at birth, becoming more rectangular as the infant grows older. The average circumference of the chest at birth is 32 cm (12.5 in.). Chest measurements should be taken with the tape measure at the lower edge of the scapulas and brought around anteriorly directly over the nipple line (Figure 22–14,B). The abdominal

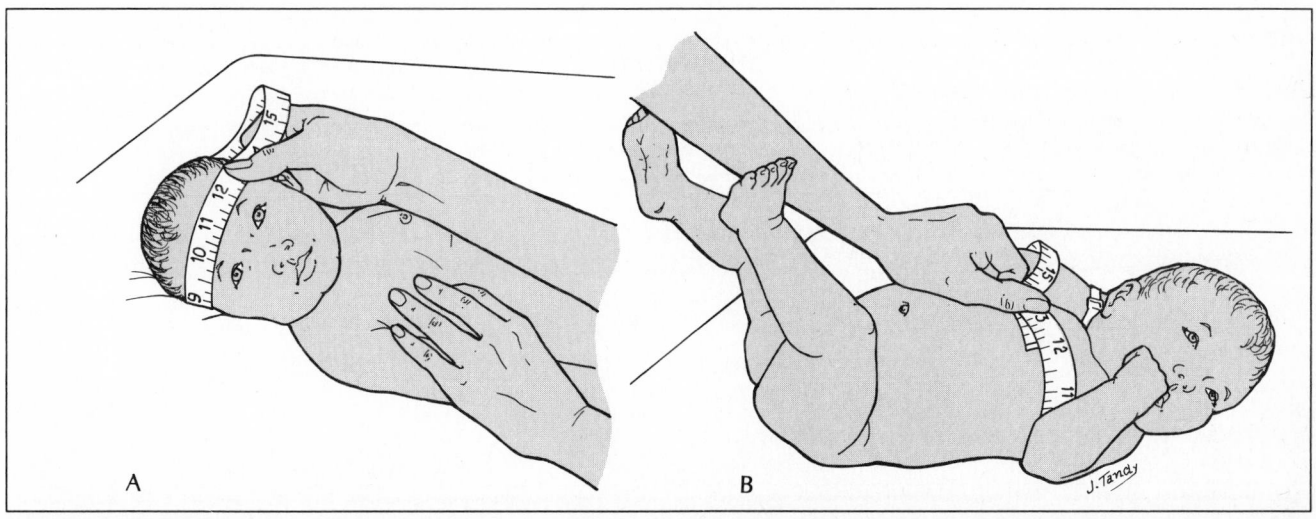

FIGURE 22–14 A, Measuring the head circumference of the newborn. **B,** Measuring the chest circumference of the newborn.

circumference or girth is also measured at this time by placing the tape around the newborn's abdomen at the level of the umbilicus with the bottom edge of the tape at the top edge of the umbilicus.

Temperature

Initial assessment of the newborn's temperature is critical. In utero, the temperature of the fetus approximates or is slightly higher than the expectant mother's. With exposure to the outside world, the newborn's temperature can suddenly drop as a result of adaptation to the extrauterine environment, exposure to cold drafts, and the skin's heat-loss mechanisms. Upon arrival in the nursery, a newborn's skin temperature may be as low as 36C (96.8F) if the newborn was not dried and placed under a radiant warmer in the delivery room (Korones, 1981). The temperature should stabilize at around 36.7C (98F) within 8–12 hours. Temperature should be monitored at least every hour until stable, then every 4 hours for 24 hours (Standards and

Recommendations for Hospital Care of Newborn Infants, 1977). Many institutions utilize a continuous probe or measurements are obtained every 15–30 minutes for the first hour, then each hour for 4 hours. (See Chapter 21 for a discussion of the physiology of temperature regulation.)

The temperature may be taken either by axilla or rectally (Figure 22–15). In some agencies the initial temperature is taken rectally; other agencies rely exclusively on axillary methods. The rectal route is not recommended as a routine method as it may predispose to rectal mucosal irritation and increase chances of perforation (Avery, 1981). If taken rectally, the thermometer should be held by the nurse for a period of 5 minutes. Care must be taken to avoid inserting the thermometer too far. It is not unusual for an imperforate anus to be diagnosed initially when the nurse is unable to take the temperature rectally.

Axillary temperature reflects skin temperature and the body's compensatory response to changes in the thermal environment. Some clinicians question the accuracy of axillary temperature in the first 24 hours of life due to poor

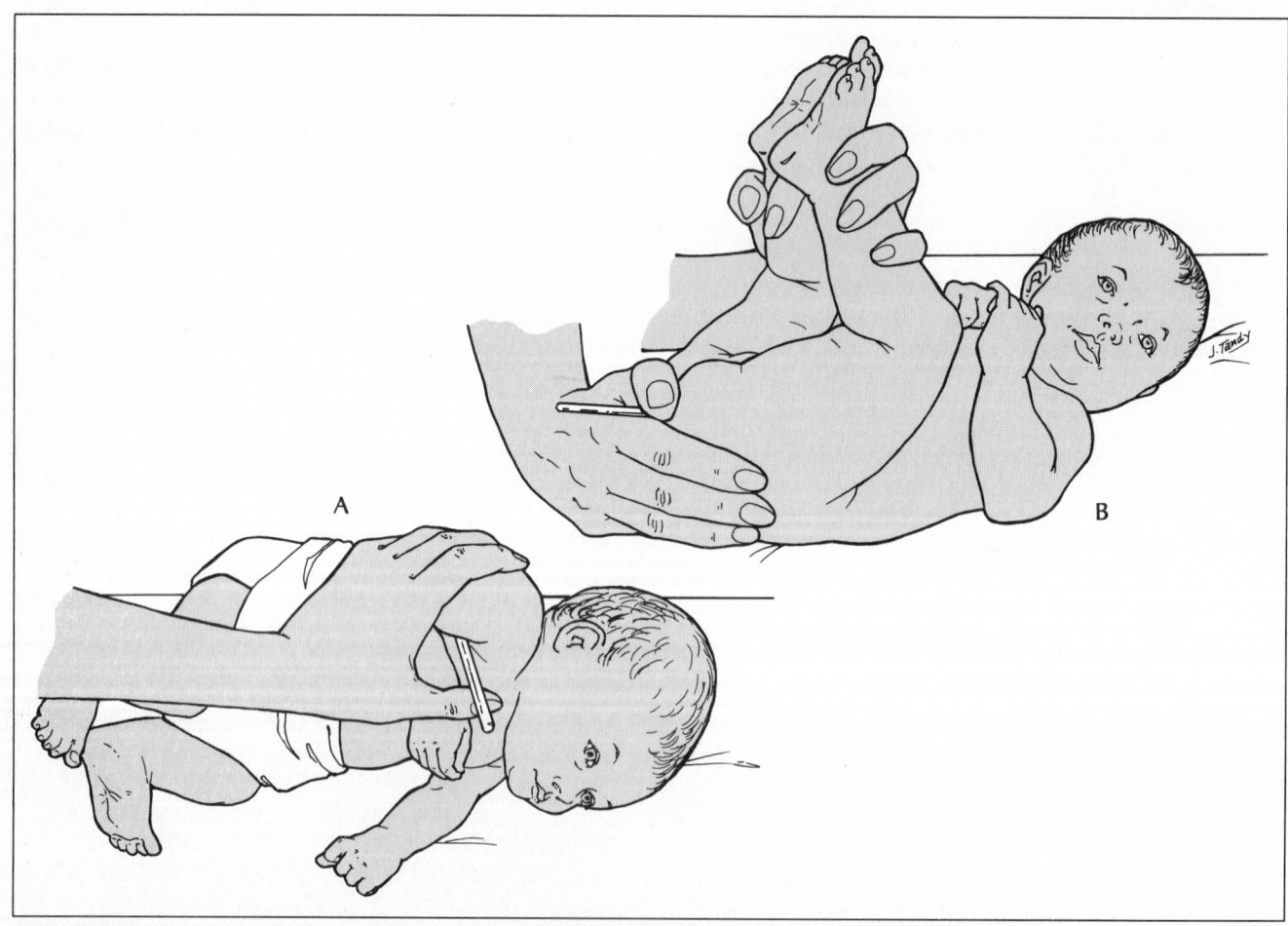

FIGURE 22–15 A, The axillary temperature should be taken for 3 minutes. The newborn's arm should be tightly but gently pressed against the thermometer and the newborn's side as illustrated. **B,** The rectal thermometer must be held in place for 5 minutes and the legs supported.

peripheral circulation. Skin temperature assessment does allow time for initiation of interventions prior to a more serious fall in the core temperature (as assessed by rectal temperatures), which is indicative of compensatory heat-regulatory mechanism failure (Korones, 1981). If the axillary method is used, the thermometer must remain in place at least 3 minutes (Standards and Recommendations, 1977) unless an electronic thermometer is used. Axillary temperatures can provide a false high reading because of friction caused by apposition of inner arm skin and upper chest wall and approximation of brown fat to the probe. The best measure of skin temperature is by means of continuous skin probe rather than axillary temperature, especially for small neonates.

Temperature instability, a deviation of more than 1C (2F) from one reading to the next, or a subnormal temperature may indicate an infection. In contrast with an elevated temperature in older children, an increased temperature in a newborn may indicate reactions to too much covering, too hot a room, or dehydration. Dehydration, which tends to increase body temperature, occurs in newborns whose feedings have been delayed for any reason. Newborns respond to overheating (temperature greater than 37.5C or 99.5F) by increased restlessness and eventually by perspiration. The perspiration is initially seen on the head and face, then on the chest (Hey and Katz, 1968). At 34–36 weeks' gestation, perspiration can appear on the lower extremities.

Skin

The skin of the newborn should be pink-tinged or ruddy in color and warm to the touch. The ruddy color results from increased concentration of red blood cells in the blood vessels and from limited subcutaneous fat deposits. *Acrocyanosis* (bluish discoloration of the hands and feet) may be present in the first 2–6 hours after birth and is due to poor peripheral circulation with resultant vasomotor instability and capillary stasis, especially when the newborn is exposed to cold. If the central circulation is adequate, the blood supply should return quickly when the skin is blanched with a finger. Occasionally a *harlequin* (clown) color change will be noted: A deep red color develops over one side of the infant's body while the other side remains pale, so that the skin resembles a clown's suit. This color aberration results from a vasomotor disturbance in which blood vessels on one side dilate while the vessels on the other side constrict. It usually lasts from 1–20 minutes. Affected neonates may have single or multiple episodes.

Suspected jaundice is evaluated by blanching the tip of the nose or the gum line. This procedure must be carried out in appropriate lighting. If jaundice is present, the area will appear yellowish immediately after blanching. This test determines the existence and, to a limited extent, the degree of jaundice. Evaluation and determination of the

cause of jaundice must be initiated immediately to prevent possible serious sequelae. The jaundice may be related to breast-feeding (small incidence), hematomas, or immature liver function, or may be caused by blood incompatibility or severe hemolytic process.

Erythema neonatorum toxicum is a perifollicular eruption that may be seen in 30%–70% of full-term infants. The peak incidence is 24–48 hours of life. The lesions are firm, vary in size from 1–3 mm, and consist of a white or pale yellow papule or pustule with an erythematous base. The rash may appear suddenly, usually over the trunk and diaper area, and is frequently widespread. The lesions do not appear on the palms of the hands or the soles of the feet. Diagnosis may be confirmed by obtaining a smear of aspirated pustule, which after staining shows numerous eosinophils and no bacteria culture. The etiology is unknown and no treatment is necessary. The lesions disappear in a few hours or days.

Skin turgor is assessed to determine hydration status, the need to initiate early feedings, and the presence of any infectious processes.

Vernix caseosa, a whitish cheeselike substance, covers the fetus while in utero and serves as a skin lubricant for the newborn. It is generally more pronounced on preterm infants. The skin of the term or postterm infant is frequently dry, and peeling is common, especially on the hands and feet. *Milia,* which are plugged sebaceous glands, appear as raised white spots on the face, especially across the nose. *Mongolian spots,* which are macular areas of bluish-black pigmentation found on the lumbar dorsal area and the buttocks, are common in Oriental and black infants and newborns of other dark-skinned races (Colorplate VII). They gradually fade during the first or second year of life.

After a difficult forceps delivery, the newborn may have reddened areas over the cheeks and jaws. It is important to reassure the mother that these will disappear, usually within 1 or 2 days. Transient facial paralysis resulting from the forceps pressure is a rare complication.

Telangiectatic nevi, or "stork bites," are thought to be superficial telangiectatic areas as opposed to new growth of tissue. They appear as pale pink or red spots and are frequently found on the eyelids, nose, lower occipital bone, and nape of the neck. These lesions are common in light-complexioned neonates and are more noticeable during periods of crying. These areas blanch easily, have no clinical significance, and usually fade by the second birthday. *Nevus flammeus,* or port-wine stain, is a capillary angioma directly below the epidermis. It is a nonelevated, sharply demarcated, red to purple birthmark (Colorplate X). The size and shape is variable but it commonly appears on the face. It does not grow in size, does not fade with time, and does not blanch. In the black infant, the nevus flammeus appears jet black in color. The birthmark may be concealed by using an opaque cosmetic cream such as "covermark." If convulsions, contralateral hemiplegia, or intracortical calcification accompanies the nevus flammeus, it is suggestive of Sturge-Weber syndrome. *Nevus vasculosus,* or "strawberry mark," is a capillary hemangioma. It consists of newly formed and enlarged capillaries in the dermal and subdermal layers. It is a raised, clearly delineated, dark red, rough-surfaced birthmark commonly found in the head region. Such marks usually grow (often rapidly) for several months and become fixed in size by 8 months of age. They then begin to regress in size and, except in rare cases, are completely gone by the time the child is 7 years old.

Birthmarks are frequently a cause of concern for the parents. The mother may be especially anxious, fearing that she is to blame ("Is my baby 'marked' because of something I did?"). Guilt feelings are common in the presence of misconceptions about the cause. Birthmarks should be identified and explained to the parents. By providing appropriate information about the cause and course of birthmarks, the nurse frequently allays the fears and anxieties of the family.

Head

GENERAL APPEARANCE

The newborn's head is large (approximately one-fourth of the body size), with soft, pliable skull bones. The head may appear asymmetrical in the newborn of a vertex delivery. This asymmetry, called *molding,* is caused by overriding of the cranial bones during labor and delivery. The degree of molding varies with the degree and length of the pressure exerted. Within a few days after delivery, the overriding usually diminishes and the suture lines become palpable. Because head measurements are affected by molding, a second measurement is indicated a few days after delivery. The heads of breech-born newborns and those delivered by caesarean birth are characteristically round and well shaped, because pressure was not exerted on them during birth. Any extreme differences in head size may indicate microcephaly or hydrocephaly. Variations in the shape, size, or appearance of the head measurements may be due to craniostenosis (premature closure of the cranial sutures) and plagiocephaly (asymmetry caused by pressure on the fetal head during gestation).

Two *fontanelles* ("soft spots") may be palpated on the infant's head. Fontanelles, which are openings at the juncture of the cranial bones, can be measured with the fingers. Accurate measurement necessitates that the examiner's finger be measured in centimeters. The diamond-shaped *anterior fontanelle* is approximately 3–4 cm long by 2–3 cm wide. It is located at the juncture of the frontal and parietal bones. The *posterior fontanelle,* smaller and triangular, is formed by the parietal bones and the occipital bone. The fontanelles will be smaller immediately after birth than several days later because of molding. The

anterior fontanelle closes within 18 months, whereas the posterior fontanelle closes within 8–12 weeks.

The fontanelles are a useful indicator of the newborn's condition. The anterior fontanelle may swell when the newborn cries or may pulsate with the heartbeat, which is normal. A bulging fontanelle usually signifies increased intracranial pressure, and a depressed fontanelle indicates dehydration. An overlapping of the anterior fontanelle occasionally occurs in malnourished or preterm neonates. The sutures between the cranial bones should be palpated for amount of overlapping.

In addition to being inspected for degree of molding and size, the head should be evaluated for soft tissue edema and bruising.

Cephalhematoma. Cephalhematoma is a collection of blood resulting from ruptured blood vessels between the surface of a cranial bone and the periosteal membrane. The scalp in these areas feels loose and slightly edematous. These areas emerge as defined hematomas between the first and second day. Although external pressure may cause the mass to fluctuate, it does not increase in size with crying. Cephalhematomas may be unilateral or bilateral, do not cross suture lines, are relatively common in vertex deliveries, and may disappear within 2–3 weeks or very slowly over subsequent months (Danforth, 1982). Figure 22–16 shows a cephalhematoma.

Caput succedaneum. Caput succedaneum is a localized, easily identifiable soft area of the scalp, generally resulting from a long and difficult labor or vacuum extraction. The sustained pressure of the presenting part against the cervix results in compression of local blood vessels, and venous return is slowed. This causes an increase in tissue fluids, an edematous swelling, and occasional bleeding under the periosteum. The caput may vary from a small area to a severely elongated head. The fluid of the caput is reabsorbed within 12 hours or a few days after birth. Caputs resulting from vacuum extractors are sharply demarcated circular areas that can reach up to 2 cm in thickness. They disappear more slowly than naturally occurring edema. It is possible to distinguish between a cephalhematoma and a caput because the caput overrides suture lines, whereas the cephalhematoma, because of its location, never crosses a suture line (Figure 22–17).

Face

The newborn's face is well designed for sucking. Sucking (fat) pads are located in the cheeks, and a labial tubercle is frequently found in the center of the upper lip. The chin is recessed, and the nose is flattened. The lips are sensitive to touch, and the sucking reflex is easily initiated. Symmetry of the eyes, nose, and ears is evaluated. See the Neonatal Physical Assessment Guide, p. 688, for deviations in symmetry and variations in size, shape, and spacing of facial features. Facial movement symmetry should be as-

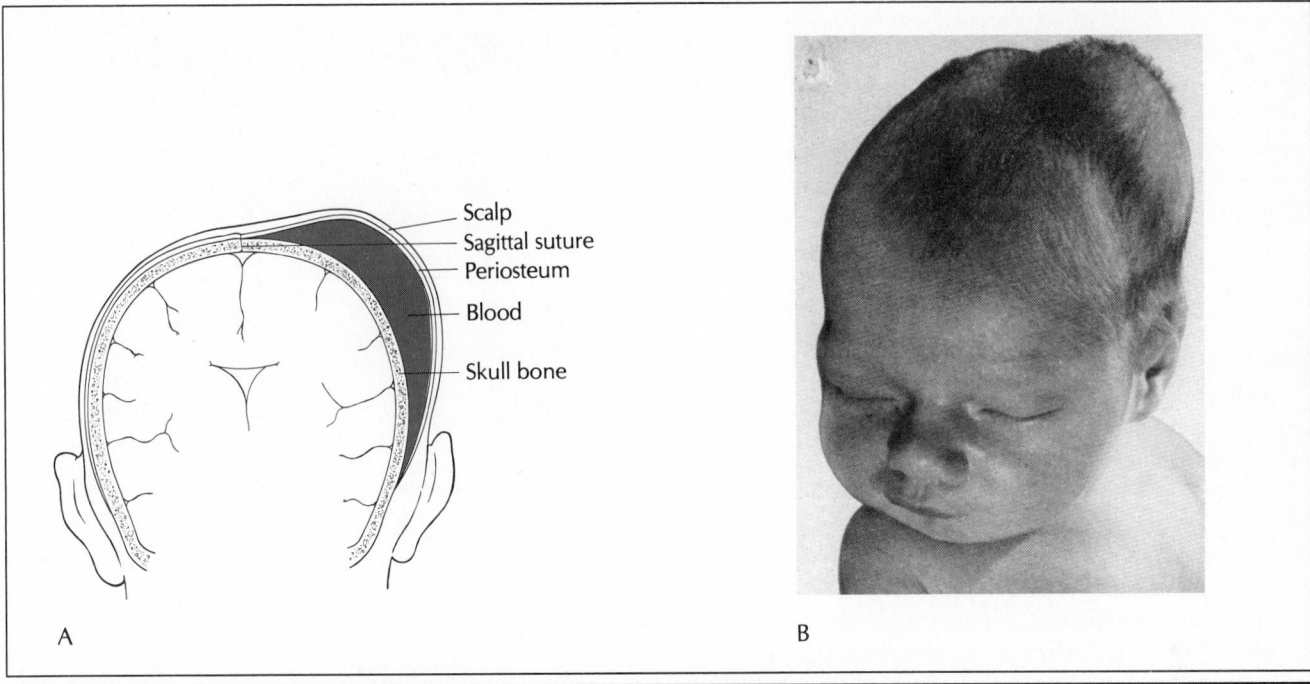

FIGURE 22–16 A, Cephalhematoma is a collection of blood between the surface of a cranial bone and the periosteal membrane. **B,** Cephalhematoma over left parietal bone. (Photo: Reproduced with permission from Potter, E. L., and Craig, J. M.: *Pathology of the fetus and infant,* 3rd ed. Copyright © 1975 by Year Book Medical Publishers, Inc., Chicago.)

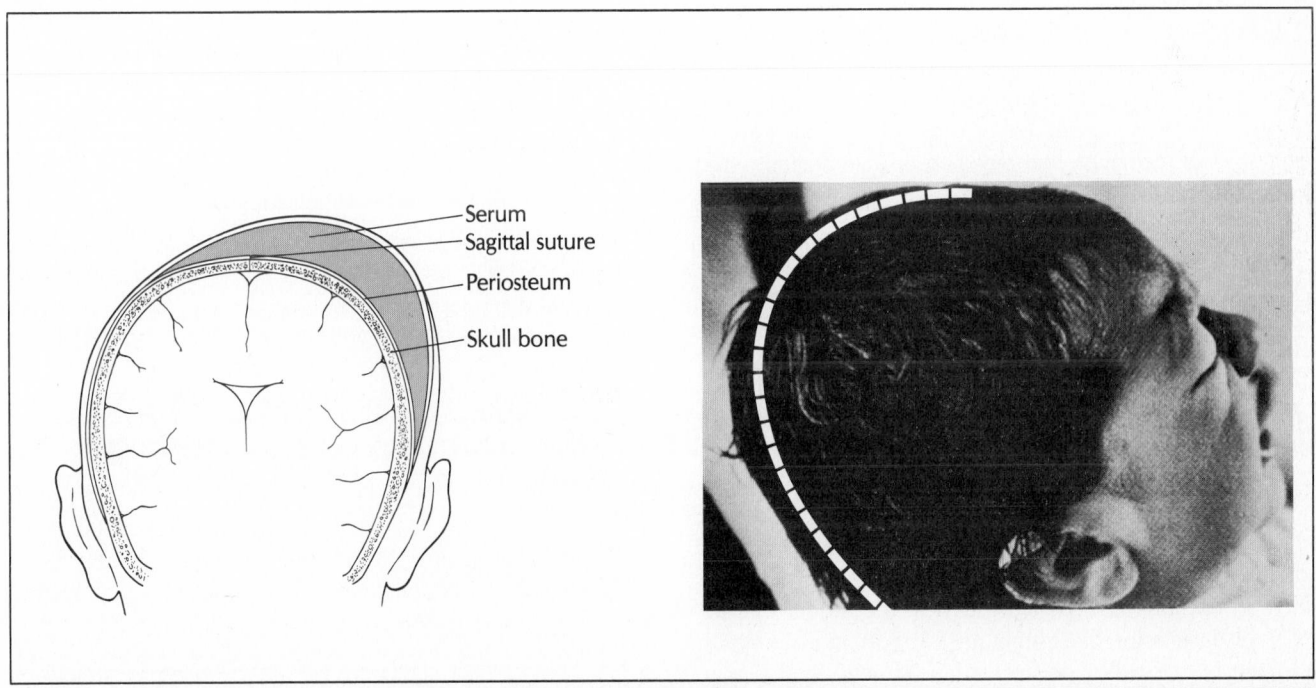

FIGURE 22–17 Caput succedaneum is a collection of fluid (serum) under the scalp. (Photo courtesy Mead Johnson Laboratories, Evansville, Ind.)

sessed to determine presence of facial palsy. Facial paralysis appears when the neonate cries; the affected side is immobile and the palpebral fissure widens (Figure 22–18). It may result from forceps delivery or pressure on the facial nerve from the maternal pelvis during the birth process. Facial paralysis usually disappears within a few days to 3 weeks.

EYES

The eyes of the neonate are a blue or slate blue-gray in color. Scleral color tends to be bluish because of its relative thinness. The infant's eye color usually is established at approximately 3 months of age, although it may change any time up to 1 year. Dark-pigmented neonates tend to have dark eyes at birth.

The eyes should be checked for size, equality of pupil size, reaction of pupils to light, blink reflex to light, and edema and inflammation of the eyelids. The eyelids are usually edematous during the first few days of life because of the delivery and the instillation of silver nitrate drops in the newborn's eyes. Chemical conjunctivitis appears a few hours after the instillation of the silver nitrate drops but disappears without treatment in 1–2 days. In infectious conjunctivitis the infant has the same purulent exudate as in chemical conjunctivitis, but it is caused by staphylococci or a variety of gram-negative rods and requires treatment with ophthalmic antibiotics. Onset is usually after the second day. Edema of the orbits or eyelids may persist for several days until the neonate's kidneys can evacuate the fluid.

Small subconjunctival hemorrhages appear in about 10% of newborns and are commonly found on the inner aspect of the sclera. These are caused by the changes in vascular tension during birth. They will remain for a few weeks and are of no pathologic significance, but parents need reassurance that this bleeding is unimportant, that the infant is not bleeding from within the eye, and that vision will not be impaired.

The neonate may demonstrate transient strabismus due to poor neuromuscular control of eye muscles (Figure 22–19). It gradually regresses in 3–4 months. The "doll's eye" phenomenon is also present for about 10 days after birth. As the newborn's head position is changed to the left and then to the right, the eyes move to the opposite direction. This results from underdeveloped integration of head-eye coordination.

The nurse should observe the neonate's pupils for opacities or whiteness and for the absence of a normal red reflex. Red reflex is a red-orange flash of color observed when an ophthalmoscope light falls on the retina. In newborns of dark color, the retina may appear more greyish. Absence of red reflex occurs with cataracts. In the newborn, congenital cataracts should be suspected in infants of mothers with a history of rubella or cytomegalic inclusion disease.

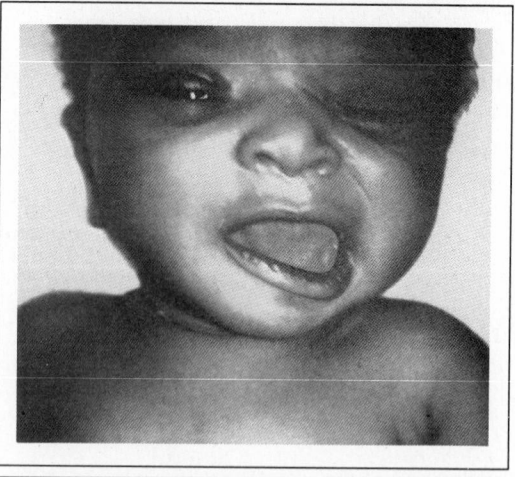

FIGURE 22–18 Facial paralysis. Paralysis of right side of face from injury to right facial nerve. (Courtesy of Dr. Ralph Platow. In Potter, E. L., and Craig, J. M.: *Pathology of the fetus and infant,* 3rd ed. Copyright © 1975 by Year Book Medical Publishers, Inc., Chicago.)

The cry of the neonate is commonly tearless because the lacrimal structures are immature at birth and do not usually become fully functional until the second month of life, although some infants may produce tears during the neonatal period.

Although the newborn's vision is not so acute as that of an adult, they do see. Poor oculomotor coordination and absence of accommodation limit visual abilities, but the newborn does have peripheral vision and can fixate on near objects (3–10 in.) for short periods of time (Kempe et al., 1982). The newborn can perceive faces, shapes, and colors and begins to show visual preferences early. The neonate blinks in response to bright lights, to a tap on the bridge of the nose (glabellar reflex), or to a light touch on

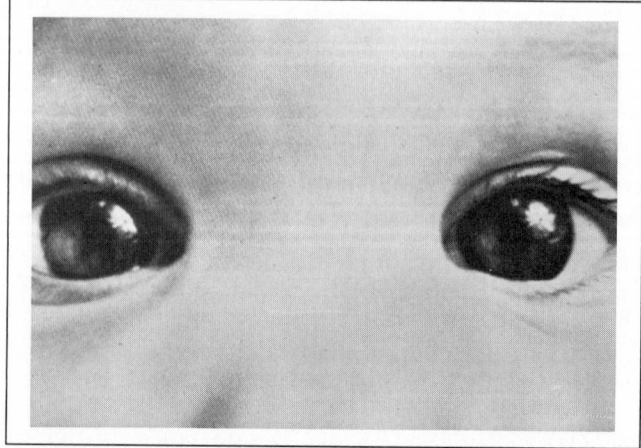

FIGURE 22–19 Transient strabismus may be present in the newborn due to poor neuromuscular control. (Courtesy Mead Johnson Laboratories, Evansville, Ind.)

the eyelids. Pupillary light reflex is also present. Examination of the eye is best accomplished by rocking the newborn from an upright position to the horizontal a few times or by other methods that will elicit an opened-eye response.

NOSE

The neonate's nose is small and narrow. Infants are characteristically nose breathers for the first few months of life. A clear passage must be maintained, free of mucus, or the neonate will suffer respiratory distress. The newborn generally removes the obstruction by sneezing. The nose may also be cleansed by gentle suction with a bulb syringe or catheter. Nasal patency is assured if the neonate breathes easily with mouth closed. If respiratory difficulty occurs, the nurse should check for choanal atresia (see p. 852).

The newborn has the ability to smell after the nasal passages are cleared of amniotic fluid and mucus. This ability is demonstrated by their search for milk. Infants will turn their head toward the milk source, whether bottle or breast.

MOUTH

The lips of the newborn should be pink, and a touch on the lips should produce sucking motions. Saliva is normally scant. The taste buds are developed prior to birth, and the newborn can easily discriminate between sweet and bitter.

The easiest way to completely examine the mouth is to gently stimulate infants to cry by depressing their tongue, thereby causing them to open the mouth fully. It is extremely important to observe the entire mouth to look for a cleft palate, which can be present even in the absence of a cleft lip. The examiner places a clean index finger along the hard and soft palate to feel for any openings.

Occasionally an examination of the gums will reveal *precocious teeth* on the lower central incisor. If they appear loose, they should be removed to prevent aspiration. Gray-white lesions (*inclusion cysts*) on the gums may be confused with teeth. On the hard palate and gum margins, *Epstein's pearls*, small glistening white specks (keratin-containing cysts) that feel hard to the touch are often present. These usually disappear in a few weeks and are of no significance. Thrush may appear as white patches that look like milk curds adhering to the mucous membranes and that cause bleeding when removed. Thrush is caused by *Candida albicans*, often acquired from an infected vaginal tract during birth, and is treated with a preparation of Mystatin.

A neonate who is *tongue-tied* has a ridge of frenulum tissue attached to the underside of the tongue at varying lengths from its base, causing a heart shape at the tip of the tongue. "Clipping the tongue," or cutting the ridge of tissue, is not recommended. This ridge does not affect speech or eating, but cutting does create an entry for infection.

Transient nerve paralysis resulting from birth trauma may be seen by asymmetrical mouth movements when the neonate cries or may be seen as difficulty with sucking and feeding.

EARS

The ears of the newborn may be crumpled or flattened against the skull and should have well-formed cartilage (one determinant of gestational age). In the normal newborn, the top of the ear should be parallel to the outer and inner canthus of the eye. The ears should be inspected for shape, size, and position. Low-set ears are characteristic of many syndromes and may indicate chromosomal abnormalities (especially trisomies 13 and 18), mental retardation, and/or internal organ abnormalities, especially bilateral renal agenesis as a result of embryologic developmental deviations (Figure 22–20). Preauricular skin tags may be present. They are ligated at the base and allowed to slough off.

Following the first cry, the newborn can hear. Hearing becomes acute as mucus from the middle ear is absorbed and the eustachian tube becomes aerated.

Downs and Silver (1972) have identified the following risk factors associated with potential hearing loss:

- The presence of hearing loss in any family member prior to the age of 50 years
- Serum bilirubin level greater than 20 mg/dL for the full-term newborn
- Suspected maternal rubella infection during pregnancy, resulting in congenital rubella syndrome
- Defects of the ear, nose, or throat
- Small neonatal size, particularly less than 1500 g at birth

The newborn's hearing is evaluated by response to loud or moderately loud noises unaccompanied by vibrations. The neonate should stir or awaken in response to the nearby sounds while asleep.

Neck

A short neck, creased with skin folds, is characteristic of the normal newborn. Because muscle tone is not well developed, the neck cannot support the full weight of the head, which rotates freely. The head lags considerably when the neonate is pulled from a supine to a sitting position, but the prone infant is able to raise the head slightly. The neck should be palpated for masses and presence of lymph nodes and should be inspected for webbing. Adequacy of range of motion and neck muscle function is determined by fully extending the head in all directions. Injury to the sternocleidomastoid muscle (congenital torticollis) must be considered in the presence of neck rigidity.

The clavicles should be evaluated for evidence of fractures, which occasionally occur during difficult deliveries or in neonates with broad shoulders. The normal clavicle is straight. If fractured, a lump and a snapping sensation during movements may be palpated along the course of the side of the break. The Moro reflex should also be elicited to evaluate bilateral equal movement of the arms. If the clavicle is fractured, the response will be demonstrated only on the unaffected side.

Chest

The thorax is cylindrical at birth, and the ribs are flexible. Chest circumference is less than head circumference and remains so until the child is about 2 years old. The general appearance of the chest should be assessed. A protrusion at the lower end of the sternum, called the *xiphoid cartilage*, is frequently seen. It is under the skin and will become less apparent after several weeks because of accumulation of adipose tissue.

As mentioned earlier, engorged breasts occur frequently in male and female newborns. This condition, which occurs by the third day, is a result of maternal hormonal influences and may last up to 2 weeks. The infant's breast should not be massaged or squeezed, because this practice may cause a breast abscess. Extra or *supernumerary nipples* are occasionally noted below and medial to the true nipples (Figure 22–21). These harmless pink spots vary in size and do not contain glandular tissue (Korones, 1981). At puberty, the accessory nipple may darken. Assessment and differentiation from a pigmented nevi (mole) are facilitated by placing the fingertips alongside the accessory nipple and pulling the adjacent tissue laterally. The accessory nipple will appear dimpled.

Cry

The neonate's cry should be strong, lusty, and of medium pitch. A high-pitched, shrill cry is abnormal and may indicate neurologic disorders or hypoglycemia. The neonate's cry is an important method of communication and alerts caretakers to changes in his condition and needs.

Respiration

Normal breathing for a term newborn is between 30 and 50 respirations/min. It is predominantly diaphragmatic, with associated rising and falling of the abdomen with inspiration and expiration. Any signs of respiratory distress—nasal flaring, intercostal or xiphoid retraction, expiratory grunt or sigh, seesaw respirations, or tachypnea—should be noted. Hyperextension (chest appears high) or hypoextension (chest appears low) of the anteroposterior diameter of the chest should also be noted. Auscultation should be done over both the anterior and posterior chest. Some breath sounds are heard better when the neonate is

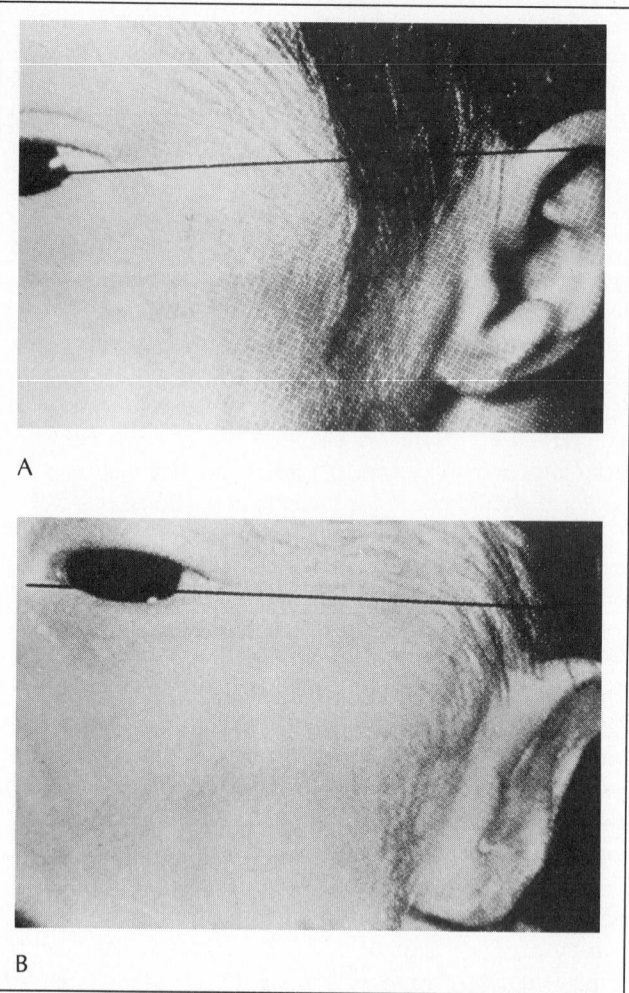

FIGURE 22–20 The position of the external ear may be assessed by drawing a line across the inner and outer canthus of the eye to the insertion of the ear. **A,** Normal position. **B,** True low-set. (Courtesy Mead Johnson Laboratories, Evansville, Ind.)

crying, but localization and identification of breath sounds are difficult in the newborn. Because sounds may be transmitted from the unaffected lung to the affected lung, the absence of breath sounds cannot be diagnosed. Air entry may be noisy in the first couple of hours until fluid resolves, especially in cesarean births.

Heart

Heart rates are rapid (100–180 beats/min) in neonates but fluctuate a great deal. Auscultation provides the nurse with valuable assessment data. The heart is examined for rate and rhythm, position of apical impulse, and heart sound intensity.

The pulse rate is labile and follows the trend of respirations in the neonatal period. The pulse rate is influenced by

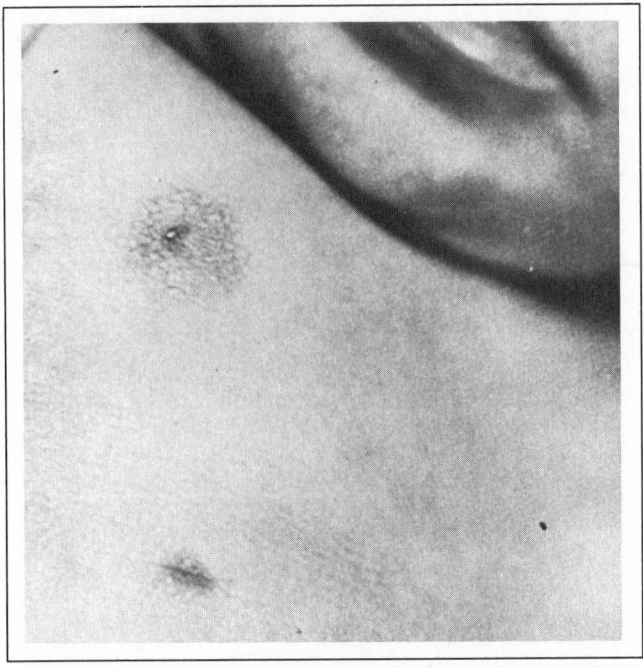

FIGURE 22-21 Extra or supernumerary nipples may appear below and medial to the true nipples. (Courtesy Mead Johnson Laboratories, Evansville, Ind.)

physical activity, crying, state of wakefulness, and body temperature. The usual rate is 120–150 beats/min. If the neonate is sleeping, the rate can be as low as 70–90 beats/min. If the neonate is crying, the pulse rate may be as high as 180 beats/min. Auscultation should be performed over the entire precordium, below the left axilla, and posteriorly below the scapula.

The placement of the heart in the chest should be determined when the neonate is in a quiet state. The heart is relatively large at birth and is located high in the chest, with its apex somewhere between the fourth and fifth intercostal space.

A shift in the mediastinum to either side may indicate pneumothorax, dextrocardia (heart placement on the right side of the chest), or a diaphragmatic hernia. These and many other problems can be diagnosed early with a stethoscope and a trained ear. Normally the heart beat has a "toc tic" sound. A slur or slushing sound (usually after the first sound) may indicate a *murmur*. Although 90% of all murmurs are transient and are considered normal (Korones, 1981), they should be observed closely by a physician. Some murmurs are evidence of a delay in closure of the fetal circulatory passages. Conversely, significant murmurs may not appear immediately after birth.

Neonatal peripheral circulation is sluggish initially, resulting in cyanosis of the extremities (acrocyanosis) for several hours after delivery. *Mottling* also occurs as a result of general circulatory lability. It may last several hours to several weeks or may come and go periodically.

Brachial pulses should be palpated bilaterally for equality and should be compared with the femoral pulses. Femoral pulses are palpated by applying gentle pressure with the middle finger over the femoral canal. Decreased or absent femoral pulses indicate coarctation of the aorta, and require additional investigation. A wide difference in blood pressure between the upper and lower extremities also indicates coarctation. Blood pressure is usually 80/40 mm Hg at birth, and by the tenth day of life, 100/50 mm Hg. It may be difficult to obtain the diastolic pressure or to hear the blood pressure with a standard sphygmomanometer. Blood pressures may not routinely be measured on newborns unless they are having distress, are premature, or are suspected of some anomaly.

Abdomen

Without disturbing the infant, one can learn a great deal about the newborn's abdomen. The shape should be cylindrical, with some protrusion. A certain amount of laxness of the abdominal muscles can be seen. The absence of abdominal contents is suggested if the abdomen has a scaphoid appearance. No cyanosis should be present, and few if any blood vessels should be apparent to the eye. There should be no gross distention or bulging. The more distended the abdomen, the tighter the skin becomes, with engorged vessels appearing. Distention is the first sign of many of the abnormalities found in the gastrointestinal tract.

Abdominal palpation should be done in a systematic manner. The nurse palpates each of the four abdominal quadrants and moves in a clockwise direction until all four quadrants have been palpated for softness or tenderness and the presence of masses.

When palpating the abdomen, one should feel for the liver and both kidneys. The newborn's liver is large in proportion to the rest of the body and can usually be felt between 1 and 2 cm below the right costal margin. Kidneys are more difficult to feel, but examination is facilitated if done within 4–6 hours after birth, before the intestines become distended with air and feedings are initiated. By placing a finger at the posterior flank and pushing upward while pressing downward with the opposite hand, each kidney may be palpated as a firm oval mass between the examiner's finger and hand. The lower pole of the kidney is usually found about 1–2 cm above the umbilicus. The spleen tip is palpated in the lateral aspect of the left upper quadrant in the normal newborn.

Initially the umbilical cord is white and gelatinous in appearance, with the two umbilical arteries and one umbilical vein readily apparent. Because a single umbilical artery is frequently associated with congenital anomalies, the vessels should be counted as part of the newborn assessment. The cord begins drying within 1 or 2 hours after delivery and is shriveled and blackened by the second or third day.

Within 7–10 days it sloughs off, although a granulating area may be evident for a few days longer.

Cord bleeding is abnormal and may result because the cord was inadvertently pulled or because the cord clamp was loosened. Foul-smelling drainage is also abnormal and is generally caused by infection. Such infection requires immediate treatment to prevent the development of septicemia. If the neonate has a patent urachus (abnormal connection between the umbilicus and bladder), moistness or draining urine may be apparent at the base of the cord.

Genitals

MALE INFANTS

The penis should be inspected to determine whether the urinary orifice is correctly positioned. *Hypospadias* occurs when the urinary meatus is located on the ventral surface of the penis. It occurs most commonly in whites in the United States (Holmes, 1976). *Phimosis* is a condition commonly occurring in newborn males in which the opening of the prepuce is narrowed and the foreskin cannot be retracted over the glans. This condition may interfere with urination, so the adequacy of the urinary stream should be evaluated.

The scrotum should be inspected for size and symmetry and should be palpated to verify the presence of both testes. Scrotal edema and discoloration are common in breech deliveries. Hydroceles are common in newborns and should be identified. The testes should be palpated separately between the thumb and forefinger, with the thumb and forefinger of the other hand placed together over the inguinal canal.

FEMALE INFANTS

The labia majora, labia minora, and clitoris should be examined, and the nurse should note the size of each as appropriate for gestational age. A vaginal tag or hymenal tag is often evident and will usually disappear in a few weeks. During the first week of life, the neonate may have a vaginal discharge composed of thick whitish mucus. This discharge, which can become tinged with blood, is referred to as *pseudomenstruation* and is caused by the withdrawal of maternal hormones. Smegma, a white cheeselike substance, is often present under the labia.

Anus

The anal area should be inspected to verify that it is patent and has no fissure. Imperforate anus and rectal atresia may be ruled out by a digital examination. The passage of the first meconium stool should also be noted. Atresia of the gastrointestinal tract or meconium ileus with resultant obstruction must be considered if no meconium has been passed in the first 24 hours of life.

Extremities

Extremities are examined for gross deformities, extra digits or webbing, clubfoot, and range of motion. The normal neonate's extremities appear short, are generally flexed, and move symmetrically.

ARMS AND HANDS

Nails are present and extend beyond the fingertips in term infants. Fingers and toes should be counted. *Polydactyly* occurs when there are extra digits on either the hands or feet. Polydactyly is more common in blacks (Holmes, 1976). It can be seen with a dominant disorder. If the infant has polydactyly and the parents do not, a dominant disorder can be ruled out. *Syndactyly* refers to fusion (webbing) of fingers or toes. Hands should be inspected for normal palmar creases. A single palmar crease, called *simian line* (see Figure 7–20) is frequently present in children with Down syndrome.

Brachial palsy, which is partial or complete paralysis of portions of the arm, results from trauma to the brachial plexus during a difficult delivery. It occurs most commonly when strong traction is exerted on the head of the neonate in an attempt to deliver a shoulder lodged behind the symphysis pubis in the presence of shoulder dystocia. Brachial palsy may also occur during a breech delivery if an arm becomes trapped over the head and traction is exerted.

The portion of the arm affected is determined by the nerves damaged. *Erb-Duchenne paralysis* involves damage to the upper arm (fifth and sixth cervical nerves) and is the most common type. Injury to the eighth cervical and first thoracic nerve roots and the lower portion of the plexus produces the relatively rare *lower arm injury*, whereas the *whole arm type* results from damage to the entire plexus.

With Erb-Duchenne paralysis, the infant's arm lies limply at the side. The elbow is held in extension, with the forearm pronated. The infant is unable to elevate the arm, and the Moro reflex cannot be elicited on the affected side (Figure 22–22). When lower arm injury occurs, paralysis of the hand and wrist results; complete paralysis of the limb occurs with the whole arm type.

Treatment involves passive range-of-motion exercises to prevent muscle contractures and to restore function. The nurse should carefully instruct the parents in the correct method of performing the exercises and provide for supervised practice sessions. In more severe cases, splinting of the arm is indicated until the edema decreases. The arm is held in a position of abduction and external rotation with the elbow flexed 90°. The "Statue of Liberty" splint is commonly used, although similar results are obtained by attaching a strip of muslin to the head of the crib and tying the other end around the wrist, thereby holding the arm up.

Prognosis is related to the degree of nerve damage resulting from trauma and hemorrhage within the nerve

FIGURE 22–22 Erb's palsy resulting from injury to fifth and sixth cervical roots of brachial plexus. (Photos: Reproduced with permission from Potter, E. L. and Craig, J. M.: *Pathology of the fetus and infant,* 3rd ed. Copyright © 1975 by Year Book Medical Publishers, Inc. Chicago.)

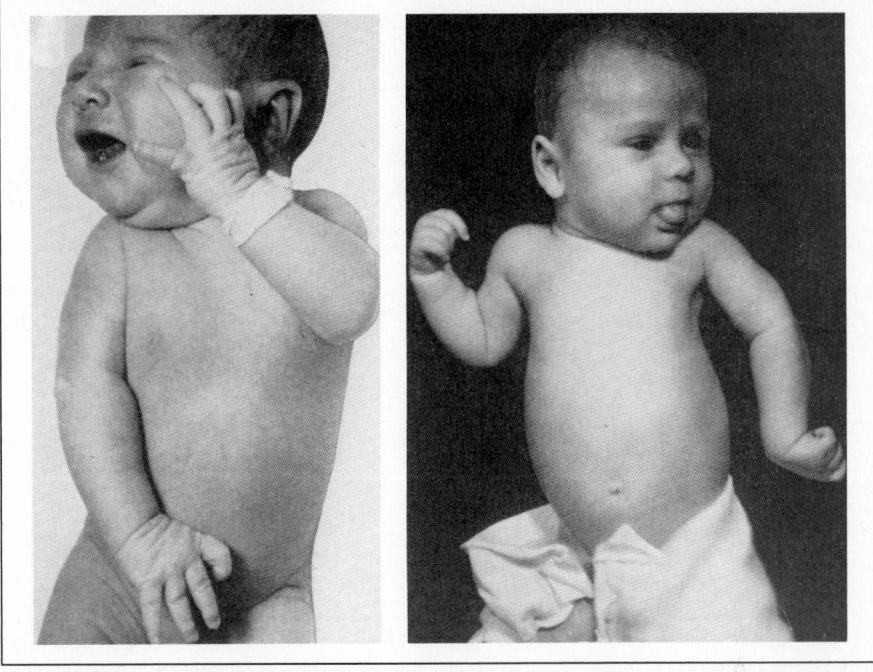

sheath. Complete recovery occurs within a few months with minimal trauma. Moderate trauma may result in some partial paralysis. Recovery is unlikely with severe trauma, and muscle wasting may develop.

LEGS AND FEET

The legs of the newborn should be of equal length, with symmetrical skin folds. *Ortolani's maneuver* (see Figure 26–12, A) is performed to rule out the possibility of congenital hip dysplasia. With the neonate supine, the nurse places thumbs on the inner thighs and fingers on the outer aspect of the neonate's leg from the knee to the head of the femur. The legs are flexed, then abducted and pressed downward. If a click is felt under the index finger, a dislocation exists.

The feet are then examined for evidence of a talipes deformity (clubfoot). Intrauterine position frequently causes the feet to appear to turn inward. If the feet can easily be returned to the midline by manipulation, no treatment is indicated. Further investigation is indicated when the foot will not turn to a midline position or align readily.

The femoral and pedal pulses should be palpated. Absence of pulses in the lower extremities is a classic sign of coarctation of the aorta and requires additional investigation.

Back

With the neonate prone, the nurse should examine the back. The spine should appear straight and flat, because the lumbar and sacral curves do not develop until the in-fant begins to sit. The base of the spine is then examined for a dermal sinus. The nevus pilosus ("hairy nerve") is only occasionally found at the base of the spine in newborns, but it is significant because it is frequently associated with spina bifida.

Neurologic Status

Neonatal tremors are common in the full-term infant and must be evaluated to differentiate them from a convulsion. A fine jumping of the muscle is likely to be a CNS disorder and requires further evaluation. Tremors may also be related to hypoglycemia or hypocalcemia. Neonatal seizures may consist of no more than chewing or swallowing movements, deviations of the eyes, rigidity, or flaccidity because of CNS immaturity.

The CNS of the newborn is immature and characterized by a variety of reflexes. Because the newborn's movements are uncoordinated, methods of communication are limited, and control of bodily functions drastically limited, the reflexes serve a variety of purposes. Some are protective (blink, gag, sneeze), some aid in feeding (rooting, sucking), and some stimulate human interaction (grasping). Neonatal reflexes and general neurologic activity should be carefully assessed.

The most common reflexes found in the normal neonate are the following:

Tonic neck reflex (fencer position). When the neonate is in the supine position, if the head is turned to one side, the extremities on the same side straighten, whereas on the opposite side they flex (Figure 22–23). This reflex may

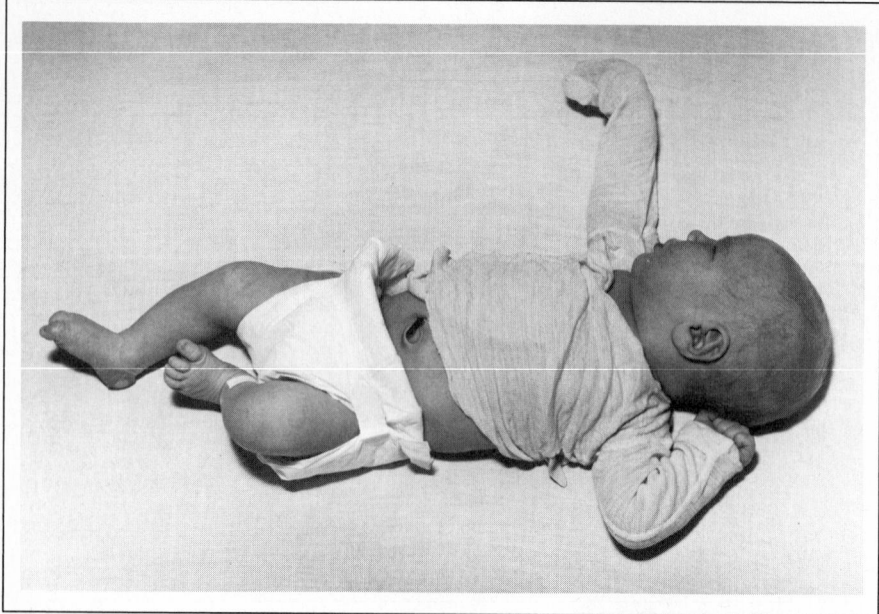

FIGURE 22–23 Tonic neck reflex.

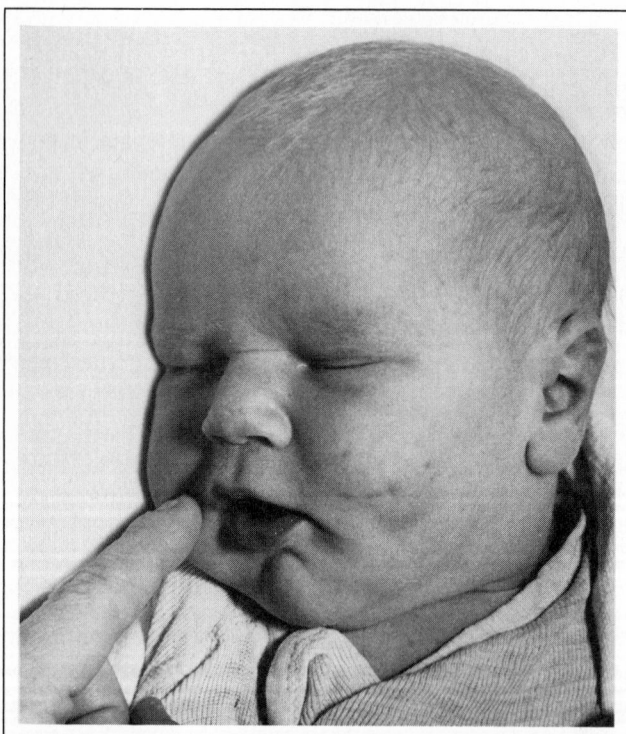

FIGURE 22–24 Rooting reflex.

the chest, as in an embrace. The fingers spread, forming a C, and the infant may cry.

Grasp reflex. If the palm is stimulated with a finger or object, the infant grasps and holds it firmly enough to be lifted momentarily from the crib.

Rooting reflex. When the side of the infant's mouth or cheek is touched, the newborn turns toward that side and opens the lips to suck (Figure 22–24).

Sucking reflex. When an object is placed in the neonate's mouth, a sucking motion begins.

Plantar grasp and *Babinski reflexes.* These are described in the Assessment Guide, p. 688.

In addition to these reflexes, the infant can blink, yawn, cough, sneeze, and draw back from pain (protective reflexes). Neonates can even move a little on their own. When placed on their stomach, they push up and try to crawl (*prone crawl*). When he or she is held upright with one foot touching a flat surface, the neonate puts one foot in front of the other and walks (*stepping reflex*) (Figure 22–25). This reflex is more pronounced at birth and is lost in 1–2 months.

Brazelton (1977) recommends the following steps as a means of assessing CNS integration:

1. Insert a clean finger into the newborn's mouth to elicit a sucking reflex.

2. As soon as the neonate is sucking vigorously, assess hearing and vision responses by noting sucking changes in the presence of a light, rattle, and a voice.

3. The neonate should respond with a brief cessation of sucking followed by continuous sucking with repetitious stimulation.

not be seen during the early neonatal period, but once it appears it persists until about the third month.

Moro reflex. When the neonate is startled by a loud noise or by being lifted slightly above the crib and then suddenly lowered, the infant straightens arms and hands outward while the knees flex. Slowly the arms return to

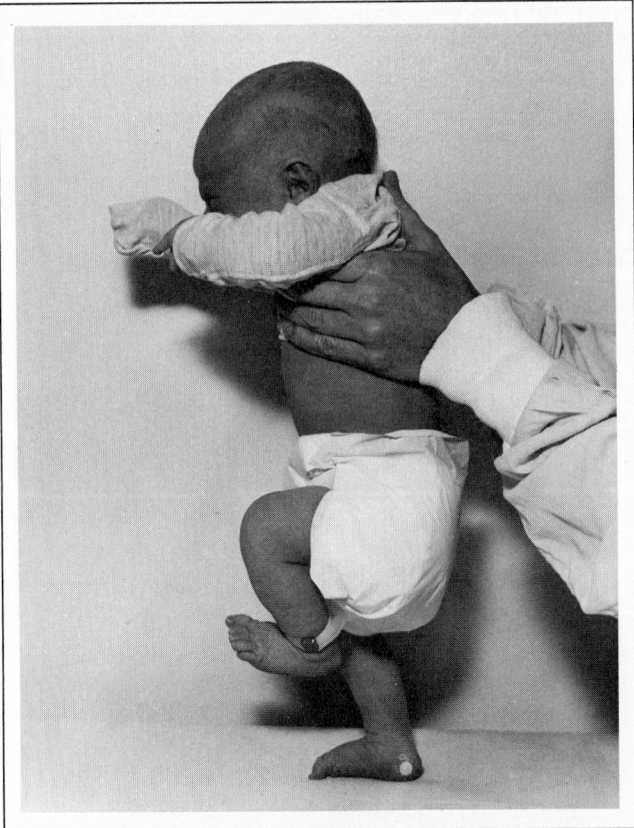

FIGURE 22-25 Stepping reflex disappears after about 1 month.

This examination demonstrates auditory and visual integrity as well as the ability for complex behavioral interactions.

NEONATAL PHYSICAL ASSESSMENT

Following is a guide (p. 688) for systematically assessing the newborn. Normal findings, alterations, and related causes are presented, in correlation with suggested nursing respon- ses. The findings are based on a full-term neonate.

NEONATAL BEHAVIORAL ASSESSMENT

Two conflicting forces influence parents' perceptions of their infant. One is the parents' preconceptions, based on hopes and fears, of what their newborn will be like. The other is their initial reaction to the infant's temperament, behaviors, and physical appearance.

Brazelton (1973) has developed a tool that has revolutionized our understanding and perception of the new-

born's capabilities and responses, permitting us to recognize each infant's individuality. This assessment tool provides valuable guidelines for assessing the newborn's state changes, temperament, and individual behavior patterns. It provides a means by which the health care provider, in conjunction with the parents (primary caregivers), can identify and understand the individual newborn's states. Parents learn which responses, interventions, or activities best meet the special needs of their infant, and this understanding fosters positive bonding experiences.

The assessment tool attempts to identify the infant's repertoire of behavioral responses to the environment and also documents the infant's neurologic adequacy. The examination usually takes 20 to 30 minutes and involves about 30 different tests and maneuvers.* The scale includes 27 behavioral items, each scored on a 9-point scale, and 20 elicited reflexes, which are scored on a 3-point scale. The behavioral items are as follows:

- Response decrement to light
- Response decrement to rattle
- Response decrement to bell
- Response decrement to pinprick
- Inanimate visual orientation
- Inanimate auditory orientation
- Animate visual orientation
- Animate auditory orientation
- Animate visual and auditory orientation
- Alertness
- General tonus
- Motor maturity
- Pull to sit
- Cuddliness
- Defensive movements
- Consolability
- Peak of excitement
- Rapidity of buildup
- Irritability
- Activity
- Tremulousness
- Startles
- Lability of skin color
- Lability of states
- Self-quieting activity
- Hand-mouth facility
- Smiles

*For a complete discussion of all test items and maneuvers, the student is referred to the original scale.

(Text continues on p. 705.)

NEONATAL PHYSICAL ASSESSMENT GUIDE

Assess	Normal findings	Alterations and possible causes*	Nursing responses to data base†
Vital signs			
Blood pressure	At birth: 80–60/45–30 mm Hg Day 10: 100/50 mm Hg (may be unable to measure diastolic pressure with standard sphygmomanometer)	Low BP (hypovolemia, shock)	Monitor BP in all cases of distress, prematurity, or suspected anomaly Low BP; refer to physician immediately so measures to support adequacy of circulation are initiated
Pulse	120–150 beats/min (if asleep 70–90/min; if crying, up to 180/min)	Weak pulse (decreased cardiac output) Bradycardia (severe asphyxia) Tachycardia (over 160/min at rest) (infection, CNS problems)	Assess skin perfusion by capillary refill test Correlate finding with BP assessments; refer to physician Carry out neurologic and thermoregulation assessments
Respirations	30–50 respirations/min. Synchronization of chest and abdominal movements Diaphragmatic and abdominal breathing Transient tachypnea	Tachypnea (pneumonia, RDS) Rapid, shallow breathing (hypermagnesemia due to large doses given toxemic mothers) Grunting expiratory, subcostal and substernal retractions, flaring of nares (respiratory distress) Apnea (cold stress, respiratory disorder) Respirations below 30/min (maternal anesthesia or analgesia)	Identify sleep–wake state, correlate with respiratory pattern Evaluate for all signs of respiratory distress; report findings to physician
Crying	Strong and lusty Moderate tone and pitch Alternate periods of excitability and quietness Cries vary in length from 3–7 min after consoling measures are used	High-pitched, shrill (neurologic disorder, hypoglycemia) Weak or absent (CNS disorder, laryngeal problem)	Discuss neonate's use of cry for communication Assess and record abnormal cries
Temperature	Axilla 36.5–37C (97.7–98.6F) Rectal 35.5–37.2C (96–99F); 36.8C (98.8F) desired Heavier neonates tend to have higher body temperatures	Elevated temperature (room too warm, too much clothing or covers, dehydration, sepsis, brain damage) Subnormal temperature (infection, brain stem involvement, cold) Swings of more than 2F from one reading to next or subnormal temperature (infection)	Attempt to identify cause; notify physician of elevation or drop Counsel parents on possible causes of elevated or low temperatures, appropriate home care measures, when to call physician Teach parents how to take rectal and/or axillary temperature; assess ability to read thermometer; provide information as needed

* Possible causes of alterations are placed in parentheses.
† This column provides guidelines for further assessment and initial nursing interventions.

NEONATAL PHYSICAL ASSESSMENT GUIDE Cont'd

Assess	Normal findings	Alterations and possible causes*	Nursing responses to data base†
Weight	2950–3515 g (6.5–7.75 lb)	< 2748 g (< 6 lb) = SGA or preterm infant > 4050 g (> 9 lb) = LGA (infants of diabetic clients)	Plot weight and gestational age to identify high-risk infants Ascertain genetic predisposition for body build Counsel parents regarding appropriate caloric intake
	Within first 3 to 4 days, normal weight loss of 5%–15% Large babies tend to lose more due to greater fluid loss in proportion to birth weight	Loss greater than 5%–15% (small fluid intake, loss of meconium and urine, feeding difficulties)	Notify physician of net losses or gains Calculate fluid intake and losses from all sources (insensible water loss, radiant warmers, and phototherapy lights) Weight gain in 8–12 hours if loss is excessive
Length	45 cm (18 in.) to 52.3 cm (20.5 in.) Grows 10 cm (4 in.) during first 3 months or approximately 2.5 cm (1 in.) per month for next 6 months	Less than 45 cm (congenital dwarf) Too long Short long bones proximally (achondroplasia) Short long bones distally (Ellis-Van Creveld)	Assess for other signs of dwarfism Determine other signs of skeletal system adequacy Plot progress at subsequent well-baby visits
Posture	Body usually flexed, hands tightly clenched, neck appears short as chin rests on chest	Only extension noted, inability to move from midline (trauma, hypoxia, immaturity) Constant motion	Record spontaneity of motor activity and symmetry of movements If parents express concern about neonate's movement patterns, reassure and evaluate further if appropriate
	Appearance: prominent abdomen with sloping shoulders, narrow hips, rounded chest In breech deliveries, feet are usually dorsiflexed		
Skin Color	Color consistent with racial background	Pallor of face, conjunctiva (anemia, hypothermia, anoxia)	Discuss with parents common skin color variations to allay fears
	Pink-tinged or ruddy color over face, trunk, extremities	Beefy red (hypoglycemia, immature vasomotor reflexes, polycythemia)	Document extent and time of occurrence of color change
	Common variations: acrocyanosis, periorbital cyanosis, circumoral cyanosis, or harlequin color change	Meconium staining (fetal distress)	Assess for respiratory difficulty Obtain Hb and hematocrit values

* Possible causes of alterations are placed in parentheses.
† This column provides guidelines for further assessment and initial nursing interventions.

NEONATAL PHYSICAL ASSESSMENT GUIDE Cont'd

Assess	Normal findings	Alterations and possible causes*	Nursing responses to data base†
		Icterus (hemolytic reaction from blood incompatibility, sepsis)	Perform differential diagnosis to determine whether deviation is physiologic or pathologic jaundice
	Mottled when undressed	Cyanosis (choanal atresia, CNS damage or trauma, respiratory or cardiac problem, cold stress)	Assess degree of (central or peripheral) cyanosis and causative condition; refer to physician
	Minor bruising over buttocks in breech presentation and over eyes and forehead in facial presentations		Discuss with parents cause and course of minor bruising related to labor and delivery
Texture	Smooth, soft, flexible; may have dry peeling hands and feet	Generalized cracked or peeling skin (SGA or postterm, blood incompatibility, metabolic kidney dysfunction)	Perform differential diagnosis
		Scalines (eczema on cheeks, behind ears, on popliteal and antecubital areas)	
		Seborrhea-dermatitis (cradle cap)	Instruct parents to shampoo the scalp and anterior fontanelle area daily; soap should be used and oil avoided; rinse well
		Large amount of lanugo (preterm)	
		Rough or dry (frequent bathing)	
		Absence of vernix (postmature)	
		Yellow vernix (bilirubin staining)	
Turgor: pinch skin (lower abdomen) in "tent shape"	Elastic, returns to normal shape after pinching	Maintains tent shape (dehydration)	Assess for other signs and symptoms of dehydration
Pigmentation	Clear; milia across bridge of nose or forehead will disappear within a few weeks		Advise parents not to pinch or prick these pimplelike areas
	Café-au-lait spots (one or two)	Six or more (neurologic disorder such as von Recklinghausen disease, cutaneous neurofibromatosis)	
	Mongolian spots or macular bluish-black pigmentation over lumbar dorsal area and buttocks; common in ethnic infants of color	Xanthoma (benign or may be associated with abnormal metabolism of lipids)	Assure parents of normalcy of this pigmentation; it will fade in first year or two
			Reassure parents that xanthoma plaques will disappear in a few weeks
	Erythema neonatorum toxicum	Impetigo (group A β-hemolytic streptococcus or *Staphylococcus aureus* infection)	If impetigo occurs, instruct parents about hand-washing and linen precautions during home care

* Possible causes of alterations are placed in parentheses.
† This column provides guidelines for further assessment and initial nursing interventions.

NEONATAL PHYSICAL ASSESSMENT GUIDE Cont'd

Assess	Normal findings	Alterations and possible causes*	Nursing responses to data base†
	Telangiectatic nevi Birthmarks	Hemangiomas: Nevus flammeus (port-wine stain) Nevus vascularus (strawberry hemangioma) Cavernous hemangiomas	Collaborate with physician Counsel parents about birthmark's progression to allay misconceptions Record size and shape of hemangiomas Refer for follow-up at well-baby clinic
	Moles	Any mole or growth that changes in color or character Rashes (infection)	Refer to physician Assess location and type of rash (macular, papular, vesicular) Obtain history of onset, prenatal history, and related signs and symptoms
	Petechiae of head or neck (breech presentation, cord around neck)	Generalized petechiae (clotting abnormalities)	Determine cause; advise parents if further health care is needed
Head General appearance, size, movement	Round, symmetrical, and moves easily from left to right and up and down; soft, pliable	Asymmetrical, flattened occiput on either side of head (plagiocephaly) Head held at angle (torticollis)	Instruct parents to change infant's sleeping positions frequently
		Unable to move head side-to-side (neurologic trauma)	Determine adequacy of all neurologic signs
	Circumference: 33–35 cm (13–14 in.); 2 cm greater than chest circumference	Extreme differences in size may be: microencephaly (Cornelia De Lange syndrome, CID, rubella, toxoplasmosis, chromosome abnormalities), hydrocephaly (meningomyelocele, achondroplasia), anencephaly (neural tube defect) Head is 3 cm or more larger than chest circumference (preterm, hydrocephaly)	Measure circumference from occiput to frontal area, using metal or paper tape Measure chest circumference using metal or paper tape and compare to head circumference
	One-fourth of body size		Record measurements on growth chart
	Size increases 2 in. during first 4 months of life		Reevaluate at well-baby visits
	Common variations: Molding—overriding of cranial bones during delivery Breech and cesarean newborns' heads are round and well shaped	Cephalhematomas (trauma during delivery, persist up to 3 weeks) Caput succedaneum (long labor and delivery, disappears in 1 week)	Reassure parents regarding common manifestations due to birth process and when they should disappear

* Possible causes of alterations are placed in parentheses.
† This column provides guidelines for further assessment and initial nursing interventions.

NEONATAL PHYSICAL ASSESSMENT GUIDE Cont'd

Assess	Normal findings	Alterations and possible causes*	Nursing responses to data base†
Fontanelles Palpation of juncture of cranial bones	Anterior fontanelle: 3–4 cm long by 2–3 cm wide, diamond-shaped, closes within 18 months Posterior fontanelle: 1–2 cm at birth, triangle-shaped, closes in 8–12 weeks	Overlapping of anterior fontanelle (malnourished or preterm infant) Premature closure of sutures (craniostenosis) Late closure (hydrocephaly)	Discuss normal closure times with parents and care of "soft spots" to allay misconceptions Refer to physician Observe for signs and symptoms of hydrocephaly
Pulsation	Slight pulsation Moderate bulging noted with crying or pulsations with heartbeat	Moderate to severe pulsation (vascular problems) Bulging (increased intracranial pressure, meningitis) Sunken (dehydration)	Refer to physician Evaluate hydration status
Hair Texture	Smooth with fine texture variations (Note: variations dependent on ethnic background)	Coarse, brittle, dry hair (hypothyroidism) White forelock (Waardenburg syndrome)	Instruct parents regarding routine care of hair and scalp
Distribution	Scalp hair high over eyebrows (Spanish-Mexican hairline begins midforehead and extends down back of neck)	Low forehead and posterior hairlines may indicate chromosomal disorders	Assess for other signs of chromosomal aberrations Refer to physician
Face	Symmetrical, normal hairline, eyebrows and eyelashes present; symmetry of facial movement; chin recessed and nose flattened; milia present on nose and forehead		Assess and record symmetry of all parts, shape, regularity of features, sameness or differences in features
Spacing of features	Eyes at same level; nostrils equal size; fullness of cheeks and sucking pads present Lips equal on both sides of midline Chin recedes when compared to other bones of face Face sensitive to light, touch, warmth, cold	Eyes wide apart—ocular hypertelorism (Apert syndrome, cri-du-chat, Turner syndrome) Abnormal face (Down syndrome, cretinism, gargoylism) Abnormally small jaw— micrognathia (Pierre Robin syndrome, Treacher Collins syndrome) Lack of facial sensation (fifth and seventh cranial nerve damage)	Observe for other signs and symptoms indicative of disease states or chromosomal aberrations Initiate surgical consultation and referral Maintain airway Initiate neurologic assessment and consultations
Movement	Makes facial grimaces	Inability to suck, grimace, and close eyelids (cranial nerve injury)	

* Possible causes of alterations are placed in parentheses.
† This column provides guidelines for further assessment and initial nursing interventions.

NEONATAL PHYSICAL ASSESSMENT GUIDE Cont'd

Assess	Normal findings	Alterations and possible causes*	Nursing responses to data base†
	Symmetrical when resting and crying	Asymmetry (paralysis of facial cranial nerve)	
Frontal and maxillary sinuses	Frontal—absent at birth Maxillary—nontender		
Eyes			
General placement and appearance	Bright and clear; even placement; slight nystagmus	Gross nystagmus (damage to third, fourth, and sixth cranial nerves)	
	Concomitant strabismus	Constant and fixed strabismus	Reassure parents that strabismus is considered normal up to 6 months
	Move in all directions Blue or slate blue-gray (permanent color established by age 3 months) Brown color at birth in ethnic infants of color	Lack of pigmentation (albinism) Brushfield spots (may indicate Down syndrome)	Discuss with parents any necessary eye precautions Assess for other signs of Down syndrome
Eyelids			
Position	Above pupils but within iris, no drooping	Elevation or retraction of upper lid (hyperthyroidism) "Setting sun" (hydrocephaly) Ptosis (congenital or paralysis of oculomotor muscle)	Assess for signs of hydrocephaly and hyperthyroidism Evaluate interference with vision in subsequent well-baby visits
	Eyes on parallel plane	Upward slant in non-Orientals (Down syndrome)	Assess for other signs of Down syndrome
	Epicanthal folds in Oriental and 20% of white newborns	Epicanthal folds (Down syndrome, cri-du-chat)	
Movement	Blink reflex in response to light stimulus		
Palpation and inspection for infection	Edematous for first few days of life, resulting from delivery and instillation of silver nitrate (chemical conjunctivitis) No lumps or redness	Purulent drainage (infection) infectious conjunctivitis (staphylococcus or gram-negative organisms) Marginal blepharitis (lid edges red, crusted, scaly)	Initiate good hand-washing Refer to physician Evaluate infant for seborrheic dermatitis; scales can be removed easily
Cornea and retina	Clear Circular red reflex Corneal reflex present	Ulceration (herpes infection) Large cornea or corneas of unequal size (congenital glaucoma) Clouding, opacity of lens (cataract)	Refer to ophthalmologist Assess for other manifestations of congenital herpes; institute nursing care measures

* Possible causes of alterations are placed in parentheses.
† This column provides guidelines for further assessment and initial nursing interventions.

NEONATAL PHYSICAL ASSESSMENT GUIDE Cont'd

Assess	Normal findings	Alterations and possible causes*	Nursing responses to data base†
Sclera	May appear bluish in newborn, then white; slightly brownish color frequent in blacks	True blue sclera (osteogenesis imperfecta)	Refer to physician
Pupils	Pupils are equal in size, round, and react to light by accommodation	Anisocoria—unequal pupils (CNS damage) Dilatation or constriction (intercranial damage, retinoblastoma glaucoma) Pupils nonreactive to light or accommodation (brain injury) Nystagmus (labyrinthine disturbance, CNS disorder)	Refer for neurologic examination
	Slight nystagmus in infant who has not learned to focus Pupil light reflex demonstrated at birth or by 3 weeks of age		
Conjunctiva	Chemical conjunctivitis (subsides in 2–7 days) Palpebral conjunctiva (red but not hyperemic) Subconjunctival hemorrhage common in newborns (disappears within 10 days)	Pale color (anemia) Inflammation or edema (infection, blocked tear duct)	Obtain hematocrit and hemoglobin Perform differential diagnosis
Vision	20/150 plus some degree of discrimination of color and pattern Tracks moving object to midline Fixes focus on objects at a distance of about 7 in.; may be difficult to evaluate in newborn	Cataracts (congenital infection)	Record any questions about visual acuity and initiate follow-up evaluation at first well-baby checkup
Lashes and lacrimal glands	Presence of lashes (lashes may be absent in preterm infants)	No lashes on inner two-thirds of lid (Treacher Collins syndrome) Bushy lashes (Hurler syndrome) Long lashes (Cornelia De Lange syndrome)	
	Cry commonly tearless because duct not functional until 2–4 weeks of age	Excessive tearing (plugged lacrimal duct, natal narcotic abstinence syndrome)	Demonstrate to parents how to milk blocked tear duct Refer to ophthalmologist if tearing is excessive before third month of life

* Possible causes of alterations are placed in parentheses.
† This column provides guidelines for further assessment and initial nursing interventions.

NEONATAL PHYSICAL ASSESSMENT GUIDE Cont'd

Assess	Normal findings	Alterations and possible causes*	Nursing responses to data base†
Nose			
Appearance			
External nasal aspects	May appear flattened as a result of delivery process	Continued flat or broad bridge of nose (Down syndrome)	Arrange consultation with specialist
	Small and narrow in midline; even placement in relationship to eyes and mouth	Low bridge of nose, beaklike nose (Apert, Treacher Collins syndrome) Upturned (Cornelia De Lange syndrome)	Initiate evaluation of chromosomal abnormalities
	Patent nares bilaterally (nose breathers)	Blockage of nares (mucus and/or secretions) Flaring nares (respiratory distress) Choanal atresia	
Internal nasal aspects	Pink and firm mucous membranes		
	Septum midline and without polyps or tumors	Deviated or perforated septum; tumors or polyps of septum	Collaborate with physician
	No swelling or nasal discharge	Swelling and erythema (infection)	Note and record characteristics of nasal discharge
Smelling and breathing abilities	Identifies odors; appears to smell breast milk	No response to stimulating odors	Inspect for obstructions of nares
	Breathes through nose (does not open mouth to breathe) Sneezing common to clear nasal passages		
Mouth			
Function of facial, hypoglossal, glossopharyngeal, and vagus nerves	Symmetry of movement and strength	Mouth draws to one side (transient seventh cranial nerve paralysis due to pressure in utero or trauma during delivery, congenital paralysis)	Initiate neurologic consultation Administer eye care if eye on affected side is unable to close
	Adequate salivation Presence of gag and swallowing and sucking reflexes	Fishlike shape (Treacher Collins syndrome) Suppressed or absent reflexes	Evaluate other neurologic functions of these nerves
	Tongue midline	Deviations from midline (cranial nerve damage)	
Palate (soft and hard)	Hard palate dome-shaped Uvula midline with symmetrical movement of soft palate	High-steepled palate (Treacher Collins syndrome)	

* Possible causes of alterations are placed in parentheses.
† This column provides guidelines for further assessment and initial nursing interventions.

NEONATAL PHYSICAL ASSESSMENT GUIDE Cont'd

Assess	Normal findings	Alterations and possible causes*	Nursing responses to data base†
	Palate intact, sucks well when stimulated Epithelial (Epstein's) pearls appear on mucosa	Clefts in either hard or soft palate (polygenic disorder)	Initiate a surgical consultation referral Assure parents that these are normal in newborn and will disappear at 2 or 3 months of age
Pharynx	Unobstructed, with no drainage in back of throat No exudate on tonsils	Exudate present (infection)	Examine for other signs of infection
	Esophagus patent; some drooling common in newborn	Excessive drooling or bubbling (esophageal atresia)	Test for patency of esophagus
Tongue	Free-moving in all directions, midline	Lack of movement or asymmetrical movement Tongue-tied	Further assess neurologic functions Test reflex elevation of tongue when depressed with tongue blade Check for signs of weakness or deviation
	Pink color, smooth to rough texture, noncoated	White cheesy coating (thrush)	Differentiate between thrush and milk curds
		Tongue has deep ridges	Reassure parents that tongue pattern may change from day to day
	Tongue proportional to mouth	Large tongue with short frenulum (cretinism, Down and other syndromes)	Evaluate in well-baby clinic to assess developmental delays Initiate referrals
Ears External ear	Without lesions, cysts, or nodules	Nodules, cysts, or sinus tracts in front of ear Adherent earlobes	Evaluate characteristics of lesions Counsel parents to clean external ear with washcloth only; discourage use of cotton-tip applicators
		Preauricular skin tags	Refer to physician for ligation
Inner canal and tympanic membrane	Bony landmarks present (may not be visible)	Bulging (infection) Discharge, disagreeable odor (infection)	Assess for other signs of infections
	Tympanic membrane light color, pearly gray Translucent, intact	Ruptured tympanic membrane	Remove wax and vernix debris with wire loop or curette under constant visualization

* Possible causes of alterations are placed in parentheses.
† This column provides guidelines for further assessment and initial nursing interventions.

NEONATAL PHYSICAL ASSESSMENT GUIDE Cont'd

Assess	Normal findings	Alterations and possible causes*	Nursing responses to data base†
Hearing	With first cry, eustachian tubes are cleared		
	Absence of all risk factors	Presence of one or more risk factors	Assess history of risk factors for hearing loss
	Attends to sounds; sudden or loud noise elicits Moro reflex	No response to sound stimuli (deafness)	Test for Moro reflex
Neck Appearance	Short, straight, creased with skin folds	Abnormally short neck (Turner syndrome) Arching or inability to flex neck (meningitis, congenital anomaly)	Report findings to physician
	Posterior neck lacks loose extra folds of skin	Webbing of neck (Turner syndrome, Down syndrome, trisomy 18)	Collect more data indicative of chromosomal aberrations
	Head moves freely from side to side	Neck rigidity (congenital torticollis, eleventh cranial nerve damage)	
	Sternocleidomastoid muscle should be symmetrical on both sides		
	If infant is held upright and body tilted, head returns to upright position		
Thyroid	Thyroid not usually palpable in newborn No masses		Palpate for lymph nodes and masses
Clavicles	Straight and intact	Knot or lump on clavicle (fracture during difficult delivery)	Obtain detailed labor and delivery history; apply figure-8 bandage
	Moro reflex elicitable	Unilateral Moro reflex response on unaffected side (fracture of clavicle, brachial palsy, Erb-Duchenne paralysis)	Collaborate with physician
	Bilateral movement of both shoulders	Hypoplasia	
Chest Appearance and size	Circumference: 32.5 cm, 1–2 cm less than head Wider than it is long		Measure at level of nipples after exhalation
	Normal shape without depressed or prominent sternum	Funnel chest (congenital or associated with Marfan syndrome)	Determine adequacy of other respiratory and circulatory signs

*Possible causes of alterations are placed in parentheses.
†This column provides guidelines for further assessment and initial nursing interventions.

NEONATAL PHYSICAL ASSESSMENT GUIDE Cont'd

Assess	Normal findings	Alterations and possible causes*	Nursing responses to data base†
	Lower end of sternum (xiphoid cartilage) may be protruding, is less apparent after several weeks	Continued protrusion of xiphoid cartilage (Marfan syndrome, "pigeon chest")	Assess for other signs and symptoms of various syndromes
	Sternum 8 cm long	Barrel chest	
Expansion and retraction	Bilateral expansion	Unequal chest expansion (pneumonia, pneumothorax respiratory distress)	Collect more data regarding respiratory effort if chest expansion is unequal (regularity, flaring of nares, difficulty on both inspiration and expiration)
Percussion	No intercostal, subcostal, or suprasternal retraction	Retractions (respiratory distress)	Record and consult physician
	Decreased percussion, note dullness found over liver, diaphragm, heart, with these areas well demarcated	Dullness in lung fields (consolidation of lungs, atelectasis)	Examine chest thoroughly using techniques of inspection, palpation, and auscultation
		Hyperresonance of chest (pneumonia, pneumothorax, distended stomach)	Report positive findings to physician
Auscultation	Breath sounds are louder in infants	Decreased breath sounds (decreased respiratory activity, atelectasis, pneumothorax)	Perform complete physical exam and report to physician any positive findings
	Heard bilaterally		
	Chest and axilla clear on crying	Increased breath sounds are heard with resolving pneumonia or in cesarean births	
Bronchial breath sounds (heard where trachea and bronchi closest to chest wall, above sternum and between scapulae)	Bronchial sounds bilaterally		
	Air entry clear	Adventitious or abnormal sounds (respiratory diseases or distress)	
	Rales may indicate normal newborn atelectasis		
	Cough reflex absent at birth, appears in 2 or more days		
Determination of point of maximal impulse (PMI)	Difficult to assess exact PMI in infant up to 2 years old, but usually lateral to midclavicular line at third or fourth interspace	Malpositioning (enlargement, abnormal placement, pneumothorax, dextrocardia, diaphragmatic hernia)	Initiate cardiac evaluation
Heart Auscultation and palpation	Location: lies horizontally, with left border extending to left of midclavicle		
	Regular rhythm and rate	Arrhythmia (anoxia)	All arrhythmia and gallop rhythms should be referred
		Tachycardia, bradycardia	

*Possible causes of alterations are placed in parentheses.
†This column provides guidelines for further assessment and initial nursing interventions.

NEONATAL PHYSICAL ASSESSMENT GUIDE Cont'd

Assess	Normal findings	Alterations and possible causes*	Nursing response to data base†
	Functional murmurs No thrills	Location of murmurs (possible congenital cardiac anomaly)	Evaluate murmur: location, timing, and duration; observe for accompanying cardiac pathology symptoms, and ascertain any family history
Trachea (palpate from top to bottom with thumb and index fingers)	Slightly right of midline	Deviated left or right (pneumothorax, tumor of chest or neck)	
Rib cage and diaphragm	Horizontal groove at diaphragm shows flaring of rib cage to mild degree	Harrison groove with marked flaring (vitamin D deficiency) Inadequacy of respiration movement	Initiate cardiopulmonary evaluation; assess pulses and blood pressures in all four extremities for equality and quality
Breasts	Breasts flat with symmetrical nipple Breast tissue diameter 5 cm or more at term Distance between nipples 8 cm	Lack of breast tissue (preterm or SGA)	
	Breast engorgement occurs on third day of life, liquid discharge may be expressed in term infants	Breast abscesses	Reassure parents of normalcy of breast engorgement
	Nipples	Supernumerary nipple Dark-colored nipples	
Abdomen Appearance	Cylindrical with some protrusion; appears large in relation to pelvis; some laxness of abdominal muscles No cyanosis, few vessels seen Observe for synchronous movement with breathing	Distention, shiny abdomen with engorged vessels (gastrointestinal abnormalities, infection, congenital megacolon) Scaphoid appearance (diaphragmatic hernia) Increased or decreased peristalsis (duodenal stenosis, small bowel obstruction)	Examine abdomen thoroughly for mass or organomegaly Measure abdominal girth Report deviations of abdominal size Assess other signs and symptoms of obstruction
	Diastasis recti—common in black infants	Localized flank bulging (enlarged kidneys, ascites, or absent abdominal muscles)	Refer to physician
Palpation	Nontender	Tense abdomen with marked rigidity or resistance to pressure (infection)	Take temperature and assess other signs and symptoms
	No palpable masses	Solid masses (Wilm's tumor)	Avoid palpation of abdomen; initiate referral

*Possible causes of alterations are placed in parentheses.
†This column provides guidelines for further assessment and initial nursing asterventions.

NEONATAL PHYSICAL ASSESSMENT GUIDE Cont'd

Assess	Normal findings	Alterations and possible causes*	Nursing responses to data base†
Umbilicus	No protrusion of umbilicus and no umbilical hernia Protrusion of umbilicus common in black infants Bluish white color Cutis navel (umbilical cord projects); granulation tissue in navel	Umbilical hernia Patent urachus (congenital malformation) Omphalocele Gastroschisis Redness or exudate around cord (infection) Yellow discoloration (hemolytic disease, meconium staining)	Measure umbilical hernia by palpating the opening and record; it should close by 1 year of age; if not, refer to physician Instruct parents on cord care and hygiene
	Two arteries and one vein apparent Begins drying 1–2 hours after birth, blackens by 3–5 days, sloughs off by 7–9 days No bleeding	Single umbilical artery (congenital anomalies)	
Liver	Liver 1–2 cm below right costal margin	Enlarged liver (sepsis, erythroblastosis)	Report and record size, consistency, and tenderness
Spleen	Tip under left costal margin	Enlarged spleen (trauma)	
Kidney	Posterior flank firm, oval mass, not enlarged, less commonly palpable	Displaced kidney (Wilm's tumor, neuroblastoma, polycystic kidney, agenesis)	Initiate nephrologic consultation
Auscultation and percussion	Soft bowel sounds heard shortly after birth; heard every 10–30 sec Normal peristalsis	Bowel sounds in chest (diaphragmatic hernia) Absence of bowel sounds Hyperperistalsis (intestinal obstruction)	Collaborate with physician Assess for other signs of dehydration and/or infection
	Abdomen has tympanic sound except over liver and spleen (dull sound)	Increased dull sound (mass or organomegaly)	Examine abdomen thoroughly by light and deep palpation
Femoral pulses	Palpable, equal, bilateral	Absent or diminished femoral pulses (coarctation of aorta)	Monitor blood pressure in upper and lower extremities
Inguinal area	No bulges along inguinal area No inguinal lymph nodes felt	Inguinal hernia	Collaborate with physician
Bladder	Percusses 1–4 cm above symphysis Emptied about 3 hours after birth; if not, at time of birth Urine—nonoffensive, mild odor	Failure to void within 24 hours after birth Exposure of bladder mucosa (exstrophy of bladder) Foul odor (infection)	
Genitals Male	Gender clearly delineated	Ambiguous genitals	Refer for genetic consultation
Penis	Slender in appearance, 2.5 cm long, 1 cm wide at birth Normal urinary orifice, urethral meatus at tip of penis	Micropenis (congenital anomaly) Meatal atresia Hypospadius, epispadius	Observe and record first voiding Collaborate with physician in presence of abnormality

*Possible causes of alterations are placed in parentheses.
†This column provides guidelines for further assessment and initial nursing interventions.

NEONATAL PHYSICAL ASSESSMENT GUIDE Cont'd

Assess	Normal findings	Alterations and possible causes*	Nursing responses to data base†
	Noninflamed urethral opening	Urethritis (infection)	Palpate for enlarged inguinal lymph nodes and record painful micturition
	Foreskin adheres to glans, prepuce can be retracted beyond urethral opening	Ulceration of meatal opening (infection, inflammation)	Evaluate whether ulcer is due to diaper rash; counsel regarding care
	Uncircumcised foreskin tight for 2–3 months	Phimosis — if still tight after 3 months	Instruct parents to retract foreskin gently for cleaning at monthly intervals after 4 months of age
	Circumcised		Teach parents how to care for circumcision
	Erectile tissue present		
Scrotum	Skin loose and hanging or tight and small; extensive rugae		
	Scrotum of normal size	Large scrotum containing fluid (hydrocele)	Shine a light through scrotum (transilluminate) to verify diagnosis
	Normal skin color	Red, shiny scrotal skin (orchitis)	
	Scrotal discoloration common in breech		
Testes	Descended by birth; not consistently found in scrotum	Undescended testes (cryptorchidism)	If testes cannot be felt in scrotum, gently palpate femoral, inguinal, perineal, and abdominal areas for presence
	Testes size 1.5–2 cm at birth	Enlarged testes (tumor)	Refer and collaborate with physician for further diagnostic studies
		Small testes (Klinefelter syndrome or adrenal hyperplasia)	
Female Mons	Normal skin color; area pigmented in dark-skinned races		
	Labia majora cover labia minora, symmetrical size appropriate for gestational age	Hematoma, lesions	Evaluate for recent trauma
Clitoris	Normally large in newborn	Hypertrophy (hermaphroditism)	
	Edema and bruising in breech delivery		
Vagina	Urinary meatus and vaginal orifice visible (0.5 cm circumference)	Inflammation; erythema and discharge (urethritis)	Collect urine specimen for laboratory examination
	Vaginal tag or hymenal tag; disappears in a few weeks	Congenital absence of vagina	Refer to physician
	Discharge: smegma under labia	Foul-smelling discharge (infection)	Collect data and further evaluate reason for discharge

*Possible causes of alterations are placed in parentheses.
†This column provides guidelines for further assessment and initial nursing interventions.

NEONATAL PHYSICAL ASSESSMENT GUIDE Cont'd

Assess	Normal findings	Alterations and possible causes*	Nursing response to data base†
	Bloody or mucoid discharge	Excessive vaginal bleeding (blood coagulation defect)	
Buttocks and anus	Buttocks symmetrical	Pilonidal dimple	Examine for possible sinus Instruct parents about cleansing this area
	Anus patent and passage of meconium within 24–48 hours after birth	Imperforate anus, rectal atresia (congenital gastrointestinal defect)	Evaluate extent of problems Initiate surgical consultation Perform digital examination to ascertain patency
	No fissures, tears, or skin tags	Fissures	
Extremities and trunk	Short and generally flexed; extremities move symmetrically through range of motion but lack full extension	Unilateral or absence of movement (spinal cord involvement) Fetal position continued or limp (anoxia, CNS problems, hypoglycemia)	
	All joints move spontaneously; good muscle tone, of flexor type, birth to 2 months	Spasticity when infant begins using extensors (cerebral palsy, lack of muscle tone, "floppy baby" syndrome)	Collaborate with physician
Arms	Equal in length Bilateral movement Flexed when quiet	Brachial palsy (difficult delivery) Erb-Duchenne paralysis Muscle weakness, fractured clavicle Absence of limb or change of size (phocomelia, amelia)	
Hands	Normal number of fingers and size of hands	Polydactyly (Ellis-Van Creveld syndrome) Syndactyly — one limb (developmental anomaly) Syndactyly — both limbs (genetic component)	Collect data to rule out possible syndromes
	Normal palmar crease	Simian line on palm (Down syndrome)	
	Nails present and extend beyond fingertips in term infant	Short fingers and broad hand (Hurler syndrome) Cyanosis and clubbing (cardiac anomalies) Nails long (postterm)	
Spine	C-shaped spine Flat and straight when prone Slight lumbar lordosis Easily flexed and intact when palpated At least half of back devoid of lanugo Full-term infant in ventral suspension should hold head 45°, back straight	Spina bifida occulta (nevus pitosus) Dermal sinus Myelomeningocele Head lag, limp, floppy trunk (neurologic problems)	Evaluate extent of neurologic damage; initiate care of spinal opening

*Possible causes of alterations are placed in parentheses.
†This column provides guidelines for further assessment and initial nursing interventions.

NEONATAL PHYSICAL ASSESSMENT GUIDE Cont'd

Assess	Normal findings	Alterations and possible causes*	Nursing responses to data base†
Hips	No signs of instability No resistance to hip abduction Hips abduct to more than 60° Iliac crests are equal	Sensation of abnormal movement, jerk, or snap of hip dislocation	Examine all newborn infants for dislocated hip prior to discharge from hospital If this is suspected, refer to orthopedist for further evaluation Reassess at well-baby visits
Legs	Legs equal in length Legs shorter than arms at birth Legs one-third overall length of body when infant supine with legs flexed at knees	Shortened leg (dislocated hips) Lack of leg movement (fractures, spinal defects)	Refer to orthopedist for evaluation Counsel parents regarding symptoms of concern and discuss therapy
Inguinal and buttock skin creases	Symmetrical inguinal and buttock creases	Asymmetry (dislocated hips)	Refer to orthopedist for evaluation; counsel parents regarding symptoms of concern and therapy
Feet	Foot is in straight line Positional clubfoot—based on position in utero Fat pads and creases on soles of feet	Talipes equinovarus (true clubfoot)	Discuss differences between positional and true clubfoot with parents Teach parents passive manipulation of foot Refer to orthopedist if not corrected by 3 months of age
Arches	Pes planus (flat foot) normal under 3 years of age		Reassure parents that flat feet are normal in infant
Neurologic—muscular Motor function	Symmetrical movement and strength in all extremities	Limp, flaccid, or hypertonic (CNS disorders, infection, dehydration, fracture)	Appraise newborn's posture and motor functions by observing activities and motor characteristics
	May be jerky or have brief twitchings	Tremors (hypoglycemia, hypocalcemia, infection, neurologic damage)	Evaluate electrolyte imbalance and neurologic functioning
	Head lag not over 45°	Delayed or abnormal development (preterm, neurologic involvement)	
	Neck control adequate to maintain head erect briefly	Asymmetry of tone or strength	
Reflexes Moro	Response to sudden movement or loud noise should be one of symmetrical extension and abduction of arms with fingers extended; then return to normal relaxed flexion	Asymmetry of body response (fractured clavicle, injury to brachial plexus) Consistent absence (brain damage)	Discuss normalcy of this reflex in response to loud noises and/or sudden movements

*Possible causes of alterations are placed in parentheses.
†This column provides guidelines for further assessment and initial nursing interventions.

NEONATAL PHYSICAL ASSESSMENT GUIDE Cont'd

Assess	Normal findings	Alterations and possible causes*	Nursing responses to data base†
	Fingers form a C Present at birth, disappears at 1-4 months of age		
Sucking and rooting	Turns in direction of stimulus to cheek or mouth; opens mouth and begins to suck; difficult to elicit after feeding; disappears by 7 months of age Sucking is adequate for nutritional intake and meeting oral stimulation needs; disappears by 12 months	Poor sucking or easily fatiguable (preterm, breast-fed infants of barbiturate-addicted mothers) Absence of response (preterm, neurologic involvement, depressed infants)	Evaluate strength and coordination of sucking Observe neonate during feeding and counsel parents about mutuality of feeding experience and neonate's responses
Palmar grasp	Fingers grasp adult finger when palm is stimulated and hold momentarily; lessens at 3-4 months of age	Asymmetry of response (neurologic problems)	Evaluate other reflexes and general neurologic functioning
Plantar grasp	Toes curl downward when sole of foot is stimulated; lessens by 8 months	Absent (defects of lower spinal column)	
Stepping	When held upright and one foot touching a flat surface, will step alternately; disappears at 7-8 months of age	Asymmetry of stepping (neurologic abnormality)	Evaluate muscle tone and function on each side of body Refer to specialist
Babinski	Hyperextension of all toes when one side of sole is stroked from heel upward across ball of foot	Absence of response (low spinal cord defects)	Refer for further neurologic evaluation
Tonic neck	Fencer position—when head is turned to one side, extremities on same side extend and on opposite side flex; this reflex may not be evident during early neonatal period; disappears at 3-4 months of age Response often more dominant in leg than in arm	Absent after 1 month of age or persistent asymmetry (cerebral lesion)	
Prone crawl	While on abdomen, neonate pushes up and tries to crawl	Absence or variance of response (preterm, weak or depressed infants)	Evaluate motor functioning Refer to specialist
Trunk incurvation	In prone position, stroking of spine causes pelvis to turn to stimulated side	Failure to rotate to stimulated side (neurologic damage)	

*Possible causes of alterations are placed in parentheses.
†This column provides guidelines for further assessment and initial nursing interventions.

Some items are scored according to the infant's response to specific stimuli; others, such as consolability and alertness, are scored as a result of continuous behavioral observations throughout the assessment.

Generally, the scales are set up so that the midpoint is the norm for most items. The Brazelton scale differs from most assessment tools in that, for all but a few items, the infant's score is determined not on the average performance but on the best. In the case of the infant who is uncoordinated for 48 hours after delivery, the behavior of the third day must be taken as the expected mean. Every effort should be made to elicit the best response. This may be accomplished by repeating tests at different times or by testing during situations that facilitate the best possible response, such as when parents are alerting their infants by holding, cuddling, rocking, and singing to them.

The assessment of the infant should be carried out initially in a quiet, dimly or softly lit room, if possible. The infant's state of consciousness should be determined, because scoring and introduction of the test items are correlated with the sleep or awake state. The newborn's state depends on physiologic variables, such as the amount of time from the last feeding, positioning, environmental temperature, and health status; presence of such external stimuli as noises and bright lights; and the wake–sleep cycle of the infant. An important characteristic of the neonatal period is the *pattern of states,* as well as the transitions from one state to another. The pattern of states is a predictor of the infant's receptivity and ability to respond to stimuli in a cognitive manner. Infants learn best in a quiet, alert state and in an environment that is supportive and protective and that provides appropriate stimuli.

The nurse should observe the newborn's sleep–wake patterns as discussed in Chapter 21, the rapidity with which the infant moves from one state to another, ability to be consoled, and ability to diminish the impact of disturbing stimuli. The following questions may provide the nurse with a framework for assessment:

Does the infant's response style and ability to adapt to stimuli indicate a need for parental interventions that will alert the newborn to the environment so that he or she can grow socially and cognitively?

Are parental interventions necessary to lessen the outside stimuli, as in the case of the infant who responds to sensory input with intensity?

Can the infant control the amount of sensory input that he or she must deal with?

The scale items and maneuvers and the *sleep–awake states* in which they are assessed are categorized as follows:

Habituation (state 1, 2, or 3). The infant's ability to diminish or shut down innate responses to specific repeated stimuli, such as a rattle, bell, light, or pinprick to heel, is assessed. The tests are continued until the infant effectively blocks out or becomes unresponsive to three consecutive stimuli. Normal newborns can filter out stimulation and stop responding, demonstrating an ability to control themselves by their responses to the external environment. Inability to habituate to these stimuli may be related to transient problems, such as medication given to the mother during labor or possible CNS damage, and warrants further evaluation. The immature or CNS-damaged infant demonstrates a failure to habituate to the pinprick stimulus by withdrawing the opposite foot from the pinprick, and the whole body responds as quickly as the stimulated foot.

Orientation to inanimate and animate visual and auditory assessment stimuli (state 4 or 5). How often and where the newborn attends to auditory and visual stimuli are observed. The infant's orientation to the environment is determined by an ability to respond to clues given by others and by a natural ability to fix on and to follow a visual object horizontally and vertically. This capacity and parental appreciation of it are important for positive communication between infant and parents; the parents' visual (*en face*) and auditory (soft, continuous voice) presence stimulates their infant to orient to them. Inability or lack of response may indicate visual or auditory problems. It is important for parents to know that their infant can turn to voices by 3 days of age and can become alert at different times with a varying degree or intensity of response to sounds.

Motor activity (maturity). Several components are evaluated. Motor tone (state 4; not to be assessed in state 6) of the newborn is assessed in the most characteristic state of responsiveness. This summary assessment includes overall use of tone as the neonate responds to being handled— whether during spontaneous activity, prone placement, or holding horizontally—and overall assessment of body tone as the neonate reacts to all stimuli.

Smooth movement of extremities and free, wide range of movement (states 4 and 5) demonstrate motor maturity. One assesses smoothness of movement versus jerkiness. In the preterm or CNS-irritated infant, an unbalanced cogwheel movement appears. One assesses freedom of arcs of movements versus restricted arcs. Preterm infants demonstrate unlimited freedom of movement (floppy) in lateral, sagittal, and cephalad areas, but the movements are jerky and coglike, overshooting the marks. The average newborn is somewhat limited in arcs of movement, especially in those above the head and some in the lateral plane. Very mature infants exhibit freedom of movement in all directions and smooth, balanced performance (not floppy).

Other items used to assess motor maturity are the ability to pull to sit (states 3 and 5) and the ability to coordinate hand-to-mouth movements. The nurse should discuss with the parents normalcy of hand-to-mouth movements as a self-control and comforting device and not necessarily an expression of hunger. Degree and frequency of startling (states 3 to 6), tremulousness (all states), and defensive movements (state 4), such as a newborn's attempts to remove a cloth placed over the head, are items that evaluate motor activity.

Variations. Frequency of alert states (state 4 only), state changes, color changes (throughout all states as examination progresses), activity, and peaks of excitement (state 6) are assessed. Periods of alertness can occur at any time during the examination period and are often best elicited while the examiner holds the infant. Infants are alert for only short periods. *Alerting* is defined as a brightening and widening of the eyes, and *orienting* is identified as the response of turning toward the direction of stimulation (Brazelton, 1973). Color changes reflect the autonomic nervous system's responses to stress, whereas rapidity of state changes reflects newborns' ability to control themselves in the presence of increasing aversive stimulation.

Self-quieting activity (states 6 and 5 to 4, 3, 2, and 1). Assessment is based on how often, how quickly, and how effectively newborns can utilize their resources to quiet and console themselves when upset or distressed. Consid-

ered in this assessment are such self-consolatory activities as putting hand to mouth, sucking on a fist or the tongue, and attuning to an object or sound. One must also consider the infant's need for outside consolation, for example, visualizing a face, rocking, holding, dressing, using a pacifier, and restraining extremities.

Cuddliness or social behaviors (states 4 and 5). This area encompasses the infant's need for and response to being held. Also considered is how often the newborn smiles. These behaviors influence the parents' self-esteem and feelings of acceptance or rejection. Schaeffer and Emerson's (1964) study indicated that cuddling also appears to be an indicator of personality. Cuddlers appear to enjoy, accept, and seek physical contact; are easier to placate; sleep more; and form earlier and more intense attachments. Noncuddlers are active, restless, have accelerated motor development, and are intolerant of physical restraint. Smiling, even as a grimace reflex, greatly influences the parent–infant feedback system. Parents identify this response as positive.

SUMMARY

The various neonatal assessments and the data obtained from them are only as effective as the degree to which the findings are shared with the parents and incorporated into the interaction between parents and infant. Parents must be included in the assessment process from the moment of their child's birth. The Apgar score and its meaning should be explained immediately to the parents. As soon as possible, the parents should be a part of the physical and behavioral assessments. The examiner should emphasize the uniqueness of their infant.

The nurse can encourage the parents to identify the unique behavioral characteristics of their infant and to learn nurturing activities. Bonding is facilitated when parents are allowed to explore their infant in private, identifying individual physical and behavioral characteristics. The nurse's supportive responses to the parents' questions and observations are essential throughout the assessment process. With the nurse's help, bonding and the beginning interactions between family members are established.

References

Avery, G. B., ed. 1981. *Neonatology*, 2nd ed. Philadelphia: J. B. Lippincott Co.

Ballard, J. L., et al. November 1979. A simplified score for assessment of fetal maturation of newly born infants. *J. Pediatr.* 95:5:769.

Brazelton, T. 1973. *The neonatal behavioral assessment scale.* Philadelphia: J. B. Lippincott Co.

Brazelton, T. 1977. Neonatal behavior and its significance. In *Diseases of the newborn*, ed. A. J. Schaeffer et al. Philadelphia: W. B. Saunders.

Damoulaki-Sfakianaki, E., et al. 1972. Skin creases on the foot and the physical index of maturity. Comparison between Caucasian and Negro infants. *Pediatrics.* 50:483.

Danforth, D. N., ed. 1982. *Obstetrics and gynecology*, 4th ed. Philadelphia: Harper & Row.

Downs, M. P., and Silver, H. K. Oct. 1972. The A, B, C, D's to H.E.A.R. Early identification in nursery, office and clinic of the infant who is deaf. *Clin. Pediatr.* 11:563.

Dubowitz, L., and Dubowitz, V. 1977. *Gestational age of the newborn.* Menlo Park, Calif.: Addison-Wesley Publishing Co.

Hey, E. N., and Katz, G. 1968. Evaporative water loss in the newborn baby. *J. Physiol.* 200:605.

Hittner, H. M., et al. 1977. Assessment of gestational age by examination of the anterior vascular capsule of the lense. *J. Pediatr.* 91:455.

Holmes, L. B. 1976. Congenital malformations: incidence, racial differences and recognized etiologies. In *Biological and clinical aspects of malformations*. Evansville, Ind.: Mead Johnson Symposium on Perinatal and Developmental Medicine, no. 7.

Kempe, C. H., et al. 1982. *Current pediatric diagnosis and treatment.* Los Altos, Calif.: Lange Medical Publications.

Korones, S. B. 1981. *High-risk newborn infants*, 3rd ed. St. Louis: The C. V. Mosby Co.

Robertson, A. November 1979. Commentary: gestational age. *J. Pediatr.* 95:5:732.

Schaeffer, H., and Emerson, P. 1964. Patterns of response to physical contact in early human development. *J. Child Psychol. Psychiatry.* 5:1.

Standards and Recommendations for Hospital Care of Newborn Infants. 1977. 6th ed. Evanston, Ill.: American Academy of Pediatrics.

Additional Readings

Affonso, D. Nov./Dec. 1976. The newborn's potential for interaction. *J. Obstet. Gynecol. Neonat. Nurs.* 5:9.

Brann, A. Oct. 1977. Determining gestational age. *Emergency Med.* 9:51.

Chinn, P. 1979. *Child health maintenance: concepts of family-centered care*, 2nd ed. St. Louis: The C. V. Mosby Co.

Clark, A. L., and Affonso, D. 1976. Infant behavior and maternal attachment: Two sides to the coin. *Mat. Child Nurs.* 1:94.

Lubchenco, L. O. 1970. Assessment of gestational age and development at birth. *Pediatr. Clin. North Am.* 17:125.

Maurer, D. M., et al. 1976. Newborn babies see better than you think. *Psych. Today.* 10:85.

Powell, M. L. 1982. *Assessment and management of developmental changes and problems in children*, 2nd ed. St. Louis: The C. V. Mosby Co.

Scanlon, J. W., et al. 1979. *A system of newborn physical examination*. Baltimore: University Park Press.

Sullivan, R., et al. Jan./Feb. 1979. Determining a newborn's gestational age. *MCN.* 4:38.

Usher, R., et al. 1966. Judgment of fetal age. II. Clinical significance of gestational age and an objective method for its assessment. *Pediatr. Clin. North Am.* 13:835.

White, P. L., et al. 1980. Comparative accuracy of recent abbreviated methods of gestational age determination. *Clin. Pediatr.* 19(5):319.

■ 23 ■

THE NORMAL NEWBORN: NEEDS AND CARE

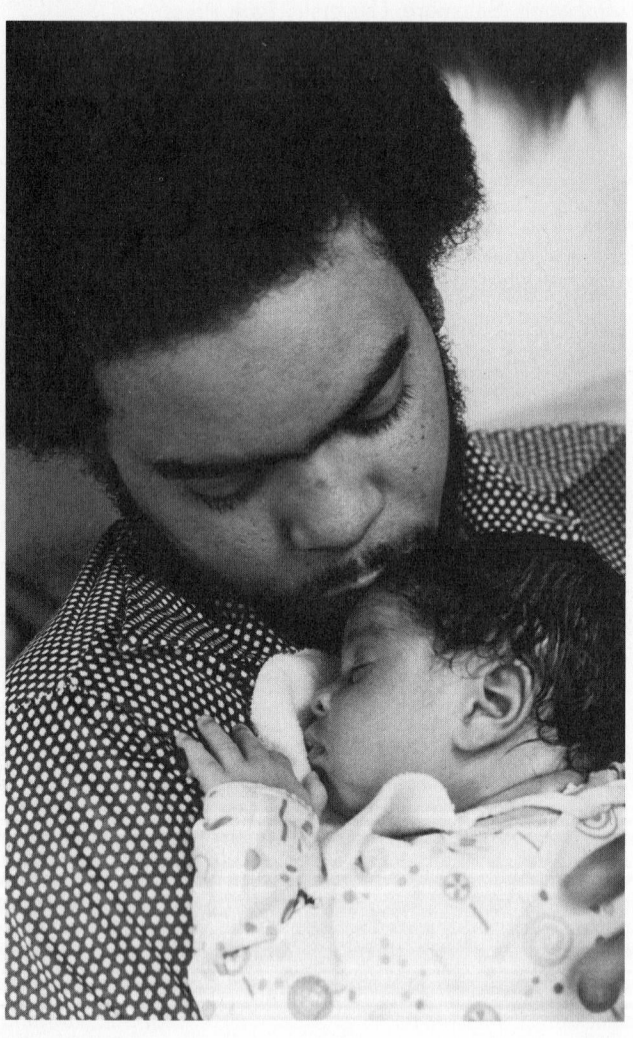

■ CHAPTER CONTENTS

NURSING OBSERVATIONS AND CARE: THE FIRST 24 HOURS

    Nursing Management of the Newborn at Admission

    Periods of Reactivity

    Subsequent Nursing Management

DAILY NEONATAL OBSERVATIONS AND CARE

    Handling and Positioning

    Nasal and Oral Suctioning

    Wrapping the Newborn

    Safety Considerations

NEWBORN FEEDING

    Initial Feeding in the Hospital

    Nutritional Needs of the Newborn

    Breast or Bottle?

    Establishing a Feeding Pattern

    Nutritional Assessment of the Infant

    Supplemental Foods

    Weaning

CIRCUMCISION

SLEEP AND ACTIVITY

    Sleep–Wake States

ENHANCING INTERACTION BETWEEN PARENT AND INFANT

    Early Experiences and Needs at Home

NEWBORN SCREENING PROGRAM

PARENT EDUCATION
    Positioning and Handling
    Oral and Nasal Suctioning
    Stools and Voids
    Bathing

Nail Care
Dressing the Newborn
Temperature Assessment
Safety
Discharge Planning

■ OBJECTIVES

- Discuss periods of reactivity after birth.

- Discuss nursing care of the newborn.

- Compare various feeding preparations and feeding techniques.

- Identify common parental concerns regarding newborns.

Nursing assessments and evaluation of the general characteristics, variations, and responses of each newborn reveal how the extrauterine adaptation process is proceeding. Based on the findings of these assessments, nurses can individualize their care to meet the needs of each newborn.

Birth also marks the beginning of the expansion of the family unit. Thus the nurse should be knowledgeable about family adjustments that need to be made as well as the health care needs of the newborn. With such a background, the nurse can provide comprehensive care and promote the establishment of a well-functioning family unit. It is important that new parents return home with a positive feeling that they have the support, information, and skills to care for their child. Equally important is the need for the family to begin a unique relationship between parents and the new child. The cultural and social expectations of individual families and communities have great implications for the specific manner in which normal newborn care is carried out. (See Chapter 3 for an in-depth view of these considerations.)

NURSING OBSERVATIONS AND CARE: THE FIRST 24 HOURS

Nursing Management of the Newborn at Admission

In many hospitals it is customary to place the infant in an observation nursery for several hours after birth. This procedure allows the nurse to carefully assess the newborn and to institute nursing care measures as needed. The ob-

servation nursery is staffed at all times and must be equipped with necessary emergency care equipment. Newborns born in alternative birthing rooms or centers may be kept in the birthing room for observation rather than being taken to an observation nursery.

When the newborn is admitted to the observation nursery after labor and delivery, identification is checked and confirmed. A concise verbal report of significant information is given to the nursery nurse. Essential data to be reported are the following:

1. *Condition of the newborn.* Essential information includes the newborn's Apgar scores at 1 and 5 minutes, resuscitative measures required in the delivery room, voidings, and passing of meconium. Complications to be noted are excessive mucus, delayed spontaneous respirations or responsiveness, abnormal number of cord vessels, and obvious physical abnormalities.

2. *Labor and delivery record.* A copy of the labor and delivery record should accompany the newborn to the nursery. The record has all significant data, for example, length and difficulty of labor; time amniotic membranes were ruptured and observations regarding color, odor, and amount of fluid; symptoms of fetal distress during labor, such as abnormal FHR patterns, or presence of meconium-stained amniotic fluid; medications, anesthetic or analgesic agents given to the woman during labor and delivery; and characteristics of the delivery such as position, length of stages, use of forceps, position of fetus at delivery, precipitous delivery, presence of nuchal cord (cord around newborn's neck at delivery). The labor and delivery nurse summarizes the data in a verbal report to the nursery nurse and takes particular care to note any variations or difficulties.

3. *Prenatal history.* Any maternal problems that may have compromised the fetus in utero, such as preeclampsia, spotting, illness, recent infections, or a history of maternal substance abuse, are of immediate concern in the assessment of the newborn. Information about maternal age, estimated day of confinement (EDC), previous pregnancies, and existing siblings is also included.

4. *Parent–infant interaction information.* Parental opportunities to hold their newborn and their desires regarding care, such as rooming-in and the type of feeding, are noted. Information about other children in the home, available support systems, and interactional patterns within each family unit assists in providing comprehensive care.

If no neonatal distress is apparent, the nurse proceeds with the admission nursery routine. The newborn's vital signs are taken, and the concerns of maintaining body tem-

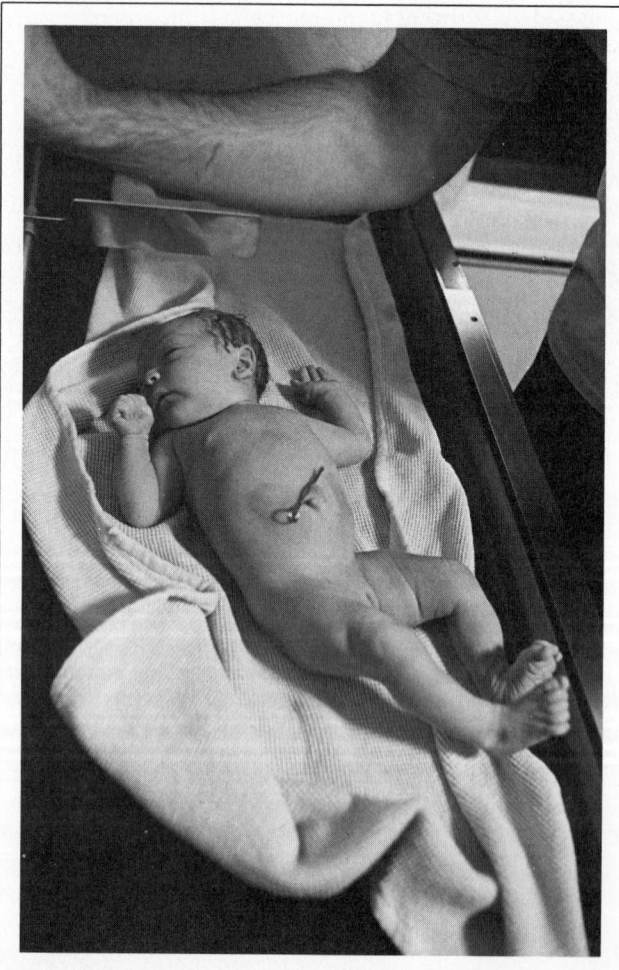

FIGURE 23–1 The scale is balanced before each weight, with the protective pad in place. The caretaker's hand is poised above the infant as a safety measure.

perature and a clear airway are addressed. The initial temperature may be taken rectally to assess patency of the anus (care should be taken to avoid inserting the thermometer too far which may perforate the intestines). Core temperature is then monitored either indirectly by obtaining an axillary temperature at intervals or by placing a skin probe on the abdomen of the newborn for continuous reading. Apical pulse and respirations are counted for a full minute and recorded. In some agencies blood pressure is assessed by auscultation, palpation, or by use of a Doppler instrument. The newborn is weighed in grams. This weight is converted to pounds for the parents' information (Figure 23–1). The scales are covered for each infant to prevent cross-infection and heat loss from conduction. The newborn is measured; the measurements are recorded in both centimeters and inches. Three routine measurements are (a) length—from top of head to heel; (b) circumference of the head; and (c) circumference of the chest. In some facilities, abdominal girth may also be determined. The nurse makes a rapid appraisal of the neonate's color, muscle tone, alertness, and general state. Basic assessments of estimating gestational age are done (for further discussion see Chapters 22 and 24).

A prophylactic injection of vitamin K is given intramuscularly in the lateral aspect of the thigh to prevent hemorrhagic problems (see Drug Guide, p. 711). The nurse is also responsible for giving the legally required prophylactic eye treatment for *Neisseria gonorrhoea,* which may have infected the neonate during the birth process if the mother is infected. The traditional drug of choice is 1% silver nitrate solution. To instill silver nitrate, the nurse punctures the wax container of 1% silver nitrate with a sterile needle, pulls down the infant's lower eyelid, and administers one or two drops in the lower conjunctival sac (Figure 23–2). The eye is closed to spread the medication. The other eye is treated in the same manner. Controversy exists as to the value of flushing the eye with sterile water following the instillation of the silver nitrate.

Some practitioners now use an antibiotic ointment such as erythromycin (Ilotycin) instead of silver nitrate. Both of these medications may cause chemical conjunctivitis, which will cause the newborn some discomfort and may interfere with the neonate's ability to focus on the parents' faces (see Drug Guide, p. 711). The resulting edema and inflammation may cause undue concern if the parents are not made aware of the need for the treatment. They should be told that the side effects will clear in 24–48 hours.

Eye-to-eye contact between the parents and child is of extreme emotional importance during the first hour after birth, and, as will be discussed later, the newborn is very alert during this time (Klaus and Kennell, 1982). To facilitate eye contact and promote bonding, prophylactic eye medication may be delayed to allow this all-important bonding opportunity.

DRUG GUIDE—
Erythromycin (Ilotycin)—Ophthalmic Ointment

OVERVIEW OF NEONATAL ACTION

Erythromycin (Ilotycin) is utilized as prophylactic treatment of ophthalmia neonatorum, which is caused by the bacteria *Neisseria gonorrhoeae*. Preventive treatment of gonorrhea in the newborn is required by law. Erythromycin is also effective against ophthalmic chlamydial infections. It is either bacteriostatic or bactericidal depending on the organisms involved and the concentration of drug.

ROUTE, DOSAGE, FREQUENCY

Ophthalmic ointment is instilled as a narrow ribbon or strand, ¼-inch long, along the lower conjunctival surface of each eye, starting at the inner canthus. It is instilled only once in each eye. Administration may be done in the delivery room or later in the nursery so that eye contact is facilitated so that the bonding process is not interrupted.

NEONATAL SIDE EFFECTS

Sensitivity reaction; may interfere with ability to focus and may cause edema and inflammation. Side effects usually disappear in 24–48 hours.

NURSING CONSIDERATIONS

Wash hands immediately prior to instillation to prevent introduction of bacteria
Do not irrigate the eyes after instillation
Observe for hypersensitivity

DRUG GUIDE—
Vitamin K₁ Phytonadione (AquaMEPHYTON)

OVERVIEW OF NEONATAL ACTION

Phytonadione is used in prophylaxis and treatment of hemorrhagic disease of the newborn. It promotes liver formation of the clotting factors II, VII, IX, and X. At birth the neonate does not have the bacteria in the colon that is necessary for synthesizing fat-soluble vitamin K_1, therefore the newborn may have decreased levels of prothrombin during the first 5–8 days of life reflected by a prolongation of prothrombin time.

ROUTE, DOSAGE, FREQUENCY

Intramuscular injection is given in the lateral thigh muscle. A one-time only prophylactic dose of 0.5–1.0 mg is given in the delivery room or upon admission to the newborn nursery. May need to repeat 6–8 hours later especially if mother received anticoagulants during pregnancy.

NEONATAL SIDE EFFECTS

Pain and edema may occur at injection site. Possible allergic reactions such as rash and urticaria. Hyperbilirubinemia may occur in newborns or preterm infants given doses greater than 25 mg.

NURSING CONSIDERATIONS

Observe for bleeding (usually occurs on second or third day). Bleeding may be seen as generalized ecchymoses or bleeding from umbilical cord, circumcision site, nose, or gastrointestinal tract. Results of serial PT and PTT should be assessed.
Observe for jaundice and kernicterus especially in preterm infants.
Observe for signs of local inflammation.

Blood work may be indicated. A hematocrit and Dextrostix evaluation is routinely ordered for SGA and LGA infants in some institutions (see Procedure 25–4, p. 817). Another routine but controversial practice in some institutions is removal of mucus from the stomach to help prevent possible aspiration. The procedure can cause bradycardia and apnea in the unstabilized neonate.

The initial admission assessment serves as a basis for establishing nursing diagnoses regarding the infant and setting priorities for care and family education needs. In many settings, the father accompanies the newborn to the nursery. This is an excellent opportunity for him to get to know his child as well as an excellent opportunity for the astute nurse to take note of the father's bonding process and comfort level with the newborn. The nurse must be aware that the father may be overwhelmed by the unfamiliar nursery setting; however, he will benefit from observing and interacting with the nurse who cares for his child.

Periods of Reactivity

The nurse must be able to appraise accurately normal behavior versus the abnormal. To do so, the nurse must be knowledgeable about the expected behavior of normal neonates.

The neonate demonstrates predictable behavior during the first several hours after birth (Figure 23–3). The first period of reactivity lasts approximately 30 minutes after birth. During this phase the newborn is awake and active, and may appear hungry and demonstrate a strong sucking

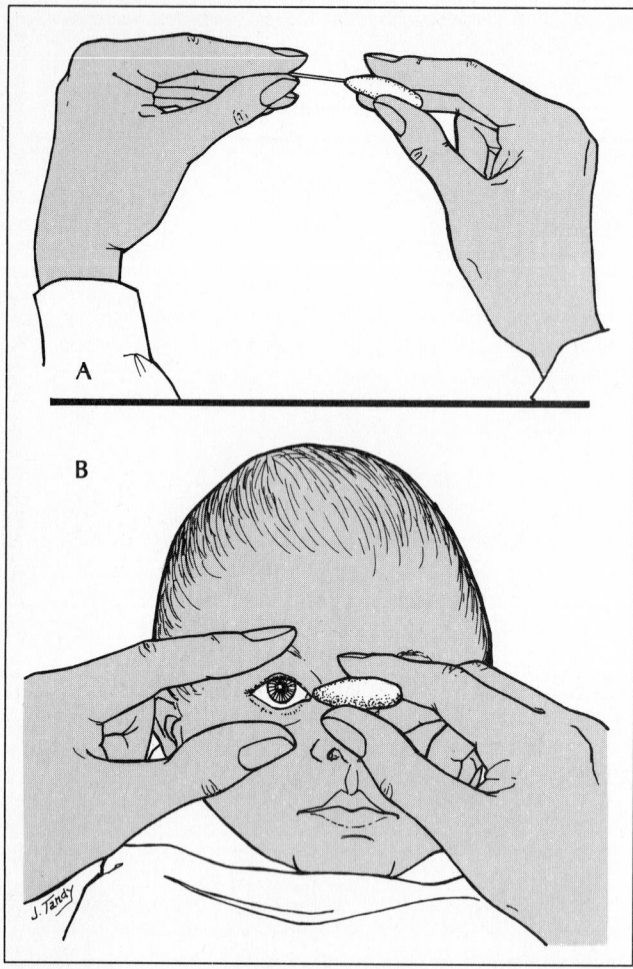

during this stage. The heart and respiratory rates accelerate; however, the nurse must be alert for apneic periods, which may cause a drop in the heart rate. The newborn must be stimulated to continue breathing during such times. The color of the newborn may become mildly cyanotic or mottled during these fluctuations. Increased respiratory and gastric mucus is produced, and the newborn responds by gagging, choking, and regurgitating.

Continued and close observation is required to maintain a clear airway. Positioning on the side and nasal suctioning with a bulb syringe or a De Lee suction may also be necessary. The gastrointestinal tract becomes active, with bowel sounds audible. The first meconium stool is frequently passed during this second active stage, and the initial voiding may also occur at this time. The newborn will demonstrate behaviors that indicate readiness for feeding, such as sucking, rooting, and swallowing reflexes. If feeding was not initiated in the first period of reactivity, it should be done at this time. See the section on feeding, p. 716, for further discussion of this first feeding.

Subsequent Nursing Management

After the initial admission assessment, the newborn's apical pulse and respirations should be taken every 15–30 minutes for 1 hour, and then every 1–2 hours until stable. During the remainder of the time the neonate is in the nursery, apical pulse and respirations should be assessed a minimum of once per shift. Apical pulse should be assessed while the neonate is at rest and heart rate, regularity, and murmurs should be noted.

The nurse must continue to closely assess the newborn's temperature and maintain body temperature in the range of 36.5–37.0C (97.7–98.6F). The axillary temperature should be monitored each hour for the first 4 hours and then once every 4 hours for the first 24 hours. When stable, it may be assessed and recorded twice daily.

The newborn is placed in a warmer just after delivery to allow his or her temperature to return to normal (about 2–4 hours). When the newborn's temperature is normal and vital signs are stable, the infant may be bathed. However, this admission bath may be postponed for some hours if the condition dictates. Temperature should be rechecked after the bath, and if stable, the newborn is dressed, wrapped, placed in a crib, and given a trial period at room temperature. If the infant does not successfully maintain his or her temperature at 36.5C (97.7F), the newborn is returned to the warmer.

The nurse should institute measures to prevent neonatal heat loss such as using heat shields, keeping the infant dry and covered, and avoiding placement on cool surfaces or the use of cold instruments. The infant should also be protected from drafts, open windows or doors, or air conditioners. Blankets and clothing should be stored in a

FIGURE 23–2 Silver nitrate instillation. **A,** Wax container is punctured with a needle. **B,** One or two drops of 1% silver nitrate solution are instilled in each lower conjunctival sac.

reflex. This is a natural opportunity to initiate breast-feeding if this is the parents' choice. Bursts of random, diffuse movements alternating with relative immobility may occur. Respirations are rapid, as high as 80/min, and there may be retraction of the chest, transient flaring of the nares, and grunting. The heart rate is rapid and irregular. Bowel sounds are absent.

Gradually activity diminishes, heart rate and respiration decrease, and the newborn enters the *sleep phase.* First sleep usually occurs an average of 3 hours after birth, and may last from a few minutes to 2–4 hours. During this period the newborn will be difficult to awaken and will show no interest in sucking. Bowel sounds become audible, and cardiac and respiratory rates return to baseline values.

The newborn is again awake and alert during the *second period of reactivity,* which lasts 4–6 hours in the normal newborn. Physiologic responses appear to be variable

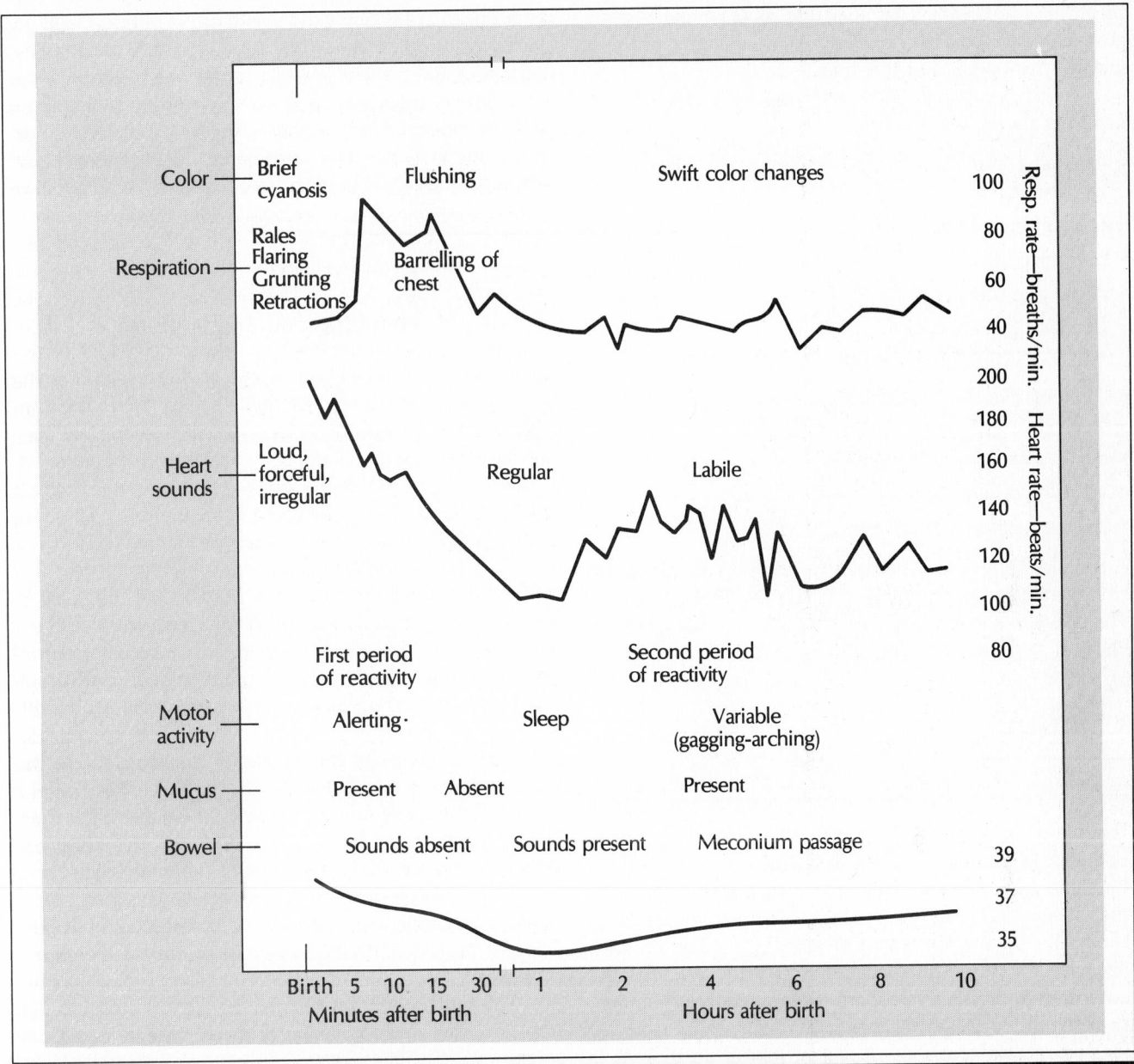

FIGURE 23–3 Example of periods of reactivity in normal newborn. (From Desmond, M. M. et al. 1966. The transitional nursery: a mechanism for preventive medicine. *Pediatr. Clin. North Am.* 13:656.)

warm place. (See discussion on nonshivering thermogenesis and the mechanism of heat loss in Chapter 21.)

When the newborn's neurologic status is normal, vital signs are stabilized, and the first feeding (usually within 5–10 hours after birth) has been tolerated, the infant is moved from the observation nursery area to the regular nursery. If rooming-in is desired, it may begin as soon as the newborn is transferred out of the observation nursery. However, some nurseries recommend that rooming-in be delayed for 24 hours. This recommendation is based on the knowledge that after 24 hours the amount of mucus in

the newborn is decreased, the chance of choking is diminished, and the initial voiding and defecation have occurred and have been assessed.

As the newborn moves through the periods of reactivity and as physiologic changes take place during the first 24 hours of life, the nurse must be constantly alert for signs of distress. If the newborn is with the parents during this period, extra care must be taken in their educational process so that they can appropriately maintain their newborn's temperature, recognize the hallmarks of physiologic distress, and know how to immediately respond to signs of respiratory problems. The nurse also must be immediately available to support the family during the bonding process, which is taking place at this time.

The most common signs of physiologic distress in the newborn are the following:

- Increased rate (more than 50/min) or difficulty of respirations
- Sternal retractions
- Excessive mucus
- Facial grimacing
- Cyanosis (generalized)
- Abdominal distention or mass
- Lack of meconium elimination within 24 hours after birth
- Inadequate urine elimination
- Vomiting of bile-stained material
- Unusual jaundice of the skin

A complete physical examination is done by the physician or pediatric nurse practitioner within the first 24 hours. The physical is then repeated on the day of discharge. (See Physical Assessment Guide in Chapter 22.)

DAILY NEONATAL OBSERVATIONS AND CARE

Routine daily care varies for each nursery and even from one shift to another. General assessment should be done on all newborns at the beginning of each shift to evaluate their health and progress. Vital signs (at least temperature) should be taken once a shift or more depending on each newborn's status. Routine laboratory work is completed according to physician's orders and procedures. The neonate should be weighed daily at the same time each day for accurate comparisons. A weight loss of up to 15% is expected. This is the result of limited initial intake and the loss of excess extracellular fluid. Parents should be informed about the expected weight loss and the reason for it. Another assessment is of the newborn's overall color. Changes in color may indicate the need for closer assessment of temperature, or hematocrit or bilirubin levels. Newborns should be kept clean and dry. Stool and voiding patterns are recorded as is the caloric and fluid intake. A notation should be made of cord care and circumcision care, if appropriate.

The nurse is responsible for assisting the mother in breast- or bottle-feeding the infant. The nurse helps the new mother by encouraging her to participate in the care of her baby, and also explains nursery routines to her. Physician visits and procedures are recorded in the nurse's notes.

A nurse in the neonatal nursery has the important re-

sponsibility of assessing the health of the newborn and providing appropriate care. The nurse's ease in handling and caring for the newborn instills confidence in the new parents. Due to today's changing family structures or possible lack of extended family, new parents often look to the nurse for guidance and information in becoming knowledgeable parents. The nurse must have a full understanding of newborn care to be able to anticipate and answer questions. The following information will provide the basic knowledge each nurse should know.

Handling and Positioning

How to pick up a newborn is one of the first concerns of anyone who has not handled many babies. When the infant is in the side-lying position, he or she is easily picked up by sliding one hand under the baby's neck and shoulders and the other hand under the buttocks or between the legs, then gently lifting the newborn from the crib. This technique provides security and support for the head (which the newborn is unable to support).

After the baby is out of the crib, one of the following holds may be used. The *cradle hold* is frequently used during feeding (Figure 23–4,A). It provides a sense of warmth and closeness, permits eye contact, frees one of the nurse's or mother's hands, and provides security because the cradling protects the infant's body. The *upright position* provides security and a sense of closeness and is ideal for burping the infant (Figure 23–4,B). One hand should support the neck and shoulders, while the other hand holds the buttocks or is placed between the newborn's legs. The *football hold* frees one of the caregiver's hands and permits eye contact (Figure 23–4, C). This hold is ideal for shampooing, carrying, or breast-feeding. It frees the mother to talk on the telephone or answer the door at home.

The newborn infant is most frequently positioned on the side with a rolled blanket or diaper behind for support (Figure 23–5). This position facilitates the drainage of mucus and allows air to circulate around the cord. It is also more comfortable for the newly circumcised male. After feeding, the infant is placed on the right side to aid digestion and to prevent aspiration. Once the cord is healed, many infants prefer to lie prone. Newborns have enough head control to turn their heads side to side to prevent suffocation. Care should be taken to periodically change the infant's position during the early months of life, because neonatal skull bones are soft, and flattened areas may develop if the newborn consistently lies in one position.

Nasal and Oral Suctioning

The infant generally maintains his or her air passage patency by coughing or sneezing. During the first few days of life, the newborn has increased mucus, and gentle suction-

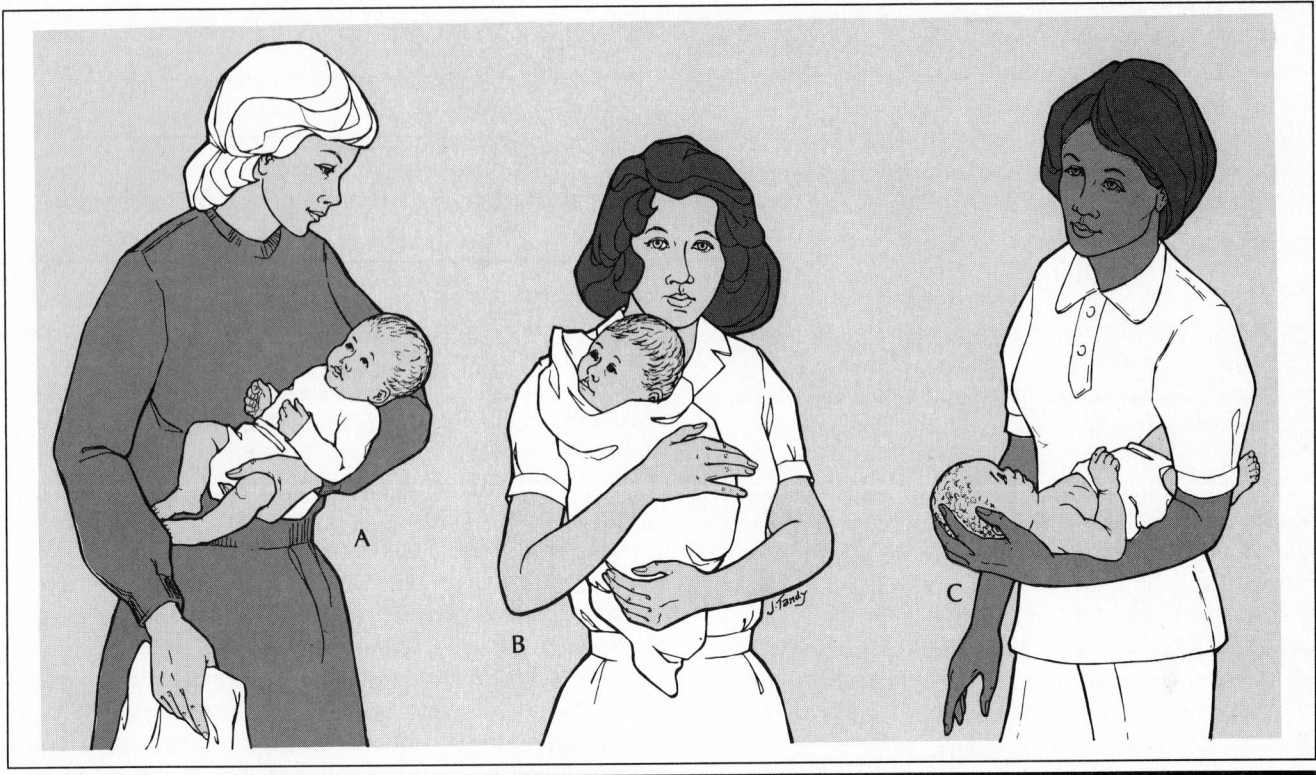

FIGURE 23–4 Various positions for holding an infant. **A,** Cradle hold. **B,** Upright position. **C,** Football hold.

ing with a bulb syringe may be indicated. The bulb is compressed, then the tip is placed in the nostril, and the bulb is permitted to slowly reexpand as the nurse or mother releases the compression on the bulb. The drainage is then compressed out of the bulb onto a tissue. The bulb syringe may also be used in the mouth if the newborn is spitting up and unable to handle the excess secretions. The bulb is compressed, then the tip of the bulb syringe is placed about 1 inch in one side of the infant's mouth, and compression is released. This will draw up the excess secre-

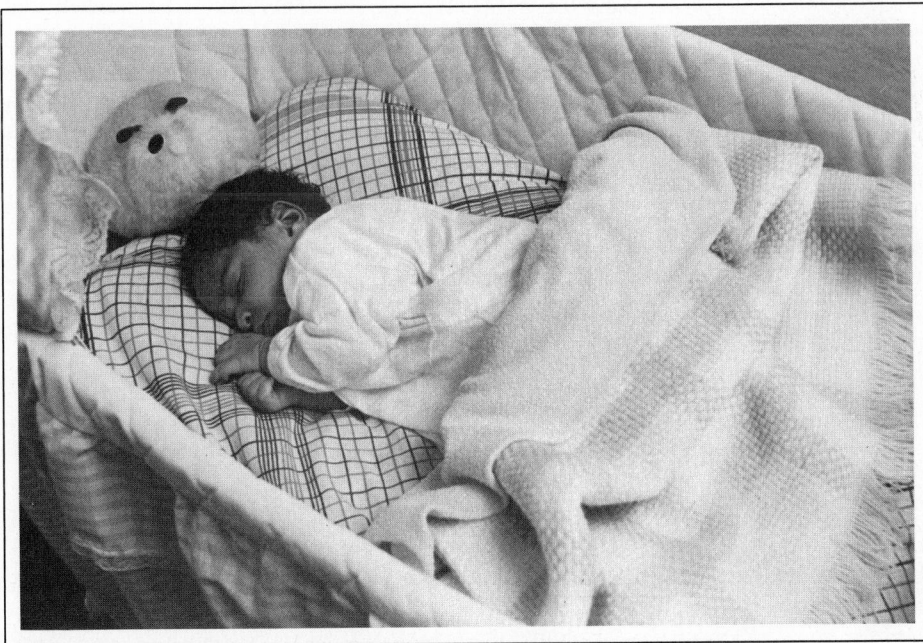

FIGURE 23–5 The most common sleeping position of the newborn is on the side. The little girl shown here does not need the additional support provided by a rolled blanket.

tions. The procedure is repeated on the other side of the mouth. The center of the infant's mouth is avoided for this might stimulate the gag reflex. The bulb syringe should be washed in warm, soapy water and rinsed in warm water after each use. The bulb syringe should always be kept near the infant, and the mother should be given a demonstration of its use (Figure 23–6).

Wrapping the Newborn

Wrapping helps the newborn maintain body temperature and soothes him or her by providing a feeling of closeness and sense of security. When wrapping, a blanket is placed on the crib (or secure surface) in the shape of a diamond. The baby's body is placed with the head at the upper corner of the diamond. The left corner of the blanket is wrapped around the right side and tucked under the right side (not too tightly—newborns need a little room to move). The bottom corner is then pulled up to the chest, and the right corner is wrapped around the baby's left side. This wrapping technique can be shared with a new mother so she will feel more skilled in handling her baby.

Safety Considerations

The nurse can be an excellent role model for parents in the area of safety. Newborns should always be positioned on the stomach or side with a blanket rolled up behind them. Correct use of the bulb syringe must be demonstrated. The baby should never be left alone anywhere but in the crib. The mother is reminded that while she and the newborn are in the hospital, she should not leave the baby alone because newborns spit up frequently the first day or two after birth. More safety information will be discussed under parent education in this chapter.

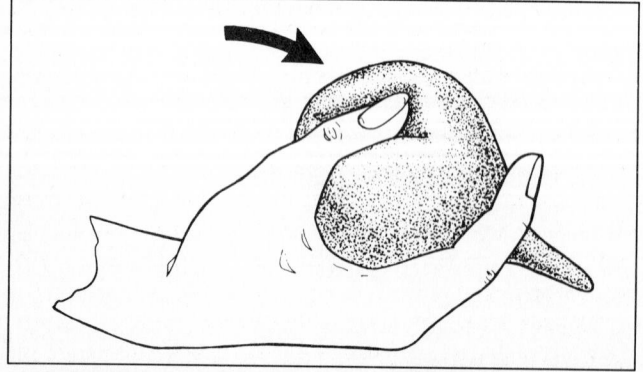

FIGURE 23–6 Nasal and pharyngeal suctioning. The bulb is compressed, then the tip is placed either in the nostril or mouth; the bulb is allowed to reexpand as the compression of the bulb is released.

NEWBORN FEEDING

Initial Feeding in the Hospital

It is the practice in most institutions to offer the newborn an initial feeding of plain sterile water approximately 1–4 hours after birth. Parents of breast-fed infants need to be informed of this practice, of the rationale for it, and of the fact that it will not hinder the newborn's intake of breast milk. If aspiration should occur, the water is readily absorbed by the lung tissue. Glucose water should not be used, as it is damaging to the newborn's lung tissue if aspirated (Avery, 1981). The sterile water provides an opportunity for the nurse to assess the effectiveness of the newborn's suck, swallow, and gag reflexes. A softer nipple made for preterm infants may be used if the newborn appears to tire easily. Extreme fatigue coupled with rapid respiration and circumoral cyanosis may indicate cardiovascular complications and should be assessed further. This initial feeding also provides an opportunity to assess the newborn for symptoms of tracheoesophageal fistula or esophageal atresia (see Chapter 26 for further discussion). In cases of atresia, the esophagus ends in a blind pouch. Consequently the feeding is taken well initially, but as the esophageal pouch fills, the feeding is quickly regurgitated unchanged by stomach contents. When a fistula is present, the infant gags, chokes, regurgitates mucus, and may become cyanotic as fluid passes through the fistula into the lungs.

It is not unusual for the neonate to regurgitate some mucus and water following a feeding even though it was taken without difficulty. Consequently the newborn should be positioned on the side after a feeding to facilitate drainage and should be observed carefully. To decrease this mucus, some nurseries routinely aspirate the stomach contents and do gastric lavage when the neonate is admitted from labor and delivery. Inability to successfully pass the gastric tube suggests the possibility of atresia. The procedure should be stopped and the newborn assessed further.

Some mothers who plan to breast-feed will ask to nurse their newborns immediately following birth, while on the delivery table. This practice provides stimulation for milk production and aids in maternal–newborn bonding. If the newborn appears to have difficulty nursing, the sterile water feeding by the nurse allows an opportunity for assessment. If the water feeding is taken without difficulty and retained, the mother may resume breast-feeding. In formula-fed newborns, after a few successful swallows of sterile water, glucose water may be substituted to give needed sugar and prevent hypoglycemia. The newborn may take 15–30 mL at this first feeding. The newborn's stomach will be filled within 3–5 minutes of sucking at the breast or bottle.

Feeding their newborn presents decisions and problems for most new parents. The nurse provides information to assist them in the decision and can recommend an appropriate diet for the newborn. The information should include (a) an assessment of newborn nutritional needs; (b) adequate facts about the choice between breast- and bottle-feeding; and (c) suggestions about when to add supplemental foods.

Nutritional Needs of the Newborn

The newborn's diet must supply nutrients to meet the rapid rate of physical growth and development. A neonatal diet should include protein, calories, carbohydrate, fat, water, vitamins, and minerals. Recommendations shown in Table 23-1 are all based on limited research data but give generalizations about requirements for optimal nutrition for the first year of life. The calories (110–120 cal/kg/day) in the newborn's diet are divided among protein, carbohydrate, and fat and should be adjusted according to the infant's weight. The essential amino acids are needed for rapid cellular growth and maintenance. The fat portion of the diet provides calories, regulates fluid and electrolyte balance, and develops the neonatal brain and neurologic system. Water requirements are high (140–160 mL/kg/day) in the newborn because of an inability to concentrate urine. Fluid needs will be further increased in illness or hot weather. The iron intake of the infant will be affected by accumulation of iron stores during the fetal life, and the mother's iron, and other food intake if she is breast-feeding. Ascorbic acid (usually in the form of fruit juices) and meat are known to enhance absorption of iron in the mother. Adequate minerals and vitamins are needed by the newborn to prevent deficiency states such as scurvy, cheilosis, and pellagra (Eckstein, 1980).

Breast or Bottle?

DECISION MAKING

Women will usually make the decision between formula or breast-feeding during pregnancy. Frequently the decision is based on the influences of relatives, friends, and social customs rather than on knowledge about nutritional and psychologic needs of herself and her newborn. With the technologic advances in formula production and the availability of knowledge about breast-feeding techniques, the mother should be confident that the choice she makes will promote normal growth and development of her newborn. The nurse's role is to provide information on the nutritional needs of the infant for growth and development and the advantages and disadvantages of both methods.

BREAST MILK: NUTRITIONAL ASPECTS

The American Academy of Pediatrics (1980) recommends breast milk as the optimal food for the first 4–6 months of life. All factors being equal, breast milk is probably the best

Table 23-1 Nutritional Needs of the Normal Newborn*

	At birth	At 1 year
Calories	120/kg	100/kg
Protein	1.9 g/100 kcal[†]	1.7 g/100 kcal[†]
Fat	30%–55% of total calories	30%–50% of total calories
Carbohydrate	35%–55% of total calories	35%–55% of total calories
Water	330 mL[‡]	700 mL
Calcium	388 mg	299 mg
Phosphate	132 mg	110 mg
Magnesium	16 mg	13.5 mg
Iron	7 mg	7 mg
Copper	Not established	Not established
Zinc	Not established	Not established
Vitamins		
A	100–200 IU[†]	100–200 IU[†]
D	0.4 mg/dL[†]	0.4 mg/dL[†]
E	0.4 mg/dL[†]	0.4 mg/dL[†]
K	75 mg/day[†]	75 mg/day[†]
C	10 mg/day[†]	10 mg/day[†]
Thiamine	0.2 mg/100 kcal[†]	0.2 mg/100 kcal[†]

* Adapted from information contained in Eckstein, E. F. 1980. *Food, people, and nutrition.* Westport, Conn.: A V. Publishing Co.
† Estimated to be approximately equivalent to levels in breast milk.
‡ Approximately.

food for a newborn. The advantages are that it contains antibodies to disease, it is nonallergenic, it aids maternal–child bonding, and it is not affected by unsafe water or insect-carried disease (Joseph, 1981). Breast milk and all its components are delivered to the infant in an unchanged form, and vitamins are not lost through processing and heating. Breast milk is composed of lactose, lipids, polyunsaturated fatty acids, and amino acids, especially taurine. Larger amounts of lactose are in breast milk than in formula milk. Some researchers feel the balance of amino acids in breast milk makes it the optimal food for neurologic development. Colostrum (the first milk) contains macrophages that appear to protect the newborn against respiratory infections, vomiting, allergy, and unexplained mortality (Palma and Adcock, 1981). Breast milk also contains an antiinfective organism called *Lactobacillus bifidus,* a natural protector against virulent disease strains in the gastrointestinal tract.

The American Academy of Pediatrics states that there is generally no need to give supplemental iron to breast-fed newborns before the age of 6 months. In fact, supplemental iron may be detrimental to the natural ability of breast milk to protect the newborn against infectious processes. The newborn already has enough iron stores and a further build-up of iron in breast-fed newborns may interfere with lactoferrin, an iron-binding protein that enhances the absorption of iron and has antiinfective properties.

If the breast-feeding mother is taking daily multivitamins the newborn does not usually need extra vitamins. When the mother's diet or vitamin intake is inadequate or questionable, most pediatricians prescribe vitamins for the infant. Breast-fed newborns receive minerals in a more acceptable dose than do formula-fed infants (Riordan and Countryman, 1980).

Before 6 months of age the infant does not produce immunoglobulins to protect against allergic responses. Introduction of foreign-produced proteins in formula may cause an allergy. Breast-fed newborns do not seem to develop allergies. Breast milk also contains thyroid hormone so the newborn who has hypothyroidism is protected against mental retardation.

One disadvantage of breast-feeding is that most drugs taken by the mother are transmitted through breast milk and may cause harm to the newborn (see Chapter 27 for specific drugs and their possible effect on the neonate). A mother's poor nutritional, physical, or mental health may be contraindications for breast-feeding. Difficulty in maintaining milk supply, sore nipples, and constant demands on her time may be other reasons not to breast-feed. Jaundice caused by breast milk is a rare phenomenon but may be yet another reason to not breast-feed.

FORMULA: NUTRITIONAL ASPECTS

Numerous types of commercially prepared formulas meet the nutritional needs of the infant. Modified cow's milk formulas contain different amounts of amino acids: tryosine and phenylalanine are more prevalent in formula milk and the taurine present in breast milk is absent in cow's milk formula. Bottle-fed babies do gain weight a little faster than breast-fed babies because of the higher protein in commercially prepared formula than in human milk. Formula-fed infants generally double their weight within 3½–4 months, whereas nursing infants double their weight at about 5 months.

Formulas contain mostly saturated fatty acids, whereas breast milk is higher in unsaturated fatty acids. The minerals calcium, sodium, and chloride occur in higher concentrations in some commercially made formulas, which may be detrimental to the newborn's kidneys as their immature state may not be ready to handle such high loads of solutes. This high solute load may also lead to thirst in the formula-fed infant, causing overfeeding and possible obesity (Evans and Glass, 1979).

Clinicians recommend iron-fortified formulas or supplements to those mothers who are bottle-feeding with non–iron fortified formulas as iron deficiency anemia is still very prevalent. Seven milligrams of iron per day is the recommended iron dosage. However, it is necessary for the nurse to be aware that too much iron in the form of the extra cereal or a too high formula iron content may interfere with the infant's natural ability to defend against disease (Picciano and Deering, 1980). Parents also need to be informed about the constipation that sometimes results from iron-enriched formula and about various methods of alleviating the constipation.

Table 23–2 compares the components of breast milk, unmodified cow's milk, and a commercially standardized formula. Many companies make an enriched formula that is similar to breast milk. These formulas all have sufficient levels of carbohydrate, protein, fat, vitamins, and minerals to meet the newborn's nutritional needs. Opinion about the use of vitamin supplements for newborns varies. Recommended amounts of vitamins A, D, and C, thiamine, niacin, riboflavin, and ascorbic acid may be obtained from commercially prepared cow's milk or soy-based formulas. Whichever method of feeding is chosen, formula or breast milk, newborns should be given one of these feedings until 9 months to 1 year of age.

Neither unmodified cow's milk nor skim milk is an acceptable alternative for newborn feeding. The protein content in cow's milk is too high (50%–75% more than human milk), is poorly digested, and may cause bleeding of the gastrointestinal tract. Cow's milk is also inadequate in vitamins. Skim milk lacks adequate calories, fat content, and essential fatty acids necessary for proper development of the neonate's neurological system. It provides excessive protein and also causes problems as a result of altered osmolarity. Nutritionists advise against use of unmodified cow's milk or skim milk for children under 2 years of age.

Establishing a Feeding Pattern

Following the initial feeding, hospitals frequently establish artificial 4-hour time frames for feedings. This scheduling may present difficulties for the new mother trying to establish lactation. Breast milk is rapidly digested by the newborn, who may desire to nurse every 2–3 hours initially, with one to two feedings during the night.

Rooming-in permits the mother to feed as needed. When rooming-in is not available, a supportive nursing staff and flexible nursery policies will allow the mother to feed when the infant is hungry. Nothing is more frustrating to a new mother than attempting to nurse a newborn who is sound asleep because he or she is either not hungry or exhausted from crying. Once lactation is established and the family is home, a feeding pattern agreeable to both mother and child is usually established.

Formula-fed newborns may awaken for feedings every 2–5 hours but are frequently satisfied with feedings every 3–4 hours. Because formula is digested more slowly, the bottle-fed infant may go longer between feedings and may begin skipping the night feeding within about 6 weeks. This is very individualized depending on the size and development of the infant.

Both breast-fed and bottle-fed infants experience growth spurts at certain times and require increased feeding. The mother of a breast-fed infant may meet these in-

Table 23-2 Composition of Mature Breast Milk, Cow's Milk, and a Routine Infant Formula*

Composition/dL	Mature breast milk	Cow's milk	Routine formula (20 cal) with iron
Calories	75.0	69.0	67.0
Protein, g	1.1	3.5	1.5
Lactalbumin %	80	18	
Casein %	20	82	
Water, ml	87.1	87.3	
Fat, g	4.0	3.5	3.7
Carbohydrate, g	9.5	4.9	7.0
Ash, g	0.21	0.72	0.34
Minerals			
Na, mg	16.0	50.0	25.0
K, mg	51.0	144.0	74.0
Ca, mg	33.0	118.0	55.0
P, mg	14.0	93.0	43.0
Mg, mg	4.0	12.0	9.0
Fe, mg	0.1	Tr.	1.2
Zn, mg	0.15	0.1	0.42
Vitamins			
A, IU	240.0	140.0	158.6
C, mg	5.0	1.0	5.3
D, IU	2.2	1.4	42.3
E, IU	0.18	0.04	0.83
Thiamin, mg	0.01	0.03	0.04
Riboflavin, mg	0.04	0.17	0.06
Niacin, mg	0.2	0.1	0.7
Curd size	Soft	Firm	Mod. firm
	Flocculent	Large	Mod. large
pH	Alkaline	Acid	Acid
Anti-infective properties	+	±	−
Bacterial content	Sterile	Nonsterile	Sterile
Emptying time	More rapid		

* From Avery, G. B. 1981. *Neonatology.* 2nd ed. Philadelphia: J. B. Lippincott Co., p. 1020.

creased demands by nursing more frequently to increase her milk supply. A slight increase in feedings will meet the needs of the formula-fed infant.

Providing nourishment for her newborn is a major concern of the new mother. Her feelings of success or failure may influence her self-concept as she assumes her maternal role. With proper instruction, support, and encouragement from professional persons, feeding becomes a source of pleasure and satisfaction to both parents and child. (See Chapter 27 for a discussion of methods of assisting a mother to breast-feed or bottle-feed her newborn.)

Nutritional Assessment of the Infant

During the early months of life the food offered to and consumed by infants will be instrumental in ensuring their proper growth and development.

At each well-child visit the nurse assesses the nutrition-al status of the newborn. Assessment should include four components: (a) nutritional history from the parent; (b) weight gain since the last visit; (c) growth chart percentiles; and (d) physical examination. The nutritional history reports the type, amount, and frequency of milk and supplemental foods being given to the infant on a daily basis. The infant should gain 1 ounce per day for the first 6 months of life and 0.5 ounce per day for the second 6 months. Individual charts show the infant's growth with respect to height, weight, and head circumference. The important consideration is that infants continue to grow at their individual rates. The physical examination will assist in identifying any nutritional disorders. Edema, dermatitis, cheilosis, or bleeding gums may be caused by excess protein intake, or riboflavin, niacin, or vitamin C deficiency, respectively. Iron deficiency should be suspected in a pale, diaphoretic, irritable infant who is obese and consumes more than 35-40 ounces of formula per day (Driggers, 1980).

Table 23–3   Tentative Definition of Obesity*

Age in months	Males Length (cm) less than	Males Weight (kg) more than	Females Length (cm) less than	Females Weight (kg) more than
1	51.8	4.2	51.5	4.0
	53.0	4.5	52.2	4.3
	54.2	4.7	53.5	4.6
	55.2	5.1	54.6	4.8
3	58.0	6.0	57.1	5.6
	59.2	6.4	58.0	5.9
	60.2	6.9	59.2	6.2
	61.5	7.3	60.2	6.6
6	65.6	7.7	63.3	7.5
	66.5	8.2	65.2	8.0
	67.8	9.0	66.3	8.4
	69.2	9.6	67.8	8.9
9	70.0	9.1	68.2	8.9
	70.9	9.7	69.5	9.4
	72.3	10.7	71.1	9.9
	73.6	11.2	73.1	10.4
12	73.6	10.2	72.5	9.9
	74.7	10.9	73.2	10.5
	76.4	11.6	75.1	11.1
	78.0	12.5	76.9	11.6
18	80.0	11.6	78.7	11.1
	81.7	12.6	80.2	11.8
	83.2	13.3	82.0	12.7
	85.3	14.4	84.2	13.2
24	85.0	12.8	84.2	12.3
	87.3	13.9	85.8	13.1
	88.8	14.5	87.5	14.2
	90.9	16.0	90.3	14.9
36	93.4	14.8	92.1	14.3
	95.3	15.7	94.2	15.3
	97.3	16.8	96.2	17.0
	100.6	18.6	99.0	17.7

* From Foman, S. J. 1974. *Infant nutrition*. Philadelphia: W. B. Saunders Co., p. 85.

Table 23–4   Average Recommended Levels of Caloric Intake*

Birth to 3 months	55 calories/lb
3–6 months	52 calories/lb
6–9 months	50 calories/lb
9–12 months	47 calories/lb

* From *Recommended Dietary Allowances*. 1980. 8th ed. Washington, D.C.: National Academy of Sciences.
Note: Caloric needs may vary up to 10% for individual infants on a day-to-day basis. This would amount to only a 2–3 ounce variation in amount of formula per day.

NUTRITIONAL ASSESSMENT TOOL

By using the following assessment methods, the nurse can recommend a diet that supplies appropriate nutrition for optimal infant growth and development. The methods are especially helpful in counseling mothers of infants under 6 months of age in view of the tendency to add too many supplemental foods or offer too much formula to infants of this age. By using the nutritional assessment method, identification of appropriate nutritional intake can be done by comparing the infant's dietary intake with the desired caloric intake, weight, age, and the number of calories needed by the infant. Table 23–3 shows a way of examining the appropriateness of the infant's weight in relation to age in months, length, weight and sex. This method is especially useful in breast-fed newborns, since it is not specifically known how many ounces they consume daily. Using Table 23–4, the infant's weight is used to calculate the number of calories recommended for the infant's age. Most commercial formulas prescribed for the normal healthy newborn contain 20 calories per ounce. Some formulas for smaller babies may contain 24 calories per ounce. If the infant is eating solids, the caloric value of those foods must be assessed and included in the calculation of nutritional intake. With knowledge of the amount of calories needed by the infant according to weight and using Table 23–5, the nurse can counsel the parents about how many ounces per day the child needs to meet caloric requirements. The following example shows the effectiveness of these assessments (Markesberry, 1979):

Ms. Leach brings Sue, age 1 month, to the clinic for a well-baby check-up. The baby measures 20½ inches and weighs 10 pounds. The "Tentative Definition of Obesity" table reveals the baby is obese. In relating the baby's dietary history, mother says Sue was a healthy eater from day one. She drains her bottle in 5–12 minutes and by 2 weeks seemed hungry after the bottle. At that time she was already taking a full can of Similac (20 calories/ounce) concentrate (26 ounces diluted) a day, and feeding every 3 hours, so Ms. Leach added baby cereal to her nighttime feeding. Sue didn't accept cereal at first but took it readily when sugar was added. Now she's taking four tablespoons both morning and evening and has strained peaches or bananas once a day. Her daily calorie intake is as follows:

One can Similac . . . . 520 calories
Cereal . . . . 88+ calories [formula or milk added to prepare cereal provides calories as does sugar]
Fruit . . . . 90 calories
Total Intake . . . . 698+ calories

A quick check of her caloric needs . . . (Table 23–5) shows that at 10 pounds Sue should require 550 calories per day. This would be met by 27½ ounces of Similac alone. Her intake is well above suggested levels, a common finding in infants at this age.*

Most times this tool will show that formula alone gives the infant enough calories so that solid foods can be delayed until later.

Supplemental Foods

Opinions vary widely about when to add new foods and what kinds of supplemental foods to add to the infant's diet. One study of a sample of mothers from pediatric clinics and private practices showed that the majority of mothers add solid foods to their infant's diets very early. Cereal was added by most mothers at 1–4 weeks of age followed by fruits and then vegetables. Meats and whole eggs were added between 2 and 6 months of age. The women gave as a basis for information their mothers, husbands, friends, and physicians. Information learned in school or on radio or television had no significant effect upon what they fed their children. When asked why they chose the selected foods, the women said it was to provide iron and to encourage their newborn to like foods they would receive in later life. Health care professionals need to help mothers plan their children's diet. If reasons are offered for why specific foods are given or withheld, more parental compliance may be expected (Crummette and Munton, 1980). Not only do opinions differ among parents, they differ among health care professionals as well. Standardization of recommendations for feeding would benefit health care professionals and the parents who are given information.

The proper time to add foods to the infant's diet should be determined by the physiologic ability to accept other foods besides milk. The American Academy of Pediatrics states that breast milk or formula meets all the requirements of growth for the normal infant until 6 months of age. It is only after 6 months that the child needs extra iron, water, carbohydrate, and vitamin C. Also at that age the infant can sit up and learn to use a spoon. Iron-fortified cereals are an excellent first food as they provide calories and iron. Next the breast-fed infant should be given meats to balance out the diet because breast milk is lower in protein. The infant on formula should be given vegetables and fruit as formula milk is already high in protein. Foods should be introduced one at a time to identify any food allergy, but the sequence of foods given is not critical.

Children may be offered juice when they can drink from a cup. Juice offered in a bottle tends to act as a pacifier and may cause dental decay. Extra water between

*From Markesberry, B. A. 1979. Watching baby's diet: A professional and parent guide. *Am. J. Mat. Child Nurs.* 4:177.

Table 23–5 Approximate Number of Ounces of 20 Calorie/Ounce Formula Needed to Meet Infant Caloric Needs*

Weight of infant	Caloric need (24 hr)	Ounces infant formula (24 hr)
Birth to 3 months		
6 lb	330	16.5
7 lb	385	19
8 lb	440	22
9 lb	495	25
10 lb	550	27.5
11 lb	605	30
12 lb	660	33
13 lb	715	36
14 lb	770	38.5
3-6 months		
10 lb	520	26
11 lb	572	28.5
12 lb	624	31
13 lb	676	34
14 lb	728	36.5
15 lb	780	39
16 lb	832	41.2
17 lb	884	44
18 lb	936	47
19 lb	988	49.5
20 lb	1040	52
21 lb	1092	54.5
22 lb	1144	57

* Reprinted with permission from Markesberry, B. 1979. Watching baby's diet: a professional and parent guide. *Am. J. Nurs.* 4:180.

meals is needed by the infant when solid food is added because the solute load on the infant's kidneys will be increased. Mothers should be cautioned against adding extra salt or sugar to the infant's food; their long-term effects on the infant's future growth, blood pressure, and need for salt are currently under study. Some clinicians also advocate withholding cow's milk, eggs, and wheat until the infant is 6–9 months old. These are known to be allergenic substances for many persons (American Academy of Pediatrics, 1980). Others believe that honey has a relationship to sudden infant death syndrome and counsel against its use for the first year of life. With these guidelines the nurse should be able to teach the parents proper nutrition for their newborn.

Weaning

The decision to wean an infant from breast milk may be made because the infant is 9–12 months old and can drink from a cup or because a separation of mother and infant is imminent. Whatever the reason, the weaning process may cause emotional and physical trauma for the mother and the infant. Engorgement of the breasts occurs if the milk supply is not decreased gradually. Weaning is a time of emotional separation for mother and infant: it may be difficult for them to give up the closeness of their nursing sessions. The nurse who is understanding about this possibility can help the mother to see that her infant is growing up and assist her to plan other activities to replace breast-feeding. A gradual approach is the easiest and most comforting way to wean the infant from breast-feedings. Other activities can serve to enhance the parent–infant bonding process.

During weaning, the mother should substitute one cup- or bottle-feeding for one breast-feeding session over several days so that her breasts gradually produce less milk. Over a period of several weeks she should substitute more cup- or bottle-feedings for breast-feedings. Many mothers continue to nurse once a day in the early morning or late evening for several months until the milk supply is gone. The slow method of weaning will prevent engorgement and allows infants to alter their eating methods at their own rates.

CIRCUMCISION

Circumcision is a surgical procedure in which the prepuce of the penis is separated from the glans and a portion is excised. This permits exposure of the glans and easier retraction of the foreskin for cleansing purposes.

The parents make the decision about circumcision for their newborn male child. In most cases the choice is based on cultural, social, and family tradition. To guarantee informed consent, during the prenatal period parents should be provided with the information about possible long-term medical effects of circumcision and noncircumcision. In the past, this procedure has been recommended for all newborn males. It is now recognized that in most cases this procedure is one of preference and not medically required (American Academy of Pediatrics, 1975). Originally, circumcision was a rite of the Jewish religion. Proponents of the procedure cite studies that imply the incidence of cervical cancer is less in women married to circumcised men. The incidence of cancer of the penis is also lower in circumcised men. In addition, some believe circumcision allows for improved cleanliness and individual comfort. Opponents question the statistical data about cervical carcinoma and feel that neonatal circumcisions predisposes to meatitis, which may eventually led to meatal stenosis. Those opposed to circumcision maintain that continued retraction and good hygienic practices result in comparable cleanliness and comfort. Considerable controversy still exists regarding the pros and cons of circumcision.

To decrease the incidence of cold stress, the procedure is usually not done until the day prior to discharge, when the infant is well stabilized. Sometimes an infant is brought in after discharge for circumcision.

The nurse's responsibilities during a circumcision begin with checking to see that the circumcision permit is signed. Equipment is gathered, and then the infant is prepared by removing the diaper and placing him on a circumcision board or some other type of restraint (Figure 23–7).

A variety of techniques for circumcision is available (Figures 23–8, 23–9 and 23–10) and all produce minimal bleeding. During the procedure, the nurse assesses the newborn's response. One consideration is pain experienced by the newborn. There is no question that he feels pain, but it is not known if he remembers the discomfort. Few physicians use anesthesia for this procedure. The nurse can provide comfort measures such as lightly stroking the baby's head and talking to him. Following the circumcision he should be held and comforted by his mother (Lubchenco, 1980).

After the circumcision a small Vaseline gauze strip may be applied to help control bleeding and to keep the diaper from adhering to the site. The Vaseline gauze is left in place for 1–2 days. It need not be changed unless it becomes contaminated with fecal material. The neonate's voiding should be assessed for amount, adequacy of stream, and presence of blood. If bleeding does occur, pressure is applied to the site with a sterile gauze, and the physician is notified. The neonate may be fussy for a few hours after the procedure or cry when he voids. He should be positioned on his side with the diaper fastened loosely to prevent undue pressure.

Before dismissal, the parents should be instructed to observe the penis for bleeding or possible signs of infection. A whitish yellow exudate around the glans is normal and not indicative of an infectious process. The exudate may be noted for about 2–3 days, and should not be removed, although the parents may be instructed to gently wash the penis and pat it dry. The diaper is loosely fastened for 2–3 days, because the glans remains tender for this length of time.

SLEEP AND ACTIVITY

Perhaps nothing is more unique to each neonate than the individual sleep–activity cycle. Parents must be with their newborn several hours a day to have the opportunity to observe the sleeping and active patterns of their child. Knowledge based on the research of sleep–wake cycles strongly influenced the development of flexible rooming-in arrangements and expanded visiting hours to include other significant members of the family (Klaus and Kennell, 1982). It is important for the nurse to recognize the individual variations of each newborn and to assist parents as

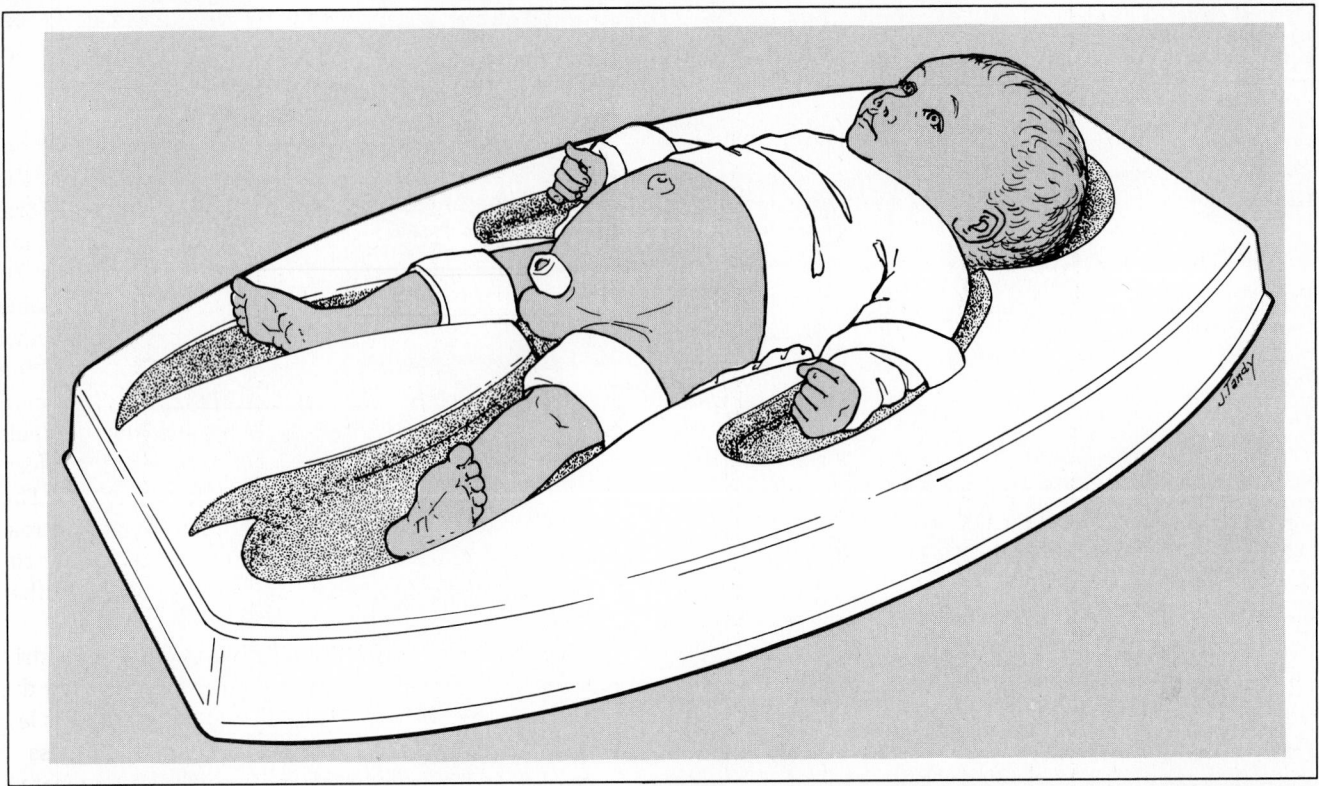

FIGURE 23–7 Proper positioning of the infant on a circumcision restraining board.

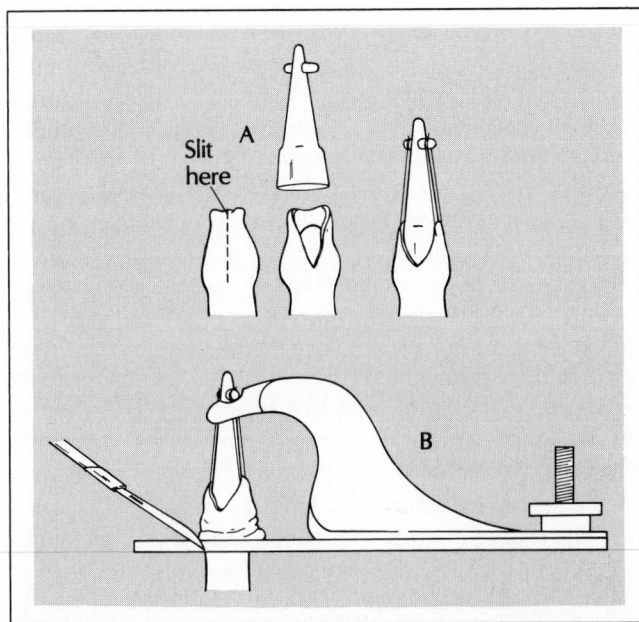

FIGURE 23–8 When the Yellen clamp is used for circumcision, the prepuce is drawn over the cone (**A**), and the clamp is applied (**B**). Pressure is maintained for 3–5 minutes, and then the excess prepuce is cut away.

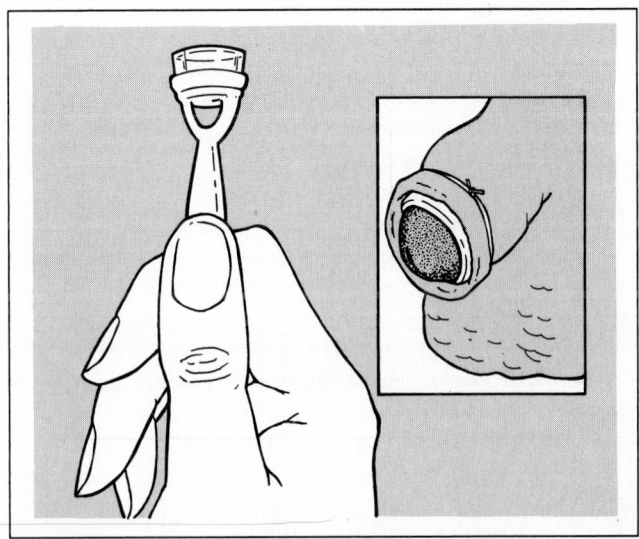

FIGURE 23–9 When the Plastibell is used for circumcision, the bell is fitted over the glans. Suture is tied around the rim of the bell and the excess prepuce is cut away. The plastic rim remains in place for 3–4 days until healing takes place. The bell may be removed or allowed to fall off.

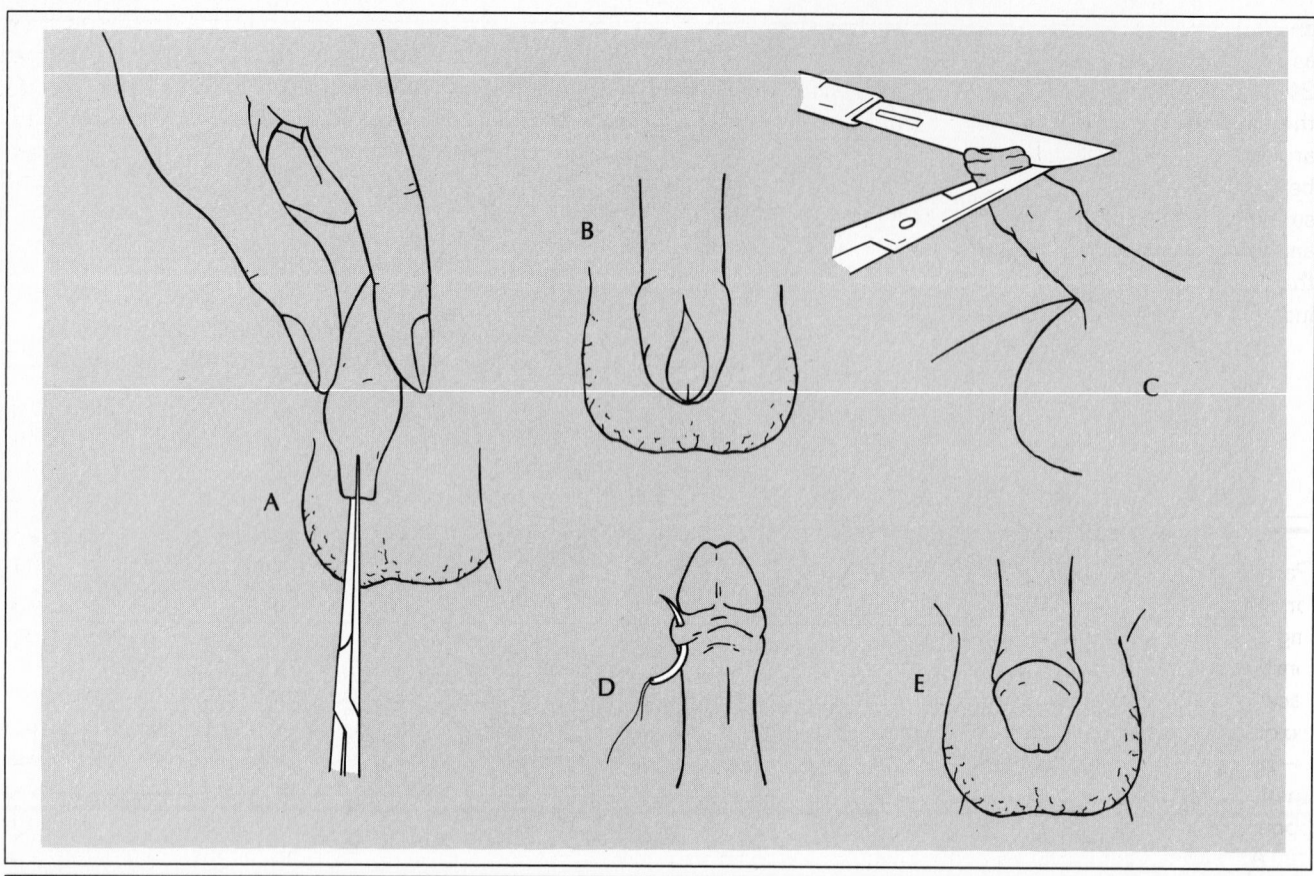

FIGURE 23–10 A and B, In this circumcision procedure, the prepuce is slit and retracted. **C,** Excess prepuce is then cut off. **D,** The prepuce is sutured in place. **E,** Circumcised penis.

they develop sensitivity to their infant's communication signals and rhythms of activity and sleep. There are clear opportunities for the nurse to be involved in this early attachment process by sharing factual information, and providing opportunities for the parent to be involved in the actual care of their newborn.

The newborn demonstrates several different sleep–wake states after the initial periods of reactivity described earlier. It is not uncommon for a neonate to sleep almost continuously for the first 2–3 days following birth, awakening only for feedings every 3–4 hours. Some newborns bypass this stage of deep sleep and may require only 12–16 hours of sleep. The parents need to know that this is normal.

Sleep–Wake States

Five sleep–wake states are observable in the newborn as discussed in Chapter 21. The length of time the newborn spends in each cycle varies with the individual. Patterns change as the child grows older. *Quiet sleep*, which correlates with non-REM sleep, is a deep sleep with regular breathing and no movement except for sudden body jerks. Normal household noise will not awaken the infant during

this time. *Regular sleep* occurs 4–5 hours a day in 15–20 minute periods. *Active sleep* correlates with active REM sleep and is typified by irregular breathing and fine muscular twitching. A newborn may cry out in sleep, but this does not mean he or she is uncomfortable or awake. Unusual household noise may awaken the infant more easily in this state; however, the newborn will quickly go back to sleep.

Wide awake is a quiet state in which newborns are quietly involved with the environment. They watch a moving mobile, smile, and as they become older, discover and play with their hands and feet. When infants become uncomfortable due to wet diapers, hunger, or cold, they enter the *active awake and crying state*. In this state, the cause of the crying should be identified and attended to. Sometimes parents are frustrated as they try to identify the external or internal stimuli that are causing the angry, hurt crying (Whaley and Wong, 1979).

CRYING

For the newborn, crying is the only means of vocally expressing needs. Parents and caregivers learn to distinguish different tones and qualities of the neonate's cry. The amount of crying is highly individual. Some will cry as little as 15–30 minutes in 24 hours or as long as 2 hours every 24 hours (Ostwald and Paltemen, 1974). When crying is the result of discomfort or hunger, once these situations are attended to, if the crying continues, the newborn may be comforted by swaddling or by rocking and other reassuring activity. If crying is excessive, this should be noted and assessed, taking other factors into consideration. After the first 2–3 days, newborns settle into patterns that are individual to each infant and family.

ENHANCING INTERACTION BETWEEN PARENTS AND INFANT

Parents develop interacting skills with their newborn as he or she responds to their voices and the stimulation of looking at their faces. Goren and coworkers (1975) have demonstrated that newborns are more attentive to the human face than to any other stimuli. The neonate also prefers color and patterns that are varied. The clearest vision is at 8–10 in. Parents need to know that their newborn can see them and that the first fleeting smile is truly a social response, and not merely a "gas bubble."

A powerful bond develops along with eye contact between the newborn and the caregivers. The importance of this early experience has been clearly documented. The nurse must incorporate this information while using nursing skills to enhance the attachment process of the new family. Strong reciprocal attachment bonds develop as parents interact with their newborn. Individual personalities and emotional needs play important roles in this developmental process. (Chapter 28 has an in-depth discussion of the bonding and attachment process.)

Early Experiences and Needs at Home

Each newborn will have variations in normal physiologic responses. Parents must learn how to interpret these changes in their newborn. It is invaluable for the parents to have a primary support system established before they take their infant home. Some physicians encourage pediatric prenatal visits so that this contact is established before the birth (Sprunger and Preece, 1981). Public health nurses have long been involved as guides in newborn care and parent education (Lauri, 1981). Hospitals are now expanding their primary care functions to the new family to include one home visit by the primary nurse who cared for the family in the hospital. The hospital nursery staff may also make themselves available as a 24-hour telephone resource for the new mother who needs additional support and consultation during the first few days at home with her newborn.

Before the newborn and mother are discharged from the hospital, parents are informed about the normal screening tests for newborns and should be told when to return to the hospital or clinic to have the tests completed. Routine well-baby visits should be scheduled with the clinic, pediatric nurse practitioner, or physician.

NEWBORN SCREENING PROGRAM

Newborn screening tests detect disorders that cause mental retardation, physical handicaps, or death if left undiscovered. Inborn errors of metabolism usually can be detected within 1–2 weeks after birth and all important treatment initiated before any damage has occurred. (Chapter 26 discusses these problems in detail.) The disorders that can be identified by a drop of blood obtained by a heel stick on the second or third day are galactosemia, homocystinuria, hypothyroidism, maple syrup urine disease, phenylketonuria (PKU), and sickle cell anemia. Parents should be instructed that a second blood specimen will be required from the newborn after 7–14 days when the newborn's metabolism is fully functioning. By this time the defects are clearly apparent and treatment initiated. Treatment of these conditions may be dietary or by administering the missing hormones. The inborn conditions themselves cannot be cured but they all can be treated. Although they are not contagious, they may be inherited.

PARENT EDUCATION

Parents may be familiar with handling and caring for infants or this may be their first time to interact with a newborn. If they are new parents, the sensitive nurse gently teaches them by example and instructions geared to their needs and previous knowledge about the various aspects of newborn care.

The nurse should spend time observing how parents interact with their infant during feeding and caregiving activities. Rooming-in, even for a short time, provides opportunities for the nurse to provide information and evaluate whether the parents are comfortable with changing diapers, wrapping, handling, and feeding their newborn. Do both parents get involved in the infant's care? Is the mother depending on someone else to help her at home? Does the mother give excuses for not wanting to be involved in her baby's care? ("I am too tired," "My stitches hurt," or "I will learn later.") All these considerations need to be taken into account when evaluating the educational needs of the parents.

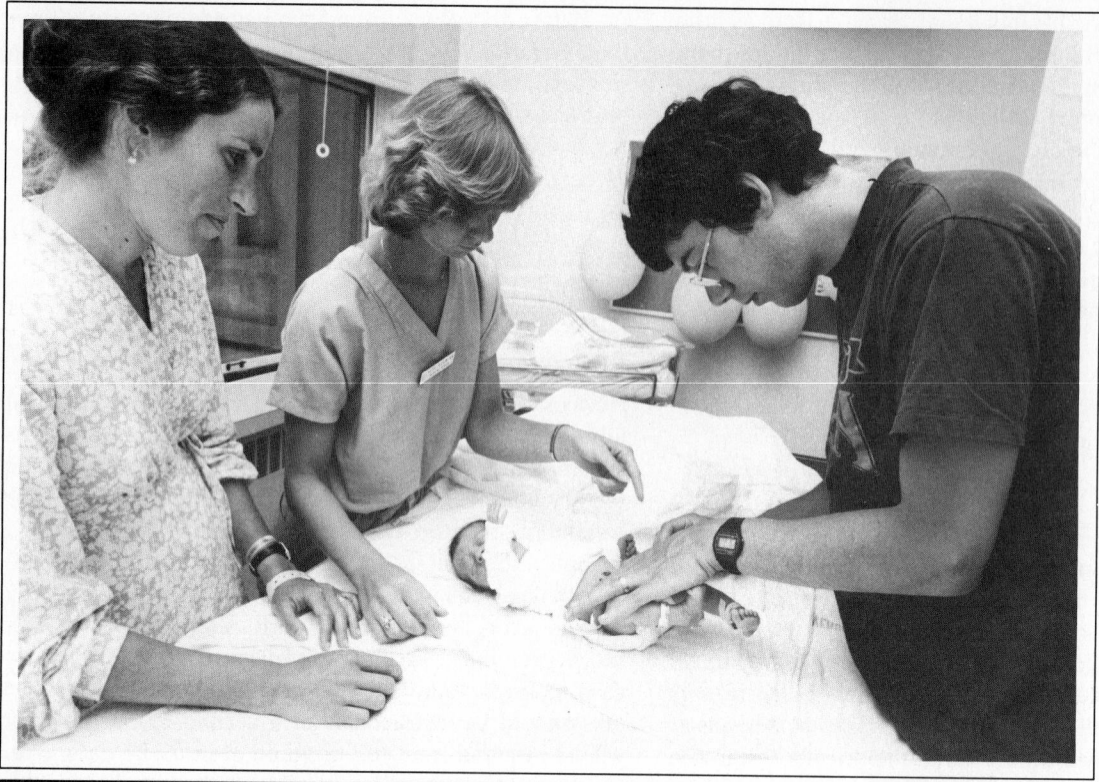

FIGURE 23–11 Individualizing parent education. Father returns demonstration of diapering his daughter.

Several methods may be used to teach parents about newborn care. Daily child care classes are a nonthreatening way to convey general information. Individual instruction is helpful to answer specific questions or to clarify an item that may have been confusing in class (Figure 23–11). Discharge planning is essential to verify the mother's knowledge when she leaves the hospital. Follow-up calls after discharge lend added support by providing another opportunity for mothers to have their questions answered. The essential areas to be covered by a nurse in educating parents before discharge are described in the following sections.

Positioning and Handling

Methods of positioning and handling the newborn are demonstrated to parents if needed. As the parents provide care, the nurse can instill parental confidence by giving them positive feedback. If the parents encounter problems, the nurse can suggest alternatives and serve as a role model (see p. 714.)

Oral and Nasal Suctioning

Parents have a great fear of their infant choking; anxiety may be relieved if they know what action to take. The use of the bulb syringe in the nose and mouth should be dem-onstrated, followed by a return demonstration. The parents should repeat this demonstration prior to discharge so they have an opportunity to feel more confident and comfortable with the procedure.

Stools and Voids

Newborn's stools can cause concern for parents unless they are prepared. The nurse discusses meconium stools, transitional stools, and the difference between breast milk and formula stools. They may be explained and highlighted with pictures. Parents should be told that breast-fed babies may have six to ten small, loose yellow stools per day, whereas formula-fed infants may have only one or two stools a day, which are more formed and brown in color.

Each baby develops his or her own stooling pattern. The parents may also be shown pictures of a constipated stool (small, pelletlike) and diarrhea (loose, green, or may be blood-tinged). Parents should understand that a green color is common in transitional stools so that transitional stools are not confused with diarrhea the first week of a newborn's life.

Infants normally void (urinate) five to eight times per day. Less than five to eight wet diapers a day may indicate the newborn needs more fluids.

Bathing

An actual bath demonstration is the best way for the nurse to teach parents. Bathing should be done every other day or twice a week because excess bathing will dry out the baby's sensitive skin. Sponge baths are recommended for the first 2 weeks or until the umbilical cord completely falls off. The following information should be included in the demonstration. Supplies can be kept in a plastic bag or some type of container to prevent hunting for supplies each time. The supplies include two washcloths, two towels, two blankets, soap (mild, without much perfume, for example, Dial or Safeguard), shampoo, A and D ointment, or petroleum jelly (Vaseline), lotion, rubbing alcohol, cotton balls, two diapers, and clean clothes. The mother may want to use a small plastic tub for water, a clean kitchen or bathroom sink, or a large bowl. Expensive baby tubs are not necessary, but some parents may prefer to purchase them.

Before starting, if no one else is at home, the parent may want to take the phone off the hook and put a sign on the door to prevent being disturbed. Having someone home during the first few baths will be helpful because that person can get items that were forgotten and provide moral support. The room should be warm and free of drafts.

SPONGE BATH

After the supplies are gathered, the tub (or any of the just mentioned containers) is filled with water that is warm to the touch. The water temperature is tested with an elbow or forearm. (Parents may also purchase a thermometer for bath water.) Soap should not be added to the water. The infant should be wrapped in a blanket, with a T-shirt and diaper on. This helps to keep the newborn warm and secure. Remove clothing to expose each new area.

To start the bath, a washcloth is wrapped once around the index finger. Each eye is gently wiped from inner to outer corner. This direction is the way eyes naturally drain and prevents irritating the eyes. A different spot on the washcloth is used for each eye to prevent cross-contamination. Some swelling and drainage may be common the first few days after birth. The ears are washed next by wrapping the washcloth once around an index finger and gently cleaning the external ear and behind the ear. Cotton swabs are never used in the ears because it is possible to put the swab too deeply in the ear and damage the ear drum. The remainder of the infant's face is then wiped with the soap-free washcloth. Many infants may start to cry at this point. The face should be washed every day and the chin wiped off after each feeding.

The neck is washed carefully but thoroughly with the washcloth. Soap may now be used. Formula or breast milk and lint collect in the skin folds of the neck, so it may be helpful to sit the baby up, supporting the neck and shoulders with one hand while washing the neck with the other hand.

The baby's T-shirt is now removed and the blanket unwrapped. The chest, back, and arms are wet with the washcloth. The mother may then lather her hands with soap and wash the baby's chest, back, and arms. Care is taken to avoid wetting the cord. Soap is rinsed off with the wet washcloth, and the upper part of the body is dried with a towel or blanket. The baby's upper body is then wrapped with a dry clean blanket to prevent a chill.

Next the infant's legs are unwrapped, wet with the washcloth, lathered, rinsed, and well dried. If the infant has dry skin, a *small* amount of lotion or ointment (petroleum jelly or A and D ointment) may be used. Ointments are better than lotions for dry cracked feet and hands. Baby oil is not used, as it clogs skin pores. Powders aggravate dry skin and are avoided also.

The genital area is cleansed daily with soap and water and with water after each wet or dirty diaper. Girls are washed from the *front* of the genital area toward the rectum to avoid fecal contamination of the urethra and thus to the bladder. Newborn girls often have a thick, white mucous discharge or a slight bloody discharge from their vaginal area. This is normal for the first 1–2 weeks of age and should be wiped off with damp cloth at diaper changes.

Parents of uncircumcised baby boys should check with the physician on caring for the penis. Baby boys who have been circumcised need daily gentle cleansing. A very wet washcloth is rubbed over a bar of soap. The washcloth is squeezed above the baby's penis, letting the soapy water run over the circumcision site. The area is rinsed off with plain warm water and patted dry. A small amount of petroleum jelly or bactericidal ointment may be put on the circumcised area, but excessive amounts may block the meatus and should be avoided.

Baby powder (or cornstarch) is not recommended for diaper rash. Baby powder may cake with urine and irritate the infant's bottom, while corn starch may lead to a fungal infection. Both products may also be inhaled by the infant while being applied. Ointments are more effective for diaper rash. If the ointment does not help the rash, mothers using disposable diapers may try another brand of diaper. If cloth diapers are used, a different detergent or fabric softener may alleviate the problem. Persistent diaper rash should always be discussed with the physician.

The umbilical cord should be kept clean and dry by cleansing it with alcohol-soaked cotton balls. The cord generally should fall off in 7–14 days. Alcohol is utilized until the cord is completely gone. The diaper should be folded down to allow air to circulate around the cord. The physician should be consulted if bright red bleeding or puslike drainage occurs.

The first or last step in bathing is washing the infant's hair with fresh water. The newborn is swaddled in a dry blanket, leaving only the head exposed and held in the football hold with the head tilted slightly downward to prevent water running in the eyes. Water should be brought to the head by a cupped hand. The hair is moistened and lathered with a small amount of shampoo. A *very* soft brush may be used to massage the shampoo over the entire head. The brush may be used over the soft spots. The hair is then rinsed and toweled dry. Oils or lotions are not used on the newborn's head. Brushing the infant's hair every day and washing the hair with a soft soapy brush during baths will prevent cradle cap.

TUB BATHS

The infant may be put in a tub after the cord has fallen off and the circumcision site is healed (approximately 2 weeks) (Figure 23–12). Older infants usually enjoy a tub bath more than a sponge bath, although newborns cry during either type. To prevent slipping, a washcloth is placed in the bottom of the tub or sink.

The newborn is placed in the tub using the cradle hold and grasping the distal thigh. The neck is supported by the parent's elbow in the cradle position. Only 3 or 4 inches of water are needed in the tub. Because wet infants are slip-

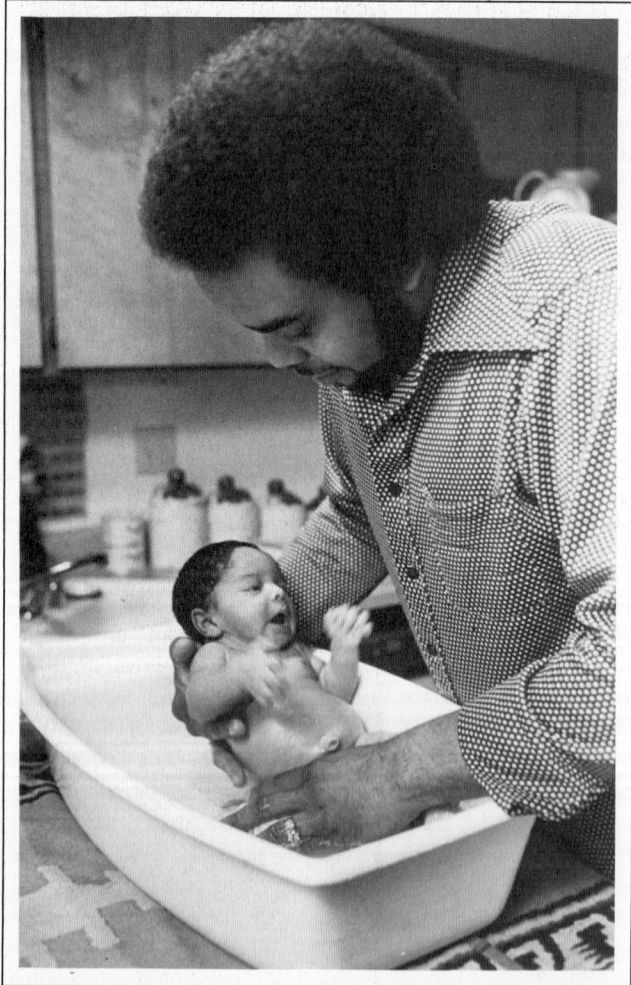

FIGURE 23–12 When bathing the infant, it is important to support her head. Note that the cord site has healed on this 2-week-old baby.

pery, some parents have found that a sweat sock with holes cut out for the fingers pulled over the arm will help prevent the baby from slipping out of one's arms. To wash the back, the infant is turned prone, and the parent places the thumb under the infant's arm closest to the parent, with the fingers on the front of the baby's chest. The infant is lifted out of the tub in the cradle position and dry well. Wrap in a dry blanket and wash the hair in the same way as for a sponge bath.

Nail Care

The nails of the newborn are seldom cut in the hospital. During the first days of life, the nails may adhere to the skin of the fingers, and cutting is contraindicated. Within a week the nails separate from the skin and frequently break off. If the nails are long or if infants are scratching themselves, the nails may be trimmed. This is most easily done while infants sleep. Nails should be cut straight across using adult cuticle scissors.

Dressing the Newborn

Newborns need to wear a T-shirt, diaper (plastic pants if using cloth diapers), a sleeper, and to be wrapped in a light blanket while being fed or on a fairly cool day. A good rule of thumb is for parents to add one more light layer of clothing than the parent is wearing. Infants should wear hats outdoors to protect their sensitive ears from drafts. Take a blanket to cover an infant in air-conditioned stores. Remember to unzip or remove a blanket when inside a warm building.

At home the amount of clothing the infant wears is determined by the temperature. Families who maintain the home at 60–65F should dress the infant more warmly than those who maintain the temperature at 70–75F. Diaper shapes vary and are subject to personal preference (Figure 23–13). Prefolded and disposable diapers are usually rectangular. Diapers may also be triangular or kite-folded. Extra material is placed in front for boys and toward the back for girls to aid in absorbency.

Infant clothing should be laundered separately using a mild soap or detergent. Diapers may be presoaked prior to washing. All clothing should be rinsed twice to remove soap and residue and to decrease the possibility of rash. Some infants may not tolerate the use of clothing treated with fabric softeners; in this case softeners should be avoided.

Temperature Assessment

The nurse must demonstrate how to take rectal and axillary temperatures for parents. A return demonstration is the only way to evaluate their understanding. The nurse shows them how to shake down a thermometer before

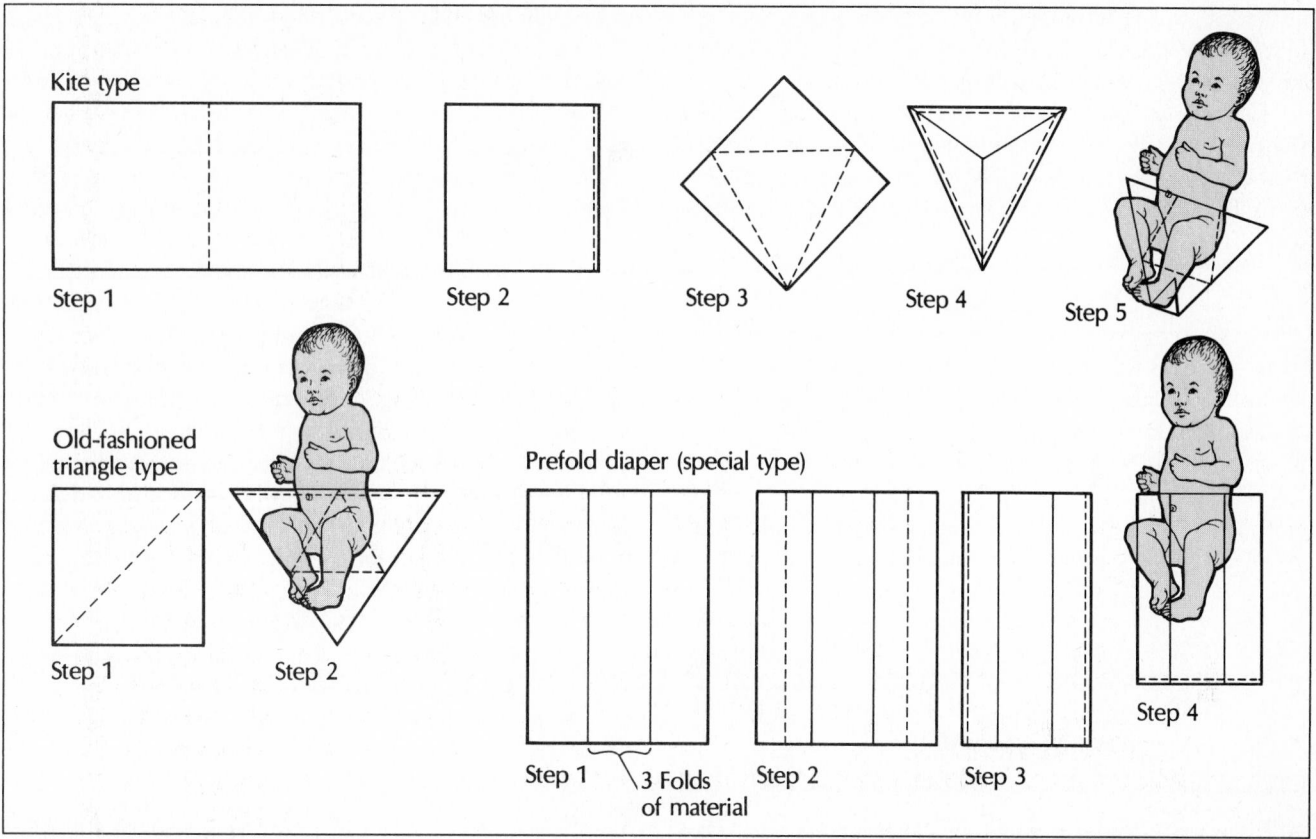

FIGURE 23-13 Three basic diaper shapes. Dotted lines indicate folds.

inserting it. When parents take a rectal temperature, the infant should be supine with the legs held up in one hand, exposing the rectum. The end of the rectal thermometer is lubricated with petroleum jelly and the thermometer is inserted just until the silver bulb is covered, approximately half an inch. The thermometer is held in place 5 minutes. A baby is never left alone with a thermometer in place. Normal rectal temperature is 97.8–99F (36.6–37.2C). Rectal temperatures are more accurate, and most pediatricians prefer temperatures taken this way by parents. To take an axillary temperature, the thermometer is placed under one of the infant's arms, making sure that the bulb of the thermometer is underneath the armpit. It is held in place 3–4 minutes (Figure 22–15). A parent needs to take the newborn's temperature when illness is suspected. *Signs of illness* include the following:

- Temperature above 101F (38.4C) or below 97F (36.1C)
- More than one episode of projectile vomiting
- Missing two feedings in a row
- Lethargy (listlessness)
- Cyanosis with or without a feeding
- Apnea

Parents are advised to call a physician immediately if any of these signs occur. Parents should also check with their physician for advice about over-the-counter medications they should have in the medicine cabinet. Flu, colds, teething, constipation, diarrhea, and other common ailments and their management should be discussed beforehand with the physician.

Safety

Accidents are the number one cause of death in children, with car accidents causing the highest number of deaths, followed by poisonings. Half of the children killed or injured in automobile accidents could have been protected by the use of federally approved car seats. Newborns should go home from the hospital in a car seat (not infant carrier seat) and always be in one whenever they are in the car until 4 years of age (depending on size of the child) no matter how short the trip. In many states, the use of car seats for children up to the age of 4 years is mandatory.

All medications must be locked up. Newborns quickly grow into toddlers who can climb to medicine cabinets. Vitamins look like candy to a toddler. Whenever medication is given, children should be told they are taking medicine instead of calling it candy. Plants should be put above a toddler's reach; many are poisonous. Move all cleaning supplies to high out-of-the-way cupboards.

Cover electrical outlets and keep electrical cords out of sight. Parents should be encouraged to think ahead before the baby becomes a toddler. Newborns do not need pillows or stuffed animals in the crib while they sleep; these items could cause suffocation.

Discharge Planning

Parents should be taught all necessary caregiving methods *before* discharge. A checklist may be helpful to see if the teaching has been completed. The nurse needs to review all areas for understanding or questions with the mother, without rushing, taking time to answer all queries. The mother should have the physician's phone number, address, and any specific instructions. Having the nursery phone number is also reassuring to a new mother. Encourage the parents to call with questions. The nurse may use this time to remind parents that normal weight loss is 5–15% the first 3–5 days of age and that they can expect the baby to regain the birth weight by 10 days of age. An infant should gain 4–6 ounces per week for the first 5 months, and then 2–4 ounces per week until the age of 1 year. The nurse may ask the mother if she is interested in having a visiting nurse help her at home.

The final step of discharge planning is documentation. Any concerns of the parents or nurse are noted. The nurse specifies exactly which demonstrations and/or classes the mother and/or father attended and their expressed understanding of the instructions given to them.

Parent education is a wonderful aspect of family-centered maternity care. The nurse who takes the time to get the family off to a good start can feel satisfied that the best care is being provided for all members of the family.

SUMMARY

At the moment of birth, numerous adaptations must take place in the newborn's body systems. The nursing care of the newborn is aimed at facilitating the child's adjustment to the new environment and ensuring his or her well-being. In addition, the nurse uses his or her teaching skills to help the parents of the newborn adjust to their new role. Caretaking activities of the nurse and parents range from feeding and bathing the infant to providing sensory stimulation and emotional comfort.

References

American Academy of Pediatrics. Committee on Fetus and Newborn. Oct. 1975. Report of the Ad Hoc Task Force on Circumcision. *Pediatrics* 56:610.

———. Committee on Nutrition. 1980. On the feeding of supplemental foods to infants. *Pediatrics.* 65:1178.

Avery, G. B. 1981. *Neonatology.* Philadelphia: J. B. Lippincott.

Benitz, W. E., and Tatro, D. S. 1981. *The pediatric drug handbook.* Chicago: Year Book Medical Publishers.

Crummette, B. D., and Munton, M. T. 1980. Mothers' decisions about infant nutrition. *Pediatr. Nurs.* 6:16.

Driggers, D. A. 1980. Infant nutrition made simple. *Am. Family Physician.* 22:113.

Eckstein, E. F. 1980. *Food, people and nutrition.* Westport, Conn.: A. V. Publishing Company.

Evans, H. E., and Glass, L. 1979. Breastfeeding: advantages and potential problems. *Pediatr. Annals.* 8:110.

Goren, C.; Sarty, M.; and Wu, P. 1975. Visual following and pattern discrimination of face-like stimuli by newborn infants. *Pediatrics.* 56:544.

Joseph, S. 1981. Anatomy of the infant formula controversy. *Am. J. Dis. Child.* 135:889.

Klaus, M. H., and Kennell, J. H. 1982. *Parent–infant bonding,* 2nd ed. St. Louis: The C. V. Mosby Company.

Lauri, S. 1981. The public health nurse as a guide in infant child care and education. *J. Advanced Nurs.* 6:297.

Lubchenco, L. O. 1980. Routine neonatal circumcision: a surgical anachronism. *Clin. Obstet. Gynecol.* 23:1135.

Markesberry, B. A. 1979. Watching baby's diet: a professional and parent guide. *Am. J. Mat. Child Nurs.* 4:177.

Ostwald, P., and Paltemen, P. March 1974. The cry of the human infant. *Sci. Am.* 230(3):84.

Palma, P. A., and Adcock, E. W. 1981. Human milk and breast-feeding. *Am. Family Physician.* 24:173.

Picciano, M. F., and Deering, R. H. 1980. The influence of feeding regimens on iron status during infancy. *Am. J. Clin. Nutrition.* 33:746.

Riordan, J. M., and Countryman, B. A. 1980. Basics of breast-feeding. Part III. *J. Obstet. Gynecol. Neonatal. Nurs.* 9:273.

Sprunger, L. W., and Preece, E. W. 1981. Use of pediatric prenatal visits by family physicians. *J. Family Pract.* 13:1007.

Whaley, L. F., and Wong, D. L. 1979. *Nursing of infants and children.* St. Louis: The C. V. Mosby Company.

Additional Readings

Dallman, P. R. 1980. Inhibition of iron absorption by certain foods. *Am. J. Disease of Child.* 143:453.

Dunn, D. M., and White, D. G. 1981. Interactions of mothers with their newborns in the first half-hour of life. *J. Advanced Nurs.* 6:271.

Gilfoyle, E. M., et al. 1981. *Children adapt.* Thorofare, N.J.: Charles B. Slack, Inc.

Osborn, L. M., et al. March 1981. Hygiene care in uncircumcised infants. *Pediatrics.* 67:365.

Rong, M. L. 1981. *Manual of newborn care plans.* Boston: Little, Brown & Co.

Siegel, E., et al. Aug. 1980. Hospital and home support during infancy: impact on maternal attachment, child abuse and neglect, and health care utilization. *Pediatrics.* 66:183.

■ 24 ■

THE HIGH-RISK NEWBORN: NEEDS AND CARE

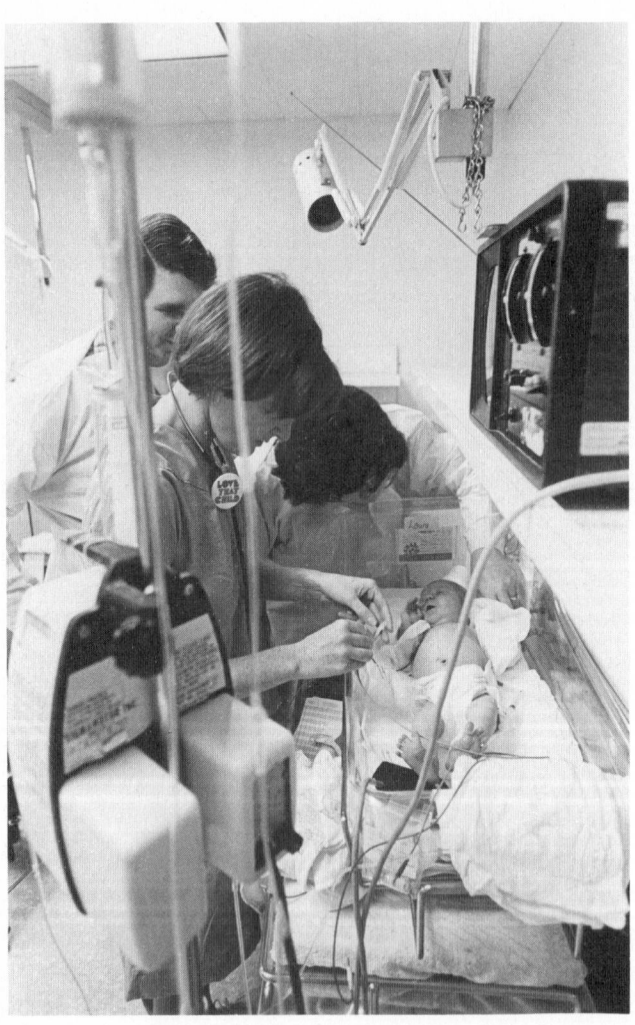

■ CHAPTER CONTENTS

IDENTIFICATION OF HIGH-RISK INFANTS

NURSING MANAGEMENT OF HIGH-RISK INFANTS

PRETERM (PREMATURE) INFANTS

    Preterm Infants' Physiologic Adaptations

    Respiratory Physiology and Considerations

    Cardiovascular Physiology and Considerations

    Nutrition and Fluid Requirements

    Renal Physiology

    Hepatic Physiology and Considerations

    Immunologic Physiology and Considerations

    Hematologic Physiology and Considerations

    Reactivity Periods and Behavioral States

    Central Nervous System Physiology and Considerations

    Long-Term Needs and Outcome

POSTTERM NEONATE

LARGE-FOR-GESTATIONAL-AGE INFANT

SMALL-FOR-GESTATIONAL-AGE INFANT

    Etiology

    Patterns of Intrauterine Growth Retardation

    Long-Term Outcome and Needs

INFANT OF DIABETIC MOTHER

INFANTS OF MOTHERS WITH CARDIAC OR HYPERTENSIVE CARDIOVASCULAR DISEASE
  Infant of Mother with Cardiac Disease
  Infant of Mother with Hypertensive Cardiovascular Disease

ALCOHOL- OR DRUG-ADDICTED NEONATES
  Alcohol Dependency
  Drug Dependency

PARENTING THE HIGH-RISK NEONATE
  Attachment
  Adjustment
  Nursing Interventions
  Predischarge Care

■ OBJECTIVES

- Discuss the physiologic differences of the preterm neonate that predispose each body system to various complications of prematurity.

- Compare the physiologic complications of the preterm, small-for-gestational-age, and large-for-gestational-age infant and the underlying etiology of the various complications.

- Explain the effects of selected maternal health problems on the high-risk neonate.

- Describe the methods used to feed a preterm infant, the criteria used to determine which method should be used, and the special nursing factors considered when feeding a preterm infant.

- Differentiate between postmaturity and placental insufficiency syndrome and explain why infants with these conditions sometimes require care similar to that for a preterm infant.

- Identify the needs and nursing support necessary for family members to deal with the crisis of a preterm birth.

- Discuss reasons why parents are now encouraged to visit and to have early contact with their preterm infant and how the nurse can best support the parents in the "mothering" process.

Within the last 20 years, the field of neonatology has broadened greatly as the findings of its research have become utilized in clinical situations. This process has led to a similar evolution in the hospital care of the neonate, so that today there are many levels of nursery care: special care, transitional care, and low-, medium-, and high-risk care. The nurse is an important caregiver in all types of nurseries. Nursing responsibilities are expanding, and the nurse is the vital link in the multidisciplinary health care communication system. The collaborative efforts of nurses, physicians, specialists, audiologists, nutritionists, inhalation therapists, laboratory personnel, physical therapists, pharmacists, social service personnel, parents, and clergy contribute to the high level of perinatal care available today.

Neonatal care has benefited from such advances in technology as monitoring devices, neonatal respirators, and microscopic laboratory techniques. Nursing and medical management stress the importance of the quality of life for high-risk survivors. Consequently, the incidence of severe sequelae such as neurologic impairment, spasticity, blindness, and hearing loss has decreased. The majority of

neonates (85%–95%) surviving in current intensive care units are normal; only 5%–10% show definite abnormalities.

Other factors besides the availability of high-level neonatal care influence the outcome. These factors include birth weight, gestational age, type and length of neonatal illness, and environmental and maternal factors.

IDENTIFICATION OF HIGH-RISK INFANTS

A high-risk infant is one whose health status renders him or her susceptible to increased morbidity or mortality because of dysmaturity, immaturity, physical disorders, or complications of birth. In the vast majority of instances the infant is the product of a pregnancy involving one or more predictable risk factors. These risk factors include low socioeconomic level of the mother, preexisting maternal conditions such as heart disease, obstetric factors such as age or parity, medical conditions related to pregnancy such as prenatal maternal infection, and obstetric complications

733

such as abruptio placentae. Various risk factors and their specific effects on the pregnancy outcome are discussed on p. 214.

Because these factors and the perinatal risks associated with them are known, the birth of many high-risk neonates can often be anticipated and prepared for through adequate prenatal care. The pregnancy can be closely monitored, treatment can be instituted as necessary, and arrangements can be made for delivery to occur at a facility with appropriate equipment and personnel to care for both mother and child.

Identification of a high-risk pregnancy is usually made during prenatal visits and is based on the history and on laboratory data such as serology, blood type, Rh factor determination (father and mother, if mother is Rh negative), and serum antibody tests for rubella and other infections. Amniocentesis may be indicated to determine the presence of chromosomal disorders or of certain inherited metabolic disorders. Bilirubin pigment tests may be required to estimate Rh isoimmunization, and the L/S ratio may be determined to evaluate fetal lung maturity prior to delivery (see p. 385). Proper follow-up observation of prenatal high-risk conditions is in order to give optimal care (medical, nursing, and psychologic) to the woman and fetus.

Intrapartally, fetal heart monitoring has played a significant role in the detection of infants in distress. Prediction of all high-risk cases cannot always be made before labor, since factors concerning labor and delivery or how the infant will withstand stress are not known prior to the actual process. One study showed that 20% of patients who were not at risk during the prenatal period became at risk during labor and delivery (Hobel et al., 1973). Intrapartal complicating factors include malpresentations, prolapsed cord, meconium-stained fluid, and abruptio placentae (Chapter 15).

Immediately after birth a valuable tool in identifying the high-risk neonate is the Apgar score. As discussed in Chapter 16, a normal infant will receive a score of 8–10, a moderately depressed infant will have a score of 3–6, and a severely depressed infant will have a score of 0–2. Infants with scores of 0–6 receive resuscitative treatment as necessary (see p. 789). It has been demonstrated that the lower the Apgar score at 5 minutes after birth, the higher the percentage of neurologic abnormalities after 1 year. This percentage also increases significantly as birth weight decreases (Korones, 1981).

The newborn classification and neonatal mortality risk chart is another useful tool in identifying newborns at risk (Figure 24–1). Before the construction of this classification tool, birth weight of less than 2500 g was the sole criterion for the determination of maturity. It was eventually recognized that an infant could weigh more than 2500 g but be immature. Conversely, an infant less than 2500 g might be functionally at term or beyond. Thus, birth weight and ges-

tational age together became the criteria used to assess neonatal maturity and mortality risk.

According to the newborn classification and neonatal mortality risk chart, *gestation* is divided as follows:

- Preterm = 0–37 (completed) weeks
- Term = 38–41 (completed) weeks
- Postterm = 42+ weeks

In Figure 24–1, intrauterine growth curves are redelineated by the tenth and ninetieth percentiles. Large-for-gestational-age (LGA) infants are those above the ninetieth percentile. Appropriate-for-gestational-age (AGA) infants are those between the tenth and ninetieth percentiles. Small-for-gestational-age (SGA) infants are those below the tenth percentile.

A newborn is assigned to one of the following nine categories depending on birth weight and gestational age:

- (Pr LGA)   Preterm (Pr), large for gestational age
- (Pr AGA)   Preterm, appropriate for gestational age
- (Pr SGA)   Preterm, small for gestational age
- (F LGA)   Term (F), large for gestational age
- (F AGA)   Term, appropriate for gestational age
- (F SGA)   Term, small for gestational age
- (Po LGA)   Postterm (Po), large for gestational age
- (Po AGA)   Postterm, appropriate for gestational age
- (Po SGA)   Postterm, small for gestational age

Neonatal mortality risk is the chance of death within the neonatal period (see Chapter 2). As indicated in Figure 24–1, the neonatal mortality risk decreases as both gestational age and birth weight increase. Infants who are preterm and small for gestational age have the highest neonatal mortality risk. Examination of the figure also reveals that two infants of the same birth weight with different gestational ages may have very different neonatal mortality risks. For example, an infant of a diabetic mother (IDM) may be born at 34 weeks' gestation with a birth weight of 3250 g. The intersection of a vertical line (from 34 weeks) and a horizontal line (from 3250 g) indicates that this infant has a mortality risk of 1%. On the other hand, a full-term infant of 40 weeks' gestation who weighs 3250 g has a mortality risk of only 0.1%. Thus, in spite of equal birth weights, the 34-week IDM has a mortality risk ten times greater than the normal full-term infant.

Neonatal morbidity can be anticipated based on birth weight and gestational age. In Figure 24–2 (p.736) the infant's birth weight is located in the vertical column, and the gestational age in weeks is found horizontally. The area where the two meet on the graph identifies commonly occurring problems and assists in determining the needs of particular infants for special observation and care. For example, an infant of 2000 g at 40 weeks' gestation should

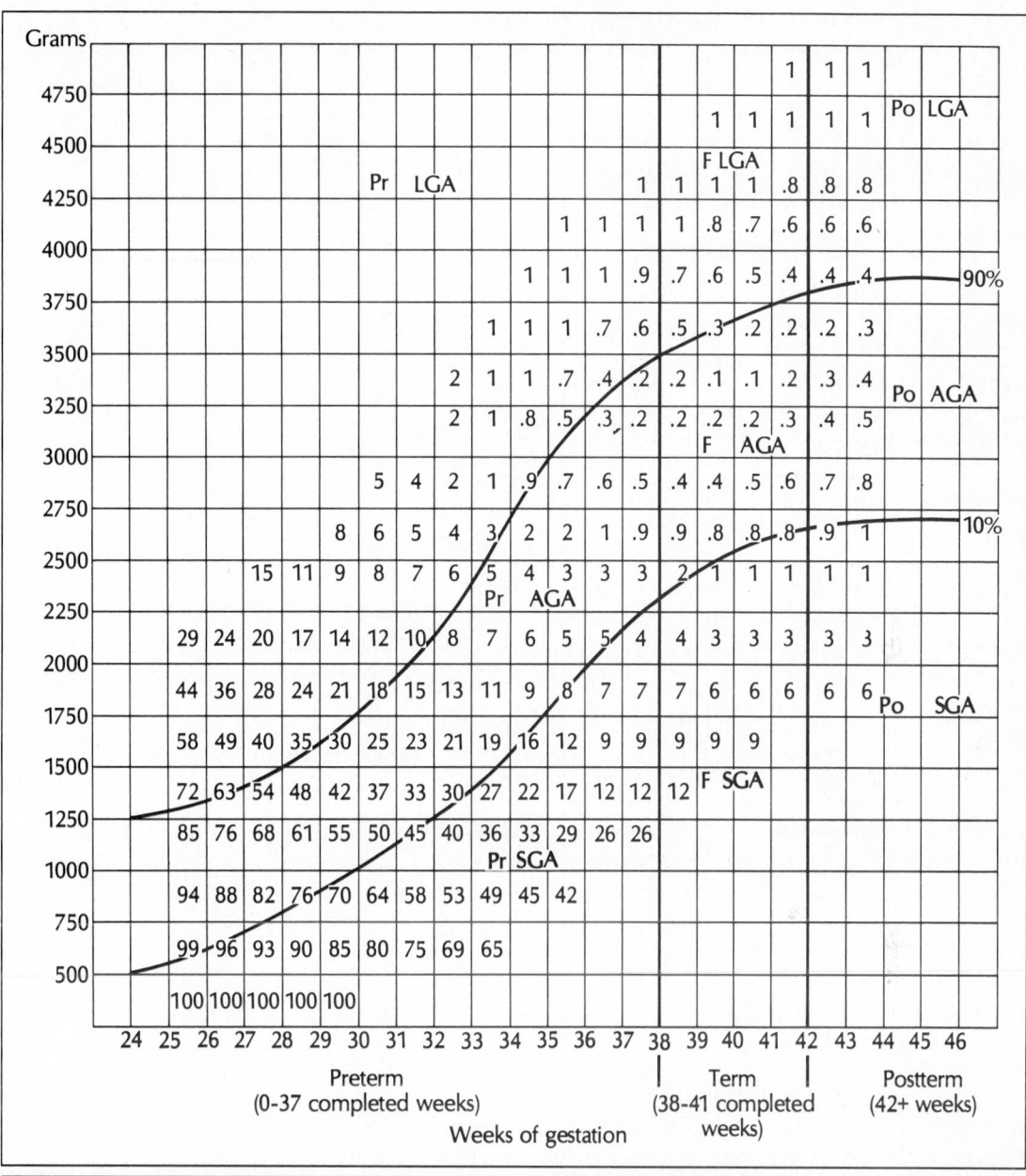

FIGURE 24–1 Newborn classification and neonatal mortality risk. (Modified from Lubchenco, L. O., et al. 1972. Neonatal mortality rate: relationship to birth weight and gestational age. *J. Pediatr.* 81:814.)

be carefully assessed for evidence of fetal distress, hypoglycemia, congenital anomalies, congenital infection, and polycythemia.

NURSING MANAGEMENT OF HIGH-RISK INFANTS

Assessment of the at-risk newborn is an ongoing process beginning with the history of the infant, which considers family and maternal history and other factors that may influence in utero development. Family history provides useful information about medical history of the parents and close relatives that can be correlated with neonatal disease. Maternal history contains data about elements of the prenatal environment—including medications and any complications of pregnancy—that can influence the infant's adaptation to extrauterine life. This historical information about the newborn enables the nurse to assess existing or potential nursing care needs and to use these factors as a basis for planning individual nursing care.

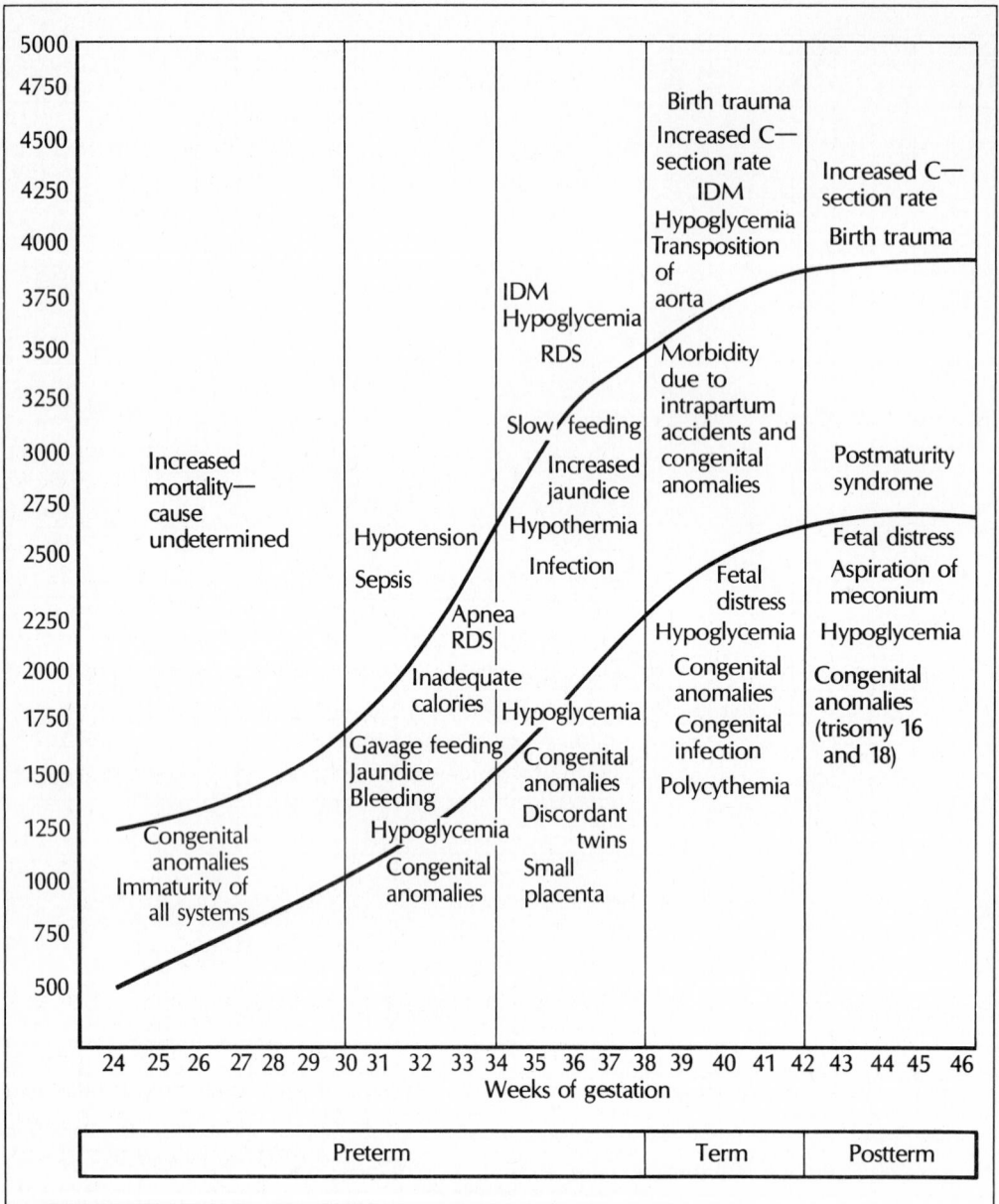

FIGURE 24-2 Neonatal morbidity by birth weight and gestational age. (From Lubchenco, L. O. 1976. *The high-risk infant.* Philadelphia: W. B. Saunders Co., p. 122.)

In the delivery room, the Apgar scores and careful observation are the basis of assessment. The scores and observed data are correlated with information such as the duration of labor, maternal analgesia and anesthesia, and any complications of labor or delivery.

Assessment continues when the newborn is admitted to the nursery. The family history, maternal history, information about the labor and delivery, Apgar scores, and treatments instituted in the delivery room are evaluated in conjunction with the physical examination of the newborn. As discussed in Chapter 22, the physical examination includes all of the following:

• Complete head-to-toe assessment, observing for cardiorespiratory function, temperature, neurologic status, and congenital anomalies

• Clinical determination of gestational age

• Consideration of the infant's classification as AGA, SGA, or LGA, based on the newborn classification and neonatal mortality risk chart (Figure 24-1) and correlated with the morbidity risks for each newborn (Figure 24-2)

When data from these various sources are incorporated, the assessment is validated and a plan for nursing intervention is formulated.

Nursing care of the high-risk neonate depends on minute-to-minute observations and changes based on physiologic parameters. The improved outcome of survivors has been traced to measures of physiologic management and support. It is essential to an infant's survival that the neonatal nurse understand the basic physiologic principles that guide nursing management of the at-risk neonate. The organization of nursing care must be directed toward:

• Decreasing physiologically stressful situations
• Constantly observing for subtle signs of change in clinical condition
• Interpreting laboratory data and coordinating interventions
• Conserving the infant's energy, especially in frail, debilitated preterm neonates
• Providing for developmental stimulation and sleep cycle
• Assisting the family in attachment behaviors

Evaluation of the plan of care is an ongoing process. It is confirmed through continuous assessments based on observations of patient behavior, communication with family and health team members, and use of diagnostic measures. As evaluation reveals a change or lack of change in the newborn's response, there should be corresponding retention or change of the care plan and approaches.

The at-risk infant is the newest member of a family, and the parents should not be excluded from the plan of care. The importance of keeping them informed of their infant's progress, involving them in the care, and providing frequent opportunities for them to interact with their newborn and to voice their fears and concerns cannot be overstressed.

PRETERM (PREMATURE) INFANT

A preterm infant is any infant born before 38 weeks' gestation. The length of gestation and thus the level of maturity are variable even in the "premature" population. Following are the four categories of prematurity.

1. *Less than 24 weeks' gestation.* These infants are very immature in their development and rarely survive.

2. *24–30 weeks' gestation.* These infants may have alveolar development, but lack of adequate surfactant precipitates severe RDS. For those of 24–27 weeks' gestation, survival is unlikely. However, with sophisticated supportive and therapeutic interventions, 28-to-30-week-old infants have a much better chance for survival today.

3. *31–34 or 36 weeks' gestation.* Supportive measures may be necessary but are not as drastic. Survival chances are improved.

4. *36–38 weeks' gestation.* These infants are said to be borderline or intermediate in their prematurity. They have characteristics of both term and preterm infants and may need minimal supportive therapy.

The incidence of preterm births in the United States ranges from 7% in white infants to 14%–15% for nonwhites.

The major problem of the preterm infant is (variable) immaturity of all systems. The degree of immaturity depends on the length of gestation. For example, infants of 32 weeks' gestation can be expected to exhibit more immaturity than infants of 36 weeks' gestation. The degree of immaturity also presents problems of management. Maintenance of the preterm infants falls within narrow physiologic parameters. "Catch-up care" is usually not possible if ground is lost in initial management. Improper physiologic management (or lack of management) adds stress and feeds the vicious cycle of physiologic deterioration. Figure 24–3 shows a preterm infant.

Preterm Infants' Physiologic Adaptations

The preterm infant must traverse the same complex, interconnected pathways from intrauterine to extrauterine life as the term infant. Because of immaturity, the preterm neonate is ill-equipped to make this transition smoothly.

Respiratory Physiology and Considerations

The preterm infant is at risk for respiratory problems because the lungs are not fully mature and ready to take over the process of oxygen and carbon dioxide exchange until 37–38 weeks' gestation. The length of time needed is variable; some infants who are born before 37–38 weeks do not develop respiratory distress, and some infants born at 37 weeks experience severe respiratory distress. The most critical influencing factor in the development of respiratory distress is the preterm infant's ability to produce adequate amounts of surfactant. Surfactant prevents alveolar collapse when the infant exhales and increases the compliance of the lung (allows the lung to fill with air easily). When surfactant is decreased, compliance is also lessened and the pressure needed to expand the lungs with air increases (see Chapter 21 for discussion of respiratory adaptation).

Besides adequate surfactant production, alveolar sacs and/or alveoli must be present in sufficient number to accomplish oxygen and carbon dioxide exchange. The term infant has about 24 million alveoli, while the adult has 200–600 million (Korones, 1981).

Lung development begins around the twenty-fourth day of fetal life when the primitive lung bud appears (Fig-

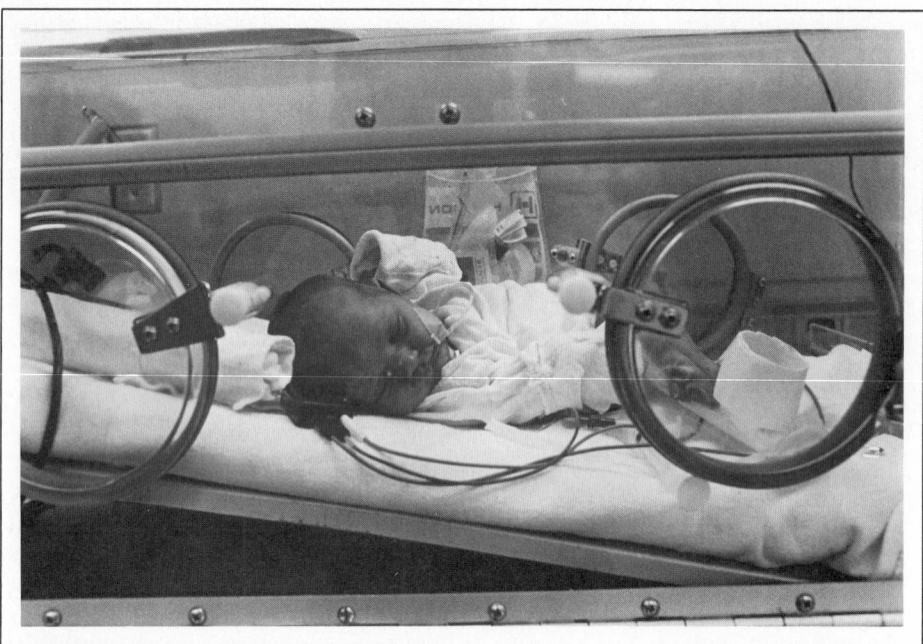

FIGURE 24–3 Preterm infant.

ure 24–4). The primitive lung bud branches at about 26–28 days to form the major right and left bronchi. Throughout gestation, growth and branching continue, forming terminal bronchioles to respiratory bronchioles, from which arise alveolar ducts. The alveolar ducts are differentiated by approximately 24 weeks' gestation and give rise to thin-walled terminal air sacs. From 24 weeks until birth, growth and development of these terminal air sacs or premature alveoli are continuous. After about 24–26 weeks of gestation, the surface area available for gas exchange is very limited (because of inadequate number and size of alveoli) and inadequate surfactant is produced, making survival at this time unlikely.

By 27–28 weeks, more alveolar sacs have developed, and more capillaries are in contact with the alveolar membrane. This allows some exchange of oxygen and carbon dioxide from the alveoli to the capillaries, and from the capillaries to the alveoli. Surfactant production at this time is unstable and inadequate, but with respiratory assistance, survival is possible. The infant is at risk, however, for many complications, such as RDS, hypoxemia, acidemia, intraventricular hemorrhage, cold stress, and metabolic imbalances, any one of which may compromise ultimate survival.

Between 29 and 30 weeks, additional differentiation of the alveolar sacs occurs and additional surfactant is released. After 30 weeks' gestation, growth of new primitive alveoli is rapid, and by 34–36 weeks, mature alveoli are present (Korones, 1981). Also by this time surfactant production increases rapidly as the second pathway (see Figure 21–2) of surfactant production begins optimal func-

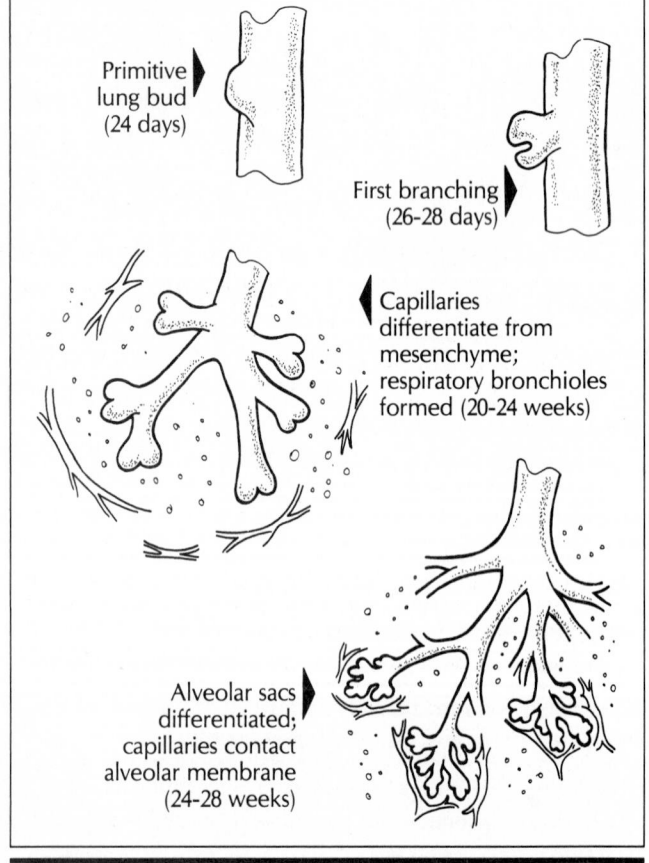

Primitive lung bud (24 days)

First branching (26-28 days)

Capillaries differentiate from mesenchyme; respiratory bronchioles formed (20-24 weeks)

Alveolar sacs differentiated; capillaries contact alveolar membrane (24-28 weeks)

FIGURE 24–4 Development of primitive lung bud and subsequent branching into surrounding mesenchyme. (From Korones, S. B., 1981. *High risk newborn infants,* 3rd ed. St. Louis: The C. V. Mosby Co., modified from Avery, M. E., and Fletcher, B. D. 1974. *The lung and its disorders in the newborn infant.* Philadelphia: W. B. Saunders Co.)

tioning. If the fetus is unstressed and without iatrogenic complications, adequate amounts of surfactant should be produced for lung expansion and gas exchange at this time. In the presence of asphyxia, hypoxemia, acidemia, or cold stress, surfactant production is impaired, resulting in increased chances of respiratory distress. The more immature the infant, the more devastating the physiologic complications.

Cardiovascular Physiology and Considerations

Fetal circulation differs from neonatal and adult circulation in several respects. The lungs of the fetus do not function in utero; a special circulatory system bypasses the blood supply to the lungs. This bypass is primarily accomplished by the foramen ovale, which allows blood to flow directly from the right atrium to the left atrium, without flowing through the pulmonary vasculature. Because the lungs are collapsed, vascular resistance within the pulmonary vasculature is high, which facilitates flow of blood into the descending aorta through the ductus arteriosus, thus bypassing the lungs and resulting in very little blood flow into the pulmonary artery. (See Chapter 8 for detailed discussion of fetal circulation.)

At birth, several changes occur within the cardiovascular system. First, loss of blood flow through the placenta increases systemic vascular resistance. This in turn raises the aortic pressure as well as the pressures in the left ventricle and left atrium, resulting in foramen ovale closure. Second, with expansion of the lungs, the pulmonary vascular resistance decreases, and blood begins to flow through the pulmonary circuit. Because of increased systemic resis-

tance and decreased pulmonary resistance, blood no longer flows from the pulmonary artery into the aorta through the ductus arteriosus. This flow of blood reverses and becomes a left-to-right shunt (from the aorta to the pulmonary artery). Under the influence of better oxygenated blood, the ductus arteriosus begins to constrict, and in the presence of adequate oxygenation and a normal pH, remains constricted and eventually becomes a ligament (Table 24–1). Similarly, the ductus venosus, which has no further function in neonatal circulation, gradually constricts and becomes a ligament in the liver.

In the preterm infant, the muscular coat of the pulmonary arterioles is incompletely developed. This muscular development occurs late in gestation; therefore the more premature the infant, the less muscular the pulmonary arterioles (Avery, 1981). With decreased pulmonary arteriole musculature, vasoconstriction is not as significant in response to increased oxygen levels. Therefore, the healthy preterm infant has a lower pulmonary vascular resistance than a full-term infant. This factor leads to increased left-to-right shunting through the ductus arteriosus, which steps up the blood flow back into the lungs. On the other hand, the preterm infant who develops respiratory distress and its complications (acidemia and hypoxemia) is at greater risk for increasing pulmonary vascular resistance (decreased Po_2 triggers vasoconstriction), which decreases blood flow through the lungs, causing additional hypoxemia and acidemia. The ductus arteriosus responds to rising oxygen levels by vasoconstriction; in the preterm infant, who has higher susceptibility to hypoxia, the ductus may remain open. A patent ductus increases the blood volume to the lungs, causing pulmonary congestion, in-

Table 24–1 Fetal and Neonatal Circulation

System	Fetal	Neonatal
Pulmonary blood vessels	Constricted with very little blood flow; lungs not expanded	Vasodilation and increased blood flow; lungs expanded; increased oxygen stimulates vasodilation
Systemic blood vessels	Dilated with low resistance; blood mostly in placenta	Arterial pressure rises due to loss of placenta; increased systemic blood volume and resistance
Ductus arteriosus	Large with no tone; blood flow from pulmonary artery to aorta	1. Reversal of blood flow. Now from aorta to pulmonary artery due to increased left atrial pressure 2. Ductus is sensitive to increased oxygen and body chemicals and begins to constrict
Foramen ovale	Patent with large blood flow from right atrium to left atrium	Increased pressure in left atrium attempts to reverse blood flow and shuts one way valve

creased respiratory effort, and higher oxygen consumption.

THERMOREGULATION

Maintaining a normal body temperature in the preterm infant presents a nursing challenge. Heat production is a factor over which the nurse has little control, yet heat loss is a major problem that the nurse can do much to prevent.

Heat production in the preterm infant is primarily a result of normal metabolic functions. Heat is produced by the oxidation of glucose and free fatty acids and also by the metabolism of brown fat. Two limiting factors in heat production, however, are the availability of glycogen in the liver (glycogen stores are primarily laid down during the third trimester) and the amount of brown fat available for metabolism (the preterm infant does not have a full complement of brown fat). If the infant is chilled after birth, both glycogen and brown fat stores are metabolized rapidly for heat production, leaving the infant with no reserves in the event of future stress. Since the muscle mass is small in preterm infants, and muscular activity is diminished (they are unable to shiver), little heat is produced.

One of the greatest threats to the preterm infant is heat loss. Heat loss occurs as a result of several physiologic and anatomic factors.

1. The preterm infant has a much larger ratio of body surface to body weight. This means that the infant's ability to produce heat (body weight) is much less than the potential for losing heat (surface area). The loss of heat in a preterm infant weighing 1500 g is five times greater per unit of body weight than in an adult (Korones, 1981). Without an adequate thermal environment, the preterm infant is at risk for excessive heat loss.

2. The preterm infant has very little subcutaneous fat, which is the human body's insulation. Without adequate insulation, heat is easily conducted from the core of the body (warmer temperature) to the surface of the body (cooler temperature). Heat is lost from the body as the blood vessels transport blood from the body core to the subcutaneous tissues. In the preterm infant, the blood vessels lie close to the skin surface, and without adequate insulation (fat) more heat is given off as the blood circulates throughout the body.

3. The posture of the preterm infant is another important factor influencing heat loss. Flexion of the extremities decreases the amount of surface area exposed to the environment; extension increases the surface area exposed to the environment and thus increases heat loss. The gestational age of the infant influences the amount of flexion, from completely hypotonic and extended at 28 weeks to strong flexion displayed by 36 weeks (Figure 22–4).

In summary, the more preterm an infant the less capable he or she is of maintaining heat balance because of disproportionate body surface area, decreased subcutaneous fat, and increased heat loss due to body posture. Prevention of heat loss by providing a neutral thermal environment is one of the most important considerations in nursing management of the preterm infant. (See Nursing Care Plan for thermoregulation, p. 752.) Cold stress, with its accompanying severe complications, can be prevented (see Chapter 25).

Nutrition and Fluid Requirements

Providing adequate nutrition and fluids for the preterm infant is a major concern of the health care team. It is now recognized that early feedings are extremely valuable in maintaining normal metabolism and lowering the possibility of such complications as hypoglycemia, hyperbilirubinemia, hyperkalemia, and azotemia. It is important to note, however, the preterm infant is at risk for complications that may develop because of immaturity of the digestive system.

DIGESTIVE PHYSIOLOGY AND ENZYMATIC ACTIVITY

Although the basic structure of the gastrointestinal (GI) tract is formed early in gestation, allowing the very preterm infant to take in suitable nourishment, maturation of the digestive and absorptive processes is more variable and occurs later in gestation. In addition, many of the problems that compromise adequate nutrition are a result of immaturity of systems other than the GI tract, such as the renal (inability to concentrate urine), respiratory (weak, or absent cough), and neurologic (poor suck and swallow reflexes) systems. Severe illness of the infant also may prevent intake of adequate nutrients (Brady et al., 1979).

The composition of the "best-suited formula" for the preterm infant is a subject of much discussion and research. Over the past decade many formulas have been tried and revised in an attempt to meet the unique nutritional needs of the preterm infant. Breast milk as the primary source of nutrition for the preterm infant has also been a topic of recent debate and research.

It is now known that the quality as well as the quantity of protein ingested is important to the small preterm infant. These neonates have limited ability to convert certain essential amino acids into other nonessential amino acids because they lack the enzymes necessary to accomplish this task (Canadian Pediatric Society, 1981). Amino acids that are known to be essential for preterm infants but are *not* essential for term infants include histidine, tyrosine, cystine, and taurine. Therefore these amino acids must be included in a preterm infant formula (Brady et al., 1979).

Another factor in protein composition is the whey-to-casein ratio. Because of immaturity of the kidneys, the preterm infant is unable to handle the increased solute load (increased osmolarity) of a protein that is high in casein. The infant requires a protein high in whey. Preterm infants fed cow's milk protein with a whey/casein ratio of 18:82 have been shown to have more complications such as azotemia and hyperammonemia than those fed a formula (or human milk) with a ratio of 60:40 (Canadian Pediatric Society, 1981).

Absorption of saturated fat, another difficulty for the preterm infant, is presumed to be a result of decreased concentration of bile salt and deficiency of pancreatic lipase. Polyunsaturated fatty acids or medium-chain triglycerides (MCTs) are well absorbed since they do not require lipase for digestion or bile salts for absorption. These fatty acids and MCTs may be added to the formula to provide additional calories for growth.

Most simple sugars are well absorbed by the preterm infant and do not present a problem in digestion. Some evidence suggests that lactose digestion may not be fully functional during the first few days of life. Polycose (glucose supplement derived from corn starch) may be added to preterm infant formulas to provide adequate calories without increasing osmolarity, which may lead to an increased incidence of necrotizing enterocolitis. When carbohydrate malabsorption does occur, one should suspect necrotizing enterocolitis (see Chapter 25), and the infant's stools should be watched carefully for reducing substances (Clinitest-positive results that indicate sugar in stools), which suggest possible carbohydrate malabsorption.

Because of the factors just discussed and the preterm infant's general immaturity, certain problems inherent in the feeding process include the following:

1. Marked danger of aspiration and its associated complications because of the infant's poorly developed gag reflex, incompetent esophageal cardiac sphincter, and poor sucking and swallowing reflexes.

2. Small stomach capacity with high caloric requirements. This limits the amount of fluid that can be introduced to meet caloric needs.

3. Decreased absorption of essential nutrients because of immaturity, malabsorption, and nutritional loss associated with vomiting and diarrhea.

4. Fatigue associated with sucking, which may lead to increased basal metabolic rate, increased oxygen requirements, and its sequelae of complications.

5. Feeding intolerance and necrotizing enterocolitis due to diminished blood flow to the intestinal tract because of shock or prolonged hypoxia at birth.

FORMULAS FOR PRETERM NEONATES

The formula of choice for feeding the preterm infant varies somewhat among institutions and areas of the country. However, most of the formulas contain protein with a whey/casein ratio of 60:40, a similar proportion to that found in breast milk, and a caloric value of 24 calories per ounce (Table 24-2). Initial feedings may be diluted to 12 calories per ounce and gradually increased, as the infant tolerates them, to 24-calorie formulas. Breast milk is widely used to feed preterm infants. Besides its many benefits for the infant, it allows the mother to contribute to her infant's well-being (Figure 24-5). It is a nursing responsibility to inform mothers of their option to breast-feed if they choose to do so. The nurse should be aware of the advantages and possible disadvantages of breast-feeding, such as decreased growth rate, hyponatremia, lactose intolerance, and rickets if breast milk is the sole source of food.

METHODS OF FEEDING

Various feeding methods are utilized for the preterm infant, depending on the infant's gestational age, health and physical condition, and neurologic status. The methods,

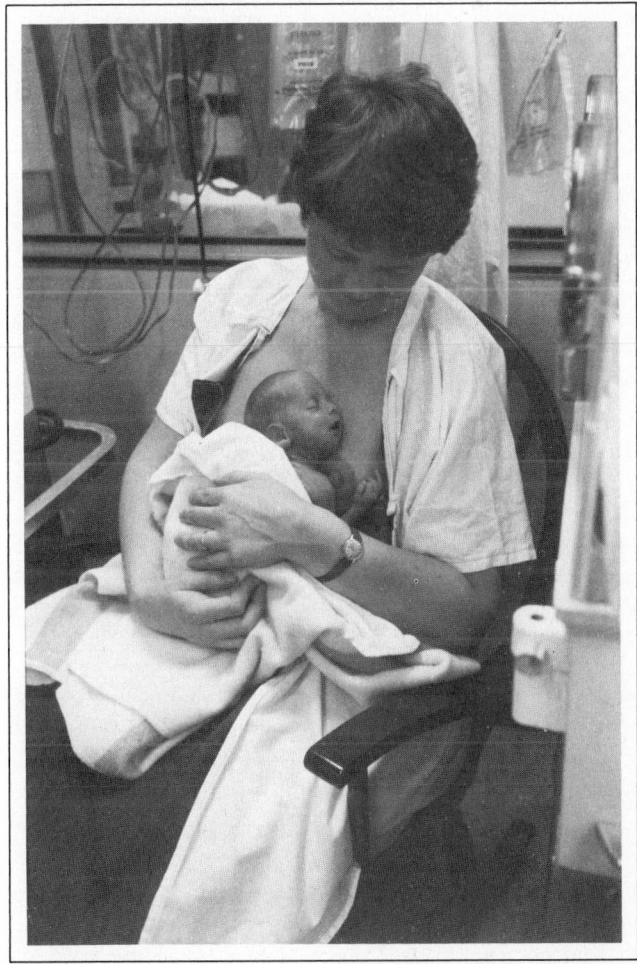

FIGURE 24–5 Mother visits intensive care unit to breastfeed her preterm infant. (© Suzanne Arms.)

Table 24–2   Commonly Used Preterm Formulas*

Formula	Caloric content	Carbohydrate		Protein		Fat		Osmolality
		g/dL	Type	g/dL	Whey/ casein ratio	g/dL	Type	mosm/kg H$_2$O
Enfamil 24 Premature Formula	81	9.1	60% polycose 40% lactose	2.4	60/40	4.1	40% MCT 40% corn	300
Enfamil 24 w/Iron	81	8.5	lactose	1.8	18/82	4.5	80% soy	355
Similac Special Care Infant Formula	81	8.6	50% lactose 50% polycose	2.2	60/40	4.4	50% MCT	290
Similac 24 w/Iron	81	8.5	lactose	2.2	18/82	4.3	60% coconut	360
Similac PM 60/40	68	6.9	lactose	1.6	60/40	3.8	60% coconut	260
SMA 24	81	4.2	lactose	1.8	60/40	4.2	oleo, soy, coconut	364

* From Avery, G. B., ed. 1981. *Neonatology.* 2nd ed. Philadelphia: J. B. Lippincott Co., p. 1026.

criteria for selection, description, and nursing responsibilities associated with each method are summarized in the following sections.

□ *NIPPLE-FEEDING* Nipple-feeding is used in infants who are 32–34 weeks' gestation and have a coordinated suck and swallow reflex or in infants who are showing consistent weight gain (20–30 g per day) because sucking requires extra energy.

Method. The infant feeds from a bottle. The feeding should take no longer than 15–20 minutes. A premature infant nipple or a regular-sized nipple may be used, depending on the infant's strength and ability (nippling requires more energy than other methods). The infant is fed in a semisitting position and burped gently after each half an ounce or ounce.

Nursing responsibilities. The infant's ability to suck is assessed. Sucking may be affected by age, asphyxia, sepsis, intraventricular hemorrhage, or other neurologic insult. Before initiating nipple feeding, the infant is observed for any signs of stress, such as tachypnea (more than 60 respirations/min), respiratory distress, or hypothermia, which may increase the risk of aspiration. During the feeding, the infant should be observed for signs of difficulty with feeding (tachypnea, cyanosis, bradycardia, lethargy, and uncoordinated suck and swallow). After the feeding, the infant is gently burped and positioned on the right side or abdomen.

□ *GAVAGE FEEDING* The gavage feeding method is used with preterm infants (less than 32–34 weeks' gestation)

who lack a coordinated suck and swallow reflex. It is also used when term or preterm infants are unable to nipple-feed due to neurologic insult, such as asphyxia or CNS depression.

Method. An orogastric tube is passed into the infant's stomach. Correct placement of the tube is verified, and formula is passed through the tube into the infant's stomach (see Procedure 24–1 for in-depth description).

Nursing responsibilities. See Procedure 24–1.

□ *TRANSPYLORIC, NASOJEJUNAL, OR NASODUODENAL TUBE FEEDING* Transpyloric, nasojejunal, or nasoduodenal feeding by tube is used with very small preterm infants who are ventilator-dependent or tachypneic, have chronic lung disease, recurrent aspiration, or repeated residuals with other methods of feeding.

Method. Transpyloric, nasojejunal, or nasoduodenal feeding involves a continuous infusion of formula into the duodenum or jejunum of the infant. An indwelling feeding tube is passed through the nostril, into the stomach and into the small intestine. Tube placement is confirmed by x-ray. A constant infusion pump is used to administer small amounts of formula continuously. The tube is left in place and changed every 3 days.

Potential risks. Although this feeding method has advantages (for example, decreased risk of aspiration), it poses risks of intestinal perforation in these infants and accidental bolus infusion by the infusion pump. In addition, formula bypasses the digestive activity of the stomach. Transpyloric method of feeding is never used in some cen-

Procedure 24–1   Gavage Feeding

Objective	Nursing action	Rationale
Ensure smooth accomplishment of the procedure	Gather necessary equipment including: 1. No. 5 or No. 8 Fr. feeding tube 2. 10–30 mL syringe 3. ¼-in. paper tape 4. Stethoscope 5. Appropriate formula 6. Small cup of sterile water Explain procedure to parents	Considerations in choosing size of catheter include size of the infant, area of insertion (oral or nasal), and rate of flow desired. The very small infant (less than 1600 g) requires a 5 Fr. feeding tube; an infant greater than 1600 g may tolerate a larger tube. Orogastric insertion is preferred over nasogastric insertion as infants are obligatory nose breathers. If nasogastric insertion is used, a No. 5 catheter should be utilized to minimize airway obstruction. The size of the catheter will influence the rate of flow. The syringe is used to aspirate stomach contents prior to feeding, to inject air into the stomach for testing tube placement and for holding measured amount of formula during feeding. Tape is used to mark tube for insertion depth as well as for securing tube during feeding. Stethoscope is needed to auscultate rush of air into stomach when testing tube placement. Sterile water may be used to lubricate feeding tube when inserted nasally. With oral insertion, there are enough secretions in the mouth to lubricate the tube adequately. The cup of sterile water may also be used to test for placement by placing the end of the tube into the water to check for air bubbles from the lungs. However, this test may not be accurate as air may also be present in the stomach (Avery, 1981).
Insert tube accurately into stomach	Position infant on back or side with head of bed elevated. Take tube from package and measure the distance from the tip of the ear to the nose to the xiphoid process, and mark the point with a small piece of paper tape (Figure 24–6). If inserting tube nasally, lubricate tip in cup of sterile water. Shake excess drops to prevent aspiration.	This position allows easy passage of the tube. This measuring technique ensures enough tubing to enter stomach. Water should be used, as opposed to an oil-based lubricant, in the event tube is inadvertently passed into lung.

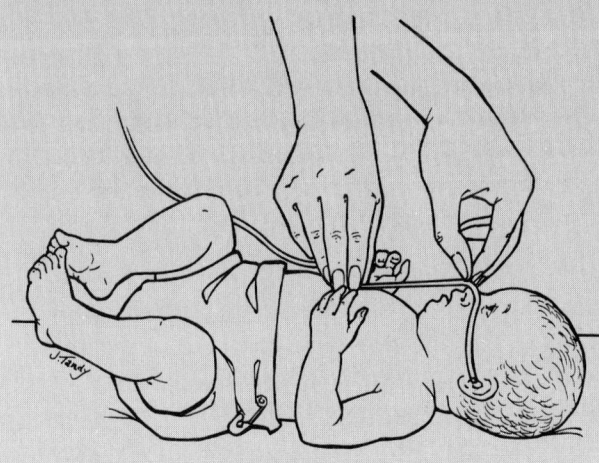

FIGURE 24–6 Measuring gavage tube length.

Procedure 24–1   Gavage Feeding Cont'd

Objective	Nursing action	Rationale
	Stabilize infant's head with one hand, and pass the tube via the mouth (or nose) into the stomach, to the point previously marked. If the infant begins coughing or choking or becomes cyanotic or aphonic, remove the tube immediately.	Any signs of respiratory distress signal likelihood that tube has entered trachea. Orogastric insertion is less likely to result in passage into the trachea than nasogastric insertion.
	If no respiratory distress is apparent, lightly tape tube in position, draw up 0.5–1.0 mL of air in syringe, and connect it to tubing. Place stethoscope over the epigastrium and briskly inject the air (Figure 24–7)	Nurse should hear a sudden rush of air as it enters stomach.
	Aspirate stomach contents with syringe, and note amount, color, and consistency. Return residual to stomach unless otherwise ordered to discard it.	Residual formula should be evaluated as part of the assessment of infant's tolerance of gavage feedings. It is not discarded, unless particularly large in volume or mucoid in nature, because of the potential for causing an electrolyte imbalance.
	If only a clear fluid or mucus is found upon aspiration and if any question exists as to whether the tube is in the stomach, the aspirate can be tested for pH.	Stomach aspirate tests in the 1–3 range for pH.

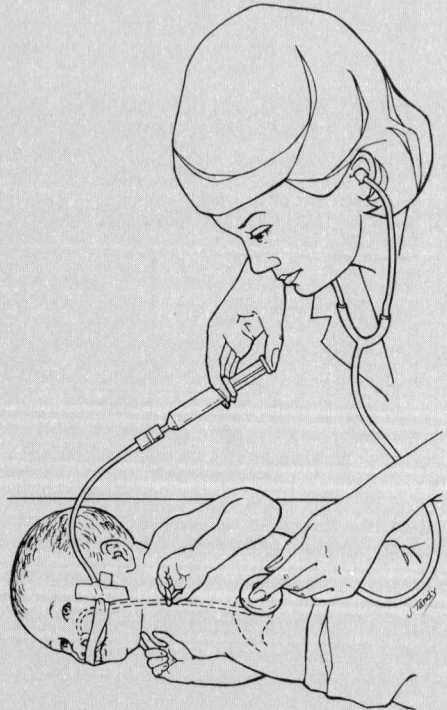

FIGURE 24–7 Auscultation for placement of gavage tube.

Objective	Nursing action	Rationale
Introduce formula into stomach without complication	Hold infant for feeding or position on right side if infant cannot be held.	Positioning on side decreases the risk of aspiration in case of emesis during feeding.
	Separate syringe from tube, remove plunger from barrel, reconnect barrel to tube, and pour formula into syringe.	Feeding should be allowed to flow in by gravity. It should not be pushed in under pressure with syringe.

Procedure 24–1 Gavage Feeding Cont'd

Objective	Nursing action	Rationale
	Elevate syringe 6–8 in. over infant's head. Allow formula to flow at slow, even rate.	Raising column of fluid increases force of gravity. Nurse may need to initiate flow of formula by inserting plunger of syringe into barrel just until formula is seen to enter feeding tube. Rate should be regulated to prevent sudden stomach distention, with possibility of vomiting and aspiration.
	Continue adding formula to syringe until desired volume has been absorbed. Then rinse tubing with 2–3 mL sterile water.	Rinsing tube ensures that infant receives all of formula. It is especially important to rinse tube if it is going to be left in place, because this decreases risk of clogging and bacterial growth in tube.
	Remove tube by loosening tape, folding it over on itself, and quickly withdrawing it in one smooth motion. If tube is to be left in, position it so that infant is unable to remove it.	Folding tube over on itself minimizes potential for aspiration of fluid, which would otherwise flow from tubing as it passes epiglottis. A tube left in place should be replaced at least every 24 hours.
Maximize feeding pleasure of infant	Whenever possible, hold infant during gavage feeding. If it is too awkward to hold infant during feeding, be sure to take time for holding afterward.	Feeding time is important to infant's tactile sensory input.
	Offer a pacifier to infant during feeding.	Infants fed for long periods by gavage can lose their sucking reflex. Sucking during feeding comforts and relaxes infant, making formula flow more easily. One study showed that infants allowed to suck during feedings were able to nipple sooner and were discharged earlier than a control group who did not suck during tube feedings (Measel and Anderson, 1979).

ters where the risks are believed to outweigh the benefits (Pereira and Lemons, 1981).

Nursing responsibilities. The nurse assists with the passing of the tube, observing the infant's vital signs and watching for any intolerance of the procedure. After feedings have begun, the nurse does the following:

- Abdominal girth is measured every 2–3 hours to check for distention
- Gastric residual is checked every 2–3 hours (by oral tube inserted into stomach along with the feeding tube)
- Rate of infusion is observed and recorded for consistency hourly to make sure the correct amount is infusing
- The infusion setup is changed every 8 hours (to decrease chances of bacterial growth in the formula)
- No more than 3 hours' worth of formula should be hung at one time; this prevents "dumping" of excess formula
- All stools are checked for blood and reducing substances (signs of necrotizing enterocolitis) (Benda, 1979).

□ *TOTAL PARENTERAL NUTRITION* Total parenteral nutrition (TPN) is used in situations that contraindicate feeding the infant through the GI tract, such as: GI anomalies requiring surgical intervention, necrotizing enterocolitis, intolerance of feedings, and extreme prematurity.

Method. TPN provides complete nutrition to the infant intravenously. Hyperalimentation gives calories, vitamins, minerals, protein, and glucose. Intralipids must also be administered to provide essential fatty acids. Hyperalimentation may be infused through either a central or peripheral line. Intralipids may only be infused peripherally, and if added as a piggy-back to the hyperalimentation, they must be piggy-backed as close to the infusion site as possible and not through the filter.

Nursing responsibilities. The nurse needs to monitor serum glucose levels carefully during TPN. Urine is checked for protein, sugar, and specific gravity at least every 8 hours. The intravenous rate is monitored hourly to maintain accurate intake (do not "catch up" if behind). The intravenous site should be observed hourly for signs of infiltration (hyperalimentation is extremely caustic and causes severe tissue destruction if it infiltrates). Fluid intake and output are carefully monitored (hyperglycemia causing an osmotic diuresis can lead to dehydration). The nurse observes for signs of reaction to intralipids, for example, dyspnea, vomiting, elevated temperature, or cyanosis.

Whichever method of feeding is selected for an infant, the nurse should carefully watch for any signs and symptoms of feeding intolerance. The signs and symptoms include (Benda, 1979):

- Increasing gastric residuals (more than 2 mL)
- Abdominal distention (measured routinely before feedings)
- Guaiac-positive stools
- Presence of reducing substances in the stools
- Vomiting
- Diarrhea

NUTRITIONAL REQUIREMENTS

Enteral caloric intake necessary for growth in an uncompromised healthy preterm infant is 120–150 kcal/kg/day. In addition to the relatively high caloric needs, the preterm infant requires more protein (3–4 g/kg/day, as opposed to 2.0–2.5 g/kg/day for the full-term infant). To meet these needs, a number of higher-calorie, higher-protein formulas are available that meet the preterm infant's nutritional demands yet do not overtax the concentration abilities of the immature kidneys.

In addition to a higher calorie and protein formula, it is recommended that preterm infants receive supplemental multivitamins and vitamin E. The requirement for vitamin E is increased by a diet high in polyunsaturated fats (those tolerated best by preterm infants). Preterm infants fed iron-fortified formulas are shown to have higher red cell hemolysis and lower vitamin E concentrations, thereby requiring additional vitamin E. Vitamin E concentrations have been shown to decrease susceptibility to hemolytic anemia and to alleviate bronchopulmonary dysplasia and retrolental fibroplasia in preterm infants (Avery, 1981).

Since two-thirds of the calcium and phosphorus in the newborn's body is deposited in the last trimester of gestation, the preterm is deficient in these minerals. Rickets and significant bone demineralization have been documented in very low-birth-weight infants and healthy preterm infants. Ziegler and coworkers (1983) recommend 210 mg of elemental calcium/kg/day for a 1000 g premature infant. For larger premature infants, 150–180 mg/kg/day may be sufficient. Few milks currently available contain sufficient calcium to meet these requirements and enteral calcium supplements are recommended. In addition to calcium supplementation, vitamin D intake should be 400–600 IU/day to facilitate retention of calcium and increase bone densities.

SCHEDULE OF FEEDINGS

Sterile water is the fluid of choice for the first few feedings, because less severe lung tissue reactions develop should aspiration occur. Feeding regimens are then established based on the weight and estimated stomach capacity of the infant (Table 24–3). In many instances it is necessary to supplement the oral feedings with parenteral fluids to maintain adequate hydration and caloric intake.

Renal Physiology

The kidneys of the preterm infant are immature in comparison with the full-term infant, which poses clinical problems in the management of fluid and electrolyte balance. Specific characteristics of the preterm infant include the following:

1. The glomerular filtration rate (GFR) is lower due to decreased renal blood flow. GFR is directly related to lower gestational age; therefore, the more preterm the infant the less the GFR, and the closer to term the greater the GFR. GFR is also decreased in the presence of diseases or conditions that decrease the renal blood flow and/or oxygen content such as severe respiratory distress, perinatal asphyxia, and congestive heart failure. Anuria and/or oliguria may be observed in the preterm infant after severe asphyxial insult with associated hypotension.

2. The kidneys of the preterm infant are limited in their ability to concentrate urine or to excrete excess amounts of fluid. This means that if excess fluid is administered, the infant is at risk for fluid retention and overhydration. If too little is administered, the infant will become dehydrated, because of the inability to retain adequate fluid.

3. The kidneys of the preterm infant begin excreting glucose (glycosuria) at a lower serum glucose level than occurs in the adult. Therefore, glycosuria with hyperglycemia is common (Oh, 1981).

4. The buffering capacity of the kidney is less, predisposing the infant to metabolic acidosis. Bicarbonate is excreted at a lower serum level, and excretion of acid is accomplished more slowly. Therefore, after periods of hypoxia or insult, the kidneys require a longer time to excrete the lactic acid that accumulates. Sodium bicarbonate is frequently required to treat the metabolic acidosis (Leake, 1977).

5. The immaturity of the renal system also affects the infant's ability to excrete drugs. Because excretion time is longer, many drugs are given at less frequent intervals in the preterm infant (that is, every 12 hours instead of every 8 hours). Urine output must be carefully monitored when the infant is receiving nephrotoxic drugs such as gentamicin, nafcillin, and others. In the

Table 24–3   Oral Feeding Schedule for the Low-Birth-Weight Infant*

Time and substance[†]	Less than 1000 g		1001–1500 g		1501–2000 g		More than 2000 g	
	Amount	Frequency	Amount	Frequency	Amount	Frequency	Amount	Frequency
First "drink": sterile H_2O, 0.45% saline, 5% glucose	1–2 mL	1 hr	3–4 mL	2 hr	4–5 mL	2–3 hr	10 mL	3 hr
Formula: Subsequent feedings, 12–72 hr	Increase 1 mL every other feeding to maximum 5 mL	1 hr	Increase 1 mL every other feeding to maximum 10 mL	2 hr	Increase 2 mL every other feeding to maximum 15 mL	2–3 hr	Increase 5 mL every other feeding to maximum 20 mL	3 hr
Formula: Final feeding schedule, 150 mL/kg	10–15 mL	2 hr	20–28 mL	2–3 hr	28–37 mL	3 hr	37–50 mL	3–4 hr

*Modified from Avery, G. B., ed. 1981. *Neonatology.* 2nd ed. Philadelphia: J. B. Lippincott Co., p. 1025.
†Supplemental IV fluids should be given to fulfill fluid requirements of 150–200 mL/kg or to give urine specific gravities of 1.005–1.008.

event of poor urine output, drugs can become toxic in the infant much more quickly than in the adult.

FLUID REQUIREMENTS

Calculation of fluid requirements takes into account both the weight of the infant and postnatal age. Fluid is normally lost through the urine, sweat, feces, and through insensible water loss (lungs and skin). In the preterm infant, more fluid is lost through the skin than in term infants because of decreased insulating fat and blood vessels close to the surface. In addition, higher environmental temperature, phototherapy, and radiant warmers may increase fluid loss an additional 50%.

Recommendations for fluid therapy in the preterm infant are approximately 80–100 mL/kg/day for the first day of life; 100–120 mL/kg/day for day 2; and 120–140 mL/kg/day by day 3 of life. These amounts may be increased up to 200 mL/kg/day if the infant is very small, receiving phototherapy, or under a radiant warmer. The infant may need less fluid if a heat shield is used, the environment is more humid, or humidified oxygen is being provided.

Parameters that indicate adequate fluid and nutritional intake in the preterm infant include:

1. Urine
   a. Volume at 1–3 mL/kg/hr
   b. Specific gravity at 1.006–1.013
   c. Absence of glycosuria when checked by Dipstix or Clinitest

2. Normoglycemic state
   a. Absence of hypoglycemia (Dextrostix value below 45 mg/dL) or clinical symptoms
   b. Absence of hyperglycemia (Dextrostix value above 130 mg/dL). Hyperglycemia may occur with glucose infusion greater than 10% or formula greater than 50% carbohydrate.

3. Continued weight gain of 20–30 g per day (initially, no gain may be noted for several days, but total weight loss should not exceed 15% of the total body weight or more than 1%–2% per day).

4. Normal blood pH (greater than 7.35).

5. Some institutions add the criteria of head circumference growth and increase in body length of 1 cm/week, once the infant is stable.

NURSING MANAGEMENT

Nursing management of the preterm infant with a fluid and electrolyte disturbance includes careful assessment and observation with attention to several parameters.

1. Observe the general state of hydration. Dehydration may be indicated by sunken fontanelle, loss of weight, poor skin turgor (skin returns to position slowly), dry oral mucous membranes, decreased urine output and an increasing specific gravity (greater than 1.013) (Nash, 1981). Overhydration is assessed by observing for edema or excessive weight gain, and by comparing urine output with fluid intake.

2. Weigh preterm infants at least once daily, using the same scales at the same time each day. Weight change is one of the most sensitive indicators of fluid balance.

3. Obtain specific gravity measurements periodically. Urine osmolality provides an indication of hydration, although this factor must be correlated with other assessments (for example, serum sodium).

4. Maintain accurate hourly intake when administering intravenous fluids. Since the preterm infant is unable to excrete excess fluid, it is important to maintain the correct amount of intravenous fluid to prevent fluid overload.

5. Accurately measure intake and output. Comparing intake and output of fluid over an 8-hour or 24-hour period provides important information about renal function and fluid balance. Assessment of a net gain or loss pattern over serial days is also essential to fluid management.

Hepatic Physiology and Considerations

Immaturity of the preterm infant's liver predisposes the infant to several problems. First, glycogen is stored in the liver throughout gestation, reaching approximately 5% of the weight of the liver by term (Klaus and Fanaroff, 1979). After birth, the glycogen stores are rapidly utilized by the newborn for energy. Glycogen deposits are affected by asphyxia in utero, and after birth by both asphyxia and cold stress. The infant born preterm has decreased glycogen stores at birth because of low gestational age, and frequently experiences stress, which uses up the glycogen rapidly. Therefore the preterm infant is at high risk for hypoglycemia and its sequelae.

Iron is also stored in the liver and the amount greatly increases during the last trimester of pregnancy. Therefore, if the preterm infant, who is born with decreased iron stores, is subject to hemorrhage, rapid growth, and excess blood sampling, the infant is likely to become iron-depleted much earlier than the term infant. Many preterm infants require transfusions of packed cells to replace the blood drawn by frequent blood sampling.

Conjugation of bilirubin in the liver is also impaired in the preterm infant until approximately 37 weeks' gestation. Thus, bilirubin levels increase more rapidly and to a higher level than in the full-term infant (Avery, 1981). Early assessment of jaundice at nontoxic bilirubin levels is more difficult in preterm infants, who lack subcutaneous fat.

Immunologic Physiology and Considerations

The preterm infant is at a much greater risk for infection than the term infant. This increased susceptibility is partial-ly attributable to low gestational age, but may also be the result of infection acquired in utero, which precipitates preterm labor and delivery.

In utero, the infant receives passive immunity from the mother via the placenta against a variety of infections (see Chapter 21). The maternal antibodies that cross the placenta (IgG immunoglobulins) provide protection for the fetus against most bacterial and viral organisms with which the mother has come in contact throughout her life. These antibodies normally provide protection until about 3 months of age, when they become depleted and infants begin synthesizing their own. Because most of this immunity is acquired in the last trimester of pregnancy, the preterm infant has decreased antibodies at birth, providing less protection, and becomes depleted earlier than does a full-term infant. This may be a contributing factor in the higher incidence of recurrent infection during the first year of life as well as in the immediate neonatal period (Korones, 1981).

The other immunoglobulin significant for the preterm infant is secretory IgA, which does not cross the placenta but is found in breast milk in significant concentrations. Breast-milk secretory IgA provides immunity to the mucosal surfaces of the GI tract, providing protection from enteric infections such as those caused by *E. coli* and *Shigella* as well as necrotizing enterocolitis. In addition, the incidence of necrotizing enterocolitis affects a higher number of formula-fed preterm infants than those receiving breast milk (Avery, 1981).

Another altered defense against infection in the preterm infant is the skin surface. In very small infants the skin is easily excoriated, and this factor, in addition to experiencing many invasive procedures, places the infant at great risk for nosocomial infections. It is of utmost importance to use good hand-washing techniques in the care of these infants to prevent unnecessary infection.

Hematologic Physiology and Considerations

The formation of red blood cells begins approximately 2 weeks after conception, with the hemoglobin and hematocrit values gradually increasing throughout gestation. Beyond 28 weeks' gestation, cord hemoglobin values increase only slightly; however, in the first few hours after birth the values increase by 10%–20%, depending on how quickly the cord was cut and the amount of placental transfusion to the infant. The hemoglobin and hematocrit levels will also be affected by blood loss (fetal-to-placental transfusion), hemorrhage, hemolytic disease, and the presence of intrauterine hypoxia. Infants who are SGA (as a result of toxemia or later-stage maternal diabetes) are generally polycythemic because the placental deficiency stimulates red cell formation in the infant. On the other hand, hemorrhage and hemolytic disease result in loss of red cells and in anemia. The normal cord hemoglobin in an infant of 34 weeks' gestation is approximately 16.8 g/dL and total blood volume ranges from 89 mL/kg to 105 mL/kg (Avery, 1981). Because of the small total blood volume, any blood loss is highly significant to the preterm infant. For this reason, all blood taken for sampling must be recorded. Blood is generally replaced when the infant has lost 10% of total blood volume.

Reactivity Periods and Behavioral States

The newborn infant's response to extrauterine life is characterized by two periods of reactivity, as discussed in Chapter 23. Because of the immaturity of all systems in comparison to those of the full-term neonate, the preterm infant's periods of reactivity are delayed. If the infant is very ill, these periods of reactivity may not be observed at all, as the infant may be hypotonic and unreactive for several days after birth.

As the preterm newborn grows and the condition stabilizes, it becomes increasingly possible to identify behavioral states and traits unique to each infant. This is a very important part of nursing management of the high-risk infant, because it facilitates parental knowledge of their infant's cues for interaction.

In general, stable preterm infants do not demonstrate the same behavioral states as term infants. Preterm infants are more disorganized in their sleep–wake cycles and are unable to attend as well to the human face and objects in the environment. Neurologically, their responses are weaker (sucking, muscle tone, states of arousal) than full-term infants' responses (Gorski et al., 1979).

By observing each infant's patterns of behavior and responses, especially the sleep–wake states, the nurse can teach parents optimal times for interacting with their infant. The parents and nurse can plan nursing care around the times when the infant is alert and best able to attend. In addition, the more knowledge parents have about the meaning of their infant's responses and behaviors, the better prepared they will be to meet their newborn's needs and to form a positive attachment with their child.

Central Nervous System Physiology and Considerations

The brain and CNS of the full-term newborn are immature at birth in comparison with the adult brain and nervous system. The reflex activity present at birth (Moro, stepping, grasping) is primarily a function of the brain stem and spinal cord, with little cerebral control over these activities. Abnormalities of the reflex responses may result from either cortical or brain stem dysfunction and are therefore difficult to localize.

The preterm infant is even less mature neurologically than the term infant, with the degree of immaturity depending on the length of gestation. Polysynaptic connections are in the early stages of development, and myelination of nerve cells is incomplete. Lining the ventricles and the spinal cord is an ependymal layer or membrane, and the germinal matrix, a structure present only until term. This germinal matrix is a highly vascular area, with very thin and fragile capillary walls. The matrix provides little supportive tissue for the fragile blood vessels. Before 32 weeks' gestation, an infant is much more susceptible to hemorrhage of these tiny vessels, because they are vulnerable to hypoxic events that damage vessel walls and cause them to rupture. Most often, hemorrhage occurs in the germinal matrix, through the ependymal wall and into the ventricles of the brain to circulate within the cerebral spinal fluid (Korones, 1981).

Because the period of most rapid brain growth and development occurs during the third trimester of pregnancy, the closer to term an infant is delivered, the better the neurologic prognosis.

APNEA AND OTHER COMPLICATIONS

Apnea is a common problem in the preterm infant (of less than 36 weeks' gestation) and is thought to be primarily a result of neuronal immaturity, a factor that contributes to the tendency for the preterm infant's irregular breathing patterns. Apnea is defined as cessation of breathing for more than 20–30 seconds. When in conjunction with cyanosis and bradycardia (heart rate less than 100 beats/min) these periods are called apneic episodes or spells (Avery, 1981). Periodic breathing is distinguished from apnea in that the cessation of breathing lasts only 5–10 seconds and is followed by a period of rapid ventilation. Neither cyanosis nor bradycardia are associated, and therapy is not required for periodic breathing.

The immaturity of the CNS in the preterm infant contributes to vulnerability to any adverse factors affecting nerve cell metabolism. Impaired nerve cell metabolism in turn can impair respiratory neurons in the brain stem. Factors that adversely affect nerve cells in the brain include hypoxia, edema, intracranial bleeding, hyperbilirubinemia, hypoglycemia, hypocalcemia, and sepsis (Schulte, 1977). Apnea may also be associated with acidosis, hypothermia or hyperthermia, RDS, patent ductus arteriosus, seizure activity, anemia, hyponatremia or hypernatremia, and pneumonia. For a discussion of nursing interventions in caring for an infant with apnea, see the Nursing Care Plan for preterm infants, p. 750. Chapter 25 discusses further the complications that pose dangers for preterm infants. The following complications are the most frequently occurring: RDS, hypoglycemia, hypocalcemia, hyperbilirubinemia, sepsis, cold stress, intraventricular hemorrhage, necrotizing enterocolitis, PDA, and anemia.

(Text continues on p. 758.)

NURSING CARE PLAN
AGA and LGA Preterm Infants

PATIENT DATA BASE

History

1. Maternal history, including general, obstetric, and events of labor and delivery. Factors frequently associated with preterm delivery include:
   a. Age — very young mothers
   b. Closely spaced pregnancies
   c. Low socioeconomic group
   d. Previous history of preterm pregnancy
   e. Abnormalities of reproductive system: uterine malformations, incompetent cervix, infections (both urinary tract and systemic)
   f. Elective cesarean delivery
   g. Obstetric complications such as abruptio placentae, placenta previa, premature rupture of membranes, amnionitis

2. Fetal conditions associated with preterm delivery include:
   a. Blood incompatibility, with resultant erythroblastosis fetalis
   b. Multiple gestations
   c. Congenital infections

Physical examination

1. Physical characteristics vary according to gestational age, but certain characteristics are frequently present:
   a. Skin — reddened, translucent, blood vessels readily apparent, lack of subcutaneous fat
   b. Nails — soft, short
   c. Lanugo — plentiful, widely distributed
   d. Small genitals (testes may not be descended)
   e. Head size — appears large in relation to body
   f. Ears — minimal cartilage, pliable, folded over
   g. Resting position — flaccid, froglike position
   h. Cry — weak, feeble
   i. Reflexes — poor sucking, swallowing, and gag

2. Gestational age determined by clinical assessment tools

3. Temperature fluctuates easily — maintenance at 97.7F (36.5C) ± 0.5F

4. Pulse taken apically — often rapid and irregular, normal range 120–160

5. Respirations — 40–60 per minute, shallow, irregular, usually diaphragmatic with intermittent periodic breathing

6. Blood pressure — determine BP for low-weight newborns using normograms (Table 24–4)

7. Color usually pink or ruddy but may be acrocyanotic; observe for cyanosis, jaundice, pallor, or plethora

8. Activity — jerky, generalized movements (Note: seizure activity is abnormal)

9. Elimination — observe for patency of anus

10. Stool — first stool meconium; stool volume may be decreased because of hypomotility of intestine

11. Voiding — first voiding within 24 hours of birth; output scanty and infrequent for 1–3 days

12. Skull — bones pliable, fontanelle smooth and flat; presence of bulging may indicate CNS problem, depressed fontanelle suggests dehydration; observe for cephalhematoma or caput succedaneum

13. Evaluate for common preterm infant morbidities (see Figure 24–2)

Laboratory evaluation

Chest x-ray (PA and left lateral) — clear with no infiltration

Complete blood count (CBC) (Table 24–5, p. 752)

Rh determination if mother RH negative and father RH positive

Urinalysis on second voided specimen

Specific gravity every voiding — normal range 1.006–1.013

Hematest and reducing substance on all stools (if positive, consider necrotizing enterocolitis)

Dextrostix every 4–6 hours

Blood glucose level drawn if Dextrostix below 45 mg/mL

NURSING PRIORITIES

1. Enhance respiratory efforts.

2. Promote homeostasis through provision of neutral thermal environment and through meeting nutrition and fluid needs.

3. Protect from infections.

4. Support psychologic well-being of parents and infant by facilitating positive parent-child bonding and sensory stimulation of infant.

5. Evaluate infant for possible complications and institute appropriate interventions.

FAMILY EDUCATIONAL FOCUS

1. Discuss the implications of having a preterm infant in regard to respiratory immaturity, caloric and fluid requirements, and thermal instability.

2. Explain treatment modalities and their rationale.

3. Explore the long term implications of such alteration on the achievement of developmental milestones for the first 2 years of life and evaluation of development based on chronological age.

4. Provide opportunities to discuss questions and individual parental concerns regarding their preterm neonate.

NURSING CARE PLAN Cont'd
AGA and LGA Preterm Infants

Problem	Nursing interventions and actions	Rationale
Respiratory distress	Maintain airway patency through judicious suctioning Position with head slightly elevated and neck slightly extended Avoid increased oxygen consumption by maintaining adequate body temperature (97.7F ± 0.5F) Observe, record, and report signs of respiratory distress, including: 1. Cyanosis — serious sign when generalized 2. Tachypnea — sustained respiratory rate greater than 60/min after first 4 hr of life. 3. Retractions. 4. Expiratory grunting. 5. Flaring nostrils. 6. Apneic episodes 7. Presence of rales or ronchi on auscultation.	Anatomic and physiological characteristics predispose preterm infant to respiratory distress because: 1. Increased danger of obstruction results from small diameter of bronchi and trachea. 2. Newborn is nose breather and prone to nasal obstruction. 3. Chest wall musculature is weak and efficiency of cough reflex is decreased. 4. Cough and gag reflexes may be absent due to immaturity. 5. Lung surfactant necessary to maintain alveolar stability and prevent collapse is inadequate (Avery, 1981).

Table 24–4 Blood Pressure of Newborns with Low Weight*

Body weight (kg)	Gestational age (weeks)													
	27	28	29	30	31	32	33	34	35	36	37	38	39	40
0.80	43	44	44	45	45	46	46	47	47	48	48	49	49	50
0.90	44	45	45	46	46	47	47	48	48	49	49	50	50	51
1.00	45	45	46	46	47	47	48	48	49	49	50	50	51	51
1.10	46	46	47	47	48	48	49	49	50	50	51	51	52	52
1.20	46	47	47	48	48	49	49	50	51	51	52	52	53	53
1.30	47	48	48	49	49	50	50	51	51	52	52	53	53	54
1.40	48	49	49	50	50	51	51	52	52	53	53	54	54	55
1.50	49	49	50	50	51	51	52	52	53	53	54	54	55	55
1.60	50	50	51	51	52	52	53	53	54	54	55	55	56	56
1.70	51	51	52	52	53	53	54	54	55	55	56	56	57	57
1.80	51	52	52	53	53	54	54	55	55	56	56	57	57	58
1.90	52	53	53	54	54	55	55	56	56	57	57	58	58	59
2.00	53	53	54	54	55	56	56	57	57	58	58	59	59	60
2.10	54	54	55	55	56	56	57	57	58	58	59	59	60	60
2.20	55	55	56	56	57	57	58	58	59	59	60	60	61	61
2.30	55	56	56	57	57	58	58	59	59	60	60	61	61	62
2.40	56	57	57	58	58	59	59	60	60	61	61	62	62	63

Add for a postnatal age of[†]

Hours	3–7	8–12	13–18	19–24	25–32	33–40	41–54	55–89	90–96
mm Hg	1	2	3	4	5	6	7	8	7

*From Bucci, G., et al. 1972. The systemic systolic blood pressure of newborns with low weight. *Acta Paediatr. Scan.* (Supp.). 229:1.
[†]Systolic blood pressure is determined based on body weight and gestational age. Additional points are added according to postnatal age in hours.

NURSING CARE PLAN Cont'd
AGA and LGA Preterm Infants

Problem	Nursing interventions and actions	Rationale
	Implement treatment plan for respiratory distress, if indicated Administer oxygen per physician order for relief of symptoms of respiratory distress	
Heat losses	Increase environmental temperature to maintain thermal neutrality Reflect principles of anatomy and physiology of temperature control and thermogenesis in planning of care Minimize heat losses and prevent cold stress by: 1. Warming and humidifying oxygen without blowing over face in order to avoid increasing oxygen consumption. 2. Maintaining skin in dry condition. 3. Keeping isolettes, radiant warmers, and cribs away from windows and cold external walls and out of drafts; utilizing heat shields with small infants.	A neutral thermal environment requires minimal oxygen consumption to maintain a normal core temperature. Body temperature fluctuates because: 1. Assuming a position of extension exposes a relatively large body surface in relation to body mass. 2. Infant lacks subcutaneous fat for adequate insulation. 3. Immature central nervous system provides poor temperature control. 4. Stores of brown fat for chemical thermogenesis are decreased; a small infant (less than 1200 g) can lose 80 cal/kg/day through radiation of body heat.

Table 24–5 Selected Normal Laboratory Values in Newborn Preterm Infants*

Laboratory test	Normal values	Laboratory test	Normal values
Hematologic		Total protein	4.8–5.3 g
Red blood cells (RBC)	4–6 million/mm^3	Albumin (first week)	3.3–4.5
White blood cells (WBC)	10,000–15,000/mm^3	Osmolality	270–285 milliosmols/L
Platelets	87,000–209,000/mm^3	pH	7.35–7.45
Reticulocytes	2.7%–8.4% of RBC	Total CO_2 content	19–20 mEq/L
Hematocrit	45%–60%	P_{CO_2}	33–38 mm Hg in Denver
Hemoglobin	15.6–20.0; mean 17–19 g/dL	Urea nitrogen (BUN)	16–22 mg/dL
Fetal Hbg	55%–85% of total Hbg	Transaminase (SGOT)	Up to 54 units in first week
Adult Hbg	15%–45% of total Hbg		of life
Plasma electrolyte		Creatinine	0.8–1.8 mg/dL
Chloride	100–104 mEq/L	Serum glucose (fasting)	40–100 mg/dL
Sodium	134–138 mEq/L	Total blood volume	80–90 mL/kg
Potassium	5.4–6.4 mEq/L	Total body water	69%–83% of body weight
Calcium	6.1–11.6 mg/dL	Extracellular body water	42% of body weight
Ionized calcium	4.1–5.4 mg/dL	Intracellular body water	35% of body weight
Phosphorus (first week)	5.4–10.9 mg/dL	Urine osmolarity	216–792

*Modified from University of Colorado School of Nursing. Adapted from Silverman, W. A. 1961. *Dunham's premature infants.* 3rd ed. New York: Paul B. Hoeber, Inc.; and from O'Brien, D., and Abbott, F. 1962. *Laboratory manual of pediatric microbiochemical techniques.* New York: Paul B. Hoeber, Inc. Values updated from Cloherty, J. P., and Stark, A. R., eds. 1980. *Manual of neonatal care.* Boston: Little, Brown & Co.
NOTE: Lab values vary depending on method of analysis used in various laboratories.

NURSING CARE PLAN Cont'd
AGA and LGA Preterm Infants

Problem	Nursing interventions and actions	Rationale
	4. Utilizing skin probe to monitor infant skin temperature at 36–37C. 5. Avoiding placing infant on cold surfaces such as metal treatment tables, cold x-ray plates. 6. Padding cold surfaces with diapers and using radiant warmers during procedures. 7. Warming blood for exchange transfusions.	Physical principles of heat loss effects include: 1. Evaporation—lungs and skin when cooling occurs as a result of water evaporation. 2. Convection—air currents. 3. Conduction—skin contact with cooler object. 4. Radiation—loss of warmth to cooler surrounding objects.
Caloric and fluid intake necessary for growth	Initiate feeding of sterile water at 2–4 hr of age in well preterm infant. Promote growth by providing caloric intake of 120–150 cal/kg/day in small amounts; increased slowly in small amounts (1–2 mL) given more frequently (every 2–3 hr). Supplement oral feedings with intravenous intake per physician orders. Feed specially formulated formulas such as Similac Special Care and Premie Enfamil formula. Utilize concentrated formulas that supply more calories in less volume, such as Similac 24 calorie Feed with soft "premie" nipple and burp frequently. Observe, record, and report signs of respiratory distress or fatigue occurring during feedings. Evaluate for signs of dehydration, including depressed fontanelle, poor skin turgor, decreased urine output, sunken eyeballs, and dry mucous membranes. Monitor daily weight, blood pH, normal urine output of 1–3 mL/kg/hour, specific gravity, Dipstix/Clinitest for evidence of glycosuria.	Sterile water is desirable for first feedings because, in the presence of gastrointestinal tract abnormalities and/or aspiration of feeding, fewer pulmonary complications will result. Adequate nutritional and fluid intake promotes growth and prevents such complications as metabolic catabolism, hypoglycemia, and dehydration. Small, frequent feedings of high caloric formula are utilized because of limited gastric capacity and decreased gastric emptying Growth is evaluated by increase in weight, length, and body measurements.
Fatigue during feedings	Utilize an orogastric or nasogastric tube or nasojejunal gavage feedings in small preterm infants not tolerating intermittent volumes of feeding. Facilitate continuous feedings and prevent vomiting by placing nasojejunal tube past pylorus. Initiate safety factors with gavage feedings: 1. Evaluate proper tube placement by aspiration of gastric contents; inject a small amount of air into stomach and auscultate with a stethoscope; place end of catheter in water and watch for continuous bubbling. 2. Allow gravity flow for feedings and never push a tube feeding.	Suck, swallow, and gag reflexes are immature at birth in preterm infant. Nipple feeding, an active rather than passive intake of nutrition, requires energy expenditure and burning of calories by infant. Gavage feedings require less energy expenditure on the part of the preterm infant. Decrease in exhaustion is an important consideration in feeding an infant who is ill, has poorly developed suck reflex, or is less than 32 weeks' gestation. Presence of residual formula in stomach is indication of intolerance to amount of feeding or to increase in amount of feeding or is indicative of obstruction, paralytic ileus, or necrotizing enterocolitis.

NURSING CARE PLAN Cont'd
AGA and LGA Preterm Infants

Problem	Nursing interventions and actions	Rationale
	Determine presence of residual formula in stomach prior to initiating feeding by aspirating from gastric tube and replacing amount before remainder of feeding is given.	Residual feeding is calculated for example by: 1. Feeding order–24 mL every 2 hours. 2. Residual–3 mL. 3. Formula this feeding – 21 mL plus 3 mL residual.
	Measure abdominal girth prior to each feeding.	Early detection of abdominal distention aids in diagnosis of necrotizing enterocolitis.
	Observe, record, and report complications of nasojejunal tube including misplacement, perforation, plugging, vomiting due to excessive volume, or sepsis.	Residual formula is readministered because digestive processes have already been initiated.
	Establish a nipple feeding program that is begun slowly and progresses slowly, such as nipple feed once per day, nipple feed once per shift, and then nipple feed every other feeding.	As infant matures, gavage feedings should be replaced with nipple feedings to assist in strengthening sucking reflexes and meeting psychologic needs.
	Monitor daily weight with anticipation of small amount of weight loss when nipple feedings start.	
	Supplement gavage or nipple feedings with intravenous therapy per physician order until oral intake is sufficient to support growth.	
	Develop a plan of care that involves parents in feeding of infant	Involvement of parents in feeding of preterm infant is essential to development of attachment and expansion of parental knowledge and coping mechanisms.
	Observe, record, and report presence of complications such as hypoglycemia or hypocalcemia.	Preterm infant requires delicate balance for homeostasis and prevention of complications.
Susceptibility to infection	Initiate a plan of care to prevent exposure to infection such as handwashing, reverse isolation, and individual equipment.	Infection is common occurrence due to immaturity of immunologic system, increased use of invasive procedures and techniques, and more prolonged hospitalization.
	Implement treatment per physician orders in presence of infection (refer to section on sepsis neonatorum, p. 841, for review of nursing care).	
Prolonged separation of infant and mother	Support emotionally the psychologic well-being of family, including positive maternal-child bonding and sensory stimulation of infant.	Maternal bonding begins in first few hours or days following birth of an infant. Preterm infants experience prolonged periods of separation from their mothers, which necessitates intervention to insure maternal-child bonding.
	Include parents in determining infant's plan of care and encourage their participation.	Related to prolonged separation of preterm infants from their mothers following delivery is increased incidence of child neglect and child abuse.
	Encourage parents to visit frequently.	
	Provide opportunities for parents to touch, hold, talk to, and care for infant.	Parents should receive same postpartum teaching as any parent taking a new infant home.
	Determine type and amount of sensory stimulation appropriate and implement sensory stimulation program.	
	Prepare for discharge by instructing parent in such areas as feeding techniques, formula preparation (including bottle sterilization), and	Mothers with preterm infants desiring to breast feed will pump their breasts to keep

NURSING CARE PLAN Cont'd
AGA and LGA Preterm Infants

Problem	Nursing interventions and actions	Rationale
	breast-feeding; bathing, diapering, and hygiene; rectal temperature monitoring; administration of vitamins; sibling rivalry; care of complications and preventing exposure to infections; normal elimination patterns, normal reflexes and activity, and how to promote normal growth and development without being overprotective; returning for continued medical care; and availability of community resources if indicated	milk flowing and in some situations to provide milk for their infant. This activity allows breast-feeding after discharge from hospital. Mothers need to understand the changes to expect in color of the infant's stool and number of bowel movements plus odor from bottle or breast-feeding in order to avoid unnecessary concern on mother's part. Preterm infants usually do not require referral to community agencies such as visiting nurse associations unless there is a specific problem requiring assistance. Infants with congenital abnormalities, feeding problems, or resolving complications with infections or mothers unable to cope with defective infants are examples of conditions requiring referral to community resources.
Possible complications Apnea	Monitor heart rate and respiratory rate continuously on all preterm infants. Check during each shift to make sure alarms are set and working properly. Document *all* episodes of apnea. Include activity at the time of apnea, length of episode, and treatment required to bring infant out of apneic spell.	Apneic onset is often insidious; however, with cardiorespiratory monitoring, early recognition and intervention prevents the need for resuscitative efforts. Apnea may occur during a feeding, during suctioning, or while stooling. On the other hand, there may be no observable activity related to the apnea. Documenting length of episode and treatment required to resolve apneic spell is also important in determining etiology and possible therapy.
	Implement treatment based on severity of apneic episode and infant's response: 1. Observe infant briefly to see if treatment is necessary or if infant will begin breathing spontaneously. 2. Begin stimulation by gently rubbing soles of feet, ankles, and up and down infant's back. 3. If the infant is dusky, cyanotic, or bradycardic, suction nasopharynx and oropharynx, provide additional oxygen and prepare for bag and mask ventilation.	The nurse must make careful observations and quickly judge the need for intervention Rubbing bony prominences is uncomfortable to the infant and therefore more stimulating than rubbing other areas of the body. Obstruction of the airway by mucus or formula may result in apnea and bradycardia. Clearing the airway while providing increased oxygen concentration and stimulation may resolve apneic episode. If the infant does not respond, bag and mask ventilation may be required to relieve cyanosis and return heart rate to normal.
	4. Prepare for intubation and use of respirator for ventilation if infant has frequent apneic episodes that require bag and mask ventilation. 5. Prepare for septic workup if infant is not on antibiotics.	Ventilatory assistance may be necessary to prevent possible sequelae of frequent apneic spells with resulting hypoxemia. Sepsis depresses CNS functioning and may be the cause of apnea.

NURSING CARE PLAN Cont'd
AGA and LGA Preterm Infants

Problem	Nursing interventions and actions	Rationale
	Administer oxygen and warm humidified air per physician order to control dyspnea and cyanosis.	Increased oxygen may alleviate episodes of apnea and bradycardia.
	Monitor and record concentration of oxygen every 2 hours	Based on recommendations by American Academy of Pediatrics.
	Evaluate and report variations in blood gases and electrolyte reports.	Apnea is associated with elevated P_{CO_2}, decreased P_{O_2}, and other metabolic disturbances.
	Administer theophylline per physician order for intractable neonatal apnea.	Theophylline is a CNS stimulant that increases respiratory drive and alveolar ventilation.
	Modify care plan to reduce or prevent apnea, including:	
	1. Gentle handling.	Prevents unnecessary stress to the infant.
	2. Indwelling orogastric or nasogastric tube rather than intermittent passage of feeding tube.	Vagal stimulation increases possibility of apnea.
	3. Gentle nasopharyngeal suction as necessary.	Nasopharyngeal stimulation may cause apnea; however, keeping airway clear is very important.
	4. Maintenance of thermal neutrality.	Temperature instability may precipitate apnea.
	Provide IV fluids as ordered to maintain adequate fluid and electrolyte balance.	Severe apnea may preclude, for a time, oral feeding, requiring nutritional maintenance with intravenous therapy. Adequate nutrition prevents catabolism of body tissues as well as biochemical aberrations such as hypoglycemia, hyperglycemia, acidosis or electrolyte imbalance.
Birth trauma	Screen and monitor all LGA infants for birth injury, including:	Disproportion between birth canal and size of LGA infant results in birth trauma and an increased rate of cesarean birth.
	1. Presence of cry that is high-pitched, weak, absent or constant, and irritable.	LGA infants are in at-risk grouping.
	2. Note activity such as flaccidity, floppiness, poor muscle tone, spasticity, hyperactivity, opisthotonos, twitching, hypertonicity, tremors, or frank convulsions.	Physical examination of LGA infant may reveal symptoms of increased intracranial pressure — with high-pitched cry — or presence of brain injury — with weak cry, absent cry, or constant, irritable crying.
	3. Observe resting posture for asymmetry resulting from intrauterine pressure or birth trauma.	CNS damage may be indicated by spasticity, hyperactivity, opisthotonos, twitching, hypertonicity, tremors, or convulsion.
	4. Evaluate fontanelles for bulging, tenseness, or fullness.	Birth trauma may result in brain damage or injury, diaphragmatic paralysis, fracture of clavicle, palsies, and/or paralysis
	5. Observe eyes for constricted pupil, unilateral, dilated fixed pupils, nystagmus, or strabismus.	
	6. Asymmetry of chest may indicate diaphragmatic paralysis.	
	7. Evaluate for fracture of clavicle, which is detected by palpable mass, crepitus, and tenderness at fracture site or by limited movements of arm such as unilateral decrease in Moro response.	

NURSING CARE PLAN Cont'd
AGA and LGA Preterm Infants

Problem	Nursing interventions and actions	Rationale
	8. Assess movement of extremities for palsies due to injury to brachial plexus, for fractures or dislocation.	
	9. Note paralysis of lower extremities.	Paralysis of both legs is due to pressure or severe trauma to spinal cord.
Congenital malformation	Complete and record results of physical examination on LGA infants of diabetic mothers for presence of congenital anomalies including: 1. Cardiac anomalies, which usually are ventricular septal defects or transposition of great vessels resulting in murmur; cardiopulmonary distress with tachypnea, tachycardia, cyanosis, or labored respiration; and/or congestive heart failure. 2. Spinal anomalies, simple or extensive, resulting in missing vertebras on palpation, pilonidal dimple or sinus, sacral agenesis, spina bifida, or myelomeningocele.	Congenital malformations in LGA infants of diabetic mothers are more frequent due to increased incidence of: 1. Abnormal intrauterine environment due to diabetes and vascular complications. 2. Drugs taken by mother during pregnancy (oral hypoglycemic agents).
Pulmonary problems, including RDS, wet lung, atelectasis, pneumothorax Cold stress, hypocalcemia, hypoglycemia Sepsis neonatorum Retrolental fibroplasia Necrotizing enterocolitis Hyperbilirubinemia or kernicterus Anemia		These additional possible complications are covered in depth in following chapters

NURSING CARE EVALUATION

Respirations are 30–50 per minute, regular, with no episodes of apnea.

Temperature is stable.

Infant is gaining weight.

Infant takes nipple feedings without developing fatigue.

Complications are controlled or absent.

Infant is active without jerky generalized movement.

Infant is free from infection or infection is controlled.

Parent–child bonding is completed.

Infant responds to sensory stimulation.

Parents understand and can demonstrate knowledge of infant care, feeding, growth projections, prevention of exposure to infections, treatment of complications, and when to return for medical care.

NURSING DIAGNOSES*	SUPPORTING DATA
1. Potential impaired gas exchange related to inadequate lung surfactant, absent or diminished cough and gag reflexes	Cyanosis Tachypnea Retractions Expiratory grunting Flaring nostrils Rales or rhonchi Nasal obstruction
2. Alteration in nutrition: potential for less than body requirements of neonate	Fatigue during feedings Immature suck, swallow, gag reflexes Hypoglycemia Residual formula in stomach Weight loss

NURSING CARE PLAN Cont'd
AGA and LGA Preterm Infants

NURSING DIAGNOSES*	SUPPORTING DATA
3. Potential fluid volume deficit	Depressed fontanelle Poor skin turgor Decreased urine output Weight loss Dry mucous membranes
4. Potential for injury related to impaired thermoregulatory mechanisms	Decreased temperature Lethargy Pallor Hypoglycemia
5. Potential anxiety in infant related to inappropriate auditory, tactile, visual stimulation	Infant separated from mother, normal stimulation decreased, for necessary medical or surgical intervention Nursery environment
6. Parental knowledge deficit concerning care of infant at home	Expressed concerns or questions regarding care of preterm infant following discharge Unaware of available community resources

* These are a few examples of nursing diagnoses that may be appropriate for AGA and LGA preterm infants. It is not an inclusive list and must be individualized for each infant.

Long-Term Needs and Outcome

The care of the high-risk infant and the family is not complete upon discharge from the nursery. Although the majority of infants requiring intensive care are at low risk for serious neurologic damage, follow-up care is extremely important because many developmental problems are not noted until the infant is older and begins to demonstrate motor delays or sensory disability.

Within the first year of life, low-birth-weight infants face higher mortality than term infants. Causes of death include sudden infant death syndrome (SIDS), which occurs about five times more frequently in the low-birth-weight infant, and respiratory infections and neurologic defects. Morbidity is also much higher among low-birth-weight infants, with those weighing less than 1500 g at highest risk for long-term complications.

The most common long-term problems observed in preterm infants include the following:

Retrolental fibroplasia (RLF). In spite of new technology and the ability to monitor arterial oxygen closely, development of RLF and resulting degrees of loss of eyesight continue to occur in the preterm infant, although the incidence has decreased to 1%–2%. Infants at highest risk are those weighing less than 1000 g at birth.

Sensorineural hearing loss. Although their rate of hearing loss has decreased since the 1940s, preterm infants at high risk include those with severe asphyxia or recurrent apnea in the neonatal period. Hyperbilirubinemia and ototoxic drugs such as gentamicin and furosemide (Lasix) are also known to contribute to hearing loss in the neonate.

Speech defects. The most frequently observed speech defects involve delayed development of receptive and expressive ability that may persist into the school-age years.

Neurologic defects. The most common neurologic defects include cerebral palsy, hydrocephalus, seizure disorders, lower IQ scores, and learning disabilities. However, the socioeconomic climate and family support systems have been shown to be extremely important factors influencing the child's ultimate intellectual ability in the absence of major neurologic defects (Fitzhardinge, 1976).

When evaluating the infant's abilities and disabilities, it is important for parents to understand that the developmental level cannot be evaluated based on chronological age. Developmental progress must be evaluated from the expected date of birth, not from the actual date of birth. In addition, the parents need the consistent support of health care professionals in the long-term management of their infant. Many new and ongoing concerns arise as the high-risk infant grows and develops; the goal is to promote the highest quality of life possible.

POSTTERM NEONATE

The postterm infant is any infant delivered after 42 weeks' gestation. It has been recommended that the term *postmaturity* be reserved for those pregnancies lasting 42 weeks or longer in which concurrent intrauterine growth retardation is documented. The incidence of postterm births has been found to be approximately 3.5%–10% in the general population. Of these, only 4%–7.3% extend beyond 43

Table 24–6   Evaluation of Fetal Status in True Prolonged Pregnancy*

Clinical parameters	Positive	Guarded	Negative
Uterine size	Increasing	No increase	Decreasing
Amniotic fluid volume	Appropriate	Diminished	Oligohydramnios
Fetal activity	Unchanged	Diminished	Absent
Maternal weight	Increasing	Decreasing	
Estriol levels	Stable/increasing	Chronically low	Decrease $\geq$ 35%
Ultrasound (growth-adjusted sonographic age)	Maintenance of growth percentile	Decrease in growth percentile	Cessation of growth
Nonstress test	Reactive	Nonreactive: spontaneous variables	Spontaneous late deceleration
Oxytocin challenge test	Negative	Ambiguous: variable decelerations	Positive
Intrapartum monitoring	Baseline 100–140 beats/min, normal pattern, variability of 6–15 beats/min	Baseline > 150 beats/min, decreased variability, variable decelerations	Baseline > 150 beats/min, absent variability, repetitive late decelerations

*From Hobart, J. M., and Depp, R., 1982. Prolonged pregnancy. In *Gynecology and obstetrics,* vol. 3. J. J. Sciarra, ed. Philadelphia: Harper & Row, p.5.

weeks (Hobart and Depp, 1982). The etiology of postterm pregnancies is not completely understood, although several conditions are known to be associated with the postterm pregnancy. Primigravidas, high parity mothers (greater than four), and a history of prolonged pregnancy are all associated with postterm deliveries (Affonso and Harris, 1980). Pregnancies in which the infant is anencephalic are also often postterm. In the latter case it is believed that certain endocrine functions important in the triggering of labor are lacking in the anencephalic (without brain tissue) fetus (Lubchenco, 1976). Many abnormally long gestations are thought to be due to delayed ovulation and subsequent delayed fertilization. Boyce, Mayaux, and Schwartz (1976) concluded that 70% of postterm pregnancies are a function of delayed ovulation.

Modern obstetric practice is faced with the dilemma of differentiating uncomplicated prolonged pregnancy from the prolonged pregnancy compounded by IUGR. Obstetric antenatal management must be directed at identifying the wrinkled, small, growth-retarded postmature infant who is at greater risk than the larger, well-nourished counterpart who has experienced an equally long gestation (Table 24–6).

Prolonged pregnancy itself is not responsible for the postmaturity. Rather, in some postdate pregnancies, the fetuses suffer from superimposed placental insufficiency. The characteristics observed in the postterm infant as described by Clifford (1957) are primarily due to advanced gestational age, placental insufficiency, and continued exposure to amniotic fluid. Because of the prolonged gestation, these infants are more alert; have decreased vernix; show cracked, peeling, and dry skin; and exhibit varying degrees of wasting (Figures 24–8). Apgar scores are fre-

quently lower (due to meconium aspiration and birth asphyxia), and these infants are frequently polycythemic with central hematocrit levels above 65.

Clifford (1957) has devised clinical criteria for the assessment of postmaturity syndrome.

Stage 1. Long, thin, infant. Loose skin (around thighs and buttocks) giving the appearance of recent weight loss. Peeling, parchmentlike skin. Decrease in or lack of vernix. Alert expression. Behavior of 1-to-3-week-old infant more mature

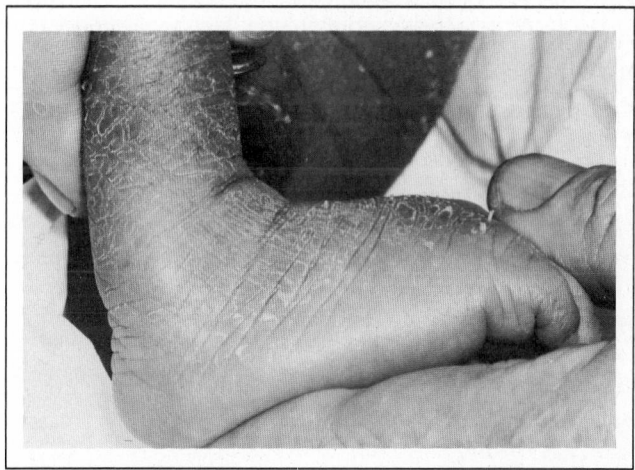

FIGURE 24–8 Postterm infant demonstrates deep cracking and peeling of skin. (From Dubowitz, L., and Dubowitz, V. 1977. *Gestational age of the newborn.* Menlo Park, Calif.: Addison-Wesley Publishing Co.)

than term newborn. Long nails—staining of nails and skin. No lanugo.

Stage II. Stage I symptoms plus meconium-stained amniotic fluid, skin, vernix, umbilical cord, and placental membranes—manifestations of fetal anoxic insult.

Stage III. Stages I and II (survived acute anoxic phase of stage II) plus nails and skin are stained a bright yellow and the umbilical cord is yellow green.*

It is important to note that Clifford's classification system applies only to those neonates who, according to clinical assessment, have suffered placental insufficiency.

The postmaturity syndrome infant is at high risk for morbidity and mortality, with a mortality two to three times greater than term infants. The majority of deaths occur during labor, as the infant has lost necessary reserves by the time labor begins. Because of decreasing placental function, oxygenation is marginal or depressed and nutrition is impaired, leaving the infant prone to hypoglycemia and asphyxia when the stresses of labor begin. Problems seen in these postmature infants are thus a result of inadequate placental function, decreased reserves, and the stress of labor. The most common disorders observed include:

1. Hypoglycemia, from nutritional deprivation and resultant depleted glycogen stores.

2. Postmaturity syndrome with intrauterine asphyxia and fetal distress. Physiologic response to hypoxia in the fetus is a relaxation of the anal sphincter and passage of meconium into the amniotic fluid. Hence, the postterm infant is meconium-stained and at risk for meconium aspiration. It is important that a postterm newborn with meconium-stained amniotic fluid be appropriately resuscitated and supported in the delivery room. Suctioning of the naso-oropharynx (while the infant is on the perineum) will help prevent meconium aspiration (Chapter 25).

3. Polycythemia. Same pathophysiology and nursing interventions as for the SGA infant with polycythemia.

4. Congenital anomalies are found more frequently in postterm infants (Chapter 26).

5. Seizure activity because of hypoxic insult. Because of chronic hypoxia, possible fetal distress in labor, and birth asphyxia, these infants have a delayed transition to extrauterine life.

6. Cold stress because of loss or poor development of subcutaneous fat. Prevention of heat loss should be ensured during the resuscitative process.

*From Clifford, S. 1957. Postmaturity. *Adv. Pediatr.* 9:13.

Nursing interventions are primarily supportive measures. They include (a) observation of cardiopulmonary parameters, since the stresses of labor are poorly tolerated and severe depression can ensue at birth; (b) provision of warmth to balance muted response to cold stress and decreased liver glycogen and brown fat stores; (c) frequent monitoring of blood glucose and initiation of early feeding (at 1 or 2 hours of age) or intravenous glucose per physician order; and (d) observation for disorders and appropriate management when possible. Nursing attention also should be directed toward facilitation of parental expression of feelings and fears regarding the infant's condition and long-term needs.

LARGE-FOR-GESTATIONAL-AGE INFANT

A large-for-gestational-age (LGA) neonate is one whose birth weight is at or above the ninetieth percentile on the intrauterine growth curve (at any week of gestation). Careful gestational age assessment is essential in identifying potential needs and problems of such infants.

An LGA infant is usually thought of as a term infant weighing 4000 g, but an infant of 3000 g at 34 weeks' gestation, although premature, also meets the criterion. The majority of infants categorized as LGA have been found to be so categorized because of miscalculation of dates because of postconceptual bleeding (Korones, 1981). The best-known condition leading to excessive fetal growth is the pregnancy of a diabetic mother; however, only a minority of large infants are born to diabetic mothers. Excessive birth weight is more reflective of the genetic predisposition of the fetus.

The etiology of the majority of LGA infants is unclear, but certain factors or situations have been found to be true.

• Genetic predisposition is correlated proportionally to the pregnancy weight and to weight gain during pregnancy. Large parents tend to have large infants.

• Multiparous women have three times the number of LGA infants as primigravidas. The second and third neonate is larger than the first but after that size does not increase predictably (Lubchenco, 1976).

• Male infants are traditionally larger than female infants.

• Infants born of diabetic mothers (IDM) or with erythroblastosis fetalis, Beckwith syndrome, or transposition of the great vessels are usually large.

Characteristically the increase in the LGA infant's body size is proportional, although head circumference and body length are in the upper limits of intrauterine growth. The exception to this rule is the infant of the diabetic mother, whose body weight increases only in proportion to length.

Common disorders of the LGA infant include the following conditions:

1. *Birth trauma because of cephalopelvic disproportion.* Often these infants have a biparietal diameter greater than 10 cm or a fundal height measurement greater than 42 cm without the presence of hydramnios. Because of their excessive size, there are more breech and shoulder dystocias, with resultant potential asphyxia, fractured clavicles, brachial palsy, facial paralysis, depressed skull fractures, and intracranial bleeding.

2. *Increased incidence of cesarean deliveries due to fetal size.* These births are accompanied by all the risk factors associated with cesarean deliveries.

3. *Hypoglycemia.* Usually the result of hyperinsulinemia, hypoglycemia is most often seen with erythroblastosis fetalis, Beckwith syndrome, and in IDMs. In these conditions the fetus is exposed to high levels of glucose, either because of breakdown of red blood cells in utero or increased circulating glucose from the mother, resulting in hyperplasia of the pancreatic islet cells.

4. *Polycythemia and hyperviscosity.* These conditions occur in the fetus when hemoglobin levels are elevated or when red blood cell mass increases (pathophysiologic mechanisms are not well known). Klaus and Fanaroff (1979) attribute the hyperviscosity of the blood to the increased rate of glucose disposal, without hyperinsulinemia. The symptomatology is caused by poor perfusion of the tissue.

The perinatal history, in conjunction with ultrasonic measurement of fetal skull and gestational age testing, is important in identifying an at-risk LGA newborn. Nursing management is directed toward early identification of the common disorders and appropriate immediate treatment. Essential components of the nursing assessment are monitoring vital signs and screening for hypoglycemia and polycythemia. For specific nursing interventions for common disorders of the LGA infant, see the Nursing Care Plan for AGA and LGA preterm infants, p. 756.

SMALL-FOR-GESTATIONAL-AGE INFANT

A small-for-gestational-age (SGA) infant is *any* infant who at birth is at or below the tenth percentile (intrauterine growth curve) on the Denver chart, or the fifth percentile on the Aberdeen chart, or two standard deviations on the Montreal chart and shows evidence of disproportionate growth. Growth retardation is possible in infants of any gestational age—preterm SGA, term SGA, or postterm SGA. Other terms used to designate a growth-retarded

neonate include intrauterine-growth-retarded (IUGR), small-for-dates (SFD), and dysmature. For this discussion, SGA and IUGR will be used interchangeably.

Between 3% and 7% of all pregnancies are complicated by IUGR. Growth-retarded infants have a fivefold increase in perinatal asphyxia and an eightfold higher perinatal mortality than normal infants (Hobbins, 1982).

Etiology

IUGR may result from maternal, placental, or fetal causes or may result without apparent cause noted antenatally. Intrauterine growth is linear in the normal pregnancy from approximately 28–38 weeks of gestation. After 38 weeks, growth is variable, depending on the growth potential of the fetus and the functioning of the placenta. The most commonly occurring causes of growth retardation are as follows:

Malnutrition. Maternal nutrition has not been found to significantly influence the birth weight of the neonate (Smith, 1947), unless starvation occurs during the last trimester of pregnancy. Before the third trimester, the nutritional supply to the fetus far exceeds its needs. By the third trimester the nutritional supply becomes a limiting factor to fetal growth. Hence, the parasitic existence of the fetus enables it to live off the nutritional stores of the pregnant woman (even if her nutritional intake is poor).

Vascular complications. Complications associated with PIH (preeclampsia and eclampsia), chronic hypertensive vascular disease, and advanced diabetes mellitus cause diminished blood flow to the uterus.

Maternal disease. Maternal heart disease, alcoholism, narcotic addiction, sickle cell anemia, phenylketonuria, and asymptomatic pyelonephritis are associated with SGA.

Maternal factors. SGA is associated with such maternal factors as small stature, primiparity, grand multiparity, smoking, lack of prenatal care, low socioeconomic class—which usually results in poor health care, poor nutritional intake, poor education, and poor living conditions—and age (very young or older).

Environmental factors. Such factors include high altitude and maternal use of drugs, such as antimetabolics, anticonvulsants, and trimethadione, which have teratogenic effects, and x rays.

Placental factors. Placental conditions such as infarcted areas, abnormal cord insertions, single umbilical artery, placenta previa, or thrombosis may affect vascular delivery to the fetus, which becomes more deficient with increasing gestational age.

Fetal factors. Congenital infections or malformations, multiple pregnancy (twins, triplets), sex (female neonate), chromosomal syndromes, and inborn errors of metabolism can predispose a fetus to IUGR.

Identification of fetuses at risk for IUGR is the first step in the identification and observation for common disorders. (See Chapter 13 for antenatal diagnosis and management.) Again, the perinatal history of maternal conditions is important in determining that a newborn is at risk. Other avenues of data collection are examination of the placenta and the newborn.

Patterns of Intrauterine Growth Retardation

Growth occurs in two ways—increase in cell number and cell size. If fetal insult occurs early during the critical period of organ development, fewer new cells are formed, organs are small, and organ weight is subnormal. In contrast, growth failure that begins later in pregnancy does not affect the total number of cells but their size. The organs are normal, but their size is diminished. Two patterns of IUGR have been described: symmetric term (proportional) IUGR and asymmetric term (disproportional) IUGR.

Symmetric term *(proportional) IUGR* is a pattern in which chronic prolonged retardation of growth in size of organs, weight, length, and, in severe cases, head circumference occurs. All body proportions are below normal for the gestational age (Figure 24–9). Causes of symmetric IUGR are long-term maternal conditions (such as chronic hypertension, severe malnutrition, chronic intrauterine infection, substance abuse, and anemia) or fetal genetic abnormalities (Bree and Mariona, 1980). Symmetric growth retardation can be noted by ultrasound in the first half of the second trimester.

Asymmetric term *(disproportional) IUGR* is an acute compromise of uteroplacental blood flow. It occurs in the majority of cases and is usually not evident before the third trimester. Weight is decreased, yet length and head circumference remain normal for the gestational age. These infants appear wasted, with loss of subcutaneous tissue and muscle mass; loose skin folds; wide-eyed faces; dry, desquamating skin; and a thin and often meconium-stained cord.

Fetuses with asymmetric IUGR are particularly at risk for perinatal asphyxia, pulmonary hemorrhage, hypocalcemia, and hypoglycemia in the neonatal period (Bree and Mariona, 1980). Birth weight is reduced below the tenth percentile, whereas cephalic size may be between the ninety-fifth and the fifteenth percentile.

As previously mentioned, IUGR is possible at any gestational age. Despite growth retardation, physiologic maturity develops according to gestational age. In the case of infants of the same weight, one preterm and one SGA, the SGA infant will be more mature in development (physiologic and neurologic) than the preterm infant. Because the SGA infant may have more physiologic maturity than the preterm AGA infant, the small-for-age infant is less predisposed to the development of respiratory distress, hyperbilirubinemia, and so on. The SGA neonate's chances for survival are better because of organ maturity, although this neonate still faces many other potential difficulties.

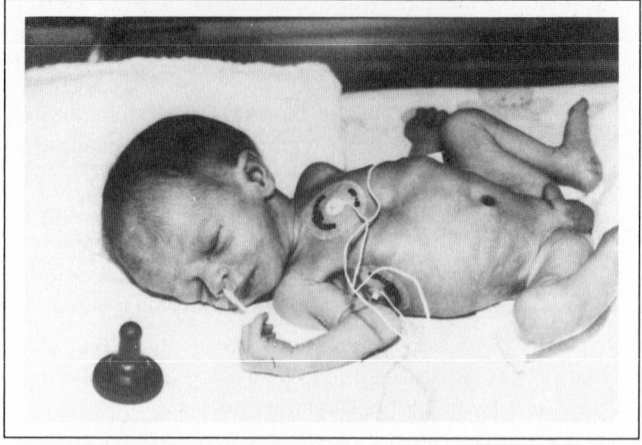

FIGURE 24–9 The infant with IUGR appears long, thin, and emaciated. The gestational age of the infant shown here is 41 weeks. He weighed approximately 1560 g at birth.

COMPLICATIONS

The complications occurring most frequently in the SGA neonate are the following:

1. Perinatal asphyxia—because of chronic hypoxia in utero, which leaves little reserve to withstand the demands of labor and delivery and increases risk of intracranial bleeding.
2. Aspiration syndromes—a physiologic response to fetal hypoxia. Gasping secondary to hypoxia can cause aspiration of amniotic fluid into the lower airways; or fetal hypoxia can lead to relaxation of the anal sphincter with passage of meconium.
3. Heat loss—decreased heat conservation ability resulting from diminished subcutaneous fat, depletion of brown fat, and large surface area.
4. Hypoglycemia—caused by high metabolic rate (secondary to heat loss) and poor glycogen stores.
5. Hypocalcemia—secondary to birth asphyxia and prematurity.
6. Polycythemia—thought to be a physiologic response to in utero chronic hypoxic stress.

Long-Term Outcome and Needs

Infants who have significant IUGR tend to have a poor prognosis, especially when born before 37 weeks' gestation. Factors contributing to poor outcome for these infants are as follows:

Congenital malformations. Usher (1970) found that congenital malformations occur 10 to 20 times more frequently in SGA infants than in AGA infants. The more severe the IUGR, the greater the chance for malformation as a result of impaired mitotic activity and cellular hypoplasia.

Intrauterine infections. When infants are exposed to intrauterine infections (rubella and cytomegalovirus), they are profoundly affected by direct invasion of the brain and other vital organs by the offending virus.

Inadequate growth. It is generally agreed that the IUGR neonate will ultimately be slimmer and shorter than neonates of the same gestational age but will have appropriate size growth. Fitzhardinge and Steven (1972) found that infants who are undergrown in all these areas (height, weight, and head circumference)—symmetric IUGRs—tend not to catch up in any parameter. Drillien (1970) concluded that if "catching up" has not occurred by 3 years of age, the child would remain small.

Learning difficulties. Because IUGR is often associated with poor brain development and subsequent failure to catch up, minimal cerebral dysfunction is not uncommon. Dysfunction is characterized by hyperactivity, short attention span, and poor fine motor coordination. Some hearing loss and speech defects also occur.

Drillien (1970) has shown that IUGR neonates born into families of high socioeconomic levels do as well as their peers at age 10–12 years while, at the same age, IUGR neonates from families of low socioeconomic levels function below their peers. This finding suggests that the environment of the IUGR neonate can play a vital role in long-term outcome.

Physiologic management. Hypoglycemia, the most common metabolic complication of IUGR, has been shown to produce such sequelae as CNS abnormalities and mental retardation. In addition to hypoglycemia, conditions such as asphyxia, hyperviscosity, and cold stress also may affect the neonate's outcome. Therefore, as with the preterm infant, meticulous attention to physiologic parameters is essential for immediate management and reduction of long-term disorders (see the Nursing Care Plan for SGA infants, p. 764).

The long-term needs of the IUGR neonate include scrupulous medical follow-up evaluation of patterns of growth and possible disabilities that may later interfere with learning or motor functioning. Long-term follow-up care is especially necessary for those infants with congenital malformations, congenital infections, and obvious sequelae from physiologic problems. In addition, the parents of the IUGR neonate need support. It has already been pointed out that a positive atmosphere can enhance the neonate's growth potential and the child's ultimate outcome.

INFANT OF DIABETIC MOTHER

Infants of diabetic mothers (IDMs) are considered at risk and require close observation the first few hours to the first few days of life. The typical IDM (type I, or White's classes B and C) is LGA (Figure 24–10). He or she is fat, macrosomic, plethoric, but not edematous, as IDMs have decreased total body water, particularly in the extracellular spaces. Their excessive weight is due to visceral organs, cardiomegaly, and increased body fat. The only organ not affected is the brain. IDMs are large in size but immature in physiologic functions, exhibiting many of the problems of the preterm infant. The cord and placenta are large. Mothers with severe diabetes or diabetes of long duration, associated with vascular complications, may give birth to infants who are SGA (type I or White's classes D–F).

The excessive fetal growth of the IDM is caused by exposure to high levels of maternal glucose, which readily crosses the placenta. The fetus responds to these high glucose levels with increased insulin production and hyperplasia of the pancreatic beta cells. The main action of the insulin is to facilitate the entry of glucose into muscle and fat cells in a function similar to a cellular growth hormone. Once in the cells, glucose is converted to glycogen and stored. Insulin also inhibits the breakdown of fat to free fatty acids, thereby maintaining lipid synthesis, increasing the uptake of amino acids and promoting protein synthesis. Insulin is an important regulator of fetal growth and metabolism.

After birth the most common problem of an IDM is hypoglycemia resulting from loss of the high maternal blood glucose supply and continued fetal hyperinsulinism, which depletes the blood glucose within hours after birth. IDMs also have less ability to release glucagon and catecholamines, which normally stimulate glucagon breakdown and glucose release. The incidence of hypoglycemia in IDMs varies from 2%–75%. The wide range in incidence is

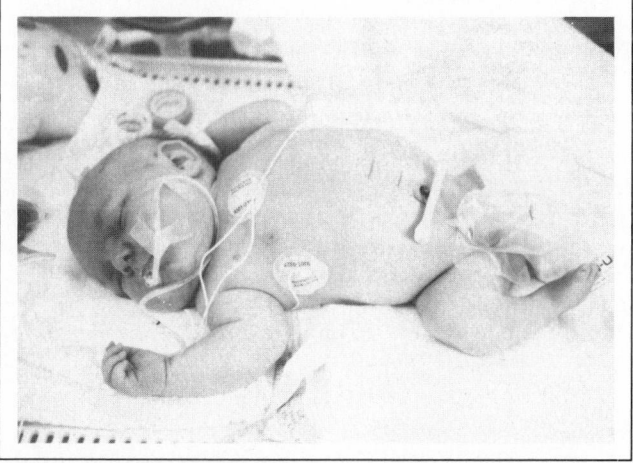

FIGURE 24–10 Macrosomic infant of diabetic mother. On x-ray, this infant was noted to have caudal regression of the spine.

(Text continues on p. 768.)

NURSING CARE PLAN
SGA Infants

PATIENT DATA BASE

History

1. Maternal history including general health, obstetric history, and events of labor and delivery; factors frequently associated with SGA infants include:

   a. Maternal malnutrition in the last trimester

   b. Vascular complications

   c. Maternal disease, including heart disease, drug addiction, alcoholism

   d. Smoking

   e. Low socioeconomic class

   f. Environmental factors, including high altitude, drugs, x-ray procedures

   g. Placental factors

   h. Congenital infections, including rubella, cytomegalic inclusion disease, toxoplasmosis, syphilis

2. Fetal-neonatal factors, including:

   a. Congenital malformations

   b. Discordant twin

3. Parents' understanding of SGA and its significance

Physical examination

1. Asymmetric term:

   a. Head appears relatively large (although it approaches normal) because chest and abdominal size are decreased

   b. Loose dry skin

   c. Scarcity of subcutaneous fat, with emaciated appearance

   d. Long, thin in appearance

   e. Sunken abdomen

   f. Sparse scalp hair (may be more plentiful in postterm infants)

   g. Anterior fontanelle may be depressed

   h. May have vigorous cry and appear deceptively alert (this is attributed to chronic marginal hypoxia in utero)

2. Symmetric term

   a. Sizes of all body parts are decreased but are in proportion, so head does not appear overly large or length excessive

   b. Generally vigorous (Korones, 1981)

3. Utilize clinical estimation of gestational age soon after birth and confirmatory neurologic examination to be done after 24 hours or soon after birth to determine gestational age

4. Physical examination findings related to gestational age include:

   a. Increased tendency to respiratory distress related to aspiration syndrome

   b. Temperature instability for increased problems of thermogenesis

   c. Neurologic manifestations indicating presence of cerebral edema that may occur, resulting in increased intracranial pressure, bulging fontanelles, or seizure activity

Laboratory evaluation

Dextrostix less than 45 mg/dL; blood glucose levels may be less than 20 mg/dL because of tendency toward hypoglycemia

Hematocrit may be greater than 65%, which is indicative of polycythemia

Calcium levels should be drawn periodically for the first 24–48 hours for evaluation of hypocalcemia (serum calcium below 7 mg/dL).

NURSING PRIORITIES

1. Maintain respirations.

2. Maintain homeostasis with neutral thermal environment and by meeting nutrition and fluid requirements.

3. Protect from infection.

4. Support psychologic well-being of parents and infant by facilitating positive parent–child bonding and sensory stimulation of infant.

5. Evaluate possible complications and initiate appropriate interventions.

FAMILY EDUCATIONAL FOCUS

1. Discuss the implications of having a SGA newborn with regard to caloric and fluid requirements, thermal instability, respiratory complications, and incidence of hypoglycemia.

2. Explain treatment modalities and their rationales.

3. Provide opportunities for parents to ask questions and discuss concerns regarding the long-term outcome for their infant.

NURSING CARE PLAN Cont'd
SGA Infants

Problem	Nursing interventions and actions	Rationale
Respiratory distress	Nursing interventions and actions are same as for preterm LGA and AGA infants (see p. 751). (See Chapter 25 for detailed nursing care and treatment on respiratory distress and infant resuscitation.)	Respiratory distress in SGA infants is not due to lung immaturity as is respiratory distress in preterm infants. Pulmonary conditions associated with SGA include: 1. Neonatal asphyxia. 2. Aspiration of meconium. 3. Aspiration pneumonia and pneumothorax.
Heat losses	Maintain skin temperature between 36–36.5C. Adjust and monitor incubator or radiant warmer to maintain skin temperature. Implement all other nursing care measures same as for temperature regulation in Nursing Care Plan for preterm LGA and AGA infants.	Neutral thermal environment charts utilized for preterm infant are not reliable for weight of SGA. Hypothermia is problem for SGA infant whose pathophysiology of thermal instability differs from that of preterm infant in the following manner: 1. Small in size, yet SGA can assume flexed position and thus decrease surface area available for heat loss. 2. Like preterm, SGA has decreased stores of brown fat available for thermogenesis, because SGA infant has utilized these stores in utero for survival. 3. Like preterm, SGA has poor insulation due to utilization of subcutaneous tissue in utero for survival. 4. SGA has mature CNS for temperature regulation. 5. SGA has ability to sweat and vasodilate in response to overheating, whereas this mechanism is unavailable to preterm infant. Other pathophysiology same as for temperature regulation in preterm infant.
Caloric and fluid intake necessary for growth	Nursing interventions and actions are same as for preterm LGA and AGA infants.	Rationale same as for preterm infant.
Fatigue during feedings	Nursing interventions and actions are same as for preterm LGA and AGA infants.	Rationale same as for preterm infant.
Susceptibility to infection	Nursing interventions and actions are same as for preterm LGA and AGA infants.	Rationale same as for preterm infant.
Prolonged separation of infant and mother	Nursing interventions and actions are same as for preterm LGA and AGA infants.	Rationale same as for preterm infant.
Possible complications Hypoglycemia	Nursing interventions and actions are same as for preterm infants	Hypoglycemia in SGA is indicated by whole blood sugar less than 20 mg/dL. Pathophysiology of hypoglycemia in SGA is due to a depletion of glycogen stores, especially hepatic glycogen stores.

NURSING CARE PLAN Cont'd
SGA Infants

Problem	Nursing interventions and actions	Rationale
		Combined with inhibited gluconeogenesis, this predisposes SGA infants to profound hypoglycemia within first 2 days of life.
Hypocalcemia	Nursing intervention and actions are the same as for the preterm neonate See further discussion of hypocalcemia in Chapter 25.	Incidence of hypocalcemia is not increased in the SGA neonate unless the newborn is preterm or has experienced birth asphyxia. Hypocalcemia is often accompanied by hyperphosphatemia (serum phosphate above 8 mg/dL) and hypomagnesemia (serum magnesium below 1.5 mg/dL).
Polycythemia	Nursing interventions and actions are same as for preterm LGA infants.	Polycythemia may occur in half of all SGA infants. Exact etiology of polycythemia in SGA is not known yet is thought to be a physiologic response to chronic hypoxia.
Congenital malformations	Complete and record results of physical examination on SGA infants for presence of congenital anomalies including: 1. Autosomal anomalies such as Down syndrome (trisomy 21), trisomy E (16–18), trisomy D (13–15). 2. Primordial short stature. 3. Inborn errors of metabolism such as Hurler syndrome, Niemann-Pick disease, Gaucher disease, maple syrup urine disease. Implement appropriate therapeutic actions.	Congenital malformations are statistically more common in SGA infants, because an anomaly of the fetus prevents normal growth (cell size and number), which results in small size of the neonate.
Congenital infections	Complete examination and identification of infected infants with clinical manifestations, including: 1. Rubella. 2. Cytomegalic inclusion disease. 3. Toxoplasmosis. 4. Syphilis. Monitor and report laboratory findings and radiographic surveys that aid in diagnosis. Institute protective measures to prevent spread of disease to other newborns, staff, or mothers. Isolate secretions and contaminated fomites. Enforce meticulous hand-washing.	Infants exposed to rubella, cytomegalic inclusion disease, toxoplasmosis, and syphilis are known to be small for their gestational age. Clinical manifestations of congenital infections include: 1. Rubella — cardiac anomalies; cataracts, retinopathy, cloudy cornea; gross anatomical abnormalities such as bone deformities and malformations, micrognathia, genitourinary anomalies, bony radiolucencies; central nervous system anomalies including encephalocele, microcephaly; hepatosplenomegaly, encephalitis; hearing loss; or "blueberry muffin" syndrome such as dermal erythropoiesis, and thrombocytopenia. 2. Cytomegalic inclusion disease —

NURSING CARE PLAN Cont'd
SGA Infants

Problem	Nursing interventions and actions	Rationale
		hepatosplenomegaly; jaundice with elevation of direct bilirubin level; thrombocytopenia with or without petechiae, or DIC (disseminated intravascular coagulopathy); microcephaly; or encephalitis.
		3. Toxoplasmosis — hepatosplen-omegaly; jaundice; meningoencephalitis with CSF changes (increased protein level); chorioretinitis; nervous system dysfunction including convulsions or calcifications.
		4. Syphilis — bone deformities; hepatosplenomegaly; jaundice with elevated direct serum bilirubin; hepatitis; or anemias.
		Precaution: No pregnant women should care for or collect specimens for infected infants because they could infect their fetus in utero.

NURSING CARE EVALUATION

Respirations are 30–50/min with no periods of apnea.	Infant shows no jerky generalized movement or other neurologic problems
Temperature is stable.	Infant responds to sensory stimulation.
Infant is gaining weight.	Parent–child bonding is completed.
Infant takes nipple feedings without developing fatigue.	Parents understand and can demonstrate knowledge of infant care, feeding, growth projections, prevention of exposure to infections, treatment of complications, and when to return for medical care.
Complications are controlled or absent.	
Infant is free from infection.	

NURSING DIAGNOSES*

	SUPPORTING DATA
1. Potential impaired gas exchange related to neonatal asphyxia, aspiration of meconium, aspiration pneumonia, or pneumothorax	Signs or symptoms of respiratory distress
2. Alteration in nutrition: potential for less than body requirements of neonate	Fatigue during feedings Immature suck, swallow, gag reflexes Hypoglycemia Residual formula in stomach Weight loss
3. Potential for injury related to impaired thermoregulation mechanisms	Lethargy Pallor Decreased temperature Hypoglycemia Increased serum bilirubin levels
4. Parental knowledge deficit concerning care of infant at home	Expressed concerns and questions about care of a SGA following discharge Unaware of available community resources

* These are a few examples of nursing diagnoses that may be appropriate for a SGA infant. It is not an inclusive list and must be individualized for each infant.

thought to be due to aspects of maternal care and success in controlling the diabetes, early versus late feedings of the infant, differences in maternal blood sugars at the time of delivery, length of labor, and the class of maternal diabetes.

In addition to hypoglycemia, other major problems may arise in the IDM during the first few hours and days of life. These include:

1. Hypocalcemia, with tremors the obvious clinical sign. This may be due to the IDM's increased incidence of prematurity and to the stresses of difficult pregnancy, labor, and delivery, which predispose any infant to hypocalcemia. Also, diabetic women tend to have higher calcium levels at term, causing possible secondary hypoparathyroidism in their infants (Tsang et al., 1975).

2. Hyperbilirubinemia, which may be seen at 48–72 hours after birth, possibly is due to slightly decreased extracellular fluid volume. This causes increased hematocrit level. Enclosed hemorrhages resulting from complicated vaginal delivery also may cause hyperbilirubinemia.

3. Birth trauma, as discussed in the section on LGA infants, p. 761.

4. Polycythemia, because of the decreased extracellular volume present in IDMs.

5. RDS, especially in newborns of classes A–C diabetic mothers. It is theorized that the high levels of fetal insulin interfere with the synthesis of the lecithin necessary for lung maturation (Frantz and Epstein, 1978). This does not appear to be a problem for infants born of diabetic mothers in classes D–F; instead the stresses of poor uterine blood supply may lead to increased production of steroids, resulting in acceleration of lung maturation.

6. Congenital birth defects, such as transposition of the great vessels, ventricular septal defect, and patent ductus (common); neurologic defects; small left colon syndrome; and caudal regression syndrome (rare).

Because the onset of hypoglycemia occurs at 2 hours of age (with a spontaneous rise to normal levels by 4–6 hours) blood glucose determinations should be done on cord blood and at 1, 2, 4, and 6 hours of age.

IDMs of classes C–F should be given 10%–15% glucose intravenously immediately after birth at the volume of fluids necessary for the hydration of the infant. The rate of 4–6 mg/kg/min usually maintains normoglycemia in the IDM (Avery, 1981). Once the blood glucose has been stable for 24 hours, the solution is then decreased in concentration with careful attention to the neonate's blood glucose level.

Twenty-five percent to fifty percent dextrose as a rapid infusion is contraindicated because it may lead to severe rebound hypoglycemia following an initial brief increase.

Glucagon has been administered to mobilize liver glycogen, but this treatment has limited use because glucagon also stimulates insulin release and causes rebound hypoglycemia.

Some hyperinsulinemic infants have been treated with 1:10,000 epinephrine given intramuscularly. Epinephrine inhibits the release of insulin from the pancreas and stimulates the release of glucose from liver and muscle cells and fatty acids from fat tissue.

Oral feedings should be begun as soon as the infant's condition permits. IDMs tend to be poor feeders, probably because of decrease in their glucose stores and their immaturity. Additional time and care in feeding may be required.

Nursing management is based on early attention to the prenatal history and assessment of maternal diabetes throughout pregnancy to identify the infant at risk. An IDM should be treated as a term or high-risk infant, and close observation in an intensive care nursery should be instituted immediately after birth. The Nursing Care Plan for AGA and LGA preterm infants has specific nursing interventions for IDMs with problems of polycythemia and birth trauma. Chapter 25 provides nursing interventions for respiratory distress syndrome, hypoglycemia and hypocalcemia.

INFANTS OF MOTHERS WITH CARDIAC OR HYPERTENSIVE CARDIOVASCULAR DISEASE

Infant of Mother with Cardiac Disease

With improvements in perinatal care, more women with cardiac disease are choosing to have children. The majority of cardiac lesions seen in pregnancy are a result of rheumatic heart disease. Women with congenital heart defects and cardiac valve prostheses are also becoming pregnant with higher frequency. See Chapter 12 for discussion of cardiac complications of pregnancy.

The antepartal presence of cardiac disease increases the risk of perinatal mortality, abortion, prematurity, stillbirth, fetal asphyxia, and IUGR. One of the most serious maternal complications is that of congestive heart failure, which diminishes maternal cardiac output and thus lowers the available circulating blood exchange through the placenta.

Of equal concern to neonatal outcome are the effects of various drugs used in maternal cardiac management. Digoxin and digitoxin both cross the placenta, although they have not been shown to adversely affect the fetus unless the drug reaches toxic levels in the pregnant woman. Thiazide diuretics also cross the placenta. Chronic thiazide administration during pregnancy causes electrolyte imbalance in the fetus resulting in marked hyponatremia and the presence of nitrogenous bodies, especially urea, in the blood at birth (Avery, 1981). Propranolol has been associated with IUGR, bradycardia, hypoglycemia, and respiratory depression in the neonatal period (Habib and McCarthy, 1977). The maternal cardiac drugs raising the most concern for fetal safety are the anticoagulants. Heparin has a relatively large molecular size and in therapeutic doses does not readily cross the placental barrier. It has little effect on the fetus, and for this reason is considered the drug of choice during pregnancy. Coumarin, although used frequently during pregnancy, can lead to neonatal hemorrhagic manifestations and death. The use of warfarin during pregnancy should be carefully evaluated, not only because of its risk of fetal hemorrhage but its potential teratogenic effects during the organogenic period. Lutz and colleagues (1978) report nineteen cases of "warfarin embryopathy." The characteristics of the syndrome include nasal hypoplasia, microcephaly, bony stippling, optic atrophy, mental retardation, spasticity, and hypotonia.

Whittemore and associates (1980) reported an increased incidence of cardiac abnormalities in the offspring of women with congenital heart defects. They suggest that careful genetic counseling be included in the long-term follow-up care of affected families.

The management and assessment of long-term needs and outcome of infants of mothers with cardiac disease should be based on evaluation of each infant for asphyxia, prematurity, and IUGR.

Infant of Mother with Hypertensive Cardiovascular Disease

Hypertensive cardiovascular disease in the pregnant woman is usually manifested in one of three ways: essential hypertension, PIH (preeclampsia and/or eclampsia), or PIH superimposed on essential hypertension or glomerulonephritis. In the presence of maternal hypertension coupled with degenerative changes that take place in the placenta secondary to the maternal disease, uteroplacental peripheral vascular resistance is increased. The long-term effects of uteroplacental vascular insufficiency causes fetal asphyxia (with meconium aspiration), prematurity, IUGR, increased incidence of abruptio placentae with stillbirths, and higher incidence of neonatal deaths.

The fetus of a woman with hypertensive cardiovascular disease is subject to the drugs used to control maternal hypertension. Reserpine has been known to produce respiratory depression in the infant at birth in addition to stuffy nose and lethargy. With prolonged maternal use, depletion of catecholamine stores has been shown to occur. The main concern with depletion of catecholamines is that they act as mediators in the cold response; thus it is possible that reserpine may block the neonate's adaptation to cold

(Avery, 1981). Diazoxide (Hyperstat) used in the treatment of severe preeclampsia readily crosses the placenta and may cause overabundant growth of lanugo or absence of hair on the neonate. Magnesium sulfate, which has been widely used to treat preeclampsia and eclampsia, has the same depressing effects on the fetus and neonate as it has on the mother. At birth the infant exhibits depressed respiratory effort and a weak cry, and is flaccid with poor deep tendon reflexes. Stone and Pritchard (1970) report that women receiving intramuscular administration of magnesium sulfate over a 24-hour period showed no deleterious effects on the fetus or newborn. Lipsitz (1971), however, using continuous intravenous infusion of magnesium sulfate for more than 24 hours, found that the neonate did manifest signs of hypermagnesemia at the time of birth.

If the mother has been maintained on intravenous magnesium sulfate for 24 hours or more preceding delivery, immediate care of the depressed newborn may require resuscitation and assisted ventilation until the respiratory depression and muscle weakness are overcome. Serum magnesium levels should be checked. If the neonate's level is higher than 5 mEq/L the infant will require this special care. Spontaneous respirations are seen within 6–48 hours.

The neonate should also be maintained on intravenous fluids to aid in excretion of the magnesium until one notes a good suck and gag reflex. After such time, oral feeding can be started. The most effective treatment of severely depressed hypermagnesemic infants is an exchange blood transfusion with citrated blood.

The neonate who has been compromised because of maternal disease processes and maternal drugs must receive special attention to prevent possible complications. Since placental insufficiency affects glycogen synthesis and storage and glucose supply, neonates are often born with low glucose levels; early depletion of cardiac glycogen has led to cardiac arrest. Antepartal administration of nitrites can cause methemoglobinemia, and thiazides have been associated with neonatal thrombocytopenia. The long-term needs and outcome for infants of mothers of hypertensive cardiovascular disease are similar to those for the growth-retarded infant. In addition, a majority of these neonates are born with respiratory and metabolic acidosis from prolonged hypoxia and from the effects of the labor process on the fetus. The neonate should be adequately ventilated with oxygen if needed, warmed, and given fluids and calories as the condition indicates.

ALCOHOL- OR DRUG-ADDICTED NEONATES

The newborn of an alcoholic or drug-addicted woman will also be alcohol- or drug-dependent. After birth, when an infant's connection with the maternal blood supply is severed, the neonate suffers withdrawal. In addition, the drugs ingested by the mother may be teratogenic, resulting in congenital anomalies.

Alcohol Dependency

The fetal alcohol syndrome (FAS) described by Jones and colleagues (1973) refers to a series of malformations frequently found in infants born to women who have been chronic severe alcoholics. It has been estimated that the complete FAS syndrome occurs in 1 or 2 live births per 1000 with a partial expression frequency at about 3–5 live births per 1000 (Cohlan, 1980).

The characteristics of FAS infants include the following: (a) persistent postnatal growth deficiency for length, weight, and brain; (b) facial abnormalities including short palpebral fissures, epicanthal folds, short upturned nose, maxillary hypoplasia, micrognathia, and thin upper lip; (c) cardiac defects such as primary septal defects; and (d) minor joint and limb abnormalities, including some restriction of movement and altered palmar crease patterns.

Controversy surrounds the exact cause of FAS. Although it is known that ethanol freely crosses the placenta to the fetus, it is still not known whether the alcohol alone or the break-down products of alcohol cause the damage. It is possible that alcohol itself may not harm the fetus but rather that the break-down product acetaldehyde, which is cytotoxic and teratogenic, is the culprit. Dunn and associates (1979) postulated that pregnant women with inherited or acquired defects of mitochondrial aldehyde dehydrogenase may have acetaldehyde levels well over the danger limit (35 mol/L) for their fetus, even after modest alcohol intake. This may explain why "social drinking" can sometimes cause adverse fetal effects, while heavy drinking may have no effect at all on the fetus. Other factors in conjunction with alcohol may contribute to the teratogenic effects. The factors include drugs (diazepam), nicotine, and caffeine, in addition to poor diet and low social-economic status (Iosub et al., 1981).

The withdrawal symptoms of the alcohol-dependent neonate are similar to those exhibited by the mother: abdominal distention, tremors, agitation, arching of the back, sweating, and seizures. The infant often has a poor sucking reflex. Signs and symptoms often appear within 6–12 hours and at least within the first 24 hours (Ostrea et al., 1978). Seizures after the neonatal period are rare. Alcohol dependence in the infant is physiologic, not psychologic. Care of the alcohol-addicted newborn ensures warmth, protection from injury during seizure, intravenous fluid therapy, reduction of environmental stimuli, and medication such as phenobarbital or diazepam to limit convulsions.

LONG-TERM OUTCOMES

The long-term prognosis for the FAS neonate is less than favorable. Most infants with FAS are growth-deficient at birth, and few infants have demonstrated postnatal catch-up growth. In fact, most FAS infants are evaluated for failure to thrive. It has been found that decreased adipose tissue is a constant feature of persons with FAS. Feeding problems are frequently present during infancy and preschool years. Many FAS infants nurse poorly and have persistent vomiting until 6–7 months. They have difficulty adjusting to solid foods and show little spontaneous interest in food (Streissguth et al., 1978).

CNS dysfunctions are the most common and serious problem associated with FAS. Most children exhibiting FAS are mildly to severely mentally retarded. The more dysmorphic the features, the lower the IQ scores. Iosub and associates (1981) found that providing a better environment for infants with FAS had no remarkable influence on IQ, which indicates that the brain damage occurred prenatally. FAS children are often hyperactive and show a high incidence of speech and language abnormalities indicative of CNS disorders. The brain is the organ most sensitive to damage from alcohol in the fetus.

The most effective treatment of FAS is early prenatal care for the pregnant woman with reduction in alcohol intake.

Drug Dependency

The infant born to a narcotic-addicted (usually heroin or methadone) woman is predisposed to a number of problems. Since almost all the narcotic drugs ingested by the woman cross the placenta and enter the fetal circulation, the fetus can develop problems in utero and/or soon after birth.

During the antenatal period, the greatest risk to the fetus is intrauterine asphyxia, with a higher incidence of stillbirths, meconium-stained amniotic fluid, fetal distress with lowered Apgar scores at birth, and aspiration pneumonia. The cause of the fetal asphyxia is often a direct result of fetal withdrawal, secondary to maternal withdrawal. Fetal withdrawal is accompanied by hyperactivity with increased oxygen consumption, which, if not adequately compensated, can lead to fetal asphyxia. Moreover, narcotic-addicted women tend to have a higher incidence of preeclampsia, abruptio placentae, and placenta previa, resulting in placental insufficiency and fetal asphyxia.

Intrauterine infection is another risk to the fetus. Because of the pregnant addict's life-style, she is often exposed to infection, particularly sexually transmitted disease and hepatitis, which can involve the fetus.

Postnatally, infants of narcotic-addicted women tend to have lower birth weights. The infant's birth weight may depend on the type of drug the mother uses. Women using predominantly heroin have infants of lower birth weight who are SGA, whereas women maintained on methadone have higher-birth-weight infants, some of whom are LGA (Ostrea et al., 1978).

These addicted infants often have low Apgar scores at

birth. Low scores may be related to the intrauterine asphyxia or the medication the woman received during labor. The use of a narcotic antagonist (nalorphine or naloxone) to reverse respiratory depression is contraindicated,
as they may precipitate acute withdrawal in the infant.

Problems of the neonate of a narcotic-addicted mother
include:

- Respiratory distress—mainly aspiration pneumonia and
transient tachypnea. Aspiration pneumonia is usually
secondary to meconium aspiration and intrauterine asphyxia. The transient tachypnea may be secondary to
the inhibitory effects of narcotics on the reflex clearing of
fluid by the lungs.
- Jaundice—due to the higher incidence of prematurity in
infants of drug-dependent mothers.
- Congenital malformations—slightly increased anomalies
of the genitourinary and cardiovascular systems.

The most significant postnatal problem of the drug-
addicted neonate is that of narcotic withdrawal. The onset
of the withdrawal manifestations usually occurs within the
first 72 hours after birth. A majority of withdrawal symptoms are seen within the first 24–48 hours. Reports of
withdrawal occurring after the first week may be secondary to other drugs besides narcotics. In most cases, the
withdrawal manifestations peak in the neonate about the
third day and subside by the fifth to seventh day.

Harper et al. (1977) and Zuspan (1978) have shown
that addicted women taking more than 20 mg of methadone daily had infants who appeared more ill than their
heroin-addicted counterparts. The number and severity of
the withdrawal symptoms are greater, and the duration is
prolonged.

The signs and symptoms of neonatal withdrawal can
be classified into five groups.

1. Central nervous system signs
   a. Hyperactivity
   b. Hyperirritability (persistent high-pitched cry)
   c. Increased muscle tone
   d. Exaggerated reflexes
   e. Tremors
   f. Sneezing, hiccups, yawning
   g. Short, nonquiet sleep
   h. Fever
2. Respiratory signs
   a. Tachypnea
   b. Excessive secretions
3. Gastrointestinal signs
   a. Disorganized, vigorous suck
   b. Vomiting
   c. Drooling
   d. Sensitive gag
   e. Hyperphagia
   f. Diarrhea
   g. Abdominal cramping

4. Vasomotor signs
   a. Stuffy nose
   b. Flushing
   c. Sweating
   d. Sudden, circumoral pallor
5. Cutaneous signs
   a. Excoriated buttocks
   b. Facial scratches
   c. Pressure point abrasions

Although many of the signs and symptoms of narcotic
withdrawal are similar to those seen with hypoglycemia
and hypocalcemia, Harper and coworkers (1977) report
glucose and calcium values to be within normal limits for
this group of infants.

Care of the newborn is based on reducing withdrawal
symptoms and promoting adequate respiration, temperature, and nutrition. Specific nursery care measures
include:

- Temperature regulation
- Careful monitoring of pulse and respirations every 15
minutes until stable; stimulation if apnea occurs
- Small frequent feedings, especially in the presence of
vomiting, regurgitation, and diarrhea
- Intravenous therapy as needed
- Medications as ordered, such as phenobarbital, parego-
ric, diazepam (Valium), or chlorpromazine hydrochloride
(Thorazine). Methadone should not be given because of
possible addiction to it
- Proper positioning on side to avoid possible aspiration of
vomitus or secretions
- Observation for problems of SGA infants
- Protection from injury
- Fostering positive mother–infant interaction to avoid potential negative feedback from infant because of abnor-
mal sleep and nutrition patterns, inability to cuddle, and
continuous crying

At the time of discharge, the mother should be instructed to anticipate mild jitteriness and irritability in the
infant, which may persist from 8–16 weeks, depending on
the initial severity of the withdrawal.

LONG-TERM OUTCOMES

The physical and mental development of infants of drug-
addicted mothers falls within normal limits up to 2 years of
age. Although these infants demonstrate higher incidence
of gastrointestinal and respiratory illnesses, it is believed
these are not related to narcotic addiction but rather to
improper infant care, feeding, and hygiene. More important is the high incidence (5.6%) of sudden infant death
syndrome or SIDS among these infants. The occurrence of
SIDS may be even higher in those infants who have had
moderate-to-severe postnatal withdrawal (Ostrea et al.,
1978).

For optimal fetal and neonatal outcome, the narcotic-addicted woman should receive complete prenatal care as soon as possible and be started on a methadone program with a reduction in dosage to 20 mg or less per day. It is not recommended that the woman be withdrawn completely from narcotics while pregnant, as this induces fetal withdrawal with poor neonatal outcomes.

PARENTING THE HIGH-RISK NEONATE

Attachment

The process by which maternal–infant attachment and bonding occurs has been the focus of intense study, because the work of earlier researchers clearly demonstrated the devastating effects of prolonged maternal–infant separation. Added impetus was provided as caregivers became increasingly aware that a disproportionately high number of battered or neglected children had been born prematurely and had required care in an intensive nursery for prolonged periods following birth. The question naturally arose as to whether interruptions in maternal contact and caregiving were significant factors in the disruption of the bonding process.

Historically, parents have been physically excluded from nurseries and isolated from care and contact with their infants. These practices are traceable to the high morbidity and mortality in hospitalized patients (circa 1900), which led to strict isolation procedures and visitor restrictions. The "incubator doctor," Dr. Martin Couney, also set an example of better newborn survival rates with parental exclusion, which served to reinforce total exclusion.

Only recently have behaviors been established as specific for development of maternal attachment, bonding, and effective mothering. Animal studies demonstrate species-specific behavior patterns in maternal behavior. Interruption of instinctive behaviors results in rejection of the offspring, inability to recognize one's offspring, and indiscriminate feeding of other young.

Studies of mother–infant interactions in human cultures have found that mother and infant remain together, usually for 3–7 days after birth, without separation. Only in the high-risk and preterm nurseries of the Western world are mothers and infants separated after birth.

The period immediately after birth has been described as the *maternal sensitive period*, during which the parents begin attachment to their infant. Research suggests that interference with this process during the early postpartal period (for example, separation because of necessary phototherapy or the need for incubator care for 24 hours or

so) can disturb the developing relationship between a mother and her newborn. It has become obvious that early maternal anxieties about the infant may have long-lasting effects (Klaus and Kennell, 1982). See Chapter 30 for a discussion of problems in attachment.

Adjustment

The events of premature labor and delivery abruptly terminate the normal adaptive processes to pregnancy. Taylor and Hall (1979) have devised a schematic representation interrelating the initiation-to-end course of the main psychologic processes that occur during pregnancy (Figure 24–11). Because pregnancy can be viewed as a developmental crisis, the pregnant woman spends much energy reworking unresolved conflicts she may have with her mother. In addition, as the pregnancy progresses to term, the mother-to-be begins voicing a desire to have the pregnancy end; these feelings usually coincide with a fetal gestation age that is maximal for extrauterine survival. It is believed that the mother's desire either to retain the preg-

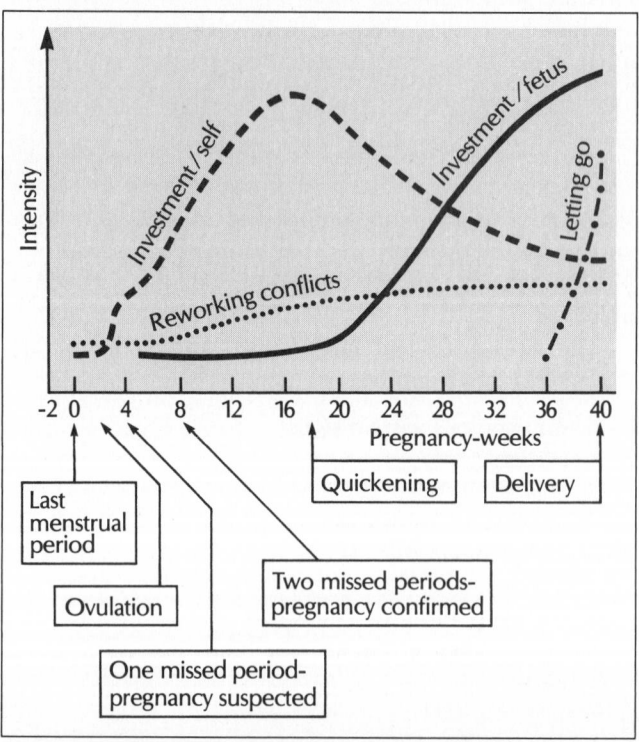

FIGURE 24–11 Relationship between basic psychologic processes and milestones of pregnancy. General agreement exists about the sequence and time courses of the processes of investment in self, investment in fetus, and letting go as represented here. The process of reworking unresolved conflicts with the woman's own mother is represented only tentatively. (From Taylor, P. M., and Hall, B. L. 1979. Parent–infant bonding: problems and opportunities in a perinatal center. *Sem. Perinatol.* 3:75.)

nancy or "let it go" might affect her attitude toward delivery and her infant. When an infant is delivered prior to term, the mother may not have had sufficient time to rework conflicts or be prepared to let the pregnancy go. As a result, the mother harbors not only feelings of anxious concern over the labor and delivery and survival of the infant, but also feelings of separation, helplessness, failure, and loss of control over the ability to produce the desired outcome.

Feelings of guilt and failure also plague the mother regarding the onset of premature labor and delivery of a preterm infant. They ask themselves "Why did labor start? What did I do (or not do)?" She may have guilt fantasies, and wonder "Was it because I had sexual intercourse with my husband (a week, three days, a day) ago?" "Was it because I carried three loads of wash up from the basement?" "Am I being punished for (something done in the past—even in childhood)?"

The birth of a defective neonate also engenders feelings of guilt and failure. As in the birth of a preterm infant, the woman may entertain ideas of personal guilt: "What did I do (or not do) to cause this?" "Am I being punished for something?"

Parental reactions and steps of attachment are altered by the birth of a preterm infant or one with a congenital anomaly. A variety of new feelings, reactions, and stresses must be recognized and dealt with before the family can work toward the establishment of a healthy parent–infant relationship.

Kaplan and Mason (1974) view maternal reactions to preterm births as an acute emotional disorder. They have identified four psychologic tasks as essential for coping with the stress and for providing a basis for the maternal–infant relationship:

1. Anticipatory grief as a psychologic preparation for possible loss of the child, while still hoping for its survival.

2. Acknowledgment of maternal failure to produce a term infant, expressed as anticipatory grief and depression and lasting until the chances of survival seem secure.

3. Resumption of the process of relating to the infant, which had been interrupted by the threat of nonsurvival. This task may be impaired by continuous threat of death or abnormality, and the mother may be slow in her response of hope for the infant's survival.

4. Understanding of the special needs and growth patterns of the preterm infant, which are temporary and yield to normal patterns.

Klaus and Kennell (1982), on the other hand, feel that with extra, sustained support and early contact with her infant a mother need not necessarily become involved in anticipatory preparation for her child's possible death.

Most authorities agree that the birth of a preterm infant or a less-than-perfect infant does require major adjust-

ments as the parents are forced to surrender the image they had nurtured for so long of their ideal child.

Solnit and Stark (1961) postulate that grief and mourning of the loss of the loved object—the idealized child—mark parental reactions to a defective child. The parents must grieve the loss of the valued object—their wish for the perfect child. Simultaneously, they must adopt the defective child as the new love object. Parental responses to a defective child may also be viewed as a staged process (Klaus and Kennell, 1982):

1. *Shock* at the reality of the birth of a defective child. This stage may be characterized by forgetfulness, amnesia of the situation, and a feeling of desperation.

2. Disbelief (*denial*) of the reality of the situation, characterized by a refusal to believe the child is defective. Assertions that "It didn't really happen!" "It isn't real!" "There has been a mistake; it's someone else's baby."

3. *Depression* over the reality of the situation comes after an acceptance of the situation and a corresponding grief reaction to its reality. This stage is characterized by much crying and sadness. Anger about the reality of the situation may also occur at this stage. A projection of blame on others or on self and feelings of "not me" are characteristic of this stage.

4. Equilibrium and *acceptance* are characteristic of a decrease in the emotional reactions of the parents. This stage is variable and may be prolonged because of a prolongation of the threat to the infant's survival. Some parents experience chronic sorrow in relation to their defective child.

5. *Reorganization* of the family to deal with the child's problems. Mutual support of the parents facilitates this process, but the crisis of the situation may precipitate alienation between the parental partners.

These stages of parental adjustment are similar to the stages of dying and of grieving. Indeed, reorganization in the face of a crisis concerning a defective child is necessary for dealing with the crisis.

In the birth of either a defective child or a preterm infant, the process of mourning is necessary for attachment to the "less-than-perfect child." *Grief work*, the emotional reaction to a significant loss, is necessary before adequate attachment to the actual child is possible. Parental detachment precedes parental attachment.

Seeing and touching the newborn appear to be species-specific behaviors for human maternal attachment. Immediate performance of these behaviors may be impossible if the infant is preterm or has a congenital anomaly. Such immediate care as resuscitation, intubation, correction of shock, and separation from the mother to an intensive care area may preclude these behaviors. With the increased attention to improved fetal outcome, maternal transports, rather than neonatal transports, are occurring more frequently. This practice gives the mother of a high-risk infant the opportunity to visit and care for her infant during the early postpartal period.

It is essential that as soon as possible after birth the mother be reunited with her infant so that:

1. She knows that her infant is alive.

2. She knows what the infant's real problems are. Fantasies of the infant's problems may be more devastating than the reality of the problem. Early acquaintance between mother and infant allows a realistic perspective of the neonate's condition.

3. She can begin the grief work over the loss of the idealized child and begin the process of the attachment of the actual child.

4. She can share the experience of the infant's problems with the father, who may have already seen and touched the infant.

The nurse should guard against indiscriminate admission of normal newborns to the intensive care unit because of prior high-risk conditions, such as cesarean birth, fetal bradycardia, or short periods of rapid breathing after birth. It has been found that while these unjustified short-term admissions to special care nurseries cause no long-term maternal–infant attachment problems, they do cause unnecessary anxiety and unhappiness for the parents.

Nursing Interventions

Before parents see their child, the nurse must prepare them to view their preterm or high-risk newborn. It is important that a positive, realistic attitude rather than a pessimistic one regarding the infant be presented to the parents. An overly negative, fatalistic attitude further alienates the parents from their infant and retards attachment behaviors. Instead of allowing attachment and bonding to develop, the mother will begin the process of anticipatory grieving, and once started, this process is difficult to reverse.

In preparing parents for the first view of their infant, it is important for a professional to look at the child, The parents should be prepared to see both the congenital anomaly and the normal aspects of their infant. All infants exhibit strengths as well as deficiencies. The nurse may say, "Your baby is small, about the length of my two hands. She weighs 2 lb, 3 oz but is very active and cries when we disturb her. She is having some difficulty breathing but is breathing without assistance and in only 35% oxygen."

INTENSIVE CARE

The equipment being used for the high-risk neonate and its purpose should be described before the parents enter the intensive care unit. Many intensive care units have booklets for parents to read before entering the unit. Through explanations and pictures, the parents can be better prepared to deal with the feelings they may experience when they see their infant for the first time. Upon entering the unit, parents may be overwhelmed by the sounds of monitors, alarms, and respirators as well as by the unfamiliar language and "foreign" atmosphere. It is more reassuring when parents are prepared and accompanied to the unit by the same person(s). The primary physician and primary nurse caring for the newborn should be with the parents when they first visit their child, taking time to describe the infant's abnormality and to point out the normal characteristics of the infant. Parental reactions are varied, but there is usually an element of initial shock. Provision of chairs and time to regain composure will assist the parents. Slow, complete, and simple explanations—first about the infant and then about the equipment—allay fear and anxiety.

As parents attempt to deal with the initial stages of shock and grief at the birth of a premature or less-than-perfect child, they may fail to assimilate new information. They may require constant repetition by the nurse to accept the reality of the situation, procedures, equipment, and the infant's condition on subsequent visits.

Misconceptions about equipment and its placement on the infant and about its potential harm are common. Such statements as "Does the fluid go into the brain?" "Does the white wire on the abdomen go into the stomach?" and "Does the monitor make the baby's heart beat?" imply much fear for the infant's safety and misconception about the machines. These worries are easily overcome by simple explanations of all equipment being used.

Concern about the infant's physical appearance is common, yet may remain unvoiced. Parents may express such concerns as "He looks so small and red—like a drowned rat." "Why do her genitals look so abnormal?" "Will that awful looking mouth [cleft lip and palate] ever be normal?" Such questions need to be anticipated by the nurse and addressed. Utilization of pictures, such as of an infant after cleft lip repair, may be reassuring to doubting parents. Knowledge of the development of a "normal" preterm infant will allow the nurse to make reassuring statements, such as, "The baby's labia may look very abnormal to you, but they are normal for her maturity. As she grows, the outer lips of the vagina will become larger and the clitoris will be covered and the genitals will then look as you expect them to. She is normal for her level of maturity."

The tone of the neonatal intensive care unit is set by the nursing staff. Development of a safe, trusting environment depends on viewing the parents as essential caregivers and not as "visitors" or "nuisances" in the unit. Pleasant, relaxed physical surroundings convey the sense of hospitality and encourage parents to "be at home here." Provision of chairs, privacy when needed, and easy access to staff and facilities are all important in developing an open, comfortable environment. An uncrowded and welcoming atmosphere lets parents know "You are welcome here." However, even in crowded physical surroundings, an attitude of openness and trust can be conveyed by the nursing staff.

A trusting relationship for collaborative efforts in caring for the infant is essential. Nurses must therapeutically use their own responses to relate on a one-to-one basis with the parents. Each individual has different needs, different ways of adaptation to crisis, and different means of support. It is essential that professionals utilize techniques that are real and spontaneous to them and avoid adopting words or actions that are "foreign" to their own spontaneity. Nurses must also gauge their interventions to match the parents' pace and needs.

Smaller hospitals may be unable to care for sick infants. Transport to a regional referral center may be necessary. These centers may be as far as 500 miles from the parents' community; it is therefore essential that the mother see and touch her infant before he or she is transported. Facilitation of this important contact may be the responsibility of the referring hospital staff as well as the transport team. Bringing the mother to the nursery or taking the infant in a warmed transport incubator to the mother's bedside will allow her to see the infant before transportation to the center.

Once the infant has reached the referral center parents also appreciate a telephone call relaying the infant's condition during the transport, safe arrival at the center, and present condition. A member of the transport team is often the best person to make the call, as the team has already begun a trusting relationship with the parents and are most knowledgeable about the infant.

Support of parents, with explanations from the professional staff, is crucial. Occasionally the mother may be unable to see the infant before transport, for example, if she is still under general anesthesia or experiencing complications such as shock, hemorrhage, or seizures. In these cases, before the infant is transported a photograph of the infant should be given to the mother, along with an explanation of the infant's condition, problems, and a detailed description of the infant's characteristics to facilitate the attachment process until the mother can visit. An additional photograph is also helpful for the father to share with siblings and/or the extended family.

TOUCHING AND CARETAKING

Mothers visiting a small or sick infant may need several visits to become comfortable and confident in their abilities to touch the infant without injuring him or her. Barriers such as incubators, incisions, monitor electrodes, and tubes may delay the mother's confidence. Knowledge of this "normal" delay in touching behavior will enable the nurse to understand parental behavior.

Klaus and Kennell (1982) have demonstrated a signifi-

cant difference in the amount of eye contact and touching behavior of mothers of preterm infants. Whereas mothers of normal newborns progress within minutes to palm contact of the infant's trunk, the mother of a preterm infant is slower in her progression from fingertip to palm contact and from touching the extremities to the infant's trunk. The progression to palm contact with the infant's trunk bay take several visits, as illustrated in Figure 24–12.

Through support, reassurance, and encouragement, the nurse can facilitate the mother's positive feelings about her ability and her importance to her infant. Utilization of touching facilitates "getting to know" her infant and thus establishing a bond with the infant. Touching, as well as seeing the infant, helps the mother to realize the "normals" and potentials of her infant.

Caretaking may be delayed for the mother of a preterm, defective, or sick infant. The variety of equipment needed for life support is hardly conducive to anxiety-free caretaking by the parents. However, even the sickest infant may be cared for, if even in a small way, by the parents. As a facilitator of parental caretaking, it is the responsibility of the nurse to promote the parents' success. Demonstration and explanation, followed by support of the parents in initial caretaking behaviors, positively reinforce this behavior. Asking the parents to change the infant's diaper, give their infant skin care or oral care, or help the nurse turn the infant may at first be anxiety-provoking. The parents increasingly become more comfortable and confident in caretaking and receive satisfaction from the child's reactions and their ability "to do something." Complimenting the parents' competence in caretaking also serves to increase their self-esteem, which has received recent "blows" of guilt and failure. It is vitally important that the mother never be given a task if there is any possibility that she will not be able to accomplish it.

NURSE–PARENT INTERACTIONS

Often mothers have ambivalent feelings toward the nurse, in the face of their own inability to provide the sophisticated care needed by the infant. As the mother watches the nurse competently perform the caretaking tasks, she feels both grateful to the nurse for the ability and expertise and jealous of the nurse's ability to care for her infant. These feelings may be acted out in criticism of the care being received by her infant, in manipulation of staff, or in personal guilt about such feelings. Instead of fostering (by silence) these inferiority feelings within mothers, nurses are in a special position to recognize these feelings and to intervene appropriately to facilitate mother–infant bonding.

Nurses who are understanding and secure will be able to support the parents' egos instead of collecting rewards for themselves. To positively reinforce parenting behaviors, professionals must first believe in the importance of the parents. The nurse could hardly convince a doubting

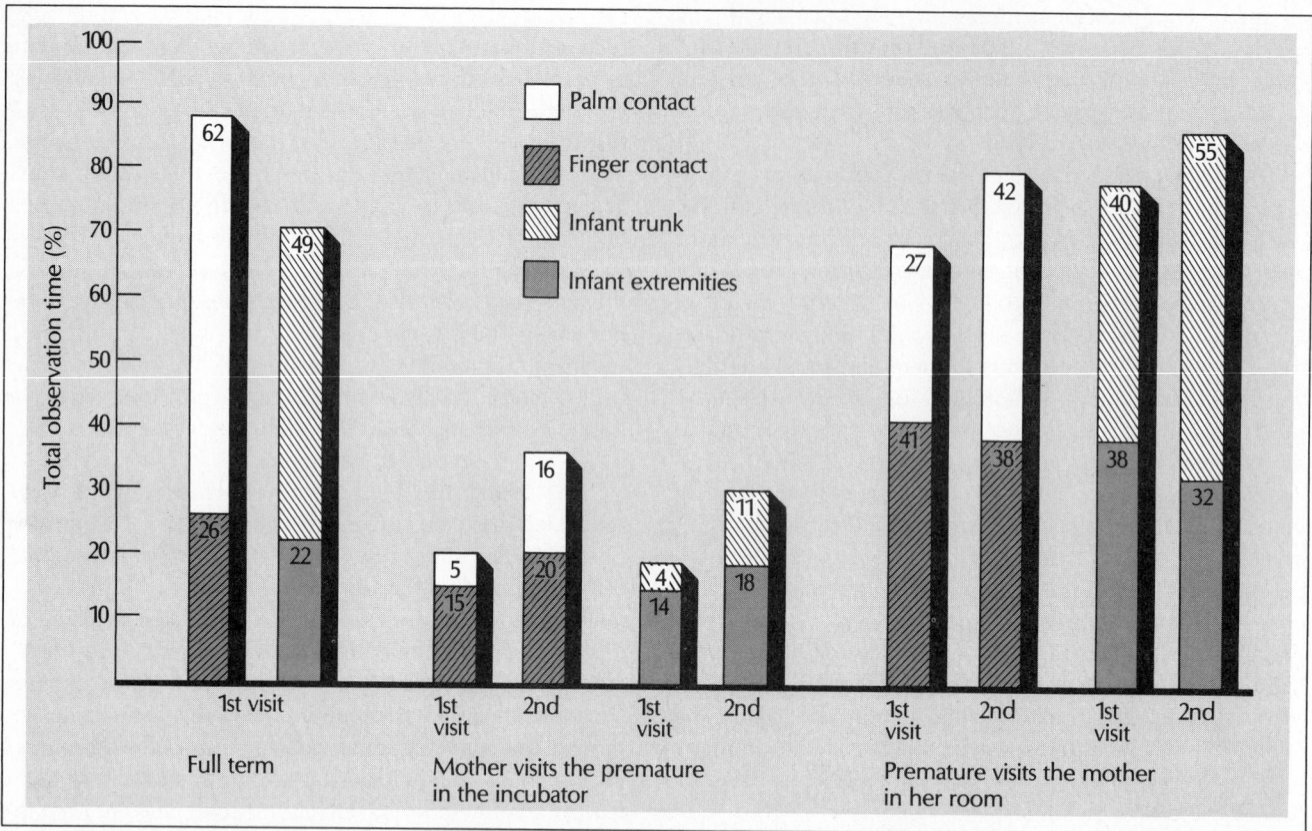

FIGURE 24–12 Fingertip and palm contact on the trunk or extremities of a newborn in three groups of mothers: (1) twelve mothers of full-term infants at their first visit; (2) nine mothers who visited their preterm infants in incubators in the intensive care unit; and (3) fourteen mothers whose preterm infants were brought to their maternity rooms and placed in their beds. (From Klaus, M. H., and Kennell, J. H. 1982. *Parent–infant bonding,* 2nd ed. St. Louis: The C. V. Mosby Co.)

parent of his or her importance to the infant unless the nurse really believes it. The attitude of the professionals communicates acceptance or rejection to the parents, regardless of what is said. During this crisis period, it is essential that attitudes *and* words say: "You are a good mother/father. You are a good person. You have an important contribution to make to the care of your infant." Unless equal care is taken in facilitating parental attachment as in providing physiologic care, the outcome will not be a healthy family.

Verbalizations by the nurse that improve parental self-esteem are essential and easily shared. Breast-feeding is possible and in many centers this is recommended for preterm or sick infants for nutrition as well as for defense against the development of necrotizing enterocolitis. In addition to physiologic use, breast milk is important because of the emotional investment of the mother. Pumping, storing, labeling, and delivering quantities of breast milk is time-consuming and a "labor of love" for mothers. Positive remarks regarding breast milk reinforce the maternal

behavior of caretaking and providing for her infant: "Breast milk is something that only you can give your baby" or "You really have brought a lot of milk today" or "Look how rich this breast milk is" or "Even small amounts of milk are important, and look how rich it is."

If the infant begins to gain weight while being fed breast milk, it is important to point this out to the mother. Parents should also be advised that initial weight loss with beginning nipple feedings is common because of the increased energy expended when the infant begins active rather than passive nutritional intake.

Within the past 20 years, increased attention has been given to the infant's need for sensory stimulation. Evidence suggests that the infant who receives tactile, kinesthetic, and auditory stimulation has fewer apneic spells, decreased stooling, improved weight gain, and advanced CNS functioning (Klaus and Kennell, 1982). Parents are ideally equipped to meet the need for stimulation. Stroking, rocking, cuddling, singing, and talking should be an integral part of the neonate's care. Visual stimulation in the form of mobiles and *en face* interaction with the caretaker are also important. Of special significance is that the parents must move at their infant's pace; overstimulation causes decreased neonatal responsibilities (Field, 1977). The nurse should work with the family to provide appropriate stimulation without sensory bombardment.

Provision of care by the parents is appropriate even for very sick or defective infants. It has been found that detachment is easier after attachment, because the parents are comforted by the knowledge that they did all they could have for their child while he or she was alive.

During crisis, maintenance of interpersonal relationships is difficult. Yet in a newborn intensive care area, the parents are expected to relate to many and varied care providers. It is important that parents have as few professionals as possible relaying information to them. A primary

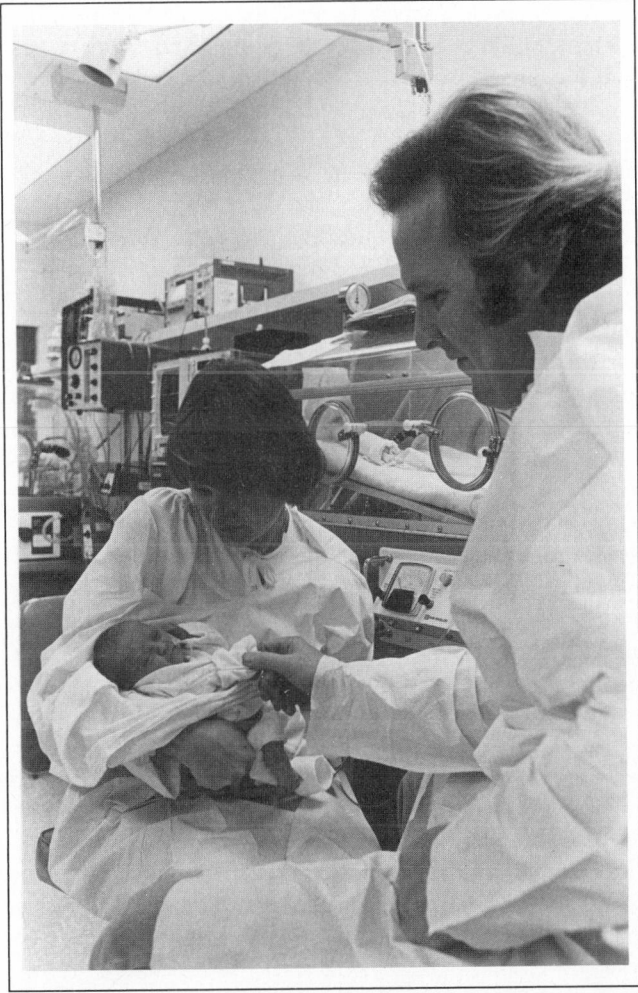

FIGURE 24–13 It is important that the parents of high-risk infants be given the opportunity to get acquainted with their children. Physical contact is extremely important in the bonding process and should be encouraged whenever possible.

nurse should coordinate and provide continuity in information-giving to parents. Care providers are individuals and thus will use different terms, inflections, and attitudes. These subtle differences are monumental to parents and only serve to confuse, confound, and produce anxiety. Several trusted relationships with professionals minimize unnecessary anxiety and concern and facilitate open communication. The nurse not only functions as a liaison between the parents and the wide variety of professionals interacting with the infant and parents; the nurse also offers clarification, explanation, interpretation of information, and support to the parents.

Bonding can be facilitated by encouraging parents to visit and become involved in their child's care (Figure 24–13). When visiting is impossible, the parents should feel free to phone whenever they wish to receive information about their child. A warm, receptive attitude is very supportive. Nursing can also facilitate parenting by personalizing a child to the parents, by referring to the infant by name or by relating personal behavioral characteristics to the parents. Remarks such as "Jenny loves her pacifier" help make the infant more individual and unique.

Development of a professional–family relationship enables information gathering in areas of concern. A concurrent illness of the mother or other family members or other concurrent stress (lack of hospitalization insurance, loss of job, age of parents) may alter the family response to the neonate. Feelings of apprehension, guilt, failure, and grief that are verbally or nonverbally expressed are important aspects of the nursing history. These observations enable all professionals to be aware of the parental state, coping behaviors, and readiness for attachment, bonding, and caretaking. Appropriate nursing observations during interviewing and relating to the family include:

1. *Level of understanding.* Observations concerning the ability to assimilate information given and to ask appropriate questions; the need for constant repetition of "the same" information.

2. *Behavioral responses.* Appropriateness of behavior in relation to information given; lack of response; "flat" affect.

3. *Difficulties with communication.* Deafness (reads lips only); blindness; dysphagia; understanding only of foreign language.

4. *Paternal and maternal education level.* Parents unable to read or write; only eighth grade completed; mother an MD or PhD; and so on.

Documentation of such information, obtained by the nurse through continuing contact and development of a therapeutic family relationship, enables all professionals to understand and utilize the nursing history in providing continuous individual care.

THE ROLE OF THE FAMILY

Development of a relationship with the family is important because parenthood or the illness of a member affects the entire family. The parents should be encouraged to deal with the crisis while utilizing their support system. The extended family attempts to meet the emotional needs and provide support for family members in crisis and stress situations. In our mobile society of isolated, nuclear families, the extended family may be the next-door neighbor, the mother's best friend, or perhaps a school chum. Biologic kin is not the only valid criterion for a support system; an emotional kinship is the most important factor. The nurse must search out the significant others in the lives of the parents and assist them in understanding so that they are able to be a constant parental support.

The impact of the crisis on the family is individual and varied. In constructing a conceptual framework for family crisis, Hill (1974) has formulated an equation to show the relationship of all elements:

A (the event) ——————> interacting with B (the family's crisis-meeting resources) —————> interacting with C (the definitions the family makes of the events) —————> produces X (the crisis).

The stressful event (A), a situation for which the family has little or no preparation, may be classified according to the source of trouble: *extra-family events*, which may solidify the family, and *intra-family events*, which may reflect negatively on the adequacy of the family.

Marked changes in the configuration, such as accession of a new member (normal or preterm infant, infant with congenital anomaly) may also be a stressful occasion for the family members. The ability of the family to adapt to changing situations is the basis of the crisis-meeting resource (B). This adaptability to events depends on the definition (C) ascribed to each event by the family. Thus, an interplay of an event, the crisis-meeting resources, and the family definition of the event produces the crisis situation.

Through the nurse–family relationship, information about the ability of the family to adapt to the situation is obtained. The event itself (normal newborn, preterm infant, infant with congenital anomaly) can then be viewed as it is defined by the family, and appropriate intervention can be instituted.

Because the family is a unit composed of individuals who must deal with the situation, it is important to encourage open interfamily communication. Secret-keeping should not be encouraged, especially between spouses, because secrets undermine the trust of their relationship. Well-meaning rationales such as "I want to protect her," "I don't want her to know," and so on can be destructive to open communication and to the basic element of a relationship—trust.

The nurse should be particularly sensitive to open communication when the mother is in an institution separate from the infant. The father is the first to visit the infant and relays information regarding the infant's care and condition to the mother. In this situation, the mother has had minimal contact, if any, with her infant. Because of her anxiety and isolation, she may mistrust all those who provide information (the father, nurse, physician, or extended family) until she can see for herself. This alone can put tremendous stress on the relationship between the spouses. The parents (and family) should be given information together. This practice helps overcome misunderstandings and misinterpretations and helps to promote "working through" together.

The entire family—siblings as well as relatives—should be encouraged to visit and receive information about the baby. Methods of intervention and assisting the family in coping with the situation include providing support, confronting the crisis, and understanding the reality. Support, explanations, and the helping role must extend to the kin network, as well as to the nuclear family, in an attempt to aid them in communication and support ties with the nuclear family.

It is also essential to meet the needs of the individuals involved. Desires and needs of the individuals must be respected and facilitated; differences are tolerable and able to exist side-by-side. Eliciting the parents' feelings is easily accomplished with the question: "How are you doing?" The emphasis is on *you*, and the interest must be sincere.

Families with children in the newborn intensive care unit become friends and support one another. To encourage the development of these friendships and to provide support, many units have established parent groups. The core of the groups consists of parents who previously have had an infant in the intensive care unit. Most groups make contact with families within a day or two of the infant's admission to the unit, either through phone calls or visits to the hospital. Garrand (1978) recently observed that early one-on-one parent contact is more beneficial in assisting families in working through their feelings than discussion groups. This personalized method gives the grieving parents an opportunity to express personal feelings about the pregnancy, labor, and delivery and their "different than expected" infant with others who have experienced the same feeling and with whom they can identify (Elsas, 1981).

Visiting and caregiving patterns give an indication of the level of (or lack of) parental attachment. A record of visits, caretaking procedures, affect (in relating to the newborn), and telephone calls is essential. Serial observations must be obtained, rather than just an isolated instance of concern. Grant (1978) has developed a conceptual framework depicting adaptive and maladaptive responses to parenting of a preterm or less-than-perfect infant (Figure 24–14).

If a pattern of distancing behaviors evolves, appropriate intervention should be instituted. Follow-up studies have found that a statistically significant number of pre-

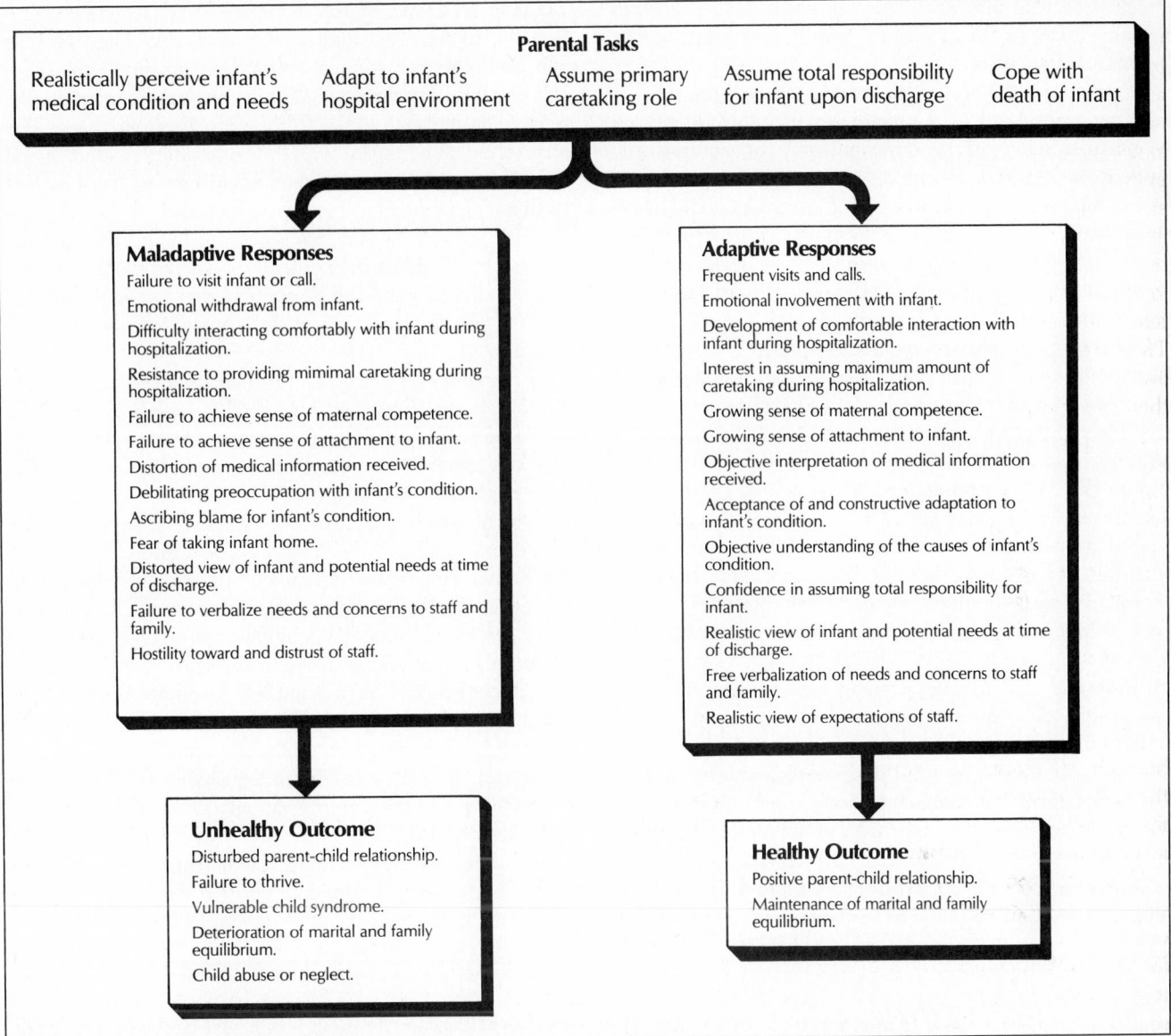

Parental Tasks

| Realistically perceive infant's medical condition and needs | Adapt to infant's hospital environment | Assume primary caretaking role | Assume total responsibility for infant upon discharge | Cope with death of infant |

Maladaptive Responses

Failure to visit infant or call.

Emotional withdrawal from infant.

Difficulty interacting comfortably with infant during hospitalization.

Resistance to providing mimimal caretaking during hospitalization.

Failure to achieve sense of maternal competence.

Failure to achieve sense of attachment to infant.

Distortion of medical information received.

Debilitating preoccupation with infant's condition.

Ascribing blame for infant's condition.

Fear of taking infant home.

Distorted view of infant and potential needs at time of discharge.

Failure to verbalize needs and concerns to staff and family.

Hostility toward and distrust of staff.

Adaptive Responses

Frequent visits and calls.

Emotional involvement with infant.

Development of comfortable interaction with infant during hospitalization.

Interest in assuming maximum amount of caretaking during hospitalization.

Growing sense of maternal competence.

Growing sense of attachment to infant.

Objective interpretation of medical information received.

Acceptance of and constructive adaptation to infant's condition.

Objective understanding of the causes of infant's condition.

Confidence in assuming total responsibility for infant.

Realistic view of infant and potential needs at time of discharge.

Free verbalization of needs and concerns to staff and family.

Realistic view of expectations of staff.

Unhealthy Outcome

Disturbed parent-child relationship.

Failure to thrive.

Vulnerable child syndrome.

Deterioration of marital and family equilibrium.

Child abuse or neglect.

Healthy Outcome

Positive parent-child relationship.

Maintenance of marital and family equilibrium.

FIGURE 24–14 Maladaptive and adaptive parental responses during crisis period, showing unhealthy and healthy outcomes. (Reprinted from Psychosocial needs of families of high-risk infants, by Grant, P. In *Fam. Comm. Health* 11:93, by permission of Aspen Systems Corporation, © 1978.)

term, sick, and congenitally defective infants suffer from failure to thrive, battering, or other disorders of mothering. Early detection and intervention will prevent these aberrations in mothering behaviors from leading to irreparable damage or death.

Predischarge Care

Predischarge planning begins once the infant's condition becomes stable and indications suggest the newborn will survive. Through adequate predischarge teaching, the parents are able to transform their feelings of inadequacy and competition with the nurse into feelings of self-assurance

and attachment. From the beginning the parents should be included in the infant's care and taught about their infant's special needs and growth patterns. This teaching and involvement is best facilitated by a nurse who is familiar with the infant and his or her family over a period of time and who has developed a comfortable and supportive relationship with them.

The nurse's responsibility is to provide instructions in an environment optimal for parental learning. Learning should take place over time, to prevent the bombardment of instructions on the day or hour before discharge.

The basic elements of predischarge care are described in the following paragraphs.

Routine well-baby care, such as bathing, temperature taking, formula preparation, and breast-feeding are learned by the parents.

Parents are trained in the special procedures specific for their newborn. These procedures may include gavage or gastrostomy feedings, tracheostomy or enterostomy care, or medications. Before discharge, the parents should be as comfortable as possible with these tasks and demonstrate independence. Written tools and instructions are useful for parents to refer to once they are home with the infant, but these should not replace actual participation in the infant's care.

Teaching and learning methods are used in assessment of parental readiness to learn. Parents often enjoy doing minimal caretaking tasks with gradual expansion of their role. Many intensive care units provide facilities for parents to room-in with their infants for a few days before discharge. This allows parents a degree of independence in the care of their infant with the security of nursing help nearby. This practice is particularly helpful for anxious parents, parents who have not had the opportunity to spend extended time with their infant, or parents who will be giving a high level of physical care at home, such as tracheostomy care.

Referrals to community health services are done before discharge. The visiting nurses' association, public health nurses, or social services can assist the parents in the traumatic transition from hospital to home by providing the necessary home teaching and support. Some intensive care nurseries have their own parent support groups to help bridge the gap between hospital and home care. Parents can also find support from a variety of community support organizations, such as Mother of Twins Groups, or Trisomy 13 Clubs, March of Dimes Birth Defects Foundation, Handicapped Children Services, and Teen Mother and Child Programs. Each community has numerous agencies capable of assisting the family in adapting emotionally, physically, and financially to the chronically ill infant. The nurse should be familiar with the community resources and help the parents identify which agencies may be of benefit to them.

The nurse helps parents recognize the growth and development needs of their infant. A development program begun in the hospital can be continued at home, or parents may be referred to an infant development program in the community.

Arrangements are made for medical follow-up care before discharge. The infant may need to be followed-up by a family pediatrician, a well-baby clinic, or a specialty clinic. The first appointment should be made before the infant is discharged from the hospital.

The nurse evaluates the need for special equipment for infant care (such as a respirator, oxygen, apnea monitor) in the home. Any extra equipment or supplies should be placed in the home before the infant's discharge. The nurse can be instrumental in helping the parents assess the newborn's needs and coordinate services.

Support cannot be given unless it can be received. Living in an emotional environment of "lots of living and lots of dying" takes its toll on staff. The emotional needs and feelings of the staff must be recognized and dealt with in order to support the parents. An environment of openness to feelings and dealing with their own human needs and emotions is essential for staff. Such techniques as group meetings, individual support, and primary care nursing may assist in maintaining staff mental health.

SUMMARY

Early identification of potential high-risk infants through assessment of prepregnant, prenatal, and intrapartal factors facilitates strategically timed nursing observations and interventions. High-risk infants, whether they are prematurely born, small or large for gestational age, postterm, or born of diabetic or substance-addicted mothers, or mothers with cardiovascular problems, have many similar problems—although their problems are based on different physiologic processes. With early recognition and intervention, the potential long-term physiologic and emotional consequences of these difficulties can be avoided or at least lessened in severity.

Resource Groups

Local visiting nurses associations, public health nurses and hospital social service departments can provide necessary home care teaching and support.

Mothers of Twins or Trisomy 13 Clubs, March of Dimes Birth Defects Foundation, Handicapped Children Services, Teen Mother and Child programs and parents' support groups assist families in adapting emotionally, physically and financially to the birth of a chronically ill infant.

References

Affonso, D. D., and Harris, T. R. 1980. Postterm pregnancy: implications for mother and infant, challenge for the nurse. *J. Obstet. Gynecol. Neonat. Nurs.* 9:139.

Avery, G. B., ed. 1981. *Neonatology.* Philadelphia: J. B. Lippincott Co.

Benda, G. I. 1979. Modes of feeding low-birth-weight infants. *Sem. Perinatol.* 3:407

Boyce A.; Mayaux, M. J.; Schwartz, D. 1976. Classical and "true" gestational postmaturity. *Am. J. Obstet. Gynecol.* 125:911.

Brady, M. S., et al. 1979. Nutritional care of the low-birthweight infant requiring intensive care. *Perinatal Press.* p. 125.

Bree, R. L., and Mariona, F. G. 1980. The role of ultrasound in the evaluation of normal and abnormal fetal growth. In *Seminars in ultrasound*, ed. H. W. Raymond, and W. J. Zwiebel. New York: Grune & Stratton.

Bucci, G., et al. 1972. The systemic systolic blood pressure of newborns with low weight. *Acta Paediatr. Scand.* (Suppl) 229:1.

Canadian Pediatric Society. Nutrition Committee. 1981. Feeding the low-birthweight infant. *CMA Journal.* 124:1301.

Clifford, S. 1957. Postmaturity. *Advances Pediatr.* 9:13.

Cloherty, J. P., and Stark, A. R., eds. 1980. *Manual of neonatal care.* Boston: Little, Brown & Co.

Collinge, J. M., et al. Nov./Dec. 1982. Demand vs scheduled feedings for premature infants. *J. Obstet. Gynecol. Neonat. Nurs.* 11:362.

Cohlan, S. O. 1980. Drugs and pregnancy. In *Progress in clinical and biological research*, ed. B. K. Young. New York: Alan R. Less, Inc.

Drillien, C. M. Feb. 1970. The small-for-dates infant: etiology and prognosis. *Pediatr. Clin. North Am.* 17(1):9.

Dunn, P. M., et al. July 1979. Metronidazole and the fetal alcohol syndrome. *Lancet.* 2:144.

Elsas, T. L. May/June 1981. Family mental health care in the neonatal intensive care unit. *J. Obstet. Gynecol. Neonatal Nurs.* 10(3):204.

Farquhar, J. W. 1965. Metabolic changes in the infant of the diabetic mother. *Pediatr. Clin. North Am.* 12:3.

Field, T. M. 1977. Effects of early separation: interactive deficits and experimental manipulations on infant–mother face-to-face interaction. *Child. Dev.* 48:763.

Fitzhardinge, P. M. 1976. Follow-up studies on the low birth weight infant. *Clin. Perinatol.* 3:503.

Fitzhardinge, P. M., and Steven, E. M. May 1972. The small-for-date infant. I. Later growth patterns. *Pediatrics.* 49(5):671.

Frantz, I. D., and Epstein, M. F. 1978. Fetal lung development in pregnancies complicated by diabetes. *Sem. Perinatol.* 2:4.

Garrand, S. Nov. 1978. A parent-to-parent program. *Fam. Com. Health.* 1(3):103.

Gorski, P. A., et al. 1979. Stages of behavioral organization in the high-risk neonate: theoretical and clinical considerations. *Sem. Perinatol.* 3:61.

Grant, P. Nov. 1978. Psychosocial needs of families of high-risk infants. *Fam. Com. Health.* 1(3):91.

Habib, A., and McCarthy, J. 1977. Effects on the neonate of propranolol administration during pregnancy. *J. Pediatr.* 91:808.

Harper, R. G., et al. 1977. Maternal ingested methadone, body fluid methadone, and the neonatal withdrawal syndrome. *Am. J. Obstet. Gynecol.* 129(4):417.

Hill, R. 1974. Generic features of families under stress. In *Crisis interventions*, ed. H. J. Parad. New York: Family Services Association of America.

Hobart, J. M., and Depp, R. 1982. Prolonged pregnancy. In *Gynecology and obstetrics*, vol. 3, ed. J. J. Siarra, Philadelphia: Harper & Row.

Hobbins, J. C. 1982. Fetoscopy. In *Protocols for high risk pregnancies*, ed. J. T. Queenan, and J. C. Hobbins. Oradell, N. J.: Medical Economics Co., Inc.

Hobel, C. J., et al. 1973. Prenatal and intrapartum high-risk screening. *Am. J. Obstet. Gynecol.* 117:1.

Iosub, S., et al. Oct. 1981. Fetal alcohol syndrome revisited. *Pediatrics.* 68(4):475.

Jones, K. L., et al. June 1973. Pattern of malformation in offspring of chronic alcoholic mothers. *Lancet.* 1:1267.

Kaplan, D. M., and Mason, E. A. 1974. Maternal reactions to premature birth viewed as an acute emotional disorder. In *Crisis interventions*, ed. H. J. Parad. New York: Family Services Association of America.

Klaus, M. H., and Fanaroff, A. A. 1979. *Care of the high-risk neonate.* Philadelphia: W. B. Saunders Co.

Klaus, M. H., and Kennell, J. H. 1982. *Maternal-infant bonding*, 2nd ed. St. Louis: The C. V. Mosby Co.

Korones, S. B. 1981. *High-risk newborn infants: the basis for intensive care nursing*, 3rd ed. St. Louis: The C. V. Mosby Co.

Leake, R. D. 1977. Perinatal nephrobiology: a developmental perspective. *Clin. Perinatol.* 8:215.

Lipsitz, P. J. March 1971. The clinical and biochemical effects of excessive magnesium in the newborn. *Pediatrics.* 47(3):501.

Lubchenco, L. 1976. *The high-risk infant.* Philadelphia: W. B. Saunders Co.

Lutz, D. J., et al. June 1978. Pregnancy and its complications following cardiac valve prostheses. *Am. J. Obstet. Gynecol.* 131(4): 460.

Measel, C. P., and Anderson, G. C. 1979. Non-nutritive sucking during tube feedings: effect on clinical course in premature infants. *J. Obstet. Gynecol. Neonat. Nurs.* 8:265.

Nash, M. A. 1981. The management of fluid and electrolyte disorders in the neonate. *Clin. Perinatol.* 8:251.

Nugent, J. Sept./Oct. 1982. Intra-arterial blood pressure monitoring in neonates. *J. Obstet. Gynecol. Neonat. Nurs.* 11:281.

Oh, W. 1981. Renal functions and clinical disorders in the neonate. *Clin. Perinatol.* 4:321.

Ostrea, E. M., et al. 1978. *The care of the drug dependent woman and her infant.* Michigan Department of Public Health.

Pereira, G. R., and Lemons, J. A. 1981. Controlled study of transpyloric and intermittent gavage feeding in the small preterm infants. *Pediatrics.* 67:68.

Schulte, F. J. 1977. Apnea. *Clin. Perinatol.* 4:65.

Smith, C. A. 1947. Effects of maternal malnutrition on fetal development. *Am. J. Dis. Child.* 73:2.

Solnit, A., and Stark, M. 1961. Mourning and the birth of a defective child. *Psychoanal. Study Child.* 16:505.

Stone, S. R., and Pritchard, J. A. 1970. Effect of maternally administered magnesium sulfate on the neonate. *Obstet. Gynecol.* 35(4):574.

Streissguth, A. P., et al. 1978. Intelligence, behavior, and dysmorphogenesis in the fetal alcohol syndrome. *J. Pediatr.* 92(3):363.

Taylor, P. M., and Hall, B. L. 1979. Parent–infant bonding: problems and opportunities in perinatal center. *Sem. Perinatol.* 3(1):75.

Tsang, R.; Chen, I.; Friedman, M.; et al. 1975. Parathyroid function in infants of diabetic mothers. *J. Pediatr.* 86:394.

Usher, R. H. Feb. 1970. Clinical and therapeutic aspects of fetal malnutrition. *Pediatr. Clin. North Am.* 17(1):169.

Whittemore, R., et al. 1980. Results of pregnancy in women with congenital heart defects. *Pediatr. Res.* 14:4.

Ziegler, E. E.; Bega, R. L.; and S. J. Fomon. 1983. Nutritional requirements of the premature infant. In *Symposium on pediatric nutrition,* ed. R. M. Suskind. New York: Raven Press.

Zuspan, F. P. 1978. Drug addiction in pregnancy: an invitational symposium. *J. Reprod. Med.* 20(6):301.

Additional Readings

Aylward, G. P. 1981. The developmental course of behavioral states in preterm infants: a descriptive study. *Child Develop.* 52:564.

Bartlett, D., and Davis, A. July/Aug. 1980. Recognizing fetal alcohol syndrome in the nursery. *J. Obstet. Gynecol. Neonat. Nurs.* 9:223.

Baumgart, S., et al. 1982. Fluid, electrolyte, and glucose maintenance in the very low birth weight infant. *Clin. Pediatr.* 21:199.

Brodish, M. S. 1981. Perinatal Assessment. *J. Obstet. Gynecol. Neonat. Nurs.* 10:42.

de Chateau, P. 1979. Effects of hospital practices on synchrony in the development of the infant–parent relationship. *Sem. Perinatol.* 3:1.

Hack, M., et al. 1980. Changing trends of neonatal and postneonatal deaths in very-low-birth-weight infants. *Am. J. Obstet. Gynecol.* 137:7.

Hill, A., and Volpe, J. J. 1981. Seizures, hypoxic-ischemic brain injury, and intraventricular hemorrhage in the newborn. *Ann. Neurol.* 10:109.

Kantor, G. Sept./Oct. 1978. Addicted mother, addicted baby: a challenge to health care providers. *MCN.* 3:281.

Lin, C. C., et al. 1980. Acid-base characteristics of fetuses with intrauterine growth retardation during labor and delivery. *Am. J. Obstet. Gynecol.* 137:51.

Miney, H. 1978. Problems and prognosis for the small-for-gestational-age and the premature infant. *MCN.* 3:4.

Noga, K. M. 1982. High-risk infants. The need for nursing follow-up. *J. Obstet. Gynecol. Neonat. Nurs.* 11:112.

Ogata, E. S. 1982. Infant of the diabetic mother. In *Gynecology and obstetrics,* vol. 3., ed. J. J. Sciarri. Philadelphia: Harper & Row.

Parke, R. D., et al. 1979. The father's role in the family system. *Sem. Perinatol.* 3:1.

Price, E., and Gyotoku, S. 1978. Using the nasojejunal feeding technique in a neonatal intensive care unit. *MCN.* 3:361.

Schraeder, B. D. 1980. Attachment and parenting despite lengthy intensive care. *Am. J. Mat. Child Nurs.* 5:1.

Stephens, C. J. 1981. The fetal alcohol syndrome: cause for concern. *Am. J. Mat. Child Nurs.* 6:4.

Trotter, C. W., et al. 1982. Perinatal factors and the developmental outcome of preterm infants. *J. Obstet. Gynecol. Neonat. Nurs.* 11:83.

■ 25 ■

COMPLICATIONS OF THE NEONATE

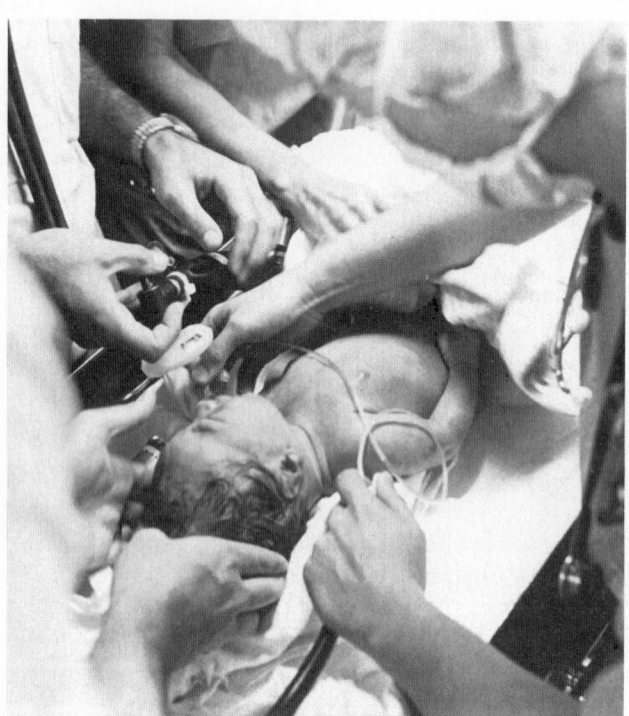

■ CHAPTER CONTENTS

ASPHYXIA
Pathophysiology
Resuscitation

RESPIRATORY DISTRESS
Idiopathic Respiratory Distress Syndrome (Hyaline Membrane Disease)
Transient Tachypnea of the Newborn (Type II Respiratory Distress Syndrome)
Meconium Aspiration Syndrome
Complications of Respiratory Therapy

COLD STRESS
Interventions

HYPOGLYCEMIA
Treatment

HYPOCALCEMIA
Diagnosis and Treatment

NEONATAL JAUNDICE
Mechanism of Bilirubin Conjugation
Pathologic Jaundice
Nursing Management

HEMOLYTIC DISEASE OF THE NEWBORN
Rh Incompatibility
ABO Incompatibility
Prognosis
Neonatal Assessment
Treatment of the Neonate and Nursing Responsibilities
Support of the Family

NEONATAL ANEMIA
    Clinical Manifestations and Diagnosis
    Management
POLYCYTHEMIA
    Therapy
HEMORRHAGIC DISEASE
INTRAVENTRICULAR HEMORRHAGE
    Interventions
DISSEMINATED INTRAVASCULAR
COAGULATION

NECROTIZING ENTEROCOLITIS
    Clinical Manifestations and Diagnosis
    Complications
    Interventions
INFECTIONS
    Sepsis Neonatorum
    Group B Streptococcus
    Syphilis
    Gonorrhea
    Herpesvirus Type 2
    Monilial Infection

■ OBJECTIVES

- Based on the labor record, Apgar score, and observable physiologic indicators, identify infants in need of resuscitation and the appropriate method of resuscitation.

- Based on clinical manifestations, differentiate the various types of respiratory distress (hyaline membrane disease, transient tachypnea, and type II respiratory distress) and meconium aspiration syndrome in the neonate.

- Identify the many components of nursing care of an infant with respiratory distress syndrome.

- Discuss the latest theory correlating the use of high concentrations of oxygen and positive pressure ventilation with development of the complications of respiratory distress.

- Differentiate between physiologic and pathologic jaundice based on onset, cause, possible sequelae, and specific management.

- Explain the set of circumstances that must be present for the development of erythroblastosis and ABO in-

compatibility and the nurse's role in the care of an infant with hemolytic disease.

- Identify the nursing responsibilities in phototherapy and exchange transfusion procedures.

- Describe the assessment of clinical manifestations that would make the nurse suspect neonatal sepsis.

- Relate the dangers of untreated syphilis, gonorrhea, or herpesvirus type 2 to management of the infant in the neonatal period.

- Explain the theories, clinical and diagnostic manifestations, nursing care, and medical treatment of necrotizing enterocolitis.

- Discuss selected metabolic abnormalities including cold stress, hypoglycemia, and hypocalcemia, and their effects on the neonate.

- Discuss selected hematologic variations and the nursing implications associated with each problem.

Marked homeostatic changes occur during the transition from fetal to neonatal life. Because the most rapid anatomic and physiologic changes of this period occur in the cardiopulmonary system, major problems of the newborn are usually related to this system. These problems include as-

phyxia, respiratory distress, jaundice, hemolytic disease, and anemia. Ideally, problems are anticipated and identified prenatally and appropriate intervention measures are begun at that time.

ASPHYXIA

Consideration of neonatal asphyxia requires knowledge of the respiratory transition from intrauterine to extrauterine life, the pathophysiology of asphyxia, the effects on circulation and biochemical status, and sequelae. The prevention or treatment for asphyxia is resuscitation.

Pathophysiology

Research studies of various species have indicated species variability in response to asphyxial insults. These research studies are not easily extrapolated to the response of the human infant, since the length of asphyxia and the possibility of subsequent anoxic brain damage are not easily estimated in the human infant. Presentation of an apneic infant in the delivery room necessitates immediate resuscitative efforts. Circulatory patterns that accompany asphyxia represent an inability to make the transition to extrauterine circulation—in effect a return to fetal-like circulatory patterns. Failure of lung expansion and establishment of respiration rapidly produces hypoxia (decreased Pao_2), acidosis (decreased pH), and hypercarbia (increased Pco_2). These biochemical changes result in pulmonary vasoconstriction, with retention of high pulmonary vascular resistance, hypoperfusion of the lungs, and a large right-to-left shunt through the ductus arteriosus. The foramen ovale opens (as right atrial pressure exceeds left atrial pressure), and blood flows from right to left.

Biochemical changes that occur in asphyxia contribute to these circulatory changes. The most profound biochemical aberration is a change from aerobic to anaerobic metabolism in the presence of hypoxia, with accumulation of lactate and the development of metabolic acidosis. A concomitant respiratory acidosis may also occur due to a rapid increase in Pco_2 during asphyxia. In response to hypoxia and anaerobic metabolism, the amounts of free fatty acids (FFA) and glycerol in the blood increase. Glycogen stores are also mobilized to provide a continuous glucose source for the brain. Rapid utilization of hepatic and cardiac stores of glycogen may occur during an asphyxial attack.

Resuscitation

The neonate is supplied with protective mechanisms against hypoxial insults. These defenses include a relatively immature brain and a resting metabolic rate less than that observed in the adult, an ability to mobilize substances within the body for anaerobic metabolism and use the energy more efficiently; and an intact circulatory system able to redistribute lactate and hydrogen ion in tissues still being perfused (Klaus and Fanaroff, 1979). Unfortunately, severe prolonged hypoxia will overcome these protective mechanisms, resulting in brain damage or death of the neonate.

The goal of resuscitation is to provide an adequate airway with expansion of the lungs, to decrease the Pco_2 and increase the Po_2, to support adequate cardiac output, and to minimize oxygen consumption by reducing heat loss (Cloherty and Stark, 1981).

IDENTIFICATION OF INFANTS IN NEED OF RESUSCITATION

As discussed in Chapter 10 and 15, knowledge of the perinatal history enables caregivers to anticipate the birth of a high-risk infant who will need resuscitative efforts from appropriate personnel. Need for resuscitation may be anticipated in any of the following antepartal or intrapartal situations:

□ *ANTEPARTAL RISK FACTORS FOR RESUSCITATION*

1. Previous obstetric history of fetal or neonatal death; premature or growth retarded infant; infant weighing 10 lb or more.
2. Maternal conditions that affect the placenta or fetus—preeclampsia-eclampsia, postterm (more than 42 weeks), preexisting hypertension, diabetes, infection, chronic renal disease, maternal obesity, and cardiac disease.
3. Maternal age—younger than 15 years or elderly primigravida (over 35 years).
4. Isoimmunization.
5. Abruptio placentae or placenta previa.
6. Multiple gestation.
7. Abnormal presentation.
8. Preterm infant.
9. Prolonged rupture of the membranes.
10. Hydramnios or oligohydramnios.
11. Abnormal estriol levels.
12. Less than mature L/S ratio.
13. Maternal drug usage (narcotic, barbiturate, tranquilizer, or alcohol).
14. Anemia (hemoglobin less than 10 mg/dL).

□ *INTRAPARTAL RISK FACTORS FOR RESUSCITATION*

1. Abnormal labor pattern—dystocia, precipitous delivery.
2. Meconium-stained amniotic fluid in cephalic presentation.
3. Fetal heart rate patterns—tachycardia (greater than 160/min without maternal temperature elevation); bradycardia (less than 120/min, particularly associated with smooth baseline, an ominous sign); irregular rate; lack of baseline variability of FHR (smooth or fixed); lack of significant variability with fetal movement; ominous patterns (moderate to severe variable deceleration and late deceleration of any magnitude).

4. Abnormal fetal presentation—breech, transverse lie, shoulder.

5. Prolapsed cord.

6. Abruptio placentae or placenta previa.

7. Indications for cesarean delivery.

□ *NEONATAL RISK FACTORS FOR RESUSCITATION*

1. Difficult delivery.

2. Fetal blood loss.

3. Apneic episode unresponsive to tactile stimulation.

4. Cardiac arrest.

5. Inadequate ventilation.

Particular attention must be paid to these pregnancies during the intrapartal period, because labor and delivery are asphyxiating processes and often the high-risk fetus has less tolerance to the stress of labor and delivery.

Biophysical (uterine contractions, FHR, ECG) and biochemical (fetal and maternal pH and blood gases) monitoring during the intrapartal period may help to identify fetal distress so that appropriate measures can be taken to deliver the fetus immediately, before major damage occurs, and to treat the asphyxiated neonate. Fetal scalp blood sampling (p.461), a valuable assessment tool, may indicate asphyxic insult and related degree of fetal acidosis if considered in relation to stage of labor, uterine contractions, and ominous FHR patterns. Normal fetal pH ranges from 7.3–7.35. The fall of pH is gradual during the first stage of labor but becomes more drastic during the second stage and delivery. The stress of labor causes an intermittent decrease in the exchange of gases in the intervillous space of the placenta and a fall in pH secondarily to the accumulation of pyruvic and lactic acid, resulting in an accumulation of hydrogen ions and the phenomenon of physiologic fetal acidosis. Physiologic fetal acidosis is metabolic rather than respiratory, because exchange of CO_2 at the placental level is more rapid than exchange of hydrogen ions. During labor, a fetal pH of 7.25 or higher is considered normal. A pH value of 7.21–7.24 is considered as "preacidosis." A pH value of 7.20 or less during first-stage labor is considered an ominous sign of fetal asphyxia (Modanlou, 1976); repeat samples should be obtained within 10–15 minutes to confirm the diagnosis, followed by immediate delivery of the fetus.

NURSE'S ROLE

Communication between the obstetric office or clinic and the labor and delivery nurse facilitates the identification of potential infants in need of resuscitation.

Upon arrival of the client in the labor area, the nurse should have the antepartal record and should note any contributory perinatal history factors and assess present fetal status. As labor progresses, nursing assessments include ongoing monitoring of fetal heartbeat and its re-

sponse to contractions, assisting with fetal scalp blood sampling, and observing for expulsion of meconium, thereby identifying fetal asphyxia and hypoxia. In addition, the nurse should alert the resuscitation team and the practitioner responsible for care of the neonate of any potential high-risk patients in the labor and delivery area.

EQUIPMENT AND MEDICATIONS

Following identification of possible high-risk situations, the next step in effective resuscitation is assembling the necessary equipment and ensuring proper functioning. Adequately trained personnel are a vital necessity in the delivery room for all high-risk and normal deliveries. Resuscitation is at least a two-person effort. The nurse should call for assistance. Adequate, well-trained personnel must always be available to assist the primary resuscitator. Systematic assembly and checking of equipment is essential for efficient resuscitation and for preventing "flail" efforts. Provision for pH and blood gas determination is desirable.

Necessary equipment includes a radiant warmer, a device that should be in every delivery room. This equipment provides an overhead radiant heat source that is servocontrolled (a thermostatic mechanism that is taped to the infant's abdomen triggers the radiant warmer to turn on or off in order to maintain a level of thermoneutrality) and an open bed for easy access to the newborn. It is essential that the nurse keep the infant warm. The infant is dried quickly to prevent evaporative heat loss and is placed under the radiant warmer.

Equipment needed is as follows:

1. Radiant warmer

2. Stethoscope

3. Bag (that can deliver 100% oxygen)

4. Mask (two mask sizes: one preterm and one newborn)

5. Tubing and pressure gauges for bag

6. Oxygen, flow meter, and provision for warmth and humidification

7. Suction equipment
  a. DeLee trap
  b. Bulb syringe
  c. Mechanical suction apparatus
  d. Suction catheters (No. 5, 6, or 8 Fr.)

8. Intubation equipment
  a. Magill forceps
  b. Portex polyvinylchloride intubation tubes—sizes 2.5, 3.0, 3.5, 4.0 mm (fitted with adapter)
  c. Wire stylets for tubes
  d. Laryngoscope handle with two blades—size 0 (premature), size 1 (newborn)
  e. Four extra batteries
  f. Two extra bulbs

9. Nasogastric tube (for decompression of stomach)

10. Infant plastic airway

11. K-Y lubricating jelly

12. Benzoin

13. Cotton applicators

14. Adhesive tape

15. Scissors

16. Safety pins (for attachments)

17. Syringes (tuberculin, 3, 5, and 10 mL)

18. Umbilical artery catheter tray (No. 3.5 and 5 Fr. catheters)

19. IV solution and tubing

20. Drugs (solutions)
    a. Sodium bicarbonate (0.5 mEq/mL)
    b. Epinephrine (1:10,000)
    c. Dextrose (10% in water for IV or 25% for hypoglycemia)
    d. Calcium gluconate (10% solution)
    e. Narcan (0.02 mg/mL neonatal solution)
    f. Volume expanders (plasma, albumin, or human plasma protein fraction (plasminate))
    g. Normal saline (for suctioning)
    h. Atropine (0.4 mg/0.5 mL)

21. Blood pressure cuff and gauge or pressure transducer

22. Doppler (to measure blood pressure)

23. ECG electrodes and heart rate monitor

Resuscitative equipment in the delivery room must be sterilized after each use. In the high-risk nursery the need for resuscitation may occur at any time. Therefore, every newborn should have his or her own bag and mask, available at the bedside. This equipment must be sterilized before use on another infant.

Equipment reliability must be maintained before an emergency arises. Inspect all equipment—bag and mask, oxygen and flow meter, laryngoscope, suction machines—for damaged or nonfunctioning parts before a delivery or assembly at the infant's bedside. A systematic check of the emergency cart and equipment should be a routine responsibility of each shift.

INITIAL RESUSCITATIVE MANAGEMENT

Initial resuscitative management of the neonate is extremely important. The infant should be kept in a head-down position prior to the first gasp to avoid aspiration of the oropharyngeal secretions. The oropharynx and nasopharynx must be suctioned immediately. After the first few breaths, the infant is kept in a flat position under a radiant heat source and dried quickly to maintain skin temperature at about 36.5C. Drying is also a good stimulation to breathing. Heat loss through evaporation is tremendous during the first few minutes of life. The temperature of a wet 1500 g baby in a 16C (62F) delivery room drops 1C

every 3 minutes. Hypothermia increases oxygen consumption and in an asphyxiated infant increases the hypoxic insult and may lead to severe acidosis and development of respiratory distress.

Appraisal of the infant's need for resuscitation begins at the time of birth. The time of the first gasp, first cry, and onset of sustained respirations should be noted in order of occurrence. The Apgar score (p. 49) is important in determining the severity of neonatal depression and the immediate course of necessary action (Table 25-1).

□ *ESTABLISH AIRWAY* A patent airway is established by clearing the nasal and oral passages of fluid that may obstruct the airway. Suction is always performed before resuscitation so that mucus, blood, meconium, or formula is not aspirated into the lungs. If the infant is flaccid, the tongue may be lying against the posterior pharyngeal wall, thereby obstructing the airway. An infant pharyngeal airway, properly inserted in the oral cavity over the tongue, will correct this obstruction (usually optional for the neonate).

□ *ESTABLISH RESPIRATIONS* To establish breathing, begin with the simplest form of resuscitative measures and, if unsuccessful, proceed to more complicated methods.

1. Simple stimulation is provided by rubbing the back.

2. If respirations have not been initiated or are inadequate (gasping or occasional respirations), the lungs must be inflated with positive pressure. The mask is positioned securely on face (over nose and mouth; avoiding the eyes) with head in "sniffing" or neutral position (Figure 25-1). Hyperextension of the infant's neck will obstruct the trachea. An airtight connection is made between the infant's face and the mask (thus allowing the bag to inflate). Inflate the lungs rhythmically by squeezing the bag. (The nurse should be familiar with the type of resuscitation bag used in the institution.) Oxygen can be delivered at 100% with an anesthesia bag and adequate liter flow, whereas an Ambu or Hope bag delivers only 40% oxygen, unless it has been adapted. In addition, it may not be possible to maintain adequate inspiratory pressure with Ambu or Hope bags. In a crisis situation it is crucial that 100% O_2 be delivered with adequate pressure.

3. The rise and fall of the chest is observed for proper ventilation. The nurse should auscultate over both lungs for air entry and check heart rate. Manual resuscitation is coordinated with any voluntary efforts. The rate of ventilation should be between 30 and 50 per minute. Pressure should be less than 30 cm of H_2O. If ventilation is adequate, the chest moves with each inspiration, bilateral breath sounds are audible, and the lips and mucous membranes become pink. If color and heart rate fail to respond to ventilatory efforts, poor or improper placement of an endotracheal tube may be the cause; if the neonate is intubated properly, pneumothorax, diaphragmatic hernia, or hypoplastic lungs

Table 25-1 Guidelines for Resuscitation of the Neonate

Apgar score	Heart rate	Arterial blood pH*	Appearance	Resuscitative measures
9 or 10	> 100	7.30-7.40 (normal)	Regular respirations; flexed extremities; cries in response to flicking of soles of feet; may be dusky or show acrocyanosis	Place under radiant heat source and dry immediately; gently suction airway.
7 or 8	60-100	7.20-7.29 (slight acidosis)	Limp, cyanotic, or dusky and dyspneic; respirations may be shallow, irregular, or gasping; heart rate is normal; fair response to flicking of sole	Dry and place under warmer; give oxygen near face.
5 or 6	60-100	7.10-7.19 (moderate acidosis)	Same as for Apgar 7 or 8	Dry and place under warmer; clear airway and stimulate through drying process. If still not improved, place in "sniff" position, insert pharyngeal airway, and begin ventilation (100% O_2) with bag and mask, using pressure of 30 cm H_2O at rate of 30-50 per min. If difficulty persists, reevaluate maternal history of drug administration, especially if heart rate responds to ventilation but there is no spontaneous respiration. Give narcotic antagonist (Narcan) if indicated. Mildly depressed newborns will usually develop regular spontaneous respirations within 5 minutes. If tracheal aspiration reveals blood or meconium, directly visualize with laryngoscope and suction as needed before administering positive pressure.
3 or 4	< 60	7.00-7.09 (marked acidosis)	Blue and limp, little or no respiratory effort. Jaw is slack during suctioning.	For Apgar 0-4: Dry under warmer; clear airway; consider immediate intubation. Hold O_2 near face during intubation. Ventilate after direct visualization with laryngoscope and appropriate suctioning. Check breath sounds. If heart rate remains low (0-40), immediately institute external cardiac massage. Correction of hypotension is usually via umbilical vein. Obtain blood gas values (pH, P_{CO_2}, P_{O_2}) and BP.
0 to 2	< 60	< 7.00 (severe acidosis)	Same as for Apgar 3 or 4	

* Correlations of Apgar score and arterial blood pH adapted from Saling, E. 1972. Technical and theoretical problems in electronic monitoring of the human fetal heart. *Int. J. Gynecol. Obstet.* 10:211, and from Korones, S. 1981. *High-risk newborn infants: the basis for intensive nursing care,* 2nd ed. St. Louis: The C. V. Mosby Co.

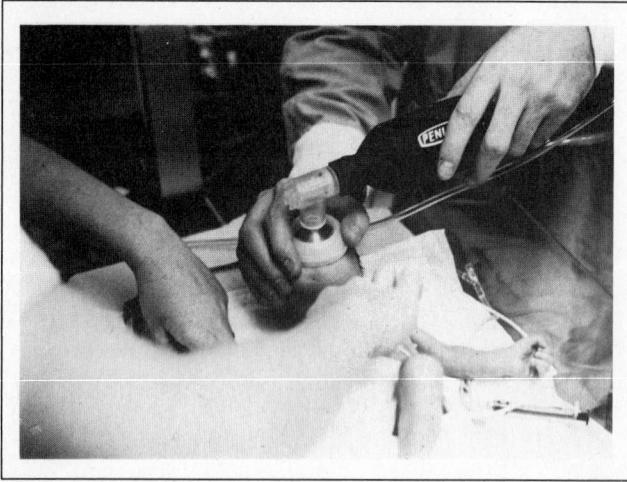

FIGURE 25-1 Resuscitation of infant with bag and mask. Note that the mask covers the nose and mouth and the head is in a neutral position.

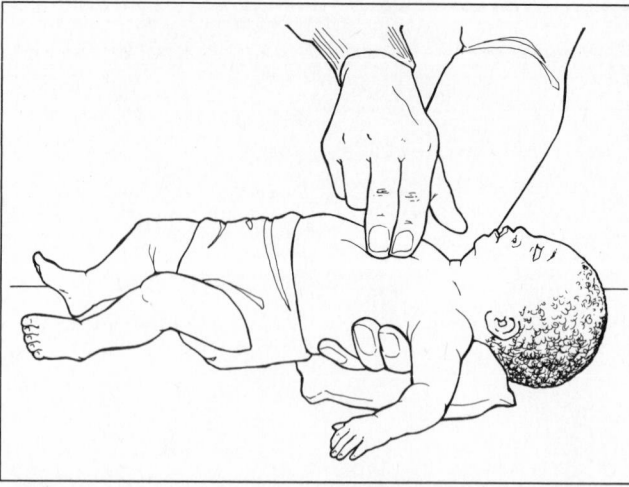

FIGURE 25-3 External cardiac massage. The midsternum is compressed with two fingertips at a rate of 80-100 beats/min.

(Potter's syndrome) may exist. Distention of the stomach is controlled by inserting a nasogastric tube for decompression.

4. Intubation (Figure 25-2, Procedure 25-1) is rarely needed, because most infants can be resuscitated by bag and mask.

□ *MAINTAIN CIRCULATION* Once breathing has been established, the heart rate should increase to over 100 beats/min. If the heart rate is less than 60 beats/min, external cardiac massage is begun. (Cardiac massage is commenced immediately if there is no detectable heart beat.)

1. The infant is positioned *properly* on a firm surface.

2. The resuscitator utilizes two fingers (Figure 25-3), or may stand at the foot of the infant and place both thumbs at the junction of the middle and lower third of the sternum, with the fingers wrapped around and supporting the back.

3. The sternum is depressed approximately two-thirds of the distance to the vertebral column (1.0-1.5 cm), at a rate of 80-100 beats/min.

4. A 3:1 ratio of heartbeat to assisted ventilation is used.

FIGURE 25-2 Endotracheal intubation is accomplished with the infant's head in the "sniff" position. The operator places the fifth finger under the chin to hold the tongue forward.

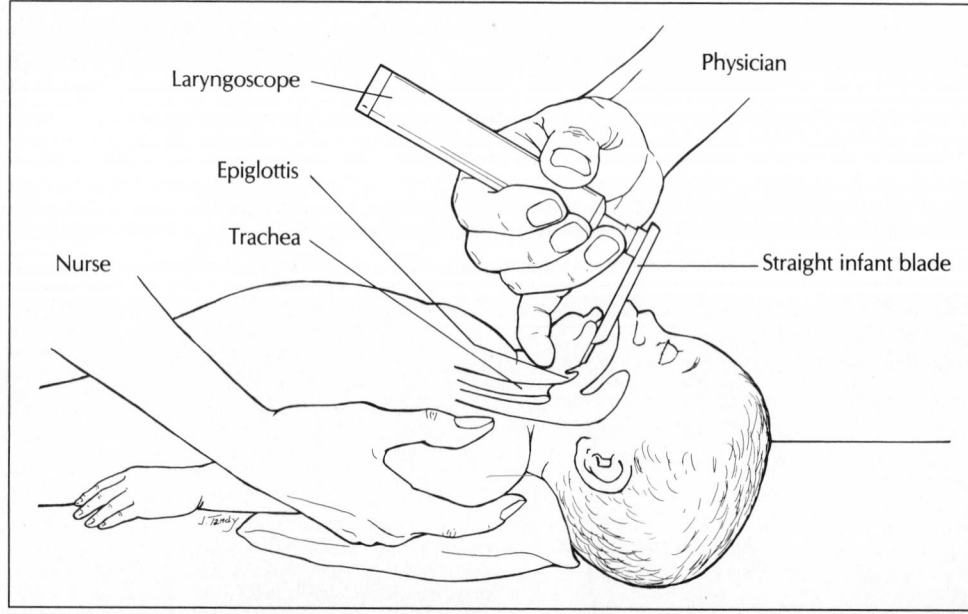

Procedure 25-1   Tracheal Intubation

Objective	Nursing action	Rationale
Facilitate atraumatic insertion of endotracheal tube in support of adequate tissue oxygenation	Gather necessary equipment, ensuring that all possible variations are available: 1. Laryngoscope handle with extra batteries and bulbs.	Intubation is usually performed as an emergency measure. It is potentially hazardous to the newborn. If prolonged, the iatrogenic effects include local orotracheal tissue damage and/or generalized hypoxia. Necessary equipment should be available on unit emergency cart.
	2. Detachable blades of curved and straight variety — infant and small child lengths	Curved blades are used when unusual tongue and jaw formations make straight blades inadequate. Smallest internal diameter endotracheal tube (3.0 mm) is used in neonates, with sizes increasing according to weight and length.
	3. Variety of uncuffed endotracheal tubes. 4. Adapters for oxygen hookup between endotracheal tube and ventilator or resuscitation bag. 5. Infant and pediatric masks and resuscitation bags. 6. Oxygen tubing and flow meter with wall outlet adapter. 7. Suction equipment (Procedure 25-3, p. 812). 8. Benzoin and 1 in. adhesive tape.	In infants, uncuffed tubes can provide adequate seal.
	Immediately set up oxygen supply system and suction equipment. Suction and preoxygenate infant by mask and bag.	Infant should be as well oxygenated as possible before intubation begins to delay onset of hypoxemia. Oropharyngeal suctioning prior to intubation can facilitate visualization of epiglottis.
	Position and immobilize infant during laryngoscopy and tube insertion (Figure 25-2). In the event of an unsuccessful intubation attempt, reoxygenate prior to next attempt	Most frequently used position is supine with very slight extension of head. Hold oxygen near neonate's face while he or she is being intubated.
	After appropriate placement of the tube has been determined (usually by portable x-ray), secure tube in that position by: 1. Applying tincture of benzoin to clean and dry upper lip and cheeks of the infant. Allow it to dry. 2. Applying overlapping split 1-in. adhesive tape around tube and onto lips and cheeks.	Tube is inserted to a point just above the carina, which ensures effective ventilation of both lungs. With poor handling techniques, it is possible to dislodge tube, causing intubation of mainstem bronchus (usually on the right) with no ventilation of other lung or causing complete extubation. Taping tube minimizes possibility of dislodgement. Some practitioners suture the tube to tape.

Procedure 25–1   Tracheal Intubation cont'd

Objective	Nursing action	Rationale
	Measure length of tube from oral exit point to its connection point every 4 hr. Assess bilateral breath sounds and chest excursion symmetry for equality every hour.	Frequent monitoring of tube length and respiratory status are measurable criteria for evaluation of tube placement.

Precautions: Only skilled practitioners should attempt to intubate newborns in an emergency situation. Intubation of unanesthetized infants is usually carried out only in a profoundly obtunded patient. Insertion and suctioning of endotracheal tubes call for use of aseptic technique to minimize pulmonary infection. Assessment for signs and symptoms of tube obstruction and/or pneumothorax (especially with mechanical ventilation) should be of utmost priority for the nurse caring for an intubated infant.

DRUG THERAPY

Drugs that should be available in the delivery room include those needed in the treatment of shock, cardiac arrest, and narcosis. Oxygen, because of its effective use in ventilation, is the drug most often used.

If by 5 minutes after delivery, the neonate has not responded to the resuscitation with spontaneous respirations and a heart rate above 100 beats/min, it may be necessary to correct the acidosis and provide the myocardium with glucose. The most accessible route for administering medications is the umbilical vein. In a severely asphyxiated neonate, sodium bicarbonate (4–5 mEq/kg) is given to correct metabolic acidosis. If bradycardia is profound, epinephrine (0.1 mL/kg of a 1:10,000 solution) is given by direct cardiac puncture or through the umbilical vein catheter. Bradycardia can also be treated with atropine (0.03 mg/kg intravenously). Calcium gluconate (1–2 mL/kg of a 10% solution intravenously) is used for severe bradycardia, arrythmias, and poor cardiac output despite adequate ventilation and for severe hypocalcemia or hyperkalemia. Dextrose (0.5–1.0 g/kg of a 25% solution) can be given to correct hypoglycemia. Usually a 10% dextrose in a water intravenous solution is sufficient to prevent or treat hypoglycemia in the delivery room. Naloxone hydrochloride (0.02 mg/mL neonatal solution intravenously or intramuscularly), a narcotic antagonist, is used to reverse narcotic depression. See Drug Guides—Sodium Bicarbonate and Naloxone on the facing page.

In the advent of shock (low blood pressure or poor peripheral perfusion) the neonate should be given a volume expander. Placental blood removed from the umbilical vein is an ideal volume expander. Fresh frozen plasma, salt-poor albumin (l g/kg; dilute 25% solution to 5%), packed red blood cells, and whole blood can also be used for volume expansion and treatment of shock.

RESPIRATORY DISTRESS

One of the prime aberrations to which the neonate is a victim is respiratory distress—an inappropriate respiratory adaptation to extrauterine life. The nursing care of a neonate with respiratory distress involves understanding of the normal pulmonary and circulatory physiology (Chapter 21), the pathophysiology of the disease process, clinical manifestations, and supportive and corrective therapies. Only with this knowledge can the nurse make appropriate observations concerning responses to therapy and development of complications. Unlike the verbalizing adult client, the newborn communicates needs only by behavior. The neonatal nurse, through objective observations and evaluations, interprets this behavior into information about the individual infant's condition. Only with basic knowledge can the observations be recognized as meaningful interpretations of the newborn's condition.

Idiopathic Respiratory Distress Syndrome (Hyaline Membrane Disease)

Respiratory distress syndrome (RDS), also referred to as *hyaline membrane disease* (HMD), is a complex disease affecting primarily preterm infants and accounts for 12,000 to 25,000 deaths per year in the United States alone. The factors precipitating the pathophysiologic changes of RDS have not been determined, but there are two main factors associated with the development of RDS:

Prematurity. All preterm infants, whether AGA, SGA, or LGA, and especially IDMs are at risk for RDS. The maternal and fetal factors resulting in preterm labor and delivery, complications of pregnancy, cesarean birth (indications for cesarean delivery rather than the type of delivery), and familial tendency are all associated with RDS.

DRUG GUIDE—Sodium bicarbonate

OVERVIEW OF NEONATAL ACTION

Sodium bicarbonate is an alkalizing agent. It buffers hydrogen ions caused by accumulation of lactic acid from anaerobic metabolism occurring during hypoxemia. Sodium bicarbonate thereby raises the blood pH, reversing the metabolic acidosis. Sodium bicarbonate should *only* be used to correct severe metabolic acidosis in asphyxiated newborns once adequate ventilation has been established (Avery, 1981).

Note: Sodium bicarbonate dissociates in solution into sodium ion and carbonic acid, which can split into water and carbon dioxide. The carbon dioxide must be eliminated via the respiratory tract.

ROUTE, DOSAGE, FREQUENCY

For resuscitation and severe asphyxiation: intravenous push via umbilical vein catheter for quick infusion. Dosage is 2 mEq/K: 4 mL of 0.5 mEq/mL (4.2%) or 2 mL of mEq/mL (8.4%). 8.4% solution diluted at least 1:1 with sterile water to decrease the osmolarity; infuse at rate no faster than 1 mEq/kg/min (Avery, 1981). Complete infusion should be given over a minimum of 10–15 minutes. Can repeat every 15 minutes if needed for total of 4 doses. For marked metabolic acidosis: a pH of less than 7.05 and a base deficit of 15 mEq/L should be corrected by 0.5 mEq of sodium bicarbonate at a rate of 1 mEq/kg/min or slower.

NEONATAL CONTRAINDICATIONS

Inadequate respiratory ventilation that causes a rise in P_{CO_2} and decrease in pH

Presence of edema, metabolic or respiratory alkalosis, and hypocalcemia, anuria, or oliguria

NEONATAL SIDE EFFECTS

Hypernatremia, hyperosmolarity, fluid overload

Intracranial hemorrhage (rapid infusion of bicarbonate increases serum osmolarity, causing a shift of interstitial fluid into the blood and capillary rupture)

NURSING CONSIDERATIONS

Assess for any contraindications
Monitor intake and output rates

Assess adequacy of ventilation by monitoring respiratory status, rate, and depth; ventilate as necessary

Dilute bicarbonate prior to administration into umbilical vein catheter (for resuscitation) or peripheral IV to prevent sloughing of tissue

Evaluate effectiveness of drug by monitoring arterial blood gases for P_{CO_2}, bicarbonate concentration, and pH determination
Incompatible with acidic solutions
Administration with calcium creates precipitates

DRUG GUIDE—Naloxone hydrochloride (Narcan)

OVERVIEW OF NEONATAL ACTION

Naloxone hydrochloride (Narcan) is used to reverse respiratory depression due to acute narcotic toxicity. It displaces morphinelike drugs from receptor sites on the neurons; therefore, the narcotics can no longer exert their depressive effects. Naloxone reverses narcotic-induced respiratory depression, analgesia, sedation, hypotension, and pupillary constriction (Berkowitz et al., 1981).

ROUTE, DOSAGE, FREQUENCY

Intravenous dose is 0.01 mg/kg, usually through umbilical vein, although naloxone can be given intramuscularly. Neonatal dose is supplied as 0.02 mg/mL solution (0.5–1.0 mL for preterms and 2 mL for full-terms). Reversal of drug depression occurs within 1–2 minutes and will last 1–2 hours. Dose may be repeated in 5 minutes. If no improvement after two or three doses, naloxone administration should be discontinued (Cloherty and Stark, 1981). If initial reversal occurs, repeat dose at 1–2 hour intervals as needed.

NEONATAL CONTRAINDICATIONS

Must be used with caution in infants of narcotic-addicted mothers as it may precipitate acute withdrawal syndrome. Respiratory depression resulting from nonmorphine drugs such as sedatives, hypnotics, anesthetics, or other nonnarcotic CNS depressants.

NEONATAL SIDE EFFECTS

Excessive doses may result in irritability and increased crying, and possibly prolongation of PTT (Benitz and Tatro, 1981). Tachycardia

NURSING CONSIDERATIONS

Monitor respirations closely—rate and depth

Assess for return of respiratory depression when naloxone effects wear off and effects of longer-acting narcotic reappear

Have resuscitative equipment, O_2, and ventilatory equipment available

Monitor bleeding studies
Incompatible with alkaline solutions

Asphyxia. Asphyxia, with a corresponding decrease in pulmonary blood flow, may interfere with surfactant production.

PATHOPHYSIOLOGY

At birth, the neonate synthesizes surfactant at an increased rate to adjust to an air-breathing existence. Development of RDS by the preterm infant indicates a failure to synthesize lecithin at the rate required to maintain alveolar stability. Alveolar instability upon expiration with increasing atelectasis causes hypoxia and acidosis, which inhibit the surfactant system and cause pulmonary vasoconstriction. Thus the central pathophysiologic defect, lung instability due to this abnormality in the surfactant system, precipitates the biochemical aberrations of hypoxemia (decreased Po_2), hypercarbia (increased Pco_2), and acidemia (decreased pH), which further increases pulmonary va-

soconstriction and hypoperfusion. The cycle of events of RDS leading to eventual respiratory failure is diagrammed in Figure 25–4.

Because of these pathophysiologic conditions, the neonate must expend increasing amounts of energy to reopen the collapsed alveoli with every breath, so that each breath becomes as difficult as the first. The progressive expiratory atelectasis upsets the physiologic homeostasis of the pulmonary and cardiovascular systems and prevents adequate gaseous exchange. Lung compliance decreases, and stiff lungs, which account for the difficulty of inflation, labored respirations, and the increased work of breathing, are the results.

Adequate gaseous exchange dependent on diffusion and ventilation/perfusion ratio is upset with RDS. Hypoxia produces physiologic complications and consequences that increase the hypoxia and decrease pulmonary perfusions:

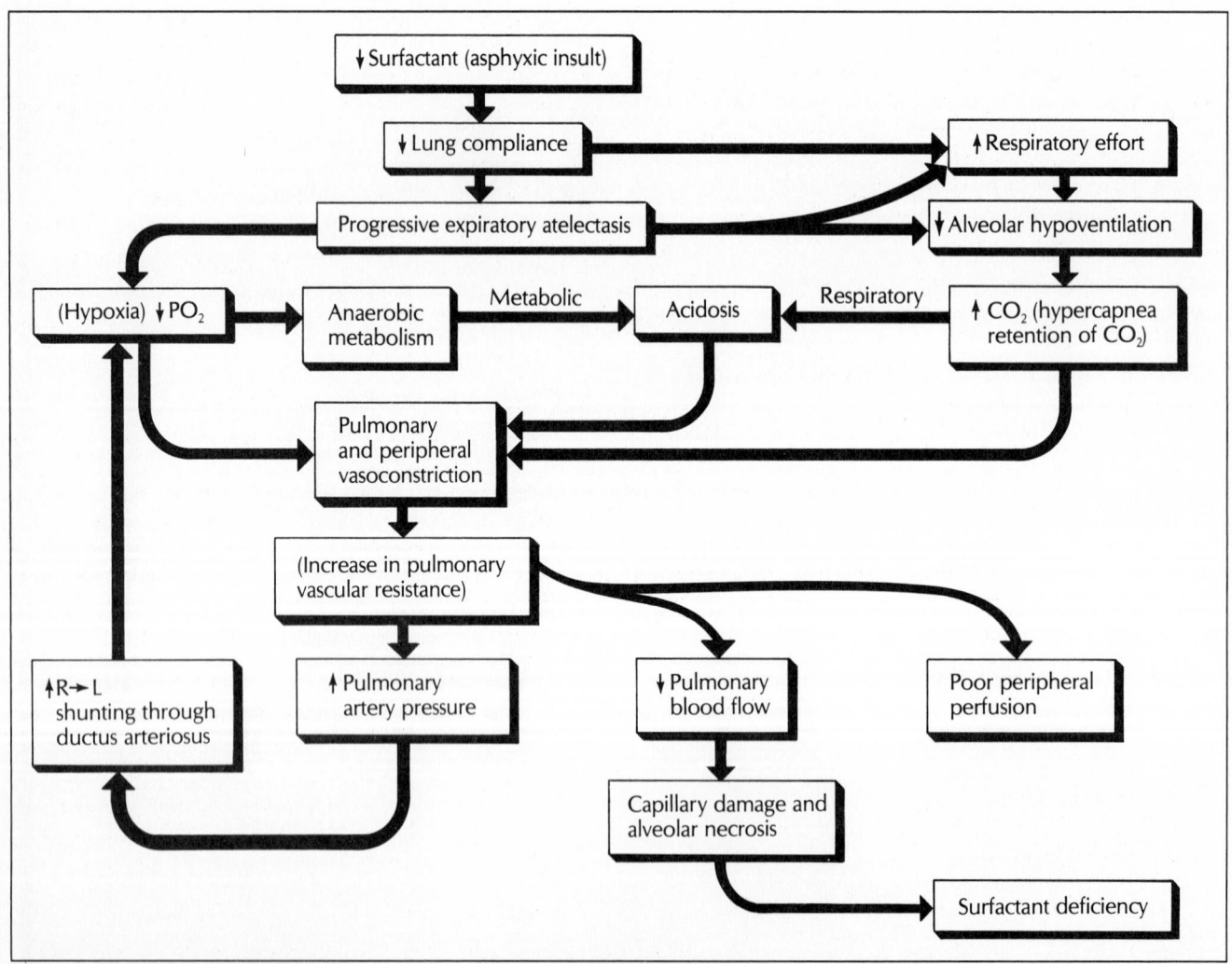

FIGURE 25–4 Cycle of events of RDS leading to eventual respiratory failure. (Modified from Gluck, L., and Kulovich, M. V. 1973. Fetal lung development. *Pediatr. Clin. North Am.* 20:375.)

1. Hypoxia causes vasoconstriction of the pulmonary vasculature, which increases pulmonary vascular resistance and further reduces pulmonary blood flow. Increased pulmonary vascular resistance may precipitate a return to fetal circulation as the ductus opens and blood flow is shunted around the lungs.

2. Hypoxia causes impairment or absence of metabolic response to cold, reversion to anaerobic metabolism, and lactate accumulation (acidosis).

   Along with hypoxia, other biochemical aberrations accompany RDS:

• *Respiratory acidosis* (increased P_{CO_2}, decreased pH) is the result of alveolar hypoventilation. Carbon dioxide retention and resultant respiratory acidosis are the measure of ventilatory inadequacy, so that persistently rising P_{CO_2} and decrease in pH are poor prognostic signs of pulmonary function and adequacy.

• *Metabolic acidosis* (decreased pH, decreased bicarbonate level) may be the result of impaired delivery of oxygen at the cellular level. Because of the lack of oxygen, the neonate begins an anaerobic pathway of metabolism, with an increase in lactate levels and a resultant base deficit. As the lactate levels increase, the pH becomes acidotic (decreased pH), and the buffer base decreases in an attempt to compensate and maintain acid-base homeostasis.

CLINICAL MANIFESTATIONS

Myriad clinical manifestations are the result of the pathophysiology of the disease process and the efforts to compensate and maintain homeostasis. Clinical symptomatology for the neonate is often nonspecific for one particular disease entity, involves many systems, may be subjective, and is nonverbal. Table 25–2 provides a review of clinical findings associated with respiratory distress (Figure 25–5).

The classic radiologic picture of RDS is diffuse reticulogranular density (bilaterally), with the air-filled tracheobronchial tube outlined by the opaque lungs (air-bronchogram). Opacification of the lung fields or "white-out" may be due to massive atelectasis, diffuse alveolar infiltrate, or pulmonary edema. The progression of radiologic findings parallels the pattern of resolution (4–7 days in uncomplicated, mild or moderate RDS) and the time of surfactant reappearance.

The gross pathologic picture at autopsy reveals lungs that are dark red-purple, airless, and liverlike in consistency. Atelectasis is widespread, and the lungs are difficult to inflate. The presence of hyaline membranes in overdistended terminal bronchioles and alveoli are representative of destruction and damage to the basement membrane of the alveolar cells.

INTERVENTIONS

The primary goal of management prenatally is the prevention of preterm delivery through aggressive treatment of

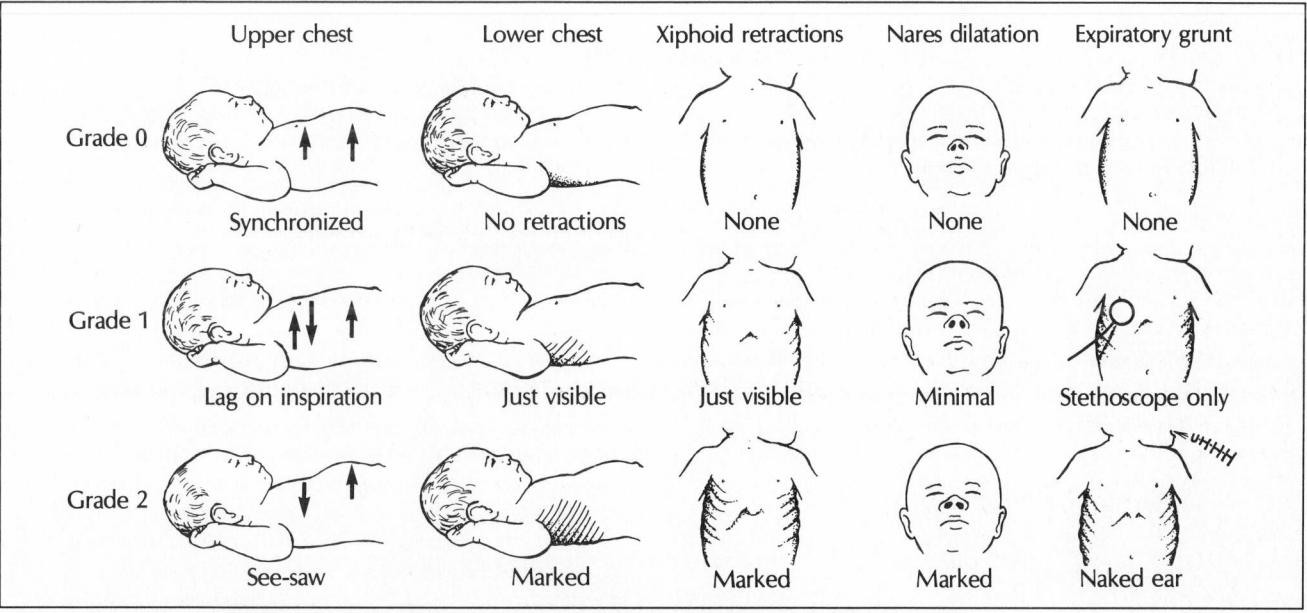

FIGURE 25–5 Evaluation of respiratory status utilizing the Silverman-Andersen index. (From Ross Laboratories, Nursing Inservice Aid no. 2, Columbus, Ohio; and Silverman, W. A., and Andersen, D. H. 1956. *Pediatrics* 17:1. Copyright © 1956 American Academy of Pediatrics.)

Table 25–2   Clinical Findings Associated with Respiratory Distress

Clinical picture	Significance
Skin	
Color	
Pallor or mottling	Represents poor peripheral circulation due to systemic hypotension and vasoconstriction and pooling of independent areas (usually in conjunction with severe hypoxia).
Cyanosis (bluish tint)	Depends on hemoglobin concentration, peripheral circulation, intensity and quality of viewing light, and acuity of observer's color vision; frankly visible in advanced hypoxia yet may be unobservable, because a large decrease in Pao_2 may be tolerated without signs of cyanosis.
Jaundice (yellow discoloration of skin and mucous membranes due to presence of unconjugated (indirect) bilirubin)	Metabolic aberrations (acidosis, hypercarbia, asphyxia) of respiratory distress predispose to dissociation of bilirubin from albumin-binding sites and deposition in the skin and central nervous system.
Edema (presents as slick, shiny skin)	Characteristic of preterm infant because of low total protein concentration with decrease in colloidal osmotic pressure and transudation of fluid; edema of hands and feet frequently seen within first 24 hours and resolved by fifth day in infant with severe RDS.
Respiratory system	
Tachypnea (normal respiratory rate 40–60/min; elevated respiratory rate 60+/min)	Increased respiratory rate is most frequent and easily detectable sign of respiratory distress after birth; a compensatory mechanism that attempts to increase respiratory dead space to maintain alveolar ventilation and gaseous exchange in the face of an increase in mechanical resistance. As a decompensatory mechanism it increases work load and energy output (by increasing respiratory rate), which causes increased metabolic demand for oxygen and thus increase in alveolar ventilation (of already over-stressed system). During shallow, rapid respirations, there is increase in dead space ventilation, thus decreasing alveolar ventilation.
Apnea (episode of nonbreathing of more than 25 sec in duration; periodic breathing, a common ''normal'' occurrence in preterm infants, is defined as apnea of 5–10 sec alternating with 10–15 sec periods of ventilation)	Poor prognostic sign; indicative of cardiorespiratory disease, central nervous system disease, and immaturity; physiologic alterations include decreased oxygen saturation, respiratory acidosis, and bradycardia.
Chest	Inspection of thoracic cage and measurement of anteroposterior diameter of chest may reveal decreased thoracic gas volume.
Labored respirations (Silverman-Andersen chart in Figure 25–5 indicates severity of retractions, grunting, and flaring, which are signs of labored respirations)	Indicative of marked increase in work of breathing.
Retractions (inward pulling of soft parts of chest cage – suprasternal, substernal, intercostal, subcostal – at inspiration)	Reflect significant increase in negative intrathoracic pressure necessary to inflate stiff, noncompliant lung; infants attempt to increase lung compliance by using accessory muscles; markedly decreases lung expansion; seesaw respirations are seen when chest flattens with inspiration and abdomen bulges; retractions increase work and O_2 need of breathing, so that assisted ventilation may be necessary due to exhaustion.
Flaring nares (inspiratory dilatation of nostrils)	Compensatory mechanism that attempts to lessen resistance of narrow nasal passage.

Table 25–2   Clinical Findings Associated with Respiratory Distress Cont'd

Clinical picture	Significance
Expiratory grunt (Valsalva maneuver in which infant exhales against closed glottis, thus producing audible moan)	Produces increase in transpulmonary pressure, which decreases or prevents atelectasis, thus improving oxygenation and alveolar ventilation; intubation should not be attempted unless infant's condition is rapidly deteriorating, because it prevents this maneuver and allows aveoli to collapse.
Rhythmic movement of body with labored respirations (chin tug, head bobbing, retractions of anal area)	Result of utilization of abdominal and other respiratory accessory muscles during prolonged forced respirations.
Auscultation of chest reveals decreased air exchange with harsh breath sounds and fine inspiratory rales, posterior lung base	Decrease in breath sounds and distant quality may indicate air or fluid occupying chest.
Cardiovascular system Continuous systolic murmur may be audible	Patent ductus arteriosus is common occurrence with hypoxia, pulmonary vasoconstriction, right-to-left shunting, and congestive heart failure.
Heart rate usually within normal limits (fixed heart rate may occur with a rate of 110–120/min)	Fixed heart rate indicates decrease in vagal control.
Hypothermia	Inadequate functioning of metabolic processes that require oxygen to produce necessary body heat.
Muscle tone Flaccid, hypotonic, unresponsive to stimuli Hypertonia and/or seizure activity	May indicate deterioration in neonate's condition and possible CNS damage, due to hypoxia, acidemia, or hemorrhage.

premature labor and possible administration of glucocorticoids to enhance fetal lung development (see p. 547). Postnatally, supportive medical management consists of ventilatory therapy, transcutaneous oxygen monitoring, correction of acid-base imbalance, environmental temperature regulation, adequate nutrition, and protection from infection. Ventilatory therapy is directed toward prevention of hypoventilation and hypoxia. Mild cases of RDS may require only increased humidified oxygen concentrations. Use of continuous positive airway pressure (CPAP) or continuous negative pressure (CNP) methods may be required in moderately afflicted infants. Severe cases of RDS require mechanical ventilatory assistance, with or without positive end-expiratory pressure (PEEP) (Figure 25–6). Criteria for instituting respirator support are included in Table 25–3.

The neonatal nurse bases the plan of care on the assessment of the clinical parameters, implements therapeutic approaches to maintain physiologic homeostasis, and provides supportive care to the neonate with RDS (see the Nursing Care Plan on respiratory distress syndrome).

Transient Tachypnea of the Newborn (Type II Respiratory Distress Syndrome)

Some newborns, primarily AGA preterm and near-term infants, develop progressive respiratory distress that re-

sembles classic RDS. These infants have usually sustained some intrauterine or intrapartal asphyxia, because of maternal oversedation, cesarean delivery, maternal bleeding, prolapsed cord, breech delivery, or maternal diabetes. The resultant effect on the neonate is failure to clear the airway of lung fluid, mucus, and other debris or an excess of fluid in the lungs due to aspiration of amniotic or tracheal fluid.

Clinical manifestations—expiratory grunting, flaring of the nares, mild cyanosis, and tachypnea—occur during the first days of life. (The expiratory grunting is an attempt to eject as much of the trapped alveolar air as possible; in true RDS the grunt is an attempt to retain as much air as possible in an effort to maintain alveolar expansion.) Rales are absent but breath sounds are decreased. After 6 hours, symptoms progressively improve.

Usually little or no difficulty is experienced at the onset of breathing. In room air, cyanosis may be noted and ambient O$_2$ concentrations as high as 70% may be required to correct the condition. Unlike infants with RDS, whose oxygen requirements increase in the first 48 hours, Type II infants are easily oxygenated during the first 8 hours and their oxygen requirements may decrease during this time.

Radiographs are characterized by generalized overexpansion of the lungs (hyperaeration of alveoli), which is identifiable principally by flattened contours of the diaphragm. Dense streaks (increased vascularity) radiate from the hilar region. These perihilar streaks may represent en-

FIGURE 25–6 Infant on respirator.

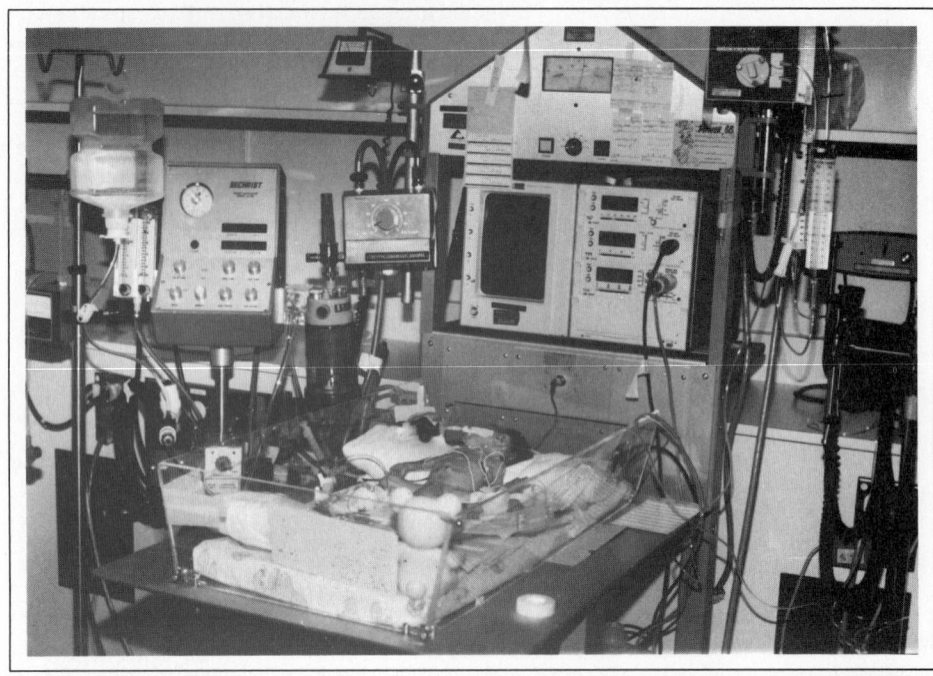

gorgement of the lymphatics, which participate in clearance of alveolar liquid upon initiation of air breathing. Occasionally one or more dense patches indicate areas of collapse and/or large fluid accumulations. Initial x-rays may be identical to those showing HMD within the first 3 hours. The infants should be improving by 24–48 hours, except for modest O_2 dependence (less than 30%). The duration of the clinical course of transient tachypnea is approximately 4 days (96 hours). Early acidosis, both respiratory and metabolic (as evidenced by a Pco_2 less than 50 mm), is easily corrected. Ventilatory assistance is rarely needed, and most of these infants survive.

Radiographs are usually normal within a week and the infant is well within 2–5 days. If progressive deterioration occurs to the extent that assisted ventilation is required, a diagnosis of superimposed sepsis must be considered and treatment measures initiated. For nursing actions, see the Nursing Care Plan on respiratory distress syndrome, p. 801.

Meconium Aspiration Syndrome

The presence of meconium in amniotic fluid is often considered a reflection of an asphyxial insult to the neonate. The physiologic response to asphyxia is increased intestinal peristalsis, relaxation of the anal sphincter, and passage of meconium into the amniotic fluid. As the victims of intrauterine asphyxia, meconium-stained neonates or newborns who have aspirated meconium are often depressed at birth and require resuscitative efforts to establish adequate respiratory effort. Prolonged labor is also associated

with meconium aspiration syndrome (MAS). MAS is a respiratory distress condition, primarily of term, SGA, and postterm infants.

CLINICAL MANIFESTATIONS

Clinical manifestations of MAS include: (a) fetal hypoxia in utero a few days or a few minutes prior to delivery, as indicated by a sudden increase in fetal activity followed by diminished activity, slowing of fetal heart rate or weak and irregular heartbeat, and meconium staining of amniotic fluid; and (b) presence of signs of distress at delivery, such as pallor, cyanosis, apnea, slow heartbeat and low Apgar scores (below 6) at 1 and 5 minutes. The literature indicates that passage of meconium in breech presentation *or* vertex presentation suggests fetal distress.

The newborn's clinical course is as follows: Blood gases indicate varying degrees of mixed respiratory acidosis and metabolic acidosis, hypoxia, and respiratory problems (usually subsiding in 48 hours, although they may persist for 6–7 days).

Presence of meconium in the lungs produces a ball-valve action (air is allowed in but not exhaled), so that alveoli overdistend; rupture with pneumonediastinum or pneumothorax is a common occurrence (Bacsik, 1977). The meconium also initiates a chemical pneumonitis in the lung with oxygen and carbon dioxide trapping and hyperinflation. Secondary bacterial pneumonias are common (Bancalari and Berlin, 1978). The chest x-ray film reveals nonuniform, coarse, patchy densities and hyperinflation (nine to eleven rib expansion) (Gregory and Gooding, 1971).

(Text continues on p. 814.)

Table 25–3 Assisted Ventilatory Methods

Types	Functions and rationale	Nursing interventions
Transpulmonary pressure maintenance	Alveolar instability and collapse are prevented by continuous application of transpulmonary pressure	Check infant for proper sealing at neck and attempt to prevent skin breakdown
Continuous negative pressure (CNP)	Applied around chest wall while neonate is able to maintain spontaneous respirations; air leaks in system pull in cool room air and cool infant Head compartment contains plastic neck sealing ring; place oxygen hood over head for deliverance of heated oxygen, easy access for suction, resuscitation, and feeding Body compartment contains thorax and rest of body exposed to negative pressure Utilization of CNP depends on deterioration in arterial blood gases and clinical condition Disadvantages include cumbersome apparatus that makes provision of care logistically difficult; may also impede venous return to heart by negative pressure about chest wall Advantages include decreased incidence of bronchopulmonary dysplasia; no increase in incidence of pneumothorax; no need for endotracheal intubation (unless positive ventilation is also used)	Maintain proper oxygen concentration by adequately sealing neck compartment and checking oxygenation concentration Check neck seal, plastic sleeve parts, and end access part for air leaks Check infant's skin temperature for indications of cold stress Organize care to decrease number of accesses to body compartment in order to decrease cold stress and maintain constant pressure Observe for alterations in cardiac functions with application or alteration of CNP: cardiac rate, rhythm, and regularity; alteration in blood pressure; peripheral circulation (color, capillary filling); metabolic acidosis
Continuous positive airway pressure (CPAP)	Application of gas with greater than atmospheric pressure to airway during spontaneous respiratory effort Infant must have spontaneous respirations, because apnea is absolute criterion for assisted ventilation; persistently low Pao_2 (below 50 while breathing 50%–60% O_2) (Avery, 1981), and repeated apneic episodes are criteria for CPAP application*	Maintain CPAP system through knowledge of elements of system and function of each
Positive end-expiratory pressure (PEEP) (application of positive pressure to airway during expiratory phase of ventilatory assistance)	Utilization of CPAP or PEEP indicated by evaluation of arterial blood gases and clinical condition	Record pressure being maintained by reading pressure gauge and filling anesthesia bag every 15 min and when necessary; monitor oxygen concentration as ordered; check patency of delivery system (orotracheal and nasotracheal tubes, nasal prongs, face mask, head hoods, etc.) Maintain water level in ''pop-off'' bottle at specified level

* The criteria for instituting CPAP or controlled ventilation are somewhat arbitrary and vary from institution to institution. Clinical assessments of severity of respiratory distress, transcutaneous monitoring of Po_2, rate of rise of Pco_2, oxygen requirements, and frequency or duration of apneic episodes are essential.

Table 25-3   Assisted Ventilatory Methods cont'd

Types	Functions and rationale	Nursing interventions
		Evaluate response of infant to CPAP application or adjustment by arterial blood gases and by clinical condition (same as for evaluation under oxygen therapy) As a general rule, first decrease concentrations of oxygen, then slowly reduce pressure until neonate is able to maintain adequate arterial oxygenation with CPAP system at 3 cm H_2O
Assisted ventilation ventilators Pressure-cycled respirators (operate by cessation of inspiratory phase when preset pressure has been reached) (see Figure 25-6)	Tidal volume and compliance of thorax and lungs is smaller in infants than adults; tidal volume is variable for newborn (20–30 mL) and preterm infant (5–12 mL)	Understand and maintain type of ventilatory support; check and record patency of system and respirator parameters (at least every hour), rate, volume, pressure, oxygen concentrations
Volume-cycled respirators (deliver predetermined volume of air with each respiratory cycle; pressure is developed within system so that delivery of a known volume to a stiff lung increases pressure within system)	Pressures needed to inflate lungs of normal infant are 5–10 cm H_2O; conditions that decrease lung compliance, such as atelectasis, respiratory distress syndrome, and meconium aspiration syndrome, require higher pressures to acquire given tidal volume; with utilization of increased pressures, there is increased incidence of complications (see p. 808)	Maintain tight seal if face mask is used for artificial ventilation (as well as CPAP) Check around face mask for air leaks Massage underlying skin every hour to prevent excoriation Check integrity of skin and note any reddened areas, any blanched or cyanotic pressure points, and naso-oropharynx suctioning
Time-cycled respirators (utilized by adjustment of inspiratory and expiratory phases of respiration)	Indications for use of mechanical ventilation are* 1. Apnea—absolute indication. 2. Hypoxia—evidenced by Pao_2 less than 50 mm Hg (torr) when breathing 60%–100% O_2 (on CPAP). 3. Hypercarbia—evidenced by $Paco_2$ greater than 65 mm Hg (torr) or rapidly rising respiratory acidosis (pH less than 7.20)	Keep bag breathing device and mask at bedside in the event of mechanical failure of ventilator or accidental or necessary extubation; if mechanical failure occurs, support neonate with bag and mask until corrections are made (an indispensable member of team is respiratory therapy department) For reintubation, keep proper size of tracheal tube at bedside Evaluate response of infant to assisted ventilation or adjustments within system by arterial blood gas determinations and by clinical condition (same as for evaluations under oxygen therapy)

NURSING CARE PLAN
Respiratory Distress Syndrome

PATIENT DATA BASE

History

Preterm delivery

Gestational history: recent episodes of fetal or intrapartal stress (that is, maternal hypotension, bleeding, maternal and resulting fetal oversedation)

Any event capable of severe fetal lung circulation compromise

Neonatal history: birth asphyxia resulting in acute hypoxia, exposure to extremes of hypothermia

Familial tendency

Physical examination

At birth or within 2 hours, rapid development initially of tachypnea (over 60 respirations/min), expiratory grunting (audible), or intercostal retractions

Followed by flaring of nares on inspiration, cyanosis and pallor, signs of increased air hunger (apneic spells, hypotonus), rhythmic movement of body and labored respirations, chin tug

Auscultation: initially breath sounds may be normal; then there is decreased air exchange with harsh breath sounds and, upon deep inspiration, rales; later there is a low-pitched systolic murmur indicative of patent ductus in infants

Increasing oxygen concentration requirements to maintain adequate Po_2 levels

Laboratory evaluation

Arterial blood gases (indicating respiratory failure): Pao_2 less than 50 mm Hg while breathing 100% O_2 and Pco_2 above 70 mm Hg.

X-ray: Diffuse reticulogranular density bilaterally, with air-filled tracheobronchial tube outlined by opaque lungs on air bronchogram; miliary atelectasis/hypoexpansion is present; in severe cases, opacification of lung fields may be seen due to massive atelectasis, diffuse alveoli infiltrates, or pulmonary edema

Clinical course worsens first 24–48 hours after birth and persists for more than 24 hours

Nursing Priorities

1. Assure adequate oxygenation.

2. Provide for assisted ventilatory exchange.

3. Determine and correct acid-base imbalances.

4. Take supportive measures to maintain homeostasis — maintain neutral thermal environment, provide for adequate fluid and electrolyte and caloric requirements, prevent infection.

5. Provide for the emotional needs of the infant with respiratory distress without overstimulation and meet the needs of the family.

6. Observe possible complications of therapy and institute appropriate nursing interventions.

FAMILY EDUCATIONAL FOCUS

1. Discuss the significance of respiratory distress syndrome for the health of their newborn.

2. Explain treatment modalities and their rationale.

3. Explore possible long-term implications of RDS, such as need for prolonged hospitalizations even after acute episode, and possible complications of respiratory management, such as bronchopulmonary dysplasia and retrolental fibroplasia.

4. Refer parents to available resources and support groups.

5. Provide opportunities to discuss questions and individual concerns about their individual neonate.

Problem	Nursing interventions and actions	Rationale
Oxygen concentration	Maintain on respiratory and cardiac monitors—note rates every 30–60 min and when necessary. Check and calibrate all monitoring and measuring devices every 8 hr. Calibrate oxygen devices to 21% and 100% O_2 concentrations. Control and monitor oxygen concentrations at least every hour. Administer oxygen by: 1. Isolette or incubator (oxygen tubing is placed inside incubator).	Stable concentration of oxygen is necessary to maintain Pao_2 within normal limits (50–70 mm). Sudden increase or decrease in O_2 concentration may result in disproportionate increase or decrease in Pao_2 due to vasoconstriction in response to oxygen. Incubators may reach 70% or more concentration but fluctuate when portholes are opened for caregiving

NURSING CARE PLAN cont'd
Respiratory Distress Syndrome

Problem	Nursing interventions and actions	Rationale
	2. Oxygen hood—a small transparent head hood that contains an inlet and carbon dioxide outlet (Figure 25-7).	Used when high concentration of oxygen (over 35%) is needed or when observations indicate that infant is unable to tolerate oxygen fluctuations. Provides a constant oxygen environment.
	Maintain infant in stable oxygen concentration by increasing or decreasing by 5%–10% increments and then obtain arterial blood gases.	
Fluctuation in oxygen environment	Response of infant to therapy is evaluated by arterial blood gases, transcutaneous oxygen monitoring and clinical assessment	
	Observe for:	
	1. Pink color, cyanosis (central or acrocyanosis), duskiness, pallor.	
	2. Respiratory effort (evaluation at rest), rate of respirations, patterns (apnea, periodic breathing), quality (easy, unlabored, abdominal, labored), auscultation (site of breath sounds—overall or part of lung fields—describe quality of breath sounds every 1–2 hr), accompanying sounds with respiratory effort (change from previous observations).	
	3. Activity—less active, flaccid, lethargic, unresponsive; increased activity, restless, irritable; inability to tolerate exertion, crying, sucking, or nursing care activity.	

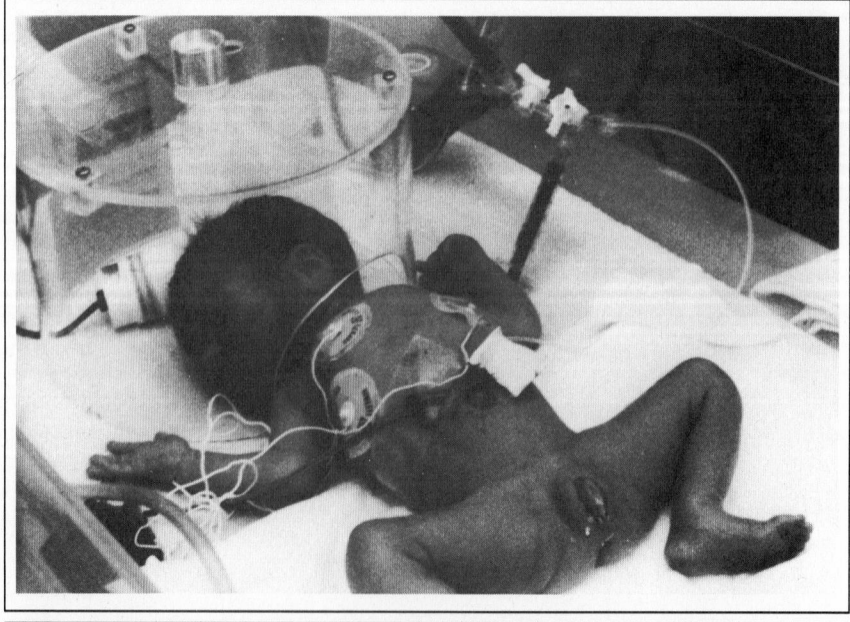

FIGURE 25–7 Infant in oxygen hood.

NURSING CARE PLAN cont'd
Respiratory Distress Syndrome

Problem	Nursing interventions and actions	Rationale
	4. Circulatory response (evaluate at rest), rate, regularity and rhythm of heart rate, periods of bradycardia, alterations of blood pressure.	
	Position infant with head slightly hyperextended.	
	Observations of clinical condition are taken serially for comparison and for changes.	
	Observations should be taken while infant is receiving oxygen and with any oxygen adjustment.	
	Return O_2 concentration to previous levels if there is deterioration in neonate's condition or drop below desired tcm levels. Repeat arterial blood gases (keep Pao_2 50–70 mm Hg). Gases should be done within 15–20 min after any change in ambient O_2 concentration or after inspiratory or expiratory pressure changes.	Any deterioration of clinical condition with oxygen adjustments (usually a decrease in ambient oxygen concentration) indicates inability of neonate to compensate for hypoxia.
	Record and report clinical observations and action taken.	
Humidification of inspired oxygen	Provide humidified gas.	Oxygen is dry gas and therefore irritating to airways.
		Evaporative water losses from skin and lungs are also decreased in high humidity (50%–65%).
	Pay careful attention to infection control by cleaning and replacing nebulizers/humidifiers at least every 24 hr; use sterile tubing and replace every 24 hr; use sterile distilled water.	The warm, moist environment found in Isolettes and with O_2 equipment promotes growth of microorganisms.
Warmed mist delivery	Provide heated mist (at the delivery site) 31–34C. Place a thermometer in the oxygen hood and monitor the temperature of the delivered gas. Oxyhood and Isolette temperature should be maintained at the same temperature.	Cold air/oxygenation blown in face of newborn is source of cold stress and is stimulus for increased consumption of oxygen and increased metabolic rate.
	Observe infant for temperature instability and signs of increased oxygen consumption (need for increased O_2 concentration) and metabolic acidosis.	
Monitoring of arterial blood gas values	Maintain stable environment prior to collection of arterial blood gas sample:	Values used to determine adequate oxygenation—normal Pao_2 50–70 mm Hg. Adequate ventilation—normal $Paco_2$ 30–45 mm. Acid-base balance—normal pH 7.35–7.45.
	1. Maintain constant O_2 concentration at least 15–20 min before sample.	Accurate arterial blood determinations are essential in management of any infant receiving oxygen, because presence or absence of cyanosis is unreliable.
	2. Avoid any disturbances of infant 15 min before gases are drawn.	Crying or struggling may cause hyperventilation or breath holding and may increase shunting of blood.
	Do not suction; if suction is absolutely necessary, delay blood sample.	

Problem	Nursing interventions and actions	Rationale
	Maintain a warm temperature (pH should be measured at body temperature).	
	Provide arterial blood gas setup (a 3 mL syringe with heparinized solution and a heparinized tuberculin syringe) to obtain blood sample.	Utilization of temporal, radial, or brachial arteries takes skill and is time-consuming; therefore, most common technique for sampling is through umbilical artery catheter (Procedure 25-2, p. 811).
	After blood sample is taken, recheck flow through line to assure patency and prevent establishment of clot.	
	Replace blood used to clear line.	Total blood volume of infant is small; blood removed to clear catheter must be returned to prevent hypovolemia, anemia.
	Use heparinized flush solution before restarting IV solution to prevent clots in the line	
Inadequate ventilation	Initial observation of respiratory effort, ventilatory adequacy — observation of chest wall movement, skin, mucous membranes, color; estimation of degree and equality of air entry by auscultation, arterial blood gases, and pH determination.	Alveoli of normal infant remain stable during expiration due to presence of surfactant. Alveoli of infant with RDS lack surfactant and collapse with expiration. Grunting, a compensatory mechanism, increases transpulmonary pressure, overcomes high surface tension, forces and prevents atelectasis, and thus enables improved oxygenation and a rise in Pao_2. Application of CPAP or PEEP produces same stabilization force on alveoli as grunting does and produces same effect — improved oxygenation and rise in Pao_2.
	Assess need for assisted ventilatory measures. Criteria for assisted ventilation: 1. Apnea. 2. Hypoxia (Pao_2 50 in 50%-60% oxygen) 3. Alert doctor if following criterion for assist is met: respiratory acidosis, pH 7.20.	
	See Table 25-3 for specific nursing management.	
Intubation (placement and patency of oral/nasal intubation tube)	Set up for endo/nasotracheal intubation and assist (see Procedure 25-1).	Delivery of CPAP or PEEP can only be done by use of nasal prongs, nasopharyngeal tube, or oral intubation.
	Apply nasal prongs, and set up with respiratory therapist.	
	Set up CPAP or PEEP (see Table 25-3) Position infant in "sniffing" position. See Figure 25-2 for intubation.	
	Attempts at intubation should not exceed 30 sec and should be terminated with evidence of hypoxia and bradycardia.	
	Determine proper placement of tube by presence and quality of breath sounds. If breath sounds are better on one side, tube may be in right main stem bronchus; slowly withdraw tube and auscultate chest for equal bilateral breath sounds.	
	Extubate if breath sounds are heard over stomach. Reoxygenate prior to another intubation attempt.	Tube is in esophagus.
	Tube is properly placed if chest moves symmetrically, infant cannot cry, color and muscle tone improve with effective oxygenation.	
	Improvement of heart rate and rhythm with effective oxygenation.	
	Chest x-ray confirmation.	

Problem	Nursing interventions and actions	Rationale
Production of and accumulation of secretion	Care of intubated neonate: 1. Observe type of secretions and ease of removal. 2. Because nasal passages are bypassed, provide humidity and moisture within system and better systemic hydration to avoid drying secretions and decreasing ciliary movement. 3. Change infant's position every 1–2 hr to maintain adequate ventilation, drain lung secretions, and promote skin integrity. 4. Secure and maintain with tape a properly positioned tube. 5. Observe nasal passage for position and deformity. Keep tube in neutral position without pulling on alae nasi. Observe for blanched area around nasal tube and reposition until blanching disappears. If oral tube is used, maintain neutral position within mouth. Observe color and integrity of gums; if blanched, reposition tube until blanching is relieved. 6. Auscultate breath sounds and observe arterial blood gas values and integrity of skin. 7. Suction to remove secretions (see Procedure 25–3). Check working order of each suction machine and pressure setting so that it will be in working order when needed.	Accumulation of humidity or secretions within tracheal tube decreases effective ventilation, increases Pco_2, and leads to clotted tube (airway). Maintenance of clear tube is especially important with pressure-cycled ventilators, because increased secretions decrease diameter of tube, increase resistance to gas flow, increase pressure within system (possibly to dangerous levels), and decrease tidal volume delivered.
	Tracheal tube suction should last no longer than 5–10 sec.	Apnea or bradycardia will occur if suction is longer than 15–20 sec.
	After each suction attempt, ventilate for a few breaths with pressures 25% above that routinely used for inspiration, to reinflate atelectatic areas. Observe and record: 1. Tolerance of neonate to suction procedure — color change, cyanosis or remains pink, cardiac changes, bradycardia, arrhythmia; evidence of spontaneous respiratory effort (or lack of) when off respirator for suction. 2. Time of suction. 3. Amount and type of secretions — thick, clear, bloody, green mucus. 4. Frequency of suction is determined by clinical assessment — amount and type of secretions in relation to frequency of suction.	Hypoxic insult with drop in Pao_2 occurs during suction efforts. Suction, the application of negative pressure to the airway, decreases pulmonary compliance by 50% and tidal volume. Suction creates pulmonary atelectasis.

Problem	Nursing interventions and actions	Rationale
	Observe for incidence of infection as noted by random culture and incidence of acquired pulmonary infection.	
	Carry out percussion and postural drainage every 2 hr with frequent turning of infant. Suction after percussion	Prevents stasis of secretions and promotes drainage.
Danger of extubation	Observe for symptoms of extubation (cyanosis, apnea, respiratory difficulty, bradycardia, no audible breath sounds). Whether accidental or symptomatic of a clogged tube, these conditions warrant *immediate* removal of ineffective tube and respiratory support with bag and mask until reintubation. Insert nasogastric tube (if not present) to decompress stomach.	
Weaning from assisted ventilation	Observe for signs of improvement in respiratory status and ability to have ventilatory support weaned and discontinued: 1. Evaluate blood gas determinations. 2. Observe toleration of lower O_2 concentrations and pressures. 3. Watch for evidence of spontaneous respirations—when ventilator is discontinued for suction; spontaneous respiratory effort against ''set rate'' of respirator; ability to assist ventilator by spontaneous respirations.	Criteria for weaning and ultimate discontinuance of ventilator: 1. Normal blood gas values—especially Pao_2, which is indicative of adequate oxygenation. 2. Decrease in ventilation pressures. 3. Decrease in O_2 concentrations. 4. Increased activity, muscle tone, and efforts at simultaneous respirations.
Maintenance of homeostasis Thermoregulation	See p. 647	Increase in respiratory rate results in chemical thermogenesis (burning brown fat to maintain body temperature), which increases O_2 needs and insensible H_2O loss in already compromised infant.
Correction of acid-base imbalance Respiratory acidosis	Maintain adequate ventilation and excretion of returned CO_2 from the lungs by monitoring blood gases and regulating ventilatory assistance mechanisms per physician's orders.	Correction of acidosis is essential to maintain homeostasis. Acidosis is powerful pulmonary vasoconstrictor, decreases pulmonary blood flow, and may upset surfactant synthesis. Acidosis dissociates bilirubin from albumin binding sites and predisposes to kernicterus at low bilirubin levels. Acidosis is a central nervous system depressant that depresses respiratory center, which causes increase in CO_2 retention and hypoxia.
Metabolic acidosis	Treat with volume replacement and cautious administration of bicarbonate	
Provision for adequate fluid, caloric, and electrolyte requirements	Maintain IV rate at prescribed level; record type and amount of fluid infused hourly. Use infusion pump. Observe vital signs for signs of too rapid infusion. Maintain normal urine output (1-3 mL/kg/hr). Maintain specific	Fluids are provided to sick neonate by intravenous route and are calculated to replace sensible and insensible water losses as well as evaporative losses due to tachypnea. Overload of circulatory system by too much

Problem	Nursing interventions and actions	Rationale
	gravity of urine between 1.006 and 1.012. Take daily weights.	or too rapid administration of fluid causes pulmonary edema and cardiac embarrassment that may be fatal.
	Manage route of IV administration	
	With umbilical catheter: Protect catheter from strain or tension (see Procedure 25-2). Restrain as necessary. Prevent dislodgement of catheter. Always keep catheter and stopcock on top of bed linens so they are easily visible.	Greater nutritional fluid is required because of energy needed to cope with stress. Stressed infants are predisposed to hypoglycemia because of increased metabolic demands as well as reduced glycogen stores and decreased ability to convert fat and protein to glucose.
	Observe for occlusion of vessels by clot and for vasospasm — discoloration of skin, discoloration of toes or feet (blanching or cyanosis). If discoloration occurs, contralateral foot may be wrapped with warm cloth, but this is controversial. Removal of catheter is preferred (Korones, 1981).	Vasospasm in unwrapped foot will be relieved by treatment, and the discoloration will disappear and toes will be pink. If discoloration persists, clot may be occluding vessel — catheter must be removed, or loss of extremity is possible.
	Observe for signs of infection or sepsis: temperature instability, drainage, redness or foul odor from cord, lethargy, irritability, vomiting, poor feeding, hypotonia.	
	Peripheral IV in scalp or extremity vein: Prepare equipment, insert IV in vein, and restrain infant.	
	Vessel chosen is artery if it pulsates. Place peripheral IV in vein (which doesn't pulsate).	Very small arteries may not pulsate and arterial area will blanch if saline is infused.
	Maintain proper placement of IV.	Ability to aspirate blood and/or easily inject small amount of saline indicates patent IV. Infiltration is evaluated by area of edema and redness about site, inability to obtain blood on aspiration, or difficulty in injecting through IV line.
	Advance as soon as possible from intravenous to oral feelings. Gavage or nipple feedings are utilized, and IV is used as supplement (discontinued when oral intake is sufficient) (see Procedure 24-1).	
	Provide adequate caloric intake: amount of intake, type of formula, route of administration, and need for supplementation of intake by other routes.	Calories are essential to prevent catabolism of body proteins and metabolic acidosis due to starvation or inadequate caloric intake.
	Plan care at minimal energy and oxygen needs.	
	Take daily weight measurement.	
	Blood pH remains normal (no metabolic acidosis).	
	Measure urine output and specific gravity.	
	Observe for hypocalcemia.	Hypocalcemia and hypoglycemia result from delayed or inadequate caloric intake and stress.
	Observe for hypoglycemia: Dextrostix below 45 mg, urine screening.	
	Observe for hyperglycemia: Dextrostix above 130 mg, urine screening: increased urine output (osmotic diuresis), sugar in urine with Dipstix and Clinitest.	

Problem	Nursing interventions and actions	Rationale
	Treatment—glucose is highest priority (calcium is next). Usually 10% calcium gluconate is administered.	
Prevention of infection	See section on sepsis nursing care, p. 842.	Decreased lung expansion predisposed to atelectasis and secondary superimposed infections.
Provision of stimulatory needs of infant	Plan care to allow for rest periods to avoid exhausting infant.	
Support of family	Explain procedures to family. Facilitate parental participation in infant's care even if critically ill.	(See p. 772 for a discussion of parenting high-risk infants.)
Complications of respiratory therapy		
Retrolental fibroplasia	Maintain O_2 at prescribed levels, usually below 70–80 mm Hg Pao_2. Make arterial blood gas determinations 15–30 min after adjustment of settings.	Oxygen toxicity results in damage to retina.
	Monitor O_2 concentration every 4 hr minimum	
	If possible, periodically check fundi during O_2 therapy; definitely check at time of discharge.	
	Perform frequent eye examination for at least 3 months.	
Residual pulmonary disease	Observe for residual pulmonary disease (usually in recovery phase from initial disease): dependence on oxygen to overcome cyanosis and remain pink; low Pao_2 in room air; inability to tolerate exertion of care, sucking, or crying; and increase in cyanosis and respiratory distress.	Positive pressure ventilation and endotracheal intubation may result in additional respiratory distress.
	Obtain chest x-ray.	Confirms diagnosis.
Bronchopulmonary dysplasia	Prevent respiratory distress attack. Maintain minimal levels of ambient O_2 concentration and minimal pressure levels.	Positive pressure ventilation may result in pathologic condition of pulmonary epithelium.
	Organize nursing care to decrease disturbance, conserve energy, and prevent increased respiratory distress and O_2 requirements.	
	Practice caution when feeding neonate.	Abdominal distention, which results in upward pressure on thoracic cavity, is prevented and thus respiratory embarrassment is prevented. Respiratory distress decreases after feeding.
	Schedule frequent, small feedings.	
	Naso-orogastric tube feeding may be utilized for respiratory distress or tachypnea associated with sucking; handle gently and maintain constant ambient oxygen concentrations.	Prevents aspiration and reduces energy requirements associated with feedings.
	Position properly to maintain open airway and to facilitate maximal chest expansion: elevate head of bed; a shoulder roll may prevent the neck from flexing on the chest and obstructing the trachea; turn head to either side; change and rotate position every 1–2 hr.	Gravitational downward position of diaphragm and abdominal contents allows for maximal lung expansion.

Problem	Nursing interventions and actions	Rationale
Interstitial pulmonary emphysema	Frequently auscultate breath sounds (presence and quality) to locate emphysema. Assemble appropriate equipment for air evacuation — needle aspiration syringe, needle, and stopcock — and for thoracotomy — tray, chest drainage, and suction apparatus. Assist with thoracentesis procedure and insertion of chest tubes.	Knowledge of location of pulmonary emphysema enables prediction and observation for impending catastrophe.
Pneumothorax	Be alert for symptoms: 1. Sudden, unexplained deterioration in clinical condition. 2. Cyanosis. 3. Cardiac abnormalities — bradycardia, arrhythmia, or decrease in height of ECG tracing. 4. Decrease in BP. 5. Mottling of skin and shocklike appearance. 6. Diminished or absent breath sounds on affected side. 7. Shift in apical cardiac sound. 8. Bulging of chest wall on affected side. 9. Hyperresponse of affected lung on percussion.	When alveoli are overdistended by excessive intraalveolar pressure, they rupture and leak air into the thoracic cavity.
	Transluminate chest wall and obtain chest x-ray films.	Confirm diagnosis of pneumothorax.
	Assist with resuscitative measures: 1. 100% O_2 by plastic oxygen hood or bag or mask. 2. Needle aspiration of pleural cavity. 3. Utilization of water-seal drainage. Assist with insertion of chest tubes.	Aids in resolution of air in pleural space and prevents further accumulation. Thoracentesis and chest tube insertion removes trapped air and fluid, returns negative pressure to thoracic cavity, removes tension, and facilitates expansion.
	Observe for oscillation of fluid level in chest tubes. Cessation of oscillation occurs if: 1. Lung has reexpanded. 2. Blood or fibrin clot occludes tube (before lung has reexpanded).	Water-seal drainage provides for escape of air and fluid into drainage bottle. Water acts as seal and keeps air from being drawn back into chest. Oscillation of water level in tubing shows that there is effective communication between pleural cavity and drainage bottle.
	Obtain serial x-rays.	Ascertains degree of lung involvement; visualizes effect of treatment.
	Observe for development of complications: 1. Hemorrhage — hourly observation of chest tube drainage for color, amount, and consistency. Observe for rapid increase in amount of drainage. Total and record amount of chest tube drainage every 8 hr. 2. Pneumothorax due to air leak into pleural cavity. Notify medical staff immediately of development of complication.	
Other pulmonary complications: pneumomediastinum, pneumopericardium, and pneumoperitoneum	Observe for signs of air dissection into the neck (pneumomediastinum); crepitus — a crackling feeling and noise of the skin when light pressure is applied; appearance of fullness to the neck (looks like a bullfrog).	Collection of air in the mediastinum either anterior to the heart or laterally compresses the mediastinal pleurae. Air may dissect into soft tissue of the neck.

NURSING CARE PLAN cont'd
Respiratory Distress Syndrome

Problem	Nursing interventions and actions	Rationale
	Observe for symptoms of compromised cardiac function.	Massive collection of air around the heart results in compression of vena cava, tachypnea, and cyanosis.
	Observe for abdominal distention and tenderness.	Collection of air in peritoneal cavity must be differentiated from perforated viscus.
Cardiac complication— patent ductus arteriosus	Observe for symptoms of alteration in cardiac output: alteration in blood pressure, peripheral circulation (color and capillary filling), metabolic acidosis.	Alteration in cardiac output is possible, because application of positive pressure may impede venous return to heart.
	Observe for clinical findings of patent ductus arteriosus: continuous murmur (most often audible in small preterms); bounding peripheral pulses; signs of congestive heart failure— tachypnea, tachycardia, cyanosis, edema (weight gain), intolerance of exertion, cardiomegaly.	Failure of ductus arteriosus to close after birth, with resultant left-to-right shunting (if ductus is large enough) and hemodynamic changes, leads to congestive heart failure.
	See Chapter 26 for care of infant with cardiac anomaly.	Persistence of ductus may occur in preterm infants (due to musculature), in preterm infants with RDS (associated with hypoxemia), and as a complication of positive pressure therapy (period of improvement followed by deterioration).

Persistent pulmonary hypertension (see discussion p. 816)

NURSING CARE EVALUATION

Oxygen therapy is discontinued and no apnea, cyanosis, or other complications are evident.	Parents understand need for continued medical supervision.
Infant is afebrile and vital signs are stable.	Parents are aware of available parent groups for assistance after discharge.
Infant is gaining weight or stabilized at desired discharge weight and tolerating food and fluids.	Referral is completed to public health nurse and other community resources.
Parent-infant bonding is appropriate.	

NURSING DIAGNOSES*	SUPPORTING DATA	
1. Impaired gas exchange related to inadequate lung surfactant	Hypoxemia Hypercarbia Acidemia Respiratory failure Altered level of infant activity	Cyanosis Increased respiratory effort Expiratory grunting Retractions
2. Potential alteration in fluid volume associated with disease process, parental fluid therapy	Abnormal urinary output Abnormal daily weights Symptoms of pulmonary edema Electrolyte imbalance	
3. Potential alteration in nutrition: Less than body requirements related to increased metabolic needs of stressed infant	Hypoglycemia Hypocalcemia Decreased daily weight	
4. Anxiety in infant related to frequent intervention, invasive techniques, intensive neonatal care environment	Signs of exhaustion in infant Failure to progress through expected behavioral states Inappropriate response to tactile, visual, auditory stimuli	
5. Parental knowledge deficit related to respiratory distress syndrome	Expressed concerns and questions about the disease process, possible long-term sequelae, and available parent support groups	

* These are a few examples of nursing diagnoses that may be appropriate for an infant. It is not an inclusive list and must be individualized for each newborn.

Procedure 25-2 Umbilical Catheterization

(Umbilical arterial catheter is used for monitoring arterial pressures, for obtaining arterial blood
for blood gas studies, and for infusion in the absence of a venous line.)

Objective	Nursing action	Rationale
Assemble equipment	Obtain the following equipment: 1. IV solution and tubing. 2. Infusion pump. 3. Umbilical arterial catheter tray. 4. Sterile stopcock. 5. Solution for skin preparation. 6. Sterile No. 4-Osille suture and umbilical tape. 7. Sterile umbilical catheter — 3½–5 Fr. 8. Heparinized sterile saline in sterile syringe. 9. Sterile gloves. 10. Nonallergic tape. 11. Spotlight.	Regulates infusion. Contains equipment for insertion. Removes bacteria that may be present. Ties around umbilical stump. Inserts in umbilical artery. Used to flush tubing as necessary. Maintain sterility. Tape is less irritating to skin. To visualize field.
Prepare infant	Place infant on restraining board and provide for warmth	Prevents sudden movement. Prevents chilling.
Prepare equipment	Attach tubing to solution and hang on IV standard. Remove all air from tubing and attach to infusion pump. Open umbilical catheter tray and add skin preparation solution, suture, cord ties. Prepare gloves.	Prepares for infusion.
Monitor procedure	The infant is draped, prepped and catheter is placed Syringe containing heparinized sterile saline is attached to catheter by stopcock. IV tubing is attached to stopcock. Set prescribed rate on infusion pump. Catheter is secured by umbilical tape and suture. Secure catheter to infant with nonallergic tape. Obtain abdominal x-ray.	Procedure done by qualified personnel. Check placement of catheter.
Assess infant	Observe the following: 1. Pulse. 2. Respiration. 3. Color of legs. Notify physician immediately in case of: 1. Blanching. 2. Mottling. 3. Cyanosis. 4. Coolness of one or both legs.	Evaluates infant's status. Blood flow to extremities is disrupted.
Maintain newborn records	Record the following: 1. IV — site, type of catheter, solution. 2. Infusion flow rate. 3. Time infusion was started. 4. Infant's response.	Maintain infant's chart.

Procedure 25–3   Endotracheal Suctioning

Objective	Nursing action	Rationale
Minimize potential for pulmonary infection through cross-contamination	Assess respiratory status to determine necessity for suctioning.	Infant should be suctioned only as often as necessary to maintain patent airways and adequate oxygenation.
	Gather all necessary equipment: catheters, suction machine, disposable sterile suction tubing, saline (no preservatives), sterile syringe/needle, and gloves (not powdered). Ensure that gloves, catheters, and liquefying solutions are sterile.	In healthy individual, lower respiratory tract is free of pathogenic organisms.
	Maintain sterile technique throughout entire suctioning procedure.	
	Discard catheter, glove, and lubricant after each procedure.	Once equipment is moistened and contaminated with body flora and mucus, it becomes a culture bed for noxious organism growth.
	Set wall suction for not more than 50 mm Hg.	Mucosal hemorrhages and tissue invagination occur more frequently when higher pressure is used.
Alleviate partial or total airway obstruction in support of cell oxygenation	Prior to suctioning, preoxygenate neonate for at least 10 min with 100% O_2 or bag at level neonate was previously receiving but at a faster rate.	Suctioning physically removes oxygen from airways. In addition, it mechanically occludes airways and therefore diminishes potential for oxygenation. It usually stimulates coughing and increased work of breathing, thereby increasing tissue demand for oxygen. Presuction elevation of PaO_2 mitigates intrasuction hypoxemia.
	Position and immobilize infant (see mummy restraint) according to desired suction site.	It is quite difficult to suction alert infant successfully without restraint. A full body restraint or an assistant should be employed to ensure effective, atraumatic suctioning in infants. To suction right main bronchus, infant's head should be turned to left. To suction left main bronchus, head should be turned to right with left shoulder slightly elevated.
	Using sterile technique, don sterile glove; hook up appropriate suction catheter; lubricate tip, position catheter angle toward desired suction site.	"Whistle-tip" catheter should be used for respiratory tract suctioning, because it tends to be less traumatizing to tissues.
		Catheter size should be no more than ½ the size of lumen to be suctioned in order to minimize hypoxemia due to airway obstruction.
	Sterile normal saline in a sterile specimen cup is used.	Prelubrication of catheter is essential to minimize tissue trauma with subsequent obstructive edema.
	If infant is intubated: 1. Disconnect source of oxygenation from infant.	Suction applied while entering airway increases removal of oxygen from airways

Procedure 25-3   Endotracheal Suctioning cont'd

Objective	Nursing action	Rationale
	2. Hold endotracheal tube while suctioning. 3. Insert catheter without applied suction into tube the distance from tube opening to anatomic location of target bronchus (this can be predetermined by measuring distance externally prior to suctioning). 4. Apply suction by placing thumb of assistive hand over vent port or Y-connector (Figure 25-8).	During suctioning, tube can be easily dislodged and increases potential for tissue invagination once catheter tip passes end of tube. Placing thumb over venting device closes negative pressure system, which allows atmospheric pressure to push secretions and debris into catheter, facilitating their removal.
	5. Slowly withdraw catheter in a pill-rolling rotation. 6. Clear catheter with sterile saline.	Rotating catheter in a slow, steady fashion maximizes catheter access to secretions while minimizing potential for tissue invagination.
	7. After each suction attempt, ventilate for a few breaths with pressures 25% above that routinely used for inspiration, to reinflate atelectatic areas. 8. Repeat procedure for opposite bronchus.	Hypoxia insult with a drop in Pao_2 occurs during suction efforts. Suction, the application of negative pressure to the airway, decreases by 50% the pulmonary compliance and tidal volume. Suction creates pulmonary atelectasis.
	9. If tenacious secretions are encountered, instill 0.5 mL of 5% sodium bicarbonate or normal saline with syringe (needle-less) into tube prior to suctioning.	Instillation of sodium bicarbonate liquefies and loosens secretions by lowering surface tension and alkalating respiratory secretions. Normal saline may also be used for liquification.

FIGURE 25-8 Suctioning with endotracheal tube.

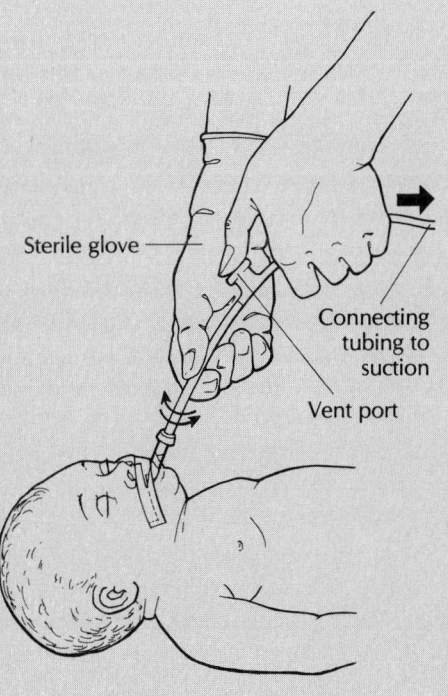

Sterile glove

Connecting tubing to suction

Vent port

Procedure 25–3 Endotracheal Suctioning cont'd

Objective	Nursing action	Rationale
	If infant is not intubated: After having failed to get infant to cough voluntarily in effective manner, follow procedure for suctioning intubated infant with these exceptions:	Suctioning to clear airways should be employed only when infant is unable to clear own airways effectively by use of cough reflex. It should be considered a last resort.
	1. Enter airway via nasopharynx, advancing catheter into trachea on inspiration.	Inspiration opens glottis and tends to entrain catheter along with inspired air.
	2. Attempt to liquefy tenacious secretions by humidification via mist tent, face mask, or hand-held nebulizer.	Achieving coordination with inspiration is often quite easy with pediatric clients, because they are frequently crying involuntarily during procedure. Instillation of liquefying agents directly into trachea in unintubated infant is not possible. Indirect means must be relied upon.
Minimize iatrogenic hypoxemia secondary to suctioning	Suction only when absolutely necessary.	Always assess need for suctioning. There should never be standing orders such as "Suction every hour."
	Limit each catheter insertion to no more than 10 sec. Reoxygenate infant with 100% O_2 between each insertion and at conclusion of procedure.	Limiting suction time and frequent reoxygenation counterbalance the mechanical obstruction of airway and removal of available oxygen.
	Remove catheter with suction applied as soon as infant begins to cough.	Holding catheter in airway while infant coughs can deprive infant of needed inspiratory volume at end of cough because of airway obstruction by catheter.
	During procedure, assess infant for signs of bradycardia.	Suctioning can cause vagal response in form of bradycardia, which, if unchecked, can lead to asystole.

The densities are associated with focal areas of irregular aeration, some of which appear atelectatic or consolidated while others appear emphysemic. These infants have massive biochemical aberrations, which include: (a) extreme metabolic acidosis resulting from the cardiopulmonary shunting and hypoperfusion; (b) extreme respiratory acidosis due to shunting and alveolar hypoventilation; and (c) extreme hypoxia, even in 100% O_2 concentrations and with ventilatory assistance. The extreme hypoxia is also caused by the cardiopulmonary shunting and resultant failure to oxygenate.

The infant may be depressed and tachypneic at birth or show no respiratory distress for several hours. Symptoms of respiratory distress, when they appear, are usually severe. Infants have tachypnea, cyanosis, hyperexpanded chest, congestive heart failure (CHF), and irregular and gasping respirations.

MANAGEMENT AT DELIVERY

The combined efforts of the obstetrician and pediatrician are needed to prevent MAS. The most effective form of preventive management is outlined as follows:

1. After the head of the neonate is delivered and the shoulders and chest are still in the birth canal, the nasopharynx and oropharynx are suctioned with a DeLee catheter. (The same procedure is followed with a cesarean delivery.)

2. Immediately after delivery of the neonate, the vocal cords should be visualized with a laryngoscope. If meconium is present, intubation and direct suctioning of the trachea through an endotracheal tube is performed.

   a. The resuscitator places his or her mouth over the endotracheal tube and sucks on the tube as it is withdrawn from the trachea (a paper mask is placed over the tube to prevent inhalation of meconium by the resuscitator).

   b. If meconium is suctioned from the trachea, the neonate is reintubated and suctioned until the airway is cleared.

   c. It is recommended that the neonate not be lavaged with normal saline once intubated, as this procedure forces the meconium into the small airways.

Failure to adequately suction on the perineum or before respiratory or resuscitative efforts are begun pushes meconium into the airway and into the lungs. Stimulation of the neonate is avoided to minimize respiratory movements. Further resuscitative efforts as indicated follow the same principles mentioned earlier in this chapter, p. 788.

MANAGEMENT IN THE NURSERY

Resuscitated neonates should be immediately transferred to the nursery for close observation and continuation of treatment. An umbilical arterial line may be used for direct monitoring of arterial blood pressures; blood sampling for pH, and blood gases; and infusion of intravenous fluids, blood, or medications.

   Treatment usually involves high ambient oxygenation and controlled ventilation. Low end-expiratory pressures (EEP) are desired to avoid air leaks. Unfortunately, high EEP pressures may be needed to cause sufficient expiratory expansion of obstructed terminal airways or stabilize airways that are weakened by inflammation so that the most distal atelectatic alveoli are ventilated. Systemic blood pressure and pulmonary blood flow must be maintained. Intravenous tolazoline (Priscoline) or isoproterenol (Isuprel) may be used to increase the pulmonary blood flow by overcoming the arterioles' vasoconstriction and pulmonary vasospasm, which has created a right-to-left cardiopulmonary shunt. Tolazoline must be used with extreme caution as dramatic falls in blood pressure can occur.

   Treatment also includes chest physiotherapy (chest percussion, vibration, and postural drainage) to remove the debris, and antibiotic therapy. Bicarbonate alkali therapy may be necessary for several days for severely ill neonates. Mortality in term or postterm infants is very high, because they are so difficult to oxygenate.

   Nursing interventions after resuscitation should include temperature regulation at 37C, Dextrostix at 2 hours of age to check for hypoglycemia, observation of intravenous fluids, calculation of necessary fluids (which may be restricted in first 48–72 hours due to cerebral edema), and provision of caloric requirements.

   The nurse carefully observes for complications such as anoxic cerebral injury manifested by cerebral edema and/or convulsions; anoxic myocardial injury evidenced by congestive heart failure or cardiomegaly; DIC resulting from hypoxic hepatic damage with depression of liver-dependent clotting factors; anoxic renal damage demonstrated by hematuria, oliguria, or anuria; fluid overload; and any signs of intestinal necrosis from ischemia, including gastrointestinal obstruction or hemorrhage.

Complications of Respiratory Therapy

Oxygen is considered a drug whose dosage and duration of administration must be regulated to prevent complications and to provide maximum benefit—reduction of hypoxia, ischemia, and infarction of vital organs. The concentration of ambient oxygen administered to the neonate must be titrated according to oxygen tension within arterial blood. Oxygen is toxic to retinal blood vessels (causing vasoconstriction, dilatation, hemorrhage, and detachment) and also to lung tissue in prolonged hyperoxic exposure. Interventions for the following conditions are explained in the Nursing Care Plan on respiratory distress syndrome, p. 801.

RETROLENTAL FIBROPLASIA

The fetal retina is unique in that its vascularization does not begin until the fourth month of gestation, with the temporal peripheral area of retinal vasculature lagging in development. Vascularization is not completed until term. Consequently, the immature vascular system is susceptible to damage in the preterm neonate and occasionally in the term neonate.

   Infants who are predisposed to developing retrolental fibroplasia are those with HMD (increased need for amount of time in oxygen and assisted ventilation) and those with multiple episodes of apnea and bradycardia even without associated RDS and other diseases such as intraventricular hemorrhage, sepsis, anemia of prematurity, and persistent pulmonary hypertension disease.

   The effect of oxygen toxicity (Po_2 over 70–100 mm Hg) on the preterm retina can be divided into two stages.

   Primary stage—vasoconstriction and vaso-obliteration. Initial response to hyperoxia is vasoconstriction. This response occurs within minutes. After a while, vessels rebound to normal caliber. Continued exposure to hyperoxia leads to endothelial cell death within the capillaries in the immature retinal vascular bed. (This is known as capillary drop-out, capillary closure, or nonperfusion.)

   Secondary stage—vasoproliferation. Following removal from the enriched oxygen atmosphere, marked proliferation of the remaining vascular elements occurs in the region of the capillary closure in the periphery of the retina. This process causes elevated arteriole venous shunts (known as demarcation lines). If the damage progresses, the A-V shunts alter the hemodynamics of the retinal vasculature, causing arteriole tortuosity and venous dilation. Intraretinal and vitreal hemorrhages may be present along with elevation of the vessels through the retina and retinal detachment due to traction and fibrous tissue formation. Eventual blindness is the end result.

BRONCHOPULMONARY DYSPLASIA

Bronchopulmonary dysplasia (BPD) is a result of direct damage to the alveolar epithelium of the lungs. The factors causing the cell destruction include: (a) positive pressure ventilation; (b) oxygen concentrations above 70%; and (c) treatment for longer than 4–5 days—although changes have been observed in neonates who have been treated for shorter periods of time. Regeneration of the epithelium begins after about 7 days of therapy, accompanied by dysplasia and changes in lung fields. This condition is rarely found in the neonate treated with negative pressure devices.

Bronchopulmonary dysplasia is characterized by airway obstruction, abnormal alveoli, pulmonary hypertension, hypoxemia, hypercarbia, and compensated respiratory acidosis. It occurs in stages (Northway et al., 1967). The first two stages are now considered by some clinicians as simply indicative of RDS with true bronchopulmonary dysplasia, or stage III, occurring on day 10–20 of respiratory distress and manifested by hypoxia and hypercarbia. On x-ray one sees generalized infiltrates and multiple cystic areas. In stage IV, the same biochemical alterations are evident, along with rales, wheezes, hepatomegaly, hypochloremia, fever without proven infection, and signs of cor pulmonale. On chest x-ray examination, hyperexpansion of the chest, cardiomegaly, and larger cystic areas alternating with streaky densities are seen.

Difficulty is often encountered in weaning the infant from the positive pressure ventilation and from long-term dependence on oxygen. Some infants may demonstrate this dependence with recurrent lower respiratory tract infections during infancy. Most infants show slow clearing of the abnormal pulmonary characteristics and have normal x-rays at 6 months to 2 years of age. A few infants develop progressive pulmonary fibrosis or cardiac disease (cor pulmonale) secondary to the pulmonary hypertension (Avery, 1981).

INTERSTITIAL PULMONARY EMPHYSEMA

Pulmonary emphysema is the pathologic accumulation of air in the tissues of the lungs. Extraalveolar air collections are most common with use of positive pressure ventilation. Air collections outside the lung are a function of compliance of the lung and utilization of increased pressures to ventilate. In interstitial pulmonary emphysema, there is air dissection along perivascular spaces but not yet into pleural space or mediastinum. This condition is a precursor of pneumothorax or pneumomediastinum.

PNEUMOTHORAX

Pneumothorax, a common complication of RDS, is an accumulation of air in the thoracic cavity between the parietal and visceral pleura (Monin and Vert, 1978). Pneumothorax occurs when alveoli are overdistended, usually by excessive intraalveolar pressure and rupture; air then leaks into the thoracic cavity. Excessive intraalveolar pressure is a result of stiff, noncompliant lungs and the use of assisted positive pressure ventilation with high inspiratory pressure. Meconium aspiration with subsequent obstruction of the airway and a ball-valve phenomenon produces poor lung compliance and trapping of air in the alveoli. In this situation, pneumothorax is a frequent complication.

Pneumothorax in the neonate causes several physiologic changes: complete collapse of the lung; compression of the heart and lungs and compromise of venous return to the right heart with mediastinal air; and development of tension in the pleural space. Symptoms of pneumothorax include a sudden unexplained deterioration in the neonate's condition, decreased breath sounds, cyanosis, increased oxygen requirements, higher P_{CO_2}, decrease in pH, mottled and shocklike appearance, and a shift in the apical cardiac impulses to the contralateral side (opposite side of pneumothorax).

X-ray examination is the main method of diagnosing a pneumothorax. Transillumination of the chest has been used in emergencies when it is not possible to obtain an x-ray series rapidly (Wyman and Kuhns, 1977). Follow-up radiographs should always be done to confirm the diagnosis and extent of the pneumothorax.

□ *TREATMENT* Pneumothorax is a life-threatening situation for the neonate and demands immediate removal of the accumulated air. Aspiration of the air, with a syringe and an 18-gauge needle inserted in the second or third intercostal space on the medial axillary line, may be done as an emergency procedure. Some institutions do thoracentesis. For complete resolution of the pneumothorax, a No. 8 or 10 Fr. thoracotomy tube should be placed appropriately in the chest wall and connected to continuous negative pressure (10–15 cm H_2O) suction with an underwater seal.

OTHER PULMONARY COMPLICATIONS

Pneumomediastinum is a massive collection of air in the mediastinum, either anterior to the heart or laterally, compressing mediastinal pleurae. This condition results in compression of the vena cava, tachypnea, cyanosis, and distant or barely audible heart sounds. Air may dissect into the soft tissues of the neck (subcutaneous emphysema).

Pneumopericardium is a collection of air about the heart with resultant tamponade and diminution of cardiac size.

Pneumoperitoneum is a collection of air in the peritoneal cavity. This condition must be differentiated from a perforated viscera.

CARDIAC COMPLICATIONS

Persistent pulmonary hypertension (PPH), or persistent fetal circulation, is a neonatal syndrome secondary to pulmonary hypertension and is not characterized by organic heart disease. Pulmonary hypertension occurs after a hypoxic insult to the fetus or neonate, resulting in pulmonary vasoconstriction and elevated pulmonary vascular resistance. Should the right ventricular and/or pulmonary arterial pressure remain greater than the systemic pressure, a right-to-left shunt develops in which blood from the right side of the heart flows primarily through the ductus ateriosus and may include the foramen ovale, causing both to remain patent (See Chapter 26 for discussion of patent ductus arteriosus). Vasoconstriction also results in pulmonary hypoperfusion and decreased oxygenation of blood in the lungs with hypoxemia (decreased oxygen in the blood), and cyanosis of the neonate.

PPH syndrome occurs in both preterm and term neonates with primary pulmonary disease (HMD, pneumonia, MAS, or transient tachypnea), polycythemia, hypoglycemia, hypocalcemia, diaphragmatic hernia, hypothermia, IDMs (etiology unknown), and neonatal asphyxia. Since muscular layers of the pulmonary arterioles develop later in gestation, PPH is more likely to occur in the term or postterm infant. Those infants who develop PPH usually show signs of cyanosis, tachypnea, and acidemia.

Diagnosis can be made by drawing simultaneous arterial blood samples from an umbilical artery catheter and the right radial or temporal artery. The vessels (right radial or temporal artery) supplying the upper extremities and head branch (or preductal) before the ductus arteriosus have a higher Po_2 than in the umbilical artery catheter (in the descending aorta or postductal) sample, which indicates right-to-left shunting (Saucier, 1980). Definitive diagnosis is achieved by cardiac catheterization and angiography.

Persistent pulmonary hypertension is usually managed through supportive measures, which include: oxygenation of the neonate, usually with a mechanically assisted ventilation; and correction of hypoglycemia, hypocalcemia, acidemia, and polycythemia. More aggressive treatment includes the use of intravenous tolazoline, a vasodilator, and hyperventilation to maintain a low Pco_2 and a high pH, thereby decreasing pulmonary hypertension. The nurse's responsibility is to monitor the neonate closely, provide a warm, well-oxygenated environment, and observe for any complication, such as hypotension, gastrointestinal bleeding, and decreased urinary output, which are seen with use of vasodilators.

COLD STRESS

Cold stress refers to excessive heat loss resulting in utilization of compensatory mechanisms (increased respirations and nonshivering thermogenesis) to maintain core body temperature. Heat loss that results in cold stress occurs in the newborn through the mechanisms of evaporation, convection, conduction, and radiation. (See Chapter 21 for a detailed discussion on thermoregulation.) Heat loss at the time of delivery that leads to cold stress can play a signifi-

cant role in the severity of RDS and the ultimate outcome of the infant.

The amount of heat loss to the environment by an infant depends to a large extent on the actions of the nurse or caretaker. An SGA infant is at risk for cold stress, and in preterm neonates, the degree of prematurity increases the risk (the smaller the infant the more susceptible to heat loss). Both preterm and SGA infants have decreased adipose tissue, brown fat stores, and glycogen available for metabolism.

As discussed in Chapter 21 (p. 647) the newborn infant's major source of heat production in nonshivering thermogenesis (NST) is brown fat metabolism. The ability of an infant to respond to cold stress by NST is impaired in the presence of several conditions:

- Hypoxemia (Po_2 less than 50)
- Intracranial hemorrhage or any CNS abnormality
- Hypoglycemia

When these conditions occur, the infant's temperature should be monitored more closely and the neutral thermal environment conscientiously maintained. The nurse must recognize these conditions and treat them as soon as possible.

The metabolic consequences of cold stress can be devastating and potentially fatal to an infant. Oxygen requirements are raised, glucose utilization increases, and surfactant production decreases. The effects are graphically depicted on p. 818.

Interventions

If cold stress occurs, the following nursing interventions should be initiated:

1. The neonate is warmed slowly as rapid temperature elevation may cause apnea.

2. Skin temperature is observed every 15 minutes. Skin temperature assessments are used because initial response to cold stress is vasoconstriction resulting in a decrease in skin temperature; therefore, monitoring rectal temperature is not satisfactory. A decrease in rectal temperature represents long-standing cold stress with decompensation in infant's ability to maintain core temperature.

3. Assess the presence of hypoglycemia, which results from the metabolic effects of cold stress. Hypoglycemia is suggested by Dextrostix values below 45 mg/mL, tremors, irritability or lethargy, apnea, or seizure activity.

4. The presence of anaerobic metabolism is assessed and interventions initiated for the resulting metabolic acidosis. Attempts to burn brown fat increase oxygen consumption, lactic acid levels, and metabolic acidosis.

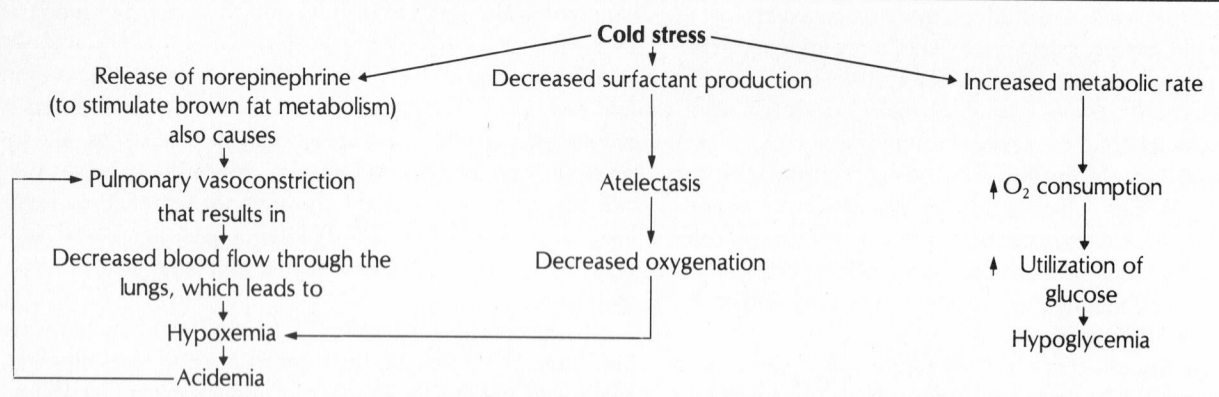

Prolonged cold stress can deplete brown fat stores, interfere with normal temperature control, and result in infant death. Prevention is of the utmost importance and is achieved by careful temperature monitoring and maintenance of a neutral thermal environment.

HYPOGLYCEMIA

Hypoglycemia is the most common metabolic disorder occurring in preterm AGA, LGA, and SGA infants. The pathophysiology of hypoglycemia differs for each classification.

AGA preterm infants have not been in utero a sufficient time to store glycogen and fat. Therefore, they have very low glycogen and fat stores and a decreased ability to carry out gluconeogenesis. This situation is further aggravated as a result of increased utilization of glucose by the tissues (especially the brain and heart) during stress and illness (chilling, asphyxia, sepsis, and RDS).

LGA preterm infants, on the other hand, are often infants of diabetic mothers (diagnosed, suspected, or gestational diabetics). These infants have increased stores of glycogen and fat. However, circulating insulin and insulin responsiveness are higher compared with other newborns. Because of the cessation of high in utero glucose loads at birth, the neonate experiences rapid and profound hypoglycemia.

SGA infants have used up their glycogen and fat stores because of intrauterine malnutrition and have a blunted hepatic enzymatic response with which to carry out gluconeogenesis.

Hypoglycemia in a preterm infant is defined as a blood glucose below 30 mg/dL whole blood (below 35 mg in plasma or serum) in the first 3 days of life and below 40 mg/dL after the first 3 days. It may also be defined as a Dextrostix result below 45 mg/dL when corroborated with laboratory blood glucose value (Procedure 25–4).

There may be no clinical symptoms, or some or all of the following may occur:

- Lethargy, irritability
- Poor feeding
- Vomiting
- Pallor
- Apnea, irregular respirations, respiratory distress
- Hypotonia, possible loss of swallowing reflex
- Tremors, jerkiness, seizure activity
- High-pitched cry

Differential diagnosis of an infant with nonspecific hypoglycemic symptoms includes determining if the infant has any of the following:

- CNS disease
- Sepsis
- Metabolic aberrations
- Polycythemia
- Congenital heart disease
- Drug withdrawal
- Temperature instability
- Hypocalcemia

Treatment

Interventions are based on knowledge of those at risk, observation for symptoms, and screening for asymptomatic occurrence. Dextrostix and urine Dipstix and urine volume (above 1–3 mL/kg/hr) are evaluated for osmotic diuresis and glycosuria.

Provision of adequate caloric intake is important. Early

Procedure 25-4   Dextrostix

Objective	Nursing action	Rationale
Ensure quick, efficient completion of procedure	Gather the following equipment: 1. Lancet (do not use needles). 2. Alcohol swabs. 3. 2 X 2 sterile gauze squares. 4. Small Band-Aid. 5. Dextrostix and bottle.	All necessary equipment must be ready to ensure that blood sample is collected at time and in manner necessary. Do not use needles because of danger of nicking periosteum. Warm heel for 5-10 sec prior to heel stick with a warm wet towel to facilitate flow of blood.
	Select clear, previously unpunctured site. Cleanse site by rubbing vigorously with 70% isopropyl alcohol swab, followed by dry gauze square. Grasp lower leg and heel so as to impede venous return slightly.	Selection of previously unpunctured site minimizes risk of infection and excessive scar formation. Friction produces local heat, which aids vasodilatation. Impeding venous return facilitates extraction of blood sample from puncture site.
Minimize trauma at puncture site	Dry site completely before lancing.	Alcohol is irritating to injured tissue and may also produce hemolysis.
	With quick piercing motion, puncture lateral heel with blade, being careful not to puncture too deeply. Avoid the darkened areas in Figure 25-9. Toes are acceptable sites if necessary.	Lateral heel is site of choice because it precludes damaging posterior tibial nerve and artery, plantar artery, and important longitudinally oriented fat pad of the heel, which in later years could impede walking. This is especially important for infant undergoing multiple Dextrostix procedures. Optimal penetration is 4 mm.

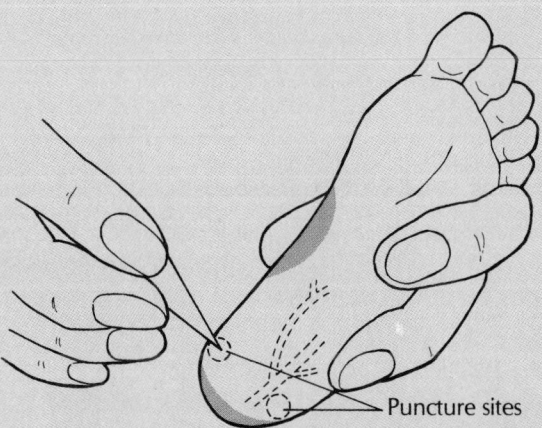

Puncture sites   **FIGURE 25-9** Dextrostix (heel prick).

Ensure accurate blood sampling	After puncture has been made, remove first drop of blood with sterile gauze square and proceed to collect subsequent drops of blood onto Dextrostix, ensuring that it is a stand-up drop of blood on Dextrostix (Figure 25-10).	First drop is usually discarded because it tends to be minutely diluted with tissue fluid from puncture.

Procedure 25–4   Dextrostix cont'd

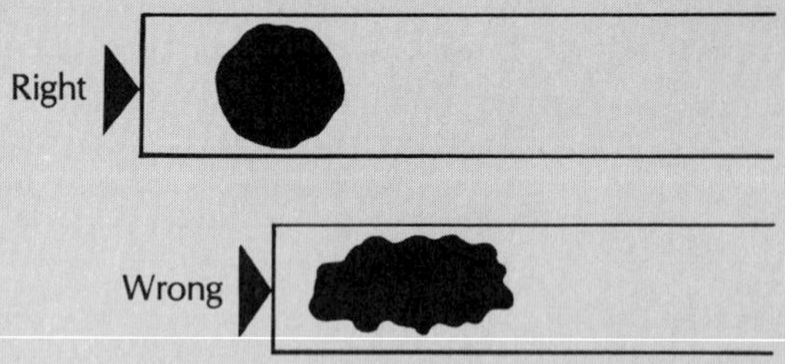

Objective	Nursing action	Rationale

FIGURE 25–10 Dextrostix test strip.

Right

Wrong

	Wait one minute (apply Band-Aid while waiting), then rinse blood gently from stick under a steady stream of running water (Figure 25–11). Compare immediately against color chart on side of bottle.	For accurate results, directions must be followed closely, and reagent strips must be fresh. False low readings may be caused by:
	Record results on vital signs sheet or on back of graph. Report immediately any findings under 45 mg/dL or over 175 mg/dL.	1. Timing. 2. Washing (chemical reaction can be washed off). 3. Squeezing foot, causing tissue fluid dilution.
Prevent excessive bleeding	Apply folded gauze square to puncture site and secure firmly with bandage.	A pressure dressing should be applied to puncture site to stop bleeding.
	Check puncture site frequently for first hour after sample	Active infants sometimes kick or rub their dressings off and can bleed profusely from puncture site, especially if bandage becomes moist or is rubbed excessively against crib sheet.

FIGURE 25–11 Dextrostix test strip rinse.

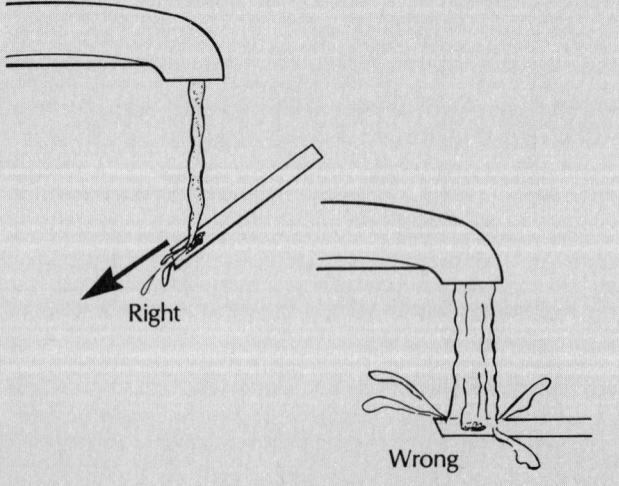

Right

Wrong

formula feeding is one of the major preventive approaches. It should be remembered that if early feedings or intravenous glucose are started to meet the recommended fluid and caloric needs, the blood glucose is likely to remain above the hypoglycemic level.

When caring for a preterm AGA infant, blood glucose levels should be monitored using Dextrostix or laboratory determinations every 4–8 hours for the first day of life, and daily or as necessary thereafter. Intravenous infusions of a dextrose solution (5%–10%) begun immediately after birth should prevent hypoglycemia. However, in the very small AGA infant, infusions of 5%–10% dextrose solution may cause hyperglycemia to develop, requiring an alteration in the glucose concentration. Infants require 6.5–8.0 mg/kg/min of glucose production to maintain normal glucose concentrations (Dodson, 1977). Therefore, an intravenous glucose solution should be calculated based on body weight of the infant, with blood glucose determinations performed to determine adequacy of the infusion treatment.

The LGA preterm infant should be monitored hourly for the first several hours after birth as this is the time when precipitous falls in glucose are most likely. If immediate oral feedings containing glucose are not possible, intravenous dextrose should be administered until serum glucose levels have stabilized and the infant is able to take adequate amounts of formula or breast milk to maintain a normal blood sugar level. LGA infants may require large doses of intravenous glucagon to promote conversion of glycogen from the liver to glucose. Hypoglycemia resulting from hyperinsulinemia may be helped by administration of long-acting epinephrine. Like glucagon, epinephrine promotes glycogen conversion to glucose; it is also an antiinsulin agent.

In the SGA infant, symptoms usually appear between 24 and 72 hours of age; occasionally they may begin as early as 3 hours of age. Infants who are below the tenth percentile (on intrauterine growth curve) should have blood sugar assessments at least every 12 hours for 24 hours and every 8 hours until 4 days of age. Treatment is similar to that for preterm AGA infants.

In more severe cases of hypoglycemia corticosteroids may be administered. It is thought that steroids enhance gluconeogenesis from noncarbohydrate protein sources (Avery, 1981).

The prognosis for untreated hypoglycemia is poor. It may result in permanent, nontreatable CNS damage or death.

HYPOCALCEMIA

Calcium is transported across the placenta in utero throughout pregnancy and in increasing amounts during the third trimester of pregnancy. This predisposes the infant who is born preterm to have lower serum calcium levels in the neonatal period. Both AGA and SGA preterm infants are at risk for the development of hypocalcemia. This risk is increased in the presence of perinatal asphyxia, trauma, hypotonia, and with the use of bicarbonate in treating acidosis. IDMs and infants of mothers with hyperparathyroidism are also at higher risk for hypocalcemia. Hypocalcemia is a common occurrence in the sick neonate due to a delay in oral feedings, which results in less intestinal absorption of calcium. Hypocalcemia is also associated with the practice of administering of low-calcium or calcium-free intravenous therapy management. Hypocalcemia is defined as "early" neonatal hypocalcemia if seen in the first 2 or 3 days of life, or "late" hypocalcemia if it appears at 6–10 days. Late hypocalcemia is related to administration of milk formulas with relatively high levels of phosphorus in relation to calcium. High levels of phosphorus depress the parathyroid gland, which results in decreased serum calcium (Korones, 1981).

The symptoms of hypocalcemia are nonspecific and are seen in conjunction with other disorders. The signs and symptoms that may be observed are:

- Apnea
- Cyanotic episodes
- High-pitched cry
- Twitching, jitteriness
- Seizures (focal or generalized)
- Abdominal distention
- Edema

Diagnosis and Treatment

Serum calcium levels should be monitored in at-risk neonatal groups. Normal serum calcium levels range from 8.0–10.5 mg/dL. Hypocalcemia refers to serum calcium levels less than 7 mg/dL. An ECG measurement of the Q-T interval will assist in the diagnosis.

Schedules for screening serum calcium levels for various at-risk groups have been recommended and are as follows: IDMs at 6, 12, 24, and 48 hours of age; infants suffering from intrapartal asphyxia at 3, 6, and 12 hours of age, and preterm infants at 12, 24, and 48 hours of age (Cloherty and Stark, 1981).

Treatment of symptomatic hypocalcemia initially is intravenous therapy. Intravenous 10% calcium gluconate may be administered as a continuous infusion or in intermittent slow pushes. However, several precautions must be taken when administering calcium gluconate intravenously.

1. When giving an intravenous push, calcium must be injected very slowly over a period of at least 10 minutes. The heart rate must be monitored and if bradycardia or

other cardiac arrhythmias occur, the infusion must be discontinued immediately.

2. When calcium is administered as a continuous drip, the heart rate must also be monitored constantly. Calcium must not be mixed with other medications such as phosphate or bicarbonate in the line as the mixture may precipitate.

3. The intravenous site must be observed closely for signs of infiltration, as calcium is very damaging to the tissues. If extravasation at the site of infusion occurs, necrosis and sloughing of the tissue is likely.

4. If the calcium is administered through an umbilical arterial catheter, the tip of the catheter should be far enough from the heart that calcium is not injected directly into the heart. If a umbilical venous catheter is used, the tip must be in the inferior vena cava or else necrosis of the liver can occur.

Maintenance calcium will be given either parentally or orally. Oral calcium chloride or calcium gluconate may be used for maintenance. High levels (greater than 2% of formula) of calcium chloride can cause gastric mucosal irritation and vomiting. Low-phosphorus milk may be used in the treatment of asymptomatic hypocalcemia.

Treatment for hypocalcemia is usually necessary for only 4 or 5 days unless other complications exist. Calcium levels should be monitored every 12–24 hours and tapered gradually. By 1 week of age, normocalcemia is maintained while receiving regular formula or breast milk without supplements.

NEONATAL JAUNDICE

The most common abnormal physical finding in neonates is *jaundice* (icterus). Jaundice develops from deposit of the yellow pigment, *bilirubin*, in lipid tissues. Unconjugated (indirect) bilirubin is a break-down product derived from hemoglobin that is released from lysed red blood cells and heme pigments found in cell elements (nonerythrocyte bilirubin).

Fetal unconjugated bilirubin is normally cleared by the placenta in utero, so total bilirubin at birth is usually less that 3 mg/dL unless an abnormal hemolytic process has been present. Postnatally, the infant must conjugate bilirubin (convert a lipid-soluble pigment into a water-soluble pigment) in the liver, producing a rise in serum bilirubin in the first few days of life. The bilirubin level at which an infant is harmed varies and depends on a number of factors; furthermore, many conditions can cause a more rapid rise in bilirubin and have the potential to produce permanent neurologic defects and even death. Management of the jaundiced infant presents unique problems that are not present in other periods of life.

Mechanism of Bilirubin Conjugation

Unconjugated (indirect, unbound) bilirubin is normally transported in the plasma firmly bound to albumin, which makes it water soluble. Albumin-bound bilirubin cannot enter intracellular compartments or cross the blood–brain barrier, so it is nontoxic. Because unconjugated bilirubin has a high affinity for extravascular tissue such as fatty tissue (subcutaneous tissue) and the brain, bilirubin not bound to albumin can cross the blood–brain barrier and damage the cells of the CNS and produce kernicterus.

Unconjugated albumin-bound bilirubin is taken up by the liver cells via a still little understood mechanism. Two intracellular nonalbumin-binding proteins, labeled Y and Z, determine the amount of bilirubin held in a liver cell for processing and consequently the potential amount of bilirubin uptake into the liver. The clearance and conjugation of bilirubin depends on the enzyme glucuronyl transferase system, which results in the attachment of unconjugated bilirubin to glucuronic acid (product of liver glycogen), producing conjugated (excretable, direct, bound) bilirubin. It is excreted into the tiny bile ducts, then into the common duct and duodenum. It then progresses down the intestines, where bacteria transform it into urobilinogen, which is not reabsorbed, and it is excreted as a yellow-brown pigment in the stools.

When the amount of bilirubin in the vascular system overwhelms the clearing capabilities of the liver, jaundice develops. Conjugated bilirubin is cleared from the body after it is processed in the liver, excreted into the bile, and eliminated with the feces. Unconjugated bilirubin is not in excretable form and is a potential toxin. Total serum bilirubin is the sum of direct and indirect bilirubin.

The rate and amount of conjugation depends on the rate of hemolysis, on the maturity of the liver, and on albumin-binding sites. The rate of hemolysis of the excess number and kind of fetal red blood cells that are no longer needed by the neonate is such that physiologic jaundice does not occur until after 24 hours of age. A normal, healthy, full-term infant's liver is usually sufficiently mature and is producing enough glucuronyl transferase so that total serum bilirubin levels do not reach pathologic levels (above 12 mg/dL blood). Too great a bilirubin level may result from polycythemia (twin-to-twin transfusion, large placental transfer of blood), enclosed hemorrhage (cephalhematoma, bleeding into internal organs, ecchymoses), increased hemolysis (sepsis, hemolytic disease of the newborn), or an excessive dose of vitamin K.

Serum albumin-binding sites are usually sufficient to meet the usual demands. However, certain conditions tend to decrease the sites available. Fetal or neonatal asphyxia decreases the binding affinity of bilirubin to albumin as acidosis impairs the capacity of albumin to hold bilirubin. Hypothermia and hypoglycemia release free fatty acids that dislocate bilirubin from albumin. Maternal use of sulfa drugs or salicylates interferes with conjugation or interferes with serum albumin-binding sites by competing with bilirubin for these binding sites.

The liver of the newborn infant, particularly that of the preterm infant, has relatively less glucuronyl transferase activity at birth and in the first few weeks of life than the adult. In 1% of breast-fed infants, some feel a substance in breast milk (3α 20β pregnanediol) can inhibit bilirubin conjugation. A number of bacterial and viral infections (cytomegalic inclusion disease, toxoplasmosis, herpes, syphilis) can also affect the liver and produce jaundice.

Even after the bilirubin has been conjugated and bound, it can be converted back to unconjugated bilirubin via the "enterohepatic circulation." In the intestines a β-glucuronidase enzyme system acts to split off (or deconjugate) the bilirubin from glucuronic acid if it has not first been reduced by gut bacteria to urobilinogen, and the free bilirubin is reabsorbed through the intestinal wall and brought back to the liver via portal vein circulation. This recycling of the bilirubin and decreased ability to clear bilirubin from the system are prevalent in the newborn and particularly in preterm infants, who have very high β-glucuronidase activity levels as well as delayed bacterial colonization of the gut.

Pathologic Jaundice

Jaundice of any origin must be considered pathologic if the serum bilirubin exceeds 6 mg/dL within the first 24 hours or persists beyond 7 days in the full-term and 10 days in the preterm infant; if serum bilirubin levels rise by more than 5 mg/dL a day or exceed 12 mg/dL in either full-term or preterm neonate; and if conjugated (direct) bilirubin is greater than 1.5–2.0 mg/dL.

High serum bilirubin levels (hyperbilirubinemia), especially bilirubin in the unconjugated state, are dangerous to the neonate. The more premature the neonate the more susceptible to tissue damage. Since the cerebral cortex and thalamus are the last to be myelinated, the nuclei of these cells are more susceptible to being infiltrated by the unconjugated bilirubin, with subsequent brain damage. The most likely causes of pathologic jaundice are hemolytic disease of the newborn (Rh incompatibility and ABO incompatibility) and sepsis. In utero infections such as toxoplasmosis, rubella, herpes, and syphilis may produce jaundice in the first 24 hours. Such affected infants also have petechiae and an enlarged liver and spleen.

The nurse is aware of the infant's prenatal and natal history and assess each neonate several times every day for color and change in behavior. Behavior changes associated with kernicterus rarely occur prior to 36 hours of age, occurring most frequently between days 3 and 10.

HYPERBILIRUBINEMIA

Neonatal *hyperbilirubinemia* (level of serum bilirubin in excess of accepted norms) is partly preventable. During pregnancy, women can be checked for conditions that may predispose to neonatal hyperbilirubinemia: hereditary spherocytosis, diabetes, infections (toxoplasmosis, cytomegalic inclusion disease, rubella, infections with gram-negative bacilli) that stimulate production of maternal isoimmune antibodies, and drug ingestion (sulfas, salicylates, novobiocin, diazepam, oxytocin). The woman who is Rh-negative or who has blood type O should be asked about outcomes of any previous pregnancies and her history of blood transfusion. Prenatal amniocentesis with spectrophotographic examination may be indicated in some cases. Cord blood from neonates is evaluated for bilirubin level, which should not exceed 5 mg/dL. Neonates of these mothers are carefully assessed for appearance of jaundice and levels of serum bilirubin.

Some neonatal conditions predispose to hyperbilirubinemia: polycythemia (central hematocrit 65% or more), pyloric stenosis, obstruction or atresia of the biliary duct or of the lower bowel, low-grade urinary tract infection, hypothyroidism, enclosed hemorrhage (cephalhematoma, large bruises), asphyxia neonatorum, hypothermia, acidemia, hypoglycemia. Hepatitis from an infectious or metabolic liver disease elevates the level of conjugated bilirubin. This type of hepatitis is associated with intrauterine infection such as rubella syndrome, cytomegalic inclusion disease, syphilis, herpesvirus type 2, or cystic fibrosis. Neonatal hepatitis (giant cell hepatitis) is a disorder of unknown etiology, which results in spontaneous cure for one-third of those affected, chronic liver disease for another third, and death for the remaining one-third. Neonates born with congenital biliary duct atresia have a poor prognosis; about 90% have an inoperable lesion and succumb during the first 3 years of life.

The goal of the management of hyperbilirubinemia regardless of cause is to treat the anemia, remove maternal antibodies and sensitized erythrocytes, increase serum albumin levels, and reduce the levels of serum bilirubin. Methods include phototherapy, exchange transfusion, infusion of albumin, and drug therapy. (These treatment techniques are discussed on p. 827.)

KERNICTERUS

Unbound (unconjugated) bilirubin, although not soluble in body fluids, is lipid soluble and capable of crossing cell membranes. *Kernicterus* (meaning "yellow nucleus") refers to the deposition of unconjugated bilirubin in the basal ganglia of the brain and to the symptoms of neurologic damage that follow untreated hyperbilirubinemia. Kernicterus (bilirubin encephalopathy) is most commonly found with blood-group incompatibility.

Kernicterus is associated with serum unconjugated bilirubin levels of over 20 mg/dL in normal term infants; safe levels for preterm infants or sick infants are lower and vary considerably. Sick preterm infants may develop kernicterus with unconjugated bilirubin levels as low as 10 mg/dL. It should be noted cases of kernicterus have been reported in term infants with unconjugated bilirubin levels below 20 mg/dL and in preterm infants with levels lower than 10 mg/dL. Determination of the (unbound) unconjugated portion of the total serum bilirubin is the most significant assessment of the potential for kernicterus.

Nursing Management

Primary nursing priorities are to identify factors that predispose to development of jaundice and to identify jaundice as soon as it is apparent. If jaundice appears, careful observation of the increase in depth of color and of the infant's behavior is mandatory. Should the infant require phototherapy (discussed on p. 829), the nurse provides the necessary care. The nurse assists with the exchange transfusion (Procedure 25–5) and observes the infant carefully following the procedure. The nurse who is working with the mother administers RhoGAM if ordered and assists the parents in coping with the situation.

As the first step in identifying impending jaundice, the nurse reviews each neonate's prenatal and perinatal history for factors that predispose to hyperbilirubinemia. The neonate's blood type, Rh, and Coombs' test results (if done) are noted. The nurse assesses each neonate for gestational age and for cephalhematoma, and notes whether the infant is breast-fed or bottle-fed.

In the presence of one or more predisposing factors, laboratory determination should be made of serum bilirubin levels (direct, indirect, and total), CO_2 combining power (decrease in CO_2 combining power is consistent with increased hemolysis), serum albumin levels and tests of bilirubin binding, if available. A new quick, reliable index of bilirubin binding as well as measure of reserve albumin capacity is the fluorescent quenching test. In addition, the nurse checks the neonate for jaundice about every 2 hours and records observations.

To check for jaundice, the nurse should blanch the skin over a bony prominence (forehead, sternum) by pressing firmly with the thumb. After pressure is released, if jaundice is present, the area appears yellow before normal color returns. The nurse should check oral mucosa and the posterior portion of the hard palate and conjunctival sacs for yellow pigmentation in darker-skinned neonates, because the underlying pigment of normal dark-skinned people can appear yellow. Assessment in daylight gives best results, as pink walls and surroundings may mask yellowish tints; yellow colors make differentiation of jaundice difficult. The time of onset of jaundice is recorded and reported.

The neonate's behavior is assessed for neurologic signs of kernicterus, especially between days 3 and 10. Kernicterus never appears before 36 hours of age, even in severe cases of hemolytic disease. Clinical features of encephalopathy appear in four stages. Kernicterus is initially evidenced by neurologic depression—hypotonia, diminished or absent Moro reflex, vomiting, absent rooting and sucking reflexes, and lethargy. During the second stage,

hyperreflexia, twitching, generalized seizures, opisthotonus, high-pitched cry, and fever may be seen. After about 1 week of age, during the third stage, all clinical manifestations may disappear. The fourth stage, appearing after the neonatal period, reveals the extent of neurologic damage. Late sequelae may include cerebral palsy (spasticity, athetosis), impaired or absent hearing, learning difficulties, and mental retardation.

HEMOLYTIC DISEASE OF THE NEWBORN

Isoimmune hemolytic disease, also known as *erythroblastosis fetalis*, occurs after transplacental passage of a maternal antibody that predisposes fetal and neonatal red blood cells to early destruction. Jaundice, anemia, and compensatory erythropoiesis result. Immature red blood cells—erythroblasts—are found in large numbers in the blood; hence the designation erythroblastosis fetalis.

Although there are more than 60 known red blood cell antigens, clinically significant hemolytic disease is associated with maternal–fetal incompatibility associated with the D factor in the Rh group and with the ABO blood types. The Rh incompatibility system is more complex.

Rh Incompatability

Those whose red blood cells contain the Rh factor (antigen) are said to be positive; those who do not are negative. Isoimmunization occurs when an Rh-negative woman carries an Rh-positive (who has the Rh factor or antigen) fetus. When fetal Rh-positive antigens (an antigenic substance on the surface of the fetal red blood cell) leak in minute amounts into maternal circulation, maternal antibodies are produced, creating a sensitization reaction.

The leakage of fetal Rh antigens into the maternal circulation most commonly occurs at the time of delivery. Other obstetric factors known to increase the likelihood of maternal Rh sensitization are PIH (pre-eclampsia-eclampsia), amniocentesis, version procedure, cesarean birth, breech deliveries, abortion, abruptio placentae, and manual removal of the placenta (see Chapter 18). In subsequent pregnancies the maternal antibodies cross the placenta and cause immediate or delayed destruction (hemolysis) of the fetal red blood cells.

Hydrops fetalis, the most severe form of erythroblastosis fetalis, results when maternal antibodies attach to the Rh antigen of the fetal red blood cells, making them susceptible to destruction by phagocytes. The fetal system responds by increased erythropoiesis within foci in the placental, extramedullary sites and hyperplasia of the bone narrow. Rapid and early destruction of erythrocytes results in a marked increase of immature red blood cells—erythroblasts—which do not have the functional capabilities of

Procedure 25–5   Exchange Transfusion
(Exchange transfusion is a therapeutic procedure for
hyperbilirubinemia of any etiology.)

Objective	Nursing action	Rationale
Prepare infant	1. Identify infant.	To prepare correct infant.
	2. Keep neonate NPO for 4 hr preceding exchange transfusion, or aspirate stomach.	Decreases chance of regurgitation and aspiration by neonate.
	3. Administer salt-poor albumin (1 g/kg body weight) 1 hr before exchange transfusion.	Increases binding of bilirubin. Do not give to severely anemic or edemic neonate or to neonate with congestive heart failure, because of hazard of hypervolemia.
	4. Assess vital signs.	Provides a baseline.
	5. Position neonate in supine position on restraining board and provide warmth (p. 829).	Provides maximum visualization, prevents chilling.
	6. Cleanse abdomen by scrubbing.	Reduces number of bacteria present.
	7. Attach monitor leads to infant.	To assess pulse and respiration.
Prepare equipment	1. Have resuscitation equipment available.	In case life support measures are necessary.
	2. Obtain blood and check it with physician.	Ensures using correct blood.
	3. Attach blood tubing.	Allows infusion.
	4. Apply blood warmer.	Reduces chill.
	5. Open trays. Pour prep solution into basins.	
	6. Prepare gown and gloves for physician.	Maintains sterility.
Monitor infant status	Assess pulse, respirations, color, activity state.	To recognize possible problems and provide data on neonate's response to treatment.
Record blood exchange and medications used	1. Using blood exchange sheet, record time, amount of blood in, amount of blood out, and medications.	Donor blood is given at rate of 170 mL/kg of body weight. It replaces 85% of infant's own blood.
	2. Inform physician when 100 mL of blood has been used.	Calcium gluconate is given IV after each 100 mL of blood to decrease cardiac irritability.
Assess neonate response after transfusion	After the exchange, carefully monitor the following for 24–48 hr:	Provides information on status of neonate and identification of complications.
	1. Vital signs. 2. Neurologic signs (lethargy, increased irritability, jitteriness, convulsion). 3. Amount and color of urine. 4. Presence of edema. 5. Signs of necrotizing enterocolitis. 6. Infection or hemorrhage at infusion site. 7. Signs of increasing jaundice. 8. Neurologic signs of kernicterus.	
Prepare blood samples	Label tubes and send to laboratory with appropriate laboratory slips.	Follow routines of your institution.
	Retype and cross-match 2 units of blood 2 hrs post exchange.	Need for possible future exchange.

mature cells. If the anemia is severe, as seen in hydrops fetalis, cardiomegaly with severe cardiac decompensation and hepatosplenomegaly occur. Severe generalized anasarca, and generalized fluid effusion into the pleural cavity (hydrothorax), pericardial sac, and peritoneal cavity (ascites) develop. Jaundice is not present until later because the bili pigments are being excreted through the placenta into the maternal circulation.

Severe anemia is also responsible for hemorrhage in pulmonary and other tissues. The hydropic hemolytic disease process is also characterized by hyperplasia of the fetal zone of the adrenal cortex and pancreatic islets. Hyperplasia of the pancreatic islets predisposes the infant to neonatal hypoglycemia similar to that of IDMs. These infants also have increased bleeding tendencies due to associated thrombocytopenia and hypoxic damage to the capillaries. Hydrops is a frequent cause of intrauterine death among infants with Rh disease. In rare cases, the grossly enlarged edemic fetal body and placenta may cause uterine rupture.

LABORATORY DATA

If the hemolytic process is due to Rh sensitization, laboratory findings reveal the following: (a) an Rh-positive neonate with a positive Coombs' test; (b) increased erythropoiesis with many immature circulating red blood cells (nucleated blastocysts); (c) anemia, in most cases; (d) elevated levels (5 mg/dL or more) of bilirubin in cord blood; and (e) a reduction in albumin-binding capacity. Maternal data may include an elevated anti-Rh titer and spectrophotometric evidence of fetal hemolytic process.

The Coombs' test can be either indirect or direct. The indirect Coombs' test measures the amount of Rh-positive antibodies in the mother's blood. Rh-positive red blood cells are added to the maternal blood sample. If the mother's serum contains antibodies, the Rh-positive red blood cells will agglutinate (clump) when rabbit immune antiglobulin is added, and the test results are labeled positive.

The direct Coombs' test reveals the presence of antibody-coated (sensitized) Rh-positive red blood cells in the neonate. Rabbit immune antiglobulin is added to the neonatal blood cells specimen. If the neonatal red blood cells agglutinate, they have been coated with maternal antibodies and the test result is positive.

The direct Coombs' test on the neonate's cells may be negative or mildly positive, but the indirect Coombs' test, when using the neonate's serum on adult red blood cells, may be strongly positive. This finding indicates that the neonate's red blood cells are not coated with the antibody; however, the antibody is present in the neonate's serum.

ABO Incompatibility

ABO incompatibility, although frequent (occurring in 20% of pregnancies), rarely results in hemolytic disease severe enough to be clinically diagnosed and treated. ABO incompatibility occurs when the woman carries a fetus with a blood type different from her own.

Anti-A and anti-B antibodies are naturally occurring; that is, women are naturally exposed to the A and B antigens through the foods they eat and through exposure to infection by gram negative bacteria. As a result, some women have high serum anti-A and anti-B titers before they become pregnant. Once the woman becomes pregnant, the maternal serum anti-A and anti-B antibodies cross the placenta and produce hemolysis of the fetal red blood cells. With ABO incompatibility the first infant is frequently involved, and no relationship exists between the appearance of the disease and repeated sensitization from one pregnancy to the next.

The most common incompatibility occurs when the mother is type O (anti-A and anti-B antibodies) and the fetus is type A or B. The fetus with type A_1 red blood cells is more affected than a fetus having type A_2 or B, as the red blood cells of these blood groups do not seem to have the same antigenicity as type A_1. The group B fetus of an A mother and a group A fetus of a B mother are only occasionally affected. Group O infants, because they have no antigenic sites on the red blood cells, are never affected regardless of the mother's blood type. The incompatibility occurs as a result of the maternal antibodies present in her serum and interaction between the antigen sites on the fetal red blood cells.

Clinically, ABO incompatibility presents as jaundice and occasionally hepatosplenomegaly. Hydrops and stillbirth are rare.

LABORATORY DATA

An increase in reticulocytes indicates the presence of a hemolytic process, but the resulting anemia is not significant during the neonatal period and is rare later on. The direct Coombs' test may be negative or mildly positive, while the indirect Coombs' test may be strongly positive. Infants with a direct Coombs' positive test have increased incidence of jaundice with bilirubin levels in excess of 10 mg/dL. Increased numbers of spherocytes (spherical, plump, mature erythrocytes) are seen on a peripheral blood smear. Increased numbers of spherocytes are not seen on smears from Rh disease infants.

Prognosis

Prognosis depends on the extent of the hemolytic process and the underlying cause. Severe hemolytic disease results in fetal and early neonatal death from the effects of anemia—cardiac decompensation, edema, ascites, and hydrothorax. Hyperbilirubinemia that is not promptly treated or adequately treated leads to kernicterus. The resultant neurologic damage is responsible for death, cerebral palsy, mental retardation, sensory difficulties, or to a lesser degree, perceptual impairment, delayed speech development, hyperactivity, muscle incoordination, or learning difficulties (Klaus and Fanaroff, 1979). Another late consequence of hyperbilirubinemia is yellowish-green tooth staining and enamel hypoplasia. The best treatment for hemolytic disease is prevention.

Neonatal Assessment

Hemolytic disease of the newborn is suspected if the placenta is enlarged (placental weight is usually only one-seventh of fetal weight), if the neonate is edematous with pleural and pericardial effusion plus ascites, if pallor or jaundice is noted during the first 24–36 hours, if hemolytic anemia is diagnosed, or if the spleen and liver are enlarged. Changes in the neonate's behavior or bleeding tendencies must be carefully assessed to determine the causative factor. Neonates who have received large doses of vitamin K or sulfonamides may have increased incidence of hyperbilirubinemia because these agents reduce the number of available binding sites by competing for them.

Treatment of the Neonate and Nursing Responsibilities

The management of the neonate is directed toward preventing anemia and hyperbilirubinemia (Figure 25–12). Exchange transfusion, phototherapy, and drug therapy are utilized. When determining the appropriate management of hyperbilirubinemia (exchange transfusion or phototherapy), the nurse must take into account three variables: (a) the serum bilirubin level; (b) the neonate's birth weight; and (c) the neonate's age in hours. If a neonate has hemolysis with an unconjugated bilirubin level of 14 mg/dL, weighs less than 2500 g (birth weight), and is 24 or less hours old, an exchange transfusion may be the best management. However, if that same neonate is over 24 hours of age, phototherapy is an adequate treatment to prevent the possible complication of kernicterus. It is generally accepted that if the neonate is preterm or at risk, phototherapy should be instituted when a bilirubin level is 10 mg/dL. Any neonate with a bilirubin level of 20 mg/dL or above should have an exchange transfusion regardless of weight or age.

EXCHANGE TRANSFUSION

Early or immediate exchange transfusion is indicated in the presence of anti-Rh titer of greater than 1:16 in the mother (see Chapter 13), severe hemolytic disease in a previous newborn, clinical hemolytic disease of the newborn at birth or within the first 24 hours, positive direct Coombs' test, cord serum of conjugated (direct) bilirubin levels greater than 3.5 mg/dL in the first week, serum unconjugated bilirubin levels greater than 20 mg/dL in the first 48 hours, hemoglobin less than 12 g/dL, or infants with hy-

Serum bilirubin mg/dL	Birth weight	<24 hrs.	24-48 hrs	49-72 hrs	> 72 hrs
<5	All				
5-9	All	Phototherapy if hemolysis			
10-14	<2500 g	Exchange if hemolysis	Phototherapy		
	>2500 g			Investigate bilirubin > 12 mg	
15-19	<2500 g	Exchange		Consider exchange	
	>2500 g			Phototherapy	
20 and +	All	Exchange			

□ Observe   ▨ Investigate jaundice

FIGURE 25–12 Therapy for isoimmune hemolytic disease in the neonate. Phototherapy is used after any exchange transfusion. If the following conditions are present, treat the neonate as if in the next higher bilirubin category: perinatal asphyxia, respiratory distress, metabolic acidosis (pH 7.25 or below), hypothermia (temperature below 35C), low serum protein (5 g/dL or less), birth weight less than 1500 g, or signs of clinical or CNS deterioration. (From Avery, G. B. 1981. *Neonatology,* 2nd ed. Philadelphia: J. B. Lippincott Co., p. 511.)

drops at birth. Infants who are at greater risk for developing kernicterus receive an exchange transfusion at lower serum bilirubin levels.

Withdrawal of neonate's blood and replacement with donor blood is used to (a) treat anemia with red blood cells that are not susceptible to maternal antibodies; (b) remove sensitized red blood cells that would be lysed soon (a two-volume exchange removes 85% of the infant's red blood cells); (c) remove serum bilirubin; and (d) provide bilirubin-free albumin and increase the binding sites for bilirubin. In Rh incompatibility, fresh (under 2 days old) group O, Rh-negative whole blood, or packed red blood cells, is chosen. This type of blood contains no A or B antigens or Rh antigens; therefore the maternal antibodies still present in the neonate's blood will not cause hemolysis of the transfused blood. Packed cells are used if the infant is anemic. CPD (citrate-phosphate-dextrose) blood is preferred because it presents less of an acid load to the infant.

In case of ABO incompatibility, group O with Rh-specific cells and low titers of anti-A and anti-B donor blood is used, not the infant's blood type, since donor blood contains no antigens to further stimulate maternal antibodies.

Every 4–8 hours after the transfusion, bilirubin determinations are made. Repeat exchange may be necessary if the serum bilirubin level rises at a rate of 0.5–1.0 mg/dL/hr (Avery, 1981) or if the bilirubin level exceeds 20 mg/dL. Daily hemoglobin estimates should be obtained until stable, and hemoglobin determinations every 2 weeks for 2 months are valuable.

□ *NURSING INTERVENTIONS* The nurse's responsibilities during exchange transfusion are to: assemble equipment, prepare the neonate, assist the physician during the procedure, maintain a careful record of all events, and observe the neonate after the procedure for complications from the transfusion and clinical signs of hyperbilirubinemia and neurologic damage (Procedure 25–5). Necessary equipment varies with the hospital, but in general, includes the following:

- Two units of donor's blood
- Sterile gown, gloves, drape, and mask
- Exchange transfusion set and record
- Monitors for temperature, pulse, and respirations
- Umbilical cut-down tray (if there is no umbilical catheter)
- Sterile umbilical cord ties or No. 4-Osille silk suture
- Intravenous standard
- Blood tubing
- Blood warmer (38C or 100F) if blood has not been prewarmed in blood bank
- Oxygen with mask and tubing
- Suction setup or DeLee trap or bulb syringe
- Umbilical catheter, No. 3½ Fr. or 5 Fr.

- Medication drawn up in syringes with No. 24 needles (10% calcium gluconate, 50% glucose, sodium bicarbonate, or trimethamine)
- Method of keeping the infant warm
- Restraining board
- Lighting to adequately visualize field
- Solution for preparing the skin (Betadine or Merthiolate)
- Laboratory tubes and slips

The neonate should not ingest anything for 4 hours or should have the stomach aspirated before the procedure. The neonate is positioned supine, restrained, and kept warm (Figure 25–13). Resuscitation equipment is assembled in an easily accessible area near the neonate in case respiratory distress occurs. Continuous monitoring equipment is used, if available. Both physician and nurse check donor blood for type, Rh, and age to minimize error. Tubing from the blood bottle (or bag) is draped through the warm bath or a blood warmer before it reaches the newborn.

The nurse assists the physician in cleansing the infusion site (usually the umbilical vein or the jugular or femoral artery) and in draping, gowning, and gloving. The catheter location should be verified by radiograph. The physician measures the central venous pressure before starting the exchange; the nurse records the time and the reading. First blood removed can be utilized for special hematologic studies, such as glucose-6-phosphate dehydrogenase (G-6-PD), virology, electrophoresis, and so on, if the neonate has a negative Coombs' test and has not been set up for ABO incompatibility or erythroblastosis fetalis.

The nurse records the time and amount of each withdrawl of fetal blood and infusion of donor blood and keeps a current tally of the total amount. The nurse alerts the physician when 100 mL has been exchanged. The physician usually administers calcium gluconate after each 100 mL is exchanged to minimize possible cardiac irritability. The nurse continues to monitor and record heart rate, respiratory rate, all medications (type, amount, time), infant response, and any other pertinent information.

Following the transfusion, the nurse observes the neonate closely for 24–48 hours for vital signs changes (temperature, pulse, respirations; bradycardia may result if calcium is injected too rapidly, pedal pulses if umbilical vein or femoral arteries were used for the exchange site), neurologic signs (lethargy, increased irritability, jitteriness, or convulsions), dark urine, and developing edema. Calcium and glucose levels may be drawn. Necrotizing enterocolitis may result from a misplaced catheter and compromised bowel circulation. Complications for which the nurse must be alert may arise from hemorrhage or infection at the infusion site or from the blood transfusion. Possible complications following any blood transfusion include heart failure, hypokalemia, hypoglycemia (result of continued an-

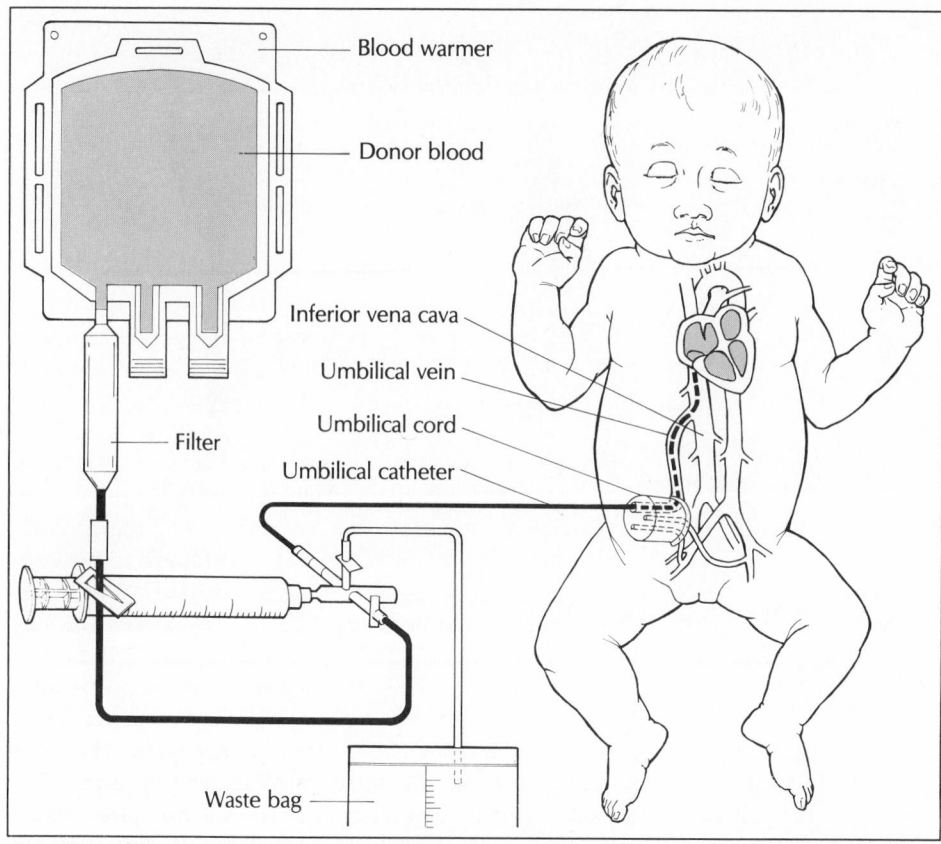

FIGURE 25-13 Infant receiving exchange transfusion.

Blood warmer

Donor blood

Inferior vena cava

Umbilical vein

Umbilical cord

Umbilical catheter

Filter

Waste bag

aerobic glycolysis within donor red blood cells), septicemia, shock, and thrombosis. The nurse remains observant for increasing jaundice and the appearance of neurologic signs that may signify kernicterus.

PHOTOTHERAPY

Phototherapy may be used alone or in conjunction with exchange transfusion to reduce serum bilirubin levels. Exposure of the neonate to high-intensity light (a bank of fluorescent light bulbs or bulbs in the blue-light spectrum) decreases serum bilirubin levels in the skin. Unbound (unconjugated) bilirubin is thought to be photo-oxidized into nontoxic compounds that are excreted in the urine and feces (via bile) (Korones, 1981). The newborn's entire skin area is exposed to the light. Phototherapy success is measured every 12 hours or with daily serum bilirubin levels. The lights must be turned off while drawing the serum bilirubin levels. Phototherapy plays an important role in preventing a rise in bilirubin levels but does not alter the underlying cause of jaundice, and hemolysis may continue and produce anemia.

□ *NURSING INTERVENTION* Currently under study is the possible effect that intensified light may have on other compounds or tissues and on biorhythms. Although it is not known whether this light injures the delicate eye structures, particularly the retina, eyes are always patched while the neonate is receiving phototherapy. The nurse applies eye patches over the neonate's closed eyes while under the lights (Figure 25–14). Phototherapy is discontinued, and the eye patches are removed at least once per shift to assess the eyes for the presence of conjunctivitis. Patches are also removed to allow eye contact during feeding (social stimulation) or when parents are visiting (parental attachment). Minimal covering is applied over the genitals and buttocks to expose maximum skin surface and to protect bedding.

The neonate's temperature is monitored to prevent hyperthermia or hypothermia. The lights should be 18 inches above the neonate. The neonate will require additional fluids to compensate for the increased water loss through the skin and loose stools. Stools and urine are evaluated for green color and amount. Loose green stools are often found with use of phototherapy and skin care is essential.

Bronzing of the skin may occur, lasting about 3 weeks after therapy is discontinued, but with no long-term sequelae if the neonate has a healthy liver. "Tanning" or deeper pigmentation of black babies has been reported during light exposure. As a side effect of phototherapy, some newborns develop a maculopapular rash.

In addition to assessing the neonate's skin color for jaundice and bronzing, the nurse examines the skin for developing pressure areas. The neonate should be reposi-

FIGURE 25–14 Infant receiving phototherapy. The phototherapy light is positioned over the Isolette. To expose as much skin surface as possible, the infant is not dressed. Bilateral eye patches are always in place.

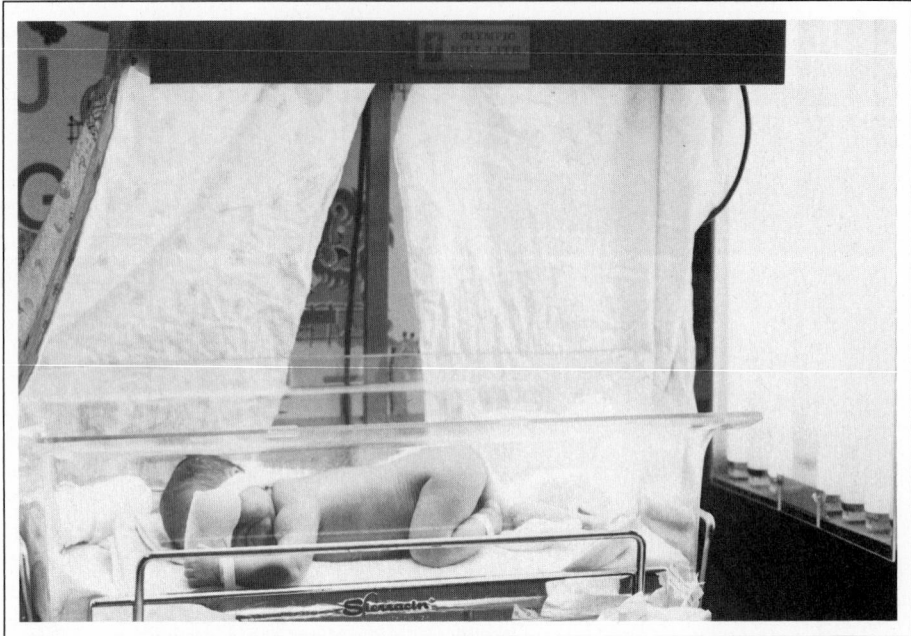

tioned at least *every* 2 hours to permit the light to reach all skin surfaces, to prevent pressure areas, and to vary the stimulation to the infant. The nurse keeps track of the number of hours each lamp is used so that each can be replaced before its effectiveness is lost.

DRUG THERAPY

Phenobarbital is capable of stimulating the liver's production of enzymes that increase conjugation of bilirubin and its excretion. This drug is only effective if given to the pregnant woman over several days prior to 2 weeks before delivery.

Postnatal drug therapy is of limited value in term infants. It takes 3–7 days to show any effect and may take much longer in preterm infants. The use of phenobarbital postnatally for the treatment of hyperbilirubinemia is controversial because the side effects (lethargy with poor feedings) may outweigh its benefits. Combining phenobarbital with phototherapy has not been shown to reduce bilirubin levels more rapidly than phototherapy alone (Valdes et al., 1971), and neonates who are already jaundiced or who are preterm may not respond at all.

Other drugs have the capacity to increase conjugation of bilirubin and to keep bilirubin at levels lower than expected. These drugs are too risky to use for the prevention and treatment of neonatal jaundice.

Support of the Family

Many parents must face the mother's discharge while the neonate remains in the hospital for treatment of hyperbilirubinemia. The terms *jaundice, hyperbilirubinemia, exchange transfusion,* and *phototherapy* may sound frightening and threatening. Some parents may feel guilty that they have caused this situation to happen. On occasion, a multidisciplinary team (nurse, obstetrician, pediatrician, clergyman, genetic counselor, psychologist, or other) may collaborate in assisting the parents to cope with the situation. Under stress, parents may not be able to "hear" or understand the physician's first explanations. The nurse must expect that the parents will need explanations repeated and clarified and that they may need help voicing their questions and fears. Early eye and tactile contact with the neonate is encouraged and planned so that the nurse can be present while the parents visit the neonate. Parents are kept informed of their infant's condition and are encouraged to return to the hospital or to telephone at any time and to be involved in the care of their infant. (See the accompanying Nursing Care Plan for jaundice.)

NEONATAL ANEMIA

Neonatal anemia is often difficult to recognize by clinical evaluation alone. Normal hemoglobin in a full term neonate is about 17 g/dL; infants with hemoglobin of less than 14 g/dL are usually considered anemic. The most common causes of neonatal anemia are blood loss, hemolysis, and impaired red blood cell production.

Blood loss (hypovolemia) occurs in utero from placental bleeding (placenta previa or abruptio placentae). Intrapartal blood loss may be fetomaternal, fetofetal, or the result of umbilical cord bleeding. Birth trauma to abdominal organs or the cranium may produce significant blood loss, and cerebral bleeding may occur due to hypoxia.

(Text continues on p. 835.)

NURSING CARE PLAN
Jaundice

PATIENT DATA BASE

History

Maternal

ABO incompatibility

Rh negative

Diabetes

Presence of infection, such as syphilis, cytomegalovirus, rubella, toxoplasmosis

Presence of familial blood dyscrasias (such as spherocytosis, G-6-PD deficiency)

Medications: use of novobiocin, sulfonamides, or salicylates interferes with conjugation or competes for serum albumin-binding sites

Number and outcome of previous pregnancies.

Condition at birth and current health status of other children.

Paternal

Rh factor — negative or positive

Delivery

Enlarged placenta (larger than one-seventh of neonate's weight)

Delayed clamping of umbilical cord

Traumatic delivery

Neonate

Enclosed hemorrhage; hematoma; large bruises; intracranial bleeding

Bacterial and/or viral infections can affect liver and thus decrease glucuronyl transferase activity

Polycythemia (central hematocrit of 65% or more)

Biliary atresia, cystic fibrosis (inspissated bile)

Congenital hypothyroidism

Conditions that decrease available albumin-binding sites:

1. Fetal or neonatal asphyxia decreases binding affinity of bilirubin to albumin.
2. Chilling and hypoglycemia create fatty acids to compete for binding sites.
3. Preterm neonates tend to have lower serum albumin levels and therefore less albumin to bind to.

Physical examination

Generalized edema with pleural and pericardial effusion

Pallor or jaundice noted in first 24-36 hours

May have enlargement of spleen or liver

Changes in behavior (lethargy, irritability)

Dark, concentrated urine

Presence of hematomas or large bruises (assess for other signs of enclosed bleeding)

Laboratory evaluation

Coombs' test

Total bilirubin level

Indications for exchange transfusion:

In ABO incompatibility, serum bilirubin levels greater than 20 mg/dL (full-term) and 15 mg/dL (preterm)

In Rh incompatibility, serum bilirubin greater than 20 mg/dL (term), greater than 15 mg/dL (large preterms), and greater than 13 mg/dL (less than 1250 g preterms).

Total serum protein (provides measure of binding capacity)

Kernlute 1+ or 2+ indication for exchange transfusion

CBC — assess anemia and polycythemia

Peripheral smear — evaluate red blood cells for immaturity or abnormality

CO_2 combining power — decrease is consistent with increased hemolysis

Blood glucose

NURSING PRIORITIES

1. Observe signs of worsening conditions.
2. Monitor levels of bilirubin during therapy.
3. Provide adequate hydration.
4. Assess for signs of dehydration.
5. Provide tactile stimulation.
6. Provide parent education.
7. Promote parent-infant bonding.

Family Educational Focus

1. Discuss the physiologic changes that occur during the newborn period predisposing the neonate to jaundice.
2. Explain the treatment modalities utilized in jaundice management and their rationale.
3. Provide parents opportunities to discuss questions and individual concerns about their newborn.
4. Discuss availability of in-home management of mild jaundice with phototherapy lights.

Problem	Nursing interventions and actions	Rationale
Prevention	Initiate feedings within 4-6 hr after delivery, if possible.	Early feeding in first 4-6 hr tends to discourage high bilirubin levels. Early feeding stimulates bowel activity and passage of bilirubin-containing meconium, thereby eliminating possibility of reabsorption of pigment from intestines.

NURSING CARE PLAN cont'd
Jaundice

Problem	Nursing interventions and actions	Rationale
	Keep infant warm.	Action necessary to prevent chill-induced acidosis, a condition that depletes serum albumin-binding sites.
	Identify risk factors (p. 823).	Presence of risk factors necessitates more frequent assessment of neonate for development of jaundice and may include determining blood levels of bilirubin.
Early identification of jaundice	Assess newborn for signs of jaundice.	Observation of jaundice may be initial sign of hyperbilirubinemia.
	1. Complete assessments in daylight, if possible.	Early detection is affected by nursery environment. Artificial lights (with pink tint) may mask beginning of jaundice.
	2. Observe sclera.	Jaundice may first be noticed as a yellowing of the sclera.
	3. Observe skin color and assess by blanching.	Blanching the skin leaves a yellow color to the skin immediately after pressure is released.
	4. Check oral mucosa, posterior portion of hard palate, and conjunctival sacs for yellow pigmentation in dark-skinned neonates.	Underlying pigment of dark-skinned people may normally appear yellow.
Elevated level of bilirubin	Maintain treatment modalities.	Method of treatment depends on level of bilirubin, time of onset, and presence of other illness (disease states).
Bilirubin levels of 10 mg/dL or greater in preterm infants. Lower levels in stressed or smaller infants	Phototherapy:	Photo-oxidation of bilirubin occurs in the skin with use of phototherapy. Photodecomposition products are largely water soluble, and can be excreted in stool and urine. Unconjugated bilirubin does not need to be bound to albumin for transport.
	1. Cover neonate's eyes with eye patches while under phototherapy light.	Protects retina from damage due to high-intensity light.
	2. Remove neonate from under phototherapy light and remove eye patches during feedings.	Provides visual stimulation.
	3. Inspect eyes for conjunctivitis and corneal abrasions.	May be caused by irritation from eye patches.
	4. Minimal coverage only (of diaper area).	Provides maximal exposure. Shielded areas become more jaundiced so maximum exposure is essential.
	5. Turn infant at regular intervals (e.g., every 2 hr).	Provides equal exposure of all skin areas and prevents pressure areas.
	6. Monitor neonate's skin and core temperature frequently until temperature is stable.	Hypothermia and hyperthermia are common complications of phototherapy. Hypothermia from exposure to lights, subsequent radiation and convection losses.

NURSING CARE PLAN cont'd
Jaundice

Problem	Nursing interventions and actions	Rationale
	7. Provide extra fluid intake.	Assures adequate hydration.
	8. Closely assess infant's daily patterns to detect notable changes in food ingestion, bowel and urination patterns, sleeping and waking rhythms, irritability.	May indicate signs of worsening condition. Neonate may develop green, watery stools.
	9. Administer thorough perianal cleansing with each stool or change of perianal protective covering.	Frequent stooling increases risk of skin breakdown.
	10. Observe for bronzing of skin.	Uncommon complication. May last for 2-4 months.
	11. Check Isolette temperature frequently	Additional heat from phototherapy lights frequently causes a rise in the Isolette temperature.
	12. Give feedings per physician order or protocol.	Increases peristalsis and excretion of bile before it can reenter enterohepatic pathway.
	13. Record number of hours that lights have been used.	Lights may become ineffective after prolonged use.

	14. Observe signs of worsening condition (kernicterus):
	  a. hypotonia, lethargy, poor sucking reflex.
	  b. spasticity and opisthotonus.
	  c. fever.
	  d. gradual appearance of extra pyramidal signs.
	  e. impaired or absent hearing.
		Deposition of bilirubin in brain leads to development of symptoms.
		NOTE: Treatment may be more aggressive in presence of neonatal complications such as asphyxia, respiratory distress, metabolic acidosis, hypothermia, low serum protein, signs of CNS deterioration (Avery, 1981).

	15. Turn phototherapy lights off when drawing blood for bilirubin levels.	Exposure of blood to phototherapy lights may result in a falsely lowered bilirubin value.
Bilirubin level rising above 20 mg/dL in term infants and 15 mg/dL in larger preterm infants (Korones, 1981)	Exchange transfusion (see Procedure 25-5):	
Dehydration	Assess dehydration: 1. Poor skin turgor. 2. Depressed fontanelles. 3. Sunken eyes. 4. Decreased urine output. 5. Weight loss. 6. Changes in electrolytes.	Phototherapy treatment may cause liquid stools and increased insensible water loss, which increases risk of dehydration. As bilirubin levels rise, neonate may become lethargic and more difficult to feed.
	Offer feedings every 3-4 hr. Offer water between feedings.	Adequate hydration facilitates elimination and execretion of bilirubin. Replace fluid losses, due to watery stools, if under phototherapy.
	Administer IV fluids:	IV fluids may be used if neonate is dehydrated or in presence of other complications. IV may be started if exchange transfusion is anticipated.

Problem	Nursing interventions and actions	Rationale
	1. Monitor flow rate.	Prevents fluid overload.
	2. Assess insertion site for evidence of infection.	Identifies infection process.
Lack of tactile stimulation	Provide tactile stimulation during feeding and diaper changes.	Neonate has normal needs for tactile stimulation.
	Provide cuddling and eye contact during feedings. Talk to neonate frequently.	Provides comforting and decreased sensory deprivation.
	Encourage parents to come into nursery for feedings and to touch neonate.	Presence of equipment may discourage parents from interacting with neonate.
Inadequate parental information	Provide explanation of:	
	1. Infant's condition.	Parents may not understand what is happening or why.
	2. Treatment modalities.	Physician preference of treatment modalities may vary. Parents may not understand why their newborn is not receiving a treatment that another with the same condition is receiving.
	3. Reasons that the mother may be asked to cease breast-feeding temporarily.	Breast milk contains pregnanediol, which may suppress the conjugation process by inhibiting glucuronyl transferase. The serum bilirubin levels begin to fall within 48 hr after discontinuation of breast-feeding. Opinion of physicians varies regarding the need for discontinuing breast-feeding.
	4. If breast-feeding is temporarily discontinued, assess mother's knowledge of pumping her breasts and provide information and support as needed.	
	5. Assist mother in reestablishment of breast-feeding.	Mother may need support and information to restart breast-feeding.

NURSING CARE EVALUATION

Kernicterus has been prevented.

Neonate has *no* or minimal residual damage.

Bilirubin levels are decreasing or normal.

Afebrile and vital signs are stable.

Adequate hydration and electrolyte balance has been achieved.

Tactile stimulation has been provided.

Parents understand the cause of the problem, the rationale for treatment, and subsequent care of the neonate.

If breast-feeding, the mother understands the reason for temporary discontinuation of breast-feeding, how to pump her breasts, and how to reinstate breast feedings.

NURSING DIAGNOSES*	SUPPORTING DATA
1. Potential for injury related to high levels of unbound bilirubin	Symptoms of neurologic damage (kernicterus) (See Patient Data Base in Nursing Care Plan for predisposing factors)
2. Potential for injury associated with treatment of hyperbilirubinemia	(See Nursing Care Plan for details of exchange transfusion, p. 833) Phototherapy
3. Potential fluid volume deficit	Lethargy in neonate causing difficulty in feeding Liquid stools Signs and symptoms of dehydration
4. Parental anxiety related to having newborn with jaundice	Expressed concerns or questions regarding infant's welfare and disease process

* These are a few examples of nursing diagnoses that may be appropriate for a newborn with jaundice. It is not an inclusive list and must be individualized for each infant.

Excessive hemolysis of red cells is usually a result of blood group incompatibilities. Bacterial and nonbacterial infections and diseases are also associated with hemolytic anemias. The most common cause of impaired red cell production is a deficiency in G-6-PD, which is genetically transmitted. Anemia and jaundice are the presenting signs.

A condition known as *physiologic anemia* exists as a result of the normal gradual drop in hemoglobin for the first 6–12 weeks of life. It is related to shorter neonatal red blood cell survival, reduced bone marrow activity, and the dilutional effect of expanded plasma on red blood cells.

Theoretically, the bone marrow stops production of red blood cells as a response to the elevated oxygenation of extrauterine respiration. When the amount of hemoglobin becomes lower, reaching levels of 10–11 g/dL at about 6–12 weeks of age, the bone marrow begins to manufacture red blood cells again, and the anemia disappears spontaneously. Rarely does the hemoglobin level fall low enough to require a transfusion. Anemia in preterm infants occurs earlier and reversal by the bone marrow is initiated at lower levels of hemoglobin (7–9 g/dL). The preterm infant's hemoglobin reaches a low sooner (5–10 weeks after delivery) than does a term infant's (6–12 weeks) because preterm red blood cell survival time is shorter compared to the term newborn, and because the rate of growth in preterms is relatively rapid. Deficiency of vitamin E, common in small preterm newborns, is another reason.

Clinical Manifestations and Diagnosis

Clinically, anemic infants are very pale in the absence of other symptoms of shock and usually are found to have abnormally low red blood cell counts. In acute blood loss, symptoms of shock may be present, such as pallor, low arterial blood pressure, and a decreasing hematocrit value. The initial laboratory workup should include hemoglobin and hematocrit measurements, reticulocyte count, examination of peripheral blood smear, bilirubin determinations, direct Coombs' test of infant's blood, and examination of maternal blood smear for fetal erythrocytes (Kleihauer–Betke preparation).

Management

Hematologic problems can be anticipated based on the obstetric history and clinical manifestations. The age at which anemia is first noted is also of diagnostic value. Management depends on severity and whether blood loss is acute or chronic. The infant should be placed on constant cardiac and respiratory monitoring. Mild or slow chronic anemia may be treated adequately with iron supplements alone or with iron-fortified formulas. Frequent determinations of hemoglobin, hematocrit, and bilirubin levels (in hemolytic disease) are essential. In severe cases of anemia, transfusions are the treatment of choice.

NURSING INTERVENTIONS

The nurse must be aware of and promptly report any symptoms and should assist in obtaining blood specimens and taking care of specimen sites. The amount of blood drawn for all laboratory tests should be recorded so that total blood removed can be assessed and blood can be replaced by transfusion when necessary. Prophylactic measures carried out by the nurse include meticulous hand-washing and careful equipment cleaning to help prevent sepsis and subsequent hemolysis.

POLYCYTHEMIA

Polycythemia is a condition in which blood volume and hematocrit values are increased. It is observed more commonly in SGA and full-term infants than in preterm neonates. An infant is considered polycythemic when the central venous hematocrit value is greater than 65%–70%, or the venous hemoglobin level is greater than 22 g/dL during the first week of life (Avery, 1981).

Several conditions predispose the neonate to polycythemia. First, at the time of birth an excessive volume of placental blood may transfuse into the infant before the cord is cut, resulting in a blood volume increase. Second, during gestation an increased amount of blood may cross the placenta to the infant (maternofetal transfusion), resulting in increased blood volume after birth. Third, a twin-to-twin transfusion may occur, in which one twin receives less blood and becomes anemic, and the other twin receives an excess amount of blood resulting in polycythemia. Fourth, increased red blood cell production may occur in utero in response to chronic fetal distress and may be seen in infants who are SGA or IDM.

Many infants are asymptomatic, but as symptoms develop they are related to the increased blood volume, hyperviscosity (thickness) of the blood, and decreased deformability of red blood cells, all of which result in poor perfusion of tissues. The most common symptoms observed include the following:

1. Tachycardia and congestive heart failure—due to the increased blood volume

2. Respiratory distress with grunting, trachypnea, and cyanosis, increased oxygen need, or hemorrhage in respiratory system

3. Hyperbilirubinemia—due to increased numbers of red blood cell hemolysed

4. Decrease in peripheral pulses, discoloration of extremity, alteration in activity or neurologic depression, renal vein thrombosis with decreased urine output, hematuria, or proteinuria due do thromboembolism

5. Seizures—due to increased perfusion of the brain as a result of sluggish blood flow

The nurse should assess, record, and report symptoms and do initial screening of hematocrit on admission to the nursery.

Therapy

The goal of therapy is to reduce the central venous hematocrit to less than 60%. To achieve this, the symptomatic infant receives a partial exchange transfusion in which blood is removed from the infant and replaced milliliter for milliliter with fresh frozen plasma.

HEMORRHAGIC DISEASE

Several transient coagulation-mechanism deficiencies normally occur in the first several days of a newborn's life. Foremost among these is a slight decrease in the levels of prothrombin, resulting in a prolonged clotting time during the initial week of life. For the liver to form prothrombin (factor II) and proconvertin (factor VII) for blood coagulation, vitamin K is required. Vitamin K, a fat-soluble vitamin, may be obtained from food, but it is usually synthesized by bacteria in the colon, and consequently, a dietary source is unnecessary.

Intestinal flora are practically nonexistent in newborns, so they are unable to synthesize vitamin K. Although cow's milk contains more vitamins than breast milk, neither is a rich source of K. Hemorrhagic disease of the newborn is more common in breast-fed babies, however. Bleeding due to vitamin K deficiency generally occurs on the second to third day of life, but it may occur earlier. Internal hemorrhage may occur. Bleeding from the nose, umbilical cord, circumcision site, gastrointestinal tract, and scalp, as well as generalized ecchymoses may be seen.

This disorder may be completely prevented by the prophylactic use of an injection of vitamin K. A dose of 1 mg of Aquamephyton is given as part of the immediate care of the newborn following delivery (see Drug Guide, p. 711). Larger doses are contraindicated because they may result in the development of hyperbilirubinemia.

INTRAVENTRICULAR HEMORRHAGE

Intraventricular hemorrhage (IVH) is the most common type of intracranial hemorrhage occurring in the small preterm infant. Those most susceptible to IVH are infants weighing less than 1500 g or of less than 35 weeks' gestation.

IVH frequently occurs after an insult to the infant that results in hypoxia but may also be related to venous pressure changes and increases in osmolality within the bloodstream. Events leading to hypoxia include respiratory distress, birth trauma, and birth asphyxia, with the more immature infants being at higher risk for both of these complications. Hypercapnia, a common complication of respiratory distress, causes vasodilatation of the cerebral blood vessels, contributing to the increased tendency for rupture to occur. Volume expanders (in this case plasma) are sometimes required to reverse hypotension, which is not uncommon in the preterm infant, and lead to increased central venous pressure. Administration of sodium bicarbonate to relieve acidosis causes an increase in osmolarity, which also contributes to rupture of the tiny blood vessels within the brain.

The most common site of hemorrhage is in the germinal matrix where there is a rich blood supply and the capillary walls are thin and fragile. Generally the hemorrhage occurs in the tissues next to the ventricles and then bursts into the ventricles themselves to circulate with the cerebrospinal fluid. In these cases (85%), a lumbar puncture will generally produce bloody spinal fluid, confirming the suspicion of IVH. However, in some cases, the hemorrhage is confined to the tissues surrounding the ventricles and does not enter the ventricular system or cerebral spinal fluid. In these cases (as well as those previously discussed) computerized axial tomography (CT) or ultrasound scanning can be used to identify both the site and extent of hemorrhage.

The clinical signs observed in an infant with IVH are variable. The infant may suddenly "crash," characterized by pallor and shocklike appearance, and die, or may show very subtle signs or no signs at all. The most common manifestations are neurologic signs (hypotonia, lethargy, hypothermia, nystagmus, bulging fontanelle, falling hematocrit, apnea, bradycardia, decreased blood pressure, and a worsening in the respiratory condition (increasing hypoxia), with metabolic acidosis. Seizures may occur, and opisthotonic posturing may be observed. Clinical diagnosis depends on results of spinal fluid analysis, which includes red blood cells, xanthochromia, or elevated protein content.

The outcome for the infant depends on the size of the bleed and the gestational age of the infant. The most severe hemorrhages may result in motor deficits, hydrocephalus, hearing loss, and blindness. Less severe bleeds may result in no observable sequelae (Hellmann and Vannucci, 1982).

Interventions

Nursing management of an infant with IVH is mainly observational and supportive. All related parameters should be monitored closely (vital signs, fontanelle tenseness, seizure activity, hematocrit, and blood pressure). The nurse should prepare the infant and assist with lumbar puncture for spinal fluid analysis.

Hypoxemia, acidemia, and hypotension should be corrected by maintaining adequate oxygenation. This is done by increasing ambient oxygen concentration or placement of the infant on continuous positive airway pressure or on a respirator. While administering replacement whole blood or albumin the nurse should closely monitor blood pressure. Thermal neutrality must be maintained.

Seizures may be controlled with phenobarbital. After a suspected bleed, the occipital frontal circumference should be checked closely as hydrocephalus may occur. Serial head ultrasounds may also be done. Although prevention of IVH is not possible, infants at high risk should be maintained in as stable physiologic condition as possible. Prevention of stress and asphyxia decrease the chances that IVH will occur.

DISSEMINATED INTRAVASCULAR COAGULATION

Disseminated intravascular coagulation (DIC) is an acquired pathologic process in the body, which results in depletion of plasma clotting factors and platelets. As a result of various clinical conditions, the clotting process is inappropriately activated, leading to coagulation and thrombi formation within the blood vessels and rapid consumption of clotting factors and platelets. As a result of clot formation within the blood vessels, tissue necrosis occurs, and when clotting factors are depleted, hemorrhage occurs throughout the body. The most common clinical signs observed include oozing of blood from previous puncture sites with inability to stop the bleeding, petechiae, and general bleeding from other body orifices (mouth and nose). Internal bleeding may also occur into the lungs (pulmonary hemorrhage) and into the brain (IVH).

The clinical conditions most commonly associated with the development of DIC include gram negative septicemia, acidosis, hypoxia, hypotension, and severe RDS.

The primary goal of therapy is to correct the underlying problem (for example, septicemia) that precipitated the DIC. Interim therapy can include administration of fresh platelets or fresh frozen plasma. Heparin therapy may be used to counteract thrombi formation, and complete exchange transfusion may be used to eliminate fibrin-degrading products and toxic factors that may cause DIC.

NECROTIZING ENTEROCOLITIS

With recent advances in the field of neonatology, severely ill infants who a decade ago would have succumbed are now surviving. With this increased survival, a group of infants are now being encountered with necrotizing enterocolitis. A previously unknown disease, *necrotizing enterocolitis* (NEC) occurs in the first weeks of life and may cause bowel perforation and ultimately death.

The occurrence of a "new" disease entity produces a flourish of theories as to the etiology. With NEC, the exact causation is not known, but some predisposing factors are associated with subsequent development of the disease. The current concept is that the etiology is multifocal involving mucosal damage, bacterial presence, and nutrient substrate available for proliferation of the organisms.

An ischemic attack to the intestine may be precipitated by any condition in which systemic shock and hypoxia occur. Such conditions as fetal distress, neonatal shock and asphyxia, low cardiac output syndrome, low Apgar score, RDS, umbilical arterial catheters, infusion of hyperosmolar solution, and prematurity are associated with NEC. It is thought that the diving reflex of the seal, in which blood is shunted to the heart and brain and away from the intestine and kidneys during prolonged dives, is analogous to the shunting of blood in asphyxial insults of the neonate.

Prolonged intestinal ischemia results in thrombosis in small intestinal vessels, infarction of affected bowels, and digestion of the mucosal lining of the intestine. Reestablishment of normal circulation enables restoration and regeneration of the damaged area if the damage is reversible.

The action of enteric bacteria on the damaged intestinal mucosa may serve to complicate the process, producing sepsis. Gram-negative organisms most frequently identified are *E. coli* and *Klebsiella*. Early feedings, advocated for promotion of adequate nutrition, provide excellent media for proliferation of intestinal bacteria. Gas formation and possible dissection of air into the portal system is a result of bacterial action upon the media provided by oral feedings. Some recent investigations have shown breast milk to be safer in feedings for the at-risk group. It is postulated that the antibodies present in breast colostrum act as a protector for the intestinal mucosa. Necrotic lesions are seen in any part of the intestine below the duodenum but are commonly seen in the lower ileum, the ascending and transverse colon, or both. The lesions are characterized by frequent mucosal ulcerations, pseudomembrane formation, and inflammation; radiologic examination reveals pneumatosis intestinalis and possible sequelae of perforation.

Clinical Manifestations and Diagnosis

The neonatal nurse, providing constant bedside care, is often the first person to observe the subtle signs and symptoms of early development of NEC. Recognition of the just-mentioned high-risk groups, careful observation for subtle, nonspecific symptoms, and prompt reporting of suspicions enable early, often life-saving treatment to begin. Onset usually occurs within the first 2–3 weeks of life, although NEC can be seen as early as the first day of life. Most cases are diagnosed by 1 month of age in all but the most debilitated patients. Systemic symptoms are those associated with sepsis—temperature instability (often hypothermia), respiratory changes (apnea, labored respirations), cardiovascular collapse, and behavioral changes such as lethargy or irritability. Gastrointestinal symptoms include abdominal distention and tenderness, feeding changes such as vomiting or increased gastric residual (bile-stained), poor feeding, abdominal wall cellulitis (development of an erythematous area on the abdominal wall), and blood (Hematest positive) and reducing substances in the stools.

Clinical findings are corroborated by radiographic findings, which include (a) pneumatosis intestinalis—air in the bowel wall (extraluminal or intramural air bubble and strips); (b) adynamic ileus—a paralytic ileus with stasis; (c) bowel wall thickening and loops of unequal size, bubbly appearance of intestine; and (d) free air—pneumoperitoneum or free air in the portal vein.

Serial anteroposterior and lateral decubitus (or crosstable lateral abdominal) radiographic evaluation is recommended every 4–6 hours for detection of progression of the disease and determination of complications indicating surgical intervention.

Complications

Complications or consequences of necrotizing enterocolitis include (a) surgical removal of the diseased intestine, leaving insufficient remaining small bowel to support life; (b) stenosis of the intestinal tract that develops secondary to NEC or surgery; (c) gastrointestinal dysfunction so that there is recurring intolerance to oral feedings, with vomiting, abdominal distention, water-loss diarrhea, and failure to gain weight; (d) parenteral hyperalimentation that predisposes to sepsis, thrombosis of major vessels, and metabolic complications such as hyperglycemia, glycosuria, acidosis, osmotic diuresis, dehydration, and hepatic damage (cholestatic jaundice), and (e) prolonged hospitalization with separation from parents and possible lack of appropriate developmental stimuli.

Interventions

Necrotizing enterocolitis is of increasing concern in the management of sick neonates. Survival of the infants depends on early recognition and treatment and meticulous nursing care.

Aggressive and early management may preclude the need for surgical intervention. Intensive nursing management consists of supportive therapy and constant observation of the neonate's condition (see the Nursing Care Plan on necrotizing enterocolitis on facing page). Gastric decompression, fluid and electrolyte replacement, correction of acidosis, correction of temperature instability, and parenteral antibiotics are common treatment techniques. Diffusion of volume expanders such as fresh frozen plasma may be necessary to correct existing hypotension and to improve peripheral perfusion, because large amounts of plasma protein are lost into the gut lumen and peritoneal cavity in the acute phase.

The nurse must be prepared to stop oral feedings and to place a gastric tube for gastric decompression and drainage and must be ready for possible instillation of antibiotics through the gastric tube and administration of parenteral fluids, calories, and antibiotics. Hyperalimentation through a central line (inserted into the superior vena cava) may be indicated if the infant is believed to have a severe form of NEC requiring total parenteral nutrition for 2 or more weeks (O'Neill, 1981).

Arterial oxygenation must be maintained. Constant observation of vital signs, oxygen concentration, development of increasing abdominal girth, and worsening clinical condition is the responsibility of the nurse.

Surgery is indicated at the development of intestinal perforation with pneumoperitoneum, intestinal infarction without perforation, progressive abdominal ascites and/or bowel wall thickening, and clinical deterioration. Even small or subtle changes may indicate rapid progression and worsening of the disease and the need for immediate surgical intervention.

Surgical intervention consists of removal of those areas of bowel that are necrotic or perforated. Intestinal areas of compromised circulation or questionable viability are usually preserved, in hopes of eventual recovery and regeneration. Primary anastomosis is not attempted because of the possibility of connecting areas of ischemic bowel. The infant may return with a gastrostomy in place to decompress the intestinal tract and an ostomy for drainage.

Meticulous nursing care is required in maintenance of skin integrity around the openings in these debilitated infants. Reestablishment of continuity of the intestines is done when the infant can tolerate oral feedings and when general health is improved.

Recovery of the intestinal mucosa and return to proper small bowel functioning (in nutritional absorption) are delayed after enterocolitis (with or without surgical intervention). The small bowel mucosa must recover from the ischemia and regenerate to resume its function of absorption of nutrients. Meanwhile, parenteral hyperalimentation is utilized to maintain positive nitrogen balance, so that healing is promoted. After rest of the gastrointestinal tract, cautious feedings are begun, using elemental formulas (such as Vivonix) to promote easy absorption.

NURSING CARE PLAN
Necrotizing Enterocolitis

PATIENT DATA BASE

History

Prematurity

Gestational history: fetal distress, asphyxia, fetal acidosis

Neonatal history: low Apgar scores, hypovolemia, RDS, asphyxia, utilization of umbilical catheters and/or infusion of hyperosmolar solution, bacterial infections; may have no clinical manifestations until about 1–2 weeks of age

Feeding patterns: changes, poor feeding, increased gastric residual

Physical examination

Hypothermia, apneic episodes, labored respirations, lethargy or irritability

Gastrointestinal signs: abdominal distention, shiny abdominal wall, tenderness, abdominal wall cellulitis, diarrheal stools; may have observable loops of bowel

Vomiting (may be bile-stained)

Absence of bowel sounds

Laboratory evaluation

Abnormal coagulation studies and platelet counts

Hematest positive stools

Reducing substances in the stools

Radiologic examination: pneumatosis intestinalis, adynamic ileus, thickening of bowel wall and bowel loops of unequal size, and pneumoperitoneum or free air in the portal vein

NURSING PRIORITIES

1. Achieve early recognition by doing Hematests and reducing substances at least once per shift.
2. Determine and correct acid-base imbalances.
3. Provide support measures to maintain homeostasis; that is, maintain neutral thermal environment and provide adequate fluid and electrolytes.
4. Observe for progression of clinical manifestations indicating surgical intervention.
5. Preoperative management: withhold feedings and maintain gastric decompression.
6. Provide for the emotional needs of the infant.
7. Provide parents with adequate explanation of treatment modalities and infant's condition, plus anticipatory information about colostomy if surgery is pending.

FAMILY EDUCATIONAL FOCUS

1. Explain treatment modalities utilized in NEC and their rationale.
2. Explore possible long-term implications of NEC such as feeding difficulties, strictures, short bowel syndrome (if surgery is necessary), and need for possible colostomy.
3. Refer family to available resource and support groups.
4. Provide opportunities for parents to discuss questions and individual concerns about their neonate.

Problem	Nursing interventions and actions	Rationale
Early recognition	Clinitest stools to check for reducing substances and Hematest positive stools at least every shift. Evaluate changes in feeding patterns: 1. Poor feeding. 2. Bile-stained emesis. 3. Increase in gastric residual.	Reducing substances in the stools indicate poor absorption of sugars and may be one of the earliest indications of NEC. Increased gastric retention is caused by prolonged gastric emptying.
	Auscultate bowel sounds. Measure abdominal girth every 2–3 hr if NEC is suspected.	May be absent due to paralytic ileus. An increase greater than 1 cm in 4 hours is significant.
Ischemia of bowel	Discontinue oral feedings.	Rests bowel.
	Insert nasogastric tube with continuous low suction	Provides for gastric decompression and drainage.
	Prevent trauma to abdomen: 1. Avoid diapers.	Diapers place pressure on lower abdomen and obstruct good observation of abdomen for any changes in condition.
	2. Pick up infant only when necessary.	Minimal handling prevents abdominal trauma.

NURSING CARE PLAN cont'd
Necrotizing Enterocolitis

Problem	Nursing interventions and actions	Rationale
	Observe for signs of perforation of bowel and peritonitis and increasing distention.	
	Take axillary temperature.	Rectal temperatures are contraindicated. Decreases trauma to rectal mucosa.
Acid-base imbalance	Administer parenteral fluid and electrolyte replacements as ordered. Observe vital signs. Monitor electrolytes.	Corrects acid-base imbalance.
Infection	Administer broad-spectrum antibiotic parenterally and intragastrically as ordered. Obtain blood, urine, CSF, and stool cultures for sepsis workup.	Combats infectious process if present.
Shock	Observe for signs of shock (temperature instability, drop in blood pressure, apneic spells, bradycardia, listlessness).	
	Administer fresh frozen plasma per order.	Improves peripheral perfusion and corrects existing hypotension caused by shift of large amounts of plasma protein into gut lumen and peritoneal cavity.
	Administer Dextran.	Dextran counters platelet adherence.
Lack of physical stimulation	Stroke hands and head. Talk to infant as often as possible, even in absence of tactile stimulation. Provide visual and auditory stimulation—mobiles, windup toys, music boxes.	Meets emotional and sensory stimulation needs.

NURSING CARE EVALUATION

Stool Hematest is negative for 3 consecutive days.	Parents understand need for continual medical supervision.
Infant is afebrile and vital signs are stable.	Parent–infant bonding is appropriate.
Infant tolerates food and fluids.	

NURSING DIAGNOSES*	SUPPORTING DATA	
1. Alteration in nutrition: Potential for less than body requirements related to prolonged gastric emptying and malabsorption	Poor feeding Bile-stained emesis Increase in gastric residual	
2. Alteration in bowel elimination related to ischemic mucous membranes of lower GI tract	Diminished or absent bowel sounds Increasing abdominal girth Hematest positive stools Significant radiologic examination (see Nursing Care Plan)	
3. Potential intravascular fluid volume deficit related to loss of plasma protein into gut lumen and peritoneal cavity	Decreased blood pressure Symptoms of electrolyte imbalance Symptoms of shock	Listness Temperature instability Apneic spells Bradycardia
4. Parental knowledge deficit related to necrotizing enterocolitis	Expressed concerns and questions about the disease process and its complications	

* These are a few examples of nursing diagnoses that may be appropriate for an infant with necrotizing enterocolitis. It is not an inclusive list and must be individualized for each infant.

INFECTIONS

Sepsis Neonatorum

Neonates up to 1 month of age are particularly susceptible to infection, referred to as *sepsis neonatorum*, caused by organisms that do not cause significant disease in older children. Incidence of severe infection is 0.5 to 2 per 1000 live newborns.

One predisposing factor is prematurity. The general debilitation and underlying illness often associated with prematurity necessitates invasive procedures such as umbilical catheterization, intubation, resuscitation, ventilatory support, and monitoring. Even the full-term infant is susceptible because of an immature immunologic system, which lacks the complex factors involved in effective phagocytosis and the ability to effectively localize infection or to respond with a well-defined recognizable inflammatory response. Maternal antepartal infections such as rubella, toxoplasmosis, cytomegalic inclusion disease, and herpes may cause congenital infections and resulting disorders within the newborn. Intrapartal maternal infections such as amnionitis and those resulting from premature rupture of membranes and precipitous delivery are sources of neonatal infection. Passage through the birth canal and contact with colonization of the vaginal flora (β-hemolytic streptococci, herpes, listeria, and gonococci) expose the infant to infection. With infection anywhere in the fetus or newborn, the adjacent tissues or organs are very easily penetrated, and the blood–brain barrier is ineffective. Septicemia is more common in males, except for those infections caused by group B β-hemolytic streptococcus.

The etiology of sepsis has changed in recent years. In the past, gram positive organisms (that is, *Staphylococcus aureus* and group A streptococcus pneumococci) were the causative agents of significant neonatal illness. At present, gram negative organisms (especially *Escherichia coli*, Aerobacter, Proteus, and *Klebsiella*) and the gram positive organism B β-hemolytic streptococci are the most common causative agents. Pseudomonas is a common contaminant of fomites used for ventilatory support and oxygen therapy.

CLINICAL MANIFESTATIONS AND DIAGNOSIS

Sepsis neonatorum is characterized by positive blood cultures and generalized clinical manifestations of illness, which are subtle and nonspecific and may be caused by other problems. Early detection of sepsis is extremely important.

Infants with a history of possible exposure to infection in utero (for example PROM more than 24 hours before delivery or questionable maternal history of infection) should have cultures taken as soon after birth as possible. A gastric aspirate and culture of external orifices (such as the ear canal) will reveal the organisms to which the infant was exposed. A high index of suspicion for the presence of sepsis is of utmost importance so that signs and symptoms of sepsis are discovered and appropriate intervention is begun immediately.

Symptoms are most often noticed by the nurse in the daily care of the neonate rather than during the infant's sporadic contact with the physician. The infant may deteriorate rapidly in the first 12–24 hours after birth if β-hemolytic streptococcal infection is present, with signs and symptoms mimicking RDS. On the other hand, the onset of sepsis may be more gradual with more subtle signs and symptoms. The most common symptoms observed include:

1. Subtle behavioral changes—infant "isn't doing well"; often lethargic or irritable, especially after first 24 hours, and hypotonic. Color changes may include pallor, duskiness, cyanosis, or a "shocky" appearance. Skin is cool and clammy.

2. Temperature instability, manifested by either hypothermia (recognized by a decrease in skin temperature) or hyperthermia (elevation of neonatal skin temperature) necessitating a corresponding increase or decrease in incubator temperature to maintain neutral thermal environment.

3. Poor feeding, evidenced by a decrease in total intake, abdominal distention, vomiting, poor sucking, lack of interest in feeding, and diarrhea.

4. Hyperbilirubinemia.

5. Onset of apnea.

Signs and symptoms may suggest CNS disease (jitteriness, tremors, seizure activity), respiratory system disease (tachypnea, labored respirations, apnea, cyanosis), hematologic disease (jaundice, petechial hemorrhages, hepatosplenomegaly), or gastrointestinal disease (diarrhea, vomiting, bile-stained aspirate, hepatomegaly). A differential diagnosis is necessary because of the similarity of symptoms to other more specific conditions.

Isolation of the causative agent is necessary to obtain the diagnosis of sepsis in a suspected case and to identify the drugs to which the pathogen is susceptible. The nurse must be prepared to assist in the aseptic collection of specimens for laboratory investigation. Before antibiotic therapy is begun, cultures are obtained.

1. Two blood cultures are obtained from different peripheral sites. They are taken from a peripheral, rather than umbilical vessel, because catheters have yielded false positives resulting from contamination. The skin is prepared by cleansing with an antiseptic solution, such as one containing iodine, and allowed to dry; the specimen is obtained with a sterile needle/syringe.

2. Spinal fluid culture is obtained following a spinal tap.

3. Urine culture is best obtained from a specimen obtained by a suprapubic bladder aspiration.

4. Skin cultures are obtained of any lesions or drainage from lesions or reddened areas.

5. Nasopharyngeal, rectal, ear canal, and gastric aspirate cultures may be obtained.

Other laboratory investigations include a complete blood count, chest x-ray examination, serology, and Gram stains of cerebrospinal fluid, urine, skin exudate, and umbilicus. White blood count with differential may indicate the presence or absence of sepsis. A level of 30,000 WBC may be normal in the first 24 hours of life, while a low WBC may be indicative of sepsis. A low neutrophil count and a high band count indicate that an infection is present. Stomach aspirate should be sent for culture and smear if a gonococcal infection or amnionitis are suspected. Serum IgM levels are elevated (normal level less than 20 mg/dL) in response to transplacental infections. Counterimmunoelectrophoresis tests for specific bacterial antigens, if available, are done. Evidence of congenital infections may be seen on skull x-rays for cerebral calcifications (cytomegalovirus, toxoplasmosis), bone x-rays (syphilis, cytomegalovirus), and serum-specific IgM levels (rubella). Cytomegalovirus infection is best diagnosed by urine cultures.

NURSING MANAGEMENT

□ *TREATMENT* Because neonatal infection causes high mortality, therapy is instituted before results of the septic workup are obtained. A combination of two broad-spectrum antibiotics in large doses is initiated until culture with sensitivities is received.

After the pathogen and its sensitivities are determined, appropriate specific antibiotic therapy is begun. Combinations of penicillin or ampicillin and kanamycin have been utilized in the past, but new kanamycin-resistant enterobacteria and penicillin-resistant staphylococcus necessitate increasing use of gentamycin. Duration of therapy varies from 7–14 days (Table 25–4). If cultures are negative and symptoms subside, antibiotics may be discontinued after 3 days.

In administration of antibiotics the nurse must be knowledgeable about: (a) the proper dose to be administered, based on the weight of the newborn; (b) the appropriate route of administration, as some antibiotics cannot be given intravenously; (c) admixture incompatibilities (some antibiotics are precipitated by intravenous solutions or by other antibiotics); and (d) side effects and toxicity.

In addition to antibiotic therapy, physiologic supportive care is essential in caring for a septic infant:

- Observe for resolution of symptoms or development of other symptoms of sepsis
- Maintain neutral thermal environment with accurate regulation of humidity and oxygen administration
- Provide respiratory support—administer oxygen and observe and monitor respiratory effort

- Provide cardiovascular support—observe and monitor pulse and blood pressure; observe for hyperbilirubinemia, anemia, and hemorrhagic symptoms
- Provide adequate calories, because oral feedings may be discontinued due to increased mucus, abdominal distention, vomiting, and aspiration
- Provide fluids and electrolytes to maintain homeostasis
- Detect and treat metabolic disturbances, a common occurrence
- Observe for the development of hypoglycemia, hyperglycemia, acidosis, hyponatremia, and hypocalcemia

□ *PREVENTION* Protection of the newborn from infections starts prenatally and continues throughout pregnancy and through delivery into the world.

Prenatal prevention should include maternal screening for sexually transmitted disease and monitoring of rubella titers in women who are negative. Intrapartally, sterile technique is essential, smears from genital lesions are taken, placenta and amniotic fluid cultures are obtained if amnionitis is suspected and if genital herpes is present toward term, and delivery by cesarean birth may be indicated. Local eye treatment with silver nitrate or an antibiotic ophthalmic ointment is given to all newborns to prevent gonococcal damage.

In the nursery, environmental control and prevention of acquired infection is the responsibility of the neonatal nurse. Being the vanguard of infection control, the nurse must promote vigorous, strict hand-washing technique for all who enter the nursery, including nursing colleagues; physicians; laboratory, x-ray, and inhalation technicians; and parents. Scrupulous care of equipment—changing and cleaning of incubators at least every 7 days, removal and sterilization of wet equipment every 24 hours, prevention of cross-utilization of linen and other equipment, periodic cleaning of sinkside equipment such as soap containers, and special care with the open radiant warmers (access without prior hand-washing is much easier than with the closed incubator)—will all prevent fomite contamination or contamination through improper hand-washing of debilitated, infection-prone newborns. An infected neonate can be effectively isolated in an incubator and receive close observation. Visitation of the nursery area by unnecessary personnel should be discouraged. Restriction of visiting parents has not been shown to have any effect on the rate of infection and may indeed be harmful for a newborn's psychologic development. With instruction and supervision from the nurse, both parents should be allowed to handle the baby and participate in the care, even inside the incubators.

Group B Streptococcus

Group B streptococcus (β-hemolytic streptococcus) has become a leading cause of septicemia in the newborn, and is

Table 25-4 Neonatal Sepsis Antibiotic Therapy

Drug	Dose	Route	Schedule	Comments
Ampicillin	50–200 mg/kg/day	IM or IV	Every 12 hours* Every 6–8 hours†	Effective against gram positive microorganisms and majority of *E. coli* strains.
Gentamycin	5.0–7.5 mg/kg/day	IM or IV	Every 12 hours* Every 8 hours†	Effective against gram negative rods and staphylococci; may be used instead of kanamycin against penicillin-resistant staphylococci and *E. coli* strains and *Pseudomonas aeruginosa*. May cause ototoxicity and nephrotoxicity. Need to follow serum levels if using more than 3 days. Must never be given as IV push. Must be given over at least 30–60 min. In presence of oliguria or anuria, dose must be decreased or discontinued.
Kanamycin	7.5–10.0 mg/kg/day	IM or IV	Every 8–12 hours	Initial sepsis therapy effective against almost all gram negative organisms with exception of pseudomonas; not to be used more than 12 days. May cause ototoxicity and nephrotoxicity. In presence of oliguria or anuria, dose must be decreased or discontinued.
Nafcillin	50–100 mg/kg/day	IM or IV	Every 12 hours* Every 8 hours†	Effective against penicillinase-resistant staphylococci.
Penicillin G (aqueous crystalline)	100,000 U/kg/day	IM or IV	Every 12 hours* Every 8 hours†	Initial sepsis therapy effective against most gram positive microorganisms except resistant staphylococci; can cause heart block in infants.
Methicillin	50–200 mg/kg/day	IM or IV	Every 12 hours* Every 6–8 hours†	Effective against penicillinase-resistant staphylococci.

* Up to 7 days of age.
† Greater than 7 days of age.

a major cause of morbidity and mortality in the neonate. Pregnant women who carry group B streptococcus are asymptomatic but harbor the organism in the birth canal, resulting in exposure of the infant to the organism during the birth process. It is estimated that 4%–6% of pregnant women have positive cervical cultures, while a larger number have positive vaginal cultures. Approximately 1%–2% of neonates are colonized with group B streptococcus but only one in ten of those colonized develops the disease (Korones, 1981).

Two clinical disease entities may result from group B streptococcus. One is an early onset form (first 24 hours) of acute septicemia. The other occurs later (several days to 3 months) presenting as meningitis without respiratory distress. The early form carries a higher mortality risk (approximately 50%) than the later onset form (20%–40%) (Avery, 1981).

The early onset form of group B streptococcus usually occurs within the first 12–24 hours of life. The infant appears to be in severe respiratory distress (grunting and cyanosis), may become apneic, and may demonstrate symptoms of shock. The chest x-ray examination may show aspiration pneumonia or may appear similar to that seen in hyaline membrane disease. Early recognition of a group B streptococcal condition is essential to the infant's intact survival, as the course is one of rapid deterioration. Cultures should be done immediately (blood, gastric aspirate, external ear canal, nasopharynx), and antibiotics should be started before results of the cultures are obtained. Antibiotic treatment usually involves aqueous penicillin or ampicillin. Some feel ampicillin combined with gentomycin is superior to ampicillin alone. It is the nurse's responsibility to be alert to all signs and symptoms suggesting sepsis, and to intervene as rapidly as possible when sepsis is suspected. There must be no delay in the administration of antibiotics, as this may determine the infant's ultimate survival.

Syphilis

Because congenital syphilis is difficult to detect at birth, all infants of syphilitic mothers should be screened to determine the necessity of treatment. Diagnostic serologic dilution tests are usually accurate between 3 and 6 months of age. Development and detection of the infant's own antibodies are essential for diagnosis.

By 3 months of age the congenitally infected infant exhibits the following signs:

- Positive serology; elevated cord serum, immunoglobulin M (IgM)
- Vesicular lesions over palms and soles
- Red rash around mouth and anus; copper-colored rash covering face, palms, and soles
- Hepatosplenomegaly
- Irritability
- Rhinitis (sniffles); fissures at mouth corners and on excoriated upper lip
- Pyrexia
- Painful extremities
- Bone lesions
- Generalized edema, particularly over joints
- Jaundice
- Small for gestational age (SGA) and failure to thrive

The nursing management of these infants and their parents requires careful physical and psychologic care. Drug treatment of choice is penicillin. After proper treatment for 48 hours, the infant should no longer be contagious. Initially, nursing care includes use of isolation techniques. However, following treatment, general care may ensue. This would include basic assessment of axillary temperature every 3 to 4 hours; intake and output record; feedings; and infant's tolerances. Infants should be swaddled for comfort, and their hands should be covered to minimize trauma to their skin from scratching. Support to the parents is crucial. They need to be informed of the infant's prognosis as treatment continues and to be involved in care as much as possible. They need to understand how infection is transmitted. It is essential to avoid judging the parents and to encourage positive parental involvement.

Gonorrhea

Gonorrhea may be contracted by the fetus during vaginal delivery. Gonorrhea is usually manifested clinically as an eye infection, ophthalmia neonatorum. This is first diagnosed as a conjunctivitis that is indistinguishable from that caused by silver nitrate instillation. However, one clue is that chemical conjunctivitis disappears within 24 hours, whereas ophthalmia neonatorum becomes more readily apparent in the neonate on the third or fourth postnatal day. Other more severe clinical signs that develop are a purulent discharge and ulcerations of the cornea, which can be prevented if treatment is instituted promptly. In some cases, gonorrhea infection may be observed as temperature instability, poor feeding response, and/or hypotonia.

For neonates of all vaginal births, a 1% silver nitrate solution or antibiotic ophthalmic ointment is instilled in the conjunctiva of the infant's eyes to prevent infection. Irrigation of the eyes following administration is controversial. (See Drug Guide, p. 711.) Penicillin may also be administered topically and systemically, in lieu of silver nitrate. If allergy to penicillin is suspected, erythromycin, a tetracycline, or chloramphenicol may be substituted. If the infant's eyes are left untreated, partial or complete loss of vision may occur as a result of corneal ulceration.

Herpesvirus Type 2

A wide variety of clinical manifestations of herpesvirus hominis (HVH) type 2 are noted in the neonate. Signs and symptoms are present at birth or by 3–4 weeks of age. The disseminated form is seen as a bleeding tendency, hepatitis with jaundice, hepatosplenomegaly, and neurologic abnormalities. About one-third of affected infants exhibit vesicular skin lesions in small clusters all over the body. The more localized form includes convulsions (focal or generalized), abnormal muscle tone, opisthotonus, a bulging fontanelle, and lethargy or coma and carries very high mortality rates. In the eyes, keratitis (cloudy corneas), conjunctivitis, and chorioretinitis are seen. Another form is asymptomatic at birth and can develop symptomatology up to 12 days after birth. Frequently the skin lesions are the only diagnostic finding.

In the absence of skin lesions, diagnosis is difficult, because the presenting clinical picture resembles septicemia (such as fever or subnormal temperature, respiratory congestion, dyspnea, cough, tachypnea, and tachycardia). It is therefore necessary to obtain cultures from the infant's lesions and throat and to identify the herpesvirus type 2 antibodies in the serum IgM fraction. Positive cultures are observable within 24 to 48 hours.

Therapy has consisted of treatment systemically with idoxuridine (IDU), which has been successful in some infants and of no avail in others (Korones, 1981). Currently, an antiviral drug, acyclovir (Z ovirax), is used for initial and recurrent mucosal and cutaneous Herpes. Other drug therapy includes cytosine arabinoside (ara-C) and adenine arabinoside (ara-A) (Amstey et al., 1976), all of which are immunosuppressive in nature. Careful hand-washing and adequate infection-control methods are essential. Isolation measures should be instituted for all infants born to mothers known to have had third trimester infections.

Monilial Infection (Thrush)

Thrush (oral moniliasis) is caused by the fungus *Candida albicans*, contracted from a yeast-infected vagina during delivery. Clinically, it appears as white plaques distributed on the buccal mucosa, on the tongue, on the gums, inside the cheeks, and even on the lips. As it resembles milk curds, differentiation should be made by using a cotton-tipped applicator to gently attempt wiping away the patches. If the plaques are thrush, a raw bleeding area beneath them will be exposed. Involvement of the diaper area skin is seen as a bright red, well-demarcated eruption. On occasion, generalized moniliasis may be seen. Lesions are most frequently seen at about 5–7 days of age. However, infants receiving long-term antibiotic therapy are also susceptible to development of thrush, which may occur at any time in the hospitalization.

Care of the neonate infected with *Candida albicans* involves:

1. Maintaining cleanliness of hands, bedding, clothing, diapers, and feeding apparatus, because *Candida albicans*

is present in the oral secretions and in the stools. Breast-feeding mothers should be instructed on treating their nipples with topical nystatin; otherwise a cycle of reinfection as well as sore nipples with breakdown of nipple tissue will occur.

2. Supporting physiologic well-being.
3. Administering drug therapy. Gentian violet (1%–2%) is swabbed on oral mucosa, usually an hour after feeding, once or twice a day; or nystatin (Mycostatin) is instilled in the oral cavity with a medicine dropper. The mouth should be cleared of milk prior to instillation. It may also be swabbed over the oral mucosa. Topical nystatin is used for skin involvement.
4. Discussing with the parents that gentian violet is a dye and will cause staining of the infant's mouth and possibly the infant's clothing if the saliva is gentian colored.

SUMMARY

The sick neonate—whether preterm, term, or postterm—must be managed within narrow physiologic parameters. These parameters (respiratory and thermal regulation) will maintain physiologic homeostasis and prevent introduction of iatrogenic stress to the already stressed infant. Maintenance of this physiologic environment must begin immediately, because lost ground is difficult or impossible to recover.

The nursing care of the neonate with special problems involves the understanding of normal physiology, the pathophysiology of the disease process, clinical manifestations, and supportive and corrective therapies. Only with this theoretical background can the nurse make appropriate observations concerning responses to therapy and development of complications. Neonates communicate needs only by their behavior; the neonatal nurse, through objective observations and evaluations, interprets this behavior into meaningful information about the infant's condition.

References

Amstey, M. S., et al. Jan. 1976. Herpesvirus infection in the newborn: its treatment by exchange transfusion and adenosine arabinoside. *Obstet. Gynecol.* (suppl.) 47:33.

Avery, G. B. 1981. *Neonatology: pathophysiology and management of the newborn.* Philadelphia: J. B. Lippincott Co.

Bacsik, R. D. 1977. Meconium aspiration syndrome. *Pediatr. Clin. North Am.* 24:3.

Bancalari, E., and Berlin, J. A. 1978. Meconium aspiration and other asphyxial disorders. *Clin. Perinatol.* 5:2.

Berkowitz, R. L., et al. 1981. Handbook for prescribing medications during pregnancy. Boston: Little, Brown, & Co.

Cloherty, J. P., and Stark, A. R., eds. 1981. *Manual of neonatal care.* Boston: Little, Brown & Co.

Dodson, W. E. 1977. Neonatal metabolic encephalopathies, hypoglycemia, hypocalcemia, hypomagnesemia, and hyperbilirubinemia. *Clin. Perinatol.* 4:131.

Gluck, L., and Kulovich, M. May 1973. Fetal lung development. *Pediatr. Clin. North Am.* 20:367.

Gregory, G. A., and Gooding, C. A. 1971. Roentgenographic analysis of meconium aspiration of the newborn. *Radiology.* 100:131.

Hansen, F. H. Jan./Feb. 1982. Nursing care in the neonatal intensive care unit. *J. Obstet. Gynecol. Neonat. Nurs.* 11:17.

Hellmann, J., and Vannucci, R. C. 1982. Intraventricular hemorrhage in premature infants. *Sem. Perinatol.* 6:42.

Jennings, C. Mar./Apr. 1982. An alternative: nasal cannula. Oxygen therapy for infants who are oxygen dependent. *MCN* 7:89.

Klaus, M. H., and Fanaroff, A. A. 1979. *Care of the high-risk neonate.* Philadelphia: W. B. Saunders Co.

Korones, S. B. 1981. *High-risk newborn infants: the basis for intensive nursing care,* 2nd ed. St. Louis: The C. V. Mosby Co.

Mason, T. N. Nov./Dec. 1982. A hand ventilation technique for neonates. *MCN* 7:366.

Modanlou, H. D. 1976. Identification and resuscitation of the high-risk infant. Lecture on Critical Care of the Neonate presented at University of Colorado Medical Center.

Monin, P., and Vert, P. 1978. Pneumothorax. *Clin. Perinatol.* 5:335.

Northway, W. H., Jr., et al. 1967. Pulmonary disease following respiratory therapy of hyaline membrane disease: bronchopulmonary dysplasia. *N. Engl. J. Med.* 276:357.

O'Neill, J. A. 1981. Neonatal necrotizing enterocolitis. *Surg. Clin. North Am.* 61:1013.

Saucier, P. H. 1980. Persistent fetal circulation. *J. Obstet. Gynecol. Neonatal Nurs.* 9:50.

Scanlon, K. B.; Grylack, L. J.; and Borten, M. Nov./Dec. 1982. Placement of umbilical artery catheters: high vs low. *J. Obstet. Gynecol. Neonat. Nurs.* 11:355.

Valdes, O. S., et al. 1971. Controlled clinical trial of phenobarbital and/or light in reducing neonatal hyperbilirubinemia in a predominately Negro population. *J. Pediatr.* 79:1015.

Wyman, M. L., and Kuhns, L. R. 1977. Accuracy of transillumination in the recognition of pneumothorax and pneumomediastinum in the neonate. *Clin. Pediatr.* 16:323.

Additional Readings

Andiman, W. A. 1979. Congenital herpesvirus infection. *Clin. Perinatol.* 6:331.

Bahr, J. E. Jan./Feb. 1978. Herpesvirus: hominis type 2 in women and newborns. *MCN.* 3:16.

Baker, C. J. 1979. Group B streptococcal infections in neonates. *Pediatrics in Review.* 1:5.

Coleman, M., and Thompson, T. R. 1979. A possible role of vitamin E in the prevention or amelioration of bronchopulmonary dysplasia. *Am. J. Pediatr. Hematol./Oncol.* 1:175.

Dallman, P. R. 1981. Anemia of prematurity. *Ann. Rev. Med.* 32:143.

Davis, V. 1980. The structure and function of brown adipose tissue in the neonate. *J. Obstet. Gynecol. Neonat. Nurs.* 9:368.

Grossman, J. H. 1980. Perinatal viral infections. *Clin. Perinatol.* 7:257.

Henrickson, P. 1979. Hyperviscosity of the blood and haemostasis in the newborn infant. *Acta Paediatr. Scand.* 68:701.

Hill, A., and Volpe, J. J. 1981. Seizures, hypoxic-ischemic brain injury, and intraventricular hemorrhage in the newborn. *Ann. Neurol.* 10:109.

McBride, B. Dec. 1979. Babies with necrotizing enterocolitis—what to watch for. *The Canadian Nurse.* 75:41.

Plenat, F., et al. 1978. Pulmonary interstitial emphysema. *Clin. Perinatol.* 5:351.

Tsang, R. C.; Steichen, J. J.; and Brown, D. R. 1977. Perinatal calcium homeostasis: neonatal hypocalcemia and bone demineralization. *Clin. Perinatol.* 4:385.

Volpe, J. J. 1977. Neonatal intracranial hemorrhage. *Clin. Perinatol.* 4:77.

ship that some immediate answer be given to the parents. Honest, simple, and positive facts can be shared: "Your baby is alive"; "Your baby is a girl"; "Your baby has a strong heartbeat but needs some help with breathing"; "Your baby is alive but needs some special care right now"; "The pediatrician is helping your baby now and will talk with you soon." The information that nurses share with parents must always be honest data that nurses can observe and document. Nurses should not make promises that they cannot fulfill and should refrain from offering empty reassurances that everything will be all right.

The period of waiting between suspected abnormality or dysfunction and the confirmation of the defect or disorder is a very anxious one for parents because it is difficult, if not impossible, to begin attachment to the infant if the newborn's future is questionable. During the "not knowing period," parents need support and acknowledgment that this is an anxious time and to be kept informed as to efforts to gather additional data and to maintain the infant's livelihood. Helfer and Kempe (1976) recommend that both parents be told about the defect at the same time, with the infant present. An honest discussion of the problem and anticipatory management at the earliest possible time by health professionals help the parents (a) maintain trust in the physician and nurse, (b) appreciate the reality of the situation by dispelling fantasy and misconception, (c) begin the grieving process, and (d) mobilize internal and external support.

Nurses need to be aware that anger is a universal response and that it is best directed outward, because holding it in check requires great energy, which is diverted away from grieving and physical recovery from pregnancy and giving birth. Anger may be directed unjustifiably at the physician and/or nurse, at the food, at nursing care, or at hospital regulations and routines. Anger with the infant is rarely demonstrated by parents, and can precipitate guilt feelings.

The heightened concern for self may erroneously be interpreted by health professionals as rejection of the newborn. Both parents need time and understanding to deal with their own feelings before they can direct concern toward the infant. In a short span of time, the parent is confronted with the loss of the idealized child, the need to accept a child who deviates from normal, and a sense of personal failure. In addition, the new mother may be suffering from fatigue and sleep deprivation from her pregnancy and labor and from discomforts arising from cesarean delivery, episiotomy, inability to void, hemorrhoids, and afterpains. In the postpartal period concern for self and dependency are normal events.

In their sensitive and vulnerable state, parents are acutely perceptive of others' responses and reactions (particularly nonverbal) to the child. Parents can be expected to identify with the responses of others. Therefore, it is imperative that medical and nursing staff be fully aware of their feelings and come to terms with those feelings so that they are comfortable and at ease with the child and the grieving family. Professional support and comfort fill the emotional bank account from which parents can draw to nurture the child and themselves so that each can develop to full potential.

Nurses may feel uncomfortable, not knowing what to say or fearing confrontation with the intensity of their own and the parents' feelings. Each nurse must work out personal reactions with instructors, peers, clergy, parents, or significant others. It is helpful to have a stockpile of therapeutic questions and statements to initiate meaningful dialogue with parents. Opening statements can be as follows: "You must be wondering what could have caused this"; "Are you thinking you (or someone else) may have done something?"; "How can I help?"; "Go ahead and cry. It's worth crying about"; or "Are you wondering how you are going to manage?" Avoid statements such as "It could have been worse"; "It's God's will"; "You have other children"; "You are still young and can have more"; and "I understand how you feel." *This* child is important *now*.

Some nurses find relief for themselves or a means of escape from painful circumstances by overzealous and unrealistic reassurance that "everything will be all right" and by avoidance of the infant and family. Another means of self-defense used by many medical and nursing staff is technical jargon and involvement in the technical aspects of the mother's care rather than taking time to talk about the situation. These approaches confuse the parents at a time when they need most to be understood and to understand.

Nurses show concern and support by planning time to spend with the parents, by being psychologically as well as physically present, by encouraging open discussion and grieving, by repetitious explanations (as necessary), by providing privacy as needed, and by encouraging contact with the newborn. Identification and clarification of feelings and fears decrease distortions in perception, thinking, and feelings. Nurses invest the child with value in the eyes of the parents when they provide meticulous care to the infant, talk and coo (especially in the face-to-face position) while holding or providing care to the infant, refer to the child by gender or name, and relate the newborn's activities ("He took a whole ounce of formula"; "She burped so loud that . . ."; "He took hold of the blanket and just wouldn't let go"; "He voided all over the doctor"). Nurses should note the "normal" characteristics and capabilities of each infant as well as the infant's needs.

Cues that the parents are ready to become involved with the child's care or planning for the future include their reference to the baby as "she" or "he" or by name and their questioning as to amount of feeding taken, appearance today, and the like.

Many physicians show parents "before" and "after" photographs of conditions requiring surgical intervention.

Parents benefit from meeting other parents who have faced the same problem, such as at amputee centers or cleft palate groups. Specialists (plastic surgeons, neurosurgeons, orthopedists, oral surgeons, dentists, and rehabilitation therapists) can be reassuring and supportive of parents in their short- and long-term goals. However, these types of interventions must be carefully timed to the readiness of the parents and the family.

Mothers may be startled or feel guilty when they do not feel motherly toward their infant. One mother, looking at her child born with an severe cleft lip and palate, said, "God help me. I can't stand looking at her. I wish she wasn't mine. What a horrid thing to say, but I can't . . . I just can't." She could not bring herself to hold or touch the child prior to cleft lip repair. She needed considerable assistance to talk of these feelings in a nonjudgmental and accepting atmosphere before she was able to hold the infant after surgery. She proceeded to learn to feed her daughter (whose cleft palate was not yet repaired) and become very "motherly" before the infant was discharged. Her husband, fortunately, facilitated the whole process by his continued love for and acceptance of his wife throughout the experience.

Occasionally a mother may become overprotective and overoptimistic shortly after the infant's birth. The nurse accepts her behavior but continues to remind the mother that it is okay and natural to feel disappointment, a sense of failure, helplessness, or anger. The overprotectiveness and overoptimism are defense mechanisms. To deny the negative feelings serves only to further entrench them, to delay their resolution, and to delay realistic planning.

Parental feelings toward the child are crucial. The child's feelings about his or her physical appearance and integrity and about personal capabilities reflect those of the parents. Before confronting society at large, the child must have developed sufficient ego strength and social, intellectual, and physical skills. It is difficult for some parents to develop realistic expectations, to provide consistent discipline, and to expose the child to a healthy amount of frustration. The handicap or defect is a fact that necessitates some behavioral and goal changes, but modifications can prepare the child for constructive, self-actualizing, and satisfying pursuits as a responsible citizen in the community.

INFANT WITH FEEDING PROBLEMS

Congenitally produced feeding problems may result from the Pierre Robin syndrome, cleft lip and palate, or choanal atresia.

Pierre Robin Syndrome

PHYSIOLOGY AND PATHOPHYSIOLOGY

Hypoplasia of the mandible occurring before the ninth week of embryonic development results in a mouth too small to allow for normal development. Reduced mandibular size forces the tongue into the nasopharyngeal space, often preventing closure of the palate in the midline (cleft palate). In addition, micrognathia (small mandible) forces the tongue backward and upward (glossoptosis), thus partially or completely obstructing the airway. Respiratory distress, which can occur especially on inspiration, when the tongue is pulled down and back to lie against the epiglottis and posterior pharyngeal wall, and feeding problems are serious threats to the neonate's well-being.

Etiology of the Pierre Robin syndrome is not clearly understood. It may be transmitted by a dominant gene with variable expressivity, or it may be the result of polygenic or multifactorial inheritance.

CLINICAL MANIFESTATIONS

Micrognathia (receding chin, small mandible), which gives the neonate a birdlike face, is apparent at birth. Cleft palate may be an associated defect. The cleft usually involves the soft palate only but, in some cases, may involve the posterior hard palate. The neonate is usually of low birth weight. Respiratory distress is apparent at birth, accompanied by cyanosis and increased respiratory effort. An x-ray film of the nasopharyngeal area demonstrates the narrowed airway.

Careful physical assessment may reveal other associated defects, especially affecting the cardiovascular system, CNS, ears, or extremities. Possible ocular defects include retinal detachment, microphthalmia, congenital glaucoma, and cataracts.

DIFFERENTIAL DIAGNOSIS

Treacher Collins syndrome (mandibulofacial dysostosis) differs from the Pierre Robin syndrome in that the mandible's overall shape is grossly deformed, it is often associated with other facial anomalies, and facial appearance does not improve as mandibular growth proceeds.

INTERVENTIONS

Neonates born with micrognathia and associated defects experience life-threatening respiratory difficulties. Immediate and intensive treatment may include positional management, resuscitation efforts, and surgical intervention. Positional management requires that the neonate be kept absolutely prone and flat, head turned to the side but neither up or down, to take advantage of the effect of gravity on the tongue (Lewis and Pashayan, 1980). Having the head tilted down or up can place the tongue in a position that produces airway obstruction. Feeding, burping, cuddling, bathing, diapering, blood drawing and so on are done with the infant in a prone position.

Oxygen, suction, and oral airway devices must be at the infant's bedside at all times. If respiratory distress or cyanosis occurs while the infant is in the prone position, the tongue position should be checked, suctioning performed, and oxygen administered. The next step is to insert an oral airway. If airway problems and hypoxia persist, other means of maintaining the airway must be instituted by the physician or nurse immediately, using endotracheal intubation or tracheotomy in some cases (Chapter 25). Following these measures, the severely affected infant is best treated in an intensive care unit.

Resuscitation efforts sometimes occur in the presence of the neonate's parents. Explanations to support the parents during these efforts are important aspects of nursing care.

Surgical suturing of the tongue to the lower lip to bring the tongue forward and away from the posterior pharynx and epiglottis may be necessary to alleviate and prevent recurring respiratory distress (Smith, 1981). The parents should be informed of their child's condition and the measures being taken for care. They are encouraged to visit the nursery, touch their infant, and participate in the care as much as possible.

Presence of the cleft palate necessitates special feeding techniques (see the Nursing Care Plan on cleft lip and palate). Occasionally the child may require feeding by gavage or gastrostomy tube, but is weaned to oral feedings as soon as possible.

PROGNOSIS

Prognosis depends on the degree of expression of this syndrome in the individual infant—on the severity of micrognathia and coexisting defects.

With adequate support of respirations and nutrition, most affected infants grow out of the condition by 3–4 months of age, at which time the mandible has grown sufficiently to allow the tongue to rest in the normal position. By the age of 4–6 years, the mandible, tongue, and air passageway are essentially normal. Distinctive characteristics, noted on x-ray, persist through adulthood, however.

If the infant has an associated cleft palate, ongoing treatment of cleft palate is necessary.

Cleft Lip and Palate

Several factors seem to be responsible for cleft lip and palate. Polygenic inheritance (combination of genes from different loci on different chromosomes), an occasional mutant gene, environmental factors (fetal viral infection, radiation, hypoxia), or interaction between genetic and environmental factors may be responsible for this malformation.

Environmental factors, such as the teratogenic insult of drugs (corticosteroid or anticonvulsant drugs) during the latter part of the first trimester, have been implicated.

Differences have been noted in the incidence of cleft palate and cleft lip. The infant born with only a cleft palate generally has a lower birth weight, has a greater incidence of malformation (such as gastrointestinal tract defects), and tends to be female. Cleft lip, with or without a coexisting cleft palate, generally occurs more often in the male. Cleft palate alone is more frequent in females.

PHYSIOLOGY AND PATHOPHYSIOLOGY

Cleft lip occurs during the second month of embryonic development as a result of incomplete fusion of the nasomedial or intermaxillary process with the more laterally placed maxillary process. Because the fusion failure occurs during a period of rapid fetal growth, the structures of the face and mouth develop without the normal encircling restraints of the muscles of the lips. The characteristic depression or flattening of the infant's midfacial contour may result from the disruption of normal antagonistic forces across the midline and concomitant disturbance of growth of the facial segments involved. Facial clefts, even when not associated with cleft palate, may affect not only the lip but also the external nose, the nasal cartilages, the nasal septum, the alveolar process, and the alae (flesh flap forming the side of the nares) (Figure 26–1). The cleft is usually just beneath the center of one nostril. The more complete the cleft, the greater the incidence of missing, supernumerary, or malformed teeth in the line of the cleft. Failure of

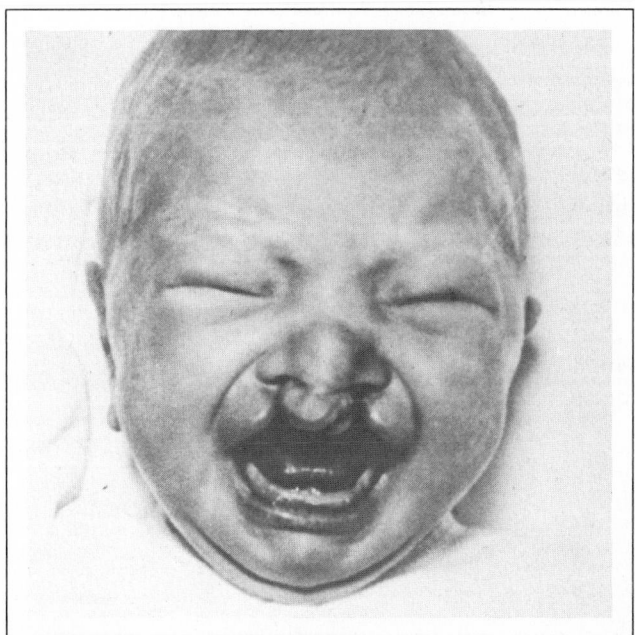

Figure 26–1 Bilateral cleft lip.

lip fusion by 35 days of gestation may impair the closure of the palatal shelves and may be a cause for cleft palate.

Palatal cleft refers to a fissure connecting the oral and nasal cavities. Cleft palate may involve the soft or soft and hard palate. The fissure is formed when embryonic fusion of the maxillary and premaxillary processes is incomplete. This abnormal development results in a complex syndrome initially involving any one or a combination of problems of respiration, feeding, or deglutition. Later consequences involve speech and hearing difficulties.

CLINICAL MANIFESTATIONS

A cleft lip is readily visible at birth. The cleft palate may first be suspected when the neonate regurgitates formula through the nose. In the absence of a visible cleft, the palate is palpated for a possible submucous cleft that decreases the competence of the velopharyngeal valve. The fissure may involve only the uvula and soft palate or may extend forward to the nostril, involving the hard palate and the maxillary alveolar ridge. It also may occupy the midline posteriorly and as far forward as the alveolar process, where it causes deviation of the involved side, usually dividing the alveolar ridge between the upper lateral incisor tooth buds and the cuspid bud (Figure 26–2). The neonate may be of low birth weight. In addition, other malformations may be noted, especially of the craniofacial structures (see the discussion of the Pierre Robin syndrome, p. 850).

INTERVENTIONS

The nursing and medical regimen focuses on repair of the lip, repair of the palate, speech development, and prevention of otitis media and dental abnormalities. The management of a cleft lip and palate is a team effort, with the nurse having an integral responsibility for fostering communications and coordinating all the various services for the parents and child.

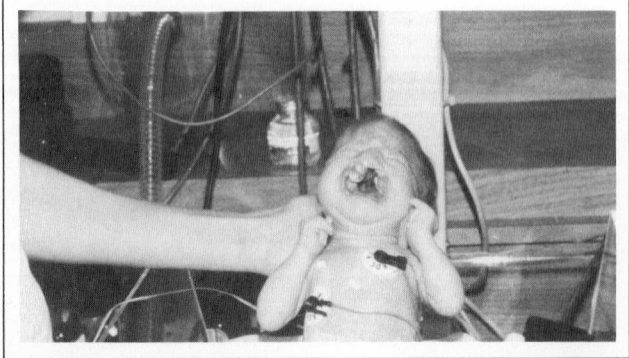

Figure 26–2 Cleft abnormality involving both hard and soft palate and unilateral cleft lip.

Repair of lip. The lip may be repaired during the first few days of life if the neonate's condition is good and weight is 2500 g. Early labial repair for cosmetic effect has a positive influence on the developing parent–child relationship and permits the neonate to strengthen circumoral musculature. If possible, surgery is delayed until the infant weighs 10 lb and has a hemoglobin of 10 g/dL, usually about 3 months of age. The most common method of repair usually uses some modification of the Z-plasty, which produces a lip of sufficient depth without sacrificing the mucocutaneous line and with minimal scar formation.

Repair of palate. The child is usually between 16 months and 2½ years of age when the palate is repaired. The aim of surgery is to obtain an airtight closure of the palatal cleft and to preserve the convexity, mobility, and length of the palate without disturbing the tooth buds. Orthodontists advocate early prosthetic treatment for neonates born with cleft palates. These prosthetic appliances may vary from simple feeding obturators to those designed to align displaced maxillary segments before definitive surgical corrections. A new obturator is constructed every 2 months to accommodate craniofacial growth. Children with prosthetic appliances are easier to feed, gain weight more quickly, and develop better palatal convexity with improved speech patterns (Jones, 1981). Speech therapy is a valuable adjunct because such infants will develop deviant speech patterns if they begin to vocalize before closure of the palate. The child with a cleft palate is particularly vulnerable to middle ear infections and consequent dysfunction because of the normal horizontal placement of the eustachian tube in children. In addition, the newborn with a cleft palate frequently has congenital eustachian tube dysfunction.

Each neonate with cleft palate is carefully examined for the existence of other malformations, especially those of the craniofacial structures, such as bifid uvula or complete absence of the hard palate. Infants with large cleft palate defects may have associated midline brain defects.

The nurse works closely with the parents in determining the most successful approach to feeding the infant with a cleft lip or palate. The difficulty parents encounter is a source of great frustration, so continued support and encouragement are essential. In addition, nursing efforts are directed to facilitating parent–infant bonding and acceptance of the defect. (See the Nursing Care Plan on cleft lip and palate.)

Choanal Atresia

Choanal atresia refers to the occlusion of the posterior nares, unilaterally or bilaterally, by either bone or membrane. Because newborns are obligatory nose breathers for at least the first few weeks of life, early symptoms include cyanosis even at rest, snorting respirations, and feeding

(Text continues on p. 857.)

NURSING CARE PLAN
Cleft Lip and Palate

PATIENT DATA BASE

History

Pertinent prenatal and perinatal information, such as genetic link or environmental factors (drugs, fetal viral infections, radiation, and hypoxia)

Complete physical assessment of neonate

Any significant respiratory difficulties at or soon after birth

Parents' reactions to defect and initial information given to them

Physical examination
Cleft lip:

Obvious unilateral or bilateral visible defect, which may involve the external nares, nasal cartilage, nasal septum, and the alveolar process

Characteristic depression or flattening of the infant's midfacial contour may be seen

Cleft palate:

Fissure connecting the oral and nasal cavity, which may involve the uvula and soft palate or may extend forward to the nostril involving the hard palate and maxillary alveolar ridge

Difficulty in sucking and feeding

May demonstrate expulsion of formula out through the nose

NURSING PRIORITIES

1. Develop safe feeding practices and prevent complications.
2. Identify coexisting defects.
3. Encourage parents to participate in and cooperate in meeting short- and long-term rehabilitation goals.

FAMILY EDUCATIONAL FOCUS

1. Discuss with parents alterations in feeding methods specific to their neonate with either a cleft lip or a cleft palate.
2. Explain treatment modalities and their rationale.
3. Provide appropriate literature about cleft lip or palate and refer family to available resources and support groups.
4. Provide opportunities for parents to discuss questions and individual concerns about their neonate.

Problem	Nursing interventions and actions	Rationale
Cleft lip Feeding preoperatively	Experiment with various nipples: soft but regular crosscut nipple, lamb's (longer and softer); asepto syringe (10 mL) with bulb and 1½ in. rubber tubing Feed slowly	Select feeding technique best suited to neonate Choose simplest method to avoid further emphasis on infant's difference to parents Approximates normal stomach filling and prevents regurgitation
	Burp frequently (after every ounce)	Prevents vomiting and discomfort from gas bubbles (neonate has greater tendency to swallow air)
	Cleanse cleft with medicine dropper full of sterile water	Prevents crusting to keep cleft in good condition for repair
	Interact with infant as with any "normal" infant	Assists in development of trust and serves as role model to mother and father
Coexisting defects	Carefully assess, especially for defects of craniofacial tissues	Assist physician to institute appropriate treatment; gather data for anticipatory guidance of parents
Eliciting parental involvement and cooperation	Provide a role model in interacting with neonate	Parents internalize others' responses to their newborn
	Provide time for and encourage parents to grieve	Grief must be resolved before parents can begin relating to this infant in positive manner and cooperating in child's total rehabilitation
	Teach parents method of feeding neonate prior to discharge if lip surgery is to be delayed	Allows time for parents to gain self-confidence

NURSING CARE PLAN Cont'd
Cleft Lip and Palate

Problem	Nursing interventions and actions	Rationale
	Review with parents ways to decrease possibility of infection, especially upper respiratory infections Encourage parents to seek prompt medical treatment for upper respiratory infections	Increases parents' self-confidence; specifies a definite course of action; precaution against development of otitis media.
Preoperative preparation	Assess for respiratory or gastrointestinal disorder and report to physician Feed infant by same method that will be used following surgery: asepto syringe with rubber catheter (a small gravy baster with 1½ in. rubber tube attached can be substituted) Place catheter in side of mouth Drip formula onto surface of tongue Apply restraints: 1. Elbow 2. Jacket In some instances, place infant in protective isolation	Avoid surgical/postsurgical complications Accustoms infant to changes in feeding method Avoids stress of sucking on suture line Avoids direct trauma to suture line Stimulates swallowing Accustoms infant to restraints to decrease postsurgical distress: 1. Prevents trauma to suture line 2. Necessary for infant who is capable of turning over Decreases possibility of cross-infection
Postoperative recovery with cosmetic and functional repair of lip		
Adequate respiration	Observe for bleeding, airway obstruction (stridor, etc.) from edema or secretions Place in croupette until respirations are normal Lay infant in supine position; prop slightly on one side	Identifies possible complications following surgery that necessitate treatment Helps liquefy secretions and reduce edema Facilitates drainage and respiration; prevents aspiration; protects suture line
Adequate nutrition	Assess for hydration: adequacy of voiding; tenseness of fontanelle and appearance of eyeballs, skin turgor over abdomen and thighs, daily weight Record intake and output Monitor IV hourly: type and amount of fluid infused, condition of infusion site Assess for adequate caloric intake; weigh daily; plot weight on chart	Aids calculation of daily fluid: type of fluid, rate of drip, total volume needed per day Assures accuracy of flow to prevent fluid overload or inadequate fluid; prevents tissue trauma Prevent inadequate intake to meet requirements of stress, surgical losses, repair and growth needs
Feeding capabilities	When infant is fully aware, offer oral fluids as ordered; later, advance to clear fluid, then formula in 3–12 hr via method utilized prior to surgery Assess response: Any chilling? Cyanosis? Abdominal distention? Type and amount of feeding? Was feeding retained? Swallowing and burping behavior? Fatigue? Activity?	Milk products increase mucous production and may cause crusting on suture line; avoid solids, nipples, pacifiers to protect suture line Determines appropriate feeding method and appropriate time to advance feeding; assists in identifying coexisting problems

NURSING CARE PLAN Cont'd
Cleft Lip and Palate

Problem	Nursing interventions and actions	Rationale
Intact suture line and even lip (vermilion) border	Feed infant in cardiac chair or infant seat or hold upright, with head and chest tilted backward slightly; feed slowly	Facilitates swallowing, burping, and retention of feeding and prevents aspiration or vomiting
	Treat suture line per physician/hospital preference: 1. Keep dressing moist with sterile saline at least every 2 hr 2. Cleanse with gauze swab moistened with sterile saline or hydrogen peroxide 3. Apply antibiotic ointment after feedings	Prevents crusting with serosanguineous drainage, mucus, or feeding and prevents excessive scar formation
	Continue use of restraints: elbow restraint pinned to shirt or mattress; jacket Remove restraints periodically; remove one at a time for massage and exercise of muscles	Prevent direct trauma to suture line
	Check and replace adhesive tape securing the Logan bar (Figure 26–3), if used; if tape is loosened, remove, paint with tincture of benzoin, and apply new tape	Maintains traction of Logan bar to prevent pull on suture line
	Feed with rubber-tipped appliance placed into corner of mouth; do not use nipple or pacifier	Prevents direct trauma to suture line and discourages sucking

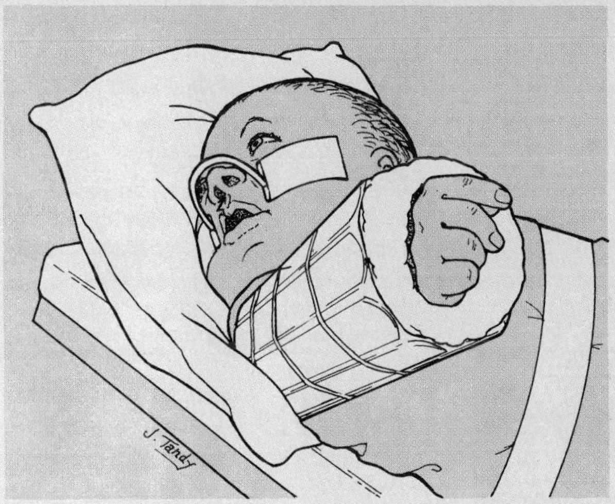

Figure 26–3 Cleft lip repair with Logan bar. Note elbow restraints on infant.

| | Prevent vomiting
Cuddle, hold, rock infant | Prevents stress on line
Prevents crying, which adds stress to suture line
Needs extra cuddling because infant cannot suck as an outlet for tension and anxiety |

NURSING CARE PLAN Cont'd
Cleft Lip and Palate

Problem	Nursing interventions and actions	Rationale
Effects of immobility	Remove one restraint at a time, exercise limb, and reapply restraint	Provides range of motion while maintaining protective restraints of unsupervised limbs; provides kinesthetic and social stimulation
	Check for reddened areas under restraints; keep all skin areas clean and dry	Prevents skin breakdown
	Turn from side to side; prop well	Prevents skin breakdown and orthostatic pneumonia; immobilization protects suture line
Infection	Administer antibiotics as prescribed by physician; carry out cleansing of suture line	
Parent education	Teach parents about feeding technique, restraining, and exercising extremities, or whatever will be expected of parents for care of infant at home	Instills self-confidence, feelings of self-worth and self-esteem — provides avenue of learning about baby and developing positive relationship between parent and infant
	Refer to community agencies as necessary, such as Homemaker's Service, visiting nurse and parent support groups	Frees mother to provide necessary care and stimulation or provides care for family that is unable to do so temporarily
Cleft palate (prior to surgery)		
Adequate respirations	Place prone or in side-lying position	Facilitates drainage
	Suction gently, as needed	Prevents aspiration or airway obstruction
	Prevent exposure to upper respiratory infections and development of otitis media	Prevents surgery delay or surgical complications since surgery is not done until infant is about 16 months of age
	Use appropriate feeding method (see section on cleft lip)	See section on cleft lip
Adequate nutrition	Choose appropriate nipple: "winged", lamb's nipple with flange cut to size, asepto syringe with bulb and 1½ in. rubber tip, and Ross' cleft palate nipple	Deemphasizes infant's "difference" to parents Decreases possibility of formula entering nasal cavities, thus discouraging aspiration and respiratory distress
	Be sure that nipples are soft and holes are slightly enlarged	Assists feeding, because infant cannot create vacuum necessary for successful nursing
	Support in upright position with head and chest tilted slightly backward	Aids swallowing and discourages aspiration
	Burp frequently — after each ounce	Aids removal of excessive air these infants tend to swallow; therefore, discourages vomiting and aspiration
	Thicken formula per physician order	Provides extra calories while utilizing gravity flow to prevent aspiration
	Begin feeding with cup or from side of spoon	Accustoms infant/toddler to postoperative situation
	Cleanse mouth with water after feedings	Prevents crusting
	Plot weight gain pattern on growth graph	Assesses adequacy of diet and readiness for surgery

NURSING CARE PLAN Cont'd
Cleft Lip and Palate

NURSING CARE EVALUATION

Infant suffers minimal emotional trauma from surgical interventions and hospitalizations

Lip is repaired with improved appearance

Otitis media is prevented or treated before hearing damage occurs

Infant is feeding well and maintaining weight

Parents develop positive relationship with the infant, demonstrating positive parenting behaviors, and are able to meet own as well as infant's needs

NURSING DIAGNOSES*	SUPPORTING DATA
1. Potential alteration in nutrition: less than body requirements related to feeding difficulties with cleft lip and/or palate	Greater tendency to swallow air Difficulty in sucking Vomiting
2. Potential for injury after surgery for cosmetic and functional repair of cleft lip and/or palate	Signs of airway obstruction from bleeding, edema, secretions Direct trauma to suture line by infant Aspiration Infection
3. Anxiety in infant related to inability to suck, restraints following surgical repair, separation from parents	Lack of normal kinesthetic and social stimulation
4. Potential alteration in parenting	Behaviors indicative of potential parental problems

* These are a few examples of nursing diagnoses that may be appropriate for an infant with cleft lip and/or palate. It is not an inclusive list and must be individualized for each infant.

difficulties because the newborn is unable to suck and breathe simultaneously. Examination of the nose for shape and function is included in the nurse's initial assessment of the newborn. Patency of the nares is assessed by listening for sounds of breathing while holding the neonate's mouth closed and alternately compressing each nostril. When the nursing evaluation indicates questionable data, patency of the nares is confirmed by passage of a catheter or feeding tube. Failure to successfully pass a feeding tube through one or both of the newborn's nares, coupled with the presence of the just-mentioned symptoms, supports a diagnosis of choanal atresia.

Surgery is required to correct this disorder. Before surgery it may be necessary to tape in place a small airway in the neonate's mouth to prevent respiratory distress. If necessary, feeding can be accomplished by orogastric tube until the infant learns to eat and breathe at the same time.

INFANT WITH INBORN ERRORS OF METABOLISM

Inborn errors of metabolism constitute a group of hereditary disorders that are transmitted by mutant genes, and result in an enzyme defect that blocks a metabolic pathway

and leads to an accumulation of metabolites that are toxic to the infant. Most of the disorders are transmitted by an autosomal recessive gene, requiring two heterozygous parents to produce a homozygous infant with the disorder. Heterozygous parents of some inborn errors of metabolism disorders can be identified by special tests, and some inborn errors of metabolism can be detected in utero.

The detection of many inborn errors of metabolism is now accomplished neonatally through newborn screening programs. These programs principally test for disorders associated with mental retardation.

Phenylketonuria

Phenylketonuria (PKU) is an inborn error of metabolism caused by autosomal recessive genes, requiring two heterozygous parents, each contributing a mutant gene to the infant. Heterozygous parents, and other carriers, can be identified by special blood tests involving high phenylalanine intake. PKU infants have a deficiency in the liver enzyme phenylalanine hydroxylase, which is necessary to convert the amino acid phenylalanine to tyrosine. Phenylalanine is an essential amino acid used by the body for growth; in the normal individual any excess is converted to tyrosine. The infant with PKU lacks this converting ability, which results in an accumulation of phenylalanine in the blood. Phenylalanine produces two abnormal metabolites, phenylpyruvic acid and phenylacetic acid, which spill into the urine, producing a musty odor. Excessive accumulation of phenylalanine and its abnormal metabolites in brain tissue leads to progressive mental retardation.

PKU is the most common of the amino acid disorders. Newborn screenings have set its incidence at about 1 in 1500 live births (Ampola, 1982). The highest incidence is noted in white populations from northern Europe and the United States. It is rarely observed in African, Jewish, or Japanese peoples.

The clinical picture involves a normal appearing newborn, most often with blond hair, blue eyes, and fair complexion. Decreased pigmentation may be related to the competition between phenylalanine and tyrosine for the available enzyme, tyrosinase. Tyrosine is needed for the formation of melanin pigment and the hormones epinephrine and thyroxin. Without treatment, the infant fails to thrive, and develops vomiting and eczematous rashes. By about 6 months of age, the infant exhibits behaviors indicative of mental retardation and other CNS involvement, including seizures and abnormal EEG patterns.

Blood testing for PKU of all hospitalized newborns is required by law in most states. The Guthrie test, done before discharge, is a simple screening tool that uses a drop of blood collected from a heel stick on filter paper. The Guthrie test should be done at least 24 hours, but preferably 72 hours, after the initiation of feedings containing the usual amounts of milk. Phenylalanine is found in milk, so its metabolites begin to build up in the PKU infant once milk feedings are initiated. With breast-fed infants, it is important to verify that the mother's milk is indeed "in" and the infant has had milk feedings before performing the test. High-risk infants should be receiving a 60% milk intake with no more than 40% of their total intake coming from nonprotein intravenous fluids. PKU testing of high-risk infants should be deferred for at least 48 hours after hyperalimentation. Hospitals and birthing centers frequently discharge mother and infant 24–48 hours after delivery. It is vital that the parents understand the need for the screening procedure, and a follow-up check is necessary to confirm that the test was done.

Because it is possible to do the testing on an infant with PKU before the phenylalanine concentration rises and thus miss the diagnosis, some states routinely request a repeat test at 4–6 weeks. When the Guthrie blood test is performed early, during the first 3–4 days of life, a phenylalanine blood level about 4–8 mg/dL is considered a presumptive positive, but only 1 in 20–30 infants with this level are true positives (Wasserman and Gromisch, 1981).

Some physicians have the parents perform a diaper test for PKU. At about 6 weeks of age, the parent should take a freshly wet diaper and press the prepared Phenistix against the wet area. They note the color of the test stick, record the color on the prepared sheet, and mail the form back to the physician. A green color reaction is positive and indicates probable PKU.

Once identified, an afflicted infant can be treated by a special diet that limits ingestion of phenylalanine. Special formulas low in phenylalanine, such as Lofenalac, are available. Special food lists are helpful for parents of a PKU child. If treatment is begun before 3 months of age, CNS damage can be minimized.

Controversy exists about when, if ever, the special diet should be terminated. Because of the rigidity and severe limitations of the low phenylalanine diet, many clinicians terminate the special diet at 6 years of age. Brain size does not dramatically increase after age 6, but myelination continues actively through adolescence and to some extent possibly through 40 years of age. The effect of high phenylalanine levels on continued development of the brain after 6 years is not known (Schuett et al., 1980).

Female children with PKU are now living longer and may bear children. There is a 95% risk of producing a child with mental retardation if the mother with PKU is not on a low-phenylalanine diet during pregnancy. It is recommended that the woman reinstate her low phenylalanine diet a few months before becoming pregnant (Mathews and Smith, 1979).

Maple Syrup Urine Disease

Maple syrup urine disease (MSUD) is an inborn error of metabolism caused by autosomal recessive genes, requiring two heterozygous parents, each contributing a mutant gene to the infant. MSUD, when untreated, is a rapidly progressing and often fatal disease caused by an enzymatic defect in the metabolism of the branched-chain amino acids: leucine, isoleucine, and valine. Affected infants have feeding problems and neurologic signs (seizures, spasticity, opisthotonus) during the first week of life. A maple syrup odor of the urine is noted and, when ferric chloride is added to the urine, its color changes to gray-green.

Some states simultaneously test all hospitalized newborns for MSUD and PKU during the first 3–4 days of life. Diagnosis is made by analyzing blood levels of leucine, isoleucine, and valine. Confirmation of the diagnosis depends on blood assay for the enzyme oxidative decarboxylase. Dietary management must be initiated immediately with a formula, such as MSUD Formula Powder by Mead Johnson, that is low in the branched-chain amino acids leucine, isoleucine, and valine (Sarett, 1979).

Homocystinuria

Homocystinuria is a disorder caused by a deficiency of the enzyme cystathionine B synthase, which produces a block in the normal conversion of methionine to cystine. This deficiency is inherited as an autosomal recessive trait with heterogenicity in its expression. The disorder varies in its presentation, but the more common characteristics are skeletal abnormalities, dislocation of ocular lenses, intravascular thromboses, and mental retardation. Abnormalities occur because of the toxic effects of the accumulation of methionine and the metabolite homocystine in the blood. Affected infants are managed on a diet that is low in methionine but supplemented with cystine and pyridoxine (vitamin B$_6$). With early diagnosis and careful management, mental retardation may be prevented.

Galactosemia

Galactosemia is an inborn error of carbohydrate metabolism in which the body is unable to utilize the sugars galactose and lactose. Galactosemia is inherited by autosomal recessive genes from two heterozygous parents. Normally, in liver cells, enzyme pathways convert galactose and lactose to glucose. In galactosemia, one step in that conversion pathway is absent, either because of the lack of the enzyme galactose 1-phosphate uridyl transferase, or because of the lack of the enzyme galactokinase. High levels of unusable galactose circulate in the blood causing cataracts, brain damage, and hepatomegaly (Smith, 1980).

In several states newborn screening includes an enzyme assay for galactose 1-phosphate uridyl transferase; this test, however, does not detect galactosemia if it is caused by a deficiency of the enzyme galactokinase. Galactosemia is treated by the use of a galactose-free formula, such as Nutramingen (a protein hydrolysate process formula), a meat-base formula, or a soybean formula. As the infant grows, parents must be educated not just to avoid giving their child milk and milk products, but to carefully read all labels and avoid any foods containing dry milk products.

Clinical manifestations of galactosemia, with the exception of mental retardation, are completely reversible when galactose is excluded from the diet. Mental retardation can be prevented by early diagnosis and careful dietary management.

Other Metabolic Disorders

There are a number of inherited errors of amino acid and carbohydrate metabolism in which an important enzyme defect blocks the metabolic pathway at a specific point and leads to an accumulation of metabolites. The incidence of metabolic errors is relatively low, but for affected infants and their families these disorders pose a threat to survival and frequently require lifelong treatment. Nursing responsibility lies in early detection, prompt and appropriate dietary management, and support for the child and family. Parents should be referred to support groups and centers that provide resources for biochemical genetics and dietary management.

Congenital Hypothyroidism

Another disorder frequently included in mandatory newborn screening blood tests is congenital hypothyroidism. An inborn enzymatic defect, lack of maternal dietary iodine, or maternal ingestion of drugs that depress or destroy thyroid tissue can cause congenital hypothyroidism. A large tongue, umbilical hernia, cool and mottled skin, low hairline, hypotonia, and large fontanelles are frequently associated with congenital hypothyroidism. Early symptoms include prolonged neonatal jaundice, poor feeding, constipation, low-pitched cry, poor weight gain, inactivity, and delayed motor development. Immediate and appropriate thyroid replacement therapy is established based on laboratory data. Management includes frequent laboratory monitoring and adjustment of thyroid medication to accommodate growth and development of the child. With adequate treatment, children remain free of symptoms, but if the condition is untreated, stunted growth and mental retardation occur.

INFANT WITH GASTROINTESTINAL DEFECT

Common congenital gastrointestinal defects include esophageal atresia and tracheoesophageal fistula, diaphragmatic hernia, omphalocele, gastroschisis, aganglionic megacolon, imperforate anus, and intestinal obstruction.

Esophageal Atresia and Tracheoesophageal Fistula

The most common high gastrointestinal tract anomaly is atresia of the esophagus with tracheoesophageal fistula, occurring in approximately 1 in 3000 births.

PHYSIOLOGY AND PATHOPHYSIOLOGY

During embryonic development, the beginning cell structures of the esophagus dorsal wall may fail to grow and thereby fail to form a continuous hollow muscular tube connecting the pharynx to the stomach, forming instead a blind pouch (*atresia*). In 87% of cases, the type III distal portion connects with the trachea (or a primary bronchus) near the bronchial bifurcation via an abnormal passageway known as *fistula* (Figure 26–4). The tracheoesophageal fistula is caused by incomplete separation between the esophagus and trachea during cleavage of the esophagotracheal groove or septum at 4 weeks' gestation.

Four other anatomic variations are less commonly seen. The upper and lower segments of the esophagus are atretic in 8% of cases (type I). The H-type of anomaly (type V, 4%) refers to a continuous esophagus that is connected by a fistulous tract to the trachea. In less than 2% of cases,

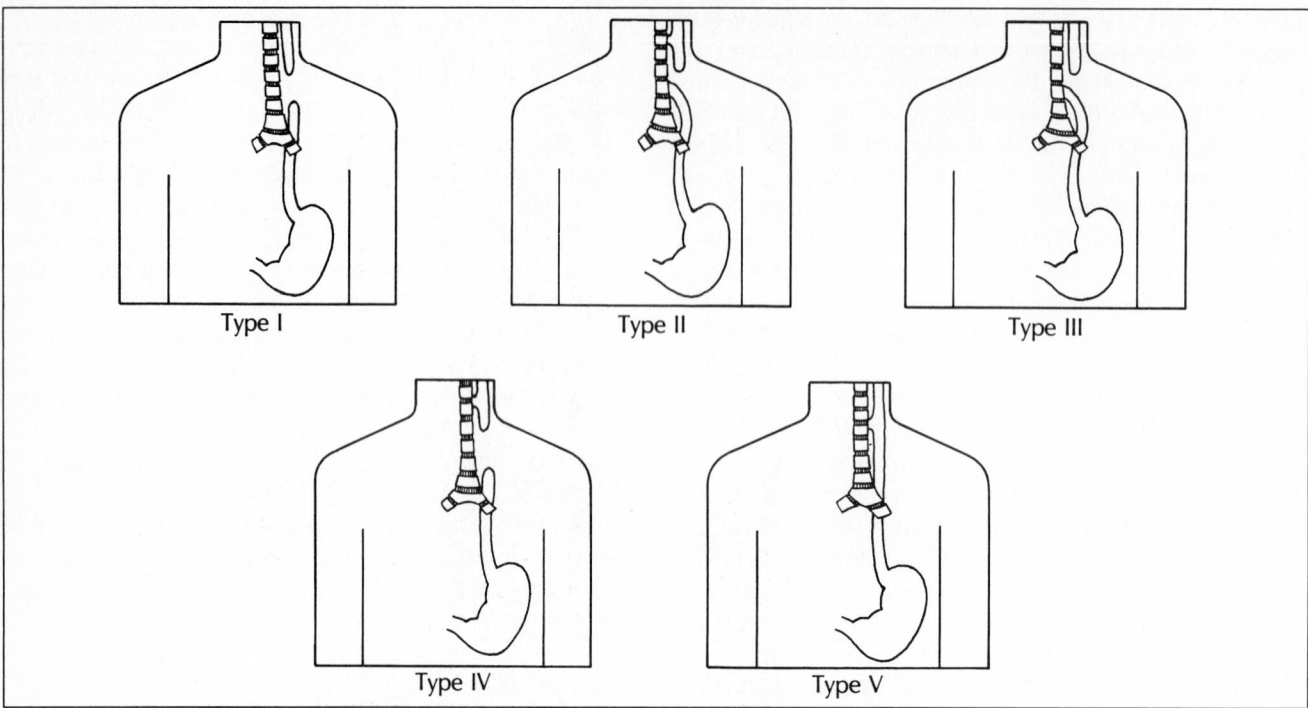

Figure 26-4 Five most frequently seen types of congenital esophageal atresia and tracheo-esophageal fistula.

the upper esophageal segment empties by a fistulous tract into the trachea, with some of these infants having the lower segment end in a blind pouch (type IV); in others it connects to the trachea (type II) (Figure 26-4).

CLINICAL MANIFESTATIONS

Maternal hydramnios is noted in about 40% of cases and is usually associated with the fetus who cannot swallow and excrete the amniotic fluid as the normal fetus does. From one-fourth to one-third of neonates with tracheoesophageal fistula (type III) anomaly are preterm (gestational age of 37 weeks or less). The neonate has excessive mucous secretions and drools almost constantly. Cyanotic episodes may occur secondary to aspiration of excessive mucus from the oropharynx. If the neonate is fed milk or formula, it is immediately regurgitated, often through the nose as well as the mouth, after one or two swallows. The neonate gags, chokes, struggles, and turns cyanotic as the fluid enters the tracheobronchial tree. Abdominal distention begins to develop soon after birth in the case of a tracheoesophageal fistula. Abdominal distention may occur, caused by air from the trachea via the fistula tract, or the neonate may pass abnormal amounts of flatus due to excess air being forced into the stomach. In contrast, the abdomen appears scaphoid (flat) if the distal segment of the esophagus does not connect to the trachea.

The neonate is examined for the presence of coexist-

ing malformations, such as intestinal atresia, urologic disorders, and cardiovascular defects (patent ductus arteriosus, coarctation of the aorta).

Symptoms of aspiration pneumonia or chemical pneumonitis may occur with respiratory distress: tachypnea, flaring of nares, cyanotic episodes, retractions, rales, rhonchi, decreased breath sounds, unstable temperature (may be subnormal). Chemical pneumonitis results from regurgitation of gastric contents into the lungs in type III. Gastric juices sear the lung tissue and may be fatal.

If routine attempts at passage of a nasogastric tube are carried out in the delivery room, 94% of the cases involving esophageal atresia could be diagnosed at birth. A well-lubricated soft no. 8 nasogastric catheter is passed through the nose into the esophagus, where it will meet resistance. Only the H-type fistula has a continuous connection to the stomach, which would accommodate the passage of a nasogastric tube. When esophageal atresia and/or tracheoesophageal fistula are not diagnosed at birth, the infant aspirates and can develop pneumonia within the first 72 hours of life (Holder and Ashcraft, 1981).

X-ray examination reveals a radiopaque catheter coiled in the esophageal pouch, demonstrating the point of resistance and the end of the pouch. H-type fistulas are particularly difficult to diagnose as they are not constantly patent. Flat x-ray film of abdomen and chest shows the presence of air in the stomach and air in the upper blind pouch. Gas in the stomach and intestines indicates the presence of a fistula from the trachea to the esophageal segment into the stomach.

INTERVENTIONS

Prompt surgical diversion or closure of the fistula is essential. Surgical correction of esophageal discontinuity is done in several stages, depending on the distance between the atresia and the lower segment as the child grows. When surgery must be postponed because of pneumonia, the absence of a lower esophageal portion, or because the distance between the lower and upper portions of the esophagus is too great, either (a) a double-lumen nasogastric tube is inserted into the blind pouch and attached to continuous suction to prevent aspiration, or (b) a cervical esophagostomy is performed and gastrostomy feeding is done until a colon transplant or esophageal replacement can be accomplished (Figure 26–5). The cervical esophagostomy provides an outlet for secretions and allows "sham" feedings. Food that enters the mouth exits through the cervical esophagostomy. Sham feedings permit the infant to be fed fluids and semisolids orally to allow for sucking needs satisfaction and development of taste. (For nursing interventions, see the Nursing Care Plan on tracheoesophageal fistula.)

Esophageal reconstruction is usually deferred until the infant is asymptomatic and between 6 months and 2 years of age. The right or transverse portion of the colon is usually used to join the upper portion of the esophagus with the stomach.

The presence of an H-type fistula without esophageal atresia may not be identified during the first month of life. This rare lesion may be diagnosed after the infant suffers repeated bouts of coughing, choking, and aspiration pneumonia. At this time, surgical obliteration of the fistula is performed.

COMPLICATIONS OF SURGERY

Complications before surgical intervention result primarily from aspiration. The infant may have a brassy cough for 6 months to 2 years and upper respiratory infections, such as recurrent pneumonitis, bronchopneumonia, and atelectasis. Postoperatively, the most common complication is ischemia, which causes total breakdown of the transplant. Another complication is difficulty swallowing. Stenosis is treated with progressive dilatation by bougie (mercury-weighted dilators). Care must be taken to avoid breaking the suture line.

PROGNOSIS

Gestational age affects the survival rate. Approximately 50% of preterm infants and 90% of term infants with tracheoesophageal atresia/fistula survive.

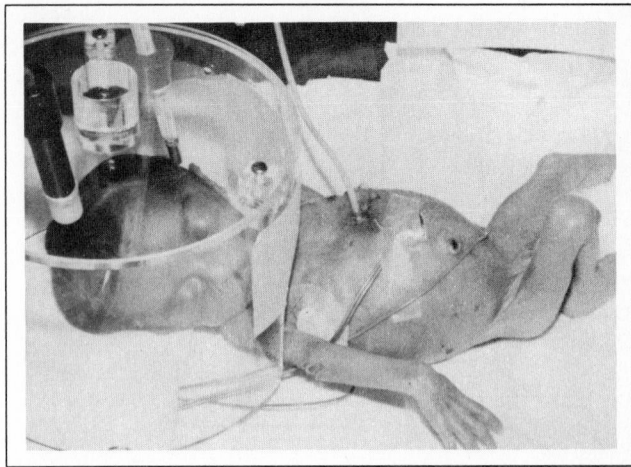

Figure 26–5 Infant with gastrostomy tube in place. Note that the tube is elevated. Oxygenation and temperature regulation are also monitored.

Diaphragmatic Hernia

Diaphragmatic hernia occurs once in every 3000 live births, and the frequency of occurrence is equal in males and females.

PHYSIOLOGY AND PATHOPHYSIOLOGY

The neonate born with a diaphragmatic hernia requires immediate surgical intervention. Herniation of abdominal contents and malrotation into the thoracic cavity are possible, because the abdominal and thoracic cavity constitute one entity due to failure of the pleuroperitoneal folds (which comprise the diaphragm) to fuse completely by the eighth week of gestation. The diaphragm usually fuses anteriorly to the posterior. This abnormal connection between the thoracic and abdominal cavities is more common through the foramen of Bochdalek on the left side, as the liver blocks movement of the gut on the right (Figure 26–6, p. 866). The size of the defect and the amount of abdominal viscera present in the thoracic cavity influence the success of surgical repair. In severe cases, the large amount of viscera in the thorax compresses lung space. The resultant pulmonary hypoplasia may be incompatible with life. The mediastinal structures are shifted to the side opposite the defect.

This otherwise normal-appearing neonate has difficulty initiating respirations. The affected side of the chest cannot expand. Absence of viscera in the abdomen gives the abdomen a scaphoid (flat) appearance. Neonates with severe herniation are hypoxic; because of their inability to take in sufficient air, they rapidly develop respiratory and metabolic acidosis.

(Text continues on p. 866.)

NURSING CARE PLAN
Tracheoesophageal Fistula/Atresia

PATIENT DATA BASE

History

Pertinent information from the prenatal and perinatal record:

    Maternal history of hydramnios

    Choking, regurgitation immediately after 1 or 2 feedings and cyanotic episodes

    In H-type, recurrent aspiration pneumonia

    Failure to pass nasogastric tube and aspiration of mucus

    Current status of neonate — free from infections

    Parental reaction to situation

Physical examination

Esophageal atresia — excessive mucous secretions

Constant drooling

Scaphoid (flat) abdomen if distal esophageal segment does not connect to trachea

Symptoms of respiratory distress

With fistula type, same as above and abdominal distention that begins soon after birth

Laboratory evaluation

X-rays — visualization of radiopaque catheter coiled in esophageal pouch; if fistula is present, flat plate of abdomen and chest shows air in stomach and upper blind pouch

NURSING PRIORITIES

1. Support respiration by preventing aspiration and aspiration pneumonia, and preventing chemical pneumonitis and entry of gastric juices into respiratory tree through specific positioning

2. Maintain adequate nutrition

3. Identify coexistent malformations

4. Maintain infant in good physical condition for stress of surgery

5. Prevent emotional trauma to infant

6. Assist parents in coping with situation

7. Prevent postoperative complications

8. Foster parent–infant bonding

FAMILY EDUCATIONAL FOCUS

1. Explain the treatment modalities and their rationale

2. Explore possible short-term and long-term implications of tracheoesophageal fistula, such as need for alterations in feeding methods (gastrostomy) and need for nonnutritive sucking

3. Discuss the growth and development needs of their infant throughout the period of hospitalization

4. Provide opportunities for parents to discuss questions and individual concerns regarding their neonate

Problem	Nursing interventions and actions	Rationale
Aspiration pneumonitis and/or reflux of gastric contents in type III T.E.F.	Do not feed until assured of esophageal patency	Decreases incidence of aspiration
	Preoperatively: Quickly assess infant before putting to breast on delivery table	
	Assess for presenting symptoms, such as excessive oral secretions and respiratory distress	Identifies anomaly prior to respiratory problems
	Use sterile water for first feeding (if aspirated, does not create chemical pneumonitis)	
	Control saliva and mucus by constant suction through a double-lumen catheter passed into pouch and attached to low intermittent suction	Prevents aspiration pneumonia, which may be fatal
	Place in warmed, humidified crib or Isolette	Liquefies mucus and facilitates its removal from trachea; protects from infection
	Elevate head of bed 20° in semi-Fowler position	Prevents reflux of gastric juices through fistula into respiratory tree and resultant chemical pneumonitis

NURSING CARE PLAN Cont'd
Tracheoesophageal Fistula/Atresia

Problem	Nursing interventions and actions	Rationale
Respiratory distress	Postoperatively: If chest tube is in place, keep tubing free of kinks and tension; reposition or move infant carefully to avoid disrupting drainage system	Promotes effective drainage of fluid from chest and facilitates lung inflation
	Place clamp at head of crib; if tubing is dislodged, clamp it close to chest wall	Prevents pneumothorax
	Measure and record amount and character of drainage	Assists physician in assessing infant's progress and instituting appropriate measures
	Do not suction or irrigate stomach	Prevents direct trauma to stomach
	Suction upper esophagus via nasal catheter as necessary	Prevents direct trauma to incision sites
	Observe patency of upper esophagus and maintain low intermittent suction	Prevents infection and crusting
	Suction oropharynx with French (no. 8 or no. 10) soft rubber catheter; watch for increasing edema	Frequent suctioning may increase already-present surgical edema
	Position head of bed at 30°; maintain position with rolled clothes or cloth sling or put infant in cardiac chair	Promotes pooling of secretions at catheter tip if indwelling nasal catheter is in use
	Reposition every 2 hr	Prevents stasis pneumonia, skin breakdown
	If gastrostomy tube has been inserted, keep open with injections of 2–4 mL of air and elevate (see Figure 26–5)	Promotes drainage
	Keep in warmed, humidified crib or isolette	Liquefies secretions and facilitates their removal
	Assess vital signs and physical appearance: color, respiratory effort; notify physician if respiratory distress persists despite suctioning	Maintains ongoing record
Adequate nutritional intake	Monitor parenteral fluids every hour preoperatively and postoperatively	Prevents overhydration or underhydration
	Assess for degree of hydration (see p.854)	
	With gastrostomy tube in place, begin feedings when bowel sounds are present	Gastrointestinal motility must be established prior to feeding
	Use IM syringe barrel, funnel, or asepto barrel to instill fluid; initially, introduce 5% dextrose water, slowly; feed with warmed formula when dextrose water is tolerated	Facilitates feeding process Tests infant's tolerance or readiness for feeding
	Gastrostomy feeding: compress the tube and fill asepto syringe barrel partially with fluid, attach to gastrostomy tube, then decompress tubing and slowly commence feeding via gravity, by raising level of feeding apparatus	Decreases amount of air introduced into stomach, thus decreasing discomfort and regurgitation Gravity flow decreases pressure on anastamosis

**NURSING CARE PLAN Cont'd
Tracheoesophageal Fistula/Atresia**

Problem	Nursing interventions and actions	Rationale
	To discontinue feeding, compress gastrostomy tube as fluid level reaches tip of feeding apparatus; for infants, suspend gastrostomy tube; keep open to air; for older children fold tubing over itself and secure with clamp or rubber band	With infant's small gastric capacity, open tubing prevents regurgitation of gastric contents up into esophagus and allows for fluctuation of feeding in tube until feeding is digested
	As stomach fills, give infant a pacifier	Meets sucking needs and helps neonate/infant associate sucking with easing of hunger and full stomach; sucking also relaxes gastrointestinal musculature
	Provide sham feedings via cervical esophagostomy	Maintains sucking mechanism and stimulates normal gastrointestinal mobility; helps infant associate pleasant sensation with feeding and avoids failure-to-thrive syndrome
	Talk or sing to infant during feeding; hold infant and cuddle during and after feeding	
	Cleanse skin around gastrostomy tube and cervical esophagostomy and apply prescribed mild ointment (aluminum paste or zinc oxide)	Prevents skin breakdown and infection
	Oral feedings: if continuity of esophagus has been achieved, begin feedings about 2 weeks postoperatively; begin by offering 5% dextrose water and feed slowly; when water is well tolerated, advance to feeding with small amounts of formula by bottle	Assess infant's tolerance for feedings and readiness for removal of gastrostomy tube Prevents possibility of coughing, choking, and regurgitation
	Record intake/output and daily weight; plot pattern of weight gain	Indicates adequacy of diet and method of feedings
Possible coexisting malformation	Assess infant's anatomic appearance and physiologic functioning	Enables physician to institute appropriate treatment; assesses readiness for surgery; provides more definitive anticipatory guidance to family
Emotional trauma to infant	Have same nurse care for infant to provide continuity of care	Facilitates development of trust
	Provide soothing environment: quiet, soft music; cuddling and talking	Facilitates rest; prevents overstimulation
	Hold whenever possible; touch, stroke; to carry infant around—pin gastrostomy asepto syringe to infant's clothing	Facilitates development of trust
	Respond to crying by stroking, talking, and cuddling	Assists infant to associate relief of hunger with sucking motions; strengthens muscles; exercises jaws; facilitates normal gastrointestinal functioning (stomach will not receive feeding if infant is upset); infant associates feeding with comfort of being held
	Offer pacifier when infant is being fed by gastrostomy	
	Feed infant while holding him or her	
	Encourage active parental participation in daily care of the infant	Facilitates positive parent–infant relationship

NURSING CARE PLAN Cont'd
Tracheoesophageal Fistula/Atresia

Problem	Nursing interventions and actions	Rationale
Parents' coping mechanisms	Keep parents informed; clarify and reinforce physician's explanations regarding malformation, surgical repair, pre- and postoperative care, and prognosis	Knowledge is ego-strengthening
	Encourage grieving for having infant with defect	Parents cannot begin positive relationship with this infant until they grieve for the loss of desired perfect infant
	Involve parents in care of infant and in planning for future; facilitate touch and eye contact	Dispels feelings of inadequacy, increases self-esteem and self-worth
		Potentiates incorporation of infant into family
	Refer family to community agencies for financial assistance (defect necessitates long hospitalizations, specialized equipment and services)	Assists family with heavy financial burden
Postoperative complications	Refer to public health nurse to continue counseling, education, and prevent pulmonary infection or stricture of esophagus	Maintains motivation and sense of hopefulness during lengthy treatment
	Teach parents signs and symptoms of complications of pneumonitis and esophageal stricture	Facilitates early identification and treatment of serious complications

NURSING CARE EVALUATION

Neonate/infant does not develop aspiration pneumonia or chemical pneumonitis	Emotional trauma is minimized in infant
Neonate's/infant's nutrition is adequate to maintain appropriate pattern of weight gain; dehydration is avoided	Parents are able to cope with needs of not only affected infant but also themselves and rest of family
Any coexisting malformations are identified and appropriate interventions taken or planned	Postsurgical complications do not occur

NURSING DIAGNOSES*	SUPPORTING DATA
1. Potential for impaired gas exchange	Symptoms of pneumonitis
2. Potential impairment of skin integrity related to gastrostomy and/or cervical esophagostomy	Redness Ulceration Edema Drainage
3. Anxiety in infant related to artificial feeding pattern, necessary interventions	Sucking reflex not stimulated Separated from parents Nursery environment Invasive procedures
4. Knowledge deficit about care of infant with GI defect	Expressed concerns and questions regarding variant feeding methods, wound care, signs of complications and possible coexisting malformations

* These are a few examples of nursing diagnoses that may be appropriate for an infant with this condition. It is not an inclusive list and must be individualized for each infant.

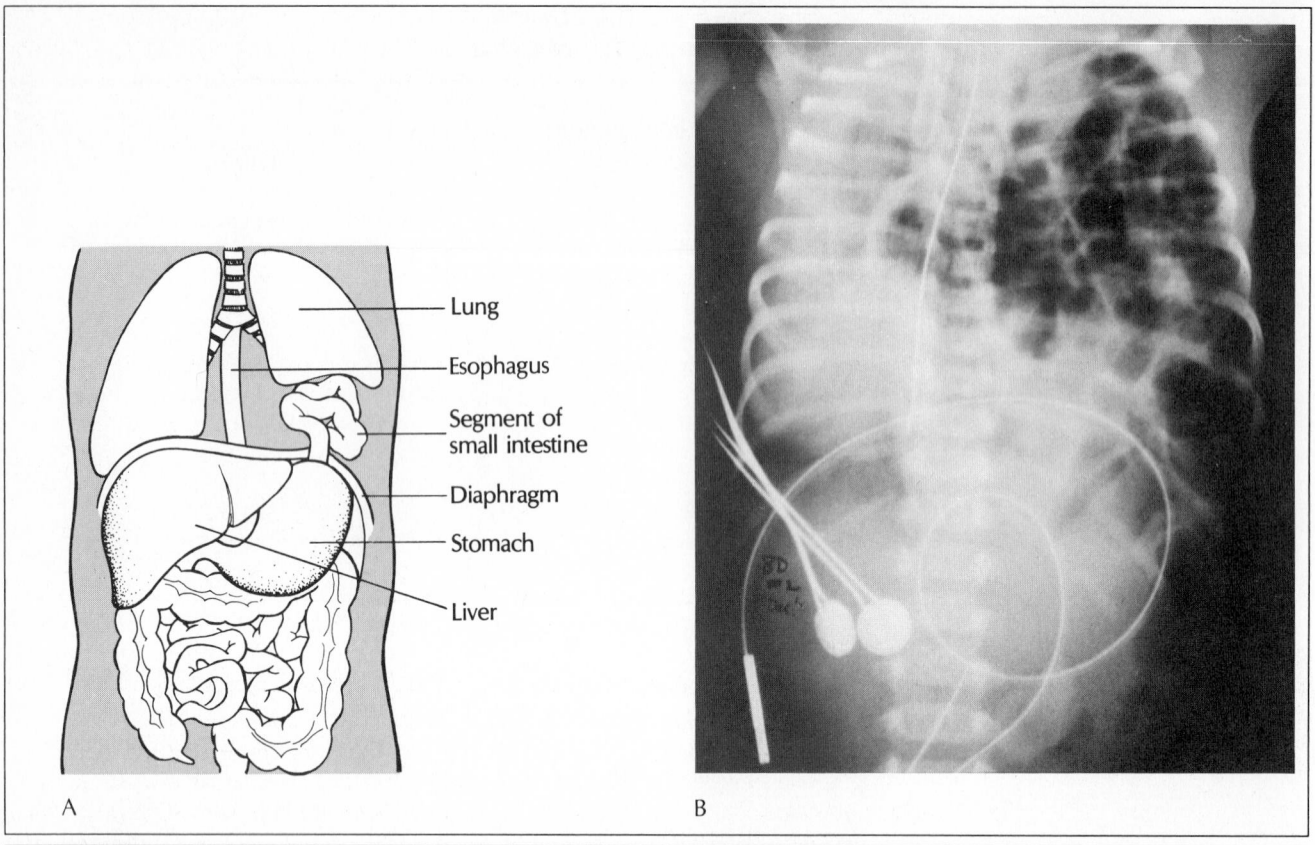

Figure 26–6 A, Diaphragmatic hernia. Note compression of the lung by the intestine on the affected side. **B,** X-ray shows bowel loops up into the left thoracic cavity.

CLINICAL MANIFESTATIONS

Breath sounds are absent on the left side. Respirations are gasping, with nasal flaring and chest retraction. Bowel sounds may soon be heard in the thoracic cavity (large barrel chest), and the abdomen appears scaphoid because of the presence of abdominal viscera in the chest. Respiratory and metabolic acidosis develop rapidly. The neonate may vomit if fed. Heart sounds displaced to the right (diagnosis of dextrocardia), a chest full to auscultation, and spasmodic attacks of cyanosis and difficulty in feeding (resulting from dyspnea) are definitive signs of herniation of diaphragm. Cardiac action and respirations are further compromised as the bowel fills with gas. Signs of intestinal obstruction due to associated malrotation of the intestines may also be seen. Radiography reveals gas-filled bowels in the thoracic cavity and a displacement of the mediastinal structures to the side opposite the diaphragmatic defect. Lung collapse and hypoplasia because of early compression also provide differential diagnosis in cases of lung hematomas, paralysis of the diaphragm, eventration of the diaphragm, and elevation in the diaphragmatic wall.

INTERVENTIONS

Immediate relief of respiratory distress is attained by administration of oxygen in high concentrations and by gas-tric decompression via insertion of a nasogastric tube. Neonates should be given nothing by mouth. Positive pressure ventilation by mask should never be used as it increases the infant's distress by adding to the air and pressure in the stomach. If positive pressure ventilation is indicated, endotracheal intubation is the treatment required. The nurse elevates the infant's head in a semi-Fowler position and turns the infant on the affected side so that the unaffected lung may expand. An umbilical catheter is inserted for monitoring blood gases and administering fluids with electrolytes as necessary for control of acidosis. Surgery is performed immediately.

The surgical procedure involves removal of the bowel from the thoracic cavity and closure of the diaphragmatic defect. The surgical approach is transthoracic when no intestinal obstruction is present and transabdominal when obstructive malrotation is present. If the defect is small, there is usually enough diaphragmatic tissue for closure; if not, a woven Teflon patch is used to close the defect.

If intestinal malrotation accompanies the hernia, this, too, must be repaired to prevent later duodenal obstruction. Because the abdominal cavity may be too small to hold all the viscera, total closure may not be possible at this time. The peritoneum and muscle layers may be left open and the viscera covered with skin or a Silastic plastic sheet, creating a ventral hernia. The compressed lung is not expanded during surgery because of the danger of a pneumothorax on the contralateral side. The compressed lung gradually expands in 7–14 days, but may remain hypoplastic.

NURSING MANAGEMENT

A nursing history contains pertinent information from the prenatal and perinatal records: a summary of the condition of the neonate prior to surgery, a description of the type of defect (minimal or extensive abdominal malformations), the preoperative clinical picture, the postsurgical condition, information about the chest tube and type of abdominal closure, and observations of the parental response to the neonate and the malformation.

Nursing priorities include maintaining adequate ventilation and nutrition, preventing postoperative complications (shock, bleeding, infection, pneumothorax), and assisting the parents to cope with the situation.

The nurse facilitates respirations by positioning the neonate in a high Fowler position (infant seat may be used) to utilize gravity to keep abdominal organ pressure off the diaphragm. A chest tube is placed on the affected side, attached to a water seal on low suction, to relieve the surgical pneumothorax and to allow for gradual reexpansion of the lung on the affected side. Positive pressure ventilation may be used for several days postoperatively to relieve pneumothorax of the affected lung. The nurse is also responsible for maintaining chest tube function (see discussion in the tracheoesophageal fistula Nursing Care Plan), placing the neonate in a warmed humidified environment, suctioning as necessary, placing the child on the affected side to facilitate lung expansion, and utilizing an appropriate feeding method. Gastric suction is continued immediately postoperatively to prevent abdominal distention and pressure on the diaphragmatic repair. Feeding may be accomplished initially by intravenous infusion and hyperalimentation, then by gavage on the second or third postoperative day to decrease air swallowing, then orally when tolerated without abdominal distention. Frequent burping is important.

The nurse assesses the neonate for adequacy of nutrition and hydration. A flexible feeding schedule is important to take advantage of the usually anorexic infant's increase in appetite and desire to eat. Care must be taken to decrease the swallowing of air, stomach compression, and predisposition to gagging and vomiting. Development of hiatal hernia is common. The parents may have difficulty coping with the situation because of the necessary rapidity of the surgery and the mechanical interventions, such as the respirator, needed to preserve their tiny infant's life.

PROGNOSIS

Prognosis depends on the severity of the defect and the degree of pulmonary hypoplasia. Surgical intervention is successful in about 50% of the affected neonates. Mortality is highest in the first 24 hours after birth. For some children, the defect is asymptomatic during infancy and may be diagnosed years later, usually following recurrent episodes of respiratory infection (from compression of the lower lobe of the lung). These children have an excellent prognosis following surgery.

Omphalocele (Exomphalos)

PHYSIOLOGY AND PATHOPHYSIOLOGY

During embryologic development, midgut development occurs outside the abdomen. By the tenth week of gestation, the intestines reenter the abdominal cavity through the umbilical opening, and the anterior abdominal wall closes. Total or partial failure of the midgut to complete this migration results in *omphalocele* anomaly. The herniated intestines are covered with a fragile, transparent amniotic membrane that will degenerate within 12 hours after birth, becoming opaque, necrotic, and malodorous because of lack of blood supply. Large omphaloceles may contain the liver and spleen as well. The incidence is 1 in every 10,000 births (Kempe et al., 1982).

In *gastroschisis* the defect occurs between the two normal rectus muscles. At 5–7 weeks in embryonic development, the intestine ruptures out at the base of the umbilical cord toward the right side where the right umbilical vein was absorbed, leaving a slight defect to the right of the umbilical cord. In gastroschisis, only the intestine is eviscerated, and because it is not covered by a sac it becomes thickened, edematous, and matted due to the irritating effect of the amniotic fluid (Klein et al., 1981).

About one-third of affected neonates with omphalocele demonstrate Beckwith syndrome: high birth weight, rapid postnatal growth, macroglossia (hypertrophy of the tongue), facial nevus flammeus, and neonatal hypoglycemia. Coexistent malformations, such as cardiac anomalies, are common. Some 65% of infants with gastroschisis are preterm but only 23% have other malformations (Mayer et al., 1980).

CLINICAL MANIFESTATIONS

The presence of an omphalocele is obvious, with small intestine, colon, liver, and stomach (or any combination) in a sac with attached umbilical cord or lying free if the sac is ruptured (Figure 26-7). Small omphaloceles may be confused with umbilical cysts or hematomas. Gastroschisis appears similar to omphalocele, as abdominal viscera protrude through an abdominal wall defect; however, gastroschisis is located lateral to the abdominal midline (usually to the right) and separate from the umbilical cord, with no sac or covering.

INTERVENTIONS

Before surgery, the nurse protects the defect from infection, drying, and rupture by either sterile gauze moistened

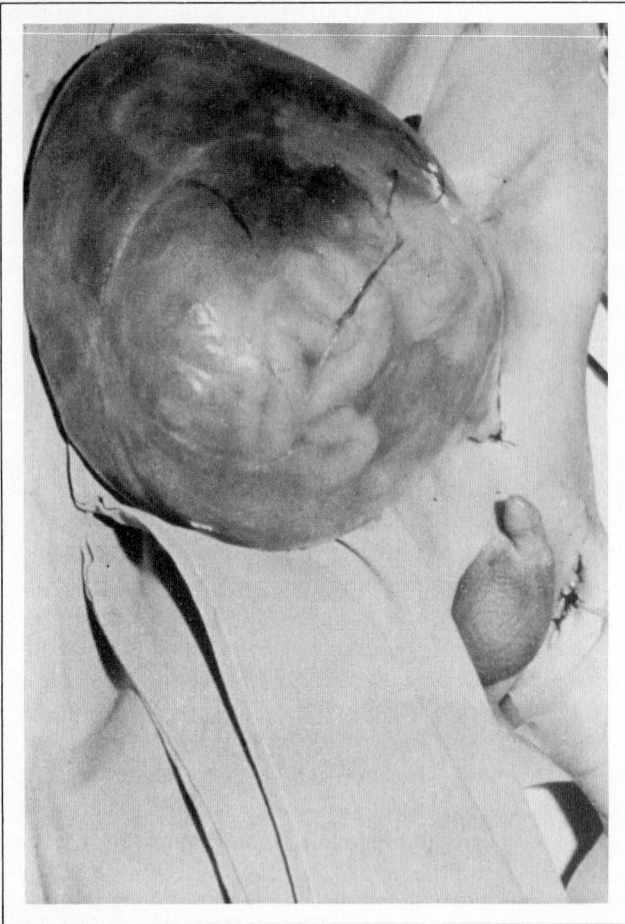

Figure 26–7 Infant with large omphalocele. The omphalocele sac is lying to the right side of the abdomen. (Courtesy Paul Winchester, M.D.)

with warmed (body temperature) sterile saline or sterile petroleum dressings and a firm (metal or plastic) shield. Sterile technique is essential. A nasogastric tube attached to low suction prevents distention of the lower bowel. Antibiotics are begun before surgery and are continued until the chance of infection has passed. Choice of corrective method depends on the general size and condition of the infant, on the presence of other abnormalities, on the size of the defect, and on the capacity of the sac.

Defects of 5 cm or less may be repaired in one procedure; larger defects require staged repairs. The viscera may not fit into the available abdominal space. Forcing the viscera into the abdominal cavity compresses the viscera, impairs venous return, and raises the diaphragm. When this occurs, within a matter of hours the infant develops respiratory distress and extreme fatigue and succumbs. Medium-sized defects are closed with skin flaps within 12 hours of birth until the peritoneal cavity has enlarged (approximately 6–12 months of age). Later a ventral umbilical herniorrhaphy is done as the final stage.

An uncommon and seldom-used nonsurgical therapy consists of treating the sac with 0.5% silver nitrate solution as an escharotic agent (Grosfeld et al., 1981), or 2% aqueous solution of Merthiolate applied two or three times a day. The restrained neonate remains in an incubator until the sac thickens and toughens and a dry eschar forms. Several weeks later, after the eschar is sufficiently toughened and contracting and the mother has learned how to continue the application of the solution, the infant may be cared for at home. The defect closes, creating a ventral herniorrhaphy in a matter of weeks or months. However, complications may include late rupture of the sac and infection.

A more common method for correcting large defects or a ruptured sac is the creation of an artificial celom (sac) using a Silastic bag (Figure 26–8). The bag forms a pouch over the abdominal contents when it is sutured to the abdominal wall fascia. Then the bag is suspended from the top of the incubator by a flexible band. Every few days, pressure is exerted on the pouch, shortening it and forcing the organs back into the abdominal cavity and stretching the abdominal cavity to allow reentry and skin flap closure within 7–10 days.

Nursing activities include observing for respiratory distress that might result from pressure of abdominal organs on the diaphragm, for fatigue, and for integrity of the operative site. The nurse should ensure that the infant is properly positioned and restrained to prevent trauma to the site. The nurse provides care of the surgical site according to physician's orders. In the nonsurgical corrective method, observations for allergic reactions to the escharotic agent should be made; signs include edema or bright red spots on the skin other than the areas being treated. The nurse also assesses for adequacy of parenteral nutrition and hydration, and assists parents (see the Nursing Care Plan for cleft lip and palate).

PROGNOSIS

The prognosis depends on the presence and severity of the defect and the coexisting malformations: intestinal malrotation, abnormal obstructing bands across the duodenum, midgut volvulus, adhesions, intestinal atresia, congenital heart disease, cleft lip, and the like. About one-third of these infants suffer the hazards imposed by prematurity as well. The poorest surgical results and increased mortality are expected if the sac is more than 7 cm wide and contains the liver.

Aganglionic Megacolon

PHYSIOLOGY AND PATHOPHYSIOLOGY

Aganglionic megacolon is also known as Hirschsprung's disease, congenital megacolon, or aganglionosis. Parasympathetic nerve–ganglion cells are absent in the submucosa

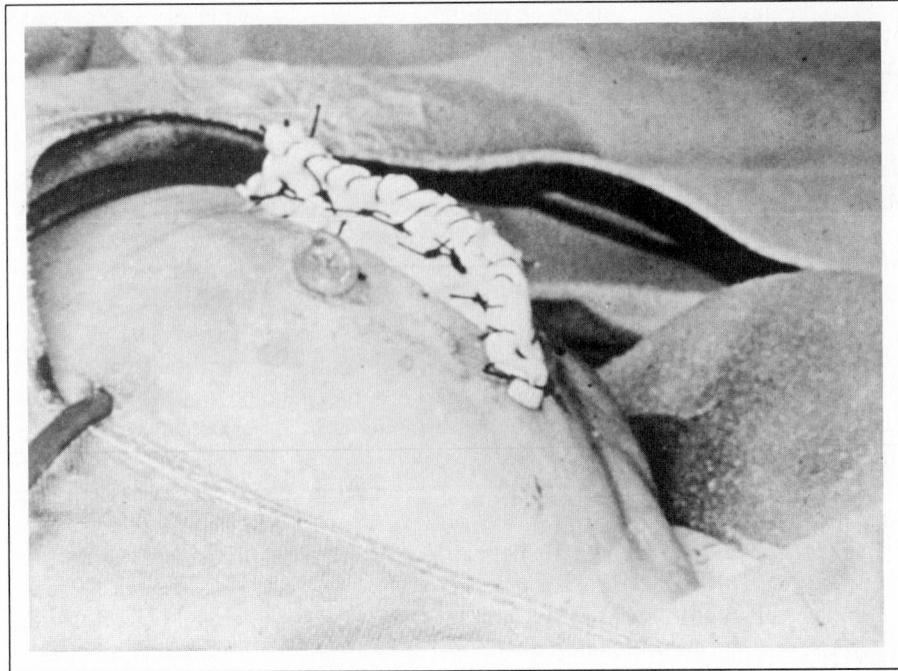

Figure 26–8 Omphalocele with Silastic mesh bag covering the abdominal contents. Note sutures in Silastic bag to decrease the size of the bag and move the abdominal organs back into the abdominal cavity. (Courtesy Paul Winchester, M.D.)

and muscles in the rectosigmoid colon. Without innervation, colonic peristalsis and passing of fecal material cannot occur in that segment. The intestine proximal to the aganglionic segment becomes grossly distended as fecal material accumulates. This motility disturbance results in intestinal obstruction, vomiting, constipation, fluid and electrolyte deficits, and hypoproteinemia. Aganglionosis is four times more common in males and is often associated with Down syndrome or with a familial predisposition.

CLINICAL MANIFESTATIONS AND DIFFERENTIAL DIAGNOSIS

Very mild cases may be undiagnosed for several years and may result in no symptoms except for persistent constipation, which is relieved by laxatives or enemas on occasion.

The neonate with this disorder may manifest the following symptoms: an absence of meconium, vomitus containing bile, constipation, increasing abdominal distention, and resultant respiratory distress (Figure 26–9). In older infants it is characterized by abdominal distention, diarrhea alternating with obstinate constipation, and large palpable fecal mass. If the condition is left untreated, the child becomes chronically ill, malnourished, anemic, and lethargic, and may suffer respiratory embarrassment. A striking foul odor to the breath and stool is significant. The rectum may be tight or collapsed. Enterocolitis may develop. Complications of hyperthermia, neurogenic shock, and severe toxicity may be fatal if not treated immediately. Crisis is heralded by profuse vomiting, fever, and offensive diarrhea progressing to rapid dehydration and collapse of the empty rectum. On rectal digital examination, the rectum is tight and conical. Often stool or gas is expelled after the examination.

An anteroposterior radiography of the abdomen reveals a distended intestinal loop. An x-ray film of a barium

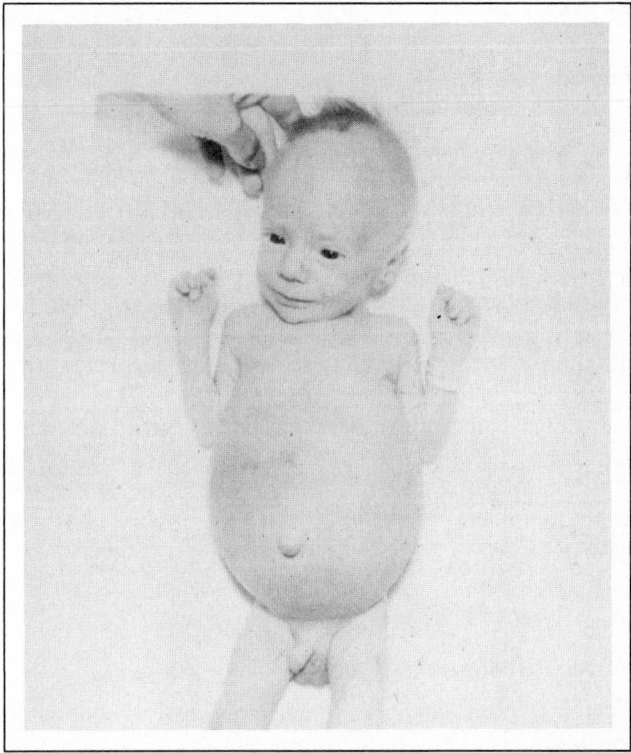

Figure 26–9 Infant with Hirschsprung's disease.

enema shows a narrow rectum and sigmoid colon and may show a zone of conversion to the distended proximal colon. Usually the barium enema fails to be expelled within 24 hours.

The newborn may not show the classic x-ray feature because there may not have been time for the size disparity to develop between the dilated proximal colon and empty distal colon segment. After abdominal decompression via gastric tube, a rectal biopsy is done to examine for absence of nerve–ganglion cells. Histology shows an absence of parasympathetic ganglion cells of the intramural plexus in the narrowed segment.

DIFFERENTIAL DIAGNOSIS

The physician must rule out meconium plug syndrome and ileus secondary to sepsis or volvulus. Diagnostic contrast enemas may be used to dislodge a meconium plug from the transverse or sigmoid colon, thus relieving this obstruction. Almost all neonates with meconium plug syndrome have ganglionic innervation to the bowel and remain well thereafter.

INTERVENTIONS

An emergency colostomy relieves the intestinal obstruction, deflates and clears the bowel, and also allows time for improvement of nutritional and general health status until the optimal time for total correction. The colostomy is placed just at the distal end of the bowel where there are ganglion cells. Until corrective surgery, the infant is placed on a low residue diet and is given stool softeners; accurate intake and output records are kept, noting frequency and nature of stools. Just prior to corrective surgery, the bowel is emptied manually and with colonic irrigations of isotonic saline solutions. Drugs such as neomycin by mouth and by rectal instillation are given to reduce normal bowel flora. A nasogastric tube is inserted to decompress the stomach, and fluid and electrolyte replacements are carried out. Electrolyte imbalances are common as a result of vomiting and intestinal dysfunction. A pull-through operation via Swenson, Duhamel, or modified Soave method is done. The procedure involves excision of the aganglionic segment and pulling the ganglionic intestines down to the anus. Final resection of the aganglionic segment and anastomosis of the proximal and distal portions are usually not done before 6 months of age and may be delayed for a year. Optimally the child is 6–12 months of age and weighs 18–20 lb (Filston, 1982).

The temporary colostomy is closed either during the total correction or usually 1 to 2 weeks later.

NURSING MANAGEMENT

The nurse plays an important role in the early diagnosis of this disorder. The nursing history contains pertinent information from the prenatal and perinatal records for familial history, the condition of the neonate from birth, and the onset of symptoms as previously described.

Nursing priorities prior to surgery include astute observations of symptoms (which assist in early diagnosis), maintenance of adequate nutrition and hydration, and assisting the parents to cope with the situation. Frequent small feedings with consideration of likes and dislikes and developmental level should be offered, because these infants tend to eat slowly, have poor appetites, and become uncomfortable after eating, resulting in difficulties in establishing proper nutritional habits.

Following colostomy surgery, the nurse's priorities include the prevention of postoperative complications, maintenance of adequate nutrition and hydration, colostomy care, and preparation of the parents for the care of the colostomy and the infant until the corrective surgery is scheduled.

Colostomy care in the neonate requires conscientious care to prevent skin irritation and possible infection. Diapers and other clothing are changed frequently to keep the neonate clean, dry, free from odor, and to minimize skin breakdown with infection. The skin around the colostomy is cleansed with warm water, dried, then protected with a thin layer of aluminum paste, karaya gum, or Maalox. Periodic exposure to air is also beneficial. Drainage from the colostomy is assessed for amount, color, consistency, and the presence of mucus or blood. Fluid replacement is partially dependent on the amount of drainage. In the early period after the colostomy is constructed, the nurse observes the neonate for abdominal distention or obstruction. Obstruction may occur from peritonitis, which is manifested by increasing abdominal tenderness, hyperthermia, vomiting, or irritability.

The thought as well as the sight of a colostomy is very difficult for parents to accept. They require considerable support while they grieve over the situation, express their anger and frustration, and then, finally, learn to care for the infant and the colostomy. The parents notice each person's reaction to the colostomy and internalize these reactions. The nurse needs to plan time to be with the parents when they are visiting with the neonate to offer support and information. It is best if the parents have some idea what a colostomy will look like prior to surgery. The parents need to learn how to keep the infant in a good nutritional state so that the infant will be ready for surgical repair later.

Postsurgical correction and the notation of feeding behaviors, pain upon elimination, and abdominal distention are important. Stools are tested for presence of bleeding and are measured to determine fluid and electrolyte losses. Initial replacement therapy based on the amount of stooling and electrolyte studies is instituted—intravenously at first until oral feedings are possible. The infant may have nothing by mouth for long periods, so to meet normal sucking needs a pacifier should be offered. Axillary temperature should be taken until rectal healing is complete. Meticulous skin care around the perineal and anal regions is essential to prevent excoriations common after pull-through operations and postoperative diarrhea. When surgical correction is achieved, the primary focus is on the establishment of normal elimination. Patterns and amount of stooling should be assessed to determine the child's progression toward this goal.

PROGNOSIS

Prognosis for normal bowel function and control depends on the length of the bowel segment that lacks the nerve-ganglia and whether the rectum can be preserved.

Imperforate Anus

PHYSIOLOGY AND PATHOPHYSIOLOGY

Imperforate anus comprises a variety of anomalies of the rectum and anus, ranging from a simple membrane at the anus to complex deformities. A brief review of embryonic development clarifies the development of this anomaly. In the normal embryonic process, a blind pouch within the abdomen moves downward to the perineum to meet another pouch invaginating upward from the anal area. The two pouches meet, fuse to form a continuous passageway, and the membrane that separates the rectum from the anus normally is absorbed during the seventh week of fetal life. Abnormality at any point in the pathway results in imperforate anus.

Imperforate anus is best classified according to the international classification of anorectal anomalies. Fistulous tracts originating in the intestinal pouch may terminate in the anal area or urinary tract in both sexes and in the vagina in females. Lesions are classified as "low" if the evidence indicates that the distal rectum transverses the puborectalis sling and terminates anterior to the external sphincter. In "high" lesions the distal rectum ends proximal to the puborectalis sling. The differentiation of these two groups is important in the operative decision and the success of surgical repair. High lesions require combined abdominal and sacroperineal operative repair, usually preceded by a colostomy. In high lesions, an increased incidence of genitourinary and vertebral anomalies exists, and normal anal continence frequently is not achievable. Low lesions do not require a colostomy and are repaired through a perineal or sacroperineal approach. Associated anomalies are less frequent in low lesions and normal anal continence is expected (Danis and Graviss, 1978). In each group the bowel ends blindly or communicates by a fistula with the nearby viscera or the perineal skin (Figure 26–10).

In all these deformities the internal anal sphincter is absent, but the external anal sphincter may be present in rudimentary form. Total sphincter absence does not necessarily produce fecal incontinence if the puborectalis sling is intact. Some slight staining may occur because the internal sphincter is absent, but the external sphincter can almost completely close the anus.

Imperforate anus is a common anomaly occurring in about 1 in 5000 births and is more common in males. In infants with high anomalies, 50% have associated neurologic defects that lessen the possibility of a well-functioning bowel after correction.

CLINICAL MANIFESTATIONS

Several variations of the anatomic appearance of the perineum are possible. The anal opening may be absent with or without the presence of a sphincter musculature (Figure 26–10). The "wink" reflex may be absent. (A "wink" is elicited when one touches the normal sphincter muscle.)

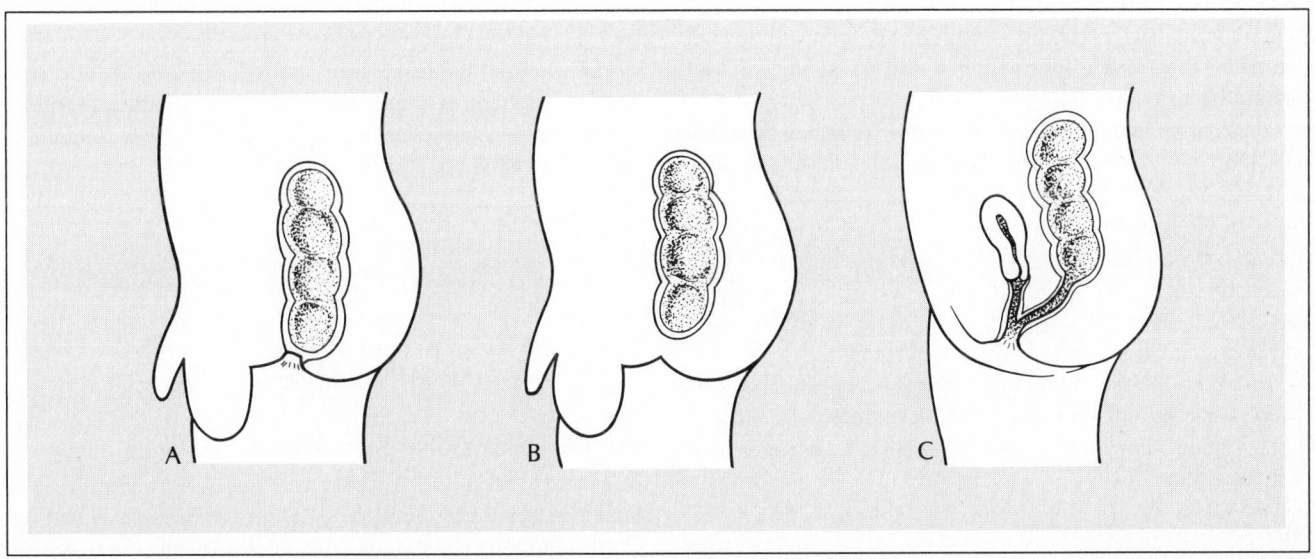

Figure 26–10 Variations in imperforate anus and anal rectal stenosis. **A,** Anal opening covered by thin membrane. **B,** Anal agenesis. **C,** Rectal vaginal fistula.

The anus may be abnormally placed. If only a thin membrane covers the anal opening, a black mass (meconium) may be seen behind the membrane. The examiner is unable to insert a lubricated thermometer (or tubing) into the anal opening. (Caution: If a rectal thermometer is used prior to the passage of meconium, the examiner must use extreme care so as not to traumatize or perforate an otherwise imperforate anus.)

The physiologic function is altered as well: No meconium is passed, and increasing abdominal distention is noted; or meconium may be passed through an ectopic opening from the vagina or urethra. Meconium in the urine of males indicates a fistula to the urinary tract.

Diagnosis is based on examinations to determine the anatomic level of the anomaly, the location of the fistula and its ectopic opening, and the presence of coexisting malformations. An invertogram roentgenogram (Wagenstein-Rice method), of the neonate tilted upside down, to determine the level of intestinal pouch is not always accurate because it takes at least 18–24 hours for air to reach the apex of the blind pouch. Lumbosacral vertebral malformations may be visualized on x-ray film, especially sacral agenesis, which affects neural pathways. A micturating cystourethrogram (MCU) identifies urologic malformations and rectourinary communication that may accompany this defect.

INTERVENTIONS

If only a simple membrane is covering the anus, it is excised or treated with a cruciate incision followed by dilatation of the anus at periodic intervals to keep the opening the size of the examiner's little finger, thereby preventing stricture and scar formation.

Low anomalies (short length of rectal agenesis—less than 1.5 cm from perineal skin) are corrected to make a continuous passageway by means of either a perineal approach "cutback" procedure or anoplasty followed by anal dilatation at periodic intervals initiated as soon as initial healing occurs.

High anomalies (those in which the blind pouch is farther than 1.5 cm away from the perineal skin) are treated in at least two stages: sigmoid colostomy above the fistulous tract to protect the urinary system from fecal contamination and corrective surgery (to make a continuous passageway) at about 9–12 months of age. Usually a sacroabdominoperineal rectoplasty is done, which exposes and delineates the puborectalis sling, then via the abdominal route the rectum is mobilized, the fistula is divided, and the bowel is brought down within the puborectalis sling to the perineum. For intermediate anomalies a sacroperineal rectoplasty is done.

NURSING MANAGEMENT

A complete nursing history based on careful observation of the neonate's anatomic appearance and physiologic func-

tioning assists in the identification and early treatment of this congenital anomaly. Notation is made of the parental reactions to the situation and the infant. Regardless of the surgical treatments, parents need assistance in coping with the birth of a neonate with a defect. Parents need to be encouraged to see and touch the neonate early and often. Postoperative care is directed toward colostomy and pull-through care (discussed in the section on aganglionic megacolon, p. 868). Immediately postoperatively, diapers are not used, and immediate cleansing of the anal area after each stool is very important. The infant should be repositioned and turned from side to side but never allowed to lie with the legs pulled up under the body, as this puts pressure on the suture area. Possible need for anal dilatations over a period of time may cause emotional trauma in the toddler because of the preoccupation with the anal area and its by-products.

Depending on the surgical procedure, parents may need to be taught to perform anal dilatation with catheters or the little finger or to perform colostomy care (see the section on aganglionic megacolon, p. 868). Parents need to be advised that even if continuity of the bowel is achieved, some infants with high anomalies will have problems with fecal incontinence throughout life, which can lead to problems in school and with peer acceptance. Toilet training is a difficult milestone to achieve; it may take months or years or may never be achieved, producing a stressful situation for both parents and child. In the case of a low anomaly, toilet training is achieved by learning to use the puborectalis muscle.

COMPLICATIONS

Anal strictures readily develop after anoplasty or rectoplasty, and anal dilatation is required at regular intervals for at least 3 months. Strictures can lead to constipation and colonic inertia, development of a large hypertrophied and dilated rectum, and incontinence. Ischemic sloughing of the rectum may result from inadequate mobilization and tension. Fistulas may recur if their initial closure was inadequate. Urinary complications and perineal or pararectal abscess may develop.

PROGNOSIS

Prognosis depends on the severity of the anomaly and on the presence of associated malformations.

Intestinal Obstruction

PHYSIOLOGY AND PATHOPHYSIOLOGY

Intestinal atresia and stenosis may result from intrauterine interferences of blood supply to the embryonic bowel or from failure to reestablish the lumen during fetal bowel development. The atresia may take the form of a septum in the lumen of the intestines, complete atresia of varying lengths, or separated multiple blind pouches. Most of these malformations occur distal to the opening of the bile and pancreatic ducts (duodenum), so that vomitus is bile-stained. The *annular pancreas* may constrict the duodenum. If the stricture is incomplete, symptoms may not occur during the first month of life. This anomaly is often coincident with Down syndrome. Duodenal and ileal atresias are most common. Atresia are not common between the duodenum and the lower ileum.

Meconium ileus refers to an obstruction of the intestine by thick, inspissated meconium. In the neonate with cystic fibrosis, a deficiency of the pancreatic enzyme trypsin causes the meconium in utero to become puttylike and to adhere to the intestinal mucosa. Meconium ileus may become complicated by rupture of the intestine proximal to the obstruction, spillage of meconium into the peritoneum, and consequent development of meconium peritonitis.

Volvulus, the twisting of the intestine, results from abnormal embryonic development. Either the colon (ileocecal structure) does not rotate properly as the intestines enter the abdomen through the umbilical area and remains in the right upper quadrant, or the mesentery does not attach properly during the tenth week of gestation, allowing the bowel to twist upon itself. Remnants of normal peritoneal attachments of the cecum to the right abdominal wall in embryonic development may exist, extending from the cecum and ascending colon across the descending duodenum, further causing obstruction. In addition to intestinal obstruction, a severe complication of volvulus is infarction and necrosis. Volvulus is possible any time during the first few years of life but is most common in early infancy.

Meconium plug syndrome results from an accumulation of meconium in the rectum. The meconium becomes inspissated and firm, thus obstructing the lower bowel. All the symptoms of intestinal obstruction are seen.

CLINICAL MANIFESTATIONS

Neonates with intestinal obstruction usually fail to pass any meconium, and prenatal hydramnios is present. Increasing abdominal distention is noted. If the distention progresses, the neonate's respiratory rate increases. Vomiting may be bilious (green) or fecal. Volvulus may be palpable. Without surgical intervention, the neonate loses weight, becomes dehydrated, and develops hypoproteinemia, hypokalemia, hyponatremia, metabolic acidosis, and shock.

DIFFERENTIAL DIAGNOSIS

With intestinal atresia, barium-contrast x-ray films show the characteristic "double bubble," indicating a large amount of barium in the stomach and a smaller amount in the duodenum only.

Ileal atresia and meconium ileus may be difficult to differentiate. Symptoms of both include abdominal distention and fecal-contaminated vomitus and absence of stooling if the condition is not diagnosed and treated soon enough. Roentgenograms show larger fluid–air levels in ileal atresia, as opposed to tiny air bubbles in viscid meconium in meconium ileus. Meconium ileus is suspected if there is a familial history of cystic fibrosis (mucoviscidosis). Volvulus is differentiated from high intestinal atresia by use of upper gastrointestinal films and barium enema. Meconium plug syndrome x-ray films show distended gaseous loops, usually without fluid levels.

INTERVENTIONS

Management of intestinal atresia or stricture of the duodenum from an annular pancreas is surgical resection of the affected intestinal segment with end-to-end anastomosis or duodenal bypass procedure (duodenoduodenostomy or duodenojejunostomy) for duodenal atresia. Treatment for jejunal or ileal atresia is excision of atretic and distended portions followed by end-to-end anastomosis (jejunojejunostomy or ileostomy). The pancreas is not incised, because this procedure is often followed by pancreatitis or fistula formation.

Management of volvulus is surgical (Ladd procedure) to relieve the twisting, to divide any constricting bands, to reduce the volvulus, and to reattach the bowel if necessary.

Management of meconium ileus is surgical, with removal of inspissated meconium after irrigations of acetylcysteine, an aproteolytic enzyme solution. The infant is assessed for cystic fibrosis, and management focuses on preventing complications of that disease if it is diagnosed.

Diagnostic tests for intestinal obstruction may relieve the meconium plug. The examiner's finger or the barium enema may force the expulsion of the meconium and pent-up gas. If the obstruction is not relieved, normal saline enemas (plain water enema should never be used, because it could lead to water intoxication), followed by an instillation of 5 mL of acetylcysteine solution, usually stimulate the expulsion of the meconium obstruction. Neonates with meconium plug syndrome are otherwise normal. To verify the accuracy of the diagnosis, neonates are observed for a time (days or months) to rule out Hirschsprung's disease, hypothyroidism, or cystic fibrosis.

NURSING MANAGEMENT

A complete nursing history with a record of day-by-day observation is invaluable in identifying symptomatology that can lead to an early definitive diagnosis and appropriate intervention.

In addition to recognizing symptomatology described in the preceding pages, the nurse needs to know how to pass an orogastric tube for aspiration; how to assess vomitus, stooling, and stools; and how to evaluate for abdominal distention.

Assessment of vomiting and vomitus. The following is noted about the vomiting:

1. Time in relation to the beginning or completion of the feeding.
2. Type:
   a. Regurgitation, or "spitting up," is usually a non-forceful "spilling out" of fluid unaccompanied by abdominal contractions. Overfeeding or inadequate burping is the probable cause.
   b. Nonprojectile vomiting is that which is mildly ejected and is often accompanied by abdominal contractions.
   c. Projectile vomiting is a forceful ejection of vomitus up to a distance of 5 feet. Pyloric stenosis or brain injury may be the underlying cause.

The nature of the vomitus is identified as follows:

1. Unchanged formula: formula that is unchanged by gastric juices and that usually occurs shortly after the feeding is started. Esophageal atresia is suspected.
2. Curdled milk: formula has been modified by gastric juices. Pyloric stenosis is suspected.
3. Greenish color: bile (turns green on exposure to air) in vomitus. Although this may be nonpathologic in nature, intestinal obstruction below the duodenum is probable.
4. Fecal contamination: obstruction of the lower gastrointestinal tract is suspected.
5. Bloody: one nonpathologic cause is swallowing of blood during birthing. Pathologic causes include a bleeding ulcer.

Assessment of stooling and stools. The following is noted:

1. Passage or lack of passage of meconium. One or two small stools can be passed even in the presence of obstruction (meconium plug).
2. Appearance of meconium:
   a. Light-colored (acholic) due to absence of bile in intestine.
   b. Inspissated (firm, thick) usually because of lack of the pancreatic enzyme trypsin.
3. Appearance of stool:
   a. Bloody. If unaccompanied by pain, may be due to a Meckel's diverticulum, a rectal polyp, or necrotizing enterocolitis.
   b. Bloody diarrhea—may be due to ulcerative colitis.
   c. Presence of mucus.
4. Pain. (Infant draws legs up to abdomen, paroxysmal bouts of crying, demonstrates facial grimaces and clenches fists.)
5. Constipation. If severe, it is accompanied by lower abdominal pain and tenderness, and the child may display anxiety and apprehension. Constipation may be due to Hirschsprung's disease.

Evaluation of abdominal distention. The location of the distention is determined:

1. Abdominal distention. Visible waves of peristalsis seen passing from left to right across the epigastrium and distention high in the abdomen indicate that the obstruction is at the level of the duodenum.
2. Marked generalized abdominal distention is commonly associated with lower intestinal tract obstruction.
3. Distention may be accompanied by respiratory distress as the diaphragm is forced upward.

Nursing priorities include identifying symptoms of intestinal obstruction prior to onset of complications (respiratory distress, fluid and electrolyte imbalance, damage to intestinal tract or other signs of toxicity), preventing postoperative complications (or the early treatment of complications to prevent untoward sequelae), and assisting the parents to cope with the situation.

INFANT WITH GENITOURINARY DEFECT

Exstrophy of the Bladder

Failure of the anterior abdominal wall and symphysis pubis to unite results in the exposure of the posterior and lateral walls of the bladder and trigone. This anomaly of unknown etiology may be accompanied by other defects of the intestinal tract and genital system. The folds of deep-red exposed bladder mucosa are sensitive when touched and are susceptible to ulceration. Urine seeps directly out over the skin, causing excoriation.

The exposed bladder mucosa with continual seepage of urine is evident at birth. Frequently associated malformations include undescended testes, inguinal hernia, vaginal agenesis, epispadias, short penis, and cleft labia (in females). When older, the child demonstrates a waddling or unsteady gait.

The objectives of treatment are continuing adequate renal function, preventing infections, and cosmetic reconstruction as needed to improve the child's appearance and meet physiologic needs. Cosmetic reconstruction is particularly important for the male child with abnormalities of the penis. Early treatment consists of collecting urine and protecting the bladder mucosa from the seeping urine with a prosthesis applied to the surrounding skin. Several weeks or months later surgery is performed. Minor defects may be corrected completely, and the infant will void normally. Major defects may require complete removal of the bladder tissue, transplantation of ureters into the colon, and plastic repair of the abdominal wall. Bladder reconstruction has been limited in its success, and treatment of choice is urinary diversion. Urinary diversion, such as ureterosigmoidostomy with antireflux urethral anastomosis is usually performed at 15–18 months of age. If chronic urethral reflux symptoms are present, this procedure frees the child from an external appliance. Complications are hydroureters, hydronephrosis, and pyelonephritis. Surgery or braces may be needed for the pelvic deformity.

Nursing priorities include protecting the exposed bladder wall and skin surrounding it from infection, as well as the respiratory and gastrointestinal tracts; preventing emotional trauma to the infant; preventing postoperative complications; and assisting the parents to cope with the situation. Convalescent priorities include control of urination and the development of an acceptable gait.

Several nursing actions help to prevent infection and direct trauma to the bladder mucosa. These include propping the neonate on his or her side, covering the defect per physician's orders (sterile petrolatum gauze or a firm covering), changing diapers frequently, cleansing the surrounding area with each diaper change, and periodically exposing the area to the air. The surrounding skin may be protected by a thin layer of aluminum paste, karaya gum, or Maalox.

Should a urine specimen be needed, the infant can be held over a sterile basin to collect the drops of urine.

Because surgery is scheduled weeks or months later, the parents are taught to care for the defect. Parents are encouraged to hold, cuddle, and assist in their newborn's care as soon after birth as they possibly can. The nurse assists the parents to grieve for the birth of an infant with a defect and provides physical and verbal support while the parents view and accept the defect.

INFANT WITH DISTURBANCE OF LOCOMOTION

Many skeletal anomalies are apparent in the neonatal period, although others are not identified until months later, usually when the child begins to walk. Early recognition and treatment is necessary for successful correction.

Two of the most common skeletal malformations apparent in the neonatal period are clubfoot and congenital dysplasia of the hip. Other disturbances of locomotion are caused by spina bifida.

Talipes Equinovarus (Clubfoot)

PHYSIOLOGY AND PATHOPHYSIOLOGY

Talipes equinovarus (clubfoot) is the most serious and most common deformity of the foot. The fixed postural deformity typically is in a position of inversion (varus) and adduction of the heel and forefoot (the bottom of the foot faces the midline), marked plantar flexion (equinus) at the ankle, and shortening of the Achilles tendon (Figure 26–11,A). Passive correction is impossible because of the tightness of the affected structures. Genetic and environmental factors (intrauterine position) are implicated. This condition occurs in 1 of every 1000 births. Recurrence in a family with one affected child is from 1 in 35 to 1 in 10. Males are affected about twice as often as females. Unilateral clubfoot is slightly more common than bilateral.

About 5% of the cases of clubfoot are classified as

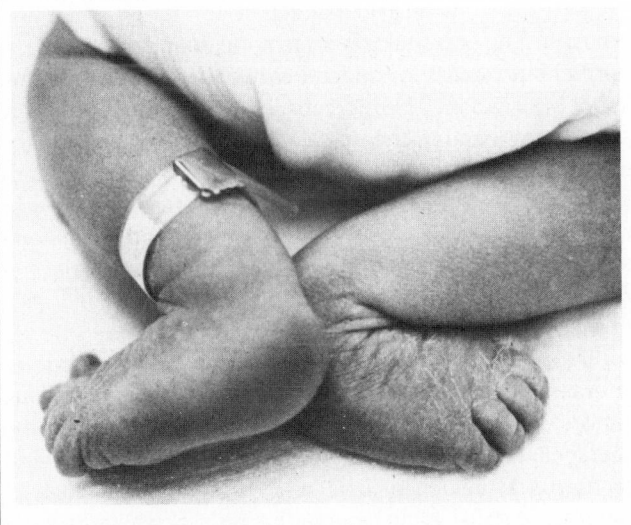
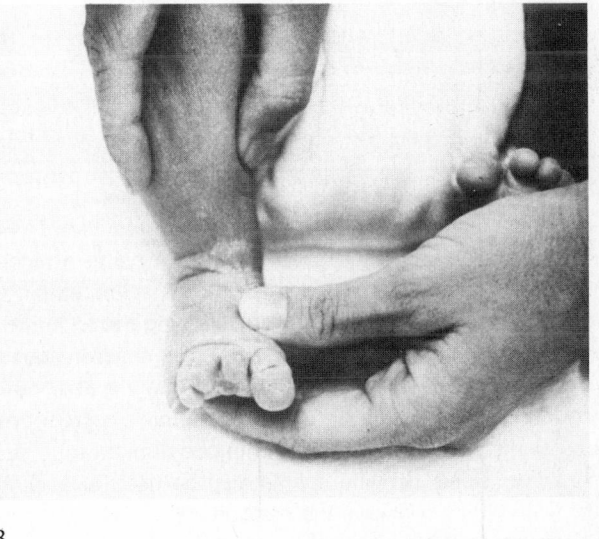

A
B

Figure 26–11 A, Bilateral talipes equinovarus seen with infant in supine position. **B,** To determine the presence of clubfoot, the nurse moves the foot to the midline. Resistance indicates true clubfoot.

talipes calcaneovalgus. The typical position is with the foot dorsiflexed (the heel turns outward and the anterior part of the foot is elevated on the outer border) and deviating laterally.

CLINICAL MANIFESTATIONS

The newborn has an obvious deformity of the foot, as just described. Calf size and degree of internal or external torsion of the tibia should be noted. In true fixed clubfoot, the calf on the affected side is smaller or atrophied; the foot lies in external torsion in relation to the knee; and the perineal muscles, stimulated by stroking the lateral side of the foot, demonstrate weakness and an inability to evert the foot. The Achilles tendon is always shortened, and the tibial tendons are contracted in proportion to the severity. When the newborn cries, the deformity is exaggerated, whereas a positional mobile "deformity" corrects itself when the newborn is crying or can be passively manipulated into correct position (Figure 26–11,B). The child must be examined for possible coexisting malformations, such as hip dysplasia, spina bifida, and meningomyelocele. Clubfoot associated with meningomyelocele is particularly resistant to correction because of the lack of nerve supply.

INTERVENTIONS

Intervention is aimed at correcting all elements of the deformity and at maintaining correction throughout the early growth years.

Plaster casts are applied in the neonatal period during the nursery stay, when the ligaments are still relaxed from maternal hormones. Depending on the severity of the deformity and physician reference, conservative methods are employed:

The *Kite method* of wedge casting is a gradual corrective measure that systematically, by means of plaster casts and wedges, deals with the different aspects of the deformity.

Manipulation and casting is the most common technique, using a series of corrective casts applied after forcible manipulation. Frequent changes of casts are required. The best results are achieved with weekly changes.

Denis Browne splints are used for infants under 1 year of age. The appliance is made of two foot plates attached to a crossbar. Feet are attached to the splint either by strapping with adhesive tape or by slipping the foot into a shoe already attached to the plates. After children start to walk, they are given special shoes with an elevated outer edge, thereby forcing them to walk in a more correct position. Denis Browne splints are continued at night for a year or longer. Denis Browne splints may be used in conjunction with other conservative methods, such as correction by casting; the splint is used to maintain correction. Lower leg braces with special shoes may be used when the child is walking. Correction by any of these methods may take up to 3 months.

Because clubfoot has a tendency to recur even following appropriate treatment, the affected child must be watched throughout childhood. Occasionally surgery may be required. Usual treatment involves lengthening of the Achilles tendon or Achilles tendon transfer, release of the medial ligaments, and ankle joint capsulotomy. Surgery on the bone (osteotomies) may be required for maximum correction in some children. Families can be referred to community agencies for financial support and to public health departments for continued moral support and supervision.

Nursing care of the child with talipes equinovarus is directed toward promoting parental acceptance of the child and the deformity and toward education of the parents regarding their infant's need for care. Care of an infant in a cast or splint is discussed, and symptoms of complications are reviewed. It is essential for a successful outcome that the parents recognize the long-term nature of the treatment program and be willing to cooperate fully.

PROGNOSIS

Repair is usually very good with proper treatment at an early age. The condition may recur later during childhood and will again require treatment. Exercises may be required for many years.

Dysplasia of the Hip

PHYSIOLOGY AND PATHOPHYSIOLOGY

Congenital dislocation of the hip in the neonatal period refers to a potential rather than a true dislocation. The term implies that the head of the femur is out of the acetabulum at birth, but this is not always true, and there are varying degrees of dysplasia of the hip joint.

Dysplasia refers to an inadequate formation of the acetabulum. The acetabulum and femoral head are potentially normal but remain in the fetal cartilaginous state with delay of ossification. The hip capsule, which ordinarily holds the femoral head in the acetabulum, is stretched, and the acetabulum is shallow and rimmed with cartilage instead of being deep and completely ossified. As a result of the capsule failure to hold the femoral head in the acetabulum, some degree of displacement occurs, and upward slant of the acetabulum roof and anteversion of the head and neck of the femur is increased.

This potentially crippling deformity is a result of an interaction between genetic influences and environmental factors such as insufficient femoral head pressure in the acetabulum during fetal life, position of the fetus in utero, or hormonal influence. It is seen four to seven times as often in females as in males (the female pelvis appears more affected by the maternal hormones, which relax maternal pelvic ligaments), involves the left hip three times more often than the right, occurs more frequently in breech presentations, and is twice as common unilaterally

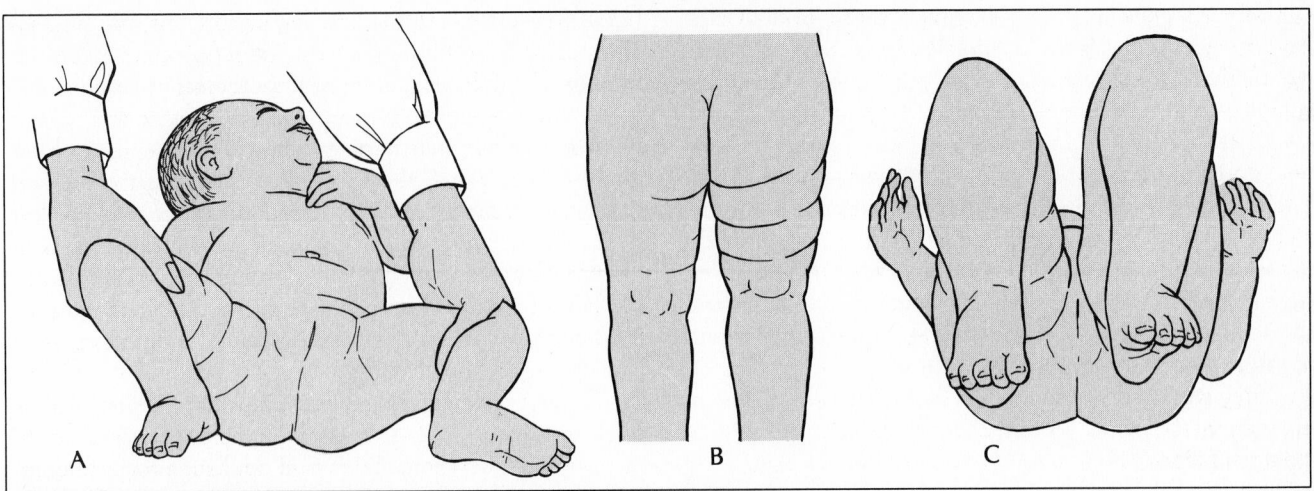

Figure 26–12 Early signs of congenital dislocation of the right hip. **A,** Limitation of abduction. **B,** Asymmetry of skin folds and prominence of trochanter. **C,** Shortening of femur. (Courtesy Ross Laboratories, Columbus, Ohio.)

as bilaterally. Early recognition and treatment is important so that the cartilaginous structures are not malformed through the muscle pull pressures and early weight bearing.

The depth of the acetabulum determines the degree of dislocation, and an infant can progress from the stage of dysplasia to subluxation to luxation or complete dislocation. *Subluxation* refers to a partial or incomplete dislocation (that is, the femoral head rides on the lateral third edge of the acetabulum, with partial displacement from the acetabulum and some degree of anteversion of the head of the femur). Subluxation is more common than dislocation but, if untreated, may result in complete dislocation. Early signs are limited abduction of the hip in a flexed position or a click sign while the hip is being abducted. Parents may note an inability to abduct the hip during diaper changes.

Luxation is present when the femoral head is completely dislocated above the acetabular rim. Anteversion of the femur is usually quite marked. It can occur during intrauterine life or can follow an untreated subluxation some time after birth. In either case, it demands early recognition, while it is possible to reduce the dislocation easily and to begin correction of the defect. Without treatment, the stretched capsule and ligaments become more rigid, the head of the femur may press a socket in the ileum above the acetabulum, and the hip abductor muscles may shorten. This development results in painful and basically untreatable crippling deformity in adulthood.

The incidence of dysplasia varies in different parts of the world. The highest incidence is among the Lapps and certain American Indian tribes, who swaddle babies for the first year of life. The next highest incidence (3 in 1000) occurs in Italy, France, and Japan. An incidence of 1 in

1000 exists in England and Sweden. Dysplasia is rarely seen among blacks.

CLINICAL MANIFESTATIONS

Upon examination, it is noted that folds on the dorsal gluteal and popliteal surfaces are asymmetrical and appear higher on the affected side. There is limited abduction of the leg at the hip on the affected side (under 60°). The greater trochanter on the affected side is prominent and elevated, and the perineum on the affected side is broadened (Figure 26–12). Marked bilateral broadening is seen if both hips are dislocated. Later, after the child has begun to bear weight, marked prominence of the greater trochanter and flattening of the buttock on the affected side can be seen. With a characteristic limp, the child lurches or sways to the affected side. The child may demonstrate lumbar lordosis and protuberant abdomen. In unilateral dislocation, there is marked shortening of the affected leg, possible functional scoliosis, and abduction and flexion contractures of the involved hip. The examiner may be unable to feel the femoral pulse over the head of the femur.

Several maneuvers assist in a definitive diagnosis:

Ortolani's maneuver. With the infant supine on a firm surface, flex hips to 90° and abduct fully; bend knees (Figure 26–12, A). As the hip is reduced during abduction, an audible click is produced by the head of the femur as it enters the acetabulum. Then, with forefinger on the greater trochanter and thumb on the lesser trochanter, adduct hip to elicit a palpable clunk. This maneuver is not always suitable in the neonatal period, because movement of the head of the femur out of the socket may be smooth and quiet or a luxated hip may not reduce and therefore not produce a click. It is best used to detect an already-dislocated hip.

Barlow's maneuver. This is a modification of the Ortolani's maneuver but is more suitable for the neonatal period and detects a potentially dislocated hip. With the infant supine on a firm surface, flex hips to 90° and flex the knee completely. With the forefingers on the greater trochanters, apply pressure posteriorly with thumbs on the lesser trochanters. The head of the femur will slip out of an unstable hip and slip back when thumb pressure is stopped.

Galeazzi's sign. With the infant supine, flex hips at right angles. Lowering of the knee length (due to apparent shortening of the thigh when the head of the femur is out of the socket) is a positive sign.

X-ray studies of the pelvis and hips are of little value in the neonatal period but may be diagnostic after 4–5 months of age.

DIFFERENTIAL DIAGNOSIS

The limited abduction characteristic of hip dysplasia is also seen in cases of voluntary resistance, spina bifida due to weak hip abductors and adduction contracture, hip joint infection, Still's disease, rickets, cerebral palsy with spastic paralysis (which causes a stretch reflex in the abductors that limits reduction), and polio. Developmental coxa vera with deformity of the femoral neck presents a clinical picture similar to congenital dysplasia but is unusual before the age of 4 years.

INTERVENTIONS

Early recognition and treatment are imperative to the successful correction of the abnormality. The longer the condition goes unrecognized, the more severe the anomaly becomes, the more difficult the treatment, and the less favorable the prognosis. The regimen depends on the age of the child and the severity of the dysplasia. The goal is prevention of dislocation and promotion of normal hip joint formation by maintaining the femoral head within the acetabulum.

Medical management of the neonate consists of reducing the head of the femur into the acetabulum and maintaining it there. A stable position of hip flexion, abduction, and external rotation is achieved by the use of appliances such as the Frejka pillow splint, orthopedic splint, or three or four diapers used at a time. The Frejka pillow splint is applied over diapers and is reapplied with each diaper change. The infant's parents or caretakers must be careful to maintain the desired position. Maintaining the hips in forced abduction or keeping them rigidly immobile can cause avascular necrosis of the femur head, both in the affected and the nonaffected hip. Some physicians (Hirsch et al., 1980) prefer to use the Pavlik harness because it avoids extreme abduction, emphasizes flexion at the hips, and permits movement of the hip joint within a limited range. The Pavlik appliance consists of shoulder harness and straps that fasten around the legs so they hold the hip and knee joints in flexion. For about 75% of infants, the

hip will revert to normal in a few weeks, but the harness should be continuously used for approximately 2–3 months and then only at night until the hip is stable.

A very unstable hip may necessitate reduction by manipulation under anesthesia and use of a hip spica cast for about a month until the capsule tightens and the femoral head pressure stimulates the development of an adequate acetabulum. Immobilization may be as long as 6–9 months, depending on hip joint development as seen on X-ray film. If treatment is begun after the first few months, traction, followed by open reduction and a hip spica cast, is used.

As with talipes equinovarus, nursing responsibilities for hip dysplasia focus on early detection, facilitation of parent–infant bonding, and parent education regarding the treatment plan. Infants in appliances or casts must have their emotional needs satisfied—the infant needs to be held and cuddled and may be allowed to sit in a high chair.

PROGNOSIS

With early and adequate treatment, adequate hip stability and movement can be achieved. When treatment is delayed for several months or even years, crippling can be anticipated despite surgical intervention.

Spina Bifida: Failure of Closure of the Neural Axis

PHYSIOLOGY AND PATHOPHYSIOLOGY

Malformations in the closure of the spinal canal are termed *spina bifida*. Defects range from a small slit in the vertebras to the absence of several spinous processes and laminae as a result of failure of the neural tube to close at around the fourth month of gestation (Figure 26–13). Three of the most common defects are spina bifida occulta, meningocele, and meningomyelocele.

Spina bifida occulta, nonclosure of the posterior arches of the spine, is found at lumbar 5 in about 30% of the normal population and is of no consequence. This defect becomes of clinical significance when its presence is associated with underlying abnormalities that may be suspected by the presence of a dimple, a tuft of hair, a hemangioma, or a lipoma in the lumbosacral area.

Meningocele is a cystic outpouching of the meninges through the spina bifida without associated abnormalities of the spinal cord and nerve roots.

Meningomyelocele is a cystic herniation of meninges that also contains spinal cord and nerve roots. There is a neurologic deficit below the level of this lesion. The lower the level (lumbar 5 to sacral 1), the greater the probability of functional ambulation, although braces may be required.

Meningomyelocele and meningocele usually communicate with the subarachnoid space and therefore contain

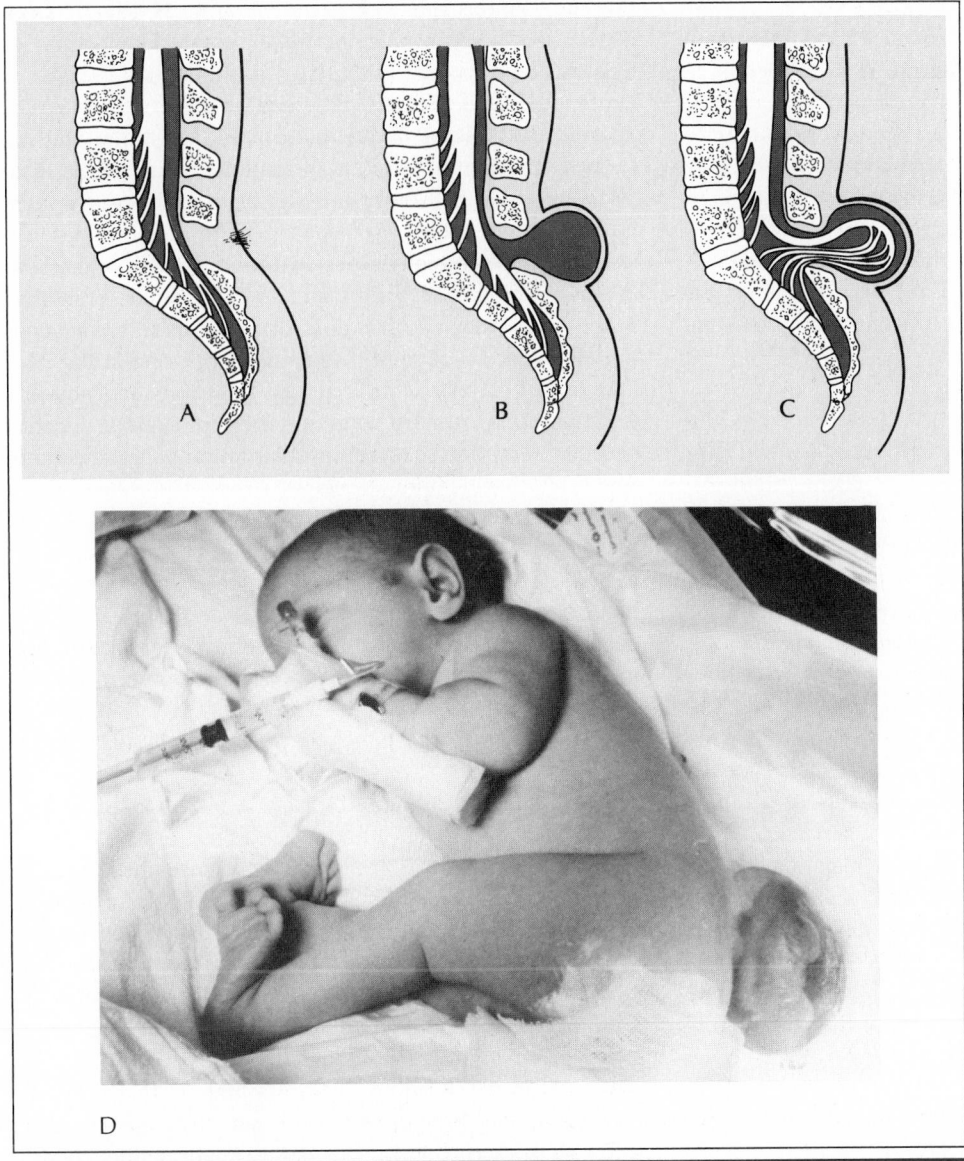

Figure 26–13 Midsagittal view of spinal column with various degrees of neural defect. **A,** Spina bifida occulta. Note posterior vertebral arches have not fused. There is no herniation of cord or meninges. **B,** Meningocele. Meninges protrude through the spina bifida forming a saclike cyst visible on the infant's back. **C,** Meningomyelocele. Meninges, elements of the cord with its nerves, and spinal fluid protrude through the spina bifida. This defect resembles a meningocele externally. **D,** Infant with lumbar myelomeningocele. (Courtesy Dr. Paul Winchester.)

cerebrospinal fluid. The pressure of the fluid enlarges the cystic sac and may cause it to rupture. This direct access to cerebrospinal fluid may predispose to meningitis.

The Arnold-Chiari lesion is frequently associated with spinal malformation such as meningomyelocele. It occurs in varying degrees of abnormality, the most serious of which is the downward displacement of the tonsils of cerebellum through the foramen magnum and the downward displacement and folding over of the medulla oblongata and fourth ventricle onto the cervical spinal cord, causing a noncommunicating type of hydrocephalus. Etiology is unknown, but it is *not* due to traction on the cord, as was first assumed. Symptoms may be absent in early life or may be expressed in the neonatal period as lower cranial nerve palsies or vocal cord paralysis. Surgical repair of the meningomyelocele may result in symptoms by compressing the

medulla and tonsils into the foramen magnum, unless ventricular drainage is also established.

Between 1 and 3 live births per 1000 have spina bifida. The lesion is more common in females but tends to be more severe in males. Spina bifida is seen more frequently in the firstborn and beyond the sixth pregnancy. It occurs with greater frequency in white populations.

At present no direct hereditary pattern has been identified, but a family who has had an infant with spina bifida faces increased risk of having a subsequent infant with an anomaly of the CNS. Families should be referred to centers for counseling regarding future pregnancies. Anomalies involving neural tube failures can be detected as early as the sixteenth or eighteenth week of intrauterine life. Because of the thinness of tissue or lack of membranes covering the spinal canal, α-fetoproteins from fetal cerebral spinal fluid escape into the amniotic fluid and are absorbed into the mother's blood stream. Pregnant women can be screened for elevation of serum α-fetoprotein concentration. The test is not definitive but serves as a referral for amniocentesis or ultrasonography. Approximately 80% of fetuses with open spina bifida can be detected by either ultrasonography or by elevation of the amniotic fluid α-fetoprotein concentration (Applegarth et al., 1978). This finding allows the physician to arrange for a cesarean birth for the baby, with less trauma to the delicate meningeal sac, or termination of the pregnancy when the parents select this alternative.

CLINICAL MANIFESTATIONS

Spina bifida occulta is asymptomatic in most cases. If the defect is associated with underlying abnormalities, the area is identifiable by the presence of a dimple, tuft of hair, hemangioma, or lipoma. Occasionally spina bifida is diagnosed in early childhood by disorders of sphincter control or muscular weakness in the lower extremities.

Meningocele is seen as a cystic outpouching in the midline over the spine. The skin may be defective as well, so that the sac is covered with a transparent fragile membrane containing the meninges. Because spinal cord or nerve roots are not involved, muscles are usually not affected. The sac may enlarge from the pressure of cerebrospinal fluid and rupture if the defect is not surgically treated. Hydrocephalus may be coincident or may occur after surgical repair of the sac. *Hydrocephalus* refers to the abnormal increase of cerebrospinal fluid in the cranial vault. It may result from obstruction of flow, faulty reabsorption, or increased production. Symptoms include enlargement of the head, "sunset" eyes, weakness, irritability, brain atrophy and retardation, and convulsions.

Meningomyelocele is also seen as a cystic outpouching in the midline, usually over the lumbosacral spine. Because

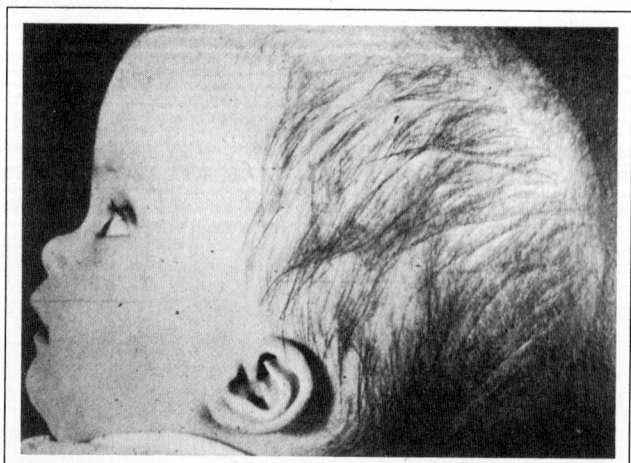

Figure 26–14 Hydrocephaly. Note enlarged occiput area and lateral view of the sunset eyes.

this sac contains spinal cord and nerve roots, several associated neurologic problems are apparent. The degree of dysfunction depends on the level of the lesion. Lesions of lumbar 3–5 and sacral 1–3 sympathetic nerve may result in musculoskeletal malformation and dysfunction (deformed feet, immobile joints of the lower extremities, flaccid paralysis of the lower extremities); proprioceptive dysfunction, and absence of sensation to the level of the lesion; or autonomic nervous system dysfunction (inability to sweat, dry and cool skin, and so on). Lesions at lumbar 1 and below may result in loss of bowel and bladder control (constant seepage of urine); stasis of urine in the malfunctioning bladder with recurrent infections and possible eventual upper urinary tract and kidney damage; incontinence or retention of feces; or obstruction of cerebrospinal fluid flow, causing hydrocephalus. Arnold-Chiari malformation may be associated with the hydrocephaly.

Surgical exposure and exploration of the lesion reveals the existence and extent of the underlying abnormality. Electromyographs identify the extent and degree of muscular denervation. Careful sensory and motor testing during early infancy predicts with a high degree of reliability the prognosis and effects of therapy.

INTERVENTIONS

There is usually no therapy for spina bifida occulta unless neurologic abnormalities appear and progress.

Meningocele is surgically corrected, usually by a fairly simple procedure within 24 hours after birth to prevent meningitis if the sac ruptures. Following surgery, the infant usually shows no neurologic deficit. However, the infant must be observed for the development of hydrocephaly.

Surgical correction of meningomyelocele is complex and difficult and often requires several procedures. Surgery is performed within 24 hours after birth to prevent continuing deterioration of nerves and to prevent infection if the sac should rupture. Coexisting abnormalities (hydrocephalus, clubfoot) must also be repaired. In addition to closure of the defect after reinserting nerve tissue, several other surgeries may be needed. These include: (a) shunting (and repetitive shunting if a high meningomyelocele exists) for hydrocephalus in 60%–75% of cases (Figure 26–14); (b) an ileal loop for urologic complications in 90% of cases; and (c) possible transplanting of muscles and tendons and casting along with braces for the orthopedic defects. Frequently, the skin above the repaired defect breaks down, necessitating further treatment and perhaps therapy for meningitis as well. About 30% of live-born infants survive past the first 2 years of life. The family is referred to support groups and social services.

A plan of care for the years succeeding the early surgical repair of the herniated sac focuses on emotional development, education, control of urinary and orthopedic complications, and physical therapy.

Preoperative nursing intervention is directed to protection of the sac, careful assessment of the infant's status and functioning, and parental support. Postoperative intervention includes careful monitoring of vital functions, observation for the development of hydrocephalus and other complications, and supportive care measures. In addition, it is vital to assist the parents in dealing with the long-term implications of this disorder and their child's rehabilitation needs. (See the Nursing Care Plan on meningocele/meningomyelocele.)

With other members of the health team, the nurse teaches parents how to provide physical care. Parents learn safe methods of holding, turning, positioning, and giving passive exercise. Techniques of feeding do not differ significantly for these infants, except that it is more difficult to burp them. Care of elimination is more complex. Parents are taught the Credé method of emptying the bladder or care of an ileostomy or indwelling catheter, if one is present. Glycerin suppositories or enemas may be needed to prevent impaction of feces. Parents are assisted in putting the child on a regular routine for bowel emptying as soon as possible. The nurse can be instrumental in developing a bowel and bladder program with the parents of the child with a meningomyelocele.

CONGENITAL HEART DEFECTS

The incidence of congenital heart defects is 2.2 per 1000 live births; they account for 33% of deaths caused by all types of congenital defects in the first year of life. Because accurate diagnosis and surgical treatment are now available, many such deaths can be prevented. Thus, it is crucial for the nurse to have comprehensive knowledge of congenital heart disease to detect deviations from normal and to initiate nursing interventions.

Overview of Congenital Heart Defects

Congenital cardiac malformations are the result of failure of the gene-directed developmental phenomenon to time each growth process at exactly the right moment for all structures to form accurately. Factors that might influence this phenomenon can be classified as environmental or genetic. Viruses, such as rubella and Coxsackie B, that affect the mother during pregnancy have been implicated. Thalidomide, and more recently, some anticonvulsants, have been shown to cause congenital malformations of the heart. Infants born with chromosomal abnormalities have a higher incidence of cardiovascular anomalies. Infants with Down syndrome and trisomy 13/15 and 16/18 frequently have heart lesions. Increased incidence and risk of recurrence of specific defects occur in families.

At the time of birth, marked changes occur in the cardiovascular system. (See p. 640 for review discussion of circulatory changes that normally occur at birth and normal heartbeat in infants.) Certain anatomic or physiologic factors in the cardiovascular system may interfere with normal circulation changes.

It is customary to divide congenital malformations of the heart into *acyanotic*—those that do not present with cyanosis—and *cyanotic*—those that do present with cyanosis. Normally, if an opening exists between the right and left sides of the heart, blood will flow from the area of greater pressure (left side) to the area of lesser pressure (right side). This process is referred to as left-to-right shunt and does not produce cyanosis because oxygenated blood is being pumped out to the systemic circulation. If pressure in the right side of the heart, due to obstruction of normal flow, exceeds that in the left side, unoxygenated blood will flow from the right side to the left side of the heart and out into the system, producing a right-to-left shunt and resulting in cyanosis. If the opening is large, there may be a bidirectional shunt with mixing of blood in both sides of the heart, also producing cyanosis.

General signs and symptoms of heart defects in infants are as follows: dyspnea, difficulty in feeding, stridor or choking spells, pulse rate over 200, recurrent respiratory infections, failure to gain weight, heart murmurs, cyanosis, cerebral vascular accidents, and anoxic attacks.

The three most common ways in which infants with congenital cardiac abnormalities first manifest their problem are cyanosis, detectable heart murmur, or congestive heart failure (a frequent sequela).

Acyanotic Lesions

Acyanotic congenital defects include patent ductus arteriosus, atrial septal defects, ventricular septal defects, endocardial cushion defects, coarctation of the aorta, and aortic stenosis.

PATENT DUCTUS ARTERIOSUS

Patent ductus arteriosus is an abnormal persistence of the fetal connection between the aorta and the pulmonary artery (Figure 26–15, p. 887). Increased incidence is noted in females, in certain families, after maternal rubella during the first trimester of pregnancy, in infants born at high altitudes, and especially in preterm infants. RDS with hypoxemia can cause persistent patency of the ductus arteriosus because of lowered oxygen saturation of blood shunted through the ductus and decreased pressure in the lungs.

About 15% of preterm infants weighing less than 1750 g and 40%–50% of preterm infants weighing less than 1500 g have persistent patent ductus arteriosus (Kaplan et al., 1978). Many preterm infants with symptomatic patent ductus arteriosus can be treated medically with maintenance of adequate hematocrit values, oxygen therapy, flu-

NURSING CARE PLAN
Meningocele/Meningomyelocele

PATIENT DATA BASE

History

Course of pregnancy and birth

Neonate's condition at birth and apparent malformations noted at birth

Assessment of neonate's anatomic appearance and physiologic functioning as described under clinical picture

Parental reactions and any teaching accomplished with parents

Physical examination

Round bulging sac on neonate's back

No response or varying response to sensation below the level of the sac

Spontaneous movement below defect is absent or minimal

May have constant dribbling of urine

Incontinence or retention of stool; anal opening may be flaccid

May develop hydrocephalus

NURSING PRIORITIES

1. Assess each neonate's anatomic and physiologic functioning to assist in identification of lesions
2. Protect herniated meningeal sac from drying and rupture
3. Protect newborn with meningomyelocele from trauma to body below lesion
4. Assess for hydrocephalus
5. Protect infant from psychologic trauma
6. Assist parents in coping with situation

FAMILY EDUCATIONAL FOCUS

1. Explain treatment modalities and their rationale
2. Discuss with parents possible long-term implications of meningomyelocele, such as development of hydrocephalus, need for hip surgery, and bladder and bowel management
3. Discussion of growth and development needs of their infant throughout the possible repeated hospitalizations
4. Provide opportunities for parents to discuss questions and concerns regarding their neonate
5. Provide for support of parents through referrals to available resources and support groups

Problem	Nursing interventions and actions	Rationale
Preoperative care: Protection of sac from drying, rupture, and infection	Position neonate on abdomen or prop on side very carefully; restrain if necessary (some hospitals use Bradford frame)	Avoids pressure and direct trauma
	Avoid touching sac with diaper, if one is used	Avoids pressure and direct trauma
	Scrupulously cleanse and dry buttocks and genitals frequently; use meningocele apron; position apron below the defect	Avoids contamination of sac from constantly dripping urine and feces and therefore decreases possibility of infection (meningitis)
	If ordered, cover defect with plastic, sterile dressing, sterile petrolatum gauze, or doughnut-shaped appliance with gauze covering (some physicians order Varidase dripped onto sac)	Prevents urine/fecal contamination

Keeps sac moist; prevents drying and cracking |
| | Observe sac for oozing of fluid or pus | Indicates rupture or infection |
| | Provide passive exercises to joints in lower extremities as ordered by physician | Prevents deformity |
| Development of hydrocephalus | Measure along suboccipital bregmatic line on admission to nursery | Provides baseline measurement of neonatal head

This may be inaccurate during the first 24 hr due to molding |
	Measure chest circumference at nipple line	Chest normally equals or is slightly smaller than head circumference
	Check fontanelle with newborn in upright position for bulging and separation of suture lines	Tenseness indicates possible increase in intracranial pressure
	Assess for change in behavior, irritability	May indicate increased intracranial pressure

NURSING CARE PLAN Cont'd
Meningocele/Meningomyelocele

Problem	Nursing interventions and actions	Rationale
Prevention of trauma to neonate's body below lesion	Evaluate urological function—note constant or intermittent dripping Does urine have good stream? If constant dripping exists, use Credé method of emptying bladder; that is, press gently but firmly starting at umbilical area, downward and under symphysis pubis toward anus, every 2 hr during day and at least once per night	Prevents stasis, which can lead to infection and damage to renal system
	Teach parents this method of evaluating anal sphincter functioning. Is there a dimple? Does it constrict to the touch—"wink"?	Determines degree of innervation to area and degree of possible incontinence
	Support parts of body with rubber pads or cloth rolls; change position from abdomen to side every 2 hr; provide passive exercises to joints in lower extremities as ordered by physician	Prevents pressure areas Prevents pressure areas and hypostatic pneumonia Prevents deformity
Postoperative care: Development of hydrocephalus	Assess frequently vital signs, color, tension of fontanelle, neurologic status, behavior (high-pitched cry, irritability or lethargy, vomiting); measure head circumference once per day	Facilitates early diagnosis and treatment of postoperative complications. Indicates increased intracranial pressure
	Raise foot of newborn's bed for first few hours	Lessens pressure of spinal fluid at site of defect and maintains pressure of cerebrospinal fluid in brain
	Change position from abdomen to side frequently	Prevents hypostatic pneumonia
	Assess for and report abdominal distention and symptoms of respiratory distress	Paralytic ileus and distention of bladder follow spinal cord surgery and embarrass respiration by upward pressure on diaphragm
Protection of surgical site from trauma and infection	Position on abdomen or prop on side	Prevents pressure and direct trauma
	Observe for signs of local infection: redness, warmth	Early treatment may prevent breakdown of skin repair
	Provide scrupulous skin care as previously described under preoperative care	Prevents contamination of operative site and prevents excoriation and infection of surrounding skin areas
Prevention of trauma to other parts of body	Same as for preoperative care	See discussion of preoperative care
Prevention of emotional trauma to neonate	In addition to content under preoperative care: 1. Hang colorful mobile or place toy where neonate can view it 2. Put musical toy in crib 3. Talk or sing to neonate while providing care	Provides visual and auditory stimulation
	4. Respond to crying by attending infant, stroking, holding, talking, or feeding	Facilitates development of parent–infant bonding
Parents' ability to cope with situation	In addition to content discussed previously: 1. Refer to community agencies: community public health, birth defect clinics with a multidisciplinary staff, physical and occupational therapy, parent groups who share the same problem	Assists with financial, emotional, and rehabilitation burden

NURSING CARE PLAN Cont'd
Meningocele/Meningomyelocele

Problem	Nursing interventions and actions	Rationale
	2. If parents are considering admitting infant to special care facility or placing for adoption, encourage expression of feelings about this; refer to social service; do not pass judgment on parents	After parents are presented with all possible alternatives other than surgical care of defect, final decision must be parents'; support parents' right to make own decision
	3. Reinforce, clarify physician's explanations of repair and prognosis	Under stress, people have difficulty hearing what is said; repetition is also needed as people work to incorporate information and its meaning for them
	4. Encourage parents to participate in infant's care; teach in small doses; stand close by as parent attempts infant's care; praise where appropriate	Facilitates development of more positive relationship with the infant; provides opportunity to see where infant is normal; builds feelings of self-worth and self-esteem, and helps parents feel less overwhelmed
	5. Prepare parents for future therapy; teach them how to check anterior fontanelle and head circumference and when to report findings	Assists parents by encouraging "grief work" and planning for rest of family as well as for affected child; assures early identification of hydrocephalus

NURSING CARE EVALUATION

All lesions are identified and appropriate treatment is instituted	Hydrocephalus is diagnosed and treated immediately if it develops
Prior to surgery, herniated sac does not rupture and does not become infected	Parents are able to come to acceptable decision regarding infant's acceptance within home or placement outside of home; parents learn to provide physical and emotional care for infant; needs of all family members are met and each has opportunity to develop to full potential
Infant's bowel and bladder function is maintained without complications and acceptable degree of ambulation is achieved	

NURSING DIAGNOSES*	SUPPORTING DATA
1. Potential for injury	Herniated meningeal sac must be protected from drying, rupture, or infection Risk of trauma to body below lesion Development of hydrocephalus Postsurgical trauma or infection (See Nursing Care Plan for details about each of these)
2. Impaired physical mobility in infant with meningomyelocele related to loss of neurologic innervation below lesion	Pressure areas Alterations in bladder and bowel elimination Joint deformities in lower extremities
3. Family coping: potential for growth associated with crisis of having infant with congenital defect	Parents and family members experience normal grief process Make plans for care of infant after discharge from hospital Provide appropriate tactile, visual, and auditory stimulation for infant Exhibit positive parenting behaviors

*These are a few examples of nursing diagnoses that may be appropriate for an infant with this condition. It is not an inclusive list and must be individualized for each infant.

id restrictions, and administration of digoxin and diuretics. Some preterm infants require early surgical ligation or pharmacologic closure of their patent ductus arteriosus.

The hemodynamics consist of a left-to-right shunting of oxygenated blood from the high-pressure system of the aorta to the lower-pressure system of the pulmonary artery. The blood is recirculated through the lungs, with eventual overloading of the left ventricle due to increased output and work load in an effort to maintain systemic circulation.

The infant with this problem is usually asymptomatic except for some impairment in growth. They tend to be small, slender, short, and susceptible to frequent upper respiratory infections. The condition is often discovered on careful auscultation. At the upper left sternal border, just beneath the left clavicle, the typical continuous murmur can be heard. It is called a machinery-type murmur and is heard throughout both systole and diastole. The infant may also show a great difference between systolic and diastolic blood pressures. This wide pulse difference is due to a low diastolic pressure, because the shunting of blood reduces peripheral resistance.

X-ray and echocardiogram findings are often normal when shunting is of a small amount. Radiographs or echocardiograms of hearts with larger shunts show left ventricular and left atrial enlargement, a dilated ascending aorta, a prominent pulmonary artery, and increased pulmonary vascularity with the increased blood flow to the lungs.

Echocardiography is a safe, noninvasive diagnostic procedure frequently used to obtain information about internal cardiac anatomy. It provides recordings of the motion of the mitral, aortic, tricuspid, and pulmonic valves, the interventricular septum and the right and left ventricular septum, and the right and left ventricular walls. It also reveals the size of the cardiac chambers and the changes of these dimensions during the cardiac cycle. Such information is valuable for diagnosing congenital heart defects or for determining the need for a cardiac catheterization. Cardiac catheterization is not necessary for diagnosis, but may be performed to rule out associated defects.

Successful constriction of the patent ductus with drugs that inhibit prostaglandin synthesis (for example, indomethacin) was first reported in 1976. Subsequent results reported in the literature show a wide range of success and failure (Friedman et al., 1980). Indomethacin is administered through an orogastric tube at a dose of 0.2 mg/kg of body weight. If closure does not occur, a second dose is administered in 12–24 hours. Potentially dangerous side effects are transient marked oliguria, gastrointestinal bleeding, or increased bilirubin levels.

Surgical ligation of the patent ductus arteriosus is the preferred treatment, especially for respirator-dependent preterm infants (O'Loughlin, 1981). This major surgery involves opening the chest, but does not require the use of a heart-lung machine. Surgery is usually done after 1 year of age unless the infant develops complications earlier.

ATRIAL SEPTAL DEFECTS

An *atrial septal defect* is an abnormal opening in the atrial septum. It is more common in females and occurs frequently in Down syndrome. Atrial septal defects are of three types. The major type of defect is within the area of the foramen ovale. Patency is caused by a short valve, a perforated valve, or an enlarged opening at the valve site. A defect high in the atrial septum, called *ostium secundum,* is less common and results from failure of the septum to develop completely. It can exist as one large or several small openings. The third type, called *ostium primum,* is caused by failure of the correct fusion of the atrial septum, the ventricular septum, and the endocardial cushions (see Figure 26–15). It is uncommon and more complicated, usually involving the mitral and tricuspid valves.

Left-to-right shunt with recirculation of oxygenated blood through the lungs produces abnormally high pulmonary blood flow. Eventually right heart failure occurs due to sustained overload. Atrial septal defects are often not detected in early infancy, because the murmur of a minimal left-to-right shunting of blood is scarcely detectable. As pressure differences become greater, the shunt becomes larger and a systolic murmur becomes audible over the second left intercostal space. With very large shunts, a diastolic rumbling murmur is present at the lower left sternal border.

The infant with a small atrial septal defect may be asymptomatic. If the defect is large, infants have frequent respiratory infections, demonstrate failure to thrive, a poor exercise tolerance, a thin build (due to abnormally high pulmonary blood flow), and poor tissue perfusion. They have episodes of congestive heart failure.

Prevention of infection and aggressive treatment with antibiotics when infections develop is essential. Open-heart surgery with the help of the heart-lung machine is required to repair atrial septal defect.

VENTRICULAR SEPTAL DEFECTS

A *ventricular septal defect* is an abnormal opening in the ventricular septum (see Figure 26–15). It is the most common congenital cardiovascular anomaly and occurs more frequently in males than in females. The abnormal opening is usually located in the membranous portion of the septum but occasionally occurs in the muscular portion of the ventricular septum. The smallest defects, called *maladie de Roger,* are associated with a minor left-to-right shunting of blood through the opening in the ventricular septum. The pressure in the right ventricle is not markedly increased and stays within normal range. At birth, pressures in the right and left ventricles are almost equal, so very little shunting occurs for the first few weeks of life.

These infants are asymptomatic, but by the end of the first month of life, a loud, blowing systolic murmur can be heard in the third and fourth left interspace. X-ray films and echocardiograms usually show the heart to be of nor-

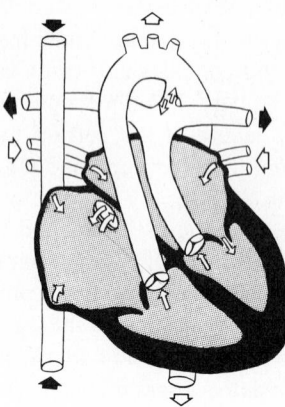

Complete Transposition of Great Vessels

This anomaly is an embryologic defect caused by a straight division of the bulbar trunk without normal spiraling. As a result, the aorta originates from the right ventricle, and the pulmonary artery from the left ventricle. An abnormal communication between the two circulations must be present to sustain life.

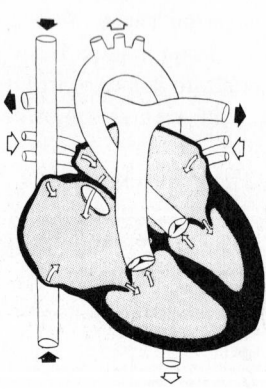

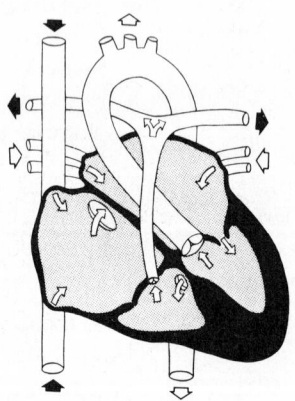

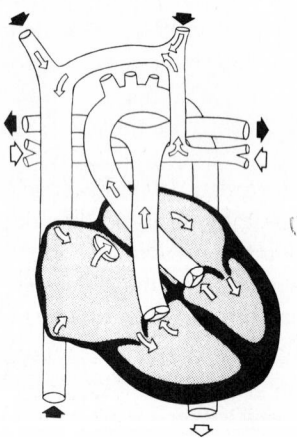

Atrial Septal Defects

An atrial septal defect is an abnormal opening between the right and left atria. Basically, three types of abnormalities result from incorrect development of the atrial septum. An incompetent foramen ovale is the most common defect. The high ostium secundum defect results from abnormal development of the septum secundum. Improper development of the septum primum produces a basal opening known as an ostium primum defect, frequently involving the atrio-ventricular valves. In general, left to right shunting of blood occurs in all atrial septal defects.

Tricuspid Atresia

Tricuspid valvular atresia is characterized by a small right ventricle, large left ventricle and usually a diminished pulmonary circulation. Blood from the right atrium passes through an atrial septal defect into the left atrium, mixes with oxygenated blood returning from the lungs, flows into the left ventricle and is propelled into the systemic circulation. The lungs may receive blood through one of three routes: 1) a small ventricular septal defect 2) patent ductus arteriosus 3) bronchial vessels.

Anomalous Venous Return

Oxygenated blood returning from the lungs is carried abnormally to the right heart by one or more pulmonary veins emptying directly, or indirectly through venous channels, into the right atrium. Partial anomalous return of the pulmonary veins to the right atrium functions the same as an atrial septal defect. In complete anomalous return of the pulmonary veins, an interatrial communication is necessary for survival.

Figure 26–15 Congenital heart abnormalities. (From Congenital heart abnormalities. Clinical Education Aid no. 7. Ross Laboratories, Columbus, Ohio.)

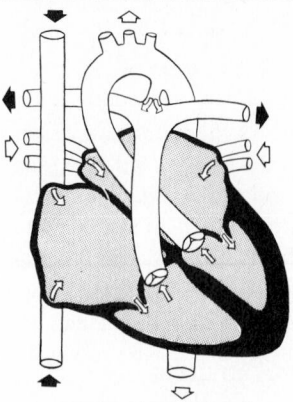

Patent Ductus Arteriosus

The patent ductus arteriosus is a vascular connection that, during fetal life, short circuits the pulmonary vascular bed and directs blood from the pulmonary artery to the aorta. Functional closure of the ductus normally occurs soon after birth. If the ductus remains patent after birth, the direction of blood flow in the ductus is reversed by the higher pressure in the aorta.

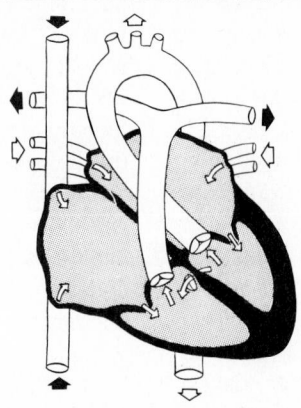

Ventricular Septal Defects

A ventricular septal defect is an abnormal opening between the right and left ventricle. Ventricular septal defects vary in size and may occur in either the membranous or muscular portion of the ventricular septum. Due to higher pressure in the left ventricle, a shunting of blood from the left to right ventricle occurs during systole. If pulmonary vascular resistance produces pulmonary hypertension, the shunt of blood is then reversed from the right to the left ventricle, with cyanosis resulting.

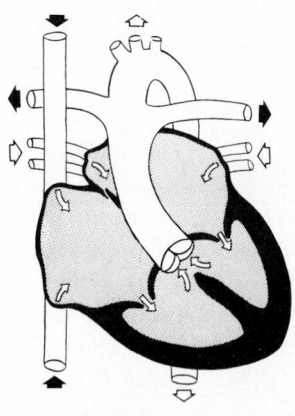

Truncus Arteriosus

Truncus arteriosus is a retention of the embryologic bulbar trunk. It results from the failure of normal septation and division of this trunk into an aorta and pulmonary artery. This single arterial trunk overrides the ventricles and receives blood from them through a ventricular septal defect. The entire pulmonary and systemic circulation is supplied from this common arterial trunk.

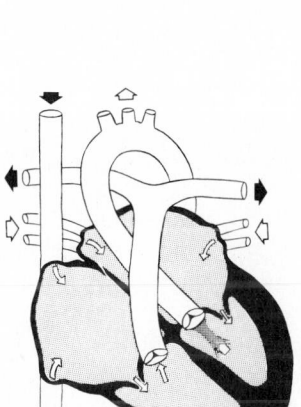

Subaortic Stenosis

In many instances, the stenosis is valvular with thickening and fusion of the cusps. Subaortic stenosis is caused by a fibrous ring below the aortic valve in the outflow tract of the left ventricle. At times, both valvular and subaortic stenosis exist in combination. The obstruction presents an increased work load for the normal output of the left ventricular blood and results in left ventricular enlargement.

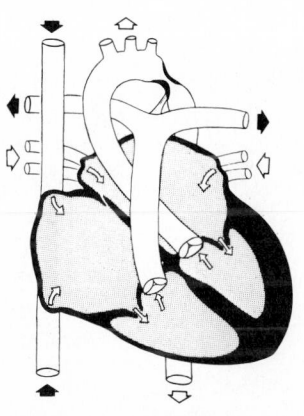

Coarctation of the Aorta

Coarctation of the aorta is characterized by a narrowed aortic lumen. It exists as a preductal or postductal obstruction, depending on the position of the obstruction in relation to the ductus arteriosus. Coarctations exist with great variation in anatomical features. The lesion produces an obstruction to the flow of blood through the aorta causing an increased left ventricular pressure and work load.

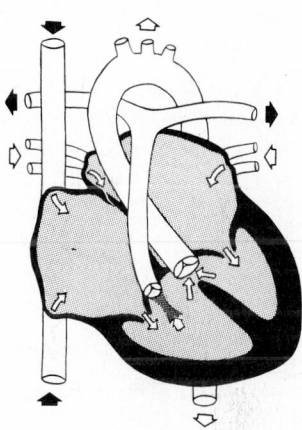

Tetralogy of Fallot

Tetralogy of Fallot is characterized by the combination of four defects: 1) pulmonary stenosis 2) ventricular septal defect 3) overriding aorta 4) hypertrophy of right ventricle. It is the most common defect causing cyanosis in patients surviving beyond two years of age. The severity of symptoms depends on the degree of pulmonary stenosis, the size of the ventricular septal defect, and the degree to which the aorta overrides the septal defect.

mal size and shape and without increased pulmonary blood flow. Cardiac catheterization is not usually done, as no treatment is required for these infants. Spontaneous closure occurs in 50% of children with ventricular septal defects.

In large membranous defects, the left-to-right shunting of blood is greater and does result in increased right ventricular pressure and right ventricular hypertrophy. There is a middiastolic murmur heard best at the left lower sternal border. Congestive heart failure may develop between 6 weeks and 2 months of age. Infants exhibit rapid respirations, growth failure, and feeding difficulties. Chest radiograph shows cardiac enlargement and increased pulmonary blood flow. Electrocardiogram demonstrates left ventricular hypertrophy and, if the defect is very large, may show combined ventricular hypertrophy.

Medications such as Lanoxin and diuretics are used to control the congestive heart failure, and the infant is usually followed for a period of time, because even large ventricular defects may close spontaneously. Cardiac catheterization reveals higher oxygen saturation in the right ventricle than in the right atrium. Pressures in the right ventricle and pulmonary artery are frequently increased.

When pressures in the right ventricle and pulmonary artery begin to approach the same pressure as the systemic pressure of the left ventricle, pulmonary hypertension due to pulmonary arterial changes is occurring and surgical intervention is necessary. Surgery may also be performed when cardiac catheterization demonstrates that the pulmo-

nary blood flow is twice the systemic blood flow. In the past, a palliative procedure called a *pulmonary artery banding* was done during the first year of life (Figure 26–16). A constricting Teflon band was placed around the pulmonary artery to reduce blood volume to the lungs. When the child was older, the band was released, the pulmonary artery was reconstructed, and the ventricular septal defect was closed with a Dacron patch. At the present time, an initial correction of the defect with a Dacron patch is being done more frequently because of the increased success of the surgery with fewer long-term complications.

ENDOCARDIAL CUSHION DEFECTS

There are four embryologic centers of growth, called *endocardial cushions* (pads of embryonic endothelium-covered connective tissue that bulge into the embryonic atrioventricular canal), that develop into the mitral valve, the tricuspid valve, a portion of the atrial septum, and a portion of the ventricular septum. When development of these growth centers is not complete, a group of cardiac lesions called *endocardial cushion defects* occurs. Endocardial cushion defects are common in infants with Down syndrome. The defect may involve the atrial septum, the ventricular septum, or both septa. The mitral valve does not completely close due to a cleft in one section of the valve, and sometimes the tricuspid valve also has a cleft with incomplete closure. These infants have left-to-right shunting of blood at the site of the defect and also leakage of blood from ventricle to atrium through the defective valves.

An apical diastolic murmur accompanies the left-to-right shunt. If a mitral defect is present, a systolic murmur is also heard, and the pulmonary hypertension causes a loud second heart sound. On chest x-ray film, the heart size is enlarged, varying with the severity of the condition. Increased pulmonary blood flow is demonstrated by extra markings in the lungs. Cardiac catheterization, vectorcardiograms, and echocardiograms are performed to study the location and severity of the defects. When there is a large ventricular defect, it is usually accompanied by pulmonary hypertension, and many of these infants are very ill. About 50% of them die from congestive heart failure and pneumonia during the first year of life.

Open-heart surgery reduces the left-to-right shunting of blood and repairs the valvular defects. Often repair is not completely successful, and many children have continuing cardiac problems and delays in height and weight maturation.

COARCTATION OF THE AORTA

Coarctation of the aorta is a congenital narrowing of a segment of the aorta (see Figure 26–15). The coarctation may involve either a short or long section of the aorta and can occur anywhere but is most often located in the aortic arch near the ductus arteriosus. Difficulties occur in infants

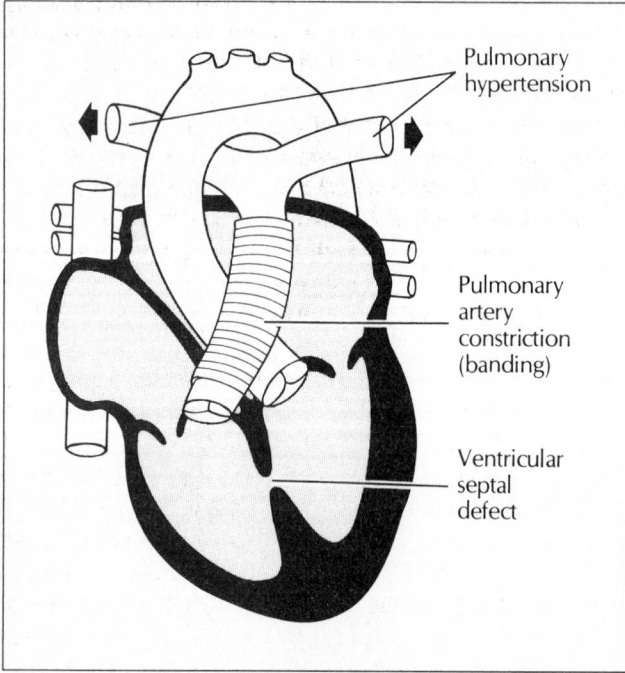

Pulmonary hypertension

Pulmonary artery constriction (banding)

Ventricular septal defect

Figure 26–16 Pulmonary banding for ventricular septal defect to decrease blood flow through the pulmonary artery.

who also have a patent ductus arteriosus or a ventricular septal defect, because of increased left-to-right shunting of blood through these defects.

Important physical findings may be detected by an astute nurse during the newborn assessment. Absent or diminished femoral pulsation should alert the nurse to listen for a late systolic heart murmur, heard best in the left interscapular region, and decreased systolic blood pressure in the lower extremities when compared with blood pressure in the upper extremities, due to increased blood volume in upper extremities and diminished blood volume in major arteries of the lower extremities. Obstruction of blood flow through the aorta causes an increased left ventricular pressure and work load. Collateral vessels arise, chiefly from the branches of the subclavian artery, and bypass the constricted aorta to supply circulation to the lower extremities. The chest x-ray film or echocardiogram shows an enlarged heart, with most of the increased size due to enlargement of the left ventricle. The indented area of the narrow segment of the aorta can usually be identified. Some infants remain generally asymptomatic, but others present in severe congestive heart failure at about 7–21 days of age.

If the coarctation is not complicated by other cardiac lesions, these infants usually respond well to medical management, and surgical correction is delayed until the child is beyond 6 years of age. Management includes monitoring left ventricular hypertrophy, observing for signs of early heart failure, and monitoring growth and development to maintain within normal parameters.

If the coarctation is accompanied by a patent ductus arteriosus or a ventricular septal defect, the response to medical management is generally poor and surgery is required. The coarctation is resected, and with short defects, the ends of the aorta are anastomosed. With longer defects, a prosthetic graft of Dacron may be inserted to bridge the gap in the aorta after resection. The patent ductus arteriosus is tied off, and a Teflon band may be placed around the pulmonary artery if pulmonary blood flow is excessive. Mortality is very low when surgery is done on older children to correct coarctation of the aorta, but it is high when the operation must be performed as an emergency measure for heart failure in infancy (Ziai et al., 1975).

AORTIC STENOSIS

Aortic stenosis is an acyanotic heart defect not frequently seen by nursery nurses. For a brief discussion of this disorder, see Figure 26–15.

Cyanotic Lesions

Cyanosis in congenital heart diseases results from shunting unoxygenated venous blood into the systemic arterial circuit. Cyanosis is defined as blue discoloration of the skin, nail beds, and mucous membranes resulting from the pres-

ence of approximately 5 g/dL of unoxygenated hemoglobin in the blood. Cyanosis depends on the total hemoglobin present as well as on the arterial oxygen saturation. In profound anemia, cyanosis may not be seen because of the insufficient amount of unoxygenated hemoglobin in the circulation. In contrast, in an infant with polycythemia peripheral cyanosis may be noted due to an increased amount of unoxygenated hemoglobin, although the degree of arterial unsaturation is minimal. Generally, cyanosis is associated with anoxia or a low arterial partial pressure of oxygen.

The nurse must differentiate between central and peripheral cyanosis. *Central cyanosis* is manifested as follows: The tongue and mucous membranes of the mouth are blue, and the blood leaving the heart contains an excess of unoxygenated hemoglobin; arterial oxygen saturation is low; arteriovenous oxygen difference is normal; extremities are warm; and cardiac output is normal. Central cyanosis is produced by the admixture of unsaturated venous blood into the systemic circulation, resulting from a large right-to-left intracardiac shunt or intrapulmonic shunt. In peripheral cyanosis, only the extremities are blue, and the central blood contains sufficient oxygenated hemoglobin. Peripheral cyanosis results from profound oxygen unsaturation of capillary blood and is seen in cases of marked vasoconstriction or advanced cardiac failure associated with low cardiac output. It is most commonly seen when cardiac output is reduced by an obstructive lesion such as mitral stenosis, pulmonic stenosis, or low-output congestive heart failure.

The usual causes of central cyanosis in the neonate are pulmonary disorders, heart defects, hematologic abnormalities, and central nervous system disorders. In CNS disorders the newborn infant is usually full term, with a history of the mother having had a difficult labor or delivery. Often some visible signs of trauma to the neonate can be seen. The infant's respirations are slow, shallow, and irregular. Administration of 100% oxygen may improve cyanosis, especially if ventilation is also increased. With hematologic abnormalities, the only differentiating factor is the laboratory analysis of the circulating hemoglobin.

The leading pulmonary disorder is respiratory distress syndrome. Neonates with RDS are born prematurely and show obvious signs of respiratory difficulties. At least at the onset of respiratory distress, placing the infant in 100% oxygen improves the cyanosis, and ventilatory assistance causes marked improvement. In contrast, infants with cyanotic heart disease are usually full term and frequently have rapid respirations with intense cyanosis but without the other signs of respiratory distress. Their cyanosis does not improve significantly with administration of 100% oxygen (Harris, 1976).

TETRALOGY OF FALLOT

Tetralogy of Fallot is thought to be the most common congenital cardiovascular defect causing cyanosis in children (see Figure 26–15). It is identified by its classic combination of four defects: pulmonary stenosis, ventricular septal defect, aorta overriding both ventricles, and hypertrophy of the right ventricle. Pulmonary stenosis may be caused by either a defective pulmonary valve or obstruction in the infundibular area of the right ventricle directly below the pulmonary valve. This obstruction decreases the outflow of blood through the pulmonary circulation and increases the work load and pressure of the right ventricle. When the pressure in the right ventricle becomes greater than the pressure in the left ventricle, a right-to-left shunting of unoxygenated blood into oxygenated blood through the ventricular septal defect occurs, and cyanosis develops. The overriding aorta is situated over the high ventricular septal defect, and much of the shunted unoxygenated blood flows directly into it and further increases cyanosis.

Infants may be cyanotic at birth or may develop cyanosis during the first months of life. The infant with this disorder is small, the growth rate is very slow due to poor nutrition caused by decreased circulation, and the infant has difficulty with feeding. The circulating blood volume tends to be sluggish and to pool in the extremities, causing clubbing of the fingers and toes. The body responds to the low oxygen saturation of the blood and attempts to compensate by increased secretion of erythropoietin, which accelerates red blood cell production. The resulting polycythemia causes increased viscosity of the blood and places the infant at risk for cerebral thrombosis. Low hemoglobin is also a constant threat, because poor nutrition and rapid red blood cell production easily deplete the infant's iron stores. A normal or low hemoglobin level may contribute to increased hypoxia and dyspnea. Anoxic spells, the result of suddenly decreased cardiac output, are usually precipitated by exertion or emotional stress. The crying infant exhibits increased cyanosis and then suddenly becomes limp and unresponsive due to decreased circulation and oxygen to the brain. Placing the infant in a knee–chest position often alleviates the anoxia somewhat. The knee–chest position decreases venous return to the heart, lessens the right side of the heart's work load, and thereby increases arterial oxygen saturation to the vital organs of the body. If the defect is severe, right ventricular hypertrophy may be extensive enough to cause protrusion of the left chest. A harsh systolic murmur can be heard along the left sternal border.

X-ray examination reveals a heart of small or normal size with a boot-shaped appearance, caused by the small pulmonary artery. Markings in the lung fields are also diminished, due to decreased pulmonary blood flow and a prominent or enlarged aorta.

The goal of medical management is to prevent dehydration and intercurrent infections and to alleviate paroxysmal dyspneic attacks. Indications for surgical intervention are severe anoxic attacks and severe dyspnea on exertion, which prevents the child from leading a normal life. The current surgical approach is for complete correction through open-heart surgery with use of the heart-lung machine. Obstructive infundibular tissue is removed from the right ventricle below the pulmonary artery, or the stenotic pulmonary valve is incised, whichever is necessary to increase pulmonary circulation. A Dacron patch is used to close the ventricular septal defect and extend the left ventricle to the right of the overriding aorta, thereby removing the right-to-left shunting of unoxygenated blood.

Palliative surgery may be done when the infant is too ill or too small to tolerate total correction. The goal of such surgical intervention is to increase blood flow to the lungs and to decrease the degree of cyanosis. The procedure that has been used for the longest period of time is the Blalock-Taussig operation, in which the subclavian artery is anastomosed to the pulmonary artery. An artificial patent ductus arteriosus is constructed to shunt blood into the pulmonary circulation for reoxygenation. In the Potts-Smith-Gibson operation, the aorta is joined to the pulmonary artery by a side-by-side anastomosis to create this shunt (Figure 26–17). A direct anastomosis of the aorta and the pulmonary artery is also done in the Waterston-Cooley procedure but at a different site. The Potts-Smith-Gibson operation creates a shunt in the descending aorta, and the Waterston-Cooley operation uses the ascending aorta. When the child is older, or when the condition is more stable, the shunt is removed and a total correction is done, using open-heart surgery.

PULMONARY STENOSIS

Pulmonary stenosis may exist alone or in combination with other cardiovascular defects. When pulmonary stenosis exists alone, the symptoms and physical findings vary from asymptomatic to dyspnea, easy tiring, cyanosis, and heart failure. There is usually a loud ejection systolic murmur, heard best at the upper left sternal border.

In mild cases, the chest x-rays and echocardiogram are normal. With severe problems, both may show right ventricular hypertrophy and right atrial hypertrophy, with decreased pulmonary blood flow. An infant with mild-to-moderate pulmonary stenosis often requires no specific treatment except for careful well-child care. More extensive stenosis requires surgical correction with the use of the heart-lung machine.

TRANSPOSITION OF THE GREAT VESSELS

In transposition of the great vessels, the aorta arises from the right ventricle and the pulmonary artery from the left ventricle. Unoxygenated venous blood from the body returns to the right side of the heart and is pumped through the aorta out to the body tissues without reoxygenation.

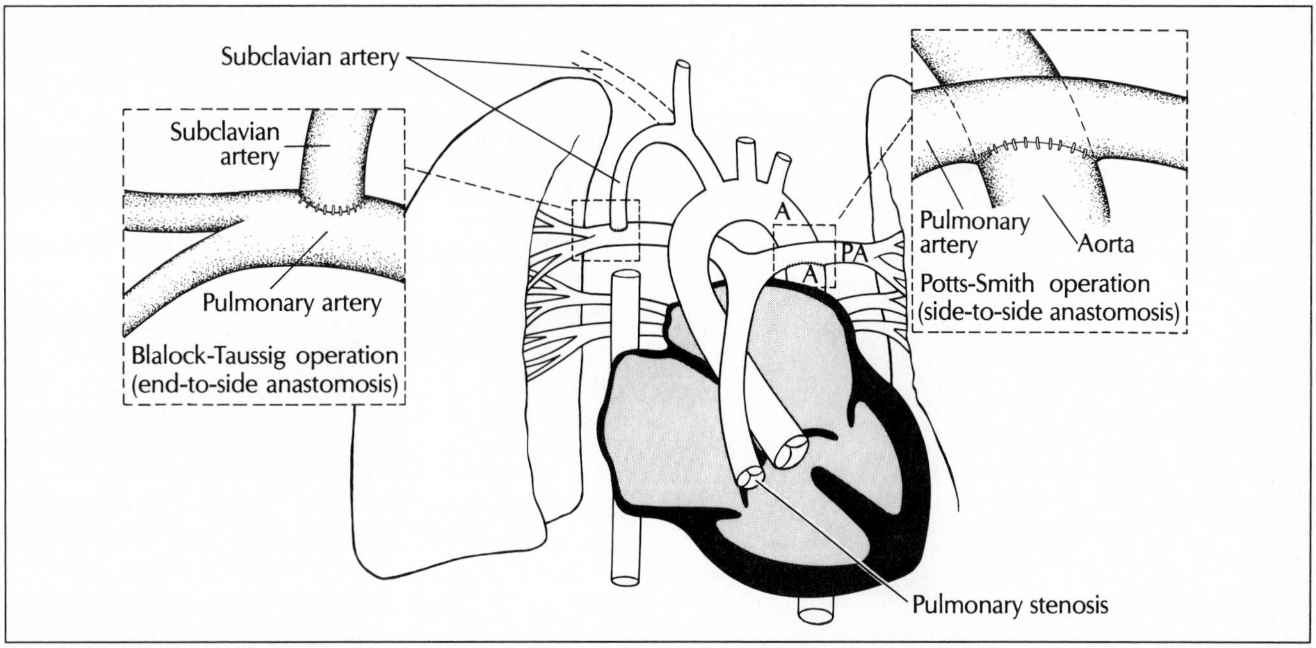
Subclavian artery
Subclavian artery
Pulmonary artery
Blalock-Taussig operation
(end-to-side anastomosis)
A
PA
A
Pulmonary artery
Aorta
Potts-Smith operation
(side-to-side anastomosis)
Pulmonary stenosis

Figure 26–17 Palliative surgery for tetralogy of Fallot.

Oxygenated blood from the lungs returns through the pulmonary veins to the left side of the heart and is pumped through the pulmonary artery back to the lungs again. The neonate cannot live unless a communication between the two circulations is present. The ductus arteriosus is usually patent during the first few days after birth and creates some mixing of blood from the two separate circulations through shunting (see Figure 26–15). If closure of the ductus begins to occur, the infant quickly enters a critical state with the threat of death from heart failure or hypoxia.

Some medical centers are using intravenous infusions of prostaglandins to inhibit or prevent closure of the ductus arteriosus. Some prostaglandins have vasoconstrictive properties, and others function as vasodilators. E-type prostaglandins appear to be able to cause vasodilatation, especially of the ductus arteriosus in the newborn (Kaplan et al., 1978). Another possible communication between the two circulations is the shunting of blood through a patent foramen ovale or an atrial septal defect. A ventricular septal defect is a commonly associated defect that creates a communication between the two separate circulations. Pulmonary stenosis may also be an associated defect.

Transposition of the great vessels occurs more frequently in males than in females and in infants of diabetic mothers. The affected infant is usually large. Transposition of the great vessels is thought to be more common than tetralogy of Fallot, but because many infants with this defect die early, more children over 2 years of age are seen with tetralogy of Fallot. Improved management is greatly increasing survival during the first year of life for infants with transposition of the great vessels, so these statistics may change soon.

Cyanosis is present at birth or occurs within 3 days. Because the infant has inadequate oxygen saturation of the systemic circulation, murmurs are present in relation to the blood flow through the various shunts—patent ductus arteriosus, ventricular septal defect, or atrial septal defect—and when present, the murmur of pulmonary stenosis can be heard. These infants have rapid respirations, tire easily, feed poorly, and fail to grow and develop at a normal rate. Hypoxia causing deep cyanosis results in polycythemia due to decreased oxygen to tissues of the kidney, which stimulates the production of erythropoietin, which in turn increases red blood cell production by the bone marrow. The infant has anoxic paroxysmal dyspneic attacks with loss of consciousness. Early clubbing of the fingers and toes also occurs.

Heart failure may occur due to overwork when pulmonary stenosis is not present because of congestion from increased pulmonary blood flow.

The chest radiograph and echocardiogram show cardiac enlargement and the classic configuration, described as an "egg on its side." When pulmonary stenosis is not present, the radiograph and echocardiogram also show evidence of increased pulmonary blood flow. An electrocardiogram demonstrates right ventricular hypertrophy,

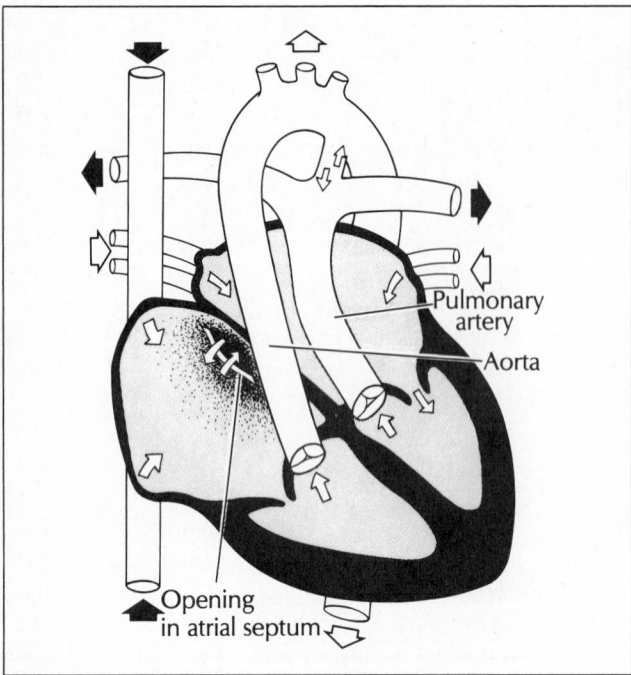

Pulmonary
artery

Aorta

Opening
in atrial septum

Figure 26–18 Palliative surgery for transposition of great vessels is accomplished by enlarging or creating an atrial septal defect.

which is considered normal for the newborn infant. A cardiac catheterization displays an increased right ventricular pressure and identifies the various defects.

If the mixing of blood does not appear to be adequate for the infant to survive, a Rashkind balloon atrial septostomy can be performed with the cardiac catheterization (Figure 26–18). A balloon-tipped catheter is passed from the right atrium through the foramen ovale into the left atrium. The balloon then is inflated with radiopaque material and forcefully withdrawn into the right atrium. This tear in the atrial septal tissue allows a bidirectional blood flow. It usually causes an immediate increase in arterial oxygen saturation and a decrease in left atrial pressure. If the balloon septostomy is not successful, a Blalock-Hanlen operation—the surgical creation of an atrial septal defect—might be performed. Open-heart surgery is done, and the tissue dividing the two atria is excised. In some infants with large ventricular septal defects and without pulmonary stenosis, increased pulmonary blood flow may require a pulmonary banding surgical procedure.

Complete repair of the total defect with open-heart surgery, the Mustard operation, is done early, even at less than 1 year of age. In this procedure, the remaining part of the atrial septum is excised, and a baffle of pericardium is sutured in place in a manner that directs the oxygenated pulmonary venous return into the right ventricle and aorta, whereas the systemic venous circulation enters the left

ventricle and pulmonary artery. Other anomalies such as patent ductus, pulmonary stenosis, or ventricular septal defect are also repaired at the same time. Selection of the proper time for the total repair varies with the child's particular defect and clinical progress and with the experience of the cardiology and surgical teams.

ANOMALOUS VENOUS RETURN OF THE PULMONARY VEINS

Anomalous return of the pulmonary veins may be either complete or partial (Figure 26–15). In complete anomalous return all the pulmonary and systemic veins empty into the right atrium. An atrial septal defect must be present for blood to reach the left side of the heart. In partial anomalous return, some of the pulmonary blood flow returns to the left atrium, and the rest is emptied into the right atrium. Part of the increased blood volume in the right atrium is shunted through an atrial septal defect into the left atrium, resulting in a mixture of unoxygenated and oxygenated blood being pumped into the systemic circulation.

The infant presents with cyanosis, fatigue, dyspnea, tachycardia, and frequent respiratory infections. Right-sided heart failure may develop due to the increased pulmonary blood flow. Chest radiography and echocardiography reveal cardiac enlargement and a large pulmonary artery with increased pulmonary circulation. The electrocardiogram shows right ventricular hypertrophy. Cardiac catheterization is done to identify all existing defects and to assess their severity. Oxygen saturation of the blood in the right atrium is higher than normal, and the pressure in the right atrium is increased.

Complete anomalous return of pulmonary veins requires surgical correction at an early age. The heart-lung machine is used to perform an open-heart procedure in which the anomalous veins are detached from the right atrium and transplanted to the left atrium, and the atrial septal defect is repaired. Partial anomalous venous return may be severe enough to require surgical correction.

HYPOPLASTIC LEFT HEART SYNDROME

Hypoplastic left heart syndrome includes aortic atresia, mitral atresia, or a combination of both lesions. In all cases, the left ventricular chamber is only a tiny, thick-walled cavity, and no blood flows through the left ventricular chamber and out the aorta in the normal manner. Systemic blood flow comes only from the output of the right ventricle into the pulmonary artery and through the ductus arteriosus into the descending aorta. Blood then flows in a retrograde fashion around the aortic arch supplying blood flow to the head and to the coronary arteries. The right ventricle is large, dilated, and hypertrophied in an attempt to maintain the entire heart action.

Infants may appear normal at birth, but within a few hours to days they develop cyanosis and shocklike congestive heart failure. As the ductus arteriosus closes, systemic flow decreases, and shock and congestive failure develop, usually by 48–72 hours of age. A nonspecific soft systolic murmur is heard just left of the sternum. Palpation of extremities reveals diminished pulses. Chest x-ray films and echocardiogram demonstrate cardiac enlargement and pulmonary venous congestion. Electrocardiogram demonstrates right axis deviation and right ventricular hypertrophy. The outcome in these cases is invariably fatal.

There is no effective treatment to correct this defect. Infants with severe defects rarely live more than 4–5 days. Infants with less severe forms of this complex may survive for longer periods. This syndrome must be differentiated from other conditions that are operable. Other cyanotic heart defects are truncus arteriosus and atresia of the tricuspid valve, discussed briefly in Figure 26–15 on p. 886.

Congestive Heart Failure

Hospitalization for congestive heart failure is one of the most common situations requiring nursing care for neonates or infants with congenital heart defects. Infants with left-to-right shunts and many with obstructive lesions may initially manifest congestive heart failure. The failure happens with greatest frequency during the first year of life but can occur at any age, prior to surgery or as a postsurgical complication.

PHYSIOLOGY AND PATHOPHYSIOLOGY

The simplest definition of heart failure is the inability of the heart to pump blood in accordance with body needs. When the *right ventricle* fails, output through the pulmonary artery is diminished, and residual blood volume in the right ventricle and right atrium is increased. Pressure rises in the right ventricle, the right atrium, and the venous circulation. Right-sided failure occurs most often in infants with tricuspid valve anomalies, pulmonary stenosis, or large atrial septal defects. Because of the systemic venous hypertension, these infants have hepatomegaly (venous engorgement of the liver) and edema due to venous pressure exceeding plasma protein pressure, with resulting loss of fluid from capillaries into surrounding tissue. Removal of interstitial fluid by the lymphatics is also impaired.

When the *left ventricle* fails, output through the aorta is diminished, and residual blood volume in the left side of the heart is increased. Decreased renal perfusion results in retention of sodium and water. Pressure increases in the left ventricle, left atrium, and the pulmonary veins, with subsequent pulmonary venous congestion. Left-sided failure occurs most frequently in infants, with hypoplastic left heart syndrome, coarctation of the aorta, or aortic stenosis. These infants have tachypnea and dyspnea, often accompanied by rales; bloody, frothy sputum; wheezing; and cyanosis.

Left- and right-sided failure often appear concomitantly in infants. They can occur as a component of transposition of the great vessels, ventricular septal defect, total anomalous venous return of the pulmonary veins, and patent ductus arteriosus. The heart dilates and enlarges in an effort to accommodate the increased residual blood volume. The dilatation at first increases the force of the heart's contraction. When this mechanism reaches its maximum, the heart's next compensatory effort is to increase its rate (tachycardia).

CLINICAL MANIFESTATIONS

In the newborn, the most common presenting signs of congestive heart failure are tachycardia, tachypnea, hepatomegaly, cardiomegaly, and diaphoresis. Preterm infants with a patent ductus arteriosus account for most of the newborns suffering from heart failure in the neonatal intensive care unit.

The alert nurse might first notice easy fatigability, which the infant frequently demonstrates as an inability to feed well, requiring many rests before finishing even 1 or 2 ounces of formula. Fatigue at feeding might be accompanied by perspiration, with beads of moisture appearing on the upper lip and forehead. Failure to gain weight may also be seen, because of their poor feeding pattern and perhaps also because of poor absorption of nutrients and the frequent respiratory infections commonly occurring in these small, weak infants. Dyspnea, if present, is caused by pulmonary venous pressure creating congested bronchial mucosa. The presence or development of rising respiratory rate reflects the increased pulmonary blood flow. Excess venous blood flow to the lungs can result not only in tachypnea but also in difficult respirations, with retraction of the chest, wheezing, and coughing. Congestion of blood flow in the liver can result in hepatomegaly, which is easily palpated in the abdomen of the small infant. Tachycardia of more than 160 beats per minute and cardiac enlargement are invariably present.

Pulsus alternans is detected by slowly releasing the sphygmomanometer until every second atrial beat is heard, as pressure drops another 5–10 mm—the number of sounds doubles suddenly and becomes equal to the apex beat. The gallop rhythm so commonly used as a sign of failure in adults is not so significant in infants and young children, because a third heart sound can frequently be heard in children with no cardiac abnormality. Edema is a late manifestation and usually does not occur in infants. If it does occur, generally periorbital edema occurs first, followed by edema of the face. The skin generally appears very pale and moist. Peripheral pulses are decreased, and if heart failure is severe, peripheral vasoconstriction can occur, resulting in low blood pressure, low urine output, acidosis, and shock.

INTERVENTIONS

Care of infants with congestive heart failure has four major goals: to reduce the energy requirements of the body, to increase cardiac efficiency, to increase oxygenation of the blood, and to reduce retention of fluids in the tissues. Rest, with the use of a sedative may be required. Morphine sulfate, a dose of 0.05 mg/kg of body weight, can be used if the infant is markedly irritable (Graham and Bender, 1980). Morphine is thought to decrease peripheral and pulmonary vascular resistance, which results in decreased tachypnea. Infants in congestive heart failure are more comfortable in a semi-Fowler's position.

Cardiac efficiency is increased by digitalization. (Digitalization will be ordered by the physician.) Digoxin (Lanoxin) is given either by mouth or intravenously. It also has a diuretic effect due to increased kidney perfusion. Digoxin is fast acting (10–30 minutes), has a short half-life of 36 hours, and is excreted mainly by the kidneys.

When the infant has dyspnea or cyanosis, oxygen must be given by an oxygen hood, tent, mask, cannula, or oxygen prongs. Mist is often ordered given with oxygen to infants, making the use of an oxygen hood or tent necessary. Oxygen administration should always be accompanied by humidity, and the air should be warmed to decrease the drying effects of cold, dry oxygen. Vital signs are carefully monitored for evidence of tachycardia, tachypnea, expiratory grunting, and retractions.

During cardiac failure, the blood supply to the kidneys is reduced, and the diminished perfusion of the glomeruli and tubules results in increased sodium and water retention. Renin is also released, which promotes aldosterone secretion and causes more sodium retention by the kidneys. Diuretics are given to block the reabsorption of sodium in the kidneys. Furosemide (Lasix) is the one most often used at the present time. The usual dose is 1 mg/kg of body weight, and it may be given either orally or intravenously. The onset of diuresis varies from about 5 minutes when given intravenously to about 2 hours when given orally.

The most common problem occurring with the use of furosemide is hypokalemia. Potassium levels should be monitored and a potassium supplement given to the infant as needed. When furosemide is taken orally by children, gastrointestinal irritation may also occur (Graef and Cone, 1974). If congestive heart failure occurs over a long period of time, sodium restriction may be necessary. Infants may be placed on low-sodium formulas, such as SMA S-26, Lonalac milk powder, or Similac PM 60/40. As long as diuretics can handle the fluid overload problems, most physicians prefer the use of regular formula; it costs less and many infants do not like the taste of low-sodium formulas (Cloutier and Measel, 1982). The infant's weight should be carefully monitored about every 8 hours, and a careful record of fluid intake and urine output should be kept.

Preparation of the parents for home care should begin early in the infant's hospitalization. Information provided should include medication administration, techniques of isolating the infant from others with infection, availability of community resources, and public health referrals. It is also essential to provide a nonjudgmental atmosphere in which the parents can express their concerns and voice their emotions of grief.

DEVELOPMENTAL CONSEQUENCES OF CONGENITAL ANOMALIES

The infant who is born prematurely, is ill, or has a malformation or disorder is at risk in emotional and intellectual, as well as physical, development. The risk is directly proportional to the seriousness of the problem and the length of treatment. For example, resolution of a meconium plug syndrome during the expected hospital stay, allowing the infant to be discharged with the mother, is not expected to alter the child's developmental course. However, the physical appearance, immediate and repeated surgeries, and complex rehabilitation problems of exstrophy of the bladder or meningomyelocele preclude a normal developmental course for the child.

Medical, surgical, and technical advances in recent years have been responsible for salvaging increasing numbers of preterm and ill neonates. The necessary physical separation of family and child and the tremendous emotional and financial burden have adversely affected the parent–child relationship. A considerable percentage of these children have been rescued only to be emotionally or physically battered by the parents. The most recent trend in many hospitals is to involve the parents with the neonate early, repeatedly, and over protracted periods of time. Early and continued involvement may only mean opportunities to look at the baby or to stroke the infant's skin. Later, when the mother's and infant's conditions warrant it, the mother participates in her baby's care (to the extent she is willing) and in planning for the future. This type of involvement facilitates early bonding, attachment, and emotional investment. The parents need a sense of personal success, self-worth, self-esteem, and confidence from knowledge that they can cope with the situation. This atmosphere aids the infant as well—the child may escape battering and may instead be assisted toward self-actualization.

Mothers of newborns who are gravely ill are often unable to chance an emotional investment in their child. These mothers need assistance in perceiving the cues and hearing the words that indicate the infant is going to survive. They need time and support to establish a positive relationship with the newborn. A mother who is unable to develop maternal feelings may reject the infant or overcompensate because of underlying guilt feelings; in either case an unproductive relationship may develop. The child may then be further handicapped by inability to relate well to others and by seeing the world as unsatisfying and painful.

The parents must have a clear picture of the reality of the handicap and the types of developmental hurdles ahead. Unexpected behaviors and responses from the child due to his or her defect or disorder can be upsetting and frightening. For example, parents find it difficult to cope with an infant's lack of motor or social responsiveness and tend to interpret the lack as a form of rejection. The parents may in return respond with rejection, and an unfortunate cycle is begun.

It is difficult for many to discipline a handicapped child, to say no, to expect the same behaviors as are expected of "normal" children. The child who is given too-free rein can feel unworthy as well as be unable to develop more mature behavior patterns. Every child requires some exposure to delayed gratification, separation, and frustration to develop mastery over the feelings aroused by such situations. If a child is aware of limit-setting for siblings, he or she feels unwanted, insecure, and unworthy of parental love and concern if he or she is denied the same limits to behavior. Such a child may be prompted to provocativeness and to testing limits to the point of irritation and possible rejection by those nearby.

The demands of care of the child and disputes regarding management or behavior stress family relationships. One or more members of the family may make a scapegoat of the child. Another may become the youngster's champion to the exclusion of others. One or the other spouse may feel pushed aside or denied attention and thus may withdraw or leave the family unit. Parents or siblings may feel that their own needs (schooling, material goods, freedom of movement) are being set aside while all assets (financial and other) go to support the one child's needs.

The child who has been overprotected has little chance to develop the intrapersonal skills needed to achieve in social situations, in school, and at work. Each child must have the opportunity to experience and explore the environment, to learn about it, to learn how to use it, and to learn how to cope with it. Deficient motor skills in particular can hamper exploration and mobility. Unless the child is motivated to explore and experience, the concept of the self and one's world is limited.

The parents and the child must confront daily an outside society that values normality. If the parents cannot develop a positive attitude toward the child, the child may see himself or herself as not good—perhaps even as responsible for the predicament.

Fortunately, many children have parents who can accept them and help them cope with their "differentness." These children can explore and grow personally without unusual amounts of frustration and anxiety.

The entire multidisciplinary team may need to pool their resources and expertise to help parents of children born with defects or disorders so that both parents and children can thrive.

SUMMARY

Early assessment and appropriate intervention to prevent possible complications are essential in the nursing management of the infant with a congenital anomaly. It is incumbent upon the neonatal nurse to be knowledgeable about possible congenital anomalies and to utilize assessment skills to identify and then initiate appropriate interventions.

The nurse should be skilled in preoperative management so that valuable time is not lost and unnecessary complications do not occur. It is imperative that the nurse understand the emotional process associated with the birth of an infant with a congenital problem, as the nurse is a key person in the establishment of the parent–infant relationship in this crucial early attachment period.

Resource Groups

Child Amputee Centers. Provide for fitting of and education on use of prostheses and carrying out activities of daily living.

March of Dimes (local chapters). Provides information on various congenital anomalies.

State Handicapped Children's Programs. Provide funds for corrective surgery and rehabilitation programs.

References

Ampola, M. G. 1982. *Metabolic diseases in pediatric practice.* Boxton: Little, Brown & Co.

Applegarth, D. A., et al. Jan. 1978. Screening for neural tube defects. *C.M.A.J.* 118:114.

Cloutier, J., and Measel, C. P. 1982. Home care for the infant with congenital heart disease. *Am. J. Nurs.* 82(1):100.

Danis, R. K., and Graviss, E. R. 1978. Imperforate anus: avoiding a colostomy. *J. Pediatr. Surg.* 13(6):759.

Ferguson, A. 1975. *Orthopedic surgery in infancy and childhood,* 4th ed. Baltimore: Williams & Wilkins Co.

Filston, H. C. 1982. *Surgical problems in children: recognition and referral.* St. Louis: C. V. Mosby Co.

Friedman, W. F., et al. 1980. The inhibition of prostaglandin and prostacyclin synthesis in the clinical management of patent ductus arteriosus. *Sem. Perinatol.* 4(2):125.

Graef, J. W., and Cone, T. E. 1974. *Manual of pediatric therapeutics.* Boston: Little, Brown & Co.

Graham, T. P., and Bender, H. W. 1980. Preoperative diagnosis and management of infants with critical congenital heart disease. *Ann. Thoracic Surg.* 29(3):272.

Grosfeld, J. L., et al. 1981. Congenital abdominal wall defects: current management and survival. *Surg. Clin. North Am.* 61(5):1037.

Harris, H. 1976. Cardiorespiratory problems in the newborn. *Postgrad. Med. J.* 60(7):92.

Helfer, R. E., and Kempe, C. H. 1976. *Child abuse and neglect: the family and the community.* Cambridge, Mass.: Ballinger Publishing Co.

Hirsch, P. J., et al. 1980. Hip dysplasia in infancy: diagnosis and treatment. *Primary Care.* 7(2):297.

Holder, T. M., and Ashcraft, K. W. 1981. Development in the care of patients with esophageal atresia and tracheoesophageal fistula. *Surg. Clin. North Am.* 61(5): 1051.

Jones, J. E. 1981. Early management of severe bilateral cleft lip and palate in an infant. *J. Dentistry Child.* 48(1):50.

Kaplan, S., et al. 1978. Therapeutic advances in pediatric cardiology. *Pediatr. Clin. North Am.* 25(4):891.

Kempe, C. H., et al. 1982. *Current pediatric diagnosis and treatment.* Los Altos, Calif.: Lange Medical Publications.

Klein, M. D., et al. 1981. Congenital defects of the abdominal wall. *J.A.M.A.* 245(16):1643.

Lewis, M. B., and Pashayan, H. M. 1980. Management of infants with Pierre Robin anomaly. *Clin. Pediatr.* 19(8):519.

Mathews, A., and Smith, A. October 1979. Presentation at NAACOG Conference on Genetics. Colorado Springs, Colorado.

Mayer, T., et al. 1980. Gastroschisis and omphalocele. *Ann. Surg.* 192(6):783.

O'Loughlin, J. E. 1981. The problem of ductal patency in prematures. *Pediatr. Ann.* 10(4):39.

Sarett, H. P. 1979. *Products for dietary management of inborn errors of metabolism and other special feeding problems.* Evansville, Ind.: Mead Johnson & Company.

Schuett, V. E., et al. 1980. Diet discontinuation policies and practices of PKU clinics in the United States. *Am. J. Public Health.* 70(5):498.

Smith, E. J. March/April 1980. Galactosemia: an inborn error of metabolism. *Nurse Pract.* 5(2):8.

Smith, J. D. July 1981. Treatment of airway obstruction in Pierre Robin syndrome. *Arch. Otolaryngol.* 107:419.

Wasserman, E., and Gromisch, D. S. 1981. *Survey of clinical pediatrics,* 7th ed. New York: McGraw-Hill Book Co.

Ziai, M., et al. 1975. *Pediatrics,* 2nd ed. Boston: Little, Brown & Co.

Additional Readings

Azarnoff, P. 1981. *The family in child health care.* New York: John Wiley & Sons.

Brown, J. W., and King, H. 1981. Cardiac surgery in the critically ill infant during the first three months of life. *Surg. Clin. North Am.* 61(5):1063.

Brueggemeyer, A. 1979. Omphalocele: coping with a surgical emergency. *Pediatr. Nurs.* 5(4):54.

Carey, W. B. 1977. Psychological sequelae of early infancy health crisis. In *Vulnerable infants,* ed. J. L. Schwartz and L. H. Schwartz. New York: McGraw-Hill Book Co.

Dennis, M., et al. 1981. The intelligence of hydrocephalic children. *Arch. Neurol.* 38:607.

Foreman, J. W., et al. 1980. Acidosis associated with dietotherapy of maple syrup urine disease. *J. Pediatr.* 96(1):62.

Fost, N. 1981. Ethical issues in the treatment of critically ill newborns. *Pediatr. Ann.* 10:383.

Hawkins-Walsh, E. Jan./Feb. 1980. Diminishing anxiety in parents of sick newborns. *MCN.* 5:30.

Levin, A. R. April 1981. Management of the cyanotic newborn. *Pediatr. Ann.* 10(4):16.

Pinelli, J. M. July 1981. A comparison of mothers' concerns regarding the care-taking tasks of newborns with congenital heart disease before and after assuming their care. *J. Adv. Nurs.* 6(4):261.

Placzek, M. M., and MacKinnon, A. E. 1980. Lateral meningocele and defect of abdominal wall. *Post Grad. Med. J.* 56:142.

Roach, E. S., et al. 1981. Neonatal cerebral ultrasonography. *North Carolina Med. J.* 42(9):642.

Rossello, P. J., and Lores, M. E. 1980. Esophageal atresia and tracheoesophageal fistula: a ten year review at the university hospital. *Bol. Asoc. Med. P. Rico.* 72(6):305.

Smith, K. M. March/April 1979. Congenital heart disease. Recognizing cardiac failure in neonates. *MCN.* 4(2):98.

Sugar, E. C. 1981. Hirschsprung's disease. *Am. J. Nurs.* 81(1):2065.

Wyatt, D. S. Sept./Oct. 1978. Phenylketonuria: the problems vary during different development stages. *MCN.* 3(5):296.

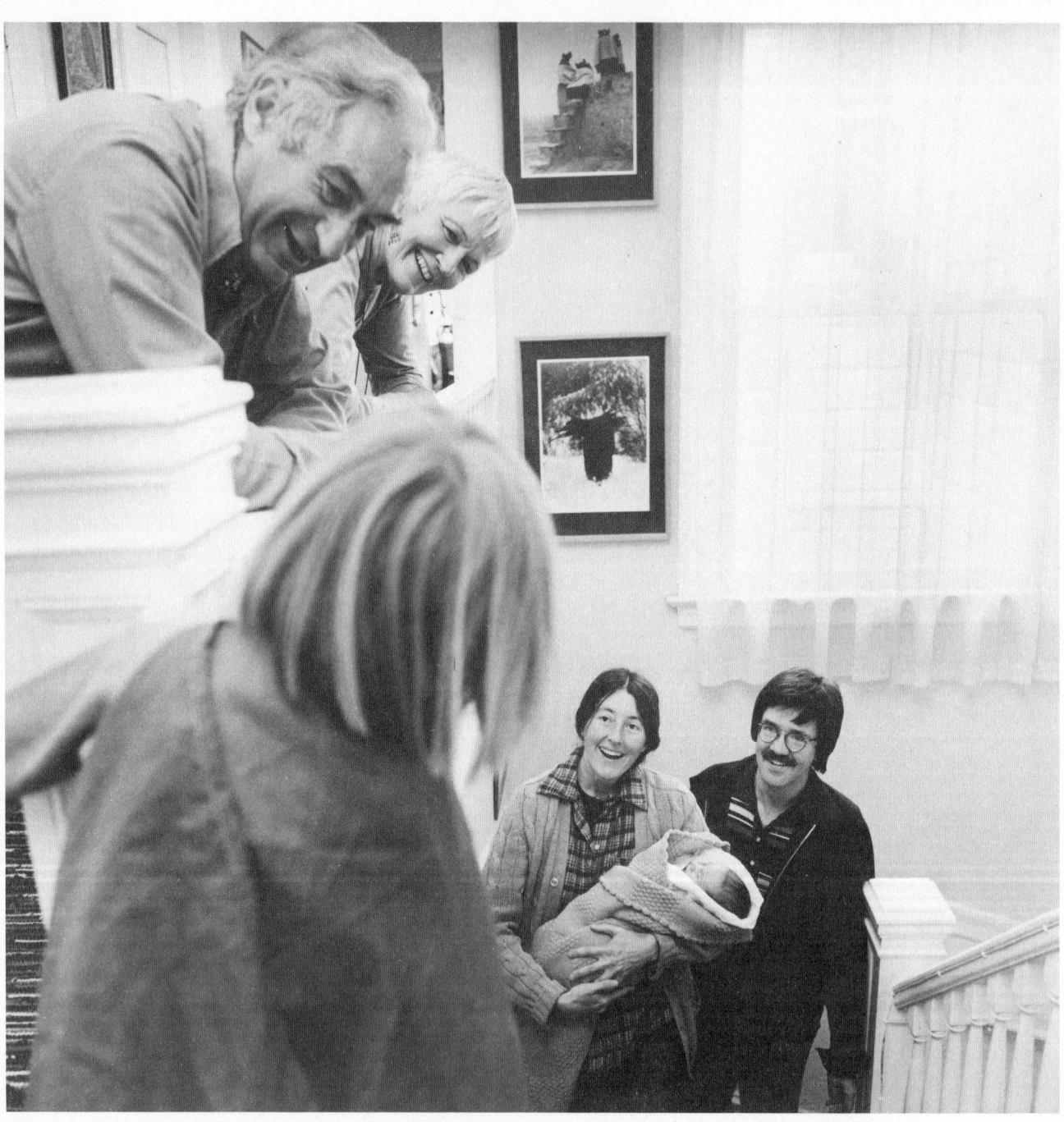

▪ VI ▪

THE PUERPERIUM

Chapter 27 ▪ The Postpartal Family: Assessment, Needs, and Care

Chapter 28 ▪ Attachment

Chapter 29 ▪ Complications of the Puerperium

Chapter 30 ▪ Families in Crisis and the Role of the Nurse

■ 27 ■

THE POSTPARTAL FAMILY: ASSESSMENT, NEEDS, AND CARE

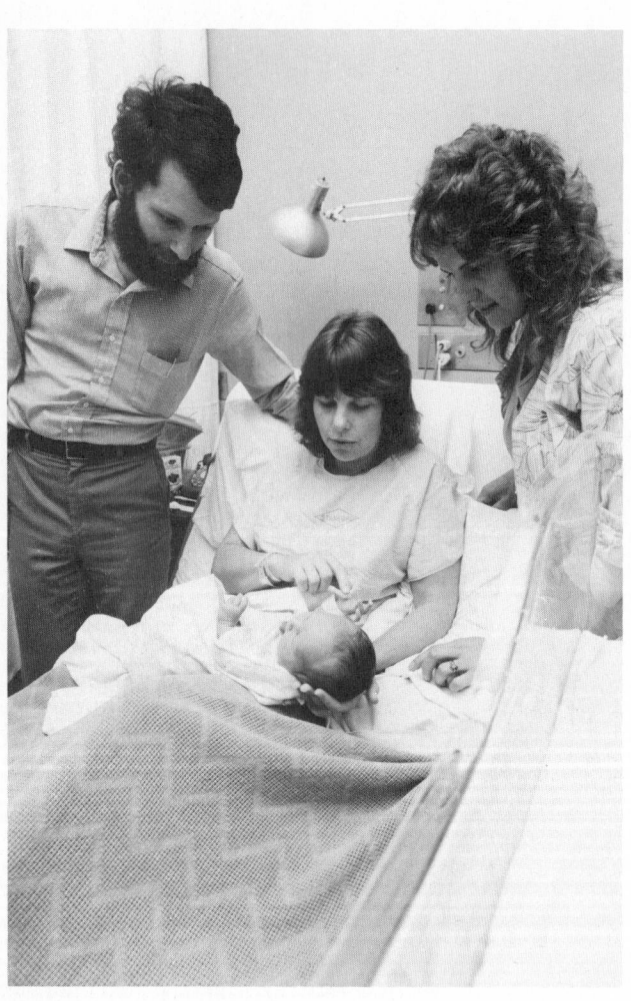

■ CHAPTER CONTENTS

PUERPERAL PHYSICAL AND PSYCHOLOGIC ADAPTATIONS

    Reproductive Organs

    Abdomen

    Lactation

    Gastrointestinal System

    Urinary Tract

    Vital Signs

    Blood Values

    Weight Loss

    Postpartal Chill

    Postpartal Diaphoresis

    Afterpains

    Puerperal Psychologic Adaptations

POSTPARTAL NURSING ASSESSMENT

    Risk Factors

    Physical Assessment

    Psychologic Assessment

    Cultural Influences

POSTPARTAL NURSING CARE

    Promotion of Comfort and Relief of Pain

    Promotion of Rest and Graded Activity

    Promotion of Maternal Psychologic Well-Being

    Promotion of Successful Infant Feeding

    Promotion of Effective Parent Education

    Promotion of Family Wellness

POSTPARTAL NURSING CARE AFTER CESAREAN BIRTH

Facilitation of Parent–Infant Interaction after Cesarean Birth

THE ADOLESCENT ON THE POSTPARTAL UNIT

THE FOURTH TRIMESTER

Nursing Management

■ OBJECTIVES

- Identify the systemic adaptations and physiologic changes of the postpartal period.

- Describe the normal psychologic changes of the postpartal family.

- Discuss assessment and nursing management of the postpartal family.

- Delineate the nursing responsibilities for client education about various newborn-feeding methods.

- Discuss the concept of the fourth trimester as it relates to the provision of nursing care for the postpartal family.

The *puerperium* (postpartum) may be described as that period of time during which the body adjusts, both physically and psychologically, to the process of childbearing. By definition, it begins immediately after delivery and proceeds for approximately 6 weeks or until the body has completed its adjustment and has returned to a near prepregnant state. Some have referred to the puerperium as "the fourth trimester," and whereas the time span does not necessarily cover 3 months, this terminology demonstrates the idea of continuity.

Postpartum does not occur as an isolated period and is significantly influenced by the processes that have preceded it. During pregnancy the body adjusted gradually to the physical changes, but now it is forced to respond more rapidly. The method of delivery and circumstances associated with the delivery alter the speed with which the body reacts. Changes in body image and assumption of new roles often influence the outcome and ultimate adaptation to childbearing. Nursing interventions during postpartum must take into account a history of the total process and reactions of all family members to effect a healthy adjustment.

Certain premises form the basis for the provision of effective nursing care during the puerperium:

1. The best postpartal care is that provided with a family-centered focus and with minimal disruption of the family unit. This approach consolidates the family's resources and enhances an early and smooth adjustment to the newborn by all family members.

2. Establishing a normative base for the physiologic as well as psychologic adaptations required during the postpartal period allows for early recognition of alterations and subsequent early intervention. Communicat-

ing this knowledge to the family facilitates their adjustment.

3. Emphasis in providing care is focused on assessment of the individual's needs and consideration of factors that could influence the outcome or nursing requirements. Nursing interventions are then planned to accomplish specific goals. It should be remembered that needs overlap, as does nursing intervention, so that one need should not be seen as being isolated from other needs.

PUERPERAL PHYSICAL AND PSYCHOLOGIC ADAPTATIONS

Comprehensive nursing assessment is first based on a sound understanding of the normal anatomic and physiologic processes of the puerperium.

Reproductive Organs

INVOLUTION OF UTERUS

Immediately following the expulsion of the placenta, the uterus contracts firmly to the size of a large grapefruit, reducing uterine size by over one-half. The fundus can be located by observation and palpation approximately halfway between the symphysis pubis and the umbilicus and is situated in the midline (Figure 27–1). The walls of the contracted uterus are in close proximity and measure approximately 4 cm $\times$ 5 cm each. In contrast to the dusky color of the congested pregnant uterus, the puerperal uterus appears more ischemic due to the compression of the uterine

901

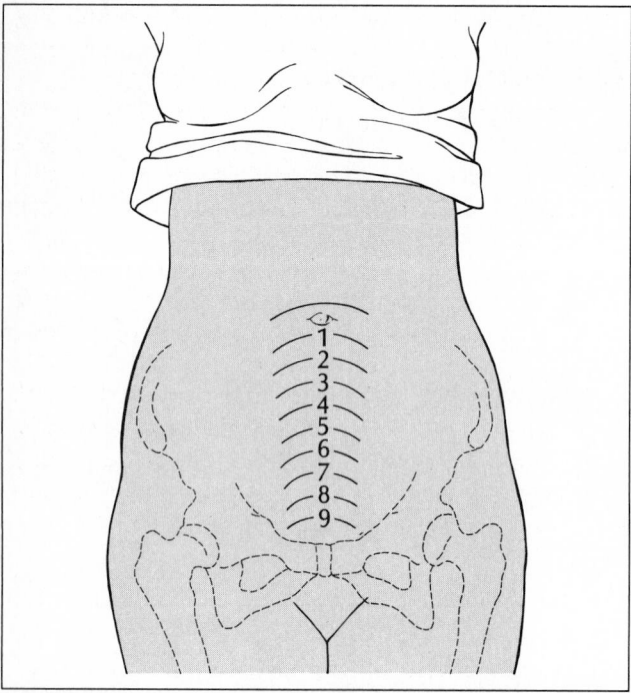

Figure 27-1 Involution of the uterus. The height of the fundus decreases about one finger breadth (approximately 1 cm) each day.

vessels by the myometrium. Within 12 hours after delivery the fundus of the uterus rises to the level of the umbilicus or one finger breadth (1.0 cm) above the umbilicus. If the uterus is higher than one finger breadth or is deviated from the midline and is boggy, the most probable cause of its displacement is a distended urinary bladder. Because the uterine ligaments are still stretched, the uterus can easily be moved by the full bladder. The uterus should be evaluated immediately after emptying the bladder and the change in height and position recorded. On each succeeding postpartal day the fundus should descend into the pelvis approximately one finger breadth. If the mother is breast-feeding, the involution of the uterus is facilitated by the release of oxytocin from the posterior pituitary as a response to suckling, and the uterus may descend more rapidly into the pelvis.

After delivery the uterus remains about the same size for 1-2 days and then begins to atrophy so rapidly that within 2 weeks postpartum, the fundus becomes a pelvic organ and is no longer palpable abdominally (Pritchard and MacDonald, 1980). Barring complications such as infection or retained secundines, the uterus approximates the nonpregnant size by 5-6 weeks. Changes in the weight of the uterus are equally dramatic. Although it weighs 1000-1200 g at term, the uterus decreases to 500 g at 1 week, 300 g at 2 weeks, and 100 g after the third week (Pritchard and MacDonald, 1980). This reduction in weight is not

due to a decreased number of muscle cells but occurs because the individual cells become thinner. With the dramatic decrease in the levels of circulatory estrogen and progesterone following placental separation, the uterine cells atrophy, and the hyperplasia of pregnancy begins to reverse. Proteolytic enzymes are released, and macrophages migrate to the uterus to promote autolysis (self-digestion). Protein material in the uterine wall is broken down and absorbed. Thus the process is basically one of cell size reduction rather than a radical decrease in cell number. The term "involution" is used to describe the rapid reduction in size and the return of the uterus to a normal condition similar to its nulliparous state.

Following separation of the placenta, the decidua of the uterus is irregular, jagged, and varied in thickness. The spongy layer of the decidua is cast off as lochia, and the basal layer of the decidua remains in the uterus to become differentiated into two layers within the first 48-72 hours after delivery. The outermost layer becomes necrotic and is sloughed off in the lochia. The layer closest to the myometrium contains the fundi of the uterine endometrial glands, and these glands lay the foundation for the new endometrium. Except at the placental site, the endometrium is formed by the proliferation of the fundi of the endometrial glands and of the stroma from the interglandular connective tissue (Pritchard and MacDonald, 1980). This process is completed in approximately 3 weeks.

Involution of the placental site follows a similar process and is generally thought to take 6 weeks for completion. Following separation, the placental site contracts to an area about 8-9 cm in diameter that appears raised and irregular. Bleeding from the larger uterine vessels is controlled by compression of the retracted uterine muscle fibers. The placental site consists of multiple thrombosed vascular sinusoids that are treated by the body as any other vascular clot. Some of these vessels are eventually obliterated and replaced by new vessels with smaller lumens (Greenhill and Friedman, 1974).

Rather than forming a fibrous scar in the decidua, the placental site heals by a process of exfoliation. This process consists of the undermining of the site by the growth of the endometrial tissue both from the margins of the site and from the fundi of the endometrial glands left in the basal layer of the site. The infarcted superficial tissue then becomes necrotic and is sloughed off.

Exfoliation is one of the most important aspects of involution in an otherwise unremarkable postpartal course for two reasons:

1. If the healing of the placental site were to leave a fibrous scar, the area available for future implantation would be limited, as would the number of possible pregnancies.

2. Failure of the placental site to undergo normal involution may result in late puerperal (delayed postpartum)

hemorrhage or subinvolution, which is characterized by persistent lochia, failure of the uterus to decrease in size progressively, lack of uterine tone, and painless fresh bleeding.

Some of the factors that retard uterine involution are prolonged labor, anesthesia or excessive analgesia, difficult delivery, grandmultiparity, a full bladder, and incomplete expulsion of the products of conception. Some factors that enhance involution include an uncomplicated labor and delivery, complete expulsion of the products of conception, breast-feeding, and early ambulation.

It is necessary to determine not only location but also consistency of the uterus, for it is the state of uterine contraction that controls bleeding, preventing hemorrhage. Following delivery the uterus should be palpated at frequent intervals: every 15 minutes times 4; every 30 minutes times 2; every hour times 2, then every 8 hours to maintain firm consistency and to evaluate the rate of involution of the uterus. Care should be taken not to overmassage, which tires the muscle, resulting in atony. The client is instructed and encouraged to gently massage the uterus at intervals to enhance uterine contraction.

The vaginally delivered client presents little difficulty for palpation of the uterus, but modifications are required for cesarean clients. Often with abdominal dressings it becomes difficult to determine the position of the fundus. If a vertical skin incision is made, firmness and position may be determined by gently palpating on each side of the incision. With the cesarean client it is essential to observe the amount of lochia to assess for relaxation of the uterus.

An oxytocic agent such as 0.2 mg methylergonovine maleate (Methergine) may be administered orally every 4 hours for the first 24–72 hours postpartum as a prophylactic measure against postpartal hemorrhage. Currently, routine use of oxytocic agents is less common. Oxytocic agents may be ordered for clients who are at risk for involution problems, such as those with prolonged labor, intrapartal hemorrhage, or overdistention of the uterus during pregnancy. (See Drug Guide—Methergine, below).

If oxytocin (Pitocin) is given after delivery, caution should be exercised. With prolonged intravenous administration, water intoxication may occur. Once the medications are discontinued, the client should be monitored closely for relaxation of the uterus.

LOCHIA

One of the most unique capabilities of the uterus is the ability to rid itself of the debris remaining after delivery. This discharge is termed lochia and is classified according to its appearance and contents. *Lochia rubra* takes its name from the dark red color of the discharge. It occurs for the first 2–3 days and contains epithelial cells, erythrocytes, leukocytes, shreds of the decidua, and occasionally fetal meconium, lanugo, and vernix caseosa. Lochia should

---

Drug Guide—Methylergonovine Maleate (Methergine)

OVERVIEW OF OBSTETRIC ACTION

Methylergonovine maleate is an ergot alkaloid that stimulates smooth muscle. Because the smooth muscle of the uterus is especially sensitive to this drug, it is used postpartally to stimulate the uterus to contract. This contraction clamps off uterine blood vessels and prevents hemorrhage. In addition, the drug has a vasoconstrictive effect on all blood vessels, especially on the larger arteries. This may result in hypertension, particularly in a woman whose blood pressure is already elevated.

ROUTE, DOSAGE, AND FREQUENCY

Methergine has a rapid onset of action and may be given intramuscularly, orally, or intravenously.

Usual IM dose: 0.2 mg following delivery of the placenta. The dose may be repeated every 2–4 hours if necessary.

Usual oral dose: 0.2 mg every 4 hours (six doses).

Usual IV dose: Because the adverse effects of Methergine are far more severe with IV administration, this route is seldom used. If Methergine is given intravenously, the rate should *not* exceed 0.2 mg/min and the client's blood pressure should be monitored continuously.

MATERNAL CONTRAINDICATIONS

Pregnancy, induction of labor, hepatic or renal disease, threatened spontaneous abortion, uterine sepsis, cardiac disease, hypertension, and obliterative vascular disease contraindicate this drug's use (Loebl and Spratto, 1980).

MATERNAL SIDE EFFECTS

Hypertension (particularly when administered IV), nausea, vomiting, headache, bradycardia, dizziness, tinnitus, abdominal cramps, palpitations, dyspnea, chest pain, and allergic reactions may be noted.

EFFECTS ON FETUS/NEONATE

Because Methergine has a long duration of action and can thus produce tetanic contractions it should never be used during pregnancy as it may result in fetal trauma or death.

NURSING CONSIDERATIONS

1. Monitor fundal height and consistency and the amount and character of the lochia.
2. Assess the blood pressure before administration.
3. Observe for adverse effects or symptoms of ergot toxicity.

not contain large clots; if it does, the cause should be discovered without delay. *Lochia serosa* follows from approximately the third until the tenth day. It is characterized by a pinkish color and serosanguineous consistency. It is composed of serous exudate (hence the name), shreds of degenerating decidua, erythrocytes, leukocytes, cervical mucus, and numerous microorganisms.

Gradually the blood cell component decreases, and a creamy or yellowish discharge persists for an additional week or two. This final discharge is termed *lochia alba* and is composed primarily of leukocytes; large, irregular round or spindle-shaped mononucleated decidual cells; both flat and cylindrical epithelial cells; fat; cervical mucus; cholesterol crystals; and bacteria. When the lochia stops, the cervix is considered closed, and chances of infection ascending from the vagina to the uterus decrease.

Lochia, similar to menstrual discharge, has a musty, stale odor that is not offensive. Microorganisms are always present in the vaginal lochia, and by the second day following delivery the uterus is contaminated with the vaginal bacteria. Researchers speculate that infection does not develop because the organisms involved are relatively nonvirulent. In addition, by the time the bacteria reach the raw, exposed surface of the uterus the process of granulation has begun, forming a protective barrier (Greenhill and Friedman, 1974). Any foul smell to the lochia or used peri-pad suggests infection and the need for prompt assessment.

The total volume of lochia discharged is approximately 240–270 mL (8–9 oz) and a gradual reduction in volume occurs. Discharge is heavier in the morning than at night, but whether this difference is real or apparent is unclear. A logical explanation would be that the recumbent position at night would tend to cause pooling of the lochia in the vagina and uterus, and this accumulation would subsequently be discharged when the upright position is achieved. The amount of lochia may also be increased by exertion or breast-feeding.

Evaluation of lochia is necessary not only to determine the presence of hemorrhage but also to assess uterine involution. The type, amount, and consistency of lochia determine the state of healing of the placental site, and a progressive change from bright red at delivery to dark red to pink to white/clear discharge should be observed. Persistent discharge of lochia rubra or a return to lochia rubra indicates subinvolution or late postpartal hemorrhage (see Chapter 29).

Caution should be exercised in the evaluation of bleeding immediately after delivery. The continuous seepage of blood is more consistent with cervical or vaginal lacerations and may be effectively diagnosed when the bleeding is evaluated in conjunction with the consistency of the uterus. Lacerations should be suspected if the uterus is firm, of expected size, and if no clots can be expressed.

CERVICAL CHANGES

Following delivery the cervix is spongy, flabby, formless, and may appear bruised. The external os has a markedly irregular outline suggestive of multiple small lacerations. The os closes slowly. It admits two fingers easily for a few days following delivery, but by the end of the first week only a fingertip opening remains.

The shape of the external os is permanently changed following the first childbearing. The characteristic dimple-like os of the nullipara changes to the lateral slit (fish-mouth) os of the multipara. After significant cervical laceration or several lacerations, the cervix may appear lopsided.

VAGINAL CHANGES

Careful inspection following delivery demonstrates that the vagina appears edematous and may be bruised. Small superficial lacerations may be evident, and the rugae have been obliterated. The hymen has been lacerated in several places. The apparent bruising of the vagina is due to pelvic congestion, and resolution takes place rapidly following the birth. The torn edges of the hymen do not reanastomose but rather stay separate and heal along the torn edges. These small tags of hymen are the carunculae myrtiformes and indicate a previous vaginal birth.

The size of the vagina decreases and vaginal rugae begin to return by 3 weeks. This facilitates the gradual return to smaller but not nulliparous dimensions. Tone and contractability of the vaginal orifice may be improved by perineal tightening exercises, which may begin soon after delivery and should be incorporated into the exercise regimen. The labia majora and labia minora are more flabby in the woman who has borne a child than in the nullipara.

PERINEAL CHANGES

During the early postpartal period the soft tissue in and around the perineum may appear edematous with some bruising. If an episiotomy is present, the edges should be approximated. Occasionally ecchymosis occurs, and this may delay healing.

RECURRENCE OF OVULATION AND MENSTRUATION

It has been generally thought that menstruation recurs in non–breast-feeding women within 6–8 weeks after delivery. However, it has been demonstrated that about 40% of non–breast-feeding women resume menstruation in 6 weeks. About 65% resume menstruation by the end of the twelfth week, and 90% within 24 weeks after delivery. At 12 weeks after delivery about 45% of lactating primiparas are menstruating. In nonnursing mothers approximately 50% ovulate during the first cycle, while 80% of the nursing mothers have one or more anovulatory cycles before the first ovulatory one. Research has suggested ovarian, pituitary, and possibly hypothalamic suppression as potential causes of the characteristic infertility of nursing mothers. Currently, however, the exact mechanisms producing this effect remain unclear (Danforth, 1982).

Abdomen

The peritoneum, if it were visible during the puerperium, would appear to drape the lower part of the uterus in uneven folds. These folds usually disappear during the first several days. Likewise, the uterine ligaments (notably the round and broad ligaments) are stretched, but they require a much longer time to recover. The abdominal wall itself has also been stretched and will appear loose and somewhat flabby for a time. Within 2–3 months, with exercise, abdominal muscle tone will improve greatly. In the grandmultipara, in the woman in which overdistention of the abdomen has occurred, or in the woman with poor muscle tone before pregnancy, the abdomen may fail to regain good tone and may remain somewhat flabby. Diastasis recti abdominis is a separation of the recti muscle, which may occur with pregnancy, especially in women with poor abdominal muscle tone. In the event of diastasis, part of the abdominal wall has no muscular support but is formed only by skin, subcutaneous fat, attenuated fascia, and peritoneum. Diastasis recti abdominis and poor muscle tone respond well to abdominal exercises. Improvement is also dependent on the physical condition of the mother, the total number of pregnancies, and the type and amount of physical exercise. Exercise may begin immediately after a vaginal delivery and within a few weeks following a cesarean delivery. See p. 922 for a discussion of postpartal exercises. If rectus muscle tone is not regained, adequate support may be lacking in the event of future pregnancies. This may result in a pendulous abdomen and increased maternal backache.

The striae (stretch marks), which occurred as a result of stretching and rupture of the elastic fibers of the skin, are red to purple at delivery. These gradually fade and after a time appear as silver or white streaks.

Lactation

During pregnancy, breast development in preparation for lactation results from the influence of both estrogen and progesterone. After delivery, the interplay of maternal hormones leads to the establishment of milk production. This process is described in detail in the section on breast-feeding, p. 927.

Gastrointestinal System

Hunger following delivery is common, and the mother may enjoy a light meal. Frequently she is quite thirsty and will drink large amounts of fluid as soon as she is permitted to do so. She may continue to drink large amounts of water to replace water lost in labor, in the urine, and through perspiration.

The bowel tends to be sluggish after delivery due to decreased muscle tone in the intestine, and decreased intraabdominal pressure. In addition, the pain from an elective episiotomy (especially a mediolateral), any lacerations, and hemorrhoids encourages women to delay elimination for fear of increasing their pain or in the belief that their stitches will be torn by the strong bearing-down pressure. In refusing or delaying the bowel movement, the client may cause increased constipation and more pain when elimination finally occurs.

Bowel elimination may become a problem after the client resumes a diet if the woman has received a cleansing enema as a part of the admission procedure in labor and has not received solid foods while in labor. Fluids and solid food are delayed for the cesarean client, until peristalsis is resumed. Generally, clear liquids are begun by the day after surgery (first postoperative day) and advances to solid food by the second or third postoperative day. It may take a few days for the bowel to regain tone. Stool softeners may be ordered to increase bulk and moisture in the fecal material and to facilitate more comfortable and complete evacuation. Constipation is avoided to prevent pressure on sutures that may increase discomfort. Encouraging ambulation, forcing fluids, and providing fresh fruits and roughage in the diet enhance bowel elimination and assist the client in reestablishing her normal bowel pattern.

Urinary Tract

An increased bladder capacity and a decreased sensitivity to fluid pressure, swelling and bruising of the tissues around the urethra, decreased sensation of bladder filling, and inability to void in the recumbent position put the puerperal woman at risk for overdistention, incomplete emptying, and buildup of residual urine. In addition, women who have had conductive anesthesia have inhibited neural functioning of the bladder and are more susceptible to bladder complications.

Urinary output increases during the early postpartal period (first 12–24 hours) due to puerperal diuresis. The kidneys must eliminate an estimated 2000–3000 mL of extracellular fluid associated with a normal pregnancy. With eclampsia and preclampsia, hypertension, and diabetes, an even greater fluid retention is experienced, and postpartal diuresis is accordingly increased.

Bladder elimination presents an immediate problem. If stasis exists, chances increase for urinary tract infection because of bacteriuria and the presence of dilated ureters and renal pelves, which persist for about 6 weeks after delivery (Danforth, 1982). A full bladder may also increase the tendency of relaxation of the uterus by displacing the uterus and interfering with its contractility, leading to hemorrhage.

The postpartal client should be encouraged to void every 4–6 hours. A careful monitoring of intake and output should be maintained and the bladder should be assessed for distention until the client demonstrates complete emptying of the bladder with each voiding. The nurse may employ techniques to facilitate voiding, such as helping the woman out of bed to void or pouring warm water on the perineum to promote relaxation of the perineum. Catheterization is required when the bladder is distended and the woman cannot void or if no voiding has occurred in 8 hours. The technique must be gentle, and when the catheter is removed, accurate measuring of the amount of urine is essential until voiding is no longer a problem. The cesarean birth client may have an indwelling catheter inserted prophylactically. The same considerations should be made in evaluating bladder emptying once the catheter is removed.

Hematuria, resulting from bladder trauma, may occasionally occur after delivery. If hematuria occurs in the second or third postpartal week, there may be a bladder infection. Acetone may be present in the urine of diabetics or of clients with prolonged labor and dehydration. Proteinuria occurs in about 40% of women following labor and may persist for about 3 days (Greenhill and Friedman, 1974). Proteinuria may be associated with an infectious process (cystitis, pyelitis) and should be further evaluated. A urine specimen contaminated with lochia may be the cause of proteinuria, so any specimen should be obtained as a midstream or a catheterized specimen. The preeclamptic patient may demonstrate proteinuria for a week or more following delivery.

In the absence of infection, the dilated ureters and renal pelves will return to prepregnant size by the end of the sixth week.

Vital Signs

During the postpartal period, with the exception of the first 24 hours, the client should be afebrile and normotensive. A temperature of 100.4F (38C) may occur after delivery as a result of the exertion and dehydration of labor. Infection must be considered in the woman with a temperature of 100.4F or above on any two of the first ten postpartal days, excluding the first 24 hours, if the temperature is taken at least four times per day.

Blood pressure readings should remain stable following delivery. A decrease may indicate physiologic readjustment to decreased intrapelvic pressure, or it may be related to uterine hemorrhage. Blood pressure elevations, especially when accompanied by headache, suggest preeclampsia, and the client should be evaluated further.

Puerperal bradycardia with rates of 50–70 beats per minute commonly occurs during the first 6–10 days of the postpartal period. It may be related to decreased cardiac strain, the decreased vascular bed following delivery, contraction of the uterus, and increased stroke volume. Tachycardia occurs less frequently and is related to increased blood loss or difficult, prolonged labor and delivery.

Blood Values

The blood values should return to the prepregnant state by the end of the postpartal period. Pregnancy-associated activation of coagulation factors may continue for variable amounts of time. This condition, in conjunction with trauma, immobility, or sepsis, predisposes the patient to development of thromboembolism. Plasma fibrinogen is maintained at pregnancy levels for a week, accounting for the higher sedimentation rate observed in the early postpartum period.

Other hemodynamic changes include leukocytosis with elevated white blood counts of 15,000–20,000, primarily due to an increased number of granulocytes. Eosinophils are rarely found, and lymphocytes may be reduced.

Blood loss averages 200–500 mL with a vaginal delivery and 700–1000 mL with cesarean birth. Because rapid red blood cell destruction does not occur following delivery, the decrease in numbers occurs gradually according to their life span. Hemoglobin and erythrocyte values vary during the early puerperium, but they should approximate or exceed prelabor values within 2–6 weeks as normal concentrations are reached. As extracellular fluid is excreted, hemoconcentration occurs, with a concomitant rise in hematocrit. A drop in values indicates an abnormal blood loss. A convenient rule of thumb: A 4-point drop in hematocrit equals 1 pint of blood loss.

Weight Loss

An initial weight loss of 10–12 lb occurs as a result of the delivery of infant, placenta, and amniotic fluid. Puerperal diuresis accounts for the loss of an additional 5 lb during the early puerperium. By the sixth to eighth week after delivery, the client has returned to approximately her prepregnant weight if she has gained the average 25–30 pounds.

Postpartal Chill

Frequently the mother experiences a shaking chill immediately after delivery, which is related to a nervous response or to vasomotor changes. If not followed by fever, it is clinically innocuous but uncomfortable for the client. Many hospitals cover the woman with warmed bath blankets to alleviate the chill. The mother may also find a warm beverage helpful. Later in the puerperium, chills and fever indicate infection and require further evaluation.

Postpartal Diaphoresis

The elimination of excess fluid and waste products via the skin during the puerperium produces greatly increased perspiration. Diaphoretic episodes frequently occur at night, and the client may awaken drenched with perspiration. The practice of covering the mattress with a protective plastic pad also contributes to the client's discomfort. This perspiration is not significant clinically, but the mother should be protected from chilling. The plastic mattress pad should be covered with both a pad and a sheet to decrease skin contact, and the bed linens and gown should be changed if diaphoresis occurs. Comfort is also enhanced with a daily shower.

Afterpains

Afterpains more commonly occur in multiparas than primiparas and are caused by intermittent uterine contractions. Although the uterus of the primipara usually remains consistently contracted, the lost tone of the multiparous uterus results in alternate contraction and relaxation. This phenomenon also occurs if the uterus has been markedly distended, as with multiple pregnancies or hydramnios, or if clots or placental fragments were retained. These afterpains may cause the mother severe discomfort for 2–3 days following delivery. The administration of oxytocic agents stimulates uterine contraction and increases the discomfort of the afterpains. Because oxytocin is released when the infant suckles, breast-feeding also increases the severity of the afterpains. The nursing mother may find it helpful to take a mild analgesic approximately one hour before feeding her infant. An analgesic is also helpful at bedtime if the afterpains interfere with the mother's rest.

Puerperal Psychologic Adaptations

Two major stages of emotional adjustment occur in the puerperium. These stages represent a reversal of the inward focusing that characterized labor. During that time the mother's energies focused increasingly inward as she drew on her personal strength to cope with the stress of labor. In the postpartal period, the focus turns outward from herself to her child, husband, other family members, and then to those in the immediate environment. Slowly she resumes her normal role and functions and also accepts the new ones resulting from the birth of her child.

Rubin (1961) describes the first period of adjustment as the *taking-in phase*. This period, lasting 2–3 days, is marked by maternal passivity and dependence. The mother follows suggestions, is hesitant about making decisions, and is still somewhat preoccupied with her own needs. Food and sleep are a major focus for her. Mealtime is eagerly awaited and food-related discussions are common

with the mothers. During this phase the new mother is talkative but passive.

The *taking-hold phase* begins on about the second or third day after delivery. The mother has had time to relive her experiences, to adjust to her new life, to rest, and to recover from childbirth. Now she is ready to resume control of her life. Initially this phase involves control of her bodily functions. She is concerned about bowel and bladder elimination. If she is breast-feeding, she may be concerned about the quality of her milk and her ability to successfully nurse her child. She requires constant reassurance that she is performing well. This desire to succeed is also apparent in concerns about her ability to be a "good" mother. If the baby is sleepy during a feeding or spits up, the mother may view this occurrence as a personal failure. The nurse who is extremely proficient in handling the child arouses feelings of inadequacy, which can be exhausting and demoralizing for the mother.

The "postpartum blues" are a transient period of depression that frequently occurs during the puerperium. It may be manifested by anorexia, tearfulness, difficulty in sleeping, and a "let-down" feeling. This depression frequently occurs during hospitalization, although it may occur at home, too. Ego adjustment and hormonal changes are both thought to be causal factors, although fatigue, discomfort, stimulation overload, or stimulation deprivation may also play a part.

POSTPARTAL NURSING ASSESSMENT

Comprehensive care is based on a thorough assessment, with identification of individual needs or potential problems.

Risk Factors

The emphasis on ongoing assessment and client education during the puerperium is designed to meet the needs of the childbearing family and to detect and treat possible complications. Table 27–1 identifies factors that may place the new mother at risk during the postpartal period. The nurse uses this knowledge during the assessment and is particularly alert for possible complications that may occur in an individual because of identified risk factors.

Physical Assessment

Several principles should be remembered in preparing for and completing the assessment of the postpartal client. First, as in any assessment, select the time that will provide the most accurate data. Palpating the fundus when the woman has a full bladder will not result in a true indica-

Table 27-1   Postpartal High-Risk Factors

Factors	Maternal implications
Preeclampsia-eclampsia	↑ Blood pressure
	↑ CNS irritability
	↑ Need for bedrest → ↑ risk thrombophlebitis
Diabetes	Need for insulin regulation
	Episodes of hypoglycemia or hyperglycemia
	↓ Healing
Cardiac disease	↑ Maternal exhaustion
Cesarean birth	↑ Healing needs
	↑ Pain from incision
	↑ Risk infection
	↑ Length of hospitalization
Overdistention of uterus (multiple gestation, hydramnios)	↑ Risk hemorrhage
	↑ Risk anemia
	↑ Stretching of abdominal muscles
	↑ Incidence and severity of afterpains
Abruptio placentae — placenta previa	Hemorrhage → anemia
	↓ Uterine contractility after delivery → ↑ infection risk
Precipitous labor (<3 hours)	↑ Risk lacerations to birth canal → hemorrhage
Prolonged labor	Exhaustion
	↑ Risk hemorrhage
	Nutritional and fluid depletion
	↑ Bladder atony and/or trauma
Difficult delivery	Exhaustion
	↑ Risk perineal lacerations
	↑ Risk hematomas
	↑ Risk hemorrhage → anemia
Extended period of time in stirrups at delivery	↑ Risk thrombophlebitis
Retained placenta	↑ Risk hemorrhage
	↑ Risk infection

tion of involution, and assessing the condition of the episiotomy following a sitz bath may produce data that would indicate complications. Second, an explanation of the purpose of regular assessment should be given to the client. Third, the woman should be as relaxed as possible, and the procedures should be accomplished as gently and smoothly as possible to avoid unnecessary discomfort. Examining the client who is experiencing afterpains only intensifies her pain, increases tension of muscles, and possibly necessitates medicinal relief. Finally, the data obtained during the assessment should be recorded and reported as clearly as possible.

A sample assessment form (Figure 27–2) has been included to assist the student nurse in organizing and charting the postpartal physical assessment. Staff nurses may want to devise a similar format as part of the client's hospital chart to assure continuity and quality of care. Nurses' notes would then concentrate on aspects of care: physical, such as the progression of involution and the establish-

ment of lactation; maternal–infant bonding; parenting behaviors; and teaching activities and return demonstrations.

While the nurse is performing the physical assessment, she should also be teaching the client. Assessing the breast provides an optimal time to discuss milk formation, the letdown reflex, and breast self-examination. Mothers are very receptive to instruction on postpartal abdominal tightening exercises when the nurse assesses the client's fundal height and diastasis. The assessment also provides an excellent time to teach her about the body's physical and anatomic changes postpartally as well as danger signs to report.

BREASTS

Beginning with the breasts, the nurse should first assess the fit and support provided by the bra. A properly fitting bra provides support to heavy breasts, thereby promoting maternal comfort. It also helps maintain the shape of the breasts by limiting undue stretching of connective tissue

NAME: _____   DATE: _____

ROOM: _____   POSTPARTUM DAY: _____   FEEDING METHOD _____

1. BREASTS
   a. General Appearance _____
   b. Nipples _____

2. DIASTASIS Rectus abdominis
   a. Length (cm) _____
   b. Width (cm) _____

3. FUNDUS
   a. Height in finger breadths in relationship
      to umbilicus _____
   b. Position _____
   c. Tenderness _____
      (1) with touch _____
      (2) constant _____

4. LOCHIA
   a. Amount _____
   b. Color _____
   c. Consistency _____
   d. Odor _____

5. PERINEUM
   a. Intact _____
   b. Episiotomy _____
      (1) type _____
      (2) healing _____
         (a) REEDA scale _____
   c. Hygiene _____

6. CVA TENDERNESS _____

7. HOMAN'S SIGN _____
   a. Superficial varicosities _____

8. BOWEL AND BLADDER HABITS _____

_____

9. SLEEP PATTERNS _____

_____

10. MENTAL OUTLOOK _____

_____

11. NUTRITIONAL INTAKE _____

_____

12. ADJUSTMENT TO INFANT _____

_____

13. EVALUATION _____

_____

_____

_____

_____

_____

_____

_____

_____

_____

_____

Figure 27–2 Postpartal physical assessment.

and ligaments. If the mother is breast-feeding, the straps of the bra should be cloth, not elastic, and they should be easily adjustable. The back should be wide and should have at least three rows of hooks to adjust for fit. Under-wires are not necessary unless the breast is large (C cup or larger). Traditional nursing bras have a fixed inner cup and a separate half cup or flap that can be unhooked to allow for breast-feeding while continuing the support of the breast. Some companies have designed the nursing flap to open and close with a plastic snap rather than the traditional loop and hook. Some women find the snap much easier and quicker to operate.

Although one brand should not be recommended, several brands of bras can be purchased by the hospital and made available as demonstrators so the woman can compare the benefits of one bra against another before investing in a brand and finding out that she would have preferred another had she known about it. Some women prefer a standard bra that hooks in front, and if the breast is not heavy this is acceptable. It is wise for mothers to purchase a nursing bra with a cup a size too large. The breast increases in size with milk production, and a bra that fits well during pregnancy will be too tight during lactation.

Once the bra has been assessed, it should be removed so that the breasts may be examined. First, the nurse should note the size and shape of the breasts and any abnormalities, reddened areas, or engorgement. One breast is usually slightly larger than the other, which is most noticeable by observing the placement of the nipples. Next, the nurse should palpate the breasts lightly, checking for heat, edema, engorgement, and caking (swelling of the lobules due to a blockage of the duct), which usually begins in the upper outer quadrant. The mother should be asked whether she has any tenderness or pain, and if so, that area should be examined carefully. The nipples should be checked for fissures, cracks and soreness. If the mother says she has problems with inverted nipples, her nipples may also be checked for erectility. This check is done by placing the thumb and first finger on each side of the nipple and gently pulling the nipple out from the breast. When released, the nipple and areola should show some signs of erectility. The procedure may need to be performed several times before results are produced.

The nursing mother needs to be reminded to keep the nipples supple, with the use of unscented lanolin-based creams, and to keep them well cleansed, avoiding a build-up of secretions that could irritate the nipples. (See discussion of nipple care, p. 931). The nonnursing mother should be assessed for evidence of breast discomfort and appropriate measures taken if necessary. (See discussion of lactation suppression in the nonnursing mother on p. 925.)

ABDOMEN AND FUNDUS

Before examination of the abdomen, the client should void. This practice assures that a full bladder is not causing any uterine atony; if atony is present, other causes must be investigated. The nurse should determine the relationship of the fundus to the umbilicus. Because of the relaxation of the abdominal wall, the uterus is usually clearly outlined, except in the most obese clients. The nurse should gently place one hand on the lower segment of the uterus to provide support and then place the first finger of the other hand on top of the fundus and should measure in finger breadths the relationship to the umbilicus. If the fundus is more than one finger breadth in either direction, the nurse should place additional fingers on the abdomen (Figure 27–3). Fundal height is recorded in finger breadths: that is, "2 FB ↓ U; 1 FB ↑ U." Once fundal height has been assessed, the nurse should check whether the uterus is deviated from the midline and should then assess the tone of the uterus. Usually the nurse has already ascertained

Figure 27–3 Measurement of descent of fundus. The fundus is located two finger breadths below the umbilicus.

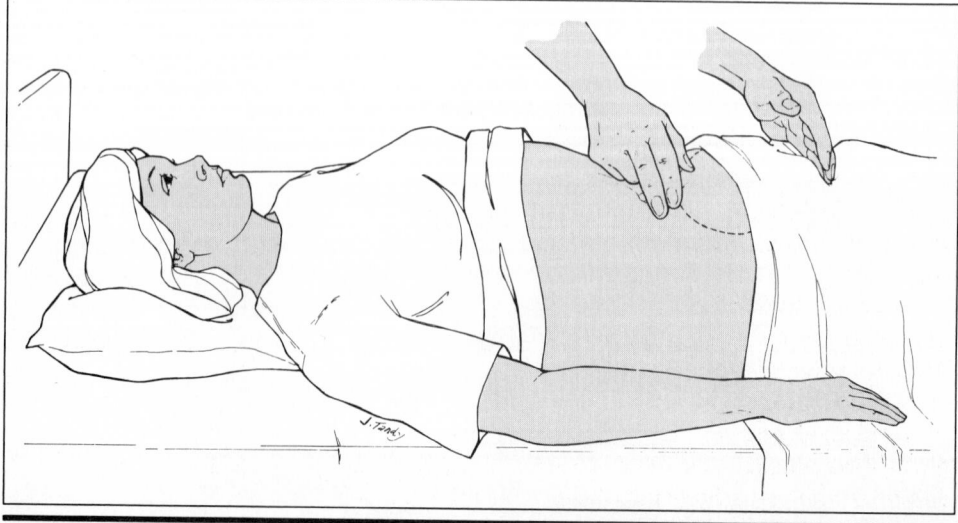

uterine tone when first palpating the fundus. If not, the fingers of the examining hand are placed gently on the fundus.

A well-contracted uterus feels as firm as the uterus does during a strong labor contraction. If handled gently, the uterus should not be tender. Excessive pain during postpartal examination should alert the nurse to possible genital tract infection. If the uterus is not firm, the nurse should gently massage the fundus with the fingertips of the examining hand, then assess the results. If the uterus becomes firm, the chart should read "Uterus: boggy → firm c̄ light massage." A good habit for the nurse to develop during the postpartal examination is to have the woman lie on her back with head comfortably elevated and legs relaxed. Then the nurse can release the peri-pad to observe the results of uterine massage based on the amount of expelled blood. Occasionally, oxytocic agents such as ergonovine maleate (Ergotrate) and methylergonovine maleate (Methergine) are administered postpartally to maintain uterine contraction and prevent hemorrhage. (See Drug Guide—Methergine, p. 903.)

The boggy uterus that does not contract with light, gentle massage may need more vigorous massage. Be sure to assess the amount and character of any expelled blood obtained while massaging the fundus. The nursing care involved with a client who has postpartal uterine atony is to:

1. Reevaluate for full bladder; if the bladder is full, have client void.

2. Question the client on her bleeding history since delivery or last examination. How heavy does her flow seem? Has she passed any clots? How frequently has she changed pads?

3. For the nursing mother, put the newborn to the mother's breast to stimulate oxytocin production.

4. Reassess the fundus; if the fundus is still boggy, alert the certified nurse-midwife or physician.

In the majority of clients the uterus will be firm; however, it is important to keep in mind the complications that cause postpartal uterine atony and the effect on the client of a postpartal hemorrhage. The alert nurse will observe, assess, plan, and implement interventions quickly.

Following the uterine assessment and prior to assessing the lochia, the nurse should examine for diastasis recti. The separation in the rectus muscle is evaluated according to its length and width. The student nurse should use a tape measure that measures in centimeters; the skilled practitioner can accurately estimate the distance visually. (A disposable paper tape measure like the one used in the nursery for measuring newborns is preferred.) The separation is palpated first just below the umbilicus, and the width is ascertained. Then the separation is palpated for length toward the symphysis pubis and toward the xiphoid process. If palpation is difficult due to abdominal relax-

ation, the client is asked to lift her head unassisted by the nurse. This action contracts the rectus muscles and more clearly defines their edges.

Methods of charting these results vary from institution to institution. Some prefer recording the diastasis measured from the umbilicus down and then from the umbilicus up:

Diastasis: U ↓ 4 cm by 1 cm
              U ↑ 2 cm by 1 cm

Others prefer recording the entire length:

Diastasis: 6 cm by 1 cm

Either method is acceptable.

LOCHIA

The next aspect to be evaluated is the lochia, which is assessed for character, amount, odor, and the presence of clots. During the first 1–3 days the lochia should be dark red, similar in appearance to menstrual flow. A few small clots are normal and occur as a result of blood pooling in the vagina. However, the passage of numerous or large clots is abnormal, and the cause should immediately be investigated. After 2–3 days, the lochia appears more pinkish or serous.

Lochia should never exceed a moderate amount, such as four to eight peri-pads daily, with an average of six. However, because this is influenced by an individual woman's pad-changing practices, she should be questioned about the length of time the current pad has been in use, whether the amount is normal, and whether any clots were passed prior to this examination, such as during voiding. If heavy bleeding is reported but not seen, put a clean peri-pad on the client and check the pad in 1 hour. If the client needs to void before the hour is up, ask her to save the pad for your inspection. Usually the flow is moderate, but the client, who is comparing it to menstrual flow, may consider it heavy. If clots are reported but not seen, ask the client to save all pads with clots or not to flush the toilet if clots were expelled during urination. Clots and heavy bleeding may be caused by uterine atony or retained placental fragments and require further assessment. Because of the manipulation of the uterine cavity during cesarean delivery, women with such surgery have less lochia after the first 24 hours than mothers who deliver vaginally. Often they need wear no pad. Therefore, amounts of lochia that would be normal in vaginally delivered women are suspect in women who have undergone cesarean delivery.

The odor of the lochia is nonoffensive and never foul. If foul odor is present, so is an infection.

The amount of lochia is charted first, followed by character. For example:

• Lochia: moderate amount rubra
• Lochia: small rubra/serosa
• Lochia: scant/serosa

PERINEUM

The perineum is observed with the client lying in a Sims position, with the top leg positioned over the bottom leg. Either side is acceptable. The buttock is lifted to expose the perineum and anus (Figure 27–4). If the perineum has not been incised, it is charted as "Perineum: intact." If an episiotomy was performed or a laceration necessitated suturing, the wound is assessed. Davidson (1974) has developed a method of evaluating the episiotomy by identifying five components that indicate the state of healing. The REEDA method allows for a systematic evaluation of the episiotomy for Redness, Edema, Ecchymosis, Discharge, and Approximation (see Table 29–1). For example, the incision should be approximated, only slightly tender, and may have some edema from the time it is repaired to 12–24 hours later. After 24 hours some edema may still be present, but the skin edges should be "glued" together so that gentle pressure does not separate them. Gentle palpation should elicit minimal tenderness, and there should be no hardened areas suggesting infection. These observations provide good evidence that the episiotomy/laceration is healing normally. Ecchymosis interferes with normal healing, as does infection.

The nurse should next assess the state of any hemorrhoids present around the anus for size, number, and pain or tenderness. Some examples of charting for this portion of the postpartal assessment:

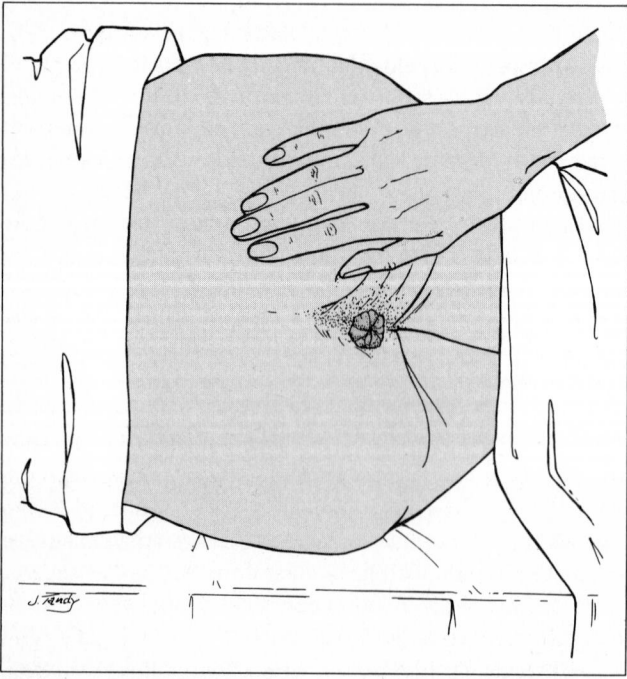

Figure 27–4 Intact perineum with hemorrhoids. Note how the examiner's hand raises the upper buttocks to fully expose the anal area.

- Perineum: intact, no hemorrhoids
- Perineum: episiotomy—skin edges approximated, slight edema; two medium-sized nontender hemorrhoids
- Perineum: laceration—nontender, nonedematous, well approximated; three large, swollen, painful hemorrhoids

In the cesarean birth client, the abdominal incision should be observed for any indications of infection. Foul odors associated with drainage from an abdominal or perineal incision indicate infection. Further observation of the incision for separation should also be made.

LOWER EXTREMITIES

Fewer than 1% of all postpartal clients develop thrombophlebitis and thromboembolic disease (Danforth, 1982). Women who are at increased risk in the postpartal period are those with dehydration, a traumatic delivery, postpartal hemorrhage, sepsis, and delivery by cesarean, and those who have received synthetic estrogens to suppress lactation (Barber and Graber, 1974).

If thrombophlebitis occurs, the most likely site will be in the woman's legs. To evaluate the client, her legs should be stretched out straight and should be relaxed. The foot is then grasped and sharply dorsiflexed. No discomfort or pain should be present. If pain is elicited, the nurse-midwife or physician is notified that the client has a positive Homan's sign. The pain is caused by inflammation of the vessel. The legs are also evaluated for edema. This may be done by comparing both legs, since usually only one leg is involved. Any areas of redness, tenderness, and increased skin temperature should also be noted.

Clients demonstrating signs of deep venous thrombosis or those considered high risk because of pelvic surgery or a history of venous thromboembolitic problems may be further evaluated using occlusive cuff impedance phlebography (IPG). (See Chapter 29 for additional discussion of this procedure.) Early ambulation is an important aspect in the prevention of thrombophlebitis. Most women are able to be up shortly after delivery. The cesarean birth client requires passive range of motion exercises until she is ambulating more freely.

VITAL SIGNS

Alterations in vital signs may be an indication of complications such as hemorrhage or infection. Blood pressure may be altered slightly as the blood volume peaks immediately after delivery, but this should not present significant problems for the client. Conversely, blood pressure may drop as a result of blood loss.

The pulse rate during the immediate postpartal period may be low but presents no cause for alarm. Rates of 56 beats/min are not unusual as the body attempts to adapt to the decreased pressures intraabdominally as well as to the reduction of the vascular bed with the contraction of the uterus. Pulse rates return to prepregnant norms very quickly unless complications arise.

Temperature elevations may be a sign of infection but must be carefully evaluated. The normal process of wound healing, as well as dehydration and breast engorgement, may also increase body temperature. Temperature elevation (less than 100.4F or 38C) from normal processes should last for only a few days and should not be associated with other clinical manifestations of infection.

Maternal risk for infections increases with the rise in invasive techniques for diagnosing and treating high-risk pregnancies, such as amniocentesis and fetal blood sampling. Gram negative pathogens are becoming more prominent as causative agents for infection. They are not as familiar as gram positive organisms, nor do they respond as effectively to the commonly used antibiotics. It is essential to evaluate temperature elevations in light of other symptomatology as well as in a careful review of history to identify factors such as premature rupture of membranes or prolonged labor, which might increase the incidence of infections in the genital tract.

NUTRITIONAL STATUS

Determination of postpartal nutritional status is based primarily on information provided by the mother and on direct assessment. During pregnancy the recommended daily dietary allowances call for increases in kilocalories, proteins, and most vitamins and minerals. After delivery, the nonnursing mother's dietary requirements return to prepregnancy levels (Food and Nutrition Board, 1980).

Visiting the mothers during mealtimes provides an opportunity for unobtrusive nutritional assessment. Which foods has a woman selected? Has she avoided fruits and vegetables? Is her diet mainly carbohydrates? Is her diet nutritionally sound? A comment focusing on a positive aspect of her meal selection may provide an opportunity for a discussion of nutrition. If the mother has a good understanding of nutritional principles, it is sufficient to advise her to reduce her daily caloric intake by about 300 kcal and to return to prepregnancy levels for other nutrients.

The dietitian should be informed of any mother whose cultural or religious beliefs require specific foods. Appropriate meals can then be prepared for her. Many women, especially those who gained excessively, are interested in losing weight after delivery. The dietitian can design weight-reduction diets to meet nutritional needs and food preferences. The nurse may also refer women with unusual eating habits or numerous questions about good nutrition to the dietitian.

The nursing mother should increase her caloric intake by 200 kcal over the pregnancy requirement (that is, a 500 kcal increase from her prepregnancy requirement). Again, simple observation and discussion will prove helpful, followed by referral as needed. In all cases literature on nutrition should be provided so that the women will have a source of appropriate information at home.

New mothers are also advised that it is common practice to prescribe iron supplements for 4-6 weeks after delivery. The hematocrit is then checked at the postpartal visit to detect any anemia.

ELIMINATION

During the hours after delivery the nurse carefully monitors a new mother's bladder status. A boggy uterus, a displaced uterus, or a palpable bladder are signs of urinary distention and require nursing intervention (see discussion of urinary tract, p. 905). In addition, during the physical assessment the nurse elicits information of a subjective nature from the woman regarding the adequacy of her fluid intake, whether she feels she is emptying her bladder completely when she voids, and any signs of urinary tract infection she may be experiencing. These data are then used to determine whether all factors are normal or whether additional evaluation is indicated.

In the same way the nurse obtains information about the new mother's intestinal elimination and any concerns she may have about it. Many mothers fear that the first bowel movement will be painful and possibly even damaging if an episiotomy has been done. Information must be provided about ways of keeping the stool soft to avoid discomfort and constipation. Often a frank discussion with the nurse does much to alleviate a new mother's anxieties about this subject.

REST AND SLEEP STATUS

As part of the postpartal assessment, the nurse evaluates the amount of rest a new mother is getting. If the woman reports difficulty sleeping at night, the cause should be determined. If it is simply the strange hospital environment, a warm drink, backrub, or mild sedative may prove helpful. Appropriate nursing measures are indicated if the client is bothered by normal postpartal discomforts such as afterpains, diaphoresis, episiotomy or hemorrhoidal pain.

A daily rest period should be encouraged and hospital activities should be scheduled to allow time for napping.

Psychologic Assessment

Adequate assessment of the mother's psychologic adjustment is an integral part of postpartal evaluation. This assessment focuses on the mother's general attitude, feelings of competence, available support systems, and caregiving skills. It also evaluates her fatigue level, sense of satisfaction, and ability to successfully accomplish her developmental tasks. See p. 916 for further discussion of emotional status of the postpartal client.

Often fatigue is a highly significant factor in a new mother's apparent disinterest in her newborn. Frequently the woman is so tired from a long labor and delivery that everything seems to be an effort. To avoid inadvertently classifying a very tired mother as one with potential bonding problem, the nurse should do the psychologic assessment on more than one occasion. After a nap the new mother is often far more receptive to her infant and her surroundings.

Some new mothers have little or no experience with infants and may feel totally overwhelmed. Women may show these feelings by asking questions and reading all available material or by becoming passive and quiet because they simply cannot deal with their feelings of inadequacy. Unless a nurse questions the woman about her plans and previous experience in a supportive, nonjudgmental way, one might conclude that the woman was disinterested, withdrawn, or depressed. Problem clues might include excessive continued fatigue, marked depression, excessive preoccupation with physical status and/or discomfort, evidence of low self-esteem, lack of support systems, marital problems, inability to care for or nurture the newborn, and current family crises (such as illness, unemployment, and so on). These characteristics frequently indicate a potential for maladaptive parenting, which may lead to child abuse or neglect (physical, emotional, intellectual) and cannot be ignored. Utilization of public health nurse referrals or other available community resources may provide greatly needed assistance and may alleviate potentially dangerous situations.

Cultural Influences

Many cultures emphasize certain postpartal routines or rituals for mother and baby. Frequently, these are designed to restore harmony or the hot–cold balance of the body. For Mexican Americans, black Americans, and Orientals, cold must be avoided after delivery. This prohibition includes cold air, wind, and all water (even if heated). Dietary changes also reflect the need to avoid cold foods and restore the balance between hot and cold (Horn, 1981).

The diet of the Mexican American reflects this concern about hot–cold balances. Chamomile tea, chicken soup, and a corn gruel are offered in the first days. Fruits, vegetables, pork, chili, garlic, beans, and chocolate are avoided (Clark, 1978). A Chinese mother may drink chicken soup that contains pigs' knuckles, vinegar, ginger, and peanuts. The vinegar in the soup helps transfer tricalcium phosphate from the bone of the pigs' knuckles into the broth, so the soup helps meet the mother's calcium requirements. The Chinese mother may also be served specially prepared noodles during a traditional celebration on the third day after delivery. This food helps her recovery process and increases lactation (Clark, 1978).

The black American new mother is offered chicken soup and sassafras tea in the early weeks to aid healing. Liver and hog chitterlings are restricted (liver has a high blood-producing function and is believed to increase lochial flow). Onions and alcohol are avoided because they affect breast milk.

The Mexican American family is concerned with balance of humors during the postpartal period. The new mother remains in bed for 3 days, begins to walk about her home after 8 days, and may go outside after 15 days. She is helped at home by family members. She avoids bathing for 15 days and carefully covers her head, body, and feet to avoid cold air because she believes that it may cause mastitis, a sudden infection (*pasmo*), a distended belly, frigidity, or sterility. A binder is worn about the abdomen and perineum to protect the body from cold (Clark, 1978).

The Vietnamese are also concerned about hot–cold imbalances; consequently the new mother remains inside for 30 days and may not wash her hair or bathe. She also wears heavy clothing and avoids all drafts.

The black American mother may have a 2- to 6-week period of confinement. Showers, tub baths, and shampoos are restricted during the "sick time" while the lochia flows.

A variety of traditions and rituals also exist in the American Indian and other cultural groups. The nurse caring for a mother during the postpartal period carefully assesses the family's beliefs and practices and adapts to them whenever possible. Family members can be encouraged to bring in preferred food and drink and some modifications in client care may be made to follow traditional beliefs.

The extended family frequently plays an essential role during the puerperium. The grandmother is often the primary helper to the mother and new newborn. She brings wisdom and experience, allowing the new mother time to rest as well as giving her ready access to someone who can help with problems and concerns as they arise. It is imperative to include members who have authority in the family. Visiting rules may be waived to allow family members or a tribal medicine man access to the mother and newborn. These practices show respect, and the nurse may gain an ally in the care of the mother and baby, especially if the mother follows the advice of her cultural mentor. Nurses can work for a blending of behaviors—the old and the new—to meet the goals of all concerned.

POSTPARTAL NURSING CARE

The physical and psychologic assessments are used as a basis for identifying normal progress and evaluating problem areas. The plan of care is based on the following objectives:

- Promotion of comfort and relief of pain
- Promotion of rest and graded activity

- Promotion of maternal psychologic well-being
- Promotion of successful infant feeding
- Promotion of effective parent education
- Promotion of family wellness
- Promotion of parent–infant bonding and attachment (see Chapter 28)

Promotion of Comfort and Relief of Pain

Pain may be present to varying degrees in the postpartal client and may be of multiple origin. The perineum is often edematous after delivery. An episiotomy presents an additional source of pain. Lacerations or extensions may further traumatize the perineum and may create sufficient pain to impede ambulation, elimination, or maintaining a comfortable position. Observations should be made for the development of hematomas, which account for pain and are also a source of blood loss not evident as overt bleeding. Clients may be taught to tighten their buttocks before sitting to avoid direct trauma to the perineum. Lateral positions may also be useful during the most painful period.

Ice packs are sometimes applied to the perineum during the first few hours after delivery, especially if there is a third- or fourth-degree laceration. Ice is effective in reducing edema and is also useful in relieving discomfort because of its numbing effect. Chemical ice bags or a disposable glove filled with ice and secured with a rubber band at the wrist of the glove may be used. The ice pack is covered with a chux pad or washcloth to avoid an ice burn on the woman's perineum.

Perineal care should be encouraged after each elimination to provide cleansing of the perineum and subsequently to promote comfort. Most agencies provide "peri-bottles," which the client fills with warm water that is squirted over the perineum following elimination. She should be instructed to cleanse from front to back to prevent contamination of the vulva from the anal area. When toilet tissue is used, the client will be more comfortable if she uses a blotting motion. She should also be instructed to apply the perineal pad from front to back so as to prevent contamination from the anal area.

Sitz baths are particularly useful with the severely traumatized perineum, as moist heat not only increases circulation to promote healing but also relaxes the tissue to promote comfort and decrease edema.

When assisting a client into a sitz bath, the nurse should be certain the water temperature is comfortable. Most clients find a temperature of 105F comfortable. In a sitz tub, the client may wear a hospital gown and drape it over the edge of the tub. This keeps her upper body from becoming chilled and provides for privacy. A call light should be available and the client instructed how to use it. Often the position and warmth during a sitz bath can cause a client to become faint; the nurse should check on her frequently. Many agencies are now using disposable sitz baths that fit inside the toilet. These are convenient for the client to use as often as she wishes both in the hospital and when she goes home.

Dry heat in the form of heat lamps may be helpful. The perineum should be cleansed before the use of the heat lamp to prevent drying of secretions on the perineum. Heat lamps generally are used for 20 minutes two or three times daily.

Topical anesthetics often relieve perineal discomfort. Nupercaine ointment, Dermoplast spray, and Americaine spray or ointment are commonly placed at the client's bedside. The woman may find it helpful to use such a product following a sitz bath or perineal care. Because of the danger of tissue burns, she must be cautioned not to apply them before using the heat lamp.

As mentioned on p. 907, afterpains are common postpartum, particularly in multiparous and breast-feeding clients. If nursing personnel are able to anticipate needs and to administer medications before the pain is excessive, greater comfort will be provided to the client. Administration of an analgesic an hour before feeding will promote comfort during the feeding and enhance the mother–infant interaction.

Some mothers experience hemorrhoidal pain after delivery. Relief measures include the use of sitz baths two to three times per day; anesthetic ointments, rectal suppositories, or witch hazel pads applied directly to the anal area. The woman may be taught to digitally replace external hemorrhoids in her rectum (see Chapter 11, p. 257). She may also find it helpful to maintain a side-lying position when possible and to avoid prolonged sitting. The mother is encouraged to maintain an adequate fluid intake, and stool softeners or laxatives should be administered to insure greater comfort with bowel movements. The hemorrhoids usually disappear a few weeks after delivery if the woman did not have them prior to this pregnancy.

Discomfort may also be caused by immobility, because the client who has been in stirrups for any length of time may experience muscular aches from such extreme positioning. It is not unusual for women to complain of joint pains and muscular pain in both arms and legs, depending on the effort they exerted during the second stage of labor.

Breast engorgement may be a source of pain for the postpartal client. Specific nursing interventions for the bottle-feeding mother are discussed on p. 926. Nursing interventions for the breast-feeding mother with engorgement are discussed on p. 936.

Nurses should be alert to both nonverbal as well as verbal manifestations of pain and should intervene with appropriate measures. The physical response to pain may be influenced by the client's level of fatigue, cultural background, possible lack of acceptance of the pregnancy and new baby, or other situational crises, which trigger psychologic crises that will ultimately affect the family's adjustment. The first alternative to pain relief may not necessarily be medication; frequently, changing positions, comfort measures such as a backrub or warm drink, or encouraging the woman to ventilate her feelings in an atmosphere of acceptance may be sufficient to promote relaxation. Drugs should be available if other measures fail. (See the Nursing Care Plan on the postpartal period).

Personal hygiene actions during the postpartal period are essential in promoting comfort. Because diaphoresis is an expected occurrence as the body attempts to dispose of the extra fluids retained during pregnancy, a daily shower is very refreshing for the client and should be strongly encouraged. Clients who have remained NPO (having nothing by mouth) for any length of time require mouth care. Assisting the client with these basic needs makes her more comfortable. During the puerperium the client is frequently thirsty as she recovers from delivery and experiences postpartal diuresis. She should have a filled pitcher of cold water within reach and should be offered milk and fruit juice frequently.

Early ambulation should be encouraged postpartally. Activity aids in promoting psychologic well-being and also in reducing the incidence of complications such as constipation and thrombus formation.

The nurse should assist the woman the first few times she gets up during the early postpartal period. Fatigue, effects of medications, loss of blood, and possibly even lack of food intake may result in feelings of dizziness or faintness when the woman stands up. Because this may be a problem during the woman's first shower, the nurse should remain in the room, checking the woman frequently, and have a chair close by in case she becomes faint. Dizziness may be aggravated by standing still and by the warmth of the water, so it is best to keep the first shower somewhat brief. Many postpartal units routinely tape ammonia inhalants to the bathroom door for use in case of fainting. During this first shower the nurse should instruct the client in the use of the emergency call button in the bathroom; if she becomes faint during a future shower, she can call for assistance.

Promotion of Rest and Graded Activity

The physical exertion experienced during labor and delivery may leave a woman exhausted and in need of rest. The client who has participated in the delivery process may be euphoric and full of psychic energy immediately after delivery, ready to relive the experience of birth repeatedly with whoever will listen. Essential nursing activities must be done frequently to adequately assess the client's condition; however, they may create an environment of constant activity, making rest a luxury and not a routine in most maternity units. Rather than becoming totally frustrated by

these circumstances, the nurse must be astute in evaluating individual needs, always with the goal of providing opportunities for rest during hospitalization. If rest is achieved while in the hospital, there is a greater likelihood that the client will arrange such opportunities at home, adjusting her schedule to meet this important need. For the excited, euphoric client, the nurse may allow a period for airing of feelings, then encourage a period of rest.

Physical fatigue often influences many other adjustments and functions with the new mother, such as reduction of milk flow, thereby increasing problems with establishing breast-feeding. Energy is required to make the psychologic adjustments to a new infant and to assume new roles. Many women are not able to anticipate their behavior and are often surprised at their response to the birth process. Adjustments to the unknown and unexpected are most smoothly accomplished when adequate rest is obtained.

The nurse may encourage rest by organizing her activities to avoid frequent interruptions for the client. Rest times should be provided before encounters with the newborn if rooming-in is not utilized.

POSTPARTAL EXERCISES

The client should be encouraged to begin simple exercises while in the hospital and continue them at home. She is advised that increased lochia or pain means she should reevaluate her activity and make necessary alterations. Most agencies provide a booklet describing suggested postpartal activities. (Exercise routines vary for clients undergoing tubal ligation following delivery or for cesarean birth clients.) See Figure 27–5 (p. 922) for a description of some commonly used exercises.

RESUMPTION OF ACTIVITIES

Ambulation and activity may gradually increase after discharge. The new mother should avoid heavy lifting, excessive stair climbing, and strenuous activity. One or two daily naps are essential and are most easily achieved if the mother sleeps when her baby does.

Many mothers find it easier to remember to avoid overdoing if they wear a robe and gown for the first few days. By the second week at home, light housekeeping may be resumed. Although it is customary to delay returning to work for 6 weeks, most women are physically able to resume practically all activities by 4–5 weeks. Delaying returning to work until after the final postpartal examination will minimize the possibility of problems.

Promotion of Maternal Psychologic Well-Being

The birth of a child, with the changes in role and the increased responsibilities it produces, is a time of emotional stress for the new mother. This stress is increased because

(Text continues on p. 920.)

NURSING CARE PLAN
Postpartal Period

CLIENT DATA BASE

History

1. Delivery information
   a. Gravida, para
   b. Date and time of delivery
   c. Anesthesia and analgesia
   d. Course of labor and delivery
2. Support people available (such as father)
3. Parenting information or beliefs
4. Condition of newborn

Physical Examination

Uterus — firm and in the midline, lochia progressing from rubra to serosa

Perineum — note presence of episiotomy or lacerations and evaluate for healing

Rectum — may have hemorrhoids

Abdomen — muscles stretched, may have striae on skin

Breast — soft, nipple erect, no reddening of tissues, colostrum with gentle expression, no nipple soreness, utilization of proper supporting bra

Pulse — may be slowed to 50 beats/min

Blood pressure — minimal fluctuation from admission

Temperature — may rise to 38C (100.4F) during first 24 hours postpartum

Weight — may have loss of 10 lb since delivery

Laboratory evaluation

Second day postpartum

Hemoglobin — not more than 2 g less than admission

Hematocrit — drop less than 3% from admission

Urine — presence of red blood cells is considered normal; no glucose; specific gravity 1.020; no bacteria

NURSING PRIORITIES

1. Restore body to approximately nonpregnant state with minimal complications.
2. Establish successful infant feeding patterns, whether breast-fed or bottle-fed.
3. Develop a healthy family–child relationship with total integration of the newly born into family unit.
4. Provide client education, including all aspects of self-care, infant care, maternal–child bonding, integration of newborn into family, and continued medical supervision for mother and child.

CLIENT/FAMILY EDUCATIONAL FOCUS

1. Discuss the physiologic changes that occur during the postpartal period.
2. Explore with the couple ways in which they can adapt their life-style to accommodate the new family member.
3. Stress the need for adequate rest and emotional support for both parents.
4. Provide opportunities to discuss questions and individual concerns.

Problem	Nursing interventions and actions	Rationale

Pain	Complete physical assessment will identify factors/conditions that may cause pain Implement specific comfort measures, including:
	 1. Episiotomy:
	   a. Sitz bath
	   b. Perineal light
	   c. Spray such as Dermoplast
	 2. Hemorrhoids:
	   a. Sitz bath
	   b. Tucks or ointment
	   c. Stool softeners to prevent constipation
	 3. Afterpains:
	   a. Administer analgesics
	   b. May administer analgesics to nursing mothers 1 hr before feeding to facilitate mother's comfort
	 4. Cesarean delivery:
	   a. Ambulation
	   b. Position changes
	   c. Analgesics
		Pain may be present in varying degrees and may be multiple in origin; pain is increased by exhaustion, and by emotional factors such as acceptance of pregnancy and of newborn Pain may interfere with ability to rest and establishment of early mother–child relationship
		
		 Infant suckling at breast stimulates release of oxytocin, which in turn stimulates uterine contractions resulting in afterpains
		
		 Cesarean birth clients may have additional pain due to interference of greater number of nerve endings; also, manipulation of abdominal contents and anesthesia lead to decreased intestinal motility

NURSING CARE PLAN Cont'd
Postpartal Period

Problem	Nursing interventions and actions	Rationale
Difficulty in elimination	Encourage voiding every 4–6 hr Monitor intake and output until complete bladder emptying is established Create positive attitude that enhances relaxation of client through: 1. Teaching 2. Assisting client to bathroom if possible 3. Pouring warm water over perineum 4. Leaving faucet running (sound of running water is suggestive) Evaluate bladder for distention Encourage increased intake of fluids Catheterize if absolutely necessary Assist client in establishing normal bowel pattern by: 1. Encouraging ambulation and fluids 2. Providing fresh fruit and roughage in diet 3. Administering stool softeners as indicated 4. Administering enema if necessary	Close proximity of urethra to birth canal results in increased trauma during delivery Pressure of larger uterus before delivery causes changes in position and capacity of bladder Medications given at delivery cause decreased sensation of bladder filling Development of diuresis postpartally causes bladder to fill more quickly Stasis leads to increased risk of urinary tract infection Full bladder increases tendency of uterus to relax by displacing uterus and intefering with its contractility, which leads to hemorrhage Bowel is sluggish due to decreased peristalsis Rectal soreness, episiotomy, extensions, and hemorrhoids create difficulty with bowel elimination Client may anticipate painful elimination and tense up Cleansing enema during labor and omission of solid foods may add to elimination problem Constipation increases pressure on sutures and increases discomfort
Fatigability	Evaluate individual rest needs Encourage rest by organizing activities to avoid frequent interruptions Provide rest periods prior to feeding times If mother is rooming-in, encourage her to rest while baby sleeps, an activity she may continue at home Initiate activities gradually with frequent rest periods Client may become overzealous in an exercise regimen if she is concerned about her protruding abdomen	Physical exertion during labor may leave client exhausted Level of physical fatigue often influences many adjustments and functions of new mother; for example, milk flow may be reduced, increasing problems with establishing breast-feeding Energy is required in order to make psychologic adjustments to new baby and to assume new roles Adjustments to unknown and unexpected are most smoothly accomplished when adequate rest is obtained
Infection	Teach and utilize measures to prevent infection including: 1. Perineal care 2. Wiping the perineum from front to back after voiding or defecation 3. Use of sitz baths or heat lamp 4. Encourage adequate fluid intake 5. Nutritious diet	Good nursing care and self-care will help prevent infection Frequent cleansing will decrease contamination and the warmth of the water used will help promote healing Prevents fecal contamination Heat increases blood flow to the area and promotes healing (the sitz bath also has a cleansing effect) Produces frequent bladder filling and elimination and thereby prevents stasis of urine in the bladder Adequate amounts of nutrients, especially protein and vitamin C, are necessary for tissue repair

NURSING CARE PLAN Cont'd
Postpartal Period

Problem	Nursing interventions and actions	Rationale
	6. Good hand-washing technique for both staff and mother	Prevents spread of contamination from client to client, self-contamination of breasts or perineum by mother, or contamination of baby
	Observe, record, and report signs and symptoms of infection, including: 1. Fever 2. Four-smelling lochia 3. Separation, edema, discharge, poor healing of episiotomy 4. Urinary urgency, frequency, pain 5. Abnormal pain in abdomen, legs, and so on Implement treatments as prescribed Document effectiveness of care	See discussion of specific infections in Chapter 29
Breast engorgement	Nursing mother: a. Increase frequency of feedings b. Warm compresses c. Manual expression of milk d. Supportive brassiere e. Ointments and exposure to air for cracked nipples f. Analgesics if necessary	Exaggeration of normal venous and lymphatic secretions produces distended, full, firm breasts
	Nonnursing mother: a. Medication to suppress lactation (such as Bromocriptine) b. Supportive brassiere c. Avoid stimulation of breast d. Cool compresses e. Do not express milk manually f. Analgesics if necessary	Breast engorgement in nonbreast-feeding mothers inhibits letdown reflex
Delayed involution	Observe, record, and report involution process, including: 1. Evaluation of fundus daily for height, position, and consistency 2. Observation of lochia for color, amount, odor	Involution is monitored to evaluate process of healing in female reproductive system following delivery of fetus
Perineal trauma	Promote healing of perineum by: 1. Assessing episiotomy for REEDA 2. Local application of heat 3. Teaching proper perineal care 4. Monitoring vital signs. Pulse may be as low as 50/min (normal); blood pressure should have minimal fluctuation; temperature may rise to 38C (100.4F) in first 24 hr but should not be elevated after that; continued temperature elevation may represent presence of infection Have client do the following several times a day for 5 min at a time: 1. Perineal tightening 2. Head raising and placing chin on chest	Perineum is traumatized during birth from stretching by baby's head, cutting during episiotomy, or tearing during delivery Application of heat promotes healing through increase of circulation Perineal area should always be cleaned from front to back or from clean to dirty area to avoid contamination with fecal material Vital sign variations alert professional staff to possible presence of complications

NURSING CARE PLAN Cont'd
Postpartal Period

Problem	Nursing interventions and actions	Rationale
	3. Pelvic rocking to strengthen muscles in lower back and abdomen 4. Leg raises 5. Defer sit-ups for approximately 2 weeks Teach client to reevaluate her activity and to make necessary alterations if she has an increase in lochia or pain	
Assimilation of new roles and tasks	Assess learning needs of client/family and readiness to learn Utilize demonstration and allow opportunity for return demonstration Suggested areas of teaching: infant feeding, burping, diapering, bathing, safety; mother's hygiene needs, care of breasts, activity, exercises, parenting skills, nutrition Support mother as she takes on mothering role; time teaching to her ability to accept new information	All postpartal clients have teaching needs (some for new information, some for review or reordering) During teaching, emphasize principles rather than encouraging mimicking of demonstrated techniques

NURSING CARE EVALUATION

Infection is absent in episiotomy (incision) site.

Infant feeding techniques are established.

Mother can care for herself and implement postpartal exercises.

Mother–infant and father–infant bonding process is established.

Parents understand infant care techniques and can demonstrate knowledge of infant care, feeding, bathing, safety, cord care, circumcision care, and continued medical supervision (including immunization schedule).

NURSING DIAGNOSES*	SUPPORTING DATA
1. Potential alteration in comfort: pain	Signs and symptoms of pain from episiotomy, hemorrhoids, afterpains, breast engorgement, cesarean delivery Evidence of maternal exhaustion
2. Potential alteration in urinary elimination related to the physiologic changes of pregnancy and the trauma of labor and delivery	Decreased sensation of bladder filling Palpable urinary bladder Inadequate urine output or inability to void Signs of urinary retention with overflow
3. Parental knowledge deficit regarding new roles and tasks	Expressed concerns or questions about parenting responsibilities and tasks Inadequate or inappropriate parenting behaviors

*These are a few examples of nursing diagnoses that might be appropriate for a person postpartally. It is not an inclusive list and must be individualized for each woman.

tremendous physiologic changes are transpiring as her body adjusts to a nonpregnant state. During the early postpartal days the mother is emotionally labile. Mood swings are common, and she may become tearful at the slightest provocation.

During the early postpartal days, the mother may repeatedly discuss her experiences of labor and delivery.

This review seems necessary to assist the mother in integrating her experiences in order to adjust to her new role. If, in her opinion, she did not cope well with labor and delivery, she may have feelings of inadequacy to work through. Reassurance from the nurse that she did well is frequently helpful. However, this reassurance is effective only if the nurse has established a warm, supportive relationship with the client. In addition, the mother must adjust to the loss of her fantasized child to deal effectively with the child she has borne. This may be more difficult if the infant is not of the desired sex or if he or she exhibits birth defects. Follow-up visits from the nurse who assisted her in labor and delivery provide additional opportunities for the mother to relive her experiences and to come to terms with them.

During the taking-in period the mother is focused on bodily concerns and teaching may not be totally effective. However, because early discharge is common, classes and information should be offered, and printed handouts provided for the client's reference when she is more ready to assume charge.

During the taking-hold phase the mother becomes very concerned about her ability to be a successful parent. Skillful intervention by the nurse, with constant reassurance that the client is a successful mother, is vital. During this time the mother is most receptive to teaching, and tactful instruction and demonstration assist her in mothering effectively. The nurse must carefully avoid "taking over" the infant. By functioning as an advisor and allowing the mother to perform the actual care, the nurse demonstrates confidence in the mother's skill and ability, which in turn increases the mother's self-confidence about her effectiveness as a parent.

Many mothers suffer from "postpartum blues" during the early postpartal period. They become depressed and weepy and frequently complain of a "let-down feeling." The mother requires reassurance that these feelings are normal and an explanation as to why they occur. A therapeutic environment that permits the mother to cry without feelings of guilt is vital. Her privacy should be protected. The nurse should also indicate her interest if the woman feels a need to talk. In rare instances initial depression leads to a pathologic condition known as postpartum psychosis (see Chapter 29).

Promotion of Successful Infant Feeding

The feeding of their newborn is the one task that parents may see as the center of the relationship between themselves and their new family member. Whether the mother has chosen to bottle-feed or breast-feed, the nurse can help the mother to have a successful experience while in the hospital and during the early days at home. Feeding and caring for newborns may be routine tasks for the nurse, but the success or nonsuccess that a mother achieves the first few times may determine her feelings about herself as an adequate mother.

As an expression of personality, the response of the newborn to caring is important. The newborn's behavior may be internalized as rejection by a parent, which may alter the progress of parent–child relationships. A parent may interpret the sleepy infant's refusal to suck or inability to retain formula as evidence of his or her incompetence as

a parent. Likewise, the breast-feeding mother may deduce that the newborn does not like her if he or she fails to take her nipple readily. Conversely, infants pick up messages from the muscular tension of those holding them.

A nurse who is sensitive to the needs of the mother can form a relationship with her that permits sharing of knowledge about techniques and emotions connected with the feeding experience. Breast-feeding women frequently express disappointment in the help given to them by hospital nurses, saying they would like more encouragement, support, and practical information about feeding their newborn (Beske, 1982). This same desire and need applies to nonnursing mothers as well. Consistency in teaching by nursing personnel is paramount. A new mother becomes very frustrated if she is shown a number of different methods of feeding her newborn. The following clinical example written by a nursing student shows that encouragement, information sharing, and follow-up care can have a positive therapeutic effect upon a breast-feeding mother and her newborn.

Ms. T. wanted to breast-feed her first baby, but she almost gave up before she got started. Her experience taught me, when I was a junior doing clinical experience, how easily nurses can encourage and discourage patients.

Ms. T. was 27 years old, single, employed, and black. She had finished high school in Puerto Rico, and her first language was Spanish. Part of the nursing care I gave was to help Ms. T. establish breast-feeding. The first time I took her baby, Jessie, to her, Ms. T. was in a chair. Just as she bared her chest, a nurse came by and gruffly ordered her to go to bed and pull the curtain. Ms. T. complied.

I asked her if she minded my sitting with her. She said that, in her country, mothers breast-feed in public without shame. Her own mother had breast-fed all six of her children.

The baby nursed a few seconds, let go, and fell asleep. "She does this all the time," Ms. T. said sadly.

"Try again. Some babies have to be encouraged," I suggested.

She tried again; and the baby sucked strongly. During this and other feeding sessions, Ms. T. and I discussed nutrition, breast care, burping, and colostrum. After a while, Ms. T. stroked the baby's cheek, and the baby turned away from her breast. I explained the rooting reflex, and after Ms. T. stroked the infant's other cheek, the baby turned toward her nipple.

The baby again let go quickly. Ms. T. wondered if she should request bottle-feeding. I told her this would discourage milk production. We talked. After 15 minutes, I asked her why she

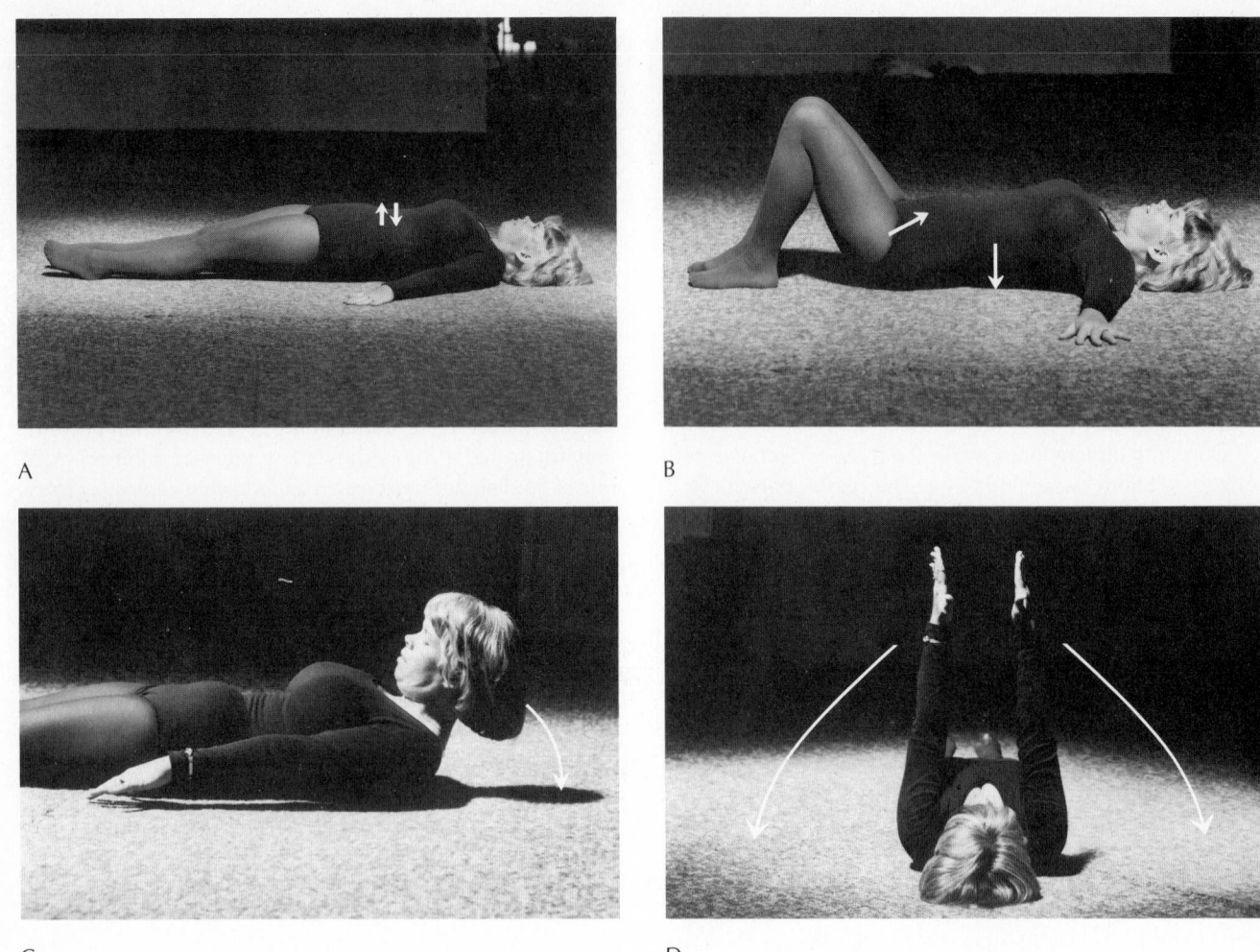

Figure 27–5 Postpartal exercises. Begin with five repetitions two or three times daily and gradually increase to ten repetitions. First day: **A,** Abdominal breathing. Lying supine, inhale deeply using the abdominal muscles. The abdomen should expand. Then exhale slowly through pursed lips, tightening the abdominal muscles. **B,** Pelvic rocking. Lying supine with arms at sides, knees bent and feet flat, tighten abdomen and buttocks and attempt to flatten back on floor. Hold for a count of ten, then arch the back, causing the pelvis to ''rock.'' On second day add: **C,** Chin to chest. Lying supine with no pillow, legs straight, raise head and attempt to touch chin to chest. Slowly lower head. **D,** Arm raises. Lying supine, arms extended at 90° angle from body, raise arms so they are perpendicular and hands touch. Lower slowly. On fourth day add: **E,** Knee rolls. Lying supine with knees bent, feet flat, arms extended to the side, roll knees slowly to one side,

had not switched to the other breast. No one had told her, she said. The nurse had showed her how to hold the baby, hold the breast with two fingers, and put the nipple into Jessie's mouth.

It seemed to me that the atmosphere of the maternity unit was not conducive to asking questions of the nursing staff. Written instructions had been placed on Ms. T.'s dining table, but she had forgotten to read them. Most verbal interactions were given by the nurses quickly, from the foot of the bed. The head nurse would ask a few questions, give a few instructions, leave the literature on the table, and depart quickly.

Ms. T. commented that the nurses seemed too busy to interrupt with questions. The most important question Ms. T. had was: Is the baby getting enough? I showed her how she could

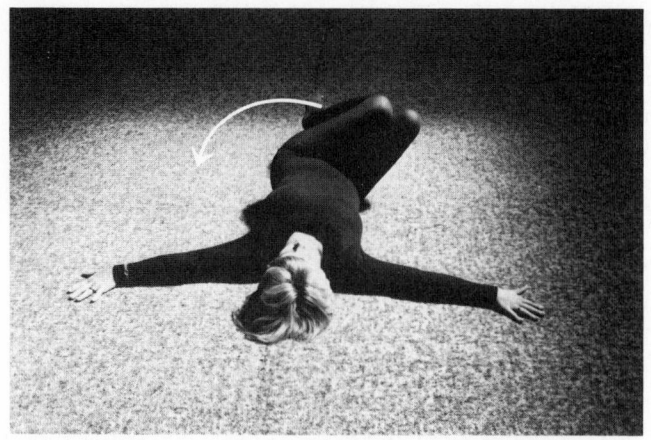

E

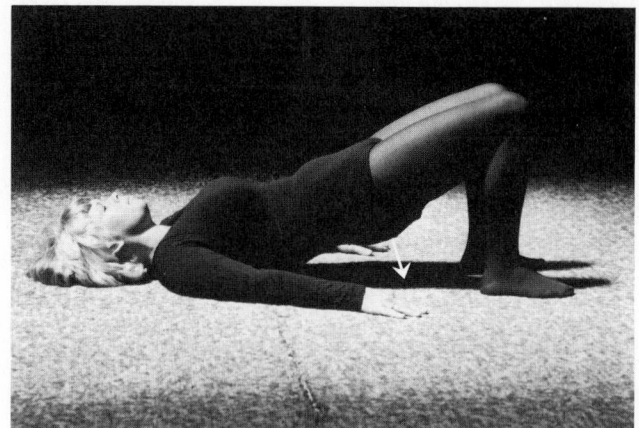

F

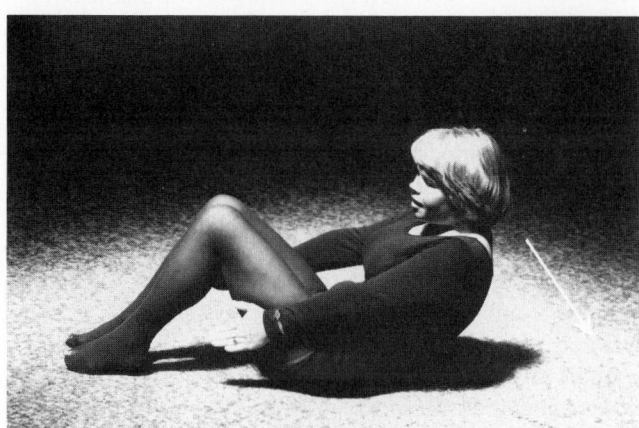

G

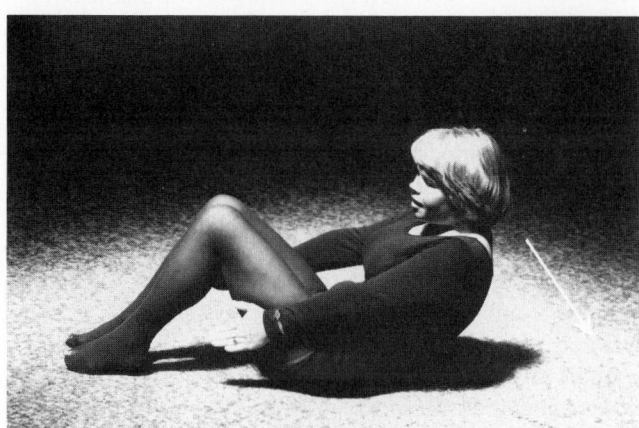

H

keeping shoulders flat. Return to original position and roll to opposite side. **F,** Buttocks lift. Lying supine, arms at sides, knees bent, feet flat, slowly raise the buttocks and arch the back. Return slowly to starting position. On sixth day add: **G,** Abdominal tighteners. Lying supine, knees bent, feet flat, slowly raise head toward knees. Arms should extend along either side of knees. Return slowly to original position. **H,** Knee to abdomen. Lying supine, arms at sides, bend one knee and thigh until foot touches buttocks. Straighten leg and lower it slowly. Repeat with other leg. After 2–3 weeks, more strenuous exercises such as sit-ups and side leg raises may be added as tolerated. Kegel exercises, begun antepartally, should be done many times daily during postpartum to restore vaginal and perineal tone.

massage her breast to express some colostrum into her baby's mouth. This way she would know she had some colostrum. Her baby had lost only two ounces, but this worried her. I assured her that this was normal, that the baby was doing fine, was sleeping well, and had a healthy cry and a strong grip.

The next time I saw Ms. T., we went over the hospital's instruction sheet together for breast-feeding. It was in English. I asked her to read it out loud. She understood the first two lines but asked questions about a bracketed sentence.

On my last day on the unit, I arranged to visit Ms. T. and Jessie when they were home. On my way home as I thought about our last hospital visit, I realized Ms. T. had never seen her baby's naked body (other than at birth) and might not be aware that the baby had a rash and dehydrated skin. I telephoned and explained that the baby's skin was normal and would look all right in a few days. She said, "You do too much for me." I was pleased because I know that in the Puerto Rican culture, this was a high compliment.

Two days after Ms. T. left the hospital, I telephoned her at home to find out how she was doing. She told me that a nurse at the hospital had given her bottle-feeding instructions, several containers of Similac, and a four-hour feeding schedule. Ms. T. said that the nurse had also told her that her baby might lose weight if she did not get enough breast milk. Ms. T. was not sure what to do. She was expressing breast milk to give by bottle and, in addition, was breast-feeding. After determining that she still wanted to breast-feed, I convinced her to try a few more days without any bottles and on a demand schedule.

Six days after Ms. T.'s discharge, I made a home visit. The baby was asleep when I got there, so I answered some questions Ms. T. had prepared for me. She said the baby slept as much as six hours between the night feedings but usually three to four hours between most feedings. After Jessie wakened, Ms. T. took her to breast, and Jessie sucked vigorously. I reinforced some of the earlier teaching, put Ms. T. in touch with the La Leche League, and complimented her on her successes with breast-feeding. The most important thing I had been able to offer her was encouragement.*

The decision by the mother about whether to breast-feed or bottle-feed is usually made by the sixth month of pregnancy and often even before conception. If the mother makes the decision to breast-feed at the time of delivery without prenatal preparation or support from her partner or other members of her family, she may encounter difficulty in having a successful experience. It is necessary for the nurse to find out before delivery whether the woman really wants to breast-feed or has made the decision based on social or family influences (Mullett, 1982).

The nurse's primary responsibility is to support the feeding-method decision and to assist the family to achieve a positive result, regardless of the method utilized. No woman should be made to feel inadequate or superior because of her choice in feeding. There are advantages and disadvantages to breast- and bottle-feeding, but positive

bonds in parent–child relationships may be developed with either method.

Immediately before feeding, the mother should be made as comfortable as possible. Preparations may include voiding, washing her hands, and assuming a position of comfort.

The cesarean delivery mother needs support so that the infant does not rest on her abdomen for long periods of time. If she is breast-feeding, she may be more comfortable lying on her side with a pillow behind her back and one between her legs. The nurse can position the newborn next to the woman's breast and place a rolled towel or small pillow behind the infant for support. The mother will initially need assistance turning from side to side and burping the newborn. She may prefer to breast-feed sitting up with a pillow on her lap and the infant resting on the pillow rather than directly on her abdomen. It may be helpful to place a rolled pillow under the arm supporting the infant's head. Bottle-feeding cesarean birth mothers frequently use the sitting position, too. If incisional pain makes this position difficult, the bottle-feeding mother may also assume the side-lying position. The infant can be positioned in a semi-sitting position against a pillow close to the mother, who can hold the bottle in her upper hand.

Depending on the newborn's level of hunger, the parents may want to use the time before feeding to get acquainted with their infant. The presence of the nurse during part of this time to answer questions and provide reinforcement of parenting skills will be helpful for the family.

For the sleepy baby, a period of playful activity—such as gently rubbing the feet and hands or adjusting clothing and loosening coverings to expose the infant to room air may increase alertness so that, when the feeding is initiated, the infant is ready and eagerly sucks. It may allow the active newborn an opportunity to calm down so that he or she can find and grasp the nipple effectively. After the feeding, when the infant is satisfied and asleep, parents may explore the characteristics unique to their newborn. Hospital routines must be flexible enough to allow this time for the family. Rooming-in offers spontaneous, frequent encounters for the family and provides opportunities to practice skills of handling, thereby increasing confidence in care after discharge. It may also allow for demand rather than scheduled feeding times, and this should be encouraged.

CULTURAL CONSIDERATIONS IN INFANT FEEDING

Breast-feeding has been the traditional feeding method for most cultures. However, bottle-feeding has become extremely popular, much to the chagrin of some older members of a culture. Navajo elders, for instance, believe that breast-feeding ensures respect and obedience because the child remains close to the mother, while the bottle-fed infant will be more disobedient (Clark, 1981).

*From Burd, B. 1981. Encouragement counts in breast feeding. *Am. J. Nurs.* 81:149. Reprinted with permission of the American Journal of Nursing, ©1981.

Western practices encourage the new mother to breast-feed as soon as possible, but in many cultures (for example, Mexican American, Navajo, Filipino, and Vietnamese) colostrum is not offered to the newborn. Breast-feeding begins only after the milk flow is established. Interestingly, when a group of Vietnamese mothers who delayed breast-feeding until the third day after delivery was studied, it was found they had no difficulty breast-feeding (Ward, Pridmore, and Cox, 1981).

In many Oriental cultures the newborn is given boiled water until the mother's milk flows. The newborn is fed on demand and cries are responded to immediately. If the crying continues, evil spirits may be blamed and a priest's blessing may be necessary. In the black American culture there is much emphasis on feeding. Solid foods are introduced early and may even be added to the infant's formula. For the traditional Mexican American, a fat baby is considered a healthy baby and infants are fed on demand. "Spoiling" is encouraged and a colicky baby may be given mint or olive oil for relief.

LACTATION

The female breast is divided into 15 or 24 lobes separated from one another by fat and connective tissue. These lobes are subdivided into lobules, composed of small units called *alveoli* where milk is synthesized by the alveolar secretory epithelium. The lobules have a system of lactiferous ductiles that join larger ducts and eventually open onto the nipple surface (see discussion of breast, p. 85). During pregnancy increased levels of estrogen stimulate breast duct proliferation and development, and elevated progesterone levels promote the development of lobules and alveoli in preparation for lactation.

Delivery results in a rapid drop in estrogen and progesterone with a concomitant increase in the secretion of *prolactin* by the anterior pituitary. This hormone promotes milk production by stimulating the alveolar cells of the breasts. When the newborn sucks on the mother's nipple, *oxytocin* is released from the posterior pituitary. This hormone increases the contractility of the myoepithelial cells lining the walls of the mammary ducts, and a flow of milk results. This is called the *letdown reflex*. Mothers have described the letdown reflex as a prickling or tingling sensation during which they feel the milk coming down. It is not unusual for the breasts to leak some milk prior to feeding (Jeffries, 1981).

The letdown reflex can be stimulated by the newborn's sucking, presence, or cry, or even by maternal thoughts about her baby. Conversely, the mother's lack of self-confidence, fear of, embarrassment about, or pain connected with breast-feeding may prevent the milk from being ejected into the duct system. Milk production is decreased with repeated inhibition of the letdown reflex. Failure to empty the breasts frequently and completely also decreases production, because as milk accumulates and is not with-

drawn, the buildup of pressure in the alveoli suppresses secretion.

Once lactation is well established, prolactin production decreases. Oxytocin and sucking continue to be the facilitators of milk production. Three types of milk are produced during the establishment of lactation: (a) colostrum, (b) transitional milk, and (c) mature milk. *Colostrum* is a yellowish or creamy-appearing fluid that is thicker than later milk and contains more protein, fat-soluble vitamins, and minerals. It also contains high levels of immunoglobulins, which may be a source of immunity for the newborn. Colostrum production begins early in pregnancy and may last for several days after delivery. However, in most cases colostrum is replaced by transitional milk within 2–4 days after delivery. *Transitional milk* is produced from the end of colostrum production until approximately 2 weeks postpartum. This milk contains elevated levels of fat, lactose, water-soluble vitamins, and more calories than colostrum.

The final milk produced, *mature milk*, has a high percentage of water. Although it appears similar to skim milk and may cause mothers to question whether their milk is "rich enough," it contains about 75 cal/dL. (For a comparison of breast milk and commercially prepared formula see Chapter 23, p. 719.)

SUPPRESSION OF LACTATION IN THE NONNURSING MOTHER

Suppression of lactation may be accomplished through drug therapy and mechanical inhibition. The drugs that suppress lactation effectively are hormones that inhibit the secretion of prolactin. Research has demonstrated, however, that the estrogen-based medications used to suppress lactation contribute to an increased incidence of thromboembolitic disease and venous thrombosis (Tindall, 1968; Niebyl et al., 1979). Therefore, most practitioners prescribe them much less frequently. The most common hormones used for lactation suppression are estradiol valerate (Deladumone) and chlorotrianisene (Tace).

A newer lactation suppressant, bromocriptine (Parlodel), is a nonhormonal ergot derivative that inhibits prolactin secretion. It is taken twice a day for 2–3 weeks. Because its primary side effect is hypotension, its use is begun after a new mother's vital signs have stabilized (Foster, 1982). See Drug Guide—Bromocriptine, p. 926.

The recognition of complications associated with drug therapy has led to renewed popularity for mechanical methods of lactation suppression. This is accomplished by applying a snug breast binder for 2–3 days post-delivery. The judicious use of analgesics and ice packs will alleviate some of the discomfort associated with tender full breasts. The mother is advised to avoid any stimulation of her breasts by her baby, herself, breast pumps, or her sexual partner until the sensation of fullness has passed, as this will increase milk production and delay the suppression process. Heat is avoided for the same reason, and the

---

DRUG GUIDE—Bromocriptine (Parlodel)

OVERVIEW OF OBSTETRIC ACTION

Bromocriptine is a dopamine agonist that acts to suppress lactation by stimulating the production of prolactin-inhibiting factor at the hypothalamic level. This results in decreased secretion of prolactin by the pituitary gland. The drug may also directly inhibit the pituitary by preventing the release of prolactin from the hormone-producing cells (Foster, 1982). When administered postpartally it helps suppress milk production and decrease breast leakage and pain. It may also be used for suppression after lactation has already begun.

ROUTE, DOSAGE, AND FREQUENCY

The usual dose is 2.5 mg orally two times per day. The total daily dose generally does not exceed 7.5 mg. The medication usually is taken for 2–3 weeks.

MATERNAL CONTRAINDICATIONS

Maternal hypotension, desire to breast-feed, pregnancy.

MATERNAL SIDE EFFECTS

Hypotension is the primary side effect. To prevent problems associated with hypotension, administration should be delayed until the new mother's vital signs are stable. Other side effects include nausea, headache, dizziness, and occasionally faintness and vomiting.

NURSING CONSIDERATIONS

Administration should be delayed until maternal blood pressure is stable. Blood pressure should be carefully monitored if bromocriptine is administered concurrently with any antihypertensives. Taking bromocriptine with meals may help decrease the possibility of nausea. Early resumption of ovulation has occurred in women taking bromocriptine; the woman should be informed of this and receive information about contraceptives (Foster, 1982).

---

mother is encouraged to let shower water flow over her back rather than her breasts. A well-fitting bra is worn continuously until lactation is suppressed. The bra provides support and eases the discomfort that may occur with tension on the breast tissue because of the fullness. In some agencies a supportive bra is recommended in lieu of breast binding, except in cases of marked engorgement and discomfort. The suppression process usually takes approximately 48-72 hours, but some milk may be produced up to a month after delivery (Benson, 1980).

BOTTLE-FEEDING

The mother who has chosen to bottle-feed her infant should be encouraged to assume a comfortable position with adequate arm support so she can easily hold her infant. Most women cradle their infants in the crook of the arm close to the body, which provides the intimacy and cuddling so essential to an infant. With the great emphasis placed on successful breast-feeding, the teaching needs of the bottle-feeding new mother may be overlooked. If she has had only limited experience in feeding infants, she may need some guidelines to successfully feed her newborn. The following important principles should be included in the teaching provided:

1. Bottles should always be held, not propped. Positional otitis media may develop when the infant is fed horizontally, because milk and nasal mucus may occlude the eustachian tube. Holding the infant provides a rest for the feeder, social and close physical contact for the baby, and an opportunity for parent–child interaction and bonding. Once feeding is initiated, the child should be held close to provide physical closeness and to facilitate eye contact (Figure 27–6).

2. The nipple should have a hole big enough to allow milk to flow in drops when the bottle is inverted. Too large an opening may cause overfeeding or regurgitation because of too-fast feeding. If feeding is too fast, the nipple should be changed and the infant should be helped to eat more slowly by stopping the feeding frequently for burping and cuddling.

3. The nipple should be pointed directly into the mouth, not toward the palate or tongue, and should be on top of the tongue. This position creates greater suction and a more controlled flow of milk. The nipple should be full of liquid at all times to avoid ingestion of extra amounts of air, which decreases the amount of feeding and increases discomfort.

4. The infant should be burped at intervals, preferably at the middle and end of the feeding. The infant who seems to swallow a great deal of air while sucking may need more frequent burping. In addition, if the infant has cried before being fed, air may have been swallowed and the infant should be burped before beginning to feed or after taking just enough to calm down. Burping is done by holding the infant upright on the mother's shoulder or by holding the infant in a sitting position on the mother's lap with chin and chest supported on her hand. The back is then gently patted or stroked.

Too-frequent burping may confuse a newborn who is attempting to coordinate sucking, swallowing, and breathing simultaneously.

5. Newborns frequently regurgitate small amounts of feedings and the mother may require reassurance that this is normal. Initially it may be due to excessive mucus and gastric irritation from foreign substances in the stomach from birth. Later, regurgitation may result when the infant feeds too rapidly and swallows air. It may also occur when the infant is overfed and the cardiac sphincter allows the excess to be regurgitated. Because this is such a common occurrence, experienced mothers and nurses generally keep a "burp cloth" available. Although regurgitation is normal, vomiting or a forceful expulsion of fluid is not. When it occurs, further evaluation may be indicated, especially if other symptoms are present.

6. A fat baby is not necessarily a healthy one. Parents should be encouraged to avoid overfeeding or feeding infants every time they cry. Infants should be encouraged but not forced to feed and should be allowed to set their own pace once feedings are established. Research suggests that mothers tend to set artificial goals—"The baby must take all five ounces"—and tend to keep feeding the child until those goals are met, even though the infant may not be hungry. Overfeeding results in infant obesity. During early feedings, however, the infant may need simple tactile stimulation—such as gently rubbing feet and hands, adjusting clothing, and loosening coverings—to maintain adequate sucking for a sufficient time to complete a full feeding.

Formula preparation and sterilization techniques are always important to discuss with families. Professional personnel frequently spend time describing detailed procedures that are time-consuming, that are not followed at home, and that are not necessary because of the milk processing required by law. However, cleanliness remains an essential component. Bottles may be effectively prepared in dishwashers (nipples may be weakened by the temperature of dishwashers and therefore should be washed thoroughly by hand with soap and water and rinsed well) or washed thoroughly in warm soapy water and rinsed well. Tap water, if from an uncontaminated source, may be used for mixing powdered formulas, which are less expensive than the concentrated or ready-to-use prepared formulas. Only one day's supply of formula should be prepared at a time. Whole or evaporated milk may be diluted with water and sweetened with a sugar source such as corn syrup, depending on the age of the infant and caloric requirements. (See Chapter 23 for a discussion of formulas, breast milk, and caloric requirements.) If the water source is questionable, the terminal heat method of sterilization or single-bottle method of preparation should be used. If more than one bottle is prepared at a time, they

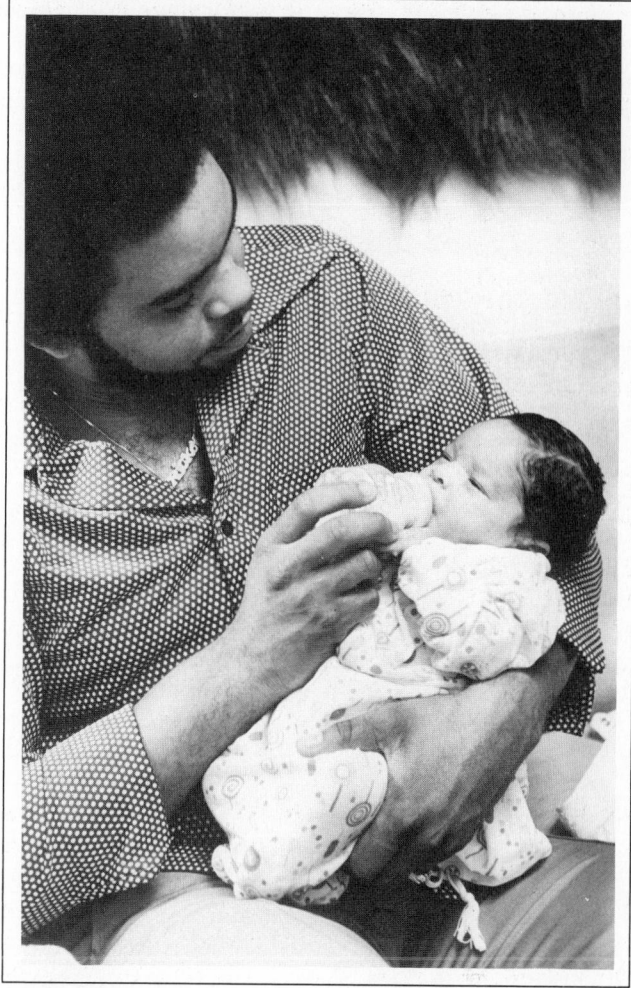

Figure 27–6 An infant is supported comfortably during bottle-feeding.

should be stored in the refrigerator and warmed slightly before feeding. (Procedure 27–1 describes techniques for bottle sterilization.)

BREAST-FEEDING

Breast-feeding has many advantages for both the mother and her infant. Because suckling stimulates the release of oxytocin, uterine involution occurs more rapidly. Breast-feeding may also contribute to increased psychologic closeness between mother and infant. Breast-feeding is convenient and economical because there is no need to purchase and prepare formula on a routine basis; and breast-feeding may offer some antibody protection to the infant. Disadvantages and contraindications are primarily related to the mother and may include maternal illness, aversion to breast-feeding, need to resume a full-time work schedule and, in some instances, another pregnancy. In the latter case, opinion varies: Some feel the nutritional demands on the pregnant mother are too great and advocate gradual

Procedure 27-1   Methods of Bottle Sterilization

Terminal sterilization	Aseptic method of sterilization
Advantages:	Advantages:
1. Safest, most efficient method	1. May be modified for use with disposable bottles
2. More easily learned	Disadvantages:
Disadvantages:	1. Difficult to learn, contamination more likely
1. Prolonged cooling period (1–2 hr)	Procedure:
2. Not suitable for disposable bottles	1. Same as steps 1 and 2 of terminal method
Procedure:	2. Place all equipment needed (bottles, nipples, caps, can opener, tongs, measuring pitcher, and spoon) in a large kettle or sterilizer; cover with water and boil for 5 min
1. Assemble equipment and wash hands	3. In another pan boil the amount of water necessary to make the formula (boil for 5 min)
2. Thoroughly wash bottles, caps, and nipples in warm soapy water; squeeze some water through the nipple holes to rid them of accumulated milk; rinse well	4. Drain the water from the sterilizer pan and let the equipment cool for a few minutes
3. Wash the lid of the formula can (if using a liquid) and prepare formula according to directions	5. Remove the measuring pitcher, being certain to touch only the handle
4. Fill the bottles with the desired amount of formula and loosely apply the nipples and caps; one or two bottles of water may be prepared at the same time	6. Using the sterilized can opener, open a can of formula after first washing the lid with soapy water and rinsing well; pour the formula into the prepared measuring pitcher and add the correct amount of boiled water, mix with the prepared spoon
5. Place the prepared bottles in a large kettle or bottle sterilizer and add the appropriate amount of water (as specified on the sterilizer or 2–3 in. if a kettle is used)	7. Using tongs, remove the bottles from the sterilizer and fill them with the desired amount of formula; (one or two bottles of water may also be prepared by boiling enough additional water)
6. Cover the sterilizer, bring the water to a gentle boil and then boil for 25 min.	8. Using the tongs set the nipples on the bottles, then touching only the edges, apply the caps
7. Remove from heat but let the bottles remain in the sterilizer with the lid on until the sides of the pan are cool to the touch	9. Refrigerate until needed
8. Remove the bottles, tighten the lids, and refrigerate until needed	To modify for disposable bottles:
	Complete all steps as directed except *do not boil the bottles* with the other equipment and allow the water to cool for 15–20 min before preparing the formula (the plastic bag may melt if the formula is too hot)

weaning. Others suggest that with adequate rest, a proper diet, and strong emotional support, continued breast-feeding during pregnancy is a valid choice. The practice of nursing one infant throughout pregnancy and then breast-feeding both infants after delivery is referred to as tandem nursing (Lawrence, 1980). When pregnancy occurs, the decision is best made on an individual basis after considering maternal health and motivation and the age of the first child.

□ *BEGINNING TO BREAST-FEED* The nurse caring for the breast-feeding mother should help the woman achieve independence and success in her feeding efforts. Prepared with a knowledge of the anatomy and physiology of the breast and lactation, the components and positive effects of breast milk, and techniques of breast-feeding, the nurse can help the woman and her family effectively use their own resources to achieve a successful experience (Riordan and Countryman, 1980a). The principles involved in breast-feeding are (a) to provide adequate nutrition, (b) to establish an adequate milk supply, and (c) to prevent trauma to the nipples. All instructions are aimed toward these goals.

The newborn who is breast-feeding should be put to breast as soon as possible, depending on the situation of birth. Some infants are not interested so soon, but for those who are, breast-feeding affords a soothing experience and has considerable physiologic and psychologic benefit for the mother. Colostrum has sufficient nutrients to satisfy the infant until milk is established in 2–4 days. Establishment of lactation depends on the strength of the infant's suck and the frequency of nursing.

Positioning of the baby at the breast is a critical factor. The entire body of the infant should be turned toward the mother's breast, with the mouth adjacent to the nipple. The mother should not have to lift her shoulder or breast to direct the nipple into the infant's mouth. The nipple should be directed straight into the mouth, not toward the palate or tongue, and as much of the areola as possible should be included so that, as the baby sucks, the jaws compress the ducts that are directly beneath the areola (Figure 27–7). To do this the mother places her index finger above the nipple and her middle finger below. She then compresses the areolar area and guides the nipple into the infant's mouth. Through the rooting reflex, the infant can locate the nipple. Avoid stimulation of both cheeks, which only confuses the hungry infant.

If the mother does not have a prominent or everted nipple, she may try rolling the nipple between her thumb and forefinger or stretching the nipple by pressing in and outward around the nipple prior to the feeding. Nurses should avoid the temptation to substitute a regular nipple shield to correct nipple positions. The shield tends to confuse the baby, as the artificial nipples on the shields are softer and easier to feed from, and the baby may refuse the human nipple when it is reoffered. This problem, termed "nipple confusion" may also be avoided if routine sterile water or dextrose and water feedings are not given to all breast-feeding infants. Following feedings, the nipples should be assessed for trauma so that corrections may be made in position and technique for the next feeding.

Breasts should be alternated at each feeding, beginning with 5 minutes on each side and progressing to 7–10 minutes by the third or fourth day and ultimately to 10 minutes on each side. A convenient way for the mother to remember which breast to use is to fasten a small safety pin to the bra cup on that side. The infant will empty the breasts during this time, and any additional time may meet an oral need for the newborn but may also cause increased breast trauma. Once feedings are established, length of nursing time on the second breast may be extended to meet this oral need, because the sucking reflex will not be so strong once the infant is partially satisfied with nourishment from the first breast. While nursing, the mother should press the breast away from the infant's nares to prevent obstruction of the nasal passageway, thus allowing the infant to breathe.

The mother should be instructed in techniques for breaking suction prior to removing the infant from the breast. By inserting a finger into the infant's mouth beside the nipple, she can break the suction, and the nipple may be removed without trauma. Burping between feedings on

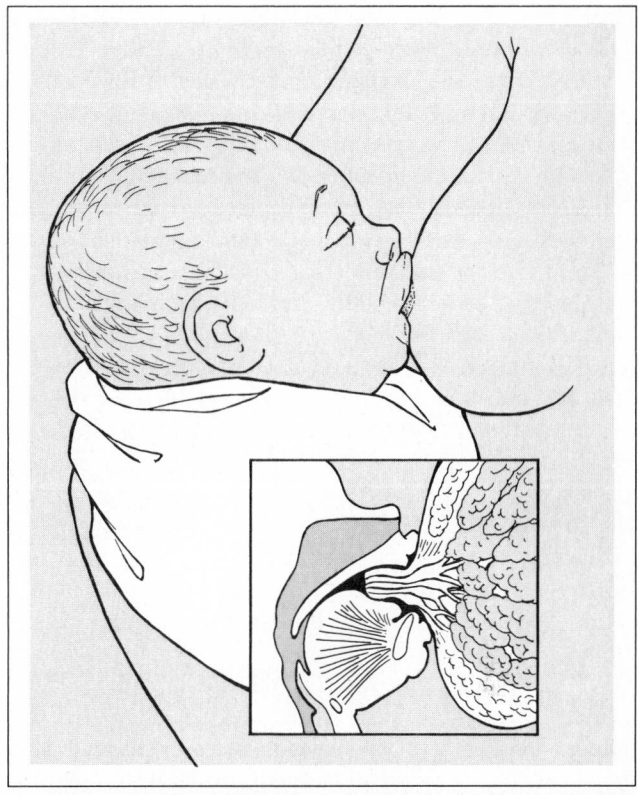

Figure 27–7 To nurse effectively, it is important that the infant's mouth covers the majority of the areola to compress the ducts below. (Courtesy Ross Laboratories, Columbus, Ohio.)

each breast and at the end of the feeding continues to be necessary. If the infant has been crying, it is also advisable to burp before beginning feeding.

Initially more milk is produced than is required by the infant (see Chapter 23). Later the amount of milk will be produced to meet nutritional need, manifested through sucking. Milk may tend to leak until supply meets demand, and the mother should expect this, utilizing breast pads in her bra to absorb the secretions. She should be cautioned to remove wet pads frequently to avoid irritation to the nipples or the possibility of infection. The mother may also be taught to apply direct pressure to the breast with her hand or forearm. This will often stop the leaking.

The use of supplementary feedings for the breast-feeding infant may weaken or confuse the sucking reflex and may interfere with successful outcome. Often parents are concerned because they have no visual assurance regarding the amount consumed. Adequacy of intake may be determined if the mother listens to the baby for sounds of swallowing while nursing. In addition, if the infant appears to gain weight and has six or more wet diapers a day, he or she is receiving adequate amounts of milk. Activity levels and intervals between feedings may also indicate how satisfied the infant is. Parents should know that, because breast milk is more easily digested than formulas, the breast-fed infant becomes hungry sooner. Thus the frequency of breast-feedings may be greater, particularly after discharge, when fatigue or excitement may decrease milk supply temporarily. Increasing the frequency of feedings alleviates problems during these periods. The parents may also expect the infant to demand more frequent nursing during periods when growth spurts are expected, such as 10 days to 2 weeks, 5–6 weeks, and 3 months. There is a lag in nursing due to increased activity and interest in surroundings at 4–6 months, 7 months, and 9 months to a year (Slattery, 1977).

The mother may be taught to manually express her milk and to freeze it for bottle-feeding if she will be absent for a scheduled feeding. Breast milk should be frozen in plastic bottles because if glass bottles are used the antibodies will adhere to the sides of the bottle and their benefits will be lost. Manual expression is also advisable if the mother must go several hours without feeding, to relieve maternal discomfort and to maintain the milk supply, which decreases unless the breasts are emptied regularly (Figure 27–8).

Many medications, when administered to the mother, are secreted in the milk. These include salicylates, bromides, antibiotics, most alkaloids, some cathartics, alcohol, and the majority of addicting drugs (Pritchard and MacDonald, 1980). The mother should receive information about this and should also be instructed to inform her physician that she is nursing, should she require medical treatment at a later time.

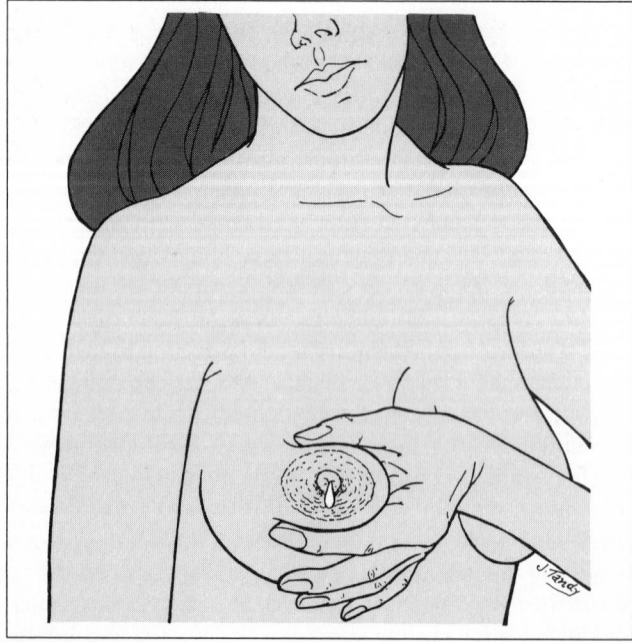

Figure 27–8 Manual expression of milk.

Numerous resources in the form of pamphlets and organized La Leche League activities are available to parents to assist with the establishment of successful breast-feeding. The mother needs the support of all family members, her pediatrician, her obstetrician, and nursing personnel, because it is often the attitudes reflected by these people that ultimately lead the mother to success or failure.

MEDICATIONS AND BREAST-FEEDING

It has long been recognized that certain medications taken by the mother may have an effect on her infant. A drug may affect the newborn in one of three ways: (a) lactation may be inhibited, thereby decreasing the supply of breast milk; (b) the newborn's physiologic processes may be directly affected by the drug if it crosses into the breast milk; and (c) the mother's physical or emotional ability to care for her newborn may be altered (Platzer, Lew, and Stewart, 1980).

Certain characteristics of a drug influence whether it passes into the breast milk, including its degree of protein binding. In general, unbound drugs enter the breast milk. Other factors are (a) the degree of ionization (drugs tend to cross in un-ionized form); (b) molecular weight (drugs with a molecular weight greater than 200 will not cross into the breast milk); (c) mechanism of transport (drugs enter breast milk by active transport, simple diffusion, or carrier-mediated diffusion); and (d) solubility of the drug (the alveolar epithelium presents a lipid barrier that tends to be more permeable when colostrum is present). The effects of the drug are also influenced by the infant's ability to absorb the drug from the gastrointestinal tract and by his or her ability to detoxify the drug and excrete it (Lawrence, 1980).

Four adjustments should be made to decrease the effects on her infant when administering drugs to a nursing mother (Lawrence, 1980):

1. The use of long-acting drug forms, which are usually detoxified in the liver, should be avoided. The infant may have problems excreting them and accumulation may be a problem.

2. Absorption rates and peak blood levels should be considered in scheduling the administration of the drugs. Less of the drug crosses into the milk if the medication is given immediately after the woman has nursed her baby.

3. The infant should be closely observed for any signs of drug reaction including rash, fussiness, or changes in sleeping habits or feeding pattern.

4. Using an appropriate table, whenever possible a drug should be selected that shows the least tendency to pass into breast milk.

The mother should be given information on the potential of most drugs to cross into breast milk. She should also be advised to tell any physician who may prescribe medications for her that she is breast-feeding. Clinicians who do not routinely care for obstetric or pediatric clients may not be familiar with the effects on breast milk of the drugs they prescribe and may need to consult the obstetrician. The positive and negative effects of the medication on the woman and her infant must be carefully considered. Table 27–2 identifies commonly used medications and their effects on the breast-fed infant.

POTENTIAL PROBLEMS IN BREAST-FEEDING

Many women stop nursing because the problems encountered seem to have no solutions. Anticipatory guidance about remedies and solutions to the problems is the nurse's role. This allows the mother to provide her infant with the nutritional and emotional experience that she has planned for during the pregnancy.

□ *ABNORMAL NIPPLES* Nipple inversion is a problem that is usually diagnosed in the prenatal period as part of the initial assessment. When a nipple is truly inverted, pressure on the areola with the examiner's thumb and forefinger causes the nipple to retract. The normal or flat nipple protrudes when this is done (Figure 27–9). When recognized during pregnancy, the woman can begin Hoffman's (1953) exercises to increase nipple protractility (Figure 27–10). If the nipple is truly inverted, she can wear special breast shields to correct the problem (for example, the Woolrich shield or the Eschmann shield) (Figure 27–11). These shields tend to absorb moisture so they should not be worn more than a few hours at a time.

□ *NIPPLE SORENESS* The mother should be told that some soreness often occurs initially with breast-feeding and that the problem will clear as soon as the letdown reflex is established. The infant should not be switched to bottle-feeding or have feedings delayed as this will only cause engorgement and more soreness.

Because the area of greatest stress to the nipple is in line with the newborn's chin and nose, nipple soreness may be decreased by encouraging the mother to rotate positions when feeding the infant. Figure 27–12 illustrates the cradle hold, football hold, and maternal side-lying positions. Changing positions alters the focus of greatest stress and promotes more complete breast emptying.

The length of time at the breast also has a significant influence on trauma and degree of comfort. Initially it is less traumatic for the mother to nurse more frequently rather than for long periods at one time. Often the mother is reluctant to terminate the feeding if an infant is sucking well, but if the infant sucks too long, by the time milk is established she will be too uncomfortable to tolerate the sucking of the infant.

Nipple soreness is especially pronounced during the first few minutes of the feeding. If the mother is not expecting this, she may become discouraged and quickly stop. The letdown reflex may take 3 minutes to activate and it may not occur if the mother stops nursing too quickly. The problem is compounded if the infant does not empty the mammary ducts; the infant is unsatisfied, and the possibility of engorgement for the mother increases.

The mother may use substances such as lanolin or A & D ointment on the nipples between feedings. These should be applied lightly after first washing the areola and nipple with water to prevent the accumulation of dried milk. If the infant objects to the taste of these substances, they may be washed off with water only (no soap) before the next feeding. After each feeding the nipples should be exposed to the air for 15–30 minutes. Exposing the nipples to the sunlight or to ultraviolet light for 30 seconds initially and gradually increasing to 3 minutes may also help. Breast pads should be changed frequently so the nipples will remain dry. (Breast pads with plastic liners interfere with air circulation—the plastic should be removed before they are used.)

Older remedies are receiving renewed acceptance. For instance, tea bags may be moistened in warm water and

(Text continues on p. 936.)

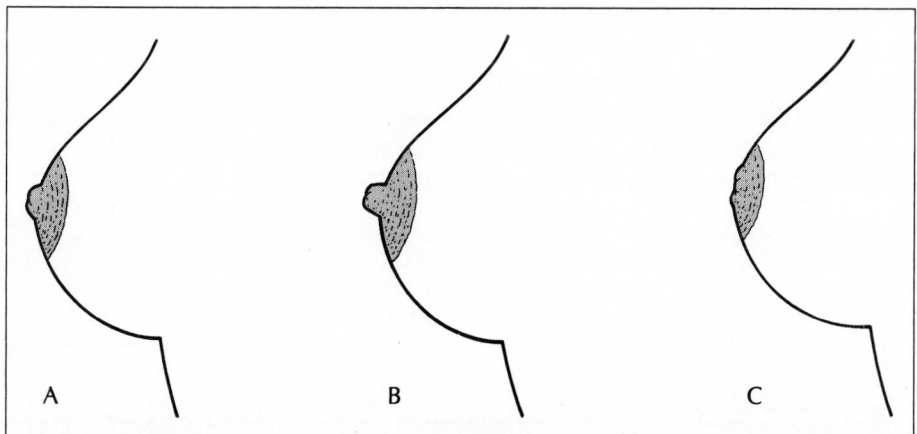

Figure 27–9 A, When not stimulated, normal and inverted nipples look alike. **B,** When stimulated, the normal nipple protrudes. **C,** When stimulated, the inverted nipple retracts.

**Table 27–2 Effects of Drugs and Substances
on the Breast-Feeding Mother and her Newborn***

Drug or substance	Small doses compatible with lactation	Harmful to new-born if taken in excess	Suppress lactation	Contra-indicated	Comments
Alcohol	X	X			Sedation of newborn Alters mother's ability to care for newborn
Analgesics (aspirin, acetominophen, mefenamic acid [Ponstel], pro-proxyphene [Darvon])	X				If the infant receives an injection of vitamin K at birth the risk of bleeding is minimal
(narcotic analgesics: codeine, meperi-dine [Demerol], pentozocaine [Talwin])	X				
Antibiotics (ampicillin, penicillin, Amoxicillin, cephalosporins)	X				Possible allergic sensitization and candidal diarrhea
(metronidazole [Flagyl])				X	Possibly carcinogenic Can interrupt nursing during treatment, manually expressing and discarding milk in the interim, and resume nursing 48 hours after the last drug A single 2-g dose is as effective as the 7-day regimen
(tetracycline)		X			Because the drug is bound to calcium in breast milk the risk of tooth staining is minimal if therapy does not exceed 10 days; whenever possible an alternative antibiotic should be administered
(chloramphenicol)				X	Possible bone marrow damage causing anemia, pancytopenia, shock, death
(sulfonamides)				X	Contraindicated for first month of life because of risk of jaundice and kernicterus; hemolytic anemia in infants of any age with G-6-PD deficiency Short-acting preparations are relatively safe after the first month of life if there are no contraindications in infant.
(erythromycin)				X	Safe after first month of life
Anticoagulants (heparin)	X				Is not excreted in breast milk

Table 27–2   Effects of Drugs and Substances
on the Breast-Feeding Mother and her Newborn* Cont'd

Drug or substance	Small doses compatible with lactation	Harmful to new-born if taken in excess	Suppress lactation	Contra-indicated	Comments
(warfarin [Coumadin])	X	X			Monitor prothrombin times of breastfeeding infants; administer vitamin K if maternal dose is high
(phenindione [Hedulin])				X	May cause bleeding in nursing infants
Antihistamines (short-acting, e.g., Benadryl)	X	X	X		May suppress lactation in large doses and may also cause drowsiness in infant
(long-acting, e.g., clemastine [Tavist])				X	
Antineoplastics (cyclophosphamide)				X	Potential for bone marrow suppression, impaired cell growth
Antithyroids (propylthiouracil,				X	Neutropenia
methimazole, [Tapazole])				X	Possibility of suppressed thyroid function with goiter, hypothyroidism, agranulocytosis
Atropine		X	X		
Barbiturates		X			May sedate newborn and mother in larger doses
Bronchodilators (epinephrine, ephedrine)	X				Drug destroyed in GI tract of newborn
Cardiac drugs (digoxin)	X				Monitor maternal serum drug levels first 2 months postpartum
(beta blockers, e.g., propranolol [Inderol])	X				
(methyldopa [Aldomet])	X				
(quinidine)				X	Arrhythmias in infant
(reserpine)				X	Cyanosis and increased respiratory tract secretions in breastfed infants
Coffee, cola (caffeine)		X			Hyperactivity, fussiness, colic
Cow's milk		X			Possible colic

Table 27–2 Effects of Drugs and Substances
on the Breast-Feeding Mother and her Newborn* Cont'd

Drug or substance	Small doses compatible with lactation	Harmful to new-born if taken in excess	Suppress lactation	Contra-indicated	Comments
Diuretics		X	X		May cause reduced total body fluid state, reducing milk formation
Ergot derivatives (bromocriptine, Ergotrate, Methergine)	X			X X	Vomiting, diarrhea, irritability, convulsions (ergotism)
Heavy metals (bismuth—contained in some dermatologic preparations, mercury)				X X	Toxic; not to be used on nipples
Herb teas		X			Diarrhea
Hormones (Oral contra-ceptives [estrogen-pro-gesterone combi-nation])			X	X	Progestin-only pills do not seem to suppress lactation; may contribute to gynecomastia in male infants
Insulin	X				Safe in therapeutic doses; destroyed in gastrointestinal tract
Laxatives (Cascara sagrada, senna, danthron [Dorbane, Modane])		X			Diarrhea
Nicotine		X	X		If started before beginning to nurse, may interfere with letdown reflex
Radioactive isotopes (Gallium citrate—^{67}Ga) (Technetium—^{99m}Tc) (Iodine 125/, 131/) (as treatment)				X X X X	Discontinue nursing until all radiation is gone from milk. Samples: gallium (about 2 weeks), technetium (about 2–3 days). Discontinue nursing until substance clears breast milk (usually 1–3 weeks) Check milk with geiger counter if necessary

Table 27-2   Effects of Drugs and Substances on the Breast-Feeding Mother and her Newborn* Cont'd

Drug or substance	Small doses compatible with lactation	Harmful to new-born if taken in excess	Suppress lactation	Contra-indicated	Comments
Recreational drugs					
Cannabis (marijuana)		X			Probably found in milk; effect not known but impaired DNA, RNA seen in animals
Methadone		X			Effects not known; withdrawal symptoms when mother stops drugs
Cocaine		X			Withdrawal symptoms when mother stops drugs
Heroin		X			Growth retardation in newborn, withdrawal symptoms when mother stops drug
LSD				X	Interferes with mother's ability to care for newborn
Sedatives and tranquilizers		X			Sedation, toxic effects
(benzodiazepines, e.g., Valium)				X	Changes in newborn ECG Drowsiness, lethargy, jaundice, failure to thrive
(phenothiazines)	X				Watch for sedation
(lithium)				X	Cyanosis, hypothermia, hypotonia, ECG changes in newborn
(tricyclic antidepressants)	X				Only scant amounts excreted in breast milk
(meprobamate [Equanil, Miltown])				X	Drowsiness
Thyroid hormone	X				Safe in therapeutic doses; check infant's thyroid function before mother on replacement therapy starts breast feeding
Vitamins (pyridoxine B$_6$)		X	X		Doses over 150–300 mg three times a day inhibit lactation

* Modified from Palma, P. A., and Adcock, E. W., III, July 1981, *Am. Fam. Physician* 24:179; and Sahub, S. Oct. 1981. *Am. Fam. Physician* 24:138.

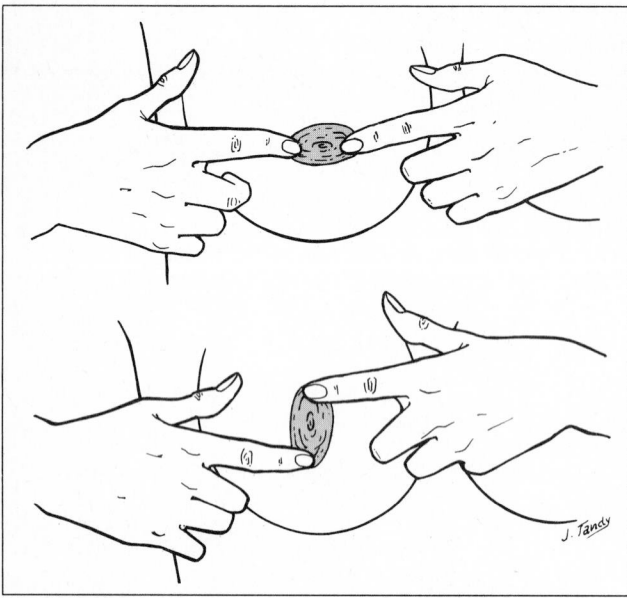

Figure 27–10 Hoffman's exercises are designed to increase nipple protractility. The client is instructed to place her thumbs or index fingers opposite each other near the edge of the areola. She then presses into the breast and stretches outward to break any adhesions. This is done both horizontally and vertically.

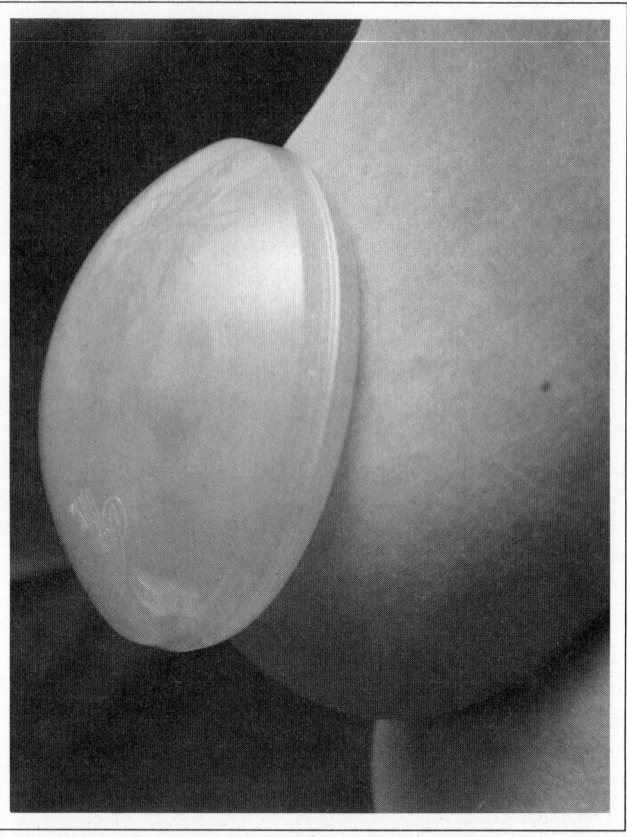

Figure 27–11 Breast shield designed to increase protractility of inverted nipples. These shields, worn the last 3–4 months of pregnancy, exert gentle pulling pressure at the edge of the areola, gradually forcing the nipple through the center of the shield. They may be used after delivery if still necessary.

applied to the nipples. The tannic acid seems to help toughen the nipples, and the warmth is soothing and promotes healing.

If the nipple soreness has a sudden onset, it may be caused by a thrush infection transmitted from the infant to the mother. White patches or streaks in the infant's mouth indicate a need for treatment of the mouth and nipple infection. If the problem is treated, the mother can usually continue breast-feeding (Riordan and Countryman, 1980b).

□ *CRACKED NIPPLES* Nipple soreness is frequently coupled with cracked nipples. Whenever a breast-feeding mother complains of soreness, the nipples must be carefully examined for fissures or cracks and the mother should be observed during breast-feeding to see whether the infant is correctly positioned at the breast. If the positioning is correct and cracks exist, interventions are necessary. The mother's first reaction may be to cease nursing on the sore breast, but this may aggravate the problem if engorgement and plugged ducts result. All the interventions described for sore nipples may be used. In addition, it may be helpful if the mother begins nursing on the less sore breast. This allows the letdown reflex to occur in the affected breast, and the infant does more vigorous sucking on the less tender breast to avoid further trauma to the cracked nipple.

Some success has been reported using a new approach that involves the application of the mother's milk to her cracked nipples. After expressing a small amount of milk, it is applied to her nipple and areola and allowed to air dry. Healing generally occurs quickly (Lawrence, 1980).

With severe cases, the temporary use of a nipple shield for nursing may be necessary. For the mother's comfort, analgesics may be taken after nursing.

□ *BREAST ENGORGEMENT* About the time their milk initially comes in, many women complain of feelings of engorgement. Their breasts are hard, painful, and warm and appear taut and shiny. At first this fullness is caused by venous congestion due to the increased vascularity in the breasts. Later the problem may be compounded by the pressure of accumulating milk.

The mother should be encouraged to wear a well-fitting nursing bra 24 hours a day. The bra supports the breasts and prevents further discomfort from tension and pulling on the Cooper's ligament. Frequent nursing is also helpful in preventing or decreasing engorgement. Breast-

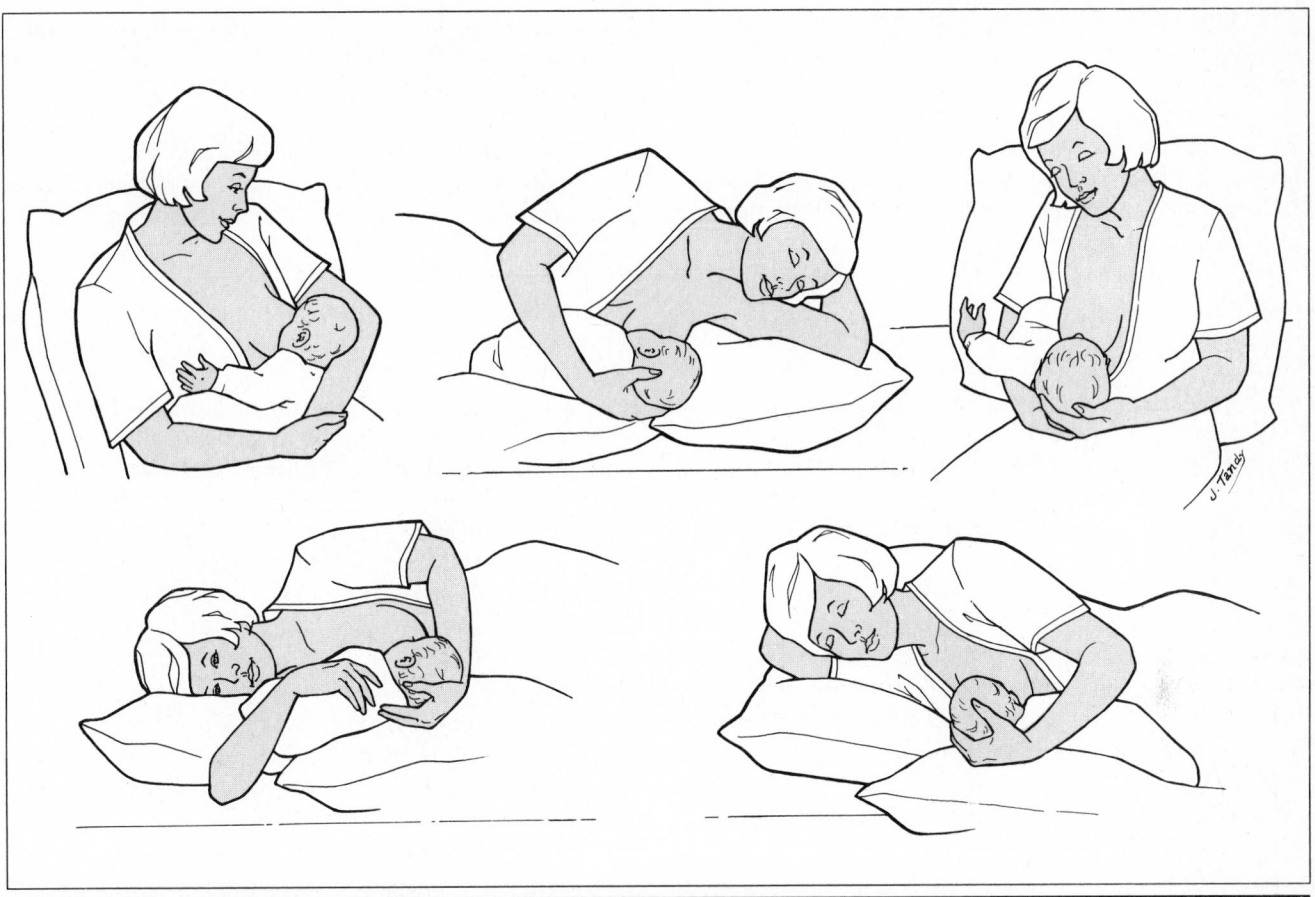

Figure 27–12. Examples of breast-feeding position changes to facilitate thorough breast empty-ing and prevent nipple soreness.

feeding every 2–3 hours initially keeps the breasts emp-tied and prevents discomfort from the vigorous suck of a ravenous infant. It also increases the circulation in the breast and helps move the fluid that might lead to engorgement.

Because the breast is quite hard, nursing may be diffi-cult for the infant and painful for the mother. Manual ex-pression of milk or the use of a nontraumatic breast pump to initiate the flow may be helpful, as is the judicious use of analgesics. Warmth is often soothing, and the mother who has problems with engorgement may find a warm shower comforting. It is also useful in stimulating the letdown reflex. The mother may find it helpful to stand in the show-er and manually express some milk before feeding. To prevent excessive stimulation, it is advisable to avoid hav-ing the spray beat directly on the nipples and breasts. Warm, moist cloths may also be used for relief. Additional relief measures include the use of ice packs between feed-ings, with hot packs applied 20 minutes prior to a feeding. The engorgement is generally relieved within 12–24 hours.

□ *PLUGGED DUCTS* Some mothers experience plugging of one or more ducts, especially in conjunction with or follow-ing engorgement. Manifested as an area of tenderness or "lumpiness" in an otherwise well woman, plugging may be relieved by the use of heat and massage. The mother can be encouraged to massage her breasts from her chest wall forward to the nipple while standing in a warm shower or following the application of hot packs to the breast (Rior-dan and Countryman, 1980b). She should then nurse her infant, starting on the unaffected breast if the plugged breast is tender. Frequent nursing will help prevent the problem and fatigue as well. In cases of repeatedly plugged ducts or caked breasts, it may be necessary for the mother to limit her fat intake to polyunsaturated fats and to add lecithin to her diet (Lawrence, 1980).

BREAST-FEEDING AND THE WORKING MOTHER

Often, although a mother returns to work, she elects to continue breast-feeding her infant. This decision requires planning on her part and family encouragement and assistance. She will find this easier to accomplish if she has 6–8 weeks at home to allow well-established lactation before returning to work. A few days before returning to work she can begin manually expressing and freezing her milk for her infant's use while she is gone. At work it will be necessary for her to pump her breasts during lunch or coffee breaks to avoid the discomfort of full breasts. Because milk production follows the principle of supply and demand, if breasts are not pumped, the milk supply will decrease.

Some mothers have flexible schedules and can return home to nurse at lunch time. If this is not possible, the infant may be fed expressed milk or a supplemental bottle of formula. If the mother is expressing milk at work for use the next day, she must be certain to keep it refrigerated and use it within 48 hours. Breast milk can be frozen in plastic bottles or bags and stored for up to 6 months (Jeffries, 1981).

Night nursing presents a dilemma in that it may help a working mother maintain her milk supply but may also contribute to fatigue. For the mother who works long hours or has a rigid work schedule, the best alternative may be to limit breast-feeding to morning and evening feedings with supplemental feedings at other times. This choice allows her to maintain a close relationship with the infant and provides some of the unique benefits of breast milk (Lawrence, 1980).

Promotion of Effective Parent Education

Meeting the educational needs of the new mother and her family is one of the primary challenges facing the postpartal nurse. Each client has educational needs that vary based on age, background, experience, and expectations. For instance, one 19-year-old mother may be very apprehensive about handling her infant while another of the same age may be quite comfortable with her baby because she is the oldest of several children and has had extensive experience with infants.

Formal schooling cannot be considered the primary criterion for assessing learning needs. It is far too easy to assume that the woman with limited education has numerous needs when, in fact, she may be very comfortable with her new role and responsibilities. By the same token, the concerns of a highly educated new mother may be overlooked either because it is assumed that she already knows the information or because a nurse with less education may find her threatening (Moss, 1981).

The steps of the nursing process provide a useful tool for identifying and meeting educational needs following delivery.

ASSESSMENT AND NURSING DIAGNOSES

Educational assessment may be accomplished in several ways. Simple observation—how a mother handles her in-

fant, the foods she selects, her hygiene practices—may provide useful information, as do listening and questioning. What areas concern the new mother? Does she seem to have misinformation or confused information? What does she already know that the nurse can build on?

Open-ended questions require a several-word reply and provide far more data for the nurse to use in the assessment than a question requiring a simple "yes" or "no." For example, asking "What plans have you made for handling things when you get home?" will elicit a more detailed response than, "Will someone be available to help you at home?"

To assess learning needs some agencies provide a client handout listing the most frequently identified areas of concern for new mothers. The mother checks those that apply to her or writes in concerns not included.

Nursing diagnoses are then formulated based on the data obtained through questioning and observation. The nurse plans educational experiences to meet the parents' specific needs.

PLANNING

In many educational settings, planning primarily involves the development of objectives that clarify what is to be taught and describe how the learner will demonstrate achievement of the objective. In planned postpartal classes, objectives are formulated and provided for the learner. However, even in nonstructured, individualized situations objectives can be identified by the nurse—"Mrs. Warren, when we are finished, you will be able to demonstrate the procedure for manually expressing your breast milk and describe appropriate methods of storing it."

IMPLEMENTATION

The educational method chosen to implement the objectives varies. Agencies with many clients and limited staff may rely heavily on structured classes while smaller units may provide more individualized instruction. Because more effective learning occurs when there is sensory involvement and active participation, television and movies (sight and hearing) are more helpful than lecture (hearing only), and demonstration—return demonstration (sight, touch, hearing, and possibly smell and taste) is even more effective (Bille, 1981).

Postpartal units use a variety of approaches—scheduled classes or demonstrations, handouts, group discussions, movies, videotapes, and individual interaction. Some agencies have access to a television channel and can show instructional films, for example, "How to Bathe Your Baby," "Dealing with Siblings' Reactions to the Baby," "Postpartal Exercises," or the like, at scheduled times during the day. Afterwards nurses are available to clarify material or answer any questions about the content.

When implementing educational activities, timing is important. The new mother is more receptive to teaching during the taking-hold phase when she is ready to assume responsibility for her own care and that of her newborn. New fathers are more likely to attend sessions planned for them if they are scheduled in the evening after visiting hours. If material is planned for siblings, perhaps late afternoon, after school or naps, would be effective.

Demonstration–return demonstration techniques offer opportunities for an individual to practice in a supervised situation. If principles are emphasized rather than simply encouraging the mimicking of techniques, transfer of the learning to the home situation is facilitated.

Teaching should not be limited to "how to" activities, however. Anticipatory guidance is essential in assisting the family to cope with role changes and the realities of a new baby. Small group discussions provide a chance for the new parents to talk about fears and expectations. New mothers may need help reconciling their actual postpartal figure with their ideal body image (Mercer, 1981). Questions may arise regarding sexuality, contraception, child care, and even the grief work associated with relinquishing the fantasized infant in order to accept the actual one.

Information is also essential for clients with specialized educational needs—the mother who had a cesarean delivery, the parents of twins, the adolescent mother, the parents of infants with congenital anomalies, and so on. They may feel overwhelmed, have difficult feelings to work through, and may not even realize what it is they need to know. Nurses who are attuned to these individual problems can begin providing guidance as soon as possible.

If the family is aware of role changes and common problems, they can anticipate possible behaviors and their origin. They are then better able to cope and less likely to evaluate expected occurrences as abnormal. Education also provides an opportunity to develop sensitivities to new modes of communication that are often required among family members.

EVALUATION

Methods of evaluation vary according to the objectives and the teaching methods. Can the woman manually express her milk? Is her description of storage methods accurate? Return demonstrations, question and answer sessions, and even programmed instruction are opportunities for evaluating learning, as are formal evaluation tools.

Evaluation of attitudinal or less concrete learning is more difficult. For example, a mother's ability to express her frustrations over an unanticipated cesarean delivery or a new mother's decision to delay for several weeks a family dinner originally scheduled for the first weekend after she arrives home, may be the nurse's only clues that learning has occurred. Follow-up phone calls after discharge may provide additional evaluative information and continue the helping process as the nurse assesses the family's current educational status and begins planning accordingly.

Promotion of Family Wellness

The promotion of family health encompasses several areas of concern, including a satisfactory maternity experience, the need for follow-up care and continued medical supervision for the mother and infant with checkups in 6 weeks, infant immunizations, and birth control. Regular health assessment of individual family members is important to maintain health and to prevent problems. Assessment of physiologic restoration should be a vital part of postpartal follow-up care. The new or expanding family may also have needs for information about adjustment of siblings, resuming sexual relations, and family planning.

ROOMING-IN

The trend to truly family-centered maternity care must, of necessity, be continued in the postpartal period. The tendency to separate the newborn from the parents is being displaced by a flexible concept—rooming-in—that provides increased opportunities for parent–child interaction.

In rooming-in, the newborn shares the mother's unit, and they are cared for together. Rooming-in provides continuous opportunities for the mother to begin to know and bond with her child and to learn how to effectively care for the infant. The newborn's crib is placed near the mother's bed, where she can easily see her baby. The crib should be a self-contained unit well stocked with items that the mother might require in providing care, including diapers, shirts, blankets, crib sheets, cotton balls, A & D ointment, and a comb or hairbrush. A bulb syringe should be readily accessible in the crib for suctioning the mouth or nares, and the mother should be familiar with its use.

Mothers are frequently extremely tired after delivery, so the responsibility for providing total infant care could be overwhelming. The rooming-in policy must be flexible enough to permit the mother to return the baby to the nursery if she finds it necessary because of fatigue or physical discomfort. Some mothers, fearing staff criticism, may be hesitant to do this and may need encouragement from the nurse. The woman with children at home may require additional rest, and a modified form of rooming-in may best meet her needs. The babies may return to the central nursery at night, allowing their mothers more time for uninterrupted rest if they desire.

Rooming-in is conducive to a self-demand feeding schedule for both breast-feeding and bottle-feeding infants. The lactating mother may find it especially beneficial to be able to nurse her child every 2–3 hours if necessary. This type of schedule meets the newborn's needs, promotes milk production, and helps prevent the nipple soreness caused by the ever-vigorous suck of the very hungry infant.

Fathers are also able to participate in the care of their infants with a rooming-in arrangement. They are asked to scrub their hands and usually wear a cover gown over their street clothes. Caps or masks are not required. Opportunities to hold and care for the child promote paternal self-confidence and foster paternal bonding. With rooming-in, father, mother, and infant have the opportunity to begin functioning as a family unit.

REACTIONS OF SIBLINGS

Sibling visitation helps meet the needs of both the siblings and their mother. A visit to the hospital reassures children that their mother is well and still loves them. It also provides an opportunity for the children to become familiar with the new baby. For the mother the pangs of separation are lessened as she interacts with her children and introduces them to the newest family member.

Although the parents have prepared their child for the presence of a new brother or sister, the actual arrival of the infant necessitates some adjustments. If small children are waiting at home, it is helpful if the father carries the baby inside. This practice keeps the mother's arms free to hug and touch her older children. She thereby reaffirms her love for them before introducing them to their new sibling. Many mothers have found that bringing a doll home with them for the older child is helpful. The child cares for the doll alongside his or her mother or father, thereby identifying with the parent. This identification helps decrease anger and the need to regress for attention. If the child is "too old" for receiving a doll, or if he is a boy to whom parents do not wish to give a doll, the child can be allowed to work alongside the parents in caring for the newborn. With constant supervision, the child may be permitted to hold the baby and to hold the bottle during feeding. In one instance, when the mother was breast-feeding, her 2½-year-old son sat next to her with his T-shirt pushed up and a doll to his breast. (Some parents may be distressed to observe this normal behavior.) The older child learns acceptable behavior toward the newborn, feels a sense of accomplishment, and learns tenderness and caring—qualities appropriate for both males and females. The nurse and parents can come up with numerous ways unique to their own environment and life-styles to show the older child or children that they too are valued, important, and have their own places in the family.

It is inevitable that an older child will at one time or another try to hurt the baby (or will hurt the baby unintentionally, not knowing his or her own strength or the effect of hitting). Parents are guided to respond by saying "I won't let you hurt (the baby) just as I won't let someone else hurt you."

The remaining umbilical cord or the unhealed stump may provoke anxiety in the older child. Parents are encouraged to point out what its function was, that it will fall off soon, and that it will look somewhat like the umbilical stump they too have.

The child, especially one of the opposite sex from the newborn, will raise queries about the appearance of the genitals as compared to his or her own. A simple explanation, such as "That's what little girls (boys) look like," is often sufficient.

SEXUAL RELATIONS BETWEEN PARENTS

Nursing intervention in the postpartal period considers the parent as a sexual person as well. An unprepared mother who experiences a sexual response (feels "turned-on") by her baby's suckling at the breast may feel abnormal or guilty. Interdiction against sexual intercourse until the sixth week postpartum is scientifically unfounded and psychologically undesirable. Episiotomies should be healed and the lochial flow abating by the end of the third week. The woman's partner can test for vaginal tenderness by inserting one clean finger (lubricated with a water-based compound such as K-Y jelly) into the vaginal orifice. If no tenderness is experienced, two fingers may be inserted. If this illicits no tenderness, the vaginal vault is almost certainly healed. Because the vaginal vault is "dry" (hormone-poor) as yet, some form of lubrication (K-Y jelly or contraceptive foam) may be necessary during intercourse. The female-superior or side-by-side positions for coitus may be preferable because they enable the woman to control the depth of penile penetration.

Breast-feeding couples need to be forewarned that, during orgasm, milk may spout from the nipples due to the release of oxytocin with sexual excitement and/or orgasm. Some couples find this pleasurable; other couples choose to have the woman wear a bra during sex. Nursing the baby prior to sexual activity may also decrease this.

Many couples have been frustrated during lovemaking by the baby's crying ("There's nothing like his crying to turn a guy off"). Some men as well as women are repulsed by the woman's changed body—the stretch marks, flabby abdominal skin, or breast changes. Maternal sleep deprivation may interfere with a mutually satisfying sexual relationship during this period. Couples may also be frustrated if there are changes in the woman's physiologic response to sexual stimulation. These changes are due to hormonal changes and may persist for about 3 months.

Anticipatory guidance during the prenatal and postnatal period can forewarn the couple of these eventualities and of their temporary nature. Anticipatory guidance is enhanced if the couple can discuss their feelings and reactions as they are experienced. Postpartal discussion groups reassure and support couples.

FAMILY PLANNING

Because research (Masters and Johnson, 1966; Hames, 1980) has demonstrated that many couples resume sexual activity before the postpartal examination, family planning information should be made available before discharge. This enables a woman or a couple to select a method that is personally acceptable and physiologically appropriate (see discussion in Chapter 6).

DISCHARGE INSTRUCTIONS

In addition to the general information a mother receives regarding her needs and care and those of her infant, she should be advised to contact her physician if any of the following develop:

- Sudden persistent or spiking fever
- Change in the character of the lochia—foul smell, return to bright red bleeding, excessive amount
- Evidence of mastitis, such as breast tenderness, reddened areas, malaise
- Evidence of thrombophlebitis, such as calf pain, tenderness, redness
- Evidence of urinary tract infection, such as urgency, frequency, burning on urination
- Continued severe or incapacitating postpartal depression.

POSTPARTAL NURSING CARE AFTER CESAREAN BIRTH

After a cesarean birth the new mother has postpartal needs similar to those of her counterparts who delivered vaginally. Because she has undergone major abdominal surgery, the client's nursing care needs also are similar to those of other surgical patients.

The chances of pulmonary infection are increased due to immobility after the use of narcotics and sedatives, and because of the altered immune response in postoperative patients. For this reason, the woman is encouraged to cough and deep breathe every 2–4 hours while awake for the first few days following cesarean delivery. This procedure may be uncomfortable because the incisional area is stretched. Optimal results are more likely if coughing and deep breathing are done after pain medication has been given and while the abdominal incision is splinted with a pillow. The client should take several deep breaths, then take another and cough at the end of inspiration.

Leg exercises are carried out every 15 minutes in conjunction with the postpartal check in the recovery room. The exercises should be continued every 2 hours throughout the first day or two until the client is ambulatory. The leg exercises indicate when the client has recovered from the anesthesia, increase circulation, and aid in the improvement of abdominal motility by tightening abdominal muscles.

Monitoring and management of the client's pain experience is carried out during the postpartum period. Sources of pain include incisional pain, gas pain, referred shoulder pain, periodic uterine contractions (afterbirth pains), and pain from voiding, defecation, or constipation. Incisional and afterbirth pains are most intense during the immediate postpartum and decrease in intensity and frequency with time.

Nursing interventions are oriented toward preventing or alleviating pain or helping the woman cope with pain. The nurse should undertake the following measures:

- Administer analgesics as needed, especially during the first 24–72 hours. Their use will improve the woman's outlook and enable her to be more mobile and active.
- Offer comfort through proper positioning, backrubs, oral care, and the reduction of noxious stimuli such as noise and unpleasant odors.
- Encourage the presence of significant others, including the newborn. This practice provides distraction from the painful sensations and is helpful in reducing the woman's fear and anxiety.
- Encourage the use of breathing, relaxation, and distraction (for example, stimulation of cutaneous tissue) techniques taught in childbirth preparation class.

Discomfort resulting from the accumulation of gas in the intestines usually reaches its peak on the third postoperative day. It is a normal physiologic phenomena resulting from (a) exposure of intestines to air; (b) slowing of gastrointestinal motility due to anesthesia and narcotics with subsequent increase in peristalsis; (c) material previously in the gastrointestinal tract contributing to gas formation; and (d) uncoordinated bowel activity. Measures to prevent or minimize gas pains are leg exercises, abdominal tightening, ambulation, avoiding carbonated or very hot or cold beverages, avoiding the use of straws, and providing a high-protein, semisolid diet for the first 24–48 hours. Medical intervention for gas pain includes the use of suppositories, enemas, and encouraging the woman to lie prone or on her left side. Lying on the left side allows the gas to rise from the descending colon to the sigmoid colon so that it can be expelled more readily. Preventive measures to avoid pain secondary to constipation include forcing fluids and administration of a stool softener and mild cathartic.

The nurse can be quite instrumental in minimizing discomfort and promoting success and satisfaction as the mother assumes the activities of her new role. Especially for the mother who has intravenous lines in place, instruction and assistance in assuming comfortable positions when holding and/or breast-feeding the infant will do much to increase her sense of competence and comfort. Sitting in a chair or tailor fashion in bed, leaning slightly forward with the infant propped on a pillow in her lap will prevent irritation to the incision. Another preferred position for breast-feeding during the first postoperative days is lying on the side with the newborn positioned along the mother's body.

Signs of depression, anger, or withdrawal may indicate a grief response to the loss of the fantasized birth experience. Fathers as well as mothers may experience feelings of "missing out," guilt, or even jealousy toward another couple who had a vaginal birth. The cesarean birth couple needs the opportunity to tell their story repeatedly to work through these feelings. The nurse as an empathetic listener can provide factual information about their situation and support the couple's effective coping behaviors.

By the second or third day the cesarean birth mother moves into the taking-hold phase and is usually receptive to learning how to care for herself and her infant. Special emphasis should be given to home management. She should be encouraged to let others assume responsibility for housekeeping and cooking. Fatigue not only prolongs recovery but interferes with breast-feeding and mother–infant interaction. Demonstration of proper body mechanics in getting out of bed without the use of a side rail and appropriate ways of caring for the infant so as to prevent strain and torsion on the incision are also indicated.

The cesarean delivery client usually does extremely well postoperatively. If delivery was accompanied by spinal anesthesia, the side effects of general anesthesia are avoided. Even after general anesthesia, however, most women are ambulating by the day after the surgery. Usually by the third postpartal day the incision can be covered with plastic wrap so the woman can shower, which seems to provide a mental as well as physical lift. Most are discharged by the fifth or sixth postoperative day, although some go home as early as the fourth day after delivery.

Facilitation of Parent–Infant Interaction after Cesarean Birth

Several factors associated with cesarean birth can promote or inhibit the participation, reciprocal feedback, and synchrony that the mother and infant bring to the initial discovery period. Contributing factors that can make the attachment process more difficult include the physical condition of the mother and her newborn and maternal reactions to separation, stress, anesthesia, and other drugs.

The mother and newborn may be separated after birth because of hospital routines, prematurity, or neonatal morbidity. Healthy neonates born by uncomplicated cesarean delivery are not more fragile than their vaginal route counterparts, although some agencies follow routines of automatically placing cesarean newborns in the high-risk nursery for a time.

A mother may react with some degree of hostility and apprehension toward an infant whose birth necessitated a major assault on her body and its subsequent discomforts. Affonso (1981) describes a series of interventions that can be carried out by birth attendants to promote the parent–infant attachment process. Called "Max-min-con" for *maximize, minimize,* and *control,* it involves *maximizing* the

parents' choices by allowing them to participate in decision making about the options available to them (for example, type of anesthesia) and giving informed consent. The nurse supports whatever positive coping behavior and abilities they have in dealing with the stresses of the event, and strengthens the client's support system through involvement and contact with significant others. The nurse can also become part of that support system by giving information, reassurance, praise, and maintaining eye, vocal, and touch contact with the client. The anticipatory guidance and support of the nurse's decisions and efforts can also *minimize* stress. The nurse can *control* the situation by providing knowledge, focusing the mother's attention on the infant (when she is ready), timing interactions to enhance the interactive opportunities between parent and infant, decreasing environmental distractions, and promoting comfort.

The presence of the father or significant other during the birth process positively influences the client's perception of the birth event (Marut and Mercer, 1979). Not only does his or her presence reduce the woman's fears, but it enhances her sense of control. It also enables the couple to share feelings and respond to one another with touch and eye contact. Later, they have the opportunity to relive the experience and fill in any gaps or lapses of memory (missing pieces). This is especially valuable if the mother has had general anesthesia. The father or significant other can take pictures, hold the infant, and foster the discovery process by directing the mother's attention to the details of the infant.

The perception of and reactions to a cesarean birth experience depend on how the client defines that experience. Her reality is what she perceives it to be. If the woman's attitude is more positive than negative, successful resolution of subsequent stressful events is more likely. Because the definition of events is transitory in nature, the possibility of change and growth is present. Often the mothering role is perceived as an extension of the childbearing role, and inability to fulfill expected childbearing behavior (vaginal birth) may lead to parental feelings of role failure and frustration. The nurse can help families alter their negative definitions of cesarean birth, and bolster and encourage positive perceptions.

THE ADOLESCENT ON THE POSTPARTAL UNIT

The adolescent presents special postpartal needs, depending on her level of maturity, support systems, and cultural background. The nurse needs to assess maternal–infant interaction, roles of support people, plans for discharge, knowledge of childrearing and plans for follow-up care. It is imperative to have a community health service be in touch with the client shortly after discharge.

Contraception counseling is an important part of teaching. As previously discussed, the incidence of repeat pregnancies during adolescence is high and the younger the adolescent, the more likely she is to become pregnant again. Often the young woman tells the nurse that she does not plan on engaging in sex again. This denial mechanism is unrealistic, and the nurse must help the young woman realize this. The nurse should make sure that the client has some method of birth control available to her, and that she understands ovulation and fertility in relation to her menstrual cycle. This is an excellent opportunity for sex education.

The nurse has many opportunities for teaching the adolescent about the newborn in the postpartal unit. It is important to remember that the nurse serves as a role model; therefore, the manner in which she handles the newborn greatly influences the young mother. The father should be included in as much of the teaching as possible.

A newborn physical exam done at the client's bedside accomplishes several goals. The mother has immediate feedback about the newborn's health; she is able to observe the many facets of her baby and sees the proper manner in which to handle the infant. The nurse can teach as the examination progresses, giving the new mother information about the fontanelles, cradle cap, shampooing the newborn's hair, and so on. The nurse might also use this time to teach the young mother about infant stimulation techniques. Because adolescent mothers tend to concentrate their interactions in the physical domain, they need to comprehend the importance of verbal, visual, and auditory stimulation for newborns as well.

Performing an examination at the bedside also gives the client permission to explore her newborn, which she may have been hesitant to do. A Brazelton neonatal assessment (see Chapter 22, p. 687) will assist the client to further understand her newborn's response to stimuli, a key factor in the client's response to the individuality of her newborn once she goes home. Parents who have some idea of what to expect from their infants will be less frustrated with the newborn's behavior.

The adolescent mother appreciates positive feedback about her fine newborn and her developing maternal responses. This praise and encouragement will increase her confidence and self-esteem.

Group classes for adolescent mothers should include infant care skills, information about growth and development, infant feeding, well-baby care, and danger signals in the ill newborn. An excellent way to incorporate neurologic development and stimulation for newborns it to teach the mothers how to make a few simple toys, such as mobiles and wall hangings. Often the child life department of a hospital may help with such classes, while the nursing staff concentrates on other areas of teaching.

Lunch groups can be organized around discussions of topics of interest to the adolescents. These are ideal times to explore the young mothers' ideas about cuddling and rocking their newborns, ways to handle crying, misbehavior, and "spoiling." The nurse can correct misconceptions. Jarrett (1982) found that young mothers were deficient in their knowledge and expectations of their newborns. In her study, nearly half of the adolescents expected their infants to be bladder trained by less than 12 months of age; three-quarters of her sample expected obedient behavior before 12 months. These findings demonstrate the need for education regarding growth and development.

Ideally, teenage mothers should visit adolescent clinics where mother and newborn are assessed for several years after birth. In this way, classes on parenting, vocational guidance, and school attendance could be followed closely. School systems that offer classes for young mothers are an excellent way of helping adolescents finish school and learn how to parent at the same time.

THE FOURTH TRIMESTER

The disparity between the quality and consistency of care provided to a woman during the intrapartal period and during the initial weeks of the postpartal period has received increased recognition by both consumers and health care providers. The term "fourth trimester" is frequently used to define this period.

During the postpartal period, the mother must accomplish certain physical and developmental tasks, including restoring physical condition, developing competence and skill in caring for and meeting the needs of her dependent infant, establishing a relationship with her new child, and adapting to altered life-styles and family structure resulting from the addition of a new member (Gruis, 1977).

Although physical restoration is fairly predictable, the new mother may have an inadequate or incorrect understanding of what to expect during the weeks following delivery. Concern over the restoration of her figure is often high, especially if she has retained some weight or had not expected a soft abdomen, stretch marks, or changes in her breasts. If her partner seems disappointed in her appearance, the problem may be compounded and the new mother may secretly fear that the physical changes in her body are permanent.

Continued physical discomfort frequently represents an unexpected element, too. Breast enlargement and nipple tenderness may produce discouragement for the breast-feeding mother, and episiotomy and hemorrhoidal pain may interfere with elimination and sexual relations and may promote fatigue. Fatigue is perhaps the most pervasive yet underestimated problem during the initial weeks.

Increased social mobility has decreased the availability of family support systems to assist a new family in adjusting. If the partner is unable to provide assistance and if there are other small children in the family, obtaining adequate rest becomes especially difficult. The constant, consistent needs of the new child for care also contribute to the problem as mother and child attempt to establish a mutually acceptable routine.

Developing competence and skill in caring for an infant may be especially anxiety-provoking for a new mother. Nurses and other health care providers have attempted to alleviate this anxiety by offering classes in child care both prenatally and in the postpartal unit. However, the psychologic changes occurring during the immediate postpartal period, coupled with the excitement and anxiety of parenthood, may serve as blocks to complete learning. Then, too, small unanticipated concerns may become monumental to a mother home alone attempting to cope. Her feelings of awkwardness or inadequacy may cause her to perceive herself as a failure. If she has family or friends nearby, she will generally ask for their assistance and advice, but many new mothers do not have adequate support systems and thus experience increased feelings of isolation.

The maternal–infant attachment process begins during pregnancy, intensifies in the period following delivery, and continues into the postpartal period. As the mother–child relationship develops, it is vital that the mother understand both normal growth and development and her child's distinct patterns of behavior, crying, eating, and sleeping. She should also be aware of the interaction capacity, behavioral response, and mood or temperament of the infant.

The woman's developmental task of adapting to the new family member involves developing a realistic acceptance of changed roles, retaining a sense of autonomy while developing a sense of "family," establishing and maintaining healthful routines, sharing parenting responsibilities, and maintaining a satisfactory personal relationship with her husband (Duvall, 1977). Efforts to achieve these tasks frequently produce stress, even if the child was planned. It is difficult to be adequately prepared for the changes a child brings, and a certain degree of grief for the lost lifestyle is to be expected. Sibling problems must be anticipated and dealt with as other children also seek to adjust to the new family member (Gruis, 1977).

Nursing Management

Nurses have been in the forefront of health providers in attempting to rectify the deficiencies in care currently existing during the postpartal period. Many obstetricians and nurse practitioners now routinely see all postpartal clients 1–2 weeks after delivery in addition to the routine 6-week checkup. This extra visit provides an opportunity for physical assessment as well as assessment of the mother's psychologic and informational needs.

TWO- AND SIX-WEEK EXAMINATIONS

The routine physical assessment, which may rapidly be made, focuses on the woman's general appearance, breasts, reproductive tract, bladder and bowel elimination, and any specific problems or complaints. (See the accompanying Postpartal Physical Assessment Guide.) In addition, conversation is used to determine nutrition patterns, fatigue level, family adjustment, and psychologic status of the mother (see the accompanying Psychologic Assessment Guide). Any problems with child care are explored, and referral to a pediatric nurse practitioner or pediatrician is made if needed. Available community resources, including Public Health Department follow-up visits, are mentioned when appropriate.

Discussion of family planning is appropriate at this time, and information regarding birth control methods is provided.

The couple may wish to resume a method that they used before the pregnancy or may require information regarding alternative birth control methods (see Chapter 6). Contraceptive methods are reinstated at various times following delivery. Vaginal foams, jellies, spermaticides, and condoms may be used as soon as sexual activity resumes. A diaphragm needs to be refitted after delivery due to possible change in the size of the vaginal vault; this is usually done at the postpartal checkup. An IUD may be inserted 3–6 weeks after delivery with no resultant increased risk of perforation of the uterus, expulsion of the device, or pregnancy. Birth control pills may be restarted at 3 weeks postpartum as long as there are no contraindications (Pritchard and MacDonald, 1980).

In ideal situations a family approach involving the father, infant, and possibly other siblings would permit a total evaluation and provide an opportunity for all family members to ask questions and express concerns. In addition, disturbed family patterns might be more readily diagnosed so that therapy could be instituted to prevent future problems of neglect or abuse.

FOLLOW-UP CARE

Follow-up care for the postpartal client may be accomplished by home visits, postpartal classes, or follow-up phone calls. A home visit 2–3 days after discharge facilitates accurate assessment and client teaching.

Postpartal classes are becoming more common as caregivers recognize the continuing needs of the childbearing family. A series of structured classes may focus on topics such as parenting, postpartal exercise, or nutrition, or there may be loosely structured group sessions that address concerns of mothers as they arise. Such classes offer chances for the new mother to socialize, share her concerns, and receive encouragement. Because babysitting arrangements may be difficult or expensive, it is desirable to provide child care for newborns and siblings, or in some instances, infants may remain with mothers in the class.

Postpartal Physical Assessment Guide: 2 Weeks and 6 Weeks After Delivery

Assess	Normal findings	Alterations and possible causes*	Nursing responses to data base†
Vital signs Blood pressure	Return to normal prepregnant level	Elevated blood pressure (anxiety, essential hypertension, renal disease)	Review history, evaluate normal baseline; refer to physician if necessary
Pulse	60–90 beats/min (or prepregnant normal rate)	Increased pulse rate (excitement, anxiety, cardiac disorders)	Count pulse for full minute, note irregularities; marked tachycardia or beat irregularities require additional assessment and possible physician referral
Respirations	16–24/min	Marked tachypnea or abnormal patterns (respiratory disorders)	Evaluate for respiratory disease; refer to physician if necessary
Temperature	36.2C–37.6C (98F–99.6F)	Increased temperature (infection)	Assess for signs and symptoms of infection or disease state
Weight	2 weeks: probable weight loss of 14–20+ lb	Little or no weight loss (fluid retention, subinvolution, poor dietary habits)	Evaluate dietary habits and nutritional state; review blood pressure to evaluate fluid retention or blood losses
	6 weeks: returning to normal prepregnant weight	Retained weight (poor dietary habits)	Determine amount of daily exercise Refer to dietitian if necessary for dietary counseling
		Extreme weight loss (excessive dieting)	Discuss appropriate diets; refer to dietitian if necessary
Breasts Nonnursing	2 weeks: may have mild tenderness; small amount of milk may be expressed; breasts returning to prepregnant size	Some engorgement (incomplete suppression of lactation)	Engorgement usually seen only when no medication has been given to suppress lactation; advise client to wear a supportive well-fitted bra, avoid hot showers, etc. (see p. 925); evaluate for signs and symptoms of mastitis (rare in nonnursing mothers)
	6 weeks: soft, with no tenderness; return to prepregnant size	Redness, marked tenderness (mastitis) Palpable mass (tumor)	
Nursing	Full, with prominent nipples; lactation established	Cracked, fissured nipples (feeding problems) Redness, marked tenderness, or even abscess formation (mastitis) Palpable mass (full milk duct, tumor)	Counsel about nipple care (see p. 931) Evaluate client condition, evidence of fever; refer to physician for initiation of antibiotic therapy, if indicated Opinion varies as to value of breast examination for nursing mothers; some feel a nursing mother should examine her breasts monthly, after feeding, when breasts are empty; if palpable mass is felt, refer to physician for further evaluation

Postpartal Physical Assessment Guide: 2 Weeks and 6 Weeks After Delivery Cont'd

Assess	Normal findings	Alterations and possible causes*	Nursing responses to data base†
			For breast inflammation instruct the mother to: 1. Keep breast empty by frequent feeding 2. Rest when possible 3. Take aspirin for pain 4. Force fluids If symptoms persist for more than 24 hours, instruct her to call her physician
Abdominal musculature	2 weeks: improved firmness, although ``bread dough'' consistency is not unusual, especially in multipara Striae pink and obvious	Marked disastasis recti (relaxation of muscles)	Evaluate exercise level; provide information on appropriate exercise program
	Cesarean incision healing	Drainage, redness, tenderness, pain, edema (infection)	Evaluate for infection; refer to physician if necessary
	6 weeks: muscle tone continues to improve; striae may be beginning to fade, they may not achieve a silvery appearance for several more weeks Linea nigra fading		
Elimination pattern Urinary tract	Return to prepregnant urinary elimination routine	Urinary incontinence, especially when lifting, coughing, laughing, and so on (urethral trauma) Pain or burning when voiding, urgency and/or frequency, pus or WBC in urine, pathogenic organisms in culture (urinary tract infection)	Assess for cystocele; instruct in appropriate muscle tightening exercises; refer to physician Evaluate for urinary tract infection; obtain clean catch urine; refer to physician for treatment if indicated
	Routine urinalysis within normal limits (proteinurea disappeared)	Sugar or ketone in urine — may be some lactose present in urine of breast-feeding mothers (diabetes)	Evaluate diet; assess for signs and symptoms of diabetes; refer to physician
Bowel habits	2 weeks: may still be some discomfort with defecation, especially if client had severe hemorrhoids or 3° extension	Severe constipation or pain when defecating (trauma or hemorrhoids)	Discuss dietary patterns; encourage fluid, adequate roughage Continue use of stool softener if necessary to prevent pain associated with straining; continue sitz baths, periods of rest for severe hemorrhoids; assess healing of episiotomy and/or lacerations; severe constipation may require administration of laxatives,

Postpartal Physical Assessment Guide: 2 Weeks and 6 Weeks After Delivery Cont'd

Assess	Normal findings	Alterations and possible causes*	Nursing responses to data base†
			stool softeners, and an enema
	6 weeks: return to normal prepregnancy bowel elimination	Marked constipation	See above
		Fecal incontinence or constipation (rectocele)	Assess for evidence of rectocele; instruct in muscle tightening exercises; refer to physician
Reproductive tract Lochia	2 weeks: lochia alba, scant amounts, fleshy odor	Foul odor, excessive in amounts (infection) Return to lochia rubra or persistence of lochia rubra or serosa	Assess for evidence of infection and/or subinvolution; culture lochia; refer to physician
	6 weeks: no lochia, or return to normal menstruation pattern	See above	See above
Pelvic examination	2 weeks: uterus no longer palpable abdominally; external os closed; uterine muscles still somewhat lax and uterus may be displaced; introitus of vagina still lacking tone—gapes when intraabdominal pressure is increased by coughing or straining Episiotomy and/or lacerations healing; no signs of infection	External cervical os open, uterus not decreasing appropriately (subinvolution, infection) Evidence of redness, tenderness, poor tissue approximation in episiotomy and/or laceration (wound infection)	Assess for evidence of subinvolution and/or infection; refer to physician if indicated
	6 weeks: almost returned to prepregnant size with almost completely restored muscle tone Cervix completely closed with only transverse slit apparent	Continued flow of lochia, some opening of cervical os, failure to decrease appropriately in size (subinvolution)	Assess for evidence of subinvolution and/or infection; refer to physician for further evaluation and for dilatation and curettage if necessary
	Good return of muscle tone to pelvic floor	Marked relaxation of pelvic floor muscles (uterine prolapse)	Assess for evidence of uterine prolapse; discuss appropriate perineal exercises; refer to physician if indicated
Papanicolaou test	Negative	Test results show atypical cells (see p. 230)	Refer to physician for further evaluation and treatment
Hemoglobin and hematocrit level	6 weeks: Hgb 12 g/dL Hct 37% ± 5%	Hgb < 12 g/dL Hct 32% (anemia)	Assess nutritional status, begin (or continue) supplemental iron; for marked anemia (Hgb 9 g/dL) additional assessment and/or physician referral may be necessary

* Possible causes of alterations are placed in parentheses.
† This column provides guidelines for further assessment and initial nursing interventions.

PSYCHOLOGIC ASSESSMENT GUIDE

Assess	Normal findings	Alterations and possible causes*	Nursing responses to data base†
Attachment	Evidence of bonding process demonstrated by soothing, cuddling and talking to infant, appropriate feeding techniques, eye-to-eye contact, calling infant by name	Failure to bond demonstrated by lack of behaviors associated with bonding process, calling infant by nickname that promotes ridicule, inadequate infant weight gain, infant is dirty, hygienic measures are not being maintained, severe diaper rash, failure to obtain adequate supplies to provide infant care (malattachment)	Provide counseling; refer to public health nurse for continued home visits
Adjustment to parental role	Parents are coping with new roles in terms of division of labor, financial status, communication, readjustment of sexual relations, and adjusting to new daily tasks	Inability to adjust to new roles (immaturity, inadequate education and preparation, ineffective communication patterns, inadequate support, current family crisis)	Provide counseling; refer to parent groups
Education	Mother understands self-care measures	Inadequate knowledge of self-care (inadequate education)	Provide education and counseling
	Parents are knowledgeable regarding infant care	Inadequate knowledge of infant care (inadequate education)	
	Siblings are adjusting to new baby	Excessive sibling rivalry	
	Parents have chosen a method of contraception	Birth control method not chosen	

* Possible causes of alterations are placed in parentheses.
† This column provides guidelines for further assessment and initial nursing interventions.

The follow-up telephone call is usually initiated by nurses from the postpartal unit of the agency where the mother delivered. The initial contact is made during the first week after discharge. If the call is delayed beyond this time, the family may have already adopted unsatisfactory methods of dealing with problems. For instance, a new nursing mother discouraged by sore nipples may elect to give up breast-feeding because she is not aware of measures she could employ to improve her comfort.

The nurse has five major functions to accomplish when telephoning:

1. Initiating contact with the family during the especially stressful first week. Frequently the family recognizes that problems exist, but they are unaware of where to seek help or are reluctant to do so.

2. Assessing the mother and family to evaluate their status.

3. Providing follow-up care as needed, utilizing all available resources.

4. Reinforcing existing knowledge and providing additional health teaching as indicated.

5. Communicating the results of the nursing assessment, intervention, and evaluation to appropriate agencies and/or health care providers (Donaldson, 1977).

The hospital identification numbers for both mother and baby are saved and utilized as a reference when phoning. Most agencies also use an assessment form to provide for consistency and information in the event that additional follow-up care is indicated.

Although the focus of concern in a follow-up call may vary, concern is frequently directed toward specific aspects of infant care. However, a written evaluation of a group of mothers by Gruis (1977) found that the group's major worry was the return of their figures to normal. Other experiences indicate that telephone follow-up support helps promote a positive breast-feeding experience (Jennings and Edmundson, 1980). Because of this variation in concerns, the nurse must be prepared to discuss physical hygiene problems or worries, basic infant care, sibling difficulties, maternal attachment, paternal engrossment, and the status of the family as a whole. The goal of the follow-up care is to promote confidence and independence while serving as a source of assistance and a guide to other resources when necessary (Donaldson, 1977).

The data obtained during the follow-up call should be preserved and incorporated into the maternal record, which is useful in providing information to the physician or community agencies and may be a helpful reference during subsequent births.

SUMMARY

The puerperium begins with the delivery of a newborn and extends through the next 6 weeks. During this period numerous changes are occurring within the mother's body. The involutional process involves changes in the majority of the body systems as they return to the prepregnant state. The addition of a new family member necessitates a reordering and restructuring of the family unit. These changes may produce a time of stress for the new family. There are many new tasks to be learned and new adjustments to be made.

Through an understanding of expected changes and assessment of numerous physical and psychologic factors, the nurse can intervene more appropriately and assist the new family as they take on the parenting role. In these times of increased mobility and lack of family members in close proximity, the new family looks to the nurse as a resource person who can assist them in learning their new tasks.

Resource Groups

Cesarean Association for Research, Education, Support and Satisfaction in Birthing, (CARESS), Burbank, CA 91510.

Cesarean Birth Council, San Jose, CA 95101.

Cesarean/Support, Education and Concern (C/Sec., Inc.), Dedham, MA 02026.

La Leche League, U.S. Headquarters, 9616 Minneapolis Avenue, Franklin, IL 60131.

Parent Education Resource Center, Box 94, Metropolitan State College, 1006 11th Street, Denver, CO 80204.

References

Affonso, D. D. 1981. *Impact of cesarean childbirth*. Philadelphia: F. A. Davis Company.

Barber, H. R., and Graber, E. A. 1974. *Surgical disease in pregnancy*. Philadelphia: W. B. Saunders Co.

Benson, R. C. 1980. *Handbook of obstetrics and gynecology*. Los Altos, Calif.: Lange Medical Publications.

Beske, J. E. May/June 1982. Important factors in breast-feeding success. *MCN*. 7:174.

Bille, D. A. 1981. *Practical approaches to patient teaching*. Boston: Little, Brown & Co.

Bowes, W. A. 1980. The effect of medications on the lactating mother and her infant. *Clin. Obstet. Gynecol.* 23:1073.

Burd, B. Aug. 1981. Encouragement counts in breast-feeding. *Am. J. Nurs.* 81:149.

Clark, A. L., ed. 1978. *Culture/child-bearing/health professionals*. Philadelphia: F. A. Davis Company.

Clark, A. L. 1981. *Culture and childrearing*. Philadelphia: F. A. Davis Company.

Danforth, D. N. 1982. *Obstetrics and gynecology*, 4th ed. Philadelphia: Harper & Row.

Davidson, N. 1974. REEDA: evaluating postpartum healing. *J. Nurse-Midwifery.* 9(2):6.

Donaldson, N. E. 1977. Follow-up at home. *Am. J. Nurs.* 77(7):1176.

Duvall, E. 1977. *Marriage and family development*, 5th ed. Philadelphia: J. B. Lippincott Co.

Food and Nutrition Board. 1980. *Recommended dietary allowances*, 9th ed. Washington, D.C.: National Academy of Sciences, National Research Council.

Foster, S. March/April 1982. Bromocriptine: suppressing lactation. *MCN*. 7:99.

Greenhill, J. P., and Friedman, E. A. 1974. *Biological principles and modern practice of obstetrics*. Philadelphia: W. B. Saunders Co.

Gruis, M. May/June 1977. Beyond maternity: postpartum concerns of mothers. *MCN*. 2(3):182.

Hames, C. T. Sept./Oct. 1980. Sexual needs and interests of postpartum couples. *J. Obstet. Gynecol. Neonatal Nurs.* 9:313.

Hoffman, J. B. 1953. A suggested treatment for inverted nipples. *Am. J. Obstet. Gynecol.* 66:346.

Horn, B. M. 1981. Cultural concepts and postpartal care. *Nurs. Health Care.* 2:516.

Jarrett, G. E. March/April 1982. Childbearing patterns of young mothers: expectations, knowledge and practices. *MCN.* 7:119.

Jeffries, R. D. 1981. A short course in breastfeeding. *Iss. Comp. Pediatr. Nurs.* 5:243.

Jennings, B., and Edmundson, M. Dec. 1980. The postpartum period: After confinement: the fourth trimester. *Clin. Obstet. Gynecol.* 23(4):1093.

Lawrence, R. A. 1980. *Breastfeeding: a guide for the medical profession.* St. Louis: The C. V. Mosby Co.

Loebl, S., and Spratto, G. 1980. *The nurse's drug handbook.* New York: John Wiley & Sons.

Marut, J., and Mercer, R. May 1979. Comparison of primiparas' perceptions of vaginal and cesarean births. *Nurs. Res.* 28:260.

Masters, W. H., and Johnson, V. E. 1966. *Human sexual response.* Boston: Little, Brown & Co.

Mercer, R. T. Sept./Oct. 1981. The nurse and maternal tasks of early postpartum. *MCN.* 6:341.

Moss, J. R. Nov./Dec. 1981. Concerns of multiparas on the third postpartum day. *J. Obstet. Gynecol. Neonatal Nurs.* 10:421.

Mullett, S. E. 1982. Helping mothers breast-feed. *MCN.* 7:178.

Niebyl, J. R., et al. 1979. The effect of chlorotrianisene as postpartum lactation suppression on blood coagulation factors. *Am. J. Obstet. Gynecol.* 134:518.

Palma, P. A., and Adcock, E. W., III. July 1981. Human milk and breastfeeding. *Am. Fam. Physician.* 24:179.

Platzer, A. C.; Lew, C. D.; and Stewart, D. Sept. 1980. Drug administration via breast milk. *Hosp. Pract.* 15:111

Pritchard, J. A., and MacDonald, P. C. 1980. *Williams obstetrics,* 16th ed. New York: Appleton-Century-Crofts.

Riordan, J. M., and Countryman, B. A. Sept./Oct. 1980a. Basics of breastfeeding. Part IV: preparation for breastfeeding and early optimal functioning. *J. Obstet. Gynecol. Neonatal Nurs.* 9:357.

————. Nov./Dec. 1980b. Basics of breastfeeding. Part VI: some breastfeeding problems and solutions. *J. Obstet. Gynecol. Neonatal Nurs.* 9:361.

Rubin, R. Nov. 1961. Basic maternal behavior. *Nurs. Outlook.* 9:683.

Sahub, S. Oct. 1981. Drugs and the nursing mother. *Am. Fam. Physician.* 24:138.

Slattery, J. S. March/April 1977. Nutrition for the normal healthy infant. *Am. J. Mat. Child Nurs.* 2(2):105.

Tindall, V. R. 1968. Factors influencing puerperal thromboembolism. *J. Obstet. Gynecol. Br. Commonw.* 75:1324.

Ward, B. G.; Pridmore, B. R.; and Cox, L. W. 1981. Vietnamese refugees in Adelaide: an obstetric analysis. *Med. J. Australia.* 1:72.

Additional Readings

Austin, S. E. J. March/April 1980. Family-centered discharge planning classes . . . postpartum instruction. *MCN.* 5:96.

Carr, K. C., and Walton, V. E. Jan./Feb. 1982. Early postpartum discharge. *J. Obstet. Gynecol. Neonatal Nurs.* 11:29.

Crowder, D. S. Jan./Feb. 1981. Maternity nurses' knowledge of factors promoting successful infant breastfeeding: a survey at two hospitals. *J. Obstet. Gynecol. Neonatal Nurs.* 10:28.

Fawcett, J. Sept./Oct. 1981. Needs of cesarean birth parents. *J. Obstet. Gynecol. Neonatal Nurs.* 10:372.

Freeman, K. March 1980. A postpartum program that really works . . . help for new mothers as near as the phone. *Can. Nurse.* 76:40.

Fuller, W. E. 1980. Family planning in the postpartum period. *Clin. Obstet. Gynecol.* 23:1081.

Harris, J. K. March 1980. Self-care is possible after cesarean delivery. *Nurs. Clin. North Am.* 15:191.

Hedahl, K. J. Sept./Oct. 1980. Working with parents experiencing a cesarean birth. *Pediatr. Nurs.* 6:21.

Inglis, T. Sept./Oct. 1980. Postpartum sexuality. *J. Obstet. Gynecol. Neonatal Nurs.* 9:28.

Leonard, L. G. May/June 1982. Breastfeeding twins: maternal–infant nutrition. *J. Obstet. Gynecol. Neonatal Nurs.* 11:148.

Lipson, J. G., and Tilden, V. P. 1980. Psychological integration of the cesarean birth experience. *Am. J. Orthopsychiatry.* 50:598.

Senie, R. T. Jan./Feb. 1982. Possible related risks to breastfeeding. *J. Obstet. Gynecol. Neonatal Nurs.* 11:34.

Sheehan, F. Jan./Feb. 1981. Assessing postpartum adjustment: a pilot study. *J. Obstet. Gynecol. Neonatal Nurs.* 10:19.

Wainwright, S. 1981. How to promote successful breastfeeding. *Nurs. Times.* 77:1397.

■ 28 ■

ATTACHMENT

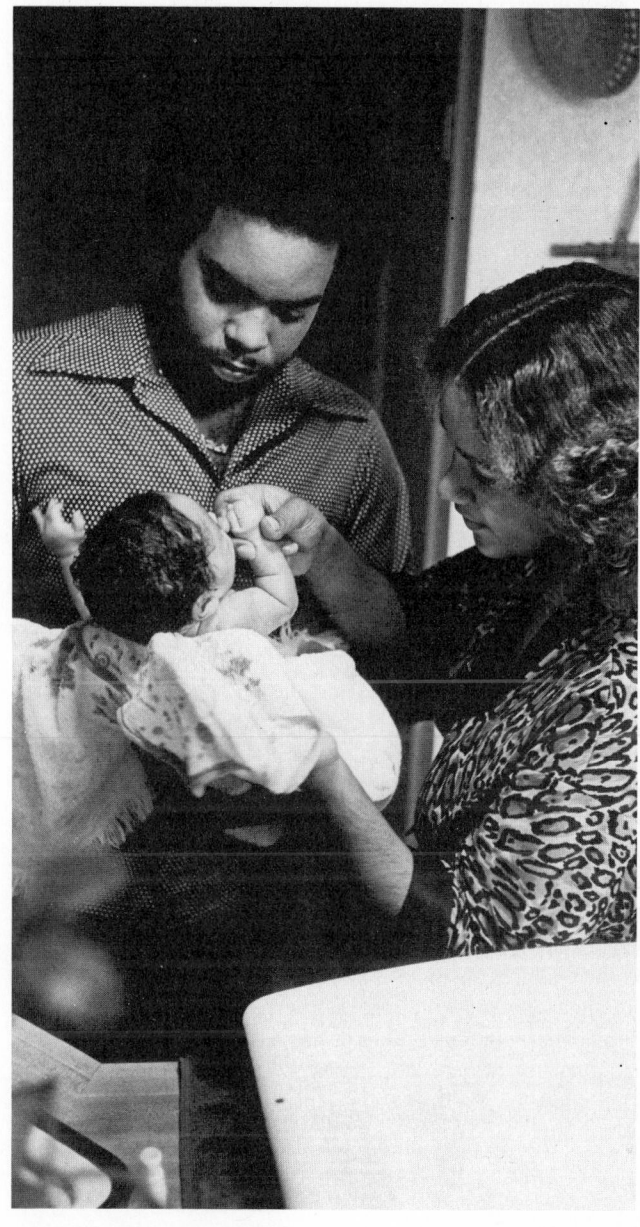

■ CHAPTER CONTENTS

NATURE OF ATTACHMENT

WHAT THE MOTHER BRINGS TO THE FIRST INTERACTION

    Life History

    Personality

    Sexual-Reproductive Experience

    Present Pregnancy

WHAT THE NEWBORN BRINGS TO THE FIRST INTERACTION

    Appearance

    Behaviors

THE SETTING

    Physical Environment

    Human Environment

    Condition of the Interactors

MOTHER-INFANT INTERACTIONS

    Introductory Bonding

    Acquaintance Phase

    Phase of Mutual Regulation

    Reciprocity

    Attachment Behaviors in the Adolescent Mother

FATHER-INFANT INTERACTIONS

SIBLINGS AND OTHERS

EVALUATION AND INTERVENTIONS IN MOTHER-INFANT RELATIONSHIPS

    Assessment of Early Attachment

    Guidelines for Intervention

    Assessment of Bonding

COMPLICATIONS OF MATERNAL-INFANT ATTACHMENT

■ OBJECTIVES

- Describe the attachment process, including the phases of maternal–infant interaction.

- List methods the nurse can use to facilitate a positive attachment process.

- Compare the factors influencing the first maternal–infant interaction.

- Explain the types of questions used for evaluating the maternal–infant relationship.

- Contrast the factors affecting family member interactions with the infant.

- List the types of complications that can affect the maternal–infant attachment process.

NATURE OF ATTACHMENT

What is the language of human attachment? How can the concept of attachment apply to so many different patterns of behavior? Those who have studied attachment in the past decades have approached the topic with different goals, out of varying professional backgrounds, and from opposite directions. Among the purposes of the research on attachment have been to describe it, to operationally define it, to relate it to outcomes in cognitive and social development, to support or refute psychologic theories, and to determine public child care policy. The background disciplines of researchers and clinicians interested in attachment include psychoanalysis, psychiatry, psychology, pediatrics, obstetrics, social work, teaching, child development, ethnology, and nursing.

The two major directions of attachment that are investigated are from mother to newborn and from newborn to mother. The early literature on attachment related primarily to the infant's tie to its mother, which was understood to occur in the second half of the first year of life when the infant was capable of recognizing the mother. This literature was derived in part from experience with maternally deprived infants. More recently, and motivated in part by disorders and failures in mothering, researchers have investigated the attachment of mothers to infants. The importance of fathers and siblings as attachers and attachees is in the early stages of exploration.

Just this brief glimpse at the past history of the concept of attachment makes it easy to understand why the language of attachment research is indeed a varied one. Definitions of the term, when found, vary in specificity and generality.

WHAT THE MOTHER BRINGS TO THE FIRST INTERACTION

It is often important in developing an understanding of a mother–newborn dyad to become aware of certain aspects of the mother's life history that may have significance for the relationship between the two. Each mother brings to the first meeting with her newborn a broad range of life experiences—pleasant, unpleasant, neutral, or mixed.

Life History

The mother brings the total of her years of experience as a participating family member in her family of origin. The number of years can vary considerably, but she has been an infant, a child, an adolescent, and probably a young adult within a particular family setting. Although the experiential content of those years, in pattern and meaning, is unique to each mother, certain aspects of the family can be viewed as potentially important to the present interaction:

1. The mother was born into a specific ordinal position in her family, which in part determined the nature of some life experiences. For example, she could have been first-born, last-born, middle child, only child, or only girl. Each position could have influenced the quality of parenting she received, limited her opportunities for practice with young infants, or shaped her feelings for a baby of similar position. For example, if the mother has sought out and experienced encounters with infants and young children, she is more likely to be aware of their abilities and therefore have realistic expectations of her own newborn. Early interest in young children has been found to be predictive of postpartal maternal adaptation (Shereshefsky and Yarrow, 1973).

2. Her family could be described as relatively stable or unstable in terms of geographic location, employment, persons available, and physical and mental health of its members. Instability in any of these areas adds situational stresses to the developmental stresses of a growing child. Poverty, poor housing, fears of unemployment, geographic mobility, and undernutrition are all environmental factors that can affect a mother's ability to relate well to her newborn or child.

3. Her family utilized communication patterns that were relatively effective or ineffective in meeting the emotional and educational needs of individual family mem-

bers or in maintaining the healthy functioning of the family system.

4. Significant persons in the family who were responsible for her nurturance had a greater or lesser capacity to express interpersonal tenderness and warmth through caring for another human being.

The constellation and characteristics of the mother's family provide the model on which she is most likely to base her mothering practices. The exact nature of the past family experiences, only suggested above, helped fashion the blueprint for family development and childrearing that the new mother carries within her. Part of the design is in conscious awareness; part lies hidden from view, waiting to be provoked in unpredictable ways by situations that arise in the course of mother–infant interaction.

Personality

The mother brings to the first interaction with her newborn the self she has become. Her genetic potential has shaped and been shaped by family and other experiences over time. She has developed into an extremely complex and unique personality with a number of characteristics of importance in her relationship with her infant.

The level of basic trust this mother has been able to develop in reaction to her life experiences. Does she view the world as a generally friendly or hostile place? Does she consider humans to be fundamentally good or evil? The feelings accompanying her views can influence her motivation for childbearing and her philosophy of childrearing, both of which are reflected in direct interactions.

A mother with adequate levels of basic trust can accept her newborn as an individual with unique and changing needs that should be gratified as much as possible. If she cannot trust that her infant is capable of expressing needs and will not make unnecessary demands, she is put in the position of deciding whether to respond to fussing or crying each time it occurs. Such a decision-making burden can delay maternal responses and can also result in inconsistencies in mothering behavior. In addition, a prevailing mistrust of others can result in unwillingness to reach out for emotional and informational support and in an inability to benefit from support when it is received (Kennedy, 1969).

Level of self-esteem. How much does she value herself as a person, as a woman, as a potential mother? Does she feel relatively competent or generally ineffective in coping with tasks, transitions, and adjustments?

Capacity for enjoying oneself. Is the mother able to find pleasure in everyday activities and in human relationships?

Interest in and adequacy of knowledge about childbearing and childrearing. A mother's beliefs about the course of pregnancy, the capacities of newborns, and the nature of

maternal emotions can set up expectations for both self and infant that may influence her behavior at first contact with the newborn and in later interactions.

Her prevailing mood, or usual feeling tone. Is the woman predominantly content, angry, depressed, or anxious? Does she tend to express or withhold her feelings, positive or negative? Is her expression appropriate and authentic, devious, oblique, or nonverbal? Is she sensitive to her own feelings and those of others? These capacities will help determine her ability to understand and accept her own needs and to obtain support in meeting them.

In an extensive study of essentially normal middle-class families, Shereshefsky and Yarrow (1973) reported that two personality factors—ego strength and nurturance—were predictive of maternal adjustment during pregnancy and in the postpartal period. *Ego strength* was described as a woman's overall level of maturity and emotional adaptation and included, among other qualities, her self-acceptance and ability to provide for her own enjoyment. *Nurturance* was a woman's ability and willingness to respond to others in a giving way. The authors concluded that a woman's "adaptation to pregnancy and maternity tends to be consistent with her characteristic patterns of response and her adaptive behavior in general." Another recent study indicates that personality qualities (self-confidence, self-image, and others) observable in early pregnancy can be predictive of overall pregnancy adjustment and adaptation to motherhood (Leifer, 1977).

Sexual–Reproductive Experience

Each mother brings to her first meeting with her newborn a mixture of past experiences related to the reproductive function. Some of the experiences are indirect or vicarious. Stories related by relatives, friends, acquaintances, and strangers have become a part of her store of information. More often than not, it is the unpleasant or fearful experiences that are remembered, exaggerated, misinterpreted, and transmitted, creating or confirming fears and negative expectations.

A mother's direct experiences with sexuality can influence her view of herself as a mother-to-be and her expectations of her newborn. If she experienced menstruation negatively—as a painful condition, a sickness, or a vulnerable state—or if she considers her genital expression of sexuality as less than adequate or normal, she might also question the outcome of her procreative efforts. A period of infertility can also reduce maternal self-confidence. A prior reproductive loss through spontaneous abortion, preterm delivery, stillbirth, or sudden infant death syndrome can diminish a mother's ability or willingness to develop an emotional tie to the next baby. Having previously delivered a genetically defective, developmentally disabled, or physically ill infant can have a similar effect.

Present Pregnancy

Each mother brings to her first visual contact with her newborn her reactions to that particular pregnancy, from conception through birth. The pregnancy evolved and developed in an emotional climate. The conception was planned or unplanned, the baby was wanted or unwanted—for any number of reasons. The course of the pregnancy was predominantly either pleasant and worry-free or filled with discomfort and anxieties. The mother felt encouraged and supported in her 9 months, or she experienced disapproval and felt isolated. Ongoing life events essentially unrelated to her pregnant condition may have enhanced her pregnancy or depleted the energy reserves and coping ability so necessary to pregnancy adjustments (Kennedy, 1969). The stresses of pregnancy, in combination with low adaptive potential, can influence the pregnancy's vulnerability to a variety of complications (Nuckolls et al., 1972).

Most important, perhaps, is the fact that each mother, by the time of expected delivery, has developed an emotional orientation of some kind toward the fetus, based on a tactile-kinesthetic awareness combined with her fantasy images and perceptions. It has been suggested that several patterns of developing maternal feeling are observable during the course of pregnancy (Leifer, 1977). One type of mother feels an emotional closeness to the fetus very early in the pregnancy. This feeling becomes deeper at quickening and grows in intensity through the second and third trimester. By the time of labor, this mother feels a close relationship and interaction between herself and the fetus. A different type of mother feels no attachment early in pregnancy, develops positive feelings shortly after feeling fetal movement, and has a well-established maternal bond by the end of pregnancy. In a third pattern, the mother experiences little or no positive feeling even by the end of the third trimester. Fetal movement is viewed as an intrusion and is reacted to with irritation. In this case the emotional orientation toward the expected newborn is essentially negative.

Leifer (1977) found that women who did not plan to become pregnant or who conceived for reasons of status or security were frequently among those who had minimal feelings of closeness to the fetus throughout the pregnancy. Those who felt well adjusted in their marriage and emotionally ready to have a baby were able to develop strong affectionate feelings and to interact with the fetus, demonstrating a positive orientation toward the infant even before the birth.

In summary, it appears that a woman's total life history, up to the time of birth, can be predictive of the nature of her adaptation to motherhood. However, a large part of her postpartal adjustment relates to the new arrival in the family, who until the moment of birth is essentially an unknown factor in the equation.

WHAT THE NEWBORN BRINGS TO THE FIRST INTERACTION

When there are two partners in an interpersonal interaction, each contributes in some way to the process. In years past, the newborn's influence on the beginning mother–infant relationship was treated as nonexistent or minimal. More recently, research on the capacities of newborns and very young neonates has shown that they are indeed active partners in the exchange and take part in shaping their own human environment from the moment of birth. Newborns do this by virtue of who they are and what they do—their appearance and behavior.

Appearance

At the moment of birth certain information about the newborn's external appearance is available to the mother. Each characteristic may have a special meaning for the mother as it relates to her hopes, fears, and expectations. The relatively obvious things are usually noted first: sex, size, shape, color, and presence or absence of abnormality or injury.

Behaviors

The newborn has, and may demonstrate at birth, certain functional behaviors, such as crying, sucking, eliminating, looking, listening, and startling. These behaviors do not occur in a random fashion. The normal newborn comes into the world programmed to respond positively to the expected maternal stimuli. For example, in the very first days of life, the infant has been shown to selectively attend to the human face, to prefer the human voice over other sounds, and to become quiet and alert when picked up and held over the shoulder (Korner and Thoman, 1970; Goren et al., 1975).

In addition to having behaviors in common with other neonates, each newborn, like the mother, is already a unique combination of genetic potential and life experience. The newborn's life experience is shorter and more limited in scope, of course, but it can have a powerful effect on observable behavior.

This simplified overview of significant background factors in the initial meeting of mother and newborn points up the fact that the exact feelings, reactions, and interactional responses of each mother at the culmination of each delivery defy prediction. The past history and present personality of each mother combine with the characteristics and behavior of her infant to influence the quality and direction of the maternal–newborn relationship. Two unique individuals are blending into an equally unique interactional system that changes with time and as the actors change and grow.

Precise prediction seems impractical, but is it feasible to develop some guidelines of normality for evaluating maternal–newborn interaction? What behaviors should alert us to watch for the disordered relationship? What behaviors should allow us to feel comfortable about the future direction?

THE SETTING

It is impossible to consider setting up behavioral norms for mother and newborn at first contact unless the variables of physical context, human environment, and condition of the interactors are first described.

Physical Environment

No drama takes place without a stage. In the case of the first dialogue between newborn and mother, the prerequisite delivery may have occurred in one of a variety of places. The most frequent setting by far is a maternity unit of a hospital. The physical surroundings are, in all probability, relatively strange to the woman as she moves from the admitting area to the labor room, delivery room, recovery area, and then to her room in the postpartal unit. She sees and comes in contact with "sickness and operation" furniture, materials, and routines. Noise levels are usually high, and many sounds are of uncertain origin and meaning for the mother. Food is usually withheld until after delivery. The strain and concomitant psychic stress of frequent accommodations to the physical environment can interfere with the progress of labor and delivery and with the comfort of mother–infant interaction.

An increasing number of women are deciding to give birth in their homes. This setting differs from the conventional hospital in that the physical environment is stable and familiar. In most instances of home birth, the mother-to-be has taken the major responsibility for selecting, furnishing, and equipping the birth environment.

Consumer and professional efforts to increase the comfort of hospital births while decreasing the risks inherent in home birth have produced an intermediate type of setting—hospital-independent birth centers or hospital birthing rooms. These facilities are more homelike in appearance and do not require moves from one module to another during the progression from labor through early recovery. Many institutions are also offering early discharge for families with support at home.

Human Environment

It appears to be a human characteristic to carry out the acts of labor and giving birth in a social setting. Very few women express the wish to be alone during parturition; most respond with distress to the idea of abandonment at such a time. Hospitals, now and in the past, have generally provided for fairly constant nursing supervision of women in active labor, in the course of delivery, and in the early hours after birth. Usually, however, there is a different caretaker present in each phase of the childbearing activities. Each nurse is relating to an unknown client at each step, and each client is relating to a series of unknown nurses. The nurse may systematically receive pertinent information about the client, but the client typically gets no help in orienting herself to interaction with each new nurse—and each has different advice, expectations, attitudes, and relating skills.

A number of hospitals have changed routines to permit the father or other significant persons to be present at labor, delivery, and after. This practice increases the possibility that a woman will have the support of one trusted person for the whole childbirth experience. The quality of support available from professionals or laypersons varies considerably according to their clinical and psychosocial skills. There are indications that a woman's perceptions of her physical care and emotional support and her reactions to the nonhuman elements of the environment can influence her mothering responses.

Condition of the Interactors

When the postbirth conditions are optimal, mother and newborn are ready to relate effectively to each other and to benefit from the interaction. The mother is emotionally high and alert, primed for maternal responsiveness by her hormonal state. The newborn is in a quiet, alert state, capable of attending to the mother's face and voice. However, several commonly occurring conditions act to diminish or divert the physical and psychologic energies available to the mother for relating with her infant. Fatigue, pain, cold, hunger, and thirst are discomforts frequently reported by mothers after delivery. Not uncommonly, the postpartal mother experiences a spell of uncontrollable shaking of the legs. In the typical labor, the mother may have received medication for relaxation and pain relief and may be encumbered in her movements by intravenous tubing.

Certain conditions in the newborn indicate lowered potential for human interaction. In addition to the physiologic adaptations immediately necessary to extrauterine existence, physical maturity, nutritional adequacy, neurologic intactness, bodily discomfort, extremes of temperature, and levels of analgesic and anesthetic agents have all been related to the infant's behavioral responses in the first hours of life—and later. Prophylactic eye treatments interfere with newborns' ability to keep their eyes open and focused on the mother's face. Generally speaking, any situation, condition, or stimulus that detracts from the energy either partner can direct toward attending to the other diminishes the probability of optimal interaction between the two.

MOTHER–INFANT INTERACTIONS

Introductory Bonding

Observers of very early mother–newborn interactions in hospital settings have presented evidence that a fairly regular pattern of maternal behaviors is exhibited at first contact with the normal newborn (Rubin, 1963; Klaus et al., 1970). In a progression of touching activities, the mother proceeds from fingertip exploration of the newborn's extremities toward palmar contact with the larger body areas

and finally to enfolding the infant with the whole hand and arms. The time taken to accomplish these steps varies from minutes to days, depending, it appears, on the timing of the first contact, the clothing barriers present, and the physical condition of the baby. Maternal excitement and elation tend to increase during the time of the initial meeting (Figure 28–1). The mother also increases the proportion of time spent in the *en face* position (Figure 28–2). She arranges herself or the newborn so that direct face-to-face and eye-to-eye contact is facilitated. There is an intense interest in having the infant's eyes open. When the eyes are open, the mother characteristically greets the newborn and talks in high-pitched tones to him or her.

Clinical observations indicate that behaviors differ somewhat in nonconventional delivery situations. Home birth and LeBoyer deliveries seem to speed up and otherwise modify the behaviors described. Often after a home birth the mother turns almost immediately to pick up and hold the newborn and to rub its cheek with her fingertip.

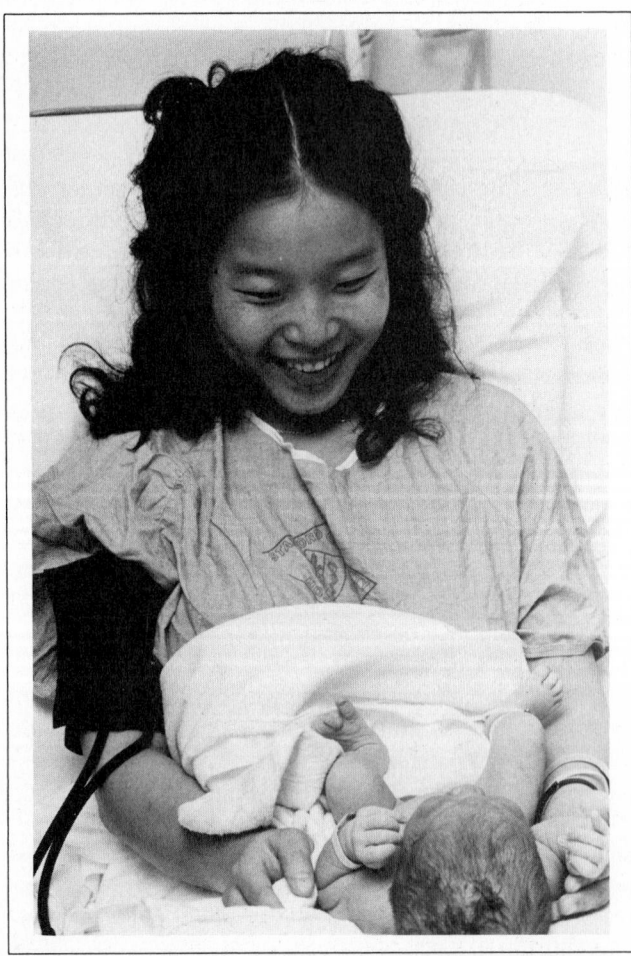

FIGURE 28–1 A new mother interacts with infant.

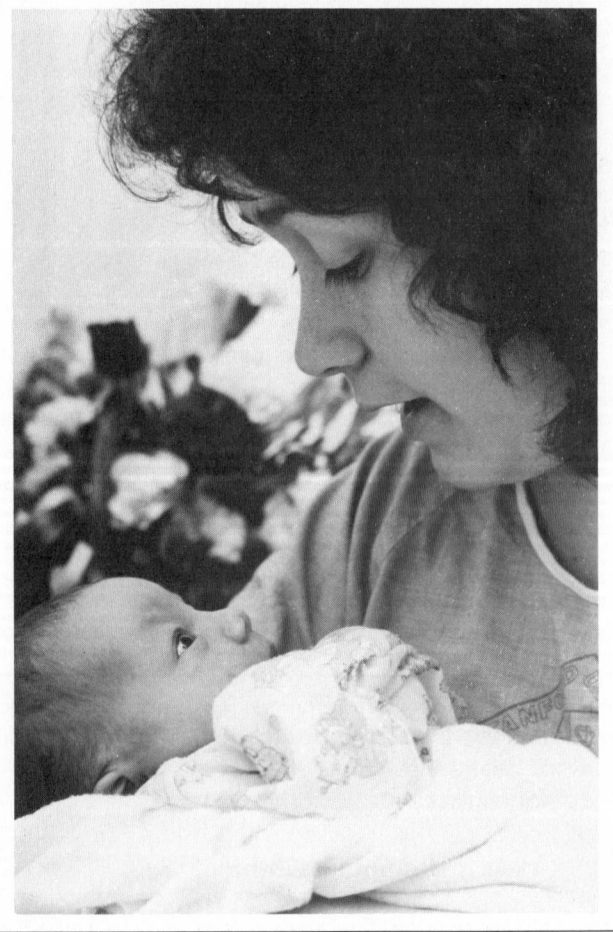

FIGURE 28–2 *En face* position.

The newborn is often offered the breast before the placenta is expelled. In a delivery patterned after the LeBoyer method, the mother, and sometimes the father, is encouraged to gently massage the infant's whole body while waiting for the placenta to be delivered.

In most instances the mother relies heavily on her senses of sight, touch, and hearing in getting to know what her baby is really like. She tends also to respond verbally to any sounds emitted by the newborn, such as cries, coughs, sneezes, and grunts. The sense of smell may also be involved, although this possibility has not been adequately studied as yet.

In addition to acting upon and interacting with the newborn, the mother is undergoing her own emotional reactions to the whole happening and, more specifically, to the baby as she perceives him or her. Sometimes direct comments and nonverbal cues clearly reflect the felt emotions; sometimes the mother reports only later on her feelings at the time. The frequency of the "I can't believe" reaction leads to the speculation that human gains as well as losses might initially be responded to with a degree of shock, disbelief, and denial. A feeling of emotional distance from the newborn is quite common: "I felt he was a stranger." On the other hand, feelings of connectedness between the newborn and the rest of the family can be expressed in positive or negative terms: "She's got your cute nose, Daddy" or "Oh, God, no! He looks just like the first one, and he was an impossible baby." A mother's facial expressions or the frequency and content of her questions may demonstrate concerns about the infant's general condition or normality, especially if her pregnancy was complicated or if a previously delivered baby was not normal.

Some of the more common emotional reactions to the newborn at birth have been noted briefly. There is, of course, a wide range of possible maternal feelings seen at delivery—positive, negative, and mixed. There are also differences in the intensity of feeling and in the mode of expression. For example, intense pleasure may be shown in smiles or in tears. In general, extremely negative feelings are predictive of later problems in the mother–infant relationship.

During the initial mother–newborn interaction the neonate, too, is continuously communicating. Although the infant behaves without conscious intent to convey interpersonal messages or to influence the behavior of others, elements of the newborn's appearance and behavior are perceived by the mother as if they represented intentionality and interpersonal dialogue, and they do influence her responses. The newborn's size says to the mother, "You nourished me well—you did a good job." Individual features say, "I am a part of you, or of my father. I belong with you." Even the time of birth can be read as a message: "I'm cooperative—or uncooperative." The intensity, timing, configuration, and other elements of the newborn's observable activity, however reflexive, are regularly responded to as a very personal communication from the baby to the mother.

What are the characteristic behaviors of a newborn? Unless care is taken to effect a gentle birth, a number of noxious stimuli impinge on the senses of the newly born neonate. The newborn is probably suctioned, held with head down somewhat, exposed to bright lights and cool air, and in some way cleaned. The infant usually responds by crying. In fact, newborns are typically stimulated to cry to reassure the caretakers that they are well and normal. When newborns no longer need to concentrate most of their energy in physical and physiologic response to the immediate crisis of birth, they are able to lie quietly with eyes open, looking about, moving limbs occasionally, making sucking motions, possibly attempting to get hand to mouth. Placed in appropriate proximity to the mother, the neonate appears to focus briefly on her face and to attend to her voice repeatedly in the first moments. When their mother is talking and neonates are attending, they are likely to move parts of their body—arms, legs, fingers, eyelids—in an exact synchrony with their mother's minute voice changes (Condon and Sander, 1974). This synchrony between rhythms of speech and body movements of an infant can clearly be seen only with stop-frame analysis of films, but the mother probably has, at some level, an awareness of its occurrence.

The introductory mother–newborn interaction proceeds on the basis of identified, mutually elicited behaviors, occurring simultaneously and in multiplicity between the partners. The significant behavioral cues that shape the dyadic interaction at the first and subsequent contacts are illustrated in Figure 28–3.

Another kind of mutuality of experience may bring the mother into emotional closeness with her infant. If the birthing has been essentially normal and the partners are not prevented from immediate contact, they share in common the experiences of surviving a traumatic event, being brought to a state of alertness, gathering information about the other through direct interaction, and, if time permits, subsiding into a sleep of recovery. Both have demonstrated to each other the heightened capacity for interaction that has been observed during the first hours after birth.

Much evidence has accumulated to show that facilitation of this apparent readiness to relate to each other results in an increased maternal responsiveness to the newborn's needs that endures over time (Lozoff et al., 1977). In a number of related studies, some groups of mothers were given earlier and/or more extended contact with their newborn than was the routine for control groups of similar mothers and then were observed in later interactions with their newborns. Mothers allowed earlier contact and/or increased in-hospital contact smiled more at their infants, showed more face-to-face behavior, and were quicker to use soothing and comforting behaviors when

FIGURE 28–3 Reciprocity system.

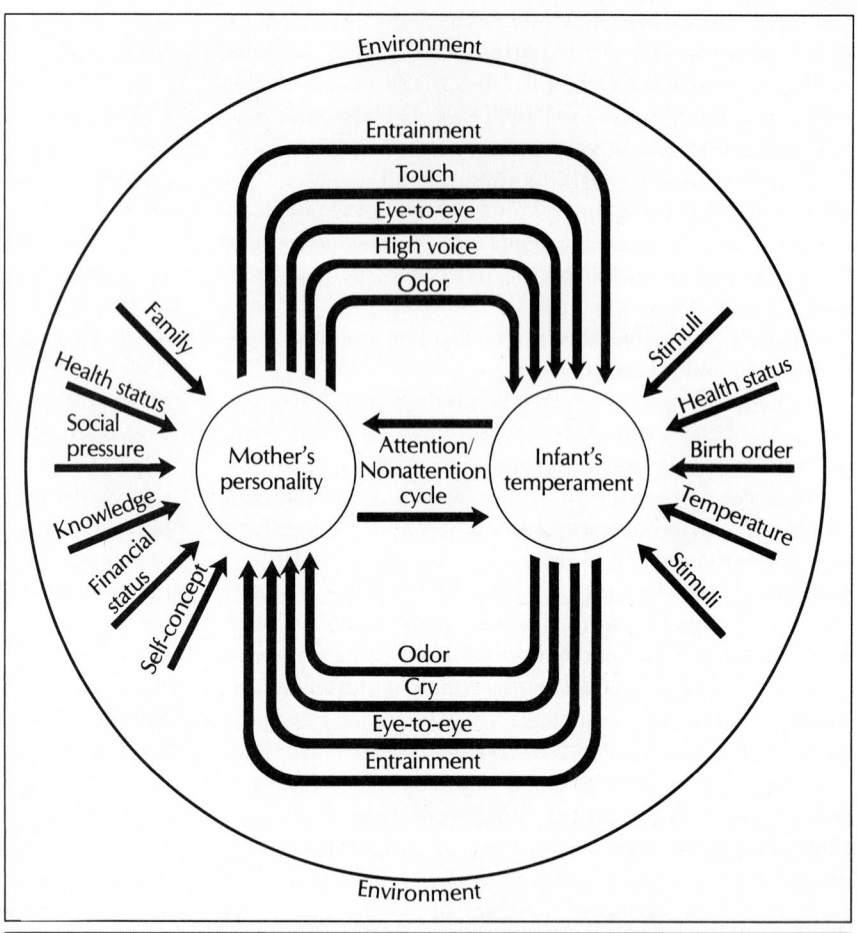

their infants exhibited distress. They appeared to enjoy subsequent contact with their infants more than the control group of mothers did. Differences between the groups were observable two years later. Klaus et al. (1970) and others have concluded that there is a period of increased maternal sensitivity in the early minutes and hours after birth, during which mother–infant contact is likely to enhance the development of the emotional bond between the mother and her newborn and to influence the nature and direction of the relationship in the early years. The term *bonding* might well be reserved for application to the time of the attraction peak immediately after birth, when first contact occurs.

Acquaintance Phase

During the introductory contact after birth, the mother gathers a certain amount of information about her baby. This learning about the partner is the first step in any interpersonal acquaintance. As described in relation to adults (Newcomb, 1961), the acquaintance process includes the following components: the acquisition of knowledge about the other, assessment of the other's attitude, and either

reinforcement or change in existing states of orientation toward the other. From the remarks, questions, and activities of a new mother in the earliest postpartal days, it is apparent that she is applying herself to the task of getting acquainted with her newborn. She wants to know what kind of newborn she is taking into her family system and what the infant's reaction to her is. She is also consciously involved in clarifying the nature of her own developing feelings toward the newborn. In part she is becoming acquainted with herself as the mother of this particular infant.

There is some indication that the degree to which a mother develops feelings of affectionate closeness or attachment to the fetus before birth is generally predictive of the course of maternal feelings toward the newborn immediately after birth and in the acquaintance phase (Leifer, 1977). Minimal closeness before birth seems to lead to less enjoyment of the newborn, less responsiveness to needs, and less empathy when the infant is in distress. Women who feel an intense attachment and interaction before birth appear to pick up the relationship at that level after delivery and to develop increased feelings of closeness in the acquaintance phase. They eagerly respond to the newborn's needs and are gratified by the newborn's apparent well-being. In addition, they are likely to be more successful at initiating and maintaining breast-feeding than are minimally attached mothers. Liking the infant at the start apparently contributes to the woman's understanding of her newborn as an individual with unique needs and adds to her willingness to respond to those needs. The positive orientation at the beginning of contact probably also influences the woman toward a positive perception of her newborn's attitude toward her as a mother. It helps her believe that her baby appreciates her.

Just as in the bonding phase, the newborn plays an important part in determining the outcome of the acquaintance phase of the mother–infant relationship. He or she can either assist or confound the mother as she attempts to learn the newborn's embryonic personality, characteristic abilities and behaviors. If he or she is relatively well organized in responses to the usual caretaking stimuli and is regular in biologic rhythms, the infant tends to be easy to understand. If he or she gives clear behavioral cues about needs, the infant's responses to mothering will be predictable. Such predictability makes a mother feel effective and competent—a pleasant feeling. If the newborn responds to motherly ministrations with a predominantly positive mood rather than with irritability, and if he or she has relatively long periods of being quietly awake and attentive, the infant is pleasant to be near and to interact with. Other behaviors that make an infant more attractive to caretakers are smiling, grasping a finger, nursing eagerly, cuddling, and being easy to console.

At the same time that the infant is unknowingly facilitating or providing obstacles to the mother's acquaintance with him or her, the newborn is also becoming acquainted. Thrust unexpectedly into a strange environment, newborns gather what information they can about their new world. They attend to sights, sounds, tastes, and smells, and experience different tactile and kinesthetic sensations. Within a few days after birth, infants show signs of recognizing recurrent situations and responding to changes in routine. To the extent that the world is their mother, it can be said that they are actively acquainting themselves with her.

The peak of the acquaintance phase appears to occur simultaneously with one of the phases of maternal puerperal restoration described by Rubin (1961). In the taking-in phase, which lasts for 2–3 days, the mother has a need to replenish her physical and emotional resources (see Chapter 27). Her inclination is to take in food, praise, information, sleep, and nurturance, in a rather undiscriminating and passive way. She seems impelled to review and to integrate every detail of her labor and delivery. So much happened in such a short time that it was difficult to take it all in while it was happening.

When the taking-in phase of rest and recuperation draws to a close and the acquaintance phase is well under way, the taking-hold phase of active maternal involvement

with self and newborn begins. The mother acts to regain control of her bodily functioning, to initiate mothering tasks, and to reintegrate herself with her family in the new role of mother with baby.

Phase of Mutual Regulation

In the performance of the necessary tasks of newborn care, such as feeding, bathing, and comforting, the new mother develops an awareness, on some level, that there is a degree of discrepancy between her wishes and needs and her baby's needs and desires. This awareness ushers in a phase of mutual regulation of behaviors. The degree of control to be exerted by each partner in the interpersonal adjustment is an issue in the early postpartal weeks. Maternal goals related to the resolution of this issue of control are, of course, variable, both among different mothers and within the same mother at different times. In some mother–infant pairs, the maternal goal is primarily to change the infant to meet the mother's needs. In other pairs it is quite apparent that the mother's intent is primarily to interpret correctly and to gratify completely all of her newborn's needs. Either of those approaches is likely to result in relational disturbances, the degree of distress and tension depending to a large extent on the newborn's reactions to the maternal behaviors used to reach the goal. For example, the mother who wishes to adjust her baby rather than adjust to him or her will have a smoother postpartal course if she is blessed with a highly adaptive infant who is positive in mood. The mother who is bent on meeting every need of her child at the same moment it arises will meet with failure very quickly if the newborn is unpredictable, is irregular in daily rhythms, and presents behavioral cues that are difficult to interpret. This kind of infant can easily take on the role of "spoiled" baby in a family.

The ideal solution to the control issue would be somewhere between the two extremes. A mother who realizes that she is a person with her own needs will be less vulnerable to the buildup of anger, frustration, anxiety, and guilt. In all but the most ideal situations, each partner must undergo disappointments, and each must at some time subordinate his or her own needs to the needs of the other. The most important consideration is that each should obtain a good measure of enjoyment from the ongoing interactions.

Generally speaking, it would seem that enjoyment is enhanced during the early months if the infant is sufficiently organized to clearly indicate his needs and if the mother's personality allows her to let him lead the interaction. Mutual maternal–infant regulation is never instantaneous; it is a process that continues to some degree throughout infancy and childhood. Fortunately, there appears to be a tendency toward improved organization of behavior in the newborn period and an increasing ability to nurture in the mother during the same time.

It is during the mutual adjustment phase that negative

maternal feelings are likely to surface or intensify. Because "everyone knows that mothers love their babies," these negative feelings often go unexpressed and are allowed to build up. If they are expressed, the response of friends, relatives, or health care personnel is often to deny the feeling to the mother: "You don't mean that"; "You can't feel that way"; "Your baby is not ugly, she is beautiful." Some negative feelings are normal in the first few days following delivery, and the nurse should be supportive when the mother vocalizes these feelings.

In the adjustment phase a mother may become ready to learn more about infants in general and about her newborn in particular (Adams, 1963). The mothering problems to be addressed have already arisen and become clarified. Information is needed to develop effective solutions. If valid information is available, the solutions will be more appropriate and more lasting than those based on inadequate data.

When mutual regulation arrives at the point where both partners have achieved a predominance of enjoyment in each other's company it is usually obvious to an observer that the relationship is good. It may be said that reciprocity has been achieved. A high degree of reciprocity is characteristic of successful mutual regulation.

Reciprocity

The mother–infant interaction process can be visualized as a system. This system is concerned with the mother–infant unit, the interactions between them, and the environment within which they operate. The interpersonal interaction is a reciprocal process that relies on cues from each member to instigate and maintain it. As in any dynamic interpersonal system, certain reactions are expected and anticipated, but individual behavioral input may vary, thus producing variations in the system's functioning.

Reciprocity within a mother–infant system may be described as an interactional cycle that occurs simultaneously between the mother and the infant (Brazelton et al., 1974). It involves mutual cuing behaviors, expectancy, rhythmicity, and synchrony. There are intimations of reciprocity in the early hours of life. The mother and her infant are like two actors who respond to each other's cues. During several weeks of interactive continuity, they establish a pattern of behavior in which they mesh with each other. When this meshing or synchrony is attained, the couple perform a reciprocal dance of cyclical attention and nonattention. Brazelton and his colleagues have studied this reciprocal process in the laboratory and have carefully analyzed the component parts. He has described five phases of the cycle: (a) initiation, (b) orientation, (c) acceleration, (d) deceleration, and (e) turning away. The first two phases establish the partner's expectations regarding the interaction. Both mother and infant utilize clusters of behaviors as the interaction develops. Feedback between partners enables them to modulate their behaviors. Sensitivity and

adjustment by the mother allows the infant to maintain a homeostatic state and to develop an expanding attention cycle. The infant may begin to develop recognizable patterning of behavior by about 2 weeks of age, and it is often well established by 6 weeks.

If the observer is aware of what to look for, the segments of an interactional cycle can be described as they are observed. The following is a hypothetical example of an interactional period, as it is likely to appear when things are going well:

Initiation: The infant is being held on the mother's knee, facing her. He looks toward her with a relaxed expression and makes slow movements with his arms and hands.

Orientation: As the infant makes eye contact with his mother, his eyes brighten and become alert, and he turns his whole body toward her, extending arms and legs in her direction. He reaches toward the mother.

State of attention: The mother smiles and talks to the infant, and he responds by smiling, moving his arms and legs in pedaling motions, cooing, and making other sounds. The eyes alternately become alert and dull as he responds to the smiles and words of his mother. The limbs move rhythmically, and if watched carefully, the ebb and flow of movement can be seen to keep time with the mother's voice. There is a constant slow smooth reaching and circular movement occurring as the tension within the infant's body rises and falls. The infant assumes the look of expectancy.

Acceleration: The infant continues to move, to wave his hands and feet about, and to increase his smiling activity. His eyes are bright and alert. He strains toward his mother in the intensity of the interaction, all the time watching her and cuing to her smile. For the most part, the body movement is smooth, but there may be occasional jerkiness.

Peak of excitement: As the infant becomes wholly involved in the interaction, his movements may become jerky and intense. He brings his hand to his mouth and tries to insert his thumb while still smiling and cooing. The other hand clutches his thigh and he leans forward to his mother as she continues to smile at him. As he endeavors to reach forward, his back arches and his body tends to twist toward one side.

Deceleration: The excitement begins to pass off as the infant's movements slow. There is a gradual decrease in body movement, the bright look dims, the eyes become dull, and the lids appear to droop. The smiles fade, and vocalization decreases. Suddenly the infant yawns and begins to suck his thumb as he leans away from his mother. His hands drop to his lap with the fingers widespread, and he appears to be relaxing.

Withdrawal or turning away: The infant's activity slows down almost completely. He slumps against his mother's hands with his body half turned away from her. His eyes are dull and focused in the direction of an object to the side. There is a faint smile on his face. The mother stops smiling and talking to the infant. She just sits holding him quietly, waiting for his next cue. The mother briefly raises her head and glances beyond the infant. This prompts a reaction in the infant. He looks toward his mother, smiles briefly, and looks away again, then turns back to the mother, ready to resume another period of interaction.

The responsibility for monitoring cues and for sensitively initiating or maintaining the interaction rests primarily with the mother. The infant uses the nonattention time to recover from the tension of interaction, to organize behavior, and to process what has been taken in during the attentive periods.

The development of reciprocity between a mother and her infant is evidence of the bond or attachment that has formed between them. It enables the mother to let go of the infant she knew as a fetus during pregnancy. A new relationship now develops with an individual who has a unique character and who evokes a response entirely different from the fantasy response of pregnancy. When reciprocity is synchronous, the interaction between mother and infant is mutually gratifying and is sought and initiated by both partners. Pleasure and delight develop in each other's company, and there is mutual development of love and growth.

Not all mothers fall in love with their newborn instantaneously. Reciprocity may take weeks to develop, and it usually requires sensitive stimuli from both actors. As infants become more organized in their behavior and as senses develop, they are able to give positive feedback to their mothers. As they transmit the appearance of listening, they follow voice and movements, and respond with intentionality to the mother as an individual whom they recognize and seek to communicate with.

In cases in which either the mother or the newborn is sick and the initial acquaintance is delayed, a concomitant delay in the development of reciprocity is likely. In some cases the lag may be so detrimental to the process that reciprocity never develops.

Overstimulation or inappropriate stimulation by the mother may interfere with the synchrony of the interaction. In the resultant dyssynchrony, the mother may be in the attention phase of the reciprocal process when the infant is in the nonattention phase. This dyssynchrony can lead to frustration on the part of either partner or both and may lead to a disharmonious relationship as both become established in their interactional patterns. In extreme instances mother and infant may cease to communicate with each other.

Infants vary in their strategies for dealing with an overload of stimulation. Four types of reaction have been described in infants responding to unpleasant and inappropriately timed stimuli (Brazelton et al., 1974): active physical withdrawal, rejection, decreased sensitivity, and communication of distress. An infant can move away from the source of stimulation, can push the stimulus away, can lapse into drowsiness or sleep, or can fuss and cry. Some of these strategies, if they become characteristic of an infant's behavior, are easier to live with than others; they interact with a mother's expectations and her personality.

The nurse may have the opportunity to observe reciprocity developing between a mother and her newborn in the early weeks of life. If nurses recognize the appearance of dyssynchrony, they may be able to initiate intervention before the dyssynchronous behaviors become firmly established.

The ultimate goals of nursing care in the maternity cycle are the continuation of life and the enhancement of the quality of that life in terms of physical and mental health. There is reason to believe that a state of mutual attachment or an enduring emotional bond between a parent (or parent surrogate) and an infant is essential to the infant's optimum health. A new mother's feelings of closeness or attachment to her infant also seem to have a positive effect on her own continued personal growth. The same is probably true of a new father. Therefore, the facilitation of parent–infant attachment is a significant goal to pursue. But what is attachment, and how is it most effectively established and maintained between members of a beginning family?

Behaviors said to indicate attachment vary. Terms such as *bond, affectional tie,* and *affiliation* are often treated interchangeably and are used as synonyms for attachment without themselves being defined.

Whichever definition or description of attachment is accepted, everyone involved in the investigation or facilitation of healthy parent–infant interaction is in agreement that the chances for optimum growth and development of both parents and newborns increase as the quality of attachment is enhanced. Because the facilitation of parent-to-infant attachment has become an accepted goal in maternal–child health nursing, an important first step toward that goal is the achievement of a clear understanding of the nature of attachment. Following is a proposed definition of parent-to-infant attachment designed to help nurses who are in direct contact with members of beginning and enlarging families. It is a tentative working definition, presented for consideration, which takes the form of an ideal outcome to be pursued.

Attachment is an attraction to and inclination to nurture one's newborn that is consistently acted upon, intelligently and sensitively, with predominately positive feeling. This definition implies a cycle of feelings that lead to mothering activities, which are in turn accompanied or followed by feelings. Ludington-Hoe (1977) has termed the physical caretaking tasks "mothering" and the emotional aspects "maternicity." She suggests *maternicity* as a nursing diagnostic term for the emotional component of the maternal role. It includes qualities that enable the mother to feel warmth, affection, attachment, protectiveness, and devotion to the child. The physical tasks of the mother's role can be observed and evaluated when the nurse is with the interacting pair. Maternicity is not as easily noted and assessed, as it can be expressed in a variety of ways at different times in the maternity cycle. However, many of the activities that provide clues to the quality of maternal bonding also provide useful guides to the degree of maternicity the mother has developed.

Attachment Behaviors in the Adolescent Mother

Differences in attachment behaviors have been observed in adolescent mothers compared with older women. The younger the adolescent, the less likely she is to display typical adult maternal behaviors of touching, synchrony with her newborn, vocalization, and proximity of mother and newborn (McAnarney, Lawrence, and Aten, 1979). It also appears that the most important domains of interaction in the early postpartal period for the adolescent are physical and motor. These mothers appear to be more attuned to these behaviors than to auditory and visual interaction.

Strong ego functioning, as demonstrated by the mother's ability to adapt to pregnancy and to plan for her future, appears to affect the mother's interaction with her newborn. The response of the newborn is also critical. Infants who are healthy are more likely to affect the relationship positively. Adolescents may have problems with parenting because they tend to have less realistic expectations of what an infant can do at a given age. In addition, cognitively immature adolescents may not foresee the consequences of their actions. Neglectful parenting may become a problem.

With these considerations in mind the nurse must be attentive to the early maternal–infant interaction, use appropriate modeling and teaching techniques, and refer adolescent mothers for follow-up care if indicated.

FATHER–INFANT INTERACTIONS

In the past 25 years, the typical perinatal experience of an expectant father has changed considerably. Many maternity nurses can remember a time when fathers-to-be kissed their wives goodbye at the admitting room door and went home to await the obstetrician's phone call announcing the new arrival. Often the father and mother were not reunited for several hours after the birth, as the mother was recovering from anesthesia. The newborn was usually viewed through the nursery window, and the father was not permitted to touch or hold him or her until all three were reunited on the day of hospital discharge. Under present, more humanized hospital practices, increasing numbers of fathers have the opportunity to become directly involved in the life of their newborn from the moment of birth.

Traditionally, the father has been seen as the primary source of support for the pregnant woman. He contributed to the growth and development of his young newborn indirectly by nurturing and supporting his partner through the pregnancy and the early postpartal weeks. As women became interested in a different kind of childbearing experience and began to attend classes to prepare themselves for more participation in the birth process, they came to value their partners and the hospital staff, as an additional support during labor. But for years, even after the father was permitted to coach his wife in labor, he was still left behind at the delivery room door to await the birth attendant's report of the birth and a brief reunion with mother and newborn as they left the delivery room. Gradually couples became less willing to be separated from each other during any part of the childbearing experience, and they became more vocal about expressing their wishes. At the same time, health care workers became more cognizant of the emotional and educational needs of the whole family and more willing to permit paternal participation during the entire hospital stay.

Out of commitment to a family-centered approach to maternity care, there developed an interest in understanding the experiences and feelings of the new father. The formerly ignored and little understood father became the willing subject of a number of research endeavors. Some of these indicate that a father experiences feelings toward his newborn that are similar to the mother's feelings of attachment. In the past the significance of any psychologic response called fatherliness has been minimized. It was implied that, because the man did not have deep physiologic roots of fatherliness, his feelings were somehow of less importance than the mother's and were weaker and longer in developing. Evidence is increasing that a father does have a strong attraction to his newborn and highly positive emotional reactions to first contact. The first hours after delivery appear to be significant in the development of the father–mother–infant bond.

Greenberg and Morris (1974) have noted the reactions of first-time fathers to early contact with their newborns. They used the term *engrossment* to label characteristic aspects of the impact of the newborn on the father—his sense of absorption, preoccupation, and interest in the infant. From this engrossment, the attachment bond between the father and his infant develops. As a result of their study of new fathers, the authors have described the characteristics of engrossment commonly found among fathers in the early postpartal days.

In general, the father is strongly attracted to his newborn and enjoys looking at him or her. He sees the baby as a unique individual with personal features and qualities that distinguish him or her from other newborns. The neonate's face is particularly attractive and beautiful. Many fathers see their newborn as perfect. The body contact involved in holding the newborn, touching the skin, and feeling the limb movements is extremely pleasurable and is sought out (Figure 28-4). The emotional reaction to first sight of the newborn and later contacts is very positive. Greenberg and Morris (1974) found that nearly all the fathers studied felt elated and gave indication of increased self-esteem.

These heightened feelings and perceptions of new fathers can be compared to those present in an infatuation. The degree of involvement in the love affair with his newborn can draw a man's time and energy away from the ongoing couple relationship. The man who has been encouraged to support his partner in her new mothering role may feel some guilt about preoccupation with the baby, and the woman may feel ignored or excluded from a significant relationship. It seems likely that couples who shared experiences, relationships, and material things before the birth will be better able to share their infant's attention after the birth and to share the responsibilities of parenting, too.

When he is pulled as if by a magnet into contact with his neonate, the new father initiates direct interaction, and the newborn responds and initiates behaviors. As with the mother–newborn interaction, the newborn contributes his or her part. The infant cries and moves, indicating aliveness and well-being. Spontaneous and reflexive movements and grimaces are interpreted by the father as personal dialogue with him, and the father responds by voice and touch. From the beginning, the father's interactive behaviors are different from the mother's, and these differences are perceptible to the infant. A father's odor, voice pitch, appearance, and touch qualities are all different from a mother's. In a face-to-face "play situation," a mother tends to use her hands to enfold and enclose her baby's body and limbs, gently modulating and smoothing out motions, whereas the father punctuates his conversation with finger pokes and more exaggerated changes in facial expression, which act to increase the baby's excitement level. Observers have noted differences in an infant's responses to interaction with mother or father as early as 2 weeks after birth.

Mothers, too, appear to notice a difference. Often in the early weeks, when asked if they play with the baby, mothers say, "No, but my husband does." It seems as if one function of the father–infant interaction is to further acquaint the mother with her baby's range of possible behaviors in the context of a shared relationship.

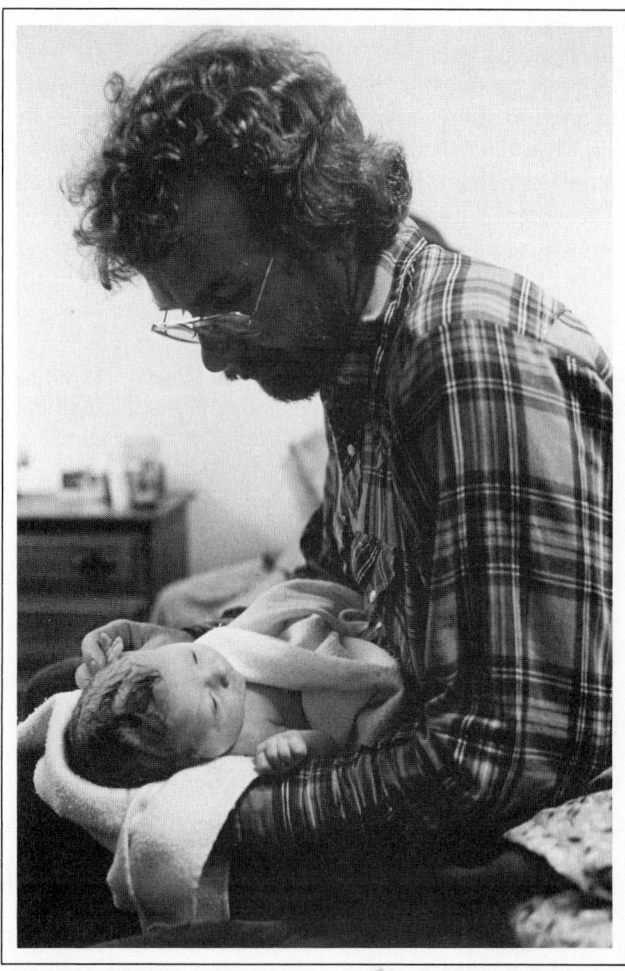

FIGURE 28-4 The bond between father and infant develops.

In families in which the couple relationship has not developed adequate stability, evidence of the baby's increased excitement and entrancement when interacting with the father can be interpreted by the mother in ways that are dangerous to the family system. For example, feelings of competition, resentment, or incompetence can arise and become detrimental to all family members.

Goals for family-centered nursing care during pregnancy should include an assessment of the couple's ability to share the experience of pregnancy through various forms of communication. Often each partner has important feelings, hopes, fantasies, and fears that have not been communicated to the other. They often unknowingly share the same concerns, which neither speaks of for fear of worrying the other. By stimulating open discussion about matters relating to the pregnancy, a nurse can help develop patterns of communication and sharing for continued use in family living.

It might be helpful if, during the pregnancy, nurses explain the potential for engrossment of the father after birth. If both parents are aware that each has needs at this time, they may be better able to support each other's growing relationship to this added family member. Many fathers in the Greenberg and Morris study were surprised and amazed at the extent of their feelings toward the newborn. The unexpectedness of the feelings seemed to increase the father's preoccupation with his relationship to the newborn. Further study is needed to describe the ways in which couples successfully cope with their own feelings and needs while continuing to support each other in the childbearing experience. To make nursing goals appropriate and intervention effective, more knowledge is also needed about the long-term effects of different levels of direct paternal involvement on the quality of the father–child relationship and other family relationships.

SIBLINGS AND OTHERS

Little is known about the components of bonding between the newborn and the siblings. Most parents endeavor to prepare their children for the advent of a new baby. Many hospitals are beginning to include sibling classes to help children learn about the newborn and become involved in the socialization of the new member into the family. The type and extent of the preparation may depend on the age of the children and the type of relationships that exist in the home. If the new baby is seen as nonthreatening to the relationships the children have with their parents, there will probably be minimal disruption, and the new baby will be accepted without serious problems.

The conventional view of the bonding or attachment process has been that the infant was capable of forming only one bond at a time and that this bond should be to the mother. Bowlby (1958) called this tie *monotropy*. More recent work with infants has shown that they are capable of maintaining a number of attachments. These attachments may include siblings, grandparents, aunts, and uncles. Some infants were found to be capable of forming attachments with five or more people simultaneously without loss of quality. The social setting and personalities of the individuals would appear to be significant factors in permitting the development of multiple attachments. The advent of "open" visiting hours and rooming-in permits siblings and grandparents to participate in the attachment process of the newborn's life.

ASSESSMENT AND INTERVENTIONS IN MOTHER-INFANT RELATIONSHIPS

Nurses come into professional contact with women and their families at any point in the maternity cycle. The nurse may be operating as a representative of an agency—such as a public health office, hospital, doctor's office, child pro-

tection center, or a childbirth education group—where objectives and priorities for care or service differ. The nurse may be an independent practitioner with her own goals to achieve. Whatever the service setting, facilitating a mother-infant relationship is usually only one of a number of concurrently operating goals of health care. This is probably a fortunate state of affairs, because much can be done during the performance of other nursing tasks to support the development of maternal attachment. A direct effort to evaluate or change feelings is often the least effective approach.

The bulk of the research that is available to guide clinical practices in the area of attachment and parent–child interaction has been carried out with groups of mothers or mother-infant dyads. Few father-infant dyads have been studied. Many studies focus on the first pregnancy of white, middle-class women with good health and an intact family. A number of other studies relate to the high-risk concept. In both instances, the research subjects, as much as possible, are asked the same questions in the same way under the same conditions. Investigators report their findings in general statements, referring to the percentage of women responding in a given way or to what is occurring in the average case or to the degree of correlation between one factor and another.

More often than not, a maternity or public health nurse is concerned with the care of a specific woman and/or her baby at a given point in time. The nurse can draw on general knowledge of norms, averages, and risk factors, but must apply what is pertinent from that store of information to a mother with a specific history and personality, in a relationship with a specific infant, and within a specific environment. It is well known that individuals classified as high risk are sometimes able to cope effectively with whatever risks are involved and to relate affectionately to a particular newborn. It also happens that what appears to be a perfect image of a potential mother can be shattered by unpredictable events occurring after the image was drawn.

A pregnancy creates emotional and behavioral reverberations throughout the family of procreation, the families of origin of the parents-to-be, and their whole social network. Reflection of these echoes back to the pregnant woman to some extent shapes her experience of maternity. Effective evaluation of a mother-infant relationship thus requires a broad understanding of a mother and newborn pair as it exists within a family and a wider social setting. This depth of understanding of a complex system within a system is in itself important, but it is also of significance in relation to its effect on a nurse's approach to nurse-client interaction.

If nurses see their task as finding facts, determining risk, and changing behaviors, their approach to a pregnant woman is different from the approach of a nurse whose goal is to understand fully the woman within her family. Although evaluation, care, and understanding of a person as a unique individual are the objectives, the assessment approach is at the same time a therapeutic measure.

In many other ways the manner in which the nurse carries out an evaluation of a mother-newborn relationship can be concurrently diagnostic, preventive, and therapeutic. A nurse is, in effect, working within one interpersonal relationship (nurse-client) to evaluate another interpersonal relationship. While interacting with a maternity client, the nurse can assess her ability to trust people and to enjoy relationships, her skills in communication, and her feeling tone. At the same time the nurse can purposefully design his or her own part of the interaction to achieve a mutually trusting relationship and an increase in maternal self-esteem and self-confidence. Through direct interaction, the nurse can also make use of his or her modeling potential. He or she can, in his or her own behaviors toward the mother, actively demonstrate forms of nurturing, communicating, and problem solving that can be unconsciously picked up and imitated or consciously studied and tested out by the mother. When feelings are expressed, the nurse can nonjudgmentally accept them. This practice enables the owner of the feelings to accept them and perhaps to examine and understand them. It also encourages the further expression of feelings. As the nurse reaches tentative conclusions about facts and feelings in the evaluation of a mother-infant relationship, it is often appropriate for him or her to share his or her ideas with the mother, both because the mother is a source of validation of the nurse's observation and because being included in the process of assessment can be ego-enhancing for the mother. Some mothers can be very accurate in predicting their own postpartal adjustment and the quality of their support network.

Assessment of Early Attachment

If attachment is accepted as a desired outcome of nursing care, a nurse in any of the various postpartal settings can periodically observe and note progress toward attachment. The following questions can be addressed in the course of nurse-client interaction:

1. Is the mother attracted to her newborn? To what extent does she seek face-to-face contact and eye contact? Is she actively reaching out or only passively holding her newborn? Has she progressed from fingertip touch, to palmar contact, to enfolding the infant close to her own body? Is attraction increasing or decreasing? If the mother does not exhibit increasing attraction, why not? Do the reasons lie primarily within her, in the baby, or in the environment?

2. Is the mother inclined to nurture her infant? Is she progressing through the stages of taking in, taking hold, and letting go in her interactions with her infant? Has she selected a rooming-in arrangement if it is available?

3. Does the mother act consistently? Is she developing a consistent and predictable approach to the care of her infant? Does she tend to respond to the same situation in the same way from day to day? If not, is the source of unpredictability within her or her infant?

4. Is her mothering intelligently carried out? Does she seek information and evaluate it objectively? Does she develop solutions based on adequate knowledge of valid data? How did she prepare herself for the parenting role? Does she evaluate the effectiveness of her maternal care and make appropriate adjustment?

5. Is she sensitive to the newborn's needs as they arise? How quickly does she interpret her infant's behavior and react to cues? Does she respond when the baby cries or fusses? Does she seem happy and satisfied with the infant's responses to her efforts? Is she pleased with feeding behaviors? How much of this ability and willingness to respond is related to the baby's nature and how much to her own?

6. Does she seem pleased with her baby's appearance and sex? Is she experiencing pleasure in interaction with her infant? What times are the most and least enjoyable? What interferes with the enjoyment? Does she speak to the baby frequently and affectionately? Does she call him or her by name? Does she point out family traits or characteristics she sees in the newborn?

7. Are there any cultural factors that might modify the mother's response? For instance, is it customary for the grandmother to assume most of the child care responsibilities while the mother recovers from childbirth?

When these questions are addressed and the facts have been assembled by the nurse, the nurse's intuitive feelings and formal background of knowledge should combine to answer three more questions: Is there a problem in attachment? What is the problem? What is its source? Each nurse can then devise a creative approach to the problem as it presents itself in the context of a unique developing mother-infant relationship.

Guidelines for Intervention

"Accentuate the positive, eliminate the negative" is an excellent motto to guide nursing intervention during the pregnancy and postpartal period. Any actions that minimize mental distress and physical discomfort or maximize feelings of well-being and pleasure have the potential of enhancing the quality of mother-infant interaction. Following are some suggested objectives and ways of achieving them:

1. Determine the childbearing and childrearing goals of the infant's mother and father and adapt them wherever possible in planning nursing care for the family. This includes giving the parents choices about their labor and delivery experience and their initial time with their new infant.

2. Arrange the health care setting so that individual nurse-client professional relationships can be developed and maintained throughout a pregnancy and during the first months of mother-infant adaptation. A consistent caregiver during the mother's prenatal experience allows a comfortable trusting relationship to develop in which the mother feels free to express concerns, ask questions, and explore choices. In the hospital a primary nurse can develop rapport and assess the mother's strengths and needs.

3. Enhance the couple's relationship and increase their communication capacity during the pregnancy. A feeling of closeness and personal satisfaction often results when the father plays an active role in the labor and delivery process by acting as the woman's coach and support person. Comfort with such a role will develop most easily if the parents attend prenatal classes. As they learn about pregnancy and delivery, anxiety decreases.

4. Use anticipatory guidance from conception through the postpartal period to prepare the parents for expected problems of adjustment. Prenatal classes often focus on possible problems a new family might encounter. In addition, literature on a variety of concerns, from feeding to sibling rivalry to infant stimulation, helps the new parents cope. If such information is available in the hospital and at the office or clinic, parents can choose according to their need.

5. Include parents in any nursing intervention planning and evaluation. Give choices whenever possible.

6. Remove barriers to voluntary contact among family members and the infant. This may be accomplished by providing time in the first hour after delivery for the new family to become acquainted with as much privacy as possible. Warmth may be maintained by placing the infant against the mother's bare chest and covering both with a warmed blanket. When the father is holding his new daughter or son, the baby may be wrapped in two or three warmed blankets. Postponing eye prophylaxis facilitates eye contact between parents and their newborn. Sibling visits also play a role in integrating the newest family member.

7. Initiate and support measures to alleviate fatigue in the parents.

8. Help parents to identify, understand, and accept both positive and negative feelings related to the overall parenting experience.

9. Support and assist parents in determining the personality and unique needs of their infant. Whenever possible rooming-in should be available. This practice gives the mother a chance to learn her infant's normal patterns

and develop confidence in caring for him or her. It also allows the father more uninterrupted time with his infant in the first days of life. If mother and baby are doing well and if help is available for the mother at home, early discharge permits the family to begin establishing their life together.

Assessment of Bonding

The Neonatal Perception Inventory (NPI), developed by Dr. Elsie Broussard (1965), is a screening tool designed to assess the adaptive potential of the mother-infant system during the newborn period. The NPI is aimed at identifying baseline perceptions of the mother in relation to her newborn and can serve as a basis for promoting growth-fostering interactions for both mother and infant. The NPI explores six behaviors: crying, feeding, spitting up, sleeping, bowel movements, and predictability.

The NPI is administered twice: first, within the first or second postpartal day, and again one month later. After the second NPI is administered, the Degree of Bother Inventory is administered to assess problems of infant behavior.

On the first or second day after delivery the nurse approaches the new mother and asks her to fill out a Neonatal Perception Inventory I (Figure 28–5,A) in regard to her perceptions of an average baby. The mother then fills out the Neonatal Inventory I on her perceptions of her own baby (Figure 28–5,B). The forms are scored between 1 and 5. One month later the new mother fills out both parts of the Neonatal Perception Inventory II (Figure 28–6). Again the scores from both forms are totaled.

The Neonatal Perception Inventory—Your Baby score is subtracted from the score of the Neonatal Perception Inventory—Average Baby. The NPI is the difference between the two scores. A positive score is identified with a positive perception of the newborn; a score of zero or minus is associated with negative perception of the newborn. If the score is positive the infant is considered at low risk; if the score is minus or zero, the newborn is at risk for developing emotional instability.

The Degree of Bother Inventory is administered when the infant is 1 month old to determine specific areas of concern for the mother (Figure 28–7). It is weighted from 1 (none) to 4 (a great deal), with possible scores of 6 to 24. The higher the score the more the mother is bothered by the infant. Each item can stand on its own; no item is weighted more than another.

Use of the NPI and Degree of Bother Inventory elicits objective data from which nursing care can be planned, implemented, and evaluated. For example, if a mother is concerned about the elimination pattern of her infant, she can keep a record of the baby's elimination for 4–5 days and validate her findings with the nurse. Together they can

How much crying do you think the average baby does?

_____   _____   _____   _____   _____
a great deal   a good bit   moderate amount   very little   none

How much trouble do you think the average baby has in feeding?

_____   _____   _____   _____   _____
a great deal   a good bit   moderate amount   very little   none

How much spitting up or vomiting do you think the average baby does?

_____   _____   _____   _____   _____
a great deal   a good bit   moderate amount   very little   none

How much difficulty do you think the average baby has in sleeping?

_____   _____   _____   _____   _____
a great deal   a good bit   moderate amount   very little   none

How much difficulty does the average baby have with bowel movements?

_____   _____   _____   _____   _____
a great deal   a good bit   moderate amount   very little   none

How much trouble do you think the average baby has in settling down to a predictable pattern of eating and sleeping?

_____   _____   _____   _____   _____
a great deal   a good bit   moderate amount   very little   none

A

How much crying do you think your baby will do?

_____   _____   _____   _____   _____
a great deal   a good bit   moderate amount   very little   none

How much trouble do you think your baby will have feeding?

_____   _____   _____   _____   _____
a great deal   a good bit   moderate amount   very little   none

How much spitting up or vomiting do you think your baby will do?

_____   _____   _____   _____   _____
a great deal   a good bit   moderate amount   very little   none

How much difficulty do you think your baby will have sleeping?

_____   _____   _____   _____   _____
a great deal   a good bit   moderate amount   very little   none

How much difficulty do you expect your baby to have with bowel movements?

_____   _____   _____   _____   _____
a great deal   a good bit   moderate amount   very little   none

How much trouble do you think that your baby will have settling down to a predictable pattern of eating and sleeping?

_____   _____   _____   _____   _____
a great deal   a good bit   moderate amount   very little   none

B

FIGURE 28–5 A, Neonatal Perception Inventory I, Average Baby; **B,** Neonatal Perception Inventory I, Your Baby. (Used with permission of Dr. Elsie R. Broussard, University of Pittsburgh, Graduate School of Public Health, Pittsburgh, PA 15261. Copyright retained.)

How much crying do you think the average baby does?

a great deal	a good bit	moderate amount	very little	none

How much trouble do you think the average baby has in feeding?

a great deal	a good bit	moderate amount	very little	none

How much spitting up or vomiting do you think the average baby does?

a great deal	a good bit	moderate amount	very little	none

How much difficulty do you think the average baby has in sleeping?

a great deal	a good bit	moderate amount	very little	none

How much difficulty does the average baby have with bowel movements?

a great deal	a good bit	moderate amount	very little	none

How much trouble do you think the average baby has in settling down to a predictable pattern of eating and sleeping?

a great deal	a good bit	moderate amount	very little	none

A

How much crying has your baby done?

a great deal	a good bit	moderate amount	very little	none

How much trouble has your baby had feeding?

a great deal	a good bit	moderate amount	very little	none

How much spitting up or vomiting has your baby done?

a great deal	a good bit	moderate amount	very little	none

How much difficulty has your baby had in sleeping?

a great deal	a good bit	moderate amount	very little	none

How much difficulty has your baby had with bowel movements?

a great deal	a good bit	moderate amount	very little	none

How much trouble has your baby had in settling down to a predictable pattern of eating and sleeping?

a great deal	a good bit	moderate amount	very little	none

B

FIGURE 28–6 **A,** Neonatal Perception Inventory II, Average Baby; **B,** Neonatal Perception Inventory II, Your Baby. (Used with permission of Dr. Elsie R. Broussard, University of Pittsburgh, Graduate School of Public Health, Pittsburgh, PA 15261. Copyright retained.)

Crying	_____	_____	_____	_____
	a great deal	somewhat	very little	none
Spitting up or vomiting	_____	_____	_____	_____
	a great deal	somewhat	very little	none
Sleeping	_____	_____	_____	_____
	a great deal	somewhat	very little	none
Feeding	_____	_____	_____	_____
	a great deal	somewhat	very little	none
Elimination	_____	_____	_____	_____
	a great deal	somewhat	very little	none
Lack of a predictable schedule	_____	_____	_____	_____
	a great deal	somewhat	very little	none
Other (specify):				
_____	_____	_____	_____	_____
	a great deal	somewhat	very little	none
_____	_____	_____	_____	_____
	a great deal	somewhat	very little	none
_____	_____	_____	_____	_____
	a great deal	somewhat	very little	none
_____	_____	_____	_____	_____
	a great deal	somewhat	very little	none

FIGURE 28–7 Degree of Bother Inventory. (Used with permission of Dr. Elsie R. Broussard, University of Pittsburgh, Graduate School of Public Health, Pittsburgh, PA 15261. Copyright retained.)

then explore ways of dealing with the problem if one exists.*

COMPLICATIONS OF MATERNAL–INFANT ATTACHMENT

The mother who experienced a high-risk labor and delivery or who has complications in the immediate postpartal period has an increased risk of encountering difficulties in attachment. She is more likely to have had medications, analgesia, or anesthesia during the intrapartal period, which may influence early interaction with her newborn. In the immediate postpartal period she may be more likely to receive medications or analgesics or face problems that limit her energy. Complications involving the mother or infant may necessitate separation during the critical early stages of attachment. Although these are only a few of the

*Permission to use the NPI and the Degree of Bother Inventory must be obtained by writing to Elsie R. Broussard, M. D., University of Pittsburgh, Graduate School of Public Health, Pittsburgh, PA 15261.

factors that may be present, they may be significant if they interfere with the bonding or attachment process.

Unfortunately, insufficient data are available in the assessment of the bonding process when the mother is ill. It would be an oversimplification to state that the effects of bonding when the mother is sick are essentially the same as the effects of early separation, because the psychologic effect of illness has not been considered. The mother may have to work through her own ambivalence about the illness and the infant's role as the possible cause of the illness. Mothers may express this anxiety in many ways. Three expressions that nurses frequently encounter are: (a) clearly blaming the infant (pregnancy) for the illness; (b) blaming herself and the infant, especially when the pregnancy was unplanned or unwanted; and (c) blaming the infant and infant's father, as if a conspiracy existed to cause the illness.

Assessment of attachment behaviors has become increasingly important in light of current theories that correlate malattachment with an increased incidence of parenting problems, failure to thrive, and child neglect or abuse. When assessing attachment behaviors, the nurse should be careful not to generalize or give too much importance to any one factor. Adaptive behavior may vary from one situation to the next. Cultural factors such as decreased eye contact should also be considered. All cultures may not recognize or value the same behaviors that members of the Western culture value.

Assessment of the mother–infant (or father–infant) interaction should be made on various occasions to avoid attaching too much significance to one behavior on a given occasion. Some behaviors that may indicate a maladaptive attachment process include refusal by the mother to see her newborn, failure to progress from fingertip to palm when holding or exploring the infant, making no attempt to establish eye-to-eye contact, inability to choose a name, or choosing a name that is so unusual that it implies hostility or ridicule (such as "Jim Beam," "Spirits," "Tornado," or the like).

The observed behaviors should be recorded objectively to validate the nursing assessment. An example of objective recording is: "At 9 A.M. mother fed her infant while holding him across her knees. She did not place her hands on the infant. During a 20-minute continuous observation the mother did not establish eye contact and did not talk to the infant. Mother refers to her infant as 'it' when talking to the nursing staff." Subjective documentation of the same situation would be: "Mother fed baby at 9 A.M. Mother does not appear to like her baby." Subjective documentation includes the observer's values or biases and is not as beneficial as objective data. (Chapter 30 considers attachment problems in depth, and describes problems that may arise if a newborn requires lengthy hospitalization.)

SUMMARY

A mother's feelings for and her behavior toward her newborn are determined by multiple factors. Past experiences, personality, pregnancy experiences, human environment, and physical setting combine to shape a mother's potential for nurturant interaction with her baby. The father is important both in his contribution to the emotional climate within which the fetus and infant are nurtured by the mother and as a nurturing and interacting figure in his own right. The infant is born with interactive capacities, which continue to develop through appropriate adult social stimulation. Generally speaking, when the lives and relationships of the procreating pair are going well, they are likely to continue in a positive direction through the course of pregnancy and adjustment to the new family member. When emotional resources and social skills are lacking in a couple and when they are generally discontent, a pregnancy and postpartal adjustment period will tend to be negatively perceived, and positive feeling for the baby will be diminished or delayed.

It would be nice if there were simple nursing measures to change negative maternal feelings to positive, but such is not the case. Instead, the nurse, who ideally has achieved emotional maturity and a measure of psychosocial skills, is challenged to understand each mother–infant pair within its unique context. Such a level of client and family knowledge is made possible only through the development of a nurse–client relationship of mutual trust, which is facilitated by continuity of interpersonal contact. In the absence of opportunity for an ongoing relationship, continuous communication of data relevant to the developing mother–infant relationship is essential to effective ma-

ternal support. Helping to initiate and maintain a healthy attachment in all its many aspects is a primary preventive goal of importance to family life. Improvement of disordered relationships is another priority goal. Nurses can support these goals through direct client care, through initiating changes in health care delivery systems, and through research for evaluation of nursing interventions.

Resource Groups

American Red Cross, National Headquarters, 17th and D Streets, Washington, D.C. 20006. Offers prenatal classes to help parents prepare for care and nurturing of infant.

References

Adams, M. 1963. Early concerns of primigravida mothers regarding infant care activities. *Nurs. Res.* 12:72.

Bowlby, J. 1958. The nature of the child's tie to his mother. *Int. J. Psychoanal.* 39:350.

Brazelton, T. B., et al. 1974. The origins of reciprocity: the early mother–infant interaction. In *The effect of the infant on its caregiver*, ed. M. Lewis and L. A. Rosenblum. New York: John Wiley & Sons.

Broussard, E. R. 1964–65. A study to determine the effectiveness of television as a means of providing anticipatory counseling to primiparae during the postpartum period. *Dissertation Abstracts*. 26:484.

Condon, W. S., and Sander, L. W. 1974. Synchrony demonstrated between movements of the neonate and adult speech. *Child Dev.* 45:456.

Goren, C. C., et al. 1975. Visual following and pattern discrimination of facelike stimuli by newborn infants. *Pediatrics.* 56:544.

Greenberg, M., and Morris, N. 1974. Engrossment: the newborn's impact upon the father. *Am. J. Orthopsychiatry.* 44:520.

Kennedy, J. C. 1969. *The little stranger: mother–infant acquaintance and the first two weeks.* PhD diss., Boston University.

Klaus, M. H., et al. 1970. Human maternal behavior at first contact with her young. *Pediatrics.* 46:187.

Korner, A. F., and Thoman, E. B. 1970. Visual alertness in neonates as evoked by maternal care. *J. Exploratory Child Psych.* 10:67.

Leifer, M. 1977. Psychological changes accompanying pregnancy and motherhood. *Genet. Psychol. Monographs.* 95:55.

Lozoff, B., et al. 1977. The mother–newborn relationship: limits of adaptability. *J. Pediatr.* 91:1.

Ludington-Hoe, S. L. 1977. Postpartum: development of maternicity. *Am. J. Nurs.* 77:1171.

McAnarney, E. R.; Lawrence, R. A.; and Aten, M. J. April 1979. Premature parenthood: a preliminary report of adolescent mother–infant interaction. *Pediatr. Res.* 13:327.

Newcomb, T. M. 1961. *The acquaintance process.* New York: Holt, Rinehart & Winston, Inc.

Nuckolls, K. B., et al. 1972. Psychological assets, life crisis and the prognosis of pregnancy. *Am. J. Epidemiol.* 95:431.

Rubin, R. 1961. Puerperal change. *Nurs. Outlook.* 9:753.

―――. 1963. Maternal touch. *Nurs. Outlook.* 11:828.

Shereshefsky, P. M., and Yarrow, L. J. 1973. *Psychological aspects of a first pregnancy and postnatal adaptation.* New York: Raven.

Additional Readings

Avant, K. C. 1981. Anxiety as a potential factor affecting maternal attachment. *J. Obstet. Gynecol. Neonat. Nurs.* 6:416.

Brody, S. 1981. The concepts of attachment and bonding. *J. Am. Psych. Psychoanal. Assoc.* 4:815.

Broussard, E. R. Winter 1976. Neonatal prediction and outcome at 10/11 years. *Child Psychiatr. Hum. Dev.* 7:85.

―――. Jan. 1979. Assessment of the adaptive potential of the mother–infant system: the neonatal perception inventories. *Sem. Perinatol.* 3:91.

Carek, D. J., et al. 1981. Mothers' reactions to their newborn infants. *J. Am. Acad. Child Psychiatry.* 1:16.

Jenkins, R. L., et al. 1981. The nurse role in parent–infant bonding: overview, assessment, intervention. *J. Obstet. Gynecol. Neonat. Nurs.* 2:114.

Johnston, M. 1980. Cultural variations in professional and parenting patterns. *J. Obstet. Gynecol. Neonat. Nurs.* 1:9.

Klaus, M. H., and Kennell, J. H. 1982. *Parent–infant bonding,* 2nd ed. St. Louis: The C. V. Mosby Co.

Kunst-Wilson, W., et al. 1981. Nursing care for the emerging family: promoting paternal behavior. *Res. Nurs. Health.* 1:201.

Reiser, S. L. 1981. A tool to facilitate mother–infant attachment. *J. Obstet. Gynecol. Neonat. Nurs.* 4:294.

Ross, G. S. 1980. Parental responses to infants in intensive care: the separation issue reevaluated. *Clin. Perinatol.* 7:47.

Taubenheim, A. M. 1981. Paternal–infant bonding in the first-time father. *J. Obstet. Gynecol. Neonat. Nurs.* 4:261.

Tracy, R. L., et al. 1981. Maternal affectionate behavior and infant–mother attachment patterns. *Child Dev.* 4:1341.

■ 29 ■

COMPLICATIONS OF THE PUERPERIUM

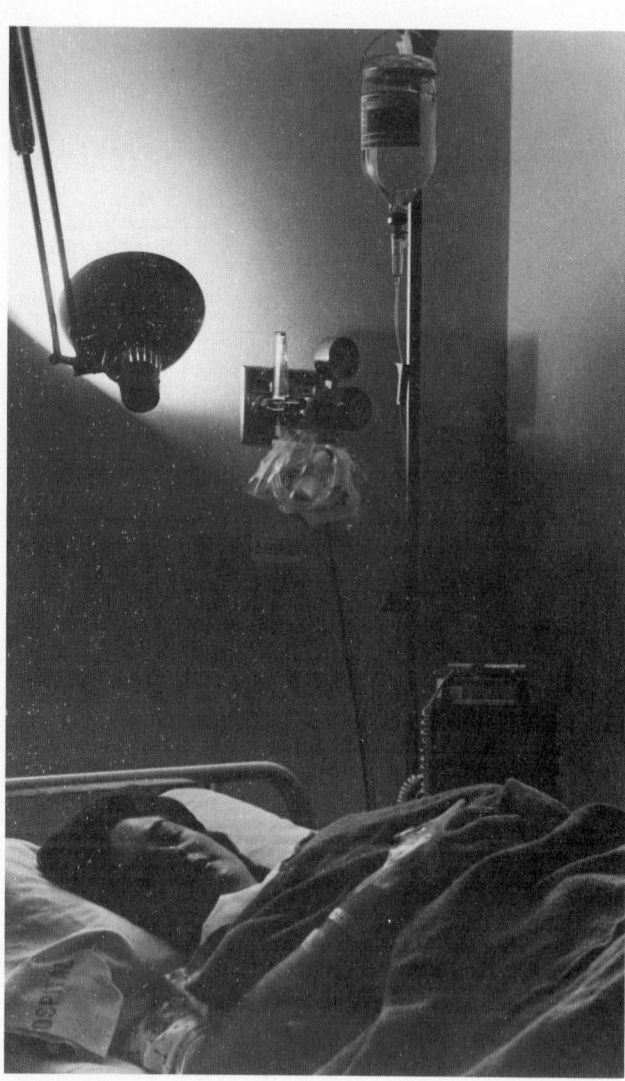

■ CHAPTER CONTENTS

PUERPERAL HEMORRHAGE AND HEMATOMAS
    Postpartal Hemorrhage
    Hematomas
    Discharge Planning

PUERPERAL INFECTIONS
    Causative Factors
    Pathophysiology
    Interventions and Nursing Care
    Discharge Planning

THROMBOEMBOLIC DISEASE
    Superficial Leg Vein Disease
    Deep Leg Vein Disease
    Pulmonary Embolism

PUERPERAL CYSTITIS AND PYELONEPHRITIS
    Overdistention
    Cystitis
    Pyelonephritis
    Interventions and Nursing Care

DISORDERS OF THE BREAST AND COMPLICA-TIONS OF LACTATION
    Mastitis
    Breast Abscess
    Persistent Abnormal Lactation
    Postdelivery Anterior Pituitary Necrosis

PUERPERAL PSYCHIATRIC DISORDERS

- List the causes and nursing interventions of hemorrhage during the postpartal period.

- Discuss the causative factors, pathophysiology, and nursing interventions of puerperal infections.

- Discuss causative factors, pathophysiology, and nursing interventions for thromboembolic disease of the puerperium.

- Describe puerperal cystitis and pyelonephritis and its implications for maternal nursing care.

- Differentiate disorders of the breast and complications of lactation.

- Identify the possible precipitating factors associated with puerperal psychiatric disorders.

A tendency exists to view the puerperium as the smooth and uneventful time that follows the anticipation of pregnancy and the excitement and work of labor and delivery—and often it is. However, the nurse must be aware of problems that may develop postpartally and their implications for the childbearing family.

This chapter deals with the broad area of complications during the puerperium and appropriate nursing intervention and care.

PUERPERAL HEMORRHAGE AND HEMATOMAS

Postpartal Hemorrhage

Puerperal hemorrhage has been divided into early and late postpartal hemorrhage. Early postpartal hemorrhage (or immediate postpartal hemorrhage) occurs when blood loss is greater than 500 mL in the first 24 hours after delivery. Late postpartal hemorrhage (delayed postpartal hemorrhage) occurs after the first 24 hours. Because of the tendency to underestimate the amount of blood lost with delivery, this figure is probably not especially accurate as a guide. Perhaps a more reliable determinant is based on a clinical assessment of excessive blood loss (usually far more than 500 mL) (Visscher and Visscher, 1982).

The main causes of early postpartal hemorrhage are uterine atony, lacerations of the vagina and cervix, and retained placental fragments. Certain factors predispose to hemorrhage: (a) overdistention of the uterus due to hydramnios, a large infant, or multiple gestation; (b) grand multiparity; (c) use of anesthetic agents (especially halothane) to relax the uterus; (d) trauma due to obstetric procedures such as midforceps delivery, any intrauterine manipulation or forceps rotation; (e) an abnormal labor pattern, either hypotonic or hypertonic; (f) use of oxytocin to induce or to augment labor; and finally, (g) maternal malnutrition, anemia, preeclampsia, or history of hemorrhage.

In most cases the clinician can predict which woman is at risk for hemorrhage. The key to successful management is prevention.

Prevention begins with adequate nutrition, good prenatal care, and early diagnosis and management of any complications that may arise. Traumatic procedures should be avoided, and delivery should take place in a facility that has blood immediately available. Any client at risk should be typed and cross-matched for blood and have intravenous lines in place. Excellent labor management and delivery technique is imperative.

During delivery, excessive pressure on the fundus or continuous vigorous kneading of the fundus when it is already contracted may result in incomplete placental separation and increased blood loss. Immediately after delivery, careful exploration of the uterus and thorough inspection of the birth canal facilitates an early diagnosis of retained placental fragments or lacerations of the cervix, vagina, or perineum. The placenta should be inspected carefully for intactness (Visscher and Visscher, 1982). (For further discussion of appropriate assessments and care see the discussion on hemorrhage during the third or fourth stage, Chapter 18, p. 578.)

Periodic assessment for evidence of bleeding is a major nursing responsibility on the postpartal unit. After the fourth stage of labor most hemorrhage is caused by retained cotyledons, retained fetal membranes, or subnormal or abnormal involution of the placental site.

Careful observation and documentation of vaginal bleeding (often by way of pad count or weighing of the peri-pad) is important if medical intervention is to be elicited. A boggy uterus that does not stay contracted without constant massage is atonic, whereas a uterus that does not involute appropriately needs to be investigated for possible retained placental tissue and infection. The most commonly employed intervention is a continuous infusion of fluids and oxytocin. If the woman is normotensive, methylergonovine or ergonovine may be employed. (Typical dosage is methylergonovine 0.2 mg every 4 hours × 6 doses.) If this treatment is not effective or if a placental fragment is retained for several days, curettage is usually indicated, together with the administration of antibiotics to prevent puerperal infection.

Occasionally, late postpartal hemorrhage occurs around the fifth to the fifteenth day after delivery when the woman is home and recovering. Bleeding most often is caused by retained placental fragments or abnormal involution of the placental site. When placental fragments are retained, they may become necrosed, fibrin may be deposited, and the fragments form a so-called placental polyp (Danforth, 1982). Brisk bleeding may occur if the "polyp" becomes detached. This type of hemorrhage usually is treated with administration of oxytocics, curettage if necessary, and prophylactic antibiotics.

SUBINVOLUTION

Subinvolution of the uterus occurs when the uterus fails to follow the normal pattern of involution but instead remains enlarged. Retained placental fragments or infection are the most frequent causes. With subinvolution the fundus is higher in the abdomen than expected. In addition, lochia often fails to progress from rubra to serosa to alba. Lochia may remain rubra or return to rubra after several days postpartum. Leukorrhea and backache may occur if infection is the cause. Subinvolution is most commonly diagnosed during the routine postpartal examination at 4–6 weeks. The woman may relate a history of irregular or excessive bleeding, or describe the symptoms listed previously. Diagnosis is made when an enlarged, softer-than-normal uterus is palpated with bimanual examination. Treatment involves oral administration of methylergonovine (Methergine) or ergonovine (Ergotrate) 0.2 mg every 3–4 hours for 24–48 hours. When metritis is present, antibiotics are also administered. If this treatment is not effective or if the cause is believed to be retained placental fragments, curettage is indicated (Pritchard and MacDonald, 1980).

Hematomas

Hematomas are usually the result of injury to a blood vessel without noticeable trauma to the superficial tissue. Hematomas occur following spontaneous as well as forceps deliveries.

The most frequently observed hematomas are of the external genitals, particularly of the vagina and vulva. The soft tissue in the area offers no resistance, and hematomas containing 250–500 mL of blood develop rapidly. The client complains of severe vulvar pain (pain that seems out of proportion or excessive), usually from her "stitches," or of severe rectal pressure. On examination, the large hematoma appears as a unilateral tense, fluctuant bulging mass at the introitus or encompassing the labia majora. The hematoma may not be as apparent as described here, so the observant nurse checks for unilateral bluish or reddish discoloration of skin of the perineum and buttocks. The area feels firm and is painful to the touch. The nurse should estimate the size of the hematoma carefully with the first assessment to better estimate increases in size and the potential blood loss.

Hematomas can develop in the upper portion of the vagina. In this case, besides pain the woman may have difficulty voiding because of pressure on the urethra or meatus. Diagnosis is confirmed through careful vaginal examination.

Hematomas may also occur upward into the broad ligament, which may be more difficult to diagnose. The client may complain of severe lateral uterine pain, flank pain, or abdominal distention. Occasionally the hematoma can be discovered with high rectal examination or with abdominal palpation. If the bleeding continues, signs of anemia may be noted.

Small vulvar hematomas may be treated with the application of ice packs and continued observation. Large hematomas generally require surgical intervention to evacuate the clot and to achieve hemostasis. General anesthesia is usually required, and if the hematoma is not accessible vaginally, a laparotomy must be performed.

Continuous assessment of the vaginal bleeding is required after surgery. If the hematoma was of the vulva or perineum, the nurse should check for recurrence. It should be standard procedure for the nurse giving report to the new shift to assist the next shift in examining the client so that baseline data can be obtained. The nurse assuming responsibility for the oncoming shift should record findings immediately and state that the client was examined by both nurses together.

Discharge Planning

In the current practice of obstetrics the mother may be discharged any time after 4 hours postdelivery. Because hemorrhage and/or hematoma may subsequently develop, she and her family or support persons should receive clear, preferably written, explanations of the normal postpartal course of readjustment, including changes in the lochia and fundus and signs of abnormal bleeding. Instruction for the prevention of bleeding should include fundal massage, ways to assess the fundus for height and consistency, and inspection of the episiotomy and lacerations, if present. The woman should receive instruction in perineal care. The client and her family are advised to contact their caregiver if any of the following occur: excessive or bright red bleeding, a boggy fundus that does not respond to massage, abnormal clots, leukorrhea, high temperature, or any unusual pelvic discomfort or backache.

PUERPERAL INFECTIONS

Puerperal infection is an infection of the reproductive tract associated with parturition and generally encompasses the time from delivery to 10 days postpartum. The most common infection is metritis/endometritis and is limited to the uterine cavity. However, infection can spread by way of the lymphatics and blood vessels to become a progressive disease resulting in peritonitis or pelvic cellulitis. The client's prognosis is directly related to the stage of the disease at the time of diagnosis, the invading organism, and the woman's state of health and ability to resist the disease state.

Because infection accounts for a large percentage of postpartal morbidity, it is useful to remember the definition of puerperal morbidity published by the Joint Committee on Maternal Welfare:

> Temperature of 100.4°F (38.0°C) or higher, the temperature to occur on any two of the first ten postpartum days, exclusive of the first 24 hours, and to be taken by mouth by a standard technique at least four times a day.

Recent research (Filker and Monif, 1979) suggests that a temperature greater than 101F in the first 24 hours is also "highly indicative of ensuing infection."

Causative Factors

Antibiotic therapy alone has not caused the decrease in morbidity and mortality that is seen today. Aseptic technique, fewer traumatic operative deliveries, a better understanding of labor dystocia, improved surgical intervention, plus a population that is generally at less risk from malnutrition and chronic debilitative disease have also contributed to this reduction.

The vagina and cervix of approximately 70% of all healthy pregnant women contain pathogenic bacteria that alone or in combination are sufficiently virulent to cause extensive infections. Why the organisms do not cause infection during pregnancy is not altogether clear; however, recent studies indicate that more than the presence of a pathogen in the woman's genital tract is necessary for infection to begin.

The uterus is essentially a sterile cavity prior to rupture of the fetal membranes. Once membranes rupture, vaginal microorganisms may ascend to the uterus so that within 24 hours after rupture, chorioamnionitis can be histologically demonstrated in about 50% of women (Vorherr, 1982). Thus, prolonged rupture of the membranes is a major factor in the development of infection postpartally. Also, the placental site, episiotomy, lacerations, abrasions, and any operative incisions are all potential portals for bacterial entrance and growth. Hematomas are easily infected and enhance the possibility of sepsis. Tissue that has been compromised through trauma is less able to marshal the necessary forces to combat infection. Other factors predisposing the woman to infection include frequent vaginal examinations, lapses in aseptic technique, anemia, intrauter-

ine manipulation, hemorrhage, cesarean delivery, retained placental fragments, and faulty perineal care.

□ *AEROBIC BACTERIAL INFECTIONS* The most common aerobic bacteria found in women with postpartal infection are group B beta hemolytic streptococci and *Escherichia coli. E. coli* may be introduced as a result of contamination of the vulva or reproductive tract from feces during labor and delivery. Though it occurs less frequently, group A beta hemolytic streptococcus is responsible for an especially virulent infection. It may be transmitted from the skin or nasopharynx of the patient herself, or more probably from an external source such as personnel or equipment. Because it is highly contagious, it presents a serious problem for hospital personnel (Vorherr, 1982). Other aerobic bacteria implicated in puerperal infections include klebsiella, *Proteus mirabilis*, pseudomonas, *Staphyloccus aureus*, and *Neisseria gonorrhoeae* (Eschenbach and Wager, 1980).

□ *ANAEROBIC BACTERIAL INFECTIONS* After delivery the amniotic fluid, blood, lochia, and decreased numbers of lactobacilli present in the reproductive tract have a neutralizing effect. The pH of the vagina changes from acid to alkaline, which is suitable for the growth of aerobic organisms. Then, approximately 48 hours after delivery, acid end-products accumulate as a result of necrosis of endometrial and placental remnants and the intrauterine environment becomes more favorable to anaerobic organisms. Consequently, approximately 70% of puerperal infections are caused by anaerobes (Vorherr, 1982). The most common anaerobes involved include bacteroides (all species), peptostreptococcus, peptococcus, and *Clostridium perfringens.*

Pathophysiology

LOCALIZED INFECTIONS

A less severe complication of the puerperium is the localized infection of the episiotomy or of lacerations to the perineum, vagina, or vulva. Wound infection of the abdominal incision site following cesarean delivery is also not infrequent. The skin edges become reddened, edematous, firm, and tender. The skin edges then separate, and purulent material, sometimes mixed with sanguineous liquid, drains from the wound (Table 29–1). The woman may complain of localized pain and dysuria and may have a low-grade fever (less than 101F or 38.3C). If the wound abscesses or is unable to drain, high temperature and chills may result.

Prevention is, of course, the first clinical goal, and is accomplished by aseptic technique, client teaching about correct perineal care, and the use of sitz baths or heat lamps to facilitate healing (see Nursing Care Plan for further discussion). The woman's perineum should be inspected at least twice each day for early signs of developing infection. When a localized infection develops, it is

Table 29–1 REEDA Scale Utilized to Evaluate Healing*

Points	Redness	Edema	Ecchymosis	Discharge	Approximation
0	None	None	None	None	Closed
1	Within 0.25 cm of incision bilaterally	Perineal, less than 1 cm from incision	Within 0.25 cm bilaterally or 0.5 cm unilaterally	Serum	Skin separation 3 mm or less
2	Within 0.5 cm of incision bilaterally	Perineal and/or vulvar, between 1 to 2 cm from incision	Between 0.25 to 1 cm bilaterally or between 0.5 to 2 cm unilaterally	Serosanguineous	Skin and subcutaneous fat separation
3	Beyond 0.5 cm of incision bilaterally	Perineal and/or vulvar, greater than 2 cm from incision	Greater than 1 cm bilaterally or 2 cm unilaterally	Bloody purulent	Skin, subcutaneous fat, and fascial layer separation
Score:	____	____	____	____	____
					Total ____

* From Davidson, N. 1974. REEDA: Evaluating postpartum healing. *J. Nurse-Midwifery.* 19:7.

treated with antibiotic creams, stiz baths, and analgesics as necessary for pain relief. If an abscess has developed or a stitch site is infected, the suture is removed and the area allowed to drain.

ENDOMETRITIS

After delivery of the placenta, the placental site provides an excellent culture medium for bacterial growth. The site (in the contracted uterus) is a 4 cm round, dark red, elevated area with a nodular surface composed of numerous veins, many of which become occluded due to clot formation. The remaining portion of the decidua is also susceptible to pathogenic bacteria because of its thinness (approximately 2 mm) and its hypervascularity. The cervix may also present a bacterial breeding ground because of the multiple small lacerations attending normal labor and spontaneous delivery.

The pathogens deposited at the cervix during vaginal examination and those already present invade the decidua and eventually involve the entire mucosa. If the infection is confined to the surface of the mucosa, this area will become necrotic and be sloughed off within 3–5 days. In this instance the discharge is scant (or profuse), bloody, and foul smelling.

In more severe cases, symptoms may include uterine tenderness and jagged, irregular temperature elevation, usually between 101F (38.3C) and 104F (40C). Tachycardia, chills, and evidence of subinvolution may be noted. Foul-smelling lochia generally is cited as a classic sign of metritis, but in the case of infection with beta hemolytic streptococcus, the lochia may be scant and odorless (Pritchard and MacDonald, 1980).

Treatment includes the administration of oxytocics in mild cases to stimulate strong uterine contractions. In more severe cases antibiotics and careful patient monitoring to prevent the development of serious pelvic infection are necessary.

SALPINGITIS AND OOPHORITIS

Occasionally, bacteria may spread into the lumen of the fallopian tubes, producing infection in the tubes and ovaries. Most often caused by a gonorrheal infection, such infection generally becomes apparent between the ninth and fifteenth postpartal day. Symptoms include bilateral (or unilateral) lower abdominal pain, high temperature, and tachycardia. If tubal closure results, then sterility may ensue (Vorherr, 1982). Treatment is basically the same as that described in the next section on parametritis.

PELVIC CELLULITIS (PARAMETRITIS) AND PERITONITIS

Pelvic cellulitis (parametritis) refers to infection involving the connective tissue of the broad ligament and, in more severe forms, the connective tissue of all the pelvic structures. It is generally spread by way of the lymphatics in the uterine wall, but may also occur if pathogenic organisms invade a cervical laceration that extends upward into the connective tissue of the broad ligament. This laceration then serves as a direct pathway that allows the pathogens already in the cervix to spread into the pelvis. *Peritonitis* refers to infection involving the peritoneum.

Pelvic abscess may form in the case of puerperal peritonitis and most commonly is found in the uterine ligaments, Douglas' cul-de-sac, and the subdiaphragmatic space. Pelvic cellulitis may be a secondary result of pelvic vein thrombophlebitis. This condition occurs when the clot becomes infected and the wall of the vein breaks down from necrosis, spilling the infection into the connective tissues of the pelvis.

As the course of pelvic cellulitis advances, a mass of exudate develops along the base of the broad ligament that may push the uterus toward the opposite wall (if the infection is unilateral), where it will become fixed. If the exudate spreads into the rectocervical septum, a firm mass develops behind the cervix instead. The abscess that results should be drained or resolved through appropriate antibiotic therapy to avoid rupture of the abscess into the peritoneal cavity and development of a possibly fatal peritonitis.

A woman suffering from parametritis may demonstrate a variety of symptoms, including marked high temperature (102–104F or 38.9–40C), chills, malaise, lethargy, abdominal pain, subinvolution of the uterus, tachycardia, and local and referred rebound tenderness. If peritonitis develops, the woman will be acutely ill with severe pain, marked anxiety, high fever, rapid, shallow respirations, pronounced tachycardia, excessive thirst, abdominal distention, nausea, and vomiting.

Interventions and Nursing Care

Management of an infectious process begins with assessment of presenting signs and symptoms. The first 24–48 hours of the infectious process may be accompanied by a temperature no higher than 38.3–38.9C (101–102F) and a white blood count that remains in the normal range. As the infection progresses, the patient has a sustained temperature elevation and may manifest other symptoms such as pain, tenderness, malaise, anorexia, and urinary complaints. Diagnosis of the infection site and causative pathogen is accomplished by a complete physical examination, blood work, cultures (particularly of lochia), and urinalysis.

Antibiotic therapy usually is implemented based on the culture and sensitivity results, with a broad-spectrum antibiotic effective against the most commonly occurring causative organisms being used in the interim. The antibiotics are administered intravenously.

The development of an abscess frequently is heralded by the presence of a palpable mass and may be confirmed with ultrasound. An abscess usually requires incision and drainage to avoid rupture into the peritoneal cavity and development of possibly fatal peritonitis.

The Nursing Care Plan on puerperal infection presents the nursing management for infections. General and specific aspects of nursing care are identified for the major patient problems.

Discharge Planning

The woman with a puerperal infection needs assistance when she is discharged from the hospital. If the family cannot provide this home assistance, a referral to the community homemakers' service is needed. The community health/visiting nurse service can also be contacted as soon as puerperal infection is diagnosed so that the nurse can meet with the client for a family and home assessment and development of a home care plan. The community health nurse is aware of the community resources available to assist the client and planning with the client/family before discharge will assure continuity of care after discharge.

The family needs instruction in the care of a newborn, including feeding, bathing, cord care, immunizations, and significant observations that should be reported. A well-baby appointment should be scheduled. Breast-feeding mothers should be instructed to inspect the infant's mouth for signs of thrush and to report the finding to their physician.

The mother should be instructed regarding activity, rest, medications, diet, and signs and symptoms of complications, and she should be scheduled for a return medical examination.

THROMBOEMBOLIC DISEASE

Thromboembolic disease occurs in approximately 1% of spontaneously delivered women and in 2%–10% of women undergoing cesarean birth (Vorherr, 1982). Although the disease may also occur antepartally, it is generally considered a postpartal complication. *Venous thrombosis* refers to thrombus formation in a superficial or deep vein with the accompanying risk that a portion of the clot might break off and result in pulmonary embolism. When the thrombus is formed in response to inflammation in the vein wall, it is termed *thrombophlebitis*. In this type of thrombosis the clot tends to be more firmly attached and therefore is less likely to result in embolism. In *noninflammatory venous thrombosis* (also called phlebothrombosis) the clot tends to be more loosely attached and the risk of embolism is greater. The main factors responsible for this type of thrombosis are venous stasis, vascular anoxia, and endothelial damage (Vorherr, 1982).

Factors contributing directly to the development of thromboembolic disease postpartally include (a) increased amounts of certain blood clotting factors; (b) postpartal thrombocytosis (increased quantity of circulating platelets) and their increased adhesiveness; (c) release of thromboplastin substances from the tissue of the decidua, placenta, and fetal membranes; and (d) the increased amounts of fibrinolysis inhibitors present. Predisposing factors are (a)

(Text continues on p. 981.)

NURSING CARE PLAN
Puerperal Infection

CLIENT DATA BASE

History

1. Predisposing health factors include:
   a. Malnutrition
   b. Anemia
   c. Debilitated condition
2. Predisposing factors associated with labor and delivery include:
   a. Prolonged labor
   b. Hemorrhage
   c. Premature and/or prolonged rupture
   d. Soft tissue trauma
   e. Invasive techniques
   f. Operative procedures

Physical examination

1. Localized episiotomy infections may present the following signs and symptoms:
   a. Complaints of unusual degree of discomfort
   b. Reddened edematous lesion
   c. May have associated purulent drainage
   d. Failure of skin edges to approximate
   e. Fever (generally below 101F)
   f. Dysuria
2. Endometritis
   a. Mild case may be asymptomatic or characterized only by low-grade fever, anorexia, and malaise
   b. More severe cases may demonstrate:
      (1) Fever of 101–103F+
      (2) Anorexia, extreme lethargy
      (3) Chills
      (4) Rapid pulse
      (5) Lower abdominal pain or uterine tenderness
      (6) Lochia — appearance varies depending on causative organism: may appear normal, be profuse, bloody, and foul smelling, may be scant and serosanguineous to brownish and foul smelling
      (7) Severe afterpains
3. Pelvic cellulitis (parametritis)
   a. Signs and symptoms of severe infection (see previous discussion of endometritis)

   b. Severe abdominal pain, usually lateral to the uterus on one or both sides and apparent with both abdominal palpation and pelvic examination
4. Puerperal peritonitis
   a. Symptoms just described plus severe abdominal pain
   b. Abdominal rigidity, guarding, rebound tenderness
   c. Vomiting and diarrhea may occur
   d. If paralytic ileus develops, marked bowel distention will be evident

Laboratory evaluation

1. Elevated white blood count (WBC), although it may be within normal puerperal limits (10,000–15,000/mm^3) initially
2. Culture of intrauterine material reveals causative organism
3. Urine culture should be normal but is done to rule out an asymptomatic urinary tract infection

NURSING PRIORITIES

1. Promote healing of perineum, uterus, and pelvic area without exposure to infectious agents
2. Assess signs and symptoms of impending infections with prompt interventions
3. Implement an appropriate client education program based on the specific needs of the woman and her partner

CLIENT/FAMILY EDUCATIONAL FOCUS

1. Provide the woman and her partner with information about the signs and symptoms, course of the condition, treatment methods, self-care measures to ensure cleanliness and promote tissue healing, and home care routines for postpartal infections
2. Provide opportunities for the couple to ask questions, express concerns and make plans for home and infant management depending on the seriousness of the infection and the amount of assistance available at home

Problem	Nursing interventions and actions	Rationale
Wound infection	Promote normal wound healing by utilizing: 1. Sitz baths 2–3 times daily for 10–15 min 2. Peri-light 2–3 times daily for 10–15 min	Warm water is cleansing, promotes healing through increased vascular flow to affected area, and is soothing to patient

NURSING CARE PLAN Cont'd
Puerperal Infection

Problem	Nursing interventions and actions	Rationale
	3. Peri-care following elimination	Peri-care promotes removal of urine and fecal contaminants from perineum
	4. Frequent changing of peri-pads	Changing pads frequently decreases the media for bacterial growth
	5. Early ambulation	
	6. Diet high in protein and vitamin C	These nutrients are essential for satisfactory wound healing
	7. Fluid intake to 2000 mL/day	
	Evaluate degree of healing by applying REEDA Scale (Table 29-1)	REEDA Scale provides consistent, objective tool for evaluation of wound healing
	Observe, record, and report signs and symptoms of wound infection, including:	Wound infection produces characteristic signs and symptoms
	1. Redness	
	2. Edema	
	3. Excessive pain	
	4. Inadequate approximation of wound edges	
	5. Purulent drainage	
	6. Fever, anorexia, malaise	
	Obtain culture from wound site and administer antibiotics, per physician order	Antibiotic therapy based on knowledge of causative organism is treatment of choice for localized infection
	Increase wound drainage by:	Abscesses may develop when infected material accumulates in closed body cavity; iodoform packing maintains patency of opening so drainage can continue
	1. Assisting physician in opening wound for drainage, when indicated	
	2. Anticipating packing of a cavity greater than 2-3 cm with iodoform gauze	
	Assess pain level and administer analgesics per physician orders if pain is not relieved through nursing measures	
	Prevent spread of infection through:	
	1. Careful hand-washing techniques by staff, patient, and visitors	
	2. Special disposal of infected materials such as disposable bed chux, peri-pads, and contaminated linen	
	Promote and maintain mother-infant interaction by:	Success at feeding infant generally enhances the patient's outlook, encourages mother-infant interaction, and prevents woman from dwelling on herself to exclusion of infant
	1. Encouraging mother to continue feeding her infant	
	2. Reassuring mother that infant is not likely to become infected by her localized infection	Breast-feeding is not affected by localized infection and should be encouraged
		Some institutions still insist on separation of the mother and infant if an infection is present; the mother must be

NURSING CARE PLAN Cont'd
Puerperal Infection

Problem	Nursing interventions and actions	Rationale
		instructed in pumping her breasts (if breast-feeding) and will need support during this separation
Metritis/endometritis	Care of the patient is essentially the same as for wound infections, including antibiotics, analgesics, and careful cleansing techniques	
	Newborn: Assess breast-feeding infant's mouth for signs of thrush, which is a common side effect of antibiotics ingested by infant in mother's milk Treatment should be initiated but breast-feeding need not be stopped	Thrush, a monilial infection caused by *Candida albicans,* often occurs when normal oral flora are destroyed by antibiotic therapy
Pelvic cellulitis	Observe, record, and report signs and symptoms of severe infection, including: 1. Fever spiking to 102–104F 2. Elevated white blood count 3. Chills 4. Extreme lethargy 5. Lower abdominal pain, especially lateral to uterus 6. Nausea and vomiting	Infection produces characteristic signs and symptoms
	Administer IV fluids and antibiotics as ordered	IV fluids maintain proper hydration of client
	Assist physician in pelvic examination for detection of abscess; be prepared for surgical incision and drainage if necessary; in cases where all management fails, removal of infected uterus, tubes, and ovaries may be necessary	
	Promote patient comfort through: 1. Adequate periods of rest 2. Emotional support 3. Judicious use of antibiotics 4. Maintenance of cleanliness and warmth	
	5. Maintainance of semi-Fowler position	Position promotes comfort and helps prevent spread of infection
Peritonitis	Observe, record, and report signs and symptoms of severe infection, such as nausea, vomiting, and abdominal rigidity	Paralytic ileus is frequently associated with peritonitis
	Maintain continuous nasogastric suction per physician order	Continuous nasogastric suction is used to decompress bowel when paralytic ileus complicates clinical course
	Administer IV fluids and antibiotics as ordered	Vigorous fluid and electrolyte therapy is necessary not only because of vomiting and diarrhea, but also because both fluid and electrolytes become sequestered in lumen and wall of bowel
	Monitor intake and output, urine specific gravity, vital signs, and level of hydration	
	Provide narcotic analgesics for alleviation of severe pain, per physician order	

NURSING CARE PLAN Cont'd
Puerperal Infection

Problem	Nursing interventions and actions	Rationale
	Transfer patient to intensive care or provide critical care services by skilled registered nurse Provide emotional support, including: 1. Anticipate maternal depression 2. Provide opportunities for mother to see, touch, and hold infant when possible, taking proper precautions to protect infant 3. Assist breast-feeding mothers to pump breasts in order to maintain milk production 4. Encourage partner/family/support persons to become involved with patient's care and with infant 5. Take pictures of the infant for the mother's bedside	Patient with peritonitis is in critical condition, and quality of nursing care this patient receives will weigh the balance between recovery and demise Critically ill patient may become very depressed not only from disease process but also because her anticipated postpartal course is now denied to her, and she may interpret this as a failure of her ability to mother her infant

NURSING CARE EVALUATION

Purulent drainage, odor, edema, elevated temperature, and wounds are controlled or relieved Wound is healing Woman is ambulating	Woman understands condition, treatment regimen, prevention of spread of infection, infant care, and necessity of continued medical supervision

NURSING DIAGNOSES* | **SUPPORTING DATA**

NURSING DIAGNOSES*	SUPPORTING DATA
1. Potential for injury to the genital tract related to infection	See Nursing Care Plan for signs and symptoms of wound infection, metritis, endometritis, pelvic cellulitis, or peritonitis
2. Knowledge deficit about the condition and its treatment	Faulty or inadequate postpartal hygiene practices Expressed concerns or questions about specific aspects of puerperal infection

* These are a few examples of nursing diagnoses that may be appropriate for a person with this condition. It is not an inclusive list and must be individualized for each woman.

obesity, increased maternal age, and high parity; (b) anesthesia and surgery with possible vessel trauma and venous stasis due to prolonged inactivity; (c) previous history of venous thrombosis; (d) maternal anemia, hypothermia, or heart disease; and (e) the use of estrogen for suppression of lactation (Vorherr, 1982).

Superficial Leg Vein Disease

Superficial thrombophlebitis is far more common postpartally than during pregnancy. Often the clot involves the saphenous veins. This disorder is more common in women with preexisting varices, although it is not limited to these women. Symptoms usually become apparent about the third or fourth postpartal day: tenderness in a portion of the vein, some local heat and redness, absent or low-grade fever, and occasionally, slight elevation of the pulse. Treatment involves application of local heat, elevation of the affected limb, bed rest and analgesics, and the use of elastic support hose. Anticoagulants are usually not necessary unless complications develop. In most cases pulmonary embolism is extremely rare. Occasionally the involved veins have incompetent valves, and as a result, the problem may spread to the deeper leg veins, such as the femoral vein.

Deep Leg Vein Disease

Deep venous thrombosis is more frequently seen in women with a history of thrombosis. Certain obstetric complications such as hydramnios, preeclampsia, and operative delivery are associated with an increased incidence. Generally, the disease occurs unilaterally; in 75% of affected women the left leg is the site (Vorherr, 1982). Clinical manifestations may include edema of the ankle and leg, and an initial low-grade fever often followed by high temperature and chills. Depending on the vein involved, the woman may complain of pain in the popliteal and lateral tibial areas (popliteal vein), entire lower leg and foot (anterior and posterior tibial veins), inguinal tenderness (femoral vein), or pain in the lower abdomen (iliofemoral vein). The Homan's sign (Figure 29–1) may or may not be positive, but pain often results from calf pressure. Because of reflex arterial spasm, sometimes the limb is pale and cool to the touch—the so-called milk leg or *phlegmasia alba dolens*—and peripheral pulses may be decreased.

Because cases are seldom clearcut, diagnosis involves a variety of approaches, such as client history and physical examination, occlusive cuff impedance phlebography (IPG), Doppler ultrasonography, and contrast venography. IPG is a relatively new, noninvasive procedure that can be used to diagnose deep venous thrombosis. This test has a high accuracy and can be performed at the bedside. An occlusive thigh cuff is placed on the client and, using electrodes on the calf, changes in the volume of venous blood are measured as electrical impedance changes (Clarke-Pearson and Creasman, 1981). Doppler ultrasonography is also noninvasive and is used to demonstrate increased circumference in the affected leg. However, in questionable cases, contrast venography provides the most accurate diagnosis of deep venous thrombosis. Unfortunately, venography is not practical for multiple examinations or prospective screening and may, in itself, induce phlebitis.

TREATMENT OF DEEP VEIN THROMBOSIS

Treatment involves the administration of intravenous heparin, using an infusion pump to permit continuous, accurate infusion of medication. Bed rest is required, and analgesics are given as necessary to relieve discomfort. If fever is present, deep thrombophlebitis is suspected and the patient is also given antibiotic therapy. The nurse monitors the patient closely for signs of pulmonary embolism, the most severe complication of deep venous thrombosis. Nurses must observe for any signs of bleeding while the woman is receiving the heparin. In most cases thrombectomy is not necessary.

Once the symptoms have subsided (usually in a few days), the woman may begin ambulation while wearing elastic support stockings. She is instructed to avoid prolonged standing or sitting, and to avoid crossing her legs. The knee gatch on the bed should never be used. Women who have deep venous thrombosis often are given warfarin (Coumadin) therapy and need careful instruction about its use, side effects, and possible interactions with other medications.

Pulmonary Embolism

A sudden onset of dyspnea accompanied by sweating, pallor, cyanosis, confusion, systemic hypotension, and increased jugular pressure may indicate the possibility of pulmonary emboli. Chest pain that mimics cardiac ischemia, coupled with the patient's verbalized fear of imminent death and complaint of pressure in the bowel and

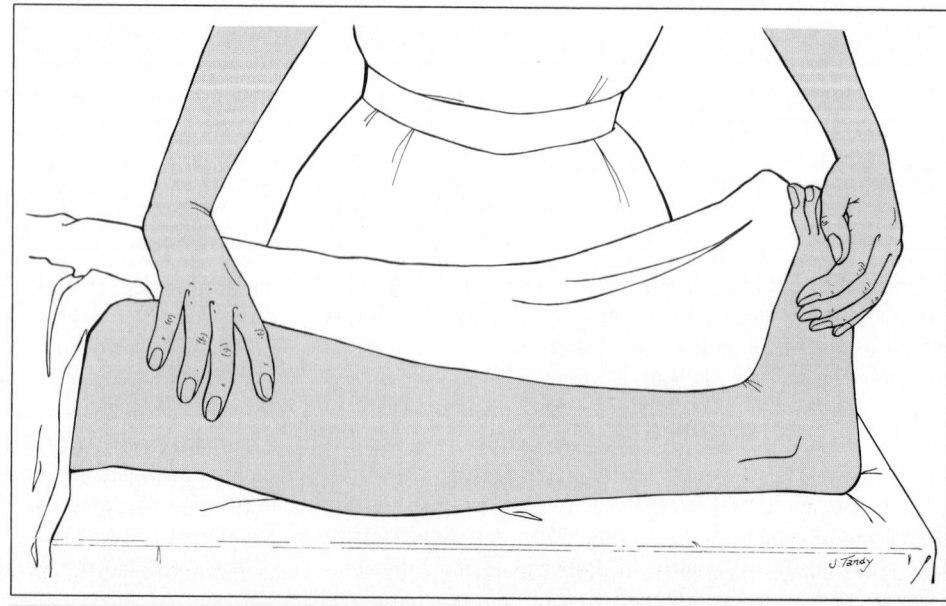

FIGURE 29–1 Homan's sign. While holding the client's knee flat, the nurse dorsiflexes the client's foot. Pain in the client's foot or leg is indicative of a positive Homan's sign.

rectum, should alert the nurse to the extensive size of the embolus. A gallop (heart) rhythm may be present even if respiratory inspiration is normal, although smaller emboli may present with only transient syncope, tightness of the chest, or unexplained pyrexia.

Even x-ray films and ECG changes and laboratory data are not always reliable. If a case of pulmonary embolism is suspected, prompt treatment should begin even in the absence of collaborative data. If the embolism is small and heparin therapy is begun quickly, the chance of survival is excellent. However, when a large thrombus occludes a major pulmonary vessel, death may occur before therapy can even begin.

Therapy involves the administration of a variety of intravenous medications, such as meperidine hydrochloride to relieve the pain, lidocaine for the correction of any arrhythmias, and drugs such as papaverine hydrochloride and aminophylline to reduce spasms of the bronchi and coronary and pulmonary vessels (Vorherr, 1982). Oxygen is administered and heparin infusion is begun. In severe cases an embolectomy may be necessary, although fibrinolytic therapy with medications (such as streptokinase) that lyse clots may be tried first.

For nursing management of thrombophlebitis and pulmonary embolism, see the accompanying Nursing Care Plan.

PUERPERAL CYSTITIS AND PYELONEPHRITIS

The puerperal woman is a likely candidate for development of urinary tract problems. Diuresis is a normal physiologic function during the immediate postpartal period. The body uses this mechanism to begin to eliminate the extra fluid volume that was accumulated during pregnancy. The bladder has a normal increase in capacity following delivery and is less sensitive to fluid retention than during pregnancy or in the nonpregnant state.

Stretching or trauma to the base of the bladder occurs to some degree in any vaginal delivery, and in rare instances the resulting edema of the trigone is great enough to obstruct the urethra and to cause acute retention. Obstruction by large hematomas is not unknown and should be investigated when other causes of acute urinary retention have been ruled out.

Modern obstetric practice has also contributed to the increased risk of puerperal urinary retention and cystitis. Routine administration of intravenous fluids increases the circulating fluid volume that must be filtered out and eliminated following delivery. General anesthesia temporarily inhibits the normal neural control of the bladder and facilitates rapid filling and overdistention. However, except in the case of emergency and cesarean sections, general anesthesia is rarely seen in enlightened obstetrics today. Conductive anesthesia, popular among some obstetricians, inhibits the normal functioning of the bladder to an even greater extent.

Emptying the bladder is vital. Women who are not sufficiently recovered from the effect of anesthesia cannot void spontaneously, and catheterization is necessary.

Retention of residual urine, bacteria introduced at the time of catheterization, and a bladder traumatized by delivery combine to provide an excellent environment for the promotion of cystitis.

Overdistention

The overdistended bladder appears as a large mass, reaching sometimes to the umbilicus and displacing the uterine fundus upward. There is increased vaginal bleeding, a boggy fundus, and the client may complain of cramping as the uterus attempts to contract.

Overdistention, if discovered in the recovery room, is often managed by draining the bladder with a straight catheter as a one-time measure. If the overdistention is recurrent or is diagnosed later in the postpartal period, an indwelling catheter is generally ordered for 24 hours. When the catheter is discontinued, normal bladder functioning is evaluated by one of the two following measures. First, the client who is able to void within 6–8 hours may be catheterized for residual urine. If the residual is greater than 100 mL, the catheter is left in for another 24 hours. Second, if the client is unable to void within 6–8 hours, the bladder is catheterized, and if the amount measured is greater than 200 mL, the catheter is retained for an additional 24 hours. If the amount is less than 200 mL, the catheter is removed and the client is given another trial of 6–8 hours. In the case of a client who is required to void within 6–8 hours after removal of an indwelling catheter, it is important to encourage fluid intake.

Diligent monitoring of the bladder during the recovery period and preventive health measures greatly reduce the number of women who need to be treated for overdistention of the bladder. Encouraging the mother to void spontaneously and assisting her to use the toilet, if possible, or the bedpan if she has received conductive anesthesia prevent the largest percentage of overdistention. If catheterization becomes necessary, an indwelling catheter should always be used, and meticulous aseptic technique should be employed.

As previously mentioned, the vagina and vulva are traumatized to some degree by vaginal delivery, and edema is common. If forceps have been used (a frequent adjunct to conductive anesthesia), the trauma is greater, and edema, especially of the vestibule, is marked. This edema may obscure the urinary meatus, and the nurse needs to be extremely careful in cleansing the vulva and inserting

(Text continues on p. 987.)

NURSING CARE PLAN
Thrombophlebitis and Pulmonary Embolism

CLIENT DATA BASE

History

1. Predisposing factors include:
   a. Increased maternal age
   b. Obesity
   c. Increased parity
   d. Prolonged labor with associated pressure of the fetal head on the pelvic veins
   e. Preeclampsia-eclampsia
   f. Heart disease
   g. Hypercoagulability of the early puerperium
   h. Anemia
   i. Immobility
   j. Hemorrhage
   k. Previous history of venous thrombosis
2. Initiating factors may include:
   a. Trauma to deep leg veins due to faulty positioning for delivery
   b. Operative delivery, including cesarean
   c. Abortion
   d. Postpartal pelvic cellulitis

Physical examination

1. Superficial thrombophlebitis
   a. Tenderness along the involved vein
   b. Areas of palpable thrombosis
   c. Warmth and redness in the involved area
2. Deep vein thrombosis
   a. Positive Homan's sign (pain occurs when foot is dorsiflexed while leg is extended)
   b. Tenderness and pain in affected area
   c. Fever (initially low, followed by high fever and chills)
   d. Edema in affected extremity
   e. Pallor and coolness in affected limb
   f. Diminished peripheral pulses
3. Pulmonary embolism
   a. Sudden onset of dyspnea, sweating, pallor, cyanosis, confusion, chest pain, and verbalized anxiety and feelings of impending doom

   b. Systemic hypotension and increased jugular pressure may be present
   c. Gallop heart rhythm

Laboratory evaluation

1. Thrombophlebitis
   a. Doppler ultrasonography demonstrates increased circumference of affected extremity
   b. Occlusive cuff impedance phlebography
   c. Venography confirms diagnosis
2. Pulmonary embolism
   a. Electrocardiogram may reveal indications of right-sided heart strain
   b. Lung scan or pulmonary angiography may reveal evidence of pulmonary embolism but may not be definitive
   c. SGOT and LDH may be elevated

NURSING PRIORITIES

1. Prevent circulatory stasis through correct positioning in delivery stirrups, early ambulation, avoiding crossing legs, leg exercise, and applications of support stockings
2. Maintain maternal-infant interrelations
3. Perform daily assessments to recognize the development of vascular complications and implement appropriate nursing care if they develop
4. Promote mental health through woman's expressions of fears, acceptance of change in body image, and alternatives to infant care when activities are restricted

CLIENT/FAMILY EDUCATIONAL FOCUS

1. Provide information about the cause of the condition, the treatment regime, medications, infant care, necessity of continued medical supervision, and means to avoid circulatory stasis.
2. Carefully review the implications, rationale, side effects, and possible problems that may develop with warfarin therapy following discharge
3. Provide opportunities for the couple to ask questions and express concerns about the diagnosis and its implications

Problem	Nursing interventions and actions	Rationale
Thrombophlebitis	Initiate and maintain actions to prevent development of thrombophlebitis, including: 1. Careful positioning of woman in stirrups for delivery 2. Early active ambulation	Prolonged pressure, resulting in venous stasis and trauma to the vein wall, is contributing factor to development of thrombophlebitis Movement and support encourage venous return and decrease tendency to venous stasis

NURSING CARE PLAN Cont'd
Thrombophlebitis and Pulmonary Embolism

Problem	Nursing interventions and actions	Rationale
	3. Use of support stockings following operative deliveries 4. Instruction as to necessity for doing leg exercises regularly when confined to bed 5. Instruction to elevate knee gatch in bed Observe, record, and report signs and symptoms of thrombophlebitis. Maintain bed rest and warm, moist soaks as ordered Administer analgesics for relief of pain per physician order	Bed rest is ordered to decrease possibility that portion of clot will dislodge and result in pulmonary embolism. Warmth promotes blood flow to affected area

	Administer intravenous heparin as ordered, by continuous intravenous drip, heparin lock, or subcutaneously, including:
	1. Monitor IV or heparin lock site for signs of infiltration
	2. Obtain Lee White clotting times per physician order and review prior to administering heparin
	3. Observe for signs of anticoagulant overdose with resultant bleeding, including:
	   a. Hematuria
	   b. Epistaxis
	   c. Ecchymosis
	   d. Bleeding gums
	4. Provide protamine sulfate, per physician order, to combat bleeding problems related to heparin overdosage
		Heparin does not dissolve clot but is administered to prevent further clotting. It is safe for breast-feeding mothers because heparin is not excreted in mother's milk
		
		Protamine sulfate is heparin antagonist, given intravenously, which is almost immediately effective in counteracting bleeding complications caused by heparin overdose

	5. Initiate progressive ambulation following the acute phase; provide properly fitting elastic stockings prior to ambulation	Elastic stockings or "Teds" help prevent pooling of venous blood in lower extremities
Pulmonary embolism	Observe, record, and report signs and symptoms of pulmonary embolism, including: 1. Sudden onset of severe chest pain, often located substernally 2. Apprehension and sense of impending catastrophe 3. Cough (may be accompanied by hemoptysis) 4. Tachycardia 5. Fever 6. Hypotension 7. Diaphoresis, pallor, weakness 8. Shortness of breath 9. Neck vein engorgement 10. Friction rub and evidence of atelectasis upon auscultation	Signs and symptoms may occur suddenly and require immediate emergency treatment; prognosis is related to size and location of embolism

NURSING CARE PLAN Cont'd
Thrombophlebitis and Pulmonary Embolism

Problem	Nursing interventions and actions	Rationale
	Initiate or support emergency treatment and additional treatment, including: 1. Combat hypoxia: a. Administer oxygen b. Assist physician with tracheal intubation if necessary 2. Monitor vital signs, ECG 3. Administer medications as ordered: a. Sedative b. Digitalis 4. Prepare patient for embolectomy if ordered 5. Additional treatment involves anticoagulants, bed rest, and analgesics and is similar to treatment for thrombophlebitis	Sedation is used to control pain and anxiety Digitalis is administered to improve myocardial function
Prevention of maternal/ infant deprivation	Maintain mother–infant attachment when mother is on bed rest by: 1. Providing frequent contacts for mother and infant; modified rooming-in possible if crib placed tangent to mother's bed or if Baby Bonding Crib is used 2. Encouraging continuation of breast-feeding or breasts may be pumped for acutely ill patients 3. Provide photos of infant if contact limited	Evidence indicates that first few days of life may be crucial to development of maternal–infant bonds, and separation during this period should be avoided Flow of milk is contingent on emptying of breast, either by placing infant to breast or pumping milk from breast; many institutions utilize milk pumped from mother's breasts for feeding infant

NURSING CARE EVALUATION

Presenting signs and symptoms are relieved or controlled

Patient is stabilized on anticoagulant medication

No inflammatory process is evident

Patient is ambulatory without pain

Patient applies elastic stocking

Patient knows to avoid constrictive clothing; to avoid placing legs in dependent positions; purposes of medications, including dosage, untoward effects of anticoagulant medications, frequency, symptoms to report to physician; and necessity of continued medical supervision

Maternal–infant bonding is established

NURSING DIAGNOSES*	SUPPORTING DATA
1. Potential alteration in tissue perfusion related to deep vein thrombosis	See physical examination in Nursing Care Plan
2. Potential fluid volume deficit related to anticoagulant treatment resulting in bleeding	Hematuria Epistaxis Ecchymoses Bleeding gums Signs or symptoms of hypovolemia
3. Impaired gas exchange related to pulmonary embolism	See signs and symptoms of pulmonary embolism in Nursing Care Plan
4. Knowledge deficit about the condition and its treatment	Expressed concerns or questions about specific aspects of thrombophlebitis and/or pulmonary embolism

* These are a few examples of nursing diagnoses that may be appropriate for a person with this condition. It is not an inclusive list and must be individualized for each woman.

the catheter. It is imperative to discard a catheter that has inadvertently been introduced into the vagina and thus contaminated. (Catheterization, an uncomfortable procedure at any time, is generally painful during the puerperium due to the trauma and edema of the tissue. Therefore, the nurse should be especially careful, considerate, and gentle not only in inserting the catheter but also in handling and cleansing the perineal area.)

If the amount of urine siphoned from the bladder reaches 900–1000 mL, the catheter should be clamped, the Foley balloon inflated, and the catheter attached firmly to the client's leg. The physician should be notified, and the procedure, including the woman's vital signs before and after the procedure and her responses, should carefully be charted. After an hour, the catheter may be unclamped and placed on gravity drainage. By following this technique, the bladder is protected, and rapid intraabdominal decompression is avoided. When the indwelling catheter is removed, a urine sample is often sent to the laboratory, and usually the tip of the catheter is removed and sent for culture.

Cystitis

E. coli has been demonstrated to be the causative agent in 73%–90% of the cases of postpartal cystitis and pyelonephritis. Aerobacter, Proteus, klebsiella, pseudomonas, and Staphylococcus are responsible for most of the remainder (Vorherr, 1982). In the vast majority of cases the infection ascends the urinary tract from the urethra to the bladder and then to the kidneys because vesiculoureteral reflux forces contaminated urine into the renal pelvis.

Symptoms of cystitis (bladder inflammation) often appear 2–3 days after delivery. The initial symptoms of cystitis may include frequency, urgency, dysuria, and nocturia. Hematuria and suprapubic pain may also be present. A slightly elevated temperature may occur, but systemic symptoms are often absent.

When cystitis is suspected in the puerperium, a clean-catch midstream urine sample is obtained for microscopic examination, culture, and sensitivity tests. A catheterized specimen is avoided when possible because of the increased risk of infection. When the bacterial concentration is greater than 100,000 microorganisms per milliliter of fresh urine, infection is generally present; counts between 10,000 and 100,000 are suggestive, particularly if clinical symptoms are noted.

Pyelonephritis

When a urinary tract infection progresses to pyelonephritis, systemic symptoms usually occur, and the women becomes acutely ill. Symptoms include chills, high fever, flank pain (unilateral or bilateral), nausea, and vomiting, in addition to all the signs of lower urinary tract infection. Costovertebral pain also may be elicited. If untreated, the renal cortex may be damaged and kidney function may be impaired.

Interventions and Nursing Care

Prevention is important in dealing with urinary tract infection. Regular, complete bladder emptying, instruction on proper wiping techniques to avoid fecal contamination of the meatus, coupled with good perineal care and frequent changing of the perineal pads all decrease chances of infection.

When cystitis is suspected, treatment is delayed until the culture and sensitivity reports are available. The appropriate antibiotic medication is then begun. In the case of pyelonephritis, bed rest, forced fluids, and broad-spectrum antibiotics are prescribed even before the culture results are available. If nausea and vomiting are severe, fluids are administered intravenously. Antispasmodics and analgesics are also given to relieve discomfort. The woman usually continues to take antibiotics for 2–4 weeks after clinical and bacteriologic response. A routine clean-catch urine culture should be obtained 2 weeks after completion of therapy and then periodically for the next 2 years.

Continuation of breast-feeding during therapy is acceptable and is only limited by the degree of the mother's malaise and clinical discomfort. For the breast-feeding mother the antibiotic chosen should be selected carefully to avoid problems for the infant via the milk. The mother is encouraged to be as actively involved with her new baby as possible to promote the maternal–infant bond and help distract the client from her problems.

DISORDERS OF THE BREAST AND COMPLICATIONS OF LACTATION

Mastitis

Mastitis refers to an inflammation of the breast generally caused by Staphylococcus aureus and primarily seen in breast-feeding mothers. Because symptoms seldom occur before the second to fourth week postpartally, nurses often are not fully aware of how uncomfortable and acutely ill the woman may be.

The infection usually begins when bacteria invade the breast tissue. Often the tissue has been traumatized in some way (fissured or cracked nipples, overdistention, manipulation, or milk stasis) and is especially susceptible to pathogenic invasion. The most common source of the bacteria is the infant's nose and throat, although other sources include the hands of the mother or hospital personnel or the woman's circulating blood.

Once the infection develops, the woman may have a

high temperature, chills, tachycardia, and headache. The breasts may be very tender, have a reddened and warm area, feel firm to the touch, or show areas of lumpiness (Figure 29–2). Diagnosis is usually based on the symptoms, physical examination, and a culture and sensitivity test of the breast milk.

Prevention is far simpler than therapy. Meticulous hand-washing by all personnel is obviously the primary measure in preventing epidemic nursery infections and subsequent maternal mastitis. Periodic nasal cultures of all nursery personnel identify bacteria carriers, who can then be treated. Prompt attention to mothers who have blocked milk ducts eliminates the stagnant milk as a growth medium for bacteria. Frequent breast-feeding of the infant usually prevents mastitis.

If a mother finds that one area of the breast feels distended (caked), several simple methods will help. First, she can rotate the position of the newborn for nursing so that the baby's gums compress different sinuses each time. Second, if the affected breast has not been emptied at a particular feeding, manual expression or a nontraumatic breast pump can be employed to assure that the breast is emptied. Third, as the infant is nursing, the mother should massage the caked area, starting from the point farthest away from the nipple and gently stroking down toward the nipple. (Be sure that the mother doesn't accidentally break the infant's suction.) This technique manually stimulates emptying the breast.

Treatment involves administration of appropriate anti-biotics, use of analgesics to ease discomfort, and local application of heat.

Opinion varies about whether breast-feeding should be discontinued in the presence of mastitis. Those advocating cessation of breast-feeding suggest that a vicious cycle of reinfection may develop as the infant ingests infected milk, becomes reinfected, and in turn, reinfects the mother. Those favoring continuation of breast-feeding raise several points in support of their beliefs. First, if the milk contains bacteria, it also contains the antibiotic that the mother is taking. Second, if infants are the initial carriers of the infections, they should also be under treatment. And third, sudden cessation of lactation will certainly cause caking and severe engorgement, which may be much more painful than continuing to breast-feed. Breast-feeding adds an additional benefit in that it stimulates circulation and moves bacteria-containing milk out of the breast, instead of leaving the affected milk to stagnate in the breast. A third alternative is considered in many agencies, which involves the temporary cessation of breast-feeding from the involved breast during the acute phase. Nursing can be resumed when the mother is afebrile and has received antibiotics for a time. To prevent recurrence the mother must completely understand the necessity to continue taking the antibiotic for the full 10 days of therapy.

Breast Abscess

Occasionally the process of mastitis may continue and a frank abscess develops. The mother's milk and any drainage from the nipple should be cultured and antibiotic therapy instituted. In addition, it is usually necessary to incise surgically and drain the abscessed area. If multiple abscesses are present, multiple incisions will be necessary, usually under general anesthesia. After incision and drainage, the area is packed with sterile gauze. The packing is gradually decreased to permit proper healing.

Because the breast is covered with a sterile surgical dressing, access to the breast will temporarily be inhibited and breast-feeding will become impossible. Once the dressings, drains, and packing have been removed and the incisions are healing well, careful breast-feeding may resume, closely supervised by the experienced nurse.

Persistent Abnormal Lactation

Persistent abnormal lactation (postdelivery galactorrhea—Chiari-Frommel syndrome) is a rare disorder characterized by galactorrhea, amenorrhea, and estrogen deficiency. Microadenomas of the pituitary gland are considered a leading cause, although primary hypothyroidism and even chronic renal disease, especially if treated with dialysis, also have been implicated (Danforth, 1982). Symptomatic treatment using medications such as bromocriptine (Parlodel) to suppress lactation have been employed, but there is no cure for the underlying disorder.

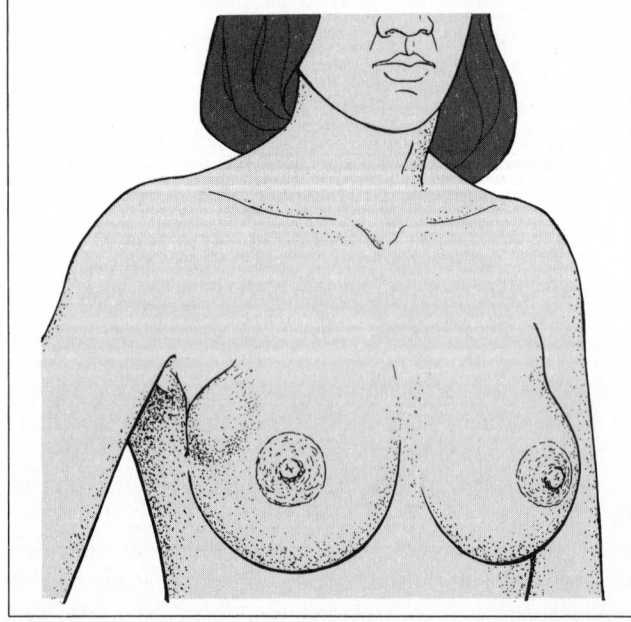

FIGURE 29–2 Mastitis. Erythema and swelling are present in the upper outer quadrant of the breast. Axillary lymph nodes are enlarged and tender.

Postdelivery Anterior Pituitary Necrosis

Postdelivery anterior pituitary necrosis (hypophyseal cachexia—Sheehan syndrome) is a rare complication of hypovolemic shock and disseminated intravascular coagulation (DIC) in women who survive postpartal hemorrhage, and is a result of infarction of the anterior pituitary. Symptoms of the disorder include failure of lactation, breast and genital atrophy, loss of pubic hair and axillary hair, amenorrhea and infertility, increased susceptibility to infection, and fatigue. The severity of the symptoms and the extent of therapy depend on the amount of damage to the hypophysis. In general, treatment involves hormone replacement as necessary.

PUERPERAL PSYCHIATRIC DISORDERS

Since Hippocrates first misdiagnosed puerperal infection for puerperal psychosis in 460 B.C., health care providers have continued to believe that there is a psychologic, physiologic, endocrine, or metabolic rationale that makes women susceptible to "mental breakdown" following childbirth. Even today, the literature continues to hypothesize a multitude of reasons to account for "the phenomenon" of puerperal psychosis.

Many different types of psychiatric problems may be encountered in the puerperium and only rarely is the disorder serious.

Approximately 60% of women experience a transient depression during the first week, which is most common on the third postpartal day (Danforth, 1982). This transient depression is usually accompanied by tearfulness and is a self-limiting, brief episode. The DSM-III (Diagnostic and Statistical Manual III) does not have a definitive heading for postpartum psychosis per se. In some instances the clinical picture will meet the criteria for Schizophreniform Disorder, Paranoid Disorder, Affective Disorder, or Organic Mental Disorder. If not, it is included under 298.20, Atypical Psychosis.

When psychiatric illness occurs after delivery, one or several of the following signs are usually present: depression, delusions, confusion, mania, delirium, hallucinations, anxiety, and sexual dysfunction (Hamilton, 1982). Occasionally, violent behavior forms part of the clinical picture; sometimes this violence is directed against the infant. Approximately 1 in 1000 term pregnancies is followed by psychiatric problems sufficiently severe to require hospitalization (Hamilton, 1982).

Depression is the most common type of psychiatric disorder seen after childbirth. It tends to peak about 6 weeks postdelivery, although symptoms may arise earlier, for example, feelings of failure, self-accusatory thoughts, depression, and exhaustion. Suicidal thinking may be present, which poses a true danger to the woman. Treatment generally is directed at relief of symptoms, and hospitalization may be indicated if the woman seems capable of harming herself.

Postpartal schizophrenic reactions may have an earlier onset—usually by the tenth day, although they may occur earlier. This disorder is manifested by delusional thinking, flight of ideas, and gross distortion of reality, often accompanied by agitation. Although the behavior of these patients may seem especially bizarre, if correctly treated their prognosis is excellent (Hamilton, 1982).

In some women postpartal psychosis has a more subtle onset and may be characterized by increasing hostility and anger, fearfulness, anxiety, and aversion to sexual activity. Unfortunately, this type of disturbance frequently culminates in an act of violence, such as child abuse.

It is important to consider contributing factors to postpartal psychiatric disorders, because one-fourth of women with a history of postpartal mental illness experience recurrence after a subsequent pregnancy. Contributing factors include (a) a chronic history of inability to deal with life's crises without decompensating; (b) a traumatic relationship with the woman's own mother, especially during childhood; (c) self-defensive or conflicting motives for the pregnancy itself; (d) external variables such as prolonged infertility prior to pregnancy, physical complications during pregnancy or labor and delivery, problems or abnormalities with the infant; (e) concomitant life stresses, such as poverty, a recent family member's death, or home or job change (Barglow, 1982).

Prevention is the main goal. The clinician should be familiar with the woman and her partner, the client's background, family, and personal history, social adjustment, level of maturity, and attitudes toward pregnancy and childrearing (Danforth, 1982). Frank and frequent discussion between the woman and her caregiver helps permit early intervention. In addition, active participation in the entire delivery process allows the woman to achieve a sense of mastery.

Treatment of mild postpartal psychiatric disorders usually is achieved on an outpatient basis, although medications or hospitalization is indicated in some cases. If the mother appears to have rejected her infant, it is never wise to compel her to care for him or her, as this forces the women to deal with feelings of guilt, shame, and hostility that may overwhelm her and endanger the infant.

Psychiatric problems often are noted first by a nurse, obstetrician, or family member. If caregivers have any doubts about the woman's stability, a referral may be made to the public health service so that follow-up care is possible. In this way one may identify problems before they become major obstacles to the woman's or her infant's emotional health.

SUMMARY

The normal puerperium is a dynamic period during which major physiologic changes must take place in order for the body to return to its nonpregnant state. When nurses are keenly aware of these normal physiologic changes, they can quickly assess whether deviations occur in the involutional process. These deviations place additional stress on the body, creating a risk situation for the mother that necessitates immediate intervention and evaluation. In addition to the dynamic physiologic changes of the postpartal period, new psychologic needs must be met as the mother and family adapt to the challenge of their new roles and responsibilities as parents and as an expanded family.

References

Barglow, P. 1982. Postpartum mental illness: detection and treatment. In *Gynecology and obstetrics*, vol. 2, ed. J. J. Sciarra. Philadelphia: Harper & Row.

Clarke-Pearson, D. L., and Creasman, W. T. July 1981. Diagnosis of deep venous thrombosis in obstetrics and gynecology by impedance phlebography. *Obstet. Gynecol.* 58:52.

Danforth, D. N., ed. 1982. *Obstetrics and gynecology*, 4th ed. Philadelphia: Harper & Row.

Eschenbach, D., and Wager, G. 1980. Puerperal infections. *Clin. Obstet. Gynecol.* 23(4):1003.

Filker, R., and Monif, G. March 1979. The significance of temperature during the first 24 hours postpartum. *Obstet. Gynecol.* 53(3):358.

Hamilton, J. A. 1982. Puerperal psychoses. In *Gynecology and obstetrics*, vol. 2, ed. J. J. Sciarra. Philadelphia: Harper & Row.

Pritchard, J. A., and MacDonald, P. C. 1980. *Williams obstetrics*, 16th ed. New York: Appleton-Century-Crofts.

Visscher, H. C., and Visscher, R. D. 1982. Early and late postpartum hemorrhage. In *Gynecology and obstetrics*, vol. 2, ed. J. J. Sciarra. Philadelphia: Harper & Row.

Vorherr, H. 1982. Puerperium: maternal involutional changes—management of puerperal problems and complications. In *Gynecology and obstetrics*, vol. 2, ed. J. J. Sciarra. Philadelphia: Harper & Row.

Additional Readings

Brinsden, P. R., and Clark, A. D. 1978. Postpartum hemorrhage after induced and spontaneous labor. *Br. Med. J.* 2:855.

Droegmueller, W. 1980. Cold sitz baths for relief of postpartum perineal pain. *Clin. Obstet. Gynecol.* 23(4):1039.

Faro, S. 1981. Group B beta hemolytic streptococci and puerperal infections. *Am. J. Obstet. Gynecol.* 139(6):686.

Friedman, C. 1980. Maternal infections: problems and prevention. *Nurs. Clin. North Am.* 15(4):817.

Hagen, D. Sept. 1975. Maternal febrile morbidity associated with fetal monitoring and cesarean section. *Obstet. Gynecol.* 46:260.

Ott, W. J. 1981. Primary cesarean section: factors related to postpartum infection. *Obstet. Gynecol.* 57(2):171.

Tentoni, S. C., and High, K. A. July/Aug. 1980. Culturally induced postpartum depression. *J. Obstet. Gynecol. Neonatal Nurs.* 9(4):246.

Vanden Bergh, R. L. 1980. Postpartum depression. *Clin. Obstet. Gynecol.* 23(4):1105.

Wager, G. P.; Martin, D. H.; Koutsky, L., et al. 1980. Puerperal infectious morbidity: relationship to route of delivery and to antepartum chlamydia trachomatis infection. *Am. J. Obstet. Gynecol.* 138:1028.

Watson, P. 1980. Postpartum hemorrhage and shock. *Clin. Obstet. Gynecol.* 23(4):985.

Wiechetek, W. J., et al. May 1974. Puerperal morbidity and internal fetal monitoring. *Am. J. Obstet. Gynecol.* 119:230.

▪ 30 ▪

FAMILIES IN CRISIS AND THE ROLE OF THE NURSE

■ CHAPTER CONTENTS

FAMILIES AND CRISIS

CRISIS INTERVENTION

    Assessment

    Planning Therapeutic Intervention

    Intervention

    Evaluation

THE ROLE OF THE MATERNITY NURSE DURING CRISIS

FAMILIES AT RISK

LOSS AND GRIEF

CRISIS INTERVENTION DURING POSTPARTAL PERIOD

    Loss of Newborn

    Preterm Birth

    Defective Newborn

CRISIS INTERVENTION DURING POSTPARTAL FOLLOW-UP CARE

    Attachment Problems

    Unwanted Pregnancy and Relinquishment

    Child Abuse

    The Adolescent Parent

    Single-Parent Families

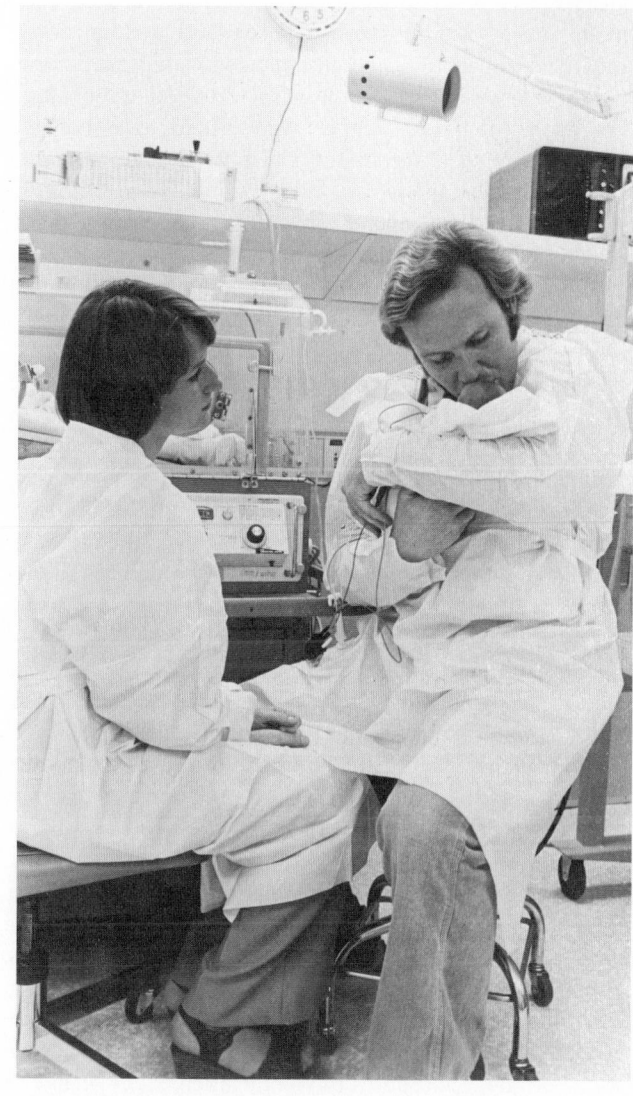

- Define the term *family crisis*.

- List the types of crises that may occur within a family.

- Compare the process of crisis intervention to the nursing process.

- Describe crisis intervention as applied to maternity nursing.

- Identify specific assessment strategies to predict which families will need additional support to avert or resolve a crisis.

- Describe nursing interventions for several postpartal crises.

Pregnancy and the birth of a baby are frequently times of stress and can be viewed as a crisis for the family. Each member experiences role changes as transitions from one life stage to another occur. Identity crises may be paramount during role transition. The structure and function of the family is becoming increasingly complex. Role differentiation is less clearcut than it was several generations ago. For example, if two women were asked to visualize a scene depicting a successful goal achievement for themselves, one woman's vision might be expressed in the following way: "I'm walking into an executive office in my gray wool suit, briefcase in hand, ready to sit down in the president's chair as the board of directors of the company meets to draft a major decision." This woman imagines feelings of power, trust, challenge, excitement, and accomplishment. Another woman may say, "I picture myself playing on the floor with my children, surrounded by laughter as the dog steps in the middle of the toys. My husband leans over and strokes my hair." She imagines feelings of love, pride, comfort, security and warmth. Even more important than the divergence between the role visualizations of these two women is that often both goals may belong to the same woman. Many women no longer see the need to decide between career and family.

Potential role conflict of women is only one of many factors that may contribute to a family crisis at the time of birth. A father may find that the increased responsibility of parenthood conflicts with the freedom and independence he enjoys. He may be jealous of the relationship between the mother and their newborn infant. Siblings may experience loss and confusion as the parents spend more time with the new baby. Adolescent parents may find themselves adjusting to the stresses of parenthood at the same time that they are trying to establish their own identities. Single parents may be trying to cope with pregnancy and birth without an adequate support system. These situations only begin to illustrate the variation in the human condition that contributes to identification of the birth of a baby as a crisis. Most of these variables are of a more or less predictive nature and plans can be made to resolve stress, conflict, and crisis. Other crises, such as the death of a newborn or even an emergency cesarean delivery, are less predictable and extremely stressful.

If the family is perceived as a system, then any change within the family affects each member of the family, whether they face an unpredictable crisis or changes in expectations of role fulfillment of one member of the family. This chapter reviews the theoretic basis for crisis theory and describes some specific crises requiring nursing intervention during pregnancy and the postpartal period.

FAMILIES AND CRISIS

A crisis can be viewed as a turning point. It has the potential to be growth promoting or emotionally destructive for those involved. During a crisis one perceives disequilibrium because of profound disruption in the usual pattern of one's life process. The individual usually strives to reestablish equilibrium, which can be accomplished in adaptive or maladaptive ways. The ordinary coping mechanisms individuals and families utilize to deal with stress are no longer adequate when a crisis occurs. Tension and anxiety increase in an emergency, and people feel helpless.

Two types of crisis are generally recognized: maturational crisis and situational crisis. Maturational crises are those related to the normal processes of growth and development. A maturational crisis generally evolves more slowly, is characterized by feelings of disequilibrium, and requires the individual to make character changes. Adolescence is seen as a common maturational crisis. A situational crisis is seen by Lindemann (1956) as an event in the life of an individual that generates intense emotional strain and stress and that requires successful adaptation to master the situation.

The breakdown in coping mechanisms associated with a crisis can result from internal or external pressures. Families with fewer resources may have more trouble coping with a crisis. Families typically feel the effects of particular pressures at certain stages of the family life cycle (see Chapter 3) more than at other times. For example, economic pressures are generally greatest in the first and last years of a marriage. In the middle years, after the children have left home, a couple usually has a higher income and fewer expenses.

Increased social pressures take their toll on families. Political and economic factors, influences by the media, governmental policies, and various other environmental variables affect family structure. Some people decry the degeneration of the institution of the family; others believe that social development has made certain changes in the family necessary. Various life-styles have made divorce and family dissolution more prevalent. In the event of a crisis, unless the individual members have values that support the integrity of the family, the crisis often becomes the stimulus for family breakdown.

Examples of family crises include:

1. Loss within family
   a. Hospitalization
   b. Loss of child
   c. Loss of spouse
   d. Loss of parents
   e. Separation (work, military service, and so on)
2. Loss of standing in community
   a. Disgrace (drug addiction, spouse or child abuse, delinquency, alcoholism)
   b. Marital infidelity
   c. Nonsupport or poverty
   d. Progressive dissention
3. Addition of new members
   a. Pregnancy and birth
   b. Adoption
   c. Relative moves in
   d. Reunion after separation
   e. Remarriage
4. Other crises
   a. Divorce
   b. Annulment
   c. Desertion by spouse
   d. Illegitimate birth
   e. Imprisonment
   f. Institutionalization
   g. Runaway child
   h. Suicide of member
   i. Homicide
   j. Birth of deformed or preterm child

The postpartal family must deal with several of these events simultaneously. For example, the birth of a healthy child, the stress of adjusting to the new member, learning new roles and responsibilities, and adapting to rearranged daily schedules and life-style changes can precipitate disruption within a family. If other factors are present, such as economic problems, the family may not have the coping mechanisms to deal with the crisis adaptively. Without adequate adjustment, these crises can prevent a family from adequately performing the task of nurturing its members.

A significant feature of the family in crisis is the phenomenon of *scapegoating*. An individual within the family becomes the focus of the underlying disturbance and carries most of the blame for the disturbance by "acting out" in certain unacceptable ways. If the family is dealt with as a unit, it can be seen that the family member who is acting out does so in the context of disturbed social relations within the family group. In other words, the individual is not the only one in need of treatment—the entire family needs to be treated. An individual acts in the context of his or her environment and in response to those nearby. For example, the woman who suffers from severe postpartal depression may be responding to a situation in which she is receiving no help from other family members or in which her spouse demands the same kind of attention that he received before the baby arrived.

Conflict about an issue may gradually erode a family if ineffective means of coping with conflict are utilized. The individual who attempts to escape the situation by desertion, divorce, or separation, who submits to domination, or who uses physical force is contributing to his or her family's crisis state (Duvall, 1975).

How a family crisis is met depends on the personalities involved, on the family structure, and on previously existing problems. It is also determined by the family's previous experience with crises and patterns of problem solving. Responses may range from defeatism and self-pity to acceptance to belief in the situation as a challenge. Situations that cause a crisis may differ from family to family. Family adjustment depends on family philosophy and outlook, family policies and practices, and personal resources of family members.

Factors that aid in the weathering of a crisis include adaptability, a value system in which family closeness is of greater importance than material gain, sharing of tasks by a couple, accurate perception of problems, the attitude that an individual's emotional problems are a family concern, problem-solving skills of the individuals, and personal adjustment of the couple (Hill et al., 1953). Constructive coping mechanisms during a family crisis include such measures as open communication of feelings and wishes among family members, empathy, competency in role playing and role reversal, negotiation until the family members are satisfied, mental health maintenance for the family as a whole, consultation with competent resource persons, and consolidation of the family's goals (Duvall and Hill, 1960).

It is important to recognize that a crisis cannot continue forever. The high anxiety level existing in a crisis state moves the individual to some action to end the crisis, and the outcome of a crisis is significantly influenced by the amount of support the family or individual receives. Several outcomes are possible for the family or individual:

- The family can return to its precrisis state. This may be the result of effective problem solving. Growth has not necessarily taken place; the family has simply returned to its previous level of functioning.

- The family may grow from the crisis experience. For example, marriage may be strengthened as a result of a difficult situation that the partners overcame together. A couple may become better parents because of a crisis with their child.

- The intolerable tension of a crisis may be reduced by neurotic behavior such as resorting to alcoholism or drug dependency. Possibly one or both of the partners in a marriage may desire dissolution of the relationship, thus seeking to end the tension of a crisis. Desertion or breakdown of a family member's mental health may occur.

The purpose of crisis intervention is to recognize the potential negative outcomes for each family and to prevent their occurrence. The utilization of crisis intervention by skilled professionals can lessen the effects of crisis and can assist the family in returning to a state of equilibrium.

CRISIS INTERVENTION

Crisis intervention is a form of psychotherapy. The main differences between crisis intervention and traditional psychoanalysis or psychotherapy are in the amount of time involved, the focus of the therapy, and the role of the therapist. Psychoanalysis may continue for a number of years before the goal of restructuring the personality is attained. The psychoanalyst is passive and nondirective. Traditional psychotherapy focuses on removing specific symptoms and preventing the development of neurosis or psychosis. The psychotherapist is more active than the psychoanalyst, but he or she still assumes an indirect role or that of a participating observer. There are up to twenty sessions in brief psychotherapy.

Crisis intervention, on the other hand, focuses on the immediate crisis. It is not necessary to know the history or the personalities of the people in crisis. The therapist's role is direct, active, and participating. Getz et al. (1974) describe the qualities necessary for crisis intervention counseling:

- Empathy, or perception of the client's feelings
- Warmth, or a communication of acceptance and an effort to understand
- Genuineness, which leads to a trusting relationship

The techniques of crisis intervention are relatively simple and do not require extensive training. Time is limited; usually one to four sessions are all that are needed, because most crises last no longer than 4–6 weeks.

Depending on the resolution of the crisis, continuing therapy of a longer duration may be necessary. The nurse in a maternity setting is frequently in an excellent position to make this referral because of the trust relationship that has been established. An in-depth knowledge of community mental health resources is a valuable asset if one is to provide comprehensive nursing care. Other health team members, such as the social worker, might be part of the referral process. A client who is functioning minimally in a crisis condition will be more likely to follow through with making an appointment if she has written information, including a phone number, in hand. In the case of serious threat to a member of the family, such as potential for suicide or child abuse, the nurse may need to initiate the contact with the appropriate mental health agency. If the client is not familiar with the agency of referral, for example, an alcohol treatment program or parent education group, the nurse can increase the client's compliance and comfort level by sharing as much information as possible about what the individual may expect from such agencies.

The primary goals of crisis intervention (Getz et al., 1974) are (a) to help the client deal with the crisis and to regain his or her equilibrium, that is, to return to the precrisis state; and (b) to enable the person to grow from the experience, to gain more self-awareness, and to improve coping skills.

Aguilera and Messick (1978) have developed a paradigm that clearly demonstrates the process whereby the perceived state of disequilibrium caused by various stressors can progress toward either a "crisis" or a "no crisis" state. The outcome depends on the presence or absence of balancing factors, such as perception of the event, situational support, and coping mechanisms. If adequate balancing factors are present, the problem can be resolved and the crisis averted. If events are misperceived, coping mechanisms absent, and situational supports lacking, then depression and anxiety deepen, and crisis may result. Figure 30–1 shows a paradigm of the crisis of the birth of a preterm infant. The following case study illustrates the use of the paradigm.

Laura and Peter experienced the preterm birth of their son shortly after being transferred to another city for Peter's employment. Laura did not feel comfortable relating her fears and concerns about the baby to her new physician and did not want to worry her husband. Since it was their second child, she thought everyone expected her to know what to do. She became physically exhausted and had episodes of crying. A visit by her mother-in-law precipitated a crisis when Pe-

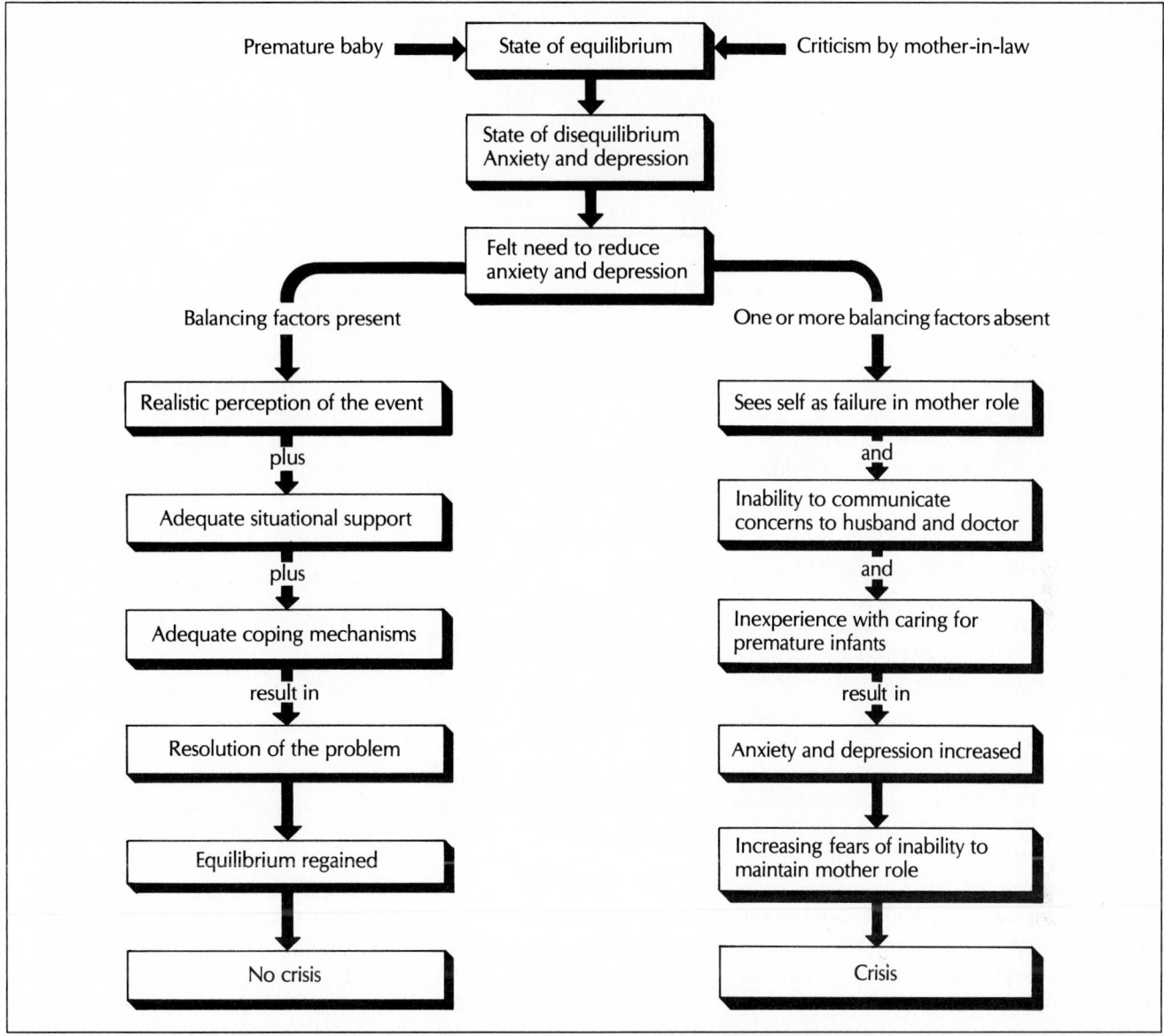

FIGURE 30–1 Paradigm of the birth of a preterm infant. (From Aguilera, D. C., and Messick, J. M. 1978. *Crisis intervention: theory and methodology,* 3rd ed. St. Louis: C. V. Mosby Co., p. 78.)

ter's mother criticized Laura's ability to care for the baby by implying she was doing something wrong because the baby cried so much. Reluctant to take sides against his mother, Peter failed to offer the support Laura needed. Laura's feeling of inadequacy intensified. She cried uncontrollably and was unable to care for the infant. A crisis resulted.

Examining the paradigm helps clarify the specific interventions that would help resolve Laura and Peter's crisis. These include discussing the couple's feelings and changing their communication patterns so that Peter is able to

offer support to his wife and Laura is able to develop a more realistic perception of her parenting competencies (Aguilera and Messick, 1978).

The specific problem-solving steps involved in the technique of crisis intervention as outlined by Aguilera and Messick (1978) are similar to the steps in the nursing process: (a) assessment, (b) planning of therapeutic intervention, (c) intervention, and (d) evaluation.

Assessment

The first step in the assessment is to clearly define the situation before any action is taken and to identify the crisis-precipitating event. The client's perception of the event is examined. What does the event mean to the client? Is the perception distorted or realistic? Assessment is then made of the person's support systems (family, friends, and values). The individual's coping skills are evaluated. How does this person usually handle tension, depression, or anxiety? Questions from the counselor may help the client remember methods he or she has used successfully in the past. At this point, the counselor may determine that the person needs more extensive therapy. For example, the person may seem suicidal, may be in danger of hurting others, or may be out of touch with reality.

Planning Therapeutic Intervention

Further data must be collected at this point. How much has the crisis disrupted the individual's life? How does the family feel about the problem? Tentative approaches are proposed to the individual and examined for their usefulness.

Intervention

The type of intervention most comfortable for the nurse working in a maternity setting depends on the nurse's knowledge base about crisis, flexibility and creativity, interpersonal skills, and the realization that referral is necessary when the limit of the nurse's skills is reached.

The nurse can be an empathetic listener, helping the client develop an understanding of the crisis. Frequently client perceptions are distorted. Emotional catharsis, such as crying, sometimes helps to release tension. Exploring coping mechanisms with clients is valuable; they may utilize coping mechanisms that were effective for them in the past or they may be able to develop new ones. Identifying and expanding the support system available to an individual or family is an important part of crisis intervention. Many times, friends and relatives wish they could help those in crisis, but the individuals involved may feel so guilty, worthless, or withdrawn that they cannot bring themselves to ask for help. The nurse may serve as the liaison between family and friends, community groups, and the client.

Crisis theory suggests that the counselor should be able to make an accurate assessment of the potential for destructive behavior toward self or others. Such problems are not usual in a maternity setting, but the situation may arise. For example, if a nurse working in a prenatal agency saw a young woman at the clinic who was so distraught over the prospect of being pregnant that she used phrases such as "I could end it all for myself," the nurse would be obligated to follow up on the assessment. The nurse should question the young woman about what she means by the statement, by asking directly, "Are you thinking of suicide?" or "Are you thinking of trying to abort the baby

yourself?" The information should be obtained in a gentle, supportive, understanding, warm, but direct way. Using words such as "suicide" will not suggest ideas to someone in crisis that are not already being entertained, as is sometimes feared. If the nurse believes that the woman will injure herself or her child, the nurse needs to notify appropriate agencies who can offer help.

Planned intervention may include one technique or a combination of several. A direct approach may help the client gain an intellectual understanding of the crisis. This approach includes interpretation and confrontation and must be used carefully to avoid further raising the client's anxiety. Allowing the person to express his or her feelings freely stimulates the person to explore these feelings. The counselor should be attentive and relaxed. A knowledge of community resources is valuable. Assertiveness training sessions may benefit the client by increasing self-esteem. When a trusting relationship has been established, reassurance based on truth and concrete evidence can be a powerful tool to alleviate anxiety and to give moral support. Feedback is important for increasing the person's confidence in the progress being made and thus hastening it.

A counselor might try self-disclosure—sharing one's own experiences with the client. This method is effective in stimulating a person in crisis to talk about the problem. The counselor must be careful that he or she does not add to the client's problem. The client is not there to resolve the counselor's crises. To determine the appropriateness of self-disclosure, the caregiver must decide whether the purpose of sharing the information is primarily client-centered or nurse-centered.

Group therapy or group process might be used by the nurse as an effective way to avert or resolve a client's crisis. The nurse working with maternity clients does not have to be a trained psychotherapist to use groups effectively. Groups often are an ideal format to provide anticipatory guidance for clients to learn about child care or to express their concerns. Sometimes a client more readily accepts a suggestion from another parent who has had a similar experience than from a caregiver. Parents who have a preterm or defective child frequently find the support and shared information from a group of parents in the same situation absolutely invaluable. Parents may continue to provide support for each other even after the formal group has ceased functioning.

Problem solving is important for the person experiencing crisis. The nurse can help the client to identify the problem and explore various solutions as well as the consequences of these solutions. The person in crisis is usually very open to suggestion and may imply that they want a caregiver to "just tell me what to do and I will." It may be tempting to give advice at this time rather than allow the client to problem solve, but except in extreme cases in which an individual is severely immobilized by a crisis, it is best to resist the temptation.

Being aware of sociocultural values of clients will make any intervention more effective. No one is able to perceive the meaning of a crisis to an individual unless one has some understanding of his or her world. Any positive coping mechanisms that can be added to the client's repertoire will help this individual handle future stressful situations more easily.

Evaluation

Evaluation is an ongoing process throughout planning and intervention. Various approaches are tried and then discarded or modified depending on their success. As the crisis is resolved, attention is turned to anticipatory planning. The adaptive coping mechanisms that the client has used successfully are reinforced. Discussion can include ways in which the present experience may help in coping with future problems.

THE ROLE OF THE MATERNITY NURSE DURING CRISIS

Nurses are in a unique position to assist the individual or family in crisis because of their helping role, varied skills, and close proximity to the clients. Society generally views nurses as people who can be trusted, are there to help, and are sensitive and professional about information disclosed to them. Nursing has traditionally stressed family-centered care and knowledge of developmental tasks and crises. Since a crisis affects the entire family, these skills are essential for effective counseling. The nurse has had experience caring for individuals at all stages of the life span. Even though a nurse may specialize in an area such as maternity nursing, the nurse is keenly aware of the interrelatedness of various developmental levels in individuals. The impact and resolution of a crisis at one stage (for example, child abuse or preterm birth) will influence other life stages.

According to Caplan (1961) nurses have a unique advantage in their role as crisis counselor because they are especially close to their clients in many ways.

Close in space. The nurse is physically close in the home, in the hospital, and at the bedside.

Close in time (contact time). The nurse is often present throughout a crisis, as during labor and delivery.

Psychologic closeness. The nurse becomes involved with the family members, forms trusting relationships, and gives emotional support.

Sociologic closeness. Communications between the nurse and family members can be open. Clients feel free to ask questions.

Nurses are in a position to make referrals, because they observe family interaction and interpersonal relationships and thus can recognize and identify crisis situations. The nurse can also motivate clients to seek help because of the unique, trusting relationship with their clients.

The nurse is in a good position to explain a client's situation to other team members or support personnel and to interpret their recommendations to the client. The nurse can serve as the primary coordinator of the crisis intervention program for the family. The nurse's teaching skills are useful for crisis resolution in maternity nursing.

Experience helps the counselor to become familiar with several other methods of intervention. For example, *modeling* might be helpful. Modeling is introducing the behavior of others as examples through role playing or by having the client talk with someone who has mastered a similar crisis. This is an especially effective strategy if the crisis concerns a mother feeling inadequate about her parenting skills. As the mother watches the nurse caring for the infant in a relaxed and comfortable way, she is encouraged to incorporate these behaviors into her way of functioning. The nurse can assess the kinds of behaviors that it would be helpful to model. Behavior modeling may be subtle, such as the tone of voice or way of sitting while holding the infant, or it may be more complex, such as a method of problem solving. On the other hand, the nurse must be very careful not to appear to be the "expert" in the area of care, which may make the mother feel more hopeless about her own abilities. The mother needs a good deal of reinforcement about her progress as she carries out specific behaviors.

The counselor can teach the client relaxation techniques as an effective means of dealing with anxiety. One that nurses have found to be helpful is an adaptation of the relaxation and breathing techniques used by women in labor.

Relaxation techniques are especially valuable for parents who respond to stress by increased tension, feelings of helplessness, withdrawal from caretaking responsibilities, or abusive behaviors. Relaxation techniques are based on the principle of *reciprocal inhibition*, meaning that it is impossible to feel relaxed and tense at the same time. With some direction from the nurse, clients can learn to do relaxation exercises on their own.

Clients should be instructed to sit or recline in a comfortable position in a quiet environment. They might close their eyes or look at a fixed object. The goal is to elicit relaxed muscle tone and attitude. Three easy-to-learn components are breathing techniques, muscle relaxation, and imagery, and all three can be combined. Instruct the client to pay attention to breathing, encouraging them to breathe in and out slowly. The nurse might say, "As you breathe in, feel the energy flow into your body. As you breathe out, feel the tension leave your body. Now breathe in, slowly. Breathe out, slowly." To teach clients muscle relaxation, one might instruct them "to be aware of the muscles in your forehead, feel the tension in it, now relax your forehead, and feel the tension draining away." The nurse continues the same process with shoulders, back, arms, and so on. Some individuals prefer to start with the feet and work up to the head. The client may return to concentrating on her breathing periodically throughout the exercise. Some clients find visualization a helpful way to relax. They may visualize the "warmth of the sun shining above them," or they might imagine a special place, such as the seashore: "As you walk along the beach, feel the sand flow between your toes. Experience the warm breeze blowing against your face. As the waves splash against the shore, they seem to whisper, you are relaxed." Others may feel soothed by imagining a mountain stream. The nurse and the client create each relaxation technique, which can last a few seconds or be lengthy. There is no magic formula, but rather each method should contain individualized components that seem to work for the client. Professionally prepared tapes can also be purchased from a number of distributors.

A major function of the nurse in the prevention of crisis is anticipatory guidance. Anticipatory guidance is valuable both for the expectant family and for families with infants. The nurse's role as health educator is good preparation for this intervention. Before birth the parents may need to discuss emotional and physical changes, myths about pregnancy, what to expect about the labor and delivery, infant bonding, family planning, economic concerns, infant caretaking, and methods of sibling preparation (Clausen, 1979). Families with infants are more concerned about parent–infant bonding, changing couple relationships, clothing, feeding, equipment, sleeping, crying, bathing, circumcision and cord care, infant stimulation, toys, safety, when to seek medical care, and other unexpected problems (McCabe, 1979).

Utilizing nursing skills, and those discussed under nursing interventions, maternity nurses will find that they are in a critical position to help identify, avert, and resolve the crises of individuals and families.

FAMILIES AT RISK

Many human experiences are predictable, such as progress through developmental stages and addition of family members. With precautionary measures, one can avoid some crises. Role changes occur when a person leaves school, attains employment, marries, becomes a parent, and eventually retires. When a person cannot or does not prepare for these events, crisis may result. For example, with adequate family planning a newly married couple need not start a family immediately but can determine the optimal time when they are economically and emotionally secure.

Unpredictable life events also occur within families, including death of a significant other, serious physical illness, natural disasters resulting in personal or financial loss, stillbirth, and birth of an infant with congenital anomalies. These, too, may result in crisis if normal coping mechanisms are not adequate.

When a diagnosis of high-risk pregnancy is made, a couple faces a unique set of problems. The uncertainty of the outcome leads them to view the pregnancy with anxiety and ambivalence rather than confidence. All members of the family may be vulnerable during this time and need additional support. Penticuff (1982) found that those couples who had emotional support at the time of the perinatal crisis and relied on realistic coping strategies eventually were able to see the events as a meaningful and significant part of their lives, even if the infant did not live.

Through the process of assessment, nurses and other health care professionals are responsible for identifying families at risk. Assessment should discover crisis states in families and identify whether a particular family or individual is in crisis.

After determination that the family is, in fact, in a crisis or precrisis state, the information obtained from careful assessment becomes the basis for the plan for crisis intervention. Hoff (1984) suggests that the following key questions be answered before formulating a plan for help:

- To what extent has the crisis disrupted the family's normal life pattern?
- Are there any family members not able to go to school or to hold a job?
- Can family members handle the responsibilities involved in the activities of daily living—for example, eating or personal hygiene?
- Has the crisis situation disrupted the lives of others?
- Is a family member suicidal, homicidal, or both?
- Does the family or a family member seem to be on the brink of despair?
- Has the high level of tension distorted one or more individual's perception of reality?
- Is the family's usual support system present, absent, or exhausted?
- What are the resources of the nurse or agency in relation to the family's assessed needs?*

Essential data are identified from the answers to these and related questions. These data are used for the intervention plan. Following are key features of an effective intervention plan (Hoff, 1984):

*Modified from, Hoff, L. A. 1984. *People in crisis: understanding and helping,* 2nd ed. Menlo Park, Calif.: Addison-Wesley Publishing Co.

- The plan is problem oriented, with a focus on the immediate concrete problem.
- The plan considers the family's functional level and dependency needs.
- The plan is appropriate to the family's culture and lifestyle.
- The plan is inclusive of all family members and their social milieu.
- The plan is practical, has a specified time frame, and is concrete.
- The plan is dynamic and renegotiable.
- The plan includes an arrangement for follow-up contact.

Active involvement of the family in the plan for crisis resolution is essential for the success of the intervention plan.

A specific prenatal assessment tool is helpful when working with couples who may need additional support to promote healthy parenting. When the tool is highly predictive of a crisis, such as neglect or abuse, interventions can begin before it occurs. Josten (1981) has published an assessment guide developed by the Minneapolis Health Department based on the developmental tasks of pregnancy, which identifies women who may need assistance with parenting skills. Table 30–1 contains the Prenatal Assessment of Parenting Guide.

Many of the crises affecting families postpartally require an intervention plan directed toward loss and grief. The family that suffers loss of an infant or that faces the task of caring for a deformed or seriously ill child is a family at risk for serious disruption.

LOSS AND GRIEF

Loss is a state of being deprived or being without something one has had. Some losses are natural and predictable, whereas others are unpredictable. Losses can be sudden or gradual, traumatic or nontraumatic.

The most serious loss is the loss of a loved one by death. Loss also can occur through divorce or separation. Serious illness can cause partial loss because of disability.

One can also lose an aspect of "self." "Self" is how we feel about ourselves, our ideas, our worth, and our capacities. Loss of health, loss of body parts, loss of pride, and loss of independence are all examples of loss of self.

Object loss refers to the loss of an object that has special value and emotional meaning to a person.

Losses are experienced throughout life. For example, there are numerous developmental losses. A mother feels a tremendous loss (of a part of herself) when giving birth and later feels a loss whenever her baby is separated from the breast. Such losses produce strong emotional responses. Other losses are hardly noticeable, but they still evoke responses. How a person responds or adapts to the resultant change contributes to the development of that person's personality.

Grief is an emotional state, a reaction to loss. Studies have shown that the grief reaction is similar whether the loss is of a loved one, a body part, or a body function (Schoenberg et al., 1970).

Grief has been studied by Freud, Deutsch, and many others in the past, but it was Lindemann's classic report, "Symptomatology and Management of Acute Grief" (1944), that brought the medical, psychologic, and sociologic implications of separation, grief, and bereavement to the attention of medical and social scientists. Lindemann observed that *acute grief* is a definite syndrome and described five features he considered to be characteristic of this syndrome:

1. Somatic distress characterized by sighing respiration, a complaint of lack of strength and of exhaustion, digestive symptoms, and lack of appetite.

2. An intense preoccupation with the image of the deceased and feelings of unreality.

3. Strong feelings of guilt, self-accusation, and feelings of negligence in relation to the deceased.

4. A disturbing loss of warmth in relationship to other people, feelings of irritability, and anger.

5. A disorganized pattern of conduct, such as restlessness.

Grief work is the inner process of working through or managing the bereavement (Schoenberg et al., 1974). The first stage of this process is disbelief, which is similar to the denial stage of dying (Kübler-Ross, 1969). It is common for people to say, "No, no . . . it can't be!" The second stage is a questioning one. The person who suffers the loss looks for reasons why the death occurred, asking "What happened?" and "How?" This search for reasons is an attempt to make the event believable. Questioning is usually followed by anger (stage 3). Anger is often manifested in questions such as "Why did this happen?" Anger at God may be expressed. The fourth stage is anger combined with desperation. The person seems resigned, dismayed, and in despair. This stage is the first indication of acceptance, which is necessary before the final stage can be reached—resolution.

The duration of grief is variable, and it can last up to 6 months or a year, but the acute stage should be over in 1 or 2 months. Brief upsurges of these feelings will occur in later months, especially when the bereaved person is faced with reminders of the loss. The best indicator of the resolution of grief is a gradual return to the preloss level of functioning. New interests and relationships are formed. Ac-

(Text continues on p. 1002.)

Table 30–1   Prenatal Assessment of Parenting Guide*

Areas assessed	Sample questions

I. Perception of complexities of mothering
  A. Baby is desired for itself.
  Positive:
    1. Feels positive about pregnancy.
  Negative:
    1. Wants baby to meet own needs such as someone to love her, someone to get her out of unhappy home.
	1. Did you plan on getting pregnant?
	2. How do you feel about being pregnant?
	3. Why do you want this baby?

B. Expresses concern about impact of mothering role on other roles (wife, career, school).
  Positive:
    1. Realistic expectations of how baby will affect job, career, school, and personal goals.
    2. Interested in learning about child care.
  Negative:
    1. Feels pregnancy and baby will make no emotional, physical, or social demands on self.
    2. No insight that mothering role will affect other roles or life-style.
  C. Gives up routine habits because "not good for baby"; e.g., quits smoking, adjusts time schedule, etc.†
  Positive:
    1. Gives up routines not good for baby—quits smoking, adjusts eating habits, etc.
	1. What do you think it will be like to take care of baby?
	2. How do you think your life will be different after you have your baby?
	3. How do you feel this baby will affect your job, career, school, and personal goals?
	4. How will the baby affect your relationship with boyfriend or husband?
	5. Have you done any reading, babysitting, or made any things for a baby?

II. Attachment
  A. Strong feelings regarding sex of baby.
    Why?
  Positive:
    1. Verbalizes positive thoughts about the baby.
  Negative:
    1. Baby will be like negative aspects of self and partner.
  B. Interested in data regarding fetus; e.g., growth and development, heart tones, etc.
  Positive:
    1. As above.
  Negative
    1. Shows no interest in fetal growth and development, quickening, and fetal heart tones.
    2. Negative feelings about fetus expressed by rejection of counseling regarding nutrition, rest, hygiene.
	1. Why do you prefer a certain sex? (Is reason inappropriate for a baby?)
	2. Note comments client makes about baby not being normal and why client feels this way.

C. Fantasies about baby.
  Positive:
    1. Follows cultural norms regarding preparation.
    2. Time of attachment behaviors appropriate to her history of pregnancy loss.
  Negative:
    1. Bonding is conditional depending on sex, age of baby, and/or labor and delivery experience.
    2. Patient only considers own needs when making plans for baby.
    3. Exhibits no attachment behaviors after critical period of previous pregnancy.
	1. What did you think or feel when you first felt baby move?
	2. Have you started preparing for the baby?
	3. What do you think your baby will look like—what age do you see your baby at?
	4. How would you like your new baby to look?

Table 30-1 Prenatal Assessment of Parenting Guide Cont'd

Areas assessed	Sample questions
4. Failure to follow cultural norms regarding preparation.	

III. Acceptance of child by significant others.
  A. Acknowledges acceptance by significant other of the new responsibility inherent in child.
  Positive:
    1. Acknowledges unconditional acceptance of pregnancy and baby by significant others.
    2. Partner accepts new responsibility inherent with child.
    3. Timely showing of experience of pregnancy with significant others.
  Negative:
    1. Significant others not supportively involved with pregnancy.
    2. Conditional acceptance of pregnancy depending on sex, race, age of baby.
    3. Decision making does not take in needs of fetus; e.g., spends food money on new Honda.
    4. Take no/little responsibility for needs of pregnancy, woman/fetus.
	1. How does your partner feel about pregnancy?
	2. How do your parents feel?
	3. What do your friends think?
	4. Does your partner have preference regarding sex of baby and why?
	5. How does partner feel about being a father?
	6. What do you think he'll be like as a father?
	7. What do you think he'll do to help you with child care?
	8. Have you and partner talked about how the baby might change your lives?
	9. Who have you told about pregnancy?

B. Concrete demonstration of acceptance of pregnancy/baby by significant others; e.g., baby shower, significant other involved in prenatal education.†
  Positive:
    1. Baby shower.
    2. Significant other attends prenatal class with client.
	1. Note if partner attends clinic with client (degree of interest); e.g., listens to heart tones, etc. Significant other plans to be with client in labor and delivery.
	2. Is partner contributing financially?

IV. Ensures physical well-being.
  A. Concerns about having normal pregnancy, labor and delivery, and baby.
  Positive:
    1. Client preparing for labor and delivery, attends prenatal classes, interested in labor and delivery.
    2. Client aware of danger signs of pregnancy.
    3. Seeks and utilizes appropriate health care: e.g., time of initial visit, keeps appointments, follows through on recommendations.
  Negative:
    1. Denial of signs and symptoms that might suggest complications of pregnancy.
    2. Verbalizes extreme fear of labor and delivery — refuses to talk about labor and delivery.
    3. Fails appointments, failure to follow instructions, refuses to attend prenatal classes.
  B. Family/client decisions reflect concern for health of mother and baby; e.g., use of finances, time.†
  Positive:
    1. As above.
	1. What have you heard about labor and delivery?
	2. Note data about client's reaction to prenatal class.

*Used with permission by the Minneapolis Health Dept., Minneapolis, MN
†When "Negative" is not listed in a section, the reader may assume that negative is the absence of positive responses.

cording to Engel (1964), the clearest indication that grieving has successfully been completed is the ability to realistically and completely remember both the pleasures and disappointments of the lost relationship.

Grief work can be helped or hindered by a person's emotional status and by the ability of family members or significant others to allow the person to express grief. If the person does not successfully complete the grief work, he or she may have prolonged or distorted grief reactions.

For example, delayed grief may occur if affected persons are maintaining the morale of others and therefore are repressing their own reactions. Or they may be attempting to respond to Western culture's expectation of controlled behavior.

Chronic grief is a response that represents a denial of the reality of the loss. There can be no resolution if there is no acceptance. One manifestation of chronic grief is retaining the lost loved one's belongings as they were during his or her lifetime.

Anticipatory grief reactions are seen when there is a threat of death or separation (Lindemann, 1944). Because the dynamics of anticipatory grief have much in common with those of acute grief, one might expect that working through anticipatory grief would diminish the acute grief when the loss finally does occur. This may be the case with some, but many people cannot work through feelings of denial. These feelings are supported by the hope that accompanies anticipatory grief. Kübler-Ross (1969) has noticed this with the dying patient. However, hope must be gone before acceptance of death can be complete. (This is especially true with parents of very ill children.)

There are often ambivalent feelings about the dying loved one that relatives find difficult to accept or to recognize. The difference in the impact of ambivalence on the anticipatory grief of family members is that the target of the ambivalent feelings is not only still alive but also particularly vulnerable (Schoenberg et al., 1974). The ambivalence may be interpreted as a death wish—which is too unacceptable to admit—and so these feelings are repressed.

The stable family, with healthy coping mechanisms and strong support both from within the family structure and from friends and other ties, can weather the crises of life. However, the high-risk family may need the help and support that crisis intervention can give.

The maternity nurse may be involved with clients who are grieving for a loss; for example, intense grief usually attends the death of a newborn. Parents grieve following the birth of a defective infant and mourn the loss of the normal infant they dreamed would be theirs. Even parents who had a strong preference for the sex of their unborn child may experience a brief period of sorrow after the birth of the "wrong sex" infant. In each of these cases couples may manifest stages of denial or disbelief, anger, resignation, and acceptance. Occasionally, a nurse who

has been caring for clients who have experienced profound losses may become frustrated with parents who mourn a minor defect or the gender of a child. The nurse may feel that the parents "should be happy that they had a healthy baby," not realizing that it may be necessary for them to mourn the idealized infant before they can begin to form a strong attachment with their actual infant. Acceptance and support by the nurse facilitates attachment between the parents and child.

CRISIS INTERVENTION DURING POSTPARTAL PERIOD

The postpartal period is a time of disequilibrium and of emotional changes. It is also a period of increased susceptibility to situational crises because of changes in roles of family members and because of the many economic and social pressures that are encountered (Caplan, 1961). Although the stable family can usually cope and even grow in strength, family members need help to handle certain highly stressful events that can occur during the maternity cycle. These include fetal death and birth of a low-birth-weight infant or of a defective child.

Loss of Newborn

The loss of a newborn evokes intense mourning reactions whether the baby lives 1 hour, lives several days, or is stillborn; whether the baby is a nonviable 500 g fetus or a 4000 g healthy infant; and whether the baby is planned or not.

Until recently, it was not realized that both parents show the same grief reactions (Klaus and Fanaroff, 1973). The father may have more difficulty expressing his grief because, while supporting and comforting the mother, he may be suppressing his own feelings and thus delaying his grief work. He may have not worked through ambivalent feelings of guilt. Thus, denial mechanisms may be persistent, with the anger being directed outward—perhaps at the woman. Disturbance in communication between the father and mother could lead to serious disturbances within the family, as one study shows (Cullberg, 1972). If the father is not included in the grief work and if his needs are not recognized, he may feel alienated from his partner at a time when she needs him the most. This alienation increases his feelings of helplessness, and he may withdraw.

The following self-reported case study of Mary, a woman who lost her newborn and then later had two healthy children, relates some of the feelings associated with the loss of an infant.

One day I was working, feeling happy and healthy and the next day I found myself in the hospital, having given birth to our baby almost 3 months early. There were no warning signs. On all my prenatal visits the doctor assured me "everything was fine." I started bleeding in the morning and when it didn't stop, the doctor advised that I be admitted to the hospital. I was terrified because I knew if I went into labor now, the baby might not live. As I lay there on the bed, with blood infusing in one arm and an intravenous line in the other, thoughts were racing through my head. Primarily I thought about whether the baby was going to live or die through all this. Certain things in my environment seemed to fade into oblivion and other things became very intense. One of the nurses caring for me had a terrible cold, and I kept thinking "I wish she would leave the room" because I was sure that on top of everything else I would catch that cold. I was feeling very vulnerable.

The bleeding continued, and contractions started. After it became obvious that the baby would be born, my concerns changed. I began to worry about whether the baby would be alright if it lived. I thought that if the baby was going to be retarded or deformed, I wanted it to die instead. I remember feeling very guilty about these thoughts, especially after Beth did not live. I wondered if we could afford long hospitalizations and care if it would be needed. During the entire time, my husband was supportive and comforting, although seemingly overwhelmed by everything.

When I was taken into the delivery room, it was as if I were progressing through a normal delivery. After Beth was born, they let me look at her and touch her very briefly before rushing her off for special care. I remember saying "She's so beautiful." That moment was the highlight of the entire experience for me. I recapture the sight frequently. The next day the doctor told me that the baby's weight was a positive factor (slightly over 3 lb), but that her lungs were not well developed. It was too early for him to talk about her prognosis. When I asked if I could go in to see her, he said he preferred that I did not. How I wish I would have had the assertiveness to take the matter into my own hands and insist, but I had no self-direction and seemed to be waiting for others to tell me what to do next. This feeling was in sharp contrast to my normal way of functioning.

In the morning the woman who takes the baby pictures came in to get permission from mothers to photograph babies. I was very excited about the prospect, but when she learned the baby wasn't in the regular nursery, she said it probably wouldn't be possible to photograph her. I was so disappointed. The mother in the bed next to me was receiving her baby for feedings, and I felt so alone and so empty during those times. We named our baby and started hoping and believing that she was going to be alright. The ambivalence was overwhelming— wanting to hold and love her, but knowing that if we became too attached, the hurt would be greater if we lost her.

I felt very angry that everyone else seemed to be having healthy babies. I was an intelligent, competent woman. Why was I so inadequate at this? When friends and relatives called I tried to tell them what a beautiful baby we had but that she was born early. My husband visited her, and I pried every bit of information out of him that I could about her progress.

Later that day, the doctor came in and told me that Beth had died. My husband came and we cried and cried. Other than having him there, nothing seemed to comfort. One of the staff came in and asked what we wanted to do with her body. That came as a shock. Somehow I never thought of having to make a decision like that. We decided to bury her near my grandparents. It was critically important to me that she had been baptized, and the nurses assured me that she had been baptized shortly after delivery.

My husband took me home from the hospital empty-armed. My feelings were very confusing. I felt guilty—thinking that perhaps if I had stopped working earlier or had called the doctor earlier things would have been different. I was angry. I was sad. I wondered if we would ever have other children. A neighbor had hand-crocheted some beautiful white baby clothes before I went to the hospital, and she told me to keep them—that was very meaningful and I got them out and looked at them many times. When I got back to work, people who knew I was pregnant but hadn't heard the outcome asked about the baby. I had to tell them.

NURSING INTERVENTION

A major goal of the nurse should be to facilitate and to encourage communication between parents who have experienced the loss of a newborn (see the accompanying Nursing Care Plan on stillbirth). If the parents are not present at the time of the infant's death, they usually are notified by the physician. Privacy should be provided for them at the hospital. The parents may want to be alone or may prefer to have the nurse stay with them for a while. The

NURSING CARE PLAN
Stillbirth

CLIENT DATA BASE

History

1. Prenatal history
   a. Uneventful? High risk?
   b. Fetal death before labor? During labor? Totally unexpected?
2. Family history
   a. Interactions, communications — are they mutually supportive? Blaming?
   b. Grief response — are normal reactions manifested?

NURSING PRIORITIES

1. Facilitate the normal grief process.

CLIENT/FAMILY EDUCATIONAL FOCUS

1. Explain the grief process and its psychologic impact
2. Provide names of local support groups the couple might find helpful when they are ready
3. Provide close family and friends with information about ways in which they can help the grieving couple cope with their loss

Problem	Nursing interventions and actions	Rationale
Communications between couple	Encourage them to express feelings, to cry Provide support	Disturbance in communication can delay resolution of grief and cause possible long-range disturbances within family
Father's needs	Include father in intervention	Both parents have same grief responses; each needs support of the other
Acceptance of reality of the situation	Listen; correct any misconceptions, answer questions	Misconceptions reinforce guilt feelings and lower self-esteem
	Make it possible for couple to see infant; explain the reasons for the infant's death, if known; prepare them fully for the experience	Acceptance is facilitated and resolution will follow more smoothly

NURSING CARE EVALUATION

There is evidence that normal grief work is in process

Disbelief phase has been worked through, followed by questioning and anger; feelings have been expressed freely, and acceptance has begun

Because crisis lasts 4–6 weeks, resolution will not be evident in the hospital; further support may be needed to help parents cope, because acute grief can be recurrent; referral can be made to community mental health agency, to appropriate parent groups, or to visiting community health nurse

A month or 6 weeks after the stillbirth, parents are regaining their equilibrium, to precrisis level; their coping skills have been strengthened, and family relationships are even closer than before

Without resolution, guilt feelings and lack of communication between parents may not only lead to abnormal grief reactions (delayed or chronic grief) but may lead to disorganization of family unit

NURSING DIAGNOSIS*

1. Potential dysfunctional grieving associated with the death of the newborn

SUPPORTING DATA

Evidence of lack of communication between parents
Inadequate support systems
Signs of overwhelming feelings of guilt or shame

* This is an example of a nursing diagnosis that might be appropriate for a couple experiencing this loss. It is not necessarily inclusive and must be individualized for each person experiencing this crisis.

nurse should encourage them not to hold back their feelings—to cry if they feel like it. Unless they are told what reactions to expect, their feelings may worry them and further interfere with their relationship.

Once denial is overcome and the questioning phase starts, the nurse can clarify the reality of situations in which mothers blame themselves for the death. It is usual for the woman to review the pregnancy over and over. The nurse should allow her to express her feelings of anger, which may be directed toward the physician, the staff, or God. The mother's feelings may be turned inward. The nurse should watch for feelings of shame and guilt, which are destructive to the mother's self-esteem and can delay her grief work. The nurse must be as positive as possible but should avoid such meaningless phrases as "Don't worry" or "Everything will be fine." Especially important is avoiding comments on future pregnancies ("You are young, you can have other babies"). Such remarks negate this baby. Good crisis intervention concentrates on the immediate problem.

A diagnosis of intrauterine death before or during labor is extremely stressful for parents and staff. Shock and disbelief plus the physical discomfort of labor produce overwhelming stresses. Denial is maintained by most women up to the moment of delivery, often combined with anger, bargaining, and depression, as described by Kübler-Ross (1969). Allowing the woman to express her feelings facilitates her working through her acute grief in a healthy manner when the death is confirmed at delivery.

The woman should not be left alone in labor. For optimal emotional support, continuity of care (one caregiver) should extend through the labor and delivery and into the immediate postpartal period.

Infant death may occur after the discharge of the mother from the hospital or after both mother and infant have been at home for some time and the attachment process with the family has been progressing. Parents may be expecting the death, as in the case of a terminal illness or serious defect that are incompatible with continued growth and development. In other cases the death may be completely unexpected, as in sudden infant death syndrome. In either situation, the loss is an overwhelming experience for the family. Nursing interventions can help the family to resolve feelings of grief, anger, confusion, guilt, and depression. Williams and colleagues (1981) have identified several "at-risk" situations that make a family more vulnerable when a child is dying. They include (a) single parents; (b) families who have recently moved to town; (c) families with another ill family member; (d) families who lack child care arrangements for children at home; (e) cases in which the ill infant is a twin; and (f) families who have experienced several deaths in the recent past.

Siblings of the dying infant need special consideration from the family and the nurse. During bereavement, parents may become so consumed by their own reactions that the children perceive the withdrawal as abandonment. Loneliness engulfs the siblings just when their needs for love and reassurance are very strong. Wong (1980) reports the shock one mother who was grieving the loss of a newborn felt when her son drew a picture of the family that did not include her. He attempted to draw her several times but erased her each time. The mother had been physically absent as well as emotionally detached from the home. Children may respond to death of a brother or sister with guilt reactions, especially young children who use magical thinking (Williams, Rivara, and Rothenberg, 1981). In some way they may feel that they are responsible for the death and need reassurance that this is not true. Young children may also view the cause of death as communicable and may develop symptoms similar to those of the deceased child. An in-depth knowledge of child development helps the nurse to plan appropriate interventions with siblings.

Being certain that a dying infant is baptized is of extreme importance to some parents. All nurses who work in the delivery room or the nursery should be aware of how to perform a baptism, in the event that the hospital chaplain is not available. If spiritual support is requested by parents, the nurse should be prepared to contact a rabbi, priest, or appropriate minister for each family.

Open, honest discussion with the parents about their dying infant is important for them. Occasionally parents who have an infant with a congenital deformity that makes death inevitable refuse to visit the nursery. It is more likely, however, that the parents will remain interested in the newborn's progress and telephone when they are unable to visit. They may be in the process of simultaneous attachment and termination of bonds. Wooten (1981) reports that it is important for parents to touch their infant and to take pictures even if he or she is surrounded by technical equipment. Parents frequently want to cradle the baby in their arms at the time of death.

Research indicates that most mothers want to see and touch their dead babies (Seitz and Warrick, 1974; Kowalski and Osborn, 1977). This is especially important when the attachment process has been incomplete (Williams, Rivara, and Rothenberg, 1981). Kowalski and Osborn (1977) suggest that even mothers of gestationally nonviable infants be given the opportunity to see and touch their dead infant to facilitate attachment and termination. It is felt that this practice facilitates grief work, because acceptance and then resolution follow more smoothly.

The nurse who has been caring for the mother and has established a trusting and therapeutic relationship with the parents is able to sense feelings and concerns that parents may have about seeing the baby. If parents wish to see the child and are denied their wish, they may imagine something far worse than the reality. If parents do not want to see their child, the nurse should support their decision. If the parents are prepared by descriptions of what they will see and by explanations of what happened when there is evidence of trauma to the fetus, the experience is less stressful. All normal and positive aspects of the infant may be pointed out. Mothers who have seen their dead babies (even those who are macerated or deformed) have stated that the reality was not so bad as they had imagined. For the mother unable to face the task, some benefit may be realized from answering her questions concerning the delivery and the child.

After the death of an infant, the family may need assistance with funeral arrangements, body or organ donation, autopsy requests, or legal problems. Many of these decisions are difficult for the family who is already experiencing a great deal of stress. Social service departments and legal services may provide information. The parents should be reassured that they are in control in making these decisions but that support is available.

If continuing assistance is needed, a couple can be informed of community agencies that offer support. Some communities have mutual support groups for couples who have lost children. Groups of this type may be especially helpful for parents who have lost an infant to SIDS. Unresolved feelings may be explored with other couples experiencing the same problems. Reaching out to help others or becoming involved in raising funds for research or treatment of a specific disorder sometimes channels energies into productive tasks and speeds the grieving process.

It is necessary for professionals to clarify their own feelings about death before they are able to work effectively with others. Nurses may be shocked at their own feelings of anger and despair and therefore find it extremely difficult to work effectively with grieving parents. Nurses who recognize that they, too, are going through the grief process must not suppress these feelings, so that they can move through the phases quickly. Nurses who suppress or deny their reactions tend to remove themselves from the situation, to increase their physical and psychologic distance from clients, and thus reduce their effectiveness. Each nurse must assess personal reactions: How am I expressing my anger? Am I venting anger on my peers or my family? With my client, am I being nonjudgmental, helpful, and approachable?

Structured groups of peers may help resolve the professional's conflicts regarding death. In areas such as intensive care nurseries where death may be a more frequent occurrence, such support groups may be especially important.

Preterm Birth

The delivery of a preterm infant is an acute crisis situation for a family. Acute grief reactions follow the loss of the perfect full-term baby they have fantasized. Also, the preterm birth has interrupted the attachment process, deny-

ing the mother the last few weeks of pregnancy that seem to prepare her psychologically for the stress of birth. Attachment at this time is fragile, and interruption of the process by separation can affect the future mother–child relationship. Many studies on the crisis of prematurity focus on this aspect. A healthy mother–infant relationship depends upon a successful resolution of the crisis.

Kaplan and Mason (1960) have identified four psychologic tasks that must be mastered for successful resolution. The first task, at time of delivery, prepares the mother for possible loss of the child. It is anticipatory grief, involving a withdrawal from the attachment process. She can still hope for the child's survival but is prepared for its death. The second task is to face the reality of the loss. The anticipatory grief and depression the mother exhibits are normal responses and show that she is mastering these tasks. When the infant's survival is certain, the third task is undertaken—the resumption of the attachment process. Her outlook is then one of hope and anticipation. The fourth task is understanding and learning the special needs of the preterm infant in preparation for assuming responsibilities of care.

Table 30–2 illustrates the maternal emotional and situational differences between term and preterm births. The factors listed may be commonly found in mothers but are by no means universal. These factors may be influenced or altered by the woman's past experiences, her personality, the specifics of her situation, and the amount of education and support she may receive concerning her situation. The following case study contains many of the factors identified in the table.*

> Eric was born 8 weeks preterm to Mrs. V. He weighed approximately 1790 g at birth and subsequently reduced to 1680 g. He remained in the neonatal intensive care unit for over 5 weeks, had abdominal surgery for pyloric stenosis, and nearly died from surgical complications.
>
> This was Mrs. V's third pregnancy. Her first son was stillborn. Her second son was born after a high-risk pregnancy, a fetus-threatening virus, and 2 months of strict maternal bed rest.
>
> Mrs. V's labor and delivery occurred before she was psychologically ready and her child physically ready for birth. Because she perceived a malfunctioning of her reproductive system, her self-esteem was lowered. She was very anxious and showed limited confidence in her ability to give birth with a good outcome. At a time that should have been filled with happiness and joy because personal expectations were being met, Mrs. V perceived yet another repro-

*Modified from material prepared by Lauri Lowen, Chairman of Parents of Prematures, Seattle, Washington.

Table 30-2 Comparison of Maternal Emotional and Situational Factors in Term and Preterm Births*

Factors	Term birth	Preterm birth
Emotional factors at time of birth	More likely to be regarded as rewarding experience	May be regarded as less than rewarding experience; frustration and a sense of missing something
	More likely to have good self-image regarding body functioning	May have poor self-image regarding imperfectly functioning body
	Pleasurable experience	Anxiety-producing experience
	Confident in ability to give birth with good outcome	Not confident in ability to give birth with good outcome
	Little fear of danger to infant	Great fear of danger to infant
	Great sense of achievement; pride in success	Little sense of achievement; no pride in failure; guilt
	Emotionally prepared for outcome as planned and expected	Shocked; emotionally unprepared for outcome, which is different from plans and expectations
	Previous pregnancy and birth experience likely to have been considered favorable	Previous pregnancy and birth experience probably considered unfavorable if previous reproductive failure occurred
	Happiness and joy	Unhappiness and grief
	Meets expectations	Disappointment; does not meet expectations
Situational factors at time of birth	Able to choose option of active role in birth	Possibly forced to play passive role by circumstances
	More in control of situation; more opportunity for voluntary decisions	Less in control of situation; decisions often made for her
	More opportunity to be independent	Dependent
	Nonemergency atmosphere	Emergency and crisis atmosphere
Postpartal emotional factors	Pleased at appearance of newborn	Shocked at appearance of newborn
	Identifies with other mothers in her chosen role	Does not identify with other mothers; did not choose this strange role; does not know exactly what her role is
	Loss of fantasized child; replaced by different but probaby equally acceptable child	Loss of fantasized child; replaced by less acceptable sick or imperfect child
	Usually under less than severe stress	Under severe stress
	Happy with successful completion of pregnancy	Regrets unsuccessful completion of pregnancy; feels "empty"
	Less anxious about newborn's health than mother of preterm infant	Very anxious about infant's health
	Sees newborn as better than average; feels proud	Sees infant as better than average preterm baby but not as good as average term baby; may feel envious
	Confident in ability to care for child	Not confident in ability to care for child
	Naturally inclined and eager to increase attachment to child	Naturally inclined to increase attachment to child, but may be hindered by question of infant's survival
	Attachment process free of many obstacles	Attachment process more difficult, with more obstacles

Table 30–2   Comparison of Maternal Emotional and Situational Factors in Term and Preterm Births* Cont'd

Factors	Term birth	Preterm birth
Postpartal situational factors	Realistic expectations	May have unrealistic expectations; less able to anticipate outcome
	Infant seems to be parents' possession	Newborn seems to be hospital's possession
	Infant is responsive to mother	Newborn is less responsive to mother
	Major caregiver; role as major caregiver begins early; caregiving requires moderate energy and effort	Not major caregiver; role as major caregiver begins late; caregiving requires more energy and effort
	Recognition by others of identity as mother	Less recognition by others of identity as mother
	Gives pregnancy up in exchange for possessing infant	Gives pregnancy up but cannot possess newborn
	Many opportunities for contact with infant	Fewer opportunities for contact with infant
	Information about parents' situation readily available	Information about parents' situation not readily available
	Family unit can be together	Family unit may be divided due to hospitalization of infant

*Copyright © 1980, Lauri Lowen, Chairman of Parents of Prematures, Seattle, Washington.

ductive failure and exhibited unhappiness, grief, and disappointment about not meeting her expectations.

During the delivery, Mrs. V was allowed to be only a passive participant. She told the health care team to do whatever was necessary to save her baby. An air of emergency filled the delivery room as additional staff hurried to assist with and to make decisions about the birth process. Immediately after delivery, her infant was rushed to the neonatal intensive care unit. Mrs. V was not given an opportunity to see or to hold him.

Postpartal stress is extremely great for Mrs. V because she is anxious about her ill infant's health. He appears small and unattractive when she compares him to full-term babies. She expresses concern about her ability to care for her son. She fears emotional attachment to her infant, because of his uncertain health. The memories of her previous stillbirth surface, which increases the stress. Mrs. V watches the nurses and physicians as they touch, feed, diaper, and care for her son. She feels that it should be she who takes care of her infant but that instead her son "belongs" to the hospital staff.

Mrs. V leaves the hospital carrying not her infant but flowers. Her role as a new mother is not recognized by others because she does not have a baby in her arms. Although she has few opportunities to have contact with the baby, she participates by bringing her breast milk for Eric and by breast-feeding him when his condition allows. She expends much time and energy traveling to the hospital and telephoning to ask about Eric's condition.

When Eric is discharged from the hospital, Eric's responsiveness to Mrs. V increases as he matures. Mrs. V begins to receive more recognition as a new mother.

Nursing intervention in Mrs. V's case requires identification of the immediate crisis situation, appropriate action directed toward each problem contributing to the crisis, and evaluation of the effectiveness of the intervention.

NURSING INTERVENTION

Nursing intervention should be family-centered, focusing on helping the parents cope with the crisis. The nurse should assess their relationship. Are they able to share their feelings? The nurse should share their concerns and encourage them to express their feelings. What is their perception of the sequence of events? The nurse should clarify and correct any misconceptions, explaining as soon as possible the status and condition of the infant and arranging for them to see and to touch their newborn. Few parents take the initiative, because persons in crisis feel helpless. Without aid and encouragement, many hours might pass, further delaying optimal resolution of the crisis.

The nurse should accompany the parents to the intensive care nursery, preparing them ahead of time as much as possible for what they will see. Not only should the newborn's appearance and condition be described but also the equipment and procedures. The nurse should encourage questions and anticipate as many as possible. Experience makes one aware of which aspects of care alarm the parents the most. The couple should be made to feel welcome so that they feel free to return whenever they wish. As soon as feasible (and depending on the infant's condition), the parents should be included in the child's care (Figure 30–2). Being a part of the team increases the mother's self-esteem. She feels less futile if she can do something useful and positive. It is especially important to include the parents in planning for the baby's care at home.

The evaluation of this intervention should be ongoing. For example, the nurse should be careful not to give the mother a caretaking task too difficult for her. Failure reinforces her feelings of inadequacy. Further evaluation after the infant has gone home is useful in determining whether the crisis has been resolved satisfactorily. The parents are usually given the intensive care nurse's telephone number to call for support and advice. It is suggested that the staff follow up each family with visits or telephone calls at intervals for several weeks to assess and evaluate the infant's (and parents') progress.

Caplan et al. (1965) identified indicators for healthy and unhealthy outcomes in parent–child relationships and in parenting skills. The best indicator, they found, was the frequency of the parents' visits to the child in the nursery. Why are some parents hesitant to visit their baby? One reason might be the staff's pessimism about the infant's chance of survival (Klaus and Fanaroff, 1973). While the bonds of affection are still forming, they can be damaged by such pessimism. If the mother abandons hope, anticipatory grief becomes acute grief and can move rapidly toward resolution, which in reality is detachment. If the infant lives, attachment will be a difficult task.

Another parental behavior signaling future problems is the inability to accept help that has been offered (DuBois, 1975). Some parents are unwilling or unable to share their fears with each other and with other family members and friends. They need these support systems and should be encouraged to express their feelings.

It is healthy for the future parent–child relationship if the new parent seeks information about the infant's condition, prognosis, and treatment. The emotionally healthy mother is aware of ambivalent and negative feelings and is willing to express them. It is unhealthy for the future rela-

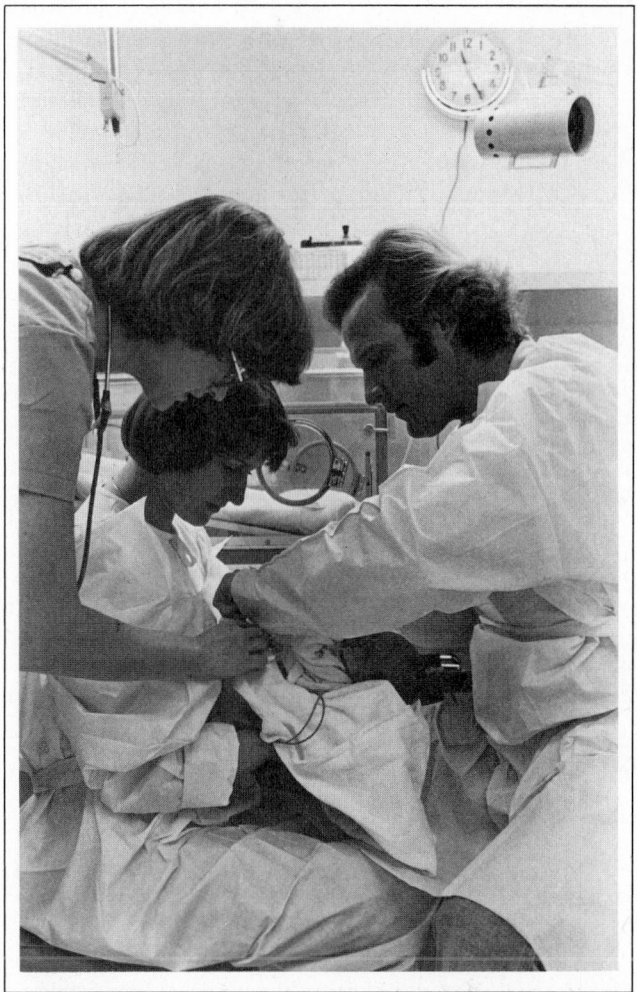

FIGURE 30–2 The parents of this preterm infant are learning how to take care of their child.

tionship if the parents do not seek information, cannot express feelings, and show no anxiety.

It is important to identify possible poor-outcome parents and to help them avoid negative patterns of behavior through prompt, active intervention. Intervention is a possibility, because persons in crisis usually have an increased desire to be helped and are more susceptible to influence (Caplan et al., 1965). Identification and assistance for these couples could reduce the incidence of parenting disorders. Consequences of parenting disorders range from minor abnormalities, such as persistent overconcern, to the most severe—the battered child syndrome. Klaus and Kennell (1970) believe that the whole range of problems may be due in part to maternal-infant separation during the early newborn period. Statistics show that 21%–41% of battered children were preterm. Green and Solnit (1964), in their report on the vulnerable child syndrome (children who are expected by their parents to die prematurely and who develop severe emotional disturbances), observed that 44% of these infants were separated from their parents in the first weeks of life because of prematurity or severe illness.

Many interesting psychologic aspects of prematurity are undergoing research. For example, a recent study suggests that stress may be a factor in the cause of prematurity (Schwartz and Schwartz, 1977). Mothers of preterm infants were compared with mothers of full-term infants. Results showed that mothers of preterm infants showed significantly higher numbers of life changes preceding and during pregnancy.

Obviously, prematurity is a psychologic as well as a medical problem. High-risk women can be identified, and early crisis intervention may be useful in reducing the levels of stress and perhaps the incidence of prematurity.

Defective Newborn

The crisis created by the birth of a defective infant is devastating. Not only is the expected normal child lost, but both parents feel a severe loss of self-esteem and self-confidence. The grief reactions become prolonged and recurrent because as long as the child lives there can be no resolution of grief. Guilt and ambivalent feelings are overwhelming. As time elapses, the unresolved grief becomes less intense. The term chronic sorrow has been used to describe the long-term effect (Young, 1977). Although there is no resolution, acceptance of the reality of the disability can be reached with either maladaptive or adaptive outcomes.

With *maladaptive responses*, acceptance can be precarious. Persistent denial can make it almost impossible to care for the infant. Or overwhelmed by guilt, the mother may spend all her time with the affected child, ignoring her other children. Social life is often restricted because of the time involved in care. Marriages or relationships, under a tremendous strain, often break down.

Olshansky (1962) has described a grief reaction in parents of defective or mentally retarded children that he terms "chronic sorrow." The parents begin this process with the birth of the child and the grieving or sorrow continues throughout the life span as they face subsequent developmental milestones that their child is unable to meet. For the first few months their child may not be very different from other children, but as their child reaches the age when the "normal child" would be walking and talking, toilet-training, going to school, or learning to drive a car, their sorrow is reinforced. The process continues until they are elderly and concerned with what will happen to their child when they die.

The goal of nursing intervention (and crisis intervention) is to enhance adaptation. With the *adaptive response*, the parents accept the reality and learn to cope with the crisis. They attempt to face the consequences of the child's defect, and they take part in his or her care. Support systems (family and friends) are mobilized. There are

many ups and downs, with parents alternating between maladaptive and adaptive responses.

Powell (1981) suggests several positive strategies that increase the effectiveness of nursing interactions with parents of children with developmental problems.

- Problem solve with the family rather than giving advice
- View the child as a total individual, rather than emphasizing only the handicap
- Observe the uniqueness of the child rather than stereotyping or labeling with phrases such as "slow," or "unmanageable."
- Avoid labeling parents as "inadequate," "rejecting," or "angry."
- Avoid a pathologic framework, stressing instead the child's similarities to other children
- Stress strengths and competencies of parents
- Help parents realize that they are in charge of their children and themselves
- Be aware of the needs of all members of the family, including siblings

Emotional support, acceptance of often intense reactions, and explanations as indicated help families toward acceptance of the child and the defect. As with the preterm infant, the rationale for early contact with the newborn is the establishment of a positive parent–child relationship. The nurse should help the couple assess their strengths and coping skills. Their perception of the problem is often distorted by strong guilt feelings. Correcting these perceptions helps relieve some of the self-blame and helps them move toward acceptance.

The needs of siblings should not be overlooked. They have been looking forward to the new baby, and so they, too, suffer a degree of loss. The siblings have grief work to do, and they are frightened and confused by their ambivalent feelings. Younger children may react with hostility and older ones with shame. Both reactions make them feel guilty. Parents, preoccupied with working through their own feelings, cannot give the other children the attention and support they need. Sometimes another child becomes the focus of family tension. Anxiety thus directed can take the form of finding fault or of overconcern. It is a form of denial; the parents cannot face the real worry—the congenital anomaly of the new child. The observant nurse could, after assessing the situation, see that another family member or friend steps in and gives the needed support to the siblings of the afflicted baby.

CRISIS INTERVENTION DURING POSTPARTAL FOLLOW-UP CARE

During the postpartal follow-up contact the nurse should be attuned to any clues indicating a family in crisis. In this section, attachment problems, child abuse, unwanted pregnancy and relinquishment, adolescent parenting, and single-parent families are discussed.

Child abuse is a tragedy, and when it is discovered, action should be taken immediately to ensure the safety of the children and to resolve the emotional problem of the parents. Single-parenthood is a situation that carries the risk of potential crisis. Economic and social factors may place intense stress on the single parent, and the problems of the parent ultimately affect his or her children. By the same token, the mother giving up her newborn for adoption may need support while grieving her loss.

Nurses often deal with families suffering from other kinds of crises (for example, alcoholism, drug dependency, poverty, and other serious problems that can contribute to the malfunctioning of a family). An in-depth discussion of all these problems is beyond the scope of this text. However, the nurse who is familiar with the basic steps of crisis intervention can identify a problem, initiate support, assess the client's coping mechanism, and make necessary referrals.

Referral to agencies for financial assistance or referral to parent groups increases the range and depth of support for the family. Again, knowledge of community resources is important. If genetic counseling is indicated, the nurse should prepare the family with thorough explanations and support to reduce possible stress and should make sure they understand the counseling.

A multidisciplinary approach is needed to adequately care for the affected child and family, including perhaps a social worker, a family counselor, medical specialists, and various agencies. This approach can be overwhelming for the family; if continuity of care is not maintained, they may feel fragmented and confused. The nurse can often interpret the many facets of care.

Parents have expressed deep appreciation of the nurse who cares, listens, and shares their feelings and concerns (Figure 30–3). As one mother of an infant born with an encephalocele said, "Someone came to my bed and identified herself as a nurse from pediatrics. She asked me if I would like to *hold* my baby. I couldn't believe it! Someone finally cared about the here and now for me and my child. This nurse seemed to realize my strong need to hold the child I had carried nine months" (Donnelly, 1974).

Many families do adapt, accept the infant as he or she is, and find fulfillment in caring for the child. For these families, even a crisis as profound as the birth of a defective child can be a strengthening experience for the individual and for the family unit.

Attachment Problems

Bonding between mother and infant is critically important if the infant is to grow and develop optimally. Much of the research in the area of attachment formation is relatively recent, and the entire process is incompletely understood.

Nevertheless, changes, such as providing increased contact between preterm infants and their mothers, have occurred in the delivery and postpartal periods because of increased understanding of this phenomenon. Occasionally mothers who are aware of the bonding process become very concerned if for reasons such as illness of the baby or themselves they are deprived of postpartal contact. This concern in itself can become a crisis for the parents, and to avoid a self-fulling prophecy the nurse can assure the couple that strong bonding can occur, even between adoptive parents and their children. Kennell and Klaus (1971) have identified several crucial steps or events in the process of attachment:

- Planning the pregnancy
- Confirming the pregnancy
- Accepting the pregnancy
- Fetal movement
- Accepting the fetus as an individual

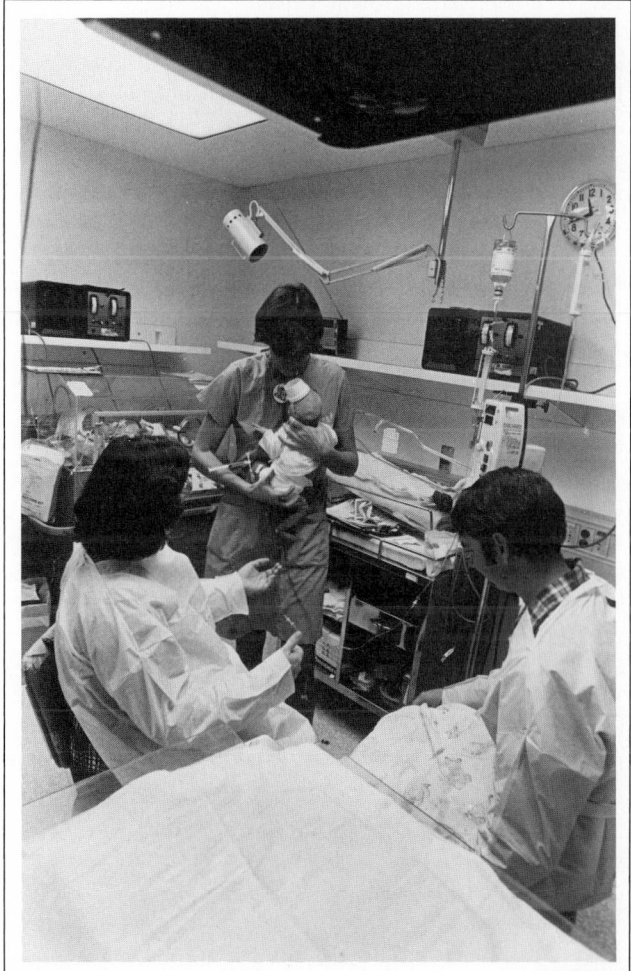

FIGURE 30–3 It is essential that the nurse recognize the emotional needs of parents of children with defects or complications.

- Birth
- Seeing the baby
- Touching the baby
- Caretaking

During the past 15 years a body of evidence has grown that clearly demonstrates that the most common element in the lives of parents who neglect or abuse their children is a "lack of empathic mothering" in their own lives (Steele and Pollack, 1968). This phrase describes inadequate responses of the caretaker to the infant, frequently beginning in the perinatal period and related to poorly developed maternal–infant attachment or insufficient bonding (Helfer and Kempe, 1976). Because of this finding, attention has been given to the promotion of adequate parent–infant bonding to prevent malattachment and its related sequelae. Factors that may retard the formation of maternal–infant attachment include "an abnormal pregnancy, an abnormal labor or delivery, neonatal separation, other separation in the first six months, illnesses in the infant during the first year of life, and illnesses in the mother during the first year of life" (Helfer and Kempe, 1976, p. 29).

In the prenatal period, warning signs that may indicate lack of acceptance of the pregnancy and a potential for malattachment include: negative maternal self-perception, excessive mood swings or emotional withdrawal, failure to respond to quickening, excessive maternal preoccupation with appearance, numerous physical complaints, and failure to prepare for the infant during the last trimester (Helfer and Kempe, 1976).

At delivery, signs of maladaptive responses may include lack of interest in seeing the newborn; withdrawal, sadness, or disappointment; negative comments such as "She's such an ugly thing"; or expressions of marked disappointment when told of the infant's sex. When shown the infant, the mother may avoid looking at the child or may regard the child without expression. She may decline to hold the infant, or if she does agree to do so, she may not touch or stroke the infant's face or extremities. The mother may also avoid asking questions or talking to the infant and may suddenly decide she does not want to breast-feed (Johnson, 1979).

During the early postpartal period, evidence of maladaptive mothering may include limited handling of or smiling at the infant, lack of preparation or questions about infant needs and care, and failure to snuggle the newborn to her neck and face. The mother may also describe her infant negatively or use animal characteristics in a hostile manner when referring to the infant: "He looks just like a withered old monkey to me!"

The father, too, may exhibit signs of malattachment to his infant. Examples of maladaptive paternal behaviors include inattentiveness and indifference toward the child, rough, unrelaxed handling, and tense, rigid posture. The father may also choose inappropriate types of play and exhibit no protective behavior toward his child (Johnson, 1979).

NURSING INTERVENTIONS

Interventions to promote healthy parent–infant attachment should begin during the prenatal period. The health history should include questions that provide the caregivers with some initial understanding of the parent's attitudes, supports, fears, and knowledge. Questions such as "Do you have family or close relatives nearby?" "How often do you see them?" and "Are there things that have happened in the past that make you worry about the baby or being pregnant?" may provide invaluable information.

As the pregnancy progresses, further information may be elicited and teaching instituted. During the third trimester the caregivers should begin looking for evidence that the parents have started to prepare for the infant. Has the mother made arrangements for the care of other infants, if any, while she is hospitalized? Have the parents chosen names or prepared a room or area for the infant? Lack of preparation suggests continued rejection of the pregnancy.

A tour of the maternity unit is often helpful in decreasing fear of the unknown and fostering confidence in the parents so that they will be able to cope.

It is essential that whenever possible, mother, father, and newborn have a period of time alone to begin getting acquainted. The infant should be undressed so that the parents can explore him or her thoroughly, and the mother may nurse if she so desires. To facilitate eye contact, eye prophylaxis may be delayed until after this parent–infant meeting (Helfer and Kempe, 1976).

When maladaptive behaviors are identified, there are various interventions that can be used. A team approach involving all three nursing shifts is advised. Any positive behaviors are communicated so that each staff member can continue to offer support and stimulate further development of such strengths.

Hospital practices should be examined for factors that may inhibit or exaggerate the maladaptive behaviors. Hospital practices such as strict adherence to 4-hour feedings, discouraging the mother from unwrapping and looking at her newborn, or prolonged separation may create a problem for some mothers.

The mother needs a supportive, understanding person she can interact with as she works through her feelings about her baby. At times, in the presence of severe emotional disorders, a referral to a psychologist or psychiatrist may be necessary. Referral to community agencies such as the Public Health Department is advised so that follow-up care can be established.

The referral should be accompanied by a summary of the hospital course, the identified strengths and maladaptive behaviors, the educational process that was accomplished in the hospital, and the mother's response. Personal or telephone contact may be maintained after dismissal so that the mother can continue to have contact with a supportive person with whom she is already acquainted. The mother should be encouraged to call the postpartal unit or newborn nursery if she has questions.

PROMOTING ATTACHMENT WHEN THE NEWBORN IS HOSPITALIZED

When infants require lengthy intensive care, special efforts by the nurse may facilitate attachment. It is important that parents believe that the child "belongs" to them rather than to the medical team. They should be encouraged to participate in care and to give suggestions about that care. Schraeder (1980) suggests establishing a care plan and in-

cluding specific nursing diagnoses such as "alteration in the parent–child relationship" or "impairment of the parent–infant bond" (p. 38). Nursing interventions are then established according to the stages of parenting behaviors as outlined in Figure 30–4. For example, if the mother entered the nursery, lowered the crib rail, and established an *en face* position while talking to the infant, she would be ready to move into stage II. If there is a specific problem, with the feeding schedule or technique, for example, the parents might be encouraged to work with the nurses to help establish the care plan.

During the postpartal period, continued family interaction should be encouraged by a supportive staff, liberal

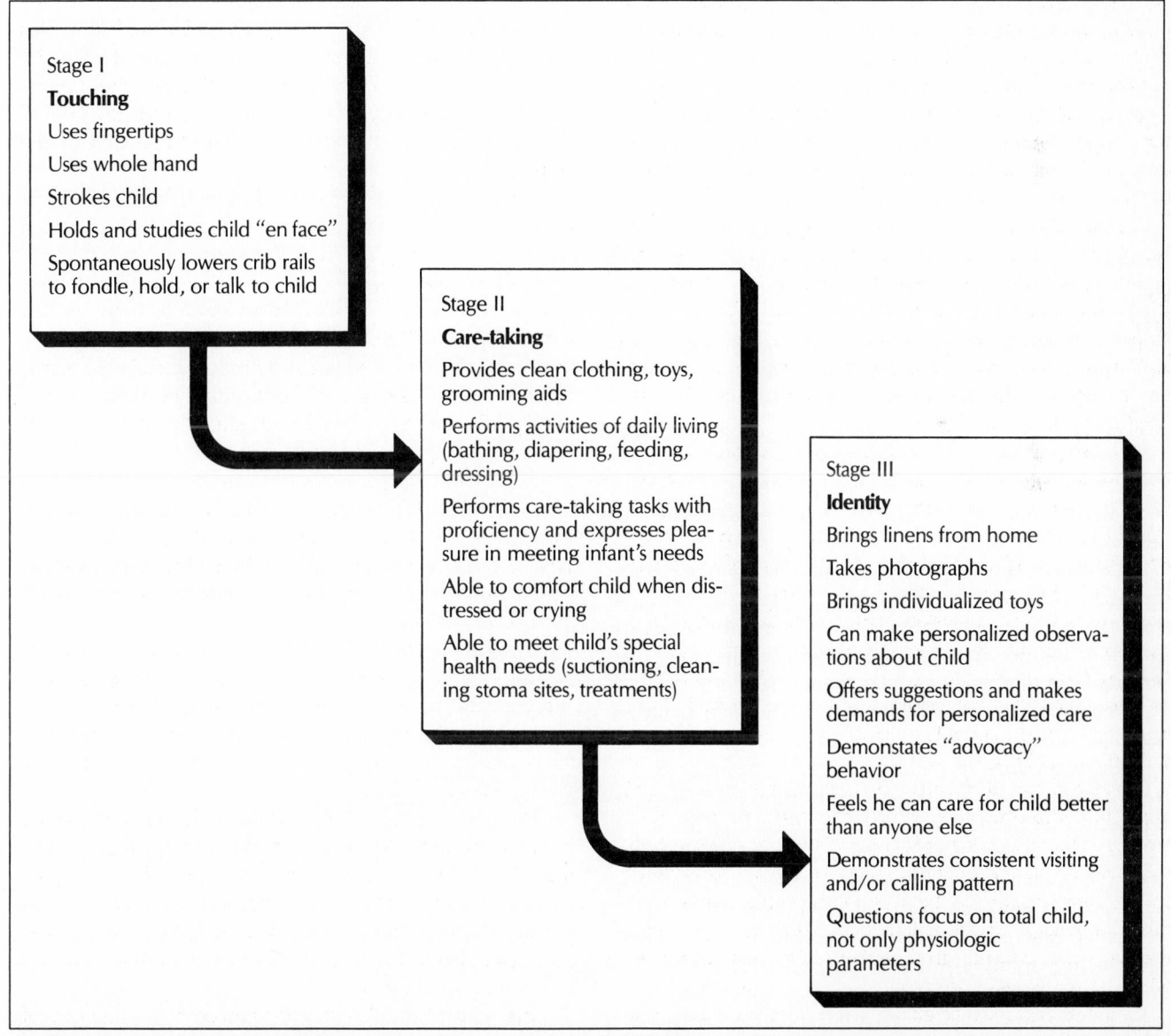

FIGURE 30–4 Stages of parenting behavior. (Adapted from the work of Rubin, Shaeffer Jay, and Schraeder by Schraeder, B. D. Jan./Feb. 1980. Attachment and parenting despite lengthy intensive care. *Am. J. Mat. Child Nurs.* 5:38.)

visiting policies, and educational offerings for both father and mother. Staff should be trained in assessment techniques and alert for evidence of malattachment, so that appropriate interventions may be initiated. If necessary, referrals to the community health nurse or social services may provide the ongoing assistance needed. Telephone hot-lines may provide a useful resource for a frustrated or worried parent, as may classes or parents' groups during the early weeks after delivery.

Unwanted Pregnancy and Relinquishment

A woman frequently feels ambivalent when she first learns she is pregnant. As the pregnancy progresses, she moves into a state of acceptance as she adjusts to the idea. She then becomes excited about the prospect of becoming a mother and shares this joy with her family. In some cases, however, the pregnancy is unwanted. The expectant woman may be an adolescent, unmarried, or economically restricted. She may dislike children or the idea of being a mother. Her partner may disapprove of the pregnancy. These and many other reasons may cause the woman to continue to reject the idea of her pregnancy. An emotional crisis arises as she attempts to resolve the problem. She may choose to have an abortion, to carry the fetus to term and keep the baby, or to have the baby and relinquish it by allowing others to adopt it. The mother should not be given direct advice during this time, but rather allowed to discuss her situation and problem solve. After she has made a decision, she needs support in that choice. When the woman has chosen an abortion, she may want to explore her feelings and express her loss to someone. Each nurse needs to explore personal attitudes about abortion to be effective therapeutically. (See Chapter 6 for a discussion of abortion.)

Unwanted children and their families are more crisis-prone than others, although in many cases, parents grow to love the child after attachment occurs. If nurses are aware of the potential for parenting problems, they may initiate crisis strategies or make appropriate referrals.

Many mothers who choose to give their infants up for adoption are young and/or unmarried. However, approximately two-thirds of children born out-of-wedlock are raised by their mothers alone. The decision of a mother to relinquish her infant is an extremely difficult one. Harvey (1977) reports that there are social pressures against giving up one's child. She states that "society in general exerts a subtle influence in that it obliges people to be responsible and pay for their mistakes" (p. 24). Some women may want to prove to themselves that they can manage on their own by keeping their infants. Mothers who choose to relinquish their infants suffer a loss and need to complete a grieving process. Nurses may neglect to provide support and preparation for this grieving process unless they are sensitive to the mother's needs.

NURSING INTERVENTION

The mother who chooses to let her child be adopted usually experiences intense ambivalence. These feelings may heighten just before delivery and upon first seeing her baby. The woman usually has made considerable adjustments in her life-style to give birth to this child. She may not have told friends and relatives about the pregnancy and so lacks an extended support system. The nurse can encourage her to express grief, loneliness, guilt, and other feelings. The mother will make the decision about whether she wants to see the newborn; seeing the infant often facilitates the grieving process. When the mother sees her baby, she may feel strong attachment and love. The nurse needs to assure her that these feelings do not mean that her decision was a wrong one. Relinquishment is frequently a painful act of love (Harvey, 1977). Table 30–3 identifies nursing interventions the nurse may use in caring for the mother who chooses to give up her newborn.

Initial denial of pregnancy by women usually moves into acceptance of the pregnant state. Occasionally, however, a nurse might encounter a woman who denies she is pregnant even as she is admitted to the maternity unit. Pregnancy and birth are crisis situations and Bascom (1977) states that "perhaps for those who lack adequate coping skill and/or support, denial is an attempt to defend themselves against a traumatic experience" (p. 174). It may seem impossible that a woman who is so obviously pregnant could maintain this delusion. It is important for the nurse to establish a trusting relationship while gently guiding the woman to accept reality. Sometimes the parents of the mother-to-be are unaware of the pregnancy; she may have adjusted her clothing style and appeared to be only gaining weight. Some women decide not to tell their families or friends about the birth and therefore lack a support system. Because no prenatal care was sought, the mother and infant may be at risk. Preparation for the birth experience may be incomplete.

Child Abuse

One of the most disastrous results of lack of parenting ability is child abuse. *Child abuse* refers to the physical, emotional, or sexual harming of a child, either by the child's parents or by older siblings. Child abuse arises in part from the cultural sanctioning of physical disciplining of children by their parents. Among the many serious effects of child abuse are physical handicaps, a poor self-image, inability to love others, antisocial or violent behavior in later life, and death.

A small number of abusing parents are seriously mentally ill, but most abusing parents have less serious problems that respond to intervention. It may be necessary to remove children temporarily from the parents' home during therapy, but the goal of treatment is to help parents

Table 30–3   Nursing Interventions for Relinquishing Mothers

Prenatal	Intrapartal	Postpartal
Assessing social and psychological support systems	Informing staff adequately of the mother's relinquishment	Allowing for a recount of the labor and delivery experience
Providing continuity of care	Giving the mother a sense of achievement	Allowing for free access to the infant
Facilitating the decision-making process	Accepting and encouraging her	Promoting anticipatory guidance for future emotions
Allowing for justification of the decision	expression of emotions	Encouraging expression of emotions and concerns
Promoting anticipatory grief	Creating a simple, honest, and direct environment	Facilitating meaningful communication with significant others
Reassuring that the mother's ambivalence is normal	Respecting special requests for delivery	Exploring the concept of sexuality and attitudes toward birth control
Preparing mother for labor and delivery	Helping significant others to deal with their loss	Arranging for follow-up care
Exploring how the woman wants her delivery handled		Helping the mother to find a meaning in her loss
Helping with the decision over whether or not to see and hold the infant		
Counseling on legal aspects		
Involving a social worker, if possible		

* From Harvey, K. Jan./Feb. 1977. Caring perceptively for the relinquishing mother, *Am J. Mat. Child Nurs.* 2:27.

and their children live together. Most children are able to return to their home after a time.

Helfer and Kempe (1972) have identified an abusing pattern in which a complex of variables interact. Three components can be studied: the parent, the child, and the crisis. The following components may lead to physical abuse of a child by his or her parents:

1. The parents' potential to abuse, which is influenced by:
   a. The way the parents were reared. Were they abused themselves? Did they have disturbed parents?
   b. Parents who are distrustful or isolated
   c. A passive spouse who cannot give love
   d. Parents who have unrealistic expectations for their child
2. The presence of a special child, who is:
   a. Perceived as different by parents
   b. Actually different (retarded, "too smart," and so on)
3. A crisis or series of crises:
   a. Personal
   b. Physical (limited resources, food, shelter, and so on)

If the home is to be made safe, early recognition of potential for abuse or actual abuse is critical. Low self-esteem and guilt are usually experienced by abusing par-

ents. The parents of an abused child are rarely malevolent and hateful. In fact, child abuse is an emotional crisis for the parents as well as for the child. In some cases the abused child is one whose behaviors provoke the parent to violent action. The parent feels shaken by hurting the child, is riddled by guilt, is in many cases fearful for the child's life, worries about being prosecuted for the act, and is afraid of future uncontrolled outbursts of anger toward the child.

The nurse must understand the emotional needs of abusive or neglectful parents to provide the proper intervention. Such parents tend to be emotionally immature, unhappily married, unsure of themselves as parents, unrealistic in their expectations for their children, themselves survivors of a deprived or abused childhood, and victims of frequent life crises.

NURSING INTERVENTION

The health professional is required by law to report cases of suspected child abuse. Not only does the law protect the nurse who in good faith reports a case of suspected child abuse that is mistaken, but if a case of abuse is known and not reported, then the individual is legally liable.

One of the most important roles of the nurse is that of assessment of the family and the child. Nurses frequently have the closest contact with the family, both emotionally and physically. As they give care in the hospital or the home they have the opportunity to observe the infant's behavior and his or her body. Helfer and Kempe (1972)

Table 30–4   Diagnosing Child Abuse*

CONSIDER PHYSICAL ABUSE WHEN THE PARENT:

1. Shows evidence of loss of control, or fear of losing control
2. Presents contradictory history
3. Projects cause of injury onto a sibling or third party
4. Has delayed unduly in bringing child in for care
5. Shows detachment
6. Reveals inappropriate awareness of seriousness of situation (either overreaction or underreaction)
7. Continues to complain about irrelevant problems unrelated to the injury
8. Personally is misusing drugs or alcohol
9. Is disliked, for unknown reasons, by the physician
10. Presents a history that cannot or does not explain the injury
11. Gives specific "eye witness" history of abuse
12. Gives a history of repeated injury
13. Has no one to "bail" her (him) out when "up tight" with the child
14. Is reluctant to give information
15. Refuses consent for further diagnostic studies
16. Hospital "shops"
17. Cannot be located
18. Is psychotic or psychopathic
19. Has been reared in a "motherless" atmosphere
20. Has unrealistic expectations of the child

WHEN THE CHILD:

1. Has an unexplained injury
2. Shows evidence of dehydration and/or malnutrition without obvious cause
3. Has been given inappropriate food, drink and/or drugs
4. Shows evidence of overall poor care
5. Is unusually fearful
6. Shows evidence of repeated injury
7. "Takes over" and begins to care for parents' needs
8. Is seen as "different" or "bad" by the parents
9. Is indeed different in physical or emotional makeup
10. Is dressed inappropriately for degree or type of injury
11. Shows evidence of sexual abuse
12. Shows evidence of repeated skin injuries
13. Shows evidence of repeated fractures
14. Shows evidence of "characteristic" x-ray changes to long bones
15. Has injuries that are not mentioned in history

* From Helfer, R. E., and Kempe, C. H. 1972. The child's need for early recognition, immediate care and protection. In *Helping the battered child and his family*, ed. C. H. Kempe and R. E. Helfer. Philadelphia: J. B. Lippincott Co.

identify a list of factors that can alert the nurse to the possibility of child abuse (Table 30–4).

Nurses who work in prenatal or postnatal settings are in a unique situation to observe parents who may have difficulty caring for their infants and present the potential for emotional or physical abuse. Parental expression of distaste or rejection upon first seeing their infant may signal difficulty. Mothers who seem unduly concerned about the "correct" appearance or the sex of the baby, as well as those who have extremely unrealistic views of motherhood or their infant, may need additional support. Some parents give the child a derisive or cruel name or fail to name the baby for an extended period of time. Parents may make many comments about "not spoiling the baby" or "controlling bad behavior." Mothers who repeatedly refer to their infants as "bad," "impossible," or use other disparaging terms may lack sufficient mothering capabilities. The mother may express pity rather than love toward her baby, or disappointment and even frank rage. Occasionally it is difficult for nurses to accept these feelings and expressions; they may need help recognizing their own reactions (Helfer and Kempe, 1972). The prenatal assessment tool in Table 30–1 may be helpful for the nurse in evaluating parenting potential. Parents who abuse each other may be at increased risk for abusing their children. Alcohol and drug abuse often intensify abusing behaviors.

Once the nurse has identified a family in need of help, crisis intervention should begin by encouraging the parents to express their feelings about the situation. Of particular value is actively involving the parents in planning the medical care for the child so that they feel that they are doing something positive and perhaps "making up" for the harm.

The attitudes of the nurse are critically important in the development of a therapeutic nurse–client relationship. Empathy, warmth, and understanding are essential. The nurse who is repulsed by the parents' behavior and projects blame or rejection will increase the parents' guilt and lower their self-esteem. If they continue to see themselves as increasingly worthless and unable to parent, the child may bear the brunt of their frustration and self-hate.

The nurse should explain to the parents the function of the child welfare authorities, pointing out that such people are there to help the parents carry out their responsibilities. The nurse can also help by referring the parents to such self-help groups as Parents Anonymous. Such groups can help parents to express their feelings and to realize that others have experienced similar situations. Additional counseling from appropriate sources can help the parents to deal with possible underlying emotional problems that contributed to their child abuse behavior.

The Adolescent Parent

Progression through adolescence is not an easy task. Neither child nor adult, the adolescent may experience inner turmoil as she struggles to establish her identity. Parents sometimes stare in amazement at the child they have lived with for years and now seem to hardly know. A teenager may be an interesting, sensitive, likable, and caring person who suddenly becomes frustrating, unreasonable, and negative. At the same time that attitudes and emotions are in rapid transition, the adolescent's body is undergoing tremendous change.

Adolescence and its associated crises pass more smoothly for some than others. Because of reproductive maturity and sexual activity the adolescent may be faced with pregnancy and parenthood. As mentioned earlier, pregnancy and the birth of a child constitute a normal developmental crisis for a family. When the parents are very young or immature, the crisis situation may be compounded. "Frequently the school-age parent is lacking the biological, educational, occupational, and social development to effectively cope with the crisis of parenthood" (Harris, Karrow, and Phillips, 1979). Approximately one-fifth of births are to mothers between 15 and 19 years old. This age group is considered a high-risk maternity population.

This group also contains a large number of single parents. The adolescent mother may be faced with other variables that complicate her situation. She may have used pregnancy to escape from an intolerable situation at home. She may come from a family in which emotional or physical abuse or incest took place. Economic conditions and poverty may be a problem. Emotional support may be lacking. The adolescent may be experiencing the pregnancy alone for fear of rejection if she tells her parents. She may feel shame and lack of self-esteem and there may be pressure for her to marry the father. Career and education plans of the teenager are threatened by the responsibility and expense of being a parent. The adolescent may view the new baby as an object—a toy or plaything—by which she can increase her own self-esteem and solidify her role identity. When the infant does not fulfill these needs for the adolescent mother, frustration and abuse may result—this may be especially true if the child is preterm or handicapped.

Adolescence is a time in which one is primarily concerned about oneself, a time for self-discovery. Harris et al. (1979) stress that it is difficult for the adolescent to delay gratification and to place her infant's needs above her own. The teenager may be grieving over loss of her own youthful fantasy life at a time when she must be concerned with child care. Her classmates may appear to be having fun while she is trapped.

NURSING INTERVENTION

Nursing involvement with the adolescent parent can be a very rewarding experience. Many adolescents have the desire and potential to provide good parenting for their child. The nurse who plans to be involved in this area should develop a complete understanding of the developmental needs of adolescents and infants. The teenager often lacks knowledge about normal infant growth and development as well as information about child care. The nurse may

utilize role modeling to carefully demonstrate care to the mother, rather than merely telling her. Having the teenager repeat the procedure is important so that the nurse can give positive feedback about her skills and abilities. As the teenage mother's confidence in her ability to care for her child increases, her self-esteem also rises.

Whenever possible the father of the child should be involved both prenatally and after the infant is born. Supportive grandparents also can provide assistance. In many families, grandparents provide child care as well as support. If possible, adolescents should be encouraged to finish high school.

The nurse may offer contraceptive counseling to the young couple. Acceptance and support are important as the nurse helps to facilitate communication between all family members. Referrals to community agencies may be appropriate, depending on the assessment of specific problems. Harris and coworkers (1979) have summarized the areas of nursing focus to ensure the following for the adolescent parent:

1. Coordination and continuity of varied resources necessary to deal with the many complex emotional, economic, social, and medical problems associated with adolescent parenting.

2. Assistance to the family or significant others (including peers) in developing a responsive long-term support system for the young parents.

3. Assistance during the phases of the childbearing cycle to involve the young mother and father in an effort to foster the development of attachment to the infant.

4. Provisions of: (a) nurturing for the parents in order to ensure their personal development through this crisis; (b) encouragement and support to the parents to build self-confidence and a sense of adequacy in their parenting abilities; (c) encouragement and assistance to the young parents in the planning and implementation of their continued education or job training; (d) assistance to parents in the arrangements for quality child care so they can continue their education and personal development; (e) practical information about child care and development, and parenting in order to help parents establish realistic expectations of themselves and of their child.*

*From Harris, D. M.; Karrow, L.; and Phillips, P. J. 1979. Adolescent parenthood. In *Family health care, vol. 2, Developmental and situational crises*, 2nd ed., ed. D. P. Hymovich and M. U. Barnard. New York: McGraw-Hill Book Co.

Single-Parent Families

In the United States in 1980, over 12 million children (19.7%) under 18 years of age lived with one parent— 1.05 million with their fathers and 11.1 million with their mothers. Single-parent homes most commonly develop as a result of divorce, desertion, or death of a spouse. Such parents are faced with problems related to maintaining their own positive self-concept in the face of depression, guilt, and lowered self-esteem. They must decide how to answer questions the children raise about family disruption and must avoid the urge to become a "superparent" in the wake of guilt associated with the effects of loss on the children.

Single-parent homes also occur when the child's parents are unmarried and the child lives with either the mother or father. The stigma of illegitimacy is decreasing, and children raised in these situations are less apt to be labeled negatively because of it. Positive acceptance of the single woman parent may be more readily available in the Chicano and black communities. Many single women rear their children with the support of their extended families.

Single-parent homes may also occur as a result of adoption. This phenomenon, although still relatively rare, is increasing. For instance, the Los Angeles County Department of Adoptions reported that from 1965 to March 1975 they placed 265 children (1.3% of all their placements) with single parents; 251 of these parents were women, and 14 were men. Single parenthood as a result of adoption requires an individual to consider the meaning not only of adoption but also of being single and a parent.

In the book *The Single-Parent Experience,* Klein (1973) lists four implications that single "expectant" parents, male or female, ought to consider prior to accepting the single-parent role:

1. What will being a single parent mean with respect to family, employment, and social relations?
2. What are the social implications for the child raised by a parent in a particular state, region, and neighborhood?
3. What child care facilities are available?
4. What are the options available with respect to sexual identity formation of the child?

Hazards to successful childrearing do exist for single-parent families. It is extremely important that, as children pass through certain developmental stages, they be provided with opportunities to relate to individuals of the same and the opposite sex to learn sex roles. In a single-parent family these opportunities may not be readily available, and provision for substitute experiences must be made. A relative or close friend may assist the single parent in providing the needed experiences. An additional drawback in a single-parent family is the lack of opportunities for the child to observe parental man–woman interactions. Furthermore, the parent in a single-parent situation is usually employed outside the home. Thus, the parent must handle the demands of job and family alone. With adequate support from the extended family, from friends and groups such as Parents Without Partners, single parents can successfully raise healthy, mature children. This task requires careful recognition of potential problems, evaluation of the needs of both child and parent, realistic planning and provision for day-to-day living, and use of available support and assistance when necessary.

NURSING INTERVENTION

Nurses will be able to counsel the single parent more effectively if they have an understanding of the stresses and demands of parenting a child. A single parent is more likely to have minimal support.

The nurse can begin by assessing the parent's educational needs and then providing information as needed. Counseling may include investigation into the availability of child care facilities and referral to single parent support groups within the community. Support groups offer opportunities for socialization, sharing of problems, and opportunities to expose the child to a group setting in which there are members of the opposite sex, which may facilitate sexual identity formation.

SUMMARY

The nurse is often in a position of first contact with families in the grip of a crisis brought about by health care problems. The death of a child, the birth of a deformed infant, and the arrival of a preterm child are various types of crises that may be seen in obstetric nursing. Successful coping on the part of the maternity client and her family can be facilitated by the health care professional skilled in crisis intervention. Even though the nurse may be unsure of personal skills in crisis intervention, the nurse may still be the person in the position to make a referral for a family in crisis. The recognition of the stresses that contribute to a crisis and the insight to make a referral to a skilled crisis intervention counselor can constitute positive nursing care for a grieving family or couple.

Recognition of the dynamics of loss and grieving are

important for the nurse practitioner, who may therefore better aid clients who experience these life situations. It is a realistic part of nursing care to assess the emotional turmoil in a client and plan intervention to aid the client in returning to a harmonious level of functioning.

Resource Groups

National Association for Mental Health, 1800 North Kent St., Arlington, VA 22209.

National Committee for Prevention of Child Abuse, Box 2866, Chicago, IL 60690.

National Organization of Mothers of Twins Clubs, 5402 Amberwood Lane, Rockville, MD 20853.

National Sudden Infant Death Syndrome Foundation, 310 S. Michigan Avenue, Chicago, IL 60604.

National Women's Health Network, 2025 I Street NW, Suite 105, Washington, D.C. 20006.

Parents Anonymous, 22330 Hawthorne Blvd., Suite 208, Torrance, CA 90505.

Parents Without Partners, Inc., 80 Fifth Ave., New York, NY 10011.

References

Aguilera, D. C., and Messick, J. M. 1978. *Crisis intervention: theory and methodology.* 3rd ed. St. Louis: The C. V. Mosby Co.

Bascom, L. May/June 1977. Women who refuse to believe: persistent denial of pregnancy. *Am. J. Mat. Child Nurs.* 2:174.

Caplan, G. 1961. *An approach to community mental health.* New York: Grune & Stratton, Inc.

Caplan, G., et al. 1965. Four studies of crisis in parents of prematures. *Community Mental Health J.* 1:149.

Clausen, J. P. 1979. Anticipatory guidance of the expectant family. In *Family health care, vol. 2, Developmental and situational crises,* 2nd ed., ed. D. P. Hymovich and M. U. Barnard. New York: McGraw-Hill Book Co.

Cullberg, J. 1972. In *Psychosomatic medicine in obstetrics and gynaecology.* 3rd International Congress, Basel. New York: S. Karger.

Donnelly, E. 1974. The real of her. *J. Obstet. Gynecol. Neonatal Nurs.* 3:48.

DuBois, D. R. 1975. Indications of an unhealthy relationship between parents and premature infants. *J. Obstet. Gynecol. Neonatal Nurs.* 4:21.

Duvall, E. M. 1975. *Marriage and family development,* 5th ed. Philadelphia: J. B. Lippincott Co.

Duvall, E., and Hill, R. 1960. *Being married.* New York: Association Press.

Engel, G. 1964. Grief and grieving. *Am. J. Nurs.* 64:93.

Getz, W., et al. 1974. *Fundamentals of crisis counseling.* Lexington, Mass.: D. C. Heath.

Green, M., and Solnit, A. J. 1964. Reactions to the threatened loss of a child: the vulnerable child syndrome. *Pediatrics.* 34:58.

Harris, D. M.; Karrow, L.; and Phillips, P. J. 1979. Adolescent parenthood. In *Family health care, vol. 2, Developmental and situational crises,* 2nd ed., ed. D. P. Hymovich and M. U. Barnard. New York: McGraw-Hill Book Co.

Harvey, K. Jan./Feb. 1977. Caring perceptively for the relinquishing mother. *Am. J. Mat. Child Nurs.* 2:24.

Helfer, R. E., and Kempe, C. H. 1972. The child's need for early recognition, immediate care and protection. In *Helping the battered child and his family,* ed. C. H. Kempe and R. E. Helfer. Philadelphia: J. B. Lippincott Co.

———. 1976. *Child abuse and neglect.* Cambridge, Mass.: Ballinger Publishing Co.

Hill, R., et al. 1953. *Eddysville's families.* Chapel Hill: University of North Carolina.

Hoff, L. A. 1984. *People in crisis: understanding and helping,* 2nd ed. Menlo Park, Calif.: Addison-Wesley Publishing Co.

Johnson, S. H. 1979. *High risk parenting: nursing assessment and strategies for the family at risk.* Philadelphia: J. B. Lippincott Co.

Josten, L. March/April 1981. Prenatal assessment guide for illuminating possible problems with parenting. *Am. J. Mat. Child Nurs.* 6:113.

Kaplan, D., and Mason, E. 1960. Maternal reactions to premature birth viewed as an acute emotional disorder. *Am. J. Orthopsychiatry.* 30:539.

Kennell, J. H., and Klaus, M. H. 1971. Care of the mother of the high-risk infant. *Clin. Obstet. Gynecol.* 14:926.

Klaus, M. H., and Fanaroff, A. A. 1973. *Care of the high-risk neonate.* Philadelphia: W. B. Saunders Co.

Klaus, M. H., and Kennell, J. H. 1970. Mothers separated from their newborns. *Pediatr. Clin. N. Am.* 17:1015

Klein, C. 1973. *The single-parent experience.* New York: Walker and Co.

Kowalski, K., and Osborn, M. R. Jan./Feb. 1977. Helping mothers of stillborn infants to grieve. *Am. J. Mat. Child Nurs.* 2:29.

Kübler-Ross, E. 1969. *On death and dying.* New York: The Macmillan Co.

Lindemann, E. 1944. Symptomatology and management of acute grief. *Am. J. Psychiatry.* 101:141.

———. 1956. The meaning of crisis in individual and family. *Teachers Coll. Rec.* 57:310.

McCabe, S. N. 1979. Anticipatory guidance for families with infants. In *Family health care, vol. 2, Developmental and situational crises,* 2nd ed., ed. D. P. Hymovich and M. U. Barnard. New York: McGraw-Hill Book Co.

Olshansky, S. 1962. Chronic sorrow: a response to having a mentally defective child. *Soc. Casework.* 43:190.

Penticuff, J. H. March 1982. Psychologic implications in high-risk pregnancy. *Nurs. Clin. North Am.* 17:69.

Powell, M. L. 1981. *Assessment and management of developmental changes and problems in children,* 2nd ed. St. Louis: The C. V. Mosby Co.

Schoenberg, B., et al. 1970. *Loss and grief: psychological management in medical practice.* New York: Columbia University Press.

———. 1974. *Anticipatory grief.* New York: Columbia University Press.

Schraeder, B. D. Jan./Feb. 1980. Attachment and parenting despite lengthy intensive care. *Am. J. Mat. Child Nurs.* 5:37.

Schwartz, J. L., and Schwartz, L. H., eds. 1977. *Vulnerable infants.* New York: McGraw-Hill Book Co.

Seitz, P. M., and Warrick, L. H. 1974. Perinatal death: the grieving mother. *Am. J. Nurs.* 74(11):2028.

Steele, B., and Pollock, C. 1968. A psychiatric study of parents who abuse infants and small children. In *The battered child,* ed. R. Helfer and C. H. Kempe. Chicago: University of Chicago Press.

Williams, H. A.; Rivara, F. P.; and Rothenberg, M. B. July/Aug. 1981. The child is dying: who helps the family? *Am. J. Mat. Child Nurs.* 6:261.

Wong, D. L. Nov./Dec. 1980. Bereavement: the empty mother syndrome. *Am. J. Mat. Child Nurs.* 5:385.

Wooten, B. July/Aug. 1981. Death of an infant. *Am. J. Mat. Child Nurs.* 6:257.

Young, R. K. 1977. Chronic sorrow: patient's response to the birth of a child with a defect. *Am. J. Mat. Child Nurs.* 2:38.

Additional Readings

Burgess, E. W. 1968. The family as a unit of interacting personalities. In *Family roles and interactions: an anthology,* ed. J. Heiss. Chicago: Rand McNally & Company.

———. 1971. *The family: from traditional to companionship.* New York: Van Nostrand Reinhold Company.

Helfer, R. E. 1975. *Child abuse and neglect: the diagnostic process and treatment programs.* DHEW Publication no. 75–69. Washington D.C.: U.S. Government Printing Office.

Holmes, T., and Rahe, R. 1967. The social readjustment rating scale. *J. Psychosom. Res.* 11:213.

Jay, S. S. Fall 1977. Pediatric intensive care: Involving parents in the care of their child. *Am. J. Mat. Child Nurs.* 6:195.

Kantor, D., and Lehr, W. 1975. *Inside the family.* San Francisco: Jossey-Bass, Inc., Publishers.

Melels, A. I. July/Aug. 1975. Role insufficiency and role supplementation: a conceptual framework. *Nurs. Res.* 24:264.

Mercer, R. T. 1977. *Nursing care for parents at risk.* Thorofare, N.J.: Charles B. Slack, Inc.

Rodgers, R. H. 1973. *Family interaction and transaction: the developmental approach.* Englewood Cliffs, N.J.: Prentice-Hall, Inc.

Rubin, R. 1967. Attainment of the maternal role. Parts 1 and 2. *Nurs. Res.* 16:237.

Selye, H. 1974. *Stress without distress.* Philadelphia: J. B. Lippincott Co.

APPENDICES

APPENDIX A THE PREGNANT PATIENT'S BILL OF RIGHTS*

The Pregnant Patient has the right to participate in decisions involving her well-being and that of her unborn child, unless there is a clearcut medical emergency that prevents her participation. In addition to the rights set forth in the American Hospital Association's "Patient's Bill of Rights," the Pregnant Patient, because she represents TWO patients rather than one, should be recognized as having the additional rights listed below.

1. *The Pregnant Patient has the right,* prior to the administration of any drug or procedure, to be informed by the health professional caring for her of any potential direct or indirect effects, risks or hazards to herself or her unborn or newborn infant which may result from the use of a drug or procedure prescribed for or administered to her during pregnancy, labor, birth or lactation.

2. *The Pregnant Patient has the right,* prior to the proposed therapy, to be informed, not only of the benefits, risks and hazards of the proposed therapy but also of known alternative therapy, such as available childbirth education classes which could help to prepare the Pregnant Patient physically and mentally to cope with the discomfort or stress of pregnancy and the experience of childbirth, thereby reducing or eliminating her need for drugs and obstetric intervention. She should be offered such information early in her pregnancy in order that she may make a reasoned decision.

3. *The Pregnant Patient has the right,* prior to the administration of any drug, to be informed by the health professional who is prescribing or administering the drug to her that any drug which she receives during pregnancy, labor and birth, no matter how or when the drug is taken or administered, may adversely affect her unborn baby, directly or indirectly, and that there is no drug or chemical which has been proven safe for the unborn child.

4. *The Pregnant Patient has the right* if cesarean birth is anticipated, to be informed prior to the administration of any drug, and preferably prior to her hospitalization, that minimizing her and, in turn, her baby's intake of nonessential preoperative medicine will benefit her baby.

5. *The Pregnant Patient has the right,* prior to the administration of a drug or procedure, to be informed of the areas of uncertainty if there is NO properly controlled follow-up research which has established the safety of the drug or procedure with regard to its direct and/or indirect effects on the physiological, mental and neurological development of the child exposed, via the mother, to the drug or procedure during pregnancy, labor, birth or lactation—(this would apply to virtually all drugs and the vast majority of obstetric procedures).

6. *The Pregnant Patient has the right,* prior to the administration of any drug, to be informed of the brand name and generic name of the drug in order that she may advise the health professional of any past adverse reaction to the drug.

7. *The Pregnant Patient has the right* to determine for herself, without pressure from her attendant, whether she will accept the risks inherent in the proposed therapy or refuse a drug or procedure.

8. *The Pregnant Patient has the right* to know the name and qualifications of the individual administering a medication or procedure to her during labor or birth.

9. *The Pregnant Patient has the right* to be informed, prior to the administration of any procedure, whether that procedure is being administered to her for her or her baby's benefit (medically indicated) or as an elec-

*Prepared by Doris Haire, Chair, Committee on Health Law and Regulation, International Childbirth Education Association, Inc., Rochester, N.Y.

1021

tive procedure (for convenience, teaching purposes or research).

10. *The Pregnant Patient has the right* to be accompanied during the stress of labor and birth by someone she cares for, and to whom she looks for emotional comfort and encouragement.

11. *The Pregnant Patient has the right* after appropriate medical consultation to choose a position for labor and for birth which is least stressful to her baby and to herself.

12. *The Obstetric Patient has the right* to have her baby cared for at her bedside if her baby is normal, and to feed her baby according to her baby's needs rather than according to the hospital regimen.

13. *The Obstetric Patient has the right* to be informed in writing of the name of the person who actually delivered her baby and the professional qualifications of that person. This information should also be on the birth certificate.

14. *The Obstetric Patient has the right* to be informed if there is any known or indicated aspect of her or her baby's care or condition which may cause her or her baby later difficulty or problems.

15. *The Obstetric Patient has the right* to have her and her baby's hospital medical records complete, accurate and legible and to have their records, including Nurses' Notes, retained by the hospital until the child reaches at least the age of majority, or to have the records offered to her before they are destroyed.

16. *The Obstetric Patient,* both during and after her hospital stay, has the right to have access to her complete hospital medical records, including Nurses' Notes, and to receive a copy upon payment of a reasonable fee and without incurring the expense of retaining an attorney.

It is the obstetric patient and her baby, not the health professional, who must sustain any trauma or injury resulting from the use of a drug or obstetric procedure. The observation of the rights listed above will not only permit the obstetric patient to participate in the decisions involving her and her baby's health care, but will help to protect the health professional and the hospital against litigation arising from resentment or misunderstanding on the part of the mother.

APPENDIX B   UNITED NATIONS DECLARATION OF THE RIGHTS OF THE CHILD

Preamble

Whereas the peoples of the United Nations have, in the Charter, reaffirmed their faith in fundamental human rights, and in the dignity and worth of the human person, and have determined to promote social progress and better standards of life in larger freedom,

Whereas the United Nations has, in the Universal Declaration of Human Rights, proclaimed that everyone is entitled to all the rights and freedoms set forth therein, without distinction of any kind, such as race, color, sex, language, religion, political or other opinion, national or social origin, property, birth or other status,

Whereas the child, by reason of his physical and mental immaturity, needs special safeguards and care, including appropriate legal protection, before as well as after birth,

Whereas the need for such special safeguards has been stated in the Geneva Declaration of the Rights of the Child of 1924, and recognized in the Universal Declaration of Human Rights and in the statutes of specialized agencies and international organizations concerned with the welfare of children,

Whereas mankind owes to the child the best it has to give

NOW THEREFORE
THE GENERAL ASSEMBLY
PROCLAIMS

This Declaration of the Rights of the Child to the end that he may have a happy childhood and enjoy for his own good and for the good of society the rights and freedoms herein set forth, and calls upon parents, upon men and women as individuals and upon voluntary organizations, local authorities and national governments to recognize these rights and strive for their observance by legislative and other measures progressively taken in accordance with the following principles:

PRINCIPLE 1

The child shall enjoy all the rights set forth in this Declaration. All children, without any exception whatsoever, shall be entitled to these rights, without distinction or discrimination on account of race, color, sex, language, religion, political or other opinion, national or social origin, property, birth or other status, whether of himself or of his family.

PRINCIPLE 2

The child shall enjoy special protection, and shall be given opportunities and facilities, by law and by other means, to enable him to develop physically, mentally, morally, spiritually and socially in a healthy and normal manner and in conditions of freedom and dignity. In the enactment of laws for this purpose the best interests of the child shall be the paramount consideration.

PRINCIPLE 3

The child shall be entitled from his birth to a name and a nationality.

PRINCIPLE 4

The child shall enjoy the benefits of social security. He shall be entitled to grow and develop in health; to this end special care and protection shall be provided both to him and to his mother, including adequate pre-natal and post-natal care. The child shall have the right to adequate nutrition, housing, recreation and medical services.

PRINCIPLE 5

The child who is physically, mentally or socially handicapped shall be given the special treatment, education and care required by his particular condition.

PRINCIPLE 6

The child, for the full and harmonious development of his personality, needs love and understanding. He shall, wherever possible, grow up in the care and under the responsibility of his parents, and in any case in an atmosphere of affection and of moral and material security; a child of tender years shall not, save in exceptional circumstances, be separated from his mother. Society and the public authorities shall have the duty to extend particular care to children without a family and to those without adequate means of support. Payment of state and other assistance toward the maintenance of children of large families is desirable.

PRINCIPLE 7

The child is entitled to receive education, which shall be free and compulsory, at least in the elementary stages. He shall be given an education which will promote his general culture, and enable him on a basis of equal opportunity to develop his abilities, his individual judgment, and his sense of moral and social responsibility, and to become a useful member of society.

The best interest of the child shall be the guiding principle of those responsible for his education and guidance; that responsibility lies in the first place with his parents.

The child shall have full opportunity for play and recreation, which shall be directed to the same purposes as education; society and the public authorities shall endeavor to promote the enjoyment of this right.

PRINCIPLE 8

The child shall in all circumstances be among the first to receive protection and relief.

PRINCIPLE 9

The child shall be protected against all forms of neglect, cruelty and exploitation. He shall not be the subject of traffic, in any form.

The child shall not be admitted to employment before an appropriate minimum age; he shall in no case be caused or permitted to engage in any occupation or employment which would prejudice his health or education, or interfere with his physical, mental or moral development.

PRINCIPLE 10

The child shall be protected from practices which may foster racial, religious and any other form of discrimination. He shall be brought up in a spirit of understanding, tolerance, friendship among peoples, peace and universal brotherhood and in full consciousness that his energy and talents should be devoted to the service of his fellow men.

APPENDIX C   EVALUATION OF FETAL WEIGHT AND MATURITY BY ULTRASONIC MEASUREMENT OF BIPARIETAL DIAMETER*

Biparietal diameter (cm)	Grams	Weight (pounds)	Ounces	Weeks of gestation
1.0	NA	NA		9
1.1	NA	NA		9
1.2	NA	NA		9.5
1.3	NA	NA		10.0
1.4	NA	NA		10.0
1.5	NA	NA		10.5
1.6	NA	NA		11.0
1.7	NA	NA		11.0
1.8	NA	NA		11.5
1.9	NA	NA		12.0
2.0	NA	NA		12.0
2.1	NA	NA		12.5
2.2	NA	NA		13.0
2.3	NA	NA		13.0
2.4	NA	NA		13.5
2.5	NA	NA		14.0
2.6	NA	NA		14.0
2.7	NA	NA		14.5
2.8	NA	NA		15.0
2.9	NA	NA		15.0
3.0	NA	NA		15.5
3.1	NA	NA		16.0
3.2	NA	NA		16.0
3.3	NA	NA		16.5
3.4	NA	NA		17.0
3.5	NA	NA		17.0
3.6	NA	NA		17.5
3.7	NA	NA		18.0
3.8	NA	NA		18.0
3.9	NA	NA		18.5
4.0	NA	NA		19.0
4.1	NA	NA		19.0
4.2	NA	NA		19.5
4.3	NA	NA		20.0
4.4	NA	NA		20.0
4.5	NA	NA		20.5
4.6	NA	NA		21.0
4.7	NA	NA		21.0
4.8	NA	NA		21.5
4.9	NA	NA		22.0
5.0	NA	NA		22.0
5.1	NA	NA		22.5
5.2	42.6		2	23.0
5.3	119.9		5	23.0
5.4	197.1		6	23.5
5.5	274.3		10	24.0
5.6	351.5		13	24.0
5.7	428.7		14	24.5
5.8	514.9	1	2	25.0
5.9	583.2	1	5	25.0
6.0	660.4	1	8	25.5
6.1	737.6	1	10	26.0
6.2	814.8	1	13	26.0
6.3	892.1	2		26.5
6.4	969.3	2	2	27.0
6.5	1046.5	2	5	27.0
6.6	1123.7	2	8	27.5
6.7	1200.9	2	10	28.0
6.8	1278.2	2	13	28.0
6.9	1355.4	3		28.5
7.0	1432.6	3	3	29.0
7.1	1509.8	3	5	29.0
7.2	1587.0	3	8	29.5
7.3	1664.3	3	11	29.5
7.4	1741.5	3	14	30.0
7.5	1818.7	4		30.5
7.6	1895.9	4	3	30.8
7.7	1973.1	4	5	31.0
7.8	2050.4	4	8	31.7
7.9	2127.6	4	11	32.0
8.0	2204.8	4	14	32.7
8.1	2282.0	5		33.0
8.2	2359.2	5	3	33.6
8.3	2436.5	5	6	34.0
8.4	2513.7	5	8	34.6
8.5	2590.9	5	11	35.0
8.6	2668.1	5	14	35.5
8.7	2745.3	6		36.0
8.8	2822.6	6	3	36.5
8.9	2899.8	6	6	37.0
9.0	2977.0	6	8	37.4
9.1	3054.2	6	11	38.0
9.2	3131.4	6	14	38.4
9.3	3208.7	7	2	39.0
9.4	3285.9	7	3	39.0
9.5	3363.1	7	6	39.8
9.6	3440.3	7	10	40.0
9.7	3517.5	7	11	40.8
9.8	3594.8	7	14	41.0
9.9	3672.0	8	2	41.7
10.0	3749.2	8	3	NA
10.1	3826.5	8	6	NA
10.2	3903.6	8	10	NA
10.3	3980.9	8	13	NA
10.4	4058.1	8	14	NA
10.5	4135.3	9	2	NA
10.6	4212.5	9	5	NA

*Data from Hellman and Kobayashi.

APPENDIX D   CLINICAL ESTIMATION OF GESTATIONAL AGE

Clinical estimation of gestational age. **A,** Physical examination. **B,** Neurologic examination. (Courtesy Mead Johnson Laboratories, Evansville, Ind.)

CLINICAL ESTIMATION OF GESTATIONAL AGE
An Approximation Based on Published Data*

► Examination First Hours

WEEKS GESTATION

PHYSICAL FINDINGS	20–36	37	38	39	40–41	42	43–48
VERNIX	COVERS BODY, THICK LAYER				SCANT, IN CREASES		NO VERNIX
BREAST TISSUE AND AREOLA	APPEARS; AREOLA & NIPPLE BARELY VISIBLE, NO PALPABLE BREAST TISSUE	1–2 MM NODULE	3–5 MM	5–6 MM	7–10 MM		?12 MM
EAR — FORM	FLAT, SHAPELESS; AREOLA RAISED (34); BEGINNING INCURVING SUPERIOR	INCURVING UPPER 2/3 PINNAE			WELL-DEFINED INCURVING TO LOBE		
EAR — CARTILAGE	PINNA SOFT, STAYS FOLDED; CARTILAGE SCANT RETURNS SLOWLY FROM FOLDING	THIN CARTILAGE SPRINGS BACK FROM FOLDING			PINNA FIRM, REMAINS ERECT FROM HEAD		
SOLE CREASES	SMOOTH SOLES ~ CREASES; 1–2 ANTERIOR CREASES (33); 2–3 ANTERIOR CREASES (34)	CREASES ANTERIOR 2/3 SOLE		CREASES INVOLVING HEEL		DEEPER CREASES OVER ENTIRE SOLE	
SKIN — THICKNESS & APPEARANCE	THIN, TRANSLUCENT SKIN, PLETHORIC, VENULES OVER ABDOMEN EDEMA; SMOOTH THICKER NO EDEMA (34)	PINK	FEW VESSELS		SOME DESQUAMATION PALE PINK	THICK, PALE, DESQUAMATION OVER ENTIRE BODY	
NAIL PLATES	AP- PEAR (20); NAILS TO FINGER TIPS					NAILS EXTEND WELL BEYOND FINGER TIPS	
HAIR	APPEARS ON HEAD; EYE BROWS & LASHES; FINE, WOOLLY, BUNCHES OUT FROM HEAD		SILKY, SINGLE STRANDS LAYS FLAT			?RECEDING HAIRLINE OR LOSS OF BABY HAIR, SHORT, FINE UNDERNEATH	
LANUGO	AP- PEARS (20); COVERS ENTIRE BODY; VANISHES FROM FACE				PRESENT ON SHOULDERS	NO LANUGO	
GENITALIA — TESTES	TESTES PALPABLE IN INGUINAL CANAL; IN UPPER SCROTUM					IN LOWER SCROTUM	
GENITALIA — SCROTUM	FEW RUGAE; RUGAE, ANTERIOR PORTION			RUGAE COVER		PENDULOUS	
GENITALIA — LABIA & CLITORIS	PROMINENT CLITORIS, LABIA MAJORA SMALL WIDELY SEPARATED; LABIA MAJORA LARGER NEARLY COVERED CLITORIS					LABIA MINORA & CLITORIS COVERED	
SKULL FIRMNESS	BONES ARE SOFT; SOFT TO 1" FROM ANTERIOR FONTANELLE; SPONGY AT EDGES OF FONTANELLE CENTER FIRM		BONES HARD, SUTURES EASILY DISPLACED			BONES HARD, CANNOT BE DISPLACED	
POSTURE — RESTING	HYPOTONIC LATERAL DECUBITUS; HYPOTONIC; BEGINNING FLEXION THIGH; STRONGER HIP FLEXION; FROG-LIKE; FLEXION ALL LIMBS			HYPERTONIC		VERY HYPERTONIC	
RECOIL — LEG	NO RECOIL; PARTIAL RECOIL; BEGIN FLEXION NO RE-COIL (34)	PROMPT RECOIL MAY BE INHIBITED				PROMPT RECOIL	
ARM	NO RECOIL		PROMPT RECOIL			PROMPT RECOIL AFTER 30" INHIBITION	

Weeks scale: 20 21 22 23 24 25 26 27 28 29 30 31 32 33 34 35 36 37 38 39 40 41 42 43 44 45 46 47 48

A

Confirmatory Neurologic Examination to be Done After 24 Hours

Mead Johnson LABORATORIES

WEEKS GESTATION: 20 21 22 23 24 25 26 27 28 29 30 31 32 33 34 35 36 37 38 39 40 41 42 43 44 45 46 47 48

PHYSICAL FINDINGS

TONE

- **HEEL TO EAR:** NO RESISTANCE → SOME RESISTANCE → IMPOSSIBLE
- **SCARF SIGN:** NO RESISTANCE → ELBOW PASSES MIDLINE → ELBOW AT MIDLINE → ELBOW DOES NOT REACH MIDLINE
- **NECK FLEXORS (HEAD LAG):** ABSENT → HEAD IN PLANE OF BODY → HOLDS HEAD
- **NECK EXTENSORS:** HEAD BEGINS TO RIGHT ITSELF FROM FLEXED POSITION → GOOD RIGHTING CANNOT HOLD IT → HOLDS HEAD FEW SECONDS → KEEPS HEAD IN LINE c̄ TRUNK >40″ → TURNS HEAD FROM SIDE TO SIDE
- **BODY EXTENSORS:** STRAIGHTENING OF LEGS → STRAIGHTENING OF TRUNK → STRAIGHTENING OF HEAD & TRUNK TOGETHER
- **VERTICAL POSITIONS:** WHEN HELD UNDER ARMS, BODY SLIPS THROUGH HANDS → ARMS HOLD BABY LEGS EXTENDED → LEGS FLEXED GOOD SUPPORT c̄ ARMS → HEAD ABOVE BACK
- **HORIZONTAL POSITIONS:** HYPOTONIC ARMS & LEGS STRAIGHT → ARMS AND LEGS FLEXED → HEAD & BACK EVEN FLEXED EXTREMITIES

FLEXION ANGLES

- **POPLITEAL:** NO RESISTANCE / 150° / 110° / 100° / 90° / 80°
- **ANKLE:** 45° / 20° / 30° / 0° — A PRE-TERM WHO HAS REACHED 40 WEEKS STILL HAS A 40° ANGLE
- **WRIST (SQUARE WINDOW):** 90° / 60° / 45° / 30° / 0°

REFLEXES

- **SUCKING:** WEAK NOT SYNCHRONIZED c̄ SWALLOWING → STRONGER SYNCHRONIZED → PERFECT → PERFECT HAND TO MOUTH
- **ROOTING:** LONG LATENCY PERIOD SLOW, IMPERFECT → HAND TO MOUTH → BRISK, COMPLETE, DURABLE
- **GRASP:** FINGER GRASP IS GOOD STRENGTH IS POOR → STRONGER → CAN LIFT BABY OFF BED INVOLVES ARMS → HANDS OPEN
- **MORO:** BARELY APPARENT → WEAK NOT ELICITED EVERY TIME → STRONGER → COMPLETE c̄ ARM EXTENSION OPEN FINGERS, CRY → ARM ADDUCTION ADDED → ?BEGINS TO LOSE MORO
- **CROSSED EXTENSION:** FLEXION & EXTENSION IN A RANDOM, PURPOSELESS PATTERN → EXTENSION BUT NO ADDUCTION → STILL INCOMPLETE → EXTENSION ADDUCTION FANNING OF TOES → COMPLETE
- **AUTOMATIC WALK:** MINIMAL → BEGINS TIPTOEING GOOD SUPPORT ON SOLE → FAST TIPTOEING → HEEL-TOE PROGRESSION WHOLE SOLE OF FOOT → A PRE-TERM WHO HAS REACHED 40 WEEKS WALKS ON TOES → ?BEGINS TO LOSE AUTOMATIC WALK
- **PUPILLARY REFLEX:** ABSENT → APPEARS → PRESENT
- **GLABELLAR TAP:** ABSENT → APPEARS → PRESENT
- **TONIC NECK REFLEX:** ABSENT → APPEARS → PRESENT AFTER 37 WEEKS
- **NECK-RIGHTING:** ABSENT → APPEARS → PRESENT AFTER 37 WEEKS

WEEKS: 20 21 22 23 24 25 26 27 28 29 30 31 32 33 34 35 36 37 38 39 40 41 42 43 44 45 46 47 48

B

*Brazie, J.V., and Lubchenco, L.O.: The Estimation of Gestational Age Chart, in Kempe, Silver and O'Brien: Current Pediatric Diagnosis and Treatment, ed. 3, Los Altos, California, Lange Medical Publications, 1974, chapter 3.

APPENDIX E   NATIONAL CENTER FOR HEALTH STATISTICS: PHYSICAL GROWTH PERCENTILES

GIRLS: BIRTH TO 36 MONTHS
PHYSICAL GROWTH
NCHS PERCENTILES*

NAME _____   RECORD # _____

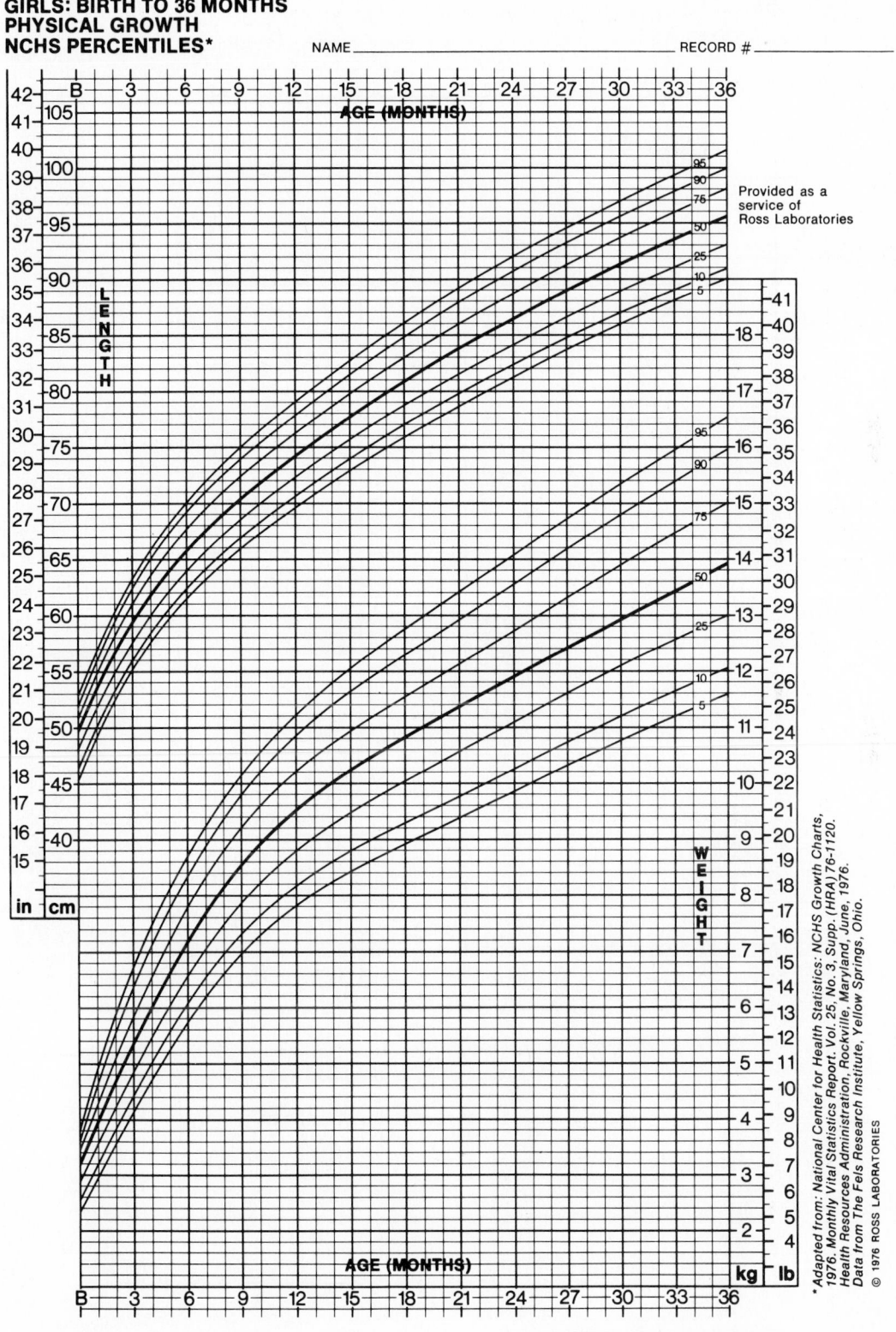

Provided as a service of Ross Laboratories

* Adapted from: National Center for Health Statistics: NCHS Growth Charts, 1976. Monthly Vital Statistics Report. Vol. 25, No. 3, Supp. (HRA) 76-1120. Health Resources Administration, Rockville, Maryland, June, 1976. Data from The Fels Research Institute, Yellow Springs, Ohio.

GIRLS: BIRTH TO 36 MONTHS
PHYSICAL GROWTH
NCHS PERCENTILES*

NAME _____ RECORD # _____

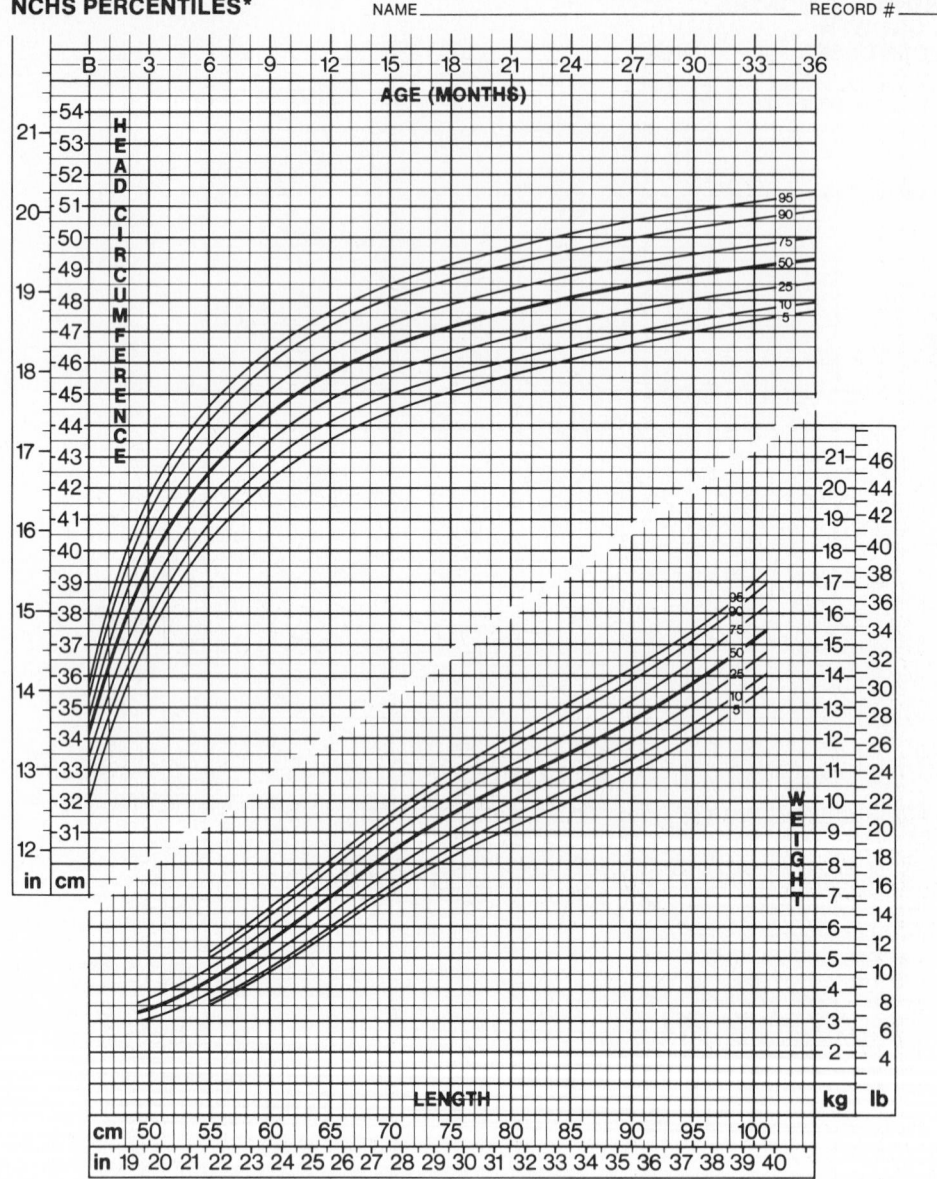

* Adapted from: National Center for Health Statistics: NCHS Growth Charts, 1976. Monthly Vital Statistics Report. Vol. 25, No. 3, Supp. (HRA) 76-1120. Health Resources Administration, Rockville, Maryland, June, 1976. Data from The Fels Research Institute, Yellow Springs, Ohio.

© 1976 ROSS LABORATORIES

DATE	AGE	LENGTH	WEIGHT	HEAD C.
	BIRTH			

DATE	AGE	LENGTH	WEIGHT	HEAD C.

BOYS: BIRTH TO 36 MONTHS
PHYSICAL GROWTH
NCHS PERCENTILES*

NAME_____ RECORD #_____

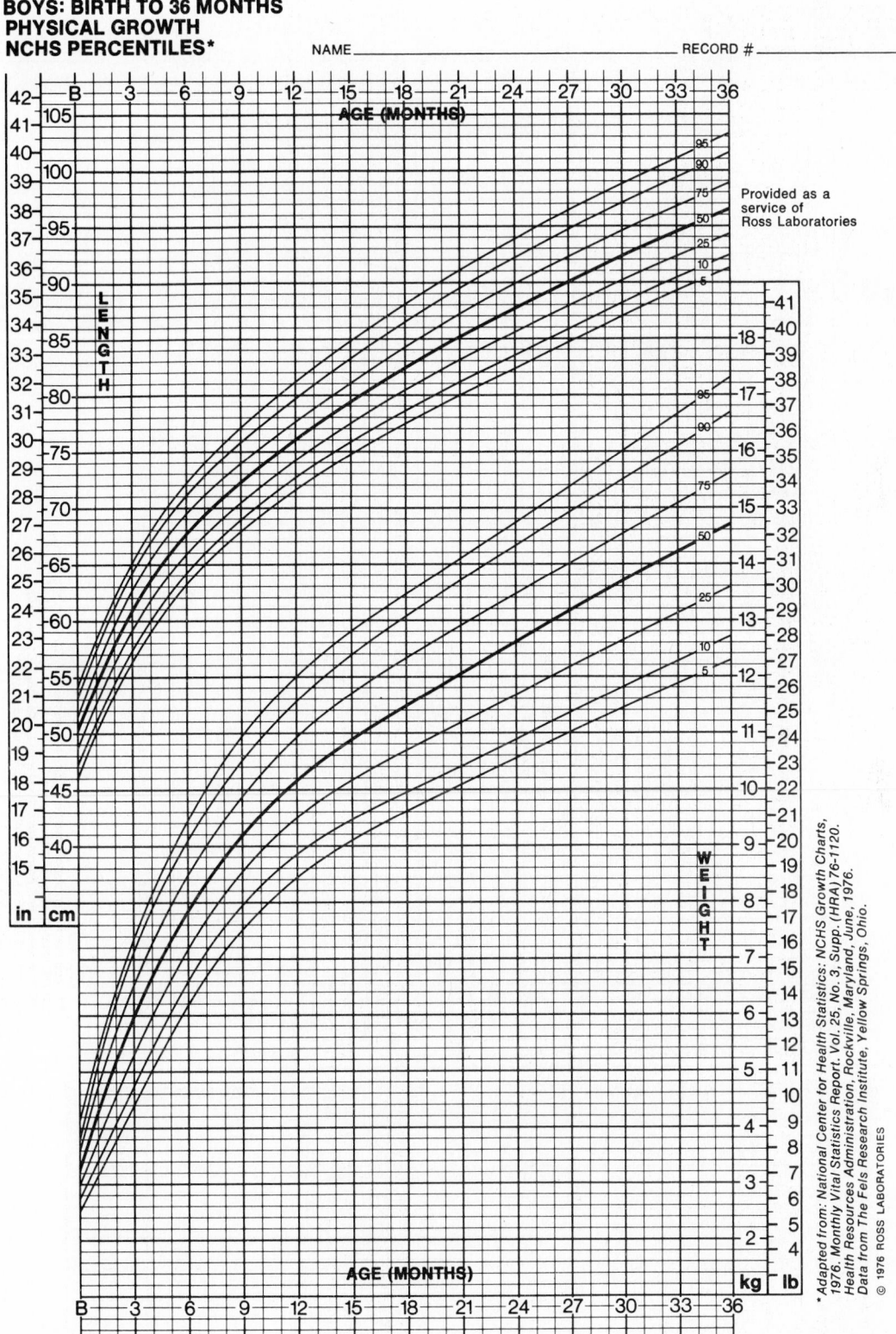

Provided as a
service of
Ross Laboratories

* Adapted from: National Center for Health Statistics: NCHS Growth Charts,
1976. Monthly Vital Statistics Report. Vol. 25, No. 3, Supp. (HRA) 76-1120.
Health Resources Administration. Rockville, Maryland, June, 1976.
Data from The Fels Research Institute, Yellow Springs, Ohio.
© 1976 ROSS LABORATORIES

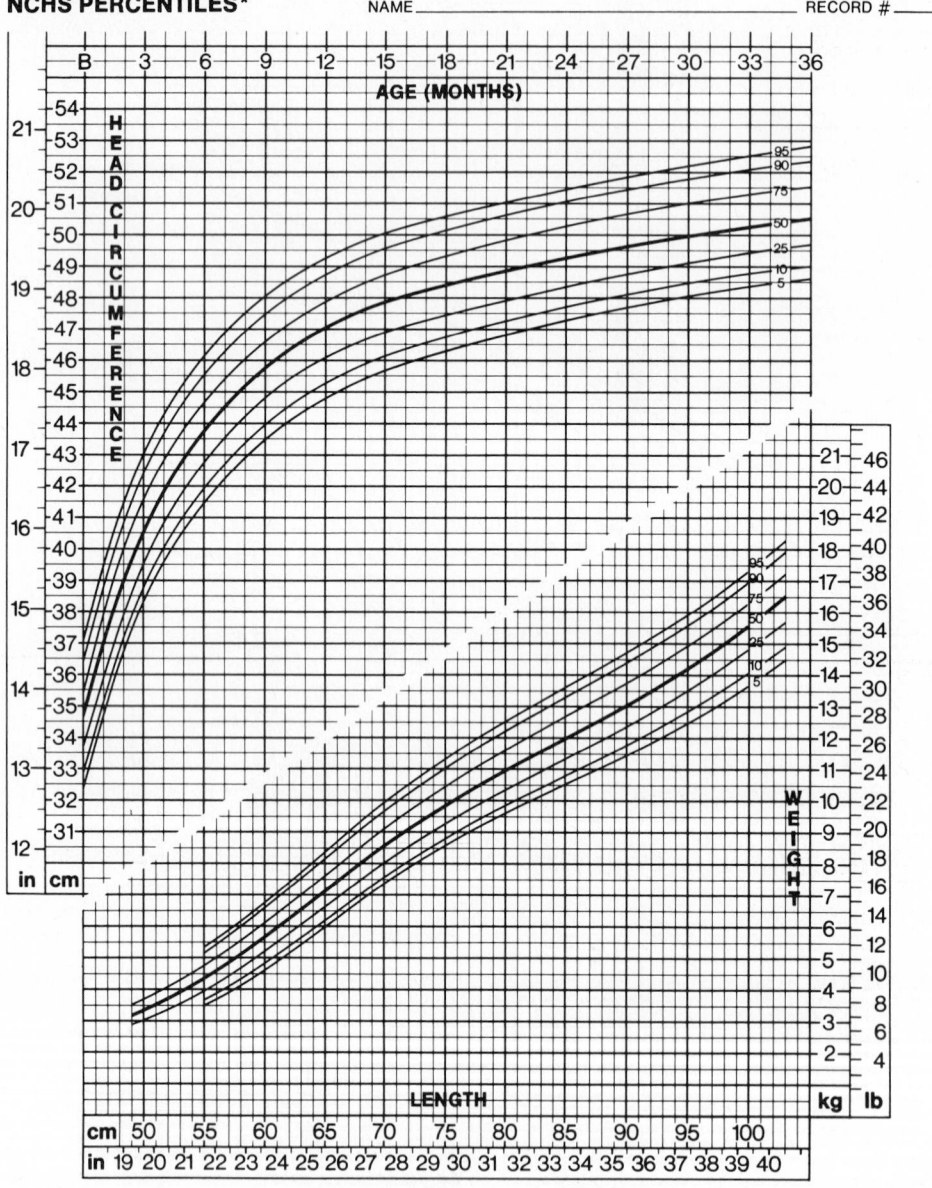

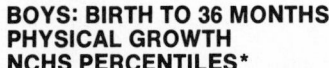

BOYS: BIRTH TO 36 MONTHS
PHYSICAL GROWTH
NCHS PERCENTILES*

NAME_____   RECORD #_____

* Adapted from: National Center for Health Statistics: NCHS Growth Charts,
1976. Monthly Vital Statistics Report. Vol. 25, No. 3, Supp. (HRA) 76-1120.
Health Resources Administration. Rockville, Maryland, June, 1976.
Data from The Fels Research Institute, Yellow Springs, Ohio.
© 1976 ROSS LABORATORIES

DATE	AGE	LENGTH	WEIGHT	HEAD C.
	BIRTH			

DATE	AGE	LENGTH	WEIGHT	HEAD C.

APPENDIX F   CONVERSIONS AND EQUIVALENTS

Temperature Conversion

(Fahrenheit temperature − 32) × $\frac{5}{9}$ = Celsius temperature
(Celsius temperature × $\frac{9}{5}$) + 32 = Fahrenheit temperature

Selected Conversions to Metric Measures

Known value	Multiply by	To find
inches	2.54	centimeters
ounces	28	grams
pounds	454	grams
pounds	0.45	kilograms

Selected Conversions from Metric Measures

Known value	Multiply by	To find
centimeters	0.4	inches
grams	0.035	ounces
grams	0.0022	pounds
kilograms	2.2	pounds

Conversion of Pounds and Ounces to Grams

POUNDS	\ OUNCES 0	1	2	3	4	5	6	7	8	9	10	11	12	13	14	15 (OUNCES)
0	–	28	57	85	113	142	170	198	227	255	283	312	340	369	397	425
1	454	482	510	539	567	595	624	652	680	709	737	765	794	822	850	879
2	907	936	964	992	1021	1049	1077	1106	1134	1162	1191	1219	1247	1276	1304	1332
3	1361	1389	1417	1446	1474	1503	1531	1559	1588	1616	1644	1673	1701	1729	1758	1786
4	1814	1843	1871	1899	1928	1956	1984	2013	2041	2070	2098	2126	2155	2183	2211	2240
5	2268	2296	2325	2353	2381	2410	2438	2466	2495	2523	2551	2580	2608	2637	2665	2693
6	2722	2750	2778	2807	2835	2863	2892	2920	2948	2977	3005	3033	3062	3090	3118	3147
7	3175	3203	3232	3260	3289	3317	3345	3374	3402	3430	3459	3487	3515	3544	3572	3600
8	3629	3657	3685	3714	3742	3770	3799	3827	3856	3884	3912	3941	3969	3997	4026	4054
9	4082	4111	4139	4167	4196	4224	4252	4281	4309	4337	4366	4394	4423	4451	4479	4508
10	4536	4564	4593	4621	4649	4678	4706	4734	4763	4791	4819	4848	4876	4904	4933	4961
11	4990	5018	5046	5075	5103	5131	5160	5188	5216	5245	5273	5301	5330	5358	5386	5415
12	5443	5471	5500	5528	5557	5585	5613	5642	5670	5698	5727	5755	5783	5812	5840	5868
13	5897	5925	5953	5982	6010	6038	6067	6095	6123	6152	6180	6209	6237	6265	6294	6322
14	6350	6379	6407	6435	6464	6492	6520	6549	6577	6605	6634	6662	6690	6719	6747	6776
15	6804	6832	6860	6889	6917	6945	6973	7002	7030	7059	7087	7115	7144	7172	7201	7228
16	7257	7286	7313	7342	7371	7399	7427	7456	7484	7512	7541	7569	7597	7626	7654	7682
17	7711	7739	7768	7796	7824	7853	7881	7909	7938	7966	7994	8023	8051	8079	8108	8136
18	8165	8192	8221	8249	8278	8306	8335	8363	8391	8420	8448	8476	8504	8533	8561	8590
19	8618	8646	8675	8703	8731	8760	8788	8816	8845	8873	8902	8930	8958	8987	9015	9043
20	9072	9100	9128	9157	9185	9213	9242	9270	9298	9327	9355	9383	9412	9440	9469	9497
21	9525	9554	9582	9610	9639	9667	9695	9724	9752	9780	9809	9837	9865	9894	9922	9950
22	9979	10007	10036	10064	10092	10120	10149	10177	10206	10234	10262	10291	10319	10347	10376	10404

GLOSSARY

abdominal   belonging or pertaining to the abdomen, its functions and disorders.

abdominal delivery   see *cesarean delivery.*

abdominal gestation   pregnancy within the abdominal cavity but outside the uterus.

abdominal hysterectomy   surgical removal of the uterus through an incision in the abdominal wall.

abduct   to draw away from the median plane of the body or one of its parts.

abortion   loss of pregnancy before the fetus is viable outside the uterus; miscarriage.

abruptio placentae   premature separation, partially or totally, of a normally implanted placenta.

abstinence   refraining voluntarily, especially from indulgence in food, alcoholic beverages, or sexual intercourse.

acceleration   periodic increase in the baseline fetal heart rate.

acini cells   secretory cells in the human breast that create milk from nutrients in the bloodstream.

acme   peak or highest point; time of greatest intensity (of a uterine contraction).

acrocyanosis   cyanosis of the extremities.

acromion   projection of the spine of the scapula, which forms the point of the shoulder.

adduct   to draw toward the main axis of the body.

adenomyoma   tumor that affects the glandular and smooth muscle tissue, such as the muscles of the uterus.

adnexa   adjoining or accessory parts of a structure, such as the uterine adnexa: the ovaries and fallopian tubes.

adolescence   period of human development initiated by puberty and ending with the attainment of young adulthood.

afibrinogenemia   absence of or decrease in fibrinogen in the blood plasma, so that the blood does not coagulate. This condition may be acquired or congenital, and it may result from such obstetric complications as abruptio placentae and retention of a dead fetus.

afterbirth   placenta and membranes expelled after the de-livery of the infant, during the third stage of labor; also called *secundines.*

afterpains   cramplike pains due to contractions of the uterus that occur after childbirth. They are more common in multiparas, tend to be most severe during nursing, and last 2–3 days.

agalactia   absence or failure of the secretion of breast milk.

alae nasi   nostrils.

albinism   a congenital absence of normal skin pigmentation.

albuminuria   readily detectable amounts of albumin in the urine.

allantois   tubular diverticulum of the posterior part of the embryo's yolk sac that passes into the body stalk. The allantoic blood vessels develop into the umbilical vein and paired umbilical arteries.

allele   one of a series of alternate genes at the same locus; one form of a gene.

alopecia   natural or abnormal loss of hair. May be partial or complete, local or generalized.

alveolus   a saclike cavity.

ambient   surrounding; that which is around us.

amblyopia   reduced vision that is not caused by visible changes in the eye or by refractive error.

amelia   absence of a limb.

amenorrhea   suppression or absence of menstruation.

amnesia   loss of memory.

amniocentesis   removal of amniotic fluid by insertion of a needle into the amniotic sac. Amniotic fluid is used for assessment of fetal health or fetal maturity and for providing information to aid in decisions about therapeutic abortion.

amniography   x-ray examination of the amniotic sac following the injection of radiopaque dye into the amniotic fluid.

amnion   the inner of the two membranes that form the sac containing the fetus and the amniotic fluid.

amnionitis   infection of the amniotic fluid.

1032

amnioscopy visualization of the amniotic fluid through the membranes with an amnioscope. This technique is used to identify meconium staining of the amniotic fluid.

amniotic relating or pertaining to the amnion.

amniotic fluid the liquid surrounding the fetus in utero. It absorbs shocks, permits fetal movements, and prevents heat loss.

amniotic sac the bag or sac formed by the amnion and containing the fetus.

anaerobic catabolism the breakdown of organized substances into simple compounds in the absence of free oxygen, with the release of energy.

analgesic drug that relieves pain and does not cause unconsciousness.

androgen substance producing male characteristics, such as the male hormone testosterone.

android pelvis male-type pelvis.

anencephaly congenital deformity in which the cerebrum, cerebellum, and flat bones of the skull are absent.

anesthesia partial or complete loss of sensation with or without loss of consciousness.

anomaly a malformation; an organ or structure that is abnormal in position, structure, or form.

anovular menstrual period cyclic uterine bleeding that is not preceded by ovulation.

anoxia deficiency of oxygen.

antenatal before birth.

antepartal before the onset of labor.

anterior pertaining to the front.

anterior fontanelle diamond-shaped area between the two frontal and two parietal bones just above the newborn's forehead.

anteroposterior repair surgical reconstruction of the upper and lower walls of the vagina to correct relaxed tissue.

anthropoid pelvis pelvis in which the anteroposterior diameter is equal to or greater than the transverse diameter.

antibody a specific protein substance developed by the body in response to specific antigens in order to restrict or destroy them.

antigen a substance formed within the body or introduced into it that induces the formation of antibodies.

antitoxin an antibody that is capable of neutralizing a specific toxin and that is produced by the body in response to the presence of the toxin.

Apert syndrome an autosomal dominant disorder characterized by mental deficiency, irregular craniosynostosis, high full forehead and flat occiput, flat facies, hypertelorism, narrow palate, and syndactyly.

Apgar score the Apgar scoring system is used to evaluate newborns at 1 minute and 5 minutes after delivery. The total score is achieved by assessing five signs: heart rate, respiratory effort, muscle tone, reflex irritability, and color. Each of the signs is assigned a score of 0, 1, or 2. The highest possible score is 10.

apnea a condition that occurs when respirations cease for more than 25 seconds, with generalized cyanosis.

areola pigmented ring surrounding the nipple of the breast.

Arnold-Chiari malformation a condition in which the inferior poles of the cerebellar hemispheres and the medulla protrude and may herniate through the foramen magnum. This is one of the causes of hydrocephaly and is usually accompanied by spina bifida or meningomyelocele.

AROM artifical rupture of (amniotic) membranes through use of a device such as amnihook or allis forceps.

articulation connection of bones in the skeleton; joint. Classified as (1) immovable, (2) slightly movable, and (3) freely movable.

artificial insemination introduction of viable semen into the vagina by artificial means for the purpose of impregnation.

Aschheim-Zondek test a test for pregnancy in which the woman's urine is injected subcutaneously into a mouse. After 5 days, the animal is killed and its ovaries examined. Enlarged ovaries and maturing follicles indicate pregnancy.

asphyxia a condition caused by a decreased amount of oxygen or an excess amount of carbon dioxide in the body.

aspiration syndrome a condition that occurs with fetal hypoxia: the anal sphincter relaxes and meconium is expelled; reflex gasping movements draw meconium and other particulate matter in the amniotic fluid into the bronchial tree, thereby obstructing air flow after birth.

asynclitism an oblique presentation of the fetal head; the pelvic planes and those of the fetal head are not parallel.

atelectasis a condition in which the lungs of a fetus remain unexpanded at birth; it involves alveolar collapse. May be partial or complete.

atony lack of normal muscle tone.

atresia congenital absence or pathologic closure of a normal anatomic opening. See also *biliary atresia; choanal atresia.*

attitude attitude of the fetus refers to the relationship of the fetal parts to each other.

auscultation process of listening for sounds produced within the body in order to detect abnormal conditions.

autosome a chromosome that is not a sex chromosome.

axis a line, real or imaginary, that a part revolves around or that runs through the center of the body.

azoospermic absence of spermatozoa in the semen.

bacteriuria existence of bacteria in the urine.

bag of waters the membrane containing the amniotic fluid and the fetus.

balanced translocation rearrangement of chromosomal material in which a piece of one chromosome is broken off and joined to another chromosome. An individual with a balanced translocation has the normal amount of genetic material but it is arranged abnormally, making the individual at risk for producing offspring with chromosomal abnormalities.

ballottement a technique of palpation to detect or examine a floating object in the body. In obstetrics, the fetus, when pushed, floats away and then returns to touch the examiner's fingers.

Bandl's ring a thickened ridge of uterine musculature between the upper and lower segments that occurs following a mechanically obstructed labor, with the lower segment thinning abnormally.

Barr body deeply staining chromatin mass located against the inner surface of the cell nucleus. Found only in normal females; also called *sex chromatin*.

Bartholin glands two small mucous glands situated on each side of the vaginal orifice that secrete small amounts of mucus during coitus.

battledore placenta placenta in which the umbilical cord is inserted on the periphery rather than centrally.

Beckwith syndrome syndrome of unknown etiology characterized by macroglossia, omphalocele, macrosomia, ear creases, neonatal polycythemia, diastasis recti, and cryptorchidism.

Bell palsy distortion of the face caused by a lesion of the facial nerve, resulting in peripheral facial paralysis.

bicornuate uterus anomalous uterus resulting from incomplete union of the müllerian ducts. May be double or single with two horns.

biliary atresia absence of the bile duct.

bilirubin orange or yellowish pigment in bile; a breakdown product of hemoglobin that is carried by the blood to the liver, where it is chemically changed and excreted in the bile or is conjugated and excreted in the stools.

bimanual performed with both hands.

bimanual palpation examination of the pelvic organs by placing one hand on the abdomen and one or two fingers of the other hand into the vagina.

biopsy excision of a small piece of tissue for microscopic examination and diagnosis.

birth rate number of live births per 1000 population.

birth stool a small wooden chair that a woman may sit on during labor and delivery.

Bishop score a prelabor scoring system to assist in predicting whether an induction of labor may be successful. The total score is achieved by assessing five components: cervical dilatation, cervical effacement, cervical consistency, cervical position, and fetal station. Each of the components is assigned a score of 0–3, and the highest possible score is 13.

blastoderm germinal membrane of the ovum.

bleeding diathesis predisposition to abnormal blood clotting.

born out of asepsis (BOA) a birth that takes place without the use of sterile technique.

brachial palsy partial or complete paralysis of portions of the arm. Results from trauma to the brachial plexus during a difficult delivery.

bradycardia slow heart rate.

Braxton Hicks sign intermittent painless contractions of the uterus that may occur every 10–20 minutes. They occur more frequently toward the end of pregnancy and are sometimes mistaken for true labor pains.

Braxton Hicks version a maneuver designed to turn the fetus from an undesirable position to a more desirable one to facilitate delivery.

breast milk jaundice yellowing of the infant's skin caused by pregnandiol in the mother's milk. Pregnandiol inhibits glucuronyl transferase, the enzyme necessary for the conjugation of bilirubin.

breech presentation a delivery in which the buttocks and/or feet are presented instead of the head. Occurs in approximately 3% of all deliveries.

bregma juncture of the coronal and sagittal sutures of the skull; the area of the anterior fontanelle of the fetus; the brow.

brim the edge of the superior strait of the true pelvis; the inlet.

bronchopulmonary dysplasia chronic pulmonary disease of multifactorial etiology characterized initially by alveolar and bronchial necrosis, which results in bronchial metaplasia and interstitial fibrosis. Appears in x-ray films as generalized small, radiolucent cysts within the lungs.

brown fat fat deposits in neonates that provide greater heat-generating activity than ordinary fat. Found around the kidneys, adrenals, and neck, between the scapulas, and behind the sternum.

Brudzinski sign in the presence of meningitis, bending the patient's neck produces flexion of the patient's lower extremities.

café-au-lait spots light brown (coffee with cream) marks that appear on the body. The presence of more than six such spots may be accompanied by a neurologic disorder.

caked breasts accumulation of milk in the secreting ducts of the breast after delivery; see also *engorgement*.

calcaneus the heel bone, which articulates with the cuboid bone anteriorly and with the astragalus bone above.

calcemia increased amount of serum calcium.

Candida albicans a fungus causing infections such as moniliasis and thrush.

caput the head; the occiput of the fetal head, which appears at the vaginal introitus prior to delivery of the head.

caput succedaneum swelling or edema occurring in or under the fetal scalp during labor.

cardinal movements of labor encompasses the positional changes of the fetus as it moves through the birth canal during labor and delivery. The positional changes are descent, flexion, internal rotation, extension, restitution, and external rotation.

carrier (1) an individual possessing an abnormal gene or chromosome who manifests no outward signs but who can pass the abnormality on to offspring. (2) A person who harbors a specific pathogenic organism in the absence of identifiable disease and is capable of spreading the disease to others.

catamenia menses.

catarrhal symptoms symptoms associated with inflammation of the mucous membranes, causing redness and mucoid drainage.

caudal anesthesia regional anesthesia used in childbirth in which the anesthetic agent is injected into the caudal area of the spinal canal through the sacral hiatus, affecting the caudal nerve roots and thereby providing anesthesia to the cervix, vagina, and perineum.

caul membranes or portions of the amnion covering the fetal head during delivery.

cautery method of destroying tissue by the use of heat, electricity, chemicals, or freezing.

centimeter unit of measurement used to describe cervical dilatation. Used interchangeably with "fingers" (one "finger" equals 2 cm).

cephalhematoma subcutaneous swelling containing blood found on the head of an infant several days after delivery. Usually disappears within a few weeks to 2 months.

cephalic pertaining to the head.

cephalic presentation delivery in which the fetal head is presenting against the cervix.

cephalopelvic disproportion (CPD) a condition in which the fetal head is of a shape, size, or position that it cannot pass through the maternal pelvis.

cerebral palsy nonprogressive form of brain damage appearing up to the third year of life and resulting in motor dysfunction.

certified nurse-midwife see *midwife*.

cervical cauterization destruction of the superficial tissue of the cervix by heat, electric current, or freezing.

cervical conization excision of a cone-shaped section of tissue from the endocervix.

cervical erosion chronic irritation or infection that causes an alteration in the epithelium of the cervix.

cervical esophagostomy surgical formation of an opening from the esophagus to the neck region.

cervical os the small opening of the cervix that dilates during the first stage of labor. See also *external os; internal os.*

cervical polyp a small tumor or a stem or pedicle attached to the inside of the cervix.

cervical stenosis narrowing of the canal between the body of the uterus and the cervical os.

cervicitis infection of the cervix.

cervix the "neck" between the external os and the body of the uterus. The lower end of the cervix extends into the vagina.

cesarean hysterectomy surgical removal of the uterus immediately after cesarean delivery.

cesarean delivery delivery of the fetus by means of an incision into the abdominal wall and the uterus; also called *abdominal delivery.*

Chadwick's sign violet bluish color of the vaginal mucous membrane caused by increased vascularity; visible from about the fourth week of pregnancy.

change of life see *climacteric.*

chignon a raised area on the vertex of the fetal head as a result of the negative pressure exerted on this area with the use of a vacuum extractor during delivery.

childbed fever see *puerperal sepsis.*

chloasma brownish pigmentation over the bridge of the nose and the cheeks during pregnancy and in some women who are taking oral contraceptives. Also called *mask of pregnancy.*

choanal atresia complete obstruction of the posterior nares by membranous or bony tissue.

chorioamnionitis an inflammation of the amniotic membranes stimulated by organisms in the amniotic fluid, which then becomes infiltrated with polymorphonuclear leukocytes.

chorioepithelioma carcinoma of the chorion, with rapid malignant proliferation of the epithelium of the chorionic villi.

chorion the fetal membrane closest to the intrauterine wall; it gives rise to the placenta and continues as the outer membrane surrounding the amnion.

chorionic villi threadlike projections growing in tufts on the external chorionic surface that project into the maternal uterine sinuses; they help form the placenta and secrete human chorionic gonadotropin.

chromatids the two longitudinal halves of each chromosome.

chromosomes the threadlike structures within the nucleus of a cell that carry the genes.

cilia   hairlike processes that project from epithelial cells and that serve to propel mucus, pus, and dust particles.

circumcision   surgical excision of the prepuce (foreskin) of the penis.

circumoral cyanosis   bluish appearance around the mouth.

circumvallate placenta   a placenta with a thick white fibrous ring around the edge.

cleavage   rapid mitotic division of the zygote; cells produced are called blastomeres.

cleft palate   incomplete closure of the roof of the mouth, producing a passageway between the mouth and nasal cavity. May be unilateral or bilateral, complete or incomplete.

climacteric   period marking the cessation of menstruation and the end of a woman's reproductive abilities; the body undergoes significant physiologic and psychologic changes. Also called *change of life* or *menopause*.

clitoris   female organ homologous to the male penis; a small oval body of erectile tissue situated at the anterior junction of the vulva.

clubfoot   see *talipes equinovarus*.

coccyx   a small bone at the base of the spinal column.

colostrum   secretion from the breast before the onset of true lactation; contains mainly serum and white blood corpuscles. It has a high protein content, provides some immune properties, and cleanses the neonate's intestinal tract of mucus and meconium.

colpectomy   surgical excision of the vagina.

colporrhaphy   suturing of the vagina.

colpotomy   incision into the wall of the vagina.

complementary feeding   additional feeding given to the infant if still hungry after breast-feeding.

complete dilatation   occurs when the cervix is sufficiently dilated for the infant to pass through; usually 10 cm or five "fingers."

conception   union of male sperm and female ovum; fertilization.

conceptional age   the number of complete weeks since the moment of conception. Because the moment of conception is almost impossible to determine, conceptional age is estimated at 2 weeks less than gestational age.

condyloma   wartlike growth of the skin, usually seen on the external genitals or anus. There are two types, a pointed variety and a broad, flat form usually found with syphilis.

congenital   present at birth.

conjoined twins   twins attached to each other, either at one small part of the body or in varying degrees up to complete sharing of the body with two heads. One twin may be small and underdeveloped, attached to the other twin parasitically.

conjugate   important diameter of the pelvis, measured from the center of the promontory of the sacrum to the back of the symphysis pubis. The diagonal conjugate is measured and the true conjugate estimated.

conjunctivitis   inflammation of the mucous membrane lining the eyelids.

consanguinity   blood relationship by descent from a common ancestor.

contraception   the prevention of conception or impregnation.

contraction   tightening and shortening of the uterine muscles during labor, causing effacement and dilatation of the cervix; contributes to the downward and outward descent of the fetus.

Coombs' test   a test for antiglobulins in the red cells. The indirect test determines the presence of Rh-positive antibodies in maternal blood; the direct test determines the presence of maternal Rh-positive antibodies in fetal cord blood.

copulation   sexual intercourse; coitus.

Cornelia DeLange syndrome   characterized by micromelia, a down-turning upper lip, shortness of stature, mental retardation, microbrachycephaly, bushy eyebrows, long curly eyelashes, high-arched palate, micrognathia, hirsutism, simian crease. Etiology unknown.

corona radiata   a ring of elongated cells surrounding the zona pellucida.

corpus luteum   a small yellow body that develops within a ruptured ovarian follicle; it secretes progesterone in the second half of the menstrual cycle and atrophies about three days before the beginning of menstrual flow. If pregnancy occurs, it continues to produce progesterone until the placenta takes over this function.

cotyledon   one of the rounded portions into which the placenta's uterine surface is divided, consisting of a mass of villi, fetal vessels, and an intervillous space.

couvade   in some cultures, the male's observance of certain rituals and taboos to signify the transition to fatherhood.

Couvelaire uterus   purplish discoloration and boardlike rigidity of the uterus caused by accumulation of blood in the interstitial myometrium of the uterus from premature separation and subsequent hemorrhage of the placenta.

CPD   see *cephalopelvic disproportion*.

cradle cap   an oily, yellowish crust that may appear on the newborn's scalp and that is caused by excessive secretion of the sebaceous glands in the scalp; also called *seborrhea dermatus*.

craniosynostosis   premature closure of cranial sutures.

Credé's maneuver   an obsolete method of expelling the placenta by downward manual pressure on the uterus through the abdominal wall.

crepitus (1) sound produced when pressure is applied to tissues containing abnormal amounts of air; (2) grating sound heard when broken bone ends are moved; (3) noise of gas being expelled from intestines.

cretinism condition caused by congenital lack of thyroid gland secretion; characteristics include arrested physical and mental development.

cri-du-chat syndrome chromosomal disorder characterized by microcephaly, downward slant of palpebral fissures, catlike cry, low birth weight, mental deficiency, hypotonia, and simian crease. Caused by partial deletion of the short arm of chromosome number 5.

crisis any naturally occurring turning point, such as courtship, marriage, pregnancy, parenthood, death.

Crouzon syndrome an autosomal dominant disorder of variable expression characterized by premature craniosynostosis, maxillary hypoplasia, and shallow orbits.

crowning appearance of the presenting fetal part at the vaginal orifice during labor.

CST contraction stress test. A method for assessing the reaction (or response) of the fetus to the stress of the uterine contractions. This test may be utilized when contractions are occurring spontaneously or when contractions are artifically induced by OCT (oxytocin challenge test) or BSST (breast self-stimulation test).

cul-de-sac of Douglas retrouterine pouch formed by an extension of the peritoneal cavity that lies between the rectum and the posterior wall of the uterus.

culture the ideas, customs, traditions, arts, and so on of a particular group of people.

curettage removal of the contents of the uterus by scraping of the endometrial lining with a curette. Done to obtain specimens for diagnostic purposes or following an abortion.

cutis marmorata purplish discoloration of skin on exposure to cold. A transient vasomotor response occurring primarily over the extremities of the infant; occasionally seen in an infant in respiratory distress.

cyesis pregnancy.

cystocele hernia of the bladder. Injury to the vesicovaginal fascia during delivery may allow herniation of the bladder into the vagina.

cytogenetics branch of genetics dealing with the study of chromosomes and associated gene behavior.

deceleration periodic decrease in the baseline fetal heart rate.

decidua endometrium or mucous membrane lining of the uterus in pregnancy that is shed after giving birth.

decidua basalis the part of the decidua that unites with the chorion to form the placenta. It is shed in lochial discharge after delivery.

decidua capsularis the part of the decidua surrounding the chorionic sac.

decidua vera nonplacental decidua lining the uterus.

decrement decrease or stage of decline, as of a contraction.

deletion in genetics, the loss of a chromosomal segment.

delivery expulsion of the infant with placenta and membranes from the woman at birth.

democratic family a family in which there is a high degree of equality and mutuality.

deoxyribonucleic acid (DNA) intracellular complex protein carrying genetic information; consists of two purines (adenine and guanine) and two pyrimidines (thymine and cystosine).

dermatoglyphics study of the surface markings and skin ridge patterns on fingers, toes, palms of hands, and soles of feet; useful in identification and in genetic studies.

desquamation shedding of the epithelial cells of the epidermis.

diagonal conjugate distance from the lower posterior border of the symphysis pubis to the sacral promontory; may be obtained by manual measurement.

diaphragmatic hernia failure of the diaphragm to fuse, resulting in protrusion of the abdominal contents through the diaphragm into the thoracic cavity. May be congenital or traumatic.

diastasis recti abdominis separation of the recti abdominis muscles along the median line. In women, seen with repeated childbirths or multiple gestation. In the newborn, usually caused by incomplete development.

diathesis hereditary predisposition to some abnormality or disease. See also *bleeding diathesis*.

DIC disseminated intravascular coagulation. May also be called consumption coagulopathy.

dilatation of the cervix expansion of the external os from an opening a few millimeters in size to an opening large enough to allow the passage of infant.

dilatation and curettage (D and C) stretching of the cervical canal to permit passage of a curette, which is used to scrape the endometrium to empty the uterine contents or to obtain tissue for examination.

dilatational phase of labor phase in which active cervical dilatation takes place.

diploid containing a set of maternal and a set of paternal chromosomes. In humans the diploid number of chromosomes is 46.

discordance discrepancy in size (or other indicators) between twins.

disparate twins twins that are different from one another, as in weight or appearance; most likely fraternal twins.

dizygotic twins   fetuses that develop from two fertilized ova; also called *fraternal twins*.

Döderlein bacillus   gram positive bacterium found in normal vaginal secretions.

dominant gene   a gene that is expressed in the heterozygous state. In a dominant disorder the mutant gene overshadows the normal gene.

Down syndrome   an abnormality resulting from the presence of an extra chromosome number 21 (trisomy 21); characteristics include mental retardation and altered physical appearance. Formerly called Mongolism or Mongoloid idiocy.

dry labor   lay term referring to labor in which amniotic fluid has already escaped. In reality, there is no such thing as a "dry labor."

ductus arteriosus   a communication channel between the main pulmonary artery and the aorta of the fetus. It is obliterated after birth by a rising Po_2 and changes in intravascular pressure in the presence of normal pulmonary functioning. It normally becomes a ligament after birth but sometimes remains patent (patent ductus arteriosus), a treatable condition.

ductus venosus   a fetal blood vessel that carries oxygenated blood between the umbilical vein and the inferior vena cava, bypassing the liver; it becomes a ligament after birth.

Duncan's mechanism   occurs when the maternal surface of the placenta presents upon delivery rather than the shiny fetal surface.

dyscrasia   incompatible mixture, such as fetal and maternal blood incompatibility.

dysfunctional uterine bleeding   abnormal bleeding from the uterus for reasons that are not readily established.

dysmenorrhea   painful or difficult menstruation; may be primary or secondary.

dyspareunia   painful sexual intercourse.

dyspnea   difficult or labored breathing.

dystocia   difficult labor due to mechanical factors produced by the fetus or the maternal pelvis, or due to inadequate uterine or other muscular activity.

ecchymosis   bleeding into tissue caused by direct trauma, serious infection, or bleeding diathesis.

eclampsia   a major complication of pregnancy of unknown cause. It occurs more often in the primigravida and is accompanied by elevated blood pressure, albuminuria, oliguria, tonic and clonic convulsions, and coma. May occur during pregnancy (usually after the twentieth week of gestation) or within 48 hours after delivery.

ectoderm   outer layer of cells in the developing embryo that give rise to the skin, nails, and hair.

ectopic   in an abnormal position.

ectopic pregnancy   implantation of the fertilized ovum outside the uterine cavity; common sites are the abdomen, fallopian tubes, and ovaries; also called *oocyesis*.

EDC   estimated date of confinement.

effacement   thinning and shortening of the cervix that occurs late in pregnancy or during labor.

effleurage   gentle stroking used in massage.

EFM   electronic fetal monitoring.

ejaculation   ejaculation of the seminal fluids from the penis.

Ellis-Van Creveld syndrome   autosomal recessive syndrome characterized by small stature with disproportionally short extremities, polydactyly of fingers and/or toes, hypoplastic nails, and short upper lip. One half the patients also have a cardiac defect.

embolus   undissolved matter present in a blood vessel brought there by the blood or lymph current; may be solid, liquid, or gaseous.

embryo   the early stage of development of the young of any organism. In humans, the period from about 2–8 weeks' gestation, which is characterized by cellular differentiation and predominantly hyperplastic growth.

empathy   objective awareness of and insight into the emotions, feelings, and behavior of another person and their meaning and significance.

en face   an assumed position in which one person looks at another and maintains his or her face in the same vertical plane as that of the other.

enanthem   eruption of the mucous membrane, such as Koplik's spots.

endocervical   pertaining to the interior of the canal of the cervix of the uterus.

endocrine glands   glands that secrete special substances (hormones) that regulate body functions.

endoderm   the inner layer of cells in the developing embryo that give rise to internal organs such as the intestines.

endometriosis   ectopic endometrium located outside the uterus in the pelvic cavity. Symptoms may include pelvic pain or pressure, dysmenorrhea, dyspareunia, abnormal bleeding from the uterus or rectum, and sterility.

endometrium   the mucous membrane that lines the inner surface of the uterus.

engagement   the entrance of the fetal presenting part into the superior pelvic strait and the beginning of the descent through the pelvic canal.

engorgement   vascular congestion or distention. In obstetrics, the swelling of breast tissue brought about by an increase in blood and lymph supply to the breast, preceding true lactation.

enuresis   involuntary urination; may be complete or partial, diurnal or nocturnal, depending upon pathologic or functional causes.

enzygotic developed from one fertilized ovum.

epicanthus a fold of skin that extends from the top of the nose to the median end of the eyebrow, covering the inner canthus.

episiotomy incision of the perineum to facilitate delivery and to avoid laceration of the perineum.

epispadias congenital opening of the urethra on the dorsum of the penis, or opening by separation of the labia minora and a fissure of the clitoris (rare).

Epstein's pearls small, white blebs found along the gum margins and at the junction of the soft and hard palates; commonly seen in the newborn as a normal manifestation.

Erb's palsy paralysis of the arm and chest wall as a result of a birth injury to the brachial plexus or a subsequent injury to the fifth and sixth cervical nerves.

ergot a drug that stimulates the smooth muscles of blood vessels and the uterus, causing vasoconstriction and uterine contractions. Obtained from *Claviceps purpurea,* a fungus.

erythema toxicum innocuous pink papular rash of unknown cause with superimposed vesicles that appears within 24–48 hours after birth and resolves spontaneously within a few days.

erythroblastosis fetalis hemolytic disease of the newborn characterized by anemia, jaundice, enlargement of the liver and spleen, and generalized edema. Caused by isoimmunization due to Rh incompatibility or ABO incompatibility.

escutcheon pattern of distribution of pubic hair.

esophageal atresia a malformation in which the esophagus ends in a blind pouch or narrows into a thin cord, failing to form a passage to the stomach.

estrangement in obstetrics, a condition that occurs when the mother is diverted from establishing a normal relationship with her newborn because of separation caused by illness or preterm birth.

estriol metabolic product of estrone and estradiol found in the urine of pregnant women.

estrogen the hormones estradiol and estrone, produced by the ovary.

estrus cyclic period of sexual activity in female mammals.

eugenics the science that deals with the improvement of the human race through control of genetic factors.

euthenics the science that deals with the improvement of the human race through control of environmental factors.

exanthem any eruption of the skin; frequently accompanies infectious diseases.

exchange transfusion the replacement of 70%–80% of circulating blood by withdrawing the recipient's blood and injecting a donor's blood in equal amounts, for the purpose of preventing the accumulation of bilirubin or other byproducts of hemolysis in the blood.

exostosis benign cartilage-covered bony growth on the surface of a bone, often caused by chronic irritation.

exotoxin a toxin produced by microorganisms and excreted into the surrounding medium.

expiratory grunt a sign of respiratory distress indicative of the newborn's attempt to hold air in the alveoli for better gaseous exchange.

expressivity the extent to which a gene is expressed in an individual.

expulsive contractions labor contractions that are effective in contracting the uterine muscle; characteristic of the second stage of labor.

exstrophy of the bladder exposure and eversion of the posterior and lateral walls of the bladder and trigone because of failure of the anterior wall and symphysis pubis to unite.

external os the opening between the cervix and the vagina.

extraperitoneal occurring or located outside the peritoneal cavity.

extrauterine occurring outside the uterus.

extrauterine pregnancy ectopic pregnancy in which the fertilized ovum implants outside the uterus.

facies pertaining to the appearance or expression of the face; certain congenital syndromes typically present with a specific facial appearance.

failure to thrive (FTT) term used to describe the infant or child whose growth and development pattern falls below the norms for his or her age.

fallopian tubes tubes that extend from the lateral angle of the uterus and terminate near the ovary; they serve as a passageway for the ovum from the ovary to the uterus and for the spermatozoa from the uterus toward the ovary. Also called *oviducts* and *uterine tubes.*

false labor contractions of the uterus, regular or irregular, that may be strong enough to be interpreted as true labor but that do not dilate the cervix.

familial the presence of a trait or disorder in more than one member of a family; not necessarily inherited.

family a group of people united by marriage, blood, or adoption, residing in the same household, maintaining a common culture, and interacting with each other on the basis of their roles within the group. See also *democratic family; nuclear family; traditional family.*

fecundation impregnation; fertilization.

ferning Formation of palm-leaf pattern by the crystallization of cervical mucus as it dries at midmenstrual cycle. Helpful in determining time of ovulation. Observed via microscopic examination of a thin layer of cervical mucus on a glass slide. This pattern is also observed when amniotic fluid is allowed to air dry on a slide and is a useful and quick test to determine whether amniotic membranes have ruptured.

fertility ability to reproduce.

fertility rate number of births per 1000 women age 15–44 in a given population per year.

fertilization impregnation of an ovum by a spermatozoon.

fetal pertaining or relating to the fetus.

fetal alcohol syndrome (FAS) syndrome caused by maternal alcohol ingestion and characterized by microcephaly, intrauterine growth retardation, short palpebral fissures, and maxillary hypoplasia.

fetal alveoli terminal pulmonary sacs that in fetal life are filled with fluid that is a transudate of fetal plasma.

fetal death death of the developing fetus after 20 weeks' gestation. Also called *fetal demise.*

fetal distress evidence that the fetus is in jeopardy, such as a change in fetal activity or heart rate.

fetal heart rate (FHR) the number of times the fetal heart beats per minute; normal range is 120–160 beats per minute.

fetal heart tones (FHTs) the fetal heartbeat as heard through the mother's abdominal wall.

fetal lie relationship of the long axis of the fetus to the long axis of the mother.

fetotoxic destructive or poisonous to the fetus.

fetoscope an adaptation of a stethoscope that facilitates auscultation of the fetal heart rate.

fetus the child in utero from about the seventh to ninth week of gestation until birth.

FHTs see *fetal heart tones.*

fibroid See *leiomyoma.*

fimbria any structure resembling a fringe; the fringelike extremity of the fallopian tubes.

first stage of labor period of time extending from the onset of regular contractions to the complete dilatation of the cervix.

fissure an open crack or groove in tissue.

fistula an abnormal tubelike passage that forms between two normal cavities or to a free surface; may be congenital or caused by trauma, abscesses, or inflammatory processes.

flaccid flabby, relaxed; absent or defective muscle tone.

flaring of nostrils widening of nostrils during inspiration in the presence of air hunger; a sign of respiratory distress.

flexion in obstetrics, a situation that occurs when resistance to the descent of the infant down the birth canal causes its head to flex, or bend, the chin approaching the chest, thus reducing the diameter of the presenting part.

follicle a small secretory cavity or sac.

follicle-stimulating hormone (FSH) hormone produced by the anterior pituitary during the first half of the menstrual cycle, stimulating development of the graafian follicle.

fontanelle in the fetus, an unossified space or soft spot consisting of a strong band of connective tissue lying between the cranial bones of the skull.

footling a breech presentation in which one or both feet present.

foramen ovale septal opening between the atria of the fetal heart. Normally, the opening closes shortly after birth; if it remains open, it can be surgically repaired.

forceps obstetric instruments occasionally used to aid in delivery.

Fordyce spots yellowish white papules on the oral mucosa; may be present at birth.

foreskin loose skin covering the end of the penis or clitoris; prepuce.

fornix a body with a vaultlike or arched shape.

fornix of the vagina the anterior and posterior spaces into which the upper vagina is divided; formed by the protrusion of the cervix into the vagina.

fossa shallow depression or furrow.

fourchette transverse fold of mucous membranes at the posterior angle of the vagina that connects the posterior ends of the labia minora.

fraternal twins see *dizygotic twins.*

fremitus vibratory tremors felt through the chest wall by palpation.

frenulum thin ridge of tissue extending from the floor of the mouth to the inferior surface of the tongue along its midline.

Friedman graph a method of describing and recording labor progress.

Friedman's test modification of the Aschheim-Zondek pregnancy test in which the woman's urine is injected into a mature, unmated female rabbit. After 2 days, the rabbit's ovaries are examined; the presence of fresh corpora lutea or hemorrhagic corpora constitutes a positive test.

FSH see *follicle-stimulating hormone.*

fundus the upper portion of the uterus between the fallopian tubes.

funic souffle hissing sound synchronous with the fetal heartbeat and considered to be produced in the umbilical cord.

funis a cordlike structure, such as the umbilical cord.

furuncle a boil.

galactagogue an agent that causes the flow of milk to increase.

galactorrhea excessive secretion of milk.

gamete   a mature germ cell; an egg or sperm.

Gardnerella vaginalis   a bacterial infection of the vagina, formerly called *Hemophilus vaginalis*, characterized by a foul-smelling, grayish vaginal discharge that exhibits a characteristic fishy odor when 10% potassium hydroxide (KOH) is added. Microscopic examination of a vaginal wet prep reveals the presence of ''clue cells'' (vaginal epithelial cells coated with gram negative organisms).

gargoylism   a hereditary condition, associated with Hurler syndrome, characterized by deformed limbs and hands and grotesque facies, with thickening of the lips, nostrils, and ears.

gastroschisis   congenital herniation of the bowel or other abdominal viscera through an extraumbilical defect in the abdominal wall with no external covering membrane.

gastrula   the stage in early embryonic development that follows the blastula.

gavage   feeding by means of a tube passed into the stomach.

gene   smallest unit of inheritance; genes are located on the chromosomes.

generative   involved in reproduction of the species.

genetic compound   a situation in which an individual has two different mutant alleles at a given locus.

genetic heterogeneity   a situation that occurs when a trait or disease can be caused by gene pairs located at different loci but presenting a similar clinical picture.

genetics   the science that deals with the genetic transmission of characteristics from parents to offspring.

genocopy   a mutant gene that produces a phenotype indistinguishable from that produced by a different mutant gene.

genotype   the genetic composition of an individual.

gestation   period of intrauterine development from conception through birth; pregnancy.

gestational age   the number of complete weeks in fetal development, calculated from the first day of the last normal menstrual cycle.

glycosuria   presence of glucose in the urine.

gonad   sex gland; the ovaries in the female and the testes in the male.

gonadotropin   a hormone that stimulates the sex glands.

Goodell's sign   softening of the cervix that occurs during the second month of pregnancy.

graafian follicle   the ovarian cyst containing the ripe ovum; it secretes estrogens.

gravid   pregnant.

gravida   a pregnant woman.

gynecoid pelvis   typical female pelvis in which the inlet is round instead of oval.

gynecology   study of the diseases of the female, especially of the genital, urinary, and rectal organs and the breasts.

habitus   physical appearance indicating a tendency or predisposition to disease or abnormal conditions.

haploid   half the diploid number of chromosomes. In humans, there are 23 chromosomes, the haploid number, in each germ cell.

harlequin fetus   a newborn with skin that resembles a thick horny armor; the skin is divided into areas by deep red fissures. These infants die within a few days.

harlequin sign   a rare color change that occurs between the longitudinal halves of the newborn's body, such that the dependent half is noticeably pinker than the superior half when the newborn is placed on one side; of no pathologic significance.

hCG   see *human chorionic gonadotropin.*

Hegar's sign   a softening of the lower uterine segment found upon palpation in the second or third month of pregnancy.

hematoma   a swelling or collection of blood in the tissues; a bruise or blood tumor.

hemianopsias   blindness for half the field of vision in one or both eyes.

hemizygous   having only one allele for a given trait instead of a pair.

hemoconcentration   increase in the number of red blood cells resulting from a decrease in plasma volume or from increased erythropoiesis.

hemorrhagic disease of newborn   hemorrhaging during the first few days of life caused by inadequate supply of prothrombin or by a delay in the production of vitamin K.

hemorrhoids   varicose veins of the rectum; may be external or internal.

hereditary   able to be passed from one generation to the next through the gametes of the parents.

herpesvirus   a family of viruses characterized by the development of clusters of small vesicles. The infection is recurring and is frequently found about the lips and nares; a genital form also exists that is primarily sexually transmitted.

heterozygous   a genotypic situation in which two different alleles occur at a given locus on a pair of homologous chromosomes.

high risk   having an increased possibility of suffering harm, damage, loss, or death.

hirsutism   excessive growth of hair or growth of hair in unusual places.

Homan's sign   pain in the calf when the foot is passively dorsiflexed; an early sign of phlebothrombosis of the deep veins of the calf.

homiothermic   warm-blooded.

homologous similar in origin or structure but not necessarily in function.

homologous chromosomes a matched pair of chromosomes.

homozygous a genotypic situation in which two similar genes occur at a given locus on homologous chromosomes.

hormone a substance produced in an organ or gland and conveyed by the blood to another part of the body in order to exert an effect.

human chorionic gonadotropin (hCG) a hormone produced by the chorionic villi and found in the urine of pregnant women; also called *prolan*.

human placental lactogen (hPL) a hormone synthesized by the syncytiotrophoblast that functions as an insulin antagonist and promotes lipolysis to increase the amounts of circulating free fatty acids available for maternal metabolic use.

Hurler syndrome lipochondrodystrophy.

hyaline membrane disease respiratory disease of the newborn characterized by interference with ventilation at the alveolar level, thought to be caused by the presence of fibrinoid deposits lining the alveolar ducts. Also called *respiratory distress syndrome (RDS)*.

hydatidiform mole degenerative process in chorionic villi, giving rise to multiple cysts and rapid growth of the uterus with hemorrhage.

hydramnios an excess of amniotic fluid, leading to overdistention of the uterus. Frequently seen in diabetic pregnant women even if there is not coexisting fetal anomaly. Also called *polyhydramnios*.

hydrocele accumulation of serous fluid in a saclike cavity, especially in the sac that surrounds the testicle, causing the scrotum to swell.

hydrocephalus increased accumulation of cerebrospinal fluid within the ventricles of the brain, resulting from interference with normal circulation and absorption of the fluid and especially from destruction of the foramens of Magendie and Lushka; caused by congenital anomalies, infection, injury, or brain tumors.

hydrops fetalis see *erythroblastosis fetalis*.

hymen membranous fold that normally partially covers the entrance to the vagina.

hymenal tag normally occurring redundant hymenal tissue that protrudes from the floor of the female newborn's vagina; disappears spontaneously a few weeks after birth.

hyperbilirubinemia excessive amount of bilirubin in the blood; indicative of hemolytic processes due to blood incompatibility, intrauterine infection, septicemia, neonatal renal infection, and other disorders.

hypercapnia an increased amount of carbon dioxide in the blood; acts as a respiratory depressant.

hypercholesterolemia excessive amount of cholesterol in the blood.

hyperemesis gravidarum excessive vomiting during pregnancy, leading to dehydration and starvation.

hyperlipidemia excessive amount of fat in the blood.

hypermagnesemia excessive amount of magnesium in the blood.

hyperplasia excessive increase of normal cells in the normal tissue arrangement of an organ.

hypersomnia excessive need for sleep.

hypertelorism abnormal width between two paired organs.

hypertrophy increase or enlargement in size of existing cells; usually applies to any increase in size as a result of functional activity.

hypofibrinogenemia lowered levels of fibrinogen in the blood.

hypogalactic pertaining to deficient secretion of milk.

hypogastric arteries branches of the right and left iliac arteries that carry deoxygenated blood from the fetus through the umbilical cord (where they are known as umbilical arteries) to the placenta.

hypoglycemia abnormally low level of sugar in the blood.

hypomagnesemia abnormally low amount of magnesium in the blood.

hypospadias abnormal congenital positioning of the male urethra on the undersurface of the penis or a urethral opening into the vagina.

hypotensive drugs drugs that lower blood pressure.

hypovolemic shock a condition in which the patient exhibits lowered blood pressure and increased pulse rate; caused by a decrease in the volume of circulating blood in the body.

hypoxemia insufficient oxygenation of the blood, resulting in metabolic acidosis.

hypoxia insufficient availability of oxygen to meet body tissue metabolic needs.

hysterectomy surgical removal of the uterus. See also *abdominal hysterectomy; panhysterectomy; subtotal hysterectomy; total hysterectomy*.

hysterotomy surgical incision into the uterus.

icterus neonatorum jaundice in the newborn.

ideopathic respiratory distress syndrome see *hyaline membrane disease*.

iliopectineal line bony ridge on the inner surface of the ilium and pubis, dividing the true and false pelvis.

immature infant considerably underdeveloped newborn weighing less than 1134 g (2½ lb) at birth.

imperforate anus congenital closure of the anal opening, usually by a membranous septum; may be associated with a fistulous tract.

impetigo a skin disease caused by streptococci or staphylococci and characterized by pustules.

implantation embedding of the fertilized ovum in the uterine mucosa 6 or 7 days after fertilization; also called *nidation*.

impotence inability of the male to perform sexual intercourse.

impregnate to make pregnant or to fertilize.

inanition condition of malnutrition caused by lack of sufficient food; may be due to lack of food supply or to malabsorption.

inborn error of metabolism a hereditary deficiency of a specific enzyme needed for normal metabolism of specific chemicals.

incompetent cervix a mechanical defect in the cervix making it unable to remain closed throughout pregnancy; produces dilatation and effacement leading to abortion, usually during the second trimester or early third trimester.

increment increase or addition; to build up, as of a contraction.

incubation (1) care of a preterm infant in an incubator; (2) the development of an impregnated ovum; (3) interval between exposure to an infection and the appearance of first symptoms.

incubator apparatus used for preterm infants in which the temperature can be regulated.

induction the process of causing or initiating labor by use of medication or surgical rupture of membranes.

inertia inactivity or sluggishness; absence or weakness of uterine contractions during labor.

infant child under 1 year of age.

infant death rate number of deaths of infants under 1 year of age per 1000 live births in a given population per year.

infantile uterus failure of the uterus to attain adult characteristics.

infertility diminished ability to conceive.

infiltration process of substance being passed into or being deposited within a tissue, such as a local anesthetic drug.

inlet passage leading to a cavity.

inlet of the pelvis upper opening into the pelvic cavity.

innominate bone the hip bone, ilium, ischium, and pubis.

internal os an inside mouth or opening; the opening between the cervix and the uterus.

interspinous diameter a transverse diameter of the pelvis that is the distance between the ischial spines. Also referred to as bi-ischial diameter.

intervillous spaces irregular spaces in the maternal portion of the placenta that are filled with maternal blood, serving as sites of maternal–fetal gas, nutrient, and waste exchange.

intrathecal within the subarachnoid space.

intrauterine device (IUD) small metal or plastic form that is placed in the uterus to prevent implantation of a fertilized ovum.

intrauterine growth retardation (IUGR) fetal undergrowth due to any etiology, such as intrauterine infection, deficient nutrient supply, or congenital malformation.

introitus opening or entrance into a cavity or canal, such as the vagina.

intromission insertion or placing of one part into another, such as insertion of the penis into the vagina.

in utero within or inside the uterus.

inversion of the uterus condition in which the fundus of the uterus protrudes through the cervix and sometimes through the vaginal introitus; may occur immediately postpartum as a result of too vigorous placental expression while the placenta is still fixed in the uterus.

involution rolling or turning inward; the reduction in size of the uterus following delivery.

ischium lower portion of the hip bone.

ischogalactic causing suppression of breast milk.

IUD see *intrauterine device.*

IUGR see *intrauterine growth retardation.*

jaundice yellow pigmentation of body tissues caused by the presence of bile pigments. See also *pathologic jaundice; physiologic jaundice.*

Kahn test test used for diagnosing syphilis.

kalemia the level of potassium in the blood.

karyotype the set of chromosomes arranged in a standard order.

kernicterus an ecephalopathy caused by deposition of unconjugated bilirubin in brain cells; may result in impaired brain function or death.

Kernig's sign nuchal rigidity; stiffness of the neck.

Klinefelter syndrome a chromosomal abnormality caused by the presence of an extra X chromosome in the male; characteristics include tall stature, sparse pubic and facial hair, gynecomastia, small firm testes, and absence of spermatogenesis.

labia external folds of skin on either side of the vulva.

labia majora the larger outer folds of skin on either side of the vulva.

labia minora   the smaller inner folds of skin on either side of the vulva.

labor   the process by which the fetus is expelled from the maternal uterus; also called childbirth, confinement, or parturition.

laceration   in obstetrics, a tear in the perineum, vagina, or cervix as a result of stretching of the tissues during childbirth.

lactation   process of producing and supplying breast milk.

lactiferous ducts   tiny tubes within the breast that conduct milk from the acini cells to the nipple.

lactogenic hormone   hormone produced by the anterior pituitary to promote growth of breast tissue and to stimulate the production of milk.

lactosuria   excretion of lactose in the urine during late pregnancy and lactation.

lambdoidal suture   line forming the base of the triangular posterior fontanelle, separating the occipital bone from the two parietal bones.

lanugo   fine, downy hair found on all body parts of the fetus after 20 weeks' gestation, with the exception of the palms of the hands and the soles of the feet.

large for gestational age (LGA)   excessive growth of a fetus in relation to the gestational time period.

lay midwife   a person who gives care during the prenatal, labor and delivery, and postpartal periods. Education varies from apprenticeship to self-teaching to short-term programs. Skills may be passed from one midwife to another.

LBW   see *low-birth-weight infants.*

leiomyoma   a benign tumor of the uterus composed primarily of smooth muscle and connective tissue. Also referred to as a myoma or a fibroid.

Leopold's maneuvers   series of four maneuvers designed to provide a systematic approach whereby the examiner may determine fetal presentation and position.

letdown reflex   pattern of stimulation, hormone release, and resulting muscle contraction that forces milk into the lactiferous ducts, making it available to the infant; milk ejection reflex.

leukorrhea   mucous discharge from the vagina or cervical canal that may be normal or pathologic, as in the presence of infection.

LGA   see *large for gestational age.*

LH   see *luteinizing hormone.*

lie   relationship of the long axis of the fetus and the long axis of the pregnant woman. The fetal lie may be longitudinal, transverse, or oblique.

ligation   suturing or tying shut, as in the suturing closed of the fallopian tubes to prevent pregnancy *(tubal ligation).*

lightening   moving of the fetus and uterus downward into the pelvic cavity; engagement.

linea nigra   line of darker pigmentation extending from the pubis to the umbilicus noted in some women during the later months of pregnancy.

linkage   occurs when genes for different traits are located near one another on the same chromosome.

lithotomy position   position in which the client lies on her back with thighs drawn up toward her chest and with her knees flexed and abducted.

lochia   maternal discharge of blood, mucus, and tissue from the uterus that may last for several weeks after birth.

lochia alba   white vaginal discharge that follows lochia serosa and that lasts from about the tenth to the twenty-first day after delivery.

lochia rubra   red, blood-tinged vaginal discharge that occurs following delivery and lasts 2–4 days.

lochia serosa   pink, serous, and blood-tinged vaginal discharge that follows lochia rubra and lasts until the seventh to tenth day after delivery.

locus   the position that a gene occupies on a chromosome.

low-birth-weight infant (LBW)   infant weighing 2500 g or less at birth independent of gestational age assessments.

L/S ratio   the ratio of the phospholipids lecithin and sphingomyelin produced by the fetal lungs; useful in assessing fetal lung maturity.

LTH   see *luteotropin.*

lunar month   a 28-day cycle corresponding to the phases of the moon. A normal pregnancy lasts 10 lunar months.

lung compliance   degree of distensibility of the lung's elastic tissues.

lutein cells   yellow ovarian cells involved in the formation of the corpus luteum.

luteinizing hormone (LH)   anterior pituitary hormone responsible for stimulating ovulation and for development of the corpus luteum.

luteotropin (LTH)   lactogenic hormone; prolactin.

lysis of adhesions   surgical procedure to release organs tied together by bands of tissue.

lysozyme   enzyme with antiseptic properties found in blood cells, saliva, sweat, tears, and breast milk.

maceration   wasting away, degeneration, or breaking down of fetal skin, as seen with postterm infants or a fetus retained in the uterus after its death.

macroglossia   hypertrophy of the tongue, as in infants with Down syndrome, or a tongue too large for present oral cavity development, as seen in some preterm neonates.

macrosomia   condition seen in some neonates of large body size and high birth weight, as those born of prediabetic and diabetic mothers.

macule   a flat, discolored skin lesion smaller than 1 cm.

magnesemia   level of magnesium in the blood.

malpresentation   a presentation of the fetus into the birth canal that is not "normal," that is, brow, face, shoulder, or breech.

mammary glands   compound glandular elements of the breast that in the female secrete milk to nourish the infant.

maple syrup urine disease   a genetic disorder resulting in the failure to metabolize the amino acids leucine, valine and isoleucine. The name is derived from the characteristic odor of the urine, and the disease is marked by progressive mental deterioration.

Marfan's syndrome   an inherited disorder characterized by abnormally long, thin extremities, spidery fingers and toes, defects of the spine and chest, and congenital heart disease.

MAS   see *meconium aspiration syndrome.*

mask of pregnancy   see *chloasma.*

mastalgia   breast pain or tenderness.

mastitis   inflammation of the breast.

maternal mortality   number of deaths from any cause during the pregnancy cycle per 100,000 live births.

maturation   in reproduction, the process of cell division that reduces the number of chromosomes in the sperm and ova to one half the number carried in the somatic cells of the species.

meatus   external opening for a passageway to an internal organ, such as the urethral meatus.

mechanism   process by which results are obtained, as in labor and delivery of a fetus.

meconium   dark green or black material present in the large intestine of a full-term infant; the first stools passed by the newborn.

meconium aspiration syndrome (MAS)   respiratory disease of term, postterm, and SGA newborns caused by inhalation of meconium or meconium-stained amniotic fluid into the lungs; characterized by mild to severe respiratory distress, hyperexpansion of the chest, hyperinflated alveoli, and secondary atelectasis.

meconium-stained fluid   amniotic fluid that contains meconium because fetal distress has caused increased intestinal activity and relaxing of the fetus's anal sphincter.

meiosis   the process of cell division that occurs in the maturation of sperm and ova that decreases their number of chromosomes by one half.

membrane   thin, pliable layer of tissue that covers an organ or that divides structures, as in the amnion and chorion surrounding the fetus.

menarche   beginning of menstrual and reproductive function in the female.

meningomyelocele   a defect in the spinal column with resulting protrusion of the spinal cord and membranes.

menopause   see *climacteric.*

menorrhagia   excessive or profuse menstrual flow.

menstrual cycle   cyclic buildup of the uterine lining, ovulation, and sloughing of the lining occurring approximately every 28 days in nonpregnant females.

menstruation (menses)   shedding of the uterine lining at the end of the menstrual cycle, resulting in a bloody discharge from the vagina.

mentum   the chin.

mesoderm   the intermediate layer of germ cells in the embryo that give rise to connective tissue, bone marrow, muscles, blood, lymphoid tissue, and epithelial tissue.

metrorrhagia   abnormal uterine bleeding occurring at irregular intervals.

microcephalic   having an abnormally small head in relation to total body size.

micrognathia   abnormally small lower jaw.

midwife   see *lay midwife; nurse-midwife.*

migration   in obstetrics, movement of the ovum from the ovary down the fallopian tube to the uterus.

milia   tiny white papules appearing on the face of a neonate as a result of unopened sebaceous glands; they disappear spontaneously within a few weeks.

milk-leg   phlebitis and thrombosis of the femoral vein, resulting in venous obstruction and edema of the affected leg.

miscarriage   see *spontaneous abortion.*

mitochrondria   slender filament or granular component of cytoplasm in which oxidative reactions occur that provide the cell with energy.

mitosis   process of cell division whereby both daughter cells have the same number and pattern of chromosomes as the original cell.

molding   shaping of the fetal head by overlapping of the cranial bones to facilitate movement through the birth canal during labor.

Mongolian spot   dark flat pigmentation of the lower back and buttocks noted at birth in some infants; usually disappears by the time the child reaches school age.

Mongolism   see *Down syndrome.*

moniliasis   yeastlike fungus infection caused by *Candida albicans.*

monosomy   the presence of only a single chromosome of a homologous pair.

monozygotic twins   two fetuses that develop from a single divided fertilized ovum; identical twins.

Montgomery's glands   small nodules located around the nipples that enlarge during pregnancy and lactation.

mons veneris   fleshy tissue over the symphysis pubis of the female from which hair develops at puberty.

morbidity   incidence of diseased persons in relation to a specific population.

morning sickness   nausea and vomiting occurring during the first trimester of pregnancy; may occur at any time during the day.

Moro reflex   flexion of the newborn's thighs and knees accompanied by fingers that fan then clench as the arms are simultaneously thrown out and then brought together as though embracing something. This reflex can be elicited by startling the newborn with a sudden noise or movement; also called the *startle reflex*.

mortality   incidence of deaths in relation to a specific population.

morula   developmental stage of the fertilized ovum in which there is a solid mass of cells.

mosaic   an individual who has two or more cell lines different from each other in chromosome number or morphology; generally some cells are normal while others contain chromosomal aberrations.

mottling   discoloration of the skin in irregular areas; may be seen with chilling, poor perfusion, or hypoxia.

mucous membrane   mucous-secreting tissue layer lining cavities and canals of the body.

mucous plug   a collection of thick mucus that blocks the cervical canal during pregnancy; also called *operculum*.

mucus   thick, viscid fluid.

multigravida   female who has been pregnant more than once.

multipara   female who has had more than one pregnancy in which the fetuses were viable.

multiple pregnancy   more than one fetus in the uterus at the same time.

mutagen   an environmental agent, either physical, chemical, or biologic, capable of inducing mutation.

mutation   change or alteration in gene or chromosome structure that may be transmitted to offspring.

myometrium   uterine muscular structure.

nadir   the lowest point.

Nägele's rule   a method of determining the estimated date of confinement (EDC): after obtaining the first day of the last menstrual period, one subtracts 3 months and adds 7 days.

natal   relating to birth.

natural childbirth   prepared childbirth, in which the couple attends a prenatal education program and learns exercises and breathing patterns that are used during labor and childbirth.

navel   area of the abdomen where the umbilical cord emerged from the fetus; the *umbilicus*.

neonatal mortality rate   number of deaths of infants in the first 28 days per 1000 live births.

neonate   infant from birth through the first 28 days of life.

neurofibromatosis syndrome   autosomal dominant syndrome characterized by café-au-lait spots, freckling in the axilla, and subcutaneous dyplastic tumors that may appear along the nerves or in the meninges or eye.

nevus   mole, blemish, or mark.

nevus cavernosus   a blemish or mark that may be well circumscribed and elevated or with poorly defined borders and that is composed of large venous channels; the overlying skin has a red-blue discoloration. The nevus enlarges when the infant cries or strains.

nevus flammeus   large port-wine stain.

nevus vasculosus   "strawberry mark"; raised, clearly delineated, dark red, rough-surfaced birth mark commonly found in the head region.

nidation   see *implantation*.

nondisjunction   failure of separation of paired chromosomes during cell division.

NST   nonstress test. An assessment method by which the reaction (or response) of the fetal heart rate to fetal movement is evaluated.

nuclear family   family group consisting of one or more adults and one or more children.

nulligravida   female who has never been pregnant.

nullipara   female who has not delivered a viable fetus.

nurse-midwife   a certified nurse-midwife (CNM) is an RN who has received special training and education in the care of the family during childbearing and the prenatal, labor and delivery, and postpartal periods. After a period of formal education, the nurse-midwife takes a certification test to become a CNM.

nystagmus   involuntary rhythmic oscillation of the eyeball in any direction.

obstetrics   the branch of medicine concerned with the care of women during pregnancy, childbirth, and the postpartal period.

occiput   posterior part of the skull.

OCT   see *oxytocin challenge test*.

ocular hypertelorism   abnormal width between the eyes.

oligohydramnios   Decreased amount of amniotic fluid, which may indicate a fetal urinary tract defect.

oliguria   decrease in urine secretion by the kidney (100–400 mL/24 hr).

omphalic   concerning the umbilicus.

omphalitis   infection of the umbilicus.

omphalocele   congenital herniation or protrusion of the abdominal contents into the base of the umbilicus.

oocyesis   see *ectopic pregnancy*.

oophorectomy   surgical removal of the ovary.

operculum   see *mucous plug*.

ophthalmia neonatorum purulent infection of the eyes or conjunctiva of the newborn, usually caused by gonococci.

opisthotonis backward flexion of the head and feet due to tetanic spasm.

orifice normal outlet of a body cavity.

Ortolani's maneuver a manual procedure performed to rule out the possibility of congenital hip dysplasia.

os opening, mouth. See also *cervical os.*

ossification conversion into bone.

osteogenesis imperfecta a dominant inherited disease characterized by blue sclerae and hypoplasia of osteoid tissue and collagen, which results in bone fractures with slight trauma.

outlet dystocia inadequate pelvic size, causing the fetal head to be pushed backward toward the coccyx, making extension of the head difficult.

ovary female sex gland in which the ova are formed and in which estrogen and progesterone are produced. Normally there are two ovaries, located in the lower abdomen on each side of the uterus.

oviducts see *fallopian tubes.*

ovulation normal process of discharging a mature ovum from an ovary approximately 14 days prior to the onset of menses.

ovum female reproductive cell; egg.

oxygen toxicity excessive levels of oxygen therapy that result in pathologic changes in tissue.

oxytocics drugs that accelerate childbirth and lessen postnatal hemorrhage by stimulating uterine contractions.

oxytocin hormone normally produced by the posterior pituitary, responsible for stimulation of uterine contractions and the release of milk into the lactiferous ducts.

oxytocin challenge test (OCT) also called the contraction stress test (CST), the test is designed to evaluate the circulatory-respiratory status of the fetoplacental unit to determine the ability of the fetus to withstand the stress of labor. While externally monitoring uterine contractions and FHR, oxytocin is administered to stimulate contractions. The FHR pattern is then assessed for evidence of a late deceleration pattern. The test is negative when there are three contractions in a 10-minute period without late deceleration.

palpation use of fingers or hands to manually determine the characteristics of tissues or organs; see also *bimanual palpation.*

palsy loss of or decreased ability to initiate or control muscle movement; paralysis.

panhysterectomy removal of the entire uterus, the ovaries, and the fallopian tubes.

Papanicolaou (Pap) smear procedure to detect the presence of cancer of the uterus by microscopic examination of cells gently scraped from the cervix.

papule a small, raised, sharply circumscribed lesion less than 1 cm in size that may be colored or flesh tone.

para a woman who has borne offspring who reached the age of viability.

parabiotic syndrome anomaly occurring in a small percentage of identical twins, in which one twin is anemic and the second suffers polycythemia as a result of a fetofetal blood transfer via placental vascular anastomoses.

parametritis inflammation of the parametrial layer of the uterus.

parametrium layer of muscle and connective tissue extending between the broad ligaments and surrounding the uterus.

parity the condition of having borne offspring who had attained the age of viability.

parturient pertaining to the act of childbirth.

parturition the process of giving birth.

pathologic jaundice jaundice that occurs within 24 hours of birth, secondary to an abnormal condition such as ABO–Rh incompatibility.

patulous open widely or spread apart.

pedigree a graphic picture using symbols representing an individual's family tree.

pelvic pertaining to the pelvis.

pelvic axis imaginary curved line that passes through the centers of all the anteroposterior diameters of the pelvis.

pelvic phase of labor the deceleration phase, in which active descent occurs.

pelvimeter instrument for the measurement of the diameters and capacities of the pelvis.

pelvis the lower portion of the trunk of the body bounded by the hip bones, coccyx, and sacrum.

pemphigus neonatorum impetigo bullosa.

penis the male organ of copulation or reproduction.

perforation of the uterus a hole made in the uterus.

perinatal mortality both neonatal and fetal deaths per 1000 live births.

perinatal period the time frame extending from the twenty-eight week past conception to the twenty-eighth day past birth.

perinatologist a physician specializing in fetal and neonatal care.

perineal body wedge-shaped mass of fibromuscular tissue found between the lower part of the vagina and the anal canal.

perineorrhaphy suturing of the perineum, usually performed following a laceration.

perineotomy a surgical incision through the perineum.

perineum   the area of tissue between the anus and scrotum in the male or between the anus and vagina in the female.

periodic breathing   sporadic episodes of apnea, not associated with cyanosis, which last for about 10 seconds and commonly occur in preterm infants.

peritoneum   a serous membrane that lines the abdominopelvic walls.

persistent fetal circulation   see persistent pulmonary hypertension.

persistent pulmonary hypertension   a neonatal syndrome secondary to pulmonary hypertension; seen in preterm infants but more common in term and postterm newborns; characterized by cyanosis, tachypnea, and acidemia.

pessary   a device inserted into the body to support an organ or structure, such as a pessary inserted into the vagina to support the uterus in place.

petechia   pinpoint, raised, round, purplish red spot caused by minute capillary hemorrhage.

phenocopy   an environmentally induced phenotype mimicking one usually produced by a specific genotype.

phenotype   the whole physical, biochemical, and physiologic makeup of an individual as determined both genetically and environmentally.

phenylalanine   a naturally occurring amino acid essential for optimal growth and nitrogen balance in humans.

phenylketonuria (PKU)   a recessive hereditary metabolic error that causes the buildup of phenylalanine, leading to mental retardation, brain damage, light pigmentation, and other characteristics. Can be treated with a low-phenylalanine diet.

phimosis   abnormal tightness of the foreskin so that it cannot be retracted over the glans; analogous to tightening of the clitoral hood.

phlebitis   inflammation of a vein.

phlebothrombosis   presence of a clot within a vein without associated symptoms of vein inflammation.

phlegmasia alba dolens   postpartal ileofemoral thrombosis (milk-leg).

phocomelia   absence of or incomplete formation and development of arms, forearms, thighs, and legs. Hands and feet are present but may be abnormally developed.

phototherapy   the treatment of disease by exposure to light.

physiologic   pertaining to normal or expected functioning of a body or organ.

physiologic jaundice   a harmless condition caused by the normal reduction of red blood cells, occurring 48 or more hours after birth, peaking at the fifth to seventh day, and disappearing between the seventh to tenth day.

pica   the eating of substances not ordinarily considered edible or to have nutritive value.

Pierre-Robin syndrome   syndrome characterized by mandibular hypoplasia that occurs prior to the ninth week of embryologic development. The mandibular hypoplasia results in micrognathia, glossoptosis, and possibly a cleft in the soft palate. The infant's mandible generally shows normal growth catch-up by 12–24 months of age.

pigeon chest   chest deformity in which the sternum is prominent. Transverse diameters may be shortened.

PIH   pregnancy-induced hypertension. See *preeclampsia.*

pilonidal cyst   a hair-containing cavity in the sacrococcygeal area.

pinna   the part of the ear that lies outside the skull.

PKU   see *phenylketonuria.*

placenta   specialized disk-shaped organ that connects the fetus to the uterine wall for gas and nutrient exchange; also called *afterbirth.*

placenta accreta   partial or complete absence of the decidua basalis and abnormal adherence of the placenta to the uterine wall.

placenta previa   abnormal implantation of the placenta in the lower uterine segment. Classification of type is based on proximity to the cervical os: *total*—completely covers the os; *partial*—covers a portion of the os; *marginal*—in close proximity to the os.

placental   pertaining to the placenta.

placental dysfunction   placental insufficiency; the placenta fails to meet fetal requirements.

placental dystocia   difficulty in the delivery of the placenta.

placental souffle   soft blowing sounds produced by blood coursing through the placenta; has the same rate as the maternal pulse.

platypelloid pelvis   an unusually wide pelvis, having a flattened oval transverse shape and a shortened anteroposterior diameter.

plethora   a reddened florid complexion, usually caused by an excessive amount of blood in the area.

pneumomediastinum   accidental or diagnostically introduced air or gas into the mediastinal area, which could lead to pneumothorax, pneumopericardium, or pneumoperitoneum.

pneumothorax   air within the chest cavity between the lung tissue and chest wall, creating a positive pressure space instead of negative pressure.

podalic version   a technique designed to produce a change in fetal position or polarity in order to convert an abnormal presentation to a breech presentation.

polycythemia an abnormal increase in the number of total red blood cells in the body's circulation.

polydactyly a developmental anomaly characterized by more than five digits on the hands or feet.

polygenic determined by the action of more than one gene.

polyhydramnios see *hydramnios*.

polymorphous pertaining to lesions in various stages of change.

polyuria passage of excessive amounts of urine within a given time period.

popliteal angle the angle formed at the knee when the thigh of the supine infant is flexed on the chest and the leg is extended by pressure behind the ankle.

position attitude or posture assumed to achieve comfort or purpose.

positive signs of pregnancy indications that confirm the presence of pregnancy.

posterior back or dorsal surface of a body or body part.

posterior fontanelle small triangular area between the occipital and parietal bones of the skull; generally closed by 8–12 weeks of life.

postmature infant a newborn that is overly developed or that is more than 42 gestational weeks of age.

postnatal occurring after birth.

postnatal period period from 28 days following birth to 11 months of age.

postpartal hemorrhage loss of blood greater than 500 mL following delivery. The hemorrhage is classified as *early* or *immediate* if it occurs within the first 24 hours and *late* or *delayed* after the first 24 hours.

postpartum after childbirth or delivery.

precipitate delivery (1) unduly rapid progression of labor, one that lasts less than 3 hours; (2) a delivery in which no physician is in attendance.

precocious teeth small unrooted teeth found in the newborn.

preeclampsia toxemia of pregnancy, characterized by hypertension, albuminuria, and edema. See also *eclampsia*.

preembryonic stage the first 14 days of human development; also called *stage of the ovum*.

pregnancy the condition of having a developing embryo or fetus in the body after fertilization of the female egg by the male sperm.

premature infant see *preterm infant*.

premonitory serving as a warning.

prenatal before birth.

preparatory phase of labor the latent phase of labor.

prepuce a covering or fold of skin.

presentation the fetal body part that enters the maternal pelvis first. The three possible presentations are cephalic, shoulder, or breech.

presenting part the fetal part present in or on the cervical os.

pressure edema accumulation of excessive fluid, primarily in the lower extremities. In obstetrics, caused by pressure of the pregnant uterus on the larger veins.

presumptive signs of pregnancy symptoms that suggest pregnancy but that do not confirm it, such as cessation of menses, quickening, Chadwick's sign, and morning sickness.

preterm infant any infant born before 38 weeks' gestation.

priapism persistent abnormal erection of the penis, usually occurring without sexual desire and accompanied by pain and tenderness.

primigravida a woman who is pregnant for the first time.

primipara a woman who has given birth to her first child (past the point of viability), whether or not that child is living or was alive at birth.

primordial original or primitive; being the simplest form of development.

probable signs of pregnancy manifestations that strongly suggest the likelihood of pregnancy, such as a positive pregnancy test, enlarging abdomen, and positive Goodell's, Hegar's, and Braxton Hicks signs.

progesterone a hormone produced by the corpus luteum, adrenal cortex, and placenta whose function it is to stimulate proliferation of the endometrium to facilitate growth of the embryo.

projectile vomiting emesis that appears to have been propelled out of the mouth by extreme force.

prolactin a hormone secreted by the anterior pituitary that stimulates and sustains lactation in mammals.

prolan see *human chorionic gonadotropin (hCG)*.

prolapsed cord umbilical cord that becomes trapped in the vagina before the fetus is delivered.

PROM premature rupture of amniotic membranes.

promontory of the sacrum projecting eminence or process of the sacrum corresponding to the junction of the sacrum and L5.

prophylactic pertaining to a preventive measure or to a measure used to ward off a disease or event.

proteinuria the presence of an excessive amount of serum protein in the urine.

pseudocyesis a condition in which the woman has symptoms of pregnancy but in which hormonal pregnancy tests are negative; false pregnancy.

pseudomenstruation blood-tinged mucus from the vagina

in the newborn female infant; caused by withdrawal of maternal hormones that were present during pregnancy.

pseudopregnancy see *pseudocyesis.*

pseudoprematurity see *intrauterine growth retardation (IUGR).*

psychologic miscarriage maternal lack of love for the infant; emotional detachment.

psychoprophylaxis psychophysical training aimed at preparing the expectant parents to cope with the processes of labor and to avoid concentration on the discomforts associated with childbirth.

ptyalism excessive salivation.

puberty the period of time during which the secondary sexual characteristics develop and the ability to procreate is attained.

pubic pertaining to the pubes or pubis.

pudendal block injection of an anesthetizing agent at the pudendal nerve to produce numbness of the external genitals and the lower one-third of the vagina to facilitate childbirth and permit episiotomy if necessary.

pudendum the external genitals of humans.

puerperal morbidity a maternal temperature of 100.4F (38.0C) or higher on any two of the first 10 postpartal days excluding the first 24 hours. The temperature is to be taken by mouth at least four times per day.

puerperal sepsis infection of the reproductive organs caused by unsterile childbirth conditions; also called *childbed fever* and *puerperal fever.*

puerperium the period or state of confinement after completion of the third stage of labor until involution of the uterus is complete, usually 6 weeks.

pustule a small, raised, sharply circumscribed lesion filled with purulent material; less than 1 cm in size.

quickening the first fetal movements felt by the pregnant woman, usually between 16 and 18 weeks' gestation.

rabbit test see *Friedman's test.*

rales an abnormal respiratory sound heard usually with the aid of a stethoscope; caused by air passing through fluid in the alveoli and terminal bronchioles.

RDS see *hyaline membrane disease.*

recessive trait a trait that is expressed only when no dominant genes are present.

recoil to spring back; to return to a starting point; for example, to return to a position of flexion after involuntary extension.

rectocele herniation of part of the rectum into the vagina.

reflex an involuntary response.

relaxin a water-soluble protein secreted by the corpus lu-

teum that causes relaxation of the symphysis and cervical dilatation.

residual related to that which is remaining as a residue, for example, formula and gastric secretions present in an infant's stomach prior to the next feeding.

residual urine urine left in the bladder after voiding.

respiratory distress syndrome see *hyaline membrane disease.*

restitution in obstetrics, turning the fetal presenting part either right or left after it has fully exited the birth canal so that the spine is once again in a straight line.

resuscitation restoration of life or consciousness by means of artificial respiration and cardiac massage.

retained placenta placenta that fails to be expelled after childbirth because of adherence or incarceration.

retraction to be drawn up or back.

retroflexion of the uterus the bending back of the body of the uterus toward the cervix, resulting in a sharp angle at the point of bending.

retrolental fibroplasia formation of fibrotic tissue behind the lens; associated with retinal detachment and arrested eye growth, seen with hyperoxemia in preterm infants.

retroversion of the uterus the turning backward of the entire uterus in relation to the pelvic area.

Rh factor antigens present on the surface of blood cells that make the blood cell incompatible with blood cells that do not have the antigen.

rhonchi coarse, abnormal auscultatory sounds made by the passage of air over mucous plugs.

rhythm method the timing of sexual intercourse to avoid the fertile time associated with ovulation.

ribonucleic acid (RNA) the complex protein responsible for transfering genetic information within a cell.

ripe being in a state of optimal readiness or consistency.

Ritgen maneuver a procedure used to control delivery of the head.

role a cluster of interpersonal behaviors, attitudes, and activities associated with an individual in a certain situation or position.

ROM rupture of (amniotic) membranes. Rupture may be PROM (premature rupture of membranes), SROM (spontaneous rupture of membranes), AROM (artificial rupture of membranes). Some clinicians may use the abbreviation RBOW (rupture of bag of waters).

rooming-in unit a hospital unit where the infant can reside in the same room with the mother after delivery and during their postpartal stay.

rooting reflex an infant's tendency to turn the head and open the lips to suck when one side of the mouth or the cheek is touched.

rotation   turning of the fetal head as it follows the pelvic curves during childbirth.

Rubin's test   tubal insufflation with a gas, usually carbon dioxide, to test the patency of the tubes or to clear small obstructions.

sacroiliac   the joints or articulation between the sacrum and ilium and their associated ligaments.

sacrum   five fused vertebras that form a triangle of bone just beneath the lumbar vertebras and between the hip bones.

saddle block anesthesia   sensory and motor anesthesia of the buttocks, perineum, and inner aspects of the thighs, produced by spinal or entrathecal injection of an anesthetic agent at approximately L3–L5.

sagittal suture   band of connective tissue that separates the parietal bones and extends anteriorly and posteriorly.

salpingo-oophorectomy   surgical removal of a fallopian tube and an ovary.

scalines   eczema on the cheeks, behind the ears, and on the popliteal and antecubital areas.

Scanzoni's maneuver   rotation of the presenting fetal head from a posterior position to an anterior position through double forceps application.

scaphoid abdomen   abdomen with a sunken interior wall, giving it a small, empty appearance.

scarf sign   the position of the elbow when the hand of a supine infant is drawn across to the other shoulder until it meets resistance.

Schultze's mechanism   delivery of the placenta with the shiny or fetal surface presenting first.

sclerema   patchy or generalized progressive hardening of subcutaneous fat in infants; lesions are cold, yellow, and very firm.

sebaceous glands   oil-secreting glands in the skin.

seborrhea dermatus   see *cradle cap.*

secondary areola   increased area of pigmentation surrounding the areola that occurs during pregnancy as a result of hormonal influences; becomes apparent at about the third month.

second stage of labor   stage lasting from complete dilatation of the cervix to expulsion of the fetus.

secundines   see *afterbirth.*

segmentation   the process of division of the fertilized ovum into many cells before differentiation into layers.

semen   thick whitish fluid ejaculated by the male during orgasm and containing the spermatozoa and their nutrients.

sensitization   initial exposure to a substance that results in an immune response.

septic abortion   a serious uterine infection that occurs most commonly after an abortion performed by an unskilled person outside an appropriate facility.

sex chromatin   see *Barr body.*

sex chromosomes   the X and Y chromosomes, which are responsible for sex determination.

sex-limited trait   a characteristic that is expressed in only one sex.

sex-linked trait   a characteristic that is determined by genes on the X chromosome.

sexually transmitted disease (STD)   refers to diseases ordinarily transmitted by direct sexual contact with an infected individual.

show   a pinkish mucous discharge from the vagina that may occur a few hours to a few days prior to the onset of labor.

simian line   a single palmar crease frequently found in children with Down syndrome.

singleton   pregnancy with a single fetus.

small for gestational age (SGA)   inadequate weight or growth for gestational age; birth weight below the tenth percentile.

sole creases   lines caused by folds covering the underpart of the foot. Distribution and number of creases contribute to determining gestational age.

souffle   a soft blowing sound made by blood turbulence in the vessels.

spermatogenesis   process by which mature spermatozoa are formed, during which chromosome number is reduced by half.

spermatozoa   mature sperm cells of the male animal produced by the testes.

sphincter muscle   a ringlike band of muscle fibers that constricts or closes a passage or orifice.

spina bifida occulta   a defect in the vertebras of the spinal column without protrusion of neural components; may be completely asymptomatic.

spinnbarkeit   describes the elasticity of the cervical mucus that is present at ovulation.

spontaneous abortion   abortion that occurs naturally; a *miscarriage.*

square window   the angle formed at the wrist when the infant's hand is flexed toward the ventral forearm.

SROM   spontaneous rupture of (amniotic) membranes.

startle reflex   see *Moro reflex.*

station   relationship of the presenting fetal part to an imaginary line drawn between the pelvic ischial spines.

steepled palate   high palate that rises to an angle instead of the more normal round shape.

sterility   inability to conceive or to produce offspring.

stillbirth   the delivery of a dead infant.

strabismus   an eye condition in which the visual axis does not converge on a desired object; incoordinate action of the extrinsic ocular muscles.

striae gravidarum   stretch marks; shiny reddish lines that appear on the abdomen, breasts, thighs, and buttocks of pregnant women as a result of stretching the skin.

Sturge-Weber syndrome   syndrome of unknown etiology characterized by flat facial hemangiomata and meningeal hemangiomata with seizures.

subinvolution   failure of a part to return to its normal size after functional enlargement, such as failure of the uterus to return to normal size after pregnancy.

subluxation   incomplete or partial dislocation.

subtotal hysterectomy   removal of the fundus and body of the uterus, leaving the cervical stump.

succedaneum   see *caput succedaneum.*

sucking reflex   the infant's tendency to suck on any object placed in the mouth.

superfecundation   successive fertilization of two or more ova during the same menstrual cycle as the result of more than one act of intercourse.

superfetation   fertilization and development of an ovum while a developing fetus is already in the uterus.

supernumerary nipples   excess number of nipples, varying from small pink spots to normal size and pigmentation, usually present along an imaginary line from midclavicle to groin.

surfactant   a surface-active mixture of lipoproteins secreted in the alveoli and air passages that reduces surface tension of pulmonary fluids and contributes to the elasticity of pulmonary tissue.

suture   fibrous connection of opposed joint surfaces, as in the skull. Also, the uniting of edges of a wound.

symphysis pubis   fibrocartilagenous joint between the pelvic bones in the midline.

synclitism   when the biparietal diameter of the fetal head is parallel to the planes of the maternal pelvis.

syndactyly   malformation of the fingers or toes in which there may be webbing or complete fusion of two or more digits.

tachycardia   abnormally rapid heart rate.

tachypnea   *excessively rapid respirations.*

talipes equinovarus   congenital defect of the foot with changes in the ligament and tendons consisting chiefly of contractures and anomalous insertions. The forefoot is adducted and supine and there is inversion of the heel and fixed plantar flexion of the foot. Also known as *clubfoot.*

Tay-Sachs disease   a genetic disorder transmitted as an autosomal recessive that occurs primarily among Ashkenazi Jews. The disease produces progressive neurologic damage and is fatal within 18 months to 2 years. No known treatment exists but the condition can be diagnosed with amniocentesis.

telangiectatic nevi   small clusters of pink-red spots appearing on the nape of the neck and around the eyes of infants; localized areas of capillary dilatation. Also referred to as *stork bites.*

teratogen   a nongenetic factor that can produce malformations of the fetus.

term infant   a live born infant of 38–42 weeks' gestation.

testes   the male gonads, in which sperm and testosterone are produced.

testosterone   the male hormone; responsible for the development of secondary male characteristics.

tetralogy of Fallot   a combination of four congenital anomalies that together make up a specific cardiac syndrome.

therapeutic abortion   medically induced termination of pregnancy when a malformed fetus is suspected or when the woman's health is in jeopardy.

thermal neutral environment   an environment that provides for minimal heat loss or expenditure.

thermogenesis   the production of heat, especially within the body.

third stage of labor   the time from delivery of the fetus to the time when the placenta has been completely expelled.

threatened abortion   a condition in which discharge of the fertilized ovum is threatened by bleeding from the vagina, which may be accompanied by cervical dilatation.

thromboembolus   thrombotic material or clot carried by the bloodstream from one site to another vessel, causing obstruction.

thrombophlebitis   inflammation of a vein associated with thrombus formation.

thrush   a fungus infection of the oral mucous membranes caused by *Candida albicans.* Most often seen in infants; characterized by white plaques.

toco, tokos   combined word form designating childbirth.

tocodynamometer   external device that can be used to estimate uterine contraction pressures during labor.

tongue tie   abnormally short frenulum of the tongue that limits its motion.

tonic neck reflex   postural reflex seen in the newborn. When the supine infant's head is turned to one side, the arm and leg on that side extend while the extremities on the opposite side flex; also called the *fencing position.*

TORCH   acronym used to describe a group of infections that represent potentially severe problems during pregnancy. TO = toxoplasmosis, R = rubella, C = cytomegalovirus, H = herpesvirus.

torticollis   contracted neck muscles, producing a twisting and contraction of the head toward the affected side; wryneck.

total hysterectomy   removal of the entire uterus, including the cervix, leaving the ovaries and fallopian tubes.

toxemia   a group of pathologic conditions, essentially metabolic disturbances, occurring in pregnant women and manifested by preeclampsia and eclampsia.

tracheoesphageal fistula   a congenital anomaly in which there is a communication between the trachea and the esophagus.

traditional family   a family type that draws its strength from the autocratic and authoritarian patriarchal line.

transient tachypnea of the newborn   respiratory condition theorized to be caused by excess lung fluid production or failure to remove normal (fetal) lung fluid; characterized by signs of respiratory distress, reduced air entry, and mild hypercarbia. Usually does not require assisted ventilation and newborns are well in 2–5 days.

transition   the period during labor when the cervix becomes approximately 8 cm dilated, contractions are very strong, and the laboring woman may feel that she cannot go on.

translocation   the occurrence of a chromosome segment at an abnormal site.

transverse lie   a lie in which the fetus is positioned crosswise in the uterus.

Treacher-Collins syndrome   mandibulofacial dysostosis.

Trichomonas vaginalis   a parasitic protozoan that may cause inflammation of the vagina characterized by itching and burning of vulvar tissue and by white, frothy discharge.

trimester   3 months, or one-third of the gestational time for pregnancy.

trisomy   the presence of three homologous chromosomes rather than the normal two.

trophoblast   the outer layer of the blastoderm that will eventually establish the nutrient relationship with the uterine endometrium.

TTN   see *transient tachypnea of the newborn.*

tubal ligation   see *ligation.*

Turner syndrome   a number of anomalies that occur when a female has only one X chromosome; characteristics include short stature, little sexual differentiation, webbing of the neck with a low posterior hairline, and congenital cardiac anomalies.

twins   two offspring produced by the same pregnancy. See also *dizygotic twins; monozygotic twins.*

type II respiratory distress syndrome   see *transient tachypnea of the newborn.*

ultrasound   high-frequency sound waves that may be directed, through use of a transducer, into the maternal abdomen. The ultrasonic sound waves reflected by the underlying structures of varying densities allow various maternal and fetal tissues, bones, and fluids to be identified.

umbilical cord   the structure connecting the placenta to the umbilicus of the fetus and through which nutrients from the woman are exchanged for wastes from the fetus.

umbilical vasculitis   inflammation of the umbilical cord and its contents.

umbilicus   see *navel.*

urachus   a canal connecting the fetal bladder with the allantois; at birth it collapses and becomes mostly fibrotic, forming the median umbilical ligament.

urinary meatus   external opening of the urethra.

uterine souffle   a soft sound made by the blood within the arteries of a gravid uterus.

uterine tetany   prolonged or continuous uterine contractions.

uterine tubes   see *fallopian tubes.*

uterus   hollow muscular organ in which the fertilized ovum is implanted and in which the developing fetus is nourished until birth.

vagina   the musculomembranous tube or passageway located between the external genitals and the uterus of the female.

valgus   bent outward.

variable expressivity   the differences in severity of a trait produced by the same gene in different individuals.

varicose veins   permanently distended veins.

vasectomy   surgical removal of a portion of the vas deferens (ductus deferens) to produce infertility.

venereal disease (VD)   see *sexually transmitted disease.*

venous   referring to veins or to unoxygenated blood.

vernix caseosa   a protective cheeselike whitish substance made up of sebum and desquamated epithelial cells that is present on the fetal skin.

version   a change of position, usually to alter the presenting fetal part and facilitate delivery.

vertex   the top or crown of the head.

vesical blastoderm   a stage in the development of the mammalian embryo consisting of a hollow sphere of cells enclosing a cavity.

vesicular   composed of or relating to small saclike structures filled with fluid.

vestibule   a space or cavity at the entrance to a canal.

viable   capable of living.

villi   short vascular processes or protrusions appearing on some membranes. See also *chorionic villi.*

vulva   the external structure of the female genitals, lying below the mons veneris.

vulvectomy   surgical removal of the vulva.

Waardenburg syndrome   a congenital syndrome transmitted as an autosomal recessive trait and characterized by cochlear deafness, wide bridge of the nose, lateral displacement of the medial canthi, confluent eyebrows, eyes of different colors, white eyelashes, white forelock, and leukodermia.

wet lung   see *transient tachypnea of the newborn.*

Wharton's jelly   yellow-white gelatinous material surrounding the vessels of the umbilical cord.

witch's milk   whitish secretion from the infant's mammary glands for approximately 7 days after delivery; caused by influence of the mother's hormones.

womb   see *uterus.*

xanthoma   yellow-white plaque on the skin as a result of lipid deposition.

X chromosome   female sex chromosome.

X linkage   genes located on the X chromosome.

Y chromosome   male sex chromosome.

zona pellucida   transparent inner layer surrounding an ovum.

zygote   a fertilized egg.

INDEX

NOTE: Letters following page numbers refer to:
d   drug guide
f   figure
g   assessment guide
n   nursing care plan
p   procedure
t   table

A and D ointment, 727, 931
A-streptococcus pneumococci, sepsis neonatorum from, 841
Abdomen, of fetus, ultrasound for measuring, 370
Abdomen, of mother
  assessing
    in fourth trimester, 946g
    with preeclampsia/eclampsia, 343, 344
    in puerperium, 910–11, 917, 919n
  injury to, as preterm labor cause, 548
  pain in, from appendicitis in pregnancy, 351
  postpartal changes in, 905
Abdomen, of neonate
  assessing, 683–84, 699–700g
    in delivery room, 496
    at nursery admission, 710
  distention of. See Abdominal distention
  hemorrhage in, from breech delivery, 554
  necrotizing enterocolitis signs in, 838, 839
  scaphoid appearance to, from diaphragmatic hernia, 861, 866
  SGA, 764
  tenderness in
    as pneumoperitoneum sign, 810n
    with necrotizing enterocolitis, 838, 839
  with tracheoesophageal atresia/fistula, 862
Abdominal cramps, as Methergine side effect, 903d
Abdominal distention
  in mother. See also Abdominal enlargement
    from postpartal hematoma, 973
    with puerperal peritonitis, 976, 977
  in neonate
    from aganglionosis, 869
    assessing, 699g
    as distress sign, 714
    as hypocalcemia sign, 821
    from intestinal obstruction, 873, 874
    after meningocele/meningomyelocele surgery, 883n
    with necrotizing enterocolitis, 838, 839
    as pneumoperitoneum sign, 810n
    preterm, assessing for, 754n

as preterm infant feeding intolerance sign, 746
as sepsis neonatorum sign, 841
with tracheoesophageal atresia/fistula, 860, 862
Abdominal effleurage. See Effleurage
Abdominal enlargement
  nonpregnancy causes of, 192t
  as pregnancy change, 193
Abdominal hemorrhage in neonate, 554
Abdominal injury, as preterm labor cause, 548
Abdominal mass, in neonate, as distress sign, 714
Abdominal measurement
  of fetus, ultrasound for, 370
  at nursery admission, 710
Abdominal pain
  from appendicitis in pregnancy, 351
  from ectopic pregnancy, 333
  as puerperal infection sign, 975, 976, 977
  severe, as hemorrhage sign, 569
  from sickle cell anemia, 327
Abdominal pregnancy, 333, 334f
Abdominal prep, before cesarean delivery, 608
Abdominal rigidity, as puerperal peritonitis sign, 977, 979n
Abdominal striae. See Stretch marks
Abdominal surgery, as preterm labor cause, 548
Abdominal wall cellulitis, as necrotizing enterocolitis sign, 838, 839
ABO incompatibility
  exchange transfusion for, 828, 831
  hemolytic disease of the newborn from, 824, 826
  as pathologic jaundice cause, 823
  spontaneous abortion caused by, 329
Abortion
  defined, 210, 328–29
  induced; see also therapeutic
    of adolescent pregnancy, family reaction and, 302
    ambivalence and, 203
    for contraception, 128–31, 130t
    controversy about, 128
    defined, 328–29
    methods of, 129–31, 130t
  infertility from, 110
  previous, as hemorrhage risk factor, 569
  Rh sensitization affected by, 349–50, 824
  spontaneous, 328–33, 332t, 332f
    ambivalence and, 203
    cardiac disease in mother and, 768
    causes of, 183, 329, 333
    from chromosomal defects, 134
    classifications of, 329–31, 332t, 332f
    complete, 330, 332t, 332f
    corpus luteum and, 168
    defined, 328–29
    from herpes infecton, 359, 360

from hypothyroidism, 201, 215t, 326
imminent, 330, 332t, 332f
incomplete, 330, 332t, 332f
interventions for, 332–33
iron deficiency anemia and, 327
late, from circumvallate placenta, 574
listeriosis as cause of, 357
from maternal drug abuse, 361t
from maternal syphilis, 354
in medical personnel, 351
missed, 330–31, 332t
multiple gestation and, 558
nursing interventions with, 333
progesterone prevents, 169, 202
risk factors for, 215t
from sickle cell anemia, 328
statistics about, 329
threatened, 329–30, 332t, 332f
from toxoplasmosis, 357
spontaneous, habitual, 329, 331, 332t, 333
  from incompetent cervix, 335
  interventions for, 332–33
  as risk factor, 215t
therapeutic
  after amniocentesis, 148
  for rubella in first trimester, 358
  for toxoplasmosis, 357
thromboembolic disease risk with, 983
Abrasions, puerperal infection risk from, 974
Abruptio placentae. See also Placental separation
  as amniotomy risk, 587
  assessing for signs of, 240g, 339
    with preeclampsia/eclampsia, 343, 344
  bleeding caused by, 329
  cesarean delivery for, 600
  as CST contraindication, 375
  danger signs of, 240g
  defined, 335
  DIC from, 567–68, 568f
  fetal distress interventions for, 540
  fetal implications of, 425t, 560, 563
  as hydramnios risk, 577
  hemorrhage evaluation with, 571–72n
  induction of labor for, 587
    risk with, 590, 591
  from maternal drug abuse, 70, 361t
  maternal hypertension and, 339, 769
  maternal implications of, 425t
  multiple gestation and, 558
  neonatal implications of, 425t, 563, 830
  PIH increases risk of, 339, 343, 344
  placental transport affected by, 170
  postpartal risks with, 908t
  resuscitation risk with, 786, 787
  Rh sensitization affected by, 824
  as risk factor, 215t

intrapartal, 425t
labor induction, 590, 591
statistics about, 329
as vacuum extraction indication, 598
Abscesses
  breast, 987
  puerperal, 975, 976
Acceleration phase of labor, 417, 417f
Acceptance
  in grief process, 999, 1002
  as pregnancy emotion, 203–4
Accidents
  with neonates, preventing, 729–30
  during pregnany, 352–53
Acetone, in urine
  during first stage labor, 429g
  postpartal, causes of, 906
Acetone precipitable fraction test, 321
Achilles tendon, with clubfoot, 875, 876
Achondroplasia
  assessing neonate for, 689g
  hydrocephaly from, 691g
Achondroplastic dwarfism, inheritance of, 143
Acidemia, in neonate
  hyperbilirubinemia risk with, 823
  as PPH sign, 817
  as prematurity risk, 738, 739
  with RDS, 794
Acidosis, in mother. See also Electrolyte imbalances
  assessment of, 460–63, 462f
  FHR with, 452
  from hemorrhage, 570
  from hyperemesis gravidarum, 328
  in labor, 409
    identifying, 787
  as ritodrine side effect, 549
  supine hypotensive syndrome and, 409
Acidosis, in neonate. See also Electrolyte imbalances
  apnea associated with, 749
  asphyxia leads to, 786
  blood bicarbonate concentration and, 653
  from cold stress, 646, 817, 818
  with congestive heart failure, 894
  DIC and, 837
  from diaphragmatic hernia, 861, 866
  drug therapy for, 792, 793d
  hyperbilirubinemia risk from, 822
  from intestinal obstruction, 873
  intraventricular hemorrhage and, 836
  with MAS, 798, 814
  oxygen dissociation curve and, 643
  physiologic jaundice encouraged by, 649
  as prematurity risk, 746
  with RDS, 794, 794f, 795, 796t, 801n, 803n, 804
    correcting, 797, 806n

Acidosis (Cont'd)
    with transient tachypnea of new-
        born, 798
Acme phase of contractions, 404,
    404f
Acquaintance phase of attachment,
    957–58
Acrocentric chromosomes, 157, 157f
Acrocyanosis, in neonate, 677, 683
    as normal, 495, 688g
    with RDS, 802n
Acromegaly, diabetes secondary to,
    315
Acrosomal reaction, 161, 162
Acrosome, 160
    fertilization role of, 161–62
ACTH. See Adrenocorticotropic
    hormone
Actin. See Contractile substances
Active acquired immunity, 654
Active awake state, in neonate, 657
Active listening, 290
Active phase. See Labor
Active transport, in placenta, 170
Activity
    of mother
        with cardiac disease, 311, 312,
            313
        lochia increased by, 904
        postpartal, 916, 920n
    of neonate
        assessing, 687, 706
        congenital hypothyroidism
            affects, 859
        lack of, as illness sign, 729
        patterns of, 657, 722, 724–25
        polycythemia alters, 835
        preterm, 749, 750
        RDS affects, 802n
Acute asphyxic insult, intrapartal
    fetal heart aberrations and,
    425t
Acute grief, 999
Acute respiratory obstruction,
    medical interventions for, 531
Acyanotic heart defects, 881. See
    also specific defects
Acyclovir (Zovirax), for herpes
    infection, 360
Adaptive responses
    to defective birth, 1010
    of family in crisis, 993
Adenine arabinoside (ara-A), for
    neonatal herpesvirus, 844
Adenomyosis, infertility from, 111t
Adenosine triphosphate (ATP)
    as energy source for contractions,
        407
    released in brown fat, 647
Adenylcyclase, role of, 96
Adhesions
    fetal, as oligohydramnios risk, 577
    infertility from, 111t
Adipose tissue. See Fat
Adlosterone levels, betamethasone
    and, 547
Admission, hospital
    from home birth, nursing role in,
        631
    to nursery, 709–13
    in labor, 466–69, 472–73n
        advanced, immediate interven-
            tions for, 488t
Adnexa
    adhesions of, spontaneous abortion
        caused by, 329
    evaluating, in infertility workup,
        114
Adolescence. See also Adolescents
    as maturational crisis, 992
    physical changes in, 91–92, 91f,
        92f, 296

pregnancy in. See Adolescent
    pregnancy
psychosocial effects of, 296–97,
    298–99t
sexual development in, 89–90
Adolescent pregnancy, 296–305,
    298–300t
    adoption as resolution to, 482
    counseling to decrease, 106
    as crisis, 992, 1017
    factors leading to, 90
    family in, 301–2, 305
    fatherhood resulting from, 300,
        301
    labor and delivery experience,
        467, 471, 482
    mother's role in, 302, 305
    nursing practice tools applied to,
        28–29
    parents' reactions to, 301–2
    physiologic risks of, 297, 299
        PIH, 336
    postpartal care, 942–43
    prenatal care, 302–5
    prenatal education, 304f, 305,
        939
    psychologic motivations for, 297
    psychologic risks of, 298–99t,
        299, 300t
    rate of, 296
    repeated, 300
    school attendance during, 305
    sociologic risks of, 299–301
Adolescent spurt, 91
Adolescents. See also Adolescence
    as parents. See also Adolescent
        pregnancy
        attachment behaviors of, 961
        crisis intervention for, 1016–
            1017
        learning needs of, 939
        response to parents' pregnancy of,
            251
    sex education for, 105–6
Adoption
    bonding with, 1011
    as genetic risk alternative, 151
    as infertility alternative, 119
    relinquishing baby for
        factors affecting decision, 302
        grieving process, 482
        nursing interventions with,
            1014, 1015t
    by single parents, 1018
Adrenal cortex
    estrogens secreted by, 93
    pregnancy changes in, 202
Adrenal function tests, after abruptio
    placentae, 564
Adrenal glands
    estrone produced postmeno-
        pausally by, 101
    pregnancy changes in, 202
    puberty role of, 91, 92
Adrenal hyperplasia, small neonatal
    testes with, 701g
Adrenocorticotropic hormone
    (ACTH), puberty and, 92
Adrenotropin, pregnancy role of, 202
Adulthood, sexual development in,
    90–91
Aerobacter
    postpartal urinary tract infection
        from, 986
    sepsis neonatorum from, 841
Aerobic bacteria, puerperal infections
    from, 974
Affonso, D. D., 942
Afterpains, 907
    as puerperal infection sign, 977
AGA neonates. See Appropriate-
    forgestational-age neonates

Aganglionic megacolon, 868–71,
    869f
Age, infertility and, 110, 112
Age of mother
    birth center use and, 618
    birth statistics and, 22, 22t, 24t,
        25t
    cesarean delivery incidence and,
        600
    Down syndrome and, 101
    genetic amniocentesis and, 147
    hemorrhage risk and, 569
    home birth and, 629
    induction of labor and, 587
    oxytocin contraindication and, 590
    PIH risk and, 336
    resuscitation risk and, 786
    as risk factor, 214t
    SGA neonates and, 761
    thromboembolic disease risk and,
        980, 983
Agenesis, in neonate, kidney
    displacement with, 700g
Agnathia, vulnerability to, 183t
Aguilera, D. C., crisis paradigm by,
    994, 995f
AID (artificial insemination with
    donor's semen), 119, 152
AIH (artifical insemination with
    husband's semen), 119
Airway, for eclampsia client, 344
Airway, in neonate
    establishing, as priority, 498, 788
    maintaining
        with apnea, 755n
        at nursery admission, 710
        with Pierre Robin syndrome,
            850, 851
        during reactivity period, 712
    obstruction of, with broncho-
        pulmonary dysplasia, 816
Aladjem, S., 336
Albinism, eye color lacking with,
    693g
Albumin
    placental transport of, 170
    in preterm infant, normal values,
        752t
    in urine, with mild or severe pre-
        eclampsia, 341
Alcohol
    in breast milk, 930
    infertility from, 111t, 112, 114
    pregnancy intake of, 362
        by adolescents, 304
        excessive, 360–62, 361t. See
            also Alcoholism
        as risk factor, 214t
    umbilical cord care with, 727
Alcoholism
    fetal/neonatal implications of,
        362, 769–70
        fetal alcohol syndrome (FAS),
            214t, 268, 770
        IUGR, 761
        withdrawal syndrome, 770
    maternal implications of, 362
Aldosterone, increased in pregnancy,
    198
Alert states, in neonate, 657
    assessing, 657
        in behavioral assessment, 687,
            705–6
        at nursery admission, 710
        in postpartal home visit, 627
        immediately after birth, 711–12,
            713f
        postterm, 759
        preterm, 749
        reactivity periods, 657
        SGA, 764
Alerting, assessing neonate for, 706

Alimentary tract atresias, hydramnios
    increases risk of, 425t
Alkali therapy, for MAS, 815
Alkaloids, in breast milk, 930
Alkalosis
    from hyperemesis gravidarum,
        328
    oxygen dissociation curve and,
        643
Alleles, 142
Allelic genes, 157, 157f
Allergic reactions. See also Allergies
    to labor anesthesia, 515–16
    to Methergine, 903d
    to vitamin K in nursery, 711d
Allergies. See also Allergic reactions
    to anesthetic agents, general
        anesthesia for, 529
    breast-feeding and, 717, 718
    in infants, supplemental foods and,
        720
    milk (lactose intolerance), 272,
        281
Alpha-receptors, uterine contractions
    stimulated by, 407
Alternative birth. See Birthing
    alternatives
Altitude, patent ductus arteriosus
    and, 881
Alveolar instability, with RDS, 794,
    794f
Alveolar sacs, in preterm infant,
    737–38, 738f
Alveoli, of neonate
    abnormal, with bronchopulmonary
        dysplasia, 816
    preterm, 737–38, 738f
    respiratory role of, 638
Ambivalence
    about pregnancy, 203
    relinquishment for adoption, 1014,
        1015t
Ambulation
    at labor admission, 467, 468
    during labor
        advantages of, 474, 617
        contraindications, 474
        decision making about, 467
        first stage latent, 474n
        omitted during active phase,
            475
    postpartal, 916
        cesarean delivery, 603–4, 917n
        elimination encouraged by,
            918n
        with epidural anesthesia, 520
        thromboembolic disease
            prevention by, 983, 984
        thrombophlebitis prevention by,
            912
        uterine involution affected by,
            903
Amelia, assessing neonate for, 702g
Amenorrhea, 100
    from contraception, 125, 127
    nonpregnancy causes of, 191t
    postdelivery
        with postdelivery galactorrhea,
            987
        with Sheehan syndrome, 988
    as pregnancy symptom, 191
    primary or secondary, 100
American Social Help Association,
    herpes information from, 360
American Academy of Husband-
    Coached Childbirth, 295
American Indians
    health beliefs among, 206
    lactose intolerance among, 281
    modesty among, 469
    physiologic jaundice of neonates
        in, 649

pregnancy and cultural values among, 205, 288–89t
labor customs, 469, 471
postpartal customs, 914
American Society for Prophylaxis in Obstetrics, 294
Amide types of anesthesia, 514
Amino acids. *See also* Protein
neonatal disorders involving
homocystinuria, 858–59
maple syrup urine disease, 858
PKU, 857–58
placental transport of, 170
for preterm infants, 740
Amnesia, about delivery, ketamine may induce, 530
Amnihook, use of, 587
Amniocentesis, 146f, 146, 147–48, 381–87, 382f, 383p
clinical applications of, 382, 384–87
complications of, 381
for diabetic client, 316
for fetal maturity evaluation, 384–87
with PIH, 342
with PROM, 546
genetic screening with, 146, 146f, 147–48, 387
herpes virus shown by, 359
as hydramnios intervention, 577
hyperbilirubinemia risk assessment with, 823
meconium staining shown by, 387
placental grading as alternative to, 372
procedure, 381–82, 383p
locating placenta before, 368, 371
for Rh evaluation, 147, 349, 382, 384, 384f
Rh sensitization affected by, 349–50, 824
risk identification with, 734
risks of, 381, 913
spina bifida detection by, 880
Amniography, 147
Amnion, 167, COLOR PLATE
as caul, 418
formation of, 164–65, 166f
Amnionitis
assessing neonate for, 842
as premature rupture of membranes risk, 425t
sign of at labor onset, 431g
Amnioscopy, 147, 387
hemoglobinopathies diagnosed by, 148
Amniotic cavity, 164, 164f, 166f
Amniotic fluid
amnioscopy to examine, 387
assessing fetal lung maturity with, 384
before induction of labor, 588
in prolonged labor, 542
after PROM, 547
aspiration of, transient tachypnea of newborn after, 797
composition of, 165
creatinine levels in, 386–87
cytologic examination of fetal cells in, 387
embolism in, 576
expulsion of before labor, 416
formation of, 165
greenish, immediate interventions for, 488t
increased volume of. *See* Hydramnios
infection in, from maternal urinary tract, 353
inspecting after amniotomy, 587

leakage of during labor, comfort and, 483
L/S ratio in, 385, 385f
lung profile of, 385–86, 386f
meconium staining in, 387. *See also* Meconium aspiration syndrome
as intrapartal risk factor, 425t
portwine, with abruptio placentae, 569
problems associated with, 575–77
role of, 165
swallowing of, neonatal vomiting from, 651
volume of, 165
in prolonged pregnancy, 759t
Amniotic fluid analysis, 381. *See also* Amniocentesis, Amnioscopy
Amniotic fluid embolism, as precipitous labor risk, 543
Amniotomy, 586–87
as abruptio placentae intervention, 564, 571
defined, 586
FHR assessment after, 574
as hypertonic labor intervention, 537
as hypotonic labor intervention, 541
induction of labor with, 588–89
for placenta previa, 567
premature, transverse lie after, 556
as prolonged labor intervention, 542
in trial labor, with CPD, 578
Amphetamines, abuse of in pregnancy, 360–62, 361t
Ampicillin
for cystitis in pregnancy, 353
fir group B streptococcus in neonate, 843
for sepsis neonatorum, 842
Ampulla of fallopian tube, 82f, 82–83
fertilization in, 160, 163f
mucosal layer in, 83
Amylase, pancreatic, neonates lack, 651
Anaerobic bacterial infections, puerperal, 974
Anaerobic metabolism in neonates, 768
with cold stress, 817, 818
with RDS, 794f, 795
Anal fissures, assessing neonate for, 684, 702g
Anal sphincter, meningomyelocele affects, 882, 883n
Anal strictures, as imperforate anus complication, 872
Analgesia
afterpains relieved by, 907, 915, 917n
attachment problems from, 968
for breast engorgement, 919n, 937
cesarean delivery, 609
postpartal pain relief, 941
for cracked nipples, 936
for culdoscopy, 117
for episiotomy discomfort, 596
for mastitis, 987
in labor and delivery
administration of, 511–13, 512d
ambulation contraindicated by, 474
for cardiac client, 313
effects on fetus of, 452, 510–11
factors affecting use of, 510–11
five cardinal C's for use of, 532

goal for use of, 510
induced, 589, 592n
methoxyflurane for, 529
in neonatal assessment, 660
neonatal response to, 511, 648, 688g
nitrous oxide for, 529, 530
preterm labor as contraindication for, 550
prolonged labor caused by, 542
record keeping about, 480n
regional, 513–16. *See also* specific types
self-administered, 529
self-esteem and, 413
twins and, 559
uterine involution affected by, 903
during lactation suppression, 925
for localized infection pain relief, 975, 978n
for puerperal pyelonephritis, 986
for pulmonary embolism, 985n
for venous thrombosis, 980, 981, 984n, 985n
Analgesic sprays, for episiotomy relief, 596
Anaphase, 158, 158f, 159f
Anaphylactoid reactions, to vitamin K, 711d. *See also* Allergic reactions
Anasarca, with hydrops fetalis, 826
Anatomic fibrosis in neonate, 641
Anchoring villi in placenta, 167
Anderson, B. G., on health beliefs, 205, 206
Androgens
in females, role of, 93
prepubertal rise in, 92
puberty role of, 93
Android pelvis, 396, 397f
Anemia. *See also* Iron-deficiency anemia
fetal
assessing, 349
intrauterine transfusion for, 349, 350p
from Rh hemolytic disease, 347
risk factors for, 214–15t
sinusoidal FHR patters and, 457
symmetric IUGR from, 762
tachycardia caused by, 450
maternal
as adolescent pregnancy risk, 297, 303
assessing for
after cesarean, 603
in fourth trimester, 947g
birth center screening for, 618
in diabetic client, 316
dysfunctional labor with, interventions for, 536
estriol levels affected by, 380
megaloblastic, 326, 327
microangiopathic, with PIH, 340–41
multiple gestation and, 558
physiologic, of pregnancy, 198
pica related to, 281–82
as placenta previa risk, 566
postpartal hemorrhage risk with, 972
as pregnancy complication, 214t, 326–28
resuscitation risk with, 786
risk factors for, 214t
sickle cell. *See* Sickle cell anemia
symmetric IUGR from, 762
thromboembolic disease risk with, 980, 983
neonatal, 830, 835

from aganglionosis, 869
apnea associated with, 749
assessing preterm infants for, 757n
causes of, 830
clinical manifestations of, 826, 830, 835
from congenital CMV, 358
from congenital toxoplasmosis, 357
conjunctiva with, 694g
cyanosis and, 889
hemoglobin values defining, 830
hemolytic, vitamin E to prevent, 746
from hemolytic disease of the newborn, 823, 826
with hydrops fetalis, 824, 826
interventions for, 835
iron-deficiency, umbilical cord controversy and, 491
multiple gestation and, 558
physiologic, 644, 835
from placenta previa, 566
as prematurity risk, 749, 757n
retrolental fibroplasia risk with, 815
risk factors for, 214–15t
skin pallor with, 689g
Anencephaly
amniotic fluid density and, 384
assessing neonate for, 691g
breech presentation and, 554
estriol levels with, 380
face presentation with, 553
hydramnios associated with, 576
postmaturity with, 759
prenatal diagnosis of, 146, 148
recurrence risk of, 145t
ultrasound to detect, 368, 370, 577
Anesthesia. *See also* specific types of anesthesia
for cesarean delivery, 609
mortality from, 605
parent choice for, 606
technologic advances in, 600
for D&C abortion, 129
during labor and delivery
anesthesia of choice, 518
attachment problems from, 968
balanced, 529, 530
cesarean; see for cesarean delivery
for drug abusers, 362
fetal effects of, 452, 456–57
five cardinal C's for, 532
as forceps delivery indication, 597
general. *See* General anesthesia
goal of, 528
hypnosis for, 295–96
inhalation, 529
local, 514–15, 528, 528f
in neonatal assessment, 660
neonatal effects of, 648, 688g
nursing care plan, 521–24
parental decision making about, 613
physiologic, 408
with PIH, 346
postpartal bladder complications from, 905, 982
postpartal hemorrhage risk with, 972
prolonged labor caused by, 542
record keeping about, 480n
regional. *See* Regional anesthesia
twins and, 559
thromboembolic disease risk with, 980

Anesthesia (Cont'd)
  urinary problems from, 905, 982
  uterine atony from, 579
  uterine involution affected by, 903
gas for, placental transport of, 170
general. See General anesthesia
"glove," 295
local
  allergy to, 515–16, 529
  for amniocentesis, 382
  for cardiac client delivery, 313
  for drug abusers in pregnancy, 362
  for episiotomy and repair, 528, 528f
  for labor and delivery, 514–15, 528, 528f
  toxic effects of, 514–16, 528
  for vasectomy, 127
in pregnancy
  spinal, 198
  for surgery, 351
regional. See Regional anesthesia; specific types of regional anesthesia
topical, perineal pain relief with, 915, 917n
for vacuum aspiration abortion, 129
Anger
  after cesarean birth, 607, 608, 941–42
  as defective birth response, 849
  in grief process, 999
  with postpartal psychosis, 988
Angiography, PPH diagnosis with, 817
Angioma, capillary, in neonate, 677–78
Angiomatous tumors of the placenta, 568
Angiotensin II
  PIH and, 336, 340
  role of in pregnancy, 340
Animals, listeriosis and, 356, 357
Aninophylline, for pulmonary embolism, 982
Anisocoria, assessing in neonate, 694g
Ankle dorsiflexion, gestational age and, 663f, 669, 671f
Ankle ulcers, from sickle cell anemia, 327
Anomalous venous return of pulmonary veins, 886f, 892
  congestive heart failure with, 893
Anorexia
  with postpartum blues, 907
  as puerperal infection sign, 977, 978n
Anorexia nervosa, 284–85
  amenorrhea from, 100
Anoxia
  fetal peristalsis stimulated by, 651
  in neonate
    arrythmia as sign of, 698g
    body position as sign of, 702g
    skin pallor with, 689g
    with tetralogy of Fallot, 890
Antacids, administering during labor, 531
Antenatal genetic screening, amniocentesis for, 387
Antenatal nursing assessment. See Antepartal nursing assessment
Antenatal nursing management. See Antepartal nursing management
Antepartal nursing assessment, 210–43. See also Assessment

baseline blood pressure, 341
child abuse potential identification, 1016
client history, 210–13, 212f, 214–15t
  diabetes mellitus and, 322
  family crisis risk as part of, 999, 1000–1001t
  high-risk screening, 213, 214–15t
  for home birth, 629
  of hyperthyroidism, 326
  multiple gestation identification in, 558
  of nutrition, 285, 286–87f
  of PIH
    eclampsia, 344
    severe preeclampsia, 343
  parenting disorder identification, 1012, 1016
  physical
    initial, 213, 216–26g, 227f, 228–30g, 231–35p, 236t
    initial, adolescent pregnancy, 303
    subsequent, 238, 239–40g
  psychologic
    initial, 238, 238g
    subsequent, 240–41, 241–43g
  resuscitation risk factors, 786
  for Rh sensitization, 347–49
Antepartal nursing management, 243, 285–92
  of adolescents, 302–5
    importance of, 297
  alcohol intake and, 269, 770
  assessment as part of, 285, 286–87f. See also Antepartal nursing assessment
  attachment affected by, 963–64, 964–65
  attachment problem identification by, 1012
  of cardiac client, 311–12
  classes for family members, 291–92
  cultural considerations, 204–7, 288–89t, 289
  for diabetic client, 318–21, 322–25n
  for drug-addicted client, 360, 361–62, 772
  early pregnancy detection and, 368
  education as part of. See Parent education
  federal support for, 5
  frequency of, with mild preeclampsia, 342
  home birth preparation, 629–30
  hyperbilirubinemia prevention during, 823
  of hyperemesis gravidarum, 328
  nutrition as part of. See Pregnancy, nutrition in
  with PIH, 337–40n
  postpartal hemorrhage risk and, 972
  postpartal anticipatory guidance as part of, 289–90
  pregnancy discomforts and, 253f, 259–60
  relinquishment for adoption, 1015t
  for Rh sensitization, 347–49, 350p
  risk factors in, 214–15t
  single parents, 1018
Anterior fontanelle
  assessing, 678, 692g
  depressed, on SGA neonate, 764
Anterior pituitary gland
  female reproductive cycle role of, 96, 97f
  postdelivery necrosis of, 988

puberty role of, 92, 92f
Anterior pituitary hormones, pregnancy role of, 202
Anthropoid pelvis, 396, 397f
Antianxiety drugs, fetal/neonatal effects of, 361t
Antibiotic cream, for localized postpartal infection, 975
Antibiotic ointment, for neonatal eye prophylaxis, 499n, 505, 710, 711d, 844
Antibiotics
  in breast milk, 930
  for cardiac client, 312, 313
  for group B streptococcus in neonate, 843
  intravenous, after PROM, 546
  for mastitis, 987
  moniliasis with, 845
  for puerperal infections, 975, 976, 978–79n
    thrush and, 979n
    urinary, 986
  for retained placental fragments, 972, 973
  for sepsis neonatorum, 842
  for subinvolution, 973
Antibodies, in neonate, 654
Antibody screen, for Rh sensitization, 348
Anticipatory grief, 1002
  with defective birth, 849
  with high-risk neonate, 773
  with preterm birth, 1006, 1009
Anticipatory guidance
  cesarean birth eased by, 942
  crisis prevention with, 998
  high-risk pregnancy requires, 998–99
  in groups, 996
  in latent phase labor, 474
  parent-infant attachment aided by, 965
  as postpartal teaching method, 939
  postpartal sexual relations, 940
  as part of prenatal education, 291
  prenatal parenting assessment, 999, 1000–1001t
  for relinquishing mothers, 1015t
Anticoagulants. See also Heparin; Warfarin
  for cardiac client, 312
  neonatal effects of, 769
  overdose signs, 984ncp
  for pulmonary embolism, 985n
Anticonvulsants
  cleft lip and palate from, 851
  congenital heart defects from, 881
  IUGR associated with, 761
  for severe preeclampsia, 344, 345d
Antidiuretic hormones, in pregnancy, 202
Antigen-antibody response, in neonates, 654
Antihistamines, for anesthesia reactions, 516
Antihypertensives, for preeclampsia/ eclampsia, 343, 344
Antimetabolic drugs, IUGR associated with, 761
Antispasmodics, for puerperal pyelonephritis, 986
Anuria, in neonate
  as MAS complication, 815
  preterm, 746
Anus of neonate
  assessing, 684, 702g
    in delivery room, 496
    by temperature taking, 710
  imperforate, 871f, 871–72

Anxiety
  with abruptio placentae, 563
  about cesarean delivery, 608
    interventions for, 602, 607
  crisis creates, 992, 993
  with DIC, interventions for, 573n
  extreme, as pulmonary embolism sign, 981, 983, 984n, 985n
  fetal tachycardia caused by, 450
  from hemorrhage, 571n, 572n
  hyperventilation from, 570
  during labor
    anesthesia as cause of, 521n
    complications from, 535–36
    coping mechanisms and, 405, 406, 413
    evaluating and managing, 435g, 484
    first stage, 417, 418, 428g
    hypertonic labor patterns increase, 537
    medications to relieve, 513
    preterm, 550
    prolonged, 542
  in neonate
    with cleft lip or palate, 855n, 857n
    preterm, sample nursing diagnosis, 758
    with tracheoesophageal atresia/ fistula, 864n
  physiologic signs of, 608
  positive role of, 484
  pregnancy complications and, 405
  of pregnant adolescent, 303
  with preterm or defective birth, 774
  PROM as cause of, 547
  with puerperal peritonitis, 976
  with puerperal psychosis, 988
  relaxation techniques for, 997–98
Aorta, of neonate
  abnormalities of, gestational age and, 183t
  coarctation of, 887f, 888–89
    assessing lower extremities for, 685
    femoral pulse with, 700g
    left-sided heart failure with, 893
    signs of, 683
  overriding, in tetralogy of Fallot, 887f, 890
  pregnancy with, 313
  transposition of, 886f, 890–92, 892f
    risk factors for, 736f
Aorta, coarctaction of, in pregnancy, 310
Aortic atresia, in hypoplastic left heart syndrome, 892–93
Aortic pressure, increased at birth, 640
Aortic stenosis
  heart murmur in neonate from, 642
  left-sided heart failure with, 893
Apert syndrome
  nose with, 695g
  ocular hypertelorism with, 692g
Apgar, Dr. Virginia, 492
Apgar scores, 492t, 492, 495
  as assessment tool, 660
    explaining to parents, 706
    implications of, 495
    in immediate neonatal nursing care plan, 498
    risk identification with, 734, 788, 789t
  blood pH correlated with, 461, 789t
  drug addiction affects, 770–71

electronic fetal monitoring and, 459

fetoscopic auscultation and, 459

FHR patterns and, 375, 461

high-risk assessment with, 736

in postterm infant, 759

MAS affects, 798

necrotizing enterocolitis and, 837, 839n

neurologic abnormalities and, 734

paracervical block and, 517

psychic factors and, 535–36

resuscitative needs assessment with, 788, 789t

Apical pulse, monitoring in nursery, 712. See also Pulse, of neonate

Apnea, fetal episodes of, as normal, 371

Apnea, in neonate
  assessing for, 688g
  in reactivity period, 712
  defined, 749
  with group B streptococcal infection, 843
  as hypocalcemia sign, 821
  with hypoglycemia, 817, 818
  as illness sign, 729
  with intraventricular hemorrhage, 836
  with MAS, 798
  with necrotizing enterocolitis, 838, 839
  normal periods of, 639
  periodic breathing vs., 796t
  preterm
    hearing loss risk from, 758
    nursing care plan for, 755–56
    as respiratory distress sign, 751
    as risk, 749
    with RDS, 796t, 801n
    resuscitation risk with, 787
    retrolental fibroplasia risk with, 815
    risk factors for, 736f
    as sepsis neonatorum sign, 841
  theophylline for, 756n
  ventilatory assistance indicated by, 800t

Appendectomy, infertility from, 112

Appendicitis, during pregnancy, 351

Appropriate-for-gestational-age (AGA) neonates
  categories of (Pr, F, Po), 734, 735f
  preterm
    hypocalcemia risk in, 821
    hypoglycemia in, 818, 821
    nursing care plan vor, 750–58
    risk identification for, 734, 735–36f
  transient tachypnea in, 797–98

Approximation of wound edges
  evaluating episiotomy for, 912
  healing assessment by, 975t

Apresoline (hydralazine), for preeclampsia, 344, 347

Aquamephyton See Vitamin K

Ara-A (adenine arabinoside), for neonatal herpesvirus, 844

Ara-C (cytosine arabinoside), for neonatal herpesvirus, 844

Arab Americans, labor support for, 412

Arachidonic acid, in labor onset theory, 407

Arachnoiditis, as spinal anesthesia complication, 526

Arches, assessing in neonate, 703g

Areola
  of neonate, gestational age and, 661, 665f, 669f
  pigmentation changes in

nonpregnancy causes of, 192t
  from pregnancy, 192, 193, 199
  pregnancy changes in, 197; see also pigmentation changes in

Argininosuccinicaciduria, prenatal diagnosis of, 147

Arm recoil, gestational age and, 663f, 665f, 672

Arms, of neonate
  assessing, 684–85, 685f, 702g
  brachial palsy of, 684
  Erb-Duchenne paralysis of, 684–85, 685f

Arnold-Chiari lesion, 879
  meningomyelocele and, 880

Arrhythmias, in neonate
  assessing, 698g
  calcium gluconate for, 792
  as pneumothorax sign, 809n

Arterial blood gas values, with RDS, 803–4, 811p

Arteries. See also Blood supply
  in uterine layers, 79
  PIH changes in, 340, 340f

Arteriosclerosis, pregnancy with, 347

Arthritis, with secondary syphilis, 354

Artifical insemination, 113f, 119
  as alternative to genetic risk, 152
  by donor (AID), 119, 152
  by husband, 119

Aschheim-Zondek pregnancy test, 194–95

Ascites
  intrauterine transfusion for, 349
  in neonate
    from hemolytic disease of the newborn, 826, 827
    with hydrops fetalis, 826
    localized flank bulging with, 699g
  pregnancy signs caused by, 192t
  ultrasound to detect, 368, 370

Ascorbic acid, neonatal requirements, 717, 717t. See also Vitamin C

Aseptic technique, puerperal infection and, 974. See also Handwashing

Asepto syringe feeding, for cleft lip, 853n, 854n, 856n

Ash, in breast milk, cow's milk, and formula, 719t

Asian Americans. See also Oriental Americans
  labor support for, 412
  postpartal customs, 914
  neonates
    epicanthal folds in, 693g
    Mongolian spots on, 677
    physiologic jaundice in, 649
    feeding customs, 925

Asphyxia
  fetal
    chronic, intrapartal fetal heart aberrations and, 425t
    hyperbilirubinemia risk from, 822, 831
    identifying risk of, 375, 425t
    intrapartal risk factors for, 425t
    maternal cardiac disease and, 768
    as maternal drug addiction risk, 770
    from maternal hypertension, 769
    nursing care plan, 538–39
    necrotizing enterocolitis from, 839n
    with oxytocin induction, 594n
    as prolonged labor risk, 542
    surfactant production impaired by, 739

from transverse lie, 556
  transient tachypnea of newborn from, 797
  from vasa previa, 575–76
  neonatal, 786–92, 789t, 790f, 791–92p, 792
    bradycardia as sign of, 688g
    as breathing onset stimulus, 636
    hearing loss risk from, 758
    hyperbilirubinemia risk with, 822, 823
    intrapartal risk factors for, 425t
    jaundice and, 831
    necrotizing enterocolitis from, 837, 839n
    pathophysiology of, 786
    PPH syndrome with, 817
    RDS risk with, 794
    severe, delay in clearing lungs from, 637
  perinatal
    GFR decreased by, 746
    hypocalcemia risk increased with, 821
    IVH from, 836
    as LGA neonatal risk, 761
    as postmaturity risk, 759, 760
    as SGA neonatal risk, 761, 762, 765p
    sinusoidal FHR pattern with, 457
    transient tachypnea of newborn from, 797

Aspiration pneumonia
  group B streptococcal infection vs., 843
  with tracheoesophageal atresia/fistula, 860

Aspiration, problems from
  as SGA neonatal risk, 762, 765
  with tracheoesophageal atresia/fistula, 860, 861, 862n
  transient tachypnea of newborn, 797

Assessment. See also Assessment guides
  of adolescents, sexuality and, 105–6
  antepartal. See Antepartal nursing assessment
  before abortion, 129
  of bleeding in pregnancy, 329
  of crisis situation, 995–96, 998–99
  of diabetic client, 318, 322
  of ectopic pregnancy, 333–34
  family as part of, 47–49
    with high-risk neonate, 777
  of fetus. See Assessment of fetus
  intrapartal. See Intrapartal assessment; Intrapartal maternal assessment
    at labor admission, 467–68
    of adolescent, 471
  of labor pain, 483
  of neonate. See Assessment of neonate
  objective vs. subjective, 969
  of parenting readiness, 725–26, 1000–1001t
  of PIH, 337
  postpartal. See Postpartal nursing assessment
  of preeclampsia, severe, 343
  of psychiatric problems, 988
  of resuscitation risk, 786–87
  sexual history as part of, 106

Assessment of fetus, 366
  of FHR tracings, 460t, 460–61
  intrapartal. See Intrapartal fetal assessment
  IUGR risk, 761–62
  with maternal PIH, 341–42

by mother, 372–73

Assessment guides
  format of, 236
  initial antepartal, 216–36
  intrapartal physical, first stage labor, 428–32
  intrapartal psychologic, 435
  neonatal physical, 688–704
  postpartal examinations, 945–48
  postpartal home visit, 624–27

Assessment of neonate
  adolescent mother and, 943
  aganglionic megacolon, 869–70
  anemia, 830, 835
  anomalous venous return, 892
  Apgar scoring system for. See Apgar scores
  atrial septal defects, 885
  bases for, 660
  behavioral, 687, 705–6
  cardiac disease in mother and, 769
  choanal atresia, 852, 857
  after circumcision, 722
  cleft lip and palate, 852, 853n
    after surgery, 854n
  coarctation of aorta, 889
  congenital hypothyroidism, 859
  congestive heart failure, 893–94
  as continual process, 660
  cyanosis, 889
  by delivery room nurse, 495–97, 496f
  diaphragmatic hernia, 866
  DIC, 837
  endocardial cushion defects, 888
  during exchange transfusion, 825p, 828–29
  general appearance, 674–75
  for gestational age, 660–74, 662–74f, APPENDIX D
  gonorrhea, 844
  hemolytic disease of the newborn, 826, 827
  hemorrhagic disease, 836
  herpesvirus type 2 infection, 844
  high-risk, 735–37. See also specific risks
  LGA, 761
  hip dysplasia, 877f, 877–78
  hypoglycemia, 818–21, 819–20p
  for hyperbilirubinemia, 824; see also for jaundice
  hypoplastic left heart syndrome, 893
  immediately after delivery, 498n
  imperforate anus, 871–72
  for IUGR, 762
  intestinal obstruction, 873–74
  intraventriculr hemorrhage, 836
  jaundice, 824, 831n; see also for hyperbilirubinemia
    pathologic, 823, 824
    physiologic, 649
  meconium aspiration syndrome, 798, 814
  meningocele/meningomyelocele, 880, 882
  moniliasis (thrush), 844–45
  by mother, during acquaintance phase, 957–58
  necrotizing enterocolitis, 839n
  neurologic, 657, 663–65f, 669, 671–73f, 672
  at nursery admission, 709–13
  in nursery routine care, 714
  nutritional, 719–21, 720–21t
  in observation nursery, 709–13
  parents' role in, 706
  patent ductus arteriosus, 885
  during phototherapy, 829–30
  physical assessment guide, 688–704g

Assessment of neonate (Cont'd)
  physical examination as part of, 674–87
  PKU, 858
  after placenta previa emergency delivery, 567
  postterm, 759–60
  preterm, 750n
  for respiratory distress, 792
  during respiratory therapy, 802–3n
    for complications, 809–10n
  for resuscitation need, 786–87
  risk identification with, 736–37
  for sepsis neonatorum, 841–42
  SGA, 764n
  sleep-wake patterns, 705
  spina bifida, 880, 882
  states of consciousness, behavior and, 705–6
  stool, 874
  during suction efforts, 805–6n
  talipes equinovarus (clubfoot), 875f, 876
  tetralogy of Fallot, 890
  with tracheoesophageal atresia/fistula, 860–61, 862n
  transient tachypnea of newborn, 797–98
  transposition of the great vessels, 891–92
  after vacuum extraction delivery, 599
  ventricular septal defects, 885, 888
  vomiting, 873–74
Asthma, labor anesthesia with, 530
Asynclitism, engagement with, 403
Ataractics, during labor, 513. See also Tranquilizers
Atelectasis
  in mother, as pulmonary embolism sign, 984n
  in neonate
    breath sounds decreased with, 698g
    with cold stress, 817
    lung assessment for, 698g
    with MAS, 814, 815
    preterm, assessing for, 757n
    suctioning creates, 805n, 813
    with RDS, 794, 794f, 795
    with tracheoesophageal atresia/fistula, 861
Athletic regimens, amenorrhea from, 100
ATP. See Adenosine triphosphate
Atresia
  aortic, 892–93
  of biliary duct, neonatal jaundice and, 831
  choanal, 695g, 852, 857
  defined, 859
  esophageal, 859–61, 860f, 861f, 862–65n
    assessing for, 696g, 716
  of gastrointestinal tract, assessing neonate for, 684
  intestinal. See Intestinal obstruction
  meatal, assessing neonate for, 700g
  mitral, 892–93
  tricuspid, 886f, 893
Atretic follicles, in ovarian cortex, 83
Atrial pressure, birth changes in, 640, 641f
Atrial septal defects, 885, 886f
  pregnancy with, 310
  right-sided heart failure from, 893
  transposition of great vessels and, 891

Atropine
  fetal heartbeat and, 171, 451, 452
  for neonatal bradycaria, 792
Attachment process, 951, 960–61. See also Bonding
  acquaintance phase, 957–58
  adolescent mother, 961
  assessing, 948g, 963–68, 966–68f, 968–69
    in postpartal home visit, 627
  breast-feeding aids, 927
  complications of, 968–69
  with congenital anomalies, 773–74, 1010, 1011f, 1013f
    crisis intervention for, 1011–14
  culture affects, 964, 968–69
  defective birth and, 849–50
  dyssynchrony in, 960
  engrossment of father, 961–62
  environment affects, 954
  facial appearance of infant and, 553, 706
  facilitating, 494f, 499n, 502–3, 503f, 725
    with bladder exstrophy, 875
    with bottle-feeding, 926, 927f
    after cesarean delivery, 608, 942
    with cleft lip and palate, 853n, 856n
    with defective neonate, 1010
    in delivery room, 500–501
    with high-risk neonates, 737, 774–79
    with imperforate anus, 872
    in intensive care, 1013f, 1013–14
    with malattachment signs, 1012–13
    with meningocele/meningomyelocele, 883–84n
    with phototherapy, 829
    with preterm infant, 749, 774–79
    with puerperal infection, 978n
    with required bed rest, 985n
    with SGA neonate, 764, 765n
    with thromboembolic disease, 985n
    with tracheoesophageal atresia/fistula, 862n, 864–65n
  factors affecting, 951–55
  with family members, 963
  father's role in, 961–63, 962f
  in fourth trimester, 944
  grief process and, 1002, 1005–6
  with high-risk neonates, 737, 772, 773–79
  importance of, 960–61, 968
  introductory bonding, 955f, 955–57, 961–63, 962f
  maladaptive, 960, 968, 969, 1012–13
    crisis intervention for, 1011–14
  mother's role in, 951–53
  mutual regulation phase, 958–59
  nature of, 951
  neonate's role in, 706, 953–54
  nursing role in, 724, 964–65
  parenting behavior affected by, 968
  pregnancy course affects, 953
  prenatal, importance of, 953, 957–58
  preterm birth affects, 772–74, 1006, 1007–8t, 1009, 1011f, 1013f; see also facilitating, with preterm infant
  previous pregnancies affect, 952
  puerperal peritonitis and, 980n
  readiness for, 951–53
  reciprocity, 957f, 959–61

separation impedes, 968
sexual experiences affect, 952
Auditory capacity of neonate, 655
  assessing, 686–87, 697g, 705
  congenital CMV and, 358
Auerbach, A., 291
Auscultation
  electronic fetal monitoring vs., 459
  of fetal heart tones
    during labor, 424, 443f, 443–44, 445t, 480n
    Leopold maneuver before, 441
  of maternal chest, pulmonary embolism signs on, 982, 983, 984n
  multiple gestation identification by, 558
  of neonatal abdomen, 700g
  of neonatal chest, 682
    diaphragmatic hernia evidence on, 866
    lungs, 698g
    RDS assessment by, 797t, 801n, 802n
  of neonatal heart, 682, 683, 698–99g
    atrial septal defect detection by, 885
    coarctation of the aorta detected by, 889
    patent ductus arteriosus heard on, 885
Autoimmunity to semen, infertility from, 111t
Automobile safety, 729
Autonomic nervous system dysfunction, with meningomyelocele, 880
Autosomal anomalies, 136–40
  assessing for, 766n
  maternal age and, 147
Autosomal dominant inheritance, 142f, 142–43
  AID as alternative to, 152
Autosomal nondisjunction, 159
Autosomal recessive diseases, prenatal diagnosis of, 147–48
Autosomal recessive inheritance, 143f, 143–44
  AID as alternative to, 152
  of galactosemia, 859
  genetic counseling referral for, 151
  of homocystinuria, 858–59
  of maple syrup urine disease, 858
  of metabolic disorders, 857–59
Autosomes, 135, 157
Awake states, in neonate, 657. See also Sleep-wake states
Axillary hair, loss of with Sheehan syndrome, 988
Axillary temperature, of neonate
  assessing, 676f, 676–77
  in nursery, 710
  teaching parents about, 728, 729
Azotemia, feeding to prevent, 740, 741

B-adrenergic (sympathetic) blocking agents, fetal bradycardia from, 452
B-hemolytic streptococcus. See Beta-hemolytic streptococci
Babinski reflex, assessing in neonate, 704g. See also Reflexes
Baby Bonding Crib, 985n
Baby oil or powder, avoiding, 727
Babysitting, anticpatory guidance about, 289, 290
Back, of neonate, meningocele/meningomyelocele on, 878, 879f, 880, 882

Back pain, during labor. See also Backache
  birthing chair relieves, 617
  deceleration phase, 477–78n
  intense, malposition as cause of, 551
  relieving, 485. See also Back rub
Back rub, during labor
  active phase, 476n
  hypertonic, 537
  induced, 592n
  latent phase, 474
Backache
  abdominal muscle tone and, 905
  fetal position and, 404
  as impending labor sign, 416
  low, in pregnancy, 200
  with multiple gestation, 558
  with subinvolution, 973
Bacteria
  in breast milk, cow's milk, and formula, 719t
  gram negative enteric, neonatal susceptibility to, 654
  in neonatal urine, 652
Bacterial infection
  in mother
    mastitis, 986–87, 987f
    postpartal, aerobic and anerobic, 974
  in neonate
    hemolytic anemia caused by, 835
    hyperbilirubinemia risk from, 823, 831
    necrotizing enterocolitis, 837–38, 839–40n
    sepsis neonatorum, 841
  neonatal immunity to, 654
Bag and mask, resuscitating with, 788, 790f
Balanced translocation carriers, repeated abortion and, 329
Ballard, J. L., gestational age estimation tool by, 660, 661
Balloon septostomy, 892, 892f
Ballottement, 193–94
  nonpregnancy causes of, 192t
Bandl rings, 545, 545f
Baptism of dying infant, 1005
Barbiturates
  in pregnancy, 360–62, 361t
  neonatal sucking reflex affected by, 704g
  neonatal withdrawal from, 361, 361t
  intravenous, for obstetric anesthesia, 529–30
  nonstress test results after, 373
Bard, Samuel, 5
Barium enema. See X-rays
Barlow maneuver, hip dysplasia diagnosis with, 878
Barton forceps, 597, 597f
Basal metabolism rate (BMR)
  decreased, as hypothyroidism sign, 326
  increase in, thermogenesis by, 647
  pregnancy changes in, 201
Bascom, L., on denial of pregnancy, 1014
Baseline changes in fetal heart rate. See Fetal heart rate
Basophils, development of in fetus, 644
BAT. See Brown adipose tissue
Bathing
  for breast engorgement relief, 937
  infertility and, 114
  neonates
    evaporative heat loss from, 646

Leboyer method, 617, 618
    in nursery, 712
    rough or dry skin from, 690g
    teaching parents about, 727–28, 728f
    postpartal, 481n, 916
    culture and, 914
Battered child syndrome, prematurity and, 1009–10. See also Child abuse
Battledore placenta, 568, 574, 574f
Beckwith syndrome, 867
    birth weight with, 760
    hypoglycemia with, 761
    omphalocele and, 867
Bed, birthing stool vs., 4
Bed linens, during labor, 483
Bed rest
    for hypertonic labor, 537
    for PIH, 342, 343
    for placenta previa expectant management, 566–67
    preterm labor requires, 549
    for puerperal pyelonephritis, 986
    for pulmonary embolism, 985n
    umbilical cord prolapse prevention with, 574
    for venous thrombosis, 980, 981, 984n
Behavior of neonate, 654–57, 656f
    assessing. See Behavioral assessment
    attachment process affected by, 953–54
    maternal nutrition and, 654
    of preterm infants, 749
    sensory capacities, 655, 656f
Behavioral assessment
    of high-risk neonate's family, 777
    of neonate
        jaundice signs, 831
        for kernicterus, 823, 824
        necrotizing enterocolitis, 838, 839
        in neurologic examination, 657
        parents' role in, 706
        polycythemia signs, 835
        sepsis neonatorum signs, 841
Bellevue Hospital, midwifery school at, 6
Beta hemolytic strepotococci
    neonatal infection from, 841, 842–43
    puerperal infection from, 974
    lochia with, 975
Beta sympathomietic drugs, fetal tachycardia caused by, 450
Beta-lactose suppositories, for non-specific vaginitis, 356
Beta-receptors, uterine contractions slowed by, 407
Betamethasone (Celestone), 546, 547, 547d
    gestational age and, 550
    side effects of, 547
Bicarbonates (HCO₃), in neonatal blood, renal threshold controls, 652–53
Bikini incision, 605
Bile ducts, in neonate
    development of, 650
    fat absorption role of, 651
    obstruction of. See Biliary duct atresia
Bile-stained vomiting, as neonatal distress sign, 714
Biliary duct atresia, in neonate
    prognosis for, 823
    hyperbilirubinemia risk with, 823, 831
Bilirubin, 822
    conjugation of, 822–23

defective, physiologic jaundice from, 648, 649
    detecting in amniotic fluid, 382, 384, 384f
    neonatal levels of
        delayed cord clamping nd, 618
        low, from maternal drug use, 214t
        physiologic jaundice and, 648–50. See also Hyperbilirubinemia
Bilirubin binding test, 824
Bilirubin determinations
    hyperbilirubinemia risk assessment with, 824
    neonatal anemia assessment with, 835
    neonatal jaundice assessment with, 831n, 832, 833
Bilirubin pigment tests, risk identification with, 734
Bilirubin staining, vernix color with, 690g
Bimanual uterine compression, 579
Bing, Elizabeth, 294
Bioassay pregnancy tests, 194–95
Biologic sex, 88
    as component of sexuality, 88
    determination of, 89
Biparietal diameter of fetal head (BPD)
    determining, 368f, 369
    hydrocephaly and, 370
    IUGR diagnosis and, 369, 370–71
    ultrasound to measure, with PROM, 546
Birth
    alert state after, 657
    as crisis, 992
    cardiovascular adaptations at, 640–43, 641–43f
    neonatal reactivity after, 711–12, 713f
    respiratory adaptations at, 635–39, 637f, 639f
    vitamin K injection on day of, 650
Birth control, defined, 110
Birth control pills. See Oral contraceptives
Birth trauma
    cephalhematomas, 691g
    cerebral, as forceps delivery risk, 598
    cyanosis as sign of, 690g
    federally funded care to prevent, 5
    head movement problems from, 691g
    hypocalcemia risk increased with, 821
    as IDM risk, 768
    in LGA neonates, 761
    mouth signs of, 695g
    neonatal anemia caused by, 830
    preterm infant nursing care plan for, 756–57
    puerperal infection risk from, 974, 977
    risk factors for, 425t, 736f
    spleen enlargement from, 700g
Birth weight. See Weight at birth
Birthing alternatives, 613–31
    attachment and, 954
    birth centers, 618–19
        attachment facilitated in, 954
        delivery photos from, 620–23
        neonatal observation in, 709
        PKU screening in, 858
    birthing chair, 616–17, 617f; see also birthing stool
    birthing positions, 614–17, 615–17f

birthing room
    attachment facilitated in, 954
    delivery position in, 489
    delivery preparation in, 487
    neonatal observation in, 709
    newborn care in, 487
    reasons for using, 487
    siblings in, 292
    birthing stool, 3, 4
    case study, 619, 628
    sibling attendance, 292, 613–14
Birthmarks, assessing, 691g
Bishop, E. H., 588, 588t
Black Americans
    health beliefs among, 206
    lactose intolerance among, 281
    neonates
        diastasis recti in, 699g
        feeding customs for, 925
        protrusion of umbilicus in, 700g
        sole creases in, 661
    pain expression among, 470
    pallor signs in, 570
    pregnancy and cultural values among, 205, 288–89t
        birth attendants, 471
        labor customs, 469, 470, 471
        postpartal customs, 914
        prenatal nutriti?n for, 283–84
Bladder
    of mother
        assessing, in fourth stage labor, 481n
        catheterizing, with cesarean, 603, 608
        hypotonia of, in fourth stage of labor, 420
        injury to, as cesarean complication, 605
        labor and delivery stresses on, 409–10, 982
        postpartal assessment of, 481n, 913
        postpartal changes in, 905–6
        pregnancy changes in, 199
    of neonate, 652
        assessing, 496, 700g
        defects in, 874–75
        exstrophy of, 700g, 874–75
        meningocele/meningomyelocele and, 880, 883
        volume of, 652
Bladder distention
    assessing for, 982
        after cesarean, 603
        during labor, 474, 476, 478, 481
        postpartal, 913, 918n
    as hypotonic labor risk, 541
    interventions for, 906, 982, 986
    postpartal risk of, 905–6
    postpartal, uterine displacement by, 902
    preventing during labor, 483
    uterine involution affected by, 902, 903
Bladder infection, hematuria as sign of, 906
Bladder irritation, in pregnany, 199
Blalock-Hanlen operation, 892
Blalock-Taussig operation, 890, 891f
Blastocyst
    hCG secreted by, 98
    implantation of, 99, 100f
Bleeding. See also Bleeding, in neonate
    antepartal, 328–35
        as danger sign, 240g
        differential diagnosis of, 566
        as abruptio placentae sign, 563, 563t

complications associated with, 328–35, 567–68, 568f
    as DIC sign, 568
    as hemorrhage sign, 563t, 569, 572n
    from ectopic pregnancy, 333
    at labor admission, as vaginal exam contraindication, 468
    in labor
        excessive, immediate actions required by, 488t
        ketamine for anesthesia with, 530
        record keeping about, 480n
        third stage, 419, 420f
        transient tachypnea of newborn after, 797
    midcycle, 98, 100
    at ovulation, 98
    from placenta previa, 564, 565
    postpartal
        assessing, 904
        with bladder distention, 982
        from hemorrhage, 569, 572n
        late, from retained placental fragments, 579
        with PIH, 346
        with subinvolution, 903
        uterine contractions control, 902, 903
    in third trimester
        as birth center contraindication, 618
        as cephalic version contraindication, 585
        as CST indication, 375
        drug addiction and, 360
        from umbilical cord vasa previa, 574, 575
Bleeding, in neonate
    disseminated intravascular coagulation, 837
    enclosed, neonatal jaundice and, 831n
    with herpesvirus type 2, 844
    with hydrops fetalis, 826
    as PPH complication, 817
    risk factors for, 736f
    vaginal, assessing, 702g
    vitamin K and, 711d, 836
Blepharitis, marginal, in neonate, 693g
Blind pouch, with imperforate anus, 871, 872
Blind spots (scotomata), with PIH, 341
Blindness
    from intraventricular hemorrhage, 836
    from ophthalmia neonatorum, 844
    as prematurity risk, 758
    preventing. See Eye prophylaxis
    from retrolental fibroplasia, 815
Blinking reflex, assessing in neonate, 693g
Blood
    formation of in fetus, 643–44
    labor changes in, 409
    pregnancy changes in, 197t, 198
Blood assays
    for galactosemia, 859
    for maple syrup urine disease assessment, 858
Blood bicarbonate concentration, in neonates, 652–53
Blood chemistry, normal neonatal values, 645t
Blood clotting problems
    as cesarean complication, 605
    coagulation factor, postpartal, 906
    hemorrhage risk with, 569
    in neonate, 836

Blood clotting problems (Cont'd)
  DIC, 837
    liver and, 650, 650t
    petechiae as sign of, 691g
    vaginal bleeding with, 702g
Blood component therapy, for DIC,
  567–68, 573n
Blood cultures
  for group B streptococcus in
    neonate, 843
  in sepsis neonatorum assessment,
    841
Blood flow, pregnancy changes in,
  197t, 198
Blood gases, of neonate
  apnea affects, 756n
  assessing, with RDS, 801n, 803–
    4n, 811p
  pneumothorax effects on, 816
  umbilical arterial line for
    monitoring, 811p
Blood glucose, neonatal levels of,
  648
  assessing
    for hypoglycemia, 818, 819–
      20p, 821, 831n
    for IDM, 768
  monitoring
    in postterm infant, 760
    in SGA neonates, 821
  normal values, 645t
Blood glucose determinations, for
  pregnant diabetic, 320. See
  also Glucose tolerance tests
Blood group sensitization, as risk
  factor, 215t
Blood hyperviscosity, in LGA
  neonates, 761
Blood imcompatibility, skin texture
  with, 690g. See also ABO
  incompatibility
Blood loss. See also Hypovolemia
  assessing amount of, 571n
    after cesarean, 603
    by hematocrit drop, 906
    with hemorrhage 569–71n
  during delivery
    normal, 420, 906
    resuscitation risk with, 787
    tachycardia after, 906
  in fetus, neonatal anemia caused
    by, 830
  in neonate
    causes of, 830
    preterm, significance of, 749
  from postpartal hemorrhage, 972
  signs of, 346
  during surgery in pregnancy, 351
Blood on diaper, causes of, 652
Blood pH
  with acidosis, 794, 795
  Apgar score correlated with, 789t
  labor changes in, 409
  in preterm infant
    monitoring, 753n
    normal values, 747, 752t
  pneumothorax effects on, 816
Blood pressure, in mother
  assessing; see also monitoring
    in fourth trimester, 945g
    with hematoma, 580
    before induction, 589, 590,
      591n
    during labor, 428g, 473, 475n,
      479, 481n, 497, 501
    before Methergine administra-
      tion, 903d
    with mild preeclampsia, 342
    at postpartal home visit, 624
    postpartum, 906, 912, 917,
      919n
    with severe preeclampsia, 343

baseline, importance of, 342
after cesarean, medications affect,
  603
change in, birth center transfer for,
  618
decreased, as shock sign, 569
after delivery, normal changes in,
  420
increased, as anxiety sign, 608
labor changes in, 409
monitoring; see also assessing
  during delivery, 490
  during external version, 586
  in hemorrhage nursing care
    plan, 569, 570
  with induced labor, 589, 591n,
    592n
  with PIH, 338
  with severe preeclampsia, 341,
    343
  with preterm labor, 549
  with ritodrine administration,
    549
  with severe preeclampsia, 344
  with uterine inversion, 580
pain response of, 483
with preeclampsia/eclampsia, 338,
  341, 342, 343
pregnancy changes in, 197t, 198
pulmonary embolism effects on,
  981, 983
Blood pressure, in neonate, 641,
  642f
  assessing, 641
    at nursery admission, 710
  blood loss lowers, 835
  coarctation of the aorta affects,
    889
  with congestive heart failure, 894
  IVH risk and, 836
  patent ductus arteriosus affects,
    885
  pneumothorax decreases, 809n
  umbilical arterial line for monitor-
    ing, 811p
Blood sampling
  fetal. See Fetal blood sampling
  neonatal
    arterial, with RDS, 803–4ncp,
      811p
    PPH diagnosis with, 817
    from preterm infants, affect on
      volume, 749
    site of, hematologic values
      affected by, 644
    umbilical arterial catheterization
      for, 811p
Blood smear
  neonatal anemia assessment with,
    835
  neonatal jaundice assessment with,
    831n
Blood supply, to endometrium, 94,
  95, 95f, 99
Blood tests. See also Screening;
  specific tests
  DIC confirmation with, 567
  before induction of labor, 591n
  for pregnant diabetic, 317–18,
    319
Blood transfusions. See also
  Exchange transfusions
  for abruptio placentae
    hemorrhage, 572
  incompatible, renal failure from,
    563
  for amniotic fluid embolism, 576
  blood volume expanders, for
    neonate, 792
  for DIC, 568
  with ectopic pregnancy surgery,
    334

for hemorrhage, 571n
for hypermagnesemic infant, 76
intrauterine, 8, 349, 350p
preparing for, with placenta
  previa, 567
for preterm infants, 748
religious preference and, 569
sickle cell anemia pregnancy and,
  328
twin-to-twin, hyperbilirubinemia
  with, 822
umbilical arterial catheterization
  for, 811p
for uterine atony hemorrhage, 579
for uterine inversion, 580
Blood type
  ABO incompatibility and. See
    ABO incompatibility
  neonatal anemia and, 835
  neonatal hyperbilirubinemia and,
    823, 824
Blood typing
  before cesarean delivery, 601
  in hemorrhage nursing care plan,
    569
  with hemorrhage risk, 972
  before induction of labor, 591n
  at labor admission, 472
    high-risk, 469
  risk identification with, 734, 824
  of umbilical cord sample, 480n
  for uterine inversion, 580
Blood urea, normal neonatal values,
  645t
Blood urea nitrogen (BUN) test, in
  PIH assessment, 337
  with severe preeclampsia, 343
Blood uric acid, in PIH assessment,
  337
Blood values, postpartal changes in,
  906
Blood volume
  increase in. See Polycythemia
  of neonate, 644, 645
    delayed cord clamping and, 645
    preterm, blood sampling affect
      on, 749
  postpartal, with PIH, 346
  pregnancy changes in, 197t, 198,
    310, 336, 340
  reduction in. See Blood loss;
    Hypovolemia
Blood volume expanders
  for resuscitation, 788
  for shock in neonate, 792
Bloody show
  assessing, 473n
  during first stage of labor, 475n,
    477n
  as impending labor sign, 415
  during second stage of labor,
    418
Blurred vision, with PIH, 341
BMR. See Basal metabolism rate
Body boundary, pregnancy changes
  in, 204
Body image, pregnancy changes in,
  204
Body mechanics, with multiple
  gestation, 558
Body position
  of mother
    after accidents in pregnancy,
      353
    for bottle-feeding, 926, 927f
    for breast-feeding, 929, 929f,
      937f
    after cesarean delivery, 609,
      917
    for contraction stress test, 376
    for deep leg vein disease, 981,
      984n

for delivery. See Delivery,
  positions for
for eclampsia, 344
for gas pain, 941
for handling neonate, 714, 715f
for hemorrhage, 571n
for hemorrhoidal relief, 915
for infant feeding, 924, 927f,
  937f
during labor. See Labor, body
  positions during
for nonstress test, 374
after oxytocin overdose, 543
for pelvic cellulitis, 979n
for PIH clients, 342, 343
for postpartal cardiac client,
  313
for surgery in pregnancy, 351
of neonate, 714, 715f
  assessing, 657, 702g
  with bronchopulmonary dys-
    plasia, 808n
  for cleft palate, 856n
  with congestive heart failure,
    894
  in crib, 716
  for diaphragmatic hernia inter-
    vention, 866, 867
  after feeding, 716
  with intubation, 805n, 806n
  for meningocele/meningomyelo-
    cele, 882n, 883n
  for mucus drainage, 492
  for narcotic withdrawal, 771
  for Pierre Robin syndrome,
    850–51
  preterm, heat loss and, 740
  for RDS, 803n
  teaching parents about, 726
  after tracheoesophageal
    surgery, 863n
Body temperature. See Temperature
Bonding, 955f, 955–57, 961–63,
  962f. See also Attachment
  process
  by adolescent mother, 300t
  adoption and, 1011
  assessing, 913–14, 964, 965–69,
    966–68f
    with father in nursery, 711
  eye prophylaxis and, 710, 11d
  facilitating, 492, 494f
    with behavioral assessment,
      706
    birthing options for, 613
    with bottle-feeding, 926, 927f
    for cardiac clients, 313
    after cesarean, 602, 603, 604,
      607
    with cleft palate, 852
    for diabetic client, 321
    with maternal drug addiction,
      771
    with preterm infant, 754n
    with SGA neonate, 764n
  factors affecting, 951–55
  importance of, 725
    with high-risk neonates, 772
  mother's readiness for, 951–53
  nursing support during, 714
Bone demineralization, in preterm
  infants, 746
Bone lesions
  from rubella, 215t
  with congenital syphilis, 844
Bone marrow
  fetal development of, 643–44
  in neonates, role of, 835
Bones, postmenopausal osteoporosis
  of, 101
Bony dystocia, transverse lie and,
  555–56

Bony pelvis, 65–71, 66f, 68–70f.
See also Pelves, types of
Boston Lying-in Hospital, night
nursery in, 5
Bottle-feeding, 926–27, 927f. *See
also* Formula-feeding;
Formulas
bottle sterilization, 927, 928p
of breast milk, 930, 938
cultural discouragement of, 925
decision making about, 716, 717,
718–19, 719t
initial, 716
lactation suppression medications,
480n
of preterm infants, 742t
sucking patterns with, 655
weight gain with, 718
Bougie, for esophageal stenosis, 861
Bowel atresia in neonate, hyperbilirubinemia risk with, 823
Bowel control, meningomyelocele
and, 880, 882
Bowel distention, hypotonic labor
patterns from, 541
Bowel elimination
postpartal, 905
assessing, 913, 946–47g
encouraging, 918n
in neonate
breast-fed vs. formula-fed, 651
frequency of, 651
Bowel obstruction, in neonate
hyperbilirubinemia risk with, 823
peristalsis with, 699g
Bowel perforation, from necrotizing
enterocolitis, 837
Bowel sounds
auscultating, after cesarean, 603
in neonate
auscultating, 700g
with diaphragmatic hernia, 866
in reactivity period, 712, 713f
BPD. *See* Biparietal diameter of fetal
head; Bronchopulmonary dysplasia
Brassiere, 260
for postpartal period, 908, 910
engorgement relieved by, 936
Braces, for meningomyelocele, 880
Brachial palsy. *See also* Brachial
plexus injury
assessing neonate for, 702g
Erb-Duchenne syndrome affects,
697g
as LGA neonatal risk, 761
Moro reflex affected by, 697g
Brachial plexus injury. *See also*
Brachial palsy
Moro reflex affected by, 703g
from vaginal breech delivery, 554
Brachystasis, 407
Bradford frame, 882
Bradley, R. A., 295
Bradley (partner-coached) method,
293, 295
Bradycardia
fetal, 451–52
assessing, through auscultation,
424
causes of, 452
defined, 451–52
with forceps delivery, 598
with induction, interventions for,
590, 594n
interventions for, 451t
intrapartal fetal heart aberrations and, 425t
after paracervical block, 516,
517
as precipitous labor risk, 543
preterminal, 458

after regional anesthesia, 523n
resuscitation risk with, 786
umbilical cord compression
causes, 455–56
from umbilical cord prolapse,
574
maternal
as Methergine side effect, 903d
puerperal, 906
neonatal
apnea with, 755–56n
assessing, 698g
assessing for, while suctioning,
814p
cardiac medications in mother
and, 769
drug therapy for, 792
with intraventricular hemorrhage, 836
as pneumothorax sign, 809n
retrolental fibroplasia risk with,
815
Brain atrophy, with hydrocephalus,
880
Brain damage
from abruptio placentae, 563
from birth trauma, 756–57n
with cleft palate, 852
from fetal alcohol syndrome, 770
FHR baseline variability caused
by, 452
from galactosemia, 859
hydrocephaly and, 557, 880
from hyperbilirubinemia, 823
from maternal CMV, 358
Moro reflex absent with, 703g
from neonatal asphyxia, 786
projectile vomiting from, 874
pupils with, 694g
from undetected CPD with
malposition, 552
Braun von Fernwald's sign, 192,
193f
nonpregnancy causes of, 192t
Braxton Hicks, John, 4
Braxton Hicks contractions, 196
as impending labor sign, 415
as pregnancy change, 193
nonpregnancy causes of, 192t
Brazelton neonatal assessment,
adolescent mother aided by,
943
Breast abscesses, assessing in
neonate, 699g
Breast cancer, during pregnancy,
352
Breast changes, as pregnancy
symptom, 192
Breast engorgement, 936–37
assessing for, 910
during lactation suppression, relief
for, 925
nursing care plan for, 919
pain from, 915, 919ncp
as pregnancy symptom, 192
temperature increases with, 913
Breast milk. *See also* Breast-feeding
composition of, 717–18, 719t
neonatal fat absorption from,
651
Breast pads, 929, 931
Breast pump, 937
Breast self-examination, 232p
by males, 64
for nursing mothers, 945g
Breast self-stimulation test (BSST),
376
Breast shields, for inverted nipples,
931, 936f
Breast tenderness
as pregnancy symptom, 192
nonpregnancy causes of, 191t

Breast-feeding, 927–38, 929f, 931f,
937f
advantages of, 927
afterpains with, 907
analgesia for, 915, 917n
alcoholism and, 362
assessing
in fourth trimester, 945–46g
at postpartal home visit, 624
for cardiac client, 313
after cesarean delivery, 941
facilitating, 607
medications and, 603
positions for, 924
colostrum. *See* Colostrum
contraindications, 718, 927–28
decision making about, 716–17,
717–19, 719t
by diabetic mother, 318, 321
encouragement needed for, 921–
24
engorgement with, 919n, 936–37
establishing pattern for, 718–19
follow-up phone call and, 948, 949
for high-risk neonates, 776
frequency of, 929–30
engorgement and, 936–37
nipple soreness and, 931
hemorrhagic disease of the newborn and, 836
heparin and, 984
with herpes infection, 360
hyperbilirubinemia risk with, 823;
see also neonatal jaundice and
hyperthyroidism and, 326
infertility with, 904–5
initial, after delivery, 613, 716
initiating, 928–30
in reactivity period, 712
leaking milk, 929
letdown reflex, 925
lochia increased by, 904
manual expression of milk, 930,
930f
engorgement relief by, 937
by working mother, 938
mastitis and, 986–87, 987f
mature milk, 925
medications and, 930–31, 932–
35t
menstruation resumption and,
904–5
necrotizing enterocolitis risk
lessened by, 837
neonatal jaundice and, 649–50,
823, 834n
nipple soreness from, 931, 936
nutritional aspects of, 717–18,
719t
nutritional assessment with, 720,
720t
passive immunity through, 654
physiology of, 925
PKU screening and, 858
plugged ducts, 937
positions for, 929, 929f, 937f, 941
nipple soreness and, 931
prenatal attachment facilitates,
958
for preterm infants, 740, 740,
741f, 776
immunity and, 748
nursing care plan, 754–55
problems in, 931, 931f, 936f,
936–37
mastitis, 986–87, 987f
in public, 921
puerperal infections and 976,
978n, 979n
rooming-in facilitates, 939
sexual relations and, 940
stools with, 651, 726

sucking patterns with, 655
supplementing, 929–30
supply vs. demand, 929–30
with thromboembolic disease,
984n, 985n
with thrush, 845
tradition of, in U.S., 4
transitional milk, 925
types of milk produced by, 925
with urinary tract infection, 986
uterine involution aided by, 902,
903
weaning from, 721–22
weight gain with, 718
by working mother, 937–38
Breasts, of mother
abscesses in, 987
assessing
in initial prenatal exam, 221g
at labor onset, 428g
in fourth trimester, 945–46g
at postpartal home visit, 624
postpartum, 908, 910, 917
atrophy of, with Sheehan
syndrome, 988
binding, for lactation suppression,
925
lactation preparation in, 925
plugged ducts in, mastitis and, 987
postpartal complications of, 986–
87, 987f
postpartal nursing care for, 919
pregnancy changes in, 197
hormones and, 202
pigmentation, 199
progesterone's effects on, 94, 202
puberty changes in, 91, 91f
sexual response of, 103t
Breasts, of neonate
assessing, 699g
in delivery room, 496
discharge from, 653
gestational age and, 661, 662f,
665f, 669f
swelling of, 653
Breath odor, from aganglionosis, 869
Breath sounds, in neonate
assessing, 698g
with bronchopulmonary dysplasia,
816
with diaphragmatic hernia, 866
with pneumothorax, 809n, 816
with RDS, 797t, 801n
with tracheoesophageal atresia/fis-
tula, 860
with transient tachypnea of newborn, 797
Breathing
by fetus, 636
by neonate
initiation of, 636–39, 637f, 639f
periodic, 639
pregnancy changes in, 197
Breathing exercises
after cesarean delivery, 941
in childbirth preparation, 293,
294, 295. *See also* Breathing
methods
as crisis intervention, 997–98
postpartal, 922f
Breathing methods, 472, 485–86,
487f
advantages of, 485
for first stage active phase, 475,
476
for first stage deceleration phase,
477, 478
with forceps delivery, 598
with induced labor, 591n, 592n
for precipitous labor, 544
to prevent pushing, 478, 484, 544
for rapid learning, 486, 544

Breathing methods (Cont'd)
  for second stage, 479n, 490
  Valsalva, during delivery, 490
Breckinridge, Mary, 7
Breech delivery, 554–55. See also
    Breech presentation
  bruising from, 690g
  clitoral edema or bruising from,
    701g
  head shape with, 691g
  Mauriceau mechanism for, 4
  petechiae from, 691g
  Piper forceps for, 597, 598
  Rh sensitization and, 824
  transient tachypnea of newborn af-
    ter, 797
Breech presentation, 400, 401f, 404,
    552, 554–55, 555f. See also
    Breech delivery
  cesarean delivery for, 550, 600,
    605
  engagement in, 402
  external version of, 585, 586,
    586f
  frank, 555f
  hip dysplasia and, 876
  with hydrocephaly, 557
  incidence of, 554
  incomplete (footling), 554, 555f
  as induction of labor contraindi-
    cation, 587
  internal or podalic version to,
    585–86
  by LGA neonate, 761
  management of, 554–55
  palpating during labor, 438p
  position notation for, 40, 404
  preterm labor with, cesarean for,
    550
  prolapsed umbilical cord with, 574
  PROM and, 546
  twins in, 559, 559f
  as vacuum extraction contraindica-
    tion, 598
Brethine (terbutaline sulfate), for
    preterm labor, 548
"Brick dust spots," 652
British midwifery, 4, 6
Bromides, in breast milk, 930
Bromocriptine (Parlodel), 925, 926d
  for lactation suppression, 919n
  for postdelivery galactorrhea, 987
Bronchial breath sounds, in neonate,
    698g
Bronchial obstruction in neonate, 637
Bronchopneumonia, with tracheoeso-
    phageal atresia/fistula, 861
Bronchopulmonary dysplasia (BPD),
    816
  interventions for, 808n
  in preterm infants, vitamin E to
    prevent, 746
  as respiratory therapy complica-
    tion, 801, 808n, 816
  signs of, 816
Broussard, Dr. Elsie R., 965
Brow presentation, 400, 400f
  management of, 552–53
Brown adipose tissue (BAT)
  depleted
    in postterm infant, 760
    in SGA neonate, 762, 765
  thermoregulation role of, 647–48,
    647f, 817
  prematurity and, 740
Brown fat. See Brown adipose tissue
Bruising, in neonate
  from labor and delivery, 690g
  hyperbilirubinemia and, 823,
    831
Brushfield spots, in neonatal eyes,
    693g

BSST (Breast self-stimulation test),
    376
Bulb syringe
  care of, 716
  for routine nursery care, 714–16,
    716f
  parent education with, 726
  suctioning newborn with, 636–37
    in reactivity period, 712
Bulging, assessing neonatal ears for,
    696g
BUN. See Blood urea nitrogen
Burning, vaginal, postmenopausal,
    101
Burping
  with bottle-feeding, 926–27
  after breast-feeding, 929
  with cleft lip, 853n
  with cleft palate, 856n
  after diaphragmatic hernia
    surgery, 867
  positioning infant for, 926
  regurgitation lessened by, 651
Buttocks
  postpartal hematoma signs on,
    973
  of neonate, assessing, 702g, 703g

C-Sec, 607
Café-au-lait spots, assessing, 690g
Caffeine, pregnancy intake of, 304,
    361t
Calcifications, placental, 372, 574
Calcium
  in breast milk, cow's milk, and
    formula, 719t
  lactation requirements, 270t
  lactose intolerance and intake of,
    281
  neonatal levels of. See also Hypo-
    calcemia
    normal values, 645t
    normal preterm values, 752t
    SGA neonate, 764n
  neonatal requirements, 717t
    preterm, 746
  placental transport of, 170
  pregnancy requirements, 199,
    201, 270t, 273
    leg cramps and, 255t, 258–59
  vitamin D and, 275
Calcium chloride, for neonatal hypo-
    calcemia, 822
Calcium gluconate
  as antidote for magnesium sulfate,
    339
  for neonatal hypocalcemia, 821–
    22
  in resuscitative therapy, 788, 792
Calcium lactate, as pregnancy sup-
    plement, 259
Caldwell, W. E., 70
Caldwell-Moloy classification of
    pelves, 70–71, 396–97,
    397
Calendar rhythm method of contra-
    ception, 120–21, 121
Calories
  in breast milk, 925
    cow's milk and formula
    compared with, 719t
  defined, 270
  lactation requirements, 913
  neonatal requirements, 652, 717,
    717t, 720–21, 720–21t
    preterm, 741, 746, 753n
  postpartal requirements, 913
  pregnancy requirements, 270,
    270t
  in preterm infant formulas, 742t
  recommended dietary allowances
    for women, 270t

Cambodian families, 46
  labor customs in, 469
Canada
  birth and fertility rates, 21t
  birth weight statistics or, 23, 25t
  infant mortality in, 23, 25t
  live births statistics, 21t, 25t
  maternal mortality in, 23
Cancer. See also specific types of
    cancer
  genetic counseling referral for, 151
  pelvic, potential lodging places of,
    75
  during pregnancy, surgery for,
    352
  signs of in initial prenatal exam,
    221g
  smoking and risk of, 214t
Candida albicans, 355
  adolescent pregnancy and, 304
  in neonates
    assessing for, 681
    thrush from, 681, 844–45
Capacitation process, of sperma-
    tozoa, 161–62
Capillaries, neonatal blood sampling
    from, 644
Capillary angioma, in neonates, 677–
    78
Capillary hemangioma, in neonate,
    678
Caplan, G., 997, 1009
Caput succedaneum, 541f
  assessing for, 678, 679f, 691g
    in prolonged labor, 542
  described, 678, 679f
  from face presentation, 553
  from hypertonic labor patterns,
    537
  pelvic inlet contractures and, 578
  as uterine rupture sign, 550
  from vacuum extraction, 599
Car seats, importance of, 729
Carbohydrate metabolism
  altered, types of, 314–15. See also
    Diabetes mellitus
  galactosemia affects, 859
  neonatal liver's role in, 648
  pregnancy alterations in, 198, 314
Carbohydrates
  in breast milk, cow's milk, and for-
    mula, 719t
  lactation requirements, 271t, 272t
  metabolism of. See Carbohydrate
    metabolism
  neonatal digestion of, 651
  neonatal requirements, 717, 717t
    preterm, 741
  pregnancy requirements, 201,
    271t, 272t, 273
  in preterm infant formulas, 742t
Carbon dioxide
  combining power, hyperbilirubine-
    mia and, 824, 831n
  with maternal cardiac decompen-
    sation, 311
  normal preterm infant values, 752t
  placental transport of, 170
Carbon dioxide laser treatments, for
    condylomata accuminata in
    pregnancy, 355
Carcinoma. See Cancer
Cardiac anomalies, in neonate, 881,
    886–87f. See also Cardiac
    problems; specific anomalies
  acyanotic, 881, 885, 886–87f,
    888–89
  central cyanosis from, 889
  cyanotic, 881, 886–87f, 889–93
  from extended rubella syndrome,
    358
  incidence of, 881

LGA preterm IDM assessment for,
    757n
  maternal alcoholism and, 361t,
    362, 770
  maternal heart disease and, 769
  nails with, 702g
  omphalocele and, 867
  as pneumothorax sign, 809n
  as polygenetically inherited, 145
  signs of, 881
Cardiac arrest, in neonate
  of hypertensive mother, 769
  resuscitation risk with, 787
Cardiac arrhythmias, with induction,
    as water intoxication sign,
    590, 593
Cardiac catheterization, as diagnostic
    tool, 885
  for endocardial cushion defect,
    888
  for PPH, 817
  for transposition of the great
    vessel, 892
  for ventricular septal defect, 888
Cardiac decompensation
  in neonate
    with hemolytic disease of the
      newborn, 824, 826
    with hydrops fetalis, 824
  in pregnancy
    risk of, 214t
    signs of, 311
Cardiac disorders, maternal. See also
    Cardiac anomalies; Cardiac
    problems; specific cardiac dis-
    orders
  birth center screening for, 618
  cesarean delivery mortality from,
    605
  as CST indication, 375
  effects of, 310–13
  as forceps delivery indication, 597
  during labor, first stage, 428g
  neonatal effects of, 761, 768–69
  postpartal exhaustion with, 908t
  as preterm labor cause, 548
  resuscitation risk with, 786
  as risk factor, 214t, 310–13
  as ritodrine contraindicaton, 549
  signs of in initial prenatal exam,
    222g, 239g
  signs of at postpartal home visit,
    624
  thromboembolic disease risk with,
    980, 983
Cardiac examination, in initial prena-
    tal exam, 222, 233–34p,
    234f
Cardiac monitoring, for neonatal ane-
    mia, 835
Cardiac output
  in neonate, 642
    decrease in. See Cardiac output
      deficiency
    oxygen capacity and, 643
    respiratory therapy effects on,
      810n
  pregnancy changes in, 310
Cardiac output deficiency. in neonate
  assessing for, 688g
  calcium gluconate for, 792
  with necrotizing enterocolitis,
    837
  peripheral cyanosis from, 889
Cardiac problems, in neonate. See
    also Cardiac anomalies; specif-
    ic problems
  from bronchopulmonary dysplasia,
    816
  cyanosis as sign of, 690g
  as respiratory therapy complica-
    tion, 809–10n, 816–17

skin color with, 690g
Cardiac sphincter
   incompetent, in preterm infants,
      741
   pregnancy changes in, 197t, 198
      heartburn and, 254t,256
Cardiac sphincter, in neonate, 651
Cardiac stenosis, pregnancy with,
   310
Cardinal ligaments, 77, 82
Cardiomegaly
   with bronchopulmonary dysplasia,
      816
   with hydrops fetalis, 824, 826
   as MAS complication, 815
   as patent ductus arteriosus sign,
      810n
Cardiopulmonary adaptation, physiology of, 638
Cardiopulmonary disease, as vacuum
   extraction indication, 598
Cardiopulmonary problems of neonates, 785. See also specific
   problems
   assessing postterm infant for, 760
Cardiopulmonary resuscitation (CPR),
   for amniotic fluid embolism,
      576
Cardiorespiratory distress, LGA preterm IDM assessment for,
      757n
Cardiovascular adaptation in neonates, 639–43, 641–4
Cardiovascular collapse, with
   necrotizing enterocolitis, 838
Cardiovascular disease. See Cardiac
   disease
Cardiovascular problems, as ritodrine
   side effect, 549
Cardiovascular system
   assessing, in initial prenatal exam,
      216t, 217g, 218g
   fetal-neonatal transition circulation,
      640–41, 641f
   pregnancy changes in, 197t, 198,
      310
   disorders in, pregnancy with, 310–
      13
Cardiovascular system, fetal
   development of, 173, 174t, 176t,
      178t, 178–82
   teratogenic damage to, 183t
Cardiovascular system, in neonate,
   639–43, 641–43f
   assessing, 682–83
   birth changes in, 739, 739t
   maternal drug addiction and,
      771
   preterm, 739t, 739–40
   Pierre Robin syndrome and, 850
   RDS effects on, 794f, 795, 797t,
      801n
   respiratory system interrelated
      with, 638
Caring role of nurse
   abortion and, 131
   cesarean delivery, 601–3, 604
   crisis intervention as, 1011
   infertility and, 112, 119
   with menopausal women, 102
   sex education and, 106
Carotene. See Vitamin A
Carpal ablation, 183t
Carriers
   of autosomal recessively inherited
      disorders, 143f, 143–44
   genetic counseling referral for,
      150–54
   of X-linked recessive disorders,
      144
Carunculae myrtiformes, 73
Casein, in breast and cow's milk, 719

Casting
   for clubfoot, 876
   for hip dysplasia, 878
   for meningomyelocele, 880
Casts, in urinalysis
   initial prenatal, 230g
   at labor onset, implications of,
      432g
   neonatal, 652
Cataracts
   congenital, assessing for, 680,
      693g, 694g
   from congenital rubella, 215t, 358
   from galactosemia, 859
   lenticular, 183t
   nuclear, 183t
   with Pierre Robin syndrome, 850
   vulnerability to, gestational age
      and, 183t
Catecholamine depletion, from
   maternal reserpine use, 769
Catecholamines
   anxiety affects release of, 535,
      572
   nonshivering thermogenesis role
      of, 647, 648
   released with blood loss, 569, 570
Cathartics, in breast milk, 930
Catheterization. See also Catheters
   cardiac. See Cardiac catheteriza-
      tion
   esophageal atresia assessment
      with, 860
   for measuring CVP, 571
   for meningomyelocele, 881
   for monitoring urine output, with
      hemorrhage, 570n
   for postpartal bladder distention,
      906, 918n
   after cesarean, 603
   after uterine inversion, 580
   after tracheoesophageal surgery,
      863n
   umbilical, 811p
   PPH diagnosis with, 817
Catheters. See also Catheterizaton
   feeding with, for cleft lip, 854n
   for gavage feeding, 743p
   indwelling, before cesarean
      delivery, 608
   intrauterine, for monitoring
      contractions, 447, 449f
   ripening cervix with, 588
   suctioning neonate's nose with,
      681
   Swan-Ganz, in eclampsia interven-
      tion, 344
   umbilical artery, for calcium
      gluconate, 822
Cats, toxoplasmosis transmitted by,
   357
Caudal anesthesia. See Spinal
   anesthesia
Caudal regression syndrome, in IDM,
   768
Cauterization, for condylomata
   accuminata in pregnancy, 355
Cauterization of cervix, incompetent
   cervix after, 335
Cavernous hemangiomas, assessing
   in neonate, 691g
CBC. See Complete blood count
CC. See Umbilical cord compression
Cecum, palpation of, 74
Celestone. See Betamethasone
Cellular differentiation, 163–65,
   164f, 166f
Cellular division, 157–59, 158f, 159f
Cellular multiplication, 162, 163f
Cellulitis, in initial prenatal exam,
   225g
Central Midwives Board, 6

Central nervous system (CNS)
   depressed, fetal breathing move-
      ments affected by, 636
   insult to, sinusoidal FHR patterns
      with, 457
   irritability in, from hypertension,
      214t
   nonshivering thermogenesis role
      of, 647
   PIH effects on, 341
   puberty role of, 92, 92f
   testosterone's effects on, 92f, 93
Central nervous system (CNS)
   damage. See also Central ner-
      vous system disorders
   anisocoria, eye signs with, 694g
   from birth trauma, 756–57n
   cyanosis as sign of, 690g
   habituation failure with, 705
   motor activity with, 705
   from neonatal hypoglycemia,
      821
   spina bifida, 878–81, 879–80f,
      882–84n
   from unconjugated bilirubin,
      822, 823–24
Central nervous system disorders.
   See also Central nervous sys-
      tem damage
   assessing in neonate, 685–87,
      686–87f
      body postiion as sign of, 702g
   central cyanosis from, 889
   cold stress aggravated by, 817
   from fetal alcohol syndrome,
      770
   myelocele, oligohydramnios
      increases risk of, 425t
   neonatal hypoglycemia and,
      763, 818
   neonatal motor function with,
      703g
   Pierre Robin syndrome affects,
      850
   PKU, 858
   in preterm infant, physiology
      and considerations, 749
   pupils with, 694g
Central venous pressure (CVP)
   monitoring
      with amniotic fluid embolism,
         576
      with eclampsia, 344
      in hemorrhage nursing care
         plan, 571, 572
      in neonate, IVH and, 836
Centriole, in mitosis, 158
Centromeres, 157, 159
Cephalhematoma
   assessing for, 678, 679f, 691g
   after prolonged labor, 542
   hyperbilirubinemia and, 822, 823
   from hypertonic labor patterns,
      537
   from macrosomia, 557
   from vacuum extraction, 598
Cephalic or external version, 585,
   586, 586f
Cephalic presentations, 400, 400–
   403f
   engagement of, 402, 403
   four types of, 400, 400f
   position notation for, 403
Cephalopelvic disproportion (CPD)
   as adolescent pregnancy risk, 297,
      303, 482
   birth center screening for, 618
   breech presentation danger with,
      554
   as cephalic version contraindica-
      tion, 585
   cesarean delivery for, 600

determining, in initial prenatal
   exam, 228g
   in diabetic client, 316
   dysfunctional labor and, 536
   face presentation with, 553
   from fetal macrosomia, 556, 557
   as forceps delivery contraindica-
      tion, 598
   from hydrocephaly, 557
   hypotonic labor patterns from, 541
   induction of labor and, 587, 590,
      591n
   neonatal trauma from, 552, 761
   obstructed labor from, 545
   passage contractures resulting in,
      577–78
   prolonged labor caused by, 542
   signs of in initial prenatal exam,
      224g
   risk factors for, 214t
   as vacuum extraction contraindica-
      tion, 598
Cerclage (Shirodkar-Barter operation), 336
   as CST contraindication, 376
   as ritodrine contraindication, 548
Cerebral bleeding, neonatal anemia
   from, 830
Cerebral compression, from brow
   presentation, 552
Cerebral damage. See Cerebral trauma; specific traumas
Cerebral disturbances, with severe
   preeclampsia, 341
Cerebral edema
   as MAS complication, 815
   as oxytocin induction risk, 594n
Cerebral hemorrhage, assessing for
   with eclampsia, 344
Cerebral lesion, tonic neck reflex
   affected by, 704g
Cerebral nerve damage, signs of in
   initial prenatal exam, 225g
Cerebral palsy
   assessing neonate for, 702g
   from congenital CMV, 359
   from congenital rubella, 358
   from kernicterus, 824, 826
   as prematurity risk, 758
   spastic paralysis with, hip dyspla-
      sia vs., 878
Cerebral thrombosis, as tetralogy of
   Fallot risk, 890
Cerebral trauma
   fetal macrosomia and, 556
   as forceps delivery risk, 598
   in precipitous labor, 543
   as prolonged labor risk, 542
   from undetected CPD with malpo-
      sition, 552
   as vacuum extraction risk, 599
Certified nurse-midwives (CNMs), 7
   maternity care roles of, 14
   as primary caregivers, 243
Cervical cancer
   genital herpes and, 360
   as induction of labor contraindica-
      tion, 587
   location of, 79
   from maternal DES use, 265–66
   during pregnancy, 352
   signs of in initial prenatal exam,
      226g
Cervical cap, 121f, 123–24
Cervical consistency, assessing before
   induction, 588, 588t
Cervical dilatation, 408, 408f, 417,
   417f, 417–18
   arrest of, malposition as cause of,
      551
   assessing, 430g, 432t, 434, 436–
      37p, 437f, 439f, 440–41, 441f

Cervical dilatation (Cont'd)
    with abruptio placentae
        hemorrhage, 572
    in active phase labor, 475n
    in deceleration phase labor,
        477c
    before induction, 588, 588t
    during induction, 590, 592n
    at labor admission, 469, 472
    in labor nursing care plan, 473,
        475, 479
    in latent stage labor, 475n
    failure of, assessing, 430g
    forceps application requires, 598
    labor time elapsed and, abnormal
        patterns, 544, 544t
    maximum slope rate of, disorders
        of, 544, 544t
    monitoring, in prolonged labor, 542
    pain caused by, 411
    pelvic floor muscles during, 67
    pelvic inlet contractures and, 578
    precipitous labor and, 543
    prolonged labor and, 542
    as ritodrine contraindication, 548,
        549
    slow, CPD as cause of, 578
    as true labor sign, 416
    uterine contractions correlated
        with, 432t
    vacuum extraction requires, 598
Cervical edema, during labor, 430g
    interventions for, 430g
    preventing, 478n
Cervical effacement, 407, 408f
    assessing, 430g, 434, 436–37p,
        437f, 473n, 475n
    with abruptio placentae
        hemorrhage, 572
    in active phase labor, 475n
    in deceleration phase, 477n
    before induction, 588, 588t
    at labor admission, 469, 472
    in latent stage labor, 473n
    failure of, assessing, 430g
    monitoring, in prolonged labor,
        542
    slow, CPD as cause of, 578
Cervical esophagostomy, 861, 864n
Cervical hyperemia, pregnancy sign
    caused by, 192t
Cervical incompetence. See Cervix,
    incompetent
Cervical lacerations, 579
    as adolescent labor risk, 482
    incompetent cervix after, 335
    as induction risk, 589, 590, 592n,
        594n
    postpartal bleeding as sign of, 904
    postpartal hemorrhage from, 579,
        972
    as precipitous labor risk, 543
Cervical mucosa, cyclic changes in,
    98, 99
Cervical mucus, 79
    assessing, for contraception, 121f,
        121–22
    "hostile," 111t, 117
    fernlike pattern of, 98
    fertiliztion aided by, 160
    infertility and, 111t, 114, 116f,
        116–17
    in pregnancy, 196
    progesterone effects on, 202
Cervical os
    assessing, fourth trimester, 947g
    assessing, in initial prenatal exam,
        226g, 227f
    incompetent. See Incompetent
        cervix
Cervical polyps, in initial prenatal
    exam, 226g

Cervical pregnancy, 333, 334f
Cervical stenosis
    dysmenorrhea from, 100
    infertility from, 111t
Cervicitis
    chlamydial, 355
    infertility from, 111t
Cervix, 74f, 77f, 78, 79
    anatomy of, 79
    assessing
        in fourth trimester, 947g
        before induction, 588, 588t,
            590, 591
        in initial prenatal exam, 226g,
            227f
    carcinoma in situ. See Cervical
        cancer
    evaluating in infertility workup,
        114
    fusiform, 78
    incompetent, 78
        as CST contraindication, 376
        after delivery, 335
        as pregnancy complication,
            335–36
        as preterm labor cause, 548
        spontaneous abortion caused
            by, 329, 333
    lacerations affect appearance of,
        904
    mucosa in, 79
    postpartal changes in, 904
    pregnancy changes in, 192, 196,
        226g
    protective role of, 79
    ripe
        precipitous labor with, 543
        after PROM, with induced
            labor, 546f
    ripe vs. unripe, described, 591n
    ripening, PG gel for, 595
    sexual response of, 103t
    squamocolumnar junction, 79, 79f
    stenosis of, infertility from, 111t
    strawberry appearance to, from
        trichomonas, 356
    uterine rupture signs in, 550
Cesarean delivery, 599–609
    abnormal presentation and, 425t
    ambulation after, 603–4
    as amniotomy induction risk, 589
    analgesia and anesthesia for, 609
        balanced, 530
    antacid therapy before, 531
    anticipated, preparation for, 601–
        2
    blood loss amount during, 906
    bonding after, facilitating, 603,
        604, 942
    breast-feeding after, 924
        medications and, 603
    for breech presentation, 554
    for brow presentation, 552
    for cardiac clients, 313
    after cerclage, 336
    childbirth preparation for, 606–7
    classic incision for, 605, 606, 606f
        uterine rupture and, 550
    complications from, maternal, 605
    as CST indication in succeeding
        pregnancy, 375
    CST results and, 379
    defined, 599
    for diabetic client, 316, 318
    early termination of pregnancy for,
        384
    elective repeat, 601–2, 606
        preparation for, 607
    elimination problems after, 905
    emergency, preparation for, 602n,
        607–8
    emotional preparation for, 601–2

external cephalic version to
    prevent, 585
for face presentation, 553, 554f
factors affecting increase in, 600
father's participation in, 603, 607,
    608
feeding positions after, 924
for fetal malformations, 557
fetal monitoring and, 9
    head shape with, 691g
for hydrocephaly, 557
incidence of, 9, 599, 600
    electronic fetal monitoring and,
        459
incision care after, 603n, 604n
indications for, 600, 605
    acidosis, 451t, 462, 462f, 463
    from monitoring, 451t, 454,
        456
    outcomes and, 600, 605
    repeat cesareans and, 606
    as resuscitation risk, 787
infection from, 605
learning needs after, 939
for LGA neonate, 761
lochia assessment after, 911
low-segment transverse incision,
    605, 606, 606f
as malposition alternative, 551
for maternal gonorrhea, 355
for maternal herpes infection,
    359–60
maternal mortality and morbidity
    from, 605
molding absent after, 678
neonatal breath sounds after, 698g
nursing care plan, 601–4
nursing interventions for, 601–4n,
    606–9
outcomes of, statistics about,
    600
pain after
    management of, 917n
    repeat anticipation of, 607
passive exercises after, 912
pathologic retraction rings require,
    545
for pelvic contractures, 578
pelvic measurements and, 228g
pelvis types requiring, 396, 397,
    397f
podalic version vs., 586
position for, with PIH, 346
postpartal incision evaluation, 912
postpartal nursing management,
    603–4, 941–42
    uterine assessment, 903
postpartal retelling of, 602, 608
postpartal risks with, 908t
prenatal classes for, 291
prep for, 608
preparation for, 601–2n, 606–8,
    318
    with fetal distress, 538n, 539n
    preterm labor indications for, 550
    previous
        birth center screening for, 618
        as induction contraindication,
            587
        as uterine rupture cause, 550
    as prolonged labor intervention,
        542
    after PROM, 546
    RDS risk and, 792
    repeat
        controversy about, 606
        incidence of, 600
        preparation for, 607
    Rh sensitization and, 824
    risk factors for, 214t
        birth weight and gestational age,
            736f

as risk factor, 215t
scar from, uterine rupture caused
    by, 550
shoulder presentation requires,
    402
site of, 78
for spina bifida, 880
surgical techniques for, 600
technologic advancements aiding,
    600
for threatened uterine rupture,
    550, 551
transient tachypnea of newborn
    after, 797
for transverse lie, 556
types of, 605–6, 606f
for umbilical cord prolapse, 574,
    575
urinary catheterization after, 906
for uterine relaxation after general
    anesthesia, 530
after uterine rupture, 551
x-ray pelvimetry before, 433
Chadwick's sign, 192, 196
    in cervix, 196
    in initial prenatal exam, 226g
    nonpregnancy causes of, 192t
    in vaginal mucosa, 197
Chamberlen, Peter, 4
Change of life, 101–2
Cheilosis, in infant
    niacin deficiency as cause of, 719
    preventing, 717
Chemical conjunctivitis in neonates,
    680
    assessing neonate for, 680, 693g,
        694g
    ophthalmia neonatorum vs., 844
    as prophylactic treatment risk,
        710, 711d
Chemical pneumonitis, in neonate
    with MAS, 798
    with tracheoesophageal atresia/
        fistula, 860
Chemical stimuli to breathing, 636,
    638
Chemical thermogenesis, 647
    preventing, with RDS, 806n
Chemicals, gene mutations and, 157
Chemoreceptors in fetal heart, 171
Chemotherapeutic agents, as terato-
    gens, 267t
Chemotherapy, for hydatidiform
    mole, 335
Chest
    assessing in initial prenatal exam,
        220g, 231p
    of neonate
        assessing, 682, 683f, 697–99g
        circumference of. See Chest cir-
            cumference of neonate
        hyperexpansion of, with
            bronchopulmonary dysplasia,
            816
        with MAS, 814
        pneumothorax signs in, 809n
        with RDS, 795f, 796–97t, 801n
        transilluminaton of, for pneumo-
            thorax assessment, 816
Chest circumference of neonate
    assessing, 675f, 675–76, 682,
        691g, 697g
    at nursery admisson, 710
    hydrocephalus and, 882n
Chest drainage
    for pneumothorax in neonate,
        809n
    postural. See Postural drainage
    for pulmonary emphysema in neo-
        nate, 809n
Chest expansion, assessing in neo-
    nate, 698g

Chest pain
  from amniotic fluid embolism, 576
  interventions for during labor, 576
  as Mendelson syndrome symptom, 531
  as Methergine side effect, 903d
Chest percussion, for MAS, 815
Chest retractions. *See* Retractions
Chest tube
  after diaphragmatic hernia surgery, 867
  insertion of, for pneumothorax, 809n
  for pulmonary emphysema in neonate, 809n
  after tracheoesophageal atresia/fistula repair, 863n
Chest x-ray
  in initial prenatal exam, 230g
  in sepsis neonatorum assessment, 842
  of preterm neonate, in nursing care plan, 750
Cheyne-Stokes respirations, in initial prenatal exam, 220g
CHF. *See* Congestive heart failure
Chignon, from vacuum extraction, 598, 599
Child abuse
  crisis intervention and, 1011, 1014–16, 1016t
  defined, 1014
  diagnosing, 1016t
  malattachment and, 968, 1012
  postpartal psychosis and, 988
  preterm birth and, 1009–10
Childbearing
  decision making about, 42–43
  family development and, 37–38
Childbearing families
  developmental tasks of, 39–40
  environmental factors affect, 46
Childbirth. *See also* Delivery; Labor
  complications in, effects on family of, 580–81
  defined, 395
  fear of, 248–49
  preparation for. *See* Childbirth preparation
  trauma during, 73. *See also* Birth trauma
Childbirth preparation, 293–96. *See also* Prenatal education
  as adaptive response, 249
  for adolescents, 471
  assessing extent of, at labor onset, 435g
  for birth center use, 619
  Bradley (partner-coached) method, 293, 295
  breathing exercise use and, 472
  for cesarean delivery, 318, 601–2, 606–7
  Dick-Read (natural childbirth) method, 12, 293–94, 295
  hypnosis, 293, 295–96
  importance of to father, 965
  importance of to couple, 247
  induction of labor and, 591n
  Kegel's, 263, 264f
  Lamaze (psychoprophylactic) method, 293, 294–95
  postpartal classes, 944
  in prenatal assessments, 242g
  prenatal exercises, 262–63, 263–64f
  for siblings, 613–14
  stress reduced by, 535–36
Childhood, sexual development in, 89
Children. *See also* Siblings
  American Indian, status and role of, 45

care and rearing of, as family function, 35
  as maternity ward visitors, 292
  reactions to pregnancy of, 250–51, 251f
  roles of in family, 35–36
    Asian American, 46
    Black American, 45
    Mexican American, 44
  sexuality counseling for, 105
  value of to families, 42–43
Chills, postpartal, 481n, 906
Chin tug, with RDS, 801
Chinese American families
  food practices of, 282t
  pregnancy valued among, 205
  prenatal nutrition for, 282t, 283–84
Chlamydia trachomatis, infection from, 355
  in pregnancy, 355
  in neonatal eyes, erythromycin ointment for, 711d
Chloasma ("mask of pregnancy"), 193
  nonpregnancy cause of, 192t
Chloramphenicol, for gonorrhea in neonate, 844
Chloride, normal neonatal values, 645t
  preterm, 752t
Chloride of lime, for hand-scrubbing, 4
Chloroform, Queen Victoria received, 4
Chlorotrianisene (Tace), 925
Chlorpromazines, amenorrhea from, 100
Choanal atresia, 852, 857
  assessing neonate for, 681
  described, 852
  signs of, 690g, 695g
Choking
  in neonatal reactivity period, 712
  suctioning to prevent, teaching about, 726
Cholecystitis, during pregnancy, 351–52
Cholelithiasis, during pregnancy, 351–52
Cholera immunization, during pregnancy, 266t
Cholestasis, symptoms of in pregnancy, 199
Cholesterol
  estrogens and, 93
  maternal/infant nutrition and, 273
  placenta synthesizes, 170
Chorioamnionitis
  from herpes infection, 359
  after PROM, intervention for, 546f
  as ritodrine contraindication, 549
Choriocarcinoma
  hydatidiform mole and, 335
  positive pregnancy test caused by, 192t
Chorion
  developed from trophoblast, 162
  fetal portion of placenta from, 169f
  formation of, 163–64, 164f
Chorionic cavity. *See* Extraembryonic coelom
Chorionic epithelium, in placenta, 168
Chorionic membrane, cysts in, 568
Chorionic villi, 164, 166–67, 166f, 167f
  in ectopic pregnancy, 333
  fetal portion of placenta in, 167, 167f
  hydatidiform mole derived from, 334

in placenta accreta, 579
  placental formation role of, 166–67, 167f
Chorioretinitis
  from congenital CMV, 359
  from congenital toxoplasmosis, 357
  with herpesvirus type 2 infection, 844
Chromatids, 157, 159
Chromatin, in mitosis, 158
Chromosomal analysis, 135–36
  postnatal, 150
Chromosomal anomalies, 136–41. *See also* Congenital anomalies
  additions and/or deletions, 139–40
  assessing neonatal face for, 692g
  cardiac anomalies and, 881
  chemical exposure can induce, 157
  diagnosing, 135–36, 148–50, 734
  genetic counseling referral for, 151
  hair and scalp signs of, 692g
  IUGR associated with, 761
  low-set ears as sign of, 681
  from maternal drug addiction, 360
  meiotic process and, 159
  microencephaly from, 691g
  neck with, 697g
  nose shape and, 695g
  of number, 136–38
  postnatal diagnosis of, 148–50
  prenatal identification of, 734
  risk factors for, 214t
  satellites and, 157
  in sex chromosomes, 140–41, 140f, 141f
  spontaneous abortion caused by, 329
  of structure, 138–40
  translocation, 138–39, 139f, 140f
Chromosomes, 135–36, 135–36f, 157, 157f
  homologous, gene pairs on, 142
  meiotic division of, 158–59, 159f
  mutations in, 159
  pictorial analysis of. *See* Karotypes
  reduced through meiosis, 158
  role of in genetic processes, 157, 160
  translocation of, 138–39, 139f, 140f
Chronic asphyxia, intrapartal fetal heart aberrations and, 425t
Chronic hypertension. *See also* Chronic hypertensive vascular disease
  as CST indication, 375
  as pregnancy complication, 346
  symmetric IUGR from, 762
Chronic hypertensive vascular disease. *See also* Chronic hypertension
  indicated induction of labor for, 587
  IUGR associated with, 761
  pregnancy with, 347
Chronic obstructive pulmonary disease (COPD), 220g
Chronic grief, 773, 1002
CID. *See* Cytomegalic inclusion disease
Ciliary action, in fallopian tube, 83
Cimetidine (Tagamet), use of during labor, 531
Circadian rhythm, in fetal breathing, 371
Circulation. *See also* Circulatory system
  in placenta, 167–68, 167f, 169f

maternal-placental-fetal, 167–68, 169f
Circulatory failure
  from amniotic fluid embolism, 576
  assessing for, with eclampsia, 344
Circulatory system. *See also* Circulation
  fetal. *See* Fetal circulation
  fetal-neonatal transition, 640–41, 641f
  in neonate. *See* Neonates, circulatory system in
Circumcision, 60, 722, 723–24f
  bathing after, 727
  bloody spotting caused by, 652
  infertility from, 112
Circumcision care, 722
Circumference of chest. *See* Chest circumference of neonate
Circumference of head. *See* Head, of neonate
Circumoral cyanosis, in neonate, 689g, 716
Circumvallate placenta, 568, 573–74, 574f
Class
  families influenced by, 41–43
  pregnancy and, 205
Classic incision, 605, 606, 606f
Clavicle, fracture of
  assessing neonate for, 702g
  as LGA neonatal risk, 761, 756–57n
  Moro reflex affected by, 703g
Clavicles, assessing in neonate, 681–82, 697g
Cleavage, of zygote, 162, 163f
Cleft lip, 851f, 851–52, 853–57n, 857
  embryonic development of, 851
  nursing care plan, 853–57
  nursing diagnoses, examples, 857
  prenatal diagnosis invalid for, 148
Cleft palate, 851, 852, 852f, 856
  assessing neonate for, 681, 696g
  embryonic development of, 852
  emotional reactions to, 850
  from fetal vitamin A overdose, 275
  from maternal drug abuse, 361t
  nursing care plan, 853, 856–57
  nursing diagnoses, examples, 857
  with Pierre Robin syndrome, 850, 851
  as polygenetically inherited, 145
  vulnerability to, gestational age and, 183t
Client, family as, 47
Client advocacy, as nursing role, 13
Client history. *See* History
Client profile, 211–13, 212f
Client-health care professional relationship, 13–14
Clifford, S., postmaturity described by, 759–60
Climacteric, 101–2
  sexual activity in, 102
Clinical nurse specialists, maternity care roles of, 14
Clinical pelvimetry
  CPD assessment with, 577
  in pregnant adolescent's first prenatal exam, 303
Clinics, nurse practitioners as heads of, 15
Clinitest, for preterm infants, 753n
Clitoris, 71f, 72–73
  assessing in initial prenatal exam, 225g
  development of, 59, 653, 653f
  evaluating in infertility workup, 114

Clitoris (Cont'd)
  of neonate, assessing, 684, 701g
  sexual response of, 103t
Clomiphene citrate (Clomid), 118
Clonus
  assessing for
    in initial prenatal exam, 225g
    with severe preeclampsia, 343
Clothing
  brassiere, 260
  cotton underwear, for herpes
    infection, 359
  for neonates, 728
  in pregnancy, 258, 260–61
  support stockings. See Support
    stockings
Clots, in lochia, 911
Clotting abnormalities. See Blood
  clotting problems; Blood coagulation defects
Clown (harlequin) color change in
  neonate, 677
Clubbing of fingers and toes
  with tetralogy of Fallot, 890
  with transposition of the great ves-
    sels, 891
Clubbing of nails
  as cardiac anomaly sign, 702g
  as hypoxia sign, 224g
Clubfoot (talipes equinovarus), 875f,
  875–76
  assessing neonate for, 685, 703g
  as polygenically inherited, 145
  positional vs. true, 703g
CMV. See Cytomegalovirus
CNMs. See Certified nurse-midwives
CNP (Continuous negative pressure),
  797, 799t
CNS. See Central nervous system
CO₂. See Carbon dioxide
Coagulation factors. See Blood
  coagulation
Coarctation of the aorta. See Aorta
Cobalamin. See Vitamin B12
Cocaine, fetal/neonatal effects of,
  361t
Coccygeal muscle, 66, 67t
Coccyx, 65, 66
Cognitive development, in adolescence, 297
Cognitive grasp
  anxiety affects, 608
  with cesarean delivery, 602
Coital lubricants, infertility from,
  111t
Coitus, 102–5
  age of first, 90
  as aspect of physical sex behavior,
    89
  optimal direction for, 74
  physiology of sexual response,
    103–4, 103t-4t, 105f
  pooling of semen after, 74
  psychosocial aspects of, 102–3
Coitus interruptus (withdrawal), 121f,
  122
Cold
  neonatal motor activity and, 654
  neonatal skin response to, 677
Cold intolerance, as hypothyroidism
  sign, 326
Cold stress, in neonates, 817–18
  apnea as sign of, 688g
  cyanosis as sign of, 690g
  maternal reserpine affects adapta-
    tion to, 769
  nursing interventions for, 817–18
  as postmaturity risk, 760
  as prematurity risk, 738, 739, 749
  preventing, in preterm infant,
    752–53n
  jaundice and, 831, 832n

skin color with, 690g
temperature with, 688g
Colds, in neonates, parental prepara-
  tion for, 729
Collagen, vitamin C and, 276
Colman, A., 203, 247
Colman, L., 203, 247
Colon, palpation of, 74
Color blindness, inheritaance of, 144,
  160
Colostomy
  for aganglionic megacolon, 870
  for imperforate anus, 872
Colostomy care, for neonate, 870
Colostrum, 197, 925, 929. See also
  Breast-feeding
  assessing for, postpartal home
    visit, 624
  before birth, 260
  IgA immunoglobulins in, 654
  leakage of, 197
  necrotizing enterocolitis prevention
    with, 837
  protective role of, 717
Coma
  in mother
    from diabetes, 319t
    from eclampsia, 341
  in neonate
    from congenital toxoplasmosis,
      357
    with herpesvirus type 2 infec-
      tion, 844
Comforting role of nurse
  during circumcision, 722
  during labor, 483–84
    prolonged, 542
  postpartal, 915–16
Comforting, assessing neonatal
  responses to, 687, 705–6
Common-law family structure, 34
Communal family structure, 34
Communicating role of nurse
  maternity care, 19, 20
  resuscitation risk identification,
    787
  with parents of high-risk infant,
    777, 778
Communication
  childbearing family stage, in, 39
  cultural differences in, 43
    American Indian, 45
    Black American, 45
    Mexican American, 44
    Oriental, 46
  family development and, 37–38
  in family, assessing, 48–49
Communication skills
  active listening, 290
  no-lose problem solving, 290
  sending I-messages, 290
  teaching as part of prenatal care,
    290–91
Community resources. See Referral
Compadre system, 44
Compensatory erythropoiesis, 824
Complete blood count (CBC)
  before abortion, 129
  in infertility workup, 114
  of mother
    at labor admission, 472
    at labor onset, 431g
    before cesarean delivery, 601
    before induction, 591n
    in initial prenatal exam, 216g,
      229g
  of neonate
    jaundice assessment with, 831n
    preterm, in nursing care plan,
      750
    in sepsis neonatorum assess-
      ment, 842

Complete breech presentation, 400
Compound or racemouse glands,
  breasts as, 85
Compound presentation, 552, 556
Compression of fetal head, as
  amniotomy induction risk, 589
Computerized axial tomography
  (CT), IVH assessment with,
  836
Conception. See also Fertilization
  calculating gestational age from,
    173
  cellular division after, 157–59,
    158f, 159f
Conditioned reflexes, in childbirth,
  295
Condoms, 121f, 122, 122f
  postpartal use of, 944
Conduct and Utilization of Research
  in Nursing (CURN) Project,
  26
Conduction, heat loss by, 646–47,
  753
Condylomata, from syphilis, 354
Condylomata accuminata, in pregnancy, 355
Confidentiality, in genetic counseling,
  153
Confinement, defined, 395
Conflicts
  in marriage, 37
  between nurses and clients, 290
Confusion, with puerperal psychosis,
  988
Congenital anomalies. See also
  specific anomalies
  amenorrhea from, 100
  assessing for, LGA preterm
    infants, 757n
  crisis intervention after birth with,
    1010
  death from, parental reactions to,
    1005
  developmental consequences of,
    894–85
  family's reactions to, 580, 581,
    773–74, 848–50
    parent education needs, 939
  feeding problems, 850
  FHR baseline variability caused
    by, 452
  gastrointestinal, 859
  genitourinary defects, 874–75
  heart defects, 881, 886–87. See
    also specific defects
  hydramnios associated with,
    576, 577
  as hypothyroidism risk, 326
  infertility from, 111t
  intrapartal risk factors for, 425t
  IUGR and, 761, 762
  LGA preterm IDM assessment for,
    757n
  male role in, 59
  maternal diabetes and, 316, 757n,
    768
  from maternal drug abuse, 360,
    361t, 771
  maternal epilepsy and, 331t
  medical personnel and, 351
  medications and, 266–68, 267t
  metabolic disorders, 857–59
  neck stiffness, 697g
  as polygenic traits, 145
  prenatal diagnosis of, 146–48
  in preterm infants, 757n
  in postterm infants, 760
  risk factors for, 214–15t, 736f
    intrapartal, 425t
  in SGA neonates, 766n
  statistics about, 134–35
  teratogenic causes of, 183t, 266

from toxoplasmosis, 357
ultrasonography to assess, 8
umbilical cord abnormalities and,
  575
of uterus, 77, 77f
of vagina, 75
Congenital cataracts, assessing for,
  680
Congenital cytomegalic inclusion
  disease, 358–59
Congenital disabilities
Congenital heart block, bradycardia
  with, 452
Congenital heart defects, 881, 886–
  87f. See also specific defects
  acyanotic, 881, 885. 886–87f,
    888–89
  cyanotic, 881, 886–87f, 889–93
  incidence of, 881
  inheritance of, 15
  from maternal PKU, 331t
  signs of, 881
Congenital heart disease
  bilirubin level rises with, 649
  in Down syndrome, 137
  hypoglycemia differentiation from,
    818
  intrapartal fetal heart aberrations
    and, 425t
  murmurs with, 699g
  pregnancy with, 310–13
    neonatal problems associated
      with, 768–69
  from rubella, 215t, 358
  vulnerability to, gestational age
    and, 183t
Congenital herpes, corneal signs of,
  693g
Congenital infection. See also specific
  infections
  assessing SGA neonate for,
    766–67n
  IUGR associated with, 761
Congenital megacolon. See
  Aganglionic megacolon
Congenital rubella, 358
Congenital syphilis, 215t, 354
Congenital torticollis, 681
Congenital listeriosis, 357
Congestive heart failure (CHF)
  from atrial septal defects, 885
  from coarctation of the aorta, 889
  from endocardial cushon defects,
    888
  GFR decreased by, 746
  in LGA preterm IDM, assessing
    for, 757n
  as MAS complication, 814, 815
  peripheral cyanosis with, 889
  with polycythemia, 835
  in pregnancy
    fetal distress nursing care plan
      for, 540
    neonatal problems with, 768
    progressive symptoms of, 311
  from pulmonary stenosis, 890
  as RDS complication, 810n
  from transposition of the great ves-
    sels, 891
  from ventricular septal defects,
    888
Conization, 335, 352
Conjunctiva, assessing in neonate,
  694g
  jaundice evidence in, 824, 832n
Conjunctivitis, in neonate
  assessing, 693g, 694g
  chemical, from neonatal prophy-
    laxis, 680, 710, 711d
  with herpesvirus type 2 infection,
    844
  infectious, in neonate, 680

ophthalmia neonatorum, 844
Consanguineous matings, autosomal recessive inheritance and, 143
Consciousness, states of
hemorrhage monitoring, 571n
in neonate, 655, 657
assessing, 688g
behavioral assessment and, 705–6
Consoling, assessing neonatal responses to, 687, 706
Constipation
in mother
after cesarean delivery, 941
fourth trimester, interventions for, 946–47
hemorrhoids from, 257
as hypothyroidism sign, 326
iron supplements and, 274
as pregnancy discomfort, 253f, 255t, 257–58
postpartal, ambulation discourages, 916
in neonate
assessing, 874
from aganglionosis, 869
with congenital hypothyroidism, 859
iron supplements and, 718
parental preparation for, 729
Constriction rings, 545, 545f
Consumer-health care provider relationship, 13–14
Consumers, patients as, 13, 14, 16
Continuing education, about sexuality, 105
Continuous negative pressure (CNP), 797, 799t
Continuous positive airway pressure (CPAP)
for IVH, 837
method, 799t
for RDS, 797, 799t, 800t, 804n
Contraception, 120–31
for adolescents, 90
postpartal, 943, 1017
defined, 110
diabetes and methods of, 318–19
discussing at postpartal exams, 944
factors affecting choice of, 120
fertility awareness methods, 120–22
injectable, 125, 127
male role in, 59
mechanical methods of, 122f, 122–25, 123f, 124f
operative sterilization 121f, 127–28, 127f, 128f
oral. See Oral contraceptives
postmastectomy, 352
postpartal planning for, 940, 943
spermicides, 121f, 127
Contracted inlets. See Pelvic inlet contractures
Contraction stress test (CST), 374–79
abnormal, as induction of labor contraindication, 587
clinical application of, 376–79, 377t, 377–78f
flow chart for, 378f
indications and contraindications for, 375–76
with maternal PIH, 342
negative, 377t, 377f
positive, 377t, 378f
procedure for, 376
as reason for delivery, 388
Contractions. See Uterine contractions
Contralateral hemiplegia, nevus flammeus with, 677–78

Convection, heat loss by, 646, 647, 753
Convulsions. See also Seizures
in mother
as danger sign of pregnancy, 240t
eclampsia, interventions for, 339, 344
as hypertension risk, 214t
during labor, interventions for, 530, 540n
with PIH, 341, 343–44
in neonate
from congenital toxoplasmosis, 357
with herpesvirus type 2 infection, 844
with hydrocephalus, 880
LGA, from birth trauma, 756n
as MAS complication, 815
neonatal tremors vs., 685
with nevus flammeus, 677–78
Coomb's test
indirect
during prenatal care, 347
for Rh sensitization screening, 347, 348
of neonatal blood
ABO incompatibility assessment with, 826
with hemolytic disease of the newborn, 826, 827
hyperbilirubinemia assessment with, 824, 831n
neonatal anemia assessment with, 835
Cooper's ligaments, in breast, 84f, 85
Coordinating role of nurse, in family health care, 49
COPD. See Chronic obstructive pulmonary disease
Coping mechanisms
after sponaneous abortion, 333
anxiety as aid or hindrance to, 484
bleeding in pregnancy requires, 329
for cesarean delivery, 601, 602
complicated childbirth and, 580
crisis adaptation affected by, 992, 994, 995, 995f, 996
of families of high-risk neonates, 778–79, 779f
for family crisis, constructive examples, 993
identifying, in family assessment, 49
during labor, 405, 406
assessing, 435, 474
hypertonic patterns as test of, 537
preterm, 550
postpartal assessment of, 948g
with preterm or high-risk neonate, 778–79, 779f
Copper, neonatal requirements, 717t
Copper 7 IUD, 124f, 124–25
Cord compression. See Umbilical cord compression
Core-gender identity (sexual identity), 88
Cornea, of neonate
assessing, 693g
ulcerated
as herpesvirus sign, 693g
from ophthalmia neonatorum, 844
Cornelia De Lange syndrome
lashes with, 694g
microencephaly from, 691g
nose shape with, 695g
Cornua of uterus, 77f, 78

Corona radiata of ovum, 160
Coronary artery disease, estrogens and, 93
Corpora albicantia, in ovarian cortex, 83
Corpora cavernosa penis, 59, 59f, 60, 60f
Corpora lutea, in ovarian cortex, 83
Corpulmonale
from amniotic fluid embolism, 576
in neonate, with bronchopulmonary dysplasia, 816
Corpus cavernosum urethra, 60
Corpus luteum
creation of in FRC, 96, 97f, 98, 98f
hCG prevents involution of, 168
in pregnancy, 196, 228g
progesterone secreted by, 94
Corpus of uterus, 77, 78
Corpus spongiosum penis, 59, 59f, 60, 60f
Cortex, ovarian, 83
Corticosterioids
for neonatal hypoglycemia, 821
during pregnancy, cleft lip and palate from, 851
Cortisol levels
lowered, as betamethasone risk, 547
pregnancy increases levels of, 202
released during shock, 570
Costovertebral angle tenderness, in initial prenatal exam, 225g
Cotyledons of placenta, 167, 168
Cough reflex, in neonates, 698g
Coughing
by mother
with cardiac disease, 311
after cesarean, 603, 604, 608
by neonate, 686
with herpesvirus type 2 infection, 844
from tracheoesophageal atresia/fistula, 861
Coumadin. See Warfarin
Counseling role of nurse. See also Crisis intervention
abortion and, 128–29, 131
habitual, 332–33
spontaneous, 333
adolescent pregnancy and, 297, 298–99t, 299, 300t, 303–5, 1017
with father, 301
antepartal, 243, 246, 285–92
psychologic, 238, 238g, 240–41, 241–43g
attachment facilitated by, 964–65
about birthmarks, 678, 691g
bleeding in pregnancy and, 329
for cardiac client, 312, 313
children's sexuality counseling, 105–6
circumcision decision, 722
communication skills, 290–91
congenital disabiities and, 581
congenital syphilis, 844
for diabetic client, 324
after ectopic pregnancy, 334
electronic fetal monitoring and, 460
factors disposing to, 997
family care, 49–50, 51–52
financial problems and, 581
fourth trimester, 948g
for genetic disorders, 150–54
for herpes clients, 360
for high-risk infants, predischarge, 780
after hydatidiform mole, 335

in infertility management, 112, 119–20
infant feeding process, 704g
infant nutrition, 689g
with meningocele/meningomyelo-cele, 883–84n
for menopausal women, 102
parental sharing aided by, 962–63
for PIH client, 337
postpartal, 917, 939, 948g
with prenatal diagnosis, 146, 148
relinquishment for adoption, 1014, 1015t
sexual relations in pregnancy and, 265
sexuality and, 105–6
single-parent families, 1018
Couvade, 250
Couvelaire uterus, postpartal hemorrhage risk with, 572
Cow's milk
fat absorption from, 651
in formulas, 718
as inadequate for infant feeding, 718, 719t
recommended age for use of, 718
Coxa vara, developmental, hip dysplasia vs., 878
Coxsackie B virus, congenital heart defects and, 881
CPAP. See Continuous positive airway pressre
CPD. See Cephalopelvic disproportion
CPR (Cardiopulmonary resuscitation), for amniotic fluid embolism, 576
Cradle cap (seborrhea-dermatitis), 690g, 728
Cradle hold , 714, 715f
for breast-feeding, 931, 937f
for tub bath, 728
Cranial nerve damage, in neonate
facial sensitivity with, 692g
neck rigidity from, 697g
eyes with, 693g
Cranial nerves, assessing in neonate, 695g
Cranial sutures, premature closing of, 678
Craniospinal defects, prenatal diagnosis of, 146
Craniostenosis
head measurements with, 678
premature closure of sutures with, 692g
Crawling, by neonate, 686
Creatinine level assessment, 386–87
before induction of labor, 591n
normal values, preterm infant, 752t
with preeclampsia/eclampsia, 342, 343
in pregnancy, renal function and, 199
Credé, Karl, 4
Credé method of emptying bladder, 881, 883n
Cremaster muscle, spermatic cord enclosed by, 3
Cremasteric muscle, 61, 61f
Cretinism
face signs of, 692g
maternal hypothyroidism and, 215t, 326
tongue signs of, 696g
Cri-du-chat (cat cry) syndrome, 140
epicanthal folds with, 693g
ocular hypertelorism with, 692g
Cricoid pressure, preventing vomiting during emergence with, 531

Crisis. See also Crisis intervention
abortion as, 131
adolescent pregnancy as, 296, 1017
cesarean delivery as, cognitive grasp alteration in, 602
defective birth as, 848–50
defined, 246
duration of, 993, 994
families at risk for, 998–99
family system in, 992–94
labor as, 405–6
maturational, 992
pregnancy and birth as, 246–47, 992
preterm birth as, 1006–10, 1007–8t
situational, 992
in postpartal period, 1002
types of, 992
Crisis intervention, 994–97
adolescent parents, 1016–17
attachment problems, 1011–14
child abuse, 1014–16, 1016t
culture and, 997
defective birth, 1010
goals of, 994
neonatal death, 1002–6, 1004n
during postpartal follow-up, 1010–19
preterm birth, 1008–10
single-parent families, 1018
unwanted pregnancy, 1014, 1015t
Crisis theory. See Crisis intervention
Crossing over, in meiosis, 159, 159f
Crown-to-rump length (CRL) of fetus, ultrasound to determine, 369–70
Cry
birth trauma affects, 756n
with congenital hypothyroidism, 859
with hypocalcemia, 821
with hypoglycemia, 818
with kernicterus, 824
maternal magnesium sulfate affects, 769
of preterm infant, 750n
of SGA neonate, 764
weak, from fetal hemorrhage, 573
Crying, by neonates, 724–25
as alert state, 657
assessing, 682, 688g
in neurologic examination, 657
blood pressure rises with, 641
breathing irregularity with, 639
facial paralysis seen with, 680, 680f
functions of, 657, 682
tearless, 680
Cryosurgery, for cervical cancer, 352
Cryptorchidism
assessing male neonate for, 701g
infertility from, 111t, 112
CST. See Contraction stress test
Cuddliness, assessing neonate for, 687, 706
Cuddling
after cleft lip surgery, 855n
with tracheoesophageal atresia/fistula, 864n
Cul-de-sac. See Pouch of Douglas
Culdoscopy, 73
in ectopic pregnancy assessment, 333
for assessing tubular function, 117
Culture. See also specific cultures
antenatal nursing management and, 204–7, 288–89t, 289
attachment process affected by, 964, 968–69
crisis intervention and, 997

defined, 43
families influenced by, 34f, 34–35, 43–46
food practices in pregnancy and, 282t, 283–84
health care behavior influenced by, 43
hip dyslpasia incidence and, 877
infant feeding and, 924–25
labor management and, 469–71
of nurse, labor pain management and, 471
postpartal customs and, 914
Curandero, 206
Curd size, in breast milk, cow's milk, and formula, 719t
Curettage, for retained placental fragments, 972. See also Dilatation and curettage
CURN (Conduct and Utilization of Research in Nursing Project), 26
Cushing's syndrome
amenorrhea from, 100
diabetes secondary to, 315
sign of in initial prenatal exam, 217g, 222g, 230g
Cutaneous neurofibromatosis, 690g
CVA, from hypertension, as risk, 214t
CVP. See Central venous pressure
Cyanosis, 889
defined, 889
maternal
from amniotic fluid embolism, 576
assessing, 570
congenital heart disease, pregnancy risk, 311
with eclampsia seizures, 341
during labor, interventions for, 576
as Mendelson syndrome sign, 531
with severe preeclampsia, 341
neonatal, 880
apnea with, 749
assessing, 688g, 689–90g
causes of, 889
central vs. peripheral, 889
with choanal atresia, 852
circumoral, during feeding, 716
defined, 889
from diaphragmatic hernia, 866
of fingernails, as cardiac anomaly sign, 702g
generalized, as distress sign, 714
with group B streptocccal infection, 843
as hypocalcemia sign, 821
as illness sign, 729
LGA preterm IDM, assessing for, 757n
with MAS, 798, 814
mild, with transient tachypnea of newborn, 797
normal variations, 689g
oxygen levels before signs of, 643
as patent ductus arteriosus sign, 810n
with pneumomediastinum, 816
as pneumopericardium sign, 810n
as pneumothorax sign, 809n, 816
with polycythemia, 835
with PPH syndrome, 817
from pulmonary stenosis, 890
during reactivity period, 712, 713f

as respiratory distress sign, 639, 751, 796t, 801n, 802n
shunting and, 881
from succenturiate placenta, 573
from tetralogy of Fallot, 890
with tracheoesophageal atresia/fistula, 860
with transposition of the great vessels, 891
Cystic fibrosis
as autosomal recessively inherited, 143f,144
diabetes secondary to, 315
hyperbilirubinemia with, 823
intestinal obstruction with, 873
jaundice and, 831
meconium ileus and, 873
prenatal diagnosis of, 148
Cystinosis, prenatal diagnosis of, 147
Cystitis
during pregnancy, 353
postpartal, proteinuria as sign of, 906
sign of in initial prenatal exam, 230g
Cystocele
assessing for, fourth trimester, 946g
sign of in initial prenatal exam, 225g
Cysts
Epstein pearls, in neonatal mouth, 681
follicular, pain caused by, 84
inclusion, on neonate's gums, 681
as induction of labor contraindication, 587
sebaceous, on labia minora, 72
Cytomegalic inclusion disease (CID), 358–59
assessing SGA neonate for, 766–67n
congenital, clinical manifestations of, 767
cataracts, 680
hyperbilirubinemia risk from, 823
Cytomegalovirus (CMV)
in pregnancy, 358–59, 654
in neonate
diagnosing, 842
low IgM levels and, 654
microencphaly from, 691g
screening for, 150
Cytosine arabinoside (ara-C), for neonatal herpesvirus type 2, 844
Cytotrophoblast, 166–67, 167f, 168

Dairy products
in lactation, 271t
in pregnancy, 271t, 272
leg cramps and, 258, 259
Danazol (danocrine), 118–19
Danger signs in pregnancy, 240g, 253f
Dartos muscle, 60, 61, 61f, 72
Dartos muliebris muscle, 72
Data base requirements. See also History
for adolescent pregnancy assessment, 302–3
for AGA and LGA preterm infants, 750
for antepartal assessment, 285
for cesarean delivery care, 601
for cleft lip and palate care, 853
for family assessment, 48
for fetal distress care, 538
for hemorrhage, 569
for labor and delivery care, 472
induced, 591

for meningocele/meningomyelocele, 882
for necrotizing enterocolitis, 839
for neonatal immediate care, 498
for neonatal jaundice care, 831
for postpartal nursing care, 917
for puerperal infection, 977
for RDS, 801
for regional anesthesia, 521
for SGA neonatal care, 764
for stillbirth care, 1004
for thromboembolic disease, 983
for tracheoesophageal atresia/fistula, 862
Data gathering, about nutrition, 285, 286–87f
Daughter cells, 158, 159
Davidson, N., 912
Davies, D. P., 268
Day of birth, mortality and morbidity risk during, 660
Decadron (Dexamethasone), 550
Deceleration phase of labor, 417, 417f, 418. See also Transition
Decelerations in FHR. See Fetal heart rate
Decidua, 163, 163f
postpartal changes in, 902
prostaglandins present in, 202
Decidua basalis, 163, 163f
placenta formed in, 166, 167, 167f, 169f
Decidua capsularis, 163, 163f
Decidua vera (parietalis), 163
Decision making
about cesarean delivery, 601–2, 942
parents' role in, 607
about feeding method, 716–17, 717–19, 719t
during labor, preparation and, 406
in marriage, 37
Decrement phase of contractions, 404, 404f
Deep leg vein disease, 981
nursing care plan, 983–84, 985
Deep tendon reflexes, with severe preeclampsia, 343
Defective birth. See Congenital anomalies
Defensive movements by neonate, 655, 667, 705–6
Defensive obstetrics, cesarean delivery rate and, 600
Degree of Bother inventory, 965, 968f
Dehydration
maternal
assessing for in initial prenatal exam, 217g
body temperature increased by, 913
from hyperemesis gravidarum, 328
at labor admission, hematocrit and, 469
during labor, 428g, 473, 536
postpartal, acetone in urine from, 906
supine hypotensive syndrome and, 409
thrombophlebitis risk with, 912
neonatal
abdominal signs of, 700g
with aganglionosis, 869
depressed fontanelles indicate, 678, 692g
from intestinal obstruction, 873
jaundice treatment and, 831n, 833–34n
motor function with, 703g
as prematurity risk, 746, 753

signs of, 833n
skin turgor with, 690g
temperature with, 677, 688g
as TPN risk, 746
Deladumone (estradiol vaerate), 925
Delayed grief, 1002
DeLee suctioning, 500p, 501f, 636
for MAS prevention, 814
during reactivity period, 712
Deletion, chromosomal, 159
Delirium, with puerperal psychosis, 988
Delivery, 416, 418–19
amnesia about, 530
analgesia during. See Analgesia
anesthesia during. See Anesthesia
attendance at, options for, 471, 613
bed vs. stool for, in history, 4
birth centers ofr, 618–19
breast-feeding immediately after, 613
with cardiac client, 313
death during, crisis intervention for, 1005
difficult
amniotic fluid embolism with, 576
attachment problems after, 968
brachial palsy after, 684, 702g
clavicle fractures from, 697g
effects on family, 580–81
in neonatal assessment, 660
neonatal jaundice and, 831
postpartal risks from, 908t
in preterm infant history, 750
resuscitation risk with, 787
tachycardia after, 906
uterine involution affected by, 903
discomfort after, attachment and, 954–55
emergency, out-of-hospital, 505–7
emergency pack for, 503
by forceps. See Forceps delivery
fossa naviculais laceration during, 73
fourth stage of labor after, 420
general anesthesia for, 528–31
heat loss during, RDS severity and, 817, 818
heat loss following, 646, 647
with herpes infection, 359, 360
hunger after, 905
immediate. See also Cesarean delivery
for abruptio placentae hemorrhage, 572
for fetal hemorrhage, 575
internal or podalic version for, 586
preparing for, with fetal distress, 538n, 539n
induced, indications for, 378f, 379, 388
informed consent during, 15
IUGR and timing of, 370
labor room for, 613
Leboyer method for, 617–18
in less-than-ideal circumstances, 503–7
lighting for, alternative, 613, 617, 618
MAS and, 798, 814–15
by maternity nurse, 503–5
neonatal reactivity after, 711–12, 713f
nursing care plan, 472–82
operative, thromboembolic disease and, 981, 983
out-of-hospital, 505–7
perineal laceration in, 73

as PIH cure, 343, 344
physical changes after, 901–7
of placenta. See Placenta
positions for, 469, 489f, 489–90
alternative, 614–17, 615–17f
culture and, 469
of fetus. See Fetal position
thromboembolic disease risk and, 983
postpartum influenced by, 901
precipitous, 503–5, 543
with oxytocin induction, interventions for, 594n
resuscitation risk with, 786
prenatal testing for, 366, 388
preparation for. See Childbirth preparation
preterm labor, decision making about, 550
prolonged, caput succedaneum from, 691g
resuscitation at, 788–92, 789t, 790f, 791–92p, 793d
risk identification during, 734
siblings at, 613–14
spontaneous, vertex presentation, described, 418
sterile technique during, importance of, 842
supportive environment for, 613
time of, recording, 480n
type of, with malpositions, 551, 552
umbilical cord prolapse and method of, 574, 575
by vacuum extraction, 598–99
Delivery date
determining, 191, 236–37, 237f
in adolescent pregnancy, 305
incorrect
estriols indicate, 380
sign of in subsequent prenatal exams, 239g
induction readiness and, 588
interval between engagement and, 415
Delivery pack, emergency, 506
Delta optical density analysis (ΔOD), 348
Delusions, with puerperal psychosis, 988
Demerol. See Meperidine hydrochloride
Demonstration-return demonstration, as teaching method, 938, 939
Denis Browne splints, for clubfoot, 876
Denmark, nurse-midwifery in, 6
Dental care, in pregnancy, 199, 265
Deodorants, vaginal, 75
Deoxyribonucleic acid (DNA), role of, 157, 158, 165
Depomedroxyprogesterone acetate (Depo-Provera), 127
Depression
fetal, from maternal drug abuse, 360
with high-risk pregnancy, 342
neonatal
midforceps delivery and, 597–98
prone crawl with, 704g
puerperal, 907, 988, 993
after cesearean birth, 608, 941–42
danger signs of, 941
with PIH, 346
with puerperal peritonitis, 980n
Dermal sinus, assessing neonate for, 685, 702g
Dermatitis, in infant, from riboflavin deficiency, 719

Dermatoglyphic analysis, 149f, 149–50
Descent. See Fetal descent
Descriptive statistics, 20–26
Developmental problems
congenital anomalies and, 894–95
inheritance and, 146
as labor and delivery complication, 536, 556–57
macrosomia, 556–57
postnatal diagnosis of, 149, 150
from postnatal insult, 146
Developmental stages, in family theory, 36–41
pregnancy, 246, 247
Developmental tasks
of adolescents, 296–97, 298–99t
pregnancy and, 301, 304
maturational crises and, 992
of pregnancy, 247
adolescent and, 296–97, 300t, 304
fourth trimester, 943, 944
Deviant behavior, gender identity and, 89
Dewees, William, 5
Dexamethasone (Decadron), 550
Dextrocardia, in neonate, 683
with diaphragmatic hernia, 866
point of maximal impulse with, 698g
Dextrose
for hypoglycemia prevention, 821
in delivery room, 792
for resuscitation, 788
Dextrostix test
for hypoglycemia assessment, 817, 818, 819–20p
for MAS neonates, 815
at nursery admission, 711
for prenatal urinalysis, 317
for preterm infant, 747, 750
procedure, 819–20
for SGA neonates, 764n
Diabetes mellitus
breast-feeding with, 318
classification of, 314t, 314–15
as CST indication, 375
described, 313–14
genetic counseling referral for, 151
gestational, 314
infertility from, 111t, 112
latent, glycosuria as sign of, 468
as polygenically inherited, 145
in pregnancy, 101, 202, 202, 313–21, 314t, 315t, 319t
carbohydrate needs and, 201, 273
classifications of, 315, 315t
diet and, 318, 320
effect on disease course, 315
as hemorrhage risk, 569
hydramnios associated with, 577
induction of labor with, 587
labor and, 321, 536
L/S ratio with, 639
lung profile for, 386
neonatal effects of, 689g, 761, 823. See also Infants of diabetic mothers
nursing care plan for, 322–26
placental transport affected by, 170–71
postpartum period, 321, 905, 906, 908t
as ritodrine contraindication, 549
signs of in prenatal exams, 230g, 240g
as risk factor, 214t, 336
postmenopausal, 101

signs and symptoms of, 314
tests for, 316–18, 319t
Diabetic mother, infants of. See Infants of Diabetic Mothers (IDMs)
Diabetogenic effect of pregnancy, 314
Diagnosis. See also Assessment; Nursing diagnoses
of appendicitis in pregnancy, 351
of CMB in pregnancy, 358
of congenital rubella, 358
of ectopic pregnancy, 333–34
genetic counseling and, 152–53
of genital herpes simplex, 359
of hyperemesis gravidarum, 328
of incompetent cervix, 335
of placenta previa, 565–66, 565p
of sepsis neonatorum, 841–42
of spontaneous abortion, 331–32
of toxoplasmosis, 357
Diaper rash, caring for, 727
Diaper test for PKU, 858
Diapers, 728m 729f
laundering, 728
stains on, 652
Diaphoresis. See Sweating
Diaphragm
assessing in neonate, 699g
pregnancy positions of, 197
Diaphragm, for contraception, 121f, 122–23, 123f
for diabetic client, 319
postpartal refitting for, 944
Diaphragmatic hernia, 861, 866f, 866–67
clinical manifestations of, 699g, 700g, 861, 866
heart location with, 683, 698g
incidence of, 861
interventions for, 866–67
PPH syndrome with, 817
ventilation problems with, 788
Diaphragmatic paralysis, from birth trauma, 756n
Diarrhea
in mother
as hyperthyroidism sign, 326
as impending labor sign, 416
with puerperal peritonitis, 977
in neonate
from aganglionosis, 869
preterm, as feeding intolerance sign, 746
as sepsis neonatorum sign, 841
transitional stools vs., 716
Diastasis recti
assessing for, 223g
in black infants, 699g
postpartum, 905, 911, 946g
Diazepam (Valium)
during labor, 510, 513
fetal/neonatal effects of, 361t
neonatal hyperbilirubinemia and, 823
for preeclampsia/eclampsia, 344
Diazoxide (Hyperstat), neonatal effects of, 769
DIC. See Disseminated intravascular coagulation
Dick-Read, Dr. Grantly, 12, 293
Diet. See also Nutrition
for galactosemia, 859
for homocystinuria, 859
for maple syrup urine disease, 858
for PKU infant, 858
for preeclampsia, 342, 343
plugged ducts and, 937
postpartal
assessment of, 913
cultural influences on, 914
elimination and, 918n

Diet, postpartal, *(Cont'd)*
    infection prevention and, 918n
Diethylstilbestrol (DES), 265–66
Dieting, amenorrhea from, 100. *See
    also* Weight loss
Differential, in initial prenatal exam,
    229g
Diffusion
    in placenta, 170
    oxygenation in neonate and, 639
Digestive system
    fetal development of, 650–51
    of preterm infant, 740–41
Digital ablation, 183t
Digital stunting, 183t
Digitalis
    for cardiac client, 312, 313
    for circulatory failure with eclamp-
        sia, 344
    for pulmonary embolism, 985n
Digitalization, for congestive heart
    failure, 894
Digitoxin, effects on fetus of, 768–69
Digoxin (Lanoxin), 885
    for congestive heart failure, 894
    effects on fetus of, 768–69
Dihydrotestosterone, 59
Dilantan (Diphenylhydantoin), 650
Dilatation and curettage
    as abortion method, 129, 130t
    after hydatidiform mole, 335
    incompetent cervix after, 335
    after spontaneous abortion, 332
Dilatation of the cervix. *See* Cervical
    dilatation
Dilators, Greeks used, 3
Dilts, P. V., 170
Diphenhydramine (Benadryl), for an-
    esthesia reaction, 516
Diphenylhydantoin (Dilantin), 650
Diphtheria, neonatal immunity to,
    654. *See also* Immunizations
Diploid number of chromosomes, 135
    at fertilization, 161f, 162
Dipping of presenting part, 402, 402f
Dipstix test, for neonatal hypoglyce-
    mia, 753n, 818. *See also*
    Dextrostix; Urinalysis
Dirty Duncan, 419
Disaccharides, digestion of by neo-
    nate, 651
Disc disease, sign of in prenatal
    exam, 225g
Discharge
    after cesarean birth, 942
    early. *See* Early discharge
    evaluating episiotomy for, 912
    postpartal instruction, 941
Discharge planning, 730
    for cardiac client, 313
    danger signs, 941, 973
    hemorrhage or hematoma and,
        973
    for preterm or defective neonate,
        779–80
    puerperal infections and, 976
    wound healing assessment and,
        975t
Dislocated hips, inheritance of, 145
Disposal of contaminated items,
    puerperal infection and, 978n
Disseminated intravascular coagula-
    tion (DIC), 567–68, 568f
    from abruptio placentae, 563,
        564, 572n
    from amniotic fluid embolism, 576
    fibrinogen replacement for, 576
    hemorrhage with, 573n
    hypovolemic shock with, in
        Sheehan syndrome, 988
    in neonate, 837
        as MAS complication, 815

with severe eclampsia, 343
    signs and symptoms of, 567,
        568
Distention theory of labor onset, 407
Diuresis, postpartal, 905, 982
Diuretics
    for cardiac client, 312, 313
    for chronic hypertension in preg-
        nancy, 347
    for congestive heart failure, 888,
        894
    for patent ductus arteriosus, 885
    for preeclampsia, 342
Diversity, recognizing, 47
Dizygotic twins, 185, 557–58
Dizziness
    as bromocriptine side effect, 926d
    as danger sign, 240g
    menopausal, 101
    as Methergine side effect, 903d
    postpartal, nursing care for,
        916
DNA (Deoxyribonucleic acid), role of,
    157, 158, 165
Döderlein's bacilli, 75, 76f, 101
    antibiotics or steroids reduce, 355
    beta-lactose suppositories to
        encourage, 356
Dogiel corpuscles, 73
"Doll's eye" phenomenon, 680
Doppler ultrasonography
    for deep vein thrombosis assess-
        ment, 981, 983
    for fetal heartbeat auscultation,
        237, 237f
        detection time reduced by, 195
        emotional acceptance and, 203
    during labor, 444, 445t, 445–46,
        446f
    for neonatal blood pressure
        assessment, 641
    umbilical cord prolapse use of,
        574
Doptone, assessing fetal heartbeat
    with, 223g
Dorsal recumbent position for labor,
    disadvantages of, 614–15
Double setup examination, 567
Double vision, as danger sign, 240g
Douching
    as contraceptive method, 121f,
        122
    contraindicated in pregnancy, 356
    infertility from, 112
    for nonspecific vaginitis, 356
    for *Trichomonas* infection, 356
    vaginal environment altered by, 75
Douglas' cul-de-sac. *See* Pouch of
        Douglas
Down syndrome, 137f
    aganglionosis and, 869
    Brushfield spots with, 693g
    cardiac malformations with, 881
        atrial septal defects, 885
        endocardial cushion defects,
            888
    chromosomal description of, 136,
        137
    clinical features of, 137
    cost of, 134
    cost of preventing, 134–35
    dermatoglyphic patterns with, 149,
        149f
    eye signs of, 693g
    face signs of, 692g
    intestinal obstruction with, 873
    "Johns Hopkins case" 10
    karotype of male with, 137f
    maternal age and, 101, 147
    mosaicism with, 138
    neck with, 697g
    nose sign of, 695g

in SGA neonates, assessing for,
    766n
simian line with, 684, 702g
tongue signs of, 696g
from translocation, 138–39, 139f,
    140f
Dressing, neonatal responses to, 706
Drooling, by neonate
    assessing, 696g
    with tracheoesophageal atresia/
        fistula, 860, 862
Drowsy state, in neonate, 657
Drug excretion, by preterm infants,
    746–47
Drug abuse
    infertility from, 112, 114
    in pregnancy, 360–62, 361t
        by adolescents, 299, 304,
            482
        assessing for in prenatal exam,
            242g
        IUGR associated with, 761, 762
        neonatal withdrawal from. *See*
            Withdrawal
        resuscitation risk from, 786
        as risk factor, 214t
Drug guides
    betamethasone (Celestone), 547
    bromocriptine (Parlodel), 926
    erythromycin (Ilotycin) ointment,
        711
    magnesium sulfate, 345
    methylergonovine maleate (Meth-
        ergine), 903
    naloxone hydrochloride (Narcan),
        793
    oxytocin (Pitocin), 590
    ritodrine (Yutopar), 549
    sodium bicarbonate, 793
    vitamin K (AquaMEPHYTON),
        711
Drug withdrawal. *See* Withdrawal
Drugs. *See* Medications
"Dry birth" oligohydramnios and,
    425t
Dry mouth
    as anxiety sign, 608
    during labor, alleviating, 483–84
Dry skin, as hypothyroidism sign,
    326
Dubowitz, L., 660, 661
Dubowitz, V., 660, 661
Ductus arteriosus
    changes in at birth, 640, 641f,
        739, 739t
        transient murmur and, 641
    in fetus, 171, 172f, 642f, 739,
        739t
    patent. *See* Patent ductus
        arteriosus
Ductus deferens, 58f. *See also* Vas
    deferens
Ductus venosus
    changes in at birth, 640–41, 641f,
        739
    in fetus, 171, 172f
Duhamel pull-through operation
    method, 870
Duncan mechanism of placental
    delivery, 419, 420f
Duodenal atresia, in neonate, 873.
    See also Intestinal obstruction
Duodenal bypass procedure, 873
Duodenal stenosis in neonate, peri-
    stalsis with, 699g
Duodenum
    fetal development of, 650, 651
    neonatal fat absorption role of,
        651
Duration of contractions, 404, 404f,
    405. *See also* Uterine
    contractions

Duskiness, in neonate, with RDS,
    802n
Duvall, Evelyn M.
    developmental theory of, 36–41,
        40t
    on postpartal developmental tasks,
        944
    on pregnancy, 247
Dwarfism
    achondroplastic, 143
    assessing neonate for, 689g
    metatropic, prenatal diagnosis of,
        146–47
Dysmaturity. *See* Small-for-
    gestational-age neonates
Dysmenorrhea, 82, 100
Dyspareunia, 73, 101
    from monilial vaginitis, 355
    from *Trichomonas* infection, 356
Dysplasia
    hip, 876–78, 877f
    renal, prenatal diagnosis of, 146
Dyspnea
    from amniotic fluid embolism, 576
    in cardiac client, 311
    during labor, interventions for,
        576
    from hydramnios, 577
    as Methergine side effect, 903d
    as normal pregnancy discomfort,
        253f, 255t, 259
    as pulmonary embolism sign, 981,
        983, 984n
    in neonate, 639
        with diaphragmatic hernia, 866
        with herpesvirus type 2 infec-
            tion, 844
        with pulmonary stenosis, 890
        with tetralogy of Fallot, 890
        with transposition of the great
            vessels, 891
Dystocia. *See* Labor, dysfunctional
Dysuria
    as cystitis sign, 986
    as danger sign in pregnancy,
        240g
    from genital herpes simplex, 359
    from monilial vaginitis, 355
    as puerperal infection sign, 974,
        976, 977
    from *Trichomonas* infection, 356

E. coli. *See Escherichia coli*
Ear culture, from neonate
    for group B streptococcus infec-
        tion, 843
    in sepsis neonatorum assessment,
        842
Ear infection, in neonate
    with cleft palate, 852
    signs of, 696g
Early detection. *See* Prenatal diagno-
    sis; Screening
Early discharge, 31
    attachment aided by, 965
    from birth center, 619
    PKU screening and, 858
Ears
    of fetus
        development of, 173, 175t,
            177t, 178, 179t, 180
        teratogenic damage to, 183t
    of mother, assessing in prenatal
        exam, 219g
    of neonate
        assessing, 681, 682f, 696–97g
        care of, 696g, 727
        gestational age and, 662f, 665f,
            668, 670f
        Pierre Robin syndrome affects,
            850
        preterm, 750

Ecchymosis
  in mother
    as anticoagulant overdose sign, 984n
    evaluating episiotomy for, 912
    signs of in initial prenatal exam, 217g
    wound healing assessment by, 975t
  in neonate
    from congenital CMV, 359
    from congenital toxoplasmosis, 357
    hyperbilirubinemia with, 822
    vitamin K deficiency, 836
ECG. See Electrocardiogram
Echocardiography, for cardiac assessment of neonates, 885
  coarctation of the aorta, 889
  endocardial cushion defects on, 888
  patent ductus arteriosus, 885
  pulmonary stenosis on, 890
  transposition of the great vessels on, 891
  ventricular septal defects on, 885, 888
Eclampsia. See also Preeclampsia-Eclampsia;
  Pregnancy-induced hypertension
  as chronic hypertension risk, 347
  as CST indication, 375
  danger signs of, 240g
  described, 336, 341
  drug guide for, 345
  edema of mons pubis with, 72
  fetal distress care with, 540
  as hemorrhage risk, 569
  incidence of, 336
  induction of labor and, 587, 590
  interventions for, 344, 345d
  as preterm labor cause, 548
  as risk factor, 215t
  as ritadrine contraindication, 548, 549
Ectoderm, 165, 165t, 166f
Ectomelia, 183t
Ectopia cordis, 183, 183t
Ectopic pregnancy, 333–34, 334f
  bleeding caused by, 329
  defined, 333
  diagnostic test for, 194
  incidence of, 333
  infertility from, 111t
  RhoGAM after, 349–50
  signs of in initial prenatal exam, 223g, 228g
  statistics about, 329
  ultrasonography to assess, 8
Ectromelia, 183t
Eczema, assessing in neonate, 690g
EDC. See Delivery date; Estimated date of confinement
Edema, in mother
  of ankle
    from deep leg vein disease, 981
    as pregnancy discomfort, 254t, 256
  assessing for
    after episiotomy, 912
    during first stage labor, 428g, 429g
    at labor admission, 472
    postpartum, 624, 912
    at postpartal home visit, 624
    with severe preeclampsia, 343
    in prenatal exams, 216g, 220g, 224g, 239g
  with cardiac disease, 311
  cervical, 430g, 478n
  as danger sign of pregnancy, 240g
  in labia majora, 72

  at labor admission, hematocrit and, 469
  of lower extremities
    from deep leg vein disease, 981
    from hydramnios, 577
  of mons pubis, in pregnancy, 72
  with PIH, 336, 338
  in pregnancy, reason for, 198
  with severe preeclampsia, 341, 343
  vaginal and vulval, catheterization with, 982, 986
  wound healing assessment by, 975t
Edema, in neonate
  with congenital syphilis, 844
  from hemolytic disease of the newborn, 826, 827
  as hypocalcemia sign, 821
  as jaundice sign, 831n
  as patent ductus arteriosus sign, 810n
  preterm
    apnea from, 749
    as overhydration sign, 747
    protein excess as cause of, 719
    with RDS, 796t
  urinary output and, 652
Educational needs, assessing in prenatal exams, 238g, 241g
EEP. See End-expirator pressure
Effacement of the cervix. See Cervical effacement
Efferent ductules, in testes, 61, 62f
  embryologic development of, 57, 58f
Effleurage, 484–85, 486f
  as hypertonic labor intervention, 537
  with induced labor, 592n
  in latent phase labor, 474
Ego integrity vs. despair, 40t, 41
Ego strength, attachment readiness requires, 952
Egophony, in initial prenatal exam, 221g
Egypt, ancient, obstetrics in, 3
Eisenmenger's syndrome, pregnancy risk and, 311
Ejaculation, 102
  amount of, 64, 161
  premature, infertility from, 111t
  retrograde
    infertility from, 111t
    medications cause, 114
Ejaculatory ducts, 63
  development of, 57, 653
EKG. See Electrocardiogram
Elastic support stockings. See Support stockings
Elderly, sexuality among, 91, 102
Electrocardiogram (ECG; EKG)
  of fetus, positive pregnancy diagnosis with, 195
  of mother
    in initial prenatal exam, 222g
    pulmonary embolism signs on, 982, 983, 985n
  of neonate
    with PKU, 858
    pneumothorax signs on, 809n
    transposition of great vessels seen on, 891–92
    ventricular septal defect seen on, 888
Electrolyte imbalances. See also Acidosis; Fluid and electrolyte balance
  in mother
    from prolonged labor, interventions for, 536
    with severe preeclampsia, 343

  from sodium bicarbonate in pregnancy, 256
  in neonate
    from aganglionic megacolon, 869, 870
    blood bicarbonate concentration and, 653
    as intestinal obstruction complication, 874
    from maternal cardiac medications, 769
    with necrotizing enterocolitis, 840n
    with RDS, correcting, 797, 806n
    tremors with, 703g
Electrolytes
  administering with oxytocin, 500
  assessing
    with ritodrine administration, 549
    with severe preeclampsia, 343
  labor changes in, 407, 409
  in preterm infant, 746–48
    normal values, 752t
  placental transport of, 170
Electromyography, meningomyelocele assessment with, 880
Electronic fetal monitoring, 8. See also Fetal heart rate, monitoring
  advantages of, 444, 445t, 446, 450, 458–59
  ambulation and, 617
  with analgesia or anesthesia
    analgesia, 510, 511
    paracervical block, 517
    regional anesthesia, 522n
  attitudes toward, 459–60
  auscultation vs., 459
  baseline variability and type of, 452
  birth center transfer for, 618
  cesarean delivery decision and, 600, 605
  with CPD assessment, 578
  in delivery room, 480n
  for diabetic client, 321
  disadvantages of, 9, 444 445, 445t, 446, 447, 447–49f
  documentation with, 460
  evaluating tracings from, 460t, 460–61
  external (indirect), 444–46, 445t, 446f, 448f
    fetal electrocardiography, 444–45
    ultrasound, 444, 445t, 445–46, 446f
  fetal electrocardiography, 444–45
  fetoscope vs., 459
  FHR patterns, 450f, 450–58, 451t, 452–53f, 455–58f
  indications for, 444
  with induction of labor, 589, 592n
  internal (direct), 444, 445t, 446–50, 447–50f
    procedure for, 446
    baseline variability shown by, 452
  with macrosomia, 557
  management interventions, 451t
  methods of, 444–50, 445t, 446–50f
  nursing role in, 459–61, 460t
  optional vs. routine, 613
  for prolonged pregnancy, 759t
  psychologic reactions to, 459–60
  risk identification with, 734
  with ritodrine administration, 549
  telemetry, 445t, 447, 450

  umbilical cord prolapse signs in, 574
  uses of, 8
Electronic monitoring, of uterine contractions, 434, 440f
Electronic thermometer, 677
Elimination
  fetal, as placental function, 168
  maternal
    during labor, 474–75n, 476, 478
    postpartal assessment of, 913, 946–47g
    postpartal difficulty with, 905–6
    postpartal management of, 918n
  neonatal
    meningomyelocele and, 880, 881, 882, 883n
    preterm, nursing care plan for, 750
    spina bifida and, 880, 881, 883n
Elliot forceps, 597, 597f
Ellis-Van Creveld syndrome, assessing neonate for, 689g, 702g
Embolectomy, 982, 985n
Embolism
  amniotic fluid, 576
  pelvic, potential lodging places of, 75
  pulmonary. See Pulmonary embolism
Embryo
  cardiovascular development in, 639–40
  cleft lip development in, 851
  cleft palate development in, 852
  defective, spontaneous abortion caused by, 333
  develops from blastocyst, 162
  diaphragmatic hernia formation in, 861
  esophageal atresia development in, 859
  factors affecting development of, 183t, 183–85
  gastrointestinal development in, 650
  gestational age of, 173
  hematopoiesis in, 643
  imperforate anus formation in, 871
  lung development in, 635
  omphalocele formation in, 867
  organ development in, 173, 174–77t, 178–79
  primary cell layers in, body structures and, 165t
  reproductive system development in, 57–59, 58f
    breasts, 84
    ovarian ligaments, 81
    ovaries, 83
    uterus, 77
    vagina, 75
  TORCH diseases and, 357–60
  tracheoesophageal fistula development in, 859
Embryonic membranes, formation of, 162, 163–65, 164f, 166f
Emergence
  from general anesthesia, 529, 530
  vomiting danger at, 531
Emergency delivery, 503–7
  cesarean, preparation for, 602n, 607–8
  out-of-hospital, 505–7
Emergency delivery pack, 503
  precipitous labor risk and, 543
Emotional distress, as risk, 215t

Emotional support. *See* Support
  groups; Supporting role of
  nurse
Emotions
  complicated childbirth, 580–81
  defective birth, 580–81, 772–74,
    848–50
  grief. *See* Grief
  infertility and, 112, 119–20
    management techniques and,
      118
  labor and, 405–6
  of neonate, meningocele/meningo-
    myelocele and, 881, 883n
  of nurse
    about defective birth, 849
    after neonatal death, 1006
  pain relief and, 513
  postpartal assessment of, 913–14
  postpartal changes in, 907
  in pregnancy, 203–4
  with preterm birth, 772–74, 1006,
    1007–8t, 1008
Empathy, as assessment tool, 48
Emphysema
  signs of in initial prenatal exam,
    220g
  interstitial pulmonary, as respira-
    tory therapy complication,
  809n, 816
Employment, during pregnancy, 261
Emptying time, of breast vs. bottle,
  719t
Encephalitis
  from congenital CMV, 359
  with extended rubella syndrome,
    358
Encephalopathy
  from cytomegalovirus, 215t
  with kernicterus, 823, 824
End-expirator pressures (EEP), for
  MAS, 815
Endocardial cushion defects, 888
Endocardial cushions, formation of,
  640
Endocervical glands, pregnancy
  changes in, 196
Endocrine functions of placenta,
  168–71
Endocrine medications, teratogenic
  effects of, 267t
Endocrine pregnancy tests, 194–95
Endocrine system
  disorders of. *See also* Diabetes
    mellitus
    dysfunctional labor from, 536–
      37
    infertility from, 114
    spontaneous abortion and,
      329
  fetal development of, 173, 175t,
    177t, 179t
  labor role of, 407
  pregnancy changes in, 201–2, 314
Endoderm, 165, 165t, 166f
Endometrial biopsy, in infertility
  workup, 115f, 116
Endometrial stroma, development of,
  57
Endometriosis
  dysmenorrhea from, 100
  infertility from, 111t, 112, 118–19
  menopause and, 101
Endometritis
  infertility from, 111t
  postpartal, 975, 977, 979n
    from cesarean delivry, 605
Endometritis/metritis, with subinvolution, 973
Endometrium, 77, 78–79
  blood supply to, in menstrual
    cycle, 94, 95, 95f

cyclic changes in, 97f, 98–99, 99f
implantation in, 162–63, 163f
infertility and, 111t, 112, 115f,
  116, 118–19
postpartal formation of, 902
pregnancy changes in, progesterone and, 202
Endopelvic fascia, 67
Endotracheal intubation of neonate,
  788, 790f, 791–92p
  for diaphragmatic hernia, 866
  for MAS prevention, 812–13p,
    813f, 814–15
  for Pierre Robin syndrome, 851
Endotracheal suctioning procedure,
  812–13, 813f
Enemas
  diagnostic contrast, for meconium
    plug, 870
  for intestinal obstruction interven-
    tion, 873
  at labor admission, 467, 468
    contraindications, 468
    decision making about, 467,
      468, 613
    postpartal elimination and, 905
  postpartal, 918n
Energy status, assessing during first
  stage labor, 428g
Energy burst, as impending labor
  sign, 416
Engagement, 402f, 402–3, 403f
  assessing during labor, 439f, 439–
    40p, 474n
  delayed, CPD as cause of, 578
  forceps delivery requires, 598
  interval before delivery of, 415
  placenta previa and, 565
Engel, G., 1002
England, midwifery in, 4, 6
English Midwives Act, 6
Engorgement of breasts
  maternal. *See* Breast-feeding
  in neonate, 699g
Engrossment, 961–62
Enterocolitis. *See* Necrotizing
  enterocolitis
Enterocytes, amino acid transfer by,
  651
Enterohepatic circulation, neonatal
  jaundice and, 823
Environment
  assessing neonatal responses to,
    687, 705–6
  attachment process affected by,
    954
  cleft lip and palate causes in, 851
  congenital heart defects caused
    by, 881
  crisis adaptation affected by, 993
  families influenced by, 34f, 34–35,
    46, 48
  fetal responses to, 654
  IUGR and, 761
  neonatal responses to, 654–57,
    656f, 657
  nongenetic conditions and, 145–46
  polygenic traits and, 145
  SGA neonates' outcomes and, 763
  as teratogenic factor, 266
Enzymatic deamination by placenta,
  170
Enzyme assays, postnatal, 150
Enzymes, in neonate, 651
Eosinophils
  development of in fetus, 644
  in neonate, 645
Epicanthal folds, in neonate
  assessing, 693g
  from fetal alcohol syndrome, 770
Epicanthus, vulnerability to, 183t
Epididymides, 59f, 62f, 62–63

Epididymis
  embryologic development of, 57,
    58f
  infertility and, 112, 114
Epidural block. *See* Lumbar epidural
  block
Epidural space, 517f, 517–18
Epigastric pain
  as danger sign of pregnancy, 240g
  with severe preeclampsia, 341
Epilepsy, pregnancy and, 267t, 331t
Epinephrine
  as additive to local anesthesia, 515
  for cardiovascular collapse, 516
  for IDM, 768
  increased with blood loss, 570
  labor role of, 407
  labor stress and, 535, 536–37
  for neonatal bradycardia, 792
  for neonatal hypoglycemia, 821
  placenta breaks down, 170
  for resuscitation, 788
  signs of reaction to, 515
  uteroplacental blood flow
    decreased by, 515
Episioprototomy, 596
Episiorrhaphy, 596
Episiotomy, 595–96, 596f
  for breech vaginal delivery, 555
  defined, 595
  early use of, 4
  extension of, from fetal malposi-
    tion, 551
  infection of, 974–75, 975t, 977–
    79n
  lithotomy position increases need
    for, 615
  optional vs. routine, 613
  perineal care after, 919n
  postpartal assessment of, 908,
    912, 919n, 947g
  for preterm delivery, 550
  record keeping about, 480n
  relief measures after, 502, 596
  repair of, 411, 596
  site of, 73
  types of, 595–96, 596f
    occiput-posterior position and,
      551
Episirectomy, 596
Epispadias, 60
  assessing neonatal male for, 700g
Epistaxis
  as anticoagulant overdose sign,
    984n
  as DIC sign, 568
  as pregnancy discomfort, 197,
    252, 254, 254t
Epithelial (Epstein) pearls, in neonatal
  mouth, 681, 696g
Epithelium, embryologic development
  of, 57
Equipment. *See also* Catheters;
  Forceps
  care of, sepsis neonatorum
    prevention by, 842
  delivery pack, 488
  emergency delivery pack, 503
    for out-of-hospital delivery, 506
  exchange transfusion, 828
  resuscitative, 787–88
  for vacuum extraction delivery,
    598, 599
Equivalents, APPENDIX F
Erb-Duchenne paralysis, 684–85,
  685f
  assessing neonate for, 702g
  as forceps delivery risk, 598
  from macrosomia, 557
  Moro reflex affected by, 697g
Ergonovine maleate (Ergotrate), postpartal administration of, 911

for hemorrhage, 500, 572n, 972
for subinvolution, 973
Erikson, Erik, developmental theory
  of, 38, 39, 40t, 40–41, 296
Eroded cervix, 226g, 227f
Erythema neonatorum toxicum, 677,
  690g
Erythroblastosis fetalis. *See* Hemolytic disease of the newborn
Erythrocytes. *See* Red blood cells
Erythromycin (Ilotycin)
  for eye prophylaxis, 499n, 505,
    710, 711d
  for gonorrhea in neonate, 844
Erythropoiesis, compensatory, 824
Erythropoietin
  fetal, 644
  neonatal, increased secretion of
    with tetralogy of Fallot, 890
    with transposition of the great
      vessels, 891
Escharotic agent, for omphalocele,
  868
Escherichia coli (E. coli)
  breast-feeding protects against,
    748
  neonatal susceptibility to, IgM lev-
    els and, 654
  puerperal infections caused by,
    974, 986
  sepsis neonatorum from, 841
  urinary tract infections from, 353
  vaginal infections from, 356
  vitamin K synthesized by, 275
Eschmann shield, 931
Escutcheon, evaluating in infertility
  workup, 114
Esophageal atresia, 859–61, 860f,
  861f
  assessing with first water feeding,
    716
  in fetus, ultrasound to identify,
    577
  hydramnios increases risk of, 425t
  nursing care plan, 862–65
  signs of, 696g
Esophagostomy, cervical, 861, 864n
Essential hypertensive vascular
  diseases, spontaneous abortion from, 329
Ester types of anesthesia, 514
Estimated date of confinement
  (EDC). *See* Delivery date
Estradiol, ovaries secrete, 169
Estradiol vaerate (Deladumone), 925
Estriol
  metabolism of, 379
  placenta secretes, 169
  pregnancy excretion of, 379f,
    379–80
  pregnancy role of, 202
Estriol determinations, 342, 379f,
  379–81
  betamethasone and, 547
  critical levels, 380, 388
  CST indicated by, 375
  patterns of excretion, 379f, 379–
    80
  in prolonged pregnancy, 759t
  resuscitation risk and, 786
  serial, 380–81
  with severe preeclampsia, 343
Estrogen. *See also* Estrogenic
  hormones
  basal body temperature and,
    115
  breast development and, 85
  endometrial changes from, 98, 99
  female reproductive cycle role of,
    96
  fertilization aided by, 160
  graafian follicle produces, 96

hCG stimulates production of, 202
infertility and, 116, 118
labor role of, 407
lactation preparation role of, 925
for lactation suppression, thrombo-
    embolic disease risk with, 980
as medication in pregnancy,
    teratogenic effects of, 267t
menopause and, 101, 102
placental, 168, 169–70
postdelivery galactorrhea and, 987
postpartal decrease in, 902
pregnancy effects of
    on adrenals, 202
    on breasts, 197, 202, 254t, 255
    on cardiovascular system, 198
    on cervix, 196
    on gums, 220g
    on liver, 199
    on nasal mucosa, 197
    on skin, 199
    on thryoid, 201
    on uterus, 196, 202
    on vagina, 196
    pregnancy role of, 160, 168, 169–
        70, 202, 407
Estrogen assays, in infertility workup,
    116
Estrogen stimulation theory, 407
Estrogenic hormones, 93. See also
    Estrogen
    breast development and, 85
    in oral contraceptives, 125, 126–
        27t
    placental and maternal, genital de-
        velopment role of, 653
    role of, 93
    target organs for, 73
    vaginal lining affected by, 75
Estrogens. See Estrogen; Estrogenic
    hormones
Estrone, postmenopausal production
    of, 101
Ether, as obstetric anesthetic, 510,
    529
Ethical issues
    abortion, 10
    passive euthanasia, 10–11
    scientific advances and, 9–11
Ethnicity, physiologic jaundice and,
    649. See also Culture
Europe
    nurse-midwifery in, 6
    obstetrics in, overview of, 3–4
Eustachian tube dysfunction, with
    cleft palate, 852
Euthanasia, passive, as ethical issue,
    10–11
Evaluation
    of AGA and LGA care, 757
    of attachment process, 963–68,
        966–68f
    of cesarean delivery care, 604
    of cleft lip and palate care, 857
    of crisis intervention process, 997
    of family care, 50
    family case example, 52
    of fetal distress care, 540
    of hemorrhage care, 573
    of high-risk infant care, 737
    of immediate neonatal care, 499n
    of induced labor care, 594
    of meningocele/meningomyelocele
        care, 884n
    of necrotizing enterocolitis care,
        840n
    of neonatal jaundice care, 834
    of parent education
        antepartal, 291, 292
        postpartal, 939
    as part of nursing process, 20
    of PIH care, 339

postpartal, 481–82, 920
    of puerperal infection care, 980
    of RDS care, 810
    of regional labor anesthesia, 524n
    statistics for, 20–26
    of stillbirth care, 1004
    of thromboembolic disease care,
        985
    of tracheoesophageal atresia/
        fistula care, 865
Evaporation, neonatal heat loss by,
    646, 647, 648, 753
Everted cervix, 226g, 227f
Evil spirits, pregnancy beliefs about,
    205–6
Exchange transfusions, 824, 825p
    for ABO incompatibility, 828, 831
    for DIC, 837
    equipment for, 828
    for hemolytic disease, 825p, 827f,
        827–29, 829f
    for hyperbilirubinemia, 827f, 827–
        29, 829f, 831, 833n
    indications for, 827f, 827–28,
        831, 833n
    for neonatal polycythemia, 836
    nursing interventions, 825p, 828–
        29
    phototherapy vs., 827, 827f
Excretion. See Elimination; Urination
Exercise. See also Exercises
    infertility from, 112
    during pregnancy, 261, 262–63,
        263–64f
    fetal breathing pattern influ-
        enced by, 636
    strenuous, shown in urinalysis,
        230g
Exercises
    postpartal, 905, 919–20n, 922–
        23f
    after cesarean delivery, 912,
        941
    encouraging, 916
    overzealousness in, 918n
    perineal tightening, 919n
    prenatal, 262–63, 263–64f
    Kegel's, 255, 263, 264f, 294
    leg cramps and, 258
    pelvic tilt, 258
Exercises for True Natural Childbirth
    (Hartman), 29
Exertion, patent ductus arteriosus
    and, 810n
Exfoliation, placental site heals by,
    902–3
Exhaustion
    as forceps delivery indication, 597
    from prolonged labor, 425t, 541,
        542
    in preterm infant, preventing,
        753n
Exomphalos. See Omphalocele
Exophthalmos, as hyperthyroidism
    sign, 326
Expectant families, developmental
    tasks of, 38–39
Expiratory grunts or sighs
    assessing in neonate, 682
    with RDS, 795f, 796t, 797t, 801n
    with transient tachypnea of new-
        born, 797
Expulsion of fetus during labor, 415
Extended family, assessing, 49
Extended family structure, 32, 33f
    cultural preferences for, 43
    subextended, 45
Extended rubella syndrome, 358
Extension of fetal head, during labor,
    414f, 415
External cardiac massage, of neo-
    nate, 790, 790f

External or cephalic version, 585,
    586, 586f
    for transverse lie, 556
External genitals
    female, 71–73, 71f
        cancer signs in, in prenatal
            exam, 225g
        male, 59–61, 59–61f
External os, 77f, 78
    postpartal changes in, 904
External rotation of fetus, during
    labor, 415
Extraembryonic coelom, 164, 164f,
    166f
Extremities
    of mother
        assessing in initial prenatal
            exam, 224g
        postpartal evaluation of, 912
        trauma to, with regional labor
            anesthesia, 523–24n
    of neonate
        assessing, 684–85, 685f, 702g,
            703g, 705
        cyanosis of, after delivery, 683
        discolored, with polycythemia,
            835
        fractured, from vaginal breech
            delivery, 554
        LGA, assessing, 756–57n
        meningomyelocele affects, 880
        painful, with congenital syphilis,
            844
        Pierre Robin syndrome affects,
            850
Extubation, observing intubated neo-
    nate for, 806n
Eye contact
    cesarean delivery preparation
        with, 602, 608
    during labor, deceleration phase,
        479
    of parents and neonate, 499n,
        502, 503
    bonding and, 954, 955
    facilitating after cesarean, 607
    neonatal eye treatment and,
        503, 710, 711d, 965
Eye prophylaxis
    Credé introduced, 4
    delaying, 503, 954, 965
        after cesarean, 607
    erythromycin for, 499n, 505, 710,
        711d
    silver nitrate for, 710, 712f
        edematous eyelids from, 680
Eye movements by neonate, 655,
    656f, 657
Eyelids, of neonate
    assessing, 693g
    edematous, from silver nitrate,
        680
Eyes
    of fetus
        development of, 173, 175t,
            177t, 178–79, 179t, 180,
            181
        teratogenic damage to, 183t
    of mother
        assessing in initial prenatal
            exam, 218–19g
        assessing, with severe pre-
            eclampsia, 343
        hyperthyroidism sign in, 326
        jaundiced sclerae in, from sickle
            cell anemia, 327
    of neonate
        assessing, 680f, 680–81, 693–
            94g
        bathing, 727
        color of, 680, 693g
        homocystinuria affects, 859

IgA protects, 654
    ophthalmia neonatorum in, 844
    Pierre Robin syndrome affects,
        850
    preterm, sight loss in, 758
    prophylaxis for. See Eye
        prophylaxis
    respiratory therapy damage to,
        815. See also Retrolental fi-
        broplasia
    "sunset" from hydrocephalus,
        880, 880f
    visual response of, 655, 656f
Fabry's disease, prenatal diagnosis
    of, 147
Face
    neonatal response to, 655, 656f,
        725
    of neonate
        assessing, 678, 680, 680f, 692–
            93g
        cleft lip effect on, 851, 851f,
            852, 853
        fetal alcohol syndrome signs on,
            770
        nevus flammeus on, 677–78
        telangectati nevi on, 677
        washing, 727
Face presentation, 400, 400f, 552,
    553–54, 553–54f
    bruising from, 690g
    for forceps delivery, 598
    management of, 553–54
    palpating, 438p
    position notation for, 403
    as vacuum extractor contraindica-
        tion, 598
Facial clefts, 183t
Facial edema
    as danger sign of pregnancy,
        240g
    of newborn, from malpresentation,
        553
Facial grimaces, as neonatal distress
    sign, 714
Facial nerve, in neonate
    assessing, 695g
    birth trauma to, 680
Facial nevus flammeus, 867
Facial palsy, assessing neonate for,
    678, 680
Facial paralysis
    assessing neonate for, 680, 680f,
        693g
    as LGA neonatal risk, 761
    transient, after forceps delivery,
        677
Facilitated transport, 170
FAD (Fetal activity diary), 373
Fad dieting, amenorrhea from, 100
Failure to thrive
    with congenital syphilis, 844
    with PKU, 858
Faintness
    postpartal, 916
    as pregnancy discomfort, 255t,
        259
Fallopian (uterine) tubes, 74f, 82f,
    82–83
    anatomy of, 78, 82–83
    development of, 57, 653, 653f
    fertilization in, 160, 161, 163f
    function of, 83
    infertility and, 111t
    inflammation recovery process in,
        83
    palpation of, 74
    psychologic effects on, 83
    testing patency of, 117–18
    transport time in, 83
False labor, 415, 416, 416t

False (major or greater) pelvis, 68, 68f
Familism, 32
  in Mexican American families, 44
  in Oriental families, 46
Family
  assessment of, 47–49, 50, 51f
  birth as expansion of, 709
  as client, 47
  conceptual framework of, 34f, 34–35
  contemporary, described, 31–35, 34f
  crises in
    defective birth as, 848–50
    examples, 993
    factors affecting, 992–95
    interventions for, 994–98, 1002–18
    postpartal, 993
    risk of, 998–99, 1000–1001t
  cultural influences on, 43–46. See also specific cultures
  defined, 32
  developmental approach to, 36–41
  environmental factors affect, 46
  evaluating care of, 50
  factors affecting, 34f, 34–35, 41–46
  father-infant role in, 962–63
  functions of, 35, 41–46
  health care role of, 31
  handicapped child in, 894–95
  of high-risk neonate, 737, 773, 778–79, 779f
  high-risk pregnancy effects on, 343, 344
  information about, in nursery records, 710
  mothering preparation in, 951–52
  neonatal hyperbilirubinemia effects on, 830
  in nursing process, 47–51
    example, 50–52, 51f
  nursing support for, 286–88
  postpartal focus on, 901
  postpartal role of, culture and, 914
  postpartal wellness care for, 939–40
  of pregnant adolescent, 301–2, 305
  of preterm neonate, 750, 778–79, 779f
  psychosocial development in, 40t, 40–41
  RDS therapy role of, 808n
  religion influences, 41
  responses to pregnancy of, 38–40, 246–52, 247–52, 248t, 251f
    with adolescent pregnancy, 301–2, 305
  roles in, 35–36, 992
  societal factors affecting, 42–43
  socioeconomic factors affecting, 41–42
  structures, 32–35, 33f
    factors affecting, 41–46
  systems approach to, 41
  theoretical approaches to, 36–41
  value of children in, 42–43
  wellness of as nursing goal, 969
  women's status affects, 42
Family development, 36–41
Family history, in adolescent pregnancy assessment, 302
Family nurse practitioner. See Nurse practitioners
Family pedigree, 48
  for genetic counseling, 150, 152, 153f

Family planning. See also Contraception
  defined, 110
  family development and, 40
  nursing role in, 105, 110
  postpartal, 940
  reasons for, 110
Family planning clinics, nurse practitioners in, 15
Family planning nurse, genetic counseling referral by, 151
Family size, adolescent pregnancy and, 299, 300
Family-centered health care
  development of, 12–13
  increase in, 31
  for maternity clients, goal of, 46
FAS. See Fetal alcohol syndrome
Fascia penis, 60, 60f
Fasting blood sugar rates, in pregnancy, 201
Fasting blood sugar (FPG) test, 317
Fasting plasma glucose (FPG) test, 317
Fat
  FAS affects, 770
  on SGA neonate, 762, 764
Fat cells, brown vs. white, 647
Fat metabolism in neonate, 648
Fat-soluble vitamins, 274–75
Father. See also Males; Parents; Partner
  adolescent, 300, 301, 1017
  attachment behaviors of, 961–63, 962f
  bonding with neonate by, 499n, 502, 503, 503f
    birth participation and, 954
    facilitating, 964, 965
    high-risk neonate, 773, 774
    with out-of-hospital emergency birth, 507
    with precipitous delivery, 505
  cesarean birth participation by, 602–3, 607, 608, 942
  childbirth role of, 471
  complicated childbirth effects on, 580, 581
  family-centered care role of, 12, 13
  grief process in, after neonatal death, 1002
  high-risk pregnancy problems of, 342
  labor and delivery participation by, 294, 295, 412, 613
    active phase role of, 417
    attachment and, 954
    Bradley and, 295
    culture and, 471
    delivery room preparation, 479n
    Dick-Read and, 12, 294
    evaluating support by, 435
    Leboyer method, 618
    pain reduced by, 413
  nurse's role with, 287
  nursery role of, 711
  postpartal exam role of, 944
  postpartal rest needed by, 502
  prenatal care participation by, 213, 242g
  psychologic assessment of, 242–43g
  relationship with parents of, 251–52
  responses to pregnancy of, 246–47, 248t, 249–50
  rooming-in and, 939–40, 965
  stillbirth nursing care plan for, 1004
  stress felt by, 992

Fatigue, in mother
  backache from, 255t, 258
  as hyperthyroidism sign, 326
  pain perception and, 413
  postpartal
    breast-feeding and, working mother, 938
    as fourth trimester problem, 943–44
    nursing care and, 916, 918n
    psychologic status and, 913–14
  as pregnancy symptom, 192
Fatigue, in neonate
  during feeding
    implications of, 716
    in preterm infant, 753–54n
    SGA neonates, 765n
  as prematurity risk, 741
  from pulmonary stenosis, 890
  with transposition of great vessels, 891
Fats
  absorption of, deficiencies and, 275
  in breast milk, cow's milk, and formula, 719t
  digestion of, in neonates, 651–52
  in formulas, 718, 719t
    preterm, 741, 742t
  neonatal requirements, 717, 717t
  pregnancy changes in metabolism of, 201
  pregnancy requirements, 272t, 273
Fatty acids, placenta synthesizes, 170
FBS (Fasting plasma glucose test), 317
Fear. See also Anxiety
  about emergency cesarean, 607–8
  in labor, 470t, 471
    during active phase, 417–18
    about anesthesia, 521n
    precipitous, 503
    risk factors for, 425t
  with out-of-hospital emergency delivery, 505, 507
  with postpartal psychosis, 988
  as pulmonary embolism sign, 981, 983, 984n
Fecal elimination
  in neonates, teaching parents about, 726
  postpartal assessment of, 913
Fecal incontinence
  maternal, in fourth trimester, 947g
  in neonate
    from imperforate anus, 872
    with meningomyelocele, 880, 882
Fecal mass, from aganglionosis, 869. See also Intestinal obstruction
Federal government, maternal-child health care role of, 5
Feeding, 716–22, 717t, 719–21t. See also Bottle-feeding; Breast-feeding; Feeding problems
  with aganglionosis, 870
  amount needed by neonate, 716
  assessing quality of, 929–30
  breast vs. bottle, 717–18, 924
  with bronchopulmonary dysplasia, 808n
  with cleft lip, 853n, 854–55n
  with cleft palate, 851, 856n
  with congestive heart failure, 894
  cultural considerations in, 924–25
  demand vs. schedule, 924, 929–30
  after diaphragmatic hernia surgery, 867

  fatigue of neonate during, 716, 753–54n
  folic acid requirements, 277
  gastrointestinal functioning, 651
  growth spurts affect, 718–19
  hypoglycemia prevention with, 818, 821
  IDMs, 768
  initial, 716–17, 928–29
  initiating in reactivity period, 712
  jaundice prevention with, 831n
  MAS neonates, 815
  missed, as illness sign, 729
  during narcotic withdrawal, 771
  necrotizing enterocolitis encouraged by, 837
  nursing role in, 714
  nutritional assessment, 719–21, 720–21t
  nutritional needs of newborns, 717, 717t
  pattern of, 718–19
  physiologic jaundice and, 649
  with Pierre Robin syndrome, 851
  postpartal learning about, 920n, 921–24
  postterm infants, 760
  preparation for, 924
  preterm infants, 740–46, 741f, 742t, 743–45p, 747t
    intolerance signs, 753
    fatigue during, 753–54n
    methods, 741–46, 743–45p, 753–54n
    nursing care plan, 753–54
    nutritional requirements, 746
    residual formula, 753–54
    schedule for, 12, 746, 747t
  with RDS, 806–8n
  regurgitation patterns, 927
  rooming-in facilitates, 939
  SGA neonates, 765n
  "sham" 861
  sterile water, after birth, 716
  supplemental foods, 720
  with tracheoesophageal atresia/fistula, 861, 861f, 863–64n
  weaning, 721–22
Feeding problems
  with choanal atresia, 852, 857
  from cleft lip or palate, 852, 853
  congenital, 850–57
  from congential herpes, 359
  with congenital hypothyroidism, 859
  from fetal alcohol syndrome, 362, 770
  with hypoglycemia, 818
  with diaphragmatic hernia, 866
  with maple syrup urine disease, 858
  maternal methadone maintenance and, 360
  as necrotizing enterocolitis sign, 838, 839
  from Pierre Robin syndrome, 853–54
  preterm, sample nursing diagnosis for, 757
  risk factors for, 736f
  as sepsis neonatorum sign, 841
  with tetralogy of Fallot, 890
  from transient nerve paralysis, 681
  with transposition of great vessels, 891
  with ventricular septal defects, 888
  weight loss and, 689g
Feet, edema of, as pregnancy danger sign, 240g

Feet, of neonate
  assessing, 685, 703g
  deformed, with meningomyelocele, 880
  lesions on, with congenital syphilis, 844
  talipes equinovarus (clubfoot), 875f, 875–76
Female frogtest, 195
Female neonates
  atrial septal defects in, 885
  bathing, 727
  cleft palate in, 851
  genitals of, assessing, 684, 701–2g
  hip dyslpasia in, 876
  IUGR in, 761
  patent ductus arteriosus in, 881
  pseudomenstruation in, 652
  size of, 760
Female reproductive cycle (FRC), 96–99, 97–99f. See also Menstrual cycle
  abnormal length of, 100
  cervical mucosal changes in, 98, 99
  endometrial changes in, 98–99, 99f
  pain with, 100
  premenstrual tension syndrome (PMT), 99–100
  variations in, 100
Female reproductive system, 65–85
  assessing
    in fourth trimester, 947g
    in initial prenatal exam, 225–28g, 235
  bony pelvis, 65–71, 66f, 68–70f
  embryologic development of, 57–59, 58f, 81, 83
  estrogens' role in, 93
  external genitals, 71–73, 71f
  hormonal development in, 92f, 93–94
  infertility causes in, 111t
  internal genitals, 73–84, 74f, 77–82f
  malignancy in, estrogen therapy and, 102
  maturation of gametes in, 160, 161f
  observation techniques for, 73
  ovarian hormones's role in, 93–94
  pelvis types in, 396–97, 397f
  postpartal adaptations in, 901–7
  pregnancy changes in, 195–97
  progesterone's role in, 94
  prostaglandins' role in, 94
  puberty changes in, 91f, 91–92, 92f, 93–94
  sexual response in, 103t, 103–5
  spontaneous abortion causes in, 329
Female sterilization, 121f, 127–28, 128f
Females
  climacteric in, 101–2
  sex chromosome abnormalities in, 140–41, 140–41f
  sexual identity development in, 88, 89
  sexual response in, 103–5, 103t, 105f
Femoral pulse, assessing in neonate, 683, 685, 700g
Femur length (FL) of fetus, ultrasound to measure 368, 370
Fencer position. See Tonic neck reflex
Ferguson reflex, 407
Ferning of cervical mucus, 114, 116, 116f
  in contraceptive method, 121, 122

Ferrous fumarate, as supplement, 274
Ferrous gluconate, as supplement, 274
Ferrous sulfate, as supplement, 274
Fertility
  cervical mucus and, 114, 116f, 116–17, 121, 122
  components of, 110–11
  male role in, 69, 64
  ovum transport and, 98
Fertility awareness methods of contraception, 120–22
Fertility rates, 21, 21t
Fertilization
  cellular division after, 157–59, 158f, 159f
  human chorionic gonadotropin (hCG) after, 98
  ovarian role in, 84
  process of, 160–62, 161f, 162f, 163f
  second meiotic division after, 96
  site of, 82–83
  in surrogate childbearing, 11
  in vitro, 9, 11
Fetal abnormalities. See Fetal anomalies
Fetal acidosis
  adverse long-term outcomes and, 459
  FHR baseline variability caused by, 452
Fetal activity
  in prolonged pregnancy, 759t
  tachycardia caused by, 451
Fetal activity diary (FAD), 373
Fetal age, ultrasound to determine, 368–70
Fetal alcohol syndrome (FAS), 214t, 268, 361t, 362, 770
  incidence of, 770
Fetal anemia. See Anemia, fetal
Fetal anomalies
  as ritodrine contraindication, 548
  transverse lie and, 556
  ultrasound to determine, 368, 369f, 370
Fetal apnea, patterns of, 371
Fetal arrhythmias. See Fetal heart rate
Fetal asphyxia. See Asphyxia, fetal
Fetal assessment. See Assessment of fetus
Fetal attitude, 399
Fetal axis pressure, 408
Fetal bleeding, from folic acid deficiency, 276
Fetal blood pressure, labor role of, 414
Fetal blood sampling, 8, 461–63, 462f
  asphyxia sign in, 538
  for fetal distress, 539n
  infection risk with, 913
  during labor, indications for, 451t, 461, 463
  with maternal hemorrhage, 572n
  procedure for, 461–62
  resuscitation risk assessment with, 787
  tests done with, 539n
Fetal bradycardia. See Bradycardia, fetal; Fetal heart rate
Fetal breathing movements (FBM), 636
  ultrasound detection of, 371
Fetal cells, cytologic examination of, 387
Fetal circulation, 171, 172f, 642f
  glucose in, 648
  hematology and, 644

persistent. See Persistent pulmonary hypertension
  prematurity and, 739t, 739–40
  transition of at birth, 640–41, 641f
Fetal congenital adrenal hypoplasia, 380
Fetal cortisol theory, 407
Fetal death. See also Fetal mortality
  from abruptio placentae, 563
  apnea preceding, 371
  as cesarean delivery contraindication, 605
  from circumvallate placenta, 574
  effects on family of, 580–81
  fibrinogen depletion follows, 573n
  grief process after, 561
  hemolytic disease and, 826
  history of, as resuscitation risk, 786
  induction of labor for, 587
  from listerial infection, 357
  podophyllin associated with, 355
  retention after, DIC from, 567–68, 568f
  risk factors for, 214–15t
  as ritodrine contraindication, 549
  signs of, 240g
    in initial prenatal exam, 223–24g
    in subsequent prenatal exams, 239g
  from transverse lie, 556
  with umbilical cord prolapse, 574
Fetal depression
  as anesthesia danger, 529, 530
  labor analgesia and, 510–11, 512
  signs of. See Fetal heart rate
Fetal descent, 414, 414f
  accelerated, as precipitous labor sign, 543
  during active phase labor, 417
  arrest of, from malposition, 551
  assessing, 430g, 434, 436–40p, 438–39f, 440–41, 441f
  failure of, assessing, 430g
  labor time elapsed and, 544, 544t
  lightening with, 415
  maximum slope rate of, disorders, 544, 544t
  protracted, problems from, 578
  rate of, 417
  during second stage, 418
Fetal development, 171, 172f
  behavior responses and, 654
  brown adipose tissue (BAT), 647
  cardiovascular, 171, 172f, 639–40
    prematurity and, 739t, 739–40
  embryonic stage, 173, 174–77t, 178–79
  factors influencing, 183t, 183–85
  FHR and, 374
  gastrointestinal system, 650–51
  genitals, 653, 653f
  hematopoiesis in, 643–44
  immune system, 653–54
  kidneys, 652
  lungs, 737–39, 738f
  placenta and, 165–71, 167f, 169f
  preembryonic stage, 162–65, 173
  respiratory system, 635, 638–39, 639f
  vulnerability timetable for, 183t
Fetal distress
  amniotic fluid signs of during labor, 430g
  assessing for, See Fetal heart rate; Fetal well-being
  from battledore placenta, 574
  cesarean delivery for, 529, 600
  during delivery, with MAS, 798
  estriol levels as sign of, 380

as forceps delivery indication, 597
from hypotonic labor patterns, 537, 541
induction of labor and, 587, 590, 591, 594n
late decelerations indicate, 451t, 454–55, 455f
from maternal cardiac decompensation, 311
as maternal drug addiction risk, 770
necrotizing enterocolitis from, 837, 839n
neonatal polycythemia as response to, 835
neonatal skin color from, 689g
nursing care plan, 538–40
nursing diagnoses for, 540
paracervical block contraindicated by, 516
as postmaturity risk, 760
as prolonged labor risk, 542
after regional anesthesia, 523n
resucitation risk with, 787
risk factors for, 736f
sinusoidal FHR patterns indicate, 457
with umbilical cord prolapse, 574
as vacuum extraction indication, 598
Fetal electrocardiography, 444–45
  as pregnancy proof, 195
Fetal exsanguination, intrapartal risk factors for, 425t
Fetal growth, evaluating, 8, APPENDIX E
  in adolescent pregnancy, 305
  impaired. See Intrauterine growth retardation
  ultrasound for, 368f, 369–70, 370–71
Fetal head
  biparietal diameter of. See Biparietal diameter of fetal head
  identifying position of, 398
  in labor, 398f. 398–99, 399f
  measuring, 398–99, 399f
  molding of, 398
  pressure on, plagiocephaly from, 678
  trauma to
    episiotomy to prevent, 595
    as induction risk, 594n
    as vaginal breech delivery risk, 554
Fetal heart, 171, 172f
  aberrations in, as intrapartal risk factor, 425t
  auscultation of
    in adolescent pregnancy, 305, 305f
    as positive pregnancy sign, 195
    determining delivery date by, 237, 237f
    in labor, 424, 443f, 443–44
    by siblings, 251, 251f
  development of, 173, 174t, 176t
  teratogenic damage to, 183t
Fetal heart rate (FHR)
  absent, as abruptio placentae sign, 563
  accelerations in, 454, 457
  acidosis signs in, 543
  assessing. See also Contraction stress test; Nonstress test
    after amniocentesis, 382, 383p
    by auscultation, 424, 441, 443f, 443–44, 445t

Fetal heart rate, assessing *(Cont'd)*
  before cesarean delivery, 601, 608
  before induction, 589, 590, 591n, 592n
  in initial prenatal exam, 223g
  at labor admission, 467, 468, 469, 472, 473
  during labor, 424, 443–50, 443–44f, 445t, 446–50f, 473–74, 479, 480n
  with rupture of membranes, 574
  in subsequent prenatal exams, 239g
  auscultation of, with amniotomy, 587
  asphyxia signs in, 538
  baseline variability of, 171, 450, 452–58, 452–53f, 455–58f
    interventions for, 451t
  changes in, as hemorrhage sign, 569
  decelerations in, 375, 451t, 454–58, 455–58f; *see also* late decelerations in; variable decelerations in
    as distress indicator, 9
    factors affecting, 171
  faint, as abruptio placentae sign, 563
  fetal scalp pH and, 462, 463
  funic souffle and, 168
  interpreting, 460t, 460–61
  labor changes in, 414, 424, 450–58, 452–53f, 455–58f
    managing, 451t, 460–61
  late decelerations in, 451t, 454–55, 455f, 456f, 458, 786
    in CST, 376, 377t, 378f, 379
    with induction, interventions for, 590
    as nonreassuring, 458
  location of
    with breech presentation, 554
    with face presentation, 553
    with malposition, 551
    with transverse lie, 555
  lumbar epidural anesthesia and, 519
  maternal environmental experiences and, 654
  mixed patterns in, 456–57
  monitoring. *See also* Electronic fetal monitoring
    with brow presentation, 552
    in deceleration phase, 477n
    for diabetic client, 321, 325
    with DIC risk, 568
    with eclampsia, 339, 344
    during external version, 585, 586
    with forceps delivery, 598
    with hypotonic labor patterns, 541
    with induction of labor, 589, 590, 592n, 593n, 594n
    during labor, 431g, 443–60, 443–44f, 445t, 446–50f, 475n
    with maternal hemorrhage, 572
    methods, 443–50, 443–44f, 445t, 446–50f
    with PIH, 339
    with placenta previa, 566
    in prolonged labor, 542
    with preterm labor, 549
    psychologic reactions to, 459–60
    with regional anesthesia, 522, 523n
    with severe preeclampsia, 343, 344

  with vaginal bleeding, 575
  during vaginal breech delivery, 555
  value of, 458–59
  "overshoot" in, 456, 458
  paracervical block affects, 517, 523n
  patterns of, 450f, 450–58, 451t, 452–53f, 455–58f
  peridural block affects, 518
  placenta previa and, 565, 566
  precipitous labor effects on, 543
  preterminal patterns, 458
  reassuring and nonreassuring patterns, 57–58
  resuscitation risk and, 786
  sinusoidal patterns in, 457, 458, 458f
  umbilical cord length and, 575
  umbilical cord prolapse signs in, 574
  after uterine rupture, 550
  variability lack in
    implications of, 454
    as nonreassuring, 458
    preterminal, 458
    reassuring vs. nonreassuring, 457–58
    resuscitation risk with, 786
  variable decelerations in, 451t, 455f, 455–57, 457f, 458
    with induction, interventions for, 590
    preterminal, 458
    resuscitation risk, 786
Fetal hemolytic disease. *See* Hemolytic disease
Fetal hemorrhage. *See* Hemorrhage
Fetal hyperactivity
  as abruptio placentae sign, 563
  as distress sign, 538
Fetal hypertension, from umbilical cord compression, 455–56, 457f
Fetal hypoxemia, tachycardia caused by, 450
Fetal hypoxia. *See* Hypoxia
Fetal kidney maturity, creatinine levels show, 386–87
Fetal lie, 399
  determining, 441–42, 442f
  transverse, in shoulder presentation, 400, 402
Fetal lung maturity. *See also* Fetal maturity
  assessing
    methods for, 385, 385f, 386, 638–39, 639f
    after PROM, 546
    betamethasone (Celestone) to accelerate, 546f, 547, 547d
  delayed, reasons for, 385
  delaying induction to aid, 547
  determining, 384–86
  diabetes and, 320–21, 768
  perinatal mortality and, 384
  placental grading and, 372
  preterm labor accelerates, 548
  RDS risk and, 384
  as reason for early delivery, 388
  resuscitation risk and, 786
  stress accelerates, 385
  surfactant synthesis and, 635
Fetal macrosomia, from maternal diabetes, 316
Fetal malformations. *See also* Congenital anomalies
  from folic acid deficiency, 276
  labor problems from, 557
Fetal malnutrition, risk factors for, 214t

Fetal manipulation, uterine rupture from, 550
Fetal maturity
  abruptio placentae outcome and, 563
  amniotic fluid density and, 384
  assessing
    amniocentesis for, 384–87
    before cesarean delivery, 601
    creatinine level for, 386–87
    before induction of labor, 587, 588, 591n
    ultrasound for, APPENDIX C
    x-ray examination for, 387
  FHR and, 374
  lungs. *See* Fetal lung maturity
  prematurity risk and. *See* Prematurity; Preterm infants
  tests of, 366, 388. *See also specific tests*
Fetal membrane phospholipid-arachidonic acid-prostaglandin theory, 407
Fetal measurement, ultrasound for, 368, 369–70
Fetal metabolic acidosis, late decelerations of FHR and, 375
Fetal monitoring. *See also* Fetal heart rate, monitoring
  after accidents, 353
  instantaneous vs. average, 444, 444f
  methods of, 443f, 443–50, 445t, 446f, 449f
  with surgical procedures in pregnancy, 351
Fetal mortality. *See also* Fetal death; Perinatal mortality
  from automobile accidents, 352
  betamethasone and, 547
  brow presentation and, 552
  from chronic uteroplacental insufficiency, 455
  from cytomegalic inclusion disease, 358
  estriol excretion patterns and, 380
  from hemolytic disease, 826
  from hydrops fetalis, 826
  from hyperemesis gravidarum, 328
  malpositions and, 552
  from maternal diabetes mellitus, 314, 315, 316
  from maternal drug abuse, 360
  maternal hypothyroidism and, 326
  from PIH, 339
  from Rh hemolytic disease, 347
  risk factors for, 214–15t
  from rubella, 358
  from sickle cell anemia, 328
  from syphilis, 354
  thyroid dysfunction and, 321
  from uterine rupture, 550
  from vasa previa, 576
Fetal movement
  absent, as danger sign, 240g
  assessing
    in adolescent pregnancy, 305
    in initial prenatal exam, 224g
    with maternal PIH, 341
  children's response to, 251
  excessive, as abruptio placentae sign, 563
  father's response to, 248t, 249, 250
  FHR accelerations caused by, 454
  maternal assessment of, 372–73
  perception of, emotions and, 203
  as positive pregnancy sign, 195
  reassurance about, 373
  after uterine rupture, 550

Fetal movement records (FMR), 373
Fetal narcosis, pregnancy diabetes and, 324
Fetal organ enlargement, labor problems from, 557
Fetal outline, palpation of, as pregnancy sign, 193
Fetal position, 399, 401f, 403–4
  ambulation and, 474
  assessing
    by inspection, 441
    at labor admission, 469, 472
    during labor, 431g, 441–42, 442f
    by palpation, 441–42, 442f
    by ultrasound, 442
    by vaginal examination, 437–38p, 437–38f, 442
    x-ray pelvimetry for, 433
  forceps used to rotate, 596
  labor changes in, 414f, 414–15
  malpositions, 551–52
    obstructed labor from, 545
    as oxytocin contraindication, 590
    prolonged labor caused by, 542
    as vacuum extraction indication, 598
  peridural anesthesia and, 518
Fetal presentation, 399–404, 400–403f
  abnormal, as intrapartal risk factor, 425t
  ambulation and, 474
  assessing
    at labor admission, 469, 472
    during labor, 431g, 441–42, 442f
    in prolonged labor, 542
    by ultrasound, 442
    by vaginal exam, 437–38p, 437–38f, 442
  breech, 400, 401d, 404, 552, 554–55, 555f
    engagement in, 402
    precipitous delivery, 505
  brow, 552f, 552–53
  cephalic, 400, 400–403f
  compound, 552, 556
  cord prolapse and, 539
  face, 552, 553–54, 553–54f
  fetal attitude and, 399
  fetal/neonatal implications of, 425t
  forceps delivery and, 598
  functional role of, 402–3
  hydrocephaly and, 557
  induction of labor and, 587
  malpresentations, 552–56, 552–56f. *See also specific presentations*
    as birth center contraindication, 618
    with hydramnios, 577
    intrapartal risk and, 425t
    oxytocin contraindication and, 590
    prolonged labor from, 542
  palpating, in vaginal exam, 437–39f, 438–40p
  preterm labor, delivery type and, 550
  PROM and, 546
  resuscitation risk and, 786, 787
  shoulder; *see* transverse lie
  sinciput, 552
  transverse lie (shoulder), 400, 402, 404, 552, 555–56, 556f
  for vacuum extraction, 598
  version of, 585–86, 586f
  vertex, abnormal, 552–54, 552–54f

precipitous delivery, 504
Fetal respiration
  breathing movements, 371, 636
  as placental function, 168
Fetal rotation, spontaneous, 552
Fetal scalp blood sampling. See Fetal
  blood sampling
Fetal scalp pH
  guidelines for using, 451t, 461–63,
    462f
  late decelerations of FHR and,
    375
Fetal sex, determining
  amniocentesis for, ethics of, 11
  in ancient Egypt, 3
Fetal size
  assessing before delivery, 557
    before cesarean delivery,
      601
    before induction, 591n
  birth center screening for, 618
  macrosomia, implications of, 556–
    57
  precipitous labor and, 542
  pregnancy diabetes and, 324
  prolapsed umbilical cord risk and,
    574
Fetal sleep
  FHR baseline variability caused
    by, 452
  nonstress test results with, 373
Fetal station, assessing, 402–3, 403f,
  588, 588t
Fetal status. See Fetal well-being; Labor, fetal response to
Fetal surgery, 8–9
Fetal tachyarrhythmias, tachycardia
  caused by, 450
Fetal tachycardia. See Tachycardia
Fetal trauma, as oxytocin induction
  risk, 590, 594n
Fetal thyroid problems, maternal
  hyperthyroidism and, 326
Fetal wastage, risk factors for, 214–
  15t
Fetal weight, assessing, 8
Fetal weight gain
  maternal cardiac decompensation
    and, 311
  maternal PIH and, 341
Fetal well-being
  alcoholic mother and, 362
  assessing. See also Assessment of
    fetus; Fetal heart rate, moni-
    toring
    with abruptio placentae, 572n
    by blood sampling, 461–63,
      462f
    by fetal breathing movements,
      (FBM), 636
    with hemorrhage 569n, 572n
    by mother, 372–73
    with oxytocin induction, 590,
      592n
  delivery timing and, 371
  drug use and abuse affects, 360–
    61, 361t
  maternal infections and, 353
  PIH jeopardizes, 339, 341
  in postterm pregnancies, 759,
    759t
  pregnancy diabetes and, 320,
    324
  tests of, 366. See also specific tests
Fetal-neonatal transition circulation,
  640–41, 641f
Feto-fetal transfusion, multiple
  gestation and risk of, 425t
Fetogram, in hydramnios assessment,
  577
Fetoscopy, 223g, 388
  electronic monitoring vs., 459

evaluating FHR with, 443f, 443–
  44, 445t
  risks of, 388
Fetotoxic hazards, employment during pregnancy and, 261. See
  also Teratogenic substances
Fetus
  death of. See Fetal death
  gestational age of, 173
  iron stored in liver of, 201
  labor response of, 413–15. See
    also intrapartal fetal
    assessment
  labor role of, 407, 408
  placental functions for, 168–71
  teratogenic substances affecting.
    See Teratogenic substances
  Fever
    in mother
      from appendicitis in pregnancy,
        351
      with deep leg vein disease, 981
      fetal tachycardia caused by,
        450
      from gallbladder disease in
        pregnancy, 351
      with mastitis, 987
      as Mendelson syndrome sign,
        531
      with postpartal infection, 919n,
        941, 974–77
      as pulmonary embolism sign,
        984n
      as pyelonephritis sign, 353, 986
    in neonate
      with bronchopulmonary dyspla-
        sia, 816
      from congenital herpes, 359
      with herpesvirus type 2, 844
      with kernicterus, 824
FHR. See Fetal heart rate
FHTs. See Fetal heart rate
Fibrinogin, semen viscosity and, 63
Fibrinogen levels
  decrease in
    determining cause of, 572n
    from DIC, 567, 568f
    from hemorrhage, 573n
  evaluating, with hemorrhage, 569n
  monitoring, with abruptio placen-
    tae, 564
  normal values, 572
  pregnancy changes in, 197t, 198
  postpartal, 906
Fibrinogen replacement, for amniotic
  fluid embolism DIC, 576
Fibrinolysin, 64
Fibrinolytic therapy, for pulmonary
  embolism, 982
Fibroid tumors
  fundal height and, 237
  as induction of labor contraindica-
    tion, 587
  menopause increases tendency
    toward, 101
  spontaneous abortion caused by,
    329
Fibromas, signs of in initial prenatal
  exam, 228g
Filipino Americans, infant feeding
  customs, 925
Fimbria (infundibulum) of fallopian
  tube, 82, 82f, 83
Financial problems, pregnancy complications and, 342, 581
  as pregnancy risk, 215t
  severe preeclampsia, 344
Finger sucking, by fetus and neonate,
  655
Fingers
  tremor of, as hyperthyroidism sign,
    326

of neonate
  assessing, 684, 702g
  clubbed, 890, 891
Finland, nurse-midwifery in, 6
Firshein, S. I., 148
Fissures, oral, with congenital
  syphilis, 844
Fistula
  defined, 859
  from maternal soft tissue damage,
    578
  postpartal, from malpositions, 552
  signs of in initial prenatal exam,
    225g
  tracheoesophageal, 859–61, 860f,
    861f, 862–65n
FL. See Femur length
Flaccidity, in LGA infant, from birth
  trauma, 756
Flagyl. See Metronidazol
Flank pain, as pyelonephritis sign,
  986
Flaring nostrils
  with diaphragmatic hernia, 866
  as respiratory distress sign, 751
  with transient tachypnea of new-
    born, 797
Flat foot (pes planus), as normal,
  703g
Flatus, passage of with tracheoesophageal fistula, 860
Flexion, of fetus during labor, 414,
  414f
  breech presentation, 505
  palpation of, 439f
Floating of presenting part, 402,
  402f
"Floppy baby" syndrome
  in LGA infant, from birth trauma,
    756n
  sign of, 702g
Flow charts, CST management
  protocol, 378f
Flu
  listeriosis mistaken for, 356
  in neonates, preparation for, 729
Fluid and electrolyte balance. See
  also Electrolyte imbalances
  hyperemesis gravidarum and, 328
  in labor, 409, 536
  of neonate
    aganglionic megacolon affects,
      869
    managing, for preterm infant,
      746–48, 756n
    normal values, 645t
Fluid intake. See Fluids
Fluid intake and output, maternal
  decreased, as danger sign, 240g
  monitoring
    with abruptio plaerium, 918n
    with ritodrine administration,
      549
    with uterine inversion, 580
  puerperal infection requirements,
    978n, 979n
Fluid intake and output, of neonate
  assessing 652, 689g
  concentration of urine and, 652
  intestinal obstruction and, 874
  monitoring, in preterm infants,
    747–48
  during TPN, 746
  with RDS, 806–7n
  with tracheoesophageal atresia/
    fistula, 863n
  prematurity and, 746
Fluid overload, as MAS complication,
  815
Fluid requirements, for preterm
  infants, 740, 746, 747
  sample nursing diagnosis, 758

Fluids
  hemorrhoids relieved by, 915
  intravenous. See Intravenous fluids
  neonatal requirements, 717, 717t
  postpartal
    assessment of, 913
    importance of, 918n
  with PIH, 342, 343
Fluorescent quenching test, 824
Flulike illness in pregnancy, vaginal
  culture for, 357
Fluothane (Halothane), 529
FMR (fetal movement records), 373
Foam stability index (FSI), 386
Fogel, C. I., 101
Foley catheter, monitoring urine output with, 570n
Folic acid, 276
  cooking methods and, 327
  deficiency effects, 276
  food sources of, 277, 277t
  lactation requirements, 270t
  megaloblastic anemia and, 327
  physiologic anemia of infancy and,
    644
  pregnancy requirements, 270t,
    276–77
  role of, 276
  sickle cell anemia requires, 328
Follicle-stimulating hormone (FSH)
  anterior pituitary secretes, 96, 97f
  female reproductive cycle role of,
    96, 97f
  male puberty role of, 92f, 93
  at menopause, 101
  postmenopausal levels of, 102
  pregnancy role of, 202
  puberty role of, 92, 92f
Follicle stimulating hormone-releasing
  hormone (FSHRH), 96
Follicular cysts, pain caused by, 84
Follow-up
  in genetic counseling, 154
  postpartal, 944, 948–49
Fontanelles, 398, 398f
  assessing, 678, 692g
  bulging
    with herpesvirus type 2 infec-
      tion, 844
    with intraventricular hemor-
      rhage, 836
  closure of, 678, 692g
  with congenital hypothyroidism,
    859
  hydrocephalus and, 882n
  on SGA neonate, 764
  sunken, as dehydration sign, 747
Football hold, 714, 715f
  for breast-feeding, 931, 937f
  for washing hair, 727
Footling breech presentation, 400,
  555f
  prolonged labor from, 554
Foramen ovale, 171, 172f
  atrial septal defects and, 885,
    886f
  closure of at birth, 640, 641f
  fetal circulatory role of, 642f, 739
  formation of, 640
  in PPH syndrome, 817
  transposition of great vessels and,
    891
Forceps, 4, 5, 596, 597, 597f
Forceps bruise, 598
Forceps delivery, 596–98, 597f,
  599f
  for breech presentation, 555
  cesarean delivery preferred to,
    600
  CNS damage to neonate by, 578
  complications of, 597–98
  constriction ring may allow, 545

Forceps delivery (Cont'd)
facial paralysis from, 680
fetal skull damage from, 578
high, 596
indications for, 597
lithotomy position increases need for, 615
low
for cardiac client, 313
psychic causes of, 535–36
for malpositions, 551, 552
maternal soft tissue damage from, 578
midforceps
for brow presentation, 552
complications with, 597–98
contractures of midpelvis and, 578
described, 596
for malpositions, 552
nursing interventions with, 598
with occiput-posterior position, 551
outlet forceps, described, 596
parental control over, 613
pediatrician attendance at 552
Piper forceps, for breech presentation, 555
postpartal hemorrhage risk with, 972
prerequisites for, 598
for preterm labor, 550
as prolonged labor intervention, 542
regional anesthesia may require, 523n
skin assessment after, 677
transient facial paralysis after, 677
for transverse arrest, 551, 552
trial or failed, 598
types of, 596
from uterine relaxation after general, 530
Foreskin (prepuce), 60, 60f. See also Circumcision
Formula-feeding. See also Bottle-feeding
establishing pattern for, 718–19
hypocalcemia and, 821
stools with, 651, 726
Formulas
calories from, 720, 721t
for congestive heart failure, 894
initial, 716
for galactosemia, 859
iron-fortified, for neonatal anemia, 835
for maple syrup urine disease, 858
after necrotizing enterocolitis, 838
nutrition in, 718, 719t
for PKU infants, 858
preparation of, 927
for preterm infants, 740–41, 742t, 753n
Fossa navicularis, 60
childbirth trauma to, 73
Foster, G. M., on health beliefs, 205, 206
Fourchette, 71f, 72
FPG. (Fasting plasma glucose test), 317
Fractures, during delivery
of clavicle, 681–82, 697g
Moro reflex affected by, 703g
in LGA infants, 756–57n, 761
motor function with, 703g
of leg, assessing neonate for, 703g
Frank breech presentation, 400, 555f
vaginal delivery with, 554–55
Fraternal twins, 185, 557–58
FRC (functional residual capacity), of first breath, 63

Free thyroxine index, 326
Frejka pillow splint, for hip dysplasia, 878
Frenulum of clitoris, 71f, 72
Frequency of contractions, 404, 404f, 405. See also Uterine contractions
Frequency of urination, as cystitis sign, 986
Friction rub
defined, 231p
as pulmonary embolism sign, 984n
Friedman, E. A., labor described by, 417
dysfunctional, 544–45, 544t
Friedman, M. M., 43, 47
Friedman graph, 434, 440–41, 441f
abnormal labor patterns seen on, 545
for adolescents in labor, 482
CPD assessment with, 578
labor analgesia effects shown on, 510
in nursing care plan, 473, 475
precipitous labor risk seen on, 543
using with macrosomia, 557
Friedman's test, for pregnancy, 195
Frog tests, 195
Fromm, E., 103
Frontier Graduate School of Midwifery, 7
Frontier Nursing Service, 7
Frontier School of Midwifery and Family Nursing, 7
Frothy sputum
during labor, interventions for, 576
from amniotic fluid embolism, 576
Fructose, neonatal digestion produces, 651
FSH. See Follicle-stimulating hormone
FSHRH (follicle stimulating hormone-releasing hormone), 96
FT. See Term neonates
Full-term neonates See Term neonates
Functional residual capacity (FRC), of first breath, 637
Fundal height
calculating gestational age with, PROM, 546
fetal size estimation by, 557
postpartal assessment of, 910f, 910–11, 919n
Fundal progression, clinical surveillance of, for IUGR, 375
Fundus, 77f, 78
abruptio placentae and, 563
assessing
in adolescent pregnancy, 305
after cesarean, 604, 609
in fourth stage labor, 481n
in initial prenatal exam, 223g
at labor onset, 428g
at labor admission, 472
postpartum, 624–25, 901–2, 902f, 907–8, 910f, 910–11, 919n
in third stage labor, 579
bladder distention affects, 982
in fourth stage of labor, 420, 502f
massage of, 501
height changes in with pregnancy, 194f
gestational age and, 236–37, 237g
hydramnios and, 577
massaging
postpartal, 481, 482n
for uterine atony, 579
subinvolution signs in, 973
Funic souffle, 168

Funis, 167. See also Umbilical cord
Funnel chest, assessing neonate for, 697g
Furosemide (Lasix)
for congestive heart failure, 894
for pulmonary edema with eclampsia, 344
hearing loss risk from, 758
Fusiform cervix, 78
Fussiness, in neonate, purposes of, 657

G-6-PD deficiency, effect of on neonate, 831, 835
Gag reflex
assessing neonate for, 695g, 716
prematurity risk and, 741
in preterm infants, feeding methods and, 753
Gagging, in neonatal reactivity period, 712
Gait, with bladder exstrophy, 874, 875
Galactorrhea, postdelivery, 987
Galactose
neonatal digestion produces, 651
placental transport of, 170
Galactosemia, 859
dietary treatment for, 135
inheritance of, 144
neonatal screening for, 150, 725
prenatal diagnosis of, 147
Galeazzi sign, 878
Gallbladder
in neonate, 650, 651
pregnancy changes in, 197t, 199
problems with, during pregnancy, 199, 351–52
Gallop
assessing in neonate, 698g
as pulmonary embolism sign, 982, 983
Gametogenesis, 158–60, 160, 161f
Gamma globulins, placental transport of, 170
Gardnerella vaginalis (Hemophilus vaginalis), 356
adolescent pregnancy and, 304
signs of, in prenatal exam, 226g, 227f
Gargoylism
face signs of, 692g
Gastric acidity
in neonate, 651
pregnancy changes in, 197t, 198
Gastric aspirate culture
for group B streptococcus in neonate, 843
in sepsis neonatorum assessment, 842
Gastric emptying, in utero, 651
Gastric mucus, in neonate, 712, 713f
Gastric residuals
as feeding intolerance sign, 746
as necrotizing enterocolitis sign, 838, 839
Gastric secretions. See Gastric acidity; Gastric mucus
Gastrointestinal (GI) tract. See Gastrointestinal system
Gastrointestinal system
fat-soluble vitamin overdose affects, 274
fetal
development of, 173, 174t, 176t, 178–80, 650–51
malformed, prenatal diagnosis of, 146
teratogenic damage to, 183t

maternal
bleeding in, as betamethasone side effect, 547
cesarean delivery effects on, 941
labor changes in, 409
postpartal changes in, 905
pregnancy changes in, 197t, 198–99
neonatal, 650–52
abdominal assessment and, 683
adaptation of, 650–52
assessing, 699–700g
bleeding in, as PPH complication, 817
breast milk protects, 717
congenital defects of, 702g, 859. See also specific defects
cow's milk risk to, 718
IDM, 768
IgA protects, 654
MAS damage to, 815
necrotizing enterocolitis in. See Necrotizing enterocolitis
preterm, 740–41
problems in, TPN for, 745–46
in reactivity period, 712, 713f
Gastroschisis, 867
assessing neonate for, 700g
prenatal diagnosis of, 146
Gastrostomy feeding
for tracheoesophageal atresia/fistula, 861, 861f, 863–64n
Gate-control theory of pain, 410, 410f
distraction and, 413
Gaucher's disease
assessing SGA neonate for, 766n
prenatal diagnosis of, 148
Gavage feeding, 742, 743–45, 743–44f
after diaphragmatic hernia surgery, 867
for Pierre Robin syndrome, 851
in preterm infant care, 753–54n
procedure, 742, 743–45
with RDS, 807n
risk factors for, 736f
Gender behavior, 88, 89
Gender identity, 88–89
Gender role behavior, 88, 89
Gender roles, pregnancy values and, 205
Gene mutation, 157
General anesthesia. See also Anesthesia
acute respiratory obstruction from, 531
for cesarean delivery, 609
dangers of, 530–31
emergence from, 529, 530
vomiting danger, 531
for episiotomy, 596
inhalation anesthetics, 529
intravenous anesthetics, 529–30
for labor and delivery, 528–31
balanced, 530
dangers of, 528, 530–31
hyperactive, 543–44
indications for, 529
nursing implications of, 529
puerperal urinary problems from, 982
for laparoscopy, 117, 118
for postpartal hematoma surgery, 973
for tubal ligation, 127, 128
for uterine inversion intervention, 580

General appearance, assessing neonate for, 674–75, 698g, 691g
  abdomen, 699g
  chest, 697–98g
  eyes, 693g
  neck, 697g
  SGA, 762, 762f, 764
Generalizations, avoiding, 47
Generativity vs. stagnation, as developmental stage, 38, 40t, 41
Genes, 157, 157f
Genetic amniocentesis, 146f, 146, 147–48
Genetic counseling, 134–54
  defined, 150
  for congenital heart disease, 769
  family assessment as part of, 48
  goals of, 150
  nurse's role in, 15, 134–35, 146, 148, 150–54
  pedigree and history as part of, 150, 152, 153f
  principles in, 152–54
  for spina bifida, 879
Genetic disorders. See also specific disorders
  amniocentesis to diagnose, 387
  for chromosomal abnormalities, 135–41
  counseling for, 150–54
  ethnic background and, 152
  patterns of inheritance for, 141–46
  postnatal diagnosis of, 148–50
  prenatal diagnosis of, 146f, 146–48
  Rh sensitivity, 347, 348, 348f
  statistics about, 134–35
Genetic engineering, 11
Genetic predisposition, birth weight and, 760
Genetic processes, overview of, 157–60
Genetics Research Group, Hastings Center, 11
Genetic screening. See Screening
General herpes. See Herpesvirus
Genital lesions
  from genital herpes simplex, 359
  intrapartal, sepsis prevention and, 842
Genital warts (Condylomata accuminata), 355
Genitals. See also External genitals
  development of, 57–59, 58f, 653, 653f
  of neonate
    assessing, 684, 700–702g
    atrophy of, with Sheehan syndrome, 988
    bathing, 727
    gestational age and, 662f, 665f, 668, 670–71f
    preterm, 750
Genitourinary system
  fetal
    development of, 175t, 177t, 179–83
    teratogenic damage to, 183t
  maternal, prenatal assessment of, 229–30g
  neonatal, 652–54, 653f
    defects in, 874–75
    maternal drug addiction risk to, 771
Genotype, 142
Gentamycin
  for group B streptococcal infection, 843
  hearing loss risk from, 758
  for sepsis neonatorum, 842

Gentian violet, for thrush, 845
Germinal epithelium, 83, 84
Gesell, Arnold, rooming-in supported by, 12
Gestation
  defined, 210
  gastrointestinal development during, 650–51
  genital development during, 653, 653f
  immune system during, 653–54
  length of, 191
    iron stores and, 648
  reproductive system development during, 57–59, 58f
  respiratory system development during, 635, 638–39, 639f
Gestational age, 173
  assessed at nursery admission, 710
  betamethasone and, 547
  blood pressure values according to, 751t
  classifications of, 660, 734, 737
  clinical estimation of, 660–74, 662–74f, APPENDIX D
  determining, in preterm infant nursing care plan, 750
  ear cartilage as indicator of, 681
  estriol excretion patterns and, 380
  fetal cell examination and, 387
  fetal lung maturity and, 384
  FHR and, 374
  flexion of extremities and, 740
  hematologic values affected by, 644
  importance of, 660
  IVH outcome and, 836
  methods of determining, 660–74, 662–74f
    with PROM, 546
    ultrasound, 8, 368–70
    x-ray, 387
  neonatal mortality and, 548
  PROM interventions and, 546f, 546–47
  risk identification with, 734–35, 735–36f
  ritodrine and, 549
  ultrasonography to assess, 8
  vulnerability to teratogens and, 183t
  weight and, 689g
Gestational diabetes mellitus (GDM), 314, 314t, 315
Gestational sac, ultrasound can detect, 368–69
Getz, W., on crisis intervention, 994
GI tract. See Gastrointestinal system
Glabellar reflex, in neonates, 680
Glands
  breasts as, 85
  endometrial, 79
Glans of clitoris, 71f, 72, 73
Glans penis, 59, 59f, 60, 60f
Glaucoma, congenital
  assessing for, 693g, 694g
  with Pierre Robin syndrome, 850
Glomerular filtration rate (GFR)
  in neonates, 652
    preterm, 746
  pregnancy changes in, 197t, 199, 254
    glycosuria and, 201
    PIH and, 340
Glomerulonephritis, in pregnancy
  neonatal problems associated with, 769
  nonhypertensive, fetal lung maturity and, 385
  sign of in prenatal exam, 230g

Glossopharyngel nerve, assessing in neonate, 695g
Glossoptosis, with micrognathia, 850
"Glove anesthesia," 295
Glucagon
  for IDM, 768
  for neonatal hypoglycemia, 821
Glucocorticoids
  betamethasone (Celestone), 547
  ritodrine with, caution about, 549
Glucose. See also Blood glucose
  in fetus, 648
  depletion of, in neonate of hypertensive mother, 769
  for IDM, 768
  need for during labor, 536
  neonatal digestion produces, 651
  for neonatal hypoglycemia, 821
  normal neonatal values, 645t
  placental transport of, 170
  in resuscitative therapy, 792
  in urine, See Glycosuria
Glucose tolerance test
  in infertility workup, 114
  prenatal, 201, 316–17
    for diabetic client, 317–18
Glucose water, for initial bottle-feeding, 716
Glucuronyl transferase, 649, 822–23
Glycogen
  placenta synthesizes, 170
  vaginal environment role of, 75, 75f
Glycogen stores
  depleted, with postmaturity syndrome, 760
  neonatal hypoglycemia and, 818
  in placenta, 170
  prematurity and, 740, 748
  in SGA neonates, 762
  used in asphyxial attack, 786
Glycosuria
  at labor onset, 468
    implications of, 432g
  in pregnancy, 199, 201, 314
    carbohydrate intake and, 273
    with diabetes mellitus, 313
    glucose tolerance test indicated by, 316–17
    in initial prenatal exam, 230g
    in subsequent prenatal exams, 240g
  in preterm infant, 746, 753n
GnRF (gonadotropin-releasing factor), 92, 92f
GnRH (gonadotropin-releasing hormone), role of, 96
Goals. See also Nursing goals
  of family care, 49, 969
  family development, 36–37
Goat's milk, 272, 277
Goiter, congenital, 215t, 326
Golbus, M. S., 148
Gonadal failure, 84
Gonadostat. See Hypothalamic-pituitary complex
Gonadotropic hormones, role of, 96, 97f, 98
Gonadotropin-releasing factor (GnRF), 92, 92f
Gonadotropin-releasing hormone (GnRH), role of, 96
Gonadotropins, testosterone and, 62
Gonads, 57
  development of, 91–92, 92f, 653, 653f
Gonorrhea, 354. See also Sexually transmitted diseases
  adolescent pregnancy and, 299, 304
  assessing neonate for, 842

blindness from, preventing, 4. See also Eye prophylaxis
  culture for
    before abortion, 129
    in infertility workup, 114
    in initial prenatal exam, 229g
    precontraception, 120
  in pregnancy, 354–55
    detecting, 229g
    at labor onset, 429g
    puerperal infection caused by, 974, 975
    signs of in initial prenatal exam, 226g
  Skene's ducts as site of, 73
  spermicides protect against, 127
Goodell's sign, 192, 226g
  nonpregnancy causes of, 192t
Gordon, T., 290
Gout, sign of in initial prenatal exam, 224g
Graafian follicles
  development of, 96, 97f, 98, 98f
  in ovarian cortex, 83
Gram negative pathogens, postpartal infection caused by, 913
Grandmultiparity
  abdominal muscle tone and, 905
  as birth center contraindication, 618
  breech presentation and, 554
  as hemorrhage risk, 569, 972
  hypotonic labor patterns from, 541
  as induction of labor contraindication, 587
  macrosomia with, 556
  malposition less crucial with, 551
  SGA neonates with, 761
  shoulder presentation with, 402
  transverse lie and, 555
  uterine involution affected by, 903
Grandparents
  attachment with, 963
  in adolescent pregnancy, 301–2, 305, 1017
  prenatal classes for, 292
  responses to pregnancy of, 251–52
Grant, P., 778
  on response to high-risk infant, 778–79, 779f
Granular leukocytes, fetal development of, 644
Granulocytes, fetal development of, 644
Granulomatous disease, fetoscopy to diagnose, 388
Grasp reflex, 657, 686
Gravida, defined, 210
Greece, ancient, obstetrics in, 3
Green, M., on vulnerable child syndrome, 1009–10
Greenberg, M., fathers studied by, 961–63
Grief. See also Grief process
  defined, 999
  infertility causes, 119
Grief process, 999, 1002
  after abortion, 131
    spontaneous, 333
  acute stage, 999
  anticipatory, with high-risk neonate, 773
  attachment as part of, 777
  after cesarean delivery, 941–42
  with cleft lip, 853n
  defective birth, 773, 848, 1010
  duration of, 999, 1002
  factors affecting, 1002
  with fetal malformations, 557
  with hydrocephaly, 557
  for idealized infant, 773, 1002

Grief process *(Cont'd)*
after neonatal death, 1002–6, 1004n
with preterm birth, 773, 1006
relinquishment for adoption requires, 1014
stages in, 999, 1002
after stillbirth, 561
facilitating, 580, 581
with tracheoesophageal atresia/fistula, 865n
with uterine rupture, 550
Grief work. *See* Grief process
Grimacing, as neonatal distress sign, 714
Group A or Group B beta hemolytic streptococci. *See* Beta-hemolytic streptococci
Group marriage, family structure in, 34
Group practice, pregnant client and, 242g
Group teaching, prenatal, 291–92
Group therapy, in crisis intervention, 996. *See also* Support groups
Growth chart percentiles, in neonatal nutritional assessment, 719
Growth hormone (somatotropin), breast changes and, 85
Growth rate
with Beckwith syndrome, 867
cardiac defects and
tetralogy of Fallot, 890
transposition of great vessels, 891
ventricular septal defects, 888
fetal alcohol syndrome affects, 770
in SGA neonates, 763
Growth spurts, breast-feeding increases during, 930
Grunting
with group B streptococcal infection, 843
with polycythemia, 835
as respiratory distress sign, 751
Guaiac-positive stools, as feeding intolerance sign, 745, 746
Guarding, as puerperal peritonitis sign, 977n
Gums
assessing in initial prenatal exam, 220g
assessing in neonate, 681
bleeding
as anticoagulant overdose sign, 984n
as DIC sign, 568
vitamin C deficiency as cause of, 719
pregnancy changes in, 198, 265
Guthrie test, PKU screening with, 858
Guttmacher, A. F., 205
Gynecoid pelvis, 70, 396, 397f
Gynecomastia, in male adolescents, 64

Habituation, in neonatal responses, 655, 687, 705
Habitus, or fetal attitude, 399
Hair
assessing, in initial prenatal exam, 217g
fetal, 177t, 179t, 180–82. *See also* Lanugo
loss of, from vitamin overdose, 274
of neonate
assessing, 692g
SGA, 764
washing, 727–28
Hairlip, gestational age and, 183t

Hall, B. L., on prematurity adjustment, 772–73
Hallucinations, with puerperal psychosis, 988
Hallucinogens, in pregnancy, 360–62, 361t
Halogenated anesthetics, obstetric use of, 529
Halothane (Fluothane)
obstetric use of, 529
postpartal hemorrhage risk with, 972
Hand-to-mouth movements
assessing neonate for, 687, 705
neonatal self-quieting by, 706
Hand-washing
mastitis prevention by, 987
with neonatal herpesvirus infection, 844
with neonatal moniliasis, 845
for preterm infant care, 748, 754n
puerperal infection and, 4, 5, 919n, 978n
sepsis neonatorum prevention by, 835, 842
for SGA neonatal care, 766n
Handicapped Children Services, 780
Handling newborns, 714, 715f
teaching parents about, 726
Hands
assessing, in initial prenatal exam, 224g
edema of, as danger sign, 240g
of neonate
assessing, 684, 702g
lesions on, with congenital syphilis, 844
Haploid cells, 159, 160, 161f
Haploid number of chromosomes, 135
Hard palate, neonatal jaundice evidence on, 824, 832n
Harlequin (clown) color change, 677, 689g
Harris, D. M., 1017
Harrison's groove, in neonate, 699g
Hartman, Rhonda, 295
Harvey, K., on relinquishment, 1014, 1015t
Harvey, William, 4
Hastings Center, Genetics Research Group, 11
Hb A$_{1c}$ levels, 320
HC. *See* Head compression
hCG *See* Human chorionic gonadotropin
HCO$_3$. *See* Bicarbonates
hCS (Human chorionic somatomammotropin). *See* Human placental lactogen
Head
assessing, in initial prenatal exam, 217–18g, 219g
of fetus. *See* Fetal head
of neonate
assessing, 675, 675f, 678, 679f, 691–92g
enlarged, with hydrocephalus, 880, 880f, 882n
measuring, 675, 675f, 678, 691g
at nursery admission, 710
preterm, 747, 750
SGA, 764
Head compression (HC), early decelerations caused by, 454, 455f, 456f
Head lag, in neonate
assessing, 702g, 703g
gestational age and, 663f, 672
muscle tone and, 681

Head lice, signs of in initial prenatal exam, 218g
Head-eye coordination, "doll's eye" syndrome, 680
Head-to-abdomen ratios, ultrasound to determine, 370
Headache
as bromocriptine side effect, 926d
as hypothyroidism sign, 326
with mastitis, 987
as Methergine side effect, 903d
with PIH, 341
postpartal, with blood pressure increase, 906
severe preeclampsia, assessing for, 343
after regional anesthesia, 524n
spinal, 526–27
lumbar epidural, 520
as ritodrine side effect, 549
severe, as danger sign of pregnancy, 240g
as terbutaline sulfate side effect, 548
as tocolytic side effect, 548, 549
Healers, cultural beliefs about, 206
Healing of intrapartal wounds, 974–75, 975t, 977–78n
Health beliefs, pregnancy and, 205–6
Health care behaviors, cultural influences on, 43. *See also* specific cultures
Health care environment changes, nursing role and, 12–16
Health maintenance, as nurse practitioner role, 15
Health team
attachment problem interventions by, 1012
crisis referral by, 994
defective birth role of, 849, 850, 895
emotions of, complicated childbirth, 580–81
federal support for use of, 5
genetic counseling role of, 154
high-risk infant care role of, 780
meningocele/meningomyelocele role of, 883n
neonatal hyperbilirubinemia role of, 830
nurse-midwives as part of, 14
perinatal care, 733
resuscitative, 787
spina bifida role of, 881
Heardman, Helen, 293
Hearing, assessing neonate for, 681, 686, 687, 697g, 705
Hearing loss, in neonate
from intraventricular hemorrhage, 836
as IUGR outcome, 763
kernicterus as cause of, 824
from maternal rubella, 358
as prematurity risk, 758
risk factors for, 681
Heart
fetal. *See* Fetal heart
maternal
assessing in initial prenatal exam, 222g, 233–34p, 234f
assessing at labor onset, 428g
pulmonary embolism signs, 982, 983, 984n
neonatal
assessing, 682–83, 698–99g, 712
congenital defects of, 881, 886–87f. *See also* Cardiac anomalies; specific defects
MAS damage to, 815

patent ductus arteriosus signs in, 885
Heart defects. *See* Cardiac anomalies; specific defects
Heart disease. *See* Cardiac disorders; specific disorders
Heart murmurs
in neonate, 641–42
assessing, 683, 699g
from atrial septal defects, 885
with coarctation of the aorta, 889
with endocardial cushion defects, 888
functional or innocent, 641–42
with pulmonary stenosis, 890
with tetralogy of Fallot, 890
with transposition of the great vessels, 891
with ventricular septal defects, 885, 888
in pregnancy with cardiac disease, 311
Heart rate. *See also* Pulse
gallop, as pulmonary embolism sign, 982, 983
of neonate, 641
with MAS, 798
monitoring in nursery, 712
monitoring, in preterm infant, 755n
with RDS, 797t
in reactivity period, 712, 713f
pregnancy changes in, 310
Heart sounds, in neonate. *See also* Murmurs
with diaphragmatic hernia, 866
with endocardial cushion defects, 888
with pneumomediastinum, 816
pneumothorax effects on, 809n
Heartburn (pyrosis), as pregnancy discomfort, 198, 253f. 254t, 256
Heat applications
for breast engorgement, 937
for mastitis, 987
plugged ducts relieved by, 937
for superficial leg vein disease, 980
for thrombophlebitis, 984n
Heat lamps
perineal pain relief with, 915, 917n
postpartal infection prevention with, 918n, 974, 977n
Heat loss, in neonates, 646–47, 753
cold stress from, 817–18
preterm, 740, 742–53n, 765
preventing in nursery, 712–13
SGA, 762, 764, 765n
Heat production. *See* Thermogenesis
Heat sensitivity, as hyperthyroidism sign, 326
Heat shields, for preterm infants, 752
Heel-to-ear maneuver, gestational age and, 663f, 665f, 672
Hegar, Alfred, 4
Hegar's sign, 192, 193f
in initial prenatal exam, 226g
nonpregnancy causes of, 192t
Height, assessing at labor admission, 472
HELP program, 360
Hemagglutination-inhibition test (pregnosticon R), 1, 195
Hemangiomas, in neonate, 678, 691g
Hematest, for preterm infant, 750n
with necrotizing enterocolitis, 838, 839n

Hematocrit
  maternal
    abruptio placentae and, 564
    before and after cesarean
      delivery, 601, 603
    decrease in, from ritodrine, 549
    elevated, as risk factor, 215t
    with fetal distress, 538
    fourth trimester, 947g
    hemorrhage and, 569n, 571n
    before induction of labor, 591n
    in initial prenatal exam, 229g
    at labor onset, 431, 469, 472
    postpartal, 906, 917, 947g
    with preeclampsia/eclampsia,
      337, 343
    pregnancy changes in, 198, 274
    precontraception assessment of,
      120
  neonatal
    anemia assessment with, 835
    blood loss decreases, 835
    for conjunctiva pallor, 694g
    decrease in, with IVH, 836
    in IDM, 768
    at nursery admission, 711
    polycythemic values, 835
    preterm infants, 748–49, 752t
    SGA, 764n
Hematologic abnormalities in neo-
    nate, central cyanosis from,
    889
Hematologic agents, teratogenic
    effects of, 267t
Hematologic tests
  in initial prenatal exam, 228–29g
  at labor onset, 431g
Hematology, neonatal, 644–45, 645t
  of preterm infant, 748–49, 752t
Hematomas
  genital
    in initial prenatal exam, 225g
    as third stage labor complica-
      tion, 580
  in labia majora, 72
  in neonate
    cephalhematoma, 678, 679f
    jaundice and, 677, 831
    of mons, 701g
  postpartal, 973
    from paracervical block, 516,
      517
    from pudendal block, 528
    infection risk from, 974
  in third stage labor, 419, 580
Hematometra, Braxton Hicks con-
    tractions from, 192t, 193
Hematopoietic system, in neonates,
    643–45, 645t
Hematuria
  in neonate
    as MAS complication, 815
    polycythemia, 835
  postpartal, 906
    as anticoagulant overdose sign,
      984n
    as cystitis sign, 986
Hemiplegia, contralateral, nevus
    flammeus with, 677–78
Hemiplegic patients, uterine contrac-
    tions in, 80
Hemivertebra, 183, 183f
Hemizygous traits, 144
Hemoglobin
  fetal, 171, 425t, 643
  maternal
    assessing in prenatal exams,
      228g, 239g
    before and after cesarean
      delivery, 601, 603
    decrease in, from ritodrine, 549
    elevated, risk of, 214t

with fetal distress, 538
fourth trimester, 947g
hemorrhage and, 569, 571n
before induction of labor, 591n
at labor admission, 431g, 469,
  472
normal pregnancy drop in, 274
postpartal assessment of, 917,
  947g
postpartal changes in, 906
neonatal, 643, 644
  anemia assessment with, 830,
    835
  assessing, after placenta previa,
    567
  for conjunctiva pallor, 694g
  iron stores and, 648
  normal values, 830, 835
  oxygen transport role of, 642–
    43
  polycythemic values, 835
  preterm, 748–49, 752t
  tetralogy of Fallot lowers, 890
  unoxygenated, cyanosis from,
    889
  precontraception assessment of,
    120
Hemoglobinopathies, prenatal diagnosis of, 148
Hemoglobinuria, sign of in prenatal
  exam, 229g
Hemolytic anemia, in preterm
  infants, preventing, 746. See
  also Hemolytic disease of the
  newborn
Hemolytic crisis, from sickle cell
  anemia, 327, 328
Hemolytic disease. See also Hemolytic disease of the newborn
  amniocentesis to evaluate, 384,
    384f
  fetal mortality from, 347
  induction of labor for, 587
  from Rh sensitization, incidence of,
    347
Hemolytic disease of the newborn,
  347, 824, 826–30, 827f,
  829–30f
  ABO incompatibility as cause of,
    826
  assessing for, 826, 827
    with ultrasound, 370
  birth weight with, 760
  described, 824, 826
  hyperbilirubinemia with, 822
  hypoglycemia with, 761
  interventions for, 825p, 827f,
    827–30, 829–30f
  liver enlargement from, 700g
  maternal phenobarbital to prevent,
    830
  as pathologic jaundice cause, 823
  in preterm infant, hematologic
    effect of, 748–49. See also
    Hemolytic disease
  prognosis with, 826–27
  Rh incompatibility as cause of,
    826
  umbilical cord discoloration from,
    700g
Hemolysis, in neonate
  anemia caused by, 830
  jaundice from, 677
  from maternal CMV, 358
Hemophilia
  fetoscopy to diagnose, 388
  inheritance of, 144, 160
  prenatal diagnosis of, 147, 148
Hemophilus vaginalis. See Gardnerella vaginalis
Hemopoietic system, labor changes
  in, 409

Hemorrhage, fetal
  as induction of labor risk, 594n
  intracranial, as CPD risk, 578
  from succenturiate placenta, 573
  uterine rupture and risk of, 425t
  from vasa previa, 575–76
  from velamentous insertion of um-
    bilical cord, 575
Hemorrhage, maternal
  antepartal
    from abruptio placentae, 563
    from amniotic fluid embolism,
      576
    from circumvallate placenta,
      574
    neonatal hematocrit decreased
      by, 644
    from hyperemesis gravidarum,
      328
  degree of, 562t, 569
  determining presence of, 571–72n
  as DIC sign, 567, 568f
  intrapartal
    as cesarean complication, 600,
      604, 605
    before delivery of placenta, 579
    during first stage labor, 429g
    general anesthesia for, 528
    as induction of labor risk, 591
    after internal version, 586
    interventions for, 576
    postpartal oxytocic agents for,
      903
    as prolonged labor risk, 542
    risk factors for, 425t
    as ritodrine contraindication,
      548, 549
  as ectopic pregnancy risk, 333,
    334
  evaluating blood loss from, 569–
    71n
  history of, as risk factor, 569,
    972
  mortality from, 206
  nursing care plan, 569–73
  postpartal, 578–79, 972–73
    from abruptio placentae, 563,
      564
    bladder distention and, 905–6
    blood pressure decrease with,
      906
    causes of, 578
    controlling, 500
    defined, 578
    as diabetes risk, 325
    from DIC, 568
    from fetal macrosomia, 556
    as hydramnios risk, 577
    as hyperthyroidism risk, 326
    as hypotonic labor risk, 541
    infection risk from, 974
    late, 902–3, 973
    lochia signs of, 904
    malpositons as cause of, 552
    midforceps delivery increases
      risk of, 598
    as multiple gestation risk, 425t
    oxytocic agents to prevent, 903,
      903d
    from placenta accreta, 579
    as placenta previa risk, 566
    as precipitous labor risk, 543
    preventing, 480, 481n, 972
    after prolonged labor, 542
    from retained placental frag-
      ments, 579
    Sheehan syndrome after, 988
    from succenturiate placenta,
      568, 573
    thromboembolic disease risk
      with, 983
    from uterine atony, 579

uterine contractions prevent,
  903
from uterine inversion, 579–80
from uterine rupture, 550
vital signs as indicator of, 912–
  13
risk factors for, 214–15t, 425t
supine hypotensive syndrome and,
  409
Hemorrhage, in neonate
  cerebral, as prematurity risk, 749
  disseminated intravascular coagu-
    lation, 837
  gastrointestinal, as MAS complica-
    tion, 815
  with hydrops fetalis, 826
  hyperbilirubinemia and, 822, 823
  intraventricular, 738, 836–37
  jaundice and, 831
  from maternal anticoagulant,
    769
  perinatal, hematocrit decreased
    by, 644
  as pneumothorax therapy compli-
    cation, 809n
  with polycythemia, 835
  preterm hematology with, 748–49
  subconjunctival, 680
  vitamin K deficiency, 836
Hemorrhagic anemia, from maternal
  folic acid deficient, 276
Hemorrhagic disease of the newborn,
  836
  vitamin K to prevent, 710, 711d
Hemorrhagic disorders, signs of in
  prenatal exam, 217g
Hemorrhagic shock, from abruptio
  placentae, 561, 563
Hemorrhoids
  described, 257
  as pregnancy discomfort, 198,
    252, 255t, 257
  signs of in prenatal exam, 228g
  pain relief for, 915, 917n
  postpartal assessment of, 912,
    912f
    fourth trimester, 946g
Hemostasis, with cesarean delivery,
  605
Heparin. See also Anticoagulants
  for amniotic fluid embolism DIC,
    576
  for deep vein thrombosis, 981,
    984n
  for DIC, 567, 568
    in neonate, 837
  as drug of choice during preg-
    nancy, 769
  overdose interventions, 984n
  placenta not crossed by, 170
  for pulmonary embolism, 982
Hepatitis
  as fetal/neonatal risk, 215t
  neonatal (giant cell), 823
    with herpesvirus type 2, 844
    hyperbilirubinemia risk with,
      823
  in pregnancy, as drug addiction
    risk, 770
Hepatitis-A immunization, in pregnancy, 266t
Hepatogmegaly, in neonate
  from galactosemia, 859
  with jaundice, 823, 831
Hepatosplenomegaly
  ABO incompatibility as cause of,
    826
  from congenital CMV, 359
  from congenital rubella, 358
  from congenital syphilis, 844
  from congenital toxoplasmosis,
    357

Hepatosplenomegaly *(Cont'd)*
  with herpesvirus type 2 infection, 844
  with hydrops fetalis, 824, 826
  with jaundice, 831
Herbalists, 206
Hermaphroditism, assessing female neonate for, 701g
Hernia
  diaphragmatic. *See* Diaphragmatic hernia
  infertility from, 112
  inguinal, assessing neonate for, 700g
  umbilical
    assessing neonate for, 700g
    with congenital hypothyroidism, 859
    cord length and 575
Herniation, sign of in initial prenatal exam, 223g
Heroin addiction in pregnancy, 360–62, 361t
  neonatal effects of, 361, 361t, 770–72
Herpesvirus type 2
  adolescent pregnancy and, 299, 304
  counseling for clients with, 360
  in initial prenatal exam, 220g
  in neonate, 844
    hyperbilirubinemia risk from, 823
    risk of, 215t
    screening for, 150
    sepsis neonatorum and, 842
    ulcerated cornea as sign of, 693g
  in pregnancy, 359–60
    birth center screening for, 618
    cesarean delivery for, 600
    fetal exposure to, IgM levels and, 654
    as induction of labor contraindication, 587
    as risk factor, 215t
Hesseltine clamp, 504
Heterozygous, defined, 142
Heterozygous traits, in autosomal dominant inheritance, 142–43
Heterozygous vs. homozygous genes, 157, 157f
Hexaprenaline, for preterm labor, 548
Hexosaminidase A, Tay-Sachs disease and, 144
High-risk neonates. *See also specific risks*
  assessment of, 735–37
  attachment with, 774–79, 968
    breast-feeding and, 776
    transport and, 773–74
  breast milk for, 776
  factors affecting, 733
  identification of, 733–35, 734–35f
  outcomes for, 733, 758
    parental responses to and, 778–79, 779f
  parental caretaking for, 772–80, 777f, 779f
  physical contact with, 775–77, 776–77f
  PKU screening for, 858
  sensory stimulation for, 776–77
High-risk obstetrical care, 8
  federal funding for, 5
  prenatal screening as part of, 213, 214–15t
  regional centers for, 389
High-risk pregnancy
  crisis intervention for, 998–99
  early delivery of, 388–89

postpartal risks, 907, 908t
Hill, R., 778
Hilum, ovarian, 83, 84
Hip, of neonate
  assessing, 703g
  dislocated, 145, 703g
  dysplasia of, 685, 876–78, 877f
  joint infection in, dysplasia vs., 878
Hippocratic oath, abortion forbidden by, 3
Hirschsprung disease (aganglionic megacolon), 868–71
  intestinal obstruction vs., 873, 874
Hirsutism, assessing, in initial prenatal exam, 217g
Hispanic culture. *See* Mexican American families
Histamine, placenta breaks down, 170
Historical data base. *See* Data base History
Historical view of maternity care, 3–7
History. *See also* Data base
  for adolescent pregnancy assessment, 302–3
  before abortion, 129
  for AGA and LGA preterm infant nursing care plan, 750
  aganglionosis assessment by, 87
  before cesarean delivery, 601
  for cleft lip and palate nursing care plan, 853
  for contraception screening, 120
  diabetes in pregnancy and, 322
  diaphragmatic hernia, 867
  family, importance of assessing, 48
    in high-risk neonatal care, 777
  in fetal distress nursing care plan, 538
  for genetic counseling, 150, 152, 153f
    postnatal, 148
  in hemorrhage nursing care plan, 569
  for high-risk infant assessment, 735–36
  imperforate anus assessment with, 872
  before induction of labor, 591
  for infertility interventions, 112, 113, 114
  intestinal obstruction assessment with, 873
  at labor admission, 472
  maternal, in neonatal assessment 660, 710
    forɴe plan, 839
  neonatal anemia assessment with, 835
  for neonatal jaundice nursing care plan, 831
  of neonate, immediate postpartal, 498n
  nutritional, at well-child visit, 719
  obstetric, 210–13, 212f, 214–15t
  in PIH assessment, 337
  in postpartal period nursing care plan, 917
  postpartal psychosis factors in, 988
  for puerperal infection nursing care plan, 977
  for RDS nursing care plan, 801
  for regional anesthesia, 521n
  resuscitation risk factors elicited in, 786
  risk identification with, 734
  before ritodrine administration, 549

for SGA neonates nursing care plan, 764
for stillbirth nursing care plan, 1004
for thromboembolic disease nursing care plan, 983
in tracheoesophageal fistula nursing care plan, 862
of woman in labor, 424–25, 425t
History taking. *See* Assessment
HMD (hyaline membrane disease). *See* Respiratory distress syndrome
hMG (Human menopausal gonadotropin), 118
Hoff, L. A., 998–99
Hoffman's exercises, for nipples, 931, 936f
Holding, assessing neonatal responses to, 706
Holmes, Oliver Wendell, 5
Homans' sign, 912, 981, 981f, 983
Home births, 13
  attachment process and, 954, 955–56
  emergency, 505–7
  nurse midwives at, 15
Home management of neonatal jaundice, 831n
Home visits
  family assessment during, 48
  planning for at discharge, 730
  postpartal, 944
    assessment guide, 624–27
    after birth center delivery, 619
    for high-risk neonates, 780
    after pretem birth, 1009
    supporting function of, 725
Homemaker's Service, cleft lip referral for, 856n
Homeothermic, newborns as, 645
Homocystinuria, 858–59
  described, 858–59
  newborn screening for, 150, 725
  prenatal diagnosis of, 148
Homograft, placenta as, 170
Homologous chromosomes, 135, 142
Homologous vs. heterozygous genes, 157, 157f
Homosexual family structure, 34
Homosexuality, 89
Homozygous, defined, 142
Homozygous traits, in autosomal recessive inheritance, 143–44
Hormonal disorders, diabetes secondary to, 315
Hormones. *See also* Endocrine system; *specific hormones*
  androgens, 61
  female reproductive cycle role of, 96, 97f, 98
  gonadotropins, 62
  imbalances in, amenorrhea from, 100
  lactation role of, 925
  lactation suppression with, 925
  male
    as androgens, 61
    effect of, 92f, 93
  menopausal changes in, 101, 102
  as oral contraceptives, 121f, 125, 126–27t
  ovarian, effects of, 92f, 93–94
  of pregnancy
    joint relaxation induced by, 66
    neonatal breast engorgement from, 682
    produced in placenta, 168–71
  pubertal role of, 91, 92, 92f
  testosterone, 61, 62
Hospital birth centers, 618–19

Hospital care
  birth alternatives in, 13
  family-centered, 12–13
  rarity of in 18th century, 5
  traditional, 12
Hospitalization
  for acute pyelonephritis, 353
  anxiety from, labor pain and, 413
  attachment process and, 954, 1012
  birth options available with, 613, 618–19
  for cardiac client, 312
  for diabetic client, 320, 324
  discharge planning, 730
    infant care and, 726
  extended, as risk, 215t
  group A streptococcal infection risk with, 974
  for hydramnios, 577
  for hyperemesis gravidarum, 328
  at labor onset, 466–69, 472–73n
  of neonate. *See also* Nursery
    for physiologic jaundice, 649
  premature labor and risk of, 425t
  for placenta previa, 566–67
  "postpartum blues" during, 907
  after PROM, 546
  for puerperal psychiatric disorders, 988
  for severe preeclampsia, 343
  for spontaneous abortion, 332
  for thyroid storm, 326
  for withdrawal during pregnancy, 362
Hossiter clamp, in precipitous delivery, 504
Hot compresses. *See* Heat applications
Hot flashes, 101
Hot weather, neonatal fluid requirements in, 717
hPL. *See* Human placental lactogen
Human chorionic gonadotropin (hCG), ("pregnancy hormone"), 168–69, 202
  cellular immunity suppressed by, 170
  decrease in, spontaneous abortion caused by, 329
  in ectopic pregnancy, 333
  function of, 98, 168–69, 202
  with hydatidiform mole, 334–35
  infertility management with, 118
  pregnancy nausea and, 191, 252, 254t
  pregnancy tests based on, 194–95
  production of, 98
Human chorionic somatomammotropin. *See* Human placental lactogen
Human menopausal gonadatropin (hMG), infertility management with, 118
Human placental lactogen (hPL), 168, 169–70, 202
  effect on diabetic patient of, 315
  endocrine balance role of, 314
  as fetal well-being test, 381
  glomerular filtration rate and, 199
  insulin requirements increased by, 202
Humidity, neonatal heat loss modified by, 647
Hunger, in fourth stage labor, 420, 905
Hunter, William, 4
Hunter syndrome, prenatal diagnosis of, 148
Huntington's chorea, 142f, 143

Hurler syndrome
assessing neonate for, 702g, 766n
lashes with, 694g
prenatal diagnosis of, 148
Husband-coached natural childbirth,
295
Hutchinson, Anne, 6
Hyaline membrane disease. *See* Respiratory distress syndrome
Hyaluronic acid, 160, 162
Hyaluronidase, 162
Hydatidiform mole, 334–35, 335f
bleeding caused by, 329
defined, 334
elevated hCG caused by, 192t,
194
incidence of, 334
PIH risk and, 336
positive pregnancy test caused by,
192t, 194
signs of in prenatal exams, 223–
24g, 239f
statistics about, 329
ultrasonography to confirm, 8
Hydatoxi lualba, 336
Hyde, J. S., 88
Hyden, Kentucky, Frontier Nursing
Service hospital in, 7
Hydralazine (Apresoline)
for chronic hypertension in pregnancy, 347
postpartal administration of, 346
for severe preeclampsia, 344, 347
Hydramnios, 576–77
breech presentation and, 554
chronic vs. acute, 577
deep leg vein disease risk with,
981
defined, 576
diabetes and, 316, 325
fetal/neonatal implications of, 577
fundal height and, 237
hemorrhage risk with, 569, 972
as induction of labor contraindication, 587
interventions for, 577
as intestinal obstruction sign, 873
as intrapartal risk factor, 425t
labor problems from, 557
maternal implications of, 577
PIH risk and, 336
placental tumors associated with,
568
as preterm labor cause, 407, 548
prolapsed umbilical cord with, 574
signs of, 239g, 577
supine hypotensive syndrome and,
409
uterine atony from, 579
Hydration
assessing
at labor admission, 472
during labor, first stage, 429g,
475, 476
hypertonic labor patterns and, 537
maintaining
with hypotonic labor pattern,
541
in prolonged labor, 542
after PROM, 547
in neonate
assessing, 677
motor activity and, 654
Hydrocele, assessing neonate for,
684, 701g
Hydrocephaly, 880f
assessing neonate for, 678, 691g,
693g
breech presentation and, 554
from congenital toxoplasmosis,
357
defined, 880

estriol levels and, 380
eyelids with, 693g
fetal surgery for, 8
head and chest circumference
with, 691g
interventions for, 880
from listeriosis, 357
from intraventricular hemorrhage,
836, 837
labor and delivery problems from,
557
late closure of sutures with, 692g
meningocele and, 880, 880f
meningomyelocele and, 879, 881,
883n
as prematurity risk, 758
prenatal diagnosis of, 146
ultrasound to detect, 368, 369f,
370
Hydrochloric acid, neonatal production of, 651
Hydrolysis of protein, in neonates,
651
Hydronephrosis, fetal surgery for, 8
Hydrops fetalis, 347, 824, 826
amniotic fluid density and, 384
fetal lung maturity and, 385
preventing, exchange transfusions
for, 349
risk factors for, 215t
ultrasound to detect, 370
Hydrostatic pressure, in placental
transport, 170
Hydrothorax, 826
Hydroxyzine (Vistaril), during labor,
513
fetal tachycardia caused by, 451
Hymen, 73, 100
Hymenal caruncles, 73
Hymenal tag, in neonate, 684, 701g
Hyperactivity
in FAS children, 362, 770
in initial prenatal exam, 225g
as IUGR outcome, 763
from kernicterus, 826
in LGA infant, from birth trauma,
756n
Hyperalimentation
after diaphragmatic hernia
surgery, 867
PKU screening and, 858
for preterm infant, 745–46
Hyperammonemia, formula type and,
741
Hyperbilirubinemia, in neonate
from congenital CMV, 358–59
from congenital rubella, 358
dangers of, 823
hearing loss risk from, 758
from hemolytic disease of the newborn, 826
from hypothyroidism, 326
in IDM, 768
interventions for, 823, 825p, 827f,
827–30, 829–30f
jaundice as first sign of, 832n
kernicterus results from, 826
long-term effects of, 826–27
from maternal drug abuse, 361t
from maternal medication, 353
with polycythemia, 835
preterm
apnea from, 749
assessing for, 757n
feeding to prevent, 740
as risk, 749
preventing, 740, 823
maternal phenobarbital for, 830
as sepsis neonatorum sign, 841
from vitamin K overdose, 711d
Hypercalcemia, from vitamin D overdose, 275

Hypercapnia, IVH from, 836
Hypercarbia, in neonate, 643, 816
asphyxia leads to, 786
as precipitous labor risk, 543
with RDS, 794
ventilatory assistance indicated by,
800t
Hypercholesterolemia, in pregnancy,
199
Hyperemesis gravidarum, 252, 328
danger sign of, 240g
Hyperemia, pregnancy sign caused
by, 192t
Hyperextension, assessing in neonate, 682
Hyperglycemia
maternal
as diabetes complication, 214t,
318, 319t
ketoacidosis from, 316
pregnancy and, 323
as ritodrine risk, 548, 549
symptoms of, 319t
neonatal
intervention for, 808n
preterm, as TPN risk, 746
with RDS, 807–8n
signs of, 807n
Hyperinsulinemia, in LGA preterm
infants, 821
Hyperkalemia, in neonate, 740
calcium gluconate for, 792
Hypermagnesemia, in neonate, from
maternal medication, 341,
769
respiratory signs of, 688g
Hypermenorrhea, 100
Hypernatremia, in preterm infants,
apnea and, 749
Hyperosmolar solutions, infusion of,
necrotizing enterocolitis and,
837, 839n
Hyperparathyroidism, neonatal
hypocalcemia risk and, 821
Hyperperistalsis
in neonate, as intestinal obstruction sign, 700g
sign of in initial prenatal exam,
223g
Hyperphosphatemia, in SGA neonate, 766n
Hyperplasia, from hydrops fetalis, 26
Hyperpnea, signs of in initial prenatal
exam, 220g
Hyperprolactinemia, infertility and,
118
Hyperreflexia
in neonate, with kernicterus, 824
with PIH, 341
interventions for, 338–39
with severe preeclampsia, 341
Hyperresonance of chest, assessing
neonate for, 698g
Hypersalivation (ptyalism), 198
Hyperstat (diazoxide), neonatal
effects of, 769
Hypertension, pregnancy and. *See
also* Pregnancy-induced hypertension
birth center screening for, 618
chronic, 347
as CST indication, 375
estriol determinations for, 379,
380
indicated induction of labor for,
587
danger signs of, 240g
in diabetic clients, 316
early termination of pregnancy for,
384
estriol determinations for, 379
as hemorrhage risk, 569

during labor, first stage, 428g
late or transient, 347
medications for, effects on neonate
of, 769
as methylergonovine maleate risk,
903d
neonatal problems associated with,
769
placental infarcts and calcifications
with, 574
placental insufficiency from, betamethasone increases, 547
placental transport affected by,
171
as polygenically inherited, 145
postpartal diuresis after, 905
at postpartal home visit, 624
resuscitation risk with, 786
as risk factor, 214t
as ritodrine contraindication, 549
signs of in initial prenatal exam,
216g
sodium intake and, 273
spontaneous abortion caused by,
329
subarachnoid block contraindicated by, 525
Hyperthermia, in neonate
from aganglionosis, 869
oxygen dissociation curve and,
643
as phototherapy complication,
832n
preterm, apnea associated with,
749
responses to, 648
Hyperthyroidism (thyrotoxicosis), in
pregnancy, 201, 218g, 321,
326
as CST indication, 375
in neonate, eyelids with, 693g
Hypertonia, in neonate, 657
in LGA infant, from birth trauma,
756n
with RDS, 797t
Hypertonic labor patterns, 537, 537f
Hypertonus, prolonged declerations
caused by, 456
Hypertrophy of clitoris, assessing
female neonate for, 701g
Hypertrophy of right ventricle, in tetralogy of Fallot, 887f, 890
Hyperventilation
from blood loss anxiety, 570
in labor, 409, 428g, 478n
for PPH syndrome, 817
in pregnancy, 197
signs and symptoms of, 478
Hyperviscosity, in LGA neonates,
761
Hypervolemia of pregnancy, 340
Hypnoreflexogenous method, 295–
96
Hypnosis, in childbirth, 293, 295–96
Hypocalcemia, in neonate, 821–22
apnea from, 749
calcium gluconate for, 792
diagnosis and treatment of, 821–
22
hypoglycemia differentiation from,
818
IDM, 768
interventions for, 821–22
IUGR and risk of, 370
narcotic withdrawal vs., 771
PPH syndrome with, 817
as prematurity risk, 749
preterm, monitoring for, 754n
as RDS risk, 807n
as ritodrine side effect, 549
SGA, 762, 764n, 766n
tremors with, 685, 703g

Hypochloremia, in neonate, 816
Hypoextension, assessing in neonate, 682
Hypofibrinogenemia
  from abruptio placentae, 563
  interventions for, 563
  from prolonged retention of dead fetus, 561
Hypoglossal nerve, assessing in neonate, 695g
Hypoglycemia
  maternal
    from diabetes, 214t, 318, 319t
    fetal breathing pattern affected by, 636
    pregnancy and, 323
    starvation ketosis from, 316
    symptoms of, 319t
  neonatal, 818–21
    apnea from, 749
    assessing for, with MAS, 815
    with Beckwith syndrome, 867
    as betamethasone risk, 547
    body position as sign of, 702g
    cardiac medications in mother and, 769
    cold stress and, 817, 818
    crying with, 682, 688g
    defined, 818
    dextrose in delivery room for, 792
    feeding to prevent, 716, 740
    with hydrops fetalis, 826
    hyperbilirubinemia risk with, 822, 823
    in IDM, 763, 768
    interventions for, 818–21, 819–20p
    IUGR and risk of, 370
    jaundice and, 831
    as LGA risk, 761
    motor activity and, 654
    narcotic withdrawal vs., 771
    pathophysiology of, 818
    as postmaturity risk, 760
    PPH syndrome with, 817
    prematurity and, 740, 748, 749
      monitoring for, 754n
    as RDS risk, 807n
    risk factors for, 214t, 215t, 736f
    as ritodrine side effect, 549
    SGA, 762, 763, 764n, 765–66n
    signs of, 817
    skin color with, 689g
    as terbutaline sulfate side effect, 548
    tremors with, 685, 703g
Hypokalemia
  as furosemide side effect, 894
  from hyperemesis gravidarum, 328
  from pica, 282
  from intestinal obstruction, 873
  as ritodrine side effect, 548, 549
Hypomagnesemia, in SGA neonate, 766n
Hypomenorrhea, 100
Hyponatremia, in neonate
  cardiac disease in mother and, 769
  from intestinal obstruction, 873
  preterm, apnea associated with, 749
Hypoparathyroidism, in IDM, 768
Hypophosphatasia, prenatal diagnosis of, 147
Hypophyseal cachexia (Sheehan syndrome), 988
Hypoplasia
  assessing neonate for, 697g
  from congential CMV, 358

with diaphragmatic hernia, 866
  of tooth enamel, from hemolytic disease, 827
Hypoplastic lungs (Potter syndrome), ventilation problems with, 788
Hypoproteinemia
  from aganglionic megacolon, 869
  from intestinal obstruction, 873
Hypospadias, 60
  assessing male neonate for, 684, 700g
  infertility from, 111t, 112
Hypotension, maternal
  from amniotic fluid embolism, 576
  from anesthesia during pregnancy, 351
  as bromocriptine side effect, 925, 926d
  fetal distress from, 540n, 539n
  from hemorrhage, 570, 571n
  with induction
    interventions for, 593n
    as water intoxication sign, 590, 593n
  as isoxsuprine side effect, 548
  in labor, 408, 409
    fourth stage, 502
    interventions for, 576
  as pulmonary embolism sign, 981, 983, 984n
  after regional anesthesia, 522–23n
    epidural, 519
    peridural block, 518
    subarachnoid block, 526
    subarachnoid block contraindicated by, 525
Hypotension, neonatal
  DIC and, 837
  IVH risk and, 836
  as PPH complication, 817
  risk factors for, 736f
  as ritodrine side effect, 549
Hypothalamic pituitary complex (gonadostat), maturation of, 91, 92, 92f
Hypothalamus
  female reproductive cycle role of, 96
  neonatal temperature control role of, 646
  puberty role of, 91, 92, 92f
Hypothermia
  maternal, thromboembolic disease risk with, 980
  neonatal
    apnea associated with, 749
    from congenital herpes, 359
    hyperbilirubinemia risk with, 822, 823
    importance of preventing, 647
    with intraventricular hemorrhage, 836
    as Leboyer bath risk, 618
    maternal medications and, 513, 648
    with necrotizing enterocolitis, 838, 839
    oxygen consumption increased by, 647
    oxygen dissociation curve and, 643
    as phototherapy complication, 832n
    PPH syndrome with, 817
    prematurity and, 749
    with RDS, 797f
    risk factors for, 736f
    as SGA risk, 765
    skin pallor with, 689g
Hypothrombinemia, from hyperemesis gravidarum, 328

Hypothyroidism
  maternal
    fetal mortality and, 321
    fetal tachycardia caused by, 451
    infertility and, 111t, 321
    postdelivery galactorrhea and, 987
    pregnancy and, 326
    signs of in initial prenatal exam, 217g, 218g, 220g
    spontaneous abortion and, 201
  neonatal
    breast-feeding for, 718
    congenital, 831, 859
    hair texture with, 692g
    hyperbilirubinemia risk with, 823
    jaundice and, 831
    newborn screening for, 150, 725
Hypotonia, in neonate
  with congenital hypothyroidism, 859
  from congenital toxoplasmosis, 357
  with hypoglycemia, 818
  with intraventricular hemorrhage, 836
  with kernicterus, 824
  maternal medications and, 512, 513
Hypovolemia. See also Blood loss
  maternal
    from abruptio placentae, 564
    CVP to assess, 571n
    from hyperemesis gravidarum, 328
    physiological effects of, 569
    PIH and, 336
    postpartal management for, 346
    as ritodrine contraindication, 549
    sign of at postpartal home visit, 624
    subarachnoid block contraindicated by, 525
    supine hypotensive syndrome and, 409
    with PIH, 336
  neonatal
    assessing for, 688g
    hemorrhage as cause of, 644
Hypovolemic shock
  DIC with, in Sheehan syndrome, 988
  from ectopic pregnancy, 333
Hypoxemia
  fetal
    late decelerations caused by, 454
    tachycardia caused by, 450
  in neonate
    with bronchopulmonary dysplasia, 816
    cold stress aggravated by, 817
    iatrogenic, after suctioning, 814p
    with PPH syndrome, 817
    as prematurity risk, 738, 739
    with RDS, 794
Hypoxia
  fetal
    from abruptio placentae, 563
    adverse long-term outcomes and, 459
    asphyxia leads to, 786
    from brow presentation, 552
    CST to monitor, 375
    developmental delays caused by, 146

from dysfunctional labor, 214t, 536
    fetal heart rate and, 171, 450, 452, 454
    glycogen stores used with, 648
    induction-tetanic contractions and, 425t
    from iron deficiency anemia, 327
    as IUGR risk, 762
    during labor, blood sampling to assess, 461–63, 462f
    labor medications and, 511
    with MAS, 798
    with maternal cardiac decompensation, 311
    from maternal drug abuse, 360
    meconimium staining from, 387, 572
    nonstress test results with, 373
    as oligohydramnios risk, 577
    as oxytocin risk, 590, 594n
    after paracervical block, 516
    physiologic effects of, 594n
    from PIH, 341
    with precipitous labor, 543
    preterm infant hematology and, 748–49
    from prolonged or difficult labor, risk of, 214t
    after regional anesthesia, 516, 523n
    as ritodrine side effect, 549
    from smoking, 268
    umbilical blood flow and, 171
  maternal
    fetal breathing pattern affected by, 636
    fetal distress care for, 540
    placental transport affected by, 171
    with pulmonary embolism, 985n
    signs of in initial prenatal exam, 224g
    of uterine muscle cells in labor, pain from, 411
  neonatal
    apnea from, 749
    bilirubin level rises with, 649
    brown fat metabolism prevented by, 648
    cerebral bleeding caused by, 830
    from diaphragmatic hernia, 861
    DIC and, 837
    difficulty of recognizing, 643
    hypocalcemia risk increased with, 821
    intraventricular hemorrhage from, 836
    with MAS, 798, 814
    necrotizing enterocolitis from, 837
    postterm, seizures from, 760
    posture with, 689g
    with RDS, 794f, 794–95, 796t
    during suctioning, 805n
    with tetralogy of Fallot, 890
    from transpositon of the great vessels, 891
    prematurity and, 748–49
    ventilatory assistance indicated by, 800t
Hysterectomy
  for cervical cancer during pregnancy, 352
  after hydatidiform mole, 335
  for placenta accreta, 579
  for puerperal infection, 979n
  for severe abruptio placentae, 564
  after uterine rupture, 550
Hysterosalpingography, 117, 128

Hysteroscope, 128
Hysterotomy
    as abortion method, 130t, 131
    as induction of labor contraindi-
        cation, 587

I-messages, 290
Ice chips
    after cesarean delivery, 603
    during labor, 474, 476, 478, 483
Ice packs
    for episiotomy relief, 596
    during lactation suppression, 925
    perineal pain relief with, 916
    for postpartal hematoma, 973
ICSH (interstitial cell-stimulating hor-
    mone), 93
Icterus, assessing in neonate, 689g.
    See also Jaundice
Icterus gravis, 347
    risk factors for, 215t
Icterus neonatorum. See Physiologic
    jaundice
Identical twins, 185, 557
Identification procedures, 499n
    confirming at nursery admission,
        709
    with precipitous delivery, 505
Identity vs. role confusion, 40t, 41
IDM. See Infant of diabetic mother
Idoxuridine (IDU), for neonatal her-
    pesvirus, 844
IgA immunoglobulins
    colustrum contains, 654
    function of, 654
    in neonate, 653, 654
IgG immunoglobulins
    in neonate, 653, 654
    preterm infants lack, 748
IgM immunoglobulins, in neonate,
    653, 654
    with congenital herpesvirus infec-
        tion, 844
    with congenital syphilis, 844
    neonatal values, implications of,
        654
    sepsis and, 842
IGTT (Intravenous glucose tolerance
    test), 317–18
Ileal atresia in neonate, 873. See also
    Intestinal obstruction
Ileostomy care, for meningomyelo-
    cele infant, 881
Ileus, in neonate
    meconium, 873
    necrotizing enterocolitis effect on,
        837, 838, 839
    paralytic, after meningocele/men-
        ingomyelocele surgery, 883n
Iliac crest, 65
Iliococcygeus muscle, 66, 67t, 67f
Ilium, 65
Illness, in neonate
    fluid requirements increased by,
        717
    signs of, 729
Ilotycin. See Erythromycin
Imagery, as crisis intervention, 997–
    98
Immobility
    postpartal discomfort from, 915
    thromboembolic disease risk with,
        983
Immunity
    breast-feeding and, 925, 927
    cellular, suppressed during preg-
        nancy, 170
    in neonates, 653–54
    placental role in, 170
Immunizations
    age to begin, 654
    in pregnancy, 265, 266t

Immunoassay pregnancy tests, 194
Immunoglobulins
    breast-feeding and, 718, 925
    with congenital syphilis, 844
    development of, 653–54
    with herpesvirus type 2 infection,
        844
    in preterm infants, 748
Immunologic infertility, 111t, 117
Impaired glucose tolerance (IGT),
    314, 314t, 315
Imperforate anus, in neonate, 871f,
    871–72
    assessing for, 684, 702g
    incidence of, 871
    prognosis, 872
Imperforate hymen, dysmenorrhea
    from, 100
Impetigo, assessing, 690g
Implantation, 162–63, 163f
    cellular differentiation after, 163–
        65, 164, 166f
    in ectopic pregnancy, 333, 334f
    endometrial changes at, 99, 100f
    progesterone and, 169
Impotence, gender identity insecurity
    and, 89
Impregnation, postcoital position and,
    74
In vitro fertilization, 9, 11, 119
Inclusion cysts, on neonate's gums,
    681
Incompetent cervix. See Cervix,
    incompetent
Incomplete (footling) breech presenta-
    tion, 555f
    umbilical cord prolapse danger
        with, 554
Incontinence, with meningomyelocele,
    880, 882
Increment phase of contractions,
    404, 404f
Incubator, radiation heat loss in, 646
India, ancient, obstetrics in, 3
Indifferent stage, 57
Indigestion, as impending labor sign,
    416
Indirect Coomb's test, 347, 348
Indomethacin, for patent ductus
    arteriosus, 885
Induction of labor. See Labor,
    induced
Induction-tetanic contractions, as
    intrapartal risk factor, 425t
Industry vs. inferiority, 40t, 41
Indwelling catheter, for bladder over-
    distention, 982, 986
Infant care, by parents of high-risk
    neonates, 774–80
Infant of diabetic mother (IDM), 763,
    768
    breast tissue in, 661
    congenital anomaly assessment
        for, 757n
    hematologic considerations in,
        748–49
    hypocalcemia risk in, 821
    hypoglycemia in, 761, 763, 768,
        818
    as LGA neonates, 760, 761
    polycythemia in, 835
    PPH syndrome in, 817
    problems in, 763, 768
    RDS risk in, 792
    risk classification for, 734, 736f
    transient tachypnea of newborn in,
        797
    transposition of great vessels in,
        891
Infant feeding. See Feeding
Infant mortality. See also Neonatal
    mortality

    from coarctation of the aorta, 889
    from endocardial cushion defects,
        888
    health care practices and, 206–7
    inferential considerations, 23
    risk of, birth weight and, 758
    statistics about, 23, 25t
Infant nutrition. See Feeding; Nutri-
    tion, for neonates
Infants. See Neonates
Infarcts, placental, 574
Infarction, intestinal, with necrotizing
    enterocolitis, 837
Infection, fetal
    as drug addiction risk, 770
    IUGR associated with, 762, 763
    as preterm labor cause, 548
    as prolonged labor risk, 542
    tachycardia caused by, 450
Infection, maternal, 353–60. See also
    specific infection
    amnionitis, risk of, 425t
    as amniotomy risk, 587, 589
    as betamethasone side effect, 547
    as cesarean complication, 600,
        605
    danger signs of, 240g
    death from, 206
    fetal breathing pattern affected by,
        636
    infertility from, 111t
    intrapartal
        as forceps delivery indication,
            597
        labor induction to prevent, 593n
        at labor onset, 428g
        signs of, 473
    pelvic/fallopian tube anatomy and,
        82
    perinatal mortality caused by,
        546
    as placenta previa risk, 566
    placental, transport affected by,
        170–71
    postpartal, 973–76, 975t
        assessing for, 624, 919n, 945–
            47g
        causes of, 974–76
        danger signs after discharge,
            941
        evaluating incisions or lacer-
            ations for, 912
        interventions for, 975, 976,
            977–80n
        localized, 974–75, 975t, 977–
            79n
        nursing diagnoses, examples,
            980
        preventive care, 918–19n
    as prolonged labor risk, 541,
        542
    from retained placental frag-
        ments, 972, 973
    signs of in lochia, 904, 911
    temperature with, 906
    vital signs as indicator of, 912–
        13
    as preterm labor cause, 548
    as PROM risk, 425t, 546, 547
        interventions for, 546, 546f
    resuscitation risk with, 786
    with Sheehan syndrome, 988
    signs of
        in initial prenatal exam, 216g,
            218g, 220g
        in subsequent prenatal exams,
            239g
        spontaneous abortion caused by,
            329
    TORCH group of, 357–60
    umbilical, in initial prenatal exam,
        223g

Infection, in neonate. See also specific
    infections
    abdominal, signs of, 699g, 700g
    acquired immunity to, 654
    congenital, clinical manifestations
        of, 766–67
    ear, signs of, 696g
    in eyes, assessing for, 680, 693g,
        694g
    hemolytic anemia caused by, 835
    hyperbilirubinemia risk from, 823
    IUGR associated with, 761
    motor function with, 703g
    nasal swelling and erythema with,
        695g
    with necrotizing enterocolitis, 840n
    preterm, susceptibility to, 754n
    preventing, 842
        anti-infective properties in feed-
            ing, 719t
        breast-feeding for, 717–18
        breast milk, cow's milk, and for-
            mula compared for, 719t
        after cleft lip surgery, 856n
        as nursing priority, 498n
        interventions for, 498–99n
        with out-of-hospital emergency
            birth, 505–6
        with RDS, 797, 808n
    as PROM risk, 425t
    with RDS
        assessing for, 807n, 808n
        preventing, 797, 808n
    risk factors for, 736f
        maternal nutrition and, 185
        prematurity as, 654, 748
    sepsis neonatorum, 841–42
    SGA, 765n, 766–67n
    signs of in pharynx, 696g
    tachycardia as sign of, 688g
    temperature with, 677, 688g
    tremors with, 703g
    urethral, assessing for, 701g
    urine odor with, 700g
    vaginal, 701g
Inferential statistics, 20–21
Inferior strait. See Pelvic outlet
Infertility, 110–20
    from amenorrhea, 100
    defined, 110
    factors affecting, 83, 110–11,
        111t
    fallopian tube dysfunction and, 83
    from hypothyroidism, 326
    in vitro fertilization, 9
    male role in, 59, 64
    management of, 113f, 118–20
        nurse's role in, 119–20
    of nursing mothers, 904–5
    ovum transport and, 98
    from pernicious anemia, 279
    preliminary investigation of, 111–
        14, 113f
    primary vs. secondary, 110
    psychological reasons for, 83
    statistics about, 111
    sterility vs., 110
    tests for, 113f, 115–18
    thyroid dysfunction and, 215t, 321
    uterine anomalies and, 77
    with Sheehan syndrome, 988
Influenza immunization, in pregnancy,
    266t
Informed consent, nursing role and,
    15
    admission in labor and, 466
Infundibulopelvic ligament, 81f, 82,
    82f, 83
Infundibulum (fimbria), 82, 82f, 83
Infusion pump
    for heparin administration, 981
    for insulin administration, 320

Infusion pump (Cont'd)
  for magnesium sulfate administration, 345, 346
  for oxytocin administration, 346, 589, 590d
    in contraction stress test, 376
    to diabetic, 321
  for preterm infant tube feeding, 742, 745
  for RDS feeding, 806-7n
Inguinal creases, assessing in neonate, 703g
Inguinal hernia, assessing neonate for, 700g
Inguinal ligament tenderness, as salpingitis sign, 223g
Inhalation anesthetics, obstetric use of, 529
Inheritance, patterns of, 142-46
  alternatives to risks from, 151-52
  autosomal dominant, 142-43, 142f
    AID as alternative to, 152
  autosomal recessive, 143f, 143-44, 147-48
    AID as alternative to, 152
    counseling for, 151
  cleft lip and palate, 851
  genetic counseling referral and, 151
  of metabolic disorders, 857
  nongenetic conditions, 145-46
  polygenic, 145
    AID as alternative to, 152
    amniocentesis for, 148
    postnatal diagnosis of, 149, 150
  postnatal diagnosis and, 148-50
  prenatal diagnosis and, 146-48
  Pierre Robin syndrome, 850
  single-gene, 142-45
  X-linked dominant, 145
  X-linked recessive, 144, 144f
    AID as alternative to, 152
    amniocentesis for, 147
Initiative vs. guilt, 40t, 41
Injectable contraceptives, 125, 127
Injection site bleeding, as DIC sign, 568
Inlet. See Pelvic inlet
Innervation
  of female reproductive system
    breasts, 85
    clitoris, 73
    fallopian tubes, 83
    labia majora, 72
    ovaries, 83, 84
    uterus, 80
  of vagina, 75
  of vaginal vestibule, 73
  of male reproductive system
    penis, 60, 60f
    scrotum, 61
    testes, 62
    vas deferens, 63
    sexual response pathways, 104-5
Innominate bones, 65
Insomnia, as hyperthyroidism sign, 326
Inspection, fetal position assessed by, 441
Insulin
  for pregnant diabetic, 320, 322
    administering, 320
    in labor, 321
    postpartum, 325
  pregnancy changes in, 201
  pregnancy requirements for, 202, 314
  role of, 313-14
  teaching administration of, in pregnancy, 318

Insulin pumps, 320
Insulin-dependent diabetes mellitus (IDDM), 314, 314
Intellectual impairment, from congenital herpes, 359. See also Learning disabilities; Mental retardation
Intensity of contractions, 404, 404f, 405
Intensive care, for puerperal peritonitis, 980n
Intensive care nursery
  goals of, 733
  for Pierre Robin syndrome care, 851
  parent involvement in, 774-77, 1009, 1009f, 1013f, 1013-14
Interactional approach to family studies, 41
Intercostal muscles, neonatal breathing with, as respiratory distress sign, 639
Intercostal retraction, assessing in neonate, 682
Intermittent positive pressure breathing (IPPB), 531
Internal hemorrhage. See Hemorrhage
Internal organ abnormalities, ears as indicator of, 681
Internal os, 77f, 78
Internal or podalic version, 585-86
Internal rotation, of fetus during labor, 414f, 414-15
Interphase
  in meiosis, 158, 159f
  in mitosis, 158, 158f
Interstitial cell-stimulating hormone (ICSH), 93
Interstitial cells of Leydig, 61, 92f, 93
Interstitial glands of pregnancy, 196
Interstitial pulmonary emphysema, as respiratory therapy complication, 809n, 816
Interventions. See also Nursing interventions
  abruptio placentae, 563-64
  aganglionic megacolon, 870-71
  amniotic fluid embolism, 576
  anemia in neonate, 835
  in antepartal care, 286-92
  bladder exstrophy, 874-75
  breech presentation, 554-55
  brow presentation, 552-53
  cardiac disease with pregnancy, 311-13
  cesarean birth facilitation, 942
  cleft lip and palate, 852
  clubfoot, 876
  coarctation of the aorta, 889
  congestive heart failure, 894
  crisis. See Crisis intervention
  diaphragmatic hernia, 866-67
  DIC, 567-68
  for drug addiction in pregnancy, 361-62
  family care, 50-52, 51f, 49-50
  fetal hydrocephaly, 557
  FHR variable decelerations, with long cord, 575
  gonorrhea in pregnancy, 355
  hemolytic disease of the newborn, 825p, 827f, 827-30m 829-30f
  hemorrhage, postpartal, 972, 973
  herpesvirus infection in neonate, 844
  herpes infection in pregnancy, 359-60
  hip dysplasia, 878

hydatidiform mole, 335
hydramnios, 577
hyperemesis gravidarum, 328
hyperthyroidism in pregnancy, 326
hypertonic labor, 537
hypothyroidism in pregnancy, 326
hypotonic labor, 541-42
imperforate anus, 872
infertility, 112, 113f, 114-20
intestinal obstruction in neonate, 873-74
intraventricular hemorrhage, 836-37
iron deficiency anemia in pregnancy, 327
labor anesthesia reactions, 516
for labor pain, 483-86
labor stress, 536
for malpositions, 550, 551-52
megaloblastic anemia in pregnancy, 327
meningocele/meningomyelocele, 880-81, 882-84n
for monilial vaginitis in pregnancy, 355-56
neonatal hyperbilirubinemia, 823
omphalocele, 867-68, 869f
patent ductus arteriosus, 881, 885
persistent pulmonary hypertension (PPH), 817
Pierre Robin syndrome, 850-51
PIH, 338-39n, 342-44, 345d
polycythemia in neonate, 836
post-cesarean gas pain, 941
postpartal hematomas, 973
postpartal hemorrhage, 578-80, 972, 973
postpartal infections, 975, 976, 977-80n
  of urinary tract, 986
precipitous labor, 504-5, 543-44
preeclampsia; see PIH
for pregnancy discomforts
  ankle edema, 254t, 256
  backache, 255t, 258f, 258
  breast tenderness, 254t, 255
  constipation, 255t, 258
  dyspnea, 255t, 259
  faintness, 255t, 259
  heartburn, 254t, 256
  hemorrhoids, 255t, 257
  increased vaginal discharge, 254t, 256
  leg cramps, 255t, 259
  nasal stuffiness, 252, 254, 254t
  nausea and vomiting, 252, 254t
  ptyalism, 254, 254t
  urinary frequency, 254t, 254-55
  varicose veins, 255t, 256-57, 257f
pregnant diabetic, 318-21, 322-25n
in prenatal group discussions, 291-92
preterm labor, 548-50, 549d
prolonged labor management, 542
PROM, 546f, 546-47
pulmonary embolism, 982, 984-85n
pulmonary stenosis, 890
RDS, 795, 797, 798f, 799-800t, 801-10n, 811-14p
retained placental fragments, 972, 973
Rh sensitization, 349-50, 350p
sickle cell anemia in pregnancy, 328
spina bifida, 880-81
spontaneous abortion, 332-33
surgical. See Surgery
syphilis in pregnancy, 354

talipes equinovarus, 876
tetralogy of Fallot, 890, 891f
tracheoesophageal atresia/fistula, 861
transverse lie, 556
Trichomonas infections, 356
umbilical cord prolapse, 574-75
umbilical cord vasa previa, 575
urinary tract infections, in puerperium, 986
uterine atony, 579
uterine inversion, 579-80
venous thrombosis, 980, 981, 983-84n, 985n
Interventricular septal defects, vulnerability to, 183t
Intestinal atresia. See Intestinal obstruction
Intestinal bleeding signs, in initial prenatal exam, 228g
Intestinal gas, after cesarean delivery, 941
Intestinal infarction, with necrotizing enterocolitis, 837
Intestinal injury, as cesarean complication, 605
Intestinal necrosis, from MAS, 815
Intestinal obstruction
  in fetus, amniotic fluid density and, 384
  in mother
    in initial prenatal exam, 222g
    from pica, 282
  in neonate, 872-74
    from aganglionic megacolon, 869, 870
    descriptions of, 872-73
    with diaphragmatic hernia, 866
    differential diagnosis, 873
    hyperbilirubinemia risk with, 823
    hyperperistalsis with, 700g
    interventions for, 873-74
    signs of, 753, 873
Intestinal rupture, from meconium ileus, 873
Intestines. See Gastrointestinal system
Intimacy vs. isolation, 40t, 41
Intra-amniotic injection, for abortion, 129, 130t
Intracervical contraceptive devices, 124
Intracortical calcification, with nevus flammeus, 677-78
Intracranial bleeding, in neonate, 836-37. See also Intracranial trauma
  apnea from, 749
  cold stress aggravated by, 817
  as LGA risk, 761
  as SGA risk, 762
  from vaginal breech delivery, 554
Intracranial calcifications, from congential toxoplasmosis, 357
Intracranial hemorrhage. See Intracranial bleeding
Intracranial pressure, signs of, 678, 692g, 756
Intracranial trauma, in neonate. See also Intracranial bleeding
  as prolonged labor risk, 425t
  pupils with, 694g
Intrapartal fetal assessment, 424, 431g, 441-63, 473-80n
  before amniotomy, 586-87
  with fetal distress, 538n
  fetal position, 441-42, 442f
  fetal presentation, 431g, 441-42, 442f
  with induction of labor, 591n

at labor admission, 469, 472
methods of, 443g, 443–50, 445t, 446f, 449f
with regional anesthesia, 521n, 522, 523n
Intrapartal maternal assessment, 424–41, 472n
abruptio placentae, 563
assessment guide, 428–32
with fetal distress, 538n
history, 424–25, 425t
with induction of labor, 591n
at labor admission, 473
labor status, 430–31g, 432t, 433–34, 436–40p, 437–40f, 440–41, 441f
malposition, 551
physical, 425–34, 436–41
pelvic adequacy, 426–27, 426f, 427f, 427g, 432–33, 433–34f, 578
precipitous labor risk assessed in, 543
psychologic, 433, 435g
before ritodrine administration, 549
uterine contractions, 430g, 432t, 433–34
Intrapartal mortality . See Perinatal mortality
Intrapartal nursing management. See also Labor; Delivery
of cardiac client, 312–13
with regional anesthesia, 522–24n
relinquishing mother, 1015t
resuscitation risk factors, 786–87
sepsis neonatorum prevention with, 842
Intrauterine asphyxia, identifying risk of, 375. See also Asphyxia
Intrauterine death. See Fetal death; Perinatal mortality
Intrauterine devices (IUDs), 121f, 124f, 124–25
diabetes and, 319
infertility from, 110, 111t, 112
in initial prenatal exam, 226g
postpartal insertion of, 944
Intrauterine growth retardation (IUGR). See also Small-for-gestational-age neonates
adolescent pregnancy and, 305
assessing for, 223g, 237
as CST indication, 375
cardiac disease in mother and, 768, 769
causes of, 370, 761–62
cesarean delivery for, 600
from chronic uteroplacental insufficiency, 455
classifications of, 370
congenital malformations associated with, 762
estriol determinations for, 379, 380
estriol excretion patterns with, 380
identifying, ultrasound for, 368, 368f, 369f, 369–70
incidence of, 370, 761
induction of labor for, 587
long-term outcome and needs, 762–63
from maternal alcohol abuse, 269, 361t, 362
maternal diabetes and, 316
from maternal drug abuse, 360, 361t
from maternal hypertension, 769
monitoring fetuses with, 375
from nutritive deficit, 374
patterns of, 762

from placental insufficiency, oligohydramnios with, 577
postterm pregnancies with, 758, 759t, 759–60
proportional vs. disproportional, 762
risk factors for, 214–15t
risks associated with, 370
as ritodrine contraindication, 549
from rubella, 358
sickle cell anemia and, 328
smoking as cause of, 268
symmetric vs. asymmetric, 762
timing delivery with, 370
Intrauterine hemorrhage. See Hemorrhage
Intrauterine infection. See Infection
Intrauterine manipulation, risks with, 973
Intrauterine organ systems, 165–71
Intrauterine surgery, 8–9, 11
Intrauterine transfusion, 349, 350p
Intravascular thromboses, with homocystinuria, 859
Intravenous antibiotics, for puerperal infections, 976, 979n
Intravenous feeding. See Total parenteral nutrition
Intravenous fluids
for abruptio placentae, 564
after cesarean delivery, 603
for hemorrhage, 571n
for hematoma, third stage labor, 580
as hypotonic labor intervention, 541
for neonates, umbilical arterial catheterization for, 811p
with oxytocin infusion, 589, 590
for placenta previa, 565p, 566, 567
postpartal hemorrhage prevention with, 972
for prolonged labor, 536, 542
for puerperal pyelonephritis, 986
puerperal urinary problems from, 982
with regional anesthesia in labor, 521n
for epidural anesthesia reaction, 519
importance of, 528
headache lessened by, 524n
for hypotension, 522n, 523n
for severe preeclampsia, 343
Intravenous glucose tolerance test (IGTT), 317–18
Intraventricular hemorrhage (IVH), in neonate, 836–37
as prematurity risk, 749
retrolental fibroplasia risk with, 815
Introductory Notes on Lying-in Institutions . . . (Nightingale), 6
Introitus, vaginal, 71f, 73
assessing in fourth trimester, 947g
dilatation of in second stage, 418, 419f
umbilical cord prolapse out of, 574–75
Introversion, as pregnancy emotion, 204
Intubation
endotracheal, with Pierre Robin syndrome, 851
for RDS, 804–6n
suctioning with, 805–6n, 812–14p, 813f
tracheal, for pulmonary embolism, 985n

Invasive hemodynamic monitoring, with eclampsia, 344
Invertogram roentgenogram, for imperforate anus assessment, 872
Involution of the uterus, 67, 901–3, 902f
Iodine
in hypothyroid pregnancy, 326
lactation requirements, 270t
placental transport of, 170
pregnancy changes in levels of, 201, 326
pregnancy requirements, 270t, 273
protein-bound, estrogens and, 93
as teratogen, 267t
Iodoform packing, for puerperal wound drainage, 978n
Ionized plasma electrolyte, normal preterm infant values, 752t
IPG. See Occlusive cuff impedance phlebography
IQ scores
fetal alcohol syndrome affects, 770
midforceps deliveries and, 598
prematurity affects, 758
Irish Americans, pain expression among, 469–70
Iritis, in secondary syphilis, 354
Iron. See also Iron supplements; Iron-deficiency anemia
absorption of, vitamin C and, 274
in breast milk, cow's milk, and formula, 719t
deficiency of in infant
irritability with, 719
as prematurity risk, 748
with tetralogy of Fallot, 890
food sources of, 274
lactation requirements, 270t
neonatal requirements, 717, 717t
physiologic anemia of infancy and, 644
placenta stores, 170
placental transport of, 170
pregnancy requirements, 198, 201, 270t, 273–74
neonatal iron stores and, 648
Iron supplements
assessing need for, fourth trimester, 947g
breast-feeding and, 717–18
in formula, 718
for neonatal anemia, 835
postpartal, 913
in pregnancy, 270t, 274
Iron-deficiency anemia
adolescent pregnancy and risk of, 297
in neonates, 644, 835
pica and, 281–82
in pregnancy, 327
Irritability
maternal
as labor response, 483
with severe PIH, 341
neonatal
with congenital syphilis, 844
with hydrocephalus, 880, 882
with hypoglycemia, 817, 818
as iron deficiency sign in infant, 719
as jaundice sign, 831
with necrotizing enterocolitis, 838, 839
from vitamin D overdose, 275
Ischemia
in mother
abdominal, danger sign of, 240g
of organs, with DIC, 567

of pituitary gland, abruptio placentae and, 564
in neonate
as MAS complication, 815
with necrotizing enterocolitis, 837–38, 839–40n
after tracheoesophageal surgery, 861
Ischemic sloughing of the rectum, 872
Ischial spines, 65, 66f
Ischiocavernosus muscle, 67f, 68
Ischium, 65
Islets of Langerhans, pregnancy stresses, 202
Isoimmune hemolytic disease. See Hemolytic disease of the newborn
Isoimmunization
preterm labor with, 548
resuscitation risk and, 786
Isolation
for congenital syphilis, 844
for neonatal herpesvirus infection, 844
with sepsis neonatorum, 842
Isoproterenol (Isuprel), for MAS, 815
Isoxsuprine (Vasodilan), for preterm labor, 548
Israel, communal family structure in, 34
Isthmus
of fallopian tube, 82, 82f
mucosal layer in, 83
of uterus, 77, 77f, 78
Italian Americans, pain expression among, 469
Itching
from genital herpes simplex, 359
from monilial vaginitis, 355
postmenopausal, 101
pruritis gravidarum, 199
from trichomonas vaginitis, 356
IUDs. See Intrauterine devices
IUGR. See Intrauterine growth retardation
IVH. See Intraventricular hemorrhage

Japanese American families
cultural patterns in, 45–46
food practices of, 282t
Jaundice, maternal
from gallbladder disease, 351
from hyperemesis gravidarum, 328
in sclerae, from sickle cell anemia, 327
Jaundice, in neonate, 822–24. See also Hyperbilirubinemia
ABO incompatibility as cause of, 826
assessing, 677, 689–90g, 824, 831n
breast-feeding and, 718
causes of, 677
with congenital herpes, 359
with congenital syphilis, 844
with congenital toxoplasmosis, 357
dehydration and, 831n, 833–34n
as distress sign, 714
from drug addiction, 771
early identification of, 832n
exchange transfusion for, 833n
with extended rubella syndrome, 358
from fetal vitamin A overdose, 275
with hemolytic disease of the newborn, 824
with herpesvirus infection, 359, 844

Jaundice, in neonate *(Cont'd)*
  with hydrops fetalis, 826
  in-home management of, 831n
  nursing care plan, 831–34
  nursing diagnosis examples, 834
  pathologic, 823–24
  phototherapy for, 832–33n
  physiologic, 648–50
  as prematurity risk, 748
  preventing, 831–32n
  prolonged, with hypothyroidism, 859
  with RDS, 796t
  risk factors for, 736f
  sulfonamides as cause of, 267
Jaw, assessing, in prenatal exam, 219g
Jejunum, development of, 651
Jerkiness, in hypoglycemic neonate, 818
Jewish families
  health care behavior in, 43
  lactose intolerance among, 281
  pain expression among, 469
  prenatal nutrition for, 282t, 283–84
  Tay-Sachs disease and, 152
Jitteriness, in hypocalcemic neonate, 821
"Johns Hopkins Case" 10
Johnson, V. E., on sexual response, 102, 103–5
Joint Commission on Accreditation of Hospitals (JCAH), 15
Joints
  assessing, in prenatal exam, 224g
  of neonate
    edema over, with congenital syphilis, 844
    fetal alcohol syndrome affects, 362, 770
    pain in
      postpartal, 915
      from sickle cell anemia, 327
Jones, K. L., 770
Josten, L., parenting assessment guide by, 999, 1000–1001t
Jugular vein, pulmonary embolism sign in, 981, 983
Juvenile-onset diabetes, 314

Kanamycin, for sepsis neonatorum, 842
Kaplan, D., on preterm birth, 1006
Kaplan, D. M., on prematurity as maternal crisis, 773
Karmel, Marjorie, 294
Karotypes, 135–36, 135f, 136f
  of balanced translocation carrier, 139f
  normal male and female, 135f
  of trisomy 21, 137f
  of Turner syndrome, 141
Kegel's exercises, 263, 264f
  in childbirth preparation classes, 294
  pregnancy bladder problems prevented by, 255
Kelly clamp, in emergency delivery pack, 503
Kempe, C. H., on child abuse, 1015–16, 1016t
Kennell, J. H.
  on attachment process, 772, 773, 1011–12
  on maternal-infant separation, 1009
Kentucky Committee for Mothers and Babies, 7
Keratitis, with neonatal herpesvirus infection, 844
Kernicterus, 347, 823–24

assessing preterm infants for, 757n
from hemolytic disease of the newborn, 826
from hyperbilirubinemia, 826–27
long-term effects of, 826–27
from maternal medication, 353
risk factors for, 215t
Kernlute, neonatal jaundice assessment with, 831n
Ketamine (Ketalar, Ketaject), obstetric use of, 530
Ketoacidosis, in pregnant diabetic, 316, 320
Ketonuria
  increased with shock, 570
  at labor onset, 468
    implications of, 432g
  monitoring
    in hypertonic labor patterns, 537
    in prolonged labor, 542
  prenatal urine tests for, 317
Ketosis
  carbohydrate intake and, 201, 273
  during labor, 536
  starvation vs. diabetic, 316
Ketosteroids, testosterone converted to, 93
Ketostix, 317
Kidney disease, dysfunctional labor with, 536
Kidneys
  of fetus, creatinine levels show maturity of, 386–87
  of mother
    assessing in prenatal exam, 225g, 229–30g
    postpartal elimination role of, 905
    pregnancy changes in, 197t, 199
  of neonate
    assessing, 683, 700g
    development and function of, 652–53
    displaced, assessing, 700g
    dysfunctional, skin texture with, 690g
    enlarged, localized flank bulging with, 699g
    formula-feeding and, 718
    MAS damage to, 815
    meningomyelocele and, 880
    polycystic, 700g
    preterm, physiology of, 746–47
Kilocalories, defined, 270
Kin network, 32, 33f
Kite method of wedge casting, 876
Kjelland forceps, 597, 597f
Klaus, M. H.
  on attachment process, 772, 773, 1011–12
  on maternal-infant separation, 1009
Klebsiella
  puerperal infections from, 974, 986
  sepsis neonatorum from, 841
Kleihauer-Betke test, 349
  neonatal anemia assessment with, 835
Klein, C., on single parents, 1018
Klinefelter syndrome, 141, 141f, 701g
Knee jerk, in neonate, 657
Knee-chest position
  decreases malposition discomfort, 551
  with umbilical cord prolapse, 574
Krabbe's disease, prenatal diagnosis of, 148
Krause corpuscles, in clitoris, 73

Kübler-Ross, E., 119
  on anticipatory grief, 1002
  on death during labor or delivery, 1005
Kupperman or rat hyperemic test, 195
Kyphosis, in initial prenatal exam, 224g, 225g

La Leche League, 924, 930
Labia majora, 71f
  anatomy of, 72
  assessing in initial prenatal exam, 225g
  development of, 59, 653
  of neonate, assessing, 684, 701g
  postpartal hematoma of, 973
  sexual response of, 103t
Labia minora (nymphae), 71f, 72
  anatomy of, 72
  development of, 59, 653, 653f
  maldevelopment or fusion of, 72
  of neonate, assessing, 684, 701g
  sexual response of, 103t
Labor
  with abruptio placentae, 563, 564
  acceleration phase during, 417, 417f
    disorders of, 544, 544t
  active phase, 417f, 417–18; see also first stage
    hypotonic uterine motility in, 541
    normal progress, 470t
    nursing care plan, 475–77
    prolonged, malposition as cause of, 551
  admisssion management, 466–69
  adolescent in, 467, 471, 482
  ambulation during, 474, 617
  analgesia. See Analgesia
  anesthesia in. See Anesthesia
  anxiety about, 247
    fetus affected by, 511
    managing, 484
  arrested, 544t, 545; see also obstructed
    plane of least importance and, 70
    x-ray examination for, 387–88
  assessing contraction intensity in, 404–5
  attendants at
    culture and, 411–12, 471
    options for, 613
  augmented, 589, 590d
    electronic monitoring with, 447
  biochemical interaction in, 407
  at birth center, 618–19
  blood pressure changes in, 409
  Braxton Hicks contractions before, 415
  of cardiac client, 312–13
  cardiac output changes in, 408–9
  cardinal movements in, 414f, 414–15
  cardiovascular system changes in, 408–9
  cerivcal changes before, 415
  childbirth preparation for. See Childbirth preparation
  comfort measures during, 483–84
  complications during
    effects on family of, 580–81
    in neonatal assessment, 660
    neonatal lung congestion and, 637
    powers as causes of, 536–51
    in preterm nursing care plan history, 750
    psyche as cause of, 535–36

contractions, 78, 404f, 404–5. See also Uterine contractions
  assessing intensity of, 404–5
  biochemical interaction in, 407
  characteristics of, 404f, 404–5
  energy source for, 407
critical factors in, 395–406
  passage, 395, 396–97, 397f
  passenger, 395, 397–404, 398–403f
  powers, 395, 404f, 404–5
  psyche, 395, 405–6
crowning, 418
cultural considerations in, 469–71
deceleration phase of; see also first stage
  adolescent in, 471
  disorders of, 544, 544t
  normal progress, 470t
  nursing care plan, 477–79
defined, 395
delivery in same room as, 613. See also Delivery
of diabetic client, 321, 325
dilatational disorders of, 544, 544t
drug addiction and, 362
duration of, in neonatal assessment, 660
dysfunctional, 536
  caput succedaneum after, 678
  cesarean delivery for, 600
  as diabetes risk, 316
  fetal conditions associated with, 536
  from fetal macrosomia, 556
  Friedman's classification of, 544t, 544–45
  hypertonic, 537, 537f
  hypotonic, 537, 541–42, 541f
  implications of, 536
  incidence of, 544–45
  intervention principles for, 536–37
  malposition as cause of, 551
  maternal implications of, 541
  from oligohydramnios, 577
  from pathologic retraction rings, 545, 545f
  patterns of, 537, 541–45, 544t
  postpartal hemorrhage risk with, 972
  prolonged; see prolonged
  psychic causes of, 535–36
  resuscitation risk with, 786
  from transverse lie, 556
  uterine atony with, 579
  x-ray pelvimetry for, 432
emotional component of, 405–6; see also psyche in; responses to
  anxiety, 247, 484, 511
  electronic monitor and, 459–60
  during first stage, 417, 418
engagement, 402f, 402–3, 403f
  assessing, 439f, 439–40p
evaluating progress of, 430g, 432t, 433–34, 436, 437–41f, 470t
  at admission, 472
  cervical dilatation, 430g, 432t, 434, 436–37p, 437f, 439f, 440–41, 441f
  cervical effacement, 430g, 434, 436–37p, 437f
  CPD assessment as part of, 578
  fetal descent, 430g, 434, 436–40p, 438–39f, 440–41, 441f
  in first stage active phase, 475n
  in first stage deceleration phase, 477n

Friedman graph for, 434, 440–41, 441f
membranes, 430–31g, 434, 436p, 437f, 439f
in nursing care plan, 473–80
in prolonged labor, 542
in second stage, 479n
uterine contractions, 430g, 432t, 433–34
expulsive stage of; see second stage
false, sedatives during, 513
false vs. true, 415, 416, 416t
fatigue from, pain response and, 413
fetal death during, crisis intervention for, 1005. See also Perinatal mortality
fetal head in, 398f, 398–99, 399f
fetal monitoring during. See Electronic fetal monitoring
fetal position in, 401f, 403–4
fetal problems in
　developmental abnormalities from, 556–57
　malpositions, 551–52
　malpresentations, 552–56, 552–56f
　multiple pregnancy, 557–60, 559f
fetal response to. See Intrapartal fetal assessment
first stage; see also active phase; deceleration phase; latent phase
　adolescent in, 471
　described, 416, 417f, 417–18, 432t
　duration of, 417, 417f
　normal progress, 470t
　nursing care plan, 472–79
　oxytocin augmentation during, 590
　pain during, 410–11, 412f, 474, 476, 477–78n
　primary power in, 404
　prolonged; see prolonged
　regional pain relief during, 513–14. See also specific relief measures
　sedatives during, 513
fluid and electrolyte balance in, 409
fourth stage
　complications of, 578–80
　defined, 416
　described, 420
　management of, 500–502, 502f. See also Postpartal nursing management
　nursing care plan, 481
　oxytocin during, 590
gastrointestinal system changes in, 409
high-risk
　adolescence and, 482
　electronic fetal monitoring for, 444, 458–59
　hydration during, 409
hypertonic patterns of, 537, 537f
hypoactive, from malpositions, 551, 552
hypotonic patterns of, 537, 541–42, 541f
hypoxia during, developmental delays from, 146
impending, signs of, 242g, 415–16, 416t
induced, 587–95
　for abruptio placentae, 563, 572n

amniotic fluid embolism with, 576
by amniotomy, 586, 588–89
assessing readiness for, 588, 588t
baseline data before, 589, 591, 592
contraindications, 587–88
defined, 587
in diabetic client, 321
elective vs. indicated, 587
electronic monitoring with, 434, 444, 447
failure of, 593n
fetal/neonatal implications of, 9, 425t
inadequate response to, 592–93n
maternal implications of, 9, 425t
methods used for, 588–89, 590
mismanagement of, uterine rupture from, 550
nursing care plan, 591–95
oxytocin infusion for, 589, 590d
pain during, 592n
with pelvic contractures, 578
PG gel for, 595
with PIH, 346
for placenta previa, 567
postpartal hemorrhage risk with, 972
precipitous, 543
prelabor scoring system, 588, 588t
after PROM, 546, 546f, 547
prostaglandin administration for, 595
as risk factor, 425t
after rupture of membranes, 416
uterine atony with, 579
informed consent during, 15
initiation of; see onset of
intraabdominal pressure in, 408
iron deficiency anemia and, 327
latent phase of, 417, 417f; see also first stage
　normal progress, 470t
　nursing care plan, 472–75
　pain during, 474n
　prolonged; see prolonged
lightening before, 415
maternal assessment during. See Intrapartal maternal assessment
maternal systemic response to, 408–13
medications during, neonatal hypothermia and, 648
mechanics of, 414f, 414–15
modesty during, 467, 475
mortality during. See Perinatal mortality
nursery retains record of, 709
nursing care plan, 472–82
nursing role in, 466, 470t. See also Intrapartal nursing management
obstructed; see also arrested
　CPD as cause of, 578
　from hydrocephaly, 557
　pathologic retraction rings from, 545
　uterine rupture from, 550
onset of
　admission procedures, 466–69
　causes of, 202, 406–7
　with eclampsia, 344
　signs of, 242g, 415–16, 416t
out-of-hospital, unplanned, 505–6

pain during, 410–13, 410–12f; see also responses to
　active phase, 476n
　culture and, 469–71, 510
　deceleration phase, 477–78n
　fatigue increases, 413
　hydramnios increases risk of, 425t
　hypertonic patterns increase, 537
　induced, 592n
　latent phase, 474n
　management of, 406, 482–86, 510. See also Analgesia; Anesthesia; Psychoprophylaxis
　nursing care plan for, 474, 476, 477–78, 480
　from oligohydramnios, 577
　physiologic basis for, 80, 411
　precipitous labor and management of, 543
　second stage, 418, 480n
　self-esteem and, 406, 413
　as stress factor, 535–36
parenteral fluids during, 409
passage role in, 395, 396–97, 397f, 525
passenger in, 398–404, 398–403f, 525
pelvic dimensions affect, 68–71
pelvic division disorders in, 544, 544t
phase of maximum slope during, 417, 417f
physiology of, 406–8
with PIH , 344, 346
placental transport affected by, 171
positions during, 474n, 475, 479n, 483, 614–17, 515–17f
　alternative, 614–17, 615f, 617f
　for cardiac client, 312–13
　for diabetic client, 321
　for fetal distress, 538, 540, 560, 594n
　first stage active phase, 475
　for hypertonic labor patterns, 537
　for hypotension, 593n
　induced, 593n, 594n
　late decelerations caused by, 451t, 454
　for malpositions, comfort with, 551
　with PIH, 346
　preterm, 549
　after regional anesthesia, for FHR decelerations, 456
　for ritodrine administration, 549
　second stage, 479n
　for umbilical cord prolapse relief, 540n, 574
　variable decelerations improved by, 456
positive experience of, 406
post-saline abortion, 131
postterm, defined, 210
powers in, 404f, 404–5, 525
　complications caused by, 536–51
　precipitous, 542–44, 543f, 544t
　as oxytocin risk, 589, 590
　defined, 425t, 542
　factors contributing to, 542–43
　fetal/neonatal implications of, 425t, 543
　induction to prevent, 587
　as intrapartal risk factor, 425t
　maternal implications of, 425t, 543
　postpartal risks from, 908t
premature, 547–50

causes of, 548
defined, 210, 547
fetal/neonatal implications of, 425t
as intrapartal risk factor, 425t
maternal implications of, 425t
medications for, 548–50, 549d
as multiple gestation risk, 425t
preventing, RDS prevention by, 795, 797
as PROM risk, 546
uterine anomalies and, 77
preparatory division disorders of, 544, 544t
preparation for. See Childbirth preparation
preterm; see premature
progress of; see evaluating progress of
prolonged, 542
　abnormal presentation and, 425t
　acetone in urine after, 906
　anxiety as reason for, 482
　birth center transfer for, 618
　from breech presentation, 554
　caput succedaneum after, 678, 691g
　causes of, 542
　from CPD, 578
　defined, 542
　exhaustion from, interventions for, 536
　from face presentation, 553
　fetal/neonatal implications of, 425t, 542
　Friedman's classifications of, 544, 544t
　implications of, 536
　incidence of, 542, 545
　as intrapartal risk factor, 425t
　labor patterns resulting in, 537, 541–42
　from malpositions, 551
　MAS associated with, 798
　maternal implications of, 425t, 541, 542; see also postpartal risks from
　neonatal implications of, 425t, 542, 678. 691g, 798
　from occiput-posterior postion, 551
　with oligohydramnios, 577
　oxytocic agents after, 903, 903d
　pelvic inlet contractures and, 578
　postpartal risks from, 903, 908t, 913, 977, 983
　psychic causes of, 535–36
　puerperal infection risk from, 913, 977
　tachycardia after, 906
　thromboembolic disease risk with, 983
　from transverse arrest, 551
　from transverse lie, 556
　underweight and, 214t
　uterine involution affected by, 903
　as vacuum extraction indication, 598
　x-ray examination for, 387–88
psyche in, 405–6, 525; see also emotional component of; responses to
　complications caused by, 535–36
pushing role in, 408
record of, 709
respiratory system changes in, 409

Labor (Cont'd)
  responses to, 470t; see also
      emotional component of; psy-
      che in
  assessing, 435g
  coping mechanisms, 405, 406
  resuscitation risk identification in,
      786–87
  ripening of cervix before, 415
  risk factors in, 425, 425t, 734
  round ligaments during, 81
  rupture of membranes before,
      415–16
  second stage. See also Delivery
    adolescent in, 471
    cardiac output changes in,
        408–9
    described, 416, 418–19,
        419f
    disorders of, 544, 544t
    emotions in, 418
    epidural anesthesia and, 520
    forceps delivery to shorten, 597
    normal progress, 470
    nursing care plan, 479–80
    oxytocin augmentation in, 590
    pain during, 411, 412f
    perineal signs of, 429g
    primary power in, 404
    pudendal block effects during,
        527
    regional pain relief methods dur-
        ing, 514, 523n. See also spe-
        cific methods
  sibling attendance at, 613–14
  sickle cell anemia and, 328
  spontaneous, contraindications to,
      587
  stages of, 416–20. See also specif-
      ic stages
  station, 402–3, 403f
  sterile technique during, impor-
      tance of, 842
  stress factors in, 425t
  support during, 405–6, 470t
    analgesia and, 511
    environment and, 613
  third stage
    abnormal bleeding in, from cir-
        cumvallate placenta, 574
    complications of, 578–80
    described, 416, 419, 420f
    genital tract trauma in, 580
    hemorrhage in, 578–79
    pain during, 411, 412f
    management of, 497,500
    nursing care plan, 480–81
    oxytocics in, 497, 500, 590
    retained placenta in, 579
    uterine atony in, 579
    uterine inversion during, 579–
        80
  transient blood pressure elevation
      in, 347
  transition; see deceleration phase
      of
  trial
    limit of, 578
    pelvic contractures and, 578
    prerequisites for, 606
    as repeat cesarean alternative,
        606
  tumultuous, amniotic fluid embo-
      lism with, 576
  uterine contractions during; see
      contractions
  vomiting in, 409
  x-ray examination during, 387–88
Labor coach. See also Father;
    Husband; Partner
  delivery room preparation by,
      479n

support for, in hypertonic labor
    patterns, 537
Laboratory evaluations. See also spe-
    cific tests
  before abortion, 129
  amniotic fluid opitcal density, 384,
      384f
  before cesarean delivery, 601
  congenital syphilis, 843–44
  for conjunctiva pallor in neonate,
      694g
  before contraception, 120
  with cystitis, puerperal, 986
  for diabetic client, 316–18, 319t,
      320
    pregnancy diabetes and, 322
  of DIC, 567
  of ectopic pregnancy, 333
  estriol determinations, 379–81
  with fetal distress, 538
  of fetal lung maturity, 385–86
  fetal scalp pH, 451t, 461–63.
      462f
  for fetal status, with Rh senstiza-
      tion, 349
  fourth trimester, 946g, 947g
  group B streptococcus in neonate,
      843
  hemolytic disease of the newborn,
      826
  hemorrhage, 569
  of human placental lactogen (hPL),
      381
  for hyperthyroidism, 326
  of hypothyroidism, 326
  for IDM, 768
  before induction, 591n
  in infertility workup, 113f, 114
  at labor onset, 431–32g, 468,
      469, 472
  lecithin/sphingomyelin (L/S) ratio,
      385, 385f
  lung profile of amniotic fluid, 385–
      86, 386f
  for mastitis, 987
  metabolic disorders, 857–59
  for mixed FHR decelerations,
      451t, 457
  necrotizing enterocolitis, 839n
  neonatal anemia, 835
  neonatal hematology, 644–45,
      645t
  neonatal hyperbilirubinemia assess-
      ment, 824
  neonatal hypoglycemia monitoring,
      821
  for neonatal icterus, 689–90g
  neonatal jaundice, 831n
  neonatal screening tests, 725
  normal neonatal blood values,
      644–45
  at nursery admission, 711
  in nursery routine, 714
  in PIH assessment, 337
  for placenta previa, 566
  for postnatal genetic diagnosis,
      150
  postpartal, 906, 917n
  pregnancy changes in, 197t, 198,
      199
  pregnancy tests, 194–95
  in prenatal exams
    EKG, 222g
    hemoglobin, 327
    initial, 216g, 223g, 228–30g
    subsequent, 239–40g
    ultrasound, 223g
  for preterm infants, 750n
    normal values, 752t
  after PROM, 546, 547
  puerperal infections, 976, 977
  pulmonary embolism, 982, 983

for RDS, 801n
  with regional anesthesia, 521n
  for Rh sensitization, 347, 348, 349
  risk identification with, 733
  with ritodrine administration,
      549
  sepsis neonatorum, 841–42
  for SGA neonates, 764n
  with severe preeclampsia, 343
  thromboembolic disease, 983
  tracheoesophageal atresia/fistula,
      862
  urinary tract infections, 353, 354
  vaginal bleeding, 575
Labyrinthine disturbance, neonatal
    pupils with, 694g
Lacerations. See also Cervical lacer-
    ations; Vaginal lacerations
  assessing, fourth trimester, 947g
  hemorrhage risk from, 569, 579
  infection risk from, 974
  as oxytocin induction risk, 594n
Lacrimal glands, assessing in neo-
    nate, 694g
Lactalbumin, in breast and cow's
    milk, 719t
Lactate
  accumulation of, with RDS, 795
  normal neonatal blood values,
      645t
Lactation, 925. See also Breast-
    feeding
  abnormal, 987
  abruptio placentae and, 564
  amenorrhea from, 100
  betamethasone and, 547
  breast cancer during, 352
  diabetes and, 318
  establishment of, 905
    hospital policy and, 718
    facilitating onset of, 503
    failure of, with Sheehan syndrome,
        988
  infertility from, 111t
  nutrition during, 269, 270t, 913
    daily food plan, 271–72t
  suppressing, 480n, 919n, 925–26,
      926d
    thromboembolic disease and,
        980
Lactic acid
  normal neonatal blood values,
      645t
  vaginal environment role of, 75,
      76f
Lactiferous ducts, in breast, 84f, 85
Lactobacillus bifidus, breast milk con-
    tains, 717
Lactoferrin, breast-feeding and, 717–
    18
Lacto-ovovegetarians, pregnancy nu-
    trition for, 278–81
Lactose
  in breast milk, 717
  digestion of by neonate, 651
Lactose intolerance, 272, 281
Lactovegetarians, pregnancy nutri-
    tion for, 278–81
Ladd procedure, for volvulus, 873
Ladies' Obstetrical College, 6
Ladin's sign, 192, 193f
  in initial prenatal exam, 226g
Lamaze, Dr. Fernand, 294
Lamaze (psychoprophylactic)
    method, 293, 294–95, 475,
    476, 477
Laminaria
  for dilating os before abortion, 129
  ripening cervix with, 588
Lanolin, for sore nipples, 910, 931
Lanoxin. See Digoxin
Lanugo, 177t, 179t, 180–82

gestationl age and, 661, 662f,
    665f
  in meconium at birth, 651
  on preterm infant, 690g, 750
Laparoscopy, 73, 117–18, 11
  in ectopic pregnancy assessment,
      333
Laparotomy, 127–28
  for ectopic pregnancy, 334
  emergency, for uterine rupture,
      550
  for postpartal hematoma, 973
Large-for-gestational-age (LGA) neo-
    nates, 760–61
  categories of (Pr, F, Po), 734, 735f
  defined, 760
  disorders of, 761
  hypoglycemia in, 818, 821
  laboratory evaluations fo, 711
  from maternal diabetes, 316,
      757n, 763, 818
  methadone addiction and, 770
  nursing care plan for, 750–58
  preterm
    birth trauma risk in, 756–57n
    of diabetic mother, assessing,
        757n
    risk identification for, 734, 735–
        36f
Larynx, of neonate
  assessing, 688g
  brow presentation may damage,
      552
Laser surgery, for cervical cancer
    during pregnancy, 352
Laser treatments, for condyloma
    accuminata, 355
Lashes, assessing in neonate, 694g
Lasix. See Furosemide
Late adolescence, sexuality in, 90
Late decelerations. See Fetal heart
    rate
Late or transient hypertension, 347
Lateral positions. See Side-lying
    positions
Latex agglutination tests (Gravidex
    and pregnosticon slide test),
    194
Lavage, for continuous regurgitation,
    651
LDH, with SGOT, 983
Learning disabilities
  from congenital CMV, 358
  IUGR associated with, 763
  from kernicterus, 824, 826–27
  from maternal drug abuse, 361t
  maternal nutrition and, 185
  midforceps delivery and, 598
  prematurity and, 758
Leboyer method, 617–18, 955–56
Lecithin (phosphatidylcholine)
  in lung profile of amniotic fluid,
      385–86
  production of in fetus, 638–39,
      639f
  synthesis of by neonate, RDS and,
      794
Lecithin/sphingomyelin (L/S) ratio
  in diabetic client, 320
  fetal lung maturity and, 638–39
  risk identification with, 734
Left lateral recumbent position. See
    Side-lying positions
Leg cramps, 253f, 255t, 258–59,
    259f
  in deceleration phase labor, 478n
  described, 258
  after lightening, 415
Leg exercises, after cesarean
    delivery, 941
Leg recoil, gestational age and, 663f,
    672

Leg tremors, in deceleration phase labor, 478
Legal aspects of maternal-newborn nursing, 14–15
  child abuse and, 1015
Legs
  assessing, in prenatal exam, 224g
  edema of, as danger sign, 240g
  of neonate, assessing, 685, 703g. *See also* Leg recoil
  postpartal assessment of, 912, 919n
  postpartal thrombophlebitis in, 980–81, 981f
  varicose veins in, 198
Leif, H. I., sexual system by, 88–89
Leiomyoma, spontaneous abortion caused by, 329
Lejeune, J., trisomy 21 described by, 136
Length of neonate
  assessing, 675, 689g, 710
  average, 675
  preterm, adequate growth in, 747
Lenticular cataract, gestational age and, 183t
Leonardo da Vinci, 3
Leopold maneuvers, 431g, 441–42, 442f
  before auscultation of FHTs, 443
  brow presentation revealed by, 552
  face presentation detected by, 553
  before induction of labor, 591
Lesch-Nyhan syndrome, prenatal diagnosis of, 148
Lesions
  assessing in initial prenatal exam, 217g, 225g
  on neonate, from congenital syphilis, 844
Letdown reflex, 925
  nipple soreness alleviated by, 931
  warm shower stimulates, 937
Lethargy
  as puerperal infection sign, 976, 977
  in neonate
    from aganglionosis, 869
    with herpesvirus infection, 844
    as hypoglycemia sign, 817, 818
    as illness sign, 729
    with intraventricular hemor-rhage, 836
    with jaundice, 831
    with necrotizing enterocolitis, 838, 839
Leukemia, childhood
  extended rubella syndrome and,358
  pregnancy radiology linked to, 266
Leukocytes
  fetal development of, 644
  labor increases, 409
  neonatal production of, 644
  placental transfer of, 170
  pregnancy changes in production of, 197t, 198
  postpartal production of, 906
Leukorrhea (increased vaginal discharge)
  as pregnancy discomfort, 253f, 254, 255–56
  with subinvolution, 973
Levallorphan (Lorfan), 512
Levator ani muscle, 66, 67t
  labor changes in, 408
Levels of consciousness
  assessing, with severe pre-eclampsia 343
  of neonate. *See* Sleep-wake patterns

Leydig's (interstitial) cells, 61, 92f, 93
LGA neonates. *See* Large-for-gestational-age neonates
LH. *See* Luteinizing hormone
LH assays, in infertility workup, 115
LHRH (luteinizing hormone- releasing hormone), 96
Libido, postmenopausal, 102
Lidocaine (Xylocaine)
  for amniocentesis, 382
  for labor anesthesia, 514, 528
    paracervical block, 516
    pudendal block, 528
  for pulmonary embolism, 982
Lie, fetal, 399
Life cycle, family development stages in, 37–40
Ligaments
  Cooper's, in breast, 84f, 85
  ovarian, 81–82, 81f, 82f
  uterine, 74f, 76–77, 77f, 78f, 80–82, 81f, 82f
Light, neonatal motor activity and, 654
Light reflex, pupillary, neonate, 681, 694g
Lightening
  dyspnea relieved by, 259
  as impending labor sign, 415
Liley, A. W., hemolytic disease evaluation by, 384, 384f
Limbs
  assessing, in initial prenatal exam, 224g
  nongenetic abnormalities of, 145–46
    with fetal alcohol syndrome, 362, 770
  prenatal assessment of, 146
Lindemann, E., on crisis, 992, 999
Linea nigra, 193, COLOR PLATE
Linen change, as hypertonic labor intervention, 537
Linkage, in chromosomes, 160
Linoleic acid, as essential nutrient, 273
Lipase, fat absorption and, 651
Lips
  assessing, in initial prenatal exam, 220g
  of neonate, assessing, 681
Listening role of nurse. *See also* Counseling role of nurse; Supporting role of nurse
  after cesarean birth, 942
  crisis intervention, 996
Listerial infection, 356
  in pregnancy, 356–57
Listlessness, as neonatal illness sign, 729
Lithium, fetal/neonatal effects of, 361t
Lithotomy position, 235f
  Dewees advocated, 5
  for delivery
    alternatives to, 614–17, 615–17f
    disadvantages of, 614–15
  for intrapartal vaginal examination, 436p
  PIH and, 346
Live births, in U.S. and Canada, 21t, 25t
Live-birth order, birth rates by, 22, 22t
Liver
  of mother
    assessing in initial prenatal exam, 223g
    pregnancy effects on, 198–99

of neonate, 648–50
  assessing, 700g
  bilirubin conjugation role of, 822–23
  development of, 650
  enlarged, 700g. *See also* Hepatomegaly
  immature functioning of, jaundice from, 677
  MAS damage to, 815
  palpating, 683
  perfusion of, anatomic fibrosis from, 641
  preterm, problems with, 748
  role of, 648
Lobenstein, Dr. Ralph W., 7
Lobenstein School, 7
Local anesthesia
  allergy to, 515–16, 529
  for amniocentesis, 382
  for delivery, 528
    absorption of, 514–15
  for drug abusers in labor, 362
  for episiotomy and repair, 528, 528f
  toxic effects of, 514–16, 528
Lochia, 903–4
  amount discharged, 904, 911
  assessing, 481n, 501, 911, 917, 919n
    after cesarean delivery, 604
    in fourth trimester, 947g
    after precipitous delivery, 505
  composition of, 902, 903–4
  danger signs in, 941
  puerperal infections signs in, 919n, 975, 976, 977
  subinvolution signs in, 903, 973
Lochia alba, 904
Lochia rubra, 903
Lochia serosa, 904
Locomotion, congenital disturbances of, 875–81
Locus of gene, 142
Lofenalac, for PKU, 858
Logan bar, 855b, 855f
Longitudinal lie, 399
Lordosis, in initial prenatal exam, 224g
Lorfan (Levallorphan), 512
Loss. *See also* Grief process
  abortion and feelings of, 1014
  crisis intevention for, 999, 1002–1006,1004n
  defined, 999
  with relinquishment for adoption, 1014, 1015t
Love, components of, 103
Low backache in pregnancy, 200
Low birth weight
  cesarean delivery indicated by, 600
  as induction of labor contraindication, 587
  with Pierre Robin syndrome, 850
  risk factors for, 214–15t
    adolescent pregnancy as, 297
    multiple gestation as, 425t
    smoking in pregnancy as, 268
Low blood pressure. *See* Hypotension
Low spinal block. *See* Subarachnoid block
L/S ratio. See Lecithin/sphingomyelin ratio
LSD, pregnancy and, 361, 361t
Lubchenco, L. O., 661
Lubricants, infertility from, 111t, 112
Ludington-Hoe, S. L., 961
Lumbar epidural block, 514, 514f, 518f, 518–20

agent for, 519
  for cesarean delivery, 609
  failure of, 519
  maternal side effects, 346, 519–20
  prolonged decelerations of FHR after, 456, 458
  for surgical procedures in pregnancy, 351
  technique, 518f, 518–19
Lumbar sympathetic block, 514, 514f
Lumbodorsal lordosis, in pregnancy, 200, 200f
Lumbodorsal spinal curve, accentuated in pregnancy, 200, 200f
Luminal. *See* Phenobarbital
Lung collapse, in neonate
  with diaphragmatic hernia, 866
  from pneumothorax, 816
Lung compliance in neonates, 638
  RDS decreases, 794, 796t
  suction decreases, 805n, 813
  surfactant and, 637
Lung profile, assessing fetal lung maturity with, 385–86, 386f
Lung scan, pulmonary embolism assessment with, 983
Lungs
  of fetus
    development of, prematurity risk and, 737–39, 738f
    placenta assumes role of, 171
  of mother, assessing
    in initial prenatal exam, 220–21g, 231p
    at labor onset, 428g
  of neonate. *See also* Respiratory system
    assessing, 698g
    delay in clearing, reasons for, 637
    physiology of, 637–39
    preterm, 737–39, 738f
Luteinizing hormone (LH)
  anterior pituitary secretes, 96, 97f
  female reproductive cycle role of, 96, 97f, 98
  hCG cross reactions with, 194
  infertility and, 115
  male puberty role of, 92f, 93
  pregnancy role of, 202
  puberty role of, 92, 92f
Luteinizing hormone-releasing hormone (LHRH), 96
Luxation of hip joint, 877
Lymph nodes, fetal role of, 644
Lymphadenopathy
  inguinal, from genital herpes simplex, 359
  posterior cervical, from toxoplasmosis, 357
Lymphatic supply
  of breasts, 85, 85f
  of cervix, 80
  of fallopian tubes, 83
  of labia majora, 72
  of ovaries, 83
  of testes, 62
  of uterus, 80
  of vagina, 75
Lymphoblasts, in fetus, 644
Lymphocytes
  development of in fetus, 44
  in neonate, 644, 645
Lyon hypothesis, 140, 144

MacDonald's sign, 192
Machismo, pregnancy and, 205
Mackenrodt's (cardinal) ligaments, 82
Macroglossia, with Beckwith syndrome, 867

Macrophages, in colostrum, 717
Macrosomia, 556–57
  in IDM, 763, 763f
  fetal, uterine atony from, 579
  risk of, 214t
Magnesium
  in breast milk, cow's milk, and formula, 719t
  calcium intake and, 273
  lactation requirements, 270t
  neonatal requirements, 717t
  pregnancy requirements, 270t, 273
Magnesium sulfate, 338–39n, 344, 345d
  antidote for, 339
  FHR baseline variability caused by, 452
  in hyperactive labor, 543–44
  neonatal effects of, 341, 769
  nonstress test results after, 373
Magnesium trisilicate, as antacid during labor, 531
Mal aire, concept of, 205, 206
Malabsorption, as preterm risk, 741
Maladie de Roger, 885
Malaise
  as parametritis sign, 976
  as toxoplasmosis symptom, 357
Malays, pregnancy beliefs of, 206
Male frog test, 195
Male neonates
  aganglionosis in, 869
  assessing genitals of, 684, 700–701g
  bathing, 727
  circumcision of, 722, 723–24f
  cleft lip and palate in, 851
  clubfoot in, 875
  imperforate anus in, 871
  septicemia in, 841
  size of, 760
  transposition of great vessels in, 891
  ventricular septal defects in, 885
Male reproductive system, 59–64, 59–62f, 65f
  accessory glands, 63–64
  development of, 57–59, 58f, 92, 92f, 93
  external, 59–61, 59–61f
    in neonates. See Male neonates
  hormonal development in, 92, 92f, 93
  infertility causes in, 111t
  internal, 61–64, 62f, 65f
  maturation of gametes in, 160, 161f
  puberty changes in, 91–93, 92f
  sexual response in, 103–5, 104t
Male sterilization, 121f, 127, 127f
Males
  American Indian, status and role of, 45
  Asian American, status and role of, 46
  climacteric in, 101
  Mexican American, status and role of, 44
  neonates. See Male neonates
  pregnancy emotions of, 204
  sex chromosome abnormalities in, 141, 141f
  sexual identity development in, 88, 89
  sexual response in, 103–5, 104t
Malignancy. See also Cancer
  estrogen therapy and, 102
  hydatidiform mole and, 335
  of labia majora, lymphatics and, 72
Malmström vacuum extractor, 598

Malnutrition. See also Nutritional deficiency
  fetal
    as IUGR cause, 761, 762
    risk factors for, 214t
  amenorrhea from, 100
  infertility from, 111t
  neonatal
    from aganglionosis, 869
    anterior fontanelle overlap from, 678, 692g
  during pregnancy
    alcoholism and, 269
    from drug abuse, 360
    megaloblastic anemia and, 327
    PIH risk and, 336
    postpartal hemorrhage risk with, 972
    risk factors for, 214t
    spontaneous abortion caused by, 329
Malpositions. See Fetal position
Malpractice, cesarean delivery and, 600
Malpresentations. See Fetal presentation
Maltose, digestion of in neonate, 651
Mammary glands, pregnancy changes in, 197
Mandible, with Pierre Robin syndrome, 850–51
Mandibulofacial dysostosis. See Treacher Collins syndrome
Mania, with puerperal psychosis, 988
Manipulation and casting, for clubfoot, 876
Manning, F. A., 371
Manual conversion, for brow presentation, 552
Manual expression of breast milk, 930, 930f
  for caked breasts, 987
  engorgement relieved by, 937
  by working mothers, 938
Manual rotation, for transverse arrest, 551
Maple syrup urine disease (MSUD), 858
  newborn screening for, 150, 725, 766n
  prenatal diagnosis of, 148
March of Dimes Birth Defects Foundation, 780
Marfan syndrome, chest appearance with, 697g, 698g
Marginal blepharitis, 693g
Marijuana
  fetal/neonatal effects of, 361t
  infertility from, 112, 114
Marriage
  developmental stages in, 37–41
  sexuality in, 90
MAS. See Meconium aspiration syndrome
Masculinity, 88, 89
"Mask of pregnancy" See Chloasma
Mason, E. A., 773, 1006
Massage
  of breasts
    caked, 987
    for plugged ducts, 937
  of fundus
    in fourth stage labor, 501
    postpartal, 903, 911
    for uterine atony, 579
  of newborn, Leboyer method, 617
Mastectomy, during pregnancy, 352
Masters, W. H., on sexual response, 102, 103–5
Mastitis, 986–87, 987f
  assessing for, 941, 945g

Masturbation
  in adolescence, 89
  in childhood, 89
  clitoris as site of, 72
  in pregnancy, 265
Maternal age. See Age of mother
Maternal deprivation, 12
Maternal medication, danger sign of, 240g
Maternal morbidity
  from cesarean delivery, 605
  from infection, of, 974
Maternal mortality, 23, 25t
  from abruptio placentae, 563
  from amniotic fluid embolism, 576
  from automobile accidents, 352
  defined, 25
  from cardiac disease, 214t, 310, 311
  from cesarean delivery, 605, 606
  from diabetes mellitus, 314, 315, 316
  from drug abuse, 360
  federal programs to reduce, 5
  health care practices and, 206–7
  from hyperemesis gravidarum, 328
  inferential considerations, 23
  perinatal, risk of, 214t
  prolonged labor increases, 536
  puerperal peritonitis and, 980n
  from pulmonary embolism, 982
  from sickle cell anemia, 327
  from uterine rupture, 425t, 550
Maternal problems, risk factors for, 214–15t
Maternal sensitive period, 772
Maternicity, 961
Maternity care
  contemporary, overview of, 8–14
  ethical issues in, 10, 11
  family-centered, 31, 46–51
  legal aspects of, 14–15
  nursing role changes in, 13–16
  overview of, 8–14
  specialization affects, 10
  technologic advances, 8–10
Maternity Center Association, 7
Maternity girdle, 258
Maternity and Infant (M&I) Care Projects, 5
Maturational crisis, 246, 992
Mature milk, 925
Maturity-onset diabetes, 314
Mauriceau, François, 4
Maxillary hypoplasia, from fetal alcohol syndrome, 770
McDonald's method for measuring fundal height, 237, 237f
  in initial prenatal exam, 223g
McDonalds cerclage modification, 336
McLaughlin, M. K., 168
MCU (micturating cystourethrogram), 872
Measles, neonatal immunity to, 654
Measurements, conversions and equivalents,
Measurement of pelvis, 68–70, 69f, 70f
Measuring neonates, 675–76, 675f, 689g, 691g, 710
Meatus, urethral, assessing in neonate, 700–701g
Meckel diverticulum, bloody stool from, 874
Meconium
  absence of, from aganglionosis, 869
  fetal swallowing evidence in, 651
  formation of in utero, 651
  lack of, as distress sign, 714

Meconium aspiration. See also Meconium aspiration syndrome
  as drug addiction risk, 360, 361t, 771
  from maternal hypertension, 769
  meconium staining of amniotic fluid and, 425t
  as postmaturity risk, 759
  risk factors for, 736f
  as SGA neonatal risk, 765
Meconium aspiration syndrome (MAS), 798, 814–15
  clinical course of, 798, 814
  complications of, 815
  management of, 814–15
  mortality from, 815
  pneumothorax from, 816
  PPH syndrome with, 817
  preventing, 812–13p, 813f, 814–15
Meconium ileus, 873
Meconium peritonitis, 873
Meconium plug syndrome, 870, 873
Meconium staining of amniotic fluid
  as abruptio placentae sign, 563
  amniocentesis shows, 387
  amnioscopy to identify, 387
  as asphyxia sign, 538
  assessing for
    with hemorrhage, 572
    with oxytocin induction, 594n
  birth center transfer for, 618
  clinical significance of questioned, 387
  as drug addiction risk, 770
  fetal/neonatal implications of, 425t
  with induction, 590, 594n
  as intrapartal risk factor, 425t
  with MAS, 798. See also Meconium aspiration syndrome
  maternal implications of, 425t
  from maternal withdrawal, 360
  neonatal skin color from, 689g
  with placenta previa, 566
  with postmaturity, 760
  resuscitation risk with, 786
  umbilical cord discoloration from, 700g
Medical disorders in pregnancy, 328–50. See also specific disorders
Medical history. See History
Medications. See also Drug guides; Drugs
  amenorrhea from, 100
  breast-feeding and, 930–31, 932–35t, 718
  for cancer during pregnancy, 352
  for cardiac client, 312, 313
    effects on fetus of, 768–69
  after cesarean, breast-feeding and, 603
  childbirth preparation and, 27, 510
  for chlamydial infections, 355
  congenital heart defects from, 881
  for DIC, 567
  estriol excretion patterns affected by, 380
  fetal apnea and, 371
  fetal death danger from, 240g
  fetal lung maturity acceleration with, 547
  FHR variability caused by, 452
  for gonorrhea in pregnancy, 355

for herpes infection in pregnancy, 359, 360
for hyperemesis gravidarum, 328
for hypertension, during pregnancy, 347; see also for PIH
neonatal effects of, 769
for hyperthyroidism in pregnancy, 326
infertility from, 111t, 112, 114
for infertility management, 118–19
IUGR associated with, 761
during labor
for cardiac client, 313
fetal bradycardia from, 452
fetal tachycardia caused by, 450, 451
hyperactive, 543–44
neonatal brown fat metabolism and, 648
neonatal hyperbilirubinemia and, 823
optional vs. routine, 613
preterm, 548–50, 549d
prolonged labor caused by, 542
for labor pain relief, 510–13, 512d
prenatal education reduces need for, 27, 510
for lactation suppression, 489, 919n, 925, 926d
for listeriosis in pregnancy, 357
maternal, affects on infant of, 930–31, 932–35t
for monilial vaginitis, 355–56
for neonates
for alcohol withdrawal, 770
for congestive heart failure, 888, 894
for drug withdrawal, 771
hyperbilirubinemia and, 823, 830
jaundice and, 831
over-the-counter, 729
for patent ductus arteriosus, 885
preterm, excretion problems in, 746–47
resuscitative, 788, 789t, 792, 793d
umbilical arterial catheterization for, 811p
nonstress test results after, 373
for PIH, 338–39n, 344, 345d; see also for hypertension
placental transport of, 170
for postpartal pain relief, 915, 916, 917n
safety with, 729–30
for severe preeclampsia, 344
for syphilis in pregnancy, 354
as teratogens, 184, 266–68, 267t
metronidazol (Flagyl), 356
podophyllin, 355
for thromboembolic disease, 981, 982, 983
for Trichomonas infections, 356
for urinary tract infections in pregnancy, 353
Mediterranean families, thalassemias and, 152
Medulla, ovarian, 83
Megacolon, aganglionic, 699g, 868–71, 869f
Megakaryocytes, development of, 644
Megaloblastic anemia, as pregnancy complication, 326, 327
Meiosis, 158–59, 159f, 161f
at fertilization, 161f, 162
mitosis vs., 158–59
Melzack, R., 410
Membranes, rupture of. See Rupture of membranes

Membranous urethra, 63, 64
Men. See Males
Menadione, given to infants, 275. See also Vitamin K
Menarche, 91, 91f
average age of, 94
factors affecting, 296
Mendelian inheritance, 142–45
Mendelson syndrome, 531
Meningitis
developmental delays caused by, 146
from late-onset listeriosis, 357
in neonate
bulging fontanelles with, 692g
from group B streptococcus, 843
meningocele/meningomyelocele and, 879, 880
neck stiffness with, 697g
as spinal anesthesia complication, 526
Meningocele
clinical manifestations of, 880, 882
described, 878, 879, 879f
interventions for, 880
Meningomyelocele
clinical manifestations of, 880, 882
clubfoot and, 876
described, 878–79, 879f
hydrocephaly from, 691g
interventions for, 880–81, 882–84n
nursing diagnoses, examples, 884
ultrasound to detect, 368, 370
Menopause, 101–2
physical aspects of, 101–2
physiological reason for, 84
positive pregnancy test and, 192t
premature, 84
psychologic aspects of, 101
Menorrhagia, 100
Menses. See Menstruation
Menstrual cycle, 94–100. See also Female reproductive cycle; Menstruation
breast changes in, 85
duration of, 94
endometrium in, 79
hormonal role in, 93, 94
ovarian ligament role in, 81–82
postpartal resumption of, 904–5
as uterine cycle, 96
Menstrual extraction, as abortion method, 129, 130t
Menstrual history
in adolescent pregnancy assessment, 303
in ectopic pregnancy assessment, 333
infertility and, 112
Menstrual problems, from contraception, 124, 125, 127
Menstruation. See also Menstrual cycle
absence of (amenorrhea), 100
cessation of, at menopause, 101–2
components of, 95
duration of, 94
abnormal, 100
excessive (menorrhagia), 100
hormonal role in, 93, 94
painful (dysmenorrhea), 100
Mental function, hyperthyroidism affects, 326
Mental illness
genetic counseling referral for, 151
as polygenically inherited, 145
Mental retardation
alcoholism as cause of, 362, 770
chromosomal abnormalities and, 136f, 136–41

from congenital CMV, 358
from congenital rubella, 358
ears as indicator of, 681
federally funded care to prevent, 5
from galactosemia, 859
genetic causes of, 134
genetic counseling referral for, 151
homocystinuria as cause of, 859
with hydrocephalus, 880
from hypothyroidism, 215t
breast-feeding prevents, 718
from kernicterus, 824, 826
from listeriosis, 357
neonatal screening for, 725, 857, 858, 859
nonspecific, prenatal diagnosis and, 148
parental reactions to, 1010
PKU as cause of, 331t, 857–58
from SGA neonatal hypoglycemia, 763
sex chromosome abnormalities and, 141
Meperidine hydrochloride (Demerol)
during labor, 510, 512, 512d
fetal apnea increased by, 371
hypotonic labor patterns from, 541
neonatal brown fat metabolism affected by, 648
with PIH, 346
for pulmonary embolism, 982
Mepivacaine (Carbocaine)
delivery anesthesia with, 528
labor anesthesia with, 514, 516
toxic reactions to, 515
Mercer, R., on adolescents' developmental tasks, 297, 298–99t
Merthiolate, for omphalocele, 868
Mesoderm, 165, 165t, 166f
Mesonephric ducts, 57, 58f
Mesosalpinx, blood supply in, 83. See also Broad ligament of uterus
Mesovarian ligament, 81f, 83
Messick, J. M., crisis paradigm by, 994, 995f
Metabolic acidosis. See also Acidosis
fetal
late decelerations of FHR and, 375
supine hypotensive syndrome and, 409
maternal
blood loss leads to, 570
as ritodrine side effect, 549
neonatal
asphyxia leads to, 786
with cold stress, 817, 818
from diaphragmatic hernia, 861, 866
drug therapy for, 792, 793d
from intestinal obstruction, 873
with intraventricular hemorrhage, 836
with MAS, 798, 814
maternal hypertension and, 769
prematurity and, 746
with RDS, 794f, 795, 806n
Metabolic alkalemia, sign of in initial prenatal exam, 229g
Metabolic activities of placenta, 170
Metabolic alkalemia, sign of in initial prenatal exam, 229g
Metabolic disorders, 857–59
apnea associated with, 756
assessing SGA neonates for, 766n
as autosomal recessively inherited, 144
genetic counseling referral for, 151
infertility from, 111t
IUGR associated with, 761

kidney dysfunction, skin texture with, 690g
neonatal hypoglycemia vs., 818
neonatal screening for, 150, 725
as prematurity risk, 738
prenatal diagnosis of, 147–48, 734
Tay-Sachs disease, 143–44
Metabolism
maternal, pregnancy changes in, 197t, 200–201
endocrine balance and, 314
hPL and, 202
neonatal
brown fat role in, 647
hyperthermia increases, 648
Metacentric chromosomes, 157, 157f
Metachromatic leukodystrophy, prenatal diagnosis of, 148
Metaphase
in meiosis, 158, 159f
in mitosis, 158, 158f
Metastatic tumors of the placenta, 568
Metatropic dwarfism, prenatal diagnosis of, 146–47
Methadone maintenance, fetal/neonatal effects of, 360, 361, 361t, 770–72
Methemaglobinemia, from maternal hypertension, 769
Methicillin, for sepsis neonatorum, 844
Methoxyflurane (Penthrane), 529
Methyldopa, for chronic hypertension in pregnancy, 347
fetal apnea increased by, 371
Methylergonovine maleate (Methergine), 903, 903d, 911
for postpartal hemorrhage control, 500
for postpartal hemorrhage prevention, 972
for subinvolution, 973
Methylmalonic aciduria, prenatal diagnosis of, 148
Metritis/endometritis. See Endometritis
Metronidazol (Flagyl), as teratogenic, 356
Metrorrhagia, 100
Mexican American families
cultural patterns in, 44
pregnancy and, 205, 206, 288–89t
feeding customs, 925
labor customs, 412, 469, 470
lactose intolerance among, 281
modesty among, 471
neonatal hair patterns in, 692g
pain expression among, 470
percent of population, 43, 44t
prenatal nutrition for, 282t, 283–84
sample menus, 283–84
postpartal customs, 914
Michelangelo Buonarroti, 3
Microbiologic studies, postnatal diagnosis with, 150
Microencephaly
assessing neonate for, 678, 691g
from congenital CMV, 359
from congenital toxoplasmosis, 357
prenatal diagnosis of, 146
Micrognathia
assessing, 692g
described, 850
from fetal alcohol syndrome, 770
gestational age and, 183t
with Pierre Robin syndrome, 850–51

Microorganisms, placental transfer of, 170
Micropenis, in neonate, 700g
Microphthalmia
   from congenital toxoplasmosis, 357
   gestational age and, 183t
   with Pierre Robin syndrome, 850
Micturating cystourethrogram (MCU), 872
Midcycle pain (mittelschmerz), 84, 98
Midcycle spotting, 98
Middle adolescence, sexuality in, 90
Middle-class families, 42
Midpelvis, contractures of, labor problems from, 578
Midwifery
   in ancient Greece, 3
   British, 4, 6
   historical overview of, 4–5, 5–7
   van Deventer and, 4
Milia, on neonate, 677, 690g, 692g
Military (median vertex) presentation, 400, 400f
Milk. See also Cow's milk; Goat's milk
   allergy to (lactose intolerance), 272, 281
   breast vs. cows, neonatal fat absorption from, 651
   leg cramps and, 258, 259
Milk leg, 981
Mims, F. H., on sexual history assessments, 106
Minerals
   in breast milk, cow's milk, and formula, 719t
   food sources of, 271t
   metabolism of, pregnancy changes in, 201
   neonatal requirements, 717, 717t
   pregnancy requirements, 271–72t, 273–74
   recommended dietary allowances, 270t
Mini-pill, 125
Miscarriage. See Abortion, spontaneous
Mitleiden, 249
Mitosis, 158, 158f, 161f
   meiosis vs., 158–59
Mitral stenosis, peripheral cyanosis from, 889
Mittelschmerz (midcycle pain), 84, 98
Modeling, in crisis intervention, 997
Modesty, during labor, 469, 475
Molding, 398, 541f
   assessing for, 691g
      in prolonged labor, 542
   causes and degree of, 678
   excessive
      as amniotomy induction risk, 589
      as CPD risk, 578
      from hypertonic labor pattern, 537, 541f
      from malpresentation, 553
   malposition increases, 551, 552
   pelvic inlet contractions and, 578
Moles, assessing in neonate, 691g
Moloy, H. C., 70
Mongolian spots, 677, 690g
Moniliasis
   oral (thrush), in neonates, 844–45
   in pregnancy, 196, 355–56
      with diabetes, 316
   signs of, 226g, 227f
Monitrices, in Lamaze method, 294
Monocytes
   development of in fetus, 644
   in neonate, 645

Monosaccharides, neonatal digestion produces, 651
Monosomies, 136, 137
Monotropy, multiple attachment vs., 963
Monozygotic twins, 195, 557
   incidence of, 558
Mons pubis, 71f, 71–72
   assessing in female neonate, 701g
   assessing in initial prenatal exam, 225g
Mons veneris. See Mons pubis
Montgomery tubercles, enlargement of in pregnancy, 193
Montgomery's follicles, pregnancy changes in, 197
Montgomery's glands, pregnancy changes in, 192
Mood swings, 204
   postpartal, 920, 921
Moore, K. L., 165
Morale, maintenance of, as expectant family task, 39, 40
Morning sickness, 252, 253f, 254t
   as pregnancy symptom, 191–92
Morning-after pill, 129
Moro reflex, 657
   assessing, 682, 686, 697g, 703–4g
   brachial palsy affects, 697g
   clavicle fracture affects, 697g
   Erb-Duchenne paralysis affects, 684
   kernicterus affects, 824
Morphine
   during labor, 511–12
   for neonates with congestive heart failure, 894
Morris, N., fathers studied by, 961–63
Morula, formation of, 162, 163f
Mosaicism, 136, 138
Mother. See also Parents
   adolescent, postpartal care for, 942–43
   attachment behaviors of, 955f, 955–61, 957f
   complicated childbirth effects on, 580, 581
   expectant
      reactions to pregnancy of, 246–49, 248t
      relationship with parents of, 251–52
   facilitating attachment with, 499n, 502–3
   out-of-hospital emergency birth, 507
   feeding role of, self-concept and, 719
   labor analgesia effects on, 510
   maladaptive signs in, 1012
   maternicity in, 961
   of pregnant adolescent, 301–2, 305
   role conflicts of, 992
   stress felt by, 992
Mother role, identification with, 247–49
Mother of Twins Groups, 780
Motor activity, of neonate, 654
   in alert states, degree of, 657
   assessing, 657, 687, 688g, 702–3g, 705–6
   birth trauma affects, 756–57n
   breathing irregularity with, 639
   fetal alcohol syndrome affects, 770
   IUGR affects, 763
   in reactivity period, 712, 713f
Motor defects, 875–81. See also specific defects

from intraventricular hemorrhage, 836
   delayed motor development, with congenital hypothyroidism, 859
Mottling, in neonates, 683
Mourning. See Grief process
Mouth
   assessing in initial prenatal exam, 220g
   assessing in neonate, 681, 695–96g
Mouth care
   as labor intervention, 542
   postpartal, 916
MSUD. See Maple syrup urine disease
Mucosal layer of fallopian tube, 83
Mucous plug, 196
   expulsion of, as impending labor sign, 242g, 415, 473n
Mucous secretions, from vulvovaginal (Bartholin's) glands, 73
Mucoviscidosis. See Cystic fibrosis
Mucus, cervical. See Cervical mucus
Mucus, in neonate
   excessive
      as distress sign, 714
      with tracheoesophageal atresia/fistula, 860, 862
   during reactivity period, 712, 713f
   suctioning, in nursery routine, 714–16, 716f
Müllerian duct, 653, 653f
Mullerian regression factor, 57
Mullerian-inhibiting factor, 653, 653f
Multigravida, 210. See also Multiparas
Multiparas. See also Grandmultiparity
   afterpains in, 907
   amniotic fluid embolism in, 576
   brow presentation in, 552
   defined, 210
   dysfunctional labor among, 544–45
   engagement in, 402
   external os shape in, 904
   external version in, 585
   face presentation in, 553
   labor length in
      active phase, 417
      latent phase, 417
      second stage, 418, 551
   LGA neonates and, 760
   as oxytocin contraindication, 590
   placenta previa more common in, 564
   postterm pregnancy and, 759
   precipitous labor with, 542
   risk factors for, 214t
   thromboembolic disease risk in, 980, 983
Multiple delivery, 185. See also Multiple pregnancy
   uterine atony after, 579
Multiple gestation. See Multiple pregnancy
Multiple pregnancy, 557–60, 559f
   as birth center contraindication, 618
   breech presentation and, 554
   connected fetuses, delivery of, 557
   cord prolapse and, 539
   as CST contraindication, 376
   fetal/neonatal implications of, 425t
   as hemorrhage risk, 569, 972
   hydramnios associated with, 576, 577
   hypotonic labor patterns with, 541
   identification of, 558

at labor onset, 428g
   in prenatal exams, 223g, 239g
   with ultrasound, 8, 367f, 368, 368f
   as induction of labor contraindication, 587
   as intrapartal risk factor, 425t
   IUGR associated with, 761
   maternal implications of, 425t
   PIH risk and, 336
   postpartal risks with, 908t
   as preterm labor cause, 407, 548
   as prolapsed umbilical cord risk, 574
   resuscitation risk with, 786
   as risk factor, 215t, 425t
   statistics about, 185
   supine hypotensive syndrome and, 409
   transverse lie with, 556
   velamentous insertion of umbilical cord with, 575
Multiple sclerosis, as pregnancy complication, 330t
Mumps
   infertility from, 111t, 112
   neonatal immunity to, 654
Mumps immunization, contraindicated in pregnancy, 266t
Murmurs. See Heart murmurs
Muscle disorders, signs of in initial prenatal exam, 217g
Muscle guarding, from appendicitis in pregnancy, 351
Muscle incoordination, from kernicterus, 826
Muscle tension, as pain response, 483
Muscle tone. See also Muscles
   abdominal, restoring postpartum, 905
   assessing in fourth trimester, 946g
   birth trauma affects, 756n
   with herpesvirus type 2 infection, 844
   prenatal exercises for, 262–63, 264f
   in neonate
      assessed at nursery admission, 710
      assessing, in neurologic examination, 657
      head lag and, 681
      with RDS, 797t
Muscles. See also Muscle tone
   in breast, 84f, 85
   in fallopian tube, 83
   of neonate, assessing, 687, 702g, 705–6
   pelvic floor, 66–68, 67t, 67f
   at perineum, 73
   of uterus, 78, 78f. See also Myometrium
   in vagina, 75
   wasting of, from hyperthyroidism, 326
Muscular activity, thermogenesis by, 647
Muscular dystrophy, Duchenne-type
   prenatal diagnosis of, 147, 148
   as X-linked recessively inherited, 144
Muscular irritability, as danger sign of pregnancy, 240g
Muscular pains, postpartal, 915
Musculoskeletal malformations, from meningomyelocele, 880, 882
Musculoskeletal system
   assessing in initial prenatal exam, 224g

fetal
development of, 173, 174t, 176t, 178t, 178–82
teratogenic damage to, 183t
Mutuality, in attachment process, 957f, 958–59, 959–61
Mutation, 142, 157
Myalgia, as toxoplasmosis symptom, 357
Myasthenia gravis, as pregnancy complication, 330t
Mycobacterium tuberculosis, 331t
Mycostatin (Nystatin), for thrush, 845
Myelomeningocele
assessing neonate for, 702g
LGA preterm IDM, 757n
hydrocephaly and, 557
prenatal diagnosis of, 148
Myomas
Braxton Hicks contractions from, 192t, 193
fetal outline vs., 192t, 193
fundal height and, 237
as induction of labor contraindication, 587
infertility from, 111t
menopause increases tendency toward, 101
palpation of, fetal outline vs., 192t, 193
spontaneous abortion caused by, 329
Myomectomy, as induction of labor contraindication, 587
Myometrial cells, hypertrophy of, 195–96, 196f
Myometrial dysfunction in labor, psychic factors and, 535–36
Myometrium, 77f, 78, 78f
embryologic development of, 57
labor role of, 406, 407
tetanic ring formation in, 545
Myosin. See Contractile substances
Myotonia, as sexual response, 103, 104
Myths, about food in pregnancy, 282–83
Myxedema, 215t, 326

Nabothian or retention cysts, 226g, 227f
Nadler, H. L., 148
Naeye, R. L., 168
Nafcillin, for sepsis neonatorum, 843t
Nägele, Franz, 4
Nagele's rule, 191, 236, 546
Nails
of mother
assessing, in prenatal exam, 224g
hyperthyroidism sign in, 326
of neonate
assessing, 684, 702g
caring for, 728
postterm, 760
preterm, 750
Naloxone hydrochloride (Narcan)
neonatal contraindications, 771, 793d
neonatal depression relieved by, 512
for resuscitation, 788, 789t, 792, 793d
Nalorphine, contradicted for addicted infants, 771
Naming, attachment indicated by, 969
Narcan. See Naloxone hydrochloride
Narcotic addiction. See Drug abuse
Narcotic analgesics, during labor, 511–12, 512d. See also Narcotics

ataractics with, 513
supine hypotensive syndrome and, 409
Narcotic antagonists, 512
contraindicated for addicted infants, 771
Narcotics
in breast milk, 930
in pregnancy, 360–62, 361t
Nares, of neonate. See also Nose
assessing, 695g
flaring
assessing, 682
with RDS, 795f, 796t, 801n
with tracheoesophageal atresia/fistula, 860
occlusion of. See Choanal atresia
Nasal bone ablation, gestational age and, 183t
Nasal stuffiness in pregnancy, 197, 252, 254, 254t
Nasal suctioning
in nursery routine care, 714–16, 716f
teaching parents about, 726
Nasoduodenal tube feeding, 742
Nasogastric intubation
for diaphragmatic hernia, 866
for omphalocele, 868
during surgery in pregnancy, 351
for tracheoesophageal atresia/fistula, 860, 861
Nasogastric tube feeding, 753–54n
Nasojejunal tube feeding, 742, 753–54n
Nasopharyngeal culture
for group B streptococcus in neonate, 843
in sepsis neonatorum assessment, 842
Nasopharyngeal suctioning, apnea prevention with, 756n
Natal narcotic abstinence syndrome. See Withdrawal
Natale, R., fetal breathing studied by, 371
National Certification Examination, 7
Native American families. See American Indian families
Natural childbirth (Read method), 293–94, 295
Nausea
from appendicitis in pregnancy, 351
as bromocriptine side effect, 926d
after cesarean, intervention for, 603
from fat-soluble vitamin overdose, 274
from gallbladder disease in pregnancy, 351
as general anesthesia side effect, 529, 530–31
with hydatidiform mole, 334–35
as impending labor sign, 416
with induction, as water intoxication sign, 590, 593n
during labor, deceleration phase, 478n
as Methergine side effect, 903d
nonpregnancy causes of, 191t
in pregnancy, 191–92, 252, 253f, 254t
reasons for, 198
with puerperal peritonitis, 976
as pyelonephritis sign, 353, 986
with regional anesthesia in labor, 524n
as ritodrine side effect, 549
Navajo
childbirth among, 411

feeding customs among, 924, 925
NEC. See Necrotizing enterocolitis
Neck
assessing in prenatal exam, 218g
of neonate
assessing, 681-82, 697g
assessing motor function in, 703g
bathing, 727
compressed, from brow presentton, 552
Neck aches in pregnancy, 200
Neck vein engorgement, as pulmonary embolism sign, 984n
Necrosis, of maternal soft tissues, as CPD complication, 578
Necrotizing enterocolitis (NEC), 837-38, 839-40n
assessing preterm infants for, 757n
breast-feeding protects against, 748, 776
complications of, 838
nursing care plan, 839-40
as prematurity risk, 749
preterm carbohydrate malabsorption and, 741
preterm formula and, 741
signs of, 753, 754n, 837-38, 839
in stool, 745, 874
TPN for, 745
Needs, physiologic and psychologic, family provides, 35
Negligence, standards of care and, 15
Neisseria gonorrhoeae, 354. See also Gonorrhea
prophylactic treat of neonate for, 710, 711d
puerperal infection from, 974.
Nembutal (pentobarbital), during labor, 513
Neonatal asphyxia. See Asphyxia, neonatal
Neonatal blood sampling, placenta previa and, 566
Neonatal bradycardia. See Bradycardia, neonatal
Neonatal complications, record keeping about, 480n
Neonatal death. See also Neonatal mortality
attachment before, importance of, 777
crisis intervention after, 1002-6, 1004n
emotional effects of, 580, 581
history of, as resuscitation risk, 786
Neonatal distress, signs of, 713-14
Neonatal hyperviscosity, as oxytocin risk, 500
Neonatal morbidity
birth weight and, 758
breech presentation and, 605
group B streptococcus as cause of, 843
postmaturity risk of, 760
risk identification for, 734-35, 736f
risk of, first 24 hours, 660
Neonatal mortality, 23, 25t. See also Neonatal death; Perinatal mortality
from accidents, 729
from asphyxia, 786
breech presentation and, 605
cesarean delivery and, 600
repeat vs. trial labor and, 606
from cold stress, 817, 818
from congenital heart defects, 881, 891
Coumarin as cause of, 769
decrease in, reasons for, 600

from diaphragmatic hernia, 861, 867
electronic fetal monitoring and, 459
from group B streptococcus, 843
from hemolytic disease of the newborn, 826
from herpesvirus infection, 359, 360, 844
hyperthyroidism and, 321
from hypoglycemia, 821
infection as cause of, 842
from intraventricular hemorrhage, 836
from kernicterus, 826
from listeriosis, 357
malpositions and, 552
from maple syrup urine disease, 858
MAS as cause of, 815
from maternal cardiac decompensation, 311
from maternal drug abuse, 361t
maternal hypertension and, 769
from necrotizing enterocolitis, 837
omphalocele as cause of, 868
postmaturity risk of, 760
prematurity increases, 548
prolonged labor increases, 536
from RDS, 792
risk of, first 24 hours, 660
screening for risk of, 725, 734-35, 735f
from toxoplasmosis, 357
from tracheoesophageal atresia/fistula, 860
from transposition of the great vessels, 891
unexplained, colostrum as protection from, 717
Neonatal Perception Inventory (NPI), 965, 966-67f
Neonatal period, defined, 635
Neonatal trauma, abnormal presentation and risk of, 425t
Neonates
abruptio placentae complications in, 563
acidosis in. See Acidosis; Metabolic acidosis
activity states in, 722, 724-25
of adolescent mothers, health of, 299, 301
alcohol-addicted, 769-70
anemia in, 830, 835
assessing. See Assessment of neonate
attachment readiness of, 954-55
attachment role of, 499n, 502-3, 953-54, 956, 957f, 958-60, 962
with family, 963
with father, 961-63
auditory capacity of, 655
bathing, 727-28, 728f
behavioral assessment for, 687, 705-6
in birth center, monitoring, 619
birth trauma to, abnormal presentation and, 425t
bladder defect in, 874-75
blood pressure in, 641, 642f
blood values, normal range, 644-45, 645t
breast-feeding, maternal drugs and, 930-31, 932-35t
carbohydrate digestion in, 651
carbohydrate metabolism in, 648
of cardiac clients, 311, 313, 768-69

Neonates *(Cont'd)*
cardiopulmonary complications in, 785. *See also specific complications*
cardiovascular adaptations in, 639-43, 641-43f
care of
basic information, 725-30, 728-29f
discharge planning for, 730
high-risk, 775-77
immediate, 498-99n, 506-7
chlamydial infections in, 355
circulatory system in
prematurity and, 739t, 739-40
RDS and, 803n
circumcision of, 722, 723-24f
clothing for, 728
cold stress in, 646-47, 817-18
colostomy care in, 870
crying by. *See* Crying
death of. *See* Neonatal death; Neonatal mortality
defense mechanisms of, 655
dehydration sign in, temperature increase as, 677
DeLee suction for, 500p
of diabetic mother. *See* Infant of diabetic mother
diapers for, 728, 729f
diaphragmatic hernia in, 861, 866-67
disease resistance in, 654
disseminated intravascular coagulation in, 837
distress signs in, 713-14
dressing, 728
drug abuse effects on, 361t, 362, 769, 770-72
eye contact with, 499n, 502, 503
eye treatment for, delaying, 503
fat digestion in, 651-52
feeding responses of, 921. *See also* Feeding
female, vaginal environment of, 75
follow-up phone assessment of, 948, 949
forceps bruise on, 598
fussiness in, purposes of, 657
gastric lavage of, after delivery, 711, 716
gastrointestinal adaptation in, 650-52
gastrointestinal defects in, 859. *See also specific defects*
genetic evaluation of, 148-50
genitourinary adaptation in, 652-54, 653f
genitourinary defects in, 874-75
gestational age assessment of. *See* Gestational age
gonorrheal infections in, 354-55, 844
group B streptococcal infections in, 842-43
growth patterns in, 675
growth spurts in, feeding patterns with, 718-19
habituation to stimuli in, 655, 687, 705
handling, 714, 715f, 726
heart defects in, 881, 886-87f. *See also specific defects*
heart rate in, 641
heat loss in, 646-47, 817-18
hematology of, 644-45, 645t
hematopoietic system in, 643-45, 645t
hemolytic disease in. *See* Hemolytic disease of the newborn
hemorrhagic disease in, 836

hepatic adaptation in, 648-50, 650t
herpesvirus infections in, 359, 844
high-risk, parenting, 772-80. *See also* High-risk neonates; *specific risks*
hypertensive disease in mother and, 769
hyperthyrodism in, 326
hypocalcemia in, 821-22
hypoglycemia in, 818-21, 819-20p
hypothyroidism in, 326
hypoxia in, difficulty of recognizing, 643
identification procedure for, 499n
with precipitous delivery, 505
illness in
emotional effect on family of, 580
signs of, 729
immediate care of, 498-99n
out-of-hospital emergency delivery, 506-7
immunologic adaptation in, 653-54
imperforate anus in, 871f, 871-72
intestinal obstruction in, 872-74
IUGR effects on, 370
jaundice in. *See* Hyperbilirubinemia; Jaundice
kidney development and function in, 652-53
labor analgesia effects on, 511
lactose digestion in, 651
laryngeal papillomas in, 355
Leboyer method of handling, 617-18
LGA. *See* Large-for-gestational-age neonates
listeriosis in, 357
macrosomia problems in, 557
measurements of
assessing, 691g. *See also specific measurements*
conversions and equivalents, APPENDIX F
metabolic disorders in, 857-59
metastatic lesions in, 568
monilial infection (thrush) in, 355, 844-45
motor activity in, 654, 657
nail care for, 728
Narcan administration to, 793d
neurologic assessment of, 657, 685-87, 686-87f, 705-6
neurologic functioning in, 654-57, 656f
nursery admission process, 709-11
nursing diagnoses for, examples, 499n
nutritional assessment of, 719-21, 720-21t
physiologic anemia and, 644
nutritional needs of, 717, 717t
olfactory capacity in, 655
pathologic jaundice definition for, 823
perceptual functioning in, 654-57, 656f
physical assessment of. *See* Assessment of neonate
physical growth percentiles for, APPENDIX E
PKU screening for, 858
pneumonia in, from chlamydial infection, 355
polycythemia in, 835-36
positioning and handling, 726
postterm, problems with, 758-60, 759t, 759f
precipitous delivery of, 504-5
preterm. *See* Prematurity; Preterm infants

protein digestion in, 651
pulmonary physiology of, 637-39
pulse in, 641
reactivity period in, 711-12, 713f
respiratory adaptations in, 635-39, 637f
respiratory distress in. *See* Respiratory distress
resuscitative management for, 788-92, 788t, 790f, 791-92p, 793d
rights of, APPENDIX B
risk classifications for, 734-35, 735-36f
risk levels for, 733
safety for, 729-30
screening tests for, 150
sensory/perceptual functioning, 654-57, 656f
sepsis in, after hypotonic labor, 541
sepsis neonatorum in, 841-42
size of, hemorrhage risk and, 972
skeletal defects in, 875-81. *See also specific defects*
sleep-activity patterns in, 655, 722, 724-25
smiling by, 725
sodium bicarbonate administration to, 793d
states of consciousness in, 655, 657
variables affecting, 705
stools and voids by, teaching about, 726
suctioning, procedure for, 500p
syphilis in, 354, 843-44
tactile capacity in, 655
taste response in, 655
temperature regulation in, 645-48, 646-47t
toxoplasmosis in, 357
transition circulation in, 640-41, 641f
urinary output in, 652
vitamin E needs of, 275
vitamin K needs of, 275
weight gain in, ideal rate of, 652
weight loss after birth, 652
weight of, conversions and equivalents, APPENDIX F
withdrawal syndrome in. *See* Withdrawal
wrapping or swaddling, 716
Neonatology, as pediatric subspecialty, 8
Neoplasm
infertility from, 111t
sign of in prenatal urinalysis, 230g
transverse lie and, 556
Nephritis, chronic, spontaneous abortion caused by, 329
Nephrons, in neonate, 652
Nephrotic syndrome, sign of in prenatal exam, 230g
Nerve blocks, during labor, 513-16
Nerve deafness, from rubella, 215t
Nerve disorders, signs of in initial prenatal exam, 217g, 219g, 220g, 225g
Nerves. *See* Innervation
Nervous system. *See* Neurologic assessment; Neurologic development
Nervousness
hyperthyroidism as cause of, 326
as ritodrine side effect, 549
as terbutaline sulfate side effect, 548
Nesacaine. *See* Chlorprocaine

"Nesting instinct," as impending labor sign, 416
Neural tube defects
anencephaly from, 691g
ethnic background and, 152
prenatal diagnosis of, 148
recurrence risk for, 145t, 148
Neurofibromatosis (von Recklinghausen's disease)
as autosomal dominantly inherited, 143
cafe au lait spots from, 217g
Neurohormonal control, male reproductive role and, 59
Neurologic abnormalities
Apgar score predicts, 734
from maternal herpesvirus type 2, 215t
weight at birth and, 734
Neurologic adaptations, in neonates, 657
Neurologic assessment
maternal, in initial prenatal exam, 219g
of neonate, 657, 685-87, 686-87f, 705-6
cranial nerve function, 692g, 693g, 695g
gestational age and, 663-65f, 669, 671-73f, 672
intraventricular hemorrhage shown by, 836
with kernicterus, 824
polycythemia, 835
pupils, 694g
SGA, 764n
spinal problems, 702g
Neurologic cord lesions, infertility from, 111t
Neurologic development
in fetus, 173, 174t, 176t, 178t, 178-82
teratogenic damage to, 183t
in neonate, breast milk aids in, 717
in preterm infant, 749
Neurologic disorders
in fetus
hydramnios associated with, 576
in neonate
from congenital toxoplasmosis, 357
crying with, 682, 688g
with herpesvirus infection, 844
IDM, 768
incidence of, birth weight and, 758
from kernicterus, 826-27
long-term, as prematurity risk, 758
with maple syrup urine disease, 858
from maternal drug abuse, 361t
neuroblastoma, kidney displacement with, 700g
neurofibromatosis, 690g
nutrition and, 740
preterm, 740, 749, 758
reflex deficits with, 703-4g
tremors with, 703g
trunk incurvation affected by, 704g
Neurologic response, in sexual activity, 104-5
Neurologic system, in neonates, 654-57, 656f
Neurologic trauma, assessing head for, 691g
Neuromuscular development, gestational age and, 660, 661, 663-65f, 669, 671-73f, 672

Neuromuscular disassociation, in Lamaze method, 294
Neutrophils, 644, 645
Nevi
  in neonates
    nevus flammeus (port-wine stain), 677-78, 691g, 867
    nevus pilosus ("hairy nerve"), 685, 702g
    nevus vasculosus ("strawberry mark"). 678
    pigmented (mole), supernumerary nipple vs., 682
    telangiectatic, 677
    spider, in pregnancy, 199. See also Spider nevi
New York City Health Department, midwifery report by, 6
Newborn nurseries. See Nursery
Newborns. See Neonates
Niacin, 276
  in breast milk, cow's milk, and formula, 719t
  deficiency of in infant, 719
  food sources of, 276
  lactation requirements, 270t, 276
  pregnancy requirements, 270t, 276
Nicotine, fetal/neonatal effects of, 361t. See also Smoking
Niemann-Pick disease
  assessing for, in SGA neonate, 766n
  prenatal diagnosis of, 148
Night sweats, postpartal, 907
Nightingale, Florence, 6
Nile blue sulfate, staining fetal cells with, 387
"Nipple confusion," avoiding, 929
Nipple shield, 929
Nipple-feeding
  for cleft lip, 853n
  for cleft palate, 856n
  for preterm infants, 742, 753n, 754n
  for RDS neonate, 807n
Nipples, 84f, 85
  anatomy of, 85
  assessing, postpartal home visit, 624
  breast-feeding problems with, 931, 931f, 936, 936f
  care of, 919n, 931, 936
    cracked, of, 936
    postpartal, 910
  extra or supernumerary, assessing neonate for, 682, 683f
  inverted, 260, 931, 931f, 936f
  of neonate, assessing, 699g
  pigmentation changes in
    with pregnancy, 192, 193, 199, 221g
    nonpregnancy-caused, 192t
  postpartal assessment of, 910
  pregnancy changes in, 197; see also pigmentation changes in
  soreness in, 931, 936
    toughening to prevent, 26-27, 260
  supernumerary, assessing neonate for, 699g
Nitrazine test
  at labor admission, 472
  PROM confirmed with, 430g, 436p, 546
Nitrites, neonatal effects of, 769
Nitrofurantoin (Furadantin), 353
Nitrogen retention in pregnancy, 197t, 201
Nitrous oxide, obstetric anesthesia with, 529
Nocturia, as cystitis sign, 986

Noise, fetal responses to, 654
No-lose problem solving, 290
Nondisjunction, 136
  abnormalities caused by, 136-38
  autosomal, mechanism of, 159
  maternal age and, 147
Nongenetic conditions, 145-46
Nongonoccocal urethritis (NGU), 355
Noninflammatory venous thrombosis, 976
Noninsulin dependent diabetes mellitus (NIDDM), 314, 314t
Nonmendelian inheritance, 142, 145
Non-REM sleep, in neonates, 724
Nonshivering thermogenesis (NST), 647, 817
Nonspecific vaginitis, 356
Nonstress test (NST), 373-74, 373-74f
  as fetal status indicator, with FBM, 636
  in hypothyroid pregnancy, 326
  with maternal PIH, 341
  nonreactive
    as CST indication, 375
    example, 374f
  procedure for, 374
  for prolonged pregnancy, 759t
  reactive, example, 373f
Nonverbal communication, labor pain behavior and, 470-71
Norepinephrine
  fetal stress and, 171
  hemorrhage effect of, 570
  labor stress and, 407, 535, 536-37
  nonshivering thermogenesis role of, 647
Norethindrone enanthate, 127
Norfolk, Virginia, in vitro fertilization clinic in, 9
Nose
  fetal development of, 173, 175t, 177t, 178, 180
  of mother, assessing in prenatal exam, 219g
  of neonate, 681, 695g. See also Nares
Nosocomial infections, as prematurity risk, 748
Novobiocin, during pregnancy, 823, 831
Novocaine. See Procaine
NPI (Neonatal Perception Inventory), 965, 966-67f
NST (Nonshivering thermogenesis), 647, 817
NST. See Nonstress test
Nuclear cataract, gestational age and, 183t
Nuclear dyad, 32, 33f
Nuclear family
  developmental stages in, 36-41, 40t
  structure of, 32, 33f, 34f, 34-35
Nulliparas. See also Primigravidas
  breech presentation in, cesarean delivery for, 600
  brow presentation in, 552
  defined, 210
  delivery room admission for, 479n
  dysfunctional labor among, 544-45
  hypertonic labor patterns in, 537
  pelvic inlet contracture risks in, 578
  prolonged labor in, 542, 551
Nurse anesthetists, 513
Nurse-client relationship, establishing in initial visit, 238
Nurse-geneticist, 154
Nurse-midwifery, development of, 5-7

Nurse-midwives
  absent from delivery, 503-5
  birth center role of, 618
  physicians' attitudes toward, 15-16
  as primary caregivers, 15
  regional anesthesia administration by, 513
Nurse Practice Acts, 14
Nurse practitioners
  expanding role of, 15
  genetic counseling referral by, 151
  maternity care roles of, 14, 243
  pediatric, nursery role of, 714
  physicians' attitudes toward, 15-16
Nursery
  admission to, 709-13
    risk assessment at, 736
  as consultant after discharge, 725, 730
  eye prophylaxis in, 710, 711d, 712f
  intensive care
    goals of, 733
    for IDM, 768
    nursing peer support in, 1006
    parents in, 774-77, 1009, 1009f, 1013f, 1013-14
    for Pierre Robin syndrome care, 851
    resuscitative equipment in, 788
  levels of care in, 733
  neonatal assessment in, 660
  neonatal feeding in, 716-17, 718
  observation, 709-13
  rooming-in vs., in first 24 hours, 713-14
  routine care in, 714-16
  sepsis prevention in, 842
  vitamin K administration in, 710, 711d
Nursery care, introduction of, 5
Nursery nurse, genetic counseling referral by, 151
Nursing assessments. See Assessment
Nursing care evaluations. See Evaluation
Nursing care plans
  AGA and LGA preterm infants, 750-58
  cesarean delivery, 601-4
  cleft lip and palate, 853-57
  for diabetic pregnancy, 322-25
  family as part of, 49
  fetal distress, 538-40
  hemorrhage, 569-73
  immediate care of newborn, 498-99
  induction of labor, 591-95
  labor and delivery, 472-82
  meningocele/meningomyelocele, 882-84
  necrotizing enterocolitis, 839-40
  neonatal jaundice, 831-34
  postpartal period, 917-20
  preeclampsia-eclampsia (PIH), 337-40
  puerperal infection, 977-80
  pulmonary embolism, 983, 984-85
  regional anesthesia, 521-24
  respiratory distress, 801-10
  SGA neonates, 764-67
  stillbirth, 1004
  thromboembolic disease, 983-85
  tracheoesophageal fistula, 862-65
Nursing diagnoses, 19-20, 340. See also Nursing process
  AGA and LGA preterm infants, 757-58

attachment problems, 1013
cesarean delivery, 604
child abuse, 1016t
cleft lip and palate, 857
of diabetes mellitus in pregnancy, 325
family care, 49, 50
fetal distress, 540
hemorrhage, 573
for immediate care of neonate, 499
induction of labor, 595
during labor, 482
medical vs., 19
meningocele/meningomyelocele, 884
necrotizing enterocolitis, 840
neonatal jaundice, 834
  at nursery admission, 711
  as part of nursing process, 19-20
of PIH, 340
postpartal period, 920, 938
puerperal infection, 980
with regional anesthesia during labor, 524
research application and, 27
respiratory distress syndrome, 810
SGA neonates, 767
stillbirth, grief process after, 1004
subinvolution, 973
thromboembolic disease, 985
tracheoesophageal atresia/fistula, 865
Nursing education, 5, 10
Nursing history. See History
Nursing interventions, 19-20. See also Assessment guides; Nursing care plans; Nursing process; Nursing role
  abortion, 131
  abruptio placentae, 563, 564
  acute respiratory obstruction, 531
  adolescent parents, 961, 1017
  aganglionic megacolon, 870-71
  alcohol-addicted neonate, 770
  with amniocentesis, 382, 383p
  attachment facilitation, 964-65
  attachment problems, 1012-14
  bladder exstrophy, 875
  bleeding in pregnancy, 329
  for brow presentation, 552-53
  cesarean delivery, 606-9
    preparation, 601-2
    recovery, 603-4
  child abuse, 1015-16
  cold stress, 817-18
  congenital syphilis, 844
  continuous regurgitation by neonate, 651
  CPD trial labor, 578
  defective birth, 1010
  diaphragmatic hernia, 867
  DIC, 568
  for dysfunctional labor, principles of, 536-37
  episiotomy, 596
  exchange transfusion, 825p, 828-29
  external or cephalic version, 586
  fetal distress, 538-40n
  fetal malformations, 557
  forceps delivery, 598
  fourth trimester, 944-49
  in group prenatal discussions, 291-92
  hemolytic disease of the newborn, 825p, 827f, 827-30, 829-30f
  hemorrhage, 569-73n
  high-risk neonates, 735-37. See also specific risks
    facilitating attachment with, 774-79

Nursing interventions (Cont'd)
hypermagnesemia in neonate, 769
hypertonic labor patterns, 537
hypotonic labor patterns, 541–42
IDM, 768
immediate care of newborn, 498–99n
imperforate anus, 872
with induction of labor, 589, 590, 590–95
internal or podalic version, 586
intestinal obstruction in neonate, 873–74
intraventricular hemorrhage, 836–37
during labor. See Intrapartal nursing management; Labor
MAS, 815
mastitis, 987
meningocele/meningomyelocele, 880–81, 882–84n
for menopausal women, 102
moniliasis, in neonate, 845
Narcan administration to neonate, 793d
necrotizing enterocolitis, 838, 839–40n
neonatal alcohol withdrawal, 770
neonatal anemia, 835
neonatal death, 1003–6, 1004n
neonatal group B streptococcal infection, 843
neonatal herpesvirus infection, 844
neonatal hyperbilirubinemia, 823, 824, 825p
neonatal hypocalcemia, 821–22
neonatal hypoglycemia, 818, 821
neonatal narcotic withdrawal, 771
omphalocele, 868
as part of nursing process, 19–20
persistent pulmonary hypertension (PPH), 817
phototherapy, 829–30, 830f
physiologic jaundice, 649
Pierre Robin syndrome, 850–51
placenta previa, 565p,, 566–67
postpartal. See Postpartal nursing management
postterm infant, 760
precipitous delivery, 504–5
pregnancy discomforts, 259–60
pregnancy-induced hypertension (PIH), 338–39n
preterm birth, 1008–10, 1009f
preterm infant feeding, 741–46, 743–45p
preterm labor, 549, 550
prolonged labor, 542
PROM, 547
puerperal infections, 976
of urinary tract, 986
pulmonary embolism, 982, 984–85n
for RDS, 797, 799–80t, 801–10ncp, 811–14p
with regional anesthesia during labor, 521–24n
relinquishment for adoption, 1014, 1015t
for respiratory obstruction after anesthesia, 531
resuscitation preparation, 787–88
sepsis neonatorum, 842
single-parent families, 1018
sodium bicarbonate administration to neonate, 793d
spina bifida, 880–81, 882–84n
talipes equinovarus, 876
thrush, in neonate, 845
transverse lie, 556
umbilical cord prolapse, 574–75
uterine inversion, 580

uterine rupture, 550
vacuum extraction delivery, 599
vomiting by neonate, 651
Nursing practice
family-centered, implications of, 46–51
research as part of, 26–27
tools applied to, 27–28
Nursing priorities
aganglionosis, 870
bladder exstrophy, 875
cesarean delivery, 601n
diaphragmatic hernia, 867
family health needs, 49
fetal distress, 538
immediate care of newborn, 498
induction of labor, 591n
intestinal obstruction, 874
at labor admission, 472
meningocele/meningomyelocele, 882
necrotizing enterocolitis, 839n
neonatal jaundice, 831n
postpartal, 917
preterm infant care, 750
puerperal infection, 977
with regional anesthesia during labor, 521n
respiratory distress syndrome, 801
with ritodrine, 549
SGA neonates, 764n
stillbirth, 1004
thromboembolic disease, 983
tracheoesophageal atresia/fistula, 862
Nursing process, 19–20. See also Nursing role; specific processes
applied, example of, 20
assessment, 19
evaluation as part of, 20
family-oriented, 47–52, 52f
as maternity care tool, 19–20
nursing diagnoses and planning, 19–20
nursing interventions, 19–20
research as part of, 19, 26–27
Nursing role. See also Nursing interventions; Nursing process
in abortion, 131
in adolescent pregnancy, 297, 298–99t, 299, 300t, 302–5
in amniocentesis, 382, 383p
antepartal, 243, 285–92
with cardiac client, 313
changing health care environment and, 12–16
client advocacy as part of, 13
client-health care professional relationship, 13–14
communication skills for, 290–91
conflict management in, 290
in contraceptive choice, 120
in crisis intervention, 997–98
in diabetic pregnancy, 321
with electronic monitoring, 446, 447
emotions and, with infant death, 1006
ethical issues and, 11
expansion in, 14–16
in genetic counseling, 134–35
in infertility management, 119–20
in labor
as backup for support person, 418
in true vs. false labor assessment, 416
legal aspects of, 14–15
physical examinations, 213
pregnancy discomforts and, 259–60

Pregnant Patient Bill of Rights, APPENDIX A
referral as, 994
Nursing, schools of. See Nursing education
Nurturance, attachment readiness requires, 952
Nutramingen, for galactosemia, 859
Nutrient metabolism in pregnancy, 201
Nutrition
amenorrhea and, 100
after cesarean delivery, 603
counseling about
assessing need for, in prenatal exams, 216g, 217g, 239g
WIC program provides, 5
dysmenorrhea and, 100
of fetus, as placental function, 168
habitual abortion and, 333
in lactation
daily food plan, 271–72t
recommended dietary allowances (RDA), 269, 270t
neonatal. See Nutrition, for neonates
in pregnancy. See Nutrition, in pregnancy
postpartal, 913
for puerperal infection, 978n
Nutrition, for neonates. See also Feeding
assessing, 719–21, 720–21t
digestive process, 651–52
folic acid requirements, 277
preterm, 740–46, 741f, 742t, 743–45p, 747t
nursing care plan, 753–54
requirements, 746
sample diagnosis, 757
with RDS, 797, 806–8n
Nutrition, in pregnancy, 269–85, 270–72t, 277t, 286–87f
adolescents and, 297, 298t, 303–4
alcohol consumption and, 269
assessing, 285, 286–87f
counseling about. See Nutrition, counseling about
daily food plan, 271–72t
diabetes and, 318, 320, 322
factors influencing, 281–85
cultural, ethnic, and religious, 282t, 283–84
psychologic, 284–85
psychosocial, 284–85
socioeconomic, 284
fetal development and, 184–85
high risk and, 214t
importance of, 269
for adolescents, 303–4
iron requirements, 327
IUGR and, 761
maternal weight gain and, 269–70
metabolic changes and, 201
neonatal behavior and, 654
neonatal iron stores and, 648
physiologic anemia of infancy and, 644
protein, for PIH, 338
recommended dietary allowances (RDA), 269, 270t
requirements, 269, 270, 270–72t, 272–79, 277t
sample menus, 278–81, 283–84
sickle cell anemia and, 328
skeletal system needs and, 199
Nymphae. See Labia minora
Nystagmus, assessing in neonate, 693g, 694g
Nystatin (Mycostatin), for thrush in neonates, 681, 845

Obesity
absent fetal movement from, 240g
amenorrhea from, 100
infant
as formula feeding risk, 718
iron deficiency with, 719g
preventing, 927
Leopold maneuvers and, 441
PIH risk and, 336
pregnancy confused with, 192t
in prenatal exams, 239g
resuscitation risk with, 786
supine hypotensive syndrome and, 409
thromboembolic disease risk with, 976, 980, 983
Object loss, 999
Objective data, 19
in POMR system, 20
Observation, of neonate
importance of, 660
in neurologic assessment, 657
Observation nursery, 709–13
Obstetric conjugate, 69
Obstetric history. See History
Obstetric trauma
labia majora hematomas from, 72
lacerations from. See Lacerations
uterine rupture from, 550
Obstetrical Society of London, midwives certified by, 6
Obturator, for cleft palate, 852
Obturator foramen, 66
Occiput-posterior position, 551, 552
Occlusive cuff impedance phlebography (IPG)
deep vein thrombosis assessment with, 981, 983
postpartal use of, 912
Occupation, infertility and, 112
OCT (Oxytocin challenge test). See Contraction stress test
Ocular abnormalities
with extended rubella syndrome, 358
hypertelorism, assessing neonate for, 692g
ocular lens dislocation, with homocystinuria, 859
Oculomotor muscle paralysis, ptosis in neonates from, 693g
Office nurse, prenatal care by, 243
OGGT (Oral glucose tolerance test), 317
Ointments
circumcision care with, 727
for diaper rash, 727
for eye prophylaxis. See Erythromycin
for hemorrhoidal pain relief, 915, 917n
for nipple care, 910, 931
perineal pain relief with, 915, 917n
skin care with, 727
"Old Americans" pain expression among, 469–70
Olfactory sense
assessing, in initial prenatal exam, 219g
in neonate, 655, 681, 695g
Oligohydramnios, 577
as cephalic version contraindication, 585
defined, 399, 577
fetal attitude with, 399
fetal implications of, 425t, 577
as intrapartal risk factor, 425t
maternal implications of, 425t, 577
neonatal implications of, 425t, 786
ultrasound to detect, 368

Oligomenorrhea, 100
Oliguria (decreased urinary output)
  maternal
    assessing, with abruptio
      placentae, 564
    as danger sign of pregnancy,
      240g
    with PIH, 340
    with severe preeclampsia, 341
  neonatal
    as MAS complication, 815
    preterm, 746
Olshansky, S., 1010
Omphalocele (exomphalos), 183t,
  867–68, 868–69f
  assessing neonate for, 700g
  developmental origin of, 650
  incidence of, 867
  prenatal diagnosis of, 146
  vulnerability to, 183t
One-to-one teaching, prenatal, 291
Oocytes, 83–84
  meiotic division in, 96, 160, 161f
  secondary, extrusion of, 98
Oogenesis, 83, 158, 160, 161f
Oogonia, formation of in embryo, 57
Oogonial cells, oocytes develop from,
  160, 161f
Oophoritis, puerperal, 975
Operative sterilization, 121f, 127–
  28, 127f, 128f
Ophthalmia neonatorum, 844
  chemical conjunctivitis vs., 844
  from chlamydial infection, 355
  drug administration to prevent,
    499n, 710, 711d, 712f
  from gonorrhea, 354–55
Opisthotonus, in neonate
  with herpesvirus infection, 844
  with kernicterus, 824
  in LGA infant, from birth trauma,
    756n
  with maple syrup urine disease,
    858
Opsonization, 654
Optic fundi evaluation, in infertility
  workup, 114
Optical density, bilirubin in amniotic
  fluid measured by, 384, 384f
Oral contraceptives, 121f, 125, 126–
  27t
  amenorrhea from, 100
  chloasma caused by, 192t
  contraindications for, 125
  diabetes and, 315, 318–19
  estrogens in, 93
  infertility from, 110
  postpartal use of, 944
    after PIH pregnancy, 346–47
  pregnancy signs caused by, 192t
  side effects of, 125
Oral glucose tolerance test (OGGT),
  317
Oral hygiene. See Mouth care
Oral moniliasis (thrush), in neonates,
  844–45
Oral mucosa, jaundice evidence on,
  824, 832n
Oral secretions, pregnancy changes
  in, 198
Oral sex
  herpes simplex from, 359
  in pregnancy, 265
Oral suctioning
  in nursery routine care, 714–16,
    716f
  teaching parents about, 726
Orbits of eyes, edema of in neonate,
  680
Orchitis
  assessing neonatal scrotum for,
    701g

infertility from, 112
Organ abnormalities, ears as
  indicator of, 681
Organ development, in embryo and
  fetus, 173–85, 174–79t
  teratogenic risk during, 266, 268–
    69
Organic phosphates in erythrocytes,
  oxygen affinity and, 643
Organs, intrauterine, 165–71
Orgasm, 102
  physiology of, 103t, 104, 104t,
    105
  pregnancy changes in, 264–65
Oriental Americans. See also Asian
  Americans
  cultural patterns among, 45–46
  health beliefs among, 206
  labor customs among, 412, 469,
    470, 471
  lactose intolerance among, 281
  modesty among, 469
  pain expression among, 470, 471
  percent of population, 44, 44t
  pregnancy customs among, 205,
    206
  prenatal nutrition for, 282t
    sample menus, 283–84
Orienting, assessing neonate for, 706
Orogastric intubation
  for choanal atresia, 857
  for intestinal obstruction, 873
  preterm infant feeding with, 753–
    54n
Orogenital sex. See Oral sex
Orthodontia, for cleft palate, 852
Orthopedic splint, for hip dysplasia,
  878
Orthostatic pneumonia, after cleft lip
  surgery, 856n
Ortolani maneuver, 685, 877
Os. See Cervical os
Osmolality
  in neonatal blood
    IVH risk and, 836
    normal preterm values, 752t
  in preterm formulas, 741, 742t
Osmotic pressure, in placental trans-
  port, 170
Osteoarthritis, signs of in initial pre-
  natal exam, 224g
Osteogenesis imperfecta, in neonate,
  694f
Osteoporosis, postmenopausal, 101
Ostium primum, 885, 886f
  persistent, gestational age and,
    183t
Ostium secundum, 885, 886f
Otitis media, in neonate
  as cleft lip or palate risk, 852,
    854n, 856n
  from propped bottles, 926
Ototoxic drugs, hearing loss risk
  from, 758
Ould, Sir Fielding, 4
Outlet dystocia, 70
Ova. See Ovum
Ovarian cancer, 83, 84
Ovarian cycle, 96, 97f, 98, 98f. See
  also Menstrual cycle
Ovarian cysts, signs of in initial pre-
  natal exam, 228g
Ovarian disorders, signs of in initial
  prenatal exam, 222g
Ovarian failure, 84
Ovarian hormones, 92f, 93–94
Ovarian lesions, amenorrhea from,
  100
Ovarian ligaments, 81–82, 81f, 82f,
  83
Ovarian trauma, as cesarean delivery
  risk, 605

Ovarian tumors
  pregnancy sign caused by, 192t
  signs of in initial prenatal exam,
    222g, 228g
Ovaries, 74f, 82f, 83–84. See also
  Adnexa
  anatomy of, 83–84
  assessing, 74
    in infertility workup, 114
    in initial prenatal exam, 222g,
      228g
  development of, 57, 58f, 653,
    653f
  FSH and LH receptor cells in, 96
  function of, 84
  hormones secreted by, 92f, 93–94
  infertility and, 111t
  position of, 83
  pregnancy changes in, 196
  size of, 83
Over-the-counter pregnancy tests,
  195
Overdue pregnancy. See Postterm
  pregnancy
Overfeeding of neonate
  avoiding, 927
  regurgitation from, 651
Overheating, neonatal response to,
  677
Overhydration, as prematurity risk,
  746, 747
Overstimulation, protecting newborn
  from, 506, 507
Oviducts. See Fallopian tubes
Ovulation
  cervical mucus at, 79, 98
  delayed, postterm pregnancies
    from, 759
  detecting, tests for, 115–17
  hormonal role in, 93, 94
  infertility and, 111t
  as ovarian cycle, 96
  pain with, 98
  pharmacologic management of,
    118
  physiologic description of, 98
  postpartal resumption of, 904–5
    bromocriptine and, 926
  prostaglandins' role in, 94
  temperature change at, 94, 98
  time of in cycle, 96, 115
    cervical mucus to assess, 98
Ovulation method of contraception,
  121f, 121–22
Ovulatory function tests, in infertility
  workup, 113f, 115–16
Ovum
  described, 160
  fertilization of, 160–62, 161f,
    162f
  imperfections in, spontaneous
    abortion from, 329
  implantation of, 163–64
  maturation of, 160, 161f
  ovarian ligament role and, 82
  stage of the, 162–65, 173
  transport of, 162, 163f
Oxygen administration
  for amniotic fluid embolism, 576
  for apnea, 755n, 756n
  bronchopulmonary dysplasia from,
    816
  for cardiac client in labor, 313
  complications of therapy with,
    815–17
  for congestive heart failure, 894
  for cyanosis, 889
  for eclampsia, 344
  during fetal bradycardia episode,
    517
  as fetal distress intervention, 538
    with induced labor, 590, 594n

for FHR aberrations during labor,
  451t
for hemorrhage, 569, 571
for intraventricular hemorrhage,
  837
for labor anesthesia reaction, 516,
  519, 522n, 523n
for MAS, 815
for neonate, guidelines for, 498
for neonate of hypertensive mother, 769
with oxytocin induction
  for fetal distress, 590, 594n
  after overdose, 543
placental transport of, 170
with positive pressure, 576
for pulmonary embolism, 982,
  985n
for RDS, 801–3n
  humidified, 797, 803n
for resuscitation, 787, 788, 789t,
  791p, 792
retinal damage from, 815
with suctioning, 812p, 814p
for supine hypotensive syndrome,
  467
for transient tachypnea of newborn, 797
for uterine atony hemorrhage, 579
Oxygen affinity, 643, 643f
Oxygen capacity, defined, 643
Oxygen consumption in neonate,
  temperature and, 648
Oxygen dissociation curve, 643,
  643f
Oxygen hood, use of, 802n, 802f
Oxygen saturation, 643, 643f
Oxygen supply. See Oxygenation of
  blood
Oxygen transport
  in fetus, 171, 172f
  in neonate, 642–43, 643f
    factors affecting, 638–39
    hemoglobin type and, 643
Oxygenation of blood
  cyanosis and, 889
  factors regulating, 643, 643f
  pregnancy changes in, 197t, 198
Oxytocic agents
  as abruptio placentae intervention,
    563, 564, 572
  augmenting labor with, monitoring
    and, 447
  breast-feeding stimulates release
    of, 902, 907, 925
  with breech presentation, mortality
    risk, 554
  after cesarean delivery, 603, 609
  contraindications, 537, 590d
  CST utilizes, 375, 376
  for diabetic client, 321
  Ferguson reflex caused by, 407
  as hypertonic labor intervention,
    537
  as hypotonic labor intervention,
    541
  for induction of labor, 589, 590d.
    See also Labor, induced
    accelerated labor from, inter-
      ventions for, 543
    decreasing or discontinuing,
      with fetal distress, 539
    inadequate response to, 592–
      93n
  with magnesium sulfate, 346
  mismanagement of, uterine rup-
    ture from, 550
  overdose, precipitous labor
    from, 543
  postpartal hemorrhage risk
    with, 972
labor role of, 406

Oxytocic agents *(Cont'd)*
  myometrial activity increased by, 407
  neonatal hyperbilirubinemia and, 823
  with pelvic contractures, 578
  postpartal use of, 590, 903
    afterpains increased by, 907
    for hemorrhage, 579, 973
    hemorrhage prevention with, 903, 903d, 972
    milk production stimulated by, 925
    for puerperal endometritis, 975
  pregnancy role of, 202
  as prolonged labor intervention, 542
  record keeping about, 480n
  risks associated with, 500, 589, 590
  in third stage labor, 497, 500
  uterine atony and, 579
  water intoxication as risk with, 500
  x-ray pelvimetry before use of, 432, 433
Oxytocin challenge test (OCT). *See also* Contraction stress test
  as fetal status indicator, with FBM, 636
  for prolonged pregnancy, 759t
Oxytocin stimulation theory, 406

Pacifier
  after aganglionosis surgery, 870
  assessing neonatal responses to, 706
  with tracheoesophageal atresia/fistula, 864n
Paget, Rosalind, 6
Pain
  from acute pyelonephritis in pregnancy, 353
  from appendicitis during pregnancy, 351
  attention and distraction affect, 413
  behavioral responses to, 483
  after cesarean delivery, 941
    interventions for, 603
    repeat, anticipation of, 607
  culture and, 411–13
  cutaneous stimulation to relieve, 413
  with deep vein thrombosis, 981, 983
  dysmenorrhea, 100
  emotions and, 513
  factors affecting response to, 411–13
  fallopian tube, 83
  from gallbladder disease in pregnancy, 351
  gate-control theory of, 410, 410f
    distraction and, 413
  from hydramnios, 577
  in iliac fossae, 83
  with intercourse, postmenopausal, 101
  intestinal, in neonate, 874
  in labor. *See* Labor, pain during
  menstrual (dysmenorrhea), 100
  midcycle (*mittelschmerz*), 84, 98
  ovarian, causes of, 84
  pattern theory of, 410
  physiologic responses to, 483
  postpartal (afterpains), 907
    management of, 915–16, 917n
  from postpartal hematoma, 973
  as puerperal infection sign, 975, 976, 977
  as pyelonephritis sign, 986
  specificity theory of, 410

theories on, 410
  from uterine rupture, 550
Pain medication, knowledge deficit and, 27. *See also* Analgesia; Anesthesia
Palatal cleft. *See* Cleft palate
Palate
  assessing in initial prenatal exam, 220g
  assessing in neonate, 695–96g
Pallor
  in mother
    as anxiety sign, 608
    assessing, 570
    as pulmonary embolism sign, 981, 983, 984n
    as shock sign, 569
  in neonate
    as anemia sign, 835
    assessing, 689g
    with hypoglycemia, 818
    with intraventricular hemorrhage, 836
    as iron deficiency sign, 719
    as jaundice sign, 831n
    with MAS, 798
    with RDS, 796t, 801n, 802n
    from succenturiate placenta, 573
Palmar creases
  assessing, 684, 702g
  fetal alcohol syndrome affects, 770
Palmar erythema in pregnancy, 199
Palmar grasp reflex, assessing in neonate, 704g
Palpation
  assessing uterine contractions by, 433–34
  fetal position assessed by, 431g, 441–42, 442f
  fetal size estimation by, 557
  FHT assessment by, 424
  of fundus after delivery, 501, 502f
  during labor, FHR baseline variability caused by, 452
  Leopold maneuvers, 431g, 441–42, 442f
  of maternal abdomen, in initial prenatal exam, 223g
  of neonatal abdomen, 683, 699g
  of neonatal heart, 698g
  of neonatal testes, 701g
  postpartal assessment by, 501, 502f, 903
  vaginal, during labor, 436–40, 437–39f
  vaginal fornices used in, 74
Palpitations
  menopausal, 101
  as Methergine side effect, 903d
  in pregnancy, 222g
    with cardiac disease, 311
  as ritodrine side effect, 549
Palsy. *See also specific palsies*
  brachial, 684, 697g, 702g
  facial, assessing neonate for, 680
  in LGA infants, from birth trauma, 756–57n
  lower cranial nerve, from Arnold-Chiari lesions, 879
Pancreas, pregnancy changes in, 202
Pancreatic disease, diabetes secondary to, 315
Pantothenic acid, 276, 277
Papanicolaou (Pap) test
  genital herpes and, 360
  in infertility workup, 114
  in initial prenatal exam, 230g
  postpartal, 947g
  precontraception, 120
  reporting results of, 230

Papaverine hydrochloride, for pulmonary embolism, 982
Para, defined, 210
Paracervical block, 514f, 516f, 516–17
  contraindications for, 516
  FHR affected by, 456, 458, 523n
  for first stage labor, 514, 516
  maternal complications with, 517
  nursing implications of, 517
  pudendal block used with, 528
  technique, 516f, 516–17
    for vacuum aspiration abortion, 129
Paralysis
  congenital, mouth signs with, 695g
  diaphragmatic, signs of in initial prenatal exam 221g
  Erb-Duchenne, of neonatal arm, 684–85, 685f
  facial
    assessing neonate for, 680, 680f
    transient, after forceps delivery, 677
  in LGA neonates, from birth trauma, 756–57n
  of lower extremities, with meningomyelocele, 880, 882
Paralytic ileus, in preterm infant, 753
Paramesonephric ducts, 57, 58f, 77
Parametritis. *See* Pelvic cellulitis
Pararectal abscess, as imperforate anus complication, 872
Parasympatholytics, FHR baseline variability caused by, 452
Parathyroid glands, pregnancy changes in, 201
Parathyroid hormone, pregnancy changes in levels of, 201
Paraurethral glands
  embryologic development of, 57
  female (Skene's ducts), 71f, 73
Parent education, 725–30, 728–29f. *See also* Teaching role of nurse
  for adolescents, 301, 305, 943, 1017
  attachment aided by, 965, 1014
  cleft lip, 853, 856n
  cleft palate, 853n
  communication skills, 290–91
  congestive heart failure, 894
  discharge planning, 730
  fourth trimester assessment of, 944, 948g
  hip dysplasia, 878
  IUGR and, importance of for outcome, 763
  meningocele/meningomyelocele, 881, 882, 883–84n
  neonatal hyperbilirubinemia, 830
  neonatal jaundice, 831n, 834n
  neonatal safety, 716
  nurses as instructors, 13
  postpartal, 917n, 920n, 944
    principles and methods of, 938–39
  with preterm infant, 750, 754–55n, 758
  puerperal infection, 976, 977
  with RDS, 801
  with SGA neonate, 764
  stillbirth, 1004n
  talipes equinovarus (clubfoot), 876
  thromboembolic disease, 983
  with tracheoesophageal atresia/fistula, 862n, 865n
Parent-infant attachment. *See* Attachment process; Bonding
Parent-infant feedback system, smiling influences, 706

Parent-infant interaction
  assessing, 964, 965–68. 966–68f, 968–69
    in follow-up phone call, 948–49
  cesarean delivery affects, 604, 942
  facilitating
    after cesarean, 942
    with high-risk neonates, 737, 774–77
    in intensive care nursery, 1012–14
    by neonatal behavioral assessment, 687
    with neonatal hyperbilirubinemia, 830
    with preterm infant, 745n, 749, 754–55n, 774–77
    in puerperium, 920n, 965
    with RDS, 808n
    with tracheoesophageal atresia/fistula, 864–65n
  father's role in, 961–63
  feeding as central to, 921
  as nursing priority, 917n
  nursing role in, 725
  postpartal assessment of, 913–14
  reported to nursery nurse, 710
  sepsis neonatorum and, 842
Parenteral fluids. *See* Intravenous fluids
Parenting, prenatal assessment of, 999, 1000–1001t
Parenting disorders
  child abuse, 1014–16, 1016t
  preterm birth and, 1009–10
Parents. *See also* Mother; Father
  assessing, 47–49
  of defective child, nursing role with, 848–50
  interaction with infant by. *See* Attachment process; Parent-infant interaction
  neonatal assessment role of, 706
  reaction to adolescent pregnancy of, 301–2
Parents Anonymous, 1016
Parents Without Partners, 1018
Parer, J. T., 170
Parlodel (bromocriptine), 925, 926d
Partial thromboplastin time (PTT) test, for DIC, 567
Partner. *See also* Father; Husband
  cesarean delivery participation by, 602–3
  delivery room preparation by, 479n
  in psychologic assessments, 238, 240
  pregnancy diabetes role of, 318
Parturition
  defined, 395
  pelvic floor muscles during, 67
Passage, 535, 577–78
Passenger, 525
  complications involving, 551–77
Passive acquired immunity, 654
Passive euthanasia, as ethical issue, 10–11
Patent ductus arteriosus, in neonate, 881, 885, 887f
  apnea associated with, 749
  coarctation of the aorta with, 889
  of diabetic mother, 768
  heart murmur from, 641, 642
  incidence of, 881
  prematurity problems with, 739–40
  with RDS, 794f, 797t, 801n, 810n
  as respiratory therapy complication, 810n, 817

with transposition of the great vessels, 891

Patent ductus arteriosis, pregnancy with, 310

Patent urachus, in neonate, 684, 700g

Pathologic jaundice of newborn, 689–90g, 823–24. *See also* Jaundice; Hyperbilirubinemia

Pathologic retraction rings, 550, 578

Patients' rights, APPENDIX A, APPENDIX B

Patrick, J. E., 371

Pattern of states, in neonate, 705

Pattern theory of pain, 410

Pavlik harness, for hip dysplasia, 878

PAWP (pulmonary artery wedge pressure), monitoring with eclampsia, 344

PCO₂
  pneumothorax effects on, 816
  in preterm infant, normal values, 752t
  with respiratory acidosis, 794, 795

PDA, as prematurity risk, 749

PDR (*Physicians Desk Reference*), teratogenic substances and, 267

Pedal ablation, 183t

Pedal pulse, assessing in neonate, 685

Pediatric care units, family participation in, 12

Pediatric examination, initial, in birth center, 619

Pediatric nurse, genetic counseling referral by, 151

Pediatrician, birth attendance of
  at cesarean, 608, 609
  with malpresentations, 553, 555
  at midforceps delivery, 598

Pediatrics, neonatology as subspecialty of, 8

Pedigree, for genetic counseling, 150, 152, 153f

PEEP. *See* Positive end-expiratory pressure

Peer support, for intensive care nursery nurses, 1006

Pellagra, preventing in neonate, 717

Pelves, types of, 70–71
  Caldwell-Moloy classification of, 70–71, 396–97, 397f
  CPD predisposition and, 577
  labor complications associated with, 577–78
  transverse arrest and, 551

Pelvic "aches and pains" muscular uterine layer and, 78

Pelvic adequacy, intrapartal assessment of, 426–27, 426f, 427f, 427g, 432–33, 433–34f

Pelvic angle of inclination, 68, 68f

Pelvic carcinoma, potential lodging places of, 75

Pelvic cavity (midpelvis), 68, 68f, 69, 69f, 70
  assessing at labor onset, 426–27, 429g

Pelvic cellulitis (parametritis)
  from puerperal infection, 974, 975–76, 977, 979n
  thromboembolic disease risk with, 983

Pelvic changes
  nonpregnancy causes of, 192t
  as probable pregnancy sign, 192, 192t

Pelvic contractures
  birth center screening for, 618
  labor problems from, 577–78
  prolapsed umbilical cord with, 574

Pelvic diaphragm, 66, 67

Pelvic division, 68–70, 68f-70f

Pelvic embolism, potential lodging places of, 75

Pelvic examination
  assisting with, 235p
  in ectopic pregnancy assessmet, 333
  first, 303
  in infertility investigation, 1131f, 114
  in initial prenatal assessment, 225–28g, 235p
  precontraception, 120
  for pregnant adolescent, 303
  vaginal fornices enhance, 74

Pelvic floor
  assessing, fourth trimester, 947g
  labor changes in, 408
  muscles of, 66–68, 67t, 67f
  weakness of, from laceration, 73

Pelvic imflammatory disease (PID)
  chlamydial, 355
  residual
    dysmenorrhea from, 100
    infertility from, 111t, 112
    spontaneous abortion caused by, 329
  sign of in initial prenatal exam, 228g

Pelvic inlet, 68, 68f, 69–70, 69f-70f
  assessing at labor onset, 426, 426–27f, 429g
  contractures of, labor complications from, 577–78
    management of, 578
    prolapsed umbilical cord, 574
  diameters of, 69, 70f

Pelvic joints, pregnancy changes in, 255t, 258

Pelvic measurements, assessing in initial prenatal exam, 228g

Pelvic outlet (inferior strait), 68, 68f, 69, 69f
  assessing at labor onset, 427, 429g, 432, 433–34f
  contractures of, labor problems from, 578
  size increases at term, 66

Pelvic planes, 68–70, 69f

Pelvic presentations. *See* Breech presenations

Pelvic tilt exercise (pelvic rock), 262, 263f
  in childbirth preparation classes, 294
  in latent phase labor, 474
  postpartal, 920n, 922f
  in pregnancy, 255t, 258

Pelvic tumors, pregnancy signs caused by, 192t

Pelvic types. *See* Pelves, types of

Pelvic vein thrombophlebitis, pelvic cellulitis from, 975–76

Pelvic veins, relieving pressure on, 257

Pelvimetry, CPD assessment with, 577
  clinical, 426–27, 426f, 427f, 429g, 432–33, 433–34f
  x-ray, 387

Pelvis, bony, 66–71. *See also* Pelves, types of
  angle of inclination, 68, 68f
  assessing in initial prenatal exam, 225–28g
  bony structure, 65–66, 66f, 68–70f
  Caldwell-Moloy classification of, 70–71, 396–97, 397f
  large, precipitous labor with, 542
  obstetric implications of, 68–70
  pelvic division, 68–70, 68f-70f

pelvic floor, 66–68, 67t, 67f

Penicillin
  for congenital syphilis, 844
  for gonorrhea in neonate, 844
  for group B streptococcus in neonate, 843
  for sepsis neonatorum, 842

Penile urethra, 63
  embryologic development of, 58f, 59
  glands in, 64

Penis, 59–60, 59f, 60f
  blood supply to, 60, 60f
  cancer of, circumcision and, 722
  circumcision of, 722, 723–24f
  embryologic development of, 59
  of neonate, assessing, 684, 700–701g

Penis muliebris, 72. *See also* Clitoris

Penistix, diaper test for PKU with, 858

Penthrane (methoxyflurane), 529

Penticuff, J. H., 998

Pentobarbital (Nembutal), 513

Pentothal. *See* Thiopental sodium

Pepsinogen, neonatal stomach secretes, 651

Peptococcus infections, puerperal, 974

Peptostreptococcus infections, puerperal, 974

Perceptual functioning, in neonate, 654–57, 656f
  impaired, from kernicterus, 826

Percussion
  of neonatal abdomen, 700g
  of neonatal bladder, 700g
  of neonatal chest, 698g
  pneumothorax signs on, 809n
  as RDS intervention, 806n

Perfusion (blood flow), alveolar ventilation and, 639

Peridural block, 517f, 517–20, 518f, 520f, 525
  advantages and disadvantages of, 518
  agents for, 519
  caudal, 520, 520f, 525
  contraindications, 518
  for first and second stage labor, 514, 517
  indications for, 518
  lumbar epidural, 518f, 518–20

Perimetrium (serosal layer of uterus), 78

Perinatal morbidity
  IUGR and risk of, 370
  midforceps delivery increases, 597
  risk factors and, 459

Perinatal mortality, 23, 25t. *See also* Fetal death; Neonatal mortality
  from abruptio placentae, 563
  breech presentation and, 554, 605
  cardiac disease of mother and, 768
  crisis intervention for, 1005
  dysfunctional labor increases, 536
  eclampsia and, 341
  electronic fetal monitoring and, 459
  ethnic origin and, 206
  FHR patterns warning of, 375, 456, 458
  hydramnios and 577
  from hydrops fetalis, 826
  infection as leading cause of, 546
  intrapartal risk factors for, 425t
  IUGR as cause of, 370
  malpositions and, 552
  from maternal drug abuse, 360

maternal epilepsy and, 331t
midforceps delivery increases, 597
pelvic inlet contractures and, 578
PIH and, 341
placental lesions and, 568
as postmaturity risk, 760
prematurity as reason for, 384
from PROM, 546
pulmonary immaturity as reason for, 384
risk factors and, 214t, 459
in SGA neonates, 761
from sickle cell anemia, 328
from uterine rupture, 550
from uteroplacental insufficiency, 455

Perinatalogy, 8, 366

Perineal abscess, as imperforate anus complicaton, 872

Perineal body, 71f, 73

Perineal bulging, as imminent delivery sign, 479n

Perineal care, postpartal, 915, 917n, 919–20n
  puerperal infection and, 974
  urinary tract infection prevention by, 986
  wound healing and, 977–78n

Perineal distention, pudendal block relieves pain of, 527

Perineal lacerations, 580
  as breech delivery risk, 554
  brow presentation causes, 552
  from fetal malposition, 551
  infection of, 974–75, 975t, 977–79n
  "ironing" to prevent, 504
  as oxytocin-induction risk, 589, 590
  postpartal assessment of, 912
  postpartal care of, 915
  postpartal hemorrhage risk with, 972
  as precipitous labor risk, 425t, 543

Perineal muscles, 67, 67f
  Kegel's exercises for, 255, 263, 264f

Perineal pads, blood loss measured by use of, 501
  after cesarean, 609

Perineal prep, 467, 468, 473
  before cesarean delivery, 608
  optional vs. routine, 468, 613

Perineal tightening exercises, 919n. *See also* Kegel's exercises

Perineotomy, 596

Perineum (perineal body), 66, 71f, 73
  assessing
    at admission, 472
    in first stage labor, 429g
    in fourth stage labor, 481n, 502
  bulging, as imminent delivery sign, 479n
  caring for during labor, 483, 504
    fourth stage, 500
  hematoma pain in, in third or fourth stage labor, 580
  inspecting, precipitous delivery, 504
  "ironing" 504
  labor changes in, second stage, 418, 419f
  lacerations of. *See* Perineal lacerations
  local anesthesia for, 528, 528f
  postpartal hematoma signs on, 973
  postpartal assessment of, 912, 912f, 917

Perineum (Cont'd)
  postpartal care of, 481, 482n,
    919–20
  postpartal changes in, 904
  postpartal pain in, managing,
    915, 917n
  surgical incision of. See
    Episiotomy
  varicosities in, in late pregnancy,
    257
Periodic breathing, in neonates, 639
  apnea vs., 749, 796t
Periorbital cyanosis, as normal, 689g
Peristalsis
  of fallopian tube, 83
  in fetal intestinal tract, 651
  in neonate, assessing, 699g, 700g
Peritoneal cavity, fluid effusion into.
    See Ascites
Peritoneum
  broad ligament and, 80
  fallopian tubes covered by, 83
  in serosal layer of uterus, 78
Peritonitis
  as colostomy complication, 870
  meconium, 873
  as postpartal infection risk, 974
  puerperal, 975–76, 977, 979–
    80n
  signs of, 870
  from uterine rupture, 550
Persistent ostium primum, gesta-
    tional age and, 183t
Persistent pulmonary hypertension
    (PPH), 816–17
  as respiratory therapy complica-
    tion, 810n, 816–17
  retrolental fibroplasia risk with,
    815
Personal hygiene, in puerperium,
    916
Perspiration. See Sweating
Pes planus (flat foot), as normal,
    703g
Pessaries, Greeks used, 3
Petechiae
  as DIC sign, 567, 568
  in initial prenatal exam 217g
  in neonate
    assessing, 691g
    from congenital CMV, 359
    from congenital rubella, 358
    with pathologic jaundice, 823
Petroleum jelly, circumcision care
    with, 727
Pfannenstiel incision, 605
PG (Phosphatidylglycerol) test,
    320–21
PGs. See Prostaglandins
PGE₂ gel
  induction of labor with, 595
  ripening cervix with, 588
pH
  of amniotic fluid, Nitrazine test
    for, 430g, 436p
  of blood. See Blood pH
  of breast milk, cow's milk, and
    formula, 719t
  of cervical mucus, 98
  fetal, during labor, 461–63, 462f
    hypoxia affects, 451t, 454
    resuscitation risk and, 787
  of prostate fluid, 64
  of saliva in pregnancy, dental
    caries and, 199
  of semen, 64
  of vagina, 75
    postmenopausal, 101

in pregnancy, 196
Phallus, embryologic development
    of, 57, 59
Pharynx
  assessing in initial prenatal exam,
    220g
  assessing in neonate, assessing,
    696g
Phase of maximum slope, 417, 417f
Phenazopyridine, sign of in
    urinalysis, 229g
Phenergan (promethazine), during
    labor, 513
Phenobarbital (Luminal)
  neonatal clotting and bleeding
    problems from, 650
  for neonatal hyperbilirubinemia
    prevention, 830
  for neonatal seizures, IVH, 837
Phenothiazines
  amenorrhea from, 100
  fetal/neonatal effects of, 267t,
    361t, 452
Phenotype, 142
Phenylketonuria (PKU), 857–58
  as autosomal recessively
    inherited, 144
  cost of, 134, 135
  cost of preventing, 135
  dietary treatment for, 135
  genetic counseling referral for,
    151
  incidence of, 858
  maternal, as pregnancy complica-
    tion, 331t, 761
    diet for, 858
  neonatal screening for, 150, 725
  prenatal diagnosis invalid for,
    148
Pheochromocytoma, sign of in initial
    prenatal exam, 230g
Phimosis, assessing male neonate
    for, 684, 701g
  infertility and, 114
Phlebothrombosis, 976
  as varicose veins complication,
    257
Phlegmasia alba dolens, 981
Phocomelia, 145–46
  assessing neonate for, 702g
Phosphates, See also Phosphorus
  inorganic, placental transport of,
    170
  neonatal requirements, 717t
  organic, in erythrocytes, oxygen
    affinity and, 643
Phosphatidylglycerol (PG), in lung
    profile, 385–86, 386f, 639
Phosphatidylglycerol (PG) test, for
    diabetic, 320–21
Phosphatidylinositol (PI), in lung
    profile, 386, 386f
Phosphatidylinositol (PI) test, for
    diabetic, 321
Phospholipids
  fetal lung maturity and, 638
  in labor onset theory, 407
Phosphorus. See also Phosphates
  in breast milk, cow's milk, and
    formula, 719t
  lactation requirements, 270t
  leg cramps and, 258, 259
  neonatal hypocalcemia and, 821
  normal neonatal values, 645t
  pregnancy requirements, 199,
    270t, 273
  in preterm infant, normal values,
    752t

preterm infant requirements, 746
  vitamin D and, 275
Phototherapy, 823, 824
  exchange transfusion vs., 827,
    827f
  fluid loss with, 747
  for hemolytic disease of the new-
    born, 827, 827f, 829–30,
    830f
  for hyperbilirubinemia, 827,
    827f, 829–30, 830f
  in-home, 831n
  nursing care plan, 832–33
  nursing interventions during,
    829–30, 830f
Physical assessment. See also
    Physical examination
  antenatal. See Antepartal nursing
    assessment
  of neonate, 688–704g
    with adolescent mother, 943
    reporting to nursery nurse,
      709
  postpartal, at 2 and 6 weeks,
    944, 945–47g
  intrapartal. See Intrapartal fetal
    assessment; Intrapartal
maternal assessment
Physical characteristics, gestational
    age determination by, 660,
    661–69, 662f, 664–71f
Physical examination
  of mother
    before cesarean delivery, 601
    determining delivery date by,
      237
    double setup, for placenta
      previa, 565p, 567
    in fetal distress nursing care
      plan, 538
    in hemorrhage nursing care
      plan, 569
    before induction of labor, 591
    in infertility investigation, 113f,
      114
    at labor admission, 472
    mastitis assessment by, 987
    by physician or pediatric nurse
      practitioner, 714
    for PIH, 337
    in postnatal genetic evaluation,
      149–50, 149f
    postpartal. See Postpartal
      nursing assessment
    postpartal wound infection
      seen on, 974, 975t, 977,
      978n
    precontraception, 120
    pregnancy diabetes and, 322
    prenatal. See Antepartal
      nursing assessment
    puerperal infection assessment
      with, 976, 977n
    pulmonary embolism signs on,
      983, 984n
    before regional anesthesia,
      521n
    subinvolution signs on, 973
    thrombophlebetis signs on,
      983
    uterine atony signs on, 972
  of neonate, 674–87, 675–76f,
    679–80f, 682–83f, 685–87f,
    688–704g
    abdomen, 683–84, 699–700g
    anus, 684, 702g
    arms, 702g
    assessment data from, 660

back, 685
bladder, 700g
blood pressure, 688g
breasts, 699g
buttocks, 702g
chest, 682, 683f, 697–98g
in cleft lip and palate nursing
  care plan, 853
clitoris, 701g
cry, 682, 688g
diaphragm, 699g
ears, 681, 682f, 696–97g
esophageal atresia assessment
  with, 862
extremities, 684–85, 685f,
  702g, 703g
eyes, 680f, 680–81, 693–94g
face, 678, 680, 680f, 692–
  93g
feet, 703g
female genitals, 701–2g
femoral pulses, 700g
general appearance, 674–75
genitals, 684, 700–702g
hair, 692g
hands, 702g
head, 678, 679f, 691–92g
heart, 682–83, 698–99g
hips, 703g, 877f, 877–78
immediate, 495–97, 496f,
  498n
inguinal area, 700g
jaundice assessment with, 831,
  832n
kidneys, 700g
labia majora, 701g
labia minora, 701g
legs, 703g
length, 689g
liver, 700g
lungs, 698g
male genitals, 700–701g
measurements, 675–76, 675f,
  689g
mons, 701g
motor function, 703g
mouth, 681, 695–96g
neck, 681–82, 697g
neurologic status, 685–87,
  686–87f, 702g, 703–4g,
  705–6
neurologic-muscular, 703–4g
nose, 681, 695g
nutritional assessment with,
  719
patent ductus arteriosus detection by, 885
penis, 700–701g
posture, 675, 689g
in preterm infant nursing care
  plan, 750
pulse, 688g
for RDS nursing care plan,
  801
respiration, 682, 688g
rib cage, 699g
risk identification with, 736
scrotum, 701g
in SGA nursing care plan,
  764
skin, 677–78, 689–91g
spine, 702g
spleen, 700g
talipes equinovarus diagnosis
  by, 875f, 876
temperature, 676f, 676–77
testes, 701g
trachea, 699g

tracheoesophageal fistula
    assessment with, 862
  trunk, 702–3g
  umbilicus, 700g
  vagina, 701–2g
  vital signs, 688g
  weight, 675–76, 675f, 689g
Physical handicaps, neonatal
    screening for, 725
Physical sex behavior, 88, 89
Physicians
  nursery role of, 714. See also
    Pediatrician
  nursing role changes and, 14,
    15–16
Physicians Desk Reference (PDR),
    on teratogenic substances,
    267
Physiologic anemia of infancy, 644
Physiologic anemia of pregnancy
    (pseudoanemia), 198, 274
Physiologic jaundice (Icterus neona-
    torum), 648–50, 689–90g.
    See also Hyperbilirubinemia;
    Jaundice
Physiologic retraction ring, 407
Physiologic weight loss in neonate,
    675
Piaget, J., 297
Pica, in pregnancy, 281–82
PID. See Pelvic inflammatory
    disease
Pierre Robin syndrome, 850–51
  micrognathia with, 692g
Pigeon chest, assessing in neonate,
    698g
Pigmentation, assessing in neonate,
    690–91g
PIH. See Pregnancy-induced
    hyptertension
Pilonidal cyst or sinus
  assessing neonate for, 702g
    LGA preterm IDM, 757n
  in initial prenatal exam, 228g
Pilonidal dimple
  assessing neonate for, 702g
  in LGA preterm IDM, 757n
Pink stains on diaper ("brick dust
    spots"), 652
Pinocytosis, in placenta, 170
Piper forceps, 597, 597f
  for breech presentation, 555,
    597, 598
Piskacek's sign, 192, 193f
  nonpregnancy causes of, 192t
Pitocin. See Oxytocic agents
Pitting edema, at labor onset, 429g.
    See also Edema
Pituitary gland
  oxytocin released by, with breast-
    feeding, 902
  postdelivery anterior pituitary
    necrosis, 988
  postdelivery galactorrhea and,
    987
  pregnancy changes in, 201–2
  puberty role of, 91, 92, 92f
Pituitary tumor, infertility from,
    111t
PKU. See Phenylketonuria
Placenta
  adherence of, 579
  battledore, 568, 574, 574f
  circulation in, 167–68, 167f,
    169f
  circumvallate, 568, 573–74,
    574f
  decidua basalis as origin of, 163

delivery of, 419, 420f, 480–81n
  with emergency out-of-hospital
    delivery, 506
  inspecting after, 972
  manual, risks accompanying,
    419, 824
  oxytocin administration with,
    497, 500
  precipitous delivery, 504
development of, 165–67, 167f
  diminished perfusion in, risk
    factors for, 214–15t
  embryonic portion of, 164
  enlarged, neonatal jaundice and,
    831
  estrogen produced by, 379
  functions of, 165, 168–71
  general anesthesia crosses, 528
  as homograft, 179
  impaired gas exchange across,
    540n
  inspecting, 480n
    importance of, 579
  labor analgesia crosses, 510–11
  locating
    before amniocentesis, 381–82,
      382f, 383p
    cephalic version and, 585
    ultrasound for, 8, 368, 371
  low-lying, prolapse risk and, 574
  maternal and fetal portions of,
    167, 167f
  permeability of, 167
  problems in, 568, 573–74, 574f
    developmental vs. generative,
      568
  regional anesthesia crosses, 514
  respiratory function of, evaluat-
    ing. See Contraction stress
    test
  retained, 419, 579
    postpartal risks from, 908t
  retained fragments of, 579
    afterpains from, 907
    as hemorrhage risk, 569, 572,
      579, 972
    as infection risk, 974
    interventions for, 572n, 972,
      973
    as placenta previa risk, 566
    from succenturiate placenta,
      568, 573
    uterine involution affected by,
      903
  separation of, in third stage
    labor, 419, 420f, 504
  site of
    infection risk in, 974. See also
      Endometritis
    involution of, 902–3
  size of, hemolytic disease of new-
    born and, 827
  small, risk factors for, 736f
  succenturiate, 568, 573, 574f
    inspecting for, 579
    velamentous insertion with,
      575
  transport mechanisms in, 170–71
  umbilical cord attachment to,
    167
  velamentous, 167, 575
  weight of, hydramnios and, 576–
    77
Placenta abruptio. See Abruptio
    placentae
Placenta accreta, 579
Placenta previa, 564f, 564–67,
    565t, 566f

as birth center contraindication,
    618
  bleeding causeed by, 329
  breech presentation and, 554
  cesarean delivery for, 600
  as CST contraindication, 375
  danger sign of, 240g
  defined, 335, 402, 564
  detecting with ultrasound, 368,
    371
  diagnosis of, 565–66, 565p
  fetal distress with, 540
  fetal/neonatal implications of,
    425t, 566, 761
  incidence of, 564
  as induction of labor contraindica-
    tion, 587
  interventions for, 566–67
  IUGR associated with, 761
  maternal implications of, 425t,
    566
  narcotic addiction increases risk
    of, 770
  neontal anemia caused by, 830
  postpartal risks with, 908t
  resuscitation risk with, 786, 787
  as risk factor, 215t, 425t
  ruling out, with hemorrhage,
    572n
  shoulder presentation caused by,
    402
  statistics about, 329
  transverse lie and, 556
  types of, 564, 564f
  ultrasound to diagnose, 368
Placental anomalies, IUGR
    associated with, 761
Placental function
  maternal drug abuse affects, 360
  nutritive vs. respiratory compo-
    nents of, 374
  tests of, 366
Placental gas exchange, impaired,
    fetal distress care for, 540
Placental grading, ultrasound for,
    368, 372, 372f
Placental hormones, 202
Placental infarcts and calcifications,
    574
  IUGR associated with, 761
Placental insufficiency
  as drug addiction risk, 770
  early termination of pregnancy
    for, 384
  estriol determinations for, 379,
    380
  induction of labor with, 587
  IUGR from, oligohydramnios and,
    577
  from maternal hypertensive
    disease, 769
  paracervical block contraindicatd
    by, 516
  in postterm pregnancies, 759–60
Placental lesions, 568
Placental membranes, meconium-
    stained, postterm infant,
    760
Placental perfusion, oxytocin may
    decrease, 589
Placental polyp, 973
Placental separation. See also
    Abruptio placentae
  assessing for
    with eclampsia, 344
    with severe preeclampsia, 343
    premature, as forceps delivery
      indication, 597

Placental sterioid sulfatase defi-
    ciency, estriol levels and,
    380
Plagiocephaly, 678, 691g
Plan of care. See also Nursing care
    plans
  antepartal, 285
  crisis intervention, 996, 998–99
  for high-risk neonates, 737. See
    also specific risks
  in POMR system, 20
  postpartal learning objectives,
    938
  for RDS, 797, 801–10n
Plantar creases. See Sole creases
Plantar flexion, in neonate, 657
Plantar grasp reflex, assessing in
    neonate, 686, 704g
Plasma, fresh frozen, for DIC, 567
Plasma albumin concentrations,
    pregnancy decreases, 199
Plasma electrolyte in preterm
    infant, normal values, 752t
Plasma estriol determinations. See
    Estriol determinations
Plasma fibrinogen. See also
    Fibrinogen
  increases during labor, 409
  pregnancy changes in, 197t, 198
Plasma progesterone tests, in infer-
    tility workup, 115f, 116
Plastibell, circumcision with, 723f
Platelets
  administering, for DIC, 568
  decrease in, from, DIC, 567,
    568f
  formation of in fetus, 643
  in neonate, 645, 650
  preterm, normal values, 752t
Platypelloid pelvis, 70, 396–97,
    397f
Pleural effusion, signs of in initial
    prenatal exam, 221g
Pleural friction rub, in initial pre-
    natal exam, 221g
Plugged ducts, mastitis and, 987
PMI (point of maximum intensity),
    233p, 698g
PMT (premenstrual tension) syn-
    drome, 99–100
Pneumatosis intestinalis, with necro-
    tizing enterocolitis, 837,
    838, 839
Pneumonediastinum
  as respiratory therapy complica-
    tion, 809n, 816
  rupture with, as MAS risk, 798
Pneumonia
  maternal
    from chlamydial infection,
      355
    fetal distress nursing care plan,
      540
  neonatal
    aspiration. See Aspiration
      pneumonia
    bacterial, with MAS, 798
    breath sounds with, 698g
    chest expansion with, 698g
    drug-addicted, 770, 771
    from endocardial cushion
      defects, 888
    group B streptococcal infection
      vs., 843
    hyperresonance of chest with,
      698g
    meconium aspiration increases
      risk of, 425t

Pneumonia, neonatal (Cont'd)
    orthostatic, preventing after
        cleft lip surgery, 856n
    PPH syndrome with, 817
    in preterm infant, apnea with,
        749
    as SGA neonatal risk, 765
    tachypnea as sign of, 688g
Pneumonitis
    from aspiration of vomitus during
        labor, 530–31
    with extended rubella syndrome,
        358
    with MAS, 798
    from tracheoesophageal atresia/
        fistula, 860, 861, 862n
Pneumopericardium, as respiratory
        therapy complication, 809,
        810n, 816
Pneumoperitoneum
    as necrotizing enterocolitis sign,
        838, 839
    as respiratory therapy complica-
        tion, 809, 810n, 816
Pneumothorax, in neonate
    causes of, 809n, 816
    chest expansion with, 698g
    as diaphragmatic hernia risk, 867
    interventions for, 809n, 816
    as MAS risk, 798
    preterm, assessing for, 757n
    as SGA neonatal risk, 765
    signs of, 683, 698g, 699n, 809n
    ventilation problems with, 788
Po. See Postterm neonates
PO₂
    decreased. See Hypoxemia
    in fetal circulation, 171
Podalic version, 3, 585–86
Podophyllin, alternatives to during
        pregnancy, 355
Point of maximal impulse (PMI),
        233p, 698g
Poisoning, preventing, 729, 730
Polar body, formation of, 160, 161f
Poliomyelitis
    hip dysplasia vs., 878
    immunization in pregnancy, 266t
    neonatal immunity to, 654
Polycystic kidney disease, 143,
        368, 700f
Polycythemia, in neonate, 835–36
    cyanosis seen with, 889
    hyperbilirubinemia with, 822,
        823
    hypoglycemia differentiation
        from, 818
    in IDM, 768
    interventions for, 836
    jaundice and, 831
    in LGA neontes, 761
    as postmaturity risk, 760
    PPH syndrome with, 817
    risk factors for, 736f
    in SGA neonates, 762, 764n,
        766n
    signs of, 835–36
    skin color with, 689g
    with tetralogy of Fallot, 890
    from transposition of the great
        vessels, 891
Polydactyly, assessing neonate for,
        684, 702g
Polydipsia, as diabetes sign, 314.
        See also Thirst
Polygenic inheritance, 142, 145,
        145t
    AID as alternative to, 152

cleft lip and palate and, 696g,
        851
    Pierre Robin syndrome and, 850
    postnatal diagnosis of, 149, 150
    prenatal diagnosis of, 148
    recurrence risk for, 145, 145t,
        148
Polyhydramnios. See Hydramnios
Polymenorrhea, 100
Polyphagia, as diabetes sign, 314
Polyps
    infertility from, 111t
    placental, 973
Polyuria. See Urinary frequency
Pompe's disease, prenatal diagnosis
        of, 148
POMR. See Problem-oriented
        medical records
Pontocaine (tetracaine), 514, 516
Popliteal angle, gestational age and,
        663f, 665f, 672
Porphyria, sign of in initial prenatal
        exam, 229g
Port-wine stain (nevus flammeus),
        677–78, 691g, 867
Positive end-expiratory pressure
        (PEEP)
    method, 799–800t
    for RDS, 797, 799–800t, 804n
Positive pressure therapy, patent
        ductus arteriosus with, 810n
Positive pressure ventilation
    complications of, 808n, 816
    for diaphragmatic hernia, 866,
        867
Positive regard, as assessment tool,
        48
Postcoital examination, 113f, 116
Postdelivery anterior pituitary
        necrosis, 988
Postdelivery galactorrhea, 987
Postdelivery period, nursing care
        plan, 480–81
Posterior fontanelle, assessing, 678,
        692g
Posterior pituitary hormones, preg-
        nancy role of, 202
Posterior vaginal column, 75
Postmaturity. See also Postmaturity
        syndrome; Postterm
        neonates
    as CST indication, 375
    definition of, 758
    estriol determinations for, 379,
        380
    estriol excretion patterns and,
        380
    incidence of, 758–59
    induction of labor for, 587
    macrosomia with, 556
    MAS risk with, 798, 815
    morbidity and mortality risk with,
        760, 815
    nails with, 702g
    nonstress testing for, 374
    oligohydramnios and, 425t, 577
    PPH risk with, 817
    resuscitation risk with, 786
    skin texture with, 690g
Postmaturity syndrome, 759–60
    risk factors for, 736f
Postnatal period, nursing care plan,
        480–82. See also Postpartal
        nursing management;
        Puerperium
Postnatal diagnosis of genetic disor-
        ders, 148–50
Postneonatal period, 23

    mortality rates in, 23, 25t
Postpartal depression, 907, 921
    family situation affects, 993
Postpartal exercises. See Exercises
Postpartal floor, transfer to, 480n,
        502
Postpartal headache, from spinal
        anesthesia, 526–27
Postpartal hemorrhage. See
        Hemorrhage
Postpartal morbidity, infection as
        cause of, 974
Postpartal home visits. See Home
        visits
Postpartal nursing assessment,
        907–14, 917n
    abdomen and fundus, 910f, 910–
        11
    of adolescent needs, 942–43
    of attachment process, 963–68,
        966–68f, 968–69
    basic principles of, 901, 907–8
    cervical changes, 904
    cultural influences, 914
    elimination, 913
    follow-up, 939, 941
    hematomas, 973
    for hemorrhage, importance of,
        972
    of learning needs, 938
    lochia, 911
    nursing care plan, 481
    nutritional status, 913
    perineum, 904, 912, 912f
    by phone, 948–49
    physical, 481n, 907–13, 908t,
        909–10f, 912f
        sample form for, 909f
        at two and six weeks, 944,
            945–47g
    psychologic, 913–14, 944, 948g
    rest and sleep status, 913
    risk factors, 907, 908t
    for subinvolution, 973
    at 2 and 6 weeks, 944, 945–48g
    vaginal changes, 904
    vital signs, 912–13
    of wound infection, 974–75,
        975t, 977, 978n
Postpartal nursing management,
        914–49. See also Postnatal
        period; Puerperium
    abruptio placentae, 564
    adolescent mother, 942–43
    anticipatory guidance, 289–90
    attachment problems, 1011–14,
        1013f
    basic principles of, 901
    in birth center, 619
    of cardiac client, 313
    after cesarean delivery, 941–42
    comfort and pain relief, 915–16,
        917–20n
    complications, 972–89
    crisis intervention, during follow-
        up, 1010–19
    defective birth, 848–50
    for diabetic client, 321, 325
    family wellness promotion, 939–
        40
    follow-up care, 944, 948–49
        crisis intervention in, 1010–
            19
    fourth trimester, 943–49, 945–
        48g
    hematomas, 973
    hemorrhage prevention, 972,
        973

    home visit assessment guide,
        624–27
    infant feeding, 921–38
    infections, 973–76, 975t, 977–
        80n
    neonatal death, 1002–6, 1004n
    nursing care plan, 917–20
    nursing diagnoses, examples, 920
    objectives of, 914–15
    parent education, 938–39
    for PIH client, 346–47
    preterm birth, 1008–10, 1009f
    relinquishing mother, 1015t
    rest and activity, 916
    for Rh sensitization, 349–50
    subinvolution, 973
    thromboembolic disease, 980,
        981, 983–85n
    two- and six-week examinations,
        944, 945–48g, 948–49
Postpartal unit, transfer to, 480n,
        502
"Postpartum blues" 907
    family and, 993
    nursing management of, 921
Postpartum period. See Puerperium
Postterm labor, defined, 210
Postterm (Po) neonates, 758–60,
        759t, 759f. See also
        Postmaturity
    birth weight classification for,
        734, 735f
    breast tissue in, 661, 668
Postural drainage
    for MAS, 815
    for RDS, 806n
Postural hypotension in pregnancy,
        198
    faintness from, 255t, 259
Posture
    of neonate
        assessing, 657, 675, 689g,
            703g
        gestational age and, 661,
            663f, 665f, 667f
        LGA, evaluating, 756n
        preterm, heat loss and, 740
    pregnancy changes in, 199–200,
        200f, 258
    urinary tract changes and, 199
Potassium
    in breast milk, cow's milk, and
        formula, 719t
    normal neonatal values, 645t
    preterm infant, 752t
Potassium supplements, with furose-
        mide, 894
Potter syndrome, ventilation prob-
        lems with, 788
Potts-Smith-Gibson operation, 890,
        891f
Pouch of Douglas (cul-de-sac or
        rectouterine pouch), 74, 78
    abscesses in, 975
    palpation of, 74
Powdering infants, 727
Powell, M. L., 1010
Powers, labor role of, 525
PPD, in initial prenatal exam, 230g
PPH. See Persistent pulmonary
        hypertension
Pr. See Preterm neonates
Preauricular skin tags, in neonate,
        696g
"Precip pack" 503
Precipitous delivery, 503–5
Precocious teeth, in neonate, 681
Preeclampsia/eclampsia. See also

Eclampsia; Pregnancy-induced hypertension
as birth center contraindication, 618
with chronic hypertension, 347
clinical manifestations of, 341
as CST indication, 375
danger signs of, 240g
decline in incidence of, 336
deep leg vein disease risk with, 981
in diabetic client, 323
drug addiction increases risk of, 770
edema of mons pubis with, 72
estriol determinations for, 379, 380
fetal distress with, 540
as hemorrhage risk, 569
postpartal, 972
as hyperthyroidism risk, 326
induction of labor for, 587
interventions for, 337–40n, 342–44, 345d
ketamine contraindicated with, 530
during labor, 428g, 429g, 536
signs of, 473
testing for, at labor admission, 468
mild
clinical manifestations of, 341
interventions for, 342
as oxytocin contraindication, 590
postpartal diuresis with, 905
postpartal proteinuria from, 906
postpartal risks with, 908t
postpartal signs of, 906
as preterm labor cause, 548
resuscitation risk with, 786
risk factors for, 214–15t
as ritadrine contraindication, 548, 549
severe
clinical manifestations of, 341
drug guide for, 345
interventions for, 343–44
sickle cell anemia increases risk of, 327
signs of, 240g, 341
in initial prenatal exam, 224g, 225g, 230g
in subsequent prenatal exams, 239g, 240g
sodium intake and, 273
thromboembolic disease risk with, 981, 983n
Preembryonic development, 162–65, 173
Pregestational medical disorders, 310–28, 330–31t. See also specific disorders
anemias, 326–28
cardiac disease, 310–13
less common, 330–31t
thyroid dysfunction, 321, 326
Pregnancy
abortion of. See Abortion
activity during, 261
adolescent. See Adolescent pregnancy
alcohol in, 267t, 268–69, 362
amenorrhea from, 100
anatomy and physiology of, 195–202
anemia in, 326–28
ankle edema in, 254t, 256

antepartal assessment. See Antepartal nursing assessment
appendicitis in, 351
attachment process affected by, 953
backache in, 253f, 255t, 258, 258f
bathing in, 261
bleeding in, 328–35
nursing interventions for, 329
bony pelvis changes in, 66
breast cancer in, 352
breast care in, 260
breast-feeding during, 927–28
breast tenderness in, 254t, 255
cardiac disease with, 310–13
cardiovascular system changes in, 197t, 198
cervical cancer during, 352
cervical changes after, 79, 80f
chlamydial infections in, 355
clothing in, 260–61
maternity girdle, 258
shoes, 255t, 258
common concerns during, 260–69
complications of
abruptio placentae, 329, 335
accidents and trauma, 352–53
anemia, 326–28
bleeding disorders, 328–35, 332f, 332f, 334f, 335f
cytomegalovirus, 358–59
ectopic pregnancy, 329, 333–34, 334f
effects on family of, 580–81
epilepsy, 331t
financial effects of, 581
herpesvirus type 2, 359–60
hydatidiform mole, 329, 334–35, 335f
hyperemesis gravidarum, 328
incompetent cervix, 335–36
infections, 353–60; see also specfic infections
maternal phenylketonuria (PKU), 331t
medical disorders, 328–50. See also specific disorders
multiple sclerosis, 330t
myasthenia gravis, 330
PIH. See Preeclampsia/eclampsia; Pregnancy-induced hypertension
placenta previa, 329, 335
pregestational medical disorders, 330–31t
Rh sensitization, 347–50, 350p
rubella, 357–58
spontaneous abortion. See Abortion, spontaneous
surgical procedures, 351–53
systemic lupus erythematosus (SLE), 330–31t
thyroid dysfunction, 321, 326
TORCH infections, 357–60
toxoplasmosis, 357
tuberculosis (TB), 331t
condylomata accuminata in, 355
constipation in, 253f, 255t, 257–58
coping mechanisms in. See Coping mechanisms
couvade, 250
as crisis, 246–47

labor as part of, 405–6
cultural considerations in, 204–7, 288–89t, 289
cytomegalic inclusion disease (CID) in, 358–59
danger signs in, 240g, 253f
delivery date, determining, 236–37, 237f
ultrasound for, 368–69
denial of, 1014
dental care in, 265
developmental tasks of, 247
adolescence and, 296–97, 300t
parenting and, 999, 1000–1001t
diabetes mellitus with, 313–21, 314t, 315t, 319t, 322–25n
diabetogenic effect of, 314
diagnostic (positive) signs of, 195
discomforts of, 252–60, 253f, 254–55t
drug use and abuse in, 360–62, 361t
duration of, 171, 173, 191
dyspnea in, 253f, 255t, 259
early detection of, ultrasound for, 368–69
early termination of, reasons for, 384, 388
ectopic. See Ectopic pregnancy
edema in
of ankles, 254t, 256
of hands, 240g
of mons pubis, 72
emotional and psychologic changes of, 203–4
employment in, 261
endocrine system changes in, 201–2
endometrial changes in, 79
exercises, 262–63, 263–64f
expectant family's responses to, 247–52, 248t
faintness in, 255t, 259
family developmental tasks in, 38–39
father's psychologic status in, 242–43g
father's reactions to, 248t, 249–50
fetal attitude in, 399
fetal status in. See Assessment of fetus
first trimester
discomforts of, 252, 253f, 254t, 254–56
emotional changes in, 203, 204
parental reactions in, 241g, 242g, 248t, 249
sexual response in, 264
teratogenic risk in, 266
food myths in, 282–83
fourth trimester, 943–49, 945–58t
gallbladder disease in, 351–52
gastrointestinal system changin, 197t, 198–99
gonorrhea in, 354–55
grandparents' responses to, 251–52
health beliefs and practices and, 205–7
heartburn in, 253f, 254t, 256
hemorrhoids in, 255t, 257
herpes in, 359–60

high-risk. See also Adolescent pregnancy; High-risk pregnancy
birth center screening for, 618
crisis intervention for, 998–99
four major concerns with, 342
high-risk infants from, 733–34
management problems with, 388–89
regional centers for, 389
resuscitation risk with, 786–87
testing fetal well-being in, 366. See also Assessment of fetus
transport for, attachment process and, 773–74
hormone of, progesterone as, 94
hospitalization in. See Hospitalization
hypertension in, late or transient, 347
immunizations during, 265, 266t
infections in, 353–60. See also specific infection
lactose intolerance in, 272, 281
leg cramps in, 253f, 255t, 258–59, 259f
listerial infection in, 356–57
medical disorders preceding, 310–28
medical disorders with, 328–50
medications during, 266–68, 267t
metabolic changes in, 197t, 200–201
nasal stuffiness and epistaxis in, 252, 254, 254t
nausea and vomiting in, 252, 253f. 254t
in nurses, specimen collection caution, 766n
nursing role in, 245–46, 259–60
nutrition in, 269–85, 270–72t, 277t, 282t, 286–87f
adolescents and, 297, 298t
assessing, 285, 286–87f
cultural factors and, 282t, 283–84
daily food plan, 271–72t
diabetes and, 318, 320
factors affecting, 281–85
importance of, 269
iron requirements, 327
neonatal iron stores and, 648
IUGR and, 761
maternal weight gain and, 269–70
neonatal behavior and, 654
for PIH, 338
psychologic factors and, 284–85
RDAs, 269, 270t
requirements, 270, 270–72t, 272–79
sample menus, 278–81, 283–84
socioecnomic factors and, 284
objective (probable) changes with, 192t, 193f, 193–94, 194f
parents' reactions to, 246–50, 248t
passenger role during, 535
patient bill of rights, APPENDIX A
physical assessmments in. See Antepartal nursing assessment
pica in, 281–82

Pregnancy *(Cont'd)*
  pregestational medical disorders and, 310–28
  progesterone's role in, 94
  prolonged, 759. *See also* Postmaturity
    fetal status evaluation in, 759t
    nonstress testing for, 374
  psychologic adaptive processes during, 772f, 772–73
  psychologic assessments in, 238, 238g, 240–41, 241–43g
  ptyalism in, 254, 254t
  reproductive system changes in, 195–97
  respiratory system changes in, 197, 197t
  rest periods in, 262, 262f
  Rh sensitization in, 347–50, 348f, 350p
  risk factors in, 366
  round ligament hypertrophies during, 81
  rubella in, 357–58
  second trimester
    discomforts of, 253f, 254–55t, 256–59
    emotional changes in, 203, 204
    parental reactions in, 242g, 248t, 249–50
    psychologic status in, 241g
    sexual response in, 264
    teratogenic risk in, 266–67
  sexual activity in, 263–65
  sexually transmitted diseases in, 354–55
  shortness of breath in, 253f, 255t, 259
  siblings' responses to, 250–51, 251f
  skeletal system changes in, 199–200, 200f
  skin changes in, 199
  smoking during, 268, 361t
  as stress, 310
  striae from, vitamin E for, 275
  subjective (presumptive) changes in, 191t, 191–92
  surgical procedures during, 351–53
  syphilis in, 354
  teenage. *See* Adolescent pregnancy
  teratogenic substances in, 265–69, 267t
    medications, 266–68, 267t
    terms used to describe, 210–11
  third trimester
    discomforts of, 253f, 254–55t, 256–59
    parental reactions in, 243g, 248t, 250
    psychologic status in, 203, 204, 241g
    sexual response in, 264–65
    teratogenic risk in, 266–67
  thyroid dysfunction in, 321, 326
  timetable for teaching needs in, 253f
  TORCH group of infectious diseases in, 357–60
  toxoplasmosis in, 357
  travel during, 261
  unwanted, crisis intervention for, 1014, 1015t
  urinary tract changes in, 197t, 199

frequency and, 253f, 254t, 254–55
  urinary tract infections in, 353–54
  uterine changes after, 79, 80f
  vaginal discharge in, 253f, 254t, 255–56
  vaginal infections in, 355–56
  varicose veins in, 253f, 255t, 256–57, 257f
  weight gain in, 200–201, 269–70
  x-ray examination during, 387–88
Pregnancy tests, 194–95
  in ancient Egypt, 3
  nonpregnancy-caused positive results, 192t, 194
  precontraception, 120
Pregnancy-induced hypertension (PIH), 336–47, 340f, 343t. *See also* Eclampsia; Preeclampsia/eclampsia
  adolescents at risk for, 297, 482
  as CST indication, 375
  danger signs of, 240g
  delivery as only cure for, 344
  diet restrictions with, 342
  drug addiction and, 360
  drug guide, magnesium sulfate, 345
  dysfunctional labor with, interventions for, 536
  IUGR associated with, 761
  neonatal problems associated with, 769
  nursing care plan, 337–40
  Rh sensitization and, 824
  risk factors for, 214–15t, 297
  signs of, at labor onset, 428g, 429g
  as vacuum extraction indication, 598
Premature ejaculation, infertility from, 111t
Premature labor and delivery, 547–50. *See also* Preterm infants
  abnormal presentation and risk of, 425t
  adolescents at risk for, 297
  arresting, 548–50, 549d
  attachment problems with, 772–74
  after automobile accident, 352
  from battledore placenta, 574
  as birth center contraindication, 618
  breech presentation and, 554
  cardiac disease in mother and, 768
  causes of, 548
  cesarean delivery for, 600
  from circumvallate placenta, 574
  continuation indications for, 548
  as crisis, 772–74, 994–95, 995f, 1006, 1007–8t
    crisis intervention for, 1006, 1008–10
  danger signs of, 240g
  defined, 210, 547
  in diabetic client, 316
  as drug addiction risk, 771
  drug guide (ritodrine), 549
  emotional and situational factors in, 1006, 1007–8t, 1008
  nursing interventions for, 1008–10
  face presentation with, 553

federally funded care to prevent, 5
  fetal/neonatal implications of, 548
  fetal tachycardia caused by, 450
  FHR baseline variability caused by, 452
  as forceps indication, 597
  general anesthesia contraindicated by, 530
  gonorrhea as cause of, 354–55
  with hemolytic disease, 349
  from herpes infection, 359
  hydramnios and, 577
  as hyperthyroidism risk, 326
  incidence of, 737
  as oxytocin contraindication, 590
  induction of labor and, 590, 593n
  as intrapartal risk factor, 425t
  iron deficiency anemia and, 327
  listeriosis as cause of, 357
  long-range consequences of, 894–95
  lung maturity and. *See* Fetal lung maturity
  from maternal cardiac decompensation, 311
  from maternal drug abuse, 360
  from maternal hypertension, 769
  maternal implications of, 548
  maternal SLE and, 330t
  maternal urinary tract infection and, 353
  medications for, 548–50, 549d
  multiple gestation and, 425t
  nonstress test results with, 373
  as oligohydramnios risk, 577
  omphalocele and, 867, 868
  paracervical block contraindicated by, 516
  patent ductus arteriosus and, 881, 885
  physiologic jaundice of newborn and, 649
  PIH and, 341
  placental lesions and, 568
  premature rupture of membranes and, 546–47, 548
  RDS associated with, 795, 798
  resuscitation risk with, 786
  with Rh sensitization, 349
  risk factors for, 214–15t
  risk of, as CST contraindication, 375
  sickle cell anemia and, 328
  stress as cause of, 1010
  with tracheoesophageal fistula, 860
  transverse lie and, 556
  uterine anomalies and, 77
Premature rupture of membranes (PROM), 546f, 546–47
  causes of, 546
  as CST contraindication, 375
  defined, 546
  as danger sign, 240g
  in diabetic client, 316
  drug guide for, 547
  early termination of pregnancy for, 384
  fetal/neonatal implications of, 425t, 542, 546
  incidence of, 546
  induction of labor for, 587
  as intrapartal risk factor, 425t
  maternal implications of, 425tm 546
  from pelvic inlet contracture, 578

postpartal infection risk from, 913, 977
  prolonged labor after, 542
  as ritodrine contraindication, 548
Premenstrual tension syndrome (PMT), 99–100
Prenatal care, reported to nursery nurse, 710. *See also* Antepartal nursing management
Prenatal diagnosis of genetic diseases, 146f, 146–48. *See also* Screening
Prenatal education, 291–92. *See also* Childbirth preparation
  for adolescent, 304f, 305
  methods of teaching, 291–92
  nurses as instructors, 13
  pain reduced by, 27
  research application example about, 27
Prenatal examinations. *See* Antenatal nursing assessment
Prenatal exercises, 262–63, 263–64f
Prep, 467, 468
  controversy about, 468
  at labor admission, 473
  procedure for, 468
  types of, 468
Prepuce (foreskin), 60, 60f
  of clitoris, 71f, 72, 73
Pressure transducer. *See* Tocodynamometer
Preterm (Pr) infants, 737–58, 738f
  anemia in, course of, 835
  anterior fontanelle overlap in, 692g
  apnea in, 749, 755–56n
  behavioral states in, 749
  birth trauma in, 756–57n
  blood pressure values for, 751t
  breast milk for, 776
  breast tissue lacking in, 699g
  cardiovascular system in, 739t, 739–40
  classification of, 737
    by birth weight, 734, 735f
  CNS physiology and considerations in, 749
  coagulation factors in, 650t
  cold stress risk in, 817
  complications in, 755–56n
  crisis paradigm with, 994–95, 995f
  definition of, 737
  dehydration signs in, 753
  developmental evaluation for, 758
  developmental problems of, 894–95
  facilitating attachment with, 774–79
  feeding, 740–46, 741f, 742t, 743–45p, 747t
    formulas for, 740–41, 742t
    methods for, 741–46, 743–45p, 747t
    nursing care plan, 753–54
    problems with, 741, 746
  fluid balance management for, 747–48
  fluid requirements, 746, 747
  glycogen stores in, 748
  head and chest circumference in, 691g
  head lag in, 703g
  heat loss risk in, 647, 740

hematologic physiology and considerations for, 748–49
hepatic physiology and considerations, 748
hyperbilirubinemia risk in, 823
hypocalcemia in, 821–22
hypoglycemia in, 818, 821
immunologic physiology and considerations, 654, 748
infection susceptibility in, 754n, 841
intraventricular hemorrhage risk in, 836
iron deficiency in, 748
with IUGR, outcome factors, 762–63
jaundice interventions for, 832n, 833n
jaundice risk in, 748, 831
kernicterus danger in, 823, 824
laboratory evaluations for, 750
normal values, 752t
lanugo in, 690g
LGA, birth trauma nursing care plan, 756–57
long-term needs and outcomes for, 758
motor activity in, 705
necrotizing enterocolitis risk in, 837, 839n
nutrition for; see feeding
nutritional adequacy signs in, 747
overlapping of anterior fontanelle in, 678
parent interaction with, providing for, 754–55, 775–80, 777f, 779f
parental responses to, outcomes and, 778–79, 779f
patent ductus arteriosus in, 810n, 881, 885
pathologic jaundice definition for, 823
physiologic adaptations by, 737; see also specific adaptation
PROM risks for, 546
prone crawl in, 704g
RDS risk in, 792
reactivity periods in, 749
resuscitation risk in, 786
rooting reflex in, 704g
reflex immaturity in, 749
renal physiology and considerations in, 746–48
respiratory distress nursing care plan for, 751–52
respiratory physiology and considerations, 737–39, 738f, 749
retinal damage risk to, 815
separation problems with, 754–55n
sepsis neonatorum risk in, 841
SGA, outcomes for, 763
sucking reflex in, 704g
support groups for parents of, 996
thermoregulation in, 645, 740
touching behavior with, 775, 776f
urine adequacy in, 747
weight of, 689g
Preterm labor. See Premature labor and delivery
Primary care, by nurses, 13–14, 15
Primary germ layers, 165, 165t, 166f
Primary spermatocyte, 160, 161f

Primigravidas. See also Nulliparas
breech presentation management in, 554
cesarean deliveries among, 600
defined, 210
effacement in, 407, 408f
engagement in, 402
engagement-to-delivery interval in, 415
labor length in, 417, 418
lightening in, 415
postterm pregnancy in, 759
SGA neonates from, 761
Primipara, defined, 210
Primordial follicles, 57
Priscoline (Tolazoline), 817
Privacy, for out-of-hospital emergency birth, 506, 507
Problem solving
in crisis intervention, 995–97
in family crisis, 993, 994
no-lose, 290
for pregnant adolescents, 304
Problem-oriented medical record (POMR) system
as maternity care tool, 20
nutritional assessment using, 285
pregnancy discomforts and, 259–60
Procaine (Novocaine)
for labor anesthesia, 514, 516
toxic reactions to, 515
Procedures
amniocentesis, 381–82, 383p
applying internal monitor, 446
auscultation of chest, 231p, 231f
bottle sterilization methods, 928
breast self-examination, 232p, 232f
cardiac examination, 233–34p, 234f
contraction stress test, 376
DeLee suction, 500
Dextrostix test, 819–20
double setup examination, 565
exchange transfusions, 825
fetal blood sampling during labor, 461–62
gavage feeding, 743–45, 743–44f
intrapartal vaginal examination, 436–40, 437–39f
intrauterine transfusion, 350
nonstress test, 374
pelvic examination assistance, 235p, 235f
prep, 468
suctioning, 500, 812–14, 813f
tracheal intubation of neonate, 791–92
ultrasound, 367–68
umbilical catheterization, 811
urinary estriol determinations, 380
Professional nurses, maternity care roles of, 14
Progesterone
basal body temperature and, 115
breast development and, 85
cellulr immunity suppressed by, 170
endometrial changes caused by, 98, 99
hCG stimulates production of, 202
labor onset and decrease of, 406, 407

in oral contraceptives, 125, 126–27t
placental, 168, 169
postpartal decrease in, 902
pregnancy effects of
on breasts, 197, 254t, 255
on gastrointestinal system, 198–99, 254t, 256
on respiratory system, 197
on skin, 199
on urinary tract, 199
on uterus, 196
pregnancy production of, 196
premenstrual tension and, 99, 100
role of, 94
in female reproductive cycle, 96
lactation preparation, 925
in pregnancy, 202
Progesterone assays, in infertility workup 115f, 116
Progesterone withdrawal theory, 406
Progesterone-releasing IUDs, 124, 124f
Progestins, oral, as teratogens, 267t
Prolactin
breast changes and, 85
delivery stimulates secretion of, 925
infertility and, 118
inhibiting secretion of, 925, 926d
lactation initiation role of, 202
stimulating release of, 503
Prolapse of umbilical cord. See Umbilical cord, prolapse of
Prolapse of uterus, in initial prenatal exam, 226g
Prolonged rupture of membranes, resuscitation risk with, 786
PROM. See Premature rupture of membranes
Promazine (Sparine), during labor, 513
Promethazine (Phenergan)
during labor, 513
teratogenic effect of, 267t
Prone crawl, by neonate, 686, 704g
Prophase, 158, 158f, 159f
Propranolol, effects on neonate of, 769
Proprioceptive dysfunction, with meningomyelocele, 880
Propylthiouracil, 326
Prostaglandins (PGs), 94, 202
as abortion method, 129, 130t
dysmenorrhea and, 100
fallopian tube function and, 83
induction of labor with, 595
prevent ductus arteriosus closure, 891
role of, 59, 64, 94
in fertilization aided by, 63, 161
labor onset, 407
ovum extrusion, 98
placental blood flow regulation, 168
in pregnancy, 202, 407
seminal fluid contains, 64
seminal vesicles secrete, 63
Prostate gland, 59f
anatomy of, 63–64
development of, 57, 59, 653f
evaluating, in infertility workup, 114
Prostatic urethra, 63

Protamine sulfate, for heparin overdosage, 984n
Protective reflexes, in neonate, 685, 686
Protein
in breast milk, cow's milk, and formula, 719
complementary, 273
excess intake of, edema in infant from, 719
in formulas, 718, 719t
lactation requirements, 270t, 271t
neonatal digestion of, 651
neonatal requirements, 717, 717t
normal neonatal values
blood, 645t
preterm infant, 752t
urine, 652
pregnancy requirements, 271t, 272–73
in preterm infant formulas, 742t
preterm infant requirements, 740–41, 746
puerperal infection and, 918n, 978n
recommended dietary allowances for women, 270t
stored during pregnancy, 197t, 201
in urine. See Proteinuria
vegetarian sources of, 272–73, 279–80
Protein drink, 272–73
Protein-bound iodine, estrogens and, 93
Proteinuria
in initial prenatal urinalysis, 230g
in labor, 410, 432g, 468
in neonate, 835
with PIH, 336, 338
postpartal, 906
in subsequent prenatal exams, 240g
Proteus species
puerperal infections from, 974, 986
sepsis neonatorum from, 841
sign of in initial prenatal exam, 229g
Prothrombin, in neonates
deficiency of, 836
vitamin K and, 711d
Prothrombin time (PT) test
before cesarean delivery, 601
for DIC, 567
Protocols, legal aspects of use of, 14–15
Protozoa, placental transfer of, 170
Pruritus gravidarum, 199
Pseudoanemia (physiologic anemia of pregnancy), 198
Pseudomenstruation, in neonate, 652, 653, 684
Pseudomonas species
puerperal infections from, 974, 986
sepsis neonatorum from, 841
Psyche
labor complications involving, 535–36
labor role described, 535
Psychiatric disorders, puerperal, 988
Psychogenic anesthesia reactions, 515

Psychologic assessment
of family during pregnancy, 246–52
during labor, 433, 435g, 475
in prenatal exams
initial, 238, 238g
subsequent, 240–41, 241–43g
postpartal, 481, 907, 913–14
puerperal psychiatric disorders, 988
at 2 and 6 weeks postpartum, 944, 948g
Psychologic maintenance during labor
first stage deceleration, 478–79n
first stage active, 476–77n
first stage latent, 475n
fourth stage, 481n
second stage, 480n
Psychologic problems
with adolescent fatherhood, 301. See also Adolescent pregnancy
of cardiac client, 312, 313
with high-risk pregnancy, 342
pregnancy nutrition and, 284–85
as pregnancy risk, 215t, 246–47
prematurity and, 1010
Psychologic tasks of pregnancy
of expectant father, 248t, 249–50
of expectant mother, 247–49
postpartal adjustment, 907
Psychologic well-being, postpartal, promoting, 916, 920–21
Psychomotor impairment, from congenital herpes, 359
Psychoprophylaxis (Lamaze method), 293, 294–95
breathing exercise with, 472
for drug abusers in labor, 362
pain responses and, 412
second stage, 418
primary goal of, 413
regional anesthesia and, 413, 513, 528
Psychosocial factors, prenatal nutrition and, 284–85
Psychotherapy, crisis intervention vs., 994
Psychotropic drugs, fetal/neonatal effects of, 361t
PT (prothrombin time) test, for DIC, 567
Ptosis, assessing in neonate, 693g
PTT (partial thromboplastin time) test, for DIC, 567
Ptyalism (hypersalivation), as pregnancy discomfort, 198, 254, 254t
Puberty
defined, 91
male, hormonal effects on, 92, 92f, 93
maturation of gametes in, 160
oogenesis in, 160
physical changes in, 91–92, 91f, 92f
sexual development in, 89–90
Pubic arch, 66, 70
Pubic hair
development of, 91, 91f
loss of, with Sheehan syndrome, 988
Pubic joint, pregnancy changes in, 199
Pubis, 65–66

Public health nurses
fourth trimester referral to, 948g
genetic counseling role of, 151, 154
high-risk infant support from, 780
midwifery taught to, 7
parent education role of, 725
tracheoesophageal fistula referral to, 865n
Public Health Service, Maternity and Infant Care Projects by, 5
Pubocervical ligament, 77
Pubococcygeus muscle, 66, 67t, 67f
Kegel's exercises to strengthen, 263, 264f
Puborectalis muscle, 66, 67t
Pubovaginalis muscle, 66, 67t
Pudendal block, 514f, 527f, 527–28
agents for, 528
for delivery with PIH, 346
for labor of drug abuser, 362
labor stages used in, 514, 527
maternal complications from, 528
technique, 527, 527f
Pudendum, 71–73, 71f
Puerperal fever, 4
Puerperal morbidity, drug addiction and, 360
Puerperium
anticipatory guidance for, 289–90
complications of, 972–89
breast disorders, 986–87, 987f
cystitis and pyelonephritis, 982, 986
hematomas, 973
hemorrhage, 972–73
infection, 973–76, 975t
postdelivery anterior pituitary necrosis, 988
psychiatric disorders, 988
thromboembolic disease, 976, 980–82, 981f
defined, 901
exercises during. See Exercises
involution during, pelvic floor muscles and, 67
nursing interventions during. See Postpartal nursing management
physical adaptations during, 901–7
Pull to sit, in neonatal assessment, 687, 705
Pull-through operation, for aganglionosis, 870, 871
Pulmonary angiography, 983
Pulmonary artery, in transposition of the great vessels, 886f, 891–92, 892f
Pulmonary artery banding, 888, 888f
Pulmonary artery pressure, decreased at birth, 640, 641f
Pulmonary artery wedge pressure (PAWP), 344
Pulmonary congestion in preterm infants, 739–40
Pulmonary disorders in neonates. See also specific disorders
assessing preterm infants for, 757n
central cyanosis from, 889

from respiratory therapy, 808–9n, 816
Pulmonary edema
with abruptio placentae, 564
acute, as forceps delivery indication, 597
assessing for, with preeclampsia/eclampsia, 343, 344
as betamethasone/tocolytic side effect, 547
maternal, as terbutaline sulfate-side effect, 548
as ritodrine side effect, 549
with severe preeclampsia, 341
Pulmonary embolism, 981–82
as venous thrombosis risk, 976
nursing care plan, 983, 984–85
Pulmonary emphysema, as respiratory therapy complication, 809n, 816
Pulmonary fibrosis, 816
Pulmonary function. See also Lungs; Respiratory system
assessing in initial prenatal exam, 220–21g, 231p
pregnancy changes in, 197, 197t
Pulmonary hemorrhage
as SGA neonatal risk, 762
IUGR and risk of, 370
Pulmonary hypertension, in neonate
with bronchopulmonary dysplasia, 816
with endocardial cushion defects, 888
persistent (PPH), 810n, 816–17
retrolental fibroplasia risk with, 815
as ritodrine contraindicaton, 549
Pulmonary hypoplasia, with oligohydramnios, 577
Pulmonary infection, as post-cesarean risk, 941
Pulmonary lesions, in prenatal exam, 230g
Pulmonary status after cesarean, interventions for, 604
Pulmonary stenosis, 887f, 890, 891f
pregnancy with, 310
in tetralogy of Fallot, 887f, 890, 891f
transposition of great vessels and, 891
vulnerability to, gestational age and, 183t
Pulmonary toilet, for MAS, 815
Pulmonary vascular resistance, in preterm infants, 739
Pulmonic stenosis in neonate
heart murmur from, 642
peripheral cyanosis from, 889
Pulsation in fontanelles, assessing, 692g
Pulse, in mother
assessing
after epidural block, 519
in fourth stage labor, 502
fourth trimester, 945g
with hematoma, 580
with hemorrhage, 569n, 570n
before induction, 589, 590, 591n
during labor, 428g, 473, 475n, 481n
after paracervical block, 517
postpartal home visit, 624
in prenatal exams, 216g, 239g
with regional anesthesia, 522n;

see also specific types of anesthesia
with severe preeclampsia, 343
with subarachnoid block, 526
hyperthyroidism and, 326
increased, as anxiety sign, 608
monitoring
with induction of labor, 589, 593n
after PROM, 547
with ritodrine administration, 549
with uterine inversion, 580
normal pregnancy changes in, 197t, 198
pain response of, 483
postpartal assessment of, 912–13, 917, 919n
postpartal changes in, 906
shock sign in, 569
Pulse, in neonate, 641
assessing, 641, 682–83, 688g
at nursery admission, 710
with coarctation of the aorta, 889
decreased, with polycythemia, 835
factors affecting, 682–83
feeble, from succenturiate placenta, 573
femoral, assessing, 700g
monitoring
with narcotic withdrawal, 771
in nursery, 712
for preterm infants, 755n
normal rates, 683
with patent ductus arteriosus, 810n, 885
with pneumothorax, 809n, 816
preterm, 750n, 755n
rapid. See Tachycardia
in reactivity period, 712, 713f
Pulsed-echo ultrasound, 366. See also Ultrasound
Pupils
assessing in neonate, 680, 694g
dilated
as anxiety sign, 608
as pain response, 483
Purpura
as DIC sign, 567, 568
with extended rubella syndrome, 358
Pushing urge, in second stage labor, 418
body positions for, 479n
breathing methods to delay, 478
difficulty in, as forceps delivery indication, 597
regional anesthesia and, 523n
epidural block, 520
pudendal block, 527
spinal, 526
Pyelitis, postpartal, proteinuria as sign of, 906
Pyelonephritis
acute, during pregnancy, 353–54
estriol levels affected by, 380
IUGR associated with, 761
puerperal, 982, 986
Pyloric stenosis
hyperbilirubinemia risk with, 823
as polygenically inherited, 145
projectile vomiting from, 874
Pyrexia
with congenital syphilis, 844
as pulmonary embolism sign, 982
Pyridoxine. See Vitamin B6
Pyrosis. See Heartburn

Queen Victoria, anesthesia used by, 4, 510
Questionnaires, nutritional, 285, 286-87f
Quickening
  determining delivery date by, 237
  emotional changes with, 203
  evaluating, in adolescent pregnancy, 305
  failure to acknowledge, 241
  nonpregnancy causes of, 191t
  as pregnancy symptom, 192
  psychologic task assisted by, 247, 248t, 249
Quinine, teratogenic effects of, 267t

Rabies immunization, in pregnancy, 266t
Racemouse or compound glands, breasts as, 85
Radiant warmers
  described, 787
  fluid loss in, 747
  use of in nursery, 712
    for preterm infants, 752, 753n
    for SGA neonates, 765
Radiation
  of heat
    defined, 646
    neonatal heat loss by, 646, 647, 752, 753
  during pregnancy
    cleft lip and palate from, 853
    as teratogen, 157, 184
Radiography, for observing internal reproductive organs, 73
Radiologic examination, as positive pregnancy sign, 195. See also X-rays
Radioreceptor assay (Biocept-G) pregnancy test, 194
Rales
  in cardiac client, 311
  defined, 231p
  in initial prenatal exam, 221g
  in neonate
    with bronchopulmonary dysplasia, 816
    preterm, as respiratory distress sign, 751
    with RDS, 797t, 801n
    with tracheoesophageal atresia/fistula, 860
Rankin, J. H. G., 168
Rapid-eye-movement (REM) sleep, in neonate, 639, 655, 724
Rash, as toxoplasmosis symptom, 357
Rashes, on neonate
  assessing, 691g
  congenital syphilis, 844
  diaper, 727
  erythema neonatorum toxicum, 677
  laundering and, 727, 728
  petechial, from congenital rubella, 358
  with PKU, 858
Rashkind balloon atrial septostomy, 892, 892f
Rat hyperemic or Kupperman test, 195
RDS. See Respiratory distress syndrome
Reactivity periods
  assessing in nursery, 711-12, 713f

after birth, 657
  in preterm infants, 749
Read (natural childbirth) method, 293-94, 295
Reality testing, in adolescent pregnancy counseling, 298t, 300t
Rebound tenderness
  from appendicitis in pregnancy, 351
  as puerperal infection sign, 976, 977
Receptaculum seminis, 74
Reciprocal inhibition, relaxation techniques based on, 997
Reciprocity, in attachment process, 957f, 959-61
Recklinghausen disease, cáfe-au-lait spots with, 690g
Recommended dietary allowances (RDA), 269, 270t
Record keeping. See also Assessment guides
  analgesia during labor, 511
  attachment assessment, 969
  cesarean birth, 609
  at discharge, 730
  with electronic fetal monitoring, 460
  episiotomy, 596
  exchange transfusion, 825p, 828
  follow-up phone call, 949
  in fourth stage labor, 501
  immediate postdelivery, 480n
  legal aspects of, 15
  in nursery routine, 709, 714
  with oxytocin induction, 590
  postpartal hematomas, 973
  precipitous delivery, 504
  problem oriented method, 19, 20. See also Problem-oriented medical records
  verbal reporting, to nursery nurse, 709-10
Recovery room, after cesarean delivery, 603, 609
Rectal atresia, assessing neonate for, 684, 702g
Rectal culture, in sepsis neonatorum assessment, 842
Rectal examination. See also Rectum, assessing
  hematoma assessment by, 580
  in infertility workup, 114
Rectal pain, from hematoma in labor, 580
Rectal polyps
  in initial prenatal exam, 228g
  in neonate, bloody stool from, 874
Rectal prolapse, in initial prenatal exam, 228g
Rectal suppositories, hemorrhoidal pain relief with, 915
Rectal temperature, assessing in neonate, 676, 676f
  at nursery admission, 710
  teaching parents about, 728-29
Rectocele
  assessing for, fourth trimester, 947g
  sign of in initial prenatal exam, 225g
Rectouterine pouch. See Pouch of Douglas
Rectovaginal examination, in infertility workup, 113f, 114
Rectum
  assessing, 74

in initial prenatal exam, 228g
  postpartum, 917
  of neonate, with aganglionosis, 869
  perforation of, from pudendal block, 528
  pressure on, as pulmonary embolism sign, 981-82
  varicose veins in, in pregnancy, 198
Rectus muscles
  diastasis of, 223g
  evaluating postpartal separation in, 911
Red blood cells (RBC)
  fetal, 644
    placental transfer of, 170
  maternal
    evaluating at labor onset, 431g
    in initial prenatal exam, 229g
    pregnancy changes in, 198
    in urine at labor onset, implications of, 432g
  in neonates, 644
    anemia and, 830
    hemolysis of, 835. See also Hemolytic disease of the newborn
    impaired production of, 830, 835
    normal preterm, 752t
    placenta previa and, 567
    with polycythemia, 835
    preterm, normal values, 752t
    production of by liver, 648
    in urine, 652
Red reflex, assessing in neonates, 680, 693g
Redness, wound healing assessment by, 975t
  episiotomy, 912
Reducing substances, testing preterm stool for, 750n
  with necrotizing enterocolitis, 839n
REEDA scale, wound healing evaluation with, 975t, 978n
  for episiotomy, 912
Referral
  adolescent parents, 1017
  assessing family's need for, 49
  for attachment problems, 1012-13, 1014
  as crisis intervention, 994, 997
  breast-feeding, 924, 930
  child abuse, 1016
  for cleft lip, 856n
  for congestive heart failure, 894
  fourth trimester, 948g
  prolonged decelerations of FHR after, 456-57
Regional anesthesia during labor, 513-16
  agents used for, 514-15
  absorption of, 514-15
  action of, 514
  allergy to, 515-16
  amide type, 516
  for cardiac client, 313
  disadvantages of, 513
  for drug abusers, 362
  ester types, 516
  fetal effects of, 456-57, 516
  nursing care plan, 521-24
  pros and cons of, 513
  supine hypotensive syndrome and, 409
  toxic effects of, 514-16

types of, 513, 514f, 516. See also specific types
Regurgitation, in neonate. See also Vomiting
  assessing, 874
  cardiac sphincter immaturity and, 651
  continuous, interventions for, 651
  of initial water feeding, 716
  in neonatal reactivity period, 712
  normal patterns of, 927
  through nose
    with cleft palate, 852, 853
    with tracheoesophageal atresia/fistula, 860
Relaxation methods
  in active phase labor, 476n
  for anxiety reduction, in crisis, 997-98
  in childbirth preparation, 293, 294, 295
  home birth importance of, 630
  in latent phase labor, 474
Relaxin, role of, 202
Religion
  American Indian, 45
  Black American families and, 45
  blood transfusion and, 569
  food practices in pregnancy and, 282t, 283-84
  health care behavior.influenced by, 43
  influence on family of, 41
  Jewish health care behavior, 43
  Mexican American families and, 44
Relinquishment for adoption, nursing interventions with, 1014, 1015t
REM (Rapid-eye-movement) sleep, in neonate, 639, 655, 724
Renal agenesis, 681
Renal damage
  from abruptio placentae, 563
  danger sign of, 240g
  from MAS, 815
  risk factors for, 214-15t
Renal disease, in pregnancy, 347
  birth center screening for, 618
  cesarean delivery mortality from, 605
  as CST indication, 375
  estriol determinations for, 379
  indicated induction of labor for, 587
  PIH risk and, 336
  postdelivery galactorrhea and, 987
  as preterm labor cause, 548
  resuscitation risk with, 786
  as risk factor, 215t, 425t
  sign of in initial prenatal exam, 229g
Renal failure
  from abruptio placentae, 563
  assessing for, with eclampsia, 344
Renal lesions, intrapartal risk factors with, 425t
Renal malformations
  from fetal vitamin A overdose, 275
  in fetus, oligohydramnios with, 577
  prenatal diagnosis of, 146
Renal plasma flow (RPF), pregnancy changes in, 197t, 199

Renal system
labor changes in, 409–10
of preterm infant
nutrition problems and, 740
physiology of, 746–47
Renal threshold in neonates, blood
bicarbonate and, 652–53
Renal tubular dysfunction, sign of in
initial prenatal exam, 229g
Renal vein thrombosis, with neonatal
polycythemia, 835
Reproductive system, embryologic
development of, 57–59, 58f.
See also Female reproductive
system; Male reproductive
system
Research, as part of nursing process,
19, 26–27
Reserpine, neonatal effects of, 648,
769
Residual pulmonary disease, 808n
Resolution, in grief process, 999,
1002
Respirations of fetus
as placental function, 168
Respirations of mother
assessing
in fourth trimester, 945g
during labor, 428g, 473, 475n,
481n
before induction of labor, 589
in prenatal exams, 216g, 239g
with ritodrine administration,
549
with severe preeclampsia, 343
labor changes in, 409
monitoring
with hemorrhage, 570n
with regional anesthesia, 522n
with subarachnoid block, 526
in preterm labor, 549
with puerperal peritonitis, 976
pain response of, 483
Respirations of neonate
assessing, 682, 688g
at nursery admission, 710
at postpartal home visit, 627
in preterm infants, 750n
with RDS, 802n
characteristics of, 639
cleft palate effects on, 856n
cold stress increases, 817
diaphragm and rib cage assessment with, 699g
with diaphragmatic hernia, 866
distress signs, 714
during feeding, 716
with hypoglycemia, 818
immediate facilitation of, 498,
500p, 501f
labored
with necrotizing enterocolitis,
838, 839
with RDS, 795f, 796–97t, 801n
with MAS, 814
maternal medications and, 510–
11, 512, 513
monitoring
with anemia, 835
with narcotic withdrawal, 771
in nursery, 712
for preterm infant, 755n
normal rate of, 639, 682
nose used for, 681
in reactivity period, 712, 713f
with transposition of the great vessels, 891
with ventricular septal defects,
888
Respirator
for intraventricular hemorrhage,
837

for RDS, 797, 798f, 800t
Respiratory acidosis, in neonate. See
also Acidosis
asphyxia leads to, 786
with bronchopulmonary dysplasia,
816
from diaphragmatic hernia, 861,
866
with MAS, 798, 814
from maternal hypertension, 769
with RDS, 794f, 795
correcting, 806
Respiratory congestion, with neonatal
herpesvirus infection, 844
Respiratory depression, from
maternal medications
cardiac medications, 769
magnesium sulfate, 769
reserpine, 769
Respiratory development in neonates, 635–39, 637f, 639f
Respiratory disease in mother, signs
of in prenatal exams, 216g,
220g, 239g
Respiratory disease, as home birth
contraindication, 618, 629
Respiratory distress in mother
from amniotic fluid embolism, 576
after regional anesthesia, 523n
Respiratory distress in neonate, 792,
794–817. See also Respira-
tory distress syndrome; Respiratory problems
from abdominal distention, 874
from aganglionosis, 869
assessment of, 792
breath sounds with, 698g
chest expansion with, 698g
chest retraction with, 698g
from diaphragmatic hernia, 861
flaring nares as sign of, 688g,
695g
GFR decreased by, 746
as group B streptococcus sign, 843
with hypoglycemia, 818
IVH from, 836
meconium aspiration syndrome,
798, 814–15
with micrognathia, 850, 851
necrotizing enterocolitis and, 837,
839n
from neonatal drug addiction, 771
nursing interventions for, 681,
751–52n
with polycythemia, 835
after precipitous delivery, 505
as prematurity risk, 751
in SGA neonates, 765n
signs of, 639, 682
Silverman-Anderson index to
assess, 795f
with tracheoesophageal atresia/fis-
tula, 860, 862, 863n
Respiratory distress syndrome (RDS),
792, 794–97
apnea associated with, 749
assessing for, 688g, 757n
betamethasone to prevent, 547d
as birth center contraindication,
618
clinical course of, 801n
clinical findings with, 714, 795,
795f, 796–97t, 801n
cold stress aggravates, 817, 818
complications of therapy for, 801,
808–10n, 815–17
cyanosis with, 889
death from, maternal diabetes
and, 316
DIC and, 837
early termination of pregnancy
risks, 384

fetal lung maturity and, 384, 385
group B streptococcal infection
vs., 843
idiopathic, lecithin development
and, 639
as IDM risk, 768
mortality from, 792
nursing care plan, 801–10
nursing diagnoses, examples, 810
patent ductus arteriosus and, 881
pathophysiology of, 794f, 794–95
PPH syndrome with, 817
predicting, lung profile for, 385–
86
prematurity and, 384, 425t, 737–
39, 749
preventing, glucocorticoids for,
549–50
previous, birth center screening
for, 618
risk of, 214–15t, 425t, 736f, 792,
794
ritodrine and, 549
signs of; see clinical findings with
tachypnea as sign of, 688g
Respiratory embarassment, as
Mendelson syndrome sign,
531
Respiratory hemorrhage, in neonate
with polycythemia, 835
Respiratory infections
colostrum protects against, 717
incidence of, birth weight and, 758
maternal nutrition and, 185
from PROM, perinatal mortality
from, 546
Respiratory mucus, during reactivity
period, 712, 713f
Respiratory obstruction, from anesthesia, 531
Respiratory problems in neonate. See
also specific problems
breath sounds with, 698g
with MAS, 79, 814
from maternal drug abuse, 361t
after meperidine, 512
with necrotizing enterocolitis, 838,
839
nursing diagnosis, example, 757n
preterm, 548, 737–39, 738f, 749
apnea, 749
LGA IDM, assessing for, 757n
nutrition and, 740
with surgery in pregnancy, 351
transient tachypnea of newborn,
797–98
Respiratory system
fetal development of, 173, 175t,
177t, 178, 179t, 180–82
in mother
labor changes in, 409
pregnancy changes in, 197,
197t
in neonate, 635–39, 637f, 639f
cardiovascular system interrelated with, 638
IgA protects, 654
Respiratory therapy, complications
of, 801, 808–10n, 815–17
Rest periods
in antenatal period, 262, 262f
for cardiac client, 312
for diabetic client, 324
elevating legs during, 254t, 256,
257, 257f
for PIH, 338
with sickle cell anemia, 328
for congestive heart failure, 894
during labor
first stage, 47474, 476, 478
prolonged, as intervention, 542
second stage, 480n

postpartal
assessment of, 913
encouraging, 916, 918n
need for, 502
reviewing need for, at home visit, 625–26
Resting posture of neonate
assessing, 657
preterm, 750
Restitution of fetus during labor, 415
Restlessness, from hemorrhage, 571n
Restraints. See also Swaddling
for cleft lip, 854n, 855n, 855f
for meningocele/
meningomyelocele, 882n
for omphalocele therapy, 868
Resuscitation, 786–92, 789t, 790f,
791–92p, 793d
equipment and medications for,
787–88, 793d
goal of, 786
initial management of 788–92,
789t, 790f, 791–92p, 793d
for meconium aspiration, 812–
13p, 813f, 814–15
out-of-hospital emergency delivery,
507
with Pierre Robin syndrome, 850,
851
with pneumothorax, 809n
risk factors for, 786–87
Rete testis, 61, 62f
Reticulocytes, in neonate, 645
ABO incompatibility increases,
826
assessing, for anemia, 835
formation of in fetus, 644
hemolytic process indicated by,
826
preterm, normal values, 752t
Retina, in neonate
assessing, 680, 693g
respiratory therapy damage to.
See Retrolental fibroplasia
Retinal detachment, with Pierre Robin syndrome, 850
Retinal hemorrhage, pregnancy with,
347
Retinoblastoma glaucoma in neonate,
pupils with, 694g
Retinochoroiditis, from
toxoplasmosis, 357
Retinol. See Vitamin A
Retractions, in neonate
with diaphragmatic hernia, 866
preterm, as respiratory distress
sign, 751
with RDS, 795f, 796t, 801n
from succenturiate placenta, 573
with tracheoesophageal atresia/fis-
tula, 860
Retroflexion of uterus, in initial prenatal exam, 226g
Retrolental fibroplasia (RLF)
assessing preterm infants for, 757n
as long-term prematurity risk, 758
as respiratory therapy complication, 801, 808n, 815
vitamin E to prevent, 746
Retrospective genetic counseling,
154
Retroversion of uterus, in initial prenatal exam, 226g
Rh determination, for neonate, 480n,
826
with hemolytic disease of newborn,
826
hyperbilirubinemia risk and, 823,
824. See also Hemolytic disease of the newborn
neonatal anemia assessment and,
831

preterm, in nursing care plan, 750
risk identification with, 734, 824
Rh incompatability, exchange transfusions for, 831n
Rh sensitization, 347–50, 348f, 350p
abortion and, 129, 332
amniocentesis for, 382, 384, 384f
as CST indication, 375
factors affecting, 824
fetal/neonatal effects of. See Hemolytic disease of newborn
hemolytic disease of the newborn and, 824
as home birth contraindication, 629
hydramnios associated with, 577
normal distribution of, by race, 236t
as risk factor, 215t, 734
sinusoidal FHR pattern and, 457
testing for
before cesarean delivery, 601
in infertility workup, 114
before induction of labor, 591n
in initial prenatal exam, 229g
in utero, implications of, 347
Rheumatic heart disease, pregnancy with, 310–13
neonatal problems associated with, 768–69
Rheumatoid arthritis, signs of in initial prenatal exam, 224g
Rhinitis, with congenital syphilis, 844
Rho (d) immune globulin (RhoGAM)
after abortion, 129
administering, 349–50, 824
after amniocentesis, 382
after ectopic pregnancy, 334
after spontaneous abortion, 332
Rhonchi
defined, 231p
in initial prenatal exam, 221g
in preterm infant, as respiratory distress sign, 751
with tracheoesophageal atresia/fistula, 860
Rhythm method of birth control, 120–21, 121f, 122
Rib cage, assessing in neonate, 699g
Ribonucleic acid (RNA), role of, 157, 165
Riboflavin (vitamin B2), 270t, 276
in breast milk, cow's milk, and formula, 719t
neonatal defeciency of, dermatitis from, 719
Ribs, assessing in neonate, 682
Richardson, S. A., 205
Rickets, 275
hip dysplasia vs., 878
in preterm infants, 746
X-linked dominantly inherited, 145
Rights of patients, APPENDIX A, APPENDIX B
Ringer's lactate. See also Intravenous fluids
in abruptio placentae management, 564
in placenta previa management, 566
Ripening of the cervix
as impending labor sign, 415
induction readiness of, 588
precipitous labor with, 543
after PROM, 546f
Risk factors in pregnancy, 213, 214–15t
intrapartal, 425, 425t
Ritodrine (Yutopar), 547, 548, 549d
with betamethasone, pulmonary edema risk, 547
contraindications, 548, 549

for external cephalic version, 585
side effects of, 548, 549
RLF. See Retrolental fibroplasia
RNA. See Ribonucleic acid
Rocking, assessing neonatal responses to, 706
Roe v. Wade, abortion issue and, 10
Roig-Garcia, Santiago, 295
Role behavior, in family assessment, 48
Role model, nurse as, 248, 943, 964
in adolescent pregnancy, 303, 1017
Role playing, in crisis intervention, 997
Roles, 35
in families, 35–36
identifying, 48
pregnancy and birth affect, 246, 992
of nurses. See Nursing role
sex/gender identity and, 88–89
sexual, 88–89
Roll-over test, for mild preeclampsia, 342
ROM. See Rupture of membranes
Rome, ancient, obstetrics in, 3
Rooming-in
advantages of, 939–40
in birth center, 619
feeding pattern aided by, 718, 924
Gesell supported, 12
importance of, 9649, 965
in intensive care nurseries, 780
neonatal sleep-activity patterns and, 722, 724
nursery vs., in first 24 hours, 713–14
parent-infant interaction evaluated by, 725
as part of family-centered health care, 31
rest periods with, 918n
with thromboembolic disease, 985n
Rooting reflex, in neonate, 655, 657
assessing, 686, 686f, 704g
kernicterus affects, 824
utilizing in feeding, 921, 929
Ross' cleft palate nipple, 856n
Rotation of fetus during labor, 414f, 414–15
forceps used to aid, 596
complications from, 598
for malposition, 551
Round ligament of uterus, 74f, 76, 77f, 80–81, 81f
palpation of, 74
Royal College of Midwives, 6
Rubella
in neonate, 358
clinical manifestations of, 766–67
screening for, 150, 842
SGA neonate, 766–67n
during pregnancy, 357–58
fetal exposure to, IgM levels and, 654
microencephaly from, 691g
neonatal effects of, 680, 681, 881
as risk factor, 215t
prenatal screening for, 842
Rubella immunization, contraindicated in pregnancy, 266t
Rubella titer, in initial prenatal exam, 230g
Rubin, R.
on attachment process, 958
on pregnancy emotions, 203, 204, 247–48

on postpartal psychologic adjustment, 907
Rubin's test, 117
Ruffini corpuscles, in clitoris, 73
Rugae vaginales, 75
Running, amenorrhea from, 100
Rupture of membranes (ROM)
ambulation vs. bed rest after, 468, 474, 574, 617
artificial, with preterm labor, 550
assessing, 430–31g, 434, 436p, 437f, 439f
birth center use after, 618
breech presentation risk with, 554
as cephalic version contraindication, 585
FHR assessment at time of, 574
during first stage of labor, 418
deceleration phase, 477n
as impending labor sign, 242g, 415–16
infection risk with, 974
premature. See Premature rupture of membranes
prolonged, cesarean delivery for, 600
umbilical cord prolapse risk and, 539, 574

Sabin-Feldman dye test, for diagnosing toxoplasmosis, 357
Sacral promontory, 66
Sacrococcygeal joints, 65, 66, 66f
pregnancy changes in, 199
Sacroiliac joints, 65, 66, 66f
pregnancy changes in, 199
Sacrum, 65, 66
Saddle block. See Subarachnoid block
Safety, for infants and toddlers, 716, 729–30
Salicylates
in breast milk, 930
during pregnancy, neonatal jaundice and, 822–23, 831
Saline, suctioning use of, 788, 813p
Saline induction, as abortion method, 130t, 130–31
Saliva
in neonate, 681
pregnancy pH of, dental caries and, 199
Salivary glands in neonate, 651
Salpingitis
infertility from, 111t
puerperal, 975
sign of in initial prenatal exam, 223g
Salpingostomy, 334
Salt retention. See Sodium retention
Sanfilippo syndrome, prenatal diagnosis of, 148
Satellites on chromosomes, 157, 157f
Scalines, assessing in neonate, 690g
Scalp, assessing in initial prenatal exam, 218g
Scalp blood sampling. See Fetal scalp blood sampling
Scandinavia, nurse-midwifery in, 6
Scanning electron microscopy, 73
Scanzoni, Friedrich Wilhelm, 4
Scapegoating, in family crisis, 993
Scaphoid appearance in neonate, 699g
Scarf sign, gestational age and, 663f, 665f, 672, 673f
Schiling differential cell count, in initial prenatal exam, 229g
Schizophrenia, postpartal, 988
School nurse, genetic counseling referral by, 151

Schools, adolescent pregnancy role of, 305
Schraeder, B. D., 1013
Schultze mechanism of placental delivery, 419, 420f
Sciatic nerve trauma, from pudendal block, 528
Sclera, of neonate
assessing, 694g
jaundice evidence in, 832n
subconjunctival hemorrhages in, 680
Scoliosis, in initial prenatal exam, 224g, 225g
Scotomata (blind spots), with PIH, 341, 343
Screening
of adolescent in labor, 482
for birth center delivery, 618
fetal movement assessment, 372
for home birth, 629
for intrapartal risk factors, 425, 425t
of neonates, 725
for congenital hypothyroidism, 859
for galactosemia, 859
for hypocalcemia, 821
for maple syrup urine disease, 858
for metabolic disorders, 857
for PKU, 857, 858
serum thyroxine levels, 326
for sickle cell anemia, 150
nonstress test as, 373
prenatal
for spina bifida, 879–80
for sickle cell anemia, 148, 230g
for Rh sensitization, 347–48
for rubella, 358, 842
for sexually transmitted diseases, 354, 842
TORCH, 150
Scrotal sac, length of, 61
Scrotum, 59f, 60–61, 61f
development of, 653
of neonate, assessing, 496, 684, 701g
Scurvy, 276
preventing in neonate, 717
Seaman, Valentine, 5
Sebaceous cysts, on labia minora, 72
Sebaceous glands
breasts as, 85
pregnancy changes in, 199
Seborrhea-dermatitis, in neonate
assessing, 690g
marginal blepharitis with, 693g
Secobarbital (Seconal), during labor, 513
Secondary oocyte, 160, 161f
Secondary spermatocytes, 160, 161f
Sedatives
for congestive heart failure in neonates, 894
during labor, 513
for cardiac client, 313
hypertonic, 537
hypotonic, 541
Levallorphan increases depression from, 512
precipitous, 543
prolonged, 542
transient tachypnea of newborn from, 797
for PIH, 338, 344
for pulmonary embolism, 985ncp
teratogenic effects of, 267t
Sedimentation rate
in infertility workup, 114
postpartal, 906

Sedimentation rate (Cont'd)
  pregnancy changes in, 198
Seeds, A. E., 165
Seesaw respirations, assessing in neo-
    nate, 682
Seizures
  in mother
    with eclampsia, 341
    inheritance and, 146
  in neonate
    assessing, 685
    from congenital herpes, 359
    as hypocalcemia sign, 821
    with hypoglycemia, 817, 818
    with intraventricular hemor-
        rhage, 836, 837
    with kernicterus, 824
    with maple syrup urine disease,
        858
    with PKU, 858
    polycythemia, 835
    postterm, 760
    as prematurity risk, 758
    preterm, apnea associated with,
        749
    with RDS, 797t
Self-disclosure, in crisis intervention,
    996
Self-esteem
  adolescent parenting success
      requires, 1017
  adolescent pregnancy and, 297,
      302
  adolescent sexuality and, 90
  antepartal care and, 286
  cesarean delivery and, 604
  child abuse and, 1015, 1016
  childhood sexuality and, 89
  defective birth and, 775, 776,
      848, 849, 1006
  environmental factors affect, 46
  grief work and, 1005
  high-risk infant caretaking and,
      775, 776, 1009, 1009f
  infertility and, 112
  labor and, 405–6, 413
  menopausal symptoms and, 102
  mothering and, 952
  of parents, neonatal behavior
      affects, 706
  preterm birth and, 775, 776,
      1006, 1009, 1009f
  promoting, in puerperium, 921
  psychosocial development and, 40
  sexuality and, 89
  single parenthood and, 1018
  spontaneous abortion and, 333
Self-fulfilling prophecy, bonding and,
    1011
Self-quieting activity, assessing neo-
    nate for, 687
Sellick maneuver, preventing
    vomiting during emergence
    with, 531
Semen, 63, 64
Semen analysis, in infertility workup,
    111t, 113f, 117
  postcoital, 116, 117
Semi-Fowler's position
  for cardiac client, 312, 313
  for contraction stress test, 376
  as delivery alternative, 616
  during labor, 467
  for nonstress test, 374
Semidozing state, in neonate, 657
Seminal fluid, 63, 64
Seminal vesicles, 63
  development of, 57, 58f, 653,
      653f
Seminiferous tubules, 61, 62f
  spermatogenesis in, 61–62
Semmelweis, Ignaz Philipp, 4

Sending I-messages, as skill, 290
Sensorineural hearing loss, as
    prematurity risk, 758
Sensory functioning, in neonate, 654,
    655, 656f
  assessing, 686, 687, 705
  kernicterus affects, 826
Sensory deprivation, in preterm or
    high-risk infant
  preventing, 754n, 764n, 776–77
  sample nursing diagnosis, 758
Sensory stimuli to breathing onset,
    636
Separation
  of high-risk neonates from parents,
      772, 773, 1006
  labor pain and, 413
  of mother and infant
    attachment impeded by, 968,
        1006
    introduction of, 5
    puerperal infection and, 978–
        89n, 980n
    as SGA neonatal problem, 765n
    thromboembolic disease and,
        985ncp
  of mother and siblings, maternity
      ward visits alleviate, 292
  parenting disorders as result of,
      1009–10
Sepsis
  DIC coagulation process initiated
      by, 567, 568f
  in fetus, after prolonged labor,
      542
  hand washing prevents, 4
  in neonate. See also Sepsis
      neonatorum
    with anemia, preventing, 835
    apnea from, 749, 755n
    hypoglycemia differentiation
        from, 818
    after hypotonic labor, 541
    liver enlargement with, 700g
    with necrotizing enterocolitis,
        837, 840n
    as pathologic jaundice cause,
        823
    as prematurity risk, 749
    after PROM, assessing for,
        546–47
    retrolental fibroplasia risk with,
        815
    risk factors for, 736f
    skin color with, 689g
    temperature with, 688g
    with transient tachypnea of new-
        born, 798
Sepsis neonatorum, 841–42. See also
    Sepsis, in neonate
  assessing preterm infants for, 757n
  group B streptococcus as cause of,
      842–45
  herpesvirus type 2 vs., 844
  preventing, in preterm infant,
      754n
  signs and symptoms of, 841–42
Septa, in testes, 61
Septal defects
  from fetal alcohol syndrome,
      770
  gestational age and, 183t
Septicemia, in neonate. See also Sep-
    sis, in neonate; Sepsis
    neonatorum
  from cord infection, preventing,
      684
  gram negative, DIC and, 837
Septum, assessing in neonate
  deviated or perforated, 695g
  polyps, 695g
  tumors, 605g

Serologic studies. See also specific se-
    rum tests in infertility workup,
    114
  at labor onset, 431g, 469, 472
  postnatal, 150
  risk identification with, 734
  in sepsis neonatorum assessment,
      842
  serologic test for syphilis (STS)
    congenital, 843, 844
    in initial prenatal exam, 229g
    at labor admission, 469
    TORCH screen, 150
Serosal layer of uterus (perimetrium),
    78
Sertoli's cells, 62
Serum albumin levels
  decrease in, from ritodrine, 549
  hyperbilirubinemia assessment
      with, 824
Serum antibody tests, risk identifica-
    tion with, 734
Serum bilirubin levels in neonate
  assessing for hyperbilirubinemia,
      824
  with kernicterus, 823–24
  pathologic, 822
Serum calcium, decreased, hypocal-
    cemia as, 821–22
Serum cholinesterase activity, preg-
    nancy decreases, 199
Serum electrolytes. See Electrolyte
    imbalances; Electrolytes
Serum estriol determinations. See Es-
    triol determinations
Serum ferritin levels, iron stores
    indicated by, 327
Serum glucose levels, in preterm
    infant
  monitoring, during TPN, 745
  normal values, 752t
Serum protein, neonatal jaundice
    and, 831n
Serum protein-bound iodine (PBI),
    pregnancy changes in, 201
Serum thyroxine tests
  for neonates, 326
  in pregnancy, 326
"Setting sun" eyelids, as hydrocepha-
    ly sign, 693g
Seventh-Day Adventists, pregnancy
    nutrition for, 278–81
Sex of fetus. See Fetal sex
Sex behavior, 88, 89
Sex chromatin, 140, 140f, 141,
    160
Sex chromosome abnormalities, 140–
    41
Sex chromosomes, 135, 157
  examining, 140
  formation of, 161
  monosomy of, 137
Sex education
  need for, 105–6
  nurse's role in, 105–6
  for pregnant adolescents, 305
Sex flush, 103t, 104, 104t
Sex roles
  gender identity and, 88–89
  nursing implications of, 105
Sex-linked disorders. See X-linked
    disorders
Sex-linked traits, 160
Sexual adjustment. See also
    Sexuality
  assessing, in prenatal vistis, 241g,
      243g
  in childbearing family stage, 39
  climacteric and, 102
  family development and, 37, 39
  penile dysfunction and, 60
  in pregnancy, 38, 263–65

Sexual behavior
  estrogens and, 93
  nursing assessment and, 106
  nursing implications of, 105
Sexual development
  of fetus, 175t, 177t, 179t, 180,
      181, 183
    teratogenic damage to, 183t
  in puberty, 91–92, 91f, 92f
Sexual differentiation in fetus, 57–
    59, 58f
Sexual dysfunction, 89
  with puerperal psychosis, 988
Sexual history assessments, 106
  infertility and, 112, 114
Sexual identity (core-gender identity),
    88
  adolescent pregnancy and, 298t
  development of, 89
Sexual inhibitions, nursing implica-
    tions of, 105
Sexual intercourse in pregnancy,
    248t, 249, 250. See also
    Coitus; Sexual response
  high-risk pregnancy and, 342
  postpartal, 940
Sexual response
  diabetes and, 318
  estrogens and, 93
  gender identity insecurity and, 89
  neurologic control of, 104–5
  physiology of, 103–5, 103t, 104t,
      105f
  in pregnancy, 248t, 249, 250,
      263–65
Sexual role, adolescent pregnancy
    and, 298t
Sexual stimulation
  of breasts, 85
  male, 64
  of clitoris, 72, 73
  of labia majora, 72
  of labia minora, 72
  of mons pubis, 72
Sexual trauma, labia majora hemato-
    mas from, 72
Sexuality. See also Sexual
    adjustment
  in adolescence, 89–90
  adolescent pregnancy and, 298t
  in adulthood, 90–91
  attachment process and, 952
  components of, 88–89
  development of, 89–91
  in infancy, 89
  infertility counseling and, 112
  masculinity vs., 89
  nursing implications of, 105–6
  postpartal, reviewing at home visit,
      627
  pregnancy as affirmation of, 246
Sexually transmitted diseases
  as adolescent labor risk, 482
  adolescent pregnancy and, 299,
      304
  condoms protect against, 122
  counseling to decrease incidence
      of, 106
  cytomegalovirus, 358–59
  as drug addiction risk, 770
  genital herpes simplex, 359–60
  infertility from, 110, 112
  in pregnancy, 354–55. see also
    specific diseases
  prenatal screening for, neonatal in-
      fection prevention by, 842
  spermicides protect against, 127
SGA neonates. See Small-for-
    gestational-age neonates
SGOT (transaminase)
  in preterm infant, normal values,
      752t

with pulmonary embolism, 983
Shaft of penis, 59–60, 60f
Shake test, 386
Sham feedings, via cervical esophagostomy, 864n
Shampooing neonates, 727–28
cradle cap and, 690g
Sheehan syndrome (hypophyseal cachexia), 988
abruptio placentae and, 564
amenorrhea from, 100
Sheppard-Towner Act of 1921, 5
Shereshefsky, P. M., 951, 952
Shigella species, breast-feeding protects against, 748
Shiny Schultze, 419
Shippen, William, midwifery school by, 4–5, 6
Shirodkar-Barter operation (cerclage), 336
as CST contraindication, 376
Shivering
postpartal, 502
thermogenesis by, 647
Shock
in mother, signs and symptoms of, 569
with abruptio placentae, 561, 563
assessing for, after prolonged labor, 542
with congestive heart failure, 894
from hematoma, 580
with hemorrhage, 569, 571
as induction of labor risk, 591
postpartal
from macrosomia, 557
lacerations as cause of, 579
from uterine inversion hemorrhage, 579–80
from uterine rupture, 550
as vacuum extraction indication, 598
in neonate
assessing for, 688g
blood volume expander for, 792
from intestinal obstruction, 873
with necrotizing enterocolitis, 840n
necrotizing enterocolitis from, 837
neurogenic, from aganglionosis, 869
with pneumothorax, 809ncp
treatment of in delivery room, 792
Shocklike appearance, in neonate
with group B streptococcal infection, 843
from intraventricular hemorrhage, 836
Shoes in pregnancy, 255t, 258, 261
Shortness of breath. *See* Dyspnea
Shoulder dystocia
brachial palsy after, 684
with LGA neonate, 761
from macrosomia, interventions for, 557
Shoulder pain
in pregnancy, 200
referred, with ectopic pregnancy, 333
Shoulder presentation, 400, 402, 403, 404
Shoulder presentation, 400, 402, 403, 404, 552, 555–56, 556f. *See also* Transverse lie
management of 555–56
Shunting, in neonate, 638, 640, 642
cyanosis and, 881, 889

with atrial septal defects, 885, 886f
with coarctation of the aorta, 887f, 889
with endocardial cushion defects, 888
with MAS, 814
with patent ductus arteriosus, 885, 887f
with persistent pulmonary hypertension, 817
preterm, 739
with RDS, 794f, 797t, 810n
as RDS complication, 810n
as respiratory therapy complication, 817
with ventricular septal defects, 885, 887f, 888
Siamese twins, 560
Sibling rivalry
preventing, 940
reviewing management of, at postpartal home visit, 626–27
Sibling visitation, 940
Siblings
attachment with, 963
birth attendance by, 13, 613–14
in birth centers, 618, 619
home birth, 628, 630
defective birth reactions of, 1010
of dying infants, crisis intervention for, 1005
postpartal exam role of, 944
prenatal care role of, 287–88, 292
reactions to newborn of, 940
responses to pregnancy of 250–51, 251f
rivalry case example, 50–52, 51f
stillbirth and, 581
stress felt by, 992
Sickle cell anemia
as CST indication, 375
ethnic background and, 152
genetic counseling referral for, 151
inheritance of, 144, 157, 327
IUGR associated with, 761
as pregnancy complication, 327–28
prenatal diagnosis of, 148, 388
screening for
in initial prenatal exam, 230g
in newborn, 150, 725
signs of, 327
statistics about, 327
Sickling, 327
Side-lying position. *See also* Sim's position, lateral
for breast-feeding, 931, 937f
for cardiac client, 313
as fetal distress intervention, 538
for hemorrhoidal relief, 915
for labor and delivery, 467, 475, 616, 616f
advantages of, 616f
epidural anesthesia during, 519
FHR improved by, 451t, 454, 538
after oxytocin overdose, 543
with PIH, 346
for malposition, 551
for neonate, 714, 715f
after feeding, 716
for occult prolapse of cord, 540n
for PIH, 342, 343, 346
Significant other. *See also* Father; Husband; Partner
birth participation by, attachment and, 954
cesarean participation by, 602–3, 607, 941, 942
importance of to high-risk parents, 778

pain response and, 413
Silver nitrate
administering, 499n, 710, 712f
chemical conjunctivitis from, 693g
Credé introduced, 4
eyelid edema from, 680
for gonorrhea prevention, 844
for omphalocele, 868
Silastic bag, for omphalocele repair, 868, 869f
Silverman-Anderson chart, 795f
Sim's position, lateral. *See also* Sidelying position
for caudal anesthesia administration, 520
for delivery with maternal PIH, 346
for umbilical cord prolapse, 574–75
Simian line, as Down sundrome sign, 684, 702g
Simpson, Sir James, 510
Simpson forceps, 597, 597f
Sims-Huhner's test, 116
Sinciput presentation, 552
Single adults, as families, 32
Single-gene disorders, postnatal diagnosis of, 149, 150
Single-gene inheritance, 142–45
Single parents
adolescents as, 1017
crisis intervention for, 1018
crisis potential with, 1011
families with, 32, 33f
interventions for, 1018
Sinuses, assessing in initial prenatal exam, 220g
Sinusoidal patterns in FHR. 457, 458f
Sitting position, as delivery alternative, 616–17, 617f, 630
Situational contraceptives, 122
Situational crisis, 992, 1002
Sitz baths
for herpes infection, 359
postpartal, 915, 917n
for episiotomy discomfort, 596
infection and, 918n, 974, 975, 977n
reviewing use of, at home visit, 626
Skeletal malformations, 875–81. *See also specific malformations*
with homocystinuria, 859
hydramnios and, 577
oligohydramnios and, 577
prenatal diagnosis of, 146
Skeletal pain, from fetal vitamin A overdose, 275
Skeletal system. *See also* Musculoskeletal system
assessing in neonate, 684–85, 689g, 702–3g
pregnancy changes in, 199–200, 200f
Skene's ducts (paraurethral glands), 71f, 73
Skim milk, 718
Skin, of fetus
development of, 177t, 179t, 180–82
malformations in, fetoscopy to diagnose, 388
Skin, of mother
assessing
with hemorrhage, 570–71n
in initial prenatal exam, 216–17g
cracking or drying
from fat-soluble vitamin overdose, 274
as hypothyroidism sign, 326

pigmentation changes in, 193
pregnancy changes in, 193, 199
prolonged labor care for, 542
Skin, of neonate
assessing, 677–78, 689–91g
in delivery room, 492t, 495, 496
for jaundice, 824, 832n
with phototherapy, 829–30
caring for, 727
color of. *See* Skin color, of neonate
with congenital hypothyroidism, 859
with congestive heart failure, 893
gestational age and, 661, 662f, 665f
lesions on, *See* Skin lesions
with meningomyelocele, 880
moniliasis on, 845
monitoring temperature of, with cold stress, 817
postterm, 759, 759f, 760
preterm, 750n
infection risk through, 748
with RDS, 796t, 801n
with sepsis neonatorum, 841
SGA, 762, 764
texture of, assessing, 690g
turgor of
assessing, 677, 690g
poor, as dehydration sign, 747
Skin color, of neonate
Apgar scoring system for, 492t, 495
assessing, 687, 689–90g, 706
at nursery admission, 710
in nursery routine, 714
at postpartal home visit, 627
gestational age and, 662f
jaundice evidence in, 832n
Mongolian spots and, 677
pneumothorax effects on, 809n
in preterm infant, 750n
with RDS, 796t, 801n
during reactivity period, 712, 713f
Skin cultures
for congenital herpesvirus detection, 844
in sepsis neonatorum assessment, 842
Skin lesions, on neonate
with congenital syphilis, 844
with herpesvirus infection, 844
from moniliasis, 845
Skin probe, temperature assessment with, 677, 710
Skin tags, preauricular, 681
Skull
fetal, 398f, 398–99, 399f
of preterm infant, 750n
neonatal fractures of
as CPD risk, 578
as LGA neonatal risk, 761
from macrosomia, 557
SLE. *See* Systemic lupus erythematosus
Sleep, fetal, FHR baseline variability caused by, 452
Sleep deprivation, pain perception and, 413
Sleep disturbances, with "postpartum blues" 907
Sleep patterns of mother, postpartal assessment of, 913
Sleep-wake patterns, of neonate, 655, 722, 724–25
after birth, 712, 713f
assessing, 688g, 705
described, 655
maternal methadone maintenance and, 360

Sleep-wake patterns (Cont'd)
  motor activity and, 654
  positioning for sleep, 714, 715f, 716
  preterm, 749
  in reactivity period, 712, 713f
  respiratory patterns affected by, 639
Small intestine. See also Gastrointestinal system
  development of, 650
  in neonate, 651
Small-for-gestational-age (SGA) neonates, 761–63, 762f, 764–67n. See also Intrauterine growth retardation
  alcohol ingestion and, 362
  birth center screening for, 618
  breast tissue in, 661, 668, 699g
  categories of (Pr, F, Po), 734, 735f
  from CMV, 358
  cold stress risk in, 817
  complications affecting, 762, 764–67n
  congenital syphilis as cause of, 844
  defined, 761
  drug abuse and, 361t, 770
  growth patterns in, 763
  hearing loss risk in, 681
  hematologic considerations in, 748–49
  hyperthyroidism and, 321
  hypocalcemia risk in, 821
  hypoglycemia in, 818, 821
  iron deficiency anemia and, 327
  laboratry evaluations for, 711
  long-term outcome and needs, 762–63
  MAS risk with, 798
  maternal myasthemia gravis and, 330t
  maternal systemic lupus erythematosus and, 330t
  multiple gestation and, 558
  nursing care plan, 764–68
  nursing diagnosis examples for, 767n
  from nutritive deficit, 374
  perinatal mortality and morbidity in, 761
  PIH causes, 341
  polycythemia in, 835
  resuscitation risk in, 786
  risk identification for, 734, 735–36f
  sign of at labor onset, 428g
  skin texture in, 690g
  symmetric vs. asymmetric, 764n
  temperature regulation for, 645
  weight of, 689g
Smallpox
  immunization against, in pregnancy, 266t
  neonatal immunity to, 654
Smegma
  clitoris produces, 73
  under labia of neonate, 684, 701g
Smell, peculiarities of in pregnancy, 198. See also Olfactory sense
Smellie, William, 4
Smiling, by neonate, 687, 706, 725
Smoking
  adolescent pregnancy and, 299, 304
  diabetes and, 319
  fetal/neonatal effects of, 361t, 636, 654
  infertility from, 111t, 112, 114
  as risk factor, 214t
  teratogenic effects of, 268
Snacks, in pregnancy, 271t, 272–73

Sneezing, by neonate, 681, 685, 686
Snorting respirations, with choanal atresia, 852
Soap, for infant care, 727
SOAP format, 20
  pregnancy discomfort described with, 260
Soave pull-through operation method, 870
Social behavior, assessing neonate for, 706
Social relationships
  environmental factors affect, 46
  family development and, 37, 40
Social Security Act, maternal-child health care and, 5
Social services, for parents of high-risk infants, 780. See also Referral
Socialization, as family function, 35
Socioeconomic factors
  in adolescent pregnancy, 297, 299
    adolescent father and, 300, 301
  assessing, in initial prenatal exam, 238g
  crisis adaptation affected by, 992–93
  families affected by, 41–43
  high risk and, 214t, 388–89
  labor coping mechanisms and, 405
  PIH risk and, 336
  pregnancy health care and, 206, 207
  prenatal nutrition and, 284
  SGA neonates and, 761, 763
Sodium. See also Electrolytes
  in breast milk, cow's milk, and formula, 719t
  normal neonatal values, 645t
    preterm infant, 752t
  PIH and, 342
  pregnancy requirements, 270t, 273
  retention of in pregnancy, 201
    estrogen and, 198
Sodium bicarbonate, 793d
  for acidosis in neonate, 746, 792, 793d
    hypocalcemia risk with, 821
  IVH risk and, 836
  neonatal contraindications, 793d
  for resuscitation, 788, 793d
  suctioning use of, 813p
Sodium pentothal (Thiopental sodium), 529–530
Sole (plantar) creases, gestational age determination by, 660, 661, 662f, 665f 668f
Solid-phase radioimmune assay or RIA, (hCG and Preg/Stat B-hCG), 194
Solnit, A. J.
  on mourning the idealized child, 773
  on vulnerable child syndrome, 1009–10
Somatotropic (growth) hormone (STH), puberty and, 92
Somatotropin, breast changes and, 85
Somite formation, in embryo, 173
Sonography, for observing internal reproductive organs, 73
Soranus, as "father of obstetrics" 3
Sore throat, chronic, in secondary syphilis, 354
Southern Americans, labor customs among, 469
Spalding sign, fetal death shown by, 560
Sparine (promazine), during labor, 513

Spasticity
  in LGA infant, from birth trauma, 756
  with maple syrup urine disease, 858
Specialization, nursing implications of, 10
Specific gravity of neonatal urine, 652
  for preterm infant, 750n
    fluid balance assessment with, 747, 748
    monitoring, 753ncp
Specificity theory of pain, 410
Speculums, vaginal. See Vaginal speculums
Speech defects
  with cleft lip and palate, therapy for, 852
  in FAS children, 770
  as IUGR outcome, 763
  from kernicterus, 826
  as prematurity risk, 758
Sperm. See Spermatozoa
Sperm adequacy tests, 117
Sperm analysis, 117
Spermatids, 160, 161f
Spermatogenesis, 61–62, 158, 160, 161f
  temperature and, 61
Spermatozoa
  anatomy of, 64, 65f
  fertilization by, 160–62, 161f, 162f
  harmed by heat, 114
  imperfections in, spontaneous abortion caused by, 329
  maturation of, 62, 63, 160, 161f
  postcoital examination of, 116, 117
  production of. See Spermatogenesis
  scanning electron micrograph of, 65f
  storage of, 63, 64
  transport of, 64, 161
  uterine assistance to, 79
Spermicides, as contraceptives, 121f, 127
  with cervical cap, 123
  with diaphragm, 121f, 122–23
  postpartal use of, 944
  with vaginal sponges, 124
Spherocytes, ABO incompatibility and, 826
Spherocytosis, hereditary, neonatal hyperbilirubinemia and, 823
Sphingomyelin. See Lecithin/sphingomyelin (L/S) ratio
Spider nevi
  assessing, in initial prenatal exam, 217g
  in pregnancy, 199
Spina bifida, 878–81, 879–80f, 882n
  described, 878–79, 879f
  hip dysplasia vs., 878
  hydrocephaly and, 557
  incidence of, 879
  in LGA preterm IDM, 757n
  nevus pilosus associated with, 685
  as polygenetically inherited, 145, 145t
  prenatal diagnosis of, 148
  risk of recurrence of, 145t
Spina bifida occulta
  assessing neonate for, 702g
  clinical manifestations of, 880
  described, 878, 879f
  interventions for, 880
Spinal anesthesia. See also Subarachnoid block
  for cesarean delivery, 609

  hypotension after, interventions for, 523n
  nerves affected by, 80
  in pregnancy, 198
  spinal problems and, 224g
  for surgical procedures in pregnancy, 351
Spinal anomalies, assessing for, 702g, 703g, 704g
  LGA preterm IDM, 757n
Spinal blockade, after regional anesthesia, 523n
Spinal cord, birth trauma to
  leg paralysis from, 757n
  from vaginal breech delivery, 554
Spinal curvature, pregancy changes in, 255t, 258
Spinal fluid
  blood in, with IVH, 836
  culture of, in sepsis neonatorum assessment, 841
Spinal headache, 523n, 526–27
Spinal meningitis, developmental delays caused by, 146
Spinal nerve damage, signs of in initial prenatal exam, 225g
Spindle, 158, 159
Spine
  assessing, in initial prenatal exam, 224–25g
  assessing in neonate, 685, 702g
Spinnbarkeit, 114, 116f, 116, 117
  assessing, in contraceptive method, 121–22
Spiral uterine arteries, placental circulatory role of, 168
Spleen
  enlarged, in secondary syphilis, 354
  of neonate
    assessing, 496, 683, 700g
    enlarged. See Splenomegaly
    palpating, 683
    with pathologic jaundice, 823
Splenomegaly, 700g
  ABO incompatibiltiy as cause of, 826
  from congenital syphilis, 844
  with herpesvirus infection, 844
  with hydrops fetalis, 826
  with jaundice, 831
  as toxoplasmosis symptom, 357
Splenomegaly. See Hepatosplnomegaly
Splinting
  for clubfoot, 876
  for hip dysplasia, 878
Sponge bath, for neonate, 727–28
Spongy urethra, 63
Spontaneous delivery, vertex presentation, 418
Spotting, from contraception, 125. See also Vaginal bleeding
Sprironolactone, for premenstrual tension, 100
Sputum, frothy, 576
  from amniotic fluid embolism, 576
  during labor, interventions for, 576
Squamocolumnar junction, 79, 79f
Squamous cells, in meconium at birth, 651
Square window sign, 663f, 665f, 669, 672f
Squatting position, delivery in, 489, 616, 630
St. Mary's Hospital, Evansville, Indiana, 12
St. Thomas School of Nursing, 6
Standards of care, 15
Standing orders, protocols as, legal aspects of, 14–15

Standing position, delivery in, 620–23f, 630
Staphyloccus aureus
mastitis caused by, 986
puerperal infections from, 974, 986
sepsis neonatorum from, 841
vaginal infections from, 356
Stark, M., 773
Startle reflex in neonate, 655
assessing, 687, 705
in drowsy or semidozing state, 657
Starvation, from hyperemesis gravidarum, 328
Starvation ketosis, at labor admission, sign of, 468
State University of New York at Downstate Medical Center, 7
States of consciousness, in neonate, 655, 657
assessing, 688g, 710
behavioral assessment and, 705–6
patterns of, 705. See also Sleep-wake patterns
Station. *See* Fetal station
Statistics
birth-related, 21–26, 21t, 22t, 24t, 25t
descriptive vs. inferential, 20–21
as maternity care tool, 19, 20–26
as part of nursing process, 23, 26
Stenosis. *See specific types of stenosis*
Stepping reflex, in neonate, 686, 687f, 704g
Stereotyping of sexual roles, 89
Sterile procedure
for delivery, 488, 489, 490
for intrapartal vaginal exam, 436p
for omphalocele interventions, 868
Sterile water, for initial feeding of preterm infant, 746, 753
Sterility
defined, 110
fallopian tube dysfunction and, 83
from hypothyroidism, 326
from salpingitis, 975
Sterilization
as birth control method, 121f, 127–28, 127f, 128f
vasectomy site, 63
after uterine rupture, 550–51
Sterilizing bottles, 927, 928p
Sternal retractions, as neonatal distress sign, 714
Sternocleidomastoid muscle, assessing in neonate, 681
Steroid hormones, placental, 168, 169–70
Steroidogenesis in fetus, hCG stimulates, 169
Steroids
diabetes secondary to, 315
in injectable contraceptives, 127
in oral contraceptives, 126–27t
STH. *See* Somatotropic (growth) hormone
Still disease, hip dysplasia vs., 878
Stillbirth
from abruptio placentae, delivery method with, 564
cardiac disease and, 768
crisis intervention for, 1002–6, 1004n
defined, 210
as drug addiction risk, 770
emotional effects of, 561, 580, 581
iron deficiency anemia and, 327
from maternal diabetes, 316
maternal hypertension and, 769
maternal SLE and, 330t
from maternal syphilis, 354

nursing care plan, 1004
previous
birth center screening for, 618
as CST indication, 375
as risk factor, 215t
Rh senstization and, 349
from toxoplasmosis, 357
Stimulants, fetal/neonatal effects of, 361t
Stimulatory needs
appliances or casts and, 878
cleft lip and palate and, 855–56n
with feeding, 927
jaundice treatment and, 831n, 834n
meningocele/meningomyelocele and, 883n
overload reactions, 960
with RDS, 808n
with tracheoesophageal atresia/fistula, 864n
Stimuli, assessing neonatal responses to, 687, 705–6, 960
Stirrups. *See* Lithotomy position
Stomach, of neonate
distended, hyperresonance of chest with, 698g
functional development of, 651
mucus removal from, 711, 716
Stool. of neonate
assessing, 759n, 874
with necrotizing enterocolitis, 839n
with phototherapy, 829
breast-fed vs. formula-fed, 651
foul odor to, from aganglionosis, 869
meconium, 651
lack of, as distress sign, 714
in reactivity period, 712, 713f
monitoring, for bilirubin, 649
necrotizing enterocolitis signs in, 838, 839
preterm, 750n
reducing substances in, 745, 746
retention of, with meningomyelocele, 880, 882
teaching parents about, 726
transitional, 726
Stool softeners, postpartal, 915, 917n, 918n
Strabismus, in neonate, 680, 680f, 693g
"Strawberry mark" (nevus vasculosus), 678
Streptococci. *See* Beta-hemolytic streptococci
Streptokinase, for pulmonary embolism, 982
Stress
adolescent fatherhood and, 301
amenorrhea from, 100
assessing neonatal responses to, 706
assessing, in family, 49
of cesarean birth, minimizing, 942
congenital anomalies as cause of, 773–74
crisis resulting from. *See* Crisis; Crisis intervention
defined, 246
fetal distress increases, 560
of hospitalization, attachment and, 954
in labor
as complication, 535–36
coping mechanisms and, 405, 406
neonatal response to, 654
prolonged labor increases, 541, 542

multiple pregnancy as cause of, 558
neural and endocrine responses to, 535
neonatal responses to, 654, 748, 818
postpartal, 916, 920–21
anticipatory guidance for, 289–90
pregnancy as, 203, 246, 992
prematurity and, 548, 550, 772–74, 1006, 1007–8t, 1008
with severe preeclampsia, 344
Striae (stretch marks)
abdominal
in initial prenatal exam, 222g
as pregnancy change, 193
nonpregnancy causes of, 192t
on breasts
in initial prenatal exam, 221g
as pregnancy change, 197
postpartal changes in, 905, 946g
purple, as Cushing's syndrome sign, 222g
vitamin E for, 275
Structural-functional approach to family studies, 41
STS (serologic test for syphilis), 229g, 431g
Sturge-Weber syndrome, 677–78
Subarachnoid block (spinal, low spinal, saddle block), 525–27, 526f
for cesarean delivery, 525, 525f, 609
contraindications, 525
levels of, cesarean or vaginal delivery, 525, 525f
nursing implications of, 526–27
for second stage labor, 514
side effects of, 526–27
for surgical procedures in pregnancy, 351
technique, 525–26, 526f
Subcutaneous fat, on SGA neonate, 762, 764, 765
Subdiaphragmatic space, puerperal abscesses in, 975
Subinvolution, 903, 973
assessing for, fourth trimester, 947g
at postpartal home visit, 624, 625
lochia signs of, 904
with puerperal infection, 975, 976
Subjective data, 19
in POMR system, 20
Subluxation of hip joint, 877
Submetacentric chromosomes, 157, 157f
Substance abuse. *See* Drug abuse
Succenturiate placenta, 568, 573, 574f
inspecting for, 579
velamentous insertion with, 575
Succinylcholine
in balanced anesthesia, 530
for convulsions after labor anesthesia, 516
placental transfer of, 170
Sucking. *See also* Sucking reflex
breathing irregularity with, 639
fatigue from, as prematurity risk, 741
milk supply adjusted by, 925, 929–30
neonatal face designed for, 678
patterns of, breast- vs. formula-feeding, 655
poor, with sepsis neonatorum, 841
as response to taste, 655
as response to touch, 681

self-quieting by, 655, 706
transient nerve paralysis and, 681
Sucking reflex, 657. *See also* Sucking
assessing, 686, 695g, 704g
with water feeding, 716
kernicterus affects, 824
in preterm infant
aspiration risk and, 741
feeding method and, 742, 753
nutrition and, 740
in reactivity period, 711–12
with tracheoesophageal atresia/fistula, 864n
Sucrose, digestion of by neonate, 651
Suction curettage, for hydatidiform mole, 335
Suction evacuation, after spontaneous abortion, 332
Suctioning, with eclampsia, 344
Suctioning of neonate
for acute respiratory obstruction, 531
for apnea, 755n
after diaphragmatic hernia surgery, 867
at delivery, 491, 788
importance of, 636–37
Leboyer method eliminates, 617
MAS prevention with, 812–13p, 813f, 814–15
for postterm infant, 760
precipitous, 504
with endotracheal tube, 812–13p, 813f
equipment for, in infant care unit, 488
in nursery routine care, 714–16, 716f
preterm infant, apnea prevention with, 756n
procedure, 500, 812–14, 813f
in RDS nursing care plan, 805–6, 812–14p, 813f
during reactivity period, 712
teaching parents about, 726
after tracheoesophageal surgery, 863n
Sudden infant death syndrome (SIDS)
crisis intervention for, 1005, 1006
low birth weight and, 758
after postnatal narcotic withdrawal, 771
Suffocation, crib safety to prevent, 730
Sulfisoxazole, for cystitis in pregnancy, 353
Sulfonamides
for cystitis in pregnancy, 353
neonatal hyperbilirubinemia and, 827

Tace (chlorotrianisene), 919n, 925
Tachycardia, fetal, 450–51
causes of, 450–51
defined, 450
FHR baseline variability with, 452
as nonreassuring, 458
from hypotonic labor patterns, 541
with induction, interventions for, 594n
interventions for, 451t
intrapartal heart aberrations and, 425t
as isoxsuprine side effect, 548
preterminal, 458
resuscitation risk with, 786
as ritodrine side effect, 549
as terbutaline sulfate side effect, 548
with uterine hypotonia, 541
Tachycardia, in mother
from amniotic fluid embolism, 576

Tachycardia, in mother (Cont'd)
  assessing by auscultation, 424
  blood loss causes, 569
  with cardiac disease, 311
  as isoxsuprine side effect, 548
  in labor, 409
    fourth stage, 502
    induced, as water intoxication
      sign, 590, 593n
    interventions for, 576
  as Mendelson syndrome sign, 531
  with mastitis, 987
  after normal delivery, 420
  puerperal, 906
  as puerperal infection sign, 975,
    976
  as pulmonary embolism sign, 982,
    984n
  as ritodrine side effect, 549
  as terbutaline sulfate side effect,
    548
Tachycardia, in neonate
  assessing, 698g
  assessing for, 688g
    in LGA preterm IDM, 757n
  with herpesvirus infection, 844
  intrapartal fetal heart aberrations
    and, 425t
  as patent ductus arteriosus sign,
    810n
  with polycythemia, 835
  from succenturiate placenta, 573
Tachypnea, in mother
  during labor, first stage, 428g
  in prenatal exams, 216g, 220g,
    239g
Tachypnea, in neonate
  assessing for, 682, 688g
    in LGA preterm IDM, 757n
  with herpesvirus infection, 844
  with MAS, 814
  as patent ductus arteriosis sign,
    810n
  with pneumomediastinum, 816
  as pneumopericardium sign, 810n
  with polycythemia, 835
  as PPH sign, 817
  preterm, as respiratory distress
    sign, 751
  with RDS, 796t, 801n
  from succenturiate placenta, 573
  with tracheoesophageal atresia/fis-
    tula, 860
  transient, 797–98, 817
    in drug-addicted neonate, 771
Tactile capacity in neonate, 655
Tactile stimulation, as need. See also
    Stimulatory needs
Tagament (Cimetidine), during labor,
    531
Tail of Spence, 85
Tailor sitting, 263, 264f
Taking-hold phase, 907
  attachment during, 958
  after cesarean delivery, 942
  learning receptivity during, 938–
    39
  self-esteem in, 921
Taking-in phase, 907
  acquaintance phase during, 958
  adjustments during, 920
Talipes calcaneovalgus, 875–76
Talipes equinovarus (clubfoot), 875f,
    875–76
  assessing neonate for, 685, 703g
Tandem nursing, 928
Taste sensation
  by neonate, 655, 681
  peculiarities of in pregnancy, 198
Taylor, P. M., on prematurity
    adjustment, 772–73
Tay-Sachs disease, 143–44

  as autosomal recessively inherited,
    144
  detection of carrier parent, 143–
    44
  ethnic background and, 152
  genetic counseling referral for, 151
  prenatal diagnosis of, 148
TB. See Tuberculosis
Teaching role of nurse. See also
    Childbirth preparation;
    Parent education
  abortion and, 131
  in adolescent pregnancy, 300t,
    304f, 305
    postpartum, 943
  AGA and LGA preterm infants,
    750n
  in antepartal care, 243, 246, 291–
    92
    communication skills, 290–91
  assessing learning needs, 938
  betamethasone and, 547
  bleeding in pregnancy and, 329
  bottle-feeding, 926–27
  breast-feeding, 921–24, 928–31
  for cardiac disease in pregnancy,
    312
  cesarean delivery, 601, 602, 606–
    8
    emergency, 607
  circumcision care, 701g, 722
  cleft lip and palate, 853–54n
  communication skills, 290–91
  crisis prevention with, 998
  danger signs of pregnancy, 240g
  in diabetic pregnancy, 318, 322,
    324
  with DIC, 568
  electronic fetal monitoring and,
    459–60
  Erb-Duchenne paralysis, 684
  family care, 49–50, 50–52
  with fetal distress, 538n
  foreskin care, 701g
  group teaching method, 291–92
  handling neonates, 726
  hemorrhage, 569
  herpes infection and, 360
  for high-risk infant, predischarge,
    779–80
  in high-risk pregnancy, 388–89
  home birth preparation, 629–30
  impetigo in neonate, 690g
  infant care, 714; see also neonatal
    care
  infant nutrition, 717
  in infertility management, 118
  informed consent and, 15
  in intensive care nursery, 774, 775
  at labor admission, 472
  during labor
    fourth stage, 481, 482n
    induced, 590, 591n
    pain management and, 484
  meningomyelocele, 881, 882,
    884n
  with menopausal women, 102
  methods, 291–92, 938–39
  necrotizing enterocolitis, 839n
  neonatal anal care, 702g
  neonatal assessment process, 706
  neonatal behavioral assessment,
    687
  neonatal care, 714, 725–30, 728–
    29f
    immediate, 498n
  neonatal distress signs, 713–14
  neonatal ear care, 696g
  neonatal elimination, 726
  neonatal hair and scalp care, 692g
  neonatal hyperbilirubinemia, 830
  neonatal jaundice, 831n, 834n

  neonatal safety, 716
  neonatal "soft spots" 692g
  neonatal tear duct blockage, 694g
  neonatal temperature assessment,
    688g, 728–29
  parenting skills, 920n
  perineal care, 918n, 919n
  PIH and, 337, 342
  postpartal care, 908, 920, 921
    elimination, 918n
    exercises, 916
    home visit, 624–27
    principles of, 938–39
  pregnancy discomforts and, 259,
    260
  prenatal nutrition, 281–85, 286–
    87f
  preterm infant care, 754–55n
  prolonged labor, 542
  psychologic assessments and,
    241g
  puerperal infection, 976, 977
    with regional anesthesia, 521n
  respiratory distress syndrome, 801
  rooming-in and, 713–14
  severe preeclampsia, 344
  sex education, 105–6
  SGA neonates, 764n
  suctioning neonates, 726
    with bulb syringe, 716, 716f
  thromboembolic disease, 983
  tracheoesophageal atresia/fistula,
    862n, 865n
  umbilical cord care and hygiene,
    700g
  wrapping the newborn, 716
Team approach. See Health team
Tear duct blockage in neonate, 694g
Tearfulness, with "postpartum blues"
    907
Tears, in neonates, 680. See also
    Crying
  absence of, 694g
Technologic advances, 8–10
  ethical questions and, 9–12
  neonatal care and, 733
"Teds"   See Support stockings
Teen Mother and Child Programs,
    780
Teenage pregnancy. See Adolescent
    pregnancy
Teenagers, response to parents'
    pregnancy of, 251
Teeth
  cleft palate affects, 851, 852
  enamel hypoplasia, from hyper-
    bilirubinemia, 827
  of fetus
    development of, 176t, 178t
    teratogenic damage to, 183t,
      267, 267t
  precocious, in neonate, 681
  pregnancy and, 199
  staining of, from hemolytic disease,
    827
Teething, parental preparation for,
    729
Telangiectatic nevi ("stork bites"),
    677, 691g
Telemetry
  ambulation allowed with, 617
  electronic monitoring with, 445t,
    447, 450
Telephoning parents, after preterm
    birth, 1009
Telophase, 158, 158f, 159f
Temperature, basal body (BBT), 115,
    115f
Temperature, maternal
  assessing in fourth trimester, 945g
  assessing during labor, 473
    active phase, 475n

  first stage, 428g
  fourth stage, 481n, 501, 502,
    974
  before induction, 589
  assessing postpartum, 906, 913,
    917, 919n
    after home birth, 630
    at home visit, 624
  assessing in prenatal exams, 216g,
    239g
  assessing, with severe pre-
    eclampsia, 343
  elevated
    as anxiety sign, 608
    birth center transfer for, 618
    as pregnancy danger sign, 240g
    with mastitis, 987
  monitoring
    after amniotomy, 587
    with oxytocin induction, 593n
    after PROM, 547
  ovulation changes, 94, 98
  with puerperal infections, 974,
    986
  with thromboembolic disease, 980,
    981, 983
Temperature, neonatal
  assessing, 676f, 676–77f, 688g
    at nursery admission, 710
    in nursery routine, 714
    at postpartal home visit, 627
  as breathing onset stimulus, 636
  with cold stress, 817–18
  environmental temperature and,
    645–46
  with herpesvirus infection, 844
  interventions to maintain, 498n
  monitoring
    in nursery, 712, 714
    with phototherapy, 829
  preterm, 750n, 752–53n
  normal rectal, 729
  physiologic jaundice and, 649
  regulation of. See
    Thermoregulation
  stabilizing, as nursing priority,
    498n
  teaching parents about, 728–29
  with tracheoesophageal atresia/fis-
    tula, 860
Temperature regulation. See Ther-
    moregulation
Temporal artery, assessing in initial
    prenatal exam, 218g
Temperomandibular, assessing in ini-
    tial prenatal exam, 219g
Tentorial tears
  from brow presentation, 552
  precipitous labor and risk of,
    425t
Teratogen, defined, 184
Teratogenic abnormalities, postnatal
    diagnosis of, 149, 150
Teratogenic illnesses, 357–60
Teratogenic substances, 265–66
  addictive drugs as, 360–62, 361t
  alcohol, 361t, 362, 770
  antiemetics as, 252
  cardiac medications, 768–69
  cleft lip and palate caused by, 851
  congenital heart defects from, 881
  counseling about, 151
  employment during pregnancy
    and, 261
  IUGR associated with, 761
  malformations related to, 145–46,
    183t, 184
  screening newborns for, 150
  medications as, 266–68, 267t
  podophyllin, 355
  spontaneous abortion caused by,
    329

Terbutaline sulfate (Brethine), 371, 548

Term (F) neonates, birth weight classifications for, 734, 735f

Terminal ampulla, role of, 63

Tes-Tape, for prenatal urinalysis, 317

"Test-tube" babies, 9

Testes, 59f, 61–62, 61f, 62f
  development of, 57, 58f, 653, 653f
  infertility and, 111t, 112, 114
  of neonate
    assessing, 684, 701g
    preterm, 750

Testicular biopsy, in infertility work-up, 114

Testosterone
  effect of, 92f, 93
  fetal
    role of, 57, 59
    hCG and, 168–69
  gonadotropins cause production of, 62
  postmenopausal, libido increased by, 102
  role of, 62
  testes secrete, 61

Tetanic contractions. See Uterine contractions

Tetanus, neonatal immunity to, 654

Tetanus-diphtheria immunization, in pregnancy, 266t

Tetracaine (Pontocaine), labor analgesia with, 514, 516

Tetracycline
  for chlamydial infections, 355
  for gonorrhea in neonate, 844
  as teratogen, 266–67, 267t

Tetrad, 159

Tetralogy of Fallot, 887f, 889–90, 891f

Thalassemias
  ethnic background and, 152
  monitoring hemoglobin for, in prenatal exams, 239g
  prenatal diagnosis of, 148

Thalidomide, 881

Thank You, Dr. Lamaze (Karmel), 294

Theca externa, 96, 98

Theca interna, 96

Thecal cells, as interstitial glands of pregnancy, 196

Theophylline, for intractable neonatal apnea, 756n

Therapeutic interaction
  in cesarean delivery preparation, 602, 608
  defective birth, 849–50
  in family care, 49

Thermal neutral zone (TNZ), establishment of in neonate, 645–46, 646f

Thermal stimuli of breathing onset, 636

Thermogenesis (heat production) in neonates, 647f, 647
  motor activity and, 654

Thermoregulation in neonates, 645–48, 646–47t
  impaired
    cold stress from, 817–18
    with drug withdrawal, 771
    hypoglycemia vs., 818
    in preterm infant, 758
    with intraventricular hemorrhage, 837
    with MAS, 815
    meperidine affects, 512
    in nursery, 712–13
    preterm, 740, 752–53n

apnea prevention with, 756n
sample nursing diagnosis, 758
with out-of-hospital emergency birth, 506, 507
RDS importance of, 797, 806n
sepsis neonatorum affects, 841
as SGA need, 764n

Thiamine. See Vitamin B₁; Vitamins

Thiazides, fetal/neonatal effects of, 769

Thiopental sodium (Pentothal), 529–30

Thirst
  excessive, as diabetes sign, 314
  in fourth stage of labor, 420
  immediately after delivery, 905
  with puerperal peritonitis, 976
  from vitamin D overdose, 275

Thoracentesis
  for interstitial pulmonary emphysema, 809n
  for pneumothorax, 809n, 816

Thorax, assessing in neonate, 682

Three-generation family structure, 32, 33f
  cultural preference for, 43

Thrills, defined 233p

Throat, of neonate, hearing loss risk and, 681

Throat cultures, for congenital herpesvirus detection, 844

Thrombocytopenia, in neonate, 215t
  from congenital CMV, 359
  with extended rubella syndrome, 358
  with hydrops fetalis, 826
  maternal hypertension and, 343, 769

Thromboembolia in neonate, with polycythemia, 835

Thromboembolic disease, 976, 980–82, 981f
  factors affecting, 976, 980
  incidence of, 976
  lactation suppression drugs and, 925
  nursing diagnoses, examples, 985
  postpartal risk of, 906, 912
  pulmonary embolism, 981–82, 983, 984–85n

Thromboembolism, from contraception, 125, 127

Thrombophlebitis
  danger signs, 941
  deep, 981
  described, 976
  nursing care plan, 983–84, 985
  pelvic vein, pelvic cellulitis from, 975–76
  postpartal risk of, 908t, 912
  superficial, 980
  from surgery during pregnancy, preventing, 351
  as varicose veins complication, 257

Thromboplastin release, DIC and, 567–68, 568f

Thrombosis
  deep leg vein disease risk and, 981
  intestinal, with necrotizing enterocolitis, 837
  intravascular, with homocystinuria, 859
  placental, IUGR associated with, 761
  venous, pregnancy risk of, 198

Thrush (oral moniliasis)
  in neonates, 355, 844–45
    assessing for, 681, 696g
    nipple soreness in mother from, 936

puerperal infection and, 976, 979n
signs of in initial prenatal exam, 220g

Thymus, fetal role of, 644

Thyroid dysfunction
  habitual abortion caused by, 333
  infertility and, 114
  as pregnancy complication, 215t, 321, 326

Thyroid function tests
  after abruptio placentae, 564
  in infertility workup, 114

Thyroid gland
  assessing in initial prenatal exam, 218g
  assessing in neonate, 697g
  enlarged, from hyperthyroidism, 326
  pregnancy changes in, 201, 321

Thyroid hormone. See Thyroxine

Thyroid medication, for congenital hypothyroidism, 859

Thyroid storm
  as pregnancy risk, 215t, 326
  symptoms of, 326

Thyrotoxicosis, from hyperthyroidism, 215t

Thyrotropin, pregnancy role of, 202

Thyroxine
  breast changes and, 85
  in breast milk, 718
  pregnancy changes in, 201, 326
  puberty and, 92
  neonatal levels of, 326

Tidal volume, suctioning decreases, 805n, 813

Tinnitus, as Methergine side effect, 903d

Tocodynamometer (pressure transducer or "toco"), 434, 440f, 445–46, 446f
  in contraction stress test, 376
  with placenta previa double setup exam, 567

Tocolytic agents
  delaying labor with, 547, 548, 549d
  for external cephalic version, 585
  for uterine inversion, 580

Tocopherol. See Vitamin E

Toddlers, safety for, 729–30

Toes, of neonate
  assessing, 684
  clubbed, with heart defects, 890, 891

Tolazoline (Priscoline)
  for MAS, 815
  for PPH syndrome, 817

Tongue
  assessing in initial prenatal exam, 220g
  of neonate
    assessing, 695g, 696g
    with congenital hypothyroidism, 859

Tongue-tied neonate, 681

Tonic neck reflex (fencer position), assessing in neonate, 685–86, 686f, 704g

Tools
  communication, 19, 20
  knowledge base, 19
  nursing process, 19–20
  research, 19, 26–27
  statistics, 19, 20–26
  use of in nursing practice, 19, 27–28

Topical anesthetics, perineal pain relief with, 915, 917n

TORCH group of infectious diseases, 357–60
  screening test for, 150

Torticollis, congenital, assessing for, 681, 691g, 697g

Total parenteral nutrition (TPN), 745–46, 753, 754
  after diaphragmatic hernia repair, 867
  with necrotizing enterocolitis, 838

Touch, sense of, 89
  pain distraction with, 484
  therapeutic, in cesarean delivery preparation, 602, 608

Touching of neonate by parents, 494f, 502–3, 503f
  with high-risk neonates, importance of, 775
  parental attachment requires, 773–74
  with preterm infants, 775, 776f

Toxemia of pregnancy, 336. See also Eclampsia; Preeclampsia/Eclampsia; Pregnancy-induced hypertension
  DIC from, 567–68, 568f
  maternal death from, 206, 605
  prematurity from, hematologic considerations, 748–49

Toxic substances, infertility from, 112, 114. See also Teratogenic substances

Toxoplasmosis
  diagnosing, 767, 842
  microencephaly from, 691g
  newborn screening for, 150
    SGA neonate, 766–67n
  neonatal hyperbilirubinemia risk from, 823
  in pregnancy, 357
  fetal IgM levels and, 654

TPAL system, 210–11

TPN. See Total parenteral nutrition

Trachea
  assessing in initial prenatal exam, 218g
  of neonate
    assessing, 699g
    brow presentation may damage, 552

Tracheal fluid aspiration, transient tachypnea of newborn after, 797

Tracheal intubation. See also Intubation
  of neonate, 788, 790f, 791–92p
  for pulmonary embolism, 985n

Tracheoesophageal fistula, 183t, 859–61, 860f, 861f
  assessing with first water feeding, 716
  nursing care plan, 862–65
  prognosis, 861

Tracheotomy, for Pierre Robin syndrome, 851

Tranquilizers
  abuse of in pregnancy, 361t
  amenorrhea from, 100
  fetal/neonatal effects of, 267t, 361t
  during labor, 513
    for cardiac client, 313
    Levallorphan increases depression from, 512

Transaminase (SGOT), normal preterm values, 752t

Transcutaneous oxygen monitoring, for RDS, 797, 802n

Transfusions. See Blood transfusions; Exchange transfusions

Transient strabismus in neonate, 680, 680f

Transient tachypnea of the newborn, 797–98, 817
  in drug-addicted infant, 771

Transillumination
  of chest, pneumothorax assessment with, 816
  of scrotum, 701g
Transition See Labor, deceleration phase of
Transitional milk, 925
Translocation, 138–39, 139f, 140f
  mechanism of, 159
Transmission electron microscopy, for observing female organs, 73
Transplacental gas exchange impairment, 540n
Transport mechanisms in placenta, 170–71
Transport of neonate, attachment process and, 773–74, 775
Transposition of the great vessels, 886f, 890–92
  birth weight with, 760
  in IDM, 768
  risk factors for, 736f
Transpyloric tube feeding, 742, 745
Transverse arrest, 551, 552
Transverse cervical (cardinal or Mackedrodt's) ligaments, 82
Transverse lie (shoulder presentation), 399, 400, 402, 552, 555–56
  external or cephalic version of, 585, 586
  incidence of, 555
  as induction of labor contraindication, 587
  internal or podalic version of, 585
  management of, 555–56
  with placenta previa, 565
  preterm labor with, cesarean for, 550
  prolapsed umbilical cord with, 574
Trauma
  during pregnancy, 352–53
  during birth. See also Birth trauma
    midforceps delivery and, 597–98
    as oxytocin induction risk, 590
    uterine rupture from, 550
Travel during pregnancy, 261
  for pregnant diabetic, 319–20
Treacher Collins syndrome, 692g, 694g, 695g
  Pierre Robin syndrome vs., 850
Trembling, during deceleration phase labor, 478
Tremors
  in mother
    postpartal, 502
    as ritodrine side effect, 549
    as terbutaline sulfate side effect, 548
  in neonate
    assessing, 685, 687, 703g, 705
    with hypoglycemia, 817, 818
    IDM, from hypocalcemia, 768
Trendelenburg position
  for epidural anesthesia reaction, 519
  hemorrhage as contraindication for, 571
  modified, for neonate, 492
  for umbilical cord prolapse, 540n, 574
Treponema pallidum, 170, 354
Trichomonas vaginalis, 356
  adolescent pregnancy and, 304
  signs of in initial prenatal exam, 226g, 227f
Triglycerides
  in cow's milk, fat absorption and, 651

nonshivering thermogenesis role of, 647
Trimethadione, IUGR associated with, 761
Triplets, 368, 560. See also Multiple pregnancy
Triplo X, 141
Trisomies, 136
Trisomy 13, 137–38, 138f
  dermatoglyphic patterns with, 149
  maternal age and, 147
Trisomy 13 Clubs, 780
Trisomy 13–15 (Trisomy D)
  assessing SGA neonate for, 766n
  cardiac malformations and, 881
Trisomy 16, risk factors for, 736f
Trisomy 16–18 (Trisomy E), assessing SGA neonate for, 766n
Trisomy 18, 137–38, 138f
  maternal age and, 147
  neck with, 697g
  risk factors for, 736f
Trisomy 21, 136, 137, 137f. See also Down syndrome
  maternal age and, 147
  recurrence risks for, 147
Trisomy D. See Trisomy 13–15
Trisomy E. See Trisomy 16–16
Trophoblast
  chorion develops from, 164
  formation of, 162, 163f
  hCG secreted by, 202
  implantation of, 162–63, 163f
  placenta formed from, 166
Trophoblastic disease
  diagnostic test for, 194
  hydatidiform mole as, 334
  ⅜Hydatoxi lualba and, 336
Trophoblastic tissue, as immunologically inert, 170
True (minor or lesser) pelvis, 68–70, 68f-70f
Trunk, assessing, 702–3g
Trunk incurvation reflex, assessing in neonate, 704g
Trust vs. mistrust, 40, 40t
Trusting relationship, of nurse and client, 997
    attachment process aided by, 964, 969
    with pregnant adolescent, 303
    in prenatal care, 238, 240, 243
Truthfulness, in genetic counseling, 153–54
Tub baths, for neonates, 728
Tubal insufflation, 117
Tubal ligation, 121f, 127–28, 128f
  for diabetic, risk of, 319
  infertility from, 111t
Tubal patency tests, in infertility workup, 113f, 117–18
Tubal pregnancy, 333. See also Ectopic pregnancy
Tube feeding
  with bronchopulmonary dysplasia, 808n
  for choanal atresia, 857
  for Pierre Robin syndrome, 851
  for preterm infants, 742, 743–45p, 745, 753–54n
  preventing apnea with, 756n
  with tracheoesophageal atresia/fistula, 863–64n
Tubercles of Montgomery, 85
Tuberculosis (TB)
  infertility from, 113t
  as pregnancy complication, 331t
  testing for in initial prenatal exam, 230g
Tucker-McLean forceps, 597, 597f
Tumors
  fibroid. See Myomas

labor blocked by, 545, 600
  pelvic, pregnancy signs caused by, 192t
  placental, 568
Tunica albuginea, 59, 60f, 61, 62f
  ovarian, 83
    midcycle pain and, 98
Tunica vaginalis, 61, 62f
Turgor of skin. See Skin
Turner syndrome, 137, 141, 141f
  neck with, 697g
  ocular hypertelorism with, 692g
Twin-to-twin transfusion, 822
  polycythemia and anemia from, 835
Twins, 185. See also Multiple pregnancy
  delivery of, general anesthesia for, 529
  discordant, risk factors for, 736f
  dizygotic or fraternal, 557–58
  dizygotic, factors affecting incidence of, 558
  fetal lung maturity in, 385
  fetal problems of, 558
  fundal height and, 237
  gray-scale ultrasound scan of, 367f
  hypotonic labor patterns with, 541
  incomplete, labor problems from, 557
  internal or podalic version of, 585–86
  iron supplementation in pregnancy with, 327
  monozygotic or identical, 557
    hydramnios with, 576
    incidence of, 558
  parabiotic, fetal lung maturity in, 385
  parent education needs with, 939
  parent support groups for, 780
  umbilical cord prolapse risk with, 574
Twitching, by neonate
  as hypocalcemia sign, 821
  with kernicterus, 824
  LGA, from birth trauma, 756n
Two-hour postprandial test, for pregnant diabetic, 317
Tympanic membrane, assessing in neonate, 696g
Typhoid immunization in pregnancy, 266t

Ulceration of urethral meatus, assessing neonate for, 701g
Ultrasonic echosound, positive pregnancy diagnosis with, 195
Ultrasonography, 8, 367–68p, 366–72, 367f, 368f. See also Doppler ultrasonography
  in adolescent pregnancy, 305
  A-mode (amplitude mode), 366, 367f
  advantages of, 367
  amniocentesis preceded by, 381–82, 382f, 383p
  B-mode (brightness mode), 366–67, 367f
  BPD measurement with, 368, 368f, 369
  calculating gestational age with, after PROM, 546
  clinical applications of, 368–72
  CPD assessment with; see pelvic adequacy assessment with
  CRL measurement with, 369–70
  for deep vein thrombosis assessment, 981, 983
  determining delivery date with, 237

for early pregnancy detection, 368–69
fetal breathing movements seen by, 371, 636
fetal maturity evaluation by, 591, APPENDIX C
fetal position assessment with, 442
fetal presentation assessment with, 442
fetal size estimation by, 557, APPENDIX C
for gallbladder evaluation in pregnancy, 352
gray-scale, 367, 367f
  of triplets, 368f
  of twins, 367f
hydramnios seen with, 577
hydrocephaly seen by, 557
in initial prenatal exam, 223g
IUGR and, 370–71, 375
IVH assessment with, 836
during labor, 444, 445t, 445–46, 446f
multiple gestation evidence with, 558
pelvic adequacy assessment with, 432, 577
placenta located with, 371
placental grading with, 368, 372, 372f
placenta previa diagnosis with, 565–66, 566f
prenatal diagnosis with, 146
procedure, 367–68
with prolonged pregnancy, 759t
puerperal abscess assessment with, 976
real-time, 367
  fetal death diagnosed with, 560–61
  for fetoscopy, 388
risks of, 372
serial
  assessing fetal maturity with, 588
  for IUGR monitoring, 375
spina bifida detection by, 880
symmetric IUGR diagnosis with, 762
with twin delivery, 559
types of, 366–67
Umbilical arteries
  assessing, 700g
  congenital absence of, 574
  in fetus, 171, 172f
  single, IUGR associated with, 761
Umbilical artery catheterization
  for calcium gluconate administration, 822
  for diaphragmatic hernia monitoring, 866
  feeding RDS neonate with, 807n, 811p
  for monitoring MAS, 815
  necrotizing enterocolitis and, 837, 839n
  PPH diagnosis from, 817
  procedure, 811p
Umbilical cord
  abnormalities of, problems associated with, 575–76
  around neck, petechiae from, 691g
  assessing, 683–84, 700g
    immediately after birth, 498n
    at postpartal home visit, 627
  attachment to placenta of, 167
  battledore placenta and, 574
  bleeding from, neonatal anemia caused by, 830
  care of, 727

immediately after birth, 495, 495f, 498n
checking after delivery of head, 491
clamping and cutting, 491–92, 495f, 498n
  after precipitous delivery, 504
compression of (CC)
  from battledore placenta, 574
  fetal distress from, 560
  from fetal macrosomia, 557
  nursing care plan, 539
  as oligohyramnios risk, 577
  variable decelerations of FHR caused by, 455f
controversy about, 491
delayed clamping of
  blood volume and, 645
  blood sample accuracy and, 644
  at home birth, 630
  Leboyer method, 617, 618
  neonatal jaundice and, 648, 831
drying of, 700g
  of fetus, funic souffle at site of, 168
  formation of, 167
  impaired blood flow through, 539–40n
  infection signs in, 684
length of
  prolapse risk and, 574
  variations in, 575
malformed, 167
meconium-stained, on postterm infant, 760
number of vessels in, 499n
prolapse of, 539–40n, 574–75, 575f
  as amniotomy risk, 587, 589
  conditions associated with, 574
  as CPD danger, 578
  cesarean delivery for, 600
  emergency interventions for, 574–75
  fetal/neonatal implications of, 425t, 452, 456, 574, 787
  as forceps delivery indication, 597
  as hydramnios risk, 577
  immediate interventions for, 488t
  as inlet contracture risk, 578
  internal or podalic version for, 585–86
  as intrapartal risk, 416, 425t
  maternal implications of, 425t, 574
  nursing care plan for, 539–40
  as podalic version risk, 586
  as prolonged labor risk, 542
  as PROM risk, 546
  resuscitation risk with, 787
  transient tachypnea of newborn after, 797
  from transverse lie, 556
  "two-vessel" 575
  vasa previa, 575–76
  velamentous insertion of, 575, 575f
  yolk sac incorporated in, 165
Umbilical cord blood
  delayed clamping and, 644
  hyperbilirubinemia risk assessment with, 823
Umbilical cord clamp, in emergency delivery pack, 503
Umbilical hernia
  assessing, 700g
  with congenital hypothyroidism, 859
  cord length and, 575

Umbilical vein, 172f
  role of, 171
Umbilical venous catheter, for calcium gluconate, 822
Underwear, male infertility and, 111t, 114
United Nations Declaration of the Rights of the Child, APPENDIX B
United States
  birth rates, 21t, 22t
  fertility rates, 21t
  infant mortality in, 23, 25t
  live births statistics, 21t
  maternal mortality in, 23, 25t
  nurse-midwifery in, 6–7
  obstetrics in, historical overview of, 5–6
United States Supreme Court, *Roe v. Wade* decision, 10
University of Colorado Health Sciences Center, intrauterine surgery at, 11
Uphold, C. R., 101
UPI. *See* Uteroplacental insufficiency
Upper-class families, 41, 43
Upper-middle-class families,, 41, 42
Upper respiratory infections
  from atrial septal defects, 885
  from patent ductus arteriosus, 885
  preventing, with cleft lip, 854n
  preventing, with cleft palate, 856n
  risk of to cardiac client, 312
  with tracheoesophageal atresia/fistula, 861
Upright position, for holding infant, 714, 715f
Urea nitrogen (BUN), normal preterm values, 752t
Ureters
  palpation of, 74
  pregnancy changes in, 197t, 199
Urethra, male, 59f, 60, 60f, 63
  membranous, 63
  penile, 59f, 59, 60f
  prostatic, 63
Urethral (Littre's) glands, 64
Urethral caruncle, in initial prenatal exam, 225g
Urethral discharge, from genital herpes simplex, 359
Urethral glands, embryologic development of, 57
Urethral meatus, 60, 60f
  evaluating, in infertility workup, 114
  female, 71f, 73
    assessing in initial prenatal exam, 225g
Urethritis
  assessing neonate for, 701g
  signs of in initial prenatal exam, 225g
Urgency, as cystitis sign, 986
  at postpartal home visit, 625
Uric acid levels, with severe preeclampsia, 343
Urinalysis, of mother. *See also* Urine culture
  before abortion, 129
  before cesarean delivery. 601
  diabetic, 316–17, 319t, 320
  with fetal distress, 538n
  with hemorrhage, 570n
  before induction of labor, 591n
  in infertility workup, 114
  in labor
    at admission, 468, 472, 473
    energy status shown by, 429g
    at onset, 429g, 432g
  postpartal, 917
    at fourth trimester exams, 946g

at home visit, 624
  lochia contamination and, 906
  puerperal infection assessment with, 976, 977
  precontraception, 120
  in prenatal exams
    initial, 213, 216g, 235, 229–30g
    subsequent, 239–40g
Urinalysis, of neonate
  female, 701g
  hypoglycemia assessment with, 818
  normal values, 652
  preterm, 747, 750n
  during TPN, 745
Urinary calculi, sign of in initial prenatal exam, 230g
Urinary catheterization
  during labor, 475n, 483
  postpartal need for, 982, 986
  with surgical procedures in pregnancy, 351
Urinary complications, from imperforate anus, 872
Urinary estriol determinations, 380–81. *See also* Estriol determinations
  IUGR monitoring with, 375
  procedure, 380
  serum vs., 381
Urinary frequency
  as diabetes sign, 314
  nonpregnancy causes of, 191t
  postpartal home visit assessment of, 625
  as pregnancy discomfort, 192, 253f, 254t, 254–55
  from *Trichomonas* infection, 356
Urinary incontinence, amniotic fluid leakage vs., 416
Urinary output of neonate, 652
Urinary problems in fetus, oligo-hydramnios with, 577
Urinary protein monitoring, with severe preeclampsia, 343
Urinary retention, postpartal, 420
  catheterization for, 982, 986
  causes of, 982
Urinary stasis, postpartal risks with, 905–6
Urinary system
  labor changes in, 409–10
  in neonate, development and function of, 652–53
  postpartal assessment of, 919n, 946g
  postpartal changes in, 905–6
  pregnancy changes in, 197t, 199
Urinary tract. *See* Urinary system
Urinary tract infection, in mother
  from cesarean delivery, 605
  with diabetes, 316
  postpartal, 982, 986
    assessing for, 906, 913, 919n, 941
    fourth trimester signs of, 941, 946g
    risk of, 905
    signs of at postpartal home visit, 625
  in pregnancy, 353–54
    as danger sign, 240g
    as preterm labor cause, 548
    preventing, 986
Urinary tract infection, in neonate
  hyperbilirubinemia risk with, 823
  meningomyelocele and, 880
Urination. *See also* Urine output
  during labor, 474–75
    first stage active phase, 476
    fourth stage, 481

with hypotonic labor patterns, 541
  importance of, 483
  by neonate, 652
    assessing, 700g
    assessing after circumcision, 722
    inadequate, as distress sign, 714
    initial, in reactivity period, 712
    preterm, 750n
    teaching parents about, 726
  postpartal, 906
    difficulty in, 905–6, 973
    encouraging, 501–2, 918n
    importance of, 905–6, 982
    lumbar epidural block and, 520
    paracervical block and, 517
Urine, fetal, 652
Urine, of neonate
  assessing, 700g
    with phototherapy, 829
  character of, 652
    with jaundice, 831
    maple syrup odor to. *See* Maple syrup urine disease
  production of, 652
  seepage of
    from exstrophy of bladder, 874–75
    with meningomyelocele, 880, 882, 883n
  stasis of, with meningomyelocele, 880
Urine culture. *See also* Urinalysis
  for puerperal infection, 977. 986
  routine, after pyelonephritis, 986
  in sepsis neonatorum assessment, 842
Urine osmolarity, normal preterm values, 752t
Urine output, of mother. *See also* Urination
  increase in after delivery, 982
  monitoring
    after cesarean, 603, 609
    with hemorrhage, 569n, 570n, 571n
    with induction, 589
    with preeclampsia/eclampsia, 343, 344
  postpartal, 905
  in pregnancy, 254
Urine output, of neonate
  with congestive heart failure, 894
  decreased
    with polycythemia, 835
    as PPH complication, 817
    preterm, monitoring, 753n
Urine pregnanediol level tests, in infertility workup, 114
Urine specific gravity
  monitoring, with severe pre-eclampsia, 343
Urobilinuria, sign of in initial prenatal exam, 229g
Urogenital triangle (diaphragm), 67, 67f
Urologic examination, in infertility workup, 114
Uterine anomalies, as preterm labor cause, 548
Uterine atony, 579
  assessing for
    after abruptio placentae, 564
    postpartum, 972
    in fourth stage labor, 502, 972
    as general anesthesia danger, 530
  hemorrhage and, 569, 572n, 579, 972
  interventions for, 579, 911
    oxytocin, 590d

Uterine atony (Cont'd)
  from macrosomia, 557
  as oxytocin induction risk, 590
Uterine congestion, with maternal
    cardiac decompensation, 311
Uterine contractions. See also Labor
  abnormal; see dysfunctional
  afterpains from, 907
  amniotomy's effects on, 587
  assessing, 430, 432t, 433–34
    in active phase labor, 475n
    in deceleration phase labor,
      477n
    during delivery, by palpation,
      490
    by electronic monitoring, 434,
      440f, 460t, 460–61
    for hemorrhage, 572
    with hypotonic labor pattern,
      541
    before induction, 591n, 592n
    at labor admission, 467–68,
      469, 472
    in labor nursing care plan, 473,
      475, 477
    by palpation, 433–34
    at postpartal home visit, 624
    postpartum, 911
    with ritodrine administration,
      549
  biochemical interaction in, 407
  breathing methods with, 485–86,
    487f
  cervical dilatation correlated with,
    432t
  cessation of, as uterine rupture
    sign, 550
  characteristics of, 404f, 404–5
  after delivery
    increased risk of, 425t
    stimulating, 504
  duration of
    in first stage, 417
    oxytocin induction and, 592n
    in second stage, 418
  dysfunctional
    atony from, 579
    hypotonic, 537, 541, 541f
    interventions for, 536
    from multiple gestation, 558
  electronic monitoring of, 444,
    445t, 445–46, 446f, 447,
    449f
    assessment with, 434, 440f,
      460t, 460–61
  factors affecting, 536
  FHR changes with, 375, 424,
    451t, 454–55, 455f
  forceps delivery timed with 598,
    599f
  frequency of
    in first stage, 417
    with induction, 590, 592n
    in second stage, 418
  general anesthesia affects. 530
  hyperactive, 542, 543f
  hypertonic patterns of, 537, 537f
    amniotic fluid embolism with,
      576
    hemorrhage risk and, 569
  hypotonic, 537, 541, 541f
    hemorrhage risk and, 569
  as impending labor sign, 242g
  intensity of
    first stage, 417
    with precipitous labor, 542,
      543f
    second stage, 418
  in labor, described
    first stage, 417–18, 473n
    fourth stage, 420, 425t
    second stage, 418

    third stage, 419
  monitoring
    with CPD possibility, 578
    with DIC risk, 568
    with induction, 589, 590, 592n
    interpretation of, 460t, 460–61
    with malposition, 552
    in preterm labor, 549
    in prolonged labor, 542
  myometrial tachysystole, 542, 543
  oxytocin-induced
    goal for, 589
    relaxation between, 589, 592
  pain with, 80. See also Labor, pain
    during
  phases of, 404, 404f
  physiology of, 407–8
  postpartal pain from, 907
  power of, 404f, 404–5
  in precipitous labor, 542, 543f
  pressure of, 407
  psychic factors affecting, 535
  record keeping about, 480n
  regional anesthesia and, 523n
  responses to, 483
  resting between, 404, 404f
  side-lying position facilitates, 474
  tetanic
    general anesthesia for, 529
    as hemorrhage sign, 569
    as induction risk, 589, 591,
      593n
    as intrapartal risk factor, 425t
  trial labor and, 578
  in true vs. false labor, 416, 416t
  uterine rupture signs in, 550
Uterine cycle, 96, 97f, 98–99, 99f.
    See also Menstrual cycle
Uterine displacement, dysmenorrhea
    from, 100
Uterine distention
  atony after, 579
  from fetal macrosomia, 556
  as hemorrhage risk, 569, 972
  as induction of labor contraindica-
    tion, 587, 590
  as multiple gestation risk, 425t
  postpartal oxytocic agents for, 903
  postpartal risks with, 908t, 972
Uterine dysfunction, as hydramnios
    risk, 577
Uterine dystocia, from pathologic re-
    traction rings, 545, 545f
Uterine fibroids. See Myomas
Uterine fundus. See Fundus
Uterine glands, embryologic develop-
    ment of, 57
Uterine incisions, types of, 605–6,
    606f
Uterine inertia, record keeping about,
    480n
Uterine infection. See also Infection,
    postpartal
  assessing for, fourth trimester,
    946g
  as placenta previa risk, 566
Uterine inversion, 579–80
Uterine lacerations, postpartal hem-
    orrhage from, 579
Uterine ligaments, 80–82, 81f, 82f
  functions of, 82
  postpartal changes in, 905
  puerperal abscesses in, 975
Uterine massage, postpartal, 911
  atony risk with, 903
  for placental fragments hem-
    orrhage, 572n
  for uterine atony hemorrhage, 572
Uterine obstructions, transverse lie
    and, 555–56
Uterine pain, from postpartal hema-
    toma, 973

Uterine perforation, rupture vs., 550
Uterine polyps, pregnancy sign
    caused by, 192t
Uterine prolapse, assessing for
  in fourth trimester, 947g
  in initial prenatal exam, 226g
Uterine relaxation. See Uterine atony
Uterine rigidity, assessing for with
    preeclampsia/eclampsia, 343,
    344
Uterine rupture, 550–51
  from Bandl retraction ring, 545
  causes of, 550
  complete vs. incomplete, 550
  CPD as cause of, 578
  defined, 550
  fetal macrosomia and, 556
  fetal/neonatal implications of,
    425t, 550
  from hydrocephaly, 557
  from hydrops fetalis, 826
  as induction of labor risk, 425t,
    589, 590, 591
  as intrapartal risk factor, 425t
  maternal implications of, 425t,
    550, 551
  pelvic inlet contractures and, 578
  placenta previa risk, 566
  as podalic version risk, 586
  as precipitous labor risk, 543
  as prolonged labor risk, 542
  risk of, as oxytocin contraindica-
    tion, 590
  signs and symptoms of, 550
  as transverse lie risk, 556
Uterine souffle, 168
  nonpregnancy causes of, 192t
  as pregnancy change, 193
Uterine surgery
  as cephalic version contraindica-
    tion, 585
  as oxytocin contraindication, 590
Uterine tenderness
  in hemorrhage assessment, 572n
  as puerperal infection sign, 975,
    977
Uterine tetany. See Uterine contrac-
    tions, tetanic
Uterine tone, lack of with subinvolu-
    tion, 903
Uterine tubes. See Fallopian tubes
Uterine tumors
  fibroid. See Myomas
  obstructed labor from, 545, 600
  pregnancy signs caused by, 192t
Uteroplacental exchange, hypertonic
    labor patterns and, 537
Uteroplacental insufficiency (UPI)
  cesarean delivery for, 600
  estriol levels affected by, 380
  late decelerations caused by, 454–
    55, 455f
Uterosacral ligaments, 77, 81f, 82,
    82f
  palpation of, 74
Uterus, 74f, 75–80
  anatomy of, 76–80, 77f-80f
    in pregnancy, 195–96
  anteverted, palpation of, 74
  assessing
    for birth center delivery, 618
    after cesarean, 604
    in infertility workup, 114
    in initial prenatal exam, 223g,
      226g, 228g
    after inversion, 580
    postpartum, 901–2, 902f, 903,
      917n, 947g; see also postpar-
      tal involution of
    after precipitous delivery, 504,
      505
  Bandl ring in, 545

  congenital anomalies of, 77, 77f
  constriction ring in, 545
  contraction of, in fourth stage
    labor, 416. See also Uterine
    contractions
  couvelaire, postpartal hemorrhage
    risk with, 572n
  embryologic development of, 77
  functions of, 80
  implantation in, 162–63, 163f
  induction of labor effects on, 425t,
    589, 590
  irritability of, as abruptio placentae
    sign, 563
  labor changes in, 407, 408
    pain caused by, 411, 411f, 412f
  layers of, 77f, 78–79
    endometrium, 77f, 78–79f
    mucosal or innermost, 77f, 78–
      79
    muscular (myometrium), 77f, 78
    serosal, 78
  lochia produced by, 903–4
  malformations of, 77, 77f
    birth center screening for, 618
  malposition signs in, 551
  myths about, 75–76
  in neonate, 653
  pathologic contraction rings in,
    CPD and, 578
  physiologic retraction ring in, 407
  placental separation signs in, 497
  positions of, 76
  postpartal involution of, 901–3,
    902f
    assessing, 903, 907–8, 910f,
      910–11, 919n; see also
      assessing, postpartum
    breast-feeding and, 927
    hemorrhage risk and, 972
  pregnancy changes in, 192–93,
    193f, 194f, 195–96
  pregnancy hormones and, 169
  retraction rings in, 545, 545f
    uterine rupture and, 550
  retroverted, palpation of, 74
  round ligament of, palpation of, 74
  sexual response of, 103t
  size of, 76
    assessing in prenatal exams,
      223g, 239g
    determining delivery date by,
      236–3w, 237f
    in prolonged pregnancy, 759t
    postpartal changes in, 901–3,
      902f
  subinvolution of, 903, 973
  supports for, 71f, 76m77, 77f,
    78f, 80–82, 81f, 82f

Vacuum extraction delivery, 598–99
  caput succedaneum after, 678
  contraindications, 598
  nursing interventions for, 599
  for transverse arrest, 551
Vagina, 74f, 74–75, 76f
  assessing
    in fourth trimester, 947g
    in initial prenatal exam, 225–
      26g
    in neonate, 701–2g
    postpartum, 481n, 497
  atrophy of in menopause, 101,
    102
  burning and itching in, postmeno-
    pausal, 101
  congenital malformations of, 75
  development of, 57, 58f, 75, 653
  estrogenic hormones affect, 75
  functions of, 75
  muscular continuity with uterus of,
    78

of neonate, assessing, 701–2g
normal environment of, 75, 76f
pH of
pregnancy infection and, 196
puerperal infection and, 974
postpartal changes in, 904
postpartal hematomas of, 973
pregnancy changes in, 196–97, 254t, 255
self-cleansing of, 75
sexual response of, 103t
size of, 74
strawberry appearance to, from trichomonas, 356
Vaginal bleeding. *See also* Bleeding
assessing for, with preeclampsia/eclampsia, 343, 344
birth center transfer for, 618
with bladder distention, 982
as danger sign of pregnancy, 240g
as hemorrhage sign, 569, 572n
as home birth contraindication, 629
home birth transfer for, 631
labor interventions required by, 488t
postpartal
as hemorrhage sign, 572n
lacerations indicated by, 579
with PIH, 346
from umbilical cord vasa previa, 574, 575
as uterine rupture sign, 550
Vaginal cervix, 79. *See also* Cervix
Vaginal delivery. *See also* Delivery
with abruptio placentae, 563, 564
blood loss amount during, 906
for breech presentation, 554–55, 605
contraindications, 587
with face presentation, 553, 553f
intrapartal pelvic assessment for, 578
macrosomia dangers with, 556–57
with occiput-posterior position, 551
pelvic contractures and, 578
placenta previa and, 566
preterm labor, indications for, 550
spinal anesthesia level for, 525, 525f
twins, 560, 561
umbilical cord prolapse and, 575
Vaginal deodorants, infertility from, 112
Vaginal discharge
during active phase labor, 475n, 476
assessing
in fourth stage labor, 501
in initial prenatal exam, 226g, 227f
from genital herpes simplex, 359
with gonorrhea, 354
monilial, 355
in neonate, 652, 653, 684
assessing, 701–2g
care of, 727
during ovulation, 98
as pregnancy discomfort, 253f, 254t, 255–56
prenatal urinalyses and, 240g
trichomonal, 356
Vaginal examinations
careless, transverse lie after, 556
hydrocephaly seen on, 557
at labor admission, 468, 472
during labor, 436–40p, 437–39f
after amniotomy, 587
fetal position and presentation assessed by, 437–38p, 437–38f, 442, 551, 552, 553

FHR decelerations after, as non-reassuring, 458
first stage active phase, 475n
home birth, 630
with hypotonic labor patterns, 541
induced, 589, 591
infection risk from, 974
preterm, minimizing, 549
second stage, 479n
transverse lie detected on, 555
for umbilical cord prolapse, 539, 574
uterine rupture signs with, 550
Vaginal fistulas, from maternal soft tissue damage, 578
Vaginal foams, postpartal use of, 944
Vaginal fornices, 74, 74f
Vaginal hematoma, as third stage labor complication, 580
Vaginal hyperemia, pregnancy sign from, 192t
Vaginal infections
during birth, thrush from, 681
lymphatic drainage of, 75
in pregnancy, 196, 355–56
in pregnant diabetic, 316
sexually transmitted, 354
Vaginal introitus, 71f, 73
Vaginal lacerations, 579. *See also* Lacerations
assessing for, 481n
at postpartal home visit, 625
as breech delivery risk, 554
infection of, 974–75, 975t, 977–79n
as oxytocin induction risk, 590
postpartal bleeding as sign of, 904
postpartal hemorrhage caused by, 579, 972
as precipitous labor risk, 543
as prolonged labor risk, 542
Vaginal mucosa, pregnancy changes in, 254t, 255
Vaginal speculums, 73
Greeks used, 3
inserting, 235p
Vaginal sponges, 124
Vaginal sprays or deodorants, 75
Vaginal suppositories, for abortion, 129, 130t
Vaginal tag, in neonate, 684, 701g
Vaginal vestibule, 73
Vaginitis. *See* Vaginal infections
Vagus nerve, assessing in neonate, 695g
Valium. *See* Diazepam
Valsalva maneuver
cardiac output during, 409
during delivery, 479, 490
with RDS, 797t
Values, crisis adaptation and, 993
Values-clarification techniques, in abortion counseling, 128–29
van Deventer, Hendrik, 4
Varicocele, infertility from, 111t
Varicose veins
ankle edema and, 254t, 256
described, 256
hemorrhoids as, 257
postpartal thrombophlebitis and, 980
as pregnancy discomfort, 252, 253f, 254t, 256–57, 257f
reason for, 198
signs of in initial prenatal exam, 217g, 224g, 225g
in vulva, 72, 198, 257
in initial prenatal exam, 225g
at labor onset, 429g
Vas deferens (ductus deferens), 59f, 62f, 63

development of, 57, 58f, 653, 653f
evaluating, in infertility workup, 114
vasectomy site in, 63
Vasa previa, 575–76
Vascular problems in neonate, pulsation in fontanelles with, 692g
Vascular spasm
as hypertension risk, 214t
postpartal, from abruptio placentae, 563
Vasectomy, 121f, 127, 127f
infertility from, 111t
site of, 63
Vasocongestion, in sexual response, 103, 103t, 104t, 105
Vasoconstriction, neonatal heat retention through, 646, 647
Vasodilan (isoxsuprine), for preterm labor, 548
Vasodilatation
neonatal heat loss through, 646, 648
for PPH syndrome, 817
Vasomotor control, neonatal thermoregulation with, 646
Vasomotor disturbances, menopausal, 101, 102
Vasomotor reflexes, neonatal skin color and maturity of, 689g
Vasopressin, pregnancy role of, 202
Vasopressors, for cardiovascular collapse, 516
Vasospasm. *See* Vascular spasm
VDRL (Venereal Disease Research Laboratory) test
before cesarean delivery, 601
false-negative results from, 354
in initial prenatal exam, 229g
at labor onset, 431g
Vectorcardiograms, 888
Vegans, pregnancy nutrition for, 278–81
Vegetarians, pregnancy nutrition for, 272–73, 278, 279–81
Veins
in labia majora, 72
in penis, 60, 60f
spermatic, 62
in vagina, 75
varicose. *See* Varicose veins
Velamentous insertion of umbilical cord, 575, 575f
Velamentous placenta, 167
Vena cava compression, from hydramnios, 577
Vena cava obstruction, signs of in initial prenatal exam, 222g
Vena caval syndrome. *See* Supine hypotensive syndrome
Venereal Disease Research Laboratory. *See* VDRL
Venereal diseases. *See* Sexually transmitted disease
Venography, 981, 983
Venous insufficiency, signs of in initial prenatal exam, 224g
Venous pressure, decreased at birth, 640, 641f
Venous stasis
after surgery in pregnancy, preventing, 351
thromboembolic disease from, 976, 980
Venous thrombosis
deep, interventions for, 981, 983–84n, 985n
described, 976
lactation suppression drugs and, 925
pregnancy risk of, 198

recurrence risk with, 980
Ventilation, in neonate
factors affecting, 638–39
inadequate, resuscitation risk with, 787
tachypnea as decompensatory mechanism in, 796t
Ventilation/perfusion ratio in neonate, oxygenation and, 639
Ventilator, 800t. *See also* Respirator
Ventilatory therapy, 788, 790f, 791–92p
for apnea, 755n
complications of, 801, 808–10n, 815–17
criteria for, 804n
for diaphragmatic hernia, 866, 867
for MAS, 815
methods, 799–800t
for RDS, 797, 799–800t, 804n
weaning neonate from, 806n
Ventral suspension, gestational age and, 663f, 672
Ventricular dilatation, in pregnancy with cardiac disease, 311
Ventricular hypertrophy, in pregnancy with cardiac disease, 311
Ventricular septal defects, 885, 887f, 888, 888f
coarctation of the aorta with, 889
heart murmur from, 642
in IDM, 768
pregnancy with, 310
in tetralogy of Fallot, 887f, 890
transposition of great vessels and, 891
Verbal reporting, at nursery admission, 709–10
Vernix caseosa, 177t, 179t, 181, 182
assessing, 496, 677, 690g
gestational age and, 661, 669
on postterm infant, 759, 760
Version, 585–86
defined, 585
external or cephalic, 585, 586, 586f
internal or podalic, 585–86
Rh sensitization affected by, 824
Vertebras, assessing in initial prenatal exam, 225g
Vertex position, internal or podalic version of, 585
Vertex presentation, 400, 400f
abnormal, 552–54, 552–54f
cephalhematoma after, 678, 679f
forceps delivery requires, 598
palpating, 438p, 438f
pelvic types and, 577
position notation for, 403
precipitous delivery in, 504
spontaneous delivery with, described, 418
twins, 559
vacuum extraction requires, 598
Vesalius, Andreas, 3
Vibration, for MAS, 815
Vietnamese American families
childbirth as "women's work" among, 471
cultural stress on, 43
feeding customs, 925
lactose intolerance among, 281
postpartal customs, 914
pregnancy beliefs among, 205, 206, 288–89t
prenatal nutrition for, 283–84
Villi
anchoring, in placenta, 167
branching, in placenta, 167
chorionic, 164, 166–67, 166f, 167f
trophoblast forms, 163

Vinegar douche, for vaginal infections, 356
Violent behavior, with puerperal psychosis, 988
Viral infections in pregnancy, 357–60
  cleft lip and palate from, 853
  congenital heart defects and, 881
  neonatal acquired immunity to, 654
  neonatal hyperbilirubinemia risk from, 823
  neonatal jaundice and, 831
  TORCH group, 357–60
Viral shedding
  with asymtomatic CMV, 358
  with genital herpes simplex, 359
  prolonged, from rubella, 215t
Viruses
  placental transfer of, 170
  as teratogens, 184
Vision
  assessing in initial prenatal exam, 218g
  disturbances in, with severe pre-eclampsia, 343
  impaired, in pregnancy, 202, 240g
  pregnancy danger signs in, 240g
  of neonate, assessing, 680–81, 686–87, 694g. See also Visual stimuli, neonatal response to
Visiting hours
  attachment process and, 1013–14
  neonatal sleep-activity patterns and, 724
  in nursery, sepsis neonatorum prevention and, 842
Visiting nurse referral
  for cleft lip, 856
  for high-risk infant, 780
  for puerperal infection, 976
Vistaril. See Hydroxyzine
Visual acuity. See Vision
Visual damage, from congenital herpes, 359
Visual field
  evaluating, in infertility workup, 114
  pregnancy changes in, 202
Visual stimuli, neonatal response to, 655, 656f, 686, 687, 705. See also Vision
Visualization, as relaxation technique, 998
Vital capacity, pregnancy changes in, 197
Vital signs
  assessing
    before antiemetics, 603
    after cesarean delivery, 603
    in fourth trimester, 945g
    before induction, 591n
    at labor admission, 469, 472, 473
    during labor, 428g, 473, 475n, 477, 479, 481n
    at postpartal home visit, 624
    postpartum, 912–13, 919n, 945g
    in prenatal exams, 213, 216, 239g
  changes in after delivery, 906
  monitoring
    in abruptio placentae hemorrhage, 572
    after cesarean delivery, 603, 609
    with DIC risk, 568
    in double setup examination, 567
    in fourth stage labor, 501, 505
    with hematoma, 580

  with hemorrhage, 569n, 570n
  during home birth, 630
  with hypotonic labor patterns, 541
  with malposition, 552
  with precipitous delivery, 505
  with preterm labor, 549
  after PROM, 547
  in puerperium, 919n
  with pulmonary embolism, 985n
  with regional anesthesia, 522n
  of neonate, assessing, 688g
    at nursery admission, 710
    in nursery routine care, 714
    at postpartal home visit, 627
Vitamin A
  in breast milk, cow's milk, and formula, 719t
  deficiency signs, in initial prenatal exam, 217g
  food sources of, 275
  lactation requirements, 270t
  neonatal requirements, 717t
  pregnancy requirements, 270t, 274–75
  role of, 274
Vitamin B. See Vitamins; specific B vitamins
Vitamin B₁ (Thiamine), 270t, 276
  in breast milk, cow's milk, and formula, 719t
  neonatal requirements, 717t
Vitamin B₂ (Riboflavin), 270t, 276
  in breast milk, cow's milk, and formula, 719t
  neonatal deficiency of, dermatitis from, 719
Vitamin B₆ (pyridoxine), 276
  food sources of, 278
  lactation requirements, 270t
  pregnancy requirements, 270t, 277–78
  for premenstrual tension, 100
Vitamin B₁₂ (cobalamin), 276
  lactation requirements, 270t
  pregnancy requirements, 270t, 278–79
  deficiency signs, in initial prenatal exam, 220g
Vitamin C
  in breast milk, cow's milk, and formula, 719t
  deficiency signs
    bleeding gums, 719
    in initial prenatal exam, 220g
  food sources of, 276
  iron absorption and, 274
  lactation requirements, 270t
  neonatal requirements, 717, 717t
  pregnancy requirements, 270t, 276
  pregnancy overdose, 276
  puerperal infection and, 918n, 978n
  role of, 276
Vitamin D, 270t, 275
  in breast milk, cow's milk, and formula, 719t
  neonatal deficiency of, Harrison's groove with, 699g
  neonatal requirements, 717t
Vitamin E
  in breast milk, cow's milk, and formula, 719t
  deficiency symptoms, 275
  food sources of, 275
  lactation requirements, 270t
  neonatal requirements, 275, 717t
    anemia and, 644, 835
    preterm, 746
  pregnancy requirements, 270t, 275

  role of, 275
Vitamin K. See also Vitamin K (AquaMEPHYTON)
  neonatal requirements, 275, 650
  pregnancy requirements, 275
  role of, 275
  as teratogen, 267t
Vitamin K (AquaMEPHYTON), at day of birth, 650, 710, 711d
  dosage of, hyperbilirubinemia and, 822, 827
  need for, 717t, 836
Vitamins
  in breast milk, cow's milk, and formula, 719t
  food sources of, 271–72t
  lactation requirements, 270t
  metabolism of, pregnancy changes in, 201
  neonatal requirements, 717, 717t
  overdose symptoms, 274
  placental transport of, 170
  pregnancy requirements, 270t, 274–79, 277t
    fat-soluble, 274–75
    water-soluble, 275–79, 277t
  preterm infant requirements, 746
  recommended dietary allowances for women, 270t
Vitamin supplements, breast-feeding and, 718
Vocal cord paralysis, from Arnold-Chiari lesion, 879
Vocalizaton during labor, 483
Voiding. See Urination
Volvulus, in neonate, 873
Vomiting, by mother
  as bromocriptine side effect, 926d
  after cesarean, intervention for, 603
  as danger sign of pregnancy, 240g
  as general anesthesia danger, 528, 529, 530–31
  as impending labor sign, 416
  during labor, 409, 478n
    induced, as water intoxication sign, 590, 593n
  as Methergine side effect, 903d
  with multiple gestation, 558
  with puerperal peritonitis, 976, 977
  as pyelonephritis sign, 986
  with regional anesthesia in labor, 524n
  as ritodrine side effect, 549
  from vitamin D overdose, 275
Vomiting, by neonate. See also Regurgitation
  from aganglionic megacolon, 869
  assessment of, 873–74
  bile-stained
    causes of, 869, 873, 874
    as distress sign, 714
  bloody, causes of, 874
  colostrum protects against, 717
  with diaphragmatic hernia, 866
  as feeding intolerance sign, 746
  from fetal alcohol syndrome, 770
  with hypoglycemia, 818
  interventions for, 651
  from intestinal obstruction, 873–74
  with kernicterus, 824
  as necrotizing enterocolitis sign, 838, 839
  with PKU, 858
  projectile
    as illness sign, 729
    nonprojectile vs., 874
  as self-limiting, 651
  as sepsis neonatorum sign, 841

Von Recklinghausen's disease (neurofibromatosis), 143
von Waldeyer, Heinrich, 76
von Willebrand disease, fetoscopy to diagnose, 388
Vulnerable child syndrome, 1009–10
Vulva, 71–73, 71f
  assessing in initial prenatal exam, 225g
  monilial vaginitis effects on, 355
  postpartal hematomas of, 973
  trichomonas infection effects on, 356
  varicosities in, from pregnancy, 198, 257
  at labor onset, 429g
Vulval cleft, 72
Vulvar hyperemia, pregnancy sign caused by, 192t
Vulvovaginal (Bartholin's) glands, 71f, 73
Vulvovaginitis, irritation from, 72

Wagenstein-Rice method, 872
Wake states in neonate. See Sleep-wake patterns
Walsh, M. M. J., 148
Warfarin (Coumadin). See also Anticoagulants
  for deep venous thrombosis, 981
  neonatal effects of, 650, 769
  in pregnancy, 170, 267, 267t
  risks of, 769
Warm soaks. See Heat applications
Warrington, Joseph, 5
Wasting
  from asymmetric IUGR, 762
  in postterm infant, 759
Water
  in breast milk, cow's milk, and formula, 719t
  as essential nutrient, 271t, 272t
  initial infant feeding with, 716
  neonatal requirements, 717, 717t
  normal preterm blood values, 752t
  placental transport of, 170
Water feeding, breast-feeding and, 929
Water intoxication, as oxytocin risk, 500, 589, 590
  assessing for, 589, 590
  preventing, with oxytocin induction, 593ncp
  postpartum, 903
Water retention in pregnancy, 198, 200–201
Water-seal drainage, for pneumothorax, 809n, 816
Water-soluble vitamins, 274
  pregnancy requirements, 275–79, 277t
Waterston-Cooley operation, 890
WBC. See White blood cells
Weakness
  menopausal, 101
  in neonate, with hydrocephalus, 880
  as pulmonary embolism sign, 984n
Weaning, 721–22
Weight. See also Weight gain; Weight loss
  assessing
    in fourth trimester, 945g
    at labor admission, 472
    at labor onset, 428g
    in prenatal exams, 216g, 239g
    with severe preeclampsia, 343
  at birth. See Weight at birth
  conversions and equivalents, APPENDIX F
  of fetus, ultrasound to evaluate, APPENDIX C

as high risk factor, 214t
home birth and, 629
of neonate, assessing, 674, 689g.
    See also Weight at birth;
    Weight
gain; Weight loss
    at nursery admission, 710, 710f
    in nursery routine, 714
    at postpartal home visit, 627
Weight at birth
    with Beckwith syndrome, 867
    blood pressure and, 641, 751t
    classification of, in neonatal
        assessment, 660
    drug addiction affects, 770
    ethnic group and, 675
    fetal lung maturity and, 384
    in IDM, 763
    maternal weight gain and, 269,
        270
    mortality risk and, 758
    neonatal behavior and, 654
    neonatal morbidity and, 758
    neurologic abnormalities and, 734
    with Pierre Robin syndrome, 850
    resuscitation risk and, 786
    risk identification by, 734–35,
        735–36f
    smoking by mother and, 268
    statistics about, 23, 24t, 25t
Weight gain
    by neonate
        assessing at well-child visit, 719
        in breast- vs. bottle-fed babies,
            718
        with congenital hypothyroidism,
            859
        feeding method affects, 718
        ideal rate of, 652
        normal rate of, 675, 730
        preterm, 747, 753n, 754n
    postmenopausal, 102
    in pregnancy, 200–201
        assessing in prenatal exams,
            239g
        normal amount, 239g
        nutrition and, 269–70
        prolonged, 759t
        smoking affects, 268
Weight loss
    in mother
        as diabetes sign, 314
        as impending labor sign, 416
        infertility from, 112
        postpartal, 906, 917, 946g
        from vitamin D overdose, 275
    in neonate
        assessing, 689g
        factors affecting, 675

from intestinal obstruction, 873
normal amount of, 652, 714,
    730
physiologic, 675
preterm, as dehydration sign,
    747
Well-baby visits
    nutritional assessment at, 719–21,
        720–21t
    scheduling at discharge, 725, 780
Westbrook, M. T., 405, 406
Wet lung, assessing preterm infants
    for, 757n
Wharton's jelly, 167
Wheezes
    defined, 231p
    in initial prenatal exam, 221g
    with bronchopulmonary dysplasia,
        816
Whispered pectoriloquy, 221g
White blood cells (WBC)
    evaluating at labor onset, 431g
        in urine, 432g
    in initial prenatal exam, 229g
    in neonates, 644, 645, 652
        normal preterm values, 752t
        in sepsis neonatorum assess-
            ment, 842
    postpartal elevation in, 906
    after PROM, 547
    with puerperal infection, 977,
        979n
WIC program, 5
Wide awake state, in neonate, 657
Williams, H. A., 1005
Wilm tumor, in neonate
    kidney displacement with, 700g
    solid abdominal masses from, 699g
Wilson's disease, copper avoidance
    prevents, 135
Winick, M., 269
"Wink" reflex, 871
    of anal sphincter, meningomyelo-
        cele and, 883n
"Witch's milk" 653
Witchcraft, midwives suspected of, 6
Withdrawal
    fetal, 770
    in infant of addicted mother, 214t,
        360, 361, 361t, 770, 771,
        772
        excessive tearing with, 694g
    in infant of alcoholic mother, 362
    neonatal hypoglycemia vs., 818
    during pregnancy, 362
Withdrawal (*coitus interruptus*), 121f,
    122
Wolffian duct, 653, 653f
Women, status and role of

American Indian, 45
Black American, 45
    changing, families affected by, 42
    Mexican American, 44
    Oriental, 46
Women, Infants, and Children pro-
    gram (WIC), 5
Wong, D. L., 1005
Woods, N. F., 101
Woolrich shield, 931
Wooten, B., 1005
Wound healing, temperature
    increases with, 913
Wound infections, puerperal, 978n
    from cesarean delivery, 605
Wrapping the newborn, 716. *See also*
    Swaddling
Wrinkling, postmenopausal, 101–2

X-linked disorders
    autosomal dominant disorders vs.,
        142
    prenatal diagnosis of, 147
X-linked dominant inheritance, 145
X-linked recessive inheritance, 144,
    144f
    AID as alternative to, 152
X-ray examinations
    anganglionic megacolon evidence
        on, 869–70
    bronchopulmonary dysplasia
        assessment with, 816
    coarctation of the aorta on, 889
    CPD assessment with, 577
    diaphragmatic hernia detection by,
        866, 866f
    endocardial cushion defects on,
        888
    esophageal atresia assessment
        with, 860
    fetal death revealed by, 560
    for fetal position assessments, 442
    hip dysplasia diagnosis with, 878
    hydramnios assessment with, 577
    imperforate anus assessment with,
        872
    infertility from, 111t, 112, 114
    intestinal obstruction assessment
        with, 873
    MAS signs on, 798, 814
    multiple gestation evidence with,
        558
    necrotizing enterocolitis signs on,
        837, 838, 839n
    with neonatal group B streptococal
        infection, 843
    patent ductus arteriosus on, 885
    Pierre Robin syndrome detection
        with, 850

pneumothorax assessment with,
    809n, 816
positive pregnancy diagnosis with,
    195
for prenatal diagnosis, 146–47
pulmonary embolism and, 982
pulmonary stenosis on, 890
RDS findings on, 795, 801n
for sepsis neonatorum, 842
teratogenic effects from, 266
tetralogy of Fallot on, 890
tracheoesophageal atresia/fistula
    assessment with, 860–61, 862
transient tachypnea of newborn
    signs on, 797–98
transposition of the great vessels
    on, 891
uses of in late pregnancy, 387–88
ventricular septal defects on, 885,
    888
X-ray pelvimetry
    fetal size estimation by, 557
    intrapartal, 426
        indications for, 433–34
Xanthochromia, as IVH sign, 836
Xanthoma in neonate, pigmentation
    with, 690g
Xiphoid cartilage, assessing in neo-
    nate, 682, 698G
Xiphoid retraction, assessing in neo-
    nate, 682
    with RDS, 795f
Xylocaine. *See* Lidocaine

Yarrow, L. J., on attachment readi-
    ness, 951, 952
Yellen clamp, circumcision with, 723f
Yellow fever immunization, in preg-
    nancy, 266t
Yolk sac, formation of, 164f, 165
Yutopar. *See* Ritodrine

Zinc, 270t, 273
    in breast milk, cow's milk, and for-
        mula, 719t
    neonatal requirements, 717t
Zona basalis of endometrium, 79
Zona compacta of endometrium, 79
Zona functionalis of endometrium, 79
Zona pellucida (oolemma)
    blastomeres held together by, 162
    development of, 96, 98f
    of ovum, 160, 163f
Zona spongiosa of endometrium, 79
Zygote
    cellular multiplication in, 162, 163f
    fallopian tube environment for, 83
    formation of, 161f, 162, 163f
    transport of to uterus, 162, 163f